Case Directory

Small Animal Clinical Nutrition

5th Edition

MARK MORRIS INSTITUTE

Hand
Thatcher
Remillard
Roudebush
Novotny

Small Animal Clinical Nutrition

5th Edition

Mark Morris Institute

Small Animal Clinical Nutrition

ISBN 0-615297-01-3

For more information about this book contact:
Mark Morris Institute
P.O. Box 2097
Topeka, Kansas 66601-2097
Phone 785-286-8101
Facsimile 785-286-8173

Last digit is the print number 9 8 7 6 5 4 3 2 1

In Memory

Since the last edition, five special veterinarians passed away who, directly or indirectly, were associated with the *Small Animal Clinical Nutrition* textbook series. These men contributed greatly to veterinary medicine, the field of veterinary nutrition and to their communities. They include Mark Morris, Jr., David Kronfeld, E. Phillip Miller, Russell Frey and John L. Mara. They are, and will continue to be, greatly missed by their families, friends and the veterinary profession.

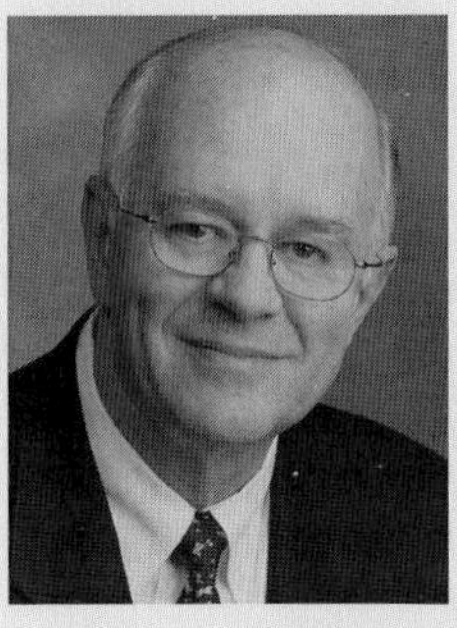

Mark L. Morris, Jr., DVM, PhD, Dipl. ACVN (1934-2007)

Mark was born in New Jersey, received his DVM from Cornell University and received a PhD in pathology from the University of Wisconsin. He returned to Topeka and joined his father at Mark Morris Associates, which was responsible for the research and development, quality control and professional education efforts supporting Prescription Diets produced by Hill's Packing Company. There, he expanded the line of Prescription Diet products and created the concept of wellness nutrition through the introduction of Science Diet pet foods. Mark also worked with the Topeka Zoo to develop ZuPreem, a line of commercial foods for exotic and endangered species. He led pet nutrition research at Theracon, a family owned private research facility and sponsored pet nutrition projects at veterinary schools throughout the U.S. Mark published widely and was invited to speak at more than 200 veterinary meetings around the world. In 1988 the Morris family sold Mark Morris Associates and Theracon to Hill's Pet Nutrition/Colgate-Palmolive. For years he provided leadership to the Morris Animal Foundation, serving as a lifetime trustee and vice president of scientific affairs. Mark was a charter diplomate of the American College of Veterinary Nutrition and a member of the Cornell University Feline Health Advisory Board. He and other members of the Morris family sponsored four faculty positions in nutrition and several graduate/residency programs in veterinary schools in the U.S. He actively contributed to his community throughout his life. Mark was an author/editor of *Small Animal Clinical Nutrition* I, II and III.

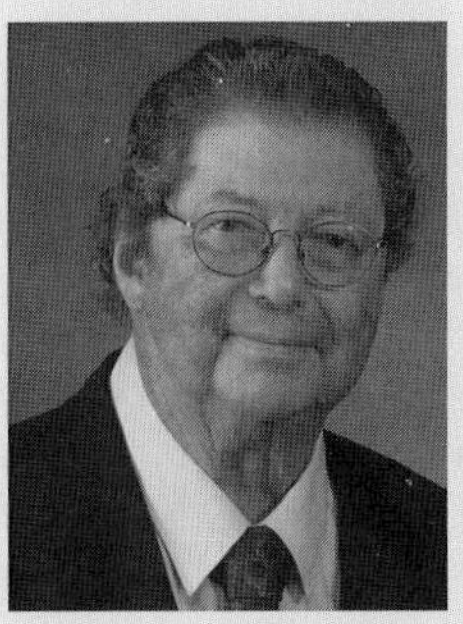

David S. Kronfeld, MVSc, MA(hc), PhD, DSc, MACVSc, Dipl. ACVIM, Dipl. ACVN (1928-2006)

David was born and raised in New Zealand. In 1952, he received his BVSc from the University of Queensland. He received his MVSc the following year. In 1959, David received a PhD in comparative physiology from the University of California, Davis. In 1972, David received his DSc from the University of Queensland for published research over the previous 20 years. He was a diplomate of the American College of Veterinary Internal Medicine and a charter diplomate of the American College of Veterinary Nutrition, serving as president. David was on the faculty at the University of Pennsylvania for 28 years where he was the Elizabeth and William Whitney Clark Professor Emeritus and Chief of Medicine at the New Bolton Center. During the subsequent 17 years he served on the faculty at Virginia Tech as the Paul Melon Distinguished Professor. David authored/coauthored more than 700 publications. He reviewed the Canine Athlete chapter in the fourth edition of *Small Animal Clinical Nutrition.*

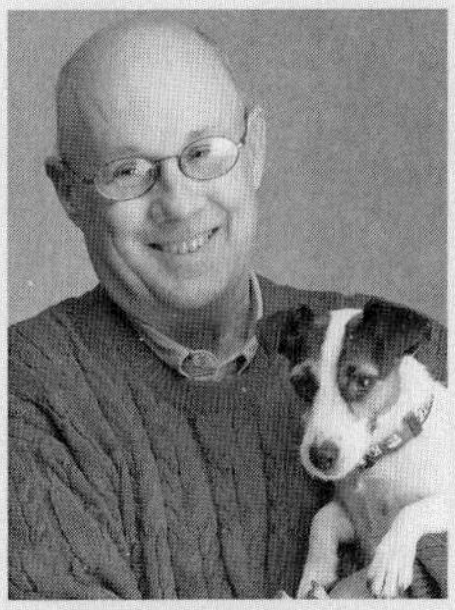

E. Phillip Miller, DVM, MS, Dipl. ABVT, Dipl. ABT (1942-2005)

Phil was born and grew up in eastern Kansas. He received his DVM from KSU in 1966. He engaged in private practice (mixed animal) in northeastern Kansas for more than 10 years. Subsequently, Phil received his MS degree in Pharmacology/Toxicology from the University of Kansas Medical Center. He was board certified in veterinary and human toxicology. After 23 years in the pharmaceutical industry, he joined Hill's Pet Nutrition, Inc., to head up the global product safety and efficacy function. Phil was active in numerous veterinary groups including the American Association of Industrial Veterinarians (Executive Board) (voted Industrial Veterinarian of the Year) and the American Board of Veterinary Toxicology (Council of Regents). He was also active in community service. Phil was an author of the Food Safety chapters in the fourth and fifth editions of *Small Animal Clinical Nutrition.*

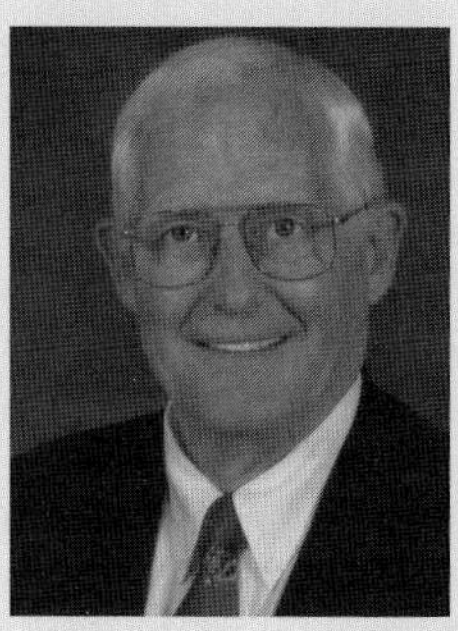

Russell A. Frey, DVM, PhD, Dipl. ACVN (1930-2003)

Russ was a veterinarian, educator and a public servant. He was born and raised outside Manhattan, Kansas. After receiving his veterinary degree from Kansas State University in 1952, Russ practiced large animal medicine and surgery in South Dakota. Upon returning to KSU in 1960, Russ received his PhD in physiology in 1970. Afterwards, he taught nutrition and physiology to 40 classes of veterinary students, twice receiving the prestigious Norden Teaching Award (1966 and 1986). He served as president of the Kansas Veterinary Medical Association (KVMA) and liaison for the KVMA to the Kansas Legislature. Russ was a delegate to the AVMA House of Delegates. He was voted Kansas Veterinarian of the Year in 1991 and twice received the KVMA President's Award (1992 and 2001). He was a charter diplomate and president of the American College of Veterinary Nutrition, served on the Board of Directors of the Mark Morris Institute and was an author in the fourth edition of *Small Animal Clinical Nutrition*.

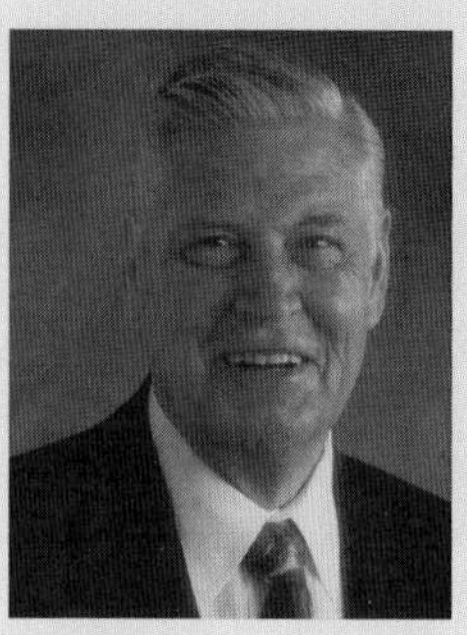

John L. Mara, DVM (1924-2003)

Jack grew up on a farm in upstate New York. He received his DVM from Cornell University and interned there in the small animal clinic. Jack took a position in a small animal practice in Long Island, but eventually built his own practice. During his years in practice he was an active community servant and politician. In 1978 he sold his practice and joined Hill's Pet Nutrition, Inc., as Professional Services Representative. Jack served for many years promoting the importance of nutrition in pet health on radio and television and at veterinary meetings. Later he became the Director of Academic Affairs at Hill's and influenced the teaching of nutrition in U.S. veterinary schools. He championed Hill's support of 19 nutrition graduate/residency programs He encouraged the establishment of the American College of Veterinary Nutrition, and in 1994 was awarded honorary ACVN diplomate status, which was one of his most treasured acknowledgements. Jack received numerous national, regional and state veterinary association awards for meritorious service. He was a trustee for the Morris Animal Foundation and worked diligently with the Delta Society and the associated Bustad Award.

Editors

Michael S. Hand, DVM, PhD
Diplomate, American College of Veterinary Nutrition
Chair, Board of Directors, Mark Morris Institute
Arroyo Hondo, New Mexico

Craig D. Thatcher, DVM, MS, PhD
Diplomate, American College of Veterinary Nutrition
Professor and Dean, Polytechnic Campus School of Applied Arts and Sciences
Arizona State University, Mesa, Arizona

Rebecca L. Remillard, PhD, DVM
Diplomate, American College of Veterinary Nutrition
Staff Nutritionist, MSPCA Angell Animal Medical Center, Boston, Massachusetts
Clinical Assistant Professor, School of Veterinary Medicine
Tufts University, North Grafton, Massachusetts

Philip Roudebush, DVM
Diplomate, American College of Veterinary Internal Medicine (Small Animal Internal Medicine)
Director, Scientific Affairs and Technical Information Services, Hill's Pet Nutrition, Inc., Topeka, Kansas
Adjunct Professor, Department of Clinical Sciences, College of Veterinary Medicine, Kansas State University, Manhattan, Kansas

Bruce J. Novotny, DVM
Owner, Managing Partner, Helios Communications, LLC, Bandon, Oregon

Contributors

Larry G. Adams, DVM, PhD, Dipl. ACVIM (Small Animal Internal Medicine)
Professor, Department of Veterinary Clinical Sciences
School of Veterinary Medicine
Purdue University
West Lafayette, Indiana
Chronic Kidney Disease

Neil W. Ahle, MBA, DVM, PhD, Dipl. ABT
Medical Director, Science and Technology
Hill's Pet Nutrition, Inc.
Topeka, Kansas
Food Safety

Hasan Albasan, DVM, MS, PhD
Veterinary Clinical Sciences Department
College of Veterinary Medicine
University of Minnesota
St. Paul, Minnesota
Canine Purine Urolithiasis: Causes, Detection, Management and Prevention, Canine Struvite Urolithiasis: Causes, Detection, Management and Prevention

Timothy A. Allen, DVM, Dipl. ACVIM (Small Animal Internal Medicine)
Technical Services Veterinarian
Dechra Veterinary Products
Overland Park, Kansas
Evidence-Based Clinical Nutrition, Chronic Kidney Disease, Feline Lower Urinary Tract Diseases

Samer Al-Murrani, PhD, MBA
Manager, Research
Science and Technology
Hill's Pet Nutrition, Inc.
Topeka, Kansas
Nutrigenomics and Nutrigenetics: Nutritional Genomics in Health and Disease

P. Jane Armstrong, DVM, MS, MBA, Dipl. ACVIM (Small Animal Internal Medicine)
Professor, Internal Medicine and Clinical Nutrition
Department of Veterinary Clinical Sciences
College of Veterinary Medicine
University of Minnesota
St. Paul, Minnesota
Introduction to Feeding Normal Cats, Feeding Young Adult Cats: Before Middle Age

Lawrence H. Arp, DVM, PhD, Dipl. ACVP, ACVM
Research Director, Discovery Pathology
Department of Inflammation & Autoimmune Diseases
Hoffman La Roche, Inc.
Nutley, New Jersey
Food Safety (case)

Joseph W. Bartges, DVM, PhD, Dipl. ACVIM (Small Animal Internal Medicine), ACVN
Professor, Medicine and Nutrition
The Acree Endowed Chair of Small Animal Research
Department of Small Animal Clinical Sciences
College of Veterinary Medicine
The University of Tennessee
Knoxville, Tennessee
Canine Purine Urolithiasis: Causes, Detection, Management and Prevention

Iveta Becvarova, DVM, MS, Dipl. ACVN
Clinical Assistant Professor
Department of Large Animal Clinical Sciences
Virginia-Maryland Regional College of Veterinary Medicine
Virginia Polytechnic Institute and State University
Blacksburg, Virginia
Introduction to Feeding Normal Cats, Feeding Young Adult Cats: Before Middle Age, Feeding Mature Adult Cats: Middle Aged and Older, Feeding Reproducing Cats, Feeding Nursing and Orphaned Kittens from Birth to Weaning, Feeding Growing Kittens: Postweaning to Adulthood

Candace Berkshire, DVM
Washington State University
Pullman, Washington
Food Safety (case)

Kiko Bracker, DVM, Dipl. ACVECC
Emergency and Critical Care
MSPCA Angell Animal Medical Center
Boston, Massachusetts
Food Safety (case)

Douglas Brum, DVM
Internal Medicine
MSPCA Angell Animal Medical Center
Boston, Massachusetts
Short Bowel Syndrome (case)

Michelle Buettner
Minnesota Urolith Center
College of Veterinary Medicine
University of Minnesota
St. Paul, Minnesota
Canine Cystine Urolithiasis: Causes, Detection, Dissolution and Prevention

William J. Burkholder, DVM, PhD, Dipl. ACVN
Division of Animal Feeds
Center for Veterinary Medicine
7519 Standish Place
Rockville, Maryland
Obesity (cases)

Kevin P. Byrne, DVM, Dipl. ACVD
Allergy Ear & Skin Care
Bensalem, Pennsylvania
Lecturer in Dermatology, School of Veterinary Medicine
University of Pennsylvania
Philadelphia, Pennsylvania
Skin and Hair Disorders (case)

James W. Carpenter, MS, DVM, Dipl. ACZM
Professor, Zoological Medicine
Department of Clinical Sciences
College of Veterinary Medicine
Kansas State University
Manhattan, Kansas
Feeding Small Pet Mammals

Maureen Carroll, DVM, Dipl. ACVIM (Small Animal Internal Medicine)
Internal Medicine
MSPCA Angell Animal Medical Center
Boston, Massachusetts
Large Bowel Diarrhea: Colitis, Large Bowel Diarrhea: Idiopathic Bowel Syndrome in Dogs, Constipation/Obstipation/Megacolon

Lori-Ann Christie, PhD
Scientist, Institute for Brain Aging & Dementia
University of California, Irvine
Irvine, California
Cognitive Dysfunction in Dogs

W. Paul Cleland, Jr., DVM, Dipl. ABVP (Canine and Feline Practice), AVDC
Veterinary Affairs Manager
Hill's Pet Nutrition, Inc.
Topeka, Kansas
Faculty Affiliate, Department of Clinical Sciences
College of Veterinary Medicine and Biomedical Sciences
Colorado State University
Fort Collins, Colorado
Periodontal Disease

Amy Cokley, BS
Minnesota Urolith Center
College of Veterinary Medicine
University of Minnesota
St. Paul, Minnesota
Canine Calcium Phosphate Urolithiasis: Causes, Detection and Prevention

Laine Cowan, DVM, MS, Dipl. ACVIM (Small Animal Internal Medicine)
Fall City, Washington
Food Safety (case)

Christopher S. Cowell, MS, PAS
Director, Regulatory Affairs/Nutrition
Néstle Purina PetCare Company
Checkerboard Square
St. Louis, Missouri
Micronutrients: Minerals and Vitamins, Commercial Pet Foods

Stephen W. Crane, DVM, Dipl. ACVS, ABLS
Chief Medical Officer and Program Director
Western Veterinary Conference
Las Vegas, Nevada
Commercial Pet Foods, Making Pet Foods at Home

Steven E. Crane, BS, BA, MBA
Associate Manager, Technical Information Service
Hill's Pet Nutrition, Inc.
Topeka, Kansas
Adjunct Professor, Baker University
School of Professional and Graduate Studies
Ottawa, Kansas
Commercial Pet Foods

James S. Cullor, DVM, PhD
Director, Veterinary Medicine Teaching and Research Center
University of California-Tulare
Tulare, California
Food Safety (case)

Deborah J. Davenport, DVM, MS, Dipl. ACVIM (Small Animal Internal Medicine)
Director, Professional Education
Hill's Pet Nutrition, Inc.
Topeka, Kansas
Adjunct Professor, Department of Clinical Sciences
College of Veterinary Medicine
Kansas State University
Manhattan, Kansas
Executive Director, Mark Morris Institute
Topeka, Kansas
Introduction to Gastrointestinal and Exocrine Pancreatic Diseases, Oral Diseases, Pharyngeal and Esophageal Disorders, Introduction to Gastric Diseases, Gastritis and Gastroduodenal Ulceration, Gastric Dilatation and Gastric Dilatation-Volvulus in Dogs, Gastric Motility and Emptying Disorders, Introduction to Small Intestinal Diseases, Acute Gastroenteritis and Enteritis, Inflammatory Bowel Disease, Protein-Losing Enteropathies, Short Bowel Syndrome, Small Intestinal Bacterial Overgrowth, Introduction to Large Intestinal Diseases, Large Bowel Diarrhea: Colitis, Large Bowel Diarrhea: Idiopathic Bowel Syndrome in Dogs, Constipation/Obstipation/Megacolon, Flatulence, Exocrine Pancreatic Insufficiency, Acute and Chronic Pancreatitis, Hepatobiliary Disease (case)

Mary C. DeBey, BS, DVM, MS, PhD, Dipl. ACVM
Consultation Clinician
Hill's Pet Nutrition, Inc.
Topeka, Kansas
Food Safety

Jacques Debraekeleer, DVM, Dipl. ECVCN, ESVCN
Associate Director, Professional and Regulatory Affairs, Europe
Hill's Pet Nutrition, Inc.
Brussels, Belgium
Macronutrients, Pet Food Labels, Introduction to Feeding Normal Dogs, Feeding Young Adult Dogs: Before Middle Age, Feeding Mature Adult Dogs: Middle Aged and Older, Feeding Reproducing Dogs, Feeding Nursing and Orphaned Puppies from Birth to Weaning, Feeding Growing Puppies: Postweaning to Adulthood, Introduction to Feeding Normal Cats, Feeding Young Adult Cats:

Before Middle Age, Feeding Mature Adult Cats: Middle Aged and Older, Feeding Reproducing Cats, Feeding Nursing and Orphaned Kittens from Birth to Weaning, Feeding Growing Kittens: Postweaning to Adulthood, Appendices

Elizabeth Dill-Macky, BVSc, MACVSc, Dipl. ACVIM (Small Animal Internal Medicine)
Technical Services Veterinarian
Hill's Pet Nutrition, Inc.
Sydney, Australia
Hepatobiliary Disease

Cheryl L. Dikeman, PhD
Department Head, Department of Nutrition
Sarah Burke, Research Assistant, Nutrition Laboratory
Henry Doorly Zoo
Omaha, Nebraska
Feeding Passerine and Psittacine Birds (cases)

Susan Donoghue, MS, VMD
President, Nutrition Support Services
Pembroke, Virginia
Nutrition of Reptiles

David A. Dzanis, DVM, PhD, Dipl. ACVN
Dzanis Consulting and Collaborations
Santa Clara, California
Pet Food Labels, Commercial Pet Foods (boxes), Obesity (box)

Martin J. Fettman, BS, DVM, PhD, Dipl. ACVP (Clinical Pathology)
Professor Emeritus of Clinical Pathology
College of Veterinary Medicine and Biomedical Sciences
Colorado State University
Fort Collins, Colorado
Private Consultant
Tucson, Arizona
Effects of Food on Pharmacokinetics

Richard B. Ford, DVM, MS, Dipl. ACVIM (Small Animal Internal Medicine), Dipl. ACVPM (Honorary)
Professor Emeritus, Department of Clinical Sciences
College of Veterinary Medicine
North Carolina State University
Raleigh, North Carolina
Disorders of Lipid Metabolism

S. Dru Forrester, DVM, MS, Dipl. ACVIM (Small Animal Internal Medicine)
Scientific Affairs
Hill's Pet Nutrition, Inc.
Topeka, Kansas
Adjunct Faculty, Department of Clinical Sciences
College of Veterinary Medicine
Kansas State University
Manhattan, Kansas
Chronic Kidney Disease, Feline Lower Urinary Tract Diseases

Kim G. Friesen, PhD, MS
Nutritionist
Elanco Animal Health
Greenfield, Indiana
Adjunct Faculty, Department of Animal Science and Industry
College of Agriculture
Kansas State University
Manhattan, Kansas
Adjunct Faculty, Department of Animal Science
University of Arkansas
Fayetteville, Arkansas
Macronutrients

Robert L. Gillette, DVM, MSE
Director, Richard G. and Dorothy A. Metcalf Veterinary Sports Medicine Program
College of Veterinary Medicine
Auburn University
Auburn, Alabama
Feeding Working and Sporting Dogs

Stephen D. Gilson, DVM, Dipl. ACVS
Sonora Veterinary Specialties
Scottsdale, Arizona
Critical Care Nutrition and Enteral-Assisted Feeding (case)

Kathy L. Gross, PhD, MS, Dipl. ACAN
Director, Research
Science and Technology
Hill's Pet Nutrition, Inc.
Topeka, Kansas
Adjunct Faculty, Department of Animal Science and Industry
College of Agriculture
Kansas State University
Manhattan, Kansas
Macronutrients, Introduction to Feeding Normal Dogs, Feeding Young Adult Dogs: Before Middle Age, Feeding Mature Adult Dogs: Middle Aged and Older, Feeding Reproducing Dogs, Feeding Nursing and Orphaned Puppies from Birth to Weaning, Feeding Growing Puppies: Postweaning to Adulthood, Introduction to Feeding Normal Cats, Feeding Young Adult Cats: Before Middle Age, Feeding Mature Adult Cats: Middle Aged and Older, Feeding Reproducing Cats, Feeding Nursing and Orphaned Kittens from Birth to Weaning, Feeding Growing Kittens: Postweaning to Adulthood

W. Grant Guilford, BPhil, BVSc, PhD, Dipl. ACVIM (Small Animal Internal Medicine), Fellow, Australian College of Veterinary Scientists
Head, Institute of Veterinary, Animal and Biomedical Sciences
Massey University
Palmerston, North, New Zealand
Adverse Reactions to Food

Michael S. Hand, DVM, PhD, Dipl. ACVN
Chair, Board of Directors
Mark Morris Institute
Topeka, Kansas
Private Consultant
Editor, Small Animal Clinical Nutrition
Arroyo Hondo, New Mexico
Small Animal Clinical Nutrition: An Iterative Process, Nutrigenomics and Nutrigenetics: Nutritional Genomics in Health and Disease, Feeding Working and Sporting Dogs, Obesity

Kenneth R. Harkin, DVM, Dipl. ACVIM (Small Animal Internal Medicine)
Associate Professor, Veterinary Clinical Sciences
College of Veterinary Medicine
Kansas State University
Manhattan, Kansas
Food Safety (case)

Herman A. W. Hazewinkel, DVM, PhD, Dipl. Royal Netherlands Veterinary Association (Companion Animal Surgery), Dipl. ECVS, ECVCN
Professor, Companion Animal Orthopedics
Head of the Clinical Nutrition Service
Department of Clinical Sciences
Utrecht University
Utrecht, The Netherlands
Developmental Orthopedic Disease of Dogs

Elizabeth Head, MA, PhD
Associate Professor, Department of Molecular and Biomedical Pharmacology Sanders-Brown Center on Aging
University of Kentucky
Lexington, Kentucky
Cognitive Dysfunction in Dogs

M. Anne Hickman, DVM, PhD, Dipl. ACVN
Pfizer, Inc.
Groton, Connecticut
Feeding Growing Kittens: Postweaning to Adulthood (case)

Hilary A. Jackson, DVM, Dipl. ACVD
Dermatology Referral Services
Glasgow, Scotland
United Kingdom
Adverse Reactions to Food

Christine C. Jenkins, DVM, Dipl. ACVIM (Small Animal Internal Medicine)
Director of Academic Affairs
Hill's Pet Nutrition, Inc.
Topeka, Kansas
Gastritis and Gastroduodenal Ulceration, Gastric Dilatation and Gastric Dilatation-Volvulus in Dogs, Gastric Motility and Emptying Disorders

Albert E. Jergens, DVM, PhD, Dipl. ACVIM (Small Animal Internal Medicine)
Associate Professor, Department of Veterinary Clinical Sciences
College of Veterinary Medicine
Iowa State University
Ames, Iowa
Inflammatory Bowel Disease, Protein-Losing Enteropathies

Dennis E. Jewell, PhD, Dipl. ACAN
Nutrition Scientist Fellow, Science and Technology
Hill's Pet Nutrition, Inc.
Topeka, Kansas
Adjunct Professor, Department of Animal Science and Industry
Kansas State University
Manhattan, Kansas
Macronutrients

Karen L. Johnston, BA, VMD, MRCVS, PhD
Director, Veterinary Strategic Initiatives
Hill's Pet Nutrition, Inc.
Topeka, Kansas
Small Intestinal Bacterial Overgrowth

Lauren Kats, MS
Senior Scientist, Science and Technology
Hill's Pet Nutrition, Inc.
Topeka, Kansas
Micronutrients: Minerals and Vitamins

Bruce W. Keene, DVM, MSc, Dipl. ACVIM (Cardiology)
Professor of Cardiology, Department of Clinical Sciences
College of Veterinary Medicine
North Carolina State University
Raleigh, North Carolina
Cardiovascular Disease

Christina Khoo, PhD
Manager, Research Sciences
Ocean Spray Cranberries, Inc.
Lakeville, Massachusetts
Adjunct Faculty, Department of Nutrition
Kansas State University
Manhattan, Kansas
Macronutrients

Claudia A. Kirk, DVM, PhD, Dipl. ACVIM (Small Animal Internal Medicine), ACVN
Professor and Head, Department of Small Animal Clinical Sciences
College of Veterinary Medicine
The University of Tennessee
Knoxville, Tennessee
Feeding Young Adult Cats: Before Middle Age (case), Feeding Mature Adult Cats: Middle Aged and Older (case), Feeding Reproducing Cats (case), Feeding Growing Kittens: Postweaning to Adulthood (case), Endocrine Disorders

Lori A. Koehler, CVT
Minnesota Urolith Center
College of Veterinary Medicine
University of Minnesota
St. Paul, Minnesota
Canine Calcium Oxalate Urolithiasis: Changing Paradigms in Detection, Management and Prevention

George V. Kollias, DVM, PhD, Dipl. ACZM
J. Hyman Professor of Wildlife Medicine
Department of Clinical Sciences
College of Veterinary Medicine
Cornell University
Ithaca, New York
Feeding Passerine and Psittacine Birds

Heidi Wearne Kollias
Research Assistant, Department of Clinical Sciences
College of Veterinary Medicine
Cornell University
Ithaca, New York
Feeding Passerine and Psittacine Birds

Christine Kolmstetter, MS, DVM
Cheyenne West Animal Hospital
Las Vegas, Nevada
Feeding Small Pet Mammals

John M. Kruger, DVM, PhD, Dipl. ACVIM (Small Animal Internal Medicine)
Professor, Associate Department Chairperson for Research
Director of the Michigan State University Center for Feline Health and Well-Being
Department of Small Animal Clinical Sciences
College of Veterinary Medicine
Michigan State University
East Lansing, Michigan
Canine Calcium Phosphate Urolithiasis: Causes, Detection and Prevention, Feline Lower Urinary Tract Diseases

Butch KuKanich, BS, DVM, PhD, Dipl. ACVCP
Assistant Professor, Department of Anatomy and Physiology
College of Veterinary Medicine
Kansas State University
Manhattan, Kansas
Effects of Food on Pharmacokinetics

Gary M. Landsberg, BSc, DVM, Dipl. ACVB
Clinician and Veterinary Behaviorist
Doncastle Animal Clinic
Thornhill, Ontario
Canada
Cognitive Dysfunction in Dogs

Michael S. Leib, DVM, MS, Dipl. ACVIM (Small Animal Internal Medicine)
C.R. Roberts Professor of Small Animal Medicine
Department of Small Animal Clinical Sciences
College of Veterinary Medicine
Virginia Polytechnic Institute and State University
Blacksburg, Virginia
Pharyngeal and Esophageal Disorders, Gastric Dilatation and Gastric Dilatation-Volvulus in Dogs (case), Large Bowel Diarrhea: Colitis (case)

Ellen I. Logan, DVM, PhD
Manager, Veterinary Consultation Service
Veterinary Business Channel
Hill's Pet Nutrition, Inc.
Topeka, Kansas
Adjunct Assistant Clinical Professor, Department of Clinical Sciences
College of Veterinary Medicine
Kansas State University
Manhattan, Kansas
Periodontal Disease, Oral Diseases

Dawn E. Logas, DVM, Dipl. ACVD
Staff Dermatologist, Veterinary Dermatology Center
Maitland, Florida
Skin and Hair Disorders (cases)

Chris L. Ludlow, DVM, MS, Dipl. ACVIM (Small Animal Internal Medicine)
Staff Internist, Animal Specialty and Emergency Center
Rockledge, Florida
Disorders of Lipid Metabolism, Short Bowel Syndrome, Small Intestinal Bacterial Overgrowth

Jody P. Lulich, DVM, PhD, Dipl. ACVIM (Small Animal Internal Medicine)
Professor, Small Animal Medicine
Veterinary Clinical Sciences Department
College of Veterinary Medicine
University of Minnesota
St. Paul, Minnesota
Canine Urolithiasis: Definitions, Pathophysiology and Clinical Manifestations, Canine Purine Urolithiasis: Causes, Detection, Management and Prevention, Canine Calcium Oxalate Urolithiasis: Changing Paradigms in Detection, Management and Prevention, Canine Calcium Phosphate Urolithiasis: Causes, Detection and Prevention, Canine Cystine Urolithiasis: Causes, Detection, Dissolution and Prevention, Canine Struvite Urolithiasis: Causes, Detection, Management and Prevention, Canine Silica Urolithiasis: Causes, Detection, Treatment and Prevention, Canine Compound Urolithiasis: Prevalence, Significance and Management, Feline Lower Urinary Tract Diseases (case)

Stanley L. Marks, BVSc, PhD, Dipl. ACVIM (Small Animal Internal Medicine, Oncology), ACVN
Professor, Department of Medicine and Epidemiology
School of Veterinary Medicine
University of California-Davis
Davis, California
Cancer (case)

Hein P. Meyer, DVM, PhD, Dipl. ECVIM (Companion Animals)
Director of Professional and Veterinary Affairs
Europe, Middle East and Africa
Hill's Pet Nutrition, Inc.
Prague, Czech Republic
Hepatobiliary Disease

Kathryn E. Michel, DVM, MS, Dipl. ACVN
Associate Professor of Nutrition, Department of Clinical Studies
School of Veterinary Medicine
University of Pennsylvania
Philadelphia, Pennsylvania
Parenteral-Assisted Feeding (case)

E. Phillip Miller, DVM, MS, Dipl. ABVT, ABVT (Deceased)
Director, Product Safety, Efficacy and Technical Information
Science and Technology
Hill's Pet Nutrition, Inc.
Topeka, Kansas
Food Safety

Jerry Millican, MS, BS
Principal Engineer, Science and Technology
Hill's Pet Nutrition, Inc.
Topeka, Kansas
Commercial Pet Foods

Edward A. Moser, BS, MS, VMD, Dipl. ACVN
Veterinary Nutrition Specialists, Inc.
Selinsgrove, Pennsylvania
Adjunct Assistant Professor of Comparative Nutrition
School of Veterinary Medicine
University of Pennsylvania
Philadelphia, Pennsylvania
Commercial Pet Foods

Richard C. Nap, DVM, PhD, Dipl. ECVS, ECVCN
Director, Uppertunity Consultants
Consultant to Animal Health Industry and Organizations
Utrecht, The Netherlands
Developmental Orthopedic Disease of Dogs

Richard W. Nelson, DVM, Dipl. ACVIM (Small Animal Internal Medicine)
Professor, Internal Medicine
Department of Medicine and Epidemiology
School of Veterinary Medicine
University of California-Davis
Davis, California
Endocrine Disorders

Bruce J. Novotny, DVM
Board of Directors, Mark Morris Institute
Editor, Small Animal Clinical Nutrition
Topeka, Kansas
Owner, Managing Partner
Helios Communications, LLC
Bandon, Oregon
Evidence-Based Clinical Nutrition, Health Literacy and Client Compliance

Gregory K. Ogilvie, DVM, Dipl. ACVIM (Small Animal Internal Medicine, Oncology)
CVS Angel Care Cancer Center
Carlsbad, California
Cancer (case)

Connie J. Orcutt, DVM, Dipl. ABVP (Avian Practice)
Staff Clinician/Service Head
Avian and Exotic Pet Medicine
MSPCA Angell Animal Medical Center
Boston, Massachusetts
Nutrition of Reptiles (case)

Carl A. Osborne, DVM, PhD, Dipl. ACVIM (Small Animal Internal Medicine)
Professor, Small Animal Medicine
Veterinary Clinical Sciences Department
College of Veterinary Medicine
University of Minnesota
St. Paul, Minnesota
Canine Urolithiasis: Definitions, Pathophysiology and Clinical Manifestations, Canine Purine Urolithiasis: Causes, Detection, Management and Prevention, Canine Calcium Oxalate Urolithiasis: Changing Paradigms in Detection, Management and Prevention, Canine Calcium Phosphate Urolithiasis: Causes, Detection and Prevention, Canine Cystine Urolithiasis: Causes, Detection, Dissolution and Prevention, Canine Struvite Urolithiasis: Causes, Detection, Management and Prevention, Canine Silica Urolithiasis: Causes, Detection, Treatment and Prevention, Canine Compound Urolithiasis: Prevalence, Significance and Management, Feline Lower Urinary Tract Diseases (case)

Inke Paetau-Robinson, PhD, MS
Senior Research Scientist, Clinical Research
Science and Technology
Hill's Pet Nutrition, Inc.
Topeka, Kansas
Micronutrients: Minerals and Vitamins

Robert W. Phillips, DVM, PhD, Dipl. ACVN
Professor Emeritus, Department of Physiology
College of Veterinary Medicine and Biomedical Sciences
Colorado State University
Fort Collins, Colorado
Distinguished Scholar
National Academies of Practice
Board of Directors, Mark Morris Institute
Topeka, Kansas
Effects of Food on Pharmacokinetics

David J. Polzin, DVM, PhD, Dipl. ACVIM (Small Animal Internal Medicine)
Professor, Small Animal Medicine
Veterinary Clinical Sciences Department
College of Veterinary Medicine
University of Minnesota
St. Paul, Minnesota
Chronic Kidney Disease (case)

Viorela Pop, PhD
Post-Doctoral Researcher, Department of Psychology
School of Science and Technology
Loma Linda University
Loma Linda, California
Cognitive Dysfunction in Dogs

Donna M. Raditic, DVM
Nutrition
MSPCA Angell Animal Medical Center
Boston, Massachusetts
Parenteral-Assisted Feeding (case), Critical Care Nutrition and Enteral-Assisted Feeding (box)

Rebecca L. Remillard, PhD, DVM, Dipl. ACVN
Staff Nutritionist
MSPCA Angell Animal Medical Center
Boston, Massachusetts
Clinical Assistant Professor, School of Veterinary Medicine
Tufts University
North Grafton, Massachusetts
Editor, Small Animal Clinical Nutrition
Mark Morris Institute
Topeka, Kansas
Small Animal Clinical Nutrition: An Iterative Process, Making Pet Foods at Home, Critical Care Nutrition and Enteral-Assisted Feeding, Parenteral-Assisted Feeding, Obesity (box), Introduction to Gastrointestinal and Exocrine Pancreatic Diseases, Oral Diseases, Pharyngeal and Esophageal Disorders, Introduction to Gastric Diseases, Gastritis and Gastroduodenal Ulceration, Gastric Dilatation and Gastric Dilatation-Volvulus in Dogs, Gastric Motility and Emptying Disorders, Introduction to Small Intestinal Diseases, Acute Gastroenteritis and Enteritis, Inflammatory Bowel Disease, Protein-Losing Enteropathies, Short Bowel Syndrome, Small Intestinal Bacterial Overgrowth, Introduction to Large Intestinal Diseases, Large Bowel Diarrhea: Colitis, Large Bowel Diarrhea: Idiopathic Bowel Syndrome in Dogs, Constipation/Obstipation/Megacolon, Flatulence, Exocrine Pancreatic Insufficiency, Acute and Chronic Pancreatitis, Hepatobiliary Disease (case)

Arleigh J. Reynolds, DVM, PhD, Dipl. ACVN
Néstle Purina PetCare
St. Louis, Missouri
Feeding Working and Sporting Dogs (case)

Daniel C. Richardson, DVM, Dipl. ACVS
Chief Executive Officer
K-State Olathe Innovation Campus, Inc.
Olathe, Kansas
Adjunct Full Professor, Surgery
College of Veterinary Medicine
North Carolina State University
Raleigh, North Carolina
Adjunct Professor, Surgery
College of Veterinary Medicine
Kansas State University
Manhattan, Kansas
Developmental Orthopedic Disease of Dogs, Nutritional Management of Osteoarthritis

Peter Romano, Jr., BS
Senior Thermal Processing Scientist, Science and Technology
Hill's Pet Nutrition, Inc.
Topeka, Kansas
Associate, Institute for Thermal Processing Specialists
Fairfax, Virginia
Commercial Pet Foods

Philip Roudebush, DVM, Dipl. ACVIM (Small Animal Internal Medicine)
Director, Scientific Affairs and Technical Information Services
Hill's Pet Nutrition, Inc.
Topeka, Kansas
Adjunct Professor, Department of Clinical Sciences
College of Veterinary Medicine
Kansas State University
Manhattan, Kansas
Editor, Small Animal Clinical Nutrition
Mark Morris Institute
Topeka, Kansas
Evidence-Based Clinical Nutrition, Macronutrients (case) Pet Food Labels, Feeding Young Adult Dogs: Before Middle Age (case), Obesity (case), Adverse Reactions to Food, Skin and Hair Disorders, Cognitive Dysfunction in Dogs (case), Cardiovascular Disease, Flatulence, Acute and Chronic Pancreatitis (case), Hepatobiliary Disease, Effects of Food on Pharmacokinetics (case)

Korinn E. Saker, MS, DVM, PhD, MSc, Dipl. ACVN
Associate Professor, Veterinary Nutrition
Department of Molecular Biomedical Sciences
College of Veterinary Medicine
North Carolina State University
Raleigh, North Carolina
Critical Care Nutrition and Enteral-Assisted Feeding, Parenteral-Assisted Feeding, Cancer

Dale Scherl, PhD
Principal Scientist, Oral Care, Clinical Research
Science and Technology
Hill's Pet Nutrition, Inc.
Topeka, Kansas
Periodontal Disease

William D. Schoenherr, PhD, MS
Principal Nutritionist, Science and Technology
Hill's Pet Nutrition, Inc.
Topeka, Kansas
Macronutrients, Obesity, Skin and Hair Disorders

Kimberly A. Selting, DVM, MS, Dipl. ACVIM (Oncology)
Assistant Professor, Oncology
Department of Veterinary Medicine and Surgery
College of Veterinary Medicine
University of Missouri
Columbia, Missouri
Cancer

Kevin J. Shanley, DVM, Dipl. ACVD
Staff Dermatologist, Metropolitan Veterinary Associates
Valley Forge, Pennsylvania
Delaware Veterinary Specialty Group
Staff Dermatologist, Newark Animal Hospital
Newark, Delaware
Assistant Professor of Clinical Dermatology
University of Pennsylvania
Philadelphia, Pennsylvania
Adverse Reactions to Food (case)

Kenny W. Simpson, BVM&S, PhD, Dipl. ACVIM (Small Animal Internal Medicine), ECVIM
Associate Professor of Medicine
College of Veterinary Medicine
Cornell University
Ithaca, New York
Exocrine Pancreatic Insufficiency, Acute and Chronic Pancreatitis

Candace A. Sousa, DVM, Dipl. ABVP (Companion Animal), ACVD
Pfizer Animal Health
El Dorado Hills, California
Skin and Hair Disorders (cases)

Scott Stahl, DVM, Dipl. ABVP (Avian)
Stahl Exotic Animal Veterinary Services
111A Center Street South
Vienna, Virginia
Adjunct Professor, Virginia-Maryland Regional College of Veterinary Medicine
Virginia Polytechnic Institute and State University
Blacksburg, Virginia
Nutrition of Reptiles

Jörg M. Steiner, Dr Med Vet, PhD, Dipl. ACVIM (Small Animal Internal Medicine)
Associate Professor and Director of the GI Lab
Small Animal Clinical Sciences
Texas A&M University
College Station, Texas
Exocrine Pancreatic Insufficiency (case)

Neil P. Stout, BS
Vice President, Pet Nutrition Global Supply Chain
Hill's Pet Nutrition, Inc.
Topeka, Kansas
Commercial Pet Foods

Laurie L. Swanson, CVT
Minnesota Urolith Center
College of Veterinary Medicine
University of Minnesota
St. Paul, Minnesota
Canine Struvite Urolithiasis: Causes, Detection, Management and Prevention

Craig D. Thatcher, DVM, PhD, Dipl. ACVN
Professor and Dean, Polytechnic Campus School of Applied Arts and Sciences
Arizona State University
Mesa, Arizona
Editor, Small Animal Clinical Nutrition
Mark Morris Institute
Topeka, Kansas
Small Animal Clinical Nutrition: An Iterative Process, Nutrigenomics and Nutrigenetics: Nutritional Genomics in Health and Disease, Effects of Food on Pharmacokinetics (case)

Philip W. Toll, DVM, MS
Associate Medical Director, Clinical Research
Science and Technology
Hill's Pet Nutrition, Inc.
Topeka, Kansas
Adjunct Faculty, Department of Anatomy and Physiology
College of Veterinary Medicine
Kansas State University
Manhattan, Kansas
Feeding Working and Sporting Dogs, Obesity, Developmental Orthopedic Disease of Dogs

Todd L. Towell, DVM, MS, Dipl. ACVIM (Small Animal Internal Medicine)
Senior Manager, Scientific Communications
Hill's Pet Nutrition, Inc.
Topeka, Kansas
Nutritional Management of Osteoarthritis

Lauren Trepanier, DVM, PhD, Dipl. ACVIM (Small Animal Internal Medicine)
Associate Professor, Department of Medical Sciences
School of Veterinary Medicine
University of Wisconsin-Madison
Madison, Wisconsin
Effects of Food on Pharmacokinetics (case)

David C. Twedt, DVM, Dipl. ACVIM (Small Animal Internal Medicine)
Professor, Department of Clinical Sciences
College of Veterinary Medicine and Biomedical Sciences
Colorado State University
Fort Collins, Colorado
Hepatobiliary Disease

Lisa K. Ulrich, CVT
Minnesota Urolith Center
College of Veterinary Medicine
University of Minnesota
St. Paul, Minnesota
Canine Urolithiasis: Definitions, Pathophysiology and Clinical Manifestations, Canine Silica Urolithiasis: Causes, Detection, Treatment and Prevention, Canine Compound Urolithiasis: Prevalence, Significance and Management

Hilary Watson, BSc
President, HW Veterinary Nutrition Inc.
Guelph, Ontario, Canada
Pet Food Labels

Charles J. Wayner, DVM
Director, Global Veterinary Practice Health
Hill's Pet Nutrition, Inc.
Topeka, Kansas
Health Literacy and Client Compliance

Karen J. Wedekind, PhD, MS
Manager, Comparative Animal Nutrition
Novus International, Inc.
St. Charles, Missouri
Micronutrients: Minerals and Vitamins, Antioxidants, Endocrine Disorders

Carroll Weiss
Director Emeritus, DCA Study Group on Urinary Stones
Sunrise, Florida
Canine Purine Urolithiasis: Causes, Detection, Management and Prevention

Robert B. Wiggs, BS, BS, DVM, Dipl. AVDC
Owner, Coit Road Animal Hospital
Dallas, Texas
Adjunct Professor, Baylor College of Dentistry
Dallas, Texas
Periodontal Disease

Karen N. Wolf, MS, DVM
College of Veterinary Medicine
North Carolina State University
Raleigh, North Carolina
Feeding Small Pet Mammals

Ryan M. Yamka, PhD, MS, MBA
Principal Nutrition Scientist, Science and Technology
Hill's Pet Nutrition, Inc.
Topeka, Kansas
Board of Directors for Friends of the Topeka Zoo
Topeka, Kansas
Macronutrients, Obesity

Shiguang Yu, PhD, MS, BM, MBA
Principal Nutritionist, Science and Technology
Hill's Pet Nutrition, Inc.
Topeka, Kansas
Micronutrients: Minerals and Vitamins

Jürgen Zentek, Dr med vet, Dipl. ECVCN
Professor, Veterinary Specialist for Animal Nutrition and Dietetics
Freie Universitat
Berlin, Germany
Developmental Orthopedic Disease of Dogs

Steven C. Zicker, DVM, PhD, Dipl. ACVIM (Large Animal Internal Medicine), ACVN
Veterinary Clinical Nutritionist, Science and Technology
Hill's Pet Nutrition, Inc.
Topeka, Kansas
Adjunct Faculty, Department of Clinical Sciences
College of Veterinary Medicine
Kansas State University
Manhattan, Kansas
Macronutrients, Antioxidants, Introduction to Feeding Normal Dogs, Feeding Young Adult Dogs: Before Middle Age, Feeding Mature Adult Dogs: Middle Aged and Older, Feeding Reproducing Dogs, Feeding Nursing and Orphaned Puppies from Birth to Weaning, Feeding Growing Puppies: Postweaning to Adulthood, Endocrine Disorders, Developmental Orthopedic Disease of Dogs, Cognitive Dysfunction in Dogs

Preface

Veterinarians are aware of the importance of pets to society. Relating and bonding to pets adds quality to our lives and improves our longevity. Children who interact with pets are better students and function better in society. Interacting with dogs and cats lowers systolic blood pressure, decreases plasma cholesterol and triglyceride concentrations and reduces anxiety–all major risk factors for cardiovascular disease. Dog owners experience fewer health problems and require fewer physician visits.

Dogs and cats are very special companions. As such, they deserve high quality health care that will ensure the length and quality of their lives. Proper dietary management is one of the most important factors in maximizing health, performance and longevity and managing numerous diseases. Also, because pet owners continue to become more aware of the importance of nutrition in their own health, they expect state-of-the-art nutritional services for their pets. For more than 20 years, improvements in the practice of veterinary nutrition have been the goal of the American College of Veterinary Nutrition (ACVN).

The ACVN was organized in 1988 and received full accreditation by the American Veterinary Medical Association in 1997. The chief objective of the ACVN is to advance the practice of veterinary nutrition. This objective is achieved primarily through enhanced veterinary nutrition education. From inception through 2009, 68 veterinarians were certified by the ACVN; most diplomates occupy positions in veterinary schools, private practice or industry. Many of these specialists have contributed to the fifth edition of *Small Animal Clinical Nutrition,* which is intended to support the goals of the ACVN.

The 5th edition introduces new authors who join many of those who contributed to the 4th edition. Also, another editor has become part of the editorial team to help manage the writing of the 5th edition. All the authors and editors are experts and reflect the intent of this textbook to cover the increasing sophistication of small animal clinical nutrition while making the textbook a more "user friendly" clinical tool.

Much has happened in the field of small animal clinical nutrition since the publication of the 4th edition in 2000. Clinical nutrition integrates the science of nutrition with the practice of medicine and surgery to optimize health. Beyond the science, however, the art of clinical nutrition successfully combines knowledge of nutrient metabolism, pathophysiology of diseases and problematic logistics into the practical day-to-day feeding of our patients. This continues to be an exciting time for those involved in the discipline of clinical nutrition because of the increased understanding by the veterinary profession of the importance of the role of nutrition in animal health and disease management, the continued interest on the part of pet owners for the best nutritional information for their pets and the continued proliferation of commercially available veterinary therapeutic foods. Veterinary health care teams have several advantages over their human medical counterparts to affect a patient's overall health through nutrition. Dietary compliance may be better among veterinary patients than among people. In human clinical nutrition, dietitians provide food and nutrient guidelines, but ultimately the patient is in control of dietary compliance and must correctly choose from a variety of foods. Although the human component is also present in compliance issues in veterinary clinical nutrition, readily available, highly palatable, convenient to use pet foods specifically designed for the treatment or prevention of specific diseases may improve compliance. These products are powerful tools in the feeding management of dog and cats. Hence, there are many opportunities for us to have a positive impact on the long-term health of pets and to assist in the medical/surgical management of numerous diseases.

Opportunities exist to expand the role of nutrition in veterinary medicine and, in the process, further improve patient care. Research shows that fewer than 5% of the dogs and cats that visit veterinary hospitals are fed veterinarian-dispensed therapeutic or wellness foods despite clinical and epidemiologic evidence that three-fourths of adult dogs and cats have periodontal disease and more than one-fourth of the pet population is overweight or obese. Nutritional answers exist for these and other clinical problems. Veterinarians and their health care teams who understand the process of clinical nutrition and conscientiously apply its principles will benefit their patients, clients and practices.

New nutritional information has led to improved commercial veterinary therapeutic and wellness foods. These foods are readily available to veterinarians; it is important that veterinarians and their health care teams understand the benefits and shortcomings of specific foods and judiciously select the best food for each patient. The concept of evidence-based clinical nutrition (Chapter 2) can assist in food selection based on rigorous assessment of evidence for or against particular management options. We have listed a variety of commercial foods in this book's product tables. These listings are dictated by quality, market share, availability of published nutrient information and space; the thousands of commercial foods and homemade recipes that are available preclude a complete listing.

The authors and editors have done their best to integrate the latest nutrition research and the current understanding of clinical nutrition into this textbook. We hope that this information will stimulate continued interest and research in small animal clinical nutrition that will benefit pets and ultimately society.

THE EDITORS

NOTICE

Companion animal practice, clinical nutrition and commercial pet foods are ever changing. The authors and editors of this textbook have carefully checked trade names, nutrient levels and recommended uses of commercial pet foods listed in *Small Animal Clinical Nutrition, 5th Edition,* to ensure that the information provided is precise and in accordance with standards accepted at the time of publication. Readers are advised, however, to check the most current product information provided by the manufacturer of each food to ensure that a product's nutrient profile, feeding guide and contraindications for feeding are accurate.

These same precautions have been taken to ensure that recommendations for drug therapy, when provided, are also accurate. And, as with foods, readers are advised to check the manufacturer's information for each drug to be used to verify that the recommended dose and the method and duration of administration are accurate and to be aware of potential contraindications.

These precautions are particularly important in regards to new or infrequently used foods or drugs. It is the responsibility of those recommending a food or administering a drug, relying on their professional skill and experience, to determine the best treatment for the patient. This includes the appropriate food and/or drug and their proper administration. Neither the publisher nor the editors assume any liability for any injury and/or damage to animals or property arising from the use of this publication.

Although this textbook is intended to be a global reference for companion animal nutrition, only North American products are listed in the food tables. Also, the regulatory guidelines used herein are those of the Association of American Feed Control Officials and the United States Food and Drug Administration. Regulatory agencies, regulation of foods, nutrients, supplements, drugs and claims may be different in geographies outside North America.

THE PUBLISHER

Features of *Small Animal Clinical Nutrition, 5th Edition*

The chief goal of this textbook is to provide basic and applied information about small animal clinical nutrition to veterinary students and practicing veterinarians worldwide. New information regarding advances in small animal nutrition is published continuously but, there is often a lack of understanding about how to apply that information to clinical patients. This book is organized not only to deliver the latest information about small animal clinical nutrition but also to teach and reinforce the process of clinical nutrition; that is, how clinical nutrition should be practiced.

Organization

The book is organized into 23 sections to facilitate location of information. Section 1 (Principles of Small Animal Clinical Nutrition) begins with an overview of the iterative process of clinical nutrition with emphasis on patient assessment, development of a comprehensive feeding plan and reassessment or monitoring the patient. The iterative process outlined in the first chapter is the foundation upon which most of the other chapters are constructed. **Figure 1** summarizes the clinical nutrition process for those chapters that directly apply to patients. The subsequent organization of these chapters emphasizes the importance of the process in addition to the clinical and nutritional information necessary for the proper dietary management of patients. The other chapters in Section 1 review basic information about dog and cat nutrition. Four new chapters are included:

- Evidence-Based Clinical Nutrition
- Health Literacy and Client Compliance
- Nutrigenomics and Nutrigenetics: Nutritional Genomics in Health and Disease
- Antioxidants.

Section 2 (Pet Foods) covers a wide range of topics about commercial and homemade pet foods. This section ends with a unique chapter on pet food safety, which is an important topic in this era of increased concerns and public debate about safety of pet and human foods. Three new cases appear in each of the Food Safety and Evidence-Based Clinical Nutrition chapters.

Sections 3 and 5 (Nutritional Management of Healthy Dogs and Cats, respectively) provide important information about how to feed dogs and cats with the goals of optimizing wellness and performance. For easier access, these chapters have been updated and subdivided according to lifestage and reproductive activity. Section 4 contains feeding information for working and sporting dogs.

Sections 6 through 21 cover dietary management of patients with clinical disorders. All chapters have been updated and two of the larger chapters from *Small Animal*

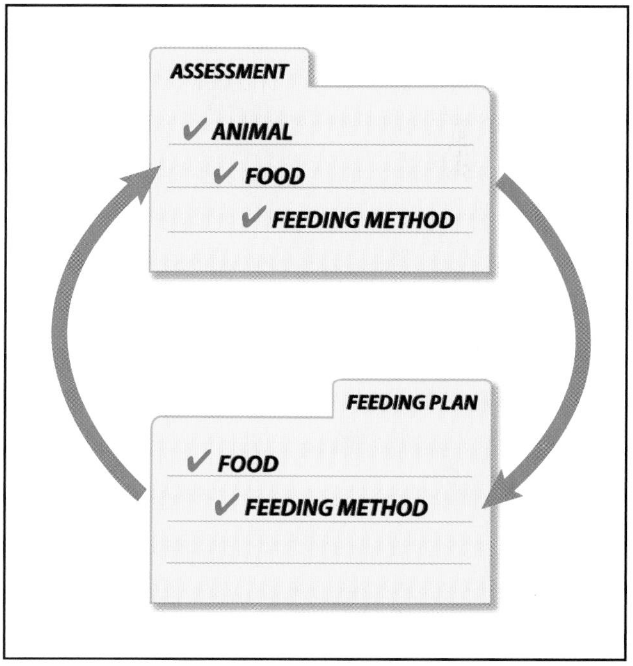

Figure 1. The iterative process of clinical nutrition.

Table 1. General format for most chapters.
Introduction/clinical importance
Patient assessment
History and physical examination
Laboratory and other clinical information
Risk factors
Key nutritional factors
Feeding plan
Assess and select the food
Assess and determine the feeding method
Reassessment
Endnotes and references
Cases

Clinical Nutrition, 4th ed. gastrointestinal/exocrine pancreatic diseases and canine urolithiasis have been subdivided based on diagnosis and urolith type, respectively. In addition to a significant amount of new information about clinical topics, two new chapters have been added:

- Nutritional Management of Osteoarthritis
- Cognitive Dysfunction in Dogs.

Thirteen new cases appear within these sections to illustrate dietary management principles.

Table 1 shows the general format for the chapters in Sections 3 through 20 that deal with nutrition of healthy patients and those with clinical problems. Most chapters follow the two-step iterative clinical nutrition process. Each chapter begins with an introduction (or clinical importance) and discussion about the goals of feeding a patient. A discussion of the first step, Patient Assessment, leads to the determination of the associated key nutritional factors. Wherever possible, key nutritional factors and their recommended levels are developed using evidence-based rules. Otherwise, information from other species and clinical experience are the basis for their determination. The second step, Feeding Plan, includes choosing an appropriate food and feeding method. The iterative process is then completed with discussion of reassessment or monitoring plans. Section 21 concludes with an updated review of the effects of food on pharmacokinetics.

Section 22 (feeding small mammals, reptiles and pet birds) is included in response to numerous requests for practical feeding information for these patients. Birds, rodents, ferrets, rabbits and reptiles were once considered exotic pets but today are common veterinary patients. Four new cases have been added to this section. Section 23 (Appendices) summarizes a broad range of useful nutritional and dietary information that supports the concepts found throughout the book. The Index is the last feature in the book.

Features

Several features are incorporated to make the book more readily accessible, including:

- Sections are divided by colors that make it easier to find content.
- The book has been prepared using full-color design and many of the medical illustrations have been redrawn in color.
- The diagram of the two-step iterative process (Patient Assessment and Feeding Plan) is found at the beginning of each section that has direct application to healthy and clinical patients.
- Separate colors are used for headings in the Patient Assessment and Feeding Plan sections so it is easier to locate the feeding plan section for quick clinical reference.
- Boxes that discuss various topics of interest are included in most chapters.
- Recommended key nutritional factor profiles are included in food tables for comparison to the key nutritional content of selected commercial foods. Commercial foods included in food tables in Sections 3 through 5 are for healthy dogs and cats, whereas those listed in food tables in Sections 6 through 20 are usually veterinary therapeutic foods. This information will help the reader select the most appropriate food for each patient.
- The key nutritional factor profiles for the foods listed in the food tables (food table information was obtained by an outside firm) will be updated periodically and these updates and Index will be available at www.markmorris.org.
- Evidence-based nutrition is used where possible to guide selection of the best food for clinical patients.
- Actual clinical cases are described at the end of most chapters and sometimes within boxes. These cases teach the key concepts outlined in the chapters through use of the two-step iterative process, guiding questions and focused discussion. A comprehensive list of cases is found inside the front cover.
- The names of journals, books and proceedings in reference lists are spelled out in full rather than using abbreviations; the references are available at www.markmorris.org.
- For the global audience, energy values are usually expressed as kilocalories and kilo- or megajoules.

Contents

Contents

Contents

Contents

Section 1

Principles of Small Animal Clinical Nutrition

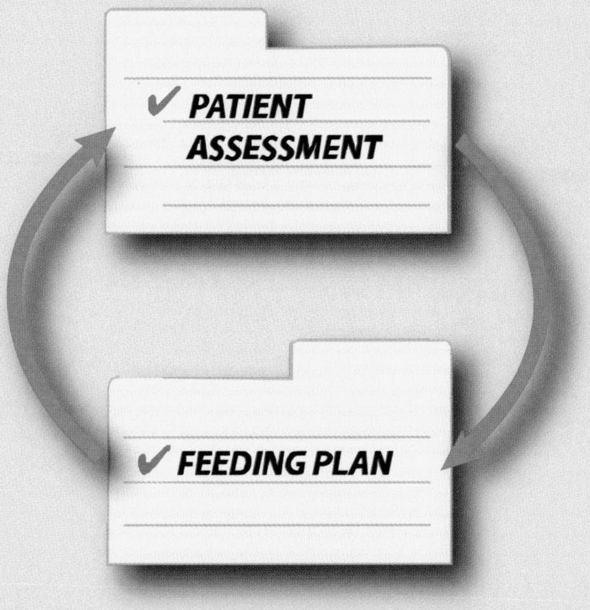

Chapter 1

Small Animal Clinical Nutrition: An Iterative Process

Craig D. Thatcher
Michael S. Hand
Rebecca L. Remillard

"Things should be made as simple as possible, but not simpler."
Albert Einstein

CLINICAL IMPORTANCE

The public has become increasingly more aware of the importance of nutrition to health during the past four decades as a result of the growing recognition that food is associated with disease processes such as coronary artery disease, hypertension, obesity, diabetes mellitus and cancer. *Healthy People 2010* is a comprehensive set of disease prevention and health promotion objectives for the United States. *Healthy People 2010* uses 10 leading health indicators that reflect the major health concerns in the nation at the beginning of the 21st century. These indicators were selected based on their importance as public health issues and their ability to motivate action and provide data to measure progress against specific goals. One of the focus areas is nutrition, especially overweight/obesity conditions (Healthy People 2010).

The discipline of veterinary nutrition and its relationship to the practice of veterinary medicine have benefited from these changes. Food animal veterinarians have long recognized that no aspect of the production enterprise has more impact on health and production than nutrition; many health problems are associated with inadequate feeding programs. Food animal veterinarians recognize that optimizing feeding programs improves food animal health and productivity and, as a result, the economic status of producers. Food animal veterinarians who provide their clients with high-quality production medicine programs become unbiased nutritional consultants.

Similarly, small animal practitioners must improve their nutritional counseling skills because they cannot truly meet their patients' health needs without optimizing nutrition. Small animal veterinarians can improve the quality of medicine delivered to their patients by knowledgeably and systematically addressing the nutritional aspects of each case, whether the goal is treating or preventing disease. Veterinarians must emphasize health maintenance and wellness strategies for companion animals to provide the most beneficial service. Total disease prevention requires lifelong dedication to proper nutrition, immunizations, dental care and parasite control programs. Nutritional factors are a cornerstone in maximizing health, performance, longevity and disease prevention. Nutritional counseling and intervention, however, are beneficial only if done properly.

Veterinarians and their health care teams have considerable influence on the foods clients feed their pets. A study conducted by *Veterinary Economics* in 1990 found that 87% of veterinarians felt that offering nutritional services improved their practices (Gants, 1990). Ninety-four percent of these veterinarians said that their clients were somewhat or very receptive to nutrition-related information. A 1995 study conducted by the American Animal Hospital Association found that 54% of pet owners interviewed sought veterinary advice on pet foods at least once and 43% had received a recommendation from their veterinarian on which manufacturer's pet food to feed their puppies or kittens. Seventy percent of the latter group fed the brand of food recommended by their veterinarian (AAHA, 1995).

The word *recommend* means to counsel or advise (American Heritage Dictionary). The implication is that the advice proceeds from actual knowledge of the subject. Veterinarians should know how food needs vary with each lifestage, with mental, physical and environmental stresses and with diseases. Causes and effects of dietary imbalances should be considered so that the resulting disorders can be prevented or diagnosed and treated. Veterinarians should also be familiar with the various pet foods available to help clients choose the most appropriate ones. Veterinarians also need to understand the benefits and shortcomings of various feeding methods. After a feeding plan has been instituted, veterinarians need the skills to monitor the program to assess and reassess outcomes and to modify the feeding plan when necessary. The primary goal of this chapter is to provide practicing veterinarians, veterinary technicians and students with the basic problem-solving processes needed to successfully manage the nutrition of companion animal patients.

The Two-Step Iterative Process of Clinical Nutrition

A brief review of instructional systems design (ISD) is in order to better understand iterative (repetitive) processes. ISD emerged after World War II as a set of recognized standard procedures used to develop well-structured materials in response to the need for more efficient training techniques (Moore and Kearsley, 1996). ISD embodies various perspectives on learning, teaching, systems theory, behavioral psychology, communications and information theory. The ISD model breaks instruction into a series of phases or steps with defined procedures; a defined service or product must be delivered at each step. Steps include: 1) design, 2) development, 3) implementation, 4) evaluation and 5) analysis. Then, the process repeats itself as a continuous loop and may involve many cycles. The American College of Veterinary Nutrition (ACVN) has recommended that nutrition problem solving include assessment of the patient, the food and the feeding method (Bauer et al, 1995).

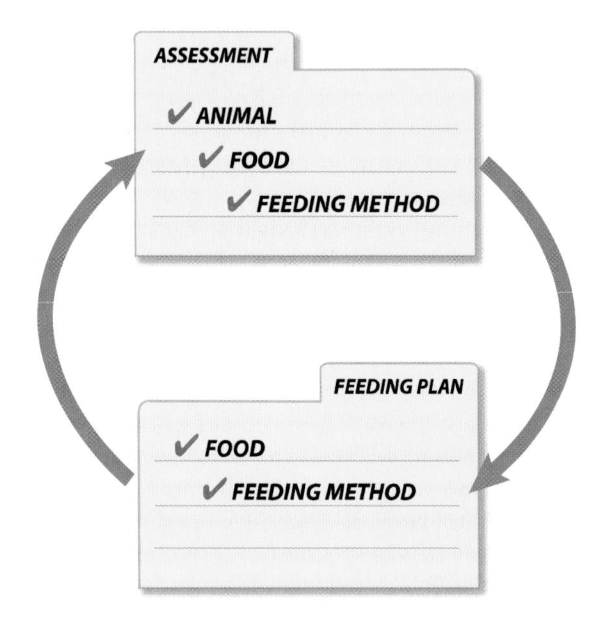

Figure 1-1. The two-step process of veterinary clinical nutrition.

Figure 1-1 depicts the iterative process used in this book. The first step is patient assessment, which allows the determination of the patient's key nutritional factors and their levels (the concept of key nutritional factors is described below). Determination of the key nutritional factors is the basis for the second step: the feeding plan. The feeding plan includes recommendations for food and feeding methods. If assessment of the current food and feeding methods indicates that they are appropriate, the current feeding plan can remain in place. However, if the assessment indicates otherwise, a new feeding plan should be formulated and implemented.

After a suitable period of time (the length of which depends on the patient's condition), the two-step process is repeated to determine the appropriateness or effectiveness of the new feeding plan. Thus, the patient is reassessed and, if necessary, a new feeding plan is developed and implemented. This is the iterative or repetitive part of the process. Any number of iterations of the two-step process can occur, depending on the needs of each patient. A critically ill patient may need to be reassessed every few hours, whereas a normal adult dog or cat may be reassessed annually. The subsequent reassessment of the patient at each cycle is also referred to as monitoring. This information is discussed under the heading of reassessment in the chapters that deal with patient assessment and feeding plans.

PATIENT ASSESSMENT

The goal of patient assessment is to establish a dog's or cat's key nutritional factors and their target levels in light of its physiologic or disease condition. The patient's key nutritional factors are the benchmark for assessing the animal's food and selecting a food. Assessment of dogs and cats to determine their key nutritional factor status should be a structured process that includes: 1) review of the history and medical record, 2) physical examination and 3) laboratory tests and other diagnostic procedures (Remillard and Thatcher, 1989). These first three steps determine the patient's physiologic state and medical diagnosis and are the basis for the fourth step, which is the determination of the key nutritional factors and the estimation of their target levels.

Obtain an Accurate History and Review the Medical Record

Obtaining the animal's history and reviewing the medical record help determine the nutritional status of the patient. The signalment is part of the history and defines the patient's physiologic state and includes: 1) species, 2) breed, 3) age, 4) gender, 5) reproductive status, 6) activity level and 7) environment.

A complete history should also include questions about the pet's weight and therapies (medical, surgical, etc.) that may affect appetite, nutrient metabolism or both. An accurate description of the current feeding plan, including the animal's food, eating and drinking habits and feeding methods should be obtained from the client. Intakes of treats and nutritional supplements should be recorded.

Review of the medical record provides objective historical information and documents the pet's previous health status, health maintenance procedures that were performed and medications that were prescribed. Veterinarians should evaluate this information to determine if any of these factors are related to the animal's current nutritional status. This review permits early nutritional intervention in the treatment of established malnutrition (under- or overnutrition) and in the prevention of malnutrition in individuals at risk (**Box 1-1**).

A patient's food is usually changed because of altered requirements or alterations in nutrient intake, digestion, absorption, metabolism, excretion or a combination of these factors. Knowledge of normal nutritional physiology and of diseases and their nutritional pathophysiology is important to identify patients at risk for malnutrition. The history and medical record are tools to help identify these risks.

Conduct a Physical Examination

A thorough physical examination can help define an animal's nutritional status and identify diseases that may have a nutritional component. Physical findings should be recorded in the patient's medical record. Veterinarians should examine each body system for problems that are responsive to nutritional intervention. An animal's body condition will likely reflect abnormalities of major organ systems.

Body condition can be subjectively assessed by a process called body condition scoring. In general, this process assesses a patient's fat stores and, to a lesser extent, muscle mass. Fat cover is evaluated over the ribs, down the topline, around the tailbase and ventrally along the abdomen. Body condition score (BCS) descriptors have been developed with respect to the species (dogs and cats) and age of the patient (**Figures 1-2** and **1-3**). Score descriptors vary due to the structural differences between species and between young and adult pets. The scores range from 1 to 5 with 1 being very thin and 5 being grossly obese. A body condition score of 3/5 is generally referred to as being ideal. An "ideal" body condition, however, depends on the dog's or cat's lifestage, lifestyle and intended use. For example, a BCS of 2/5 to 2.5/5 may be desirable for a racing greyhound, whereas a BCS of 3.5/5 might be better for a pregnant queen at the end of its first trimester to help support the upcoming lactation. A BCS of 2.5/5 to 3/5 is probably ideal for most mature dogs and cats for optimal health and resultant longevity. Thus, overall, an ideal BCS is a range of numbers rather than simply a "3/5."

Body condition scoring reasonably estimates an animal's body composition. Studies assessing scorer repeatability and variations between scorers have found agreement between 80 to 90% of the measurements (LaFlamme et al, 1994; Graham et al, 1982; Croxton and Stollard, 1976; Burkholder, 1994). Research with cats found a correlation of 0.9 or higher between BCS and body composition predicted from morphometry (LaFlamme, 1993). Veterinarians should routinely assign BCSs, obtain body weights and record both in the medical record.

The patient's body weight can be compared with breed standards (Appendix 14) or with the animal's previous body weight from the medical record. The patient's pre-illness body weight or usual body weight during health can serve as a standard for determining the effect of illness on body weight. A history of rapid weight loss and a reduced BCS may indicate a catabolic condition with a marked loss of lean tissue, dehydration or both. A history of progressive weight gain and an increased BCS may indicate an anabolic condition with an excessive accumulation of fat, water or both.

Box 1-1. Malnutrition Includes Excesses.

Malnutrition is defined as any disorder of nutrition with inadequate or unbalanced nutrition. Many veterinarians and animal owners think only of nutritional deficiencies when they hear the term malnutrition. Muscle wasting and a distended abdomen in a starving third-world child or a heavily parasitized puppy is often our first mental image of malnutrition. In first-world societies, however, malnutrition is usually due to overnutrition or excessive intake of nutrients. Obesity due to consumption of excessive levels of fat and calories is a common example of malnutrition in people and their pets. Another example of malnutrition due to unbalanced nutrition is developmental orthopedic disease seen in rapidly growing large- and giant-breed puppies as a result of excessive calcium and energy intake. Malnutrition due to either nutrient deficiencies or excesses can be harmful to dogs and cats.

Conduct Necessary Laboratory Tests and Other Diagnostics

No single laboratory test or other diagnostic procedure can accurately assess a patient's nutritional status. Routine complete blood counts, urinalyses and biochemistry profiles, however, can provide insight into the presence of metabolic disorders and other diseases. Albumin concentration, lymphocyte count, packed cell volume and serum total protein values may serve as general indicators of nutritional status. Other chapters in this textbook will discuss specific laboratory tests and other diagnostic procedures that may help assess healthy and sick patients.

Serum protein concentrations in people provide an estimate of long- and short-term changes in nutritional status and correlate with morbidity and mortality (Giner et al, 1996). For example, low serum albumin concentrations may indicate protein depletion due to chronic undernutrition or protein loss. Shorter half-life serum protein concentrations such as prealbumin, transferrin, retinol-binding protein and fibronectin are used in human medicine to assess short-term changes in nutritional status. However, these tests have not been routinely available in veterinary medicine. Although not used widely, serum creatine kinase concentrations are elevated in anorectic cats and decline after 48 hours of nutritional support. Serum

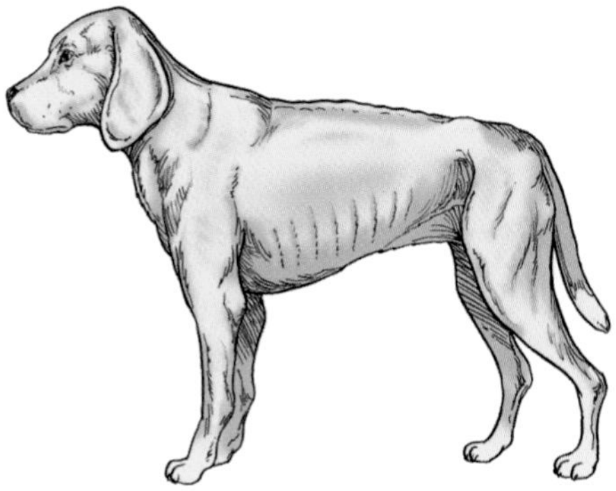

BCS 1. Very thin ▶

The ribs are easily palpable with no fat cover. The tailbase has a prominent raised bony structure with no tissue between the skin and bone. The bony prominences are easily felt with no overlying fat. Dogs over six months of age have a severe abdominal tuck when viewed from the side and an accentuated hourglass shape when viewed from above.

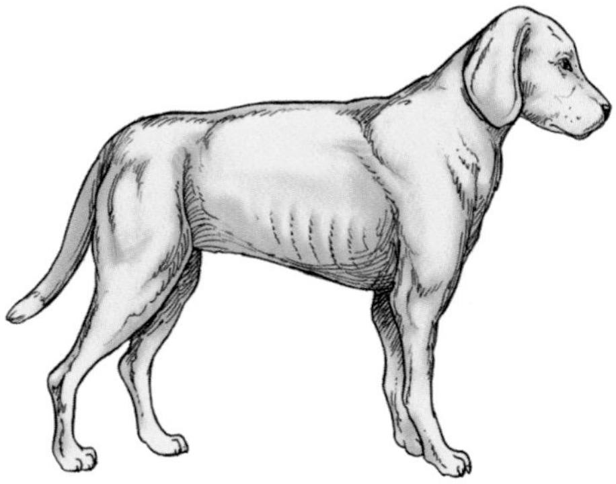

◀ BCS 2. Underweight

The ribs are easily palpable with minimal fat cover. The tailbase has a raised bony structure with little tissue between the skin and bone. The bony prominences are easily felt with minimal overlying fat. Dogs over six months of age have an abdominal tuck when viewed from the side and a marked hourglass shape when viewed from above.

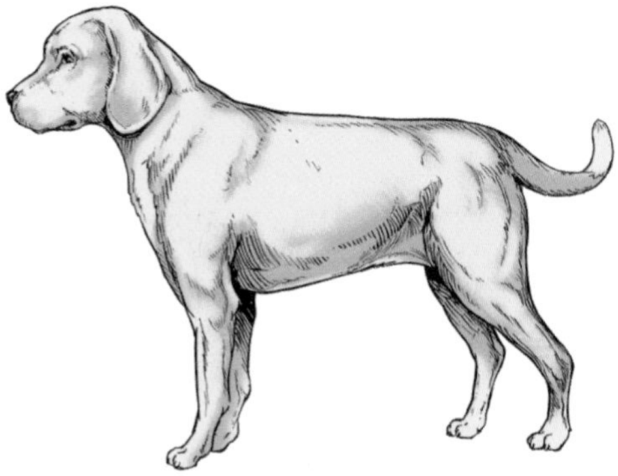

BCS 3. Ideal ▶

The ribs are palpable with a slight fat cover. The tailbase has a smooth contour or some thickening. The bony structures are palpable under a thin layer of fat between the skin and bone. The bony prominences are easily felt under minimal amounts of overlying fat. Dogs over six months of age have a slight abdominal tuck when viewed from the side and a well-proportioned lumbar waist when viewed from above.

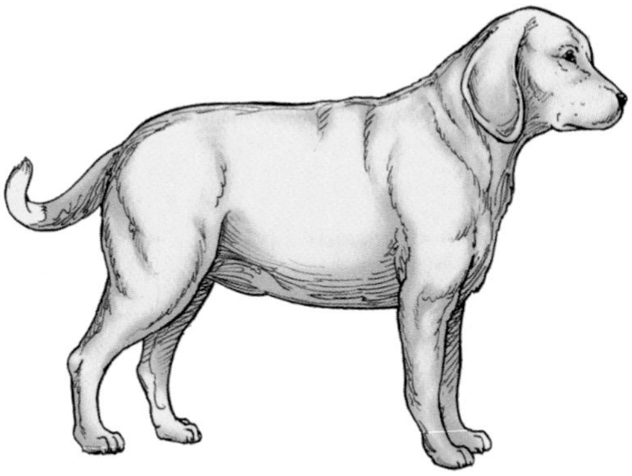

◀ BCS 4. Overweight

The ribs are difficult to feel with moderate fat cover. The tailbase has some thickening with moderate amounts of tissue between the skin and bone. The bony structures can still be palpated. The bony prominences are covered by a moderate layer of fat. Dogs over six months of age have little or no abdominal tuck or waist when viewed from the side. The back is slightly broadened when viewed from above.

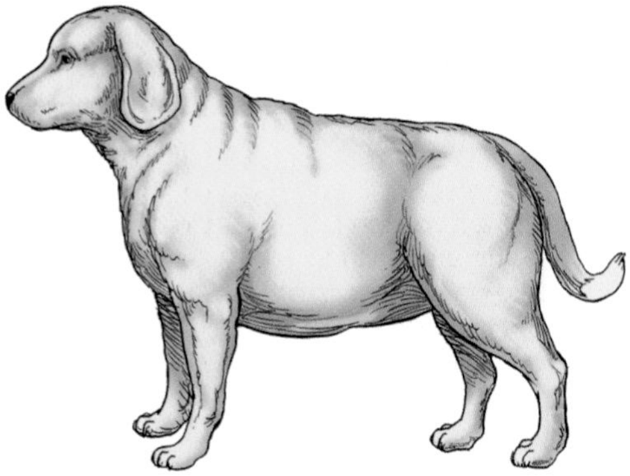

BCS 5. Obese ▶

The ribs are very difficult to feel under a thick fat cover. The tailbase appears thickened and is difficult to feel under a prominent layer of fat. The bony prominences are covered by a moderate to thick layer of fat. Dogs over six months of age have a pendulous ventral bulge and no waist when viewed from the side due to extensive fat deposits. The back is markedly broadened when viewed from above. A trough may form when epaxial areas bulge dorsally.

Figure 1-2. Body condition score (BCS) descriptors for dogs in a five-point system.

BCS 1. Very thin ▶
The ribs are easily palpable with no fat cover. The bony prominences are easily felt with no overlying fat. Cats over six months of age have a severe abdominal tuck when viewed from the side and an accentuated hourglass shape when viewed from above.

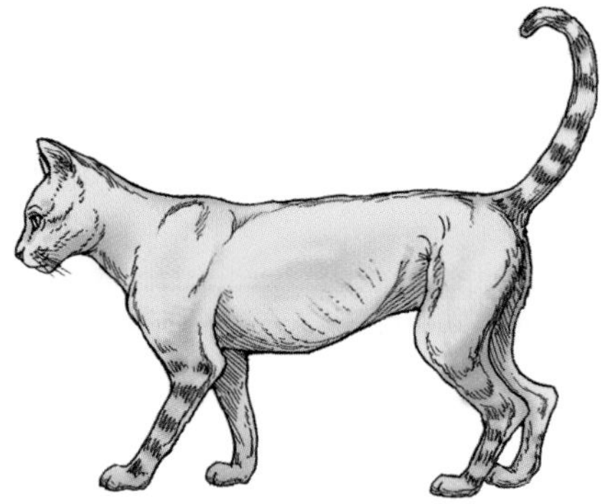

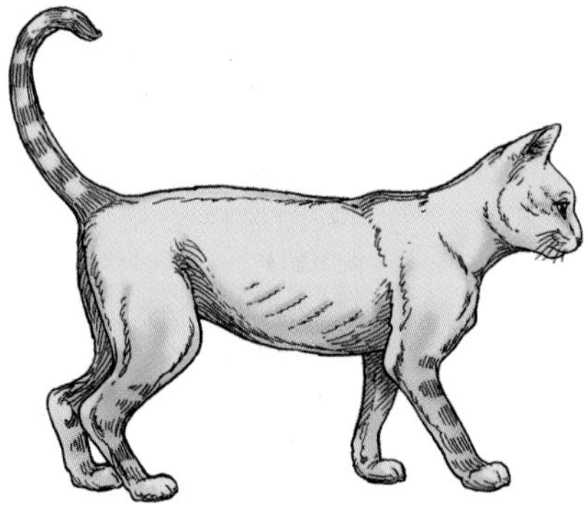

◀ BCS 2. Underweight
The ribs are easily palpable with minimal fat cover. The bony prominences are easily felt with minimal overlying fat. Cats over six months of age have an abdominal tuck when viewed from the side and a marked hourglass shape when viewed from above.

BCS 3. Ideal ▶
The ribs are palpable with a slight fat cover. The bony prominences are easily felt under a slight amount of overlying fat. Cats over six months of age have an abdominal tuck when viewed from the side and a well-proportioned lumbar waist when viewed from above.

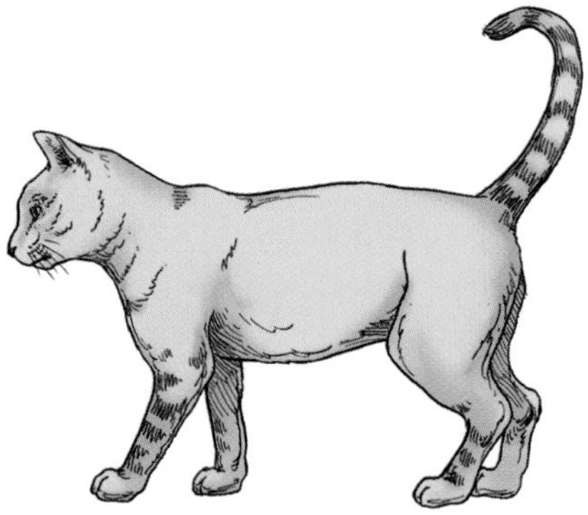

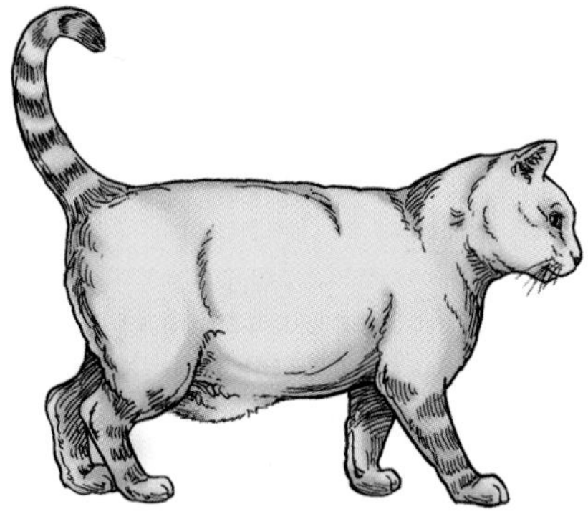

◀ BCS 4. Overweight
The ribs are difficult to feel with moderate fat cover. The bony structures can still be palpated. The bony prominences are covered by a moderate layer of fat. Cats over six months of age have little or no abdominal tuck or waist when viewed from the side. The back is slightly broadened when viewed from above. A moderate abdominal fat pad is present.

BCS 5. Obese ▶
The ribs are very difficult to feel under a thick fat cover. The bony prominences are covered by a moderate to thick layer of fat. Cats over six months of age have a pendulous ventral bulge and no waist when viewed from the side due to extensive fat deposits. The back is markedly broadened when viewed from above. A marked abdominal fat pad is present. Fat deposits may be found on the limbs and face.

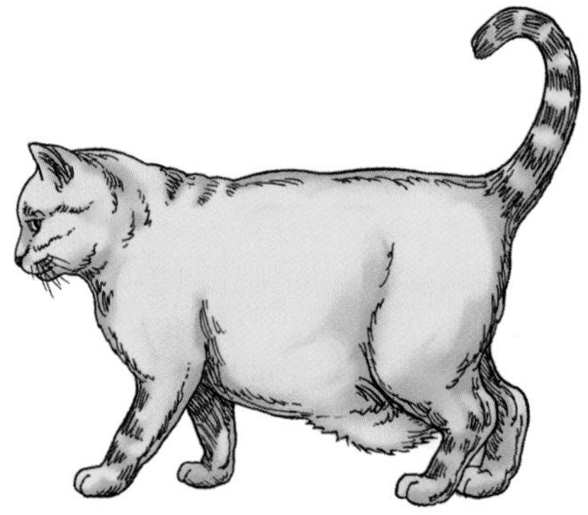

Figure 1-3. Body condition score (BCS) descriptors for cats in a five-point system.

creatine kinase concentrations may become a useful marker for assessing and monitoring nutritional status in animals (Fascetti et al, 1997).

Results of a single measurement or test must be interpreted cautiously, because over- or under-hydration can alter concentrations of these proteins. Diagnostics such as radiography and ultrasonography, including echocardiography, may be indicated to further characterize the health status of patients. Results of laboratory and diagnostic tests should always be viewed in the context of findings from the history, physical examination and the patient's medical record.

Determine the Key Nutritional Factors and Their Target Levels

The concept of key nutritional factors is fundamental to the practical application of clinical nutrition used in this text. However, to better understand the basis for this concept, a brief review of nutrient requirements vs. nutrient allowances precedes the description of key nutritional factors.

Researchers traditionally have used normal dogs and cats to determine nutrient requirements. In the United States, the primary sources for minimum nutrient requirements of healthy dogs and cats are the National Research Council (NRC) Nutrient Requirement bulletins published in 1985 and 1986, respectively and recently updated as a combined edition (NRC, 1985; NRC, 1986; NRC, 2006). The requirements published in 1985 and 1986 were determined by feeding dogs and cats purified diets rather than commercially available foods. These NRC values, therefore, were minimum nutrient requirements that had to be extrapolated to the types of foods normally fed to dogs and cats. In 1993 and 1994, the Association of American Feed Control Officials (AAFCO) published recommended nutrient profiles for dog and cat foods, respectively (Nutrient Profiles for Dog Foods, 1993; Nutrient Profiles for Cat Foods, 1994). These nutrient profiles have been republished yearly and are the official source for nutrient profiles for commercial dog and cat foods in the United States.

The AAFCO nutrient profiles include safety factors similar to those in the recommended dietary allowances (RDAs) that have been established for people (NRC, 1989). These safety factors compensate for changes in a food's nutrient availability due to ingredient and processing variables and for individual differences in nutrient requirements within dog and cat populations. Because of these safety factors, the term "allowance" is better suited to describe AAFCO values than "requirements." AAFCO values are adequate to meet the known nutrient needs of almost all healthy dogs and cats and are a better source of feeding recommendations for most dogs and cats than are minimum requirements. The earlier NRC bulletins published for dogs and cats in 1974 and 1978, respectively, also included safety factors and therefore were actually "allowances." Besides recommendations for lower limits, AAFCO prescribes upper limits for certain nutrients with the obvious implication that some nutrient excesses can be harmful. As with RDAs for people, AAFCO allowances for pet food nutrient profiles are not necessarily optimal.

Instead of separate dog and cat editions, the recently updated NRC includes information about both species. It provides nutrient requirements in three formats: minimum requirement, adequate intake and recommended allowance (2006). Minimum requirement is defined as the minimal concentration or amount of a maximally available nutrient that will support a defined physiologic state. Adequate intake is defined as the concentration or amount of a nutrient demonstrated to support a defined physiologic state when no minimum requirement has been demonstrated. Recommended allowance is defined as the concentration or amount of a nutrient in a diet formulated to support a given physiologic state. The recommended allowance is based on the minimum requirement with consideration for the normal variation in bioavailability of the nutrient in typical-quality feed ingredients. If no minimum requirement is available, the recommended allowance is based on adequate intake. Like the old editions, the more recent NRC edition also includes safe upper limit levels for a nutrient when data are available (NRC, 2006).

Neither NRC nor AAFCO has established nutrient profiles for geriatric dogs and cats and those with specific disease processes.

Key Nutritional Factors

Key nutritional factors encompass nutrients of concern and other food characteristics. The concept of nutrients of concern greatly simplifies the approach to clinical nutrition because most commercial pet foods sold in the United States provide at least AAFCO allowances of all nutrients. Thus, if a commercial food is fed, veterinarians and their health care teams need only to understand and focus on delivering the target levels for a few nutrients (nutrients of concern) rather than the 40 plus nutrients currently recognized for cats and dogs (NRC, 2006).

Nutrients of concern encompass nutritional risk factors for disease treatment and prevention as well as nutrients that are key to optimizing normal physiologic processes such as growth, gestation, lactation and physical work. The following elements must be considered in determining key nutritional factors and their target levels: 1) the patient's lifestage and physiologic state, 2) environmental conditions such as temperature, housing and pet-to-pet competition, 3) the nature of any disease or injury, 4) the known nutrient losses through skin, urine and gastrointestinal tract, 5) the interactions of medications and nutrients, if applicable, 6) the known capacity of the body to store certain nutrients and 7) the interrelationships of various nutrients.

Besides requiring specific levels of certain nutrients, some patients have other food-related needs. These needs might include management of acute or chronic systemic acid-base balance, maintenance of a specific urinary pH range, certain kibble texture, a specific range of digestibility or osmolality, avoidance of certain protein sources and presence of specific ingredients. Some nutrients and ingredients that are added to foods provide other non-nutritive functions that can be important to health and performance. Thus, specific food characteristics or factors other than the nutrient content may be important to consider. Information about such food characteristics should be available from product manufacturers. Pet food labels contain addresses and toll-free phone numbers of the manufacturer.

Chapters 12 through 24 determine and list key nutritional factors and their target levels for healthy dogs and cats. The key nutritional factors and their target levels for dogs and cats with specific disease complexes can be found in Chapters 25 through 68. For convenience, these chapters also contain levels of key nutritional factors in commercial foods typically marketed for use in patients with various medical conditions. Regardless of which nutrients are considered as key nutritional factors, the reader should understand the various ways nutrient needs are expressed. **Box 1-2** describes the methods and units for expressing an animal's nutrient needs.

In summary, the primary goal of patient assessment is to establish the patient's key nutritional factor needs. The key nutritional factors are the benchmark for assessing the adequacy of a patient's food. Additionally, the results of patient assessment are the basis for determining an appropriate feeding method.

FEEDING PLAN

The feeding plan can be developed after the key nutritional factor needs have been determined. The feeding plan includes what food or foods to feed and which feeding methods to use. Thus, the first step is to assess the current food and to select the best food to feed.

Assess and Select the Food

The primary components of food assessment should include: 1) evaluation of the current food's key nutritional factor content relative to the patient's needs (determined during Patient Assessment, above) and 2) determination whether or not feeding tests or clinical trials were conducted.

Determine the Food's Key Nutritional Factor Content

The key nutritional factors and their levels for most of the commonly used commercial foods are listed in the food tables in the individual chapters. In most instances, these profiles will provide the necessary information. If the key nutritional factor information of the food in question is not listed in the food tables, the manufacturer should be contacted for that information. Pet food labels contain addresses and toll-free phone numbers of the manufacturer.

Although much less convenient, there are other ways to determine most of a food's key nutritional factor content. Many, if not most, key nutritional factors are nutrients. **Box 1-3** describes various ways to determine the nutrient content of a food. **Box 1-2** describes methods and units used in expressing the nutrient content of food.

Key Nutritional Factor Comparison

Comparing a food's key nutritional factor content with the patient's needs will help identify any significant imbalances in the food being fed. If the patient's current food is adequate (key nutritional factors in balance with the patient's needs) then the food currently being fed can continue to be fed. However, if important excesses or deficiencies exist, the patient's current food must be "balanced."

There are numerous approaches to balancing foods. Some are rather extensive (**Boxes 1-4** and **1-5**). This section will review the most practical methods including: 1) food replacement and 2) simple mathematical ration balancing (Pearson square). Alternatively, veterinarians can contact a veterinary nutritionist who accepts referrals. Both the ACVN and the European College of Veterinary Nutrition (ECVN) have diplomates who do referral work. Contact the executive director of the ACVN to obtain a list of diplomates who do nutrition referral work. Contact information for the executive director can be found in the AVMA Directory or online at www.ACVN.org.

When comparing a food's key nutritional factor nutrient content with a patient's needs, methods of expressing nutrient content of the food and nutrient requirements of the animal must be compatible (same units). In this textbook, compatible units are used in the food tables for comparing the food's key nutritional factor content and the patient's target values. See **Box 1-2** for more details about how food content and animal needs are expressed.

Food Replacement

If food assessment indicates that an animal's key nutritional factor requirements are not being met, the most practical way to balance a food is to simply select a different food (i.e., one that does a better job of meeting the patient's requirements). The most likely application of this method occurs when one commercial food is substituted for another. If homemade foods are being used, they can be replaced by appropriate commercial foods or another homemade food if other recipes are available (Chapter 10).

The process is straightforward and simple. The nutrient content of other foods is evaluated to see which food most closely meets the animal's requirements. Assuming comparable palatability, the most acceptable food replaces the previous food. **Case 1-3** demonstrates food replacement. This process is greatly facilitated by the food tables in the feeding healthy dog and cat chapters (Chapters 12 through 17 for dogs and 19 through 24 for cats) and the feeding clinically ill patient chapters (Chapters 25 through 68). These tables list the key nutritional factor targets and the key nutritional factor contents of commercial foods commonly marketed for patients at various lifestages and those having specific diseases.

Changing foods for most healthy dogs and cats is of minor consequence. Some owners switch their pets from one food to another daily. Most dogs and cats tolerate these changes. However, vomiting, diarrhea, belching, flatulence or a combination of signs may occur with sudden, rapid switching of foods, probably because of ingredient differences. It is prudent, therefore, to recommend that owners change their pet's food over the course of at least three days. A seven-day period is even

Box 1-2. Typical Methods and Units for Expressing a Patient's Nutrient Needs and a Food's Nutrient Content and Methods for Conversion to the Same Units.

When comparing a patient's nutrient requirements to a food's nutrient content to determine adequacy of the food, the same quantifying units must be used to make the comparison meaningful. The units used for expressing food nutrient content and patient nutrient requirements are compared in **Table 1**.

PATIENT'S NUTRIENT NEEDS

The three methods for expressing an animal's nutrient needs are: 1) dry matter, energy density defined and 2) energy basis and 3) absolute basis.

Dry matter basis, energy density defined is the percentage or quantity of a nutrient in the food's dry matter that is needed by the animal. This measure is the most common method of expressing an animal's nutrient needs. It describes what is required in a food and indicates an animal's nutrient needs. Dry matter refers to that weight of the food remaining when the water content is subtracted. (**Tables 2** and **3** demonstrate methods of calculating dry matter.) Dry matter values are most meaningful if the energy density of the food's dry matter is specified because most animals eat, or are fed, to meet their energy requirements.

Energy basis refers to the quantities of nutrients per animal's energy requirement. Units of measure are typically nutrient amounts per 100 kcal or 1 MJ metabolizable energy (ME). Occasionally an animal's protein, fat and digestible (soluble) carbohydrate needs are expressed as a percentage of the animal's total energy needs (**Table 4**).

Absolute basis refers to the unit measure (usually weight) of a nutrient that is needed by an animal in a 24-hour period. These needs are expressed as quantities per kg of body weight per day.

FOOD'S NUTRIENT CONTENT

Although there are three methods for expressing an animal's nutrient needs, there are four methods for expressing a food's nutrient content: 1) as fed basis, 2) dry matter basis, 3) dry matter basis, energy density defined and 4) energy basis.

As fed basis simply refers to the quantity of nutrients in a food as it is fed. This method ignores moisture and energy content. The units of measure are percentages or quantities of nutrients per unit weight (kg) of food.

Dry matter is that weight of the food remaining after the water content has been subtracted from the as fed amount. Dry matter basis, therefore, is the amount of nutrients in the food's dry matter. It accounts for variability in water content but not variability in energy density. The units of measure are percentages or quantities of nutrients per unit weight (kg) of food dry matter. The usefulness of dry matter basis is limited because the energy density of individual foods can vary widely. This consideration will be further explained below (dry matter basis, energy density defined). **Tables 2** and **3** show the conversion from as fed basis to dry matter basis.

Dry matter basis, energy density defined is the same as dry matter but specifies a food's energy density, thus accounting for potential variability. The units of measure are the same as those used with dry matter basis but are further qualified by expressing the energy density of the food. For example, recommended nutrient values for canine and feline foods are based on an energy density of 3.5 and 4.0 kcal ME/g (14.64 and 16.74 kJ ME/g) of food dry matter, respectively. Dry matter basis, energy density defined is probably the most widely used method of expressing a food's nutrient content.

Energy basis refers simply to the amount of nutrients per 100 kcal or 1 megajoule ME of food. Occasionally, a food's protein, fat and digestible carbohydrate content is expressed as a percentage of the food's total energy content (**Table 4**).

Both dry matter basis, energy density defined and energy basis are reasonably accurate methods of expressing a food's nutrient content. However, even these methods have limitations.

Animals require less food to meet their energy requirements when foods with higher energy densities are fed. Under these circumstances, the concentrations of the other nutrients in the food need to be increased proportionately, to ensure the animal receives the minimum amount of all nutrients needed in a smaller amount of food.

When foods with lower energy densities are fed, a lower concentration of the other nutrients may be required, assuming the dog or cat could eat, or would be fed, enough of the food to meet its energy requirement. In these instances, the nutrient levels need to be decreased proportionately, so that the animal would not receive toxic levels of nutrients in a larger amount of food.

Foods of low energy density, particularly those low in fat and high in fiber, are usually intended for animals that have a tendency to be overweight. These animals should be fed fewer calories than animals with normal body weights and body condition scores. The nutrient content of foods in this category should not be corrected for their lower energy density. During weight loss, there is a disproportionately lower energy intake relative to the non-energy nutrients. Although these animals require fewer calories to lose weight, as far as is known, their requirement for other nutrients has not changed. Thus, they are essentially being fed the same amount of dry matter but fewer calories. On an energy basis (g/kcal), the food's nutrient values will be higher than if the animal had normal energy requirements.

On the other end of the spectrum are situations in which foods of high energy density are fed to animals with an unusually high need for energy-providing nutrients relative to non-energy nutrients. A working sled dog is an example. In this case, on an energy basis, the food's non-energy nutrient content could be lower than if the animal had normal energy needs.

CONVERTING TO SAME UNITS

Comparing food on an as fed basis to an animal's requirement on an absolute basis requires: 1) mathematical calculation and 2) either the energy density of the food or the amounts of the energy-supplying nutrients in the food. **Table 5** provides an example of such a calculation.

When using dry matter basis, energy density defined to compare foods or to compare foods with animal requirements, the energy densities must be the same for the comparisons to be meaningful. **Table 6** shows how to convert to the same energy density. In some cases it will be desirable to convert food nutrient content on an as fed basis to dry matter basis, energy density defined (**Case 1-1**).

Box 1-2 continued

Table 1. Comparisons of methods to express food nutrient content and animal requirements/allowances for nutritional assessment of food.

Food nutrient content (units)
As fed basis (% or amount of nutrient/kg food)
Dry matter basis (% or amount of nutrient/kg of food dry matter)
Dry matter basis, energy density defined (% or amount of nutrient/kg of food dry matter, at a specified energy density)
Energy basis (amount of nutrient/100 kcal or 1 megajoule ME of food's energy content)

Dog/cat requirements/allowances (units)
Absolute basis (amount of nutrient/kg animal)
Dry matter basis, energy density defined (% or amount of nutrient/kg of food dry matter, at a specified energy density)
Energy basis (amount of nutrient/100 kcal or 1 megajoule ME of animal's energy requirement)

Table 2. How to convert from as fed basis to dry matter basis.

Step 1. Obtain the food's dry matter content by subtracting the water content from the as fed amount of the food.

Example A: If a moist food contains 75% water, 25% of the food is dry matter:
100% as fed – 75% water = 25% food dry matter

Example B: If a dry food contains 10% water, 90% of the food is dry matter:
100% as fed – 10% water = 90% food dry matter

Step 2. Convert the percentage as fed nutrient content of the food to a dry matter basis by dividing the percentage of the nutrient content on an as fed basis by the percentage dry matter.

Example A: If the moist food above contained 10% protein on an as fed basis, on a dry matter basis it would contain 40% protein:
10% protein as fed basis ÷ 25% dry matter = 40% protein dry matter basis

Example B: If the dry food above contained 18% protein on an as fed basis, on a dry matter basis, it would contain 20% protein:
18% protein as fed basis ÷ 90% dry matter = 20% protein dry matter basis

Table 3. Shorthand method for converting from as fed basis to dry matter basis.

A less accurate, shorthand method for converting from an as fed basis to a dry matter basis is to simply multiply the percentage nutrient content on an as fed basis by four for moist foods or add 10% for dry foods. This method is based on the assumption that moist foods contain approximately 75% water and dry foods contain approximately 10% water. Check the guaranteed analysis on the product label.

Example A: If a moist food contains 10% protein on an as fed basis, on a dry matter basis it would contain 40% protein:
10% protein as fed basis x 4 (factor for moist foods) = 40% protein dry matter basis*

Example B: If a dry food contains 18% protein on an as fed basis, on a dry matter basis it would contain 20% protein:
18% protein as fed basis + 10% (factor for dry food) = approximately 20% protein dry matter basis*

*Compare these results with those obtained in **Table 2** for moist and dry foods with the same moisture content.

Table 4. How to determine the protein, fat and carbohydrate content as a percent of the food's total energy content.

Practically speaking, the available energy in foods for dogs and cats is provided by digestible carbohydrates, protein and fat; dietary fiber provides little if any energy to these species. Occasionally an animal's need for, or a food's content of, any or all of these three nutrients is expressed in terms of the fraction of the total energy they provide. The method is simply another way to express the relative amounts of these three nutrients. The following example demonstrates how to calculate the percentage of kcal and kJ from protein, fat and digestible carbohydrate of a pet food.

Nutrient	%	kcal/g of nutrient	kJ/g of nutrient	kcal/g of food**	kJ/g of food**
Protein	22	3.5*	14.64*	0.77	3.22
Fat	9	8.5*	35.56*	0.77	3.20
Digestible carbohydrate	51	3.5*	14.64*	1.79	7.47
Total	-	-	-	3.33	13.89

% kcal from protein = 0.77 ÷ 3.33 = 23.1
% kJ from protein = 3.22 ÷ 13.89 = 23.2
% kcal from fat = 0.77 ÷ 3.33 = 23.1
% kJ from fat = 3.20 ÷ 13.89 = 23.0
% kcal from digestible carbohydrate = 1.79 ÷ 3.33 = 53.8
% kJ from digestible carbohydrate = 7.47 ÷ 13.89 = 53.8

*"Modified" Atwater values.
See **Box 1-6, Table 3 for a more detailed explanation for calculation of energy density of pet foods.

Table 5. Example illustrating the mathematical process required to compare a food's nutrient content on an as fed basis to an animal's needs on an absolute basis.

Example: If an intact male cat weighing 4.5 kg requires 31 mg of magnesium (Mg) per day (recommended allowance) and the cat's food as fed contains 0.12% Mg, 20% fat, 35% protein and 27% digestible carbohydrate, does the cat receive adequate amounts of Mg? The answer is calculated as follows:

1) First find out how much food is to be fed. Because animals are fed to meet their energy requirements, the first step is to determine the energy density of the food, if it is unknown. This is done by calculating the amount of energy provided by each of the energy-supplying nutrients. Using the "modified" Atwater energy values of 3.5, 8.5 and 3.5 kcal metabolizable energy (ME)/g (14.64, 35.56 and 14.64 kJ ME/g) for protein, fat and digestible carbohydrate respectively (See **Box 1-6**, **Table 2**), multiply the percentage of each nutrient in the food (as fed basis) by 1 g of food. Then multiply the answer by the energy density of each nutrient. The sum of the three separate energy values is the energy density of the food.

In kcal ME/g of food:
35% protein x 1 g food x 3.5 kcal ME/g
= 1.23 kcal ME/g from protein

20% fat x 1 g food x 8.5 kcal ME/g
= 1.70 kcal ME/g from fat

27% digestible carbohydrate x 1 g food x 3.5 kcal ME/g
= 0.95 kcal ME/g from carbohydrate

Sum
3.88 kcal ME/g food (total)

Box 1-2 continued

2) The next step is to determine the daily energy requirement (DER) of the animal. Multiply the formula for resting energy requirement (RER) by the appropriate modifier for maintenance of an adult cat (**Box 6, Table 1**).

RER (kcal ME/day) = $70(BW_{kg})^{0.75}$
RER (kJ ME/day) = $293(BW_{kg})^{0.75}$

= $70(4.5\ BW_{kg})^{0.75}$ = 216 kcal ME/day
= $293(4.5\ BW_{kg})^{0.75}$ = 904 kJ ME/day

Modifier for feline adult maintenance = 1.4 x RER = DER
Modifier for feline adult maintenance = 1.4 x RER = DER

DER (kcal ME/day) = 1.4 x 216 kcal ME = 302 kcal ME
DER (kJ ME/day) = 1.4 x 904 kJ ME = 1,266 kJ ME

3) Determine the amount of food to be fed by dividing the cat's energy requirement by the energy density of the food.
302 kcal ME/day ÷ 3.88 kcal ME/g = 78 g food/day
1,266 kJ ME/day ÷ 16.18 kJ ME/g = 78 g food/day

4) Determine the amount of Mg provided by the food by multiplying the amount of food fed by the percentage of Mg in the food.
78 g food x 0.12% Mg = 0.090 g (90 mg) Mg
The amount of Mg provided by the food (90 mg) compared with the animal's requirement of 31 mg indicates more than an adequate (threefold) amount of Mg.

Table 6. How to convert to the same energy density.

Correcting energy densities in order to make valid nutrient comparisons, either between foods or between a food and an animal's requirement, is based on the assumption that the relationship between nutrient content and energy density is directly proportional. A simple ratio can be established to generate a multiplier that converts the units of the animal's requirements to those of the food; then the animal's requirement and the food's nutrient content can be compared. The multiplier is obtained by dividing the energy density of the food by the requirement energy density.

Example: Is a food that provides 0.72% potassium and 4 kcal (16.74 kJ)/g, on a dry matter (DM) basis, adequate for canine adult maintenance?
1) The requirement for potassium is 0.6% DM basis in an adult dog food that provides 3.5 kcal (14.64 kJ)/g.

2) Convert the requirement to the same energy density as the food by generating the multiplier.
Multiplier
= Food energy density ÷ requirement energy density
= 4.0 kcal (16.74 kJ)/g DM ÷ 3.5 kcal (14.64 kJ)/g DM
= 1.14

3) To obtain the equivalent nutrient requirement for a food providing 4 kcal (14.74 kJ)/g, on a DM basis, multiply the requirement by the multiplier.
Equivalent nutrient requirement
= 1.14 x 0.06% potassium
= 0.68% potassium, 4 kcal (14.74 kJ)/g, on a DM basis

4) The amount of potassium in the food (0.72%) is compared to the animal's equivalent nutrient requirement (0.68%) and is found to be adequate.

5) The multiplier obtained above (1.14) can be used to convert the other nutrient requirements to the same basis as the food to compare the adequacy of their levels, if desired.

After the energy densities of the food and the animal's needs are converted to the same units, the comparison is simple.

better, as owners increase the proportion of new food and decrease the proportion of old food (**Table 1-1**). Nearly all pets readily tolerate a seven-day transition period. A much longer transitional period is recommended in cases in which the food change is known to be significant, the pet has demonstrated a poor tolerance to such changes in the past or food refusal is expected (**Table 1-1**). For example, a long transition schedule is likely to be needed for an old cat recently diagnosed with kidney disease when the food must be switched from a highly palatable grocery "gourmet" food to an appropriate veterinary therapeutic food.

Table 1-1. Recommended short- and long-term food transition schedules for dogs and cats.

Short schedule* Dogs and cats (days)	Long schedule** Dogs (days)	Long schedule** Cats (weeks)	Food percentages Previous food	Food percentages New food
1,2	1-3	1	75	25
3,4	4-6	2	50	50
5,6	7-9	3	25	75
7	10	4	0	100

*Recommended for most healthy dogs and cats.
**Recommended for situations in which the food change is known to be significant, the dog or cat has demonstrated low tolerance to such changes in the past or food refusal is anticipated.

Simple Mathematical Ration Balancing (Pearson Square)

The Pearson square is another useful diet balancing tool. This handy method can be used to combine any two foods, supplements or ingredients to yield a mixture with a desired nutrient content. **Figure 1-4** shows how the Pearson square method is used to balance a diet. Here's how to use the Pearson square:

- A small square is drawn and the desired nutrient concentration of the proposed mixture is written in the middle of the square.
- The nutrient concentration of one component of the mixture is written at the upper left corner of the square.
- The nutrient concentration of the other component of the mixture is written at the lower left corner of the square.
- The nutrient values at the corners are subtracted from those in the center of the square. The smaller number is always subtracted from the larger and the differences written diagonally at the right corners of the square.
- The differences are added together and the sum is written below each difference as the denominator of a fraction.
- The fractions are converted to percentages. These percentages are the proportion of each component of the mixture in the corners directly to the left. When combined in those percentages, the constituent components will yield a mixture

Box 1-3. Four Ways to Determine the Nutrient Content of a Food.

The nutrient content of a food can be determined one of four ways:

1) Obtain the target values from the manufacturers of commercially prepared foods.
2) Order a laboratory analysis.
3) Calculate the content based on the published values for the ingredients.
4) Use the information found in the label guaranteed analysis and typical analysis (Chapter 9).

Only the first three are recommended because of the severe limitations of label guarantees and typical analyses.

Most pet food manufacturers, upon request, will supply target values for the nutrient content of their products. This approach is simple and inexpensive. Although these values usually reflect actual average nutrient levels, occasionally they vary significantly from actual values, thus this method is not always accurate. No laws govern the accuracy of target nutrient levels. In most instances, however, these values will be adequate.

The basic laboratory analysis is the proximate analysis (Figure 5-3), which provides the percentage moisture, crude protein, crude fat, ash and crude fiber in a food and allows calculation of the digestible carbohydrate fraction (also referred to as the nitrogen-free extract [NFE]). Most commercial laboratories will also conduct more expansive nutrient analyses including amino acids, fatty acids, minerals, vitamins and various fiber fractions. Analysis of food samples for nutrient content is very straightforward and usually accurate. Limitations include proper sampling, the potential issue of analytical variance for certain nutrients and the expense and time involved for a complete analysis.

Calculations require nutrient contents of ingredients and a formula for the food in question. Published average nutrient contents of ingredients can be obtained from NRC nutrient requirement booklets and listings of average nutrient contents of human foods. This approach would likely be used for determining the nutrient content of a homemade food. One limitation of this method is the time and knowledge required to do such calculations. Another limitation is accuracy (i.e., how closely the published average nutrient content of the ingredients represents the ingredient's actual nutrient content). Values can vary markedly.

The use of guaranteed analyses (United States and Canada) or typical analyses (Europe) listed on the label of commercially prepared foods as a means of establishing nutrient content has severe limitations:

In the case of guaranteed analysis, the quantities listed are minimums or maximums only.

It is only necessary to list a fraction of the nutrients in the food (e.g., guaranteed analysis only requires crude protein, crude fat, crude fiber and moisture; typical analysis only requires crude protein, crude fat, crude fiber, ash and moisture if more than 14%).

Guaranteed analysis values are not the nutrient content of the food. They are a guarantee by the manufacturer that the food contains not more, or less, than the stated amount. Label guarantees can provide a general idea of the nutrient content for a limited number of nutrients and the classification of the food (growth-type food, maintenance food, etc.).

Use caution when using guaranteed and typical analyses to compare specific nutrient levels between foods. When such comparisons are made, be sure to compare similar forms of foods (i.e., dry to dry or moist to moist). Label guarantees are listed on an as fed basis. Different forms of food can be compared if the foods are converted to the same moisture or energy content (**Tables 2, 3** and **6** in **Box 1-2**).

Box 1-4. Computerized Food Evaluation/Balancing Programs.

There are two categories of food evaluation/balancing software programs listed below. The category entitled "Veterinary Clinical Nutrition Software" is a special application designed for use by veterinarians and veterinary nutritionists. It contains commercial pet food and human food nutrient data that enable users to select foods and make feeding and weight-loss feeding plans for individual patients. Additional tools for automatic formulation of homemade pet foods from recipes are also available.

A cautionary reminder: software programs are tools intended to make the mathematical work of food evaluation/balancing/formulation easier and faster. Their accuracy depends entirely on the accuracy of the databases from which they are working and they do not account for nutrient availability regarding ingredient sourcing and cooking, nor do they ensure a palatable food.

Veterinary Clinical Nutrition Software Programs

Davis Veterinary Medical Consulting, PC
707 Fourth Street, Suite 307
Davis, CA 95616
Phone: (530) 756- 3862 or (888) 346-6362
Fax: (530) 756-3863
E-mail: info@dvmconsulting.com
www.balanceit.com
Balance IT

Commercial Formulation Software Programs

Creative Formulation Concepts, LLC
1831 Forest Drive, Suite H
Annapolis, MD 21401
Phone: (410) 267-5540
Fax: (410) 267-5542)
http://creativeformulation.com
Concept5

Feedsoft Formulation
14001 Dallas Parkway, Suite 1200
Dallas, TX 75240
Phone: (866) 363-7843
Fax: (972) 231-9096
http://feedsoft.com

Agricultural Software Consultants, Inc.
2726-600 Shelter Island Drive
San Diego, CA 92106
Phone: (619) 226-2600
Fax: (619) 226-7900
Mixit-Win 5

Format International, Ltd.
Format House
Poole Road
Woking
Surrey England GU21 6DY
Phone: +44 (0)1483 726081
Fax: +44 (0)1483 722827
www.format-international.com
New Century

Format International, Inc.
10715 Kahlmeyer Drive
St. Louis, MO 63132
Phone: (888) 628-5683
Fax: (314) 428-4102
www.format-international.com
New Century

Box 1-5. Food Formulation and Extensive Food Balancing.

It is not the intention of this book to teach complete food formulation or extensive food balancing. Few practitioners need to know how to formulate balanced foods from scratch. Nutrient requirement information is readily available; however, accurate/relevant ingredient nutrient databases, an understanding of the availability of nutrients in various ingredients, knowledge of the effect of cooking on nutrient availability and knowledge of all of these variables on palatability are complex issues. Such information is not readily available, and usually requires assimilation by a team of experts, including veterinarians, nutritionists and food scientists to ensure proper formulation of complete and balanced foods.

Fortunately, numerous complete pet food options are readily available from commercial pet food manufacturers. Many homemade food recipes have also been published. Be sure to obtain homemade food recipes from reliable sources as discussed in Chapter 10.

As an example, the Pearson square can be used to solve the following problem: How much calcium carbonate containing 36% calcium must be added to a meat-based food to increase its calcium content from 0.01% to 0.3% on an as fed basis? Assume you are making 5 kg of the mixture. The problem is set up and worked as follows:

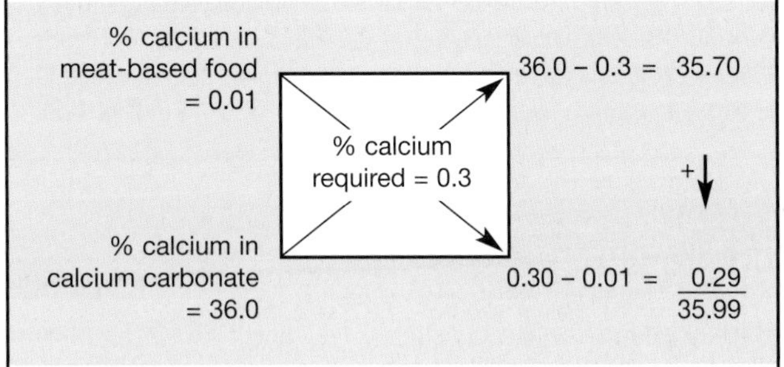

The final step converts fraction to percentages by dividing the numerator of the fractions by the denominator and multiplying by 100.

Meat-based food: (35.70 ÷ 35.99) x 100 = 99.19%

Calcium carbonate: (0.29 ÷ 35.99) x 100 = 0.81%

If the total mixture is 5 kg, then 99.19% (4.96 kg) should be a meat-based food and 0.81% (0.04 kg, or 40 g) should be calcium carbonate.

Figure 1-4. Example of how to use the Pearson square.

having the same concentration as the number in the center of the square.

Feeding Tests and Clinical Trials

Evaluation of the product label of commercial foods can provide feeding test information. Determining if a food has been evaluated in clinical trials is a more complicated matter and is covered in Chapter 9 and in various clinical chapters.

Whether or not commercial foods for healthy pets have been animal tested can usually be determined from the nutritional adequacy statement on the product's label (Chapter 9). Published clinical trials and case reports for commercial veterinary therapeutic foods can be obtained from the product's manufacturer. As mentioned above, manufacturers' addresses and toll-free phone numbers are found on pet food labels. However, some brands of these products have passed regulatory agency (AAFCO) prescribed feeding tests although the product label may not include such information.

Commercial pet foods that have undergone AAFCO-prescribed or similar feeding tests provide reasonable assurance of nutrient availability and sufficient palatability to ensure acceptability (i.e., food intake sufficient to meet nutrient needs). Feeding tests also provide some assurance that a product will adequately support certain functions such as gestation, lactation and growth. However, even controlled animal testing is not infallible.

In the United States, the AAFCO testing protocol for adult maintenance lasts six months, requires only eight animals per group and monitors a limited number of parameters (Chapter 9). Passing such tests does not ensure the food will be effective in preventing long-term nutrition/health problems or detect problems with prevalence rates less than 15%. Likewise, these protocols are not intended to ensure optimal growth or maximize physical activity. Besides feeding tests, AAFCO prescribes other methods to assure nutritional adequacy (Chapter 9). Thus, in addition to meeting AAFCO requirements, the food should be evaluated to ensure that key nutritional factors are at levels appropriate for promotion of long-term health or for optimal performance. Few, if any, homemade recipes have been animal tested according to prescribed feeding protocols.

Although not considered feeding tests, the personal observations of veterinarians and pet owners about the performance of specific foods or recipes can be valuable. Such experiences are, in a sense, uncontrolled feeding tests. Through experience, veterinarians and pet owners form impressions about a food's value in disease management, its ability to support various lifestages and work, its palatability, resultant stool quality and skin and coat benefits. Limitations of personal observations include the lack of controls and the length of time it takes (months to years) to gather sufficient information about a wide variety of products. Also, some commercial products are continuously improved; therefore, yesterday's product does not necessarily reflect the capabilities of the "same" product today. However, personal observations can augment controlled feeding tests such as published clinical trials and regulatory agency prescribed feeding protocols for healthy pets.

Physical Evaluation of the Food

Conducting a physical evaluation of the food is of limited usefulness. It can provide information about a food's consistency and whether or not there are extraneous materials in the food. It can also determine package quality, which may or may not reflect product quality. Physical evaluation of the food is probably most useful for assessing whether or not the food has spoiled (Chapter 11).

Box 1-6. A Method for Calculating the Food Dosage Estimate.

Calculations to estimate food dosage are based on the assumption that if a food contains the proper proportions of nutrients relative to its energy density, and is fed to meet an animal's energy requirement, then the animal's requirements for non-energy nutrients will automatically be met. This calculation has three steps:

1) Estimate the energy requirement of the animal (**Table 1**).
2) Determine the energy density of the food (kcal or kJ ME/g food, as fed basis). Sources include product labels, product literature, contacting the product's customer service department by phone or e-mail (phone numbers or e-mail addresses can often be found on the product label). The energy density can be calculated using Atwater values (**Tables 2** and **3**).
3) Divide the energy requirement of the patient by the energy density of the food to determine the daily amount to feed (food dosage).

Table 1. Calculation of energy requirements.

Calculation of daily energy requirement (DER) is based on the resting energy requirement (RER) for the animal modified by a factor to account for normal activity or production (e.g., growth, gestation, lactation, work). RER is a function of metabolic body size. RER is calculated by raising the animal's body weight in kg to the 0.75 power. The average RER for mammals is about 70 kcal/day/kg metabolic body size: RER (kcal/day) = $70(BW_{kg})^{0.75}$ or $30(BW_{kg}) + 70$ (if the animal weighs between 2 and 45 kg). RER values can also be obtained from Table 5-2, Part 3. Expressed in kJ, the average RER for mammals is about $293(BW_{kg})^{0.75}$. These energy requirements should be used as guidelines, starting points or estimates of energy requirements for individual animals and not as absolute requirements.

Feline DER

Maintenance (0.8 to 1.8 x RER)

Neutered adult	= 1.2-1.4 x RER
Intact adult	= 1.4-1.6 x RER
Inactive/obese prone	= 1.0 x RER
Weight loss	= 0.8 x RER
Senior adult (7-11 years)	= 1.1-1.4 x RER
Very old adult (>11 years)	= 1.1-1.6 x RER
Critical care	= 1.0 x RER
Weight gain	= 1.2-1.8 x RER at ideal weight

Gestation

Energy requirement increases linearly during gestation in cats. Energy intake should be increased to 1.6 x RER at breeding and gradually increased through gestation to 2 x RER at parturition. Free-choice feeding of pregnant queens is also recommended.

Lactation

Lactation is nutritionally demanding and the physiologic and nutritional equivalent of heavy work. Recommend 2 to 6 x RER (depending on number of kittens nursing) or free-choice feeding. The following table may also be used to estimate the DER of lactating queens:

Weeks of lactation	DER
Weeks 1-2	RER + 30% per kitten
Week 3	RER + 45% per kitten
Week 4	RER + 55% per kitten
Week 5	RER + 65% per kitten
Week 6	RER + 90% per kitten

Growth

Daily energy intake for growing kittens should be about 2.5 x RER. Free-choice feeding is recommended.

Canine DER

Maintenance (1.0 to 1.8 x RER)

Neutered adult	= 1.6 x RER
Intact adult	= 1.8 x RER
Inactive/obese prone	= 1.2-1.4 x RER
Weight loss	= 1.0 x RER
Critical care	= 1.0 x RER
Weight gain	= 1.2-1.8 x RER at ideal weight

Work

Light work	= 1.6-2.0 x RER
Moderate work	= 2.0-5.0 x RER
Heavy work	= 5.0-11.0 x RER

Gestation

First 42 days: feed as an intact adult.
Last 21 days: use 3 x RER. (This quantity may need to be increased to maintain normal body condition for some dogs, especially larger breeds.)

Lactation

Lactation is nutritionally demanding and the physiologic and nutritional equivalent of heavy work.
Recommend 4 to 8 x RER (depending on number of puppies nursing) or free-choice feeding.
The following table may also be used to estimate the DER of lactating bitches:

Puppies (No.)	DER
1	3.0 x RER
2	3.5 x RER
3-4	4.0 x RER
5-6	5.0 x RER
7-8	5.5 x RER
9	≥6.0 x RER

Growth

Daily energy intake for growing puppies should be 3 x RER from weaning until four months of age.
At four months of age energy intake should be reduced to 2 x RER until the puppy reaches adult size.

Table 2. Energy available from protein, fat and digestible carbohydrate (nitrogen-free extract).

Metabolizable energy (kcal/g)

Species	Crude protein	Crude fat	Digestible carbohydrate
All*	4.4 x digest.*	9.4 x digest.*	4.15 x digest.*
Dogs and cats**	3.5**	8.5**	3.5**

Metabolizable energy (kJ/g)

Species	Crude protein	Crude fat	Digestible carbohydrate
All*	18.41 x digest.*	39.33 x digest.*	17.36 x digest.*
Dogs and cats**	14.64**	35.56**	14.64**

Key: digest. = digestibility
*The most accurate value to use when the digestibility of the three nutrients is known. (Adapted from Lewis et al, 1987)
**"Modified" Atwater values (Dog Food Nutrient Profiles and Cat Food Nutrient Profiles). Association of American Feed Control Officials 2007.

Box 1-6 continued

Table 3. Example calculation of caloric density of a pet food.*

Analysis			**Metabolizable energy (kcal)**		
	%		kcal/g of nutrient**		kcal/g of food
Protein	22	x	3.5	=	0.77
Fat	9	x	8.5	=	0.77
Fiber***	3	x	0	=	0
Moisture	10	x	0	=	0
Ash***	5	x	0	=	0
Digestible carbohydrate†	51	x	3.5	=	1.79
Total					**3.32††**

Analysis			**Metabolizable energy (kJ)**		
	%		kJ/g of nutrient**		kJ/g of food
Protein	22	x	14.64	=	3.22
Fat	9	x	35.56	=	3.20
Fiber***	3	x	0	=	0
Moisture	10	x	0	=	0
Ash***	5	x	0	=	0
Digestible carbohydrate†	51	x	14.64	=	7.47
Total					**13.89††**

3.33 kcal/g (13.89 kJ/g) x amount of food/measuring cup = kcal/measuring cup†††

*As fed basis.
From **Table 1-8.
***If not available, these may be estimated as 3% fiber and 9% ash in dry foods, 1% fiber and 6% ash in soft-moist foods and 1% fiber and 2.5% ash in moist foods.
†Percent digestible carbohydrate (nitrogen-free extract) usually is not stated but can be calculated on an as fed basis by subtracting the percent protein, fat, fiber, moisture and ash from 100.
††If the nutrient percentages were obtained from the label guarantee, multiply the food's caloric density by 1.2 for moist pet foods and 1.1 for semi-moist and dry pet foods. In this example, 3.33 (13.89 kJ) x 1.1 = 3.66 kcal (15.28 kJ)/g of dry food.
†††An 8-oz. (volume) measuring cup holds 3 to 3.5 oz. by weight (85 to 100 g) of most dry pet foods or 3.5 to 5 oz. by weight (100 to 150 g) of most semi-moist pet foods. It is more accurate to use the average weight of three individual measuring cups of food in determining kcal or kJ/cup.

Label Evaluation

The ingredient panel of the pet food label provides general information about which ingredients were used and their relative amounts. The ingredients used in the product are listed in descending order by weight in many countries. The ingredient panel can be useful if specific ingredients are contraindicated for certain animals or an owner has an ingredient concern. However, the quality of the ingredients cannot be determined from the label and there is much misinformation and, as a result, misunderstandings about pet food ingredients (Chapter 8). As mentioned above, the presence or absence of specific protein sources or other ingredients in a food can be obtained from the product label.

Depending on the country, product labels will also provide information that indicates by what means the product has been shown to be nutritionally adequate (Chapter 9).

Assess and Determine the Feeding Method

Feeding methods relate directly to the physiologic or disease state of the animal and the food or foods being fed. Thus, the information obtained by assessing the animal and the food is fundamental to assessing the feeding method. There are at least three things to consider regarding feeding methods: 1) feeding route, 2) amount fed and 3) how the food is offered (when, where, by whom and how often). In addition, feeding factors that affect compliance should be considered, such as whether or not the animal has access to other foods and who provides the food.

Feeding Route

Whether or not the feeding route is appropriate depends on the animal's condition. Although most animals are able to feed themselves, orphans and some critical care patients may require assistance. Assisted-feeding methods are described in detail in Chapters 25 and 26. Assisted-feeding methods include enteral feeding by syringe or tube (several approaches) and parenteral feeding.

Amount Fed

The nutrient needs of an animal are met by a combination of the nutrient levels in the food and the amount of food offered and eaten. Even if a food has an appropriate nutrient profile, significant over- or undernutrition could result if too much or too little is consumed. Thus, it is important to know if the amount being consumed is appropriate.

The amount of food offered should be determined when taking the patient's history. Although many animals are fed free choice, owners should still be able to provide a reasonable estimate of the actual amount being consumed. The owner may need to return home and measure the amount the pet consumes to provide an accurate report or estimate the amount based on the purchasing frequency of bags or cans. The amount actually being consumed can then be compared with the amount that should be fed. If the animal in question has a normal BCS (3/5) and no history of weight changes, the amount fed is probably appropriate. Exceptions to this generalization include growing animals, animals that are gestating or lactating and hunting dogs and other canine athletes early in the athletic event season.

The appropriate amount to feed can be difficult to determine precisely, but can be estimated. For most commercial pet foods, food dosage estimates can be found in the feeding guidelines on the product label. However, food dosages can be calculated if guidelines are unavailable. The precision of feeding guidelines or calculated food dosages is limited because the efficiency of food use varies among individuals because of differences in physical activity, metabolism, body condition, insulative characteristics of the coat and external environment. Even when environmental conditions and physical activity are similar, sizable individual differences can exist.

Figure 1-5 contains data generated from several controlled studies about the amount of food (energy content standardized) consumed by mature, non-reproducing dogs and cats kept in kennels or runs under similar environmental conditions while maintaining body weight. The total amount of energy needed by dogs and cats for maintenance, even under similar environmental conditions can vary two- to threefold. Even when the extremes are excluded (the top and bottom 2.5%), the amount of energy needed varied more than twofold (Lewis et al, 1987). Therefore, a commercial product's amount to feed guideline or a calculated food dosage should only be considered an estimate or a starting point that may very likely need adjustment.

Calculations to estimate food dosage are based on the assumption that if a food contains the proper proportions of nutrients relative to its energy density, and is fed to meet an animal's energy requirement, then the animal's requirements for non-energy nutrients will be met automatically. This is an important concept. **Box 1-6** demonstrates the method for calculating food dosage estimates. **Case 1-2** includes an example of a food dosage problem.

How the Food is Offered

The amount fed is usually offered in one of three ways: 1) free-choice feeding (dogs and cats), 2) food-restricted meal feeding (dogs and cats) and 3) time-restricted meal feeding (dogs). The number of feedings per day must be considered when the last two methods are used.

Free-choice feeding (also referred to as ad libitum or self feeding) is a method in which more food than the dog or cat will consume is always available; therefore, the animal can eat as much as it wants, whenever it chooses. The major advantage of free-choice feeding is that it is quick and easy. All that is necessary is to ensure that reasonably fresh food is always available. Free-choice feeding is the method of choice during lactation. Free-choice feeding also has a quieting effect in a kennel and timid dogs have a better chance of getting their share if dogs are fed in a group.

Disadvantages include: 1) anorectic animals may not be noticed for several days, especially if two or more animals are fed together, 2) if food is always available, some dogs and cats will continuously overeat and may become obese (such animals should be meal fed) and 3) moist foods and moistened dry foods left at room temperature for prolonged periods can spoil and are inappropriate for free-choice feeding (Chapter 11).

When changing a dog from meal feeding to free-choice feeding, first feed it the amount of the food it is used to receiving at a meal. After this food has been consumed and the dog's appetite has been somewhat satisfied, set out the food to be fed free choice. This transitioning method helps prevent engorgement by dogs unaccustomed to free-choice feeding. Engorgement is generally not a problem when transitioning cats to free-choice feeding. Although dogs and cats unaccustomed to free-choice feeding may overeat initially, they generally stop doing so within a few days, after they learn that food is always available. Avoid taking the food away at any time during this transition period. Each time food is taken away increases the difficulty in changing the animals to a free-choice feeding regimen.

With food-restricted meal feeding, the dog or cat is given a specific, but lesser, amount of food than it would eat if the amount offered were not restricted (i.e., free choice). Time-restricted meal feeding is a method in which the animal is given more food than it will consume within a specified period of time, generally five to 15 minutes. Time-restricted meal feeding is of limited usefulness with dogs and has little if any practical application in cats. Many dogs can eat an entire meal in less than two minutes. Both types of meal feeding are repeated at a specific frequency such as one or more times a day. Some people combine feeding methods, such as free-choice feeding a

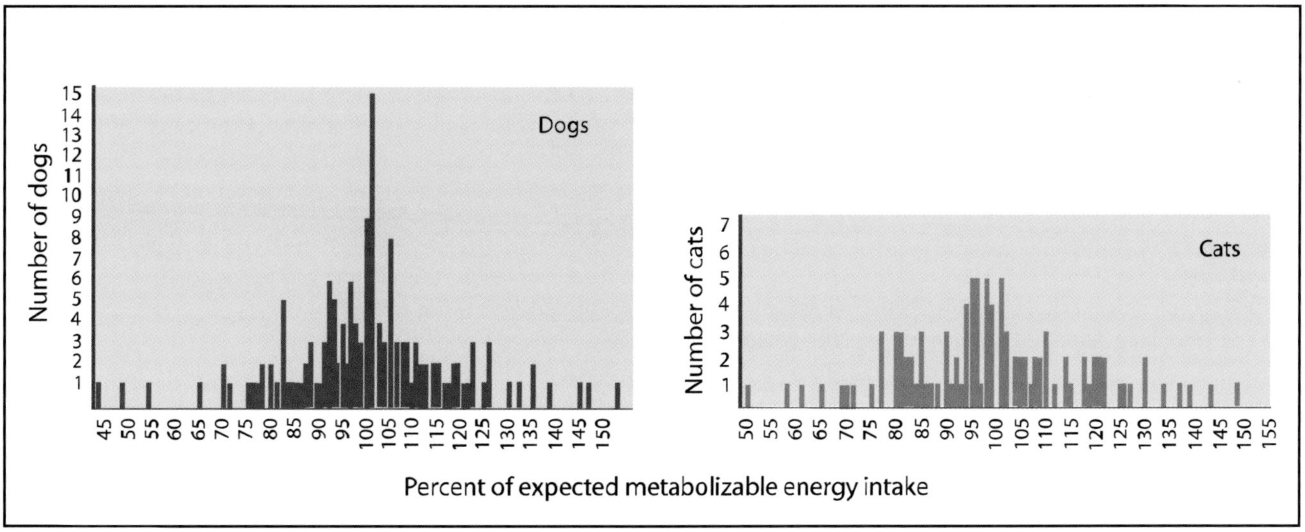

Figure 1-5. Variation in expected energy intake required to maintain optimal body weight in dogs and cats. Data were collected from 120 dogs and 76 cats kept under similar conditions and fed the amount of a variety of commercial pet foods necessary to maintain body weight (Adapted from Lewis et al, 1987).

dry or semi-moist food and meal feeding a moist food or other foods such as meat or table scraps.

Food consumption resulting from frequent meal and free-choice feeding has several advantages. Small meals fed frequently throughout the day result in a greater loss of energy due to an increase in daily meal-induced heat production. Also, providing frequent small meals generally result in greater total food intake than does less frequent feeding (Mugford and Thorne, 1980). Frequent feeding of small meals benefits animals with dysfunctional ingestion, digestion, absorption or use of nutrients.

Frequent feeding is also desirable in normal animals that require a high food intake. Puppies and kittens less than six months old, some dogs engaged in heavy work (high levels of physical activity), dogs and cats experiencing ambient temperature extremes, bitches and queens during the last month of gestation and during lactation should be fed at least three times per day to ensure that their nutritional needs are met. These animals may require one and one-half to four times as much food per unit of body weight than most normal adult dogs and cats. A reduced frequency might limit total food intake in these situations. Also, more frequent feeding during periods of variable appetite suppression, such as occurs with psychologic stress or high ambient temperatures, helps ensure adequate food intake.

Most clinically normal adult dogs that are not lactating, working or experiencing stress will have a sufficient appetite and physical capacity to consume all of the food required daily in a single 10-minute period (assuming food of typical nutrient density [about 3.5 kcal/g or 14.64 kJ/g dry matter]). Cats are less likely to eat their entire meal in one 10-minute sitting, but once-a-day feeding is adequate for most healthy adults. Although many dogs and cats are fed once daily without noticeable detrimental effects, at least twice daily feeding is generally recommended.

In summary, how the food is provided and how often it is fed depend on the animal's condition and in some cases the lifestyle of the owner. Each animal's situation will dictate which feeding method is most desirable (free choice, time-restricted meal feeding or food-restricted meal feeding). For many physiologic and disease conditions this consideration will not be important. For others it will be very important. Recommendations for the best method of providing the food and the number of times per day the food is offered are included in each individual chapter.

Compliance

Owner compliance is necessary for effective clinical nutrition. Feeding methods should reinforce or enable compliance. Enabling compliance includes limiting access to other foods and knowing who provides the food. An animal from a multi-pet household may have access to the other pets' food. If so, such access needs to be denied or limited. Restriction can be difficult in some homes. In such cases the veterinary health care team and pet owner may need to compromise.

Compliance can be eroded if everyone in the family does not support the feeding plan. Whoever feeds the pet must understand the consequences when the wrong foods are fed or even the right foods are fed in the wrong amounts. Client education is essential for the successful outcome of any feeding plan. Specific client education must be provided for feeding healthy pets and for those with specific disease problems. Both oral and written instructions encourage compliance with feeding plans.

Veterinarians and their health care teams should actively involve clients in the formulation of the feeding plan to ensure commitment to the plan. The hospital staff should strive to uncover issues that clients may have about the feeding plan and negotiate mutually acceptable solutions. Open communication about the client's and the health care team's objectives, concerns and shared responsibilities is necessary for successful implementation of the feeding plan. Authoritarian approaches are unlikely to be effective because they discount the high degree of independent decision making that clients have based on their own perceptions of nutrition. Veterinarians and their health care teams can guide clients and enable them to make informed decisions. For more about compliance see Chapter 3.

REASSESSMENT

Finally, monitoring, or reassessing the animal, should be performed at appropriate intervals to evaluate the effectiveness of the feeding plan. For patients undergoing intensive care, reassessment may need to be done every few hours, whereas pets in a health maintenance program could be reassessed annually. Reassessment signals the initiation of the iterative step of the clinical nutrition process. Involving the client in an action plan is an essential component of the veterinarian-client relationship. The reader is referred to the remaining chapters of this book for information about specific feeding plans and practices according to nutritional needs of pets in health and in specific diseases.

REFERENCES

The references for this chapter can be found at www.markmorris.org.

CASE 1-1

Calcium Supplementation in a Great Dane Puppy

Michael S. Hand, DVM, PhD, Dipl. ACVN*
Hill's Science and Technology Center
Topeka, Kansas, USA

Patient Assessment

A 10-week-old male Great Dane puppy weighing 15 kg was examined as part of its routine health maintenance procedures. The results of a physical examination were normal. The puppy's body condition score was 3/5.

Assess the Food and Feeding Method

The puppy is fed a dry lamb and rice-based commercial food. The owner feeds the puppy four 8-oz. measuring cups of food daily. The owner also provides eight calcium tablets daily as a supplement to "ensure enough calcium." A phone call to the pet food company's customer service department determined that the food's calcium content is 2.3% and that it provides 3.6 kcal/g (15.1 kJ/g) on an as fed basis (10% moisture). The customer service department also indicates that the food density is 94 g/cup. Product literature included with the calcium tablets indicates that each tablet provides 0.5 g of calcium carbonate, and that calcium carbonate contains 36% calcium (0% moisture). The owner asked if this is enough calcium for the puppy.

Questions

1. How many g of food and how many g of calcium carbonate are being fed (dry matter [DM])?
2. Determine the total amount of calcium (DM) provided by the food and supplement.
3. Determine the percentage of calcium in the DM of the combined food and supplement.
4. Convert the energy density on an as fed basis to DM.
5. Does the combination of the food and supplement meet the calcium requirement for a giant-breed puppy?

Answers and Discussion

1. Four cups x 94 g/cup = 376 g of food. Because the two components being evaluated have differing moisture contents (food = 90% DM and calcium carbonate tablets = 100% DM), it is advisable to convert the food to DM at this point: 376 g of food on an as fed basis x 90% DM = 338 g food DM.

   The owner feeds eight calcium tablets daily. The calcium carbonate source has no moisture so as fed basis equals DM: eight calcium tablets x 0.5 g calcium carbonate per tablet = 4 g calcium carbonate (as fed and DM).

2. According to the manufacturer, the food provides 2.3% calcium on an as fed basis. To convert this to DM, divide the as fed percentage by the DM percentage: 2.3% calcium as fed basis ÷ 90% DM = 2.6% calcium DM.

   We have already determined that the calcium tablets provide 4 g calcium carbonate and that calcium carbonate contains 36% calcium. To determine how much calcium is provided by each component, multiply the amount of each component being fed by the amount of calcium in each component and add them:

   338 g food dry matter x 2.6% calcium = 8.8 g calcium
   4 g calcium carbonate x 36% calcium = 1.4 g calcium
   10.2 g total calcium (DM)

3. Total food DM is the sum of the two components:

   338 g food DM + 4 g calcium carbonate DM = 342 g total food DM
   10.2 g total calcium (DM) ÷ 342 g total food DM = 3.0% calcium

4. We need to consider the effect of the supplemental calcium source on the energy density of the food and convert the energy density to DM. In this case, we ignore any dilutional effect the 4 g of calcium carbonate has on the energy density of the food because it would be inconsequential (4 g ÷ 342 g = 1%). To convert 3.6 kcal ME/g (15.06 kJ ME/g) as fed to DM, as described previ-

ously, divide the as fed basis by the DM percentage:

3.6 kcal ME/g as fed ÷ 90% DM = 4 kcal ME/g (DM), or
15.06 kJ ME/g as fed ÷ 90% DM = 16.74 kJ ME/g (DM)

Thus, the total food contains 3.0% DM calcium and provides 4 kcal ME/g (16.74 kJ) DM.

5. To compare a food's nutrient content with a recommended target level requires that the energy density of the food and that specified for the target level be similar or the same. Calcium is a key nutritional factor (nutrient of concern) for large- and giant-breed puppies. Calcium levels in foods intended for large- and giant-breed growth should not exceed 1.2% DM in foods that provide <3.8 kcal ME/g (<15.90 kJ) **(Chapter 33).** As described above, the conversion is made by generating a multiplier that converts the requirement to the same energy density as the food. This is done by dividing the food energy density by the requirement energy density and multiplying the requirement by the multiplier: 4 kcal ME/g ÷ 3.6 kcal ME/g = 1.1 (multiplier), or 16.74 kJ ME/g ÷ 15.06 kJ ME/g = 1.1 or 1.1 x 1.2% maximum = 1.32% maximum.

In this case, the combined food and supplement are providing excessive calcium for this giant-breed puppy (3% in food vs. 1.32% maximum recommended) (Chapter 33).

*Current address: Arroyo Hondo, New Mexico, USA.

CASE 1-2

Food Dosage Estimate for a Lactating Queen

Michael S. Hand, DVM, PhD, Dipl. ACVN*
Hill's Science and Technology Center
Topeka, Kansas, USA

Patient Assessment

A 4-kg, three-year-old queen is presented for weight loss. The cat is nursing five, three-week-old kittens. The queen's body condition score is 2/5 and the patient record indicates the cat has lost 1 kg since its postpartum checkup.

Assess the Food and Feeding Method

The cat is being fed one cup of a commercial dry food daily, free choice. The food is suitably balanced for feline lactation. The energy density of the food is 535 kcal metabolizable energy (ME)/cup (2,238 kJ ME/cup) on an as fed basis.

Questions

1. What is this queen's estimated daily energy requirement (DER)?
2. What should the food dosage be based on this queen's DER?

Answers and Discussion

1. Resting energy requirement (RER) (kcal ME/day) = $70(BW_{kg})^{0.75}$
   = $70(4\text{ kg})^{0.75}$ = 70(2.83) = 198 kcal ME/day, or
   = $293(4\text{ kg})^{0.75}$ = 293(2.83) = 829 kJ ME/day
   Modifier for adult feline = 1.5 x RER = DER
   DER = 1.5 x 198 kcal ME/day = 297 kcal ME/day, or
   1.5 x 829 kJ ME/day = 1,243.5 kJ ME/day
   Modifier for feline lactation = (1 + 0.25[number kittens nursing]) x DER
   = [1 + 0.25(5)] x 297 kcal ME/day
   = 2.25 x 297 kcal ME/day = 668 kcal ME/day, or
   2.25 x 1,243.5 kJ ME/day = 2,798 kJ ME/day
2. The food being fed has a nutrient profile that is satisfactory for feline lactation. The energy density of the food is 535 kcal (2,238 kJ) ME/cup. Divide the energy requirement by the energy density of the food to determine how much to feed the cat:
   668 kcal ME/day requirement ÷ 535 kcal ME/cup = 1.25 cups/day, or
   2,798 kJ ME/day requirement ÷ 2,238 kJ ME/cup = 1.25 cups/day
   According to these calculations the cat is being underfed. The amount offered free choice should be increased by at least 25%.

*Current address: Arroyo Hondo, New Mexico, USA.

CASE 1-3

Altering the Food and Feeding Method for a Young Rottweiler

Rebecca L. Remillard, PhD, DVM, Dipl. ACVN
Angell Animal Medical Center
Boston, Massachusetts, USA

Patient Assessment

A four-month-old, female Rottweiler was examined for diarrhea of five days' duration. The puppy had escaped from a fenced yard on trash pickup day and the owners suspected it had eaten garbage. The puppy appeared bright and alert, weighed 18 kg and had a body condition score of 3/5. The results of the physical examination were normal except for fluid-filled intestines on abdominal palpation. The owners described the stools as being small volume but frequent (eight to 10/day) and liquid with some bright red blood and mucus. A fecal examination was negative for intestinal parasites.

Assess the Food and Feeding Method

The puppy was fed a commercial dry puppy food three times per day until its escape. The puppy still had a good appetite, but seemed to be drinking more than usual amounts of water. On Day 1 of the diarrheic episode, the veterinarian examined the puppy and asked the owner to feed a moist commercial veterinary therapeutic food (poultry, egg and rice based) with moderate fat (13%) and low fiber (<1%) (Prescription Diet i/d Canine[a]). However, the diarrhea had not resolved after feeding the food for three days.

Question

What is the appropriate food and feeding method for this patient with large bowel diarrhea?

Answer and Discussion

The food was replaced with a moist commercial veterinary therapeutic food that contained 13% fat and 12% crude fiber on a dry matter basis (Prescription Diet w/d Canine[a]). The owners were instructed to feed the puppy at its estimated resting energy requirement (805 kcal [3,368 kJ]/day) with two cans of the new food divided into four meals per day for one to two days; then to feed at the estimated daily energy requirement (1,600 kcal/day [6,694 kJ]) with four cans of the new food divided into three to four meals per day for another two days. The owners were instructed to return for a recheck if the puppy did not have a normal stool by the fourth day. If the puppy's stool was normal, the owners were instructed to transition the food back to the original puppy food using the short schedule outlined in **Table 1-1.**

Progress Notes

No stool was produced within the first 24 hours of feeding the higher fiber food. By the end of the second day the dog had a normal bowel movement with no blood or mucus. The owners continued to feed the higher fiber food for another two days as instructed. The puppy was then switched back to the dry puppy food over seven days with no problems.

Endnote

a. Hill's Pet Nutrition Inc., Topeka, KS, USA.

Chapter 2

Evidence-Based Clinical Nutrition

Philip Roudebush
Timothy A. Allen
Bruce J. Novotny

"Each time we learn something new and surprising, the astonishment comes with the realization that we were wrong before.... In truth, whenever we discover a new fact it involves the elimination of old ones. We are always, as it turns out, fundamentally in error."
Lewis Thomas

INTRODUCTION

Practitioners should know how to determine risks and benefits of nutritional regimens, including for nutritional care, and counsel pet owners accordingly. Currently, veterinary medical education and continuing education are not based on rigorous assessment of evidence for or against particular management options. Journals and textbooks, even those designed to rapidly access decisions while patients are in a clinical situation, may not help determine specific risks and benefits of nutritional management. Consequently, veterinarians have often had to rely on clinical experience and judgment, aided by opinions of colleagues and consultants who practice similarly. Evidence-based medicine (EBM) represents a major, but still untested, intellectual advance when making clinical decisions and determining patient care (Geyman, 2000; Keene, 2000; Moriello, 2003). This chapter will apply the basic elements of EBM to veterinary clinical nutrition and provide a statistical primer to help veterinarians interpret available information.

EBM CONCEPTS

EBM and its associated concepts were first advanced by a group at McMaster University Health Sciences Centre in Canada. The first publications emerged in the early 1990s (EBM Working Group, 1992; Sackett et al, 1996). The underlying concepts are rooted in clinical epidemiology and are not new. EBM seeks to establish clinical medicine as a verifiable scientific activity (Naldi et al, 2000).

Initially, EBM was defined as the "conscientious, explicit and judicious use of current best evidence from clinical care research in making decisions about the care of individual patients" (Sackett et al, 1996). EBM was later refined to integrate the best research evidence, clinical expertise and patient values (Sackett et al, 2000). Best research evidence means clinically relevant research, especially from patient-centered clinical studies. Clinical expertise is the ability to use clinical skills and past experiences to rapidly identify each patient's unique health state, establish a diagnosis and determine the risks and benefits of potential interventions facing that patient. Patient values include unique preferences, concerns and expectations that each person brings to a clinical encounter; these must be integrated into clinical decisions that best serve the patient. Integration of these three elements supposedly helps clinicians and patients form a diagnostic and therapeutic alliance that optimizes clinical outcomes and quality of life (Sackett et al, 2000).

EBM concepts also apply to dogs, cats and other nonhuman animals. Patient values must be extended to include the unique preferences, concerns and expectations of owners and their pet (i.e., patient). Regardless of the definition, use of current best evidence should not replace clinical skills, judgment or experi-

Table 2-1. Guidelines for quality of evidence that can be used for veterinary clinical nutrition.

Evidence grade	Evidence guidelines	Examples of nutritional studies
1	Evidence obtained from at least one properly randomized, controlled, clinical study that used the nutritional product in the target species with animals that had developed the disease naturally.*	Dietary modification for treatment of cats and dogs with naturally developing chronic kidney disease.
2	Evidence obtained from randomized, controlled, clinical studies conducted in a laboratory setting that used the nutritional product in the target species with animals that had developed the disease naturally.*	Effects of a dental food on plaque accumulation and gingival health in dogs. Energy restriction in obese cats and dogs fed foods varying in protein, fat, fiber and carbohydrate content.
3	Evidence obtained from one or more of the following:* At least one appropriately designed clinical study without randomization. Cohort or case-controlled analytic studies. Studies that used acceptable models of disease or simulations in the target species. Case series. Dramatic results from uncontrolled studies.	Use of foods using novel or hydrolyzed protein sources for animals with adverse food reactions. Myocardial failure in cats associated with taurine deficiency.
4	Evidence obtained from one or more of the following: Opinions based on clinical experience (textbooks, monographs or proceedings). Descriptive studies. Studies conducted in other species. Pathophysiologic justification. Reports of expert committees.	Hepatic disease and nutritional therapy. Nutritional management of most diarrheal diseases.

*Data published in peer-reviewed journals is preferred.

ence; however, it does provide another dimension to the decision-making process that also considers the patient's and owner's preferences (Forrest and Miller, 2002). Evidence-based clinical nutrition (EBCN) attempts to efficiently integrate medical and nutritional research with clinical practice.

Figure 2-1 is a conceptual model for evidence-based clinical decisions (Hayes et al, 1996). Analysis reveals that the best evidence-based clinical decisions are made when clinical expertise, research evidence, owner or patient preferences and available resources overlap. This model can be easily adapted to veterinary clinical nutrition in which assessment of the patient, food and feeding method lead to a comprehensive feeding plan based on the best current evidence (Thatcher et al, 2000). Clinical expertise is needed to obtain a dietary history and assess a patient's nutritional and health status. This assessment must often include other pets in the household. Clinical and nutritional expertise provides individualized care for a specific patient's needs. Owners exercise their preferences for medical and nutritional care by seeking second opinions, choosing alternate treatments, exercising economic constraints and adhering (or not) to recommended feeding or therapeutic plans. Today, more clinical and nutritional information is available to pet owners than ever before. Pet preferences are most commonly recognized in veterinary clinical nutrition through palatability choices for certain types of foods.

Integrating clinical expertise with current best evidence from medical and nutritional research is complex. Veterinarians usually attempt to base their decisions on the best evidence available. This evidence often represents extrapolations of pathophysiologic principles, studies conducted in other species and logical conclusions based on data derived from patients in clinical studies (Rosenberg and Sackett, 1996). The advent and proliferation of randomized, controlled clinical studies increased the quantity and quality of clinically valid evidence. When possible, veterinarians should use information derived from systematic, rigorously controlled clinical studies (obviously, larger trials involving more patients are preferable) to make diagnostic and therapeutic decisions. EBM and EBCN do not always provide definitive answers, but they do provide a framework for making decisions and understanding the risk-benefit relationship of various feeding and therapeutic plans. Understanding the rules of evidence is necessary to understand EBM and EBCN (Sackett, 1993; Berg, 2000).

RULES OF EVIDENCE

Scientific evidence is the product of appropriately designed and carefully controlled research. A single study does not constitute evidence; rather, it contributes to knowledge derived from multiple studies that have investigated the same scientific question. Unfortunately, no central repository for clinical nutrition information exists nor is there a system for establishing quality evidence. Several classification schemes are useful for establishing rules of evidence for recommendations about clinical nutrition.

One method is to use a pyramid to rank clinical evidence (**Figure 2-2**) (Forrest and Miller, 2002; SUNY, 2003). Traditional sources of evidence include textbooks, personal journal collections, conference proceedings and clinical guidelines. Unfortunately, much of this evidence is not based on appropriately conducted clinical studies in the target species. Many clinical and nutritional interventions are used because the basic pathophysiologic rationale was reasonable, although clinical outcome data to document positive effects were lacking.

Strong EBM and EBCN evidence includes randomized, controlled clinical studies or systematic reviews of more than one study (i.e., meta-analysis). Epidemiologic studies (cohort studies or case-control studies), models of disease and case series are the next best evidence. Hierarchy of evidence is based on causation and bias control. As one ascends the pyramid, the number of studies and, correspondingly, the available literature decreases, whereas the relevance to answering clinical questions increases.

Quality of evidence guidelines, adapted from the U.S. Preventive Services Task Force, are excellent, rigorous applications of evidence-based appraisal systems (Geyman, 2000; Berg, 2000; McGowan et al, 1992; Polzin, 2003; Polzin, 2003a). Those guidelines have been modified to better fit the types of evidence encountered in veterinary clinical nutrition (**Table 2-1**) (Roudebush et al, 2004). Other classification schemes have been recommended for rules of evidence; however, they are very similar to the evidence pyramid and grades outlined here (Rosenberg and Sackett, 1996; Olivry and Mueller, 2003; Cook et al, 1995). It is beyond the scope of this chapter to describe strategies for finding clinical nutrition evidence. Numerous excellent articles, textbooks and websites provide detailed explanations about the evidence gathering process (Sackett et al, 2000; Miser, 1999; Safranek and Dodson, 2000; Hunt et al, 2000; Jahad and Haynes, 2000; Chi-Lum et al, 1997; Klemenez and McSherry, 1997; Greenhalgh, 1997).

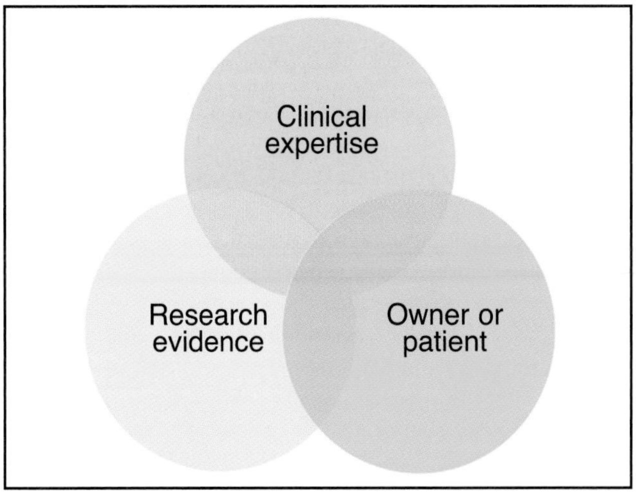

Figure 2-1. A conceptual model for making evidence-based clinical decisions. The best clinical decisions are made when clinical expertise, high-quality evidence obtained in controlled studies and owner or patient preferences overlap. (Adapted from Haynes RB, Sackett DL, Gray JMA, et al. Transferring evidence from research into practice: 1. The role of clinical care research evidence in clinical decisions. American College of Physicians Journal Club 1996; 125: A14-A16. Reprinted with permission).

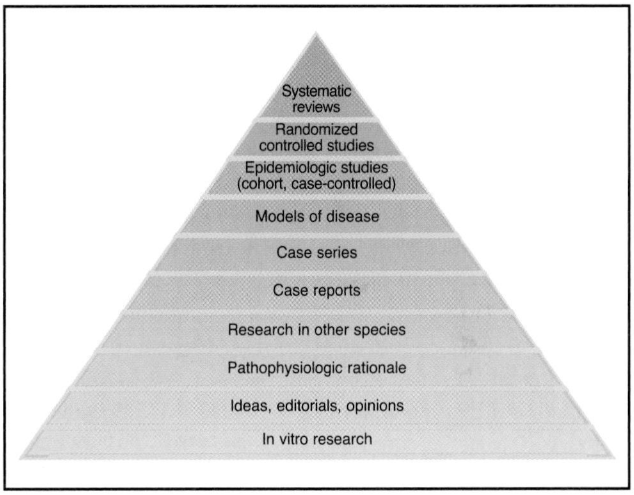

Figure 2-2. The evidence pyramid. The level of evidence for use of a diagnostic or therapeutic intervention increases as one progresses up the pyramid. (Adapted from SUNY Downstate Medical Center. Guide to research methods: the evidence pyramid. Medical Research Library of Brooklyn Web site. Available at http://library.downstate.edu/dbm. Accessed on November 2, 2003. Reprinted with permission.)

APPLYING EVIDENCE TO SPECIFIC PATIENTS

Many activities veterinarians perform in clinical medicine and nutrition have not been subjected to suitably designed scientific studies. Randomized, controlled studies are the reference criterion standard for therapeutic and nutritional interventions; however, these studies are imperfect and do not apply to studies of cause, diagnosis and prognosis (Sackett, 1993; Berg, 2000). Randomized, controlled studies are often not conducted on patients similar to those encountered in practice, and many clinical and nutritional interventions will never be subjected to such investigations. For example, randomized, controlled studies are often not conducted on patients with naturally occurring disease and many clinical and nutritional interventions will never be subjected to such investigations due to ethical or other reasons. Nonetheless, evidence from randomized, clinical studies currently is most likely to predict results in clinical practice. Randomized, clinical studies also serve as a scientific entry point for discussions with owners about therapeutic and nutritional options.

Several questions can be used to decide the applicability of evidence from clinical studies to nutritionally manage a specific patient (Strauss and Sackett, 1999; Dans et al, 1998; McAlister et al, 2000).

- Were study outcomes clinically relevant?
- Are there differences between animals in the study and my patient that may alter expected treatment response?
- Are there potential drug-nutrient interactions that may alter the expected treatment response?

- Are there differences in the nutrient contents of the food (or supplements) that may alter the expected treatment response?
- Is the food (or supplement) readily available and economically feasible?
- Is the feeding plan intervention feasible in the owner's setting?
- What are the patient's likely benefits and risks from the various nutritional management options?
- How will the owner's values and patient's preferences influence the decision about nutritional management?
- Does the patient have other health conditions that substantially alter the potential benefits and risks of nutritional management?

EVIDENCE-BASED TREATMENT DECISIONS: A FRAMEWORK FOR CLINICAL PRACTICE

EBM involves making clinical decisions by carefully identifying, evaluating and applying the most relevant information. In EBM, the first step is to identify and define the medical problem to learn what additional information is required. After the need for additional information is identified, it must be retrieved and evaluated to ensure validity. After the information is judged valid, it is next necessary to apply it to the care of your patient. This brief section will focus on how to evaluate information about treatment after it has been retrieved and conclude with a few general comments about applying treatments to individual patients.

The first step in making good treatment decisions is to decide whether the patient requires treatment or not and to identify the specific goals of treatment. Potential treatment goals include eliminating or decreasing current clinical signs, preventing recurrence of disease, slowing progression of disease and curing the disease. After the treatment goals have been identified and treatment has been initiated it is important to periodically assess progress toward these goals and to make changes as appropriate.

After the decision to treat has been made and the treatment goals identified, the next step is to decide on the specific treatment modality or modalities (pharmacologic agents, surgery and nutrition) that will achieve the treatment goals. Experienced clinicians make treatment decisions based on their own uncontrolled clinical experience. Clinicians judge the efficacy of a treatment by comparing current clinical impressions with clinical impressions before the new treatment was available. Unfortunately, this approach can lead to erroneous conclusions. Part of human nature is to remember our successes and either forget our treatment failures or attribute them to other factors (e.g., poor owner compliance). Another risk when judging the efficacy of a treatment based on clinical impressions is that neither the clinician nor the pet owner is masked to treatment so there is increased potential for bias in subjective assessments (placebo effect).

Alternatively, treatment decisions can be based on critical analysis of formal, prospective randomized clinical trials designed to determine if differences exist in clinically relevant outcomes between treatments. In clinical trials, researchers apply a treatment or intervention and observe the effect of treatment on outcome. The value of interventional compared to observational studies is the ability to determine causality.

The purpose of clinical research is to draw inferences about what really happened in the study patients and to apply those inferences to the universe of all patients with the same problem. Errors are inherent in all clinical research studies. The key issue is whether the errors change the conclusions of a study significantly. The challenge is to design and complete a study that adequately controls for random and systematic errors. Randomly assigning patients to treatment can eliminate the influence of confounding variables. Masking the veterinarian and pet owner to treatment can reduce the possibility that clinical assessments are biased. Randomized, controlled masked clinical trials are considered the gold standard of clinical research because they provide the best way to reduce bias. Bias is anything that produces results or conclusions that differ from the truth. Sources of bias can be found in the design, implementation and analysis of the study.

In general, clinical trials are expensive, time consuming and difficult to conduct. Consequently, well-designed, well-executed clinical trials are unavailable to guide every treatment decision. Nonetheless, a systematic approach to evaluating support for each treatment option is valuable to the clinician. The critical evaluation of a clinical trial depends on more than checking for appropriate randomization and the presence of a control group. The following series of questions can guide the clinician through a systematic assessment of the validity of a clinical trial.

Was Assignment to Treatment Truly Randomized?

Did every patient enrolled in the study have an equal and known probability of receiving the treatment(s) compared? Proper randomization applies a previously established method for assigning patients to a treatment group using a set of computer-generated random numbers. The random assignment of patients to treatment groups is critical for establishing the basis for statistical testing of the differences in the clinical outcomes observed between groups. In blocked randomization, age, sex and other baseline characteristics that may influence clinical outcomes are distributed equally between treatment groups and do not confound interpretation of results. When block randomization is done properly any differences in baseline characteristics between the groups are due to chance and addressed by the statistical tests. Proper random assignment guarantees that no one can influence assignment to treatment. This prevents the investigator from knowingly or unknowingly assigning a particular patient to a specific treatment because the patient seems particularly suited to receive the active or control treatment, thereby eliminating an important potential source of bias.

Are the Subjects in the Clinical Trial Adequately Described and Similar to your Patient?

Is there sufficient demographic and clinical detail provided about the study patients for you to determine similarity between them and your patient? Are the patients in the study similar enough to your patient that you are comfortable applying the study results?

Were Treatment Groups Similar at the Start of the Study?

Were there any differences in key baseline characteristics that might influence the clinical outcome between the treatment groups at the start of study? For example, in a study of spontaneous chronic kidney disease was the severity of kidney disease comparable in the treatment groups at the onset of the study?

Aside from the Investigated Treatment, were the Groups Treated Equally?

With the exception of the treatment under investigation, were all disease-related interventions identical between treatment groups? Are the details of patient management adequate to make this assessment? Could the difference in outcome be attributable to treatment differences that are not part of the stated objective of the study?

Were all Patients that Entered the Study Accounted for at the Conclusion of the Study?

Can you reconcile the number of patients in the title or methods section of the article with the tally of the final disposition of patients? If patients were lost to follow-up or dismissed from the study, were they included in the statistical analysis of the data? If yes, how were these missing data points handled? Does management of these missing data points change the study conclusions?

Are the Study Results Believable?

Was the clinical outcome of interest defined based on clear, explicit and, if possible, objective criteria? Are the results of the clinical trial consistent with those of other studies? Are the results of the clinical trial biologically plausible? Is there a biologic precedent for the putative mechanism of action?

Were Findings both Clinically and Statistically Significant?

Clinical significance refers to the medical importance of the findings. Was the magnitude of the observed treatment effect large enough to make a difference in how you manage your patient? A finding in a clinical trial can be statistically significant but clinically insignificant. Was the endpoint studied a clinical or surrogate outcome? Clinically relevant endpoints, such as survival and quality of life, are the most meaningful to veterinarians and pet owners. Surrogate markers indirectly assess the risk of a clinical outcome (e.g., serum creatinine in kidney disease and shortening fraction in heart disease). Showing a treatment causes favorable changes in surrogate markers doesn't necessarily prove better clinical outcomes. Surrogate markers are frequently used in veterinary medicine because resources are limited and studies with clinical outcomes typically take longer and are more expensive. Statistics can be viewed as a quantitative method of good clinical decision making. From a clinician's perspective, statistics provide a way to assess the level of confidence in whether the treatment described in a clinical trial will be effective in your patient. The probability of accepting an ineffective treatment (false positive) is expressed by the p value. The p value describes how often differences in the treatment effect as large or larger than those observed in the clinical trial will occur in a long series of identical trials if in fact no true treatment effect exists. If $p = 0.05$ and the identical study is repeated 20 times the same result will be obtained 19 of 20 times. The smaller the p value, the more accurate the conclusion that a treatment effect truly exists. Most articles describing veterinary clinical trials specify the likelihood of accepting an ineffective treatment (a type I error) but relatively few specify the risk of not recognizing an effective treatment (a type II error). The risk of not recognizing an effective treatment can be calculated and is known as β. In clinical trials it is typical to set the risk of accepting an ineffective treatment (p value) at 0.05 and the risk of not recognizing an effective treatment at 0.20 (20% risk). These risk levels are known as standard or conventional levels of statistical significance. If the true state of affairs is that the treatment is different than the control and the study is designed to accept the conventional levels of risk, then the power of the study is 1 - 0.20 or 80%. The power of a clinical trial is analogous to the sensitivity of a diagnostic test.

Was the Study of Sufficient Size and Duration?

The p value is influenced by group size and the variability in the measurement in question. In general, if a measurement is very precise and has nearly the same value each time it is measured it is possible to demonstrate statistical significance with smaller numbers of patients. The number of patients in a study indirectly influences clinician confidence in the results. Group size is related by square root to confidence in the research findings. In order to double confidence in the research findings, it is necessary to quadruple the number of patients in the study. The duration of a study must be adequate to assess the treatment goal. For example, if the goal is to prevent the recurrence of calcium oxalate uroliths, the duration of the study must be long enough to assess whether the treatment under investigation has a clinically significant effect.

Were Those Making Clinical Assessments (Veterinarian and Pet Owner) Masked (Blinded) to Treatment?

Masking prevents biased assessments of subjective outcomes. Unmasked clinicians may also give special attention to patients receiving the "test" material. This can take the form of additional diagnostic tests or additional treatments. This is sometimes called co-intervention. For example, an unmasked investigator consciously or unconsciously eager to demonstrate a positive "test" effect in a trial of an obesity drug might recommend increased exercise. Masking can be difficult to achieve and maintain because of logistical considerations or telltale effects of a treatment on clinical signs or laboratory tests. Logistical considerations include the physical appearance and aroma of the test material. At the conclusion of the study participants can be asked to pick the "test" material if an investigator is concerned about masking. If the percent guessing correctly is high, this should be taken into consideration when evaluating the results of the study.

REFERENCES

The references for **Chapter 2** can be found at www.markmorris.org.

CASE 2-1

Lethargy and Inappetence in a Scottish Terrier

Philip Roudebush, DVM, Dipl. ACVIM (Small Animal Internal Medicine)
Hill's Scientific Affairs
Topeka, Kansas, USA

Patient Assessment

A six-year-old intact male Scottish terrier was examined for lethargy of several days' duration and mild inappetence. The dog weighed 9.5 kg (20.9 lb), and had a normal body condition score (3 on a 5-point scale). Several peripheral lymph nodes were enlarged and splenomegaly was diagnosed. Results of per rectal palpation and ocular fundic examination were normal. Analysis of a hemogram revealed mild normocytic, normochromic, nonregenerative anemia. Results of a serum biochemistry analysis were within reference ranges, except for mild increases in hepatic enzyme activity. Thoracic radiography revealed sternal lymphomegaly. Abdominal ultrasonography revealed mesenteric lymph node enlargement; however, the liver and spleen appeared normal. Microscopic examination of a fine-needle aspirate obtained from a peripheral lymph node revealed a homogenous population of immature lymphoid cells consistent with high-grade lymphoma.

The tentative diagnosis and treatment options were discussed with the owner, who selected chemotherapy. The owner wanted to know whether nutritional therapy or dietary supplements would be appropriate for the dog.

Question

As the attending veterinarian, you must answer the following question: In dogs with lymphoma, do dietary supplements or therapeutic foods influence survival or quality of life when used in conjunction with standard treatments such as chemotherapy?

Answer

A literature search revealed two, randomized, controlled clinical studies in which clinicians used single-agent chemotherapy (i.e., doxorubicin) and a therapeutic food in dogs with lymphoma. One of these studies was published in a peer-reviewed journal, whereas the other was a research abstract at a major veterinary meeting. Both studies indicated that dogs with lymphoma that consumed a therapeutic food supplemented with fish oil and arginine, combined with doxorubicin therapy had a significantly longer disease-free interval, longer survival time and improved quality of life, compared with dogs eating a standard food while receiving similar chemotherapy. These published data are Grade 1, which is the highest quality of evidence for recommending nutritional management for dogs with lymphoma. The patient described in the case is similar to dogs enrolled in the published studies, and the food used in those studies is identical to a commercially available therapeutic food.[a]

Another literature search did not reveal published clinical studies in which nutritional supplements were effective in dogs with multicentric lymphoma. Any recommendations for use of supplements should be made on the basis of expert opinions, clinical experience, studies in other species or pathophysiologic justification. These are Grade 4 evidence, which is the weakest form of evidence for making a nutritional recommendation.

Endnote

a. Prescription Diet n/d Canine, Hill's Pet Nutrition Inc., Topeka, KS, USA.

Bibliography

Ogilvie GK, Fettman MJ, Mallinkrodt CH, et al. Effect of fish oil, arginine and doxorubicin chemotherapy on remission and survival time for dogs with lymphoma. Cancer 2000; 88: 1916-1928.

Ogilvie GK, Fettman MJ, Mallinkrodt CH, et al. Effect of fish oil, arginine and doxorubicin chemotherapy on remission and survival time for dogs with lymphoma: A double blind, randomized placebo controlled study (abstract). Proceedings. Annual Meeting, Veterinary Medical Forum 2000; 18: 766.

CASE 2-2

Polydipsia and Polyuria in a Male Domestic Shorthair Cat

Philip Roudebush, DVM, Dipl. ACVIM (Small Animal Internal Medicine)
Hill's Scientific Affairs
Topeka, Kansas, USA

Patient Assessment

A 12-year-old neutered male domestic shorthair cat was examined for routine health maintenance. The cat's body weight was 3.4 kg (7.5 lb) with a normal body condition score (3 on a 5-point scale). The owners reported a recent increase in water consumption and frequency of urination. Results of physical examination were unremarkable, except for mild periodontal disease. Laboratory tests performed included a hemogram, urinalysis and serum biochemistry profile. Azotemia was detected, with an increase in serum creatinine concentration (2.5 mg/dl; reference range, 0.4 to 1.8 mg/dl) and a urine specific gravity of 1.018. Results of other laboratory tests were within reference ranges. Subsequent microbial culture of a urine sample yielded negative results. The tentative diagnosis was naturally developing, Stage 2 chronic kidney disease.

Question

As the attending veterinarian, you must answer the following question: For cats with chronic kidney disease, does dietary management delay the onset of uremic crises, reduce the risk of future uremic crises or delay death?

Answer

A literature search found a randomized, controlled clinical study that evaluated the effect of dietary modification for treatment of cats with naturally developing chronic renal failure. Analysis of that study indicated that a food formulated for renal conditions benefited cats with uremic crises and decreased mortality in those with mild to moderate naturally developing chronic kidney disease, compared with results attained with an adult maintenance food. Cats fed the therapeutically formulated food had reduced mortality compared with cats fed the adult maintenance food.

The study represents Grade 1 evidence, which is the highest quality. Your patient is similar to cats enrolled in a published clinical study, and the food used in the study is a commercially available therapeutic food that is readily available and economically feasible.[a] Based on this evidence, use of the therapeutically formulated food and other tenets of conservative medical management should be recommended for your patient, providing owner and patient preferences are satisfied.

Endnote

a. Prescription Diet k/d Feline, Hill's Pet Nutrition Inc., Topeka, KS, USA.

CASE 2-3

Severe Halitosis and Reluctance to Eat in an Irish Setter

Philip Roudebush, DVM, Dipl. ACVIM (Small Animal Internal Medicine)
Hill's Scientific Affairs
Topeka, Kansas, USA

Patient Assessment

A seven-year-old, 30-kg (66-lb) male Irish setter was examined for severe halitosis and reluctance to eat dry food. Abnormal findings during examination of the oral cavity included moderate accumulations of plaque and calculus on both dental arcades, periodontitis, exposure of the furcation of tooth roots and loss of attachment; these findings were most prominent around the caudal mandibular premolars and molars. Results for the remainder of the physical examination were unremarkable. The dog was given antibiotics to help control infection of oral tissues while further diagnostic evaluations were performed. Results of a hemogram, serum biochemistry analysis and urinalysis were within reference ranges.

The dog was anesthetized, and supragingival scaling followed by root planing and subgingival curettage was performed. Severe periodontal disease was found around the left mandibular teeth (fourth premolar and first molar). These teeth were extracted. An osseopromotive bioactive material[a] was placed into the sockets, and extraction sites were sutured. The remaining teeth were polished. Oral antibiotics and a canned recovery-type food were dispensed. Two weeks later, the extraction sites were healed, and the owner commented that the dog is more active.

Question
As the attending veterinarian, you must answer the following question: For dogs treated to correct dental plaque and calculus, gingivitis and oral malodor, does dietary management delay the onset or reduce the severity of further dental disease?

Answer
A literature search revealed a number of randomized, controlled clinical studies that evaluated the effect of dietary modification for dogs with plaque and calculus accumulation, gingivitis and oral malodor. Those studies were conducted in a laboratory setting and involved use of a nutritional product in dogs with naturally developing oral disease. Analysis of results of those studies revealed a significant reduction of plaque, calculus, gingivitis and oral malodor when feeding a therapeutic food specially formulated for dogs with dental conditions, compared with feeding a typical dry food. This constitutes Grade 2 evidence, or the second highest quality of evidence. This patient's condition is similar to that of dogs used in the published studies; the food used was a commercially available therapeutic food[b] that is readily available and economically feasible. Based on this evidence, use of the therapeutic food specially formulated for dogs with dental conditions should be recommended for patients, providing owner and patient preferences are satisfied.

Endnotes
a. Bioglass, Nutramax Laboratories Inc., Baltimore, MD, USA.
b. Prescription Diet t/d Canine, Hill's Pet Nutrition Inc., Topeka, KS, USA.

Chapter 3

Health Literacy and Client Compliance

Bruce J. Novotny
Charles J. Wayner

"What we have here is (a) failure to communicate."
The movie Cool Hand Luke

HEALTH LITERACY

Introduction

According to the 1993 National Adult Literacy Survey (NALS), the average educational attainment of adults in the United States is above the 12th grade level (Kirsch et al, 1993). However, educational level doesn't translate into a corresponding level of reading or comprehension. Forty to 44 million adults surveyed have difficulty locating the expiration date on a driver's license, determining the location of a meeting on a form or reading a medicine label. Another 50 million Americans have only marginal literacy skills; these people have difficulty locating an intersection on a street map and identifying and entering background information on a Social Security application. Unfortunately, despite increasing education, the average reading skills of U.S. adults are between the 8th and 9th grade levels (Stedman and Kaestel, 1991).

Much of health care information, including insurance forms and advertising, is often written far above the high school level. Several studies report that the reading level of patients with various chronic diseases falls between grade levels six and 10, whereas the readability of health materials prepared for them falls between seven and 13 (IOM, 2004). More than 300 studies, conducted over three decades assessed various health-related materials (e.g., informed consent forms and medication package inserts), found that a mismatch exists between the reading levels of the materials and the reading skills of the intended audience. Most of the assessed materials exceeded the reading skills of the average high school graduate (Rudd et al, 2000). **Table 3-1** lists several problems associated with inadequate health literacy (Zarcadoolos et al, 2006).

Implications to Veterinary Medicine

For the most part, pet owners mirror the general population. That being the case, it is highly likely that the same issues the human health care system faces related to health literacy reside in the pet-owning population. Unfortunately, this has never been studied to any great degree in veterinary medicine, but the ramifications of this revelation are alarming.

Clients depend on our medical expertise and our ability to translate that skill into information they can relate to and act upon. The pet's health and well-being depend on our ability to effectively communicate our intended meaning to the owner. Although we may believe we are communicating with pet owners, we may in fact be adding substantially to their confusion, uncertainty and frustration about doing what's best for their pet.

Poor communication with clients can result in less than optimal short- and long-term care. As preventive and therapeutic medical advocates for pets, veterinarians and other health care team members have an obligation to help pet owners make informed decisions about their pet's care. Providing accurate information about proper pet nutrition is

Table 3-1. Problems caused by inadequate health literacy.*

Improper use of medications
Inappropriate use or no use of health services
Poor self-management of chronic conditions
Inadequate response in emergency situations
Poor health outcomes
Lack of self-efficacy and self-esteem
Financial drain on individuals and society

*Adapted from Zarcadoolas C, Pleasant AF, Greer DS. Advancing Health Literacy. San Francisco, CA: Jossey-Banks, 2006.

Table 3-2. Examples of skills needed for health.*

Promote and protect health and prevent disease
Understand, interpret and analyze health information
Apply health information over a variety of life events and situations
Navigate the health care system
Actively participate in encounters with health care professionals
Understand and give consent
Understand and advocate for rights

*Adapted from IOM. (Institute of Medicine.) Health Literacy: A Prescription to End Confusion. Washington, DC: National Academies Press, 2004; 1-322.

as necessary as appropriate medicine and surgery. It is a sobering thought to consider that the number of pet deaths attributable to poor communication may meet or exceed surgical or anesthetic-related deaths.

Because there is little in the way of insights about this problem in veterinary medicine, issues about the human health literacy crisis will be discussed. Readers should associate these data to the client-pet-veterinary and veterinary team interface and challenge themselves to make a concerted effort to enhance communication skills to better care for the pets and people they serve.

Definitions

Health literacy may be defined as "the degree to which individuals have the capacity to obtain, process and understand basic health information and services needed to make appropriate health decisions" (Ratzan and Parker, 2000; Healthy People 2010). A 1999 report from the Council on Scientific Affairs of the American Medical Association refers to functional health literacy as "the ability to read and comprehend prescription bottles, appointment slips and other essential health-related materials" (AMA, 1999).

Other proposed definitions include:

- Health literacy is a constellation of skills, including the ability to perform basic reading and numerical tasks required to function in the health care environment (AMA Ad Hoc Committee).
- Health literacy has three levels: 1) functional health literacy, which refers to the communication of information, 2) interactive health literacy, which deals with the development of personal skills and 3) critical health literacy, which is needed for personal and community empowerment (Nutbeam, 1998).

Understanding Health Literacy

Health literacy includes more than simply obtaining information. Health literacy embraces writing, numeracy, listening, speaking and conceptual knowledge (IOM, 2004). Health literacy emerges when expectations, preferences and skills of individuals seeking health information meet equivalent goals of those providing information and services (IOM, 2004). Education, language and culture mediate health literacy skills (IOM, 2004). Equally important are the communication and assessment skills of health care professionals. Furthermore, their patients must navigate the media, marketplace and governmental agencies to obtain health information (IOM, 2004).

Even people with strong literacy skills may have trouble obtaining, understanding and using health information; for example, an accountant may not know when to schedule a pap smear and a chef may be unable to prepare health conscious meals (IOM, 2004).

As mentioned above, 90 million adults (47% of the adult population) may lack the literacy skills to effectively use the U.S. health care system (IOM, 2004). The majority of these adults were born in the U.S. and speak English. Literacy levels are lower among elderly persons, those who have lower educational levels, those who are poor, minority populations and groups with limited English proficiency such as recent immigrants (IOM, 2004). The gap between knowledge and practice is widened by inadequate health literacy. People who lack an understanding of health care usually present with more advanced disease, receive fewer preventive care services and have poorer health outcomes (IOM, 2004). As one example, diabetics with poor health literacy were more likely than patients with adequate health literacy to have poor glycemic control and reported more retinopathies (Schillinger et al, 2002).

In its report Healthy People 2010, the U.S. Department of Health and Human Services included improved consumer health literacy as Objective 11-2, and identified health literacy as an important component of health communication, medical product safety and oral health. The 2003 Coalition for Allied Health Leadership team completed a national survey of allied health professionals and educators to assess awareness and needs concerning health literacy. Approximately one-third of all respondents were unaware of the issues surrounding health literacy, or that health literacy resources were available; denied knowledge of an impact of health literacy on patient care for their specific profession or had no institutional policy or goals to address health literacy. The article states that inadequate health literacy adversely affects health care outcomes and the quality of life of 90 million Americans. The cost to the health care system is $73 billion annually (Health Literacy Survey, 2004).

"Literacy" provides the skills that enable individuals to understand and communicate health information and concerns. As mentioned above, educators do not associate literacy

Box 3-1. Health Literacy in an Older Man.

A 64-year-old man, with a history of noncompliance, was evaluated for a routine checkup. According to the resident, he hadn't taken his medications for diabetes or a heart problem for several weeks. Before leaving he received instructions about his medications, their importance and the proper doses. He disclosed he would see his doctor for follow-up, but couldn't remember the person's name. He was given a handwritten discharge summary.

He was seen five months later at a community clinic. He said he was taking his medications, but couldn't remember their names or dosages. The regimen was reviewed a second time; dates for blood tests were provided. He was scheduled for a recheck in two weeks.

When he returned, a medical student made a diagnosis that no one had considered: illiteracy. Many of his glucose values had been written for future dates and he was unable to read his list of medications. The man lived alone, dropped out of school in the second grade and had never learned to read.

Despite avoiding jargon and use of simple language, his medical team–comprised of many doctors, nurses and social workers–had not guessed he couldn't read.

This patient's problem is not uncommon. Fourteen percent of the adults in the U.S. have substandard prose ability: "ability to use printed and written information to function in society, to achieve one's goals and potential." According to The National Assessment of Adult Literacy (NAAL), these substandard skills "are no more than the most simple and concrete literacy skills: ranging from those completely illiterate to those who can identify short phrases.

Other facts: based on NAAL data, 12% of U.S. adults have "document illiteracy." That is, they lack the ability to read and understand transportation schedules and food and drug labels. These people cannot read a television program to find what time a program will be aired. Twenty percent have below basic "quantitative literacy," the ability to perform fundamental quantitative tasks such as comparing ticket prices for two events. Older people (i.e., >64 years) fared the poorest on the NAAL; 23% had below average prose literacy, 27% below basic document literacy and 34% below basic quantitative skills.

Survey results indicate more than one-third of English-speaking patients and more than half of primarily Spanish-speaking patients at U.S. hospitals have low literacy. Often, these people present in the emergency room rather than a clinic because someone there will always write the information down so they don't have to do it themselves.

Patients with low literacy skills are often ashamed of their problem, with two-thirds never telling their spouses.

One clinician thinks that literacy screening should become a new vital sign. But that approach is controversial; no one wants to be embarrassed especially in front of his or her doctor. And there is little time to collect more information now in clinical practice. However, much has been written on the topic.

The patient described at the beginning of this case, with help, enrolled in an adult reading course, but it's still not clear if he takes all his medications as prescribed.

The Bibliography for **Box 3-1** can be found at www.markmorris.org.

with reading alone, but often consider literacy to represent a constellation of skills including reading, writing, basic mathematical calculations and speech and speech comprehension skills (Kirsch, 2001; Healthy People 2010) (**Table 3-2**).

Problems Associated with Inadequate Health Literacy

Individuals with inadequate health literacy (as currently measured) report less knowledge about their medical conditions and treatment, worse health status, less understanding and use of preventive services and a higher rate of hospitalization than those with marginal or adequate health literacy (Parker et al, 2003).

Inadequate health literacy is a hidden problem. People with limited health literacy skills may be embarrassed to discuss or even mention problems they encounter with the health care system (Baker et al, 1996; Parikh et al, 1996).

Health care personnel assume patients are telling everything, which is clearly not the case (**Box 3-1**). Studies show that a large percentage of patients are noncompliant and that health care professionals significantly underestimate how common noncompliance is (Hall et al, 1988).

Two recent studies demonstrated a higher rate of hospitalization and use of emergency services among patients with limited literacy. This higher use has been associated with higher health care costs (IOM, 2004). The Institute for HealthCare Advancement estimates that the average annual health care costs of people with very low health literacy may be four times greater than that of the general population (Sarasohn-Kahn, 2002). In a small Arizona study, patients with reading levels at or below third grade had mean Medicaid charges $7,500 higher than those who read above the third grade (Weiss and Palmer, 2004).

Inadequate health literacy is particularly common among older adults and low-income patients. More than 66% of U.S. adults age 60 and older have inadequate or marginal literacy skills and about 45% of all functionally illiterate adults live in poverty (AMA Foundation, 2000).

A study of 2,659 outpatients at two hospitals found that 42% did not understand instructions to "take medication on an empty stomach." The same study found a 52% increase in the risk of hospitalization among patients with inadequate literacy compared with patients with adequate literacy (Williams et al, 1995). In the largest study of health literacy to date, one-third of English-speaking patients at two public hospitals were unable to read basic health materials. Twenty-six percent were unable to understand information on an appointment slip and 60% did not understand a standard informed consent docu-

Box 3-2. Health Literacy and Language Barriers.

Almost 50 million Americans (~19% of U.S. residents) speak a language other than English at home. A total of more than 22 million have limited English proficiency, speaking less than "very well" by their own admission. The decade leading up to 2000 experienced a 47% (more than 15 million people) increase in the number of people who spoke a language other than English at home.

Many patients who need medical interpreters have no access to them. Results of one study showed that no interpreter was used in 46% of emergency department cases involving people with limited English proficiency. Furthermore, few clinicians receive instructions with how to work with interpreters.

Language barriers and deficits can cause great harm. Patients are often nonadherent to medications, less likely to return for follow-up visits and have higher rates of hospitalization and drug complications. Two cases follow:

Case 1: A two-year-old girl was diagnosed with an inner ear infection and was prescribed an antibiotic. Her mother understood that her daughter should receive the prescribed medication twice daily. After carefully studying the label on the bottle and deciding it didn't tell how to administer the medication, the mother filled a teaspoon and poured the antibiotic into her daughter's painful ear.

Case 2: A young Spanish-speaking man stumbled into his girlfriend's house and said he was "intoxicado." The Spanish-speaking paramedics took the work to mean "intoxicated." The patient's intended meaning was "nauseous." After 36 hours of being worked up for a drug overdose, the patient was reevaluated and found to have an intracerebellar hematoma with brainstem compression and a subdural hematoma. The young man became a quadriplegic.

Family members, friends and untrained members of the support staff are often used in these encounters, but commit more errors than those with more training. Much work needs to be done in this area given the changing dynamics of the U.S. population.

The Bibliography for **Box 3-2** can be found at www.markmorris.org.

ment (Williams et al, 1995).

Racial and ethnic differences can contribute to communication breakdowns (**Box 3-2**). As many as 20% of Spanish-speaking Latinos say they do not seek medical advice due to language barriers (IOM, 2002). A 2001 survey of 6,722 adults found that minority populations are more likely to have difficulties communicating with their health care providers compared with whites (Collins, 2001).

Even highly skilled individuals may find the health care system too complicated to understand, especially when poor health, anxiety, effects of medication, etc. make them more vulnerable. Directions, signs and official documents, including informed consent forms, social services forms, public health information, medical instructions and health education materials often use jargon and technical language that make them too difficult to use (Rudd et al, 2000).

Patients with inadequate health literacy and chronic illness have less knowledge of illness management than those with high health literacy (Kalichman and Rompa, 2000). Public hospital patients with inadequate health literacy had higher rates of hospitalization than those with adequate health literacy (Baker et al, 1996). Adults with limited health literacy have less knowledge of disease management and of health-promoting behaviors, report poorer health status and are less likely to use preventive services (IOM, 2004).

Adverse drug events are another aspect of inadequate health literacy. One report found that 10% of adverse drug events were linked to errors in the use of the drug as a result of communication failure (Leape et al, 1993).

Where do Patients Receive Health Care Information?

Socioeconomic status, education level and primary language all affect whether consumers will seek out health information, where they will look, what type of information they prefer and how they will interpret that information (IOM, 2004). There is no single reliable answer.

Between 62 and 69% of adults at all literacy levels reported obtaining information from family and friends. Between 94 and 97% of adults at all skill levels reported using radio and television to obtain information. Individuals with lower literacy levels were less likely than those with higher skills to use newspapers and magazines for health information (69.5 vs. 90%).

The National Cancer Institute conducted the Health Information Trends Survey (HINTS), one of the nation's first national surveys of health information sources in 2003 and 2005. HINTS databases are designed to provide information regarding pattern of information use and opportunities to inform Americans about cancer.

In a Gallup survey, the proportion of people who reported getting "a great deal" or "moderate" amount of health or medical information from these sources follows: doctors (70%), television (64%), books (56%), newspapers (52%), magazines (51%), nurses (49%) and the Internet (37%). The proportion of people who reported a great deal or moderate amount of trust and confidence in the health or medical information from the sources follows: doctors (93%), nurses (83%), books (82%), newspapers (64%), magazines (62%), the Internet (62%) and television (59%) (Gallup Organization, 2002).

People have more ways than ever to get information, including telephone, fax, e-mail, the Internet, television, radio, print media, family and friends, etc. More sources will be available in the future, including automated monitoring of vital signs and markers, increased use of wireless technology, among others. But how do people access information today and how accurate is that information? The National Cancer Institute sought to answer some of these questions through HINTS. Some results follow (Hesse, 2004):

- Where would you go for cancer information? Provider (50%), Internet (34%), Library (5%), Family (4%), Other (4%), Print media (3%).
- Where did you go for cancer information? Internet (49%), Print media (27%), Provider (11%), Library (6%), Other (4%), Family (3%).
- Trust information by gender? There were no gender differences. Doctors came in first, followed by television. No differences existed among family/friends, newspapers, magazines, radio, television and the Internet.
- Trust information by education? Those with no high school diploma tended to trust their doctors and television far more than family, friends, newspapers, magazines, radio and the Internet.
- When asked to agree or not with the statement "Everything causes cancer:" 51% strongly agreed or agreed; only 18% strongly disagreed.
- When asked to agree or not with the statement "There's not much people can do to lower their chances of getting cancer:" 72% strongly disagreed or somewhat disagreed.
- When asked to agree or not with the statement "There are so many different recommendations about preventing cancer, it's hard to know which ones to follow:" 77% strongly agreed or somewhat agreed.

Family and Friends

Personal stories may have the power to influence health behavior, especially in those with inadequate literary skills. One study found that many individuals with inadequate literacy more often obtained information about cancer from family and others who have had experience with a late-stage diagnosis rather than from reading about the disease (Friedell et al, 1997).

The Internet

The Internet is estimated to reach more than 70 million people living in the U.S. with health information. About 90% of 15- to 24-year-olds have been online; 75% of these have used the Internet at least once to obtain health information (Rideout, 2004). Inadequate English literacy and disparities in computer access decrease the likelihood that the information will be available to, and understood by, all health consumers (Houston and Allison, 2002). The quality and reliability of online content can be problematic. A meta-analysis of consumer health information on the Internet found that 70% of the studies analyzed concluded quality was a problem (Eysenbach et al, 2002).

Health Care Professionals

A number of studies demonstrate that patients remember and understand as little as half of what they are told by their physicians. In addition, because they have knowledge deficits, patients with inadequate health literacy may be less equipped to overcome discrepancies in understanding and memory when they are at home and experience difficulties reading or interpreting instructions (IOM, 2004).

Limited education, training, continuing education and practice opportunities to develop skills for improving health literacy exist for allied health professionals and educators at the national level (IOM, 2004).

Some evidence of a failure of communication exists with patients who have inadequate health literacy as currently measured. Patients with chronic diseases and inadequate health literacy have poor knowledge of their condition and its management, often despite having received standard self-management education (Williams et al, 1998, 1998a). Patients with inadequate health literacy have more difficulty accurately reporting their medication regimens and describing the reasons for which their medications were prescribed (Schillinger et al, 2003) and may have poorer compliance (Kalichman et al, 1999).

Communication between a health care provider and patient during outpatient visits may be hampered by several related factors. These include the relative infrequency and brevity of visits, language barriers, differences between providers' and patients' agendas and communication styles and other cultural barriers, lack of trust between the patient and provider, overriding or competing clinical problems and the complexity and variability of patients' reporting symptoms and trends in their health status (IOM, 2004).

The average patient asks only two questions during an entire medical visit lasting an average of 15 minutes, according to the Bayer Institute of Health Care Communications. Studies show that most patients are relatively uninformed about their condition or the most appropriate treatment despite the fact that most patients state they want more information. Results of one study revealed that doctors imparted information to patients for an average of a little more than a minute during interviews that lasted an average of more than 20 minutes. When asked how much time they spent on patient education, the physicians overestimated by a factor of nine. The study also found that in 65% of the cases, physicians thought patients wanted less information than they actually did (Terry, 1994).

An Institute of Medicine (IOM) report clarifies the links between miscommunication and medical and health errors and adverse events (2002). A variety of problems can result if culture and language are not accounted for including failure to obtain accurate medical histories, failure to obtain informed consent, inadequate health knowledge and understanding of health conditions, inadequate treatment adherence (compliance), medication errors, decreased use of preventive and other health care services and poor patient satisfaction. Customized and tailored care based on patient needs and values and accommodating differences in patient preferences are integral to individualized care (IOM, 2001).

The concept that no one size fits all is fundamental to the understanding of health literacy. Complex problems are rarely resolved by simple solutions. However, scientific investigations of interventions to minimize the impact of health literacy and promote the development of health literacy skills are in its infancy (IOM, 2004). Evidence-based approaches show promise for contributing to better outcomes (Chapter 2).

Health literacy must be understood and addressed in the context of culture and language (IOM, 2004). Competing sources of health information (including the national media, the Internet, product marketing, health education and consumer protection) intensify the need for improved health literacy.

Improving Health Literacy

Health literacy is fundamental to quality care (IOM, 2004). Without improvements, the effect of many advances to improve health outcomes will be diminished. Consequently, the IOM of the National Academies (U.S.) has identified improving health literacy as one of two crosscutting issues in health care requiring attention (IOM, 2003). The IOM reports that enabling patients to understand their condition and its treatment, to make the best decisions for their care and to take the right medications at the right time in the intended dose; that is, to act in their own interest remains a neglected, final pathway to high-quality health care (IOM, 2004).

A 1998 report from the U.S. Department of Health and Human Services provided evidence from accumulated studies that health, morbidity and mortality are related to income and educational factors (Pamuk et al, 1998). Life expectancy and death rates from cancer and heart disease, incidence of diabetes and hypertension and use of health services were related to family income. Death rates from chronic diseases, communicable diseases and injuries were inversely related to education (i.e., those with lower educational achievement were more likely to die of a chronic disease than those with higher educational achievement). In essence, the lower one's income or educational achievement, the worse one's health (IOM, 2004).

Approaches that appear to successfully improve health literacy include:

1. Provision of simplified/more attractive written materials
2. Technology-based communication techniques
3. Personal communication and education
4. Combined tailored approaches
5. Partnerships (collaborative measures between patient and the health care team).

In all of these, using plain language (common words, defining unusual words, writing the way people talk); simple, specific and direct sentences; active, inflective voice; sequencing ideas clearly and logically; being attentive to and respectful of culture enhance the patient's ability to understand and retain information. It is also imperative to be cognizant of overt and covert messages and to improve skills, materials and processes. This includes changing outdated approaches and encouraging professionals to improve verbal and written communication skills, including work with the adult education sector, etc. (Rudd, 2002).

Professionals are also encouraged to write legibly or type, and use simplified language with more white space, improved format and pictograms (See below.) or other graphic devices. Pictograms may be especially useful for communicating information to consumers who speak English as a second language and to those with lower reading ability levels (IOM, 2004).

The telephone can be a great means of delivering interventions such as health-related counseling and reminders, if the caller has competent verbal communication skills. Tailored print communications can improve health outcomes, but research also shows that they are less effective at influencing individuals who are not serious about making a behavioral change (Revere and Dunbar, 2001; IOM, 2002).

Arcane language and jargon that are common to health care workers are usually indecipherable to patients. Adults who have difficulty reading or understanding written materials are often embarrassed and devise ways to hide their inability to understand. If health care professionals invested more time to ask their patients to explain exactly what they understand about their diagnoses, instructions and bottle labels, the caregivers would find many gaps in knowledge, difficulties in understanding and misinterpretations (IOM, 2004). These problems are exacerbated by language and cultural variation, by technological complexity in health care and by intricate administrative documents and requirements.

Female primary care physicians tend to engage in longer visits and have more "patient-centered" consultations than their male counterparts (Roter et al, 2002). Female physicians engage in significantly more active partnership behaviors, positive talk, psychosocial counseling, psychosocial question asking and emotionally focused talk. Medical visits with female physicians are, on average, two minutes (10%) longer than those with male physicians.

Distinguishing between noncompliance and inadequate literacy may be difficult unless health care providers regularly ask patients questions such as, "Was I clear?" "Is there anything you'd like for me to go over again?" These types of questions put the burden of responsibility on the speaker rather than on the listener. Researchers and the American Medical Association advocate the importance of teachback. For example, asking "Just so we both agree, why don't you tell me what you would do if XYZ happens?" or to demonstrate how the patient would do something, like monitor blood glucose concentration.

In veterinary medicine, this simple approach of having pet owners relate back their understanding (without feeling like they've been put on the spot) can have dramatically positive ramifications for pet care. Speaking clearly and being an attentive listener can express that you care. Empathy goes a long way in building trust and establishing a relationship so that communication is successful. Focus on using basic words and making the message clear.

A meta-analysis of 41 research studies showed that giving patients more information is associated with increased patient satisfaction, better compliance and better recall and understanding of medical conditions (Rankin and Stallings, 1996).

Technology-Based Communication

It's very hard to cover all the complex information needed to make decisions in spoken and written words. Covering some information with tools such as CD-ROMs before patients meet with their doctors has increased satisfaction in at least one study in human medicine.

According to the Memorial Sloan-Kettering Cancer Center, "New technology (i.e., a CD-ROM educational tool) can save nurses' time by eliminating the need for repetitive teaching, and enrich patient teaching by allowing the nurse more time to address individual concerns" (Ginty and Sullivan, 2001). A second study conducted at the same center discussed the benefits that were realized after nurses used an educational CD-ROM to supplement their teaching to pre- and postoperative cancer patients. According to the center, "The nurse is responsible for doing preoperative teaching, much of which is standard and the same for every patient. Nevertheless, it must be repeated for each patient." The CD-ROM covering standard pre- and postoperative topics was very effective; 78% of patients who completed a follow-up quiz had one or no answers wrong. Nurses estimated that the program significantly decreased the time it took them to do standard preoperative teaching, allowing them to focus on patient-specific questions and concerns. The study concluded that "patients stated the animation, narration and photographs on the CD-ROM reinforced their understanding and decreased anxiety" (Vaziri and Gallagher, 2001).

Professional and public awareness of the health literacy issue must be increased, beginning with education of medical students and physicians and improved patient-physician skills (Schillinger et al, 2004). Such training of veterinary students, veterinarians and all health care team members would no doubt be of great benefit to pets and pet owners as well.

Pictographs

Pictographs (e.g., like simple drawings on road signs) have been used in non-literate societies to help people remember spoken instructions. Pictographs are designed to help people understand information quickly. One small study tested the hypothesis that pictographs can improve recall of spoken medical instructions. Twenty-one junior college students listened to lists of 38 actions for managing fever and 50 actions for managing sore mouths. One of the action lists was accompanied by pictographs during listening and recall whereas the other was not. Subjects did not see any written words during the intervention and therefore, relied entirely on memory of what they heard. Mean correct recall was 85% with pictographs and 14% without ($p < 0.0001$) (Houts et al, 1998).

Impact of Health Literacy on Compliance

Health literacy has only recently reached the national agenda in human medicine and for the most part, hasn't at all in veterinary medicine. Logically, many of the 90 million Americans with inadequate health literacy own pets. It would be imprudent to assume that they understand preventive protocols, diagnoses and treatments for their pets any better than they do for themselves.

There is very little information about the exact relationship between compliance and health literacy in human medicine and none in veterinary medicine. Studies show, however, that a large percentage of patients are noncompliant and that health care professionals significantly underestimate the scope of noncompliance (Hall et al, 1988). Likewise, compliance is a major problem in veterinary medicine (See below.) (AAHA, 2003).

Conclusion

Health literacy is fundamental to quality care (IOM, 2004). A former surgeon general recently stated that "health literacy can save lives, save money and improve health and well being of millions of Americans...health literacy is the currency of success for everything I am doing as Surgeon General" (Carmona, 2003).

People's prior knowledge, beliefs and experiences influence the way they interpret and use health information. Furthermore, America's increasing cultural diversity challenges health communication activities. Until now, we've known little about how people seek health information or how to bridge the substantial discrepancies between the information they want and need and what they receive (Croyle, 2004). Several books are available to provide information about improving health literacy and compliance (**Table 3-3**).

Health literacy must be actively addressed by the medical profession, and likewise, the veterinary profession should take an aggressive approach to enhance veterinary health literacy.

CLIENT COMPLIANCE

Introduction and Background

Around 400 BCE, Hippocrates supposedly observed that some of his patients failed to comply with medical instructions, thus prolonging their recovery. He subsequently counseled his students that some patients would be less than honest about taking medication. In the early 1900s, tuberculosis patients who failed to follow medical instructions were called "defaulters" (Jaret, 2001). Patients were subsequently described as "faithless," "untrustworthy" and "unreliable" over the following half century when they failed to follow their physician's orders (Steiner and Ernst, 2000). Unfortunately, noncompliance with medical instructions remains a huge problem more than 2,400 years after Hippocrates' warning.

Improving communication is an important aspect of improving compliance. The Food and Drug Administration (FDA) supports higher-quality health information for the public. An FDA study in 1999 found that 56% of people who saw a consumer-directed print advertisement for a prescription drug said they read the brief summary "not at all" or "a little." In a follow-up study in 2002, that number increased to 73%. During the same three-year span, those saying they read "almost all" or "all" decreased from 26 to 16%. Based on these data, the FDA wants manufacturers to present key risk information in consumer-directed print advertisements in more consumer-friendly ways, including use of clearer, less cluttered formats for presenting risk information. The FDA also encourages manufacturers to focus their risk disclosures on the most important and the most common risks and to do so in language easily understood by the average consumer (FDA, 2004).

Preventive and therapeutic noncompliance is a major issue in human health care and, as we'll show, in veterinary medicine. The number one problem in treating illness today is patients' failure to take prescription medications correctly, regardless of patient age (AmericanHeart.org, 2004). Failure to take medica-

Table 3-3. Additional resources for improving health literacy and compliance.

Titles	Publishers
Health literacy resources	
Health Literacy	Institute of Medicine National Academies Press 500 5th Street NW, Lockbox 285 Washington, DC 20055
Understanding Health Literacy: Implications for Medicine and Public Health	American Medical Association 800-621-8335 www.amapress.com
Health Literacy in Primary Care: A Clinician's Guide	Springer Publisher Company 11 West 42nd Street New York, NY 10036 www.springerpub.com
Health Literacy from A to Z: Practical Ways to Communicate Your Health Message	Jones and Bartlett Publishers 40 Tall Pine Drive Sudbury, MA 01776 www.jbpub.com
Advancing Health Literacy: A Framework for Understanding and Action	Jossey-Bass 800-956-7739 www.josseybass.com
Compliance resources	
The Path to High-Quality Care: Practical Tips for Improving Compliance	American Animal Hospital Association 12575 West Bayaud Avenue Lakewood, CO 80228 800-883-6301 www.aahanet.org
Veterinary Clinics of North America: Small Animal Practice (March 2006; 36(2): 419-436)	WB Saunders Co. 6277 Sea Harbor Drive Orlando, FL 32887 877-839-7126 www.usjc@elsevier.com
Journal of the American Veterinary Medical Association Evaluation of client compliance with short-term administration of antimicrobials to dogs. (Feb. 15, 2005; 226(4): 567-574)	American Veterinary Medical Association 1931 N. Meacham Rd, Suite 100 Schaumburg , IL 60173 847-925-8070

tions as directed costs the U.S. economy $100 to $300 billion annually (Fortune, 2004). In the U.S. today, the annual consequences of noncompliance include (epill.com):

- An estimated 125,000 deaths.
- 23% of nursing home admissions (380,000 patients/$31.3 billion) are the result of patients failing to take prescription medications accurately.
- 10% of hospital admissions (3.5 million patients/$15.2 billion) are the result of patients failing to take prescription medications correctly.
- Reduced productivity (absenteeism, impaired work performance [20 million workdays/$1.5 billion]).
- Lengthened hospital stays (4.2 days) due to medication noncompliance.

The American Heart Association presents the following facts on its website to further define the scope of noncompliance (AHA, 2004): Almost 49% of Americans use prescription drugs and 30% use nonprescription medications.

- Almost 29% stop taking their medicine before it runs out.
- 22% take less of the medication than is prescribed on the label.
- 12% don't fill their prescriptions at all.
- 12% don't take medication after they buy the prescription.
- At any given time, up to 59% of patients on five or more medications are taking them improperly, regardless of age.
- Adverse drug reactions may be the fourth to sixth leading cause of death. Serious adverse drug reactions occur in 6.7% of hospitalized patients.

The above data deal with health care compliance in the U.S. Similar data exist for other developed countries. The World Health Organization has published an excellent review about the difficulties of compliance: *Adherence to Long-Term Therapies: Evidence for Action* (WHO, 2003). Compliance data from developing countries is even lower.

The information that follows summarizes much of the existing knowledge about compliance in small animal veterinary practice. Promoting awareness of poor compliance rates and acknowledging our ability and obligation to improve them are the first steps in improving adherence to recommended services and products and their associated outcomes for dogs and cats.

Definitions

Compliance has been traditionally defined as "the extent to which the patient (client in veterinary medicine) follows medical instructions" (Sabate, 2001). Unfortunately, this definition promotes a paternalistic relationship and suggests patients (or clients) should be passive participants in health care. Furthermore, this concept of compliance omits many nonmedical interventions that promote health including diet, exercise, routine dental care and avoiding or minimizing behaviors that increase the risk of illness. A better definition is the extent to which a person's (or pet owner's) behavior-taking (administering) medication, following a diet and/or executing lifestyle changes-corresponds with agreed recommendations from a health care provider (WHO, 2003). Another definition used in veterinary medicine: the pets in your practice are receiving the care that you believe is best for them (AAHA, 2003). Compliance is thus a behavior and a measure (Hasford, 1999). Veterinary clients are/will become surrogates for their pets in this regard.

Compliance will be used throughout this article because the term is firmly entrenched in the medical and dental literature and is gaining in awareness in veterinary medicine. As mentioned above, compliance, as defined in human medicine, suggests a paternalistic relationship and connotes blame (as do other terms such as control, adhere, prescribe, regimen, what's best for you and will power), whether it be of patients, clients or health care providers, and is associated with the outmoded concept that the client is the sole source of noncompliance. The concept of adherence may be a better way of capturing the dynamic and complex changes required over long periods to maintain optimal health for people or pets with chronic diseases (WHO, 2004). Adherence requires that the patient (client in veterinary medicine) agree to treatment recommendations. Concordance takes the relationship further because it fosters the concept of agreement between clients and health care providers about whether, when and how medications should be taken. Adherence is used synonymously with compliance in this chapter.

Based on the 2003 AAHA Compliance Study, veterinarians strongly believe that compliance is all or mostly the client's responsibility. Forty-one percent of veterinarians said clients were responsible for noncompliance, whereas 19% said it was the veterinarians; 36% indicated that clients and veterinarians shared the responsibility (AAHA, 2003).

Compliance Research in Veterinary Medicine

The first compliance articles began to appear in the human medical literature in the 1950s. Since then, thousands of articles have been published and dozens of businesses and websites have been created to promote the concept of compliance. By comparison, only a handful of articles have appeared in the veterinary literature. A sampling of the relevant literature follows (**Boxes 3-3** through **3-5**).

In one study, 48% of the dogs visiting 36 veterinary clinics were placed on the recommended heartworm preventive program. These dogs received 78% of the medication required to fully comply with the clinics' recommendations (Cummings, 1995). In another study involving cats with stable chronic renal failure, compliance was not achieved in more than 40% of cats, although cats receiving dietary therapy (i.e., foods restricted in phosphorus and protein) were generally healthier and lived for three times longer, on average. Limited food intake by cats, owner resistance or both were cited as reasons for noncompliance (Elliott et al, 2000).

At least three studies measured compliance with short-term antibacterial therapy in dogs. In one study, investigators assessed compliance among 95 dog owners using a telephone survey. Forty-four percent reported 100% compliance with the treatment regimen and 88% reported a compliance level of 80% or more. Compliance was significantly higher when dog owners felt that the veterinarian spent enough consultation time. Compliance results were higher for dogs treated for gastrointestinal (GI) infections compared with those treated for other diseases (Grave and Tanem, 1999). In another study, electronic monitoring (e.g., Which may mean as little as the client opened a bottle with an electronic chip, whether the client gave the medication or whether the pet regurgitated the medication are variables.) showed owners administered an average of 84% (range 7 to 104%) of an antibiotic given for five to seven days. Return medication counts and client self-reports overestimated therapeutic compliance compared to electronic monitoring. The majority of owners (71%) claimed perfect compliance with the prescribed regimen (Barter et al, 1996). The third study reported that there was no difference in compliance for regimens that included twice or three times per day administration of an antibiotic (84%). However, only 34% gave doses within the designated optimal time period. Compliance tended to be better with the twice-daily regimen although the differences were insignificant (Barter et al, 1996a). It should be noted, however, that these percentages were self-reported.

In dental compliance studies, owners of dogs were given extensive instructions about brushing their dog's teeth. Six months later, 53% were still providing the minimum care necessary to prevent periodontal disease (Miller and Harvey, 1994). Another study compared three dental homecare regimens, including daily toothbrushing and two different dental foods, with a control group in 88 client-owned cats for six months after a professional cleaning. A large-sized kibble with dental properties was most efficacious in controlling calculus formation and development of gingivitis. Toothbrushing compliance was only 40% at the end of the six-month study (Theyse et al, 2002).

Box 3-3. Human Oral Health Literacy Studies.

Eight objectives in Healthy People 2010 concern the oral health of U.S. adults, including goals to reduce dental caries, gingivitis, oral cancer and tooth loss, as well as to improve use of the dental care system. The Surgeon General recognized that "the majority of people who need such information most, those in low-income groups and those with lower education levels, also are the ones who lack the information and skills (oral health literacy) to ask for and obtain specific preventive services or treatment options."

One article in this review studied the readability of 24 educational materials for dental patients. The reading levels ranged from the third to 23rd grade levels, more than 40% of which were written above the seventh to ninth grade level. Many of the materials contained grammatical errors and obscure jargon.

A second article examined the readability and distribution of 20 printed materials containing oral health educational information. Ninety-one percent of the materials were written between the 9th and 15th grade levels.

A third article assessed the difficulty of dental words and tested the readability of selected dental health education materials. Adolescents were asked to read aloud and describe the meanings of 25 commonly used dental terms. Several words were poorly understood, including "gum disease," "oral hygiene," "fluoride tablets" and "gingivitis." The four dental health education brochures studied were written from 12.4 to 17.4 reading grade levels.

Yet another study assessed the readability of 19 oral cancer educational pieces. Five pieces tested at the sixth and seventh reading grade levels, nine at the eight and ninth grade levels, and five at grades 10 through 13.

The Bibliography for **Box 3-3** can be found at www.markmorris.org.

Box 3-4. Compliance in Human Medicine.

Several types of noncompliance exist. Initial noncompliance occurs when a patient receives a written prescription or calls a pharmacy, but doesn't wait or return to pick up the filled prescription. Patients who fail to present a prescription are also initial noncompliers. Varying compliance is used to describe the process of taking a prescribed medication at a level less than recommended. Hypercompliance occurs when a patient takes a medication at a level above that prescribed. The term "white coat compliance" is used to describe behavior in which a patient who has been noncompliant takes medication at or above the prescribed level around a recheck appointment. Accordingly, both the physician and the patient may incorrectly believe the patient is receiving therapeutic benefit. "Drug holidays" refers to the behavior in which patients repeatedly and abruptly discontinue and resume taking their medication.

Studies have shown that the amount of information forgotten by patients is a linear function of the amount presented and is correlated with the patient's medical knowledge, anxiety level, and possibly age, but not with intelligence. Therefore, a phased approach is preferable in patient education. Both oral and written information should be provided (e.g., patient education booklets, medication cards, etc.) and special materials should be developed to instruct patients with low literacy (e.g., picture schedule). Formal evaluation of patient education is imperative.

Failure to attend appointments is often one of the first signs that a patient is not complying with his or her treatment. Given the difficulty of monitoring compliance directly, health care professionals may want to monitor patients' attendance at clinic appointments as a proxy measure.

Asking patients to complete diaries about medication use has the advantage of providing details about how and when the product was taken. However, whether diaries improve compliance hasn't been proven.

The Bibliography for **Box 3-4** can be found at www.markmorris.org.

The American Animal Hospital Association Compliance Study

The American Animal Hospital Association conducted the largest, most significant compliance study in veterinary medicine, which was funded by a substantial educational grant from Hill's Pet Nutrition, Inc. Results of the study were reported in the book *The Path to High-Quality Care: Practical Tips for Improving Compliance* in 2003. This comprehensive study showed that millions of dogs and cats did not receive the best care they could have. Although most practice teams thought compliance with recommendations was high, few practices actually measured compliance and the level of compliance in almost all cases was significantly less than what practice teams believed; 78% of veterinarians indicated that they were satisfied with the levels of compliance in their practices (AAHA, 2003). Researchers visited 52 practices and/or conducted in-depth interviews with practice teams. More than 1,000 pet owners were surveyed about the care they provided for their pets, their desires relative to the information and care provided by their veterinarian and their compliance with health care recommendations. Furthermore, data were gathered from the medical records of almost 1,400 cats and dogs. These data were used to quantify compliance and the opportunities that practices had to improve pet care by improving compliance (AAHA, 2003). The study quantified compliance in six areas:

- Heartworm testing and prevention
- Dental prophylaxis
- Therapeutic foods
- Senior screenings
- Canine and feline core vaccinations
- Preanesthetic testing.

Only dogs and cats seen by their veterinarian at least once during the past 12 months were included in the study; extrapolation accounts for 51 million dogs and 44.2 million cats falling into this category (AVMA, 2002). The AAHA compliance data do not include 10.6 million dogs and 22.7 million cats that were not seen at a veterinary practice during the previous year.

More than seven million dogs were not in compliance with their veterinarian's protocol for heartworm testing. Almost 21.5 million owners did not give their dog's heartworm preventive medication at all, failed to give medication for the number of days recommended by their veterinarian, or (and maybe most alarming) were never dispensed an adequate amount of preventive in the first place, or were never notified by the practice to purchase follow-up doses. In endemic areas, compliance for testing and preventive medication was 83 and 48%, respectively. The American Heartworm Association reported that more than 244,000 dogs tested positive for heartworms in 2001 (AAHA, 2003).

The AAHA Compliance Study found a dental prophylaxis compliance rate of 35% for dogs and cats with grade 2, 3 or 4 dental disease. Compliance was only 15% for those pets with grade 1 disease. The study concluded that almost 15.5 million dogs and cats with grade 2, 3 or 4 dental disease had not received dental prophylaxis. Based on chart review, 23% of those owners of pets with grade 2 or higher dental disease (3.6 million pets) did not receive a recommendation for treatment. Millions more cats and dogs had grade 1 disease. Interestingly, no grade was reported for 19% of the patients. The lack of a reported dental grade may indicate that no exam was given or poor medical record keeping (AAHA, 2003). The American Veterinary Dental College defines quality dental health care as completing a dental prophylactic procedure on any pet with grade 1 to 4 dental disease. Veterinary health care teams failed to adhere to these recommendations in a great many cases, which has resulted in less than the best care for many patients.

Compliance with feeding a therapeutic food for six canine conditions (i.e., kidney disease, bladder stones or crystals, food allergies, chronic GI disease, acute GI disease and obesity) and seven feline conditions (i.e., the same six canine topics plus feline lower urinary tract disease) was included in the survey.

Compliance with feeding therapeutic foods was 19% for dogs and 18% for cats. More than 11.6 million dogs and nine million cats with one of the diagnosed conditions were not fed an appropriate therapeutic food at all or were not fed the food for an appropriate period of time (AAHA, 2003). When all pets with diagnoses that could benefit from treatment with a therapeutic food were considered, overall compliance was 5 to 7%, which represented more than 52 million dogs and cats. The real potential for improvement for all foods combined could be as high as 20-fold. What was also disturbing is that 55% of pet owners who fed a therapeutic food also supplemented the recommended food with other foods or treats. The primary reason cited by clients was that they didn't know not to.

Thirty-five percent of the dogs and cats in a typical practice are considered senior (i.e., mature). Senior screenings minimally included blood work and a urinalysis. About 17.9 million dogs and 15.5 million cats considered to be senior had not received a diagnostic screening in the past year. Only 32 and 35% of the dogs and cats had diagnostic screening tests performed (AAHA, 2003).

Compliance for core vaccinations (i.e., distemper, hepatitis, leptospirosis, parainfluenza and parvovirus for dogs and viral rhinotracheitis, calicivirus and panleukopenia for cats) was 87%, which was higher than for any other condition studied. Still, 12.4 million dogs and cats were not protected against core diseases. Compliance with other vaccinations was not studied (AAHA, 2003).

Compliance with preanesthetic screening was 72% for dogs and 65% for cats. Compliance was 90% for practices that required preanesthetic blood work (AAHA, 2003).

Economic Aspects of Noncompliance

Poor compliance affects standards of care, overall pet health, client satisfaction and practice economics. Every veterinary health care team member and client is responsible for enhancing compliance. According to the AAHA Compliance Study, the total additional revenue opportunity per veterinarian per year is $639,700 to $660,700 for the conditions studied (2003). Other practice productivity data are available (Wayner and Heinke, 2006).

Improving Compliance

The AAHA Compliance Study concluded that compliance is related to three factors: recommendation (by the veterinarian), acceptance (by the client) and follow through (by the veterinary health care team). This can easily be remembered as CRAFT, where Compliance = Recommendation + Acceptance + Follow Through. The AAHA study noted that: 1) compliance was much lower than veterinarians believed and 2) clients would very often comply if the practice made an effort to help them comply (2003). Furthermore, a significant element of noncompliance is due to the fact that practice team members often do not make recommendations to clients. Thus a positive compliance cascade cannot happen.

As part of the study, pet owners were asked to agree with one of these statements:

- I want my veterinarian to tell me about all of the recommended treatment options for my pet, even if I may be unable to afford them.
- I want my veterinarian to tell me only about the recommended treatments for my pet that he or she thinks are not too expensive for me.

Ninety percent of respondents chose the first statement. Furthermore, only 7% declined dental care due to cost. Likewise, only 4% either discontinued or refused therapeutic foods and only 5% declined senior screenings due to cost. Cost was not a significant factor in the client's decision to accept or decline health care. Despite these findings, veterinarians overwhelmingly cited cost and insufficient client communication and education as the primary barriers to com-

Box 3-5. What Veterinarians can Learn from Physicians about Communication.

The *Journal of the American Veterinary Medical Association* published an outstanding review titled "What can veterinarians learn from studies of physician-patient communication about veterinarian-client-patient communication?" (Vol. 224 [5], March 1, 2004, pp 676-684). Several relevant points follow:

- A gold standard does not exist for assessing physician-patient interactions, nor for an accepted definition of the physician-patient relationship.
- Communication style should be tailored to the individual patient.
- The most common model for the physician-patient relationship is still paternalism. Relationship-centered care, characterized as a partnership, in which negotiation and shared decision-making is suggested as optimal. The physician's role is suggested as an advisor or counselor.
- Communication skills and dealing with clients have been listed as the most important skills for success.
- Effective communication can significantly improve medical outcomes, including patient health and satisfaction, adherence to medical recommendations and physician satisfaction.
- A controlling style including behaviors that maintain the physician's power, status, authority and professional distance negatively affects patient satisfaction.
- Factors suggested to improve client compliance include establishing two-way communication and trusting relationships, a compassionate health care team, collaborative planning of the treatment regimen, provision of specific verbal and written instructions about medications and timely encouragement.
- Medical researchers have studied physician-patient interactions for 30 years. Four basic conclusions have emerged: physician-patient interactions have an impact on patient health, patient satisfaction, adherence to medical recommendations and physician satisfaction.

The Bibliography for **Box 3-5** can be found at www.markmorris.org.

pliance (AAHA, 2003).

The AAHA study lists several follow through components to augment recommendations. These include: scheduling procedures and follow-up appointments when the recommendation is made, providing clear instructions for at-homecare and recheck exams (Almost 80% of pet owners indicated they wanted verbal and written instructions.), sending reminders (In the AAHA study, compliance was highest for core vaccinations, a service for which virtually every practice sends reminders. Few practices send reminders for medication or food refills. Sixty-five percent of pet owners said they would welcome multiple reminders by phone, mail, e-mail or a combination. Seventy-two percent said they would like to receive a phone call if they were overdue for a recommended treatment or preventive service.) and making follow-up phone calls. More than 82% of the pet owners surveyed indicated that they wanted to be able to discuss feeding and homecare instructions with other members of the health care team, not just the doctors. Practices that consistently followed-up with clients whose pets were fed a new food reported a much higher percentage of patients staying on the new food and a much higher compliance with recommended feeding guidelines (AAHA, 2003).

The AAHA Compliance Study identified six steps to improving compliance and patient care:

- Measure current compliance
- Involve the entire health care team (and establish protocols that are agreed upon)
- Set compliance goals
- Implement new protocols
- Measure and track results
- Celebrate success.

The AAHA Compliance Study found that a major cause of veterinary care providers' failure to make health care recommendations was their misjudgment of the clients' willingness to take action. The following represent reasons veterinarians cited for noncompliance (AAHA, 2003):

- Cost (60%)
- Communication and client education (55%)
- Client time or convenience (40%)
- Perceived value (25%)
- Process error at practice (15%).

Despite these perceptions 75% of pet owners agreed or strongly agreed that their veterinarian made recommendations that were good for the pet. Only 10% of pet owners agreed or strongly agreed that their veterinarian's recommendations were motivated by a desire to make money. Cost wasn't a major barrier to adherence in the AAHA Compliance Study. However, lack of an effective recommendation and lack of reinforcement by the veterinary health care team were cited by clients as important barriers to compliance. For example, veterinarians claimed that they discussed nutrition and pet food with pet owners during more than 90% of visits. Only 18 to 22% of pet owners recalled such discussions. Reasons cited for lack of client follow through include:

- Unclear diagnosis or need for follow-up care
- No one told me about the need for follow-up
- Follow-up appointment not made or was too difficult to make
- No reminders were sent.

As an example, client acceptance of dental recommendations doesn't depend on the degree of dental disease or the cost of the procedure. Clients cited these reasons for lack of compliance:

- Not enough education provided about the need for the service (45%)
- Follow-up visit not scheduled (15%)
- Veterinary health care team didn't tell me about it (8%)
- Pending appointment (5%)
- Unclear diagnosis (5%)
- Cat was too wild to catch (5%)
- Other (7%).

Several other sources bear consideration for improving compliance (**Table 3-3**).

Conclusion

It is obvious that adequate health literacy is a major obstacle to delivering optimal health care in human medicine. By extension, this issue is no less dramatic in veterinary medicine, and the processes for improved communications and health literacy cited in this chapter have direct relevance to pet care.

The health literacy issue is coupled to that of compliance/adherence. As defined in the AAHA Compliance Study, compliance in veterinary medicine is defined as, "the pets in your practice are receiving the care that you believe is best for them." That is; if you, the attending veterinarian, believe specific products and services are important for a particular pet's care, does your health care team effectively communicate your beliefs to the client in order for her/him to decide the next steps for the pet's care? Not all clients will take our recommendations, but research suggests that better communication improves medical care.

Health literacy, the degree to which individuals have the capacity to obtain, process and understand basic health information and services needed to make appropriate health decisions (Ratzan and Parker, 2000; Healthy People 2010) cannot be assumed. Effective communication is paramount to practicing great medicine (Silverman et al, 2005; Cornell et al, 2007).

REFERENCES

The references for **Chapter 3** can be found at www.markmorris.org.

Chapter 4

Nutrigenomics and Nutrigenetics: Nutritional Genomics in Health and Disease

Samer Al-Murrani
Craig D. Thatcher
Michael S. Hand

"It is from the progeny of this parent cell that we all take our looks; we still share genes around, and the resemblance of the enzymes of grasses to those of whales is in fact a family resemblance."
Lewis Thomas

INTRODUCTION

A revolution in nutrition is underway. Through newly available scientific methods and technologies, dramatic advances in understanding the role of nutrition in health and disease are within reach. These new tools include:

1. Complete or partially sequenced genomes of many animal, plant and microbial species (Bell et al, 2001; Lander et al, 2001; Waterson et al, 2002; Kirkness et al, 2003; Seshadri et al, 2006).
2. Ample historical evidence suggests nutrients provide potent dietary signals via gene control that influence cellular metabolism and homeostasis, either positively or negatively (Clarke and Abraham, 1992; Muller and Kirsten, 2003; Straus, 1994).
3. Laboratory and computer technologies that allow for the analysis of the molecular response of entire biologic systems to nutrients (Muller and Kirsten, 2003).

This chapter will acquaint readers with the current status of emerging nutritional technologies and provide insight about the future potential of these tools. When applied to nutrition, these technologies are collectively referred to as "nutritional genomics."

NUTRITIONAL GENOMICS AND OTHER "OMICS"

Because nutritional genomics is a relatively new science, the following discussion includes a review of relevant, but perhaps unfamiliar, terminology. **Table 4-1** summarizes definitions and other related terms.

"Genome" refers to the full set of an individual's genes (i.e., its genotype). "Phenotype" refers to the entire physical, biochemical and physiologic makeup of an animal as determined by its genome and the animal's environment. "Genomics" describes the mapping, sequencing and analysis of all genes present in the genome of a given species (Mutch et al, 2005). Numerous genomes are available to the public at http://www.ncbi.nlm.nih.gov/entrez/query.fcgi?db=genomeprj. The term "genomics" is sometimes used loosely to refer to sequence analysis, gene expression analysis and single nucleotide polymorphism analysis (the last two are discussed below).

Table 4-1. Glossary of nutritional genomics terminology.

Bioinformatics	The application of computerized statistical tools (informatics) to biologic data. In genome projects, informatics includes the development of methods to search databases quickly, analyze DNA sequence information and predict protein sequence and structure from DNA sequence data.
Dietary signature	The repeatable pattern of gene expression, protein expression and metabolite production in different tissues in response to one or more food components.
Gene expression	The process of converting the genetic code into mRNA and subsequently the translation of mRNA sequences into protein.
Genome	All the genetic material in the chromosomes of an organism; its size is generally given as its total number of base pairs; the term is derived from *gene* + chromo*some*.
Genomics	The mapping, sequencing and analysis of all genes present in the genome of a given species.
Genotype	The genetic makeup of an individual, in contrast to its physical appearance or phenotype.
Metabolome	The complete set of metabolites synthesized by a biologic system; all the substances except DNA, RNA and protein.
Metabolomics	The study of the influence of the genome on an organism's entire metabolite profile, at a given time.
Microarray technology	A laboratory technique that permits the simultaneous detection of thousands of genes in a small sample and analyzes the expression of those genes.
Nutrigenetics	The effect of genetic variation of an individual on the interaction between diet and disease.
Nutrigenomics	The effects of nutrients on the genome, proteome and metabolome.
Nutritional genomics	An umbrella term that includes nutrigenomics and nutrigenetics.
Phenotype	The visible properties of an organism that are produced by the interaction of the genotype and the environment.
Probes	Single stranded DNA sequences of varying lengths (depending on the technology platform) that represent individual genes that are immobilized onto a solid support.
Proteome	The entire complement of proteins, and their interactions, in cells, tissues, organs and physiologic fluids.
Proteomics	The study of the protein products of gene expression with the goal of identifying the proteins and understanding their role in the functioning of an organism.
Single nucleotide polymorphism	A variation of a gene's normal sequence, in which a single nucleotide in the genetic material is altered and the specific alteration occurs in more than 1% of the population. It is the most common form of polymorphism.
Systems biology	The study of entire biologic systems using transcriptomics, proteomics and metabolomics (**Figure 4-1**).
Transcription	The process whereby mRNA is synthesized from a DNA template.
Transcriptome	The sum of all the mRNA expressed by the genome of an organism.
Transcriptomics	The study of the relative amounts of mRNA expressed in cells or tissues at a given time.
Translation	The process of protein synthesis whereby the primary structure of the protein is determined by the nucleotide sequence in mRNA.

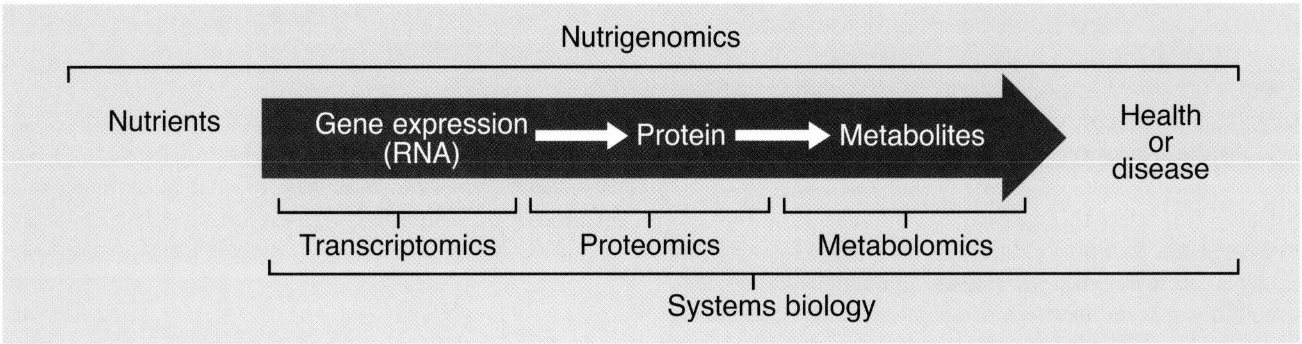

Figure 4-1. A schematic overview of the relationships between nutrigenomics, transcriptomics, proteomics, metabolomics and systems biology.

Nutritional genomics includes "nutrigenomics" and "nutrigenetics." Nutrigenetics refers to the study of how genetic variations, such as single nucleotide polymorphisms, are associated with an individual's response to nutrients or specific foods (Corella and Ordovas, 2005). That is, nutrigenetics attempts to explain how, and to what extent, nutrition-related disorders are influenced by genetic variation (Mariman, 2006). Nutrigenetics has the potential to provide for personalized dietary recommendations based on genetic makeup, by which the onset of a disorder will be prevented or delayed, thereby optimizing health. The information generated from a nutrigenetics approach can be used to identify individuals, but more importantly, groups that are most likely to benefit from a specially formulated dietary regimen.

The importance of genetic variation in the physiologic or pathophysiologic response to nutrition is already well described in principle, and examples continue to be published. A few of these examples include studies in people that link genetic variation to insulin resistance, type II diabetes mellitus and cardiovascular disease. These studies also demonstrate how an individual genotype affects appropriate dietary management for disease prevention (Mutch et al, 2005). Similar examples in animals with genetic variations that respond to special feeding regimens include obesity and diabetes mellitus (Snyder et al, 2004). It is likely that, in some cases, the increased risk for obesity in dogs may be related to breed-associated genetic variation. Another example in dogs includes large- and giant-breed puppies with genetic variation that responds to diet for the prevention of developmental orthopedic disease.

Nutrigenomics relates to the study of genome-wide influences of nutrition (**Figure 4-1**). Nutrigenomics explores the effects of nutrients on the genome, proteome and metabolome (the last two are discussed below). From a nutrigenomics perspective, nutrients are dietary signals that are detected by cellular sensor systems that influence gene and protein expression and, subsequently, metabolite production. Repeatable patterns of gene expression, protein expression and metabolite production in response to particular nutrients or foods can be viewed as "dietary signatures." Nutrigenomics studies these signatures in specific cells, tissues and complete organisms to understand how nutrition influences homeostasis and resultant health or disease (Muller and Kersten, 2003). The potential outcome from nutrigenomics research is a much clearer, more complete understanding of the effects and mechanisms of diet on health. To do this, researchers use genomics tools that include transcriptomics, proteomics and metabolomics to generate data and subsequently analyze, link and mine the data using bioinformatics tools and approaches.

Transcriptomics studies the effects of nutrients on gene expression. Because messenger RNA (mRNA) results from the process of transcription, the total pool of mRNA in a cell is referred to as the transcriptome. In nutrigenomics, transcriptomics examines nutrients that influence the expression of specific genes and the transcription of the corresponding mRNA. This is one of the first steps in the regulatory process that controls the flow of information from genes. The field of transcriptomics is based on the examination of gene expression patterns quantifying the abundance of mRNA copied from a basic nucleic acid blueprint contained in the genome (Dawson, 2006). Thus, the level of mRNA in a cell or tissue at any one time is a reflection of whether a gene is activated or inactivated. Thanks to powerful new tools that have been developed over the past decade, RNA can be measured. For example, total RNA or mRNA is extracted from a cell or tissue and used to create either a complementary labeled strand of DNA called "cDNA," or, alternatively, unlabeled cDNA can be used to generate a complementary labeled strand of RNA called "cRNA." This labeled material is then hybridized with known complementary strands of DNA sequences that are attached to a solid support such as a glass or plastic slide or a nylon substrate. These fixed sequences are called "probes." Probes are often organized as an array of small dots on the solid support matrix. In some cases, arrays of probes are called microarrays or "chips" because the probes are only micrometers apart and many of them will fit on a solid platform of only 1 to 3 cm^2. It is possible to display a whole genome on a microarray. Commercial forms of microarrays are available (**Figure 4-2**). If the original cRNA sample is labeled with a fluorescent dye, the hybridized array can be scanned with a laser scanner in which the light or signal that results from the hybrid of the labeled sample and the immobilized probes is directly related to the amount of specific mRNA present in the tissue sample and represents the level of gene expression in that tissue. Thus, it is possible to determine if a specific nutritional manipulation

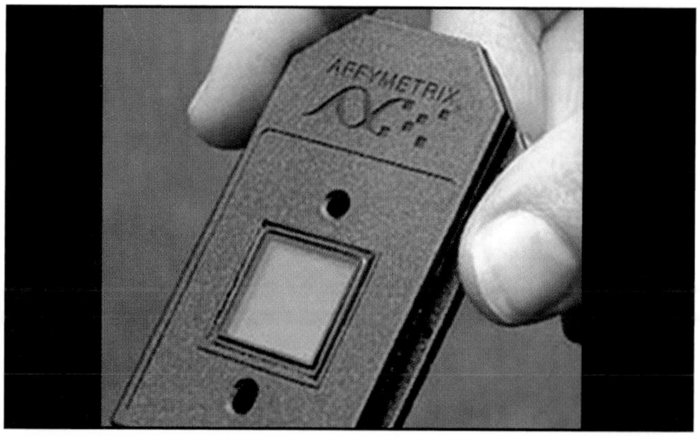

Figure 4-2. Affymetrix GeneChip probe array used for expression profiling of experimental tissues. (Courtesy Affymetrix, reprinted with permission).

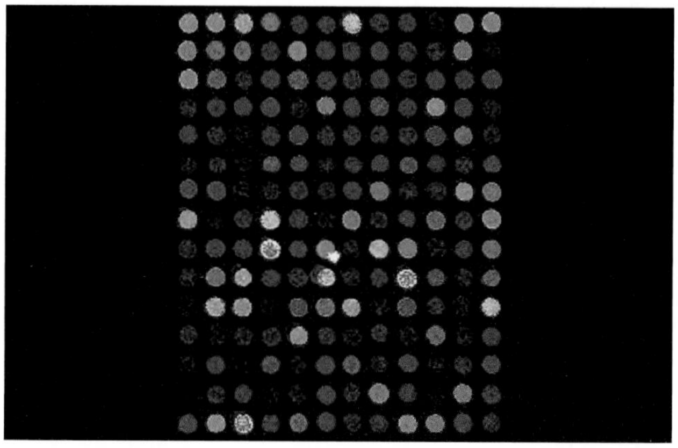

Figure 4-3. Example of the signal generated from a hybridized glass slide cDNA microarray.

switched a gene on or off using this technology (Debusk, 2005; Dawson, 2006). **Figure 4-3** shows a scanned image of a glass-based cDNA array.

However, gene transcription is only one step in the regulatory pathway that leads to functional protein formation. Thus, it is not always possible to correlate the increased or decreased presence of mRNA in tissues with specific protein changes. Even with this shortcoming, however, transcriptomics is a very powerful tool for determining and clarifying important processes in metabolic regulation because it broadly evaluates the initial regulatory steps of gene expression (Dawson, 2006).

Transcriptomics is a relatively mature technology compared with proteomics and metabolomics. Currently, it is possible to obtain an overview of the expression of essentially all genes in a single microarray or GeneChip experiment. However, it is not yet possible to measure the whole proteome or metabolome (Afman and Muller, 2006). Transcriptomic studies have already yielded exciting results, examples of which are discussed below.

"Proteome" describes the entire complement of proteins, and their interactions, in cells, tissues, organs and physiologic fluids. The number of proteins in a cell far exceeds the number of genes due to alternative gene splicing mechanisms and post-translational modifications of expressed proteins. Furthermore, because protein amounts differ widely in a cell at any given moment, with expression levels that span many orders of magnitude, there is no single technology platform that can measure all the protein in the cell. Therefore, proteomics and the corresponding proteomic technologies are not as widely used or as standardized as the gene-based studies and technologies described above. However, because protein expression is the functional outcome of gene transcription and translation, it has long been a focus of extensive research. Using proteomics tools (the analysis of the proteome), researchers can simultaneously display and determine thousands of proteins in a study sample and identify their changes in response to nutritional inputs. Research methods in proteomics are progressing rapidly. Proteome analysis holds great promise for discoveries in nutrition research (Afman and Muller, 2006).

One of the newest "omics" is metabolomics. Metabolomics technology measures the level of all substances, other than DNA, RNA or protein, present in a sample. Metabolites include such things as intermediates of metabolism and a variety of low molecular weight molecules (e.g., lactic acid, carbon dioxide, ketones, ATP, ADP, prostaglandins, prostacyclins and thromboxanes). The metabolome represents the complete set of metabolites synthesized by a biologic system. Studying metabolites is important because of the simplistic, often incorrect belief that one gene leads to the formation of one protein, which creates one metabolite (Munoz et al, 2004). The study of a cell's complete set of metabolites is much more complex than transcriptomics and proteomics. Besides the huge variety and number of potential metabolites, many cellular metabolites have a very rapid turnover. For example, ATP has a half-life of less than 0.1 second. Also, metabolites need to be determined separately in the different compartments of a cell (e.g., cytoplasm, mitochondria, extracellular matrix) (van der Werf et al, 2001).

Unlike transcriptomics, proteomics and metabolomics are not yet routinely performed, do not have standardized procedures and continue to face challenges such as sample preparation, technological sensitivity and lack of standardized statistical methods (Mutch et al, 2005). However, the potential for nutritional applications of metabolomics is considerable and a number of research teams are addressing the current shortcomings (Afman and Muller, 2006).

"Systems biology" refers to a merging of the previously discussed "omics" technologies. Together, transcriptomics, proteomics and metabolomics allow for nutrition studies to concurrently observe and quantify a significant fraction of all regulated genes, gene expression products and metabolites. Because these layers of "omics" technologies are related (e.g., genes encode RNA, which produces enzymes that catalyze the conversion of metabolites), this combination of datasets paves the way to a complete description of how a cellular system behaves in response to external stimuli (Corthesy-Theulaz et al, 2005). Although the complexity of the systems biology approach exceeds the current bioinformatics tool's capabilities, its implications for nutrition research can be enormous.

Because these genomic technologies generate an avalanche of data, there is a need for continuing developments in bioinformatics. Bioinformatics refers to the computational technologies that support the processing, clustering, dynamics, integration and storing of the enormously complex datasets like those generated from "omics" research. The challenge is to combine all these pieces of information to ensure all data can be observed coherently. To gain full access to the potential output of the new "omics" tools, it is imperative to address the enormous challenge of unifying complex and dissimilar data. The goal is to turn all these data into knowledge.

Bioinformatics software packages can be obtained through licensing arrangements with a variety of organizations, purchased from specialty software companies or are available from open sources. Open source software usually requires programming skills on the part of the user. Regardless of source, these packages generally include programs for data analysis and visualization. Visualization describes a way of qualitatively "graphing" the results; it is an important step in extracting knowledge from data. Other software go beyond data analysis and visualization to provide the means of overlaying the data generated from "omics" experiments onto knowledge-based molecular pathways and networks and provide an overview of the interactions of the genomic, proteomic and metabolomic data together in the context of the whole cell.

THE PROMISE OF NUTRITIONAL GENOMICS: EXAMPLES OF PROGRESS AND POTENTIAL

Until recently, it was thought that changes in gene expression attributed to diet were mediated through endocrine or neural pathways. However, research has shown that macronutrients, micronutrients and their metabolites can directly regulate gene expression. For example, some of the earliest evidence demonstrating direct effects of nutrients on gene expression came from studies in zinc-deficient rats. In these models, researchers found that almost 50 genes were either up- or down-regulated in the zinc-deficient group, suggesting new mechanisms for some of the signs associated with zinc deficiency (Blanchard and Cousins, 1996). Currently, many food components, including minerals besides zinc, vitamins, carotenoids, flavonoids, monoterpenes and phenolic acids are thought to act as transcriptional activator molecules affecting gene expression (Milner, 2004).

The action mechanism of dietary carbohydrates in metabolic programming and its short- and long-term effects is a macronutrients example. Studies showed that feeding rat pups a high-carbohydrate milk formula resulted in hyperinsulinemia that persisted throughout the period of dietary intervention. There was increased hexokinase activity and increased gene expression of preproinsulin and related transcription factors and kinases in the pancreatic islets. In these experiments, the predictable metabolic and genetic adaptations that occurred in rat pups during the dietary intervention continued to be expressed into adulthood. As adults, these rats demonstrated chronic hyperinsulinemia and adult onset obesity (Srinivasan et al, 2003; Swanson, 2006).

There are also nutrigenomic studies in dogs associating specific nutrients to obesity and insulin sensitivity. Dogs fed a food designed to induce obesity and insulin resistance had a decrease in the expression of uncoupling protein 1 (UCP1) and peroxisome proliferator-activated receptor gamma (PPARγ) in their adipose tissue compared to non-obese, insulin-sensitive dogs (Leray et al, 2004). PPARγ plays a role in adipocyte differentiation, lipid storage and glucose homeostasis and induces the expression of many genes including UCP1, which plays a key role in thermogenesis.

Nutrigenomic studies in dogs have also shown that obesity-related hypertension causes marked changes in gene expression in the right atrium and left ventricle. These changes were thought to contribute to early changes in heart function, hypertrophy and remodeling (Philip-Couderc et al, 2003). Other studies focusing on gene expression in the left ventricles of dogs fed normal or high-fat foods using canine cDNA arrays identified 63 differentially expressed genes involved in metabolism, cell signaling, tissue remodeling, insulin regulation, cell proliferation and protein synthesis. The results of this study further indicated that the pattern of co-regulated genes depended on the length of time that the high-fat food was fed. These findings suggested that hypertension resulting from obesity induced by high dietary fat was associated with continuous cardiac transcriptome adaptation despite stability in both body weight and blood pressure (Philip-Couderc et al, 2004).

Proteomic studies determined that supplementing rat food with genistein, a major isoflavone from soy, increased the expression of mammary gland GTP cyclohydrolase-I, a key protein related to nitrogen oxide synthesis. There was a resultant reduction in cell proliferation and susceptibility to cancer (Rowell et al, 2005). Another study showed that inadequate provision of dietary vitamin B_{12} induced profound changes in the cerebral spinal fluid proteome in rats, linking vitamin B_{12} with neurologic health (Gianazza et al, 2003).

An example of a potential indirect effect via metabolites is that of dietary fiber on transcription. One study reported increased adipocyte leptin expression in cell cultures treated with physiologic amounts of short-chain fatty acids (Xiong et al, 2004). Short-chain fatty acids from colonic microbial fermentation of dietary fibers may help protect against overeating and obesity by decreasing appetite through leptin expression (Swanson, 2006).

Through traditional methods, key nutritional factors (essential nutrients and bioactive food components) have long been established as potential modulators of health and disease (Watson, 1998; Dove, 2001; DeBoer, 2004). Understanding the ways in which foods and their components affect gene expression will further enhance use of key nutritional factors to modulate health and disease.

Box 4-1. The Value of Sequencing the Canine and Feline Genomes.

Because of the cost of sequencing mammalian genomes to completion (approximately $50 million U.S.), these projects have been restricted to a few species considered to be of greatest value to biomedical research. Knowledge of human genome function in health and disease will benefit from comparison of its structure with genomes of certain other species. The dog is a particularly good example because of its somewhat unique population structure. The physical and behavioral characteristics of approximately 300 breeds are maintained by restricting gene flow between breeds. Many modern breeds have been inbred for desired characteristics. This has led to a species with enormous phenotypic diversity but with significant homogenization of the gene pool within breeds. Many of the approximately 450 known genetic disorders in dogs resemble human conditions, and their causes may be more traceable in large dog pedigrees than in small, outbred human families. The combination of genetic homogeneity and phenotypic diversity also provides an opportunity to understand the genetic basis of many complex developmental processes in mammals. Thus, to a large part, funding of the sequencing of the canine genome and the genome of certain other mammalian species is based on their value in further understanding human health and disease.

The Bibliography for **Box 4-1** can be found at www.markmorris.org .

THE CANINE AND FELINE GENOMES: CURRENT STATUS

The primary reason for funding the sequencing of the canine and feline genomes was to provide a basis for future comparative work in human biology including development, aging, cancer, heritable diseases and immune diseases. Dogs and cats have numerous heritable diseases, many of which are homologous to human inborn errors. Furthermore, the susceptibility of cats to viruses that cause immunodeficiencies and neoplasias (feline immunodeficiency virus and feline leukemia virus, respectively) make them important models for human AIDS and leukemia research.

Canine Genome

A sequenced genome could provide the basis for valuable information to determine the molecular differences between health and disease in dogs. The dog was the first non-rodent mammalian animal chosen for genome sequencing by the National Institutes of Health (**Box 4-1**) (Swanson, 2006). The sequence was derived for a male standard poodle; investigators estimated the genome to contain approximately 2.4 billion bases (Gb), which is about the same as the mouse genome but smaller than the human genome (approximately 2.9 Gb). With private and

Box 4-2. What is Genome "Coverage?"

A genome whose DNA base pairs have been completely sequenced one time has one-fold or "1x" coverage. At 2x coverage, each nucleotide in the genome would have been sequenced twice. The more times a genome is sequenced, the less likely it is to have gaps and mistakes. Therefore, a genome that has 6x coverage would have been sequenced enough times so that each base pair was read six times, which would provide a high level of confidence that the genome was accurate.

public funding, the Canine Genome Mapping Community and the Whitehead Genome Sequencing Center at MIT recently completed a more extensive genome sequencing of a female boxer (Lindblad-Toh et al, 2005). The boxer breed was chosen because it is one of the breeds with the least amount of variability in its genome and therefore likely to provide the most reliable reference genome sequence. This study also estimated the canine genome to span about 2.4 Gb. Using evidence-based methods, the canine genome is predicted to contain sequences for approximately 19,300 genes compared to about 22,000 that are currently thought to exist in the human genome (Lindblad-Toh et al, 2005). Because these predictions are based on computer programs that use different algorithms, the reported numbers of genes per genome are expected to vary for some time.

The information obtained by sequencing the canine genome will likely have its greatest initial impact on the study of the more than 450 genetic diseases that have been identified in dogs (Zhu et al, 2003). Although genetic diseases are problematic in many canine breeds, by far most diseases affecting dogs are more complex. For many canine diseases, besides genetic factors, disease expression is also affected by pathogen exposure, age, gender, activity level and diet (Swanson, 2006).

Feline Genome

The feline genome is more similar to that of people than dogs (approximately 3.3 Gb) (Menotti-Raymond et al, 2003; Murphy et al, 2007). The existing low coverage (2x) whole genome sequence of the cat has been useful for some comparative genome studies. However, gaps in the sequence represent a major obstacle to more important in depth studies. As mentioned above, the cat is a valuable model for understanding important diseases in people. Furthermore, the feline genome has the fewest rearrangements relative to all other mammals studied (Murphy et al, 2005). This finding suggests that the feline and human genomes represent the only index ancestral genome arrangements, which is very important as a reference for genome annotation and evolutionary studies in all mammals. These considerations have led to support for a complete high coverage (6 to 7x) whole genome sequence of the cat, which is underway. This level of coverage will make the feline genome information equivalent to that from other mammalian genomes including those of people, mice, rats and dogs. **Box 4-2** explains "genome coverage."

Cats are reported to have at least 260 genetic diseases (Zhu et al, 2003). This new information should pave the way for numerous advances in nutrigenetics and nutrigenomics of cats, our most popular companion animal.

SUMMARY

The complete sequencing of the human genome has brought much attention to the value of understanding how the interplay between genes and environmental factors, such as nutrition, relate to health and disease. To enable such studies, novel technologies have been developed to monitor the activity of multiple genes simultaneously at the level of RNA by transcriptomics, the level of the proteins by proteomics and ultimately the level of metabolites by metabolomics. In addition, these technologies have boosted interest in studying the role of genetic variation to explain individual and group susceptibility for nutrition-related disorders. These new areas of science are referred to as nutrigenomics and nutrigenetics, respectively. They hold promise to increase our fundamental knowledge of the interaction between biologic processes and food/nutrition. This will, in time, help improve maintenance foods to further improve the health status of the general pet population and lead to the development of personalized diets to prevent the onset of nutrition-related disorders in genetically predisposed individuals.

REFERENCES

The references for **Chapter 4** can be found at www.markmorris.org.

Chapter 5

Macronutrients

Kathy L. Gross
Ryan M. Yamka
Christina Khoo
Kim G. Friesen
Dennis E. Jewell
William D. Schoenherr
Jacques Debraekeleer
Steven C. Zicker

"Nutriment is both food and poison.
The dosage makes it either poison or remedy."
T. B. von Hohenheim

INTRODUCTION

Proper nutrition is among the more important considerations in health maintenance and key to disease management. A basic knowledge of nutrients, requirements, availability and consequences of deficiencies or excesses is important to feed dogs and cats correctly and give advice about feeding.

A nutrient is any food constituent that helps support life. Numerous essential nutrients have been discovered over the course of history. Nutrients are essential in that they are involved in all basic functions of the body including: 1) acting as structural components, 2) enhancing or participating in chemical reactions of metabolism, 3) transporting substances into, throughout or out of the body, 4) maintaining temperature and 5) supplying energy.

Nutrients are divided into six basic categories (**Figure 5-1**). Some nutrients fulfill a number of functions. For example, water and several minerals are needed for all the functions described above except supplying energy. Carbohydrates, fats and proteins may be used for energy but they can also serve as structural components. Vitamins are involved primarily with metabolic functions.

Figure 5-2 shows how an individual nutrient can affect the health of an animal. The minimum dietary requirement has been established for most nutrients. Clinical signs of deficiency may result if a food doesn't provide this nutrient level. Similarly, the maximum tolerable levels of certain nutrients are known and toxicity may result if a food exceeds these levels. The area between deficiency and excess represents the range of safe and adequate nutrient intake. The extent of this area will change depending on the individual nutrient and overall composition of the food. What is less well known is how exposure to marginal deficiencies and excesses affects an animal over time.

The most common method of determining the nutrient content of food is the proximate analysis, which provides the percentage moisture, protein, fat, ash and crude fiber. Digestible (soluble) carbohydrate or nitrogen-free extract (NFE) can then be calculated. **Figure 5-3** shows how the determination is conducted. Many commercial laboratories conduct proximate analyses of foods.

This chapter is organized into five sections: 1) water, 2) energy, 3) carbohydrates and fiber (including prebiotic fibers, probiotics and synbiotics), 4) protein and amino acids and 5) lipids. Chapter 6 covers vitamins and minerals. The nutrients in this chapter and those in the next will be covered in the order shown in **Figure 5-1**, beginning at the base of the pyramid. Energy, a non-nutrient, but nonetheless essential for life will be covered after water.

WATER

Definition and Function

Chemically, water is the combination of hydrogen and oxygen, which are joined in the ratio of two hydrogen atoms to one oxygen (H_2O). Water is vital to life and is considered the most

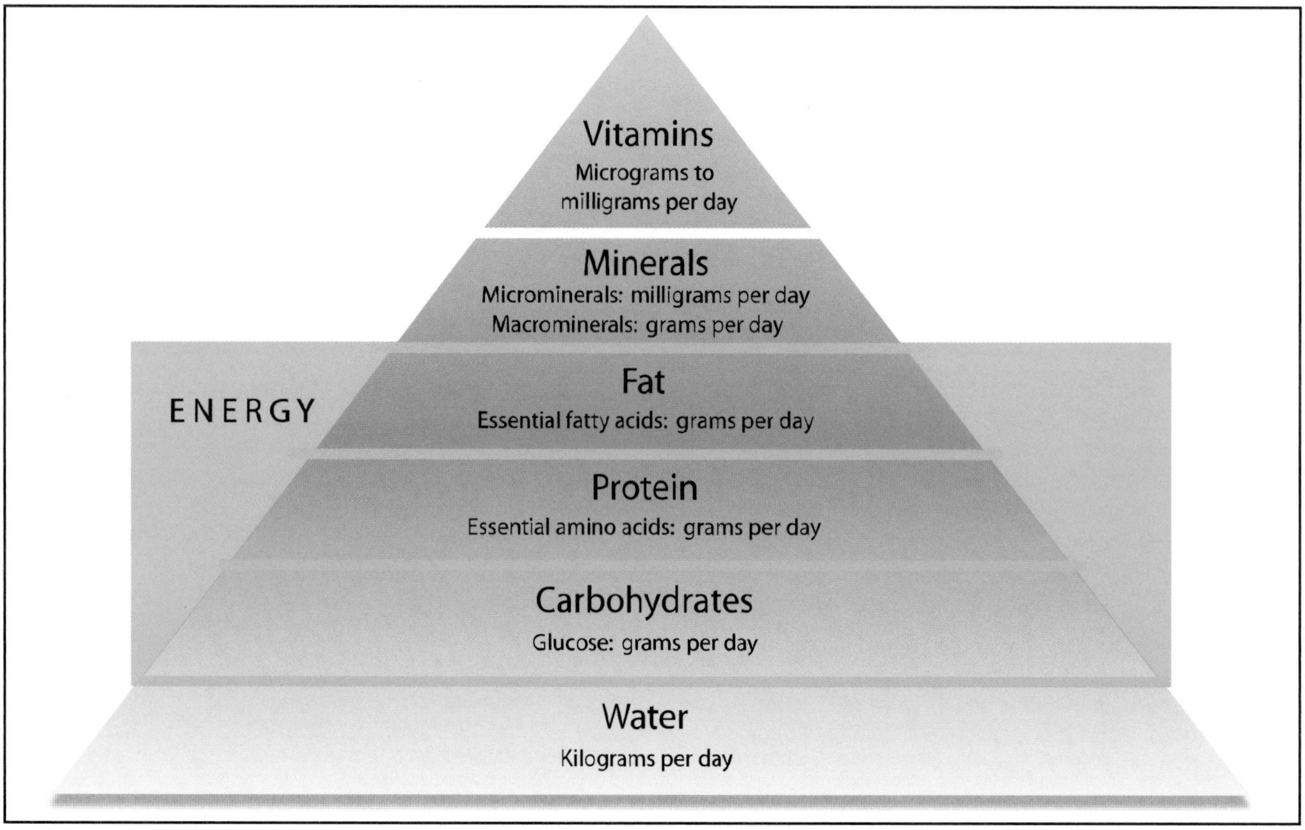

Figure 5-1. The six basic nutrients. Carbohydrates, fats and proteins may be used for energy but also serve as structural components.

important nutrient. Water performs the following important functions in animals:

1. Water is the solvent in which substances are dissolved and transported around the body. A large number of chemical compounds can be put into aqueous solution.
2. Water is necessary for the chemical reactions that involve hydrolysis (e.g., enzymatic digestion of carbohydrates, proteins and fats).
3. Water helps regulate body temperature. Water has a high specific heat (specific heat = amount of heat necessary to raise 1 g of water 1°C. Specific heat of water = 1). Large changes in heat production can take place within an animal with very little change in body temperature. This property also allows for heat to be circulated. Water has a high latent heat of vaporization. Water helps regulate body temperature when it is evaporated from the skin and respiratory tract. Large amounts of heat are required to evaporate small amounts of water; therefore, much heat can be lost with little loss of water.
4. Water provides shape and resilience to the body. Significant negative water balance can result in clinical dehydration. One manifestation of dehydration is loss of skin elasticity. As a major constituent of body fluids, water helps lubricate the joints and eyes, provides protective cushioning for the nervous system and aids in gas exchange in respiration by keeping the alveoli of the lungs moist and expanded.

Water is one of the largest constituents of the animal body, varying from 40 to more than 80% of the total. The percentage of water in an animal's body varies with species, condition and age. Generally, lean body mass contains 70 to 80% water and 20 to 25% protein, whereas adipose tissue contains 10 to 15% water and 75 to 80% fat. Younger, leaner animal contain more body water. Conversely, fatter animals have lower body water content.

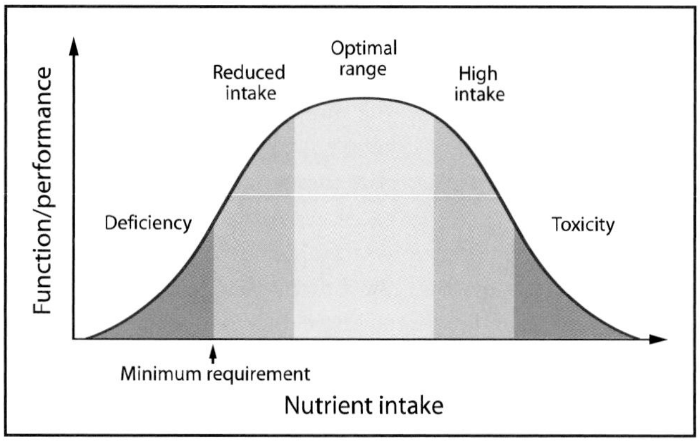

Figure 5-2. Total biologic dose-response curve. This response curve spans intakes ranging from deficiency to adequacy to toxicity. The intakes at which these three phases reside, and the width of the range between deficiency and toxicity vary widely among nutrients. (Adapted from Underwood EJ, Mertz W. Introduction. In: Mertz W, ed. Trace Elements in Human and Animal Nutrition, 5th ed. San Diego, CA: Academic Press Inc, 1987; 1.)

As animals mature, they require proportionately less water on a weight basis because they consume less food per unit of body weight; thus, there is less urinary water loss. In addition, adult animals have less surface area per unit of body weight resulting in less evaporation from skin.

Water Quality

Salinity, nitrates and nitrites, toxic organic and inorganic chemicals and microbial contamination can affect water quality. Routine measurement of water quality is the concentration of all constituents dissolved in water, referred to as "total dissolved solids" (TDS). Salinity (salt content of water) is synonymous with TDS as an indication of the total ionic concentration in fresh water. Water containing less than 5,000 parts per million (ppm or mg/l) TDS is generally considered acceptable for consumption, whereas water containing more than 7,000 ppm is considered unsuitable for livestock or poultry (NRC, 1974). Although livestock and poultry TDS values are assumed to apply to dogs and cats, water containing less than 500 ppm TDS is considered acceptable for human drinking water and is a better recommendation for dogs and cats (US EPA, 1976).

Standard water quality testing (e.g., nitrates, sulfates, bacterial contamination) typically can be addressed through local public health departments because the source of water consumed by dogs and cats is often the same as that consumed by people. Serious concerns about water quality (toxic inorganic chemicals or pesticides) need to be addressed through testing at commercial analytical laboratories capable of screening water for pesticide residues and other chemicals.

Mineral Content

Water "hardness," or the sum of calcium and magnesium salts in relation to calcium carbonate, has little effect on dog or cat well being. High levels of magnesium in hard water have been implicated as a cause of urolithiasis in cats; however, the amount of magnesium consumed in drinking water is insignificant compared with the amount consumed in food (i.e., usually a 10,000-fold difference) (Kirk et al, 1995). Cats prone to urolithiasis may benefit from consumption of distilled water rather than hard water that has been softened with a sodium chloride water softener.

Nitrates

Nitrates are widely dispersed in the environment and can be a health hazard for all animals when significant amounts are present in drinking water. Although the concentration of nitrate ions (NO_3) commonly found in drinking water is well tolerated by dogs and cats, nitrite (NO_2, the reduced form of nitrate) is readily absorbed and can be toxic. At toxic levels, nitrites oxidize iron in hemoglobin to form methemoglobin, reducing the oxygen-carrying capacity of blood.

Frequently, nitrates in the water supply indicate bacterial contamination. Bacterial reduction of nitrate to nitrite is promoted as the pH increases in the intestinal tract. Bacteria in contaminated water sources can convert nitrate to nitrite. The safe upper limits for nitrate and nitrite determined for livestock drinking water are 1,320 ppm and 33 ppm, respectively. For human drinking water, the safe upper limit is based on the total amount of nitrogen derived from the combination of nitrate (30.4% nitrogen) and nitrite (22.6% nitrogen) and is 10 ppm of nitrogen. No safe upper limits have been established for dogs or cats. The livestock limits should be used until studies are conducted to determine the upper limits for dogs and cats.

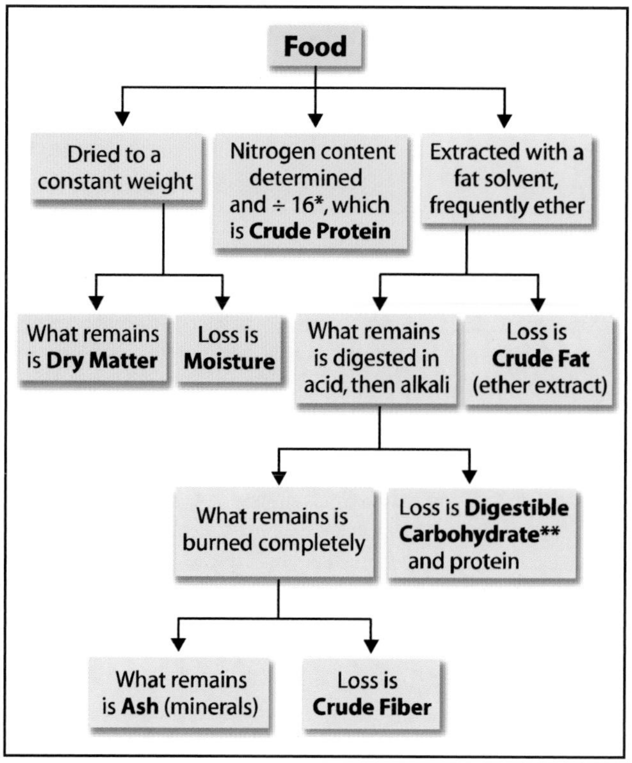

Figure 5-3. Proximate analysis of foods.
*Proteins contain 16 ± 2% nitrogen. Crude protein = nitrogen x 6.25 or nitrogen ÷ 0.16. Protein levels determined by this method will be erroneously high if the food contains non-protein nitrogen such as urea or ammonia.
**Frequently called nitrogen-free extract (NFE). NFE is determined as the difference between 100% and the amount of everything else in the food (i.e., 100% – % moisture – % crude protein – % fat – % crude fiber – % ash.) Any errors in these analyses also will appear in the NFE value.

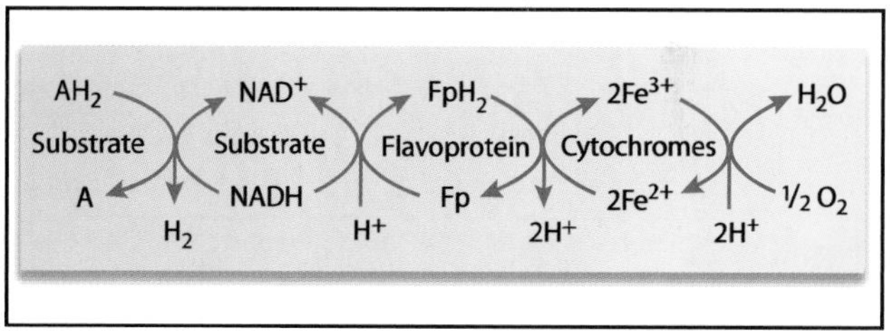

Figure 5-4. Electron transport chain and metabolic water production. Key: NAD = nicotinamide-adenine dinucleotide, NADH = the reduced form of NAD, Fe = iron, H_2O = water, O_2 = oxygen, H/H_2 = hydrogen, A = metabolite, Fp = flavoprotein.

Box 5-1. The Effect of Fasting on Water Intake: Diagnostic Implications.

Fasting eliminates water available from food, alters the amount an animal drinks and decreases total water intake. **Figure 1** shows the effect of fasting on drinking water intake, water intake from food and total water intake for dogs previously consuming moist or dry food. Total water intake decreased dramatically in both groups; however, the change in the amount consumed as drinking water was quite different. **Figure 1, Panel A** shows the response of dogs previously fed a moist food. Because most water intake for these dogs previously was from the food, only a small amount was supplied by drinking water. During fasting, water supplied by food was no longer available, thus the amount drunk increased. **Figure 1, Panel B** shows the response of dogs previously eating a dry food. Because these dogs obtained little water from the food, a large amount was supplied from drinking water. During fasting, less water was needed and the amount of drinking water consumed decreased.

The influence of the water content of the previous food on the amount of water consumed as drinking water may become important diagnostically. An owner who reports that a dog is not eating but is drinking twice as much water may be describing the normal response of a dog that has stopped eating a moist food, rather than a dog that is truly polydipsic. Conversely, dogs that had been eating dry food may appear to nearly stop drinking during periods of anorexia. These effects emphasize the importance of accurately assessing the food and feeding method.

The Bibliography for **Box 5-1** can be found can be found at www.markmorris.org.

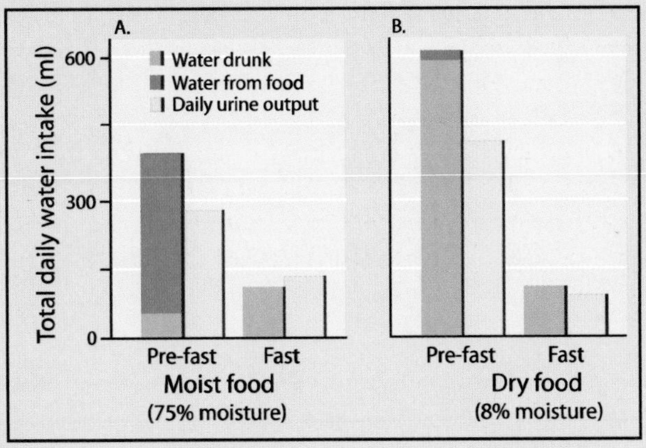

Figure 1. Effect of fasting on the amount of water consumed in the food and drunk by beagles previously consuming moist or dry foods.

Bacteria

The accepted criterion for the sanitary quality of water for people has been the absence of coliform bacteria. Although all coliform bacteria are not pathogens, many possess the potential; their presence indicates water is able to support infectious bacteria or viruses. Results of other qualitative tests made on water samples can also predict the presence of bacteria. Bacteria proportionally accompany chemical compounds such as nitrites, nitrates and phosphates. Generally, if levels of these compounds are high, the bacterial level will also be high.

Water Requirements

Water requirements are related to maintaining water balance. Body water lost by urination, defecation, evaporation and perspiration is replaced by one of two sources: 1) water derived from metabolism of nutrients and 2) water consumed as a liquid or as a portion of the food.

Oxygen is the final acceptor of hydrogen ions cleaved from energy-supplying nutrients (carbohydrates, fats and proteins) during the generation of adenosine triphosphate (ATP) (**Figure 5-4**). This combination of hydrogen and oxygen is called metabolic water. Metabolic water can account for 5 to 10% of the total water requirement. An average of 13 ml of water is produced per 100 kilocalories (kcal) of metabolizable energy (ME) ingested (Anderson, 1982). Oxidation of 1 g of glucose, fat and protein results in the production of 0.556, 1.071 and 0.396 g of metabolic water, respectively (Schmidt-Nielsen, 1964). Three to 4 g of water are released per g of glycogen used (Gosolfi, 1983).

Dogs and cats meet most of their water requirement through water ingested as food or drink. Animals consuming commercial moist foods drink less liquid than those fed dry foods because of the higher water content of moist foods (>75% water). This finding may have important diagnostic implications (**Box 5-1**). Generally, the daily water requirement of dogs and cats, expressed in ml/day, is roughly equivalent to the daily energy requirement (DER) in kcal/day (for dogs 1.6 x resting energy requirement [RER]; for cats 1.2 x RER) (Harrison et al, 1960; Haskins, 1984). The amount of water consumed by mature, healthy, nonreproducing dogs and cats at a comfortable environmental temperature is about 2.5 times the amount of dry matter (DM) consumed as food.

Domestic cats, descendants of desert animals, normally form more concentrated urine than dogs. Thus, water requirements for cats may be less than that for dogs. The need for water can be met by supplying clean, fresh water to pets at all times (**Box 5-2**).

Factors Affecting Water Requirements

Although the daily water requirements of dogs and cats are well defined, practical estimates of daily water intake are less clearly understood. In addition to metabolic needs, animals of all sizes consume water to meet a variety of needs, including physical and social. Factors such as body size (surface area), lactation, ambient temperature, type and amount of food ingested, general state of health, stress, water losses through excretion or evaporation and individual animal differences influence the absolute requirement for water.

Water Deficiency and Excess

Deficits of more than a few percent of total body water are incompatible with health, and large water deficits (i.e., 15 to 20% of body weight) lead to death. Water deprivation can lead to death within days, whereas animals may survive for weeks without food. Under normal circumstances, thirst ensures that water intake meets or exceeds the requirement. Inadequate water intake reduces food intake, which reduces production in dogs and cats (growth, lactation, reproduction and physical activity). Decreased water intake may result from reduced availability, water temperature extremes or poor quality. Water intoxication (over consumption) is extremely rare in normal, healthy dogs and cats but can be induced in animals offered water free choice after prolonged dehydration.

Box 5-2. Measuring Water Intake in Dogs and Cats.

Daily water intake in dogs and cats can be measured easily with common household tools. The following steps should allow pet owners to obtain a reasonable estimate of daily water intake.

1. Determine daily water intake requirements (in ml) by calculating the resting energy requirement of the animal and multiplying by 1.6 for dogs and 1.2 for cats.
2. Using a fluid cup measure (1 cup = 227 ml), measure the amount of water to offer the animal throughout the day in a single container.
3. Fill the water bowl with an appropriate amount of water from the single container throughout the day, ensuring fresh water is available at all times.
4. Eliminate the animal's access to other water sources (e.g., toilet bowls, sinks, etc.).
5. If more water is needed beyond the calculated amount, carefully measure more water into the container and account for the additional amount when making intake calculations.
6. Measure the water remaining at the end of the day (sum of that remaining in the water bowl and container) and determine the amount of water consumed by subtracting the remaining water from the total amount measured during the day.

ENERGY

Definition

Living organisms need energy to fuel all bodily functions. The ultimate source of all energy is the sun, which enables plants to make energy-containing nutrients from carbon dioxide and water through photosynthesis (**Figure 5-5**). A key function of dietary intake is to provide energy. Animals eat plants or other animals that have eaten plants. Although energy itself is not a nutrient, fats, carbohydrates and amino acids contain energy in the form of chemical bonds and are the energy-containing nutrients in food. Once eaten, these nutrients are digested, absorbed and transported to body cells where they are used to generate energy.

Burning nutrients and measuring the amount of released heat can determine their energy content. The body obtains energy by oxidizing nutrients to carbon dioxide and water, but does not use heat for fuel directly, although heat is used for body temperature regulation. Instead, the body captures nutrient energy in energy-containing compounds through a series of enzymatic biochemical reactions. The most important energy-containing compound is ATP.

In nutrition, the joule is the internationally recognized unit of measure for energy (Kleiber, 1972; Blaxter, 1989). The joule expresses the DER of an animal by its power needs or watts. One watt equals one joule per second. In the United States, a more commonly used energy measure is the calorie, which expresses energy in terms of heat. A calorie is the amount of heat required to raise the temperature of 1 g of water from 14.5°C to 15.5°C. A kcal is 1,000 calories and a kilojoule (kJ) is 1,000 joules. Kcal and kJ can be interconverted using the formula 1 kcal = 4.184 kJ.

Function

The biochemical reactions that take place in the body either use or release energy. Anabolic reactions require energy and, conversely, catabolic reactions release energy. ATP and other energy-trapping compounds pick up part of the energy released from one process and transfer it to the other process. For example, in the oxidation of nutrients (glucose, fatty acids and amino acids), the chemical reactions in the biochemical pathways of glycolysis, β-oxidation, deamination, tricarboxylic acid (TCA) cycle and oxidative phosphorylation simultaneously generate and consume ATP. However, the net effect of these reactions is generation of ATP. It has been estimated that the net yields for ATP are approximately 90, 75 and 55% for fat, carbohydrate and protein oxidation, respectively (Flatt, 2001). Biochemical reactions that occur in glycogen synthesis, fatty acid synthesis, protein synthesis, gluconeogenesis, protein turnover, Cori cycle, sodium-potassium ion pump, ureagenesis and muscular contractions all require ATP.

In summary, animals use energy for pumping ions, molecular synthesis and to activate contractile proteins (**Figure 5-5**). These three processes essentially describe the total use of energy by animals. Without energy supplied by food, these reactions would rapidly cease and death would occur.

Importance of Energy in the Diet of Dogs and Cats

The energy content of a food ultimately determines the quantity of food that is eaten each day and therefore affects the amount of all other nutrients that an animal ingests. Animals should be fed enough food to meet their energy requirements and the non-energy nutrients in the food should be balanced relative to energy density to ensure adequate nutrient intake. Animals eating an energy-dense food consume less of the food to meet energy needs; therefore, the concentration of other critical nutrients must be higher to ensure sufficient intake. Conversely, animals must consume more of a low-energy food to meet energy needs. Therefore, the concentration of non-energy nutrients should be lower to avoid excessive intake and maintain nutrient balance. If the energy density of the food is too low, food intake may be restricted by the physical limitations of the gastrointestinal (GI) tract. Such a food is referred

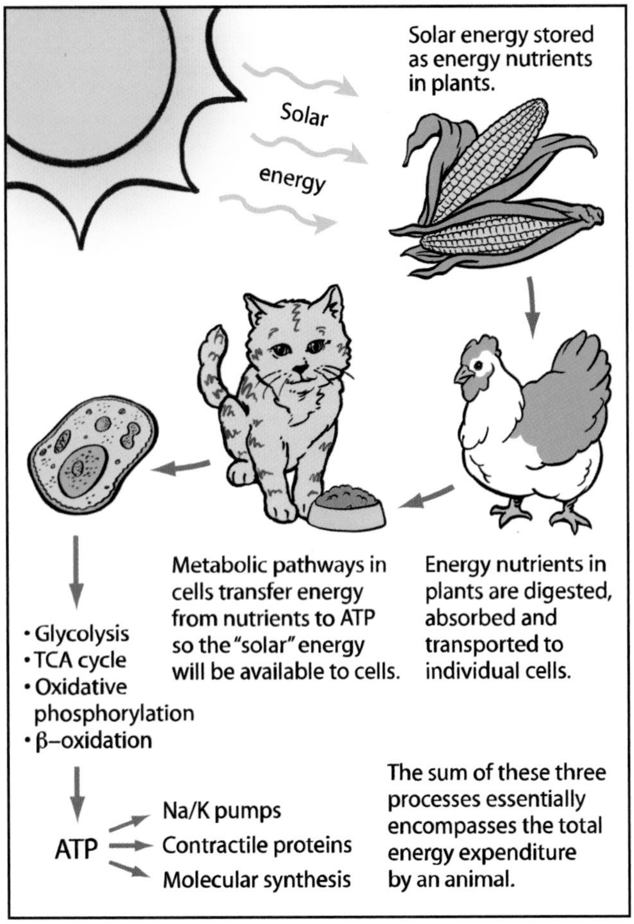
Solar energy stored as energy nutrients in plants.
Solar
energy
Metabolic pathways in cells transfer energy from nutrients to ATP so the "solar" energy will be available to cells.
Energy nutrients in plants are digested, absorbed and transported to individual cells.
• Glycolysis
• TCA cycle
• Oxidative phosphorylation
• β–oxidation
ATP
Na/K pumps
Contractile proteins
Molecular synthesis
The sum of these three processes essentially encompasses the total energy expenditure by an animal.

Figure 5-5. Schematic of how animals obtain and use energy. Plants use solar energy to produce energy-containing nutrients (i.e., proteins, fats and carbohydrates) via photosynthesis. Animals eat the energy-containing plant nutrients and other animals. Once eaten, energy-containing nutrients are digested, absorbed and metabolized by body cells to release energy that fuels the processes that sustain life.

to as being "bulk limited." Low-energy, bulk-limited foods designed for weight loss can be formulated to provide adequate intake of non-energy nutrients (Chapter 27).

Energy Metabolism

Digestion, Absorption and Excretion

Digestion and absorption of the energy-supplying nutrients (protein, carbohydrate and fat) are discussed in other sections of this chapter. The total amount of potential energy in food is termed gross energy (GE). Burning the food and measuring the heat produced in a bomb calorimeter determine GE in food. Animals are unable to use 100% of the GE in foods because some of the food energy is lost in the form of solid, liquid and gaseous excretions as well as radiant heat.

Nutritionists have partitioned dietary energy based on the losses that occur (**Figure 5-6**). Digestible energy (DE) refers to the GE content of food minus energy lost in feces (FE). Typically, ME is defined as DE minus energy lost in urine and as intestinal gaseous products of digestion (i.e., eructation and flatulence). However, because methane production is considered to be negligible in dogs and cats (McKay and Eastwood, 1984), ME can be defined in terms of DE and urinary energy losses.

Animals continuously produce heat as a result of basal metabolism and physical work. Heat production increases after a meal. This increase in heat due to food ingestion is called the heat increment of food (HI). HI consists of the heat of intestinal microbial fermentation and heat produced in intermediary metabolism as a result of using nutrients. A study in people showed that 5 to 10% of the energy consumed was lost as heat. The HI during the postprandial period was 60% greater for the protein-consuming group when compared to the isocaloric carbohydrate-consuming group. This increase in HI was attributed to the increased protein turnover observed by the protein-consuming group. The metabolic cost for protein turnover was approximately 36 and 68% for carbohydrate and protein feeding, respectively (Robinson et al, 2000). The energy of HI is normally wasted except when the environmental temperature is below an animal's critical temperature (i.e., shivering). In this situation, the HI is used to keep the body warm.

Subtracting HI from the ME gives the net energy (NE) of food. NE can also be partitioned into the amount used for maintenance (NE_m) and the amount used for production (NE_p: growth, pregnancy, lactation, exercise). NE values of foods and ingredients are typically used when discussing livestock nutrition (beef cattle, dairy cattle, swine), whereas DE and ME are more typically used in canine and feline nutrition. Although not commonly measured and used, the NE principles of partitioning energy for maintenance and production separately hold true for dogs and cats.

Energy Use

The initial biochemical reactions by which energy is derived from carbohydrates, fats and amino acids are different. However, all three nutrients eventually go through a final common pathway for energy generation (i.e., TCA cycle). Glucose derived from dietary carbohydrates is first oxidized through the glycolysis pathway to yield pyruvate and then acetyl-CoA. Acetyl-CoA is oxidized in the TCA cycle producing carbon dioxide, and electrons, which are captured by important heme-containing compounds called cytochromes (**Figure 5-7**). Electrons produced in the TCA cycle are shuttled by nicotinamide-adenine dinucleotide (NAD) and flavin adenine dinucleotide (FAD) to the electron transport chain where the cytochromes participate in electron transfer through valence changes in their heme iron (**Figure 5-4**). NAD and FAD are synthesized from the vitamins niacin and riboflavin, respectively. The electrons are passed between successive oxidation/reduction reactions to the end of the chain where oxygen accepts the final electrons and is converted to water. ATP is formed as the electrons are passed down the chain (oxidative phosphorylation). A net of 36 ATP is generated for each molecule of glucose that is oxidized to carbon dioxide and water.

Fatty acids and glycerol from dietary fats are initially oxidized to acetyl-CoA by the β-oxidation pathway (**Figure 5-8**).

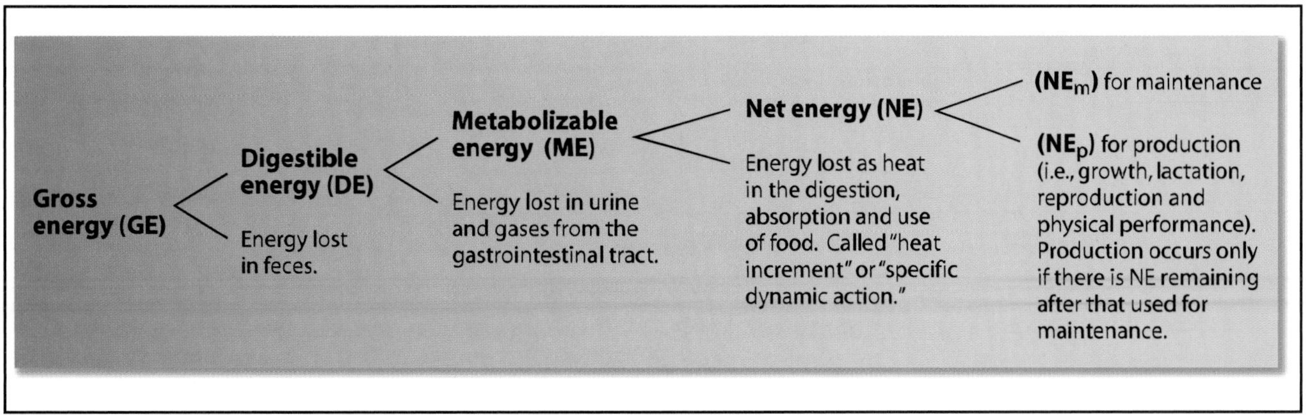

Figure 5-6. Schematic of how total gross energy of a food is partitioned into digestible energy, metabolizable energy and net energy. Net energy can be further partitioned into energy used for maintenance (NE_m) and production (NE_p).

Acetyl-CoA is then oxidized in the TCA cycle and ATP is generated via oxidative phosphorylation in the electron transport chain. The number of ATP generated from fatty acid oxidation depends on the length of the carbon chain and degree of unsaturation. For example, myristic acid (C14:0) yields 112 ATP, palmitic acid (C16:0) 129 ATP, palmitoleic acid (C16:1) 127 ATP, stearic acid (C18:0) 146 ATP and oleic acid (C18:1) 144 ATP.

Amino acids obtained from the diet and generated by endogenous protein breakdown are (re)used for protein synthesis or oxidized as an energy source. Protein synthesis requires a substantial expenditure of energy. When amino acids are oxidized, there are additional energy costs associated with gluconeogenesis and ureagenesis (Flatt, 2001). As a result the efficiency to derive energy from protein is considerably less than that from fat or carbohydrate. The amino acids used for energy are deaminated or transaminated to yield a carbohydrate moiety and ammonia; the ammonia is then converted to urea. The carbon skeleton enters the TCA cycle and ATP is formed in the electron transport chain. The number of ATP generated from oxidation of amino acids to water, carbon dioxide and urea varies, but ranges from six ATP from glycine to 42 ATP from tryptophan.

Energy Storage

ATP is the usable form of energy for body cells, but not a good energy storage molecule because it is used quickly after formation. Glycogen and triglycerides are better storage forms of energy. Production and use of ATP are equally balanced through a series of control mechanisms that monitor the amount of ATP available. After a meal containing adequate energy, the total body metabolism is generally anabolic; the body uses energy for synthetic reactions and tissue accretion (e.g., growth, reproduction). After the body has enough energy to meet demands, the pathways of glycolysis, β-oxidation, transamination, deamination and the TCA cycle are slowed. The pathways of glycogen and fat synthesis are simultaneously accelerated and excess dietary energy is stored as glycogen and body fat. These energy stores can then be used to generate ATP later when needed. Generally, in fasting animals, when the body needs energy, it uses glycogen first, fat stores second and finally, as a last resort, amino acids from body protein (Chapter 25). In fed animals, food energy is primarily used for meeting body energy needs, thus preserving body tissues by preventing catabolism. Further discussions of use and control of body energy stores during exercise can be found in Chapter 18.

Differences in the amount of energy consumed and that expended by the body can clearly result in changes in body weight, growth rate and body composition (especially body fat). Excess energy intake and storage relative to energy expenditure is a common problem in pet dogs and cats (e.g., obesity). Obese pets are at increased risk for developing a variety of health problems (Chapter 27). Excess energy intake in growing large- and giant-breed puppies may be related to developmental skeletal abnormalities (Chapter 33). Conversely, inadequate energy intake relative to expenditure may occur in animals with cancer and heart disease and resulting in cachexia (Chapters 30 and 36) and in vigorously exercising dogs such as sled dogs (Chapter 18).

Energy Analyses

The most accurate determination of the DE or ME content of food (**Figure 5-6**) is obtained through feeding studies (Yamka et al, 2007; McDonald et al, 1995; AAFCO, 2007). ME determinations involve the direct measurement of energy intake and energy lost in feces and urine obtained from digestion or metabolism studies. Energy lost as expired gases (e.g., methane) is negligible (McKay and Eastwood, 1984). As a result, energy lost as gases is typically ignored when calculating ME for dogs and cats. The Association of American Feed Control Officials (AAFCO) has published accepted protocols for the determination of ME of dogs and cat foods (2007) (**Box 5-3**). Because of the laborious nature of determining the actual ME content of dog foods, calculated ME values are used extensively for diet formulation and food labeling (Yamka et al, 2007).

Currently, AAFCO (2007) and the National Research Council (2003) recommend a predictive equation largely based on fixed energy values and digestibility coefficients for dietary components (i.e., crude protein, crude fat and carbohydrate) for estimating the ME content of dog foods. Although this predic-

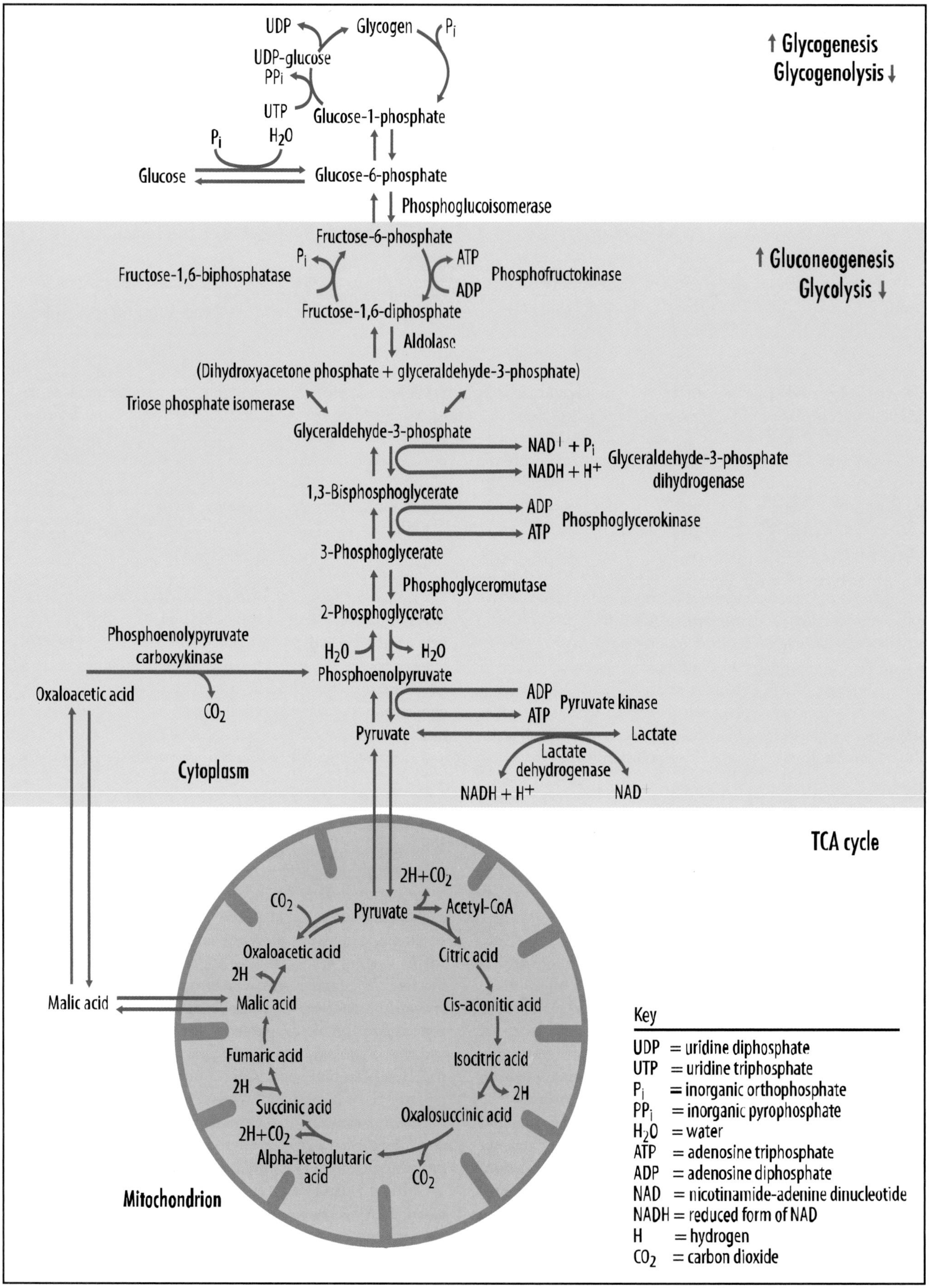

Figure 5-7. Biochemical pathways of glycogenesis, glycogenolysis, gluconeogenesis, glycolysis and the tricarboxylic acid (TCA) cycle.

tive equation reasonably provides precision for foods containing traditional ingredients, it may be inadequate for currently available commercial foods due in part to the use of new food additives/agents and diverse ingredients (Yamka et al, 2007). These methods for calculating ME can be applied to cat and dog foods and assume an average apparent digestibility of 80% for protein, 90% for crude fat and 84% for carbohydrate. The digestion coefficients are then multiplied by energy values of 4.4, 9.4 and 4.15 kcal/g for protein, fat and carbohydrate, respectively. The resulting values of 3.5, 8.5 and 3.5 kcal/g are reasonable estimates of the ME derived from protein, fat and carbohydrate in typical commercial pet foods, which range in digestibility from 75 to 85%. The method assumes no energy is derived from crude fiber, water or ash. This method overestimates the ME content of foods high in fiber or ash or foods with very low protein, fat and carbohydrate digestibility. This overestimation inadequately predicts ME for growth, lactation or trauma recovery in dogs. Likewise, the equation underestimates the ME content of highly digestible and low-fiber foods. Underestimation of the ME content could result in obesity and obesity related disorders (e.g, diabetes mellitus and arthritis) simply because the pet owner is following recommended feeding instructions for what he or she believes to be a lower calorie food (Yamka et al, 2007). Because of the inconsistency of the Atwater equation to predict ME, many researchers have attempted to identify better and more accurate methods for predicting the energy content of pet foods.

Recent research has focused on the fiber portion of the food to find a more accurate method for determining ME (Earle et al, 1998; Kienzle, 2002). This method increases ME prediction; however, the crude fiber content of most commercial dog foods accounts for approximately 3 to 5% of the food. Therefore, it becomes practical to focus on other components of the food, such as crude protein (20 to 30% of the dietary DM) or carbohydrate (20 to 50% of the dietary DM), which would contribute more to total energy content and, thus, may have a greater impact on the prediction of ME (Yamka et al, 2007). The crude protein fraction represents numerous compounds that can broadly be classified as amino acid (TAA) and non-amino acid (NAA: e.g., nucleic acids, amines, amides, etc.) compounds (Yamka et al, 2007). Digestibility (Giesecke et al, 1982; Yamka et al, 2005) and relative contribution to urinary nitrogen energy losses (Blaxter, 1989) differ among these compounds. Nucleic acids have low digestibility (approximately 57%) in dogs (Giesecke et al, 1982). Numerous studies have demonstrated that amino acids have high digestibility. (See Protein section.) With this knowledge, it becomes important to identify protein quality to further characterize crude protein. The NAA portion of crude protein has a negative impact on ME whereas the TAA influences ME directly (Yamka et al, 2007). As a result of defining protein composition (TAA:NAA), predicting ME has greatly improved for dry dog foods.

Estimation of the NE of a food requires measurement of the heat lost. Heat production can be measured directly using an animal calorimeter (direct calorimetry) or estimated indirectly

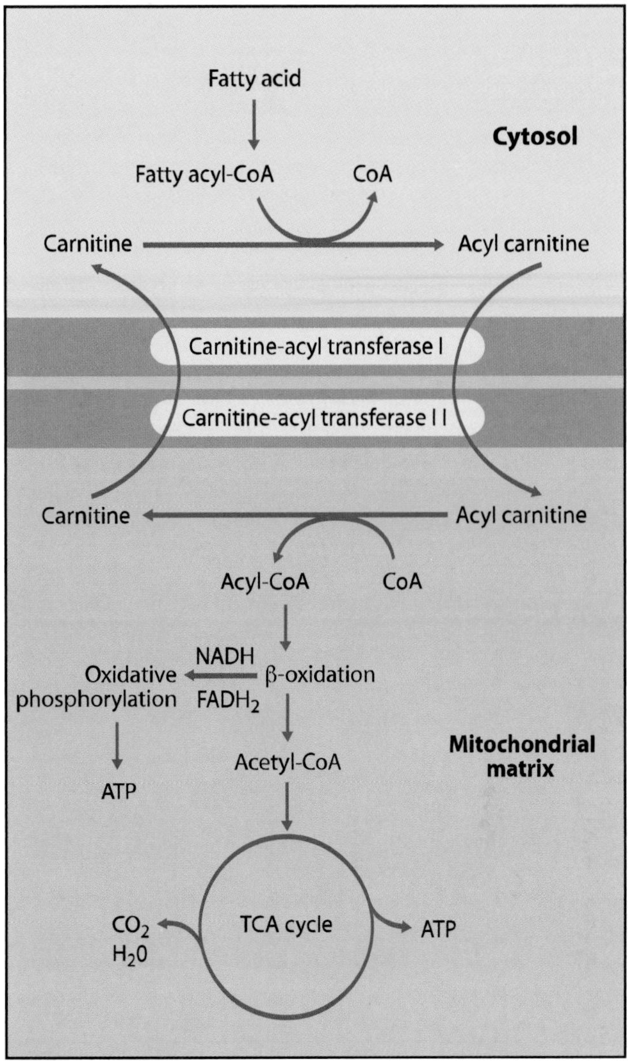

Figure 5-8. This diagram depicts metabolism of long-chain fatty acids for energy production. Entry of long-chain fatty acids into mitochondria is facilitated by carnitine-acyl transferase enzymes. Medium-chain and short-chain fatty acids bypass this important regulatory step and enter the mitochondria unaided. β-oxidation is an energy-yielding catabolic process involving fatty acids that occurs within the mitochondrial matrix. The resultant products are acetyl-CoA, which enters the TCA cycle for further metabolism (to CO_2, water and ATP) and reduced coenzymes (NADH/$FADH_2$) for ATP production by oxidative phosphorylation.

from the exchange of oxygen and carbon dioxide (indirect or respiratory calorimetry) (Kleiber, 1972; Blaxter, 1989) (**Box 5-4**). Partitioning NE into NE_m and NE_p involves estimating the energy retained by the animal and will be discussed below.

Energy Requirements

Knowledge of energy requirements is needed to determine how much food to feed to an animal. Determining energy requirements involves measuring energy expenditure of an animal under a defined set of physiologic and environmental conditions. Energy expenditure studies typically involve carefully accounting for all components of the energy budget of an ani-

Box 5-3. AAFCO Protocol for Determining Metabolizable Energy of Dog and Cat Foods.

Animal feeding studies are the most desirable means for measuring the metabolizable energy (ME) of a food. The following steps summarize what is involved when investigators conduct a ME study using dogs or cats, according to protocols established by the Association of American Feed Control Officials (AAFCO).

1. Feed a group of animals a known amount of food each day for a given number of days (typically five to seven days for dogs and between five and 15 days for cats).
2. Collect and record the weight of feces excreted on the same days as food measurements were made.
3. Analyze the gross energy (GE) content of samples of the food and feces (FE) by bomb calorimetry. Bomb calorimetry involves placing a known amount of the food or feces into a bomb compartment submerged in a water bath. Oxygen is added to the compartment and ignited with an electrical spark and the increase in water temperature that surrounds the bomb is measured as the sample burns. Urinary energy (UE) can be measured directly by collecting urine and then determining the GE of the urine. Alternatively, measuring protein digestibility and then using a factor that predicts the energy content of the urine can estimate UE. Energy from intestinal gases is typically ignored because it constitutes a very small proportion of energy lost in dogs and cats.
4. ME of the food is then calculated as GE minus FE and UE.

The Bibliography for **Box 5-3** can be found can be found at www.markmorris.org.

mal including: 1) energy consumed in food, 2) energy losses from the body via urine, feces and intestinal gases, 3) heat produced by metabolism and/or physical work, 4) retention of energy as tissue accretion and 5) secretion of energy as milk (Blaxter, 1989). Because the first law of thermodynamics states that energy is conserved, energy intake by the animal minus all energy lost must equal the energy retained or secreted as shown by the following equation:

$$RE = GE - FE - UE - GPD - HP$$

(Where GE = gross energy intake, FE = fecal energy excreted, UE = urine energy excreted, GPD = gaseous products of digestion, HP = heat production and RE = retained energy primarily in the form of lean and fat tissues or energy secreted in milk). The above equation can be simplified to three terms by substituting ME for the GE – FE – UE – GPD portion of the equation. The simplified energy budget equation is now:

$$RE = ME - HP$$

Heat production is the sum of heat lost through radiation, convection, conduction and evaporation and heat stored in the body as exemplified by an increase in body temperature. Heat is lost when food is metabolized and when physical work is performed. When no food is given, no physical work is done and an animal is in a thermoneutral environment, heat production results from basal cellular metabolism. In this case, the term basal energy expenditure (BEE) can be used as an alternative to heat production. Thus, when heat production is measured, energy expenditure is measured, and then energy expenditure is equated with energy requirements. Also, if energy retention is zero, then an animal is in energy equilibrium where heat production equals ME. In this case, ME equals NE_m. The third term can be derived if two of the three terms of the energy budget equation are known. Alternatively, if all three components are measured then there is added confidence in the energy requirement estimate.

Laboratory protocols and specialized equipment have been developed to measure the three major components of the energy budget. ME determinations have been discussed previously. **Box 5-4** provides information about whole animal calorimetry used to estimate HI. The primary forms of RE in animals are protein and fat, although a small and relatively constant proportion of carbohydrate is stored as glycogen. The gold standard method for measuring RE in farm animals is the comparative slaughter method in which the energy content of an animal is determined by bomb calorimetry on ground carcass samples (McDonald et al, 1995). Other methods have been developed that are noninvasive, less costly and allow for repeat measurements on the same subject. Underwater weighing, bioelectrical impedance, anthropometric measurements (triceps skin-fold thickness, upper arm muscle area and body mass index), stable isotopes, zoometric measurements, ultrasound and dual energy x-ray absorptiometry [DEXA]) are commonly used to estimate body compositions (fat and lean proportions) of people and other animals. Some of these methods have been further adapted for use in dogs and cats. Two-dimensional ultrasound technology has been used successfully for estimating back fat and total body fat to determine obesity in dogs (Morooka et al, 2001; Wilkinson and McEwan, 1991; Anderson and Corbin, 1982). In recent years, DEXA technology has been used to provide rapid and repeatable estimates of body composition of dogs and cats (Wedekind et al, 1992; Toll et al, 1994).

For animals under maintenance conditions, when no tissue is accreted or milk secreted, the RE component of the energy balance equation is theoretically zero; therefore, the HI is the estimate of the energy expended for maintenance of adult animals. In growing, pregnant and lactating animals, the RE portion of the energy budget is not zero; therefore, both the RE and HI should be measured to accurately predict the energy requirements for animals undergoing these production parameters.

Energy requirements have been given different names depending on the physiologic and environmental conditions under which the measurements were made (**Table 5-1**). Basal energy requirement (BER) represents energy needs for a normal, awake, fasting, resting animal in a thermoneutral environment. For dogs and cats, fasting overnight or for 12 hours is usually considered adequate. BER includes the energy needed to maintain cellular activity, respiration and circula-

Box 5-4. Calorimetry.

Calorimetry is the measurement of heat. Calorimetry has been used to understand how the body metabolizes food energy for hundreds of years. The discovery by Lavoiser and LaPlace in 1783 that heat produced by animals was related to oxygen consumption and carbon dioxide formation and was analogous to burning of a candle was revolutionary and signaled the beginning of the study of energy use by calorimetry. Because animals do not store heat, the quantity of heat lost from the animal is equal to the quantity produced. Calorimetry allows measurement of the heat lost (heat production, [HP]).

HP is one of the terms in the energy balance equation: HP = ME – RE. Because HP has been equated with energy expenditure and energy requirements, the measurement of heat really means measurement of energy requirements. HP can be measured directly (direct calorimetry) or estimated from respiratory exchange (indirect or respiratory calorimetry).

DIRECT CALORIMETRY

With direct calorimetry, an animal is placed in an airtight, insulated chamber. The heat lost from the body includes that lost by radiation, conduction and convection and by evaporation of water from skin and respiratory surfaces (e.g., lungs). The heat produced by the animal is measured as the difference in temperature between inside and outside of the chamber over time.

There are several different designs for chambers and ways to measure heat that give rise to various methods of determining HP directly. Most direct calorimetry systems are relatively expensive to construct and operate, somewhat complex to operate, require confinement of the subjects, but are very accurate and reliable.

Direct calorimetry is suited to energy expenditure measurements for research purposes and, in the clinical setting, for well patients and moderately sick patients. Direct calorimetry with an enclosed chamber is not feasible for very sick patients that are attached to ventilators or those requiring constant supervision and intervention.

INDIRECT CALORIMETRY

Indirect calorimetry involves calculation of HP by measuring respiratory exchange of oxygen and carbon dioxide. Food carbohydrates and fats are oxidized by the body to yield heat, water and carbon dioxide as shown in these example equations.

Glucose ($C_6H_{12}O_6$) + $6O_2 \rightarrow 6CO_2 + 6H_2O$ + heat (2.82MJ)

Triglyceride tripalmitin $C_3H_5O_3(C_{16}H_{31})_3 + 74O_2 \rightarrow$
$51CO_2 + 49H_2O$ + heat (32.02MJ)

The amount of heat generated from the consumption of one liter of oxygen is exactly known if only glucose or a single fat is oxidized, as well as for mixtures of the two. These thermal equivalents of oxygen are used to estimate HP from oxygen consumption. Protein is incompletely oxidized because the body cannot use nitrogen. Animals typically do not obtain energy exclusively from carbohydrate, fat or protein; rather, they oxidize mixtures. Because the ratio of the volume of carbon dioxide produced for each volume of oxygen used is different for carbohydrate, fat and protein, this ratio, known as the respiratory quotient (RQ) can be used to determine the proportions of each nutrient oxidized. The RQ is 1 ($6CO_2/6O_2$) for carbohydrate, 0.7 ($51CO_2/72.5O_2$) for fat, and 0.8 for protein. Some food energy is metabolized to hydrogen and methane by gut microflora.

The apparatus used to measure the respiratory exchange is called a respiratory chamber. As with direct calorimetry, there are several different methods for constructing chambers and measuring gas flow (oxygen and carbon dioxide) into and out of the chamber. Indirect calorimetry chambers typically are less complex and less costly to construct and maintain compared with direct calorimetry chambers. Energy expenditure calculated from indirect calorimetry measurements can be just as reliable and accurate as direct measures.

Oxygen and carbon dioxide exchange can be measured with a simple hood, canopy or expiratory collection device instead of a chamber. These systems are portable and are easier to use in clinical situations and in animals and people as they perform their daily activities. These more portable systems may not be as accurate as the chamber systems, but are less costly and highly flexible. Energy expenditure can be measured in very sick patients using a hood system when other methods are unsuitable.

Knowledge of energy use is important to make accurate estimates of energy requirements to optimize the health of animals. Energy requirements vary with nutritional, genetic and environmental influences; interactions among the factors are complex. Therefore, it is easiest to isolate and measure the specific factors that alter energy expenditure (e.g., resting energy expenditure, thermic effect of food, breed, age, gender, energy expenditure due to growth, pregnancy, lactation and work) and then develop prediction equations for total energy requirements of the animal, taking into account all the relevant factors. Although both methods of calorimetry, direct and indirect, have technical challenges, each technique is useful in research and clinical practice. Calorimetry is important to build an understanding of factors that influence energy requirements.

The Bibliography for **Box 5-4** can be found can be found at www.markmorris.org.

tion. BER is determined by measuring the energy expenditure under the stated conditions. Thus, the terms BER and BEE are synonymous.

RER represents the energy requirement for a normal animal at rest under thermoneutral but not fasted conditions (Blaxter, 1989). The amount of time between a meal and when measurements are made can affect the estimate of RER; therefore, they should be standardized between animals and experiments. RER also differs from BER because it includes energy expended for recovery from physical activity. Depending on the level of activity and time between cessation of activity and the energy expenditure determination, RER may range from almost the same value as BER to as much as 25% higher (Kleiber, 1961). Therefore, the differences between BER and RER include

Table 5-1. Commonly used measurements of energy.

Basal energy requirement (BER): BER represents the energy requirement for a normal animal in a thermoneutral environment, awake but resting and in postabsorptive (fasting) state. Other names: fasting heat production (FHP), basal metabolic rate (BMR), basal energy expenditure (BEE).
Resting energy requirement (RER): RER represents the energy requirement for a normal but fed animal at rest in a thermoneutral environment. RER differs from BER in that it includes energy expended for recovery from physical activity and feeding. Therefore, the difference between BER and RER includes energy needed for digestion, absorption and metabolism of food (heat increment) and recovery from previous physical activity. Other names: resting energy expenditure (REE).
Maintenance energy requirement (MER): MER represents the energy requirement of a moderately active adult animal in a thermoneutral environment. It includes energy needed for obtaining, digesting and absorbing food in amounts to maintain body weight, as well as energy for spontaneous activity. MER does not include energy needed to support additional activity (work, gestation, lactation and growth). Other names: maintenance energy expenditure (MEE).
Daily energy requirement (DER): DER represents the average daily energy expenditure of any animal, dependent on lifestage and activity. DER differs from MER in that it includes activity necessary for work, gestation, lactation and growth, as well as energy needed to maintain normal body temperature.
Heat production (HP): HP is the sum of heat loss through radiation, convection, conduction and evaporation and heat stored in the body as exemplified by an increase in body temperature. Heat is lost when food is metabolized (heat increment) and when physical work is performed.
Heat increment (HI): HI is heat produced from the digestion, absorption and metabolism of food. Other names: specific dynamic action (SDA), thermic effect of food, diet-induced thermogenesis.
Gross energy (GE): GE is the total heat produced by burning a food in a bomb calorimeter.
Digestible energy (DE): DE is the energy remaining after the energy lost from feces is subtracted from GE.
Metabolizable energy (ME): ME is energy available to the animal after energy from feces, urine and combustible gases has been subtracted.
Kilocalorie (kcal): One calorie is the energy needed to raise the temperature of 1 g of water from 14.5 to 15.5°C. 1 kcal = 1,000 calories = 4.184 kJ.
Kilojoule (kJ): One kilojoule equals 107 ergs, or the energy expended when 1 kg is moved 1 m by 1 newton. 1 kJ = 0.239 kcal.

energy needed for: 1) digestion, absorption and metabolism of food (heat increment) and 2) recovery from previous physical activity. An animal in a maintenance state has no net change in body composition; it produces no products and does not perform work.

Maintenance energy requirement (MER) is the energy required to keep an animal in a maintenance state. MER includes energy needed for: 1) basal metabolism, 2) obtaining, digesting and absorbing food in amounts to maintain body composition and 3) spontaneous voluntary activity (standing up, lying down, moving about to eat, drink and void feces and urine). MER does not include energy needed to support additional physical activity (e.g., exercise or work) and production (e.g., gestation, lactation, growth).

DER represents the average daily energy requirement of any animal. DER depends on lifestage and activity. It differs from MER in that it includes activity necessary for work, gestation, lactation or growth. DER equals RER plus energy needed for physical activity and production. DER will be used throughout this text because it offers a practical and immediately usable energy requirement value for veterinarians and their health care teams. **Table 5-2** summarizes energy requirements for cats and dogs.

Daily Energy Requirements

Measuring the energy expenditure of an individual animal is impractical for practicing veterinarians and pet owners. Therefore, researchers have developed prediction equations that may be used to estimate DER. Most of the equations predict RER based on the easily measured parameter of body weight. After the RER is estimated, one can calculate DER by multiplying RER by an appropriate factor. The DER for growing, pregnant, lactating and exercising animals includes energy needed for maintenance plus the additional energy for work and production, thus different multiplication factors are used for each situation (**Table 5-2**). Similarly, deviations from the RER due to breed, gender, neuter status, presence of disease and environmental conditions can be included in the multiplication factor to improve the accuracy of predicting the DER for an individual animal. In routine veterinary practice, these energy requirement equations should be used as guidelines, starting points or estimates of energy requirements for individual animals and not as absolute requirements.

SIZE

It was known as early as the eighteenth century that large animals produced more heat than small animals. Research in the nineteenth century, however, showed that small animals produced more heat per unit of body weight (body surface area) than large animals (Blaxter, 1989; Kleiber, 1961; Schmidt-Neilsen, 1984). Body surface area became the standard means of expressing energy metabolism within a species and makes sense because rate of heat loss from a body to the environment is proportional to the area of its surface.

Although use of body surface area makes sense, it is not easily determined in animals. Equations to predict body surface area from body weight were developed $(BW_{kg})^{0.67}$; however, because of different body shapes, calculated surface area did not vary with body weight to the 0.67 power in some animals (e.g., compare a Labrador retriever weighing 30 kg with an Irish setter of the same weight, or a French bulldog with a whippet) (Blaxter, 1989). In the early 1930s, Kleiber and Brody ignored the concept of body surface area and through numerous animal experiments showed that energy requirements for a variety of different species are more closely represented as metabolic rate (kcal/day) = $73.3(BW_{kg})^{0.74}$ or $70.5(BW_{kg})^{0.734}$. In an effort to simplify calculations, researchers have proposed and used modifications of Kleiber-Brody equations using different exponents or converting exponential formulas to linear formulas (Kronfeld, 1991; Hill, 1993; Burger and Johnson, 1991; Earle and Smith, 1991; Allen and Hand, 1990).

The debate about whether to use an exponential equation

Table 5-2. Calculation of energy requirements.

Calculation of daily energy requirement (DER) is based on the resting energy requirement (RER) for the animal modified by a factor to account for normal activity or production (e.g., growth, gestation, lactation, work). RER is a function of metabolic body size. RER is calculated by raising the animal's body weight in kg to the 0.75 power. The average RER for mammals is about 70 kcal/day/kg metabolic body size: RER (kcal/day) = $70(BW_{kg})^{0.75}$ or $30(BW_{kg}) + 70$ (if the animal weighs between 2 and 45 kg). Expressed in kJ, the average RER for mammals is about $293(BW_{kg})^{0.75}$. These energy requirements should be used as guidelines, starting points or estimates of energy requirements for individual animals and not as absolute requirements. This table is divided into three parts: 1) Feline DER, 2) Canine DER and 3) Resting energy requirements of adult dogs in kilocalories metabolizable energy, which may be used instead of the energy equations listed above. RER values from Part 3 still need the DER multiplication factors for dogs listed in Part 2.

Part 1. Feline	**DER**
Maintenance	**(0.8 to 1.6 x RER)**
Neutered adult	= 1.2 x RER
Intact adult	= 1.4 x RER
Active adult	= 1.6 x RER
Inactive/obese prone	= 1.0 x RER
Weight loss	= 0.8 x RER
Critical care	= 1.0 x RER
Weight gain	= 1.2-1.4 x RER at ideal weight

Gestation

Energy requirement increases linearly during gestation in cats. Energy intake should be increased to 1.6 x RER at breeding and gradually increased through gestation to 2 x RER at parturition. Free-choice feeding of pregnant queens is also recommended.

Lactation

Lactation is nutritionally demanding and the physiologic and nutritional equivalent of heavy work.
Recommend 2 to 6 x RER (depending on number of kittens nursing) or free-choice feeding.
The following table may also be used to estimate the DER of lactating queens:

Weeks of lactation	**DER**
Weeks 1-2	RER + 30% per kitten
Week 3	RER + 45% per kitten
Week 4	RER + 55% per kitten
Week 5	RER + 65% per kitten
Week 6	RER + 90% per kitten

Growth

Daily energy intake for growing kittens should be about 2.5 x RER. Free-choice feeding is recommended.

Part 2. Canine	**DER**
Maintenance	**(1.0 to 1.8 x RER)**
Neutered adult	= 1.6 x RER
Intact adult	= 1.8 x RER
Inactive/obese prone	= 1.4 x RER
Weight loss	= 1.0 x RER
Critical care	= 1.0 x RER
Weight gain	= 1.2-1.4 x RER at ideal weight

Work

Light work	= 2 x RER
Moderate work	= 3 x RER
Heavy work	= 4-8 x RER

Gestation

First 42 days: feed as an intact adult.
Last 21 days: use 3 x RER. (This quantity may need to be increased to maintain normal body condition for some dogs, especially larger breeds.)

Lactation

Lactation is nutritionally demanding and the physiologic and nutritional equivalent of heavy work.
Recommend 4 to 8 x RER (depending on number of puppies nursing) or free-choice feeding.
The following table may also be used to estimate the DER of lactating bitches:

Puppies (No.)	**DER**
1	3.0 x RER
2	3.5 x RER
3-4	4.0 x RER
5-6	5.0 x RER
7-8	5.5 x RER
≥9	≥6.0 x RER

Growth

Daily energy intake for growing puppies should be 3 x RER from weaning until four months of age.
At four months of age energy intake should be reduced to 2 x RER until the puppy reaches adult size.

Part 3. Resting energy requirements of adult dogs in kilocalories metabolizable energy*

Body weights		RER	Body weights		RER
kg	**lb**	**kcal ME/kg$^{0.75}$**	**kg**	**lb**	**kcal ME/kg$^{0.75}$**
1	2.2	70	38	83.6	1,071
2	4.4	118	39	85.8	1,092
3	6.6	160	40	88.0	1,113
4	8.8	198	41	90.2	1,134
5	11.0	234	42	92.4	1,155
6	13.2	268	43	94.6	1,175
7	15.4	301	44	96.8	1,196
8	17.6	333	45	99.0	1,216
9	19.8	364	46	101.2	1,236
10	22.0	394	47	103.4	1,257
11	24.2	423	48	105.6	1,277
12	26.4	451	49	107.8	1,296
13	28.6	479	50	110.0	1,316
14	30.8	507	51	112.2	1,336
15	33.0	534	52	114.4	1,356
16	35.2	560	53	116.6	1,375
17	37.4	586	54	118.8	1,394
18	39.6	612	55	121.0	1,414
19	41.8	637	56	123.2	1,433
20	44.0	662	57	125.4	1,452
21	46.2	687	58	127.6	1,471
22	48.4	711	59	129.8	1,490
23	50.6	735	60	132.0	1,509
24	52.8	759	61	134.2	1,528
25	55.0	783	62	136.4	1,547
26	57.2	806	63	138.6	1,565
27	59.4	829	64	140.8	1,584
28	61.6	852	65	143.0	1,602
29	63.8	875	66	145.2	1,621
30	66.0	897	67	147.4	1,639
31	68.2	920	68	149.6	1,658
32	70.4	942	69	151.8	1,676
33	72.6	964	70	154.0	1,694
34	74.8	986			
35	77.0	1,007			
36	79.2	1,029			
37	81.4	1,050			

*Use the DER multiplication factors for dogs listed above for total energy intake.

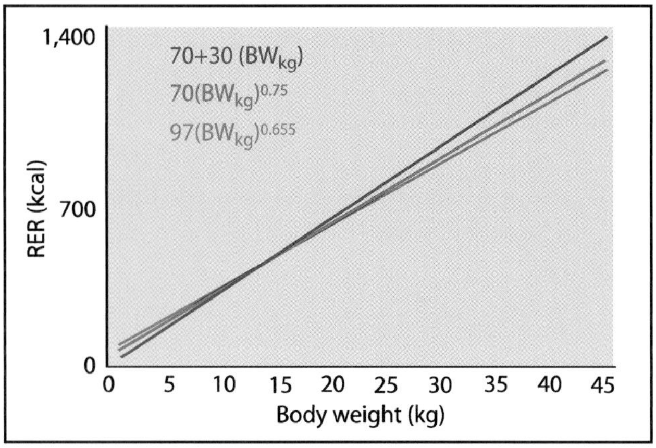

Figure 5-9. Comparison of three methods for calculating resting energy requirement (RER).

based on body surface area or metabolic body size or a linear formula to predict energy requirements for dogs and cats is largely academic (Männer et al, 1991; Männer, 1991; Kienzle and Rainbird, 1991; Finke, 1994; NRC, 2003). **Figure 5-9** compares energy requirements calculated using several different published methods. These equations yield similar estimates, especially at intermediate weight ranges. To practicing veterinarians, the differences in the energy requirement predicted by using one exponent or another or a linear equation compared to an exponential equation are small. For example, **Figure 5-10** demonstrates results among dogs and cats when the average energy consumed is set at 100%. In 95% of 120 dogs, the energy consumed varied from 65 to 135% (range 43 to 152%); in 95% of 76 cats, it varied from 61 to 139% (range 50 to 146%). Thus, the amount of food needed by dogs and cats for maintenance, even under similar environmental conditions and when kept in cages or runs, varied threefold. Even when the extremes are excluded (the top and bottom 2.5%), the amount of energy needed varied more than twofold.

The following sections discuss differences in energy requirements for different physiologic and environmental conditions.

The energy values expressed in this text are based on the exponent $(BW_{kg})^{0.75}$ because: 1) there is greater size diversity among dogs than for other species (e.g., 1 kg for a Chihuahua to 90 kg or more for a St. Bernard), 2) changes in lean body mass are of primary interest, 3) this equation works well for other mammals and 4) it can be easily calculated by cubing body weight in kg and then taking its square root twice.

LIFESTAGE

Adult Maintenance

Estimates of the DER for dogs range between 95 to 200 kcal (397 to 850 kJ) of DE per $(BW_{kg})^{0.75}$ per day (NRC, 2006; Durrer and Hannon, 1962; Leibetseder, 1978; Meyer, 1983), which represents a surprisingly wide range. Differences in activity levels of dogs account for much of this range. Other factors that contribute to differences in energy requirements include differences in breed, temperament, skin and coat insulation, age, social environment and differences in methodology used to estimate the requirement. For the average sexually intact healthy adult dog, the DER approximates 1.8 x RER.

Non-obese adult domestic cats vary in body weight from approximately 2.5 to 6.5 kg, which is a much smaller range of weight extremes than exists for dogs. The NRC recommends a DER for adult cats of 70 to 90 kcal/BW_{kg} (290 to 380 kJ/BW_{kg}) (1986). However, Earle and Smith reported that inactive cats required less energy (39 to 66 kcal/BW_{kg} or 162 to 278 kJ/BW_{kg}) and, similar to what is seen in dogs, they found that the energy intake per unit body weight was lower in heavier cats (Earle and Smith, 1991). Generally, the DER for adult intact cats is about 1.4 x RER. Energy requirements are lower for neutered animals (discussed below).

Growth

Energy needs for growth are increased above maintenance because energy is needed to form new tissue. However, growth is a dynamic process; its rate declines as animals approach maturity. Therefore, the amount of energy needed also declines

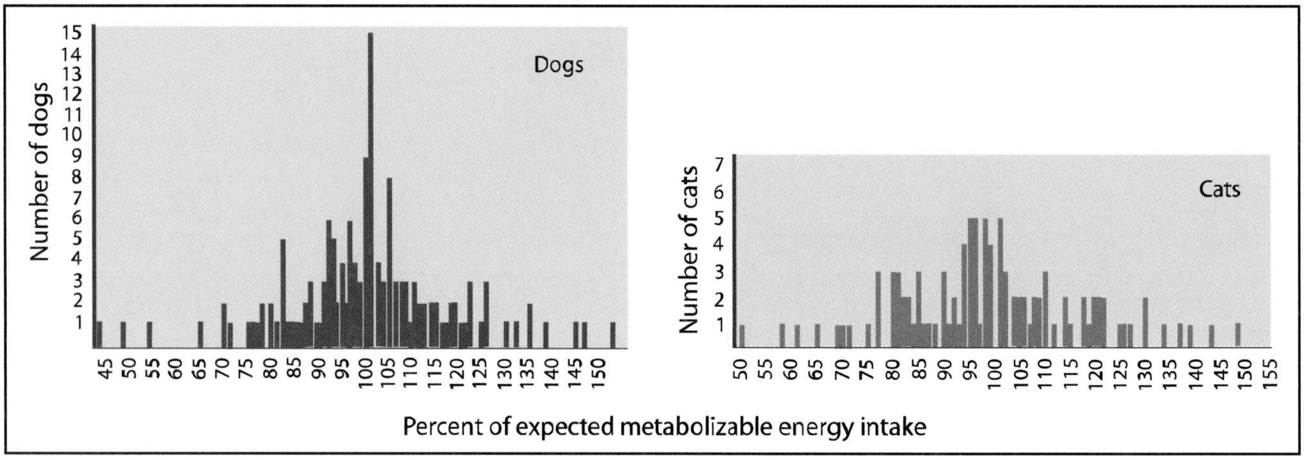

Figure 5-10. Variation in expected energy intake required to maintain optimal body weight in dogs and cats. Data were collected from 120 dogs and 76 cats kept under similar conditions and fed the amount of a variety of commercial pet foods necessary to maintain body weight. (Adapted from Lewis LD, Morris ML Jr, Hand MS. Small Animal Clinical Nutrition III. Topeka, KS: Mark Morris Associates, 1987; 1–10.)

during growth. The time taken to reach maturity in dogs increases with increasing mature body weight. The highest energy requirement for puppies occurs at weaning. Growing puppies require 3 x RER from weaning until four months of age and 2 x RER from four months of age until the puppy reaches adult size.

Much research has been done in mammals to evaluate how food energy intake affects the composition of growth (i.e., body composition, fat vs. lean). Energy consumed during growth influences the proportion of lean and fat gain during growth. The metabolic efficiency of converting dietary fat to body fat for storage is higher than the efficiency of converting dietary carbohydrate or protein to body fat. This finding has been reported to occur in puppies when comparing the effects of high-fat and low-fat foods (Romsos et al, 1976). Puppies consuming a high-fat food had similar growth in lean body mass compared with that of puppies fed foods lower in fat, but deposited more body fat (Romsos et al, 1976). The prioritization of growth results in energy being preferentially used for protein growth and secondarily for fat gain. Excess energy with resulting obesity has been incriminated as a factor contributing to degenerative joint disease (Chapters 27 and 34). Developmental orthopedic disease in growing large- and giant-breed puppies is a frequently encountered problem (Chapter 33).

The energy requirements of growing kittens follow a similar pattern as that for puppies. The highest energy requirement per unit of body weight occurs at about five weeks of age (Miller and Allison, 1958). Energy recommendations for growing kittens approximate 2.5 x RER.

Reproduction (Gestation and Lactation)

In dogs, most of the fetal weight gain occurs in the last third of pregnancy; therefore, the energy requirement of the bitch does not increase markedly until then. DER during gestation approximates 3 x RER for most breeds, although larger breeds may require more energy than this to maintain normal body condition. In cats, energy intake increases incrementally from the start of gestation and continues up to parturition (Loveridge, 1986).

Lactation is one of the most energy-demanding lifestages for animals. Depending on the size and age of the litter, DER can increase as much as 6 x RER for cats and 8 x RER for dogs. Lactation lasts approximately six weeks in dogs and cats. The energy intakes for dogs and cats during reproduction are summarized in Chapters 15 and 22.

Age

Apart from lactation and imposed activity during work or sport, age may be the single most important factor influencing DER of adult pet dogs (Finke, 1994). Three groups of adult dogs can be distinguished: 1) young (one to two years old), 2) middle aged (three to seven years old) and 3) older (more than seven years of age) (Kienzle and Rainbird, 1991; Finke, 1994; Rainbird and Kienzle, 1990). Older animals typically need fewer calories to maintain body weight and condition, primarily because of decreased activity (Meyer, 1983, 1990; Finke, 1991). This effect may also be due to increased body fat and less lean body mass resulting in reduced RER. In studies, dogs over seven years of age required 10 to 20% less energy than those three to seven years of age (Kienzle and Rainbird, 1991; Finke, 1994; Harper, 1998). It is important to note that senior dogs derive energy from their diets just as efficiently as young adult dogs. Because MER declines by approximately 15 to 20% and energy digestibility remains constant, senior dogs should be offered foods providing a 15 to 20% caloric reduction (Kienzle and Rainbird, 1991; Finke, 1994; Harper, 1998). However, it is important to realize that there are exceptions to this rule. For example, physical activity in a senior dog may offset the age-associated reduction in MER (Harper, 1998a).

Generally, people assume that senior cats are more likely to be obese because their physical activity decreases with age. As a result, it is often suggested that senior cats be fed energy-restricted foods. One study in cats ranging from one to nine years showed no apparent correlation between increasing age and changes in body composition (Munday et al, 1994). Another investigator found no significant effect of age on energy requirements of cats (Burger, 1994). Although these data indicate that energy requirements of cats do not decline with age as with dogs, the greatest proportion of overweight cats are older than four and less than 11 years (Armstrong and Lund, 1996; Kronfeld et al, 1994; Scarlett et al, 1994). There appears to be a reduction in the percentage of obese cats after age 11 and a shift towards cats being underweight. The increase in numbers of old thin cats could be the result of the early death of middle-aged obese cats (Harper, 1998a).

Dogs and cats over 11 years of age tend to be thinner and have less body fat than those between seven and 11 years old. Similar to that found in people, the lean body mass of dogs and cats declines with age (Armstrong and Lund, 1996; Harper, 1998a; Jewell et al, 1996). A study investigating the effects of

Table 5-3. Influence of low environmental temperatures on daily energy requirement (DER).

Breed	Increase in DER (%)	Environmental temperature Low	Normal
Labrador retrievers and beagles	25 (12-43)*	8.5°C (47.3°F)	15°C (59°F)
Great Danes	22**	Winter	Summer
Shorthaired dogs	95***	7.6°C (46°F)	25°C (77°F)
Longhaired dogs	59.5***	7.6°C (46°F)	25°C (77°F)
Beagles	70.5†	-17°C (1.4°F)	17°C (62.6°F)
Alaskan sled dogs	61.5†	-17°C (1.4°F)	17°C (62.6°F)

*Blaza SE. Energy requirements of dogs in cool conditions. Canine Practice 1982; 9: 10-15.

**Zentek J, Meyer H. Energieaufnahme adulter Deutscher Doggen. Berliner und Münchner Tierärztliche Wochenschrift 1992; 105: 325-327.

***Meyer H. Energie und Nährstoffe–Stoffwechsel und Bedarf. In: Ernährung des Hundes. Stuttgart, Germany: Eugen Ulmer, 1990; 99.

†Durrer JL, Hannon JP. Seasonal variations in caloric intake of dogs living in an arctic environment. American Journal of Physiology 1962; 202: 375-378.

Box 5-5. Quick Feline Feeding Guide.

Unlike dogs, most breeds of cats have a similar body size and weight (with the exception of certain large breeds like the Maine coon cat). Therefore, a starting point for feeding cats can be simplified. Assuming the ideal body weight for most cats is approximately 3.6 kg (8 lb) and apply this body weight to the equations in **Table 5-2**.

WEIGHT LOSS

Weight loss = 0.8 x RER = 0.8 x (70 x [$3.6^{0.75}$]) = approximately 150 kcal/day.*
If a wet food contains 150 kcal/can then offer the cat one can/day.
If a dry food contains 450 kcal/cup then offer the cat 1/3 cup of food/day.

PREVENTION OF WEIGHT GAIN

Weight prevention (inactive/obese-prone cats) = 1.0 x RER = 1.0 x (70 x [$3.6^{0.75}$]) = offer the cat approximately 180 kcal/day.
If a wet food contains 150 kcal/can then offer the cat 1 and 1/5 cans/day.
If a dry food contains 450 kcal/cup then offer the cat 2/5 cup of food/day.

FEEDING FOR MAINTENANCE

Maintenance = 1.2 x RER = 1.2 x (70 x [$3.6^{0.75}$]) = offer the cat approximately 200 kcal/day.
If a wet food contains 150 kcal/can then offer the cat 1 and 1/3 cans/day.
If a dry food contains 450 kcal/cup then offer the cat 1/3 cup of food per day.

Key: RER = resting energy requirement.
*These are starting points and food offerings should be adjusted to maintain or achieve the desired body weight.

aging on body composition in Labrador retrievers found that the percentage of fat mass was directly related to age ($r^2 = 0.50$). The same study also found that lean body mass was inversely related to age ($r^2 = 0.52$) (Harper, 1998a). Because energy requirements are related to lean body mass, reduced activity and lean body mass may contribute to reduced energy requirements. The reduction in lean mass and increase in fat mass associated with aging could also result from decreased levels of growth hormone (Harper, 1998a).

ACTIVITY

Activity significantly influences energy requirements (i.e., standing up requires 40% more energy than lying down) (Meyer, 1983), yet recommendations for MER do not always mention the degree of activity included. Most of the disparities in the literature for MER and RER are attributed to different activity levels of animals studied. Short bouts of intense physical exercise may cause only small increases in DER, but prolonged exercise can increase energy requirements four- to eightfold over RER. The DER for dogs with normal activity is 1.6 to 1.8 x RER. This requirement increases to 2 x RER for dogs doing light work, 3 x RER for dogs doing moderate work and 4 to 8 x RER for dogs doing heavy work. Many pets, however, are less active than their owners perceive. Many pets in the United States may have less than "normal activity;" and are overweight and obese (Chapter 27). Therefore, it may be prudent to start DER calculations lower than 1.6 and increase DER if needed to maintain body condition.

THERMOREGULATION

The influence of housing and climate should not be neglected when evaluating energy requirements. When kept outside in cold weather, dogs may need 10 to 90% more calories than during optimal weather conditions (**Table 5-3**). Heat losses are minimal at a temperature range called the thermoneutral zone. The environmental temperature range at which dogs reach their minimum metabolic rate is breed specific and is lower when the thermic insulation (e.g., coat density and length, skin insulation) is better (Kleiber, 1961; Männer, 1991; Meyer, 1983, 1990; Zentek and Meyer, 1992). The thermoneutral zone was estimated at 15 to 20°C for longhaired and 20 to 25°C for shorthaired breeds (Kleiber, 1961; Männer, 1991; Meyer, 1983, 1990). For Alaskan sled dogs, it may be as low as 10 to 15°C (Meyer, 1983, 1990).

At temperatures above the thermoneutral zone, energy is expended to dissipate heat. Conversely, at temperatures below the thermoneutral zone, energy is used to maintain core body temperature. The degree to which environmental temperature affects energy needs of an animal also depends on air movement (wind chill factor), air humidity (Meyer, 1983) and the degree of acclimatization (NRC, 1985). Animal factors including insulative characteristics of skin and coat (subcutaneous fat, hair length and coat density) (NRC, 1985; Meyer, 1983; Finke, 1991; Meyer and Heckötter, 1986) and differences in stature, behavior and activity (Finke, 1991; Meyer and Heckötter, 1986) interact and affect DER.

NEUTER STATUS

There is a paucity of information in the literature regarding the effect of neuter status on energy requirements. Neutering (castration, ovariohysterectomy) of animals is thought to be associated with the development of obesity because of a combination of factors including reduced activity and changes in BER. Data suggest that intact cats have higher energy requirements than those that have been neutered (Flynn et al, 1996; Root et al, 1996). Neutered cats may be less able to self-regulate food intake than intact cats and thus are predisposed to eat more food and to become obese (Flynn et al, 1996).

In dogs, it is unknown whether increases in body weight after neutering result from increases in appetite and thus food intake or a reduction in energy expenditure or both. In a study of six dogs, the fasting energy expenditure was reduced from 37.1 kcal/BW_{kg}/day (155 kJ) to 33.9 (142 kJ) and 35.3 (148 kJ) at

30 and 90 days postneutering, respectively (Anatharanman-Barr, 1990).

BREED

Some breeds such as Newfoundlands and huskies have relatively lower energy requirements, whereas Great Danes have energy requirements above the average (Kienzle and Rainbird, 1991; Rainbird and Kienzle, 1990; Zentek and Meyer, 1992). Breed-specific needs probably reflect differences in: 1) temperament (resulting in higher or lower activity), 2) stature, 3) insulative capacity of skin and coat (which influence the degree of heat loss) and 4) lean body mass. However, when data are corrected for age, interbreed differences become less important (Finke, 1994).

GENDER

In people, gender has a significant effect on energy requirement because of the proportionately greater muscle mass of men. (Women have a greater proportion of body fat.) No effect of gender, however, has been found in dogs (Männer, 1991; Kienzle and Rainbird, 1991) or reported to occur in cats.

DISEASE, INJURY, INFECTION AND CANCER

As a result of metabolic and physiologic changes, animals must recover from trauma, repair wounds, mount an immune response or compete with cancer to survive. These processes involve cellular work that requires energy. Energy-supplying nutrients must be provided in sufficient amounts to prevent catabolism of body tissues with resultant loss of function. However, most sick animals are inactive and anorectic and; therefore, their energy requirement is reduced. Thus, energy requirements for diseased animals logically lie somewhere between RER and DER. Although mathematical factors have been reported to multiply times RER (or MER) to estimate energy requirements for diseased dogs and cats (Kronfeld, 1991; Hill, 1993; Donoghue, 1989; Remillard and Thatcher, 1989), very few studies have verified their validity by measuring the actual energy requirements of hospitalized dogs and cats under various disease conditions (Chapters 25 and 26).

One investigator recommended a practical approach in which the RER and DER are used as references to assess whether a sick animal's voluntary food consumption is adequate or inadequate (Burkholder, 1995). Forced nutritional intervention is recommended if food consumption is less than the calculated RER. If food intake approaches DER for adult maintenance, additional nutritional support is probably not needed. Regardless of whether a sick animal consumes food voluntarily or is forced to eat, the food should have a nutrient composition that is optimized for recovery as discussed in Chapters 25 and 26.

WEIGHT LOSS/UNDERWEIGHT

The prevalence of suboptimal body condition begins to increase at about 11 years of age and rises sharply in very old animals, especially cats (Armstrong and Lund, 1996). Anorexia is common in elderly people and can also occur in older cats and dogs. Changes in appetite can be influenced by many factors including decline in acuity of taste and smell, dental problems, physical disabilities, acute or chronic diseases, drugs and other therapies including dietary modifications. Prolonged reductions in food intake ultimately lead to chronic energy deficiency. As a result, loss of body weight occurs as body energy stores are diminished (fat and muscle protein).

In people, data show that reductions in body weight are linearly related to reductions in RER and are described by the regression equation resting energy requirement (REE) (kcal/day) = -78.8 + 11.9 x weight change (kg) (Saltzman and Roberts, 1995). Decreases in lean tissue lead to decreased protein turnover, which reduces energy expenditure. Thus, reductions in RER are due in part to reductions in body protein turnover and reduced body size. Other factors such as changes in Na-K ATPase activity, hormonal changes affecting nutrient metabolism and alterations in sympathetic nervous system activity may also reduce overall RER in weight loss (Saltzman and Roberts, 1995). Data from obese dogs suggest that RER may be reduced by up to 25% following a weight loss of 17% (Brown, 1991). It is unknown whether similar reductions in

Box 5-6. Quick Canine Feeding Guide.

Unlike cats, dogs come in variable sizes from Chihuahuas to Great Danes. Therefore, the same assumptions cannot be made when simplifying food offerings for dogs. However, daily feed offerings can be simplified for the initial food offering in kcal/lb body weight (**Table 1**).

Table 1. Summary of caloric food offerings per day.*

BW (lb)	Weight loss (1.0 x RER)	Inactive/obese prone (1.4 x RER)	Maintenance (1.6 x RER)
<10	20 kcal/lb	28 kcal/lb	32 kcal/lb
10–20	15 kcal/lb	21 kcal/lb	24 kcal/lb
>20	9 kcal/lb	13 kcal/lb	15 kcal/lb

Key: BW = body weight, RER = resting energy requirement.
*Example: A 15-lb dog would require 225 kcal/day (15 lb x 15 kcal) for weight loss.
If a wet food contains 150 kcal/can then offer the dog 1 and 1/2 cans per day.
If a dry food contains 300 kcal/cup then offer the dog 3/4 cup of food per day.
These are starting points and food offerings should be adjusted to maintain or achieve the desired body weight.

RER occur in animals with normal body condition or older animals that lose weight.

WEIGHT GAIN

Weight gain occurs in growth; the energy requirements during growth have been discussed previously. Weight gain that occurs in nongrowing animals results in changes in energy requirements needed to maintain the increase in body weight (**Boxes 5-5** and **5-6**). Research in people shows that REE increases linearly with increases in body weight and gains in lean body mass (Saltzman and Roberts, 1995). Theoretical calculations of increased energy expenditure due to weight gain and actual measurements agree closely and can be described by the regression equation REE (kcal/day) = 55.6 + 16.9 x weight change (kg) (Saltzman and Roberts, 1995).

The composition of the weight gain averaged 63% body fat and 37% lean tissue in a summary of six studies involving 89 adult people (Saltzman and Roberts, 1995). The additional energy needed to support weight gain is mainly due to the amount of lean body mass that is gained and the energy required to support the increased protein turnover in the newly deposited protein.

There are no estimates supported by research using dogs and cats to correlate composition of weight gain in adults with changes in energy requirements. Therefore, in practice, dogs and cats that need to gain weight are usually fed more food, or a food with a higher energy density, until the desired weight has been achieved. The new target body weight is then used to calculate DER, and the pet is fed the amount of food necessary to maintain the new desired body weight. This method is effective, but it is difficult to predict how much of a food increase is truly needed or to estimate how long it will take for the animal to gain the needed weight. Suggested energy calculations for weight gain are summarized in **Table 5-2**.

CARBOHYDRATES INCLUDING FIBER

Simple Carbohydrates and Starches

Definition

Carbohydrates are composed of carbon, hydrogen and oxygen in the general formula $(CH_2O)_n$ (**Figure 5-11**). Carbohydrates encompass: 1) simple sugars such as monosaccharides (e.g., glucose) and disaccharides (e.g., sucrose), 2) oligosaccharides (three to nine sugar units; e.g., raffinose, stachyose) and 3) polysaccharides (more than nine sugar units). Examples of polysaccharides include starches (amylose, amylopectin, glycogen), hemicellulose, cellulose, pectins, gums, etc.

In a nutritional sense, polysaccharides, or as they are more commonly known, complex carbohydrates, can be further defined based on digestibility (**Table 5-4**). Complex carbohydrates that are digested by the animal's endogenous digestive enzymes are designated starches, whereas those polysaccharides that are resistant to enzymatic digestion and thus are fermented by intestinal microbes are labeled fibers. Starches and fibers differ chemically in that sugars in starches are linked with α-glycosidic bonds, whereas sugars in fibers are linked by β-glycosidic bonds. This small difference is important; mammalian enzymes can break α-bonds but only microbial enzymes can break β-bonds (**Figure 5-11**).

Structure

Simple sugars are divided into subgroups depending on the number of carbon atoms they contain. Three-carbon sugars (saccharides) are: 1) trioses ($C_3H_6O_3$) such as glyceraldehyde, 2) four-carbon sugars are tetroses ($C_4H_8O_4$), 3) five-carbon sugars are pentoses ($C_5H_{10}O_5$) such as ribose and xylose, 4) six-carbon sugars are hexoses ($C_6H_{12}O_6$) such as glucose, galactose and fructose and 5) seven-carbon sugars are called heptoses ($C_7H_{14}O_7$). Only one disaccharide has been found in mammals (i.e., lactose), whereas the most common plant disaccharide is sucrose. Many oligosaccharides are commonly found in plants. The trisaccharide raffinose and the tetrasaccharide stachyose are the two most common oligosaccharides found in plants (e.g., soybeans and other legume seeds, sugar beets, root crops and sugar beet molasses). Longer chain oligosaccharides can be found in a variety of plants used as food.

Starch is made up of glucose units in straight chains with α1,4 bonds (amylose) and with α1,6 bonds that form branches (**Figure 5-11**). Small intestinal digestive enzymes can break the α1,4 and α1,6 bonds. Starches in plants are called amylopectins whereas animal starch is called glycogen. Plant starches exist as semicrystalline granules that vary in size, shape and amount of other compounds (proteins) associated with the granule.

The granular structure of starch affects the ease with which it is digested (**Table 5-5**). Most starches in cooked and extruded pet foods are easily and rapidly digested. Raw or uncooked starch is typically digested more slowly than cooked starch. Some plant starches resist enzymatic digestion in the small intestine (Englyst and Cummings, 1987) and have been named resistant starch (RS). RS, by definition, is not enzymatically digested in the small intestine, thus it becomes available for microbial fermentation in the colon.

The amounts of rapidly digestible, slowly digestible and RS in foods are highly variable and depend on the starch source, type and extent of processing (BNF, 1990). **Table 5-5** shows a nutritional classification of the types of starch found in foods.

Function

The body uses simple carbohydrates and starches in foods as a source of glucose. As such, they have several major functions. First, they provide energy (ATP) via glycolysis and the TCA cycle. Second, when metabolized for energy to carbon dioxide and water, they are a source of heat for the body. Third, as they proceed through metabolic pathways, certain products can be used as building blocks for other nutrients, such as nonessential amino acids, glycoproteins, glycolipids, lactose, vitamin C, etc. Finally, simple carbohydrates and starches in excess of the body's immediate energy needs are stored as glycogen or converted to fat.

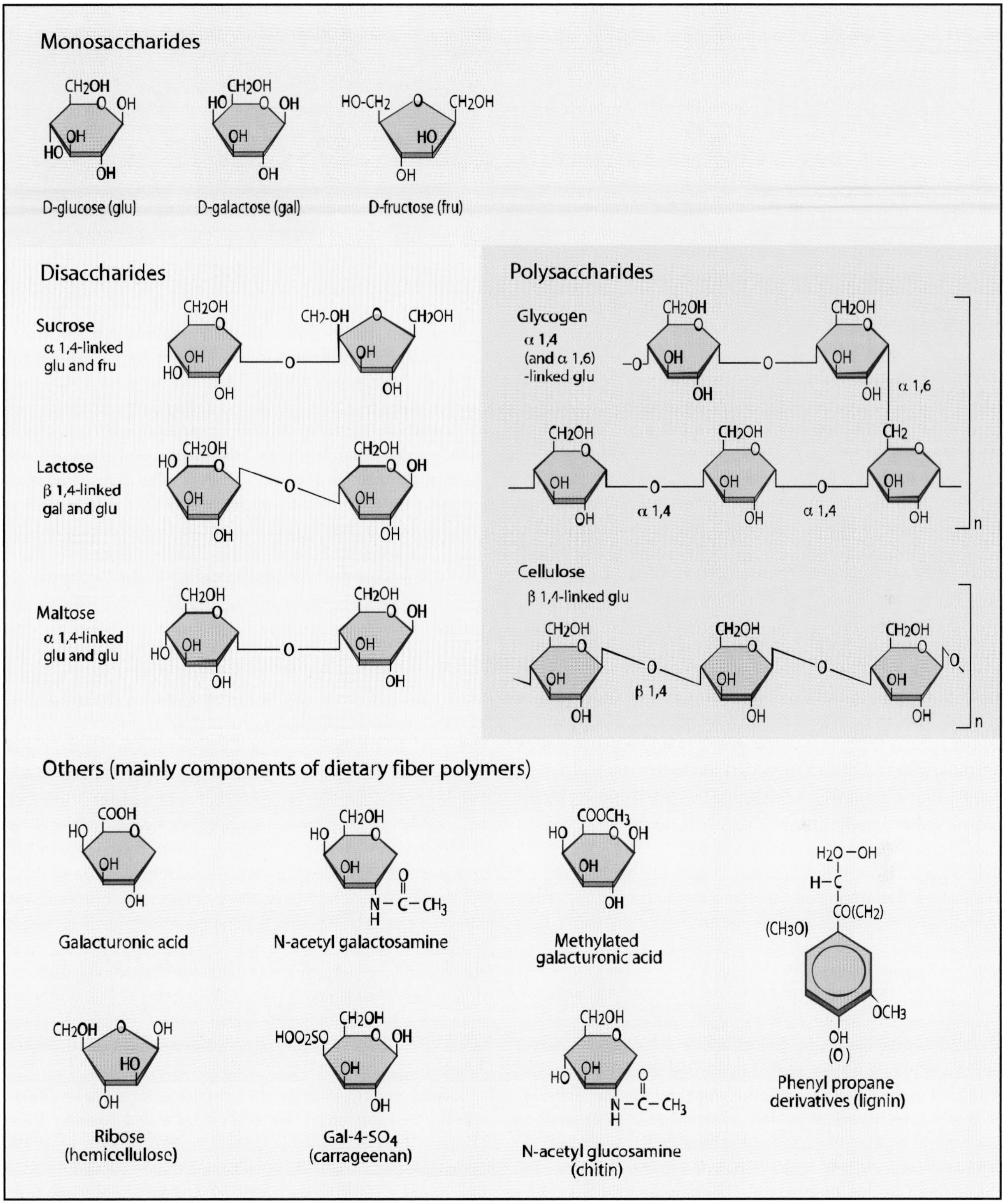

Figure 5-11. Components and classification of dietary carbohydrates. Dietary carbohydrates are usually classified as monosaccharides, disaccharides (sugars that yield two monosaccharides on hydrolysis) and polysaccharides (carbohydrates that yield nine or more monosaccharides when hydrolyzed). Other carbohydrates are primarily components of dietary fiber.

Table 5-4. Classification and digestion of complex carbohydrates.*

Complex carbohydrate type	Function	Digestion site	Digestion products
Starch, glycogen	Storage polysaccharide in plants and animals	Small intestine (enzymatic)	Mono- and disaccharides (glucose, maltose)
Hemicellulose, cellulose	Structural parts of plant cell walls	Large intestine (microbial fermentation)	Volatile fatty acids (acetate, propionate, butyrate)
Lignins, cutins, waxes	Associated cell wall substances	Not digested or fermented	Excreted in feces
Gums, mucilages, pectins	Naturally occurring polysaccharides in plants	Large intestine (microbial fermentation)	Carbon dioxide, methane, hydrogen, volatile fatty acids

*Adapted from the British Nutrition Foundation. Complex Carbohydrates in Foods. New York, NY: Van Nostrand Reinhold, 1990.

IMPORTANCE OF CARBOHYDRATES

The primary purpose for adding carbohydrates and starches to pet foods is to supply energy. Generally, assuming an average digestibility (84%), carbohydrates supply about 3.5 kcal/g. Although there is no minimum dietary requirement for simple carbohydrates or starches per se, certain organs and tissues (e.g., brain and red blood cells) require glucose for energy. Glucose can be obtained from precursor nutrients such as glucogenic amino acids or glycerol from fats via gluconeogenic pathways. The body always maintains a glucose supply to key tissues; thus, if adequate dietary carbohydrates are unavailable, amino acids will be shunted away from muscle growth, fetal growth and milk production to be used for glucose synthesis.

When energy needs are high and tissue accretion is occurring (e.g., during growth, gestation and lactation), adequate dietary carbohydrates or glucose precursors are necessary to maintain metabolic processes (Romsos et al, 1981; Kienzle et al, 1985; Meyer and Kienzle, 1991; Blaza et al, 1989). In these situations, carbohydrates become conditionally essential; therefore, foods fed to growing animals and those with high-energy needs should contain at least 20% carbohydrates.

In addition to nutritional reasons for adding carbohydrates to pet foods, carbohydrates also are important in pet food processing. Chapter 8 provides detailed information.

Metabolism

DIGESTION

Digestion of simple carbohydrates and starches occurs throughout the digestive tract and involves mechanical, enzymatic and microbial processes. Mechanical breakdown occurs primarily in the oral cavity. Because dogs and cats lack salivary α-amylase, enzymatic digestion of starch is not initiated in the mouth. In the stomach, food is mixed with gastric juices (i.e., hydrochloric acid and proteolytic enzymes). Although the stomach plays an important role in protein digestion, little carbohydrate digestion occurs here. Simple carbohydrates and starches are digested and absorbed in the small intestine. Enzymes secreted from the pancreas digest the majority of starches and sugars in the lumen of the small intestine, whereas enzymes at the small intestinal mucosal brush border are important in the final stages of carbohydrate digestion and absorption.

Starch is initially cleaved by the enzyme α-amylase, which creates branched oligosaccharides, the disaccharide maltose and the trisaccharide maltotriose. The brush border enzymes maltase, sucrase and isomaltase cleave the larger glucose chains into single glucose molecules that are then absorbed. Sucrase also splits the disaccharide sucrose into glucose and fructose units. Lactase, another brush border enzyme, splits lactose, the sugar found in milk, into glucose and galactose. Lactase activity is usually high in young, suckling animals but often declines in adults. Conversely, amylase, maltase and isomaltase display a reverse temporal pattern; concentrations of these enzymes are low in suckling animals and higher in adults (Meyer and Kienzle, 1991; Kienzle, 1988). For example, in puppies, amylase and sucrase activities increase by 21 days after birth and increase further by Day 63 postpartum. This pattern suggests that growing dogs have an increasing ability to digest carbohydrates from foods (Buddington et al, 2003).

Starch is made up of glucose units in straight chains (amylose) and with branches (amylopectin) linked with α-bonds (**Figure 5-11**). Starches are contained within granules in plants in a highly crystalline formation. As foods containing starches are heated or cooked with water, the starch crystals are melted and hydrated, a process called gelatinization (Camire et al, 1990). The extent to which starch granules are disrupted and the extent of gelatinization depend on many factors including grinding, moisture, cooking time and temperature. For most starches, digestibility increases with the degree of gelatinization. Extrusion cooking, a process used in dry pet food production, increases overall digestibility of starches in grains by gelatinizing starch. The canning process also results in gelatinization of starch.

Several reports indicate that dogs and cats readily digest starches in commercial pet foods (Meyer and Kienzle, 1991; Gross et al, 1998; Walker et al, 1994; Schunemann et al, 1989). In studies, dogs were fed foods in which 30 to 57% of the food came from extruded corn, barley, rice or oats. The starch from all grains was nearly 100% digested in the small intestine; essentially no starch passed into the colon (Walker et al, 1994).

Other studies compared the digestibility of isolated raw cornstarch, tapioca and potato starches and cooked rice starch (Meyer and Kienzle, 1991; Schunemann et al, 1989). In these studies, isolated starches contributed 40% of the DM of the food. By the time the starch reached the colon, uncooked cornstarch was digested to the same degree as cooked rice starch (>94% digested); however, uncooked potato (0%) and tapioca starches (<70%) were poorly digested in the small intestine. The uncooked tapioca starch subsequently resulted in increased bacterial fermentation rates as evidenced by high volatile fatty acid concentrations in the feces. Large amounts of easily fermentable carbohydrates (e.g., tapioca starch) in the colon increase the risk of excessive fermentation causing gas and flatulence and upsetting the balance of microflora.

In feeding trials with cats, investigators demonstrated that cooked cornstarch was nearly 100% digested when consumed by cats at 4.7 g/kg body weight per day (Meyer and Kienzle, 1991; Kienzle, 1993, 1993a). Raw cornstarch was only 60 to 70% digested and raw potato starch was 40% or less digested when consumed at 8.8 and 8.9 g/kg body weight per day. Most commercial cat foods contain approximately 30 to 35% DM carbohydrate. This level provides approximately 5 to 8 g of starch/kg body weight per day, which should pose no digestive or metabolic problems for cats (Meyer and Kienzle, 1991).

ABSORPTION

Glucose and galactose are absorbed through an active transport mechanism using specific carrier proteins and a sodium gradient. Fructose is absorbed by a separate carrier system that appears not to be sodium dependent. Absorption occurs across the small intestinal mucosa through villi. The enterocytes covering the villi contain the carbohydrate-digesting enzymes, transport proteins and other enzymes used to synthesize triglycerides and chylomicrons. Enterocytes can use absorbed sugars for energy or the sugars can be released into portal blood for transport to the liver and beyond.

Deficiency of digestive enzymes or failure of the energy-dependent transport system may cause carbohydrate intolerance or malabsorption. Many disaccharidase deficiencies result from intestinal mucosal damage induced by infections and other diseases. The resulting colonization of the lower small intestine by colonic bacteria may result in bacterial proteolysis of carbohydrate-digesting enzymes.

Unabsorbed carbohydrates in the intestinal lumen create high osmotic pressure, reduce water and mineral absorption and may result in small bowel diarrhea. In addition, excessive fermentation of unabsorbed carbohydrates leads to bacterial overgrowth, production of gas (carbon dioxide, hydrogen and methane) and short-chain fatty acids. Excessive carbohydrate fermentation can lead to flatulence, abdominal distention and diarrhea. Carbohydrate intolerance may be diagnosed by finding increased concentrations of hydrogen in the breath (breath hydrogen analysis) as a result of bacterial fermentation (Bissett et al, 1997).

USAGE

Glucose and other sugars derived from food arrive at the liver via the portal blood. The liver plays a central role in synthesizing, storing, converting and releasing glucose for use by other organs. Insulin and glucagon finely control the concentration of blood glucose. The glycemic index ranks dietary carbohydrates based on their effect on blood glucose. Carbohydrates that result in a low postprandial blood glucose response have a lower glycemic index and vice versa. Animals with impaired glucose tolerance should consume foods that have a relatively low glycemic index. Altering carbohydrate sources or adding fiber can modulate the glycemic index.

The central nervous system and erythrocytes require glucose for their energy needs, whereas other tissues can use other substrates (e.g., muscle uses fatty acids). Glucose is metabolized via glycolysis followed by the TCA cycle (**Figure 5-7**). Complete oxidation of glucose to carbon dioxide, water, ATP and heat requires oxygen and is termed aerobic metabolism. The final transfer of energy from carbohydrate to ATP occurs via the electron transport chain (**Figure 5-4**). If there is a shortage of oxygen in tissues, such as occurs with intense exercise, some ATP can be derived from glucose via anaerobic metabolism in which glucose is partially metabolized to pyruvate (via glycolysis) and then converted to lactic acid.

Glucose consumed in excess of immediate needs may be stored as glycogen. The enzyme glycogen synthetase synthesizes glycogen from glucose units. This enzyme is particularly active in liver and muscles. Endurance athletes have used carbohydrate loading (i.e., eating large amounts of carbohydrate several days before competition) to maximize muscle glycogen stores. Carbohydrate loading in canine athletes has been practiced, but has not been widely researched (Chapter 18). After glycogen stores are filled, additional dietary carbohydrates are converted to long-chain fatty acids and stored as adipose tissue.

In the hours following digestion and absorption of a carbohydrate-containing meal, the liver and other body tissues switch from glycogen storage to glycogenolysis under the influence of an increased glucagon to insulin ratio. This ratio also stimulates lipolysis, thus overall body metabolism switches toward lipid use for energy. Glucose is synthesized from carbon skeletons of amino acids, glycerol and lactic acid (gluconeogenesis) to maintain plasma glucose concentration. This function is critical to provide an adequate supply of glucose to the brain (**Figure 5-7**). The liver and kidneys, but not muscles, are the sites of gluconeogenesis; therefore, muscle cannot supply glucose to the bloodstream.

STORAGE

The body stores sugar as glycogen, a glucose polysaccharide. Its highest concentration is in the liver, but muscle tissue, because of its greater mass, stores the most glycogen.

Ribose, although not a true carbohydrate store readily available for oxidation, is found as part of nucleic acids, ATP and guanosine triphosphate (GTP). The body also has stores of sugar-protein complexes (glycoproteins, mucus and proteoglycans) and sugar-lipid complexes (glycolipids).

EXCRETION

Excreted products resulting from normal carbohydrate metabolism include carbon dioxide in the breath, heat radiating from the body and water. In cases of malabsorption of simple sugars and starches, increased intestinal fermentation may lead to more hydrogen in expired breath and flatus and short-chain fatty acids in stools. Animals with deranged carbohydrate metabolism (diabetes mellitus, ketosis, glycogen storage diseases and fructose, galactose and pyruvate enzyme deficiencies) may have elevated urinary or plasma levels of the metabolic intermediates related to the specific disease (glucose, ketones, lactic acid, oxalate, etc.). Chapter 29 discusses treatment of the most common disease of abnormal carbohydrate metabolism, diabetes mellitus.

Carbohydrates of Special Importance

XYLOSE

Xylose is a five-carbon sugar used in clinical veterinary medicine to assess intestinal absorptive capacity, alterations in GI emptying, bacterial overgrowth and exocrine pancreatic insufficiency (Chapters 54, 60 and 66). When xylose is administered orally, approximately 48% is expected to be absorbed into the bloodstream and excreted in urine (Williams and Guilford, 1996). Altered xylose absorption can be diagnostic for certain diseases. The xylose absorption test is typically only recommended for use in dogs; there is too much individual variability in results from cats (Williams and Guilford, 1996).

LACTULOSE

Lactulose is a synthetic disaccharide containing galactose and fructose connected by a β1,4 bond. Lactulose is formed when lactose (galactose and glucose) is subjected to isomerization in aqueous alkaline solutions. Lactulose is not hydrolyzed by mammalian enzymes, but can be digested by microbial enzymes; thus, it is fermented in the colon. Lactulose enhances the growth of specific types of bacteria (*Lactobacillus bifidus*), has laxative effects and acidifies the colon to aid in ammonia trapping. Fermentation of excessive amounts of lactulose may worsen flatulence and cause diarrhea. Clinically, lactulose is often given to help manage hepatic encephalopathy (Chapter 68). (It is also occasionally administered before breath hydrogen collection and used with a xylose absorption test to differentiate among small intestinal disease, bacterial overgrowth and exocrine pancreatic insufficiency (Chapters 55, 60 and 66).

GLYCOSAMINOGLYCANS

Glycosaminoglycans are complex polysaccharides associated with proteins. They form integral parts of the interstitial fluid, cartilage, skin and tendons. The primary glycosaminoglycans are chondroitin sulfate and hyaluronic acid. Chondroitin sulfate is a polymer of two alternating sugar units, glucuronic acid and N-acetylgalactosamine. Hyaluronic acid is a linear polymer of two sugars: glucuronic acid and N-acetylglucosamine. Chondroitin sulfate and other glycosaminoglycans are available as dietary supplements with alleged benefits for arthritic conditions, degenerative joint diseases and geriatric patients in general. In one study using a combination of oral chondroitin sulfate and glucosamine in human patients with osteoarthritis of the knee joint, there was no pain relief in the overall patient population, but there was some benefit for patients with moderate to severe pain (Clegg et al, 2006).

RESISTANT STARCH

RS (**Table 5-5**) is a fraction of starch found in foods that potentially resists digestion in the small intestine (Englyst and Cummings, 1987). RS is classified according to the rapidity with which glucose is released from a starch source and is a fraction of the total amount of starch that remains after a sample is incubated for 100 minutes with the enzymes pancreatin and amyloglucosidase. Four types of RS have been identified (Brown, 1996):

RS_1 = starch physically trapped within the starch granule that is released during processing and chewing.

RS_2 = starch granular structures (e.g., those found in raw potato, bananas and tapioca).

RS_3 = recrystallized starch formed after cooking, when the starch cools or is dried.

RS_4 = chemically modified starch resistant to enzymatic hydrolysis.

RS_1 and RS_2 represent the residues of starches that are digested very slowly and incompletely in the small intestine. RS_3 is highly resistant to digestion by intestinal enzymes and is fermented by colonic bacteria.

Physiologically, RS are thought to have various functions related to their dietary fiber-like properties including reducing the glycemic index of food, decreasing the glucose and insulin responses to food and improving bowel health (Brown et al, 2001). In particular, RS can be used as a source of fiber for gluten-free or hypoallergenic foods.

OLIGOSACCHARIDES

Oligosaccharides are polymers that contain up to nine sugars. Oligosaccharides that contain fructose are termed fructooligosaccharides (FOS). Although FOS are the most extensively studied oligosaccharides, other oligosaccharides include mannanoligosaccharides (MOS), galactooligosaccharides (GOS), xylooligosaccharides (XOS), isomaltooligosaccharides (IMOS), soybean oligosaccharides (SOS), pectic oligosaccharides, chitooligosaccharide, lactusucrose and lactulose or other polysaccharide/oligosaccharide-containing sources such as inulin. Oligosaccharides resist digestion by enzymes in the small intestine and enter the colon intact. In the colon, certain bacteria (bifidobacteria and *Lactobacillus* spp.) readily ferment oligosaccharides, which enhances the bacterial growth rate (Roberfroid et al, 1998, 1993; Gibson and Roberfroid, 1995; Hidaka et al, 1986; Bunce et al, 1995, Flickinger et al, 2000; Grieshop et al, 2004). Increased numbers of these bacterial species may benefit the overall health of people and other animals, including pigs, rabbits and rats (Bunce et al, 1995; Willard et al, 1994; Howard et al, 1995).

Bifidobacteria produce short-chain fatty acids that decrease the intestinal pH and inhibit the growth of pathogenic bacteria. FOS reduce fasting blood glucose levels, cholesterol and low-density lipoproteins (LDL) in people with diabetes mellitus (Yamishita et al, 1984). The benefits of oligosaccharides such as FOS, MOS and GOS in dogs, pigs, rabbits and rats include improved intestinal flora (i.e., reduced numbers of pathogens), reduced mortality, improved feed efficiency, improved weight gain, increased nitrogen digestion and retention, reduced body fat, improved stool quality and reduced fecal odor (Grieshop et al, 2004; Flickinger et al, 2003, 2000; Bunce et al, 1995; Willard et al, 1994; Delzenne et al, 1993; Morissee et al, 1992).

Analyses

The total carbohydrate content of pet foods and ingredients is not typically determined directly by analysis but indirectly by difference. NFE is the carbohydrate fraction of a proximate analysis. NFE is determined by adding the percentages of water, crude protein, crude fat, ash and crude fiber and subtracting from 100%. NFE is primarily made up of readily digestible carbohydrates (e.g., sugars and starches) (**Figure 5-3**).

Techniques such as gas-liquid chromatography and high-performance liquid chromatography can be used to separate and analyze different monosaccharides. In addition, colorimetric enzymatic assays specific for each sugar are available. The starch content of foods can be determined by heating the sample to gelatinize the starch followed by incubation with starch-digesting enzymes (amyloglucosidase and pancreatin). The amount of glucose liberated by enzymatic hydrolysis is analyzed and converted to starch content (Herrera-Saldana and Huber, 1989).

Requirements, Deficiencies and Excesses

Dogs and cats do not have an absolute dietary requirement for carbohydrates in the same way that essential amino acids or fatty acids must be provided. They do, however, have a requirement for adequate glucose or glucose precursors to provide essential fuel for the central nervous system. When energy needs are high and anabolic processes are proceeding at an active rate (e.g., during growth, gestation and lactation), it is best to supply a food containing readily digestible carbohydrates and starches. Without dietary carbohydrates, there is added strain on lipid and protein metabolic pathways to supply glucose precursors (NRC, 2006). Lipolysis must be increased to provide energy and glycerol units for gluconeogenesis. Similarly, glucogenic amino acids from dietary protein must be used for glucose formation; therefore, these amino acids are not available to meet body protein synthesis requirements.

From a practical standpoint, whether carbohydrate is essential in the food or not is of little importance because most commercially prepared pet foods contain carbohydrates well in excess of glucose requirements. Grains such as corn, rice, wheat, barley and oats provide the bulk of starch in commercial pet foods and are well digested and absorbed due to the cooking and extrusion processes used to make pet foods.

CANINE CARBOHYDRATE REQUIREMENTS

Gestation and lactation increase the need for glucose to support fetal growth and lactose synthesis in milk. In one study, pregnant bitches were fed a high-fat but carbohydrate-free (0% of energy from carbohydrate) food with 26% of ME from protein. They developed hypoglycemia the week before whelping and had reduced plasma concentrations of lactate and alanine, a reduced number of live births, lethargy and reduced mothering ability compared with bitches fed a food containing 44% of ME as starch (Romsos et al, 1981). In another study using 51% of ME as protein, pregnant bitches fed either a starch-free or starch-containing diet performed similarly (Blaza et al, 1989).

Table 5-5. Nutritional classification of starch.*

Type of starch	Example of occurrence	Probable digestion in the small intestine
Rapidly digestible starch	Freshly cooked starchy food	Rapid and complete
Slowly digestible starch	Most raw cereals	Slow and complete
Resistant starch		
Physically inaccessible starch	Partly milled grain and seeds	Resistant
Resistant starch granules	Raw potato and banana	Resistant
Recrystallized starch	Cooled, cooked potato, bread and cornflakes	Resistant

*Adapted from the British Nutrition Foundation. Complex Carbohydrates in Foods. New York, NY: Von Nostrand Reinhold, 1990.

Extensive research in dogs indicates that a starch-free food containing at least 33% of ME from protein is necessary to supply needed glucose precursors (Kienzle et al, 1985). Fetal abnormalities, embryo resorption, ketosis and reduced milk production are other possible adverse effects of providing inadequate carbohydrate during gestation and lactation (NRC, 2006).

Overall, a minimum of 23% carbohydrate is recommended in foods for gestating and lactating bitches. Excess starch in the food typically does not cause health problems in dogs. Dry extruded dog foods typically contain 30 to 60% carbohydrate, mostly starch, and cause no adverse effects. Excesses of simple sugars in commercial pet foods are also not a practical concern because sugar levels are usually low. On the other hand, carbohydrate intolerances may occur in some animals as a result of primary or secondary disaccharidase deficiencies. For animals with obesity or diabetes mellitus, foods with low glycemic indices are indicated for controlling the postprandial increase in blood glucose.

FELINE CARBOHYDRATE REQUIREMENTS

Normal cats can maintain adequate blood glucose levels when fed low-carbohydrate, high-protein foods (Kittlehut et al, 1978). Cats have some unique metabolic differences that limit their ability to efficiently use large amounts of absorbed dietary carbohydrate. For example, cats have low activities of the intestinal disaccharidases sucrase and lactase (Kienzle, 1993b); furthermore, the sugar transportation system in the feline intestine does not adapt to various levels of dietary carbohydrates. Cats

Table 5-6. Sources of dietary carbohydrates.

Carbohydrate	Sources
Amylopectin (plant starch)	Starchy plants; grains; used as thickener in processed foods
Amylose (plant starch)	Starchy plants; grains
Carrageenan	Red seaweed; used in candies and some processed foods
Cellulose	Substituent of plant cell walls; major component of wheat bran
Corn syrup	Used in processed foods
Dextrins	Used in processed foods
D-Fructose	Fruits; traces in most plant foods; honey; maple sugar
D-Galactose	Component of lactose; produced during digestion
D-Glucose (dextrose)	Fruits; traces in most plant foods; honey; maple sugar
Glycogen (animal starch)	Liver; muscle
Hemicellulose	Substituent of plant cell walls
High-fructose corn syrup	Used in processed foods
Lactose (milk sugar)	Milk; dairy products
Lignin	Substituent of plant cell walls
Maltose	Sprouted grain; produced during digestion of starches
Pectins	Fruits
Raffinose, stachyose, verbacose	Plant "antifreeze"
Sucrose	Cane sugar; beet sugar; fruits; maple sugar

produce only 5% of the pancreatic amylase that dogs produce (Kienzle, 1993). Unlike dogs, cats lack hepatic glucokinase activity, which limits their ability to metabolize large amounts of simple carbohydrates (Kienzle, 1993b; McDonald et al, 1984). Glucokinase is responsible for phosphorylating glucose to G-6-P in the pathway of glucose oxidation. Feline liver is also thought to lack fructokinase (McDonald et al, 1984).

The metabolic differences between cats and dogs support the classification of cats as strict carnivores, adapted to a low-carbohydrate diet, and dogs as omnivores. If large amounts of carbohydrates are fed to cats (e.g., more than 40% of the food's DM), signs of maldigestion occur (e.g., diarrhea, bloating and gas) (Meyer and Kienzle, 1991) and adverse metabolic effects can occur (e.g., hyperglycemia and excretion of significant amounts of glucose in urine). Despite the limitations of digestive capacity and metabolism, the starch levels found in commercial cat foods (up to 35% of the food's DM) are well tolerated. There are also differences among carbohydrate sources and their effects on blood glucose due to the glycemic index of the specific carbohydrate source. Of the cereal grains, in cats, rice has the greatest effect on postprandial blood glucose levels compared to corn, barley and sorghum (Bouchard and Sunvold, 2000).

Sources

Starches are the primary carbohydrates found in corn, wheat, rice, barley, oats and potatoes (**Table 5-6**). Meat is a poor carbohydrate source. Commercial extruded pet foods use starches in grains to provide structure, texture and form to extruded kibbles. In addition, the extrusion process gelatinizes starch, which makes it easily and rapidly digested in the small intestine of dogs and cats. Most starches from grains are easily digested in the small intestine, when fed uncooked (raw) or cooked to dogs and cats (Meyer and Kienzle, 1991; Gross et al, 1998; Walker et al, 1994). Potato starch is an exception. Raw potato starch is contained in granules that have a crystalline structure that resists digestion by people, dogs and cats (Meyer and Kienzle, 1991; Englyst and Cummings, 1987a). Freshly cooked potato starch, however, is highly digestible. A study showed that rapidly digestible starch increased from 24 to 65% when extruded (Murray, 2001). However, starch begins to recrystallize when cooled or dried. In vitro digestion studies and studies in people show that up to 13% of the recrystallized potato starch resists digestion by pancreatic amylase and thus will be fermented in the colon (Englyst and Cummings, 1987a; Cummings and Englyst, 1995).

RS in cereal grains (rice, barley, wheat, sorghum and corn) and potato flour converted to rapidly digestible forms with low or high temperature extrusion (Murray et al, 2001; Spears and Fahey, 2004). Bacteria normally present in the small intestine of dogs and cats are able to use these starches; up to 39% of their organic matter disappears after five hours of fermentation (Murray et al, 2001). An in vitro study showed that the RS concentrations of selected feed ingredients corresponded inversely to their ileal digestibility. For example legumes (various beans and peas) with an average of 25% RS had an ileal starch digestibility of 21%, whereas cereal grains had an average of 15% RS and flours with 3% RS had ileal starch digestibilities of 60 and 65% respectively (Bednar, 2001). However, the RS fraction is fermented in the large intestine, contributing to its functional properties as a fiber. Fermentation of RS in the colon produces butyrate, which is important for the health of colonocytes. Some legumes (e.g., soybeans) contain significant quantities of raffinose and stachyose, which can be digested by gut microflora but not by canine and feline digestive enzymes. These sugars allegedly cause digestive abnormalities (e.g., flatulence) due to the gaseous waste products produced by bacterial fermentation.

Sugar is sometimes added to enhance palatability of foods for dogs. Commercial semi-moist cat foods use mono- and disaccharides as functional ingredients to achieve texture and moistness and to prevent spoilage. Pet food with gravies and sauces may contain dextrins, corn syrup and other starches for texture and appearance. Sucrose does not enhance palatability of foods for cats because cats have few sucrose-sensitive taste buds (NRC, 2006; Boudreau and White, 1978). A dog's ability to taste sweetness is different from a person's because of differences in the number and type of sweetness receptors on taste buds (Boudreau and White, 1978; Boudreau, 1989). Therefore, the sweetness rankings of different sugars developed for people are not applicable to cats and dogs. Unlike in people and other primates, dietary sugars do not present a risk for dental caries in dogs and cats (Chapter 47).

Fiber

Definition

Fiber refers to a multitude of compounds categorized as complex carbohydrates (**Table 5-4**). Fibers differ from starches in that fibers resist enzymatic digestion in the small intestine. As a result, microbes in the colon usually ferment fibers. Fibers include cellulose, hemicellulose, pectin, gums and RS (See previous discussion.) and are unique because of the types of sugars they contain and the resultant chemical bonds.

Chemical Structure

Unlike starches, cellulose is a polymer of glucose units bonded by β1,4-linkages (rather than α linkages) that are only broken by microbial enzymes (**Figure 5-11**). Cellulose is the most abundant polysaccharide in plants, forming the structure of plant cell walls. In plants, hydrogen bonds closely hold straight cellulose chains to one another forming orderly and compact aggregates called fibrils. Cellulose fibrils contain regions that are highly crystalline and other regions that are more random and amorphous. Cellulose is usually associated with hemicellulose and lignin within plant cell walls. Water-soluble chemical derivatives of cellulose, including carboxymethylcellulose, methylcellulose and hydroxypropylcellulose, are used as stabilizers, thickeners and emulsifiers in pet and human foods such as ice cream, gravies, soups and beverages. Cellulose is also added to weight-reduction foods for people and pets to dilute calories and provide bulk. Cellulose is not very water soluble but can have significant water-holding capacity and is slowly fermented by microbes in the colon.

Hemicelluloses are composed primarily of glucose, galactose, mannose, xylose, arabinose and uronic acids joined together in different combinations and various linkages. Hemicelluloses are closely associated with the cellulose in the cell walls of plants. Most hemicelluloses are not water soluble because of their various structures and composition.

Pectin is a linear chain of galacturonic acid linked by α1,4-glycosidic bonds found in cell walls and intercellular regions of plants. The linear galacturonic chain of most pectins is interrupted by other sugars (e.g., galactose, arabinose and rhamnose) to form branches and kinks. Pectins are found in high levels in fruits and vegetables such as apples, strawberries, raspberries, carrots, broccoli, potatoes, sugar beet pulp and the skins of citrus fruits. Commercially, pectin is extracted from either apple or citrus waste after the manufacture of juice. Pectins are water soluble, form viscous gels and are rapidly fermented by intestinal bacteria.

Gum is a general term for the diverse group of viscous and sticky polysaccharides found in the seeds and exudates of plants. The sugars that make up gums are diverse, and the precise structural information for some gums is unknown. Gum arabic, guar gum, gellan gum, konjac gum, carrageenan gum, psyllium gum, xanthan gum, carob gum, gum ghatti and gum tragacanth are just a few of the gums used as thickening agents, water binders, stabilizers, emulsifiers and gelling agents in jams, pie fillings, confectionery products, sauces, salad dressings, canned meat products and moist pet foods. Depending on their source and processing, gums have variable viscosity and solubility in water and thus have variable fermentation rates. Intestinal bacteria moderately to rapidly ferment most gums.

Lignin is not a carbohydrate in the strictest chemical definition; however, it is often considered a fiber because it makes up the structural part of plant cell walls and is not digested by mammalian intestinal enzymes. Lignin is not a single chemical compound but a series of compounds made from derivatives of phenylpropane associated in complex cross-linked structures. Lignin is highly resistant to enzymatic (intestinal and bacterial) digestion and chemical degradation. Strong chemical bonds between lignin and plant cell wall fibers, proteins and other compounds make lignins unavailable during digestion.

Other plant polysaccharides can also be considered as fibers. These include fructans (inulin), galactans, mannans, mucilages and β-glucans with β1,3- and β1,2-glucose bonds. Amounts of these fibers in foods are usually quite low.

Carbohydrate and fiber fractions	Method	Fiber solubility	Total dietary fiber analysis	Crude fiber analysis
Fructans, galactans, mannans, mucilages	Rapidly fermentable	Soluble fiber	Total dietary fiber	
Pectin	Rapidly fermentable / Moderately fermentable	Soluble fiber	Total dietary fiber	
Hemicellulose	Moderately fermentable / Slowly fermentable	Insoluble fiber	Total dietary fiber	Crude fiber (part)
Cellulose	Slowly fermentable	Insoluble fiber	Total dietary fiber	Crude fiber
Lignin	Not digested or fermented			Crude fiber
Resistant starch	Moderately fermentable			
Starch	Enzymatically digested			
Mono- and disaccharides	Absorbed			

Figure 5-12. Physiochemical and analytical properties of dietary fiber components.

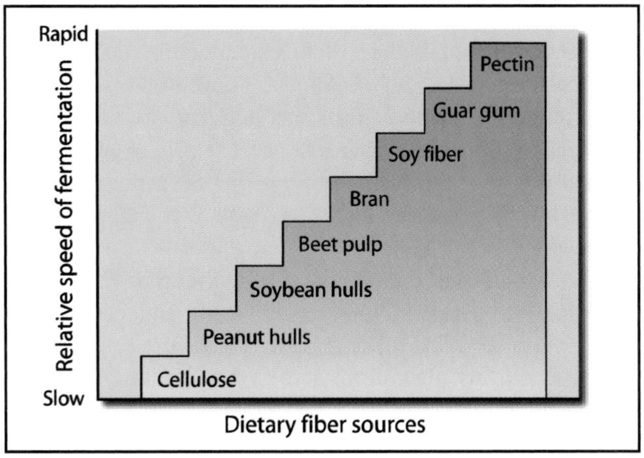

Figure 5-13. Relative degree of fermentation of various dietary fiber sources in the gastrointestinal tract of dogs and cats. At the extremes are pectin and gums, which are rapidly fermentable, and cellulose, which is slowly fermentable. Other fiber sources such as soy hulls and beet pulp are intermediate and termed moderately fermentable.

Other Classifications of Fiber

In addition to classifying fibers by their structure as described above, fibers have been classified by their rate of fermentation, digestible and indigestible fractions, solubility in water, water-holding capacity and viscosity (**Figure 5-12**). The different ways of classifying fibers allow the important physiologic functions and diverse effects of fiber in animals to be highlighted and understood.

Fiber sources can be described as rapidly to slowly fermentable (**Figure 5-13**). Rapidly fermented fibers produce more short-chain fatty acids and gases in a shorter period of time compared to fiber sources that ferment more slowly (Sunvold et al, 1994, 1994a). Slowly fermentable fiber sources used in pet foods contain primarily celluloses and hemicelluloses including purified cellulose and peanut hulls. Citrus and apple pectins and most gums are rapidly fermented. Fiber sources that contain mixtures of pectins, hemicelluloses and celluloses (e.g., rice bran, oat bran, wheat bran, soy fibers, soy hulls and beet pulp) are moderately fermentable. The rate and extent of fiber fermentation are important distinguishing characteristics when discussing physiologic functions of fiber. As the fermentation rate of fiber increases, GI transit time decreases, fecal bulk decreases and fecal bile acid excretion increases.

Fiber is also classified according to solubility, or the ability of a fiber to disperse in water. Most rapidly fermentable fibers such as pectins and gums are "soluble." Lignin and the slowly fermentable fibers such as cellulose and most hemicelluloses are "insoluble." All fibers hold water to some degree; however, the soluble fibers have a greater water-holding capacity and may form gels and viscous solutions within the GI tract. A new classification of fiber relates to the ability of certain microorganisms in the gut to use fiber as food. Fibers are classified as "prebiotic fibers," which are defined as "nondigestible food ingredients that selectively stimulate a limited number of bacteria in the colon to improve host health" (Gibson and Roberfroid, 1995). (See below.) The definition implies that prebiotic fibers are resistant to hydrolysis by mammalian enzymes, are able to support the growth of beneficial bacteria and do not support the growth of potential pathogens, although some prebiotic fibers do support growth of putative pathogens to a limited degree.

Fiber concentration, ionic concentration, pH, particle size and the hydrophobic and hydrophilic properties of polysaccharide structures affect the viscosity of fibers in water. An increase in viscosity in the GI tract can slow nutrient absorption, reduce postprandial glycemia, slow gastric emptying, delay mouth to cecum transit and reduce interactions of food particles with digestive enzymes and epithelial surfaces. The fermentation rate of a fiber interacts with its water-holding capacity and viscosity to affect the degree of fecal bulking (volume). For moderately and slowly fermentable fibers, the degree of fecal bulking is related to water-holding capacity. Slowly fermented fibers (e.g., cellulose) are the most effective stool bulking agents because they retain their structure longer and are thus able to bind water. For rapidly fermentable fibers, the increased bound water reduces fecal bulk. In fact, most fermentable fibers have laxative effects and may produce diarrhea if fed at high levels. An increase in fecal bulk has been advocated for the treatment and prevention of irritable bowel syndrome, constipation and other GI disorders (Chapters 48 to 65).

Function

The primary function and benefit of adequate dietary fiber are to increase bulk and water in the intestinal contents (Leib, 1990; Twedt, 1993; Gurr and Asp, 1994). Fiber appears to shorten intestinal transit rate in dogs with normal or slow transit time and prolong it in dogs with rapid transit rate (Burrows et al, 1982). Together, these factors help promote and regulate normal bowel function. In addition, the typical end products of microbial fermentation of fiber (acetate, propionate and butyrate) are important in maintaining colonic health. Fiber decreases luminal pH through production of short-chain fatty acids and increases the population of anaerobic flora. The antibacterial properties of short-chain fatty acids may decrease pathogenic intestinal bacteria, increase resistance of the gut to colonization by pathogenic bacteria and may be important in prevention of and recovery from intestinal disorders and cancer (Twedt, 1993; Gurr and Asp, 1994; Burrows et al, 1982; Salter et al, 1993). Dietary fibers classified as prebiotics also increase beneficial bacteria that protect the GI tract against colonization by pathogens. Prebiotic fibers may also reduce fecal odor by modifying fecal concentrations of metabolites and, via their carbohydrate residues, improve immune function by influencing gut-associated immune cells. (See below.)

Colonocytes preferentially use butyrate, an end product of fiber fermentation, as their energy source rather than glucose or amino acids (Roediger, 1982). In addition, short-chain fatty acids facilitate absorption of sodium, chloride and water in the colon. The gut microflora produce an array of compounds in addition to short-chain fatty acids, including biotin, vitamin K, carbon dioxide and methane. In cases in which short-chain fatty acids are absent (parenteral nutrition, partial bowel resection), the colonic mucosa atrophies, becomes inflamed and has decreased resistance to bacterial translocation. However, excessive fermentation and production of short-chain fatty acids may be accompanied by flatulence, abdominal distention and diarrhea. The rate and extent of fiber fermentation in the large intestine are important aspects of overall digestion and absorption of ingested nutrients. Short-chain fatty acids are an important energy source for cattle and horses (i.e., supply up to 75% of DER); however, they provide less than 5% of the energy needs of dogs and cats because of the short intestinal tract and relatively fast transit time in these species (Brody, 1994).

Importance of Fiber in Foods for Dogs and Cats

Research results demonstrate the need for some fiber in foods to maintain health and optimal function of the entire GI tract, but especially for colonocytes (BNF, 1990). In people, dietary fiber has been used to help manage diabetes mellitus, obesity, gallstones, hypercholesterolemia, irritable bowel syndrome, constipation, colonic diverticulosis, colorectal cancer, celiac disease, Crohn's disease, migraine headaches, hyperactivity in children and dental caries (BNF, 1990). Postnatal and age-related changes in bacterial flora can affect health and resistance to disease (Buddington, 2003). A study of microflora in dogs showed that potential pathogens such as *Clostridium perfringens* are present in increased numbers in elderly animals (Benno et al, 1992). However in cats, use of prebiotic fibers decreases concentrations of pathogens, including *C. perfringens* (Terada et al, 1993). Different types and specific levels of dietary fiber can be important in overall therapeutic management of specific disease conditions in dogs and cats.

OBESITY AND BODY WEIGHT MANAGEMENT

A pet food containing slowly fermentable fiber can be very effective for controlling body weight and treating obesity (Chapter 27). Slowly fermentable fibers, such as cellulose or peanut hulls, increase bulk in the stomach and intestines and help promote a feeling of satiety when fewer calories are consumed (Jewell and Toll, 1996). Pets in weight-control programs can eat more total food when the calories are diluted by fiber; thus, the dog or cat eats fewer calories and loses weight. Studies have shown that mixed fibers can also promote weight loss through several possible mechanisms including gastric distention that stimulates cholecystokinin secretion, delayed gastric emptying and longer ileal transit time. However, the ratio of slowly to rapidly fermentable fiber types is important (Kritchevsky, 2001). If rapidly fermentable fibers are included in the food at high enough levels to promote satiety, adverse effects such as loose stools and excessive gas may occur (Fahey et al, 1990). The amount of fiber in the food can be analyzed several different ways. (See Analyses below.) Because the crude fiber analysis underestimates fermentable fiber, it does not accurately represent the total fiber in a pet food. Total dietary fiber may be a better measure for weight-management foods.

DIARRHEA AND CONSTIPATION

Fiber normalizes intestinal water content, absorbing water in cases of diarrhea and adding moisture in cases of constipation (**Case 5-1**). Moderate amounts of either slowly fermentable or rapidly fermentable fiber possess this water-modulating feature. The more fermentable fibers (e.g., gums and soy fibers) can help pets with diarrhea and constipation by moderating the water content of the stool, thereby making a watery stool drier and a dry stool moister.

The binding and gelling properties of fiber also assist in managing diarrhea because the increased viscosity of the digesta is associated with slower transit and delayed gastric emptying. In constipated pets, fermentable fibers increase stool weight and moisture content, softening the stool.

Imbalances in the gut flora have been linked to diseases such as allergies, inflammatory bowel disease and diarrhea. Prebiotic fibers, in particular, can help restore or maintain a healthy balance of beneficial bacteria and prevent pathogenic organisms from increasing and contributing to disease conditions.

DIABETES MELLITUS

Management of diabetes mellitus in people, dogs and cats includes dietary changes. The glycemic index is a ranking of carbohydrates based on their effect on blood glucose. Both slowly and rapidly fermentable fiber types help control blood glucose levels in diabetic animals (Nelson et al, 1991; NRC 2006). Inclusion of fiber or changing carbohydrate sources can affect the glycemic index of the food. Clinically, pet foods that contain cellulose, soybean hulls or peanut hulls minimize blood glucose fluctuations, which can reduce or eliminate the need for insulin therapy (Chapter 29). In addition, sorghum and barley resulted in lower insulinogenic responses than rice in dogs and cats (Sunvold and Bouchard, 1998; Bouchard and Sunvold, 2000).

Metabolism

Fiber is enzymatically degraded by intestinal microbes, including bacteria, fungi and protozoa but not by intrinsic mucosal digestive enzymes. These microbes normally reside in the lower small intestine and large intestine and are referred to as anaerobes or facultative anaerobes because they can live without oxygen. They survive by producing energy through fermentation. Microorganisms colonizing the lower GI tract are similar to those found in the rumen. The proportion of different bacterial species is related to the type of fermentable substrate available. Different substrates facilitate the growth of different species. End products of different substrate and microbial combinations result in formation of different levels of short-chain fatty acids (e.g., acetate or butyrate) and/or the formation of gases such as hydrogen or methane.

Fermentation is the energy-yielding breakdown of nutrients such as sugar, starch and fiber in an environment with little or no oxygen. In this process, microbes only partially use the total

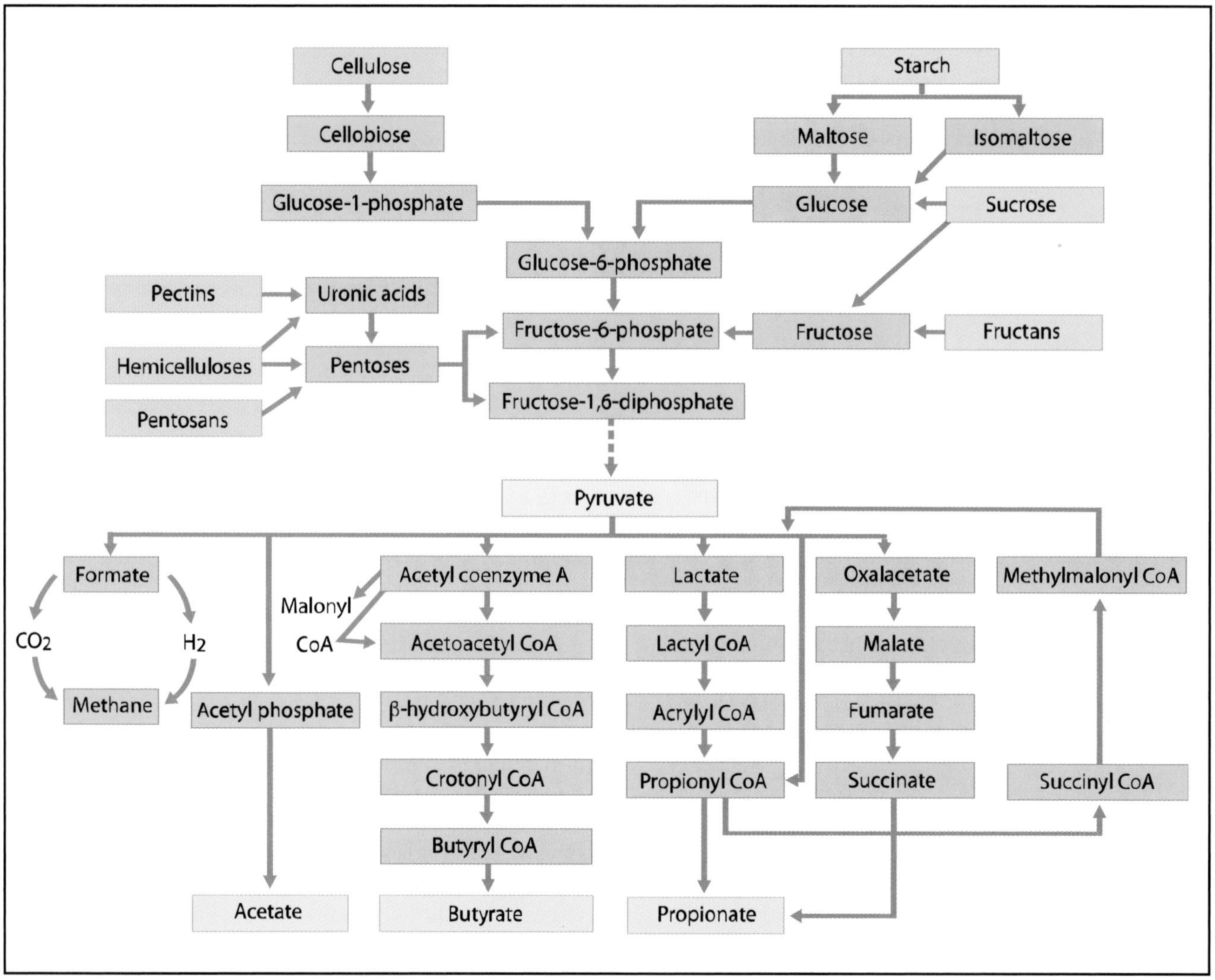

Figure 5-14. Pathways of fiber fermentation. Fibers (e.g., cellulose, pectins, hemicelluloses), starches and sugars are metabolized by intestinal microbes through various pathways to a common endpoint of pyruvate. Pyruvate is then further metabolized to yield energy for the microbe and waste products: short-chain fatty acids (e.g., acetate, propionate, butyrate) and gases (e.g., carbon dioxide, hydrogen and methane). Short-chain fatty acids are valuable substrates for the host animal that help maintain gastrointestinal tract health.

energy available. Smaller energy-containing compounds (e.g., the short-chain fatty acids acetate, propionate and butyrate), and gases (carbon dioxide, hydrogen and methane) are microbial waste products; however, short-chain fatty acids are valuable substrates for the host animal. Microbes contain enzymes that can break the chemical bonds in different fibers. For example, microbial enzymes that digest cellulose are called cellulases and common pectin-digesting enzymes include pectin esterase and pectic lyases (Robinson, 1987). **Figure 5-14** shows the major microbial pathways for fermentation of fibers through pyruvate to short-chain fatty acids.

Fermentation of fiber in the colon affects nitrogen metabolism. Fiber fermentation by bacteria increases bacterial numbers. Bacteria use ammonia as a source of nitrogen to build amino acids, proteins and DNA for reproduction. Small amounts of urea diffuse from the bloodstream into the colon where it is hydrolyzed to form ammonia (BNF, 1990; Mortensen, 1992; Younes et al, 1995).

Prebiotic Fibers, Probiotics and Synbiotics

Prebiotic Fibers

In addition to the traditional classifications for fiber such as digestibility, solubility and fermentability, an additional functional classification for fiber has emerged in the last 10 years. As mentioned above, fibers are classified as "prebiotic fibers," which are defined as "non-digestible food ingredients that selectively stimulate a limited number of bacteria in the colon to improve host health" (Gibson and Roberfroid, 1995). Prebiotic fibers are resistant to hydrolysis by enzymes, are able to support the growth of beneficial bacteria and do not support the growth of potential pathogens, although some prebiotic fibers do support limited growth of some pathogens. These traditional and new classifications are not mutually exclusive; prebiotic fibers can have different levels of fermentability or solubility.

A prebiotic is currently known as a selectively fermented ingredient that allows specific changes in the composition and/or activity in the GI flora that confers well being and health benefits to the host (Gibson, 2004). A prebiotic index (PI) may be used to quantify prebiotic effects in vitro (Palframan et al, 2003). The PI is based on changes in key bacterial groups during fermentation of prebiotic fibers with fecal material in batch cultures and is defined by the following equation:

PI = (Bifidobacteria total) - (*Bacteroides* total) + (*Lactobacillus* total) - (Clostridia total).

The above equation defines the total bacterial count in the culture. A larger PI indicates that the prebiotic fiber can increase numbers of beneficial bacterial species (bifidobacteria and *Lactobacillus* spp.) at the expense of pathogenic or less desirable bacterial species (*Bacteroides* and *Clostridium* spp.).

The mechanism by which prebiotics are selectively fermented by specific bacteria is not well understood. Two potential mechanisms have been proposed: 1) the presence of an exo-glycosidase enables bacteria to metabolize the prebiotic fiber and 2) an uptake mechanism exists on the cell walls of specific bacteria for intact oligosaccharides (Rastall et al, 2005).

Prebiotics traditional target beneficial bacteria such as bifidobacteria and *Lactobacillus* spp. However, the desirable benefits of butyrate production for the colon is recognized increasingly; thus, the potential for targeting non-clostridial butyrate producers such as gut eubacteria (Rastall et al, 2005). Prebiotic fibers are also thought to reduce fecal odor by modifying fecal concentration of metabolites and improve immune function by influencing gut-associated immune cells.

TYPES OF PREBIOTIC FIBERS

Substances that may have prebiotic activity are mainly oligosaccharides such as mannanoligosaccharide (MOS), fructooligosaccharide (FOS), galactooligosaccharide (GOS), xylooligosaccharide (XOS), isomaltooligosaccharide (IMOS), soybean oligosaccharides (SOS), pectic oligosaccharides, chitooligosaccharide, lactusucrose and lactulose or other polysaccharide/oligosaccharide-containing sources such as inulin, RS and arabinogalactans (Floch and Hong-Curtiss, 2002; Topping et al, 2003; Gibson et al, 2005). Many of these prebiotics, particularly oligosaccharides, occur naturally in foods such as artichokes, onions, bananas, wheat bran and chicory (Hussein et al, 1998). Oligosaccharides are polymers that contain up to nine sugars. Using the PI (Palframan et al, 2003), lactulose, IMOS, SOS and GOS provide significantly better prebiotic activity than FOS. An in vitro fermentation study comparing different oligosaccharides showed that XOS and lactulose produced the largest increase in bifidobacteria, whereas GOS produced the largest decrease in clostridia (Rycroft et al, 2001). All the prebiotics tested, including FOS, inulin, IMOS and SOS, increased bifidobacteria and most decreased clostridia. Although these studies show that many prebiotics are potentially useful, more feeding studies need to prove their utility in vivo. FOS is the most extensively studied prebiotic and has been shown to stimulate growth of bifidobacteria in in vivo and in vitro studies. In the colon, bifidobacteria and *Lactobacillus* spp. readily ferment FOS, which enhances bacterial growth rate (Gibson and Roberfroid, 1995; Roberfroid et al, 1993; Hidaka et al, 1986; Bunce et al, 1995). Increased numbers of these bacterial species may benefit the overall health of people and other animals, including pigs, rabbits and rats (Bunce et al, 1995; Willard et al, 1994; Howard et al, 1995; Buddington et al, 2002).

Table 5-7. Probiotic benefits and potential mechanisms.

Benefit	Proposed mechanism
Anti-allergy	Modulation of the cytokine profile
Anticarcinogenic	Metabolism and deactivation of carcinogens
Anti-diarrheal	Immunomodulation/stimulation of GI immune system, competitive exclusion, production of antimicrobials
Antiinflammatory	Stimulation of the antiinflammatory cytokine IL10
Cholesterol synthesis	Hydrolysis of bile salts, increased fermentation of end products
Immunomodulation	Stimulation of the Th1 cytokine profile to down regulate allergic responses

Data from canine feeding studies, however, are sparse and results have been mixed. Some studies showed trends towards increased bifidobacteria with FOS supplementation whereas others showed no response (Swanson, 2002, 2002a; Flickinger, 2000; Strickling et al, 2000). In a study using chicory (a source of inulin), there were no significant differences in the level of fecal bifidobacteria when dogs were fed dry, extruded food made with either 3% chicory (a non-digestible oligosaccharide) or 3% glucose, although there was a significant increase in clostridial numbers when foods with higher protein level were fed (Zentek et al, 2003).

There are even fewer feline studies and not much information is available currently. Arabinogalactan, another prebiotic polysaccharide from the Western larch tree, increased lactobacilli in dogs (Grieshop et al, 2002). Although studies in people and other species (e.g., rats and pigs) showed that prebiotics benefit GI health by promoting a healthy gut flora, it is evident that there is much that needs to be determined about the efficacy of different prebiotics in dogs and cats and the appropriate doses. Prebiotic doses that have been tested with no deleterious effects range from 0.5 to 3 g/day and 0.5 to 2% of the food on a DM basis. New and emerging prebiotics that still need to be studied in companion animals include GOS, IMOS, SOS and XOS. In addition, it would be advantageous to combine the effect of prebiotic fibers and the appropriate traditional function of fibers to obtain the best combination for improving gut flora and stool characteristics.

GUT MICROFLORA

Many studies have emerged recently about the importance of gut flora to GI health in particular and immune function health in general. The gut flora and mucosa act as barriers against invasion by gut pathogens. The gut flora also plays a significant role in modifying metabolic end products of food, detoxifying toxins in the body and competing for nutrients and colonization sites with pathogens (Gibson et al, 2005). Imbalances in the gut flora have been linked to diseases such as allergy, inflammatory bowel disease and diarrhea. Theoretically, when normal tolerance to the gut flora is disrupted, an altered response may occur in the intestinal immune system, which may initiate and maintain inflammatory bowel disease or trigger the development of allergic responses (Fedorak and Madsen, 2004; Macfarlane et al, 2005). Also, many pathogens in the GI tract, including *C. perfringens*, *C. difficile*, *Salmonella* spp. and *Escherichia coli* cause diarrhea (Marks and Kather, 2003). According to human and veterinary literature, the gut flora changes with age (Buddington, 2003; Benno et al, 1992; Reuter, 2001). Molecular techniques currently available for microbial characterization such as fluorescent in situ hybridization and denaturing gradient gel electrophoresis (DGGE) can be used to identify major groups of bacteria. Using DGGE, investigators identified *Bacteroides* spp., fusobacteria, lactobacilli and streptococci in the canine GI tract (Simpson et al, 2002). Although not quite as abundant, bifidobacteria are thought to be important for GI health. Bifidobacteria produce short-chain fatty acids that decrease intestinal pH and inhibit growth of pathogenic bacteria. Bifidobacteria are also thought to produce antibacterial substances that are active against clostridia, *E. coli* and other pathogenic bacteria. Studies have shown that bifidobacteria are found at higher levels in breast fed babies (Hoy et al, 1990) and are found at lower levels in patients with ulcerative colitis (Macfarlane et al, 2005). In young puppies, bacterial populations in the GI tract establish gradually, and can be influenced by diet and environment. Changes in the types and proportions of bacteria in puppies can influence their resistance to diseases. Total bacterial numbers in older dogs were lower than in younger dogs, whereas numbers of putative pathogens such as *C. perfringens* were higher (Benno et al, 1992). Furthermore, widespread use of antibiotics can lead to additional perturbations of the gut flora, especially in the compromised GI tracts of young and older animals. Therefore, prebiotic fibers, which support the growth of bifidobacteria, should confer benefits to the health of the host. Feeding probiotics is another approach to modulating gut flora.

Probiotics

Probiotics are live or viable bacterial cell preparations that have beneficial effects on the health of the host when administered in adequate amounts. Levels of 1×10^8 to 1×10^{11} colony forming units (cfu)/day have been tested and determined to be a desirable inclusion range although more research needs to be done. Probiotics should be nonpathogenic and resist stomach acid and bile. Some probiotics adhere to intestinal epithelial tissue and colonize the intestinal tract; adherence but not colonization may be necessary for some beneficial effects. The ability to adhere to the intestine depends on the bacterial strain rather than the host species. When administered in adequate amounts various strains of lactobacilli of human and canine origin were able to adhere to human, canine, emu, ostrich and rainbow trout intestinal or fecal mucus with no host species specific adhesion (Rinkinen et al, 2003). There was a clear trend suggesting that adhesion depended on the microorganism. Various bacteria possessing some of these attributes have been identified for potential use as probiotics, including bifidobacteria, *Saccharomyces* spp. and lactobacilli.

Table 5-7 summarizes the benefits attributed to probiotics and their potential mechanisms (Teitelbaum and Walker, 2002).

There is much literature with varying results about feeding probiotics to people and other non-human animals for GI health, immune health, diarrhea, inflammatory conditions, allergic conditions, cancer and many other disorders. As with prebiotics, many studies have not used dogs and cats. Four studies in dogs that examined four different microorganisms (fed between 1×10^8 to 1×10^9 cfu/day): *Lactobacillus GG, Enterococcus faecium, Lactobacillus acidophilus DSM 13241* and *Bacillus CIP 5832*, gave mostly neutral results (Benyacoub et al, 2003; Baillon et al, 2004; Biourge et al, 1998; Westermarck et al, 2005). *E. faecium* was the most promising organism studied; this organism improved circulating specific anti-canine distemper virus IgG (Benyacoub et al, 2003). However, use of *Enterococcus* as a probiotic must be evaluated cautiously because it was shown to significantly enhance adhesion of *C. jejuni* to the canine intestine in in vitro adhesion studies, making it a potential risk factor for infection and carriage (Rinkinen et al, 2003a). Many stability challenges exist for incorporating probiotics into pet food (Weese and Arroyo, 2003). In this study, evaluation of 19 canine and feline products claiming to contain probiotics, no product contained all the listed organisms, 11 products contained additional organisms and five products did not have any relevant growth when tested.

Synbiotics

Feeding synbiotics is a third approach to modifying gut flora. A synbiotic is "a mixture of probiotics and prebiotics that beneficially affects the host by improving the survival and implantation of live microbial dietary supplements in the GI tract" (Gibson and Roberfroid, 1995). The simplest approach includes feeding a probiotic and a prebiotic together in a food, preferably a prebiotic that can be metabolized by the probiotic, with the objective of obtaining synergistic effects. A study using this approach failed to yield significant synergistic effects (Swanson et al, 2002a). Another more targeted approach is to design a synbiotic using a probiotic and a prebiotic specifically used by the probiotic, preferably to produce an antimicrobial substance (Rabiu et al, 2001). This concept is still in its infancy and will require more research.

FIBER INTERACTIONS WITH NUTRIENT DIGESTIBILITY AND AVAILABILITY

The amount and type of fiber in a pet food have the greatest overall effect on digestibility of all nutrients. In general, foods containing slowly fermentable fiber sources have lower overall DM digestibility than foods without fiber or those containing rapidly fermentable fiber sources. Also, as the level of fiber in the food increases, the DM digestibility of the food decreases.

Apparent and true digestibility of fats, starch and energy are unaffected by the type and amount of fiber in foods (Silvio et al, 1996; Muir et al, 1996).

Apparent digestibility of protein is lower in foods containing fiber because of increased nitrogen in feces from the increased fecal biomass. Research using ileal-cannulated dogs has shown that true digestibility of protein is unaffected by dietary fiber type or content (Silvio et al, 1996; Muir et al, 1996). However, a study that evaluated varying levels of cellulose and pectin at 10% total dietary fiber (100% cellulose, 66% cellulose/34% pectin, 66% pectin/34% cellulose and 100% pectin) showed that total crude protein digestibility decreased with increasing pectin levels (Silvio et al, 2000).The discrepancy between the results obtained with total tract apparent digestibility and true digestibility can be explained by taking into account fermentation in the colon. One of the assumptions when calculating digestibility across the entire GI tract is that all fecal material is of dietary origin. Fermentation of nutrients that pass into the large intestine, however, results in significant amounts of bacterial protein in the feces. Bacterial protein is then confounded with undigested dietary protein resulting in lower apparent digestibility. Therefore, it is best to use true protein digestibility to obtain an unbiased evaluation of pet foods containing fiber. When evaluating protein digestibility data, it is essential that the fiber content of the food be known, and care must be taken when interpreting and comparing results among foods.

The main excretory product of fiber digestion is additional bacterial protein in the feces. It is typically analyzed as additional fecal nitrogen content and can confound protein digestibility measurements made using total fecal collections. Intestinal fermentation of fiber accounts for hydrogen, methane and other gases in expired breath. Some short-chain fatty acids are excreted in the stool.

Fiber affects mineral availability (BNF, 1990). Some fiber types reduce and others enhance mineral absorption and use (**Table 5-8**). It is not clear what factors in fiber are responsible for the effects on mineral availability. Water-holding capacity, viscosity, cation exchange capacity, particle size, tannin content, oxalate content and presence of phytates, uronic acid and phenolic groups are among the properties of fibers that have been evaluated to predict effects on mineral availability (BNF, 1990; Robinson, 1987; Southgate, 1987). Unfortunately, a direct relationship appears not to exist between these physiochemical properties measured on fibers in vitro and mineral availability measured in vivo. This disparity reflects the complex nature of the absorption processes within the intestine and interactions that occur with other food components.

Table 5-8. Mineral availability as affected by different fiber sources fed at 5% total dietary fiber.*

Fiber source	Zinc (%)**	Calcium (%)**	Iron (%)***	Phosphorus (%)†
Apple pectin	ND	ND	55[a]	75
Beet pulp	24[a]	44[a]	29[a]	67[a]
Cellulose	88	100	100	100
Citrus pulp cells	ND	ND	49[a]	75
Corn bran	94	92	100	ND
Guar gum	ND	ND	100	35[a]
Gum arabic	ND	ND	81	100
Pea fiber	41	58[a]	ND	ND
Peanut hulls	30[a]	100	67	58[a]
Soy cotyledon fiber	ND	ND	86	66[a]
Soy hulls	78	100	ND	64[a]
Sunflower hulls	54	100	100	ND
Wheat middlings	70	100	51[a]	ND

Key: ND = not determined.

*Availability (%) of the mineral in a food with 5% iso-total dietary fiber relative to the same food with no fiber.

**Adapted from Wedekind K, Walker L, Hancock J, et al. Bioavailability of zinc and calcium is affected by certain fiber sources. Federation of American Societies for Experimental Biology Journal 1995; 9: A450.

***Adapted from Wedekind K, Walker L, Beyer S, et al. Bioavailability of iron is affected by certain fiber sources in chicks and puppies. Ninth International Symposium on Trace Elements in Man and Animals (TEMA-9) 1996; A20.

†Adapted from Wedekind K, Beyer S, Titgemeyer E. Bioavailability of phosphorus is affected by certain fiber sources. Federation of American Societies for Experimental Biology Journal 1996; 10: A524.

[a]Within the same mineral, a superscript "a" indicates significant reductions (p <0.10) relative to the no-fiber standard.

Analyses

The fiber content of pet foods or ingredients can be measured by several different laboratory methods; the most common is the crude fiber method (**Figure 5-12**). In the United States, regulations require that the maximum amount of crude fiber be listed on the label of all pet foods (Chapter 9). Determination of crude fiber adequately represents total fiber in a pet food when most of the fiber is slowly fermentable; however, the analysis excludes the more rapidly fermentable pectins and gums. Because the crude fiber analysis underestimates fermentable fiber, it does not accurately represent the total fiber in a pet food.

Fiber can also be measured by the total dietary fiber method (Prosky et al, 1984) (**Figure 5-12**). This analysis is used to determine total fiber and is commonly used for measuring fiber content of human foods. In the total dietary fiber method, lipids are first extracted with ethanol and then the sample is digested with α-amylases to convert readily digestible starches to soluble sugars. All the water-soluble components (sugars, degraded starch, pectin, gums and most of the hemicellulose) are separated from the water-insoluble components or insoluble fibers (cellulose, lignin and a small fraction of hemicelluloses). The water-soluble components are further extracted with ethanol to remove the sugars and degraded starch. The residue that remains is termed soluble fiber, which includes pectins and gums.

The Van Soest fiber analysis system was developed as an improvement to the crude fiber method (1963). The Van Soest analysis uses detergents to more accurately estimate the different types of fiber and fractionate them into relatively digestible and indigestible fractions (**Figure 5-12**). Neutral detergent fiber (NDF) is the residue remaining after samples are boiled in a solution containing neutral pH detergent and EDTA. The residue that remains is mostly plant cell walls including hemicel-

Box 5-7. Adequate vs. Optimal Nutrient Intake.*

NUTRITIONAL ESSENTIALITY

Nutritional essentiality describes those factors in the external chemical environments of organisms specifically required for normal physiologic functions. At least 40 such factors (e.g., vitamins, minerals, amino acids, fatty acids, water) are generally considered to be nutritionally essential. Foods are considered nutritionally "adequate" if they contain amounts of each of these essential nutrients that meet or exceed known needs.

The science of nutrition has functioned for a century under the nutritional essentiality paradigm that holds nutrients are essential to prevent ill health in very specific ways. Specific prevention of nutrient deficiency diseases has been used to define nutrient essentiality and establish dietary recommendations. Indeed, unless a clinical disease has been related specifically to the deprivation of a certain nutrient, then that nutrient has not been considered "essential."

Investigators have been able to estimate nutrient requirements quantitatively based on the specific deficiency disease connotation of the nutritional essentiality paradigm. The term "required" is generally used in reference to the lowest intake that prevents disease. Such minimum requirements, while seemingly physiologically relevant, are difficult to define or measure with any reasonable precision due to inter-individual variation, which is also difficult to estimate.

Reference levels of intake ("adequate levels") are set to exceed such minimums, and thus to have acceptably low risk of deficiency. Because risk is the probability of events occurring within populations, allowances relate to populations with their characteristic food habits and inherent inter-individual variations in minimum requirements. Thus, the recommended dietary allowances (RDAs) and the reference (recommended) dietary intakes (RDIs) are implicitly intended to relate to the United States population (human) just as the Association of American Feed Control Officials (AAFCO) Dog Food and Cat Food Nutrient Profiles relate to pet populations.

CONDITIONALLY ESSENTIAL?

The nutritional essentiality paradigm does not pertain to cases in which nutrient needs of an individual or minority subgroup differ markedly from those of the general population. Under certain conditions, a dietary source of a "nonessential" nutrient can be needed to prevent physiologic dysfunction. For example, glutamine can reduce nitrogen loss and infection rate of bone marrow transplant patients. Carnitine can improve weight gain and nitrogen balance of parenterally fed infants, and helps maintain lean muscle mass in animals undergoing weight loss. The nutritional roles of these nutrients are simply not addressed by the nutritional essentiality paradigm.

NONSPECIFIC EFFECTS?

The specific deficiency disease connotation of the nutritional essentiality paradigm has become a growing problem in dealing with issues of diet and health. This is because the paradigm does not pertain to functions of nutrients that are either nonspecific or nontraditional (i.e., outside the known functions of nutrients). Such functions have been suggested by recent epidemiology, which has produced evidence linking the consumption of several nutrients (e.g., high intakes of vitamin A-containing foods, relatively high intakes or high plasma levels of vitamin E and supranutritional dietary supplements of selenium) with reduced risks of chronic diseases.

In these cases, nutrient effects do not appear to have the specificity connoted by the nutritional essentiality paradigm. For example, the complementary natures of the antioxidant functions of vitamin E, vitamin C and selenium suggest that any one "spares" the need for the others in protecting against lipid peroxidation. Thus, the antioxidant nutrients appear to be risk modifiers of disease rather than primary agents in their etiologies.

ARE NON-NUTRIENTS REQUIRED?

The nutritional essentiality paradigm relates only to nutrients (i.e., dietary factors that are absorbed and function in normal host metabolism). Yet, it has become evident that some such non-nutrients (e.g., fiber) can positively affect health through functions that are technically external to the body. Several positive physiologic responses have been associated with the consumption of isolated fiber fractions or fiber-containing foods. Epidemiology has revealed associations of fiber-rich diets with reduced risks of cancer, coronary heart disease, diabetes mellitus, diverticulosis, hypertension and gallstone formation in people. Yet, under the nutritional essentiality paradigm, these effects are not easily described.

NEW PARADIGM

A new paradigm for nutrition is emerging out of the limitations of the essentiality paradigm. It takes an individualized view of organisms. It recognizes both endogenous and exogenous conditions as determinants of the dietary needs for definable health outcomes. These outcomes are not necessarily specifically associated with single nutrients. It recognizes these factors as nutrients if their activities benefit the metabolism and/or gastrointestinal function of the host. It recognizes various outcomes as appropriate for various individuals, both within a species/population, as well as between species.

Freedom from overt physiologic dysfunction and reduced risk of chronic diseases have become important outcomes in human and pet nutrition. Nutritional needs will be based on individual genetic and metabolic characteristics to the end that foods can be prescribed on an individual basis.

Its having become rather elastic in its application indicates that the nutritional essentiality paradigm has been outgrown: Nutrients have come to be described as being required/essential for particular functions. Some are called dispensable/indispensable under certain conditions. Several are recognized as beneficial at levels greater than may be required.

Outgrowth of the old paradigm is occurring at an increasing pace with the development of the modern field of molecular biology. It is now clear that some nutrients function as gene regulators and that genetic bases can predispose to disease. The time is quickly approaching when it will be possible to identify disease predisposition, metabolic characteristics and specific dietary needs individually. Then, the population-based paradigm will be defunct and a new way of thinking about dietary needs will emerge.

*Excerpted from an article originally published by PetFood Industry in July/August 1998, pages 31-43.

lulose, cellulose and lignin; however, the pectins are lost. Acid detergent fiber (ADF) is determined by boiling the analytical sample in an acidic detergent solution. The fraction remaining contains cellulose and lignin. The result of subtracting the amounts of ADF and NDF in a particular food or ingredient approximates the hemicellulose content. Like the limitations of crude fiber determinations, NDF and ADF do not measure the more soluble fiber fractions of pectins and gums; therefore, they are not widely used to determine fiber in pet foods.

Requirements

Fiber is not considered essential in the diets of cats and dogs, although it is often included in commercial foods. Overall, dogs and cats do not derive much energy from absorbing the typical end products of bacterial fermentation; however, short-chain fatty acids are important in maintaining colonic health. Therefore, a small amount of fiber (<5%) that contains both rapidly and slowly fermentable fibers is recommended in foods for healthy pets (Chapters 13 and 20). Today, much interest exists in human and veterinary nutrition about the role of "pharmacologic doses" of certain nutrients (e.g., fiber) in preventing chronic diseases (**Box 5-7**).

Fiber also aids in managing diseases such as obesity, diabetes mellitus, diarrhea, colitis and constipation. The types and amounts of dietary fiber required to assist in the management of these diseases can be found in Chapters 27, 29, 56, 62 and 64.

Deficiencies

Total deficiency of fiber in typical pet foods is not a practical problem because many ingredients contain some fiber. Homemade foods, veterinary therapeutic foods made with more refined ingredients and purified diets used in research studies can be extremely low in fiber. Some dietary fiber that produces short-chain fatty acids is usually recommended.

Excess/Toxicity

Excess fiber may have undesirable effects. For instance, certain fiber types decrease mineral absorption. The effects on mineral absorption vary by type of fiber and the mineral. More rapidly fermentable fibers (e.g., pectins and guar gum) appear to decrease availability of some minerals, whereas fibers that contain more cellulose have little effect on mineral absorption.

Excess fiber can dilute the energy and nutrient content of the food to such an extent that an animal may have difficulty eating enough of the food to meet its needs. Controlled levels of fiber are advantageous in weight-reducing foods for dogs and cats; however, such foods are fortified so that only total energy intake is low and other nutrients are present in adequate amounts to meet daily requirements.

Sources

The maximum crude fiber content of pet foods must be listed in the guaranteed analysis section of pet food labels in the United States. Most dog and cat foods have DM crude fiber contents of less than 5%. The fiber in most pet foods comes from a variety of ingredients. Grains such as whole corn and brown rice are sources of fiber in dry extruded foods. Some pet foods contain specific ingredients added to provide fiber. Fiber sources commonly used in pet foods today include the hulls from rice, soybeans, peanuts and oats, dried beet pulp, various vegetable gums, corn bran, wheat bran, rice bran, oat bran and more purified fiber sources such as oligosaccharides, cellulose and soy fiber. AAFCO publishes official definitions of fiber ingredients (2007). **Table 5-9** lists common fiber ingredients with fiber content and general classifications of solubility and fermentability.

Table 5-9. Characteristics of selected fiber ingredients.

Fiber ingredient	Crude fiber (%)*	Total dietary fiber (%)*	Solubility in water	Fermentability rate
Apple pectin	0	95	Soluble	Rapid
Beet pulp	20	66	Insoluble	Moderate
Cellulose	80	98	Insoluble	Slow
Citrus pulp	12	77	Soluble	Rapid
Corn bran	19	90	Insoluble	Moderate
Guar gum	0	81	Soluble	Rapid
Gum arabic	0	91	Soluble	Rapid
Pea fiber	30	92	Insoluble	Moderate
Peanut hulls	57	76	Insoluble	Slow
Rice bran	44	13	Insoluble	Moderate
Soy fiber	20	83	Soluble	Rapid
Soy hulls	34	69	Insoluble	Moderate/slow
Sunflower hulls	54	80	Insoluble	Slow
Wheat bran	10	43	Insoluble	Moderate
Wheat middlings	7	46	Insoluble	Moderate

*As is basis.

PROTEIN/AMINO ACIDS

Definition

Proteins are large, complex molecules composed of hundreds to thousands of amino acids. Amino acids are composed of carbon, hydrogen, oxygen, nitrogen and sometimes sulfur and phosphorus. Four chemical groups covalently bonded to a carbon atom form the general structure of amino acids. The four groups include a hydrogen atom, a carboxyl group (COOH), an α-amino group (NH_2) and another chemical group specific for each amino acid (**Table 5-10**). Although hundreds of amino acids exist in nature, only 20 are commonly found as protein components. The amino acids found in mammalian proteins are the L-isomer of α-amino acids, which means the side chain unique to each amino acid is linked to the α-carbon atom in the L (levorotatory) position.

Structure

Proteins are linear polymers of amino acids in which the amino group of one amino acid and the carboxyl group of another amino acid are coupled together (peptide bond) (**Figure 5-15**). Amino acids arranged in chains are referred to as peptides. Two bonded amino acids form a dipeptide, three a tripeptide and more than three a polypeptide.

Proteins can be described as having a primary, secondary, tertiary or quaternary structure. The primary structure of proteins refers to the sequence (order) of amino acids along the polypeptide chain. The secondary structure of proteins refers to the configuration of the polypeptide chains resulting from hydrogen bonds between adjacent amino acids. Alpha-helices, β-pleated sheets or random coils are formed by these hydrogen bonds. The tertiary structure describes how further interactions of the amino acids cause folding and bending of the polypeptide chain giving the protein its biologic activity. Proteins have a quaternary structure if they contain more than one polypeptide chain. Hydrogen, electrostatic and ionic bonds form between the polypeptide chains and stabilize the aggregates. The primary structure of proteins is responsible for the secondary, tertiary and quaternary structures that are formed.

Other compounds bound to peptides may also classify proteins. Simple proteins are made up of only amino acids. Simple proteins are subclassified into fibrous or globular proteins according to shape, solubility and chemical composition. Fibrous proteins include collagens, elastins and keratins, which are the major structural proteins in the body. Collagens are the main proteins of connective tissues and make up about 30% of the total proteins in the body. Elastin is the protein found in tendons and arteries. Keratins are the main proteins in hair. All enzymes, hormones and antibodies that are proteins have a globular structure. Subgroups of globular proteins include the albumins, histones, globulins and protamines.

Conjugated proteins contain amino acids and carbohydrates (glycoproteins), lipids (lipoproteins) or minerals (phosphoproteins, chromoproteins). Glycoproteins are commonly found as components of cell membranes and function to modulate enzymes, receptors and immune function and to recognize cells (antigen and blood types). Glycoproteins are also components of mucous secretions that act as lubricants in many parts of the body, myelin that surrounds nervous tissue and as part of lipoproteins. Lipoproteins transport lipids in the bloodstream in a water-miscible form to tissues. Lipoproteins are typically classified into four main categories according to their density: 1) chylomicrons, 2) very low-density lipoproteins (VLDL), 3) LDL and 4) high-density lipoproteins (HDL) (Chapter 28). Proteins that contain minerals include hemoglobin (iron), cytochromes (copper) and caseins (phosphorus).

Some proteins in the body contain special amino acids that are derived from common amino acids. Collagen contains hydroxyproline and hydroxylysine, which are derivatives of proline and lysine, respectively. Triiodothyronine and tetraiodothyronine (thyroxine) are derived from tyrosine and function as hormones and part of the protein thyroglobulin. Gamma-carboxyglutamic acid is derived from glutamic acid and is key for the function of calcium binding in thrombin, which functions in blood clotting. Other amino acids such as taurine (a β-amino acid) and γ-aminobutyric acid function in specific roles in the body, but are not found as part of proteins.

Purines (adenine and guanine) and pyrimidines (cytosine, thymine, uracil) are other nitrogen-containing molecules that form nucleic acids. Nucleic acids (RNA and DNA) carry the genetic information that codes for the primary structure of proteins (the amino acid sequence).

Function

Proteins are the principal structural constituents of body organs and tissues including: 1) collagen and elastin found in cartilage, tendons and ligaments, 2) the contractile proteins actin and myosin in muscles, 3) keratin proteins in skin, hair and nails and 4) blood proteins including hemoglobin, transferrin, albumin and globulin. Proteins also function as enzymes, hormones (e.g., insulin) and antibodies. Amino acids can serve as a source of energy after the nitrogen-containing amino group is removed by deamination or transamination.

Importance of Amino Acids

Several amino acids are classified as essential or indispensable (10 for dogs and 11 for cats). These amino acids cannot be synthesized by the body in sufficient quantities and therefore must be supplied by food. The carbon skeletons of these essential amino acids are the critical component that the body cannot synthesize. Many of the remaining amino acids are nonessential or dispensable; they can be synthesized in the body from carbon and nitrogen building blocks and need not be present in the food if adequate nitrogen and energy are available. Some amino acids are conditionally essential. These amino acids ordinarily are not required in the food except during certain physiologic or pathologic conditions when they may not be synthesized in adequate quantities.

Although nonessential amino acids can be made from precursor carbon skeletons, they are just as critical to the makeup of proteins and are just as essential for metabolic reactions in the body as essential amino acids. Protein is also necessary to provide the body with a source of nitrogen for synthesis of other nitrogen-containing compounds including purines, pyrimidines, nucleotides, nucleic acids, creatinine, nitric oxide and some neurotransmitters.

Metabolism

Digestion and Absorption

Dietary proteins must be digested to be absorbed from the GI tract. Protein digestion begins in the stomach with the action of the enzyme pepsin in the presence of hydrochloric acid. The main end products of gastric protein digestion are mixtures of large polypeptides; however, little or no absorption of these molecules occurs. In the small intestine, the pancreas and cells lining the small intestine secrete other enzymes (endopeptidases and exopeptidases). These enzymes break the bonds between the amino acids of large polypeptides resulting in free amino acids, dipeptides and tripeptides that can be absorbed across the intestinal wall (Mathews, 1991). Some proteins are less readily digested than others. The rapidity of digestion is influenced by many factors, including protein structure, processing effects, other nutrients in the meal and the presence of enzyme inhibitory factors.

Absorption of amino acids is a sodium-dependent, active-transport process that requires energy (ATP). This process is mediated by four different carrier systems that transport neutral amino acids, basic amino acids, dicarboxylic amino acids and imino acids. These separate carrier systems help ensure trans-

Table 5-10. Amino acids.

Name	Structural formula	Abbreviations		Side chain	Essentiality
		3-letter	1-letter		
Alanine	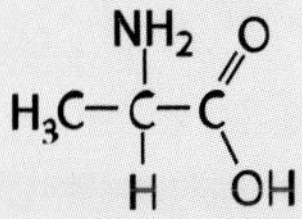	Ala	A	Aliphatic	Nonessential
Arginine	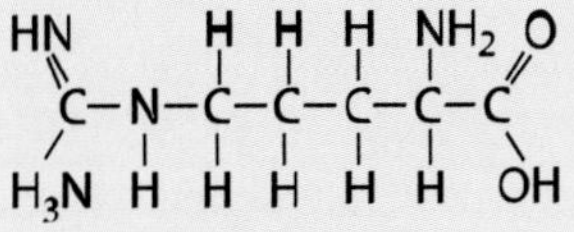	Arg	R	Basic	Essential
Asparagine	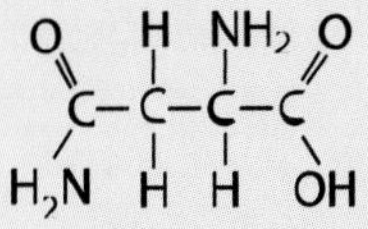	Asn	N	Acidic	Nonessential
Aspartate	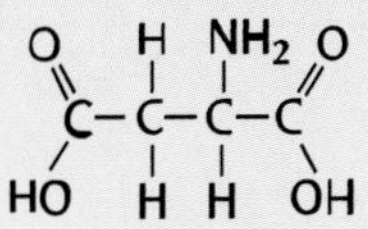	Asp	D	Acidic	Nonessential
Cysteine	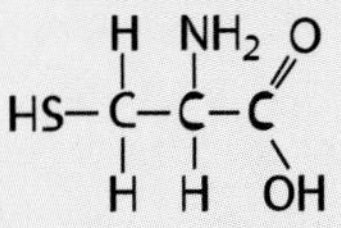	Cys	C	Sulfur containing	Nonessential, but can provide for up to 50% of methionine requirements
Glutamate	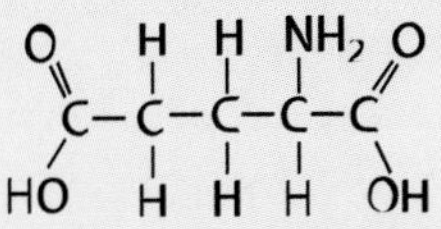	Glu	E	Acidic	Nonessential
Glutamine	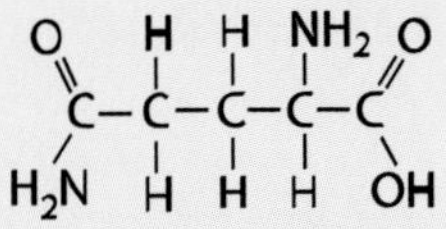	Gln	Q	Acidic	Conditionally essential
Glycine	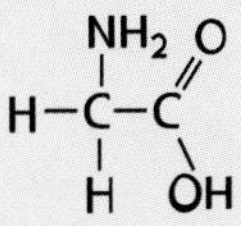	Gly	G	Aliphatic	Nonessential
Histidine	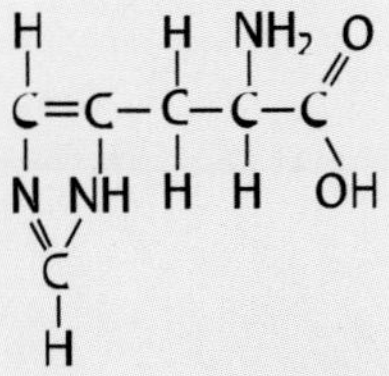	His	H	Basic and aromatic	Essential
Isoleucine	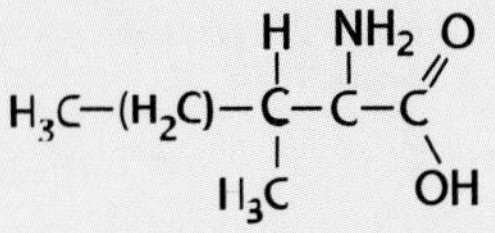	Ile	I	Aliphatic branched chain	Essential
Leucine	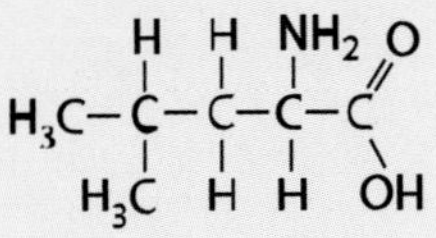	Leu	L	Aliphatic branched chain	Essential

Table 5-10. Amino acids (continued).

Name	Structural formula	Abbreviations		Side chain	Essentiality
		3-letter	1-letter		
Lysine	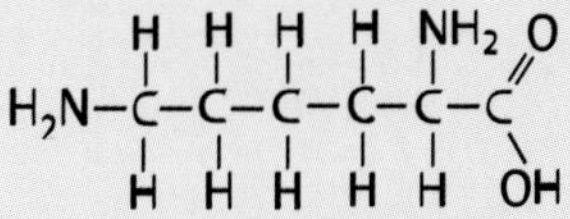	Lys	K	Basic	Essential
Methionine	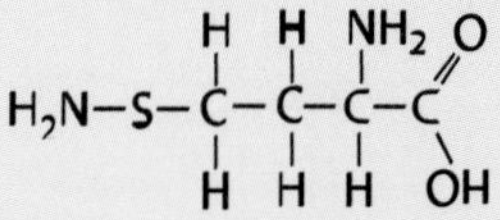	Met	M	Sulfur containing	Essential
Phenylalanine	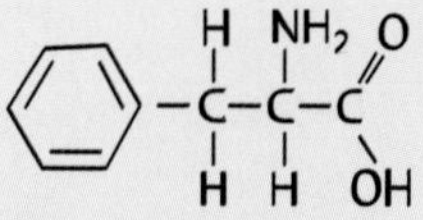	Phe	F	Aromatic	Essential
Proline	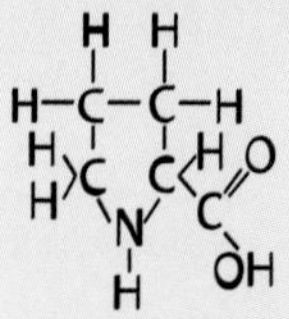	Pro	P	Imino acid	Nonessential
Serine	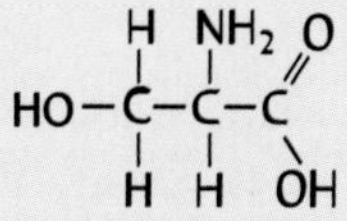	Ser	S	Aliphatic	Nonessential
Taurine	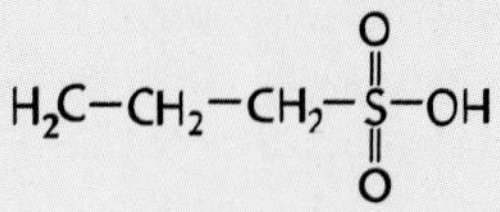	Tau		Beta-amino acid and sulfonic acid group	Essential for cats; possibly conditionally essential for dogs
Threonine	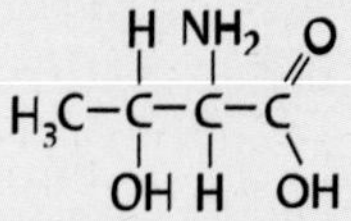	Thr	T	Aliphatic	Essential
Tryptophan	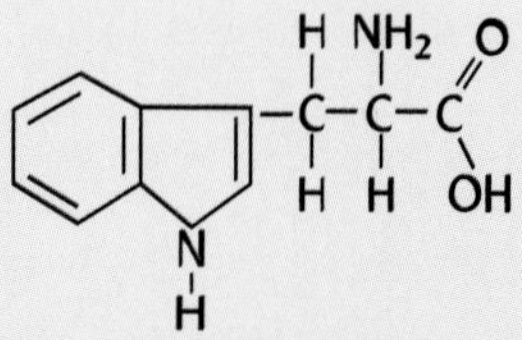	Trp	W	Aromatic	Essential
Tyrosine	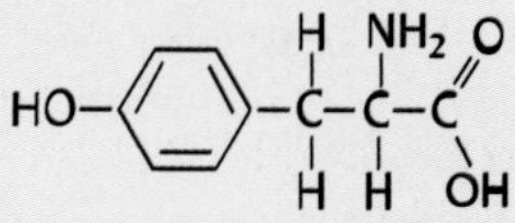	Tyr	Y	Aromatic	Nonessential, but can provide for up to 50% of phenylalanine requirements
Valine	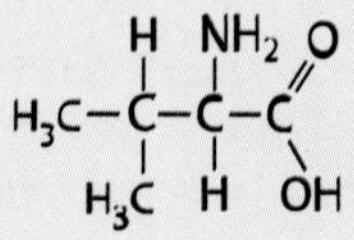	Val	V	Aliphatic branched chain	Essential

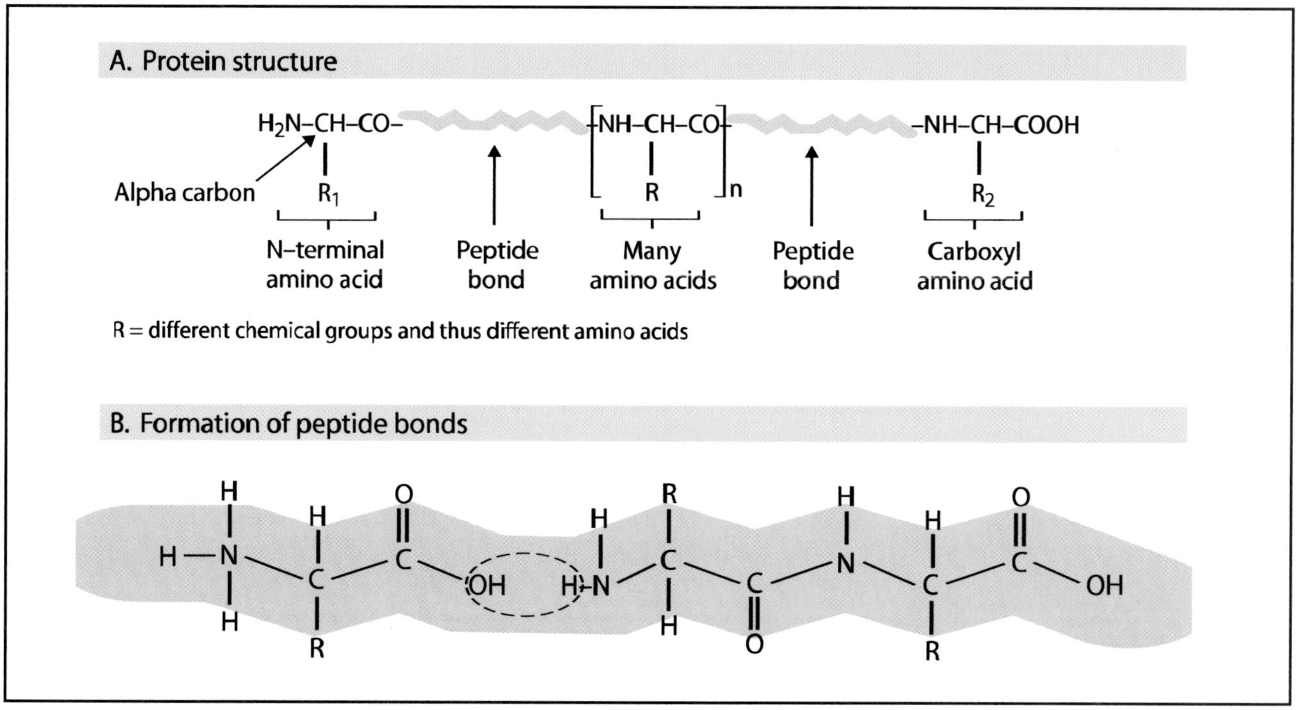

Figure 5-15. Protein structure (A) and formation of peptide bonds (B). The dotted lines show how the peptide bonds are formed, with the production of water. R = the remainder of amino acids. For example, in glycine, R = $(CH_2)_2$–COOH.

port of a well balanced mixture of amino acids from the intestinal lumen to the portal vein.

Amino acids and proteins not absorbed in the small intestine can be fermented in the hindgut and produce fecal odor compounds. These compounds are produced by bacterial enzymes during the degradation of endogenous and undigested food proteins. The fecal odor compounds include ammonia, aliphatic amines, indoles, phenols and volatile sulfur-containing compounds. These compounds not only affect fecal odors but can also seriously affect the GI health of animals (Hussein and Sunvold, 2000). The amount of dietary amino acids that reach the large intestine can alter fecal compounds. The amount of amino acids reaching the large intestine can be affected by high food DM intake, high protein foods and foods that contain low quality proteins. An increase in protein and amino acid flow to the large intestine can result in more substrate for the resident bacteria and an increase in fecal odor components (Yamka et al, 2006; Hussein and Sunvold, 2000).

Many studies investigating altering fecal odor compounds have focused on the use of prebiotics. Researchers found that feeding adult dogs FOS (0.5% of the DM) decreased putrescine, cadaverine, tyramine and total amines (Hussein and Sunvold, 2000). This study demonstrated that fecal odor could be manipulated by prebiotics; however, few studies have focused on fecal components related to protein source. Another study found that dogs consuming poultry by-product meal produced more fecal odor compounds than dogs fed soy-based foods (Yamka et al, 2006). The reduction of fecal odor compounds in soy-fed dogs was likely the result of hindgut fermentation of soluble fiber and oligosaccharides present in soy.

Apparent vs. True Digestibility

Estimations of crude protein and amino acid availabilities of most feed ingredients can be provided by determining apparent ileal protein and amino acid digestibilites. Apparent digestibilities are determined by comparing the amounts of amino acids present in the feed and digesta without determining endogenous nitrogen losses. For determining true ileal amino acid digestibilities, undigested dietary amino acids present in the ileal digesta should be differentiated from endogenous amino acids. Recent studies suggest that endogenous nitrogen losses are higher than previously estimated and that differences in apparent digestibilities between feedstuffs are attributed to differences in endogenous gut nitrogen losses rather than differences in true digestibilities (Nyachoti et al, 1997). Factors such as body weight, dietary fiber content, DM intake and the presence of anti-nutritive factors in the diet influence secretions and/or reabsorption of endogenous gut protein (Nyachoti et al, 1997).

Several methods exist for estimating the contribution of endogenous protein and amino acids at the distal ileum; three are used most commonly. The first method is a direct method for measuring endogenous protein. This method requires that animals be fed a protein-free diet. It is assumed that the recovery of endogenous protein and amino acids at the distal ileum is the same for animals fed protein-free and protein-containing diets (Nissen, 1992; Burns et al, 1982; Kendall et al, 1982). The second method is the regression method. The regression method determines endogenous protein and amino acid recoveries in digesta with the aid of regression to zero protein intake using a series of test source protein levels. However, with the regression method, no relationship is assumed between protein

Table 5-11. Glucogenic and ketogenic amino acids.

Exclusively ketogenic	Leucine, lysine
Exclusively glucogenic	Alanine, serine, glycine, cysteine, aspartate, asparagine, glutamate, glutamine, arginine, histidine, valine, threonine, methionine, proline
Ketogenic and glucogenic	Isoleucine, phenylalanine, tyrosine, tryptophan

Table 5-12. Factors for converting nitrogen to crude protein.

Food protein	Nitrogen (g/kg)	Conversion factor
Barley, oats, wheat	171.5	5.83
Corn, eggs, meat	160.0	6.25
Milk	156.8	6.38
Soybeans	175.1	5.71

intake and the recovery of endogenous protein and amino acids (Nissen, 1992). The third method for determining the recovery of endogenous protein is the ^{15}N-isotope dilution technique. The endogenous protein is labeled, secreted into the GI tract via a continuous infusion of ^{15}N-leucine. This method directly measures the contribution of endogenous to total protein recovered at the distal ileum in animals fed protein-containing foods (Grala et al, 1998; Nissen, 1992).

True, rather than apparent, ileal amino acid digestibilities should be used when formulating diets, but this requires further development of methods for routine estimation of endogenous nitrogen losses. Improvements in protein usage should be sought via reducing endogenous nitrogen losses and improving true ileal amino acid digestibilites (Nyachoti et al, 1997).

Protein Usage

Absorbed amino acids and small di- and tripeptides are reassembled into "new" proteins by the liver and other tissues of the body. Amino acids from food are transported from the liver to other tissues by serum albumin or as free amino acids. The fate of amino acids after absorption falls into three general categories: 1) tissue protein synthesis, especially in muscles and liver, 2) synthesis of enzymes, albumin, hormones and other nitrogen-containing compounds and 3) deamination and use of the remaining carbon skeletons for energy.

A high rate of protein synthesis occurs in production of red and white blood cells, epithelial cells of the skin and those lining the GI tract (i.e., intestinal mucosa, which produces exocrine secretions, such as digestive enzymes and mucus) and the pancreas. In addition, all body proteins are continuously broken down and resynthesized, a process known as protein turnover. Some proteins (muscle proteins and some plasma proteins such as albumin) have a relatively long lifetime (days to weeks). Other proteins (cytokines and enzymes) have relatively short lives (minutes to hours).

Muscle protein composes nearly 50% of total body protein, but only accounts for 30% of new protein synthesized, whereas visceral and organ proteins compose a smaller portion of total body protein but account for 50% of new proteins synthesized. Because protein turnover is the sum total of the continuous degradation and synthesis cycles of specific proteins, a measure of protein turnover is only a "snapshot" in time of protein metabolism. In addition, rates of protein synthesis and degradation for any particular protein can change under different physiologic conditions.

The body is able to synthesize new proteins and enzymes provided all the necessary amino acids are available. The source of amino acids is not important. Cells use amino acids from a variety of sources including those derived from food proteins, single amino acids added to the food and amino acids synthesized by the body. In addition, cells synthesizing new protein cannot distinguish between amino acids from grains (e.g., corn and rice) and those from meats (e.g., chicken and beef). The only criterion is that all the amino acids needed to synthesize a particular protein be present in sufficient quantities when necessary. Protein synthesis will be limited when certain amino acids are not present or available in the quantities needed.

During protein turnover, a fraction of amino acids enter catabolic pathways that lead to their permanent loss. The amount of nitrogen lost every day as a result of the body's continuous breakdown process is called obligatory nitrogen loss. Dietary protein must be consumed each day to replace amino acids lost to catabolism. Trauma, infection, severe sepsis and burns increase protein turnover and nitrogen losses, whereas nitrogen losses are reduced during long-term fasting and starvation. Nitrogen is normally lost from the body in feces (nitrogen, proteins, cells), in urine and through skin desquamation and loss of hair.

Nitrogen balance is the net difference between nitrogen consumed and lost; however, the determination is fraught with technical difficulties. Most commonly, nitrogen losses are underestimated through incomplete collection of feces, urine, hair and sloughed cutaneous cells; whereas, nitrogen intake is routinely overestimated. Thus, nitrogen balance should only be regarded as a crude estimate of body protein status and not be used to distinguish among subtleties in protein and nitrogen metabolism.

Protein Storage

Although, in effect, there is some storage of excess amino acids, they are not stored to the same degree that extra fat and carbohydrates are stored. Structural proteins in all tissues, especially in muscles and liver and serum albumin, can be considered as amino acid stores. Muscle protein represents the largest reserve from which amino acids may be drawn in times of need. Too much loss of body protein impairs muscle function. Liver and muscle protein and serum albumin synthesis increase after consumption of a protein-containing meal. After protein synthesis is maximized, excess amino acids are deaminated and transaminated to yield amino groups and carbon skeletons. The carbon skeletons can be used for many purposes including glucose precursors, which can be stored as glycogen or converted to fatty acids and acetyl-CoA, which can be used for fuel immediately. In the hours after consumption of a meal containing protein, body protein synthesis gradually declines as the amino acids from the meal are used. Because protein turnover and obligatory nitrogen losses continue to occur, muscles must convert from net uptake to net release of amino acids as fasting becomes dominant. Although glycogen and lipids are the preferred short-term and long-term energy stores, protein catabolism can supply carbon skeletons needed to maintain glucose pools and supply the body with energy (ATP). Protein degradation continues until the next meal, after which protein synthesis exceeds protein breakdown.

The carbon skeletons of catabolized amino acids can be completely oxidized to carbon dioxide or converted by the liver to glucose or ketone bodies. Thus, amino acids can be glucogenic or ketogenic. Glucogenic amino acids can be converted to glucose through pyruvate or any of the TCA cycle intermediates. Ketogenic amino acids are those that can be converted to acetyl-CoA or ketone bodies but cannot be metabolized to glucose. Some catabolized amino acids yield two different carbon skeletons, one ketogenic and the other glucogenic (**Table 5-11**).

Protein Excretion

Amino acid catabolism produces waste nitrogen, if it is not used for purine or pyrimidine synthesis. Catabolism of amino acids typically leads to formation of ammonia, which is toxic to body cells. Ammonia must be converted to a less toxic form that can be transported in blood and excreted. Ammonia formation occurs in all tissues, but is especially prevalent in the liver and kidneys during gluconeogenesis. More than 90% of the nitrogen resulting from protein degradation is converted to urea in the liver and kidneys and then excreted in urine. A smaller fraction of nitrogen is lost as ammonia, creatinine and nitrate. Hepatic and renal detoxification of ammonia via the urea cycle is a critical function. The amino acids ornithine, citrulline and arginine are key intermediates. Other amino acids (e.g., glutamate, aspartate, alanine and the amide group of glutamine) carry excess amino groups from other tissues to the liver and kidneys for conversion to urea. Catabolism of other nitrogen-containing metabolites also contributes to the waste nitrogen pool.

CLINICAL PROBLEMS ASSOCIATED WITH NITROGEN DISPOSAL

Hyperammonemia may result if any of the enzymes involved in the urea cycle are lacking or have impaired activity. Part of the therapy for any disease (e.g., liver disease) in which urea cycle function is reduced is to decrease plasma concentrations of ammonia. Reducing total protein intake, reducing intake of nonessential amino acids and substituting keto analogues of some amino acids may help reduce the ammonia load. Other measures (e.g., dialysis, transfusion, administration of drugs and other compounds that trap nitrogenous metabolites) can be used to prevent an ammonia encephalopathy crisis (Chapter 68).

Reduced renal function may also impair nitrogen disposal (i.e., urea may not be excreted efficiently). Reducing waste products of protein catabolism through dietary manipulation aids therapy for chronic renal failure (Chapter 37).

Catabolism of purines (adenine and guanine from nucleotides, ATP and GTP, RNA and DNA) may also create nitrogen disposal problems. Uric acid is the end product of purine catabolism in people, nonhuman primates, birds and Dalmatian dogs; all other mammals produce allantoin. Uric acid and allantoin are excreted in urine and feces. Accumulation of uric acid in serum can lead to gout (uric acid crystals in joints) and uric acid uroliths. Hyperuricemia can be treated with drugs (allopurinol) and with dietary intervention. Reducing total protein intake and reducing or eliminating dietary ingredients containing high levels of purines (organ meats, glandular meats, fish such as mackerel and sardines) have been successful in some dogs with urolithiasis (Chapter 39).

Protein-losing enteropathy (PLE) and protein-losing nephropathy (PLN) are two syndromes in which excessive amounts of protein are lost from the body. PLE is a group of diseases characterized by excessive loss of serum protein into the intestinal tract. Causes of PLE include lymphatic disorders (lymphangiectasia, neoplasia, congestive heart failure) and diseases associated with increased mucosal permeability or mucosal ulceration (intestinal neoplasia, granulomatous enteritis, lymphocytic-plasmacytic enteritis, intestinal parasitism, etc.).

PLN is characterized by excessive loss of serum protein into urine. Causes of PLN include glomerulonephritis and amyloidosis that develop secondary to chronic inflammatory conditions such as neoplasia, heartworm disease, ehrlichiosis, systemic mycosis, brucellosis, osteomyelitis and immune-mediated disease.

Analyses of Protein

Chemical Analyses of Protein

Protein concentration in foods (crude protein content) is typically calculated from the nitrogen content by the Kjeldahl method or Dumas combustion procedure. The Kjeldahl method involves digesting the food sample with sulfuric acid, which converts all nitrogen in amino acids to ammonia. The ammonia is distilled, collected and quantified using a colorimetric titration procedure. The Dumas combustion procedure requires no hazardous materials and involves measuring the nitrogen gas after combustion and total destruction of the sample. This method has been adopted as an acceptable method for measuring total nitrogen in animal foods (Etheridge et al, 1998). When using either method, two assumptions are made in calculating crude protein from nitrogen. First, that all nitrogen in the food sample is present as protein and second, that all protein contains 16% nitrogen. The crude protein content of the food is then calculated: crude protein in food (g/kg) = g nitrogen in food/kg x 6.25.

Neither assumption is always true. Not all nitrogen in food is present as protein; some nitrogen is present as free amino acids, amides, glycosides, alkaloids and ammonium salts. Other nitrogen is complexed with lipids. Different protein ingredients in food also have different nitrogen contents and, therefore, different conversion factors (**Table 5-12**). The use of an average conversion factor (i.e., 6.25) for all proteins in food simplifies calculations and can be rationalized by keeping in mind that most pet foods are mixtures of protein-containing ingredients. In addition, animal protein requirements are typically calculated from determination of individual amino acid requirements that are converted to nitrogen requirements and then expressed as a protein requirement by multiplying nitrogen by 6.25. Although the crude protein content of pet foods gives a measure of the amount of nitrogen available to the animal, it does not provide information about protein quality or the nutritional value of the protein source(s).

Protein Quality

Protein quality refers to the efficiency by which amino acids from food are converted into tissue. That efficiency in turn depends on the protein source, concentration of essential amino acids in the food and their availability (Brown, 1989). Proteins that provide optimal proportions of all essential amino acids are referred to as high quality proteins. When a protein lacks one or more of the essential amino acids (limiting amino acid), the quality of the protein decreases and it is referred to as a poor quality protein (Orok et al, 1975). Other amino acids may not be used when a limiting amino acid is absent. Poor protein quality can also result from an excess of certain amino acids that may interfere with usage of other amino acids. (See Imbalance and Antagonism.) Digestibility can influence protein quality and can be affected by ash content, processing time and/or temperature. The amino acids of poor quality protein cannot be properly digested and used by the animal. For example, overcooking can form indigestible nutrient forms called Maillard complexes. Processing methods and heat treatment of various feedstuffs can also affect digestibility. Researchers studied the effects of processing temperature and time on nutrient quality of moist dog food (Jamikorn et al, 2000). They demonstrated that raising the processing temperature (6°C) or increasing the processing time (25 min.) may alter nutrient content and digestion.

Other factors that can affect protein availability include fiber content, tannins, pectins, oligosaccharides and phytase or trypsin inhibitors, which can be found in plant protein sources. Proteins of plant origin generally have lower digestibility than animal proteins because plant fiber and carbohydrates lower digestion, due to a reduced degradation rate of nutrients in the gut and increased bacterial activity (Murray et al, 1997; Neirinck et al, 1991; Meyer, 1984). Feeding high-fiber diets decreases apparent protein digestibility (Kendall and Holme, 1982), presumably from increased adsorption of amino acids and peptides by fiber, and obstruction of digestive enzymes by fiber components in cell walls (Knabe et al, 1989).

Dogs use poor quality proteins less efficiently (Burns et al, 1982). Poor quality proteins can lead to profound nutritive failure, accompanied by a rapid decline in weight, loss of appetite and eventual death (Palika, 1996; Rose and Rice, 1939). Dogs and cats will increase food intake to meet their protein/amino acid requirements for maintenance if the food contains low quality protein. By understanding the availability of limiting amino acids in a particular food or protein source, nutritionists can improve the protein quality of the food through protein complementation (feeding multiple protein sources) and/or amino acid supplementation. Thus, measuring protein quality becomes necessary in formulating different feedstuffs to supply digestible amino acids or crude protein.

MEASURES OF PROTEIN QUALITY

Several methods have been used to determine the quality of protein sources for animals. Some methods involve testing the protein source by feeding it to animals (in vivo methods), whereas other methods evaluate the protein's quality by chemically analyzing its amino acid composition (in vitro methods). There are a number of ways to measure protein quality in vivo. Many of these tests are based on variations of nitrogen balance experiments.

The first and crudest method is the protein efficiency ratio (PER), which measures the ability of dietary protein to be converted into tissue. The method works only with young, growing animals and may be influenced by the level of energy or fat in the diet and by the level of dietary protein. The PER is calculated as: PER = weight gain of animal ÷ protein intake of animal (Brown, 1989; Burns et al, 1982). The typical PER value for animal proteins is 2.5 (Brown, 1989).

The most frequently used measure of protein quality is biological value (BV), which is defined as the percentage of absorbed protein retained. BV gauges the efficiency with which the body is able to convert absorbed dietary amino acids into tissues. The BV is calculated as: BV = (food nitrogen - [fecal nitrogen + urinary nitrogen]) ÷ (food nitrogen + fecal nitrogen) (Brown, 1989; Burns et al, 1982; Davidson et al, 1979). There are some practical problems using BV as a measure of protein quality. It is possible for a protein source to lack high digestibility, but have a high BV if the residue is absorbed and well used by the animal (Brown, 1989).

To account for these differences in digestibility, a new method (net protein utilization) was established for determining protein quality. This method, unlike BV, includes allowances for nitrogen losses during digestion and is equal to BV multiplied by true digestibility. Use of the coefficient allows for adjustments to determine differences in true and apparent availability of dietary amino acids for the animal (Brown, 1989; Burns et al, 1982; Davidson et al, 1979).

The amino acid score (AAS) is a chemical method for comparing the amount of the first limiting amino acid in a test protein with the level of the same amino acid found in a reference protein. The AAS is calculated as: AAS = mg of amino acid/g of test protein ÷ mg of amino acid/g of reference protein. This method for measuring protein quality is very rapid and highly reproducible. Because it is derived solely from amino acid composition, AAS does not compensate for differences in digestibility that can be caused by processing (Brown, 1989; Food and Agriculture Organization of the United Nations, 1973).

The slope ratio method is a biologic equivalent of the AAS. The slope ratio method compares the growth performance produced by a test protein with that of a reference protein such as defatted whole egg (Samonds and Hegsted, 1977). The slope ratio (SR) is calculated as: SR = slope of response curve for ani-

Table 5-13. Small intestinal and total tract crude protein and small intestinal amino acid digestibility of dog foods containing animal protein sources.*

Ingredient	% CP of dog foods	Carbohydrate source	Total tract CPD (%)	Small intestinal CPD(%)	Arg (%)	His (%)	Iso (%)	Leu (%)	Lys (%)	Met (%)	Phe (%)	Thr (%)	Try (%)	Val (%)
Beef and bone meal[1]	25	Corn/wheat	82.4	68.3	79.4	68.5	73.1	78.5	74.8	84.7	74.8	58.5	-	70.0
Beef, fresh[2]	20	Rice	89.8	80.4	92.4	84.1	88.4	88.5	87.2	91.0	80.6	77.3	-	86.3
Chicken and chicken by-product meal[3]	33	Cornstarch	85.1	73.4	86.8	76.2	77.9	78.9	80.3	86.0	75.2	69.0	-	74.7
With beet pulp inclusion (9% TDF)[3]	33	Cornstarch	83.9	70.9	87.3	75.4	78.3	79.1	80.0	87.2	72.8	67.2	-	74.7
With low-cellulose mixture inclusion (10% TDF)[3]	33	Cornstarch	83.2	66.1	83.4	68.7	71.1	74.1	68.2	86.2	69.0	62.7	-	68.9
With high-cellulose mixture inclusion (10% TDF)[3]	33	Cornstarch	82.4	76.7	87.9	77.6	79.1	81.0	78.6	86.7	77.4	72.0	-	77.2
With Solka Floc inclusion (9% TDF)[3]	33	Cornstarch	86.7	77.8	88.7	80.0	81.5	82.6	83.5	87.7	78.0	73.6	-	79.0
Egg, whole[2]	20	Rice	91.2	77.0	91.5	80.5	88.4	87.5	84.8	91.4	76.1	72.7	-	86.2
Lamb meal[6]	20	Corn	79.7	67.0	77.4	60.4	66.7	74.5	62.4	84.3	57.0	52.0	-	63.8
Meat and bone meal, rendered[2]	20	Rice	88.2	79.9	91.6	82.8	88.7	88.1	86.8	91.7	79.9	76.3	-	86.9
Meat and bone meal, high ash[6]	20	Corn	83.2	72.7	88.5	79.2	85.6	87.5	83.8	92.7	77.4	77.9	-	82.8
Meat and bone meal, low ash[6]	20	Corn	79.7	65.7	83.7	68.9	69.8	76.6	69.7	86.6	62.6	59.9	-	70.0
Meat and bone meal, low temperature[6]	20	Corn	85.2	76.4	88.8	79.4	83.7	86.0	83.4	93.3	75.5	75.8	-	82.4
Poultry by-product meal[1,5,6,7]	20	Rice	89.5	73.9	88.5	74.5	84.0	83.5	80.1	84.7	73.4	67.3	-	81.2
	25	Corn/wheat	81.6	77.2	86.8	80.1	81.8	83.9	82.2	87.6	80.4	71.3	-	70.0
	35	Rice	75.5	74.4	89.0	78.8	77.2	78.1	80.5	79.0	82.0	67.9	-	72.2
	35	Corn	77.9	63.0	75.6	60.5	66.0	68.1	65.2	77.7	66.6	52.1	-	60.0
With beet pulp inclusion (7% TDF)[7]	35	Rice	75.4	66.3	88.3	73.3	72.1	73.6	75.3	74.1	79.2	57.3	-	65.5
With soy hull inclusion I:S = 1.86 (7% TDF)[7]	35	Rice	74.1	66.2	86.8	73.2	73.0	75.0	75.2	71.8	77.6	61.1	-	69.1
With soy hull inclusion I:S = 2.65 (8% TDF)[7]	35	Rice	72.7	57.2	85.5	66.4	66.7	68.6	70.1	81.2	74.2	52.3	-	60.3
With soy hull inclusion I:S = 3.17 (9% TDF)[7]	35	Rice	78.4	59.3	85.0	65.9	65.9	67.8	69.1	69.5	74.4	52.2	-	59.4
With soy hull inclusion I:S = 5.18 (7% TDF)[7]	35	Rice	70.9	67.4	85.3	70.1	71.8	73.3	74.6	68.8	76.9	60.3	-	67.1
With soy hull inclusion I:S = 7.21 (8% TDF)[7]	35	Rice	73.9	69.5	86.7	71.7	72.7	73.8	75.5	72.3	77.7	60.7	-	67.9
With high protein corn[5]	35	Corn	75.4	64.7	80.8	64.3	70.3	72.6	69.9	82.1	70.2	59.1	-	65.5
With high protein, low-phytate corn[5]	35	Corn	76.8	57.0	76.6	56.2	63.6	64.8	64.4	74.3	63.7	51.9	-	58.3
With high amylose corn[5]	35	Corn	69.7	65.4	76.1	56.5	65.4	66.9	64.7	78.9	65.8	54.0	-	60.8
With amylomaize starch[5]	35	Corn	72.6	62.9	76.1	53.8	64.8	64.6	63.8	82.8	64.2	51.7	-	69.5
Poultry by-product meal, low ash[6]	20	Corn	80.1	68.0	78.0	63.6	69.8	75.0	65.5	83.4	56.7	54.2	-	65.5
Poultry by-product meal, high ash[6]	20	Corn	82.3	68.4	78.3	61.8	67.7	74.4	64.1	84.7	55.0	52.7	-	63.2
Poultry, fresh[2]	20	Rice	89.8	82.8	93.6	86.1	90.8	91.0	89.5	93.4	84.2	81.4	-	89.3
Poultry meal, low ash[4,8,9]	10	Cornstarch/rice	81.0	76.3	88.5	81.7	53.7	78.3	77.1	86.3	78.7	70.2	86.6	72.8
	10	Cornstarch/rice	84.5	73.4	86.2	75.5	78.7	80.2	76.8	92.6	79.0	64.7	83.9	72.3
	15	Cornstarch/rice	84.5	79.3	91.3	86.5	71.4	83.5	83.0	89.0	83.7	77.3	84.7	79.3
	20	Cornstarch/rice	86.3	79.4	90.7	84.4	74.9	83.5	83.0	90.3	83.8	76.8	80.8	78.8
	20	Cornstarch/rice	86.4	72.9	73.4	77.5	83.2	81.3	80.5	86.3	81.9	70.5	72.0	78.0
	25	Cornstarch/rice	86.6	78.1	89.9	83.0	75.4	82.6	82.0	89.0	83.2	75.5	77.2	77.7
Poultry meal, regular ash[1,10,11]	25	Corn/wheat	87.5	73.9	86.9	74.3	78.7	82.0	79.7	86.5	78.7	67.4	-	74.9
	30	Corn	77.2	65.1	80.0	66.5	69.3	73.4	74.9	67.3	60.6	56.7	-	65.9
	30	Potato starch/rice	76.9	72.7	88.3	75.9	79.5	80.3	81.0	79.4	71.6	71.9	-	75.6
Minimum digestibility (%)	-	-	69.7	57.0	73.4	53.8	53.7	64.6	62.4	67.3	55.0	51.7	72.0	58.3
Maximum digestibility (%)	-	-	91.2	82.8	93.6	86.5	90.8	91.0	89.5	93.4	84.2	81.4	86.6	89.3
Average digestibility (%)	-	-	81.2	70.9	85.1	72.9	74.9	78.0	76.2	83.7	73.8	65.0	80.9	72.4

Key: CP = crude protein, CPD = crude protein digestibility, Arg = arginine, His = histidine, Iso = isoleucine, Leu = leucine, Lys = lysine, Met = methionine, Phe = phenylalanine, Thr = thyronine, Try = tryptophan, Val = valine, TDF = total dietary fiber, I:S = insoluble fiber:soluble fiber.

*Adapted from [1]Bednar GE, Patil AR, Murray SM, et al. Starch and fiber fractions in selected food and feed ingredients affect their small intestinal digestibility and fermentability and their large bowel fermentability in vitro in a canine model. Journal of Nutrition 2001; 131: 276-286. [2]Murray SM, Patil AR, Fahey GC Jr, et al. Raw and rendered animal by-products as ingredients in dog diets. Journal of Animal Science 1997; 75: 2497-2505. [3]Muir HE, Murray SM, Fahey GC Jr, et al. Nutrient digestion by ileal cannulated dogs as affected by dietary fibers with various fermentation characteristics. Journal of Animal Science 1996; 74: 1641-1648. [4]Yamka RM, Kitts SE, True AD, et al. Evaluation of maize gluten meal as a protein source in canine foods. Animal Feed Science and Technology 2004; 116: 239-248. [5]Gajda M, Flickinger EA, Grieshop CM, et al. Corn hybrid affects in vitro and in vivo measures of nutrient digestibility in dogs. Journal of Animal Science 2005; 83: 160-171. [6]Johnson ML, Parsons CM, Fahey GC Jr, et al. Effects of species raw material source, ash content, and processing temperature on amino acid digestibility of animal by-product meals by cecectomized roosters and ileally cannulated dogs. Journal of Animal Science 1998; 76: 1112-1122. [7]Burkhalter TM, Merchen NR, Bauer LL, et al. The ratio of insoluble to soluble fiber components in soybean hulls affects ileal and total tract nutrient digestibilities and fecal characteristics in dogs. Journal of Nutrition 2001; 131: 1978-1985. [8]Yamka RM, Jamikorn U, True AD, et al. Evaluation of low-ash poultry meal as a protein source in canine foods. Journal of Animal Science 2003; 81: 2279-2284. [9]Yamka RM, Kitts SE, Harmon DL. Evaluation of low-oligosaccharide and low-oligosaccharide low-phytate whole soya beans in canine foods. Animal Feed Science and Technology 2005; 120: 79-91. [10]Zuo Y, Fahey GC Jr, Merchen NR, et al. Digestion responses to low oligosaccharide soybean meal by ileally-cannulated dogs. Journal of Animal Science 1996; 74: 2441-2449. [11]Clapper GM, Grieshop CM, Merchen NR, et al. Ileal and total tract digestibilities and fecal characteristics of dogs as affected by soybean protein inclusion in dry, extruded diets. Journal of Animal Science 2001; 79: 1523-1532.

Table 5-14. Small intestinal and total tract crude protein and small intestinal amino acid digestibility of dog foods containing plant protein sources.*

Ingredient	% CP of dog foods	Carbohydrate source	Total tract CPD (%)	Small intestinal CPD (%)	Arg (%)	His (%)	Iso (%)	Leu (%)	Lys (%)	Met (%)	Phe (%)	Thr (%)	Try (%)	Val (%)
Corn gluten meal[3]	15	Cornstarch/rice	84.7	75.0	85.3	76.6	78.8	85.6	76.6	92.6	83.0	66.0	80.9	74.4
	20	Cornstarch/rice	87.8	79.3	85.2	80.5	80.9	88.9	77.8	91.7	86.4	71.9	79.9	78.1
	25	Cornstarch/rice	90.3	82.5	87.6	84.3	82.9	91.2	80.4	92.8	89.1	75.1	82.9	81.5
	30	Cornstarch/rice	91.1	81.3	86.5	80.4	83.2	90.9	76.4	90.7	88.5	73.9	76.8	79.7
Soybean meal, 48% CP[1,4,5,6,7,8]	10	Cornstarch/rice	68.1	65.4	88.3	82.0	70.1	76.7	79.0	75.6	80.7	57.0	72.9	66.4
	15	Cornstarch/rice	68.6	66.2	88.3	81.0	71.6	75.5	81.2	76.5	80.5	59.6	65.3	66.3
	20	Cornstarch/rice	64.3	59.8	85.2	76.0	63.9	68.8	76.4	70.2	75.4	47.8	51.8	56.4
	20	Cornstarch/rice	78.2	84.8	73.9	81.6	89.1	86.5	86.6	91.2	90.2	75.6	76.7	83.7
	20	Cornstarch/rice	83.2	82.0	72.8	79.2	77.9	77.6	75.5	80.3	81.6	69.9	81.2	69.4
	25	Cornstarch/rice	65.5	51.1	83.5	70.4	59.2	64.0	71.4	63.5	71.7	39.6	39.3	50.3
	25	Corn/wheat	88.4	79.2	89.3	82.0	82.9	85.5	82.9	88.2	82.8	70.7	-	78.1
	30	Corn	84.6	77.4	90.5	83.0	83.9	84.6	85.6	72.6	73.2	70.1	-	78.7
	30	Potato starch/rice	83.9	85.3	93.2	87.3	89.1	88.0	89.3	85.7	83.9	80.1	-	85.3
Soybean meal, low oligo[7]	30	Corn	83.2	78.3	90.5	83.0	83.9	84.6	85.6	72.6	73.2	70.1	-	78.7
Soybean meal, low oligo and low phytate[4]	20	Cornstarch/rice	83.8	79.2	75.7	78.5	76.1	78.2	77.0	79.0	82.6	65.4	74.2	69.7
Soybeans, whole[4]	20	Cornstarch/rice	76.8	69.8	66.4	69.9	67.5	69.0	69.5	75.1	72.8	58.5	77.3	59.0
Soybeans, whole, low oligo[5]	20	Cornstarch/rice	81.8	71.7	67.5	76.9	83.2	78.6	79.2	85.4	83.6	66.4	62.3	73.7
Soybeans, whole, low oligo and low phytate[4,5]	20	Cornstarch/rice	82.4	75.1	75.3	82.5	86.1	82.9	83.6	89.4	86.9	70.6	66.0	79.6
	20	Cornstarch/rice	76.7	68.8	65.6	61.9	63.3	65.4	65.4	74.0	74.6	54.8	58.7	58.3
Soy flour[8]	30	Potato starch/rice	87.3	87.2	94.1	88.7	90.1	89.1	91.0	88.2	85.9	82.7	-	86.8
Soy flour, defatted[2]	20	Rice	88.3	79.5	91.5	82.1	87.6	86.7	86.3	90.1	78.6	74.0	-	85.5
Soy protein concentrate, aqueous alcohol extracted[8]	30	Potato starch/rice	86.5	82.6	93.2	86.7	87.2	86.2	89.3	79.4	81.0	72.6	-	82.4
Soy protein concentrate, extruded[8]	30	Potato starch/rice	84.7	84.5	93.5	86.0	87.7	86.9	88.8	87.1	83.6	78.0	-	83.6
Soy protein concentrate, modified molecular weight (low antigen)[8]	30	Potato starch/rice	89.3	85.9	94.3	88.5	89.5	88.6	91.1	82.3	84.2	79.5	-	85.6
Minimum digestibility (%)	-	-	64.3	51.1	65.6	61.9	59.2	64.0	65.4	63.5	71.7	39.6	39.3	50.3
Maximum digestibility (%)	-	-	91.1	87.2	94.3	88.7	90.1	91.2	91.1	92.8	90.2	82.7	82.9	86.8
Average digestibility (%)	-	-	81.6	76.3	84.1	80.4	79.8	81.7	81.1	82.3	81.4	67.9	69.7	74.6

Key: CP = crude protein, CPD = crude protein digestibility, Arg = arginine, His = histidine, Iso = isoleucine, Leu = leucine, Lys = lysine, Met = methionine, Phe = phenylalanine, Thr = thyronine, Try = tryptophan, Val = valine.

*Adapted from [1]Bednar GE, Patil AR, Murray SM, et al. Starch and fiber fractions in selected food and feed ingredients affect their small intestinal digestibility and fermentability and their large bowel fermentability in vitro in a canine model. Journal of Nutrition 2001; 131: 276-286. [2]Murray SM, Patil AR, Fahey GC Jr, et al. Raw and rendered animal by-products as ingredients in dog diets. Journal of Animal Science 1997; 75: 2497-2505. [3]Yamka RM, Kitts SE, True AD, et al. Evaluation of maize gluten meal as a protein source in canine foods. Animal Feed Science and Technology 2004. [4]Yamka RM, Hetzler BM, Harmon DL. Evaluation of low-oligosaccharide low-phytate whole soybeans and soybean meal in canine foods. Journal of Animal Science 2005; 83: 393-399. [5]Yamka RM, Kitts SE, Harmon DL. Evaluation of low-oligosaccharide and low-oligosaccharide low-phytate whole soya beans in canine foods. Animal Feed Science and Technology 2005; 120: 79-91. [6]Yamka RM, Jamikorn U, True AD, et al. Evaluation of soyabean meal as a protein source in canine foods. Animal Feed Science and Technology 2003; 109: 121-132. [7]Zuo Y, Fahey GC Jr, Merchen NR, et al. Digestion responses to low oligosaccharide soybean meal by ileally-cannulated dogs. Journal of Animal Science 1996; 74: 2441-2449. [8]Clapper GM, Grieshop CM, Merchen NR, et al. Ileal and total tract digestibilities and fecal characteristics of dogs as affected by soybean protein inclusion in dry, extruded diets. Journal of Animal Science 2001; 79: 1523-1532.

mals fed the test protein ÷ slope of response curve for animals fed the reference protein. The slope ratio method usually uses growth as the response and may be sensitive to different levels of energy (Brown, 1989).

Ileal-cannulated dogs can also be used to determine protein quality (Walker et al, 1994). Protein digestibility coefficients based on collection and analyses of digesta from the terminal ileum give a more accurate measure of protein nitrogen absorbed than those based on fecal collections. Values determined from terminal ileal digesta exclude endogenous protein secretion from the GI tract and contributions from intestinal microflora. Ileal collection eliminates the large intestine and bacterial fermentation as sources of error. Use of ileal-cannulated dogs has enabled researchers to study the effects of feeding various protein sources and carbohydrates on digestibility and protein quality. **Tables 5-13** and **5-14** summarize recent work with ileal-cannulated dogs and demonstrate the differences in quality among various protein sources. Because of the complications involved with using ileal-cannulated cats (Mawby et al, 1999), no published studies have investigated protein quality using this model. As a result, only total tract crude protein digestibility data are available for cats (**Table 5-15**).

Finally, stable isotopes have been used to study protein quality. Whole body nitrogen flux can be determined using ^{15}N-glycine and ^{13}C-leucine. These markers have been used extensively in human pediatrics (Bolster et al, 2001; Zello et al, 2003), human geriatrics (Chevalier et al, 2003; Gibson et al, 2002) and in young-adult/aging dogs (Williams et al, 2001).

Protein quality varies with the animal species; poor quality proteins for one monogastric species may not be poor quality in other monogastrics (e.g., dogs vs. cats). The sensitivity of quality depends on the rate of growth or the level of demand to synthesize proteins for needs such as lactation, trauma, athletic performance and stress. Animals that are relatively inactive, mature and under no stress may not be very sensitive to moderate differences in protein quality (Brown, 1989).

Table 5-15. Total tract crude protein (CP) digestibility of cat foods containing plant and animal protein sources.*

Protein source	Carbohydrate source	Total tract CP digestibility (%)
Fish meal[1]	Corn	78
Meat meal[2,4]	Corn	91
Soy protein	-	-
With 25% butter[3]	Cornstarch	91
With 25% lard[3]	Cornstarch	92
With 25% unbleached tallow[3]	Cornstarch	90
With 25% bleached tallow[3]	Cornstarch	90
With 25% chicken fat[3]	Cornstarch	90
With 25% yellow grease[3]	Cornstarch	90
Corn gluten meal[1,2,4]	Corn	74
	Corn	70
	Corn	86
Chicken and chicken by-product[5]	Cornstarch	87
With 12.49% beet pulp[5]	Cornstarch	83
With 8.07% Solka Floc[5]	Cornstarch	88
With 3.91% citrus pectin, 3.34% locust bean gum, 2.22% carob bean gum, 1.66 guar gum[5]	Cornstarch	59
With 6.26% Solka Floc, 2.08% gum arabic[5]	Cornstarch	86
With. 9.04% beet pulp, 3.26% rice bran, 1.51% citrus pectin, 1.22% carob bean gum[5]	Cornstarch	83
Chicken meal[4]	Corn	86
Poultry meal[6]	Not available	94
With 10% peanut hulls[6]	Not available	84
With 10% beet pulp[6]	Not available	93
With 10% alfalfa meal[6]	Not available	92

*Adapted from [1]Funaba M, Tanaka T, Kaneko M, et al. Fish meal versus maize gluten meal as a protein source for dry cat food. Journal of Veterinary Medical Science 2001; 63: 1355-1357. [2]Funaba M, Matsumoto C, Matsuki K, et al. Comparison of maize gluten meal and meat meal as a protein source in dry foods formulated for cats. American Journal of Veterinary Research 2002; 63; 1247-1251. [3]Kane E, Morris JG, Rogers QR. Acceptability and digestibility by adult cats of diets made with various sources and levels of fat. Journal of Animal Science 1981; 53: 1516-1523. [4]Funaba M, Oka Y, Kobayashi S, et al. Evaluation of meat meal, chicken meal and corn gluten meal as dietary protein sources of protein in dry cat food. Canadian Journal of Veterinary Research 2005; 69: 299-304. [5]Sunvold GD, Fahey JC Jr, Merchen NR, et al. Dietary fiber for cats: In vitro fermentation of selected fiber sources by cat fecal inoculum and in vivo utilization of diets containing selected fiber sources and their blends. Journal of Animal Science 1995; 73: 2329-2339. [6]Fekete SG, Hullar I, Andrasofszky E, et al. Effect of different fibre types on the digestibility of nutrients in cats. Journal of Animal Physiology and Animal Nutrition 2004; 88: 138-142.

Protein/Amino Acid Requirements

Factors Affecting Requirements

New proteins can be synthesized from dietary amino acids or nonessential amino acids that were previously synthesized by the body. By definition, essential amino acids used in protein synthesis must be provided by food. Therefore, animals do not have a requirement for protein per se but have an amino acid requirement. The amount of each amino acid that an animal requires varies based on factors such as growth, pregnancy, lactation and some disease states. In addition to requiring specific essential amino acids, dogs and cats have a requirement for building blocks (carbon skeletons and nitrogen) for nonessential amino acids. The building blocks for nonessential amino acids can either be derived from excess essential amino acids that are broken down and reassembled into nonessential amino acids or from other nonessential amino acids in food. Thus, a complete statement of amino acid requirements should include all the essential amino acids and an amount of amino nitrogen that can be used for synthesis of nonessential amino acids.

The amount of protein or amino acids that must be included in a pet food also depends on how much food the animal consumes. It is easy to understand why animals that are growing, pregnant or lactating require dietary protein to support new tissue growth and milk production. If an animal only consumes small quantities of food to meet its energy requirement then the food needs to have a greater protein concentration to meet the animal's protein requirement. For example, high-calorie pet foods should have more protein as a percentage of the

Table 5-16. Ideal amino acid profiles (relative to lysine) for dogs and cats.*

Amino acids	Dogs	Cats
Lysine	1.00	1.00
Methionine + cystine	0.64	1.00
Tryptophan	0.22	0.19
Threonine	0.67	0.87
Arginine	0.71	1.12
Isoleucine	0.57	0.63
Valine	0.75	0.75
Leucine	1.00	1.50
Histidine	0.29	0.38
Phenylalanine + tyrosine	1.00	1.12

*Baker DH, Czarnecki-Maulden GL. Comparative nutrition of cats and dogs. Annual Review of Nutrition 1991; 11: 239-263.

food than low-calorie foods. The opposite is also true. Larger portions of low-calorie foods are typically consumed; therefore, animals can adequately meet their daily requirements with a food that has a lower percentage of protein.

Adult animals also need dietary protein to replace the amino acids that enter pathways of amino acid catabolism and are permanently lost. Healthy adults also have a daily requirement for protein to replace nitrogen lost as urea, ammonia, creatinine, nitrate in urine and feces, sloughing of epithelial cells in skin and the GI tract, sweat, hair, nasal secretions, semen from males and secretions due to reproductive cycles in females. Dietary protein that must be consumed each day to replace the obligatory nitrogen loss is termed the maintenance protein requirement.

Adult and growing animals have maintenance requirements for protein, but only growing animals have the additional protein requirement for growth. The additional protein required by pregnant and lactating animals really supports growth. An animal's physiologic state also may result in increased or decreased protein catabolism and nitrogen losses. For example, patients with cancer, burns and trauma may have increased daily protein requirements.

Nitrogen balance is the difference between the nitrogen consumed and the amount lost each day. Growing animals, pregnant females and any animals that are replenishing or rebuilding tissue are in positive nitrogen balance. Zero nitrogen balance occurs in normal healthy adults receiving minimally adequate or more than adequate dietary protein when nitrogen output equals nitrogen intake. Negative nitrogen balance can occur during lactation, starvation or fasting when there is inadequate or no protein intake. Excessive body protein catabolism due to burns, injury, fever, infections, hormonal imbalance or psychological causes can also cause negative nitrogen balance. Amino acid imbalances and antagonisms can cause negative nitrogen balance even when adequate amounts of protein are consumed.

IMBALANCE AND ANTAGONISM

Essential amino acids must be provided in adequate amounts and in proper balance. When amino acids are used for protein synthesis, all the amino acids necessary to synthesize each protein must be present. The amino acid in shortest supply relative to demand is called the "first limiting amino acid." An imbalance occurs when one or more amino acids needed for protein synthesis are not available in the quantity needed, but at least one other amino acid is provided in excess (Harper et al, 1970). Amino acid antagonism occurs when amino acids have similar chemical structures (Harper et al, 1970). Typically, an excess of one of these amino acids increases the requirement of one or more chemically similar amino acids (antagonism). Amino acid imbalance or antagonism does not typically occur in animals consuming commercial pet foods because most foods use complementary proteins (plant and animal sources). However, even use of complementary protein sources can result in imbalances or deficiencies of other amino acids. Therefore, it becomes important to understand the optimal levels and ratios of the essential amino acids necessary for animals.

The ideal or perfect protein concept was first established in swine. This concept defines the ideal ratio of essential amino acids necessary to maximize tissue growth and diet usage. Researchers used the same concept for dogs and cats by extrapolating data from requirement studies using foods with purified amino acids (Baker and Czarnecki-Maulden, 1991). The requirement of each amino acid was determined by feeding graded levels of essential amino acids (with the same metabolizable energy) to puppies and kittens. These amino acids were then compared to the lysine requirement. Thus, the ideal protein concept creates ratios of the essential amino acids to lysine and is independent of total dietary nitrogen (crude protein of the food) and energy levels (**Table 5-16**). This ratio assures the protein in the food is "perfect" by containing optimal levels of amino acids (no imbalances or deficiencies).

Protein Requirements for Dogs and Cats

The absolute minimum dietary protein requirement can be estimated by feeding extremely high-quality protein or commonly used protein sources. If the estimate is based on feeding high-quality protein (e.g., lactalbumin), a growing dog requires approximately 18% DM protein and an adult dog about 8% DM protein (NRC, 2003). AAFCO has established that canine foods containing commonly used protein ingredients should contain at least 22% DM protein for growth, and 18% DM protein for adult maintenance (2007). It is important to note that AAFCO recommendations should be interpreted as daily allowances, not as absolute minimum requirements.

Growing kittens and adult cats have higher protein requirements than most other domestic species. The minimum protein requirement has been estimated to be about 18% DM for kittens and 16% DM for adult cats, assuming use of extremely high-quality protein sources (NRC, 2003). For commercial foods using commonly available protein sources, AAFCO has recommended that foods for kittens and adult cats contain at least 30 and 26% DM protein, respectively (2007). Again, AAFCO recommendations for protein should be interpreted as daily allowances, not as an absolute minimum requirement.

Amino Acids of Special Importance

Several amino acids have important roles in the nutrition and health of dogs and cats. Among these are taurine, arginine and glutamine/glutamate.

Taurine

Taurine is a sulfur-containing β-amino acid. The amino group resides on the second (β) carbon rather than the first (α) carbon as with other amino acids. Taurine also has a sulfonic acid (SOOH) rather than a carboxylic acid group. Taurine is not incorporated into proteins synthesized by the body because of its structure. Rather, taurine is found as a free amino acid in many tissues, including brain, retina, myocardium, skeletal muscle, liver, platelets, leukocytes, and in fluids such as milk and in complexes with bile salts (Zelikovic and Chesney, 1989).

Taurine is conjugated to bile acids to form water-soluble bile salts that assist in absorption of dietary fats. Taurine also serves as a neurotransmitter and neuromodulator in the central nervous system and is involved with body temperature regulation, brain development, maintenance of normal retinal structure and normal heart function (Zelikovic and Chesney, 1989). Taurine is also thought to conjugate toxic compounds, serve as an antioxidant, stabilize cell membranes and regulate cell volume and osmolarity (Zelikovic and Chesney, 1989).

Taurine is an essential amino acid because cats have minimal ability to synthesize it and have obligatory losses due to the necessity for conjugating bile acids to taurine. Unlike other animals, cats conjugate bile acids only to taurine and not to glycine. Furthermore, cats have an obligatory loss of taurine in the feces due to bacterial degradation in the intestine and intestinal losses of taurine through enterohepatic circulation. This obligatory loss coupled with a minimal capacity for cats to synthesize taurine makes it an essential amino acid for this species.

Documented signs of taurine deficiency include reproductive failure in queens, developmental abnormalities in kittens, central retinal degeneration and dilated cardiomyopathy (Pion et al, 1987; Morris et al, 1994). Taurine deficiency is more likely to occur in cats that are fed dog foods, homemade foods and vegetarian foods that are not supplemented with taurine.

Taurine requirements in cats are highly dependent on ingredient sources and processing. The requirement increases slightly with increased dietary protein. Certain proteins (e.g., isolated soya protein) and the canning process increase the dietary taurine allowance compared with freezing or using casein as the protein source. Processing neither destroys nor binds appreciable quantities of taurine; however, processing apparently alters food so that enhanced numbers of intestinal bacteria degrade taurine. The specific biochemical alteration of food responsible for this change has not been described. Current recommendations are to include at least 1 g of purified crystalline taurine/kg (0.1% DM) in dry foods and at least 2 g of purified crystalline taurine/kg for moist foods (0.2% DM) (AAFCO, 2007).

There is no evidence that taurine is an essential amino acid for dogs; however, research indicates that it may be conditionally essential. In one study, investigators showed that feeding a high-fat food (24% DM) significantly reduced plasma taurine concentrations. Taurine values for some dogs were marginally deficient (Sanderson et al, 1996). Dilated cardiomyopathy in American cocker spaniels and golden retrievers has also been associated with plasma taurine deficiency and low myocardial taurine concentrations (Kramer et al, 1995) (Chapter 36).

Arginine

Arginine is a basic amino acid that is essential for dogs and cats of all ages. Cats develop signs of deficiency rapidly. Within three hours after consuming a meal devoid of arginine, cats develop hyperammonemia, vomiting, ataxia, vocalization (moaning) and hyperactivity; death may occur. Similar signs of ammonia toxicity such as tremors, vomiting, profuse salivation and hyperglycemia appear quickly in dogs following a meal that lacks arginine. Arginine is a key intermediate in the urea cycle, which is the major metabolic pathway that detoxifies nitrogenous wastes, such as ammonia (Milner, 1989). Ornithine and citrulline can substitute for arginine and prevent hyperammonemia because they are also urea cycle intermediates. However, they cannot restore growth rates (Morris et al, 1979). Ornithine and citrulline are not present in high enough quantities to substitute for arginine in typical commercial foods for dogs and cats.

Most protein sources provide adequate arginine; therefore, most commercial pet foods are not supplemented with arginine. Supplements, such as milk replacers, or products intended for other species, such as some human enteral products, should be evaluated carefully for their arginine content before being administered to dogs and cats. In studies, the minimum arginine content of food that maximized growth in kittens was 0.83% (DM) (Anderson et al, 1979; Morris and Rogers, 1978; Costello et al, 1980). AAFCO recommends that foods for growing kittens and adult cats contain at least 1.25 and 1.04% DM arginine, respectively (2007).

For growing puppies, a dietary arginine content of 0.4 to 0.56% (DM) supported maximum weight gain (Czarnecki and Baker, 1984); however, 0.56% DM supported optimal growth and nitrogen balance (Ha et al, 1978). AAFCO recommends that foods for growing puppies and adult dogs contain at least 0.62 and 0.51% DM arginine, respectively (2007).

The role of arginine in the formation of nitric oxide in the body has been investigated. Nitric oxide is classified as a hormone that helps regulate flow through blood vessels and is thought to be involved with blood pressure regulation. Nitric oxide is synthesized by the endothelial cells lining blood vessels and by macrophages to assist in infection control.

Glutamine/Glutamate

Glutamine and glutamate are five-carbon amino acids that are structurally similar and play key metabolic roles in the citric acid cycle, transamination reactions, generation of NADPH, γ-aminobutyric acid (GABA), the antioxidant glutathione and as folic acid cofactors. The carboxyl group of glutamate is replaced by an amide nitrogen in glutamine. The two amino acids are interconverted by the enzymes glutaminase (glutamine to glutamate + ammonia) and glutamine synthetase (glutamate + ammonia to glutamine).

For many years, glutamine and glutamate were considered nonessential amino acids; however, numerous studies have demonstrated that endogenous glutamine storage and synthesis may not be adequate to meet the body's needs in certain situations, such as critical illness, infection, cancer chemotherapy, low birth weight infants, diarrhea, human immunodeficiency virus infection, bone marrow transplantation and cardiac surgery (Neu et al, 1996; Souba et al, 1990; Klimberg et al, 1990; Furst et al, 1989; Lacy and Yost, 1990). Glutamine is also the preferred fuel of the small intestinal mucosa. Therefore, glutamine has been reclassified as a conditionally essential amino acid (Neu et al, 1996; Lacy and Yost, 1990).

Supplementation of pet foods or any food product with L-glutamine is difficult because the amino acid is unstable through heating and cooking processes. Glutamine breaks down into glutamate and ammonia. The latter can be toxic when ingested. L-glutamine can be added safely to powdered amino acid mixtures that are reconstituted with water and administered immediately to the animal. In complete pet foods, glutamine is best supplied by a high-quality, high-protein food.

Protein Deficiency

Clinical signs of protein deficiency include reduced growth rate, anorexia, anemia, infertility, reduced milk production, alopecia, brittle hair and a poor coat (Harper et al, 1970) (**Case**

Table 5-17. Summary of protein quality of common pet food ingredients.

Ingredient	Protein (%)*	Amino acid (protein) quality**	Other comments
Egg (dried)	45-49	Good High quality, the standard to which many other sources are compared CS = 100, BV = 94, NPU = 94, PER = 3.92	Also contains lecithin
Casein	80	Good High tryptophan, lysine CS = 58, BV = 80, NPU = 72, PER = 2.86	
Whey	12	Good High lysine, isoleucine, threonine, tryptophan	
Beef, lamb, pork, chicken	29	Good Low tryptophan CS = 69, BV = 74, NPU = 67, PER = 2.30	May be variable in fat and connective tissue content
Liver	20	Good	Also a good source of vitamin A
Fish meal	59	Good High tryptophan, lysine, methionine	Highly variable
Meat and bone meal	45-50	Good	Highly variable, may contain high levels of bone that contribute to excess calcium, phosphorus and magnesium in food
Lamb meal	55	Good	Highly variable, may contain high levels of bone that contribute to excess calcium, phosphorus and magnesium in food
Chicken/poultry by-product meal	58	Good High lysine, methionine	Mineral levels can be variable
Soybean meal	48	Good High tryptophan, lysine CS = 47, BV = 73, NPU = 61, PER = 2.32	Good complementary protein source for meats, fish meal and corn
Corn gluten meal	60	Good	Good complementary protein source for meats and fish meal
Corn (whole)	8	Adequate Low tryptophan, lysine, methionine CS = 41, BV = 59, NPU = 51, PER = 1.12	Also good source of linoleic acid
Rice (white)	7	Adequate CS = 56, BV = 64, NPU = 57, PER = 2.18	Low-mineral levels
Wheat	14	Adequate Low tryptophan, lysine CS = 43, BV = 65, NPU = 40, PER = 1.53	Contains gliadin
Barley	12	Adequate Low tryptophan, methionine	Contains gliadin
Collagen (gelatin)	88	Poor Totally deficient in tryptophan CS = 0, BV = 0, NPU = 0, PER = 0	

Key: CS = chemical score, BV = biological value, NPU = net protein utilization, PER = protein efficiency ratio.
*Feedstuffs Ingredient Analysis Table: 1996 Edition. (As is basis.)
**Adapted from Brody T. Protein. In: Nutritional Biochemistry. San Diego, CA: Academic Press Inc, 1994; 295-352. Jurgens MH, Animal Feeding and Nutrition, 6th ed. Dubuque, IA: Kendall/Hunt Co, 1988; 172. National Research Council. Improvement of Protein Nutrition. Committee on Amino Acids, Food and Nutrition Board. National Academy of Sciences, Washington, DC, 1974; 70. Robinson DS. The nutritional value of food proteins. In: Food Biochemistry and Nutritional Value. New York, NY: Wiley & Sons Inc, 1987; 117-151.

5-2). If specific essential amino acids are deficient, the clinical signs can be similar to those of general protein deficiency. A deficiency of calories (energy) and essential amino acids (protein-energy malnutrition) increases catabolism of muscle and other body proteins (e.g., albumin and immunoglobulins). Continued failure to consume protein results in muscle atrophy and decreased blood levels of albumin, transferrin, thyroxine-binding protein and retinol-binding protein because carbon skeletons from these proteins are used as an energy source to supply glucose through gluconeogenesis.

Albumin concentrations in serum are not a particularly sensitive indicator of short-term protein malnutrition because the turnover rate is relatively long. Fatty liver can also be a sign of protein deficiency because specific apolipoproteins needed by VLDL to package and export fat from the liver are not synthesized in adequate quantities or at all during protein deficiency.

Protein Toxicity/Excess

Although not a practical problem, amino acid toxicity can occur if any amino acid is fed at a very high level. It is very hard to create an amino acid toxicity by feeding protein sources from plants or animals; however, synthetic amino acids mistakenly added to foods at very high levels can cause toxicity (Harper et al, 1970). Synthetic amino acids currently added to some pet foods include L-methionine or D,L-methionine, L-lysine, L-arginine and taurine.

The minimum dietary protein requirement for healthy adult dogs is about 8% (DM) (NRC, 2003); however, AAFCO recommends that dog foods contain a minimum of 18% DM protein (2007). Healthy adult cats require a minimum of 16% DM protein (NRC, 2003); however, AAFCO recommends that foods contain at least 26% DM protein (2007). Commercial dog foods contain three to seven times the minimum protein requirement. Some commercial cat foods contain two to four times the minimum protein requirement (Chapter 20).

Excess dietary protein can be problematic for dogs and cats with specific disease conditions. For example, any disease that affects organs involved with conversion of ammonia to urea and waste nitrogen disposal can result in accumulation of toxic by-products of protein metabolism. In particular, protein intake above requirement should be carefully monitored in any animal with impaired renal or liver function (Chapters 37 and 68). In other situations, such as struvite urolith dissolution in dogs and adverse food reactions in cats and dogs, minimizing excess dietary protein is a beneficial part of therapy (Chapters 31 and 43). In these cases, excess dietary protein could be considered "conditionally toxic."

Feeding protein above requirements or recommendations for healthy dogs and cats does not result in a true toxicity because the excess amino acids from the protein are catabolized and the waste nitrogen is excreted. However, not all dogs and cats that appear healthy are free of disease. Dogs and cats with chronic renal disease are usually subclinical until the disease has progressed to the point that two-thirds or more of functional renal tissue is lost (Osborne and Stevens, 1981). Protein excess may contribute to progression of the disease. In addition to any direct effects protein excess might have on the progression of subclinical renal disease (Klahr, 1989), excess protein may contribute to acidemia (Chapter 37). This development is especially important in older cats with marginal renal function. Thus, even in apparently healthy dogs and cats, excess dietary protein may at times be conditionally toxic.

Protein excesses are found in pet foods for several reasons. Cats are strict carnivores (Chapter 19) and have a higher protein requirement than dogs, which are omnivores (Chapter 12). However, some pet food companies have perpetuated the myth that dogs are carnivores and that meat-based, high-protein foods are more natural and thus better than lower protein foods that contain both animal and plant sources of protein. Other fallacies, such as high levels of dietary protein build more muscle or a thicker coat, have contributed to pet owners' mistaken perception that higher protein is indicative of a higher quality pet food.

Excess protein adds unnecessary cost to foods. Excess protein is used for energy. As an energy source, protein is no better than digestible carbohydrate; however, protein is a more expensive energy source. The increased costs associated with increased dietary protein are invariably passed on to pet owners.

There are no nutritional reasons that support providing excessive amounts of dietary protein. After the protein/amino acid requirements are met, additional protein provides no additional benefits. Thus, dog foods for adult maintenance should not exceed 30% DM protein. Cat foods for adult maintenance should not exceed 45% DM protein.

Sources

Many ingredients supply protein/amino acids to pet foods (**Table 5-17**). Typical pet food ingredients that have high-protein concentrations are animal tissues from chicken, turkey, fish, beef and lamb and viscera such as livers, lungs and spleens. Grains also supply protein to pet foods. In fact, a large portion of the protein in cereal-based dry pet foods typically comes from grains, including rice, corn, wheat and barley. Some plant products (e.g., soybean meal and corn gluten meal) are concentrated sources of plant protein.

Multiple protein sources are often combined to improve the overall quality and amino acid profile when foods are formulated. This method of improving protein quality is termed protein complementation (Zapsalis and Beck, 1985). Protein sources are combined based on their amino acid excesses and deficiencies so that the nutritional weaknesses of each source will be counterbalanced by the strengths of other sources, resulting in a food with high-quality protein. Corn and soybean meal are typically used in animal food formulations to take advantage of protein complementation. Corn protein is low in lysine and tryptophan, whereas soybean meal is adequate in both amino acids. When used together in one food, these two protein sources provide a well-balanced amino acid profile.

Amino acid fortification is another method for improving the protein quality of foods (Zapsalis and Beck, 1985). Here, one or more individual amino acids are added to a food when

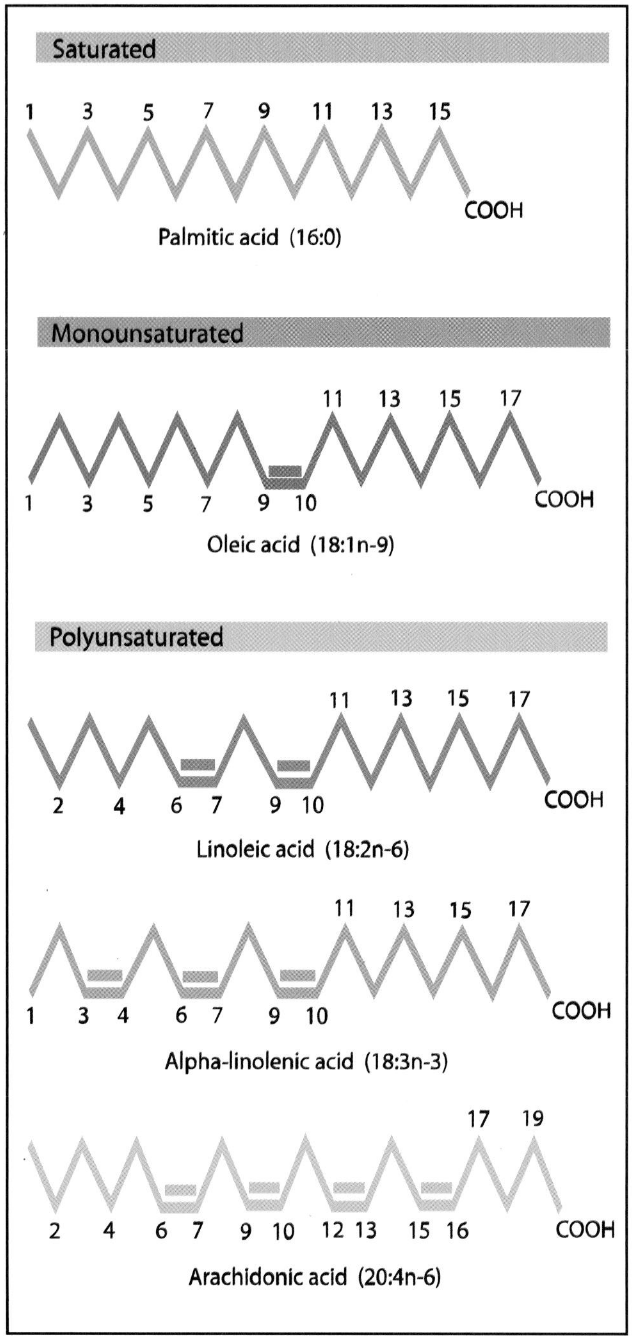

Figure 5-16. Fatty acids consist of hydrocarbon chains with a carboxylic acid group (COOH) on one terminus and a methyl group on the opposite terminus. Fatty acids with no double bonds in the hydrocarbon chain are referred to as saturated, one double bond as monounsaturated and more than one double bond, polyunsaturated. The carbon on the opposite terminus from the carboxylic acid group is designated the number one carbon and given the symbol n-1. Nomenclature specifies the number of carbons and the location and number of double bonds. For example, an 18-carbon polyunsaturated fat with three double bonds, the first of which is between carbons 6 to 7 is designated 18:3n-6 (γ-linolenic).

the main protein source of the food may be limiting. Methionine and lysine are typically used to fortify pet foods.

LIPIDS

Definition

Lipids are high energy compounds that supply nutritional and functional requirements in mammals. Generally, lipids share the physiochemical property of being insoluble (hydrophobic) in polar solvents such as water. Lipids that are solid at room temperature are commonly called fats whereas those that are liquid at room temperature are referred to as oils. In a nutrient analysis, the ether extract of a food contains primarily lipids and represents the crude fat content (**Figure 5-3**).

Structure

The structure of lipids ranges from simple to complex although any one classification scheme is difficult to impose. The basic subunits of lipids are hydrocarbon molecules linked by covalent bonds in various manners to themselves and other molecules in a vast assortment of permutations that result in the myriad of functions and structures observed in nature. **Table 5-18** and **Figures 5-16** and **5-17** will be helpful for reference throughout this chapter and the text.

Function

Dietary intake of lipids benefit the animal by supplying energy, essential fatty acids (EFA) and a positive environment for fat-soluble vitamin absorption. Dietary fats are the most concentrated forms of energy sources in pet foods, supplying 2.25 times the metabolizable energy of proteins and carbohydrates. Excess dietary lipids may be assimilated and stored as fat in adipocytes, whereas additional lipids are incorporated into functional lipid or catabolized for fuel, depending on the energy status of the animal. Triglycerides compose the majority of fat found in adipocytes, which may be synthesized de novo from nonfat precursors such as carbohydrate or protein during periods of positive energy balance.

Some lipids required for adequate physiologic function, such as certain long-chain fatty acids, cannot be synthesized de novo and are thus required in food. These fatty acids are called EFA because a lack of them in foods results in classic signs of deficiency. A small amount of lipid (1 to 2% of total food) of no specific structure is also required in foods for proper absorption of fat-soluble vitamins (A, D, E and K).

Fatty Acids

Structure

Nonesterified fatty acids (NEFA) consist of hydrocarbon chains ranging from two to 24 carbons or more, with a carboxylic acid group on one terminus and a methyl group on the opposite terminus. NEFA that contain 14 to 24 carbons are classified as long chain, eight to 12 medium chain and two to six short chain. **Figure 5-17** shows fatty acid chemistry and structure.

Lipid may be either in liquid or solid state depending on

Box 5-8. Cis and Trans Fatty Acids.

When carbons are connected by a double bond, rotation around the bond is not possible resulting in fatty acids that are either cis (with the carbons being on the same side) or trans (with the carbons being on the opposite side). Most polyunsaturated fatty acids are in the cis configuration. Fatty acids can be converted, however, to the trans configuration during excessive heating or through partial hydrogenation (i.e., the production of margarine from oil). Although trans fatty acids are metabolized for energy and incorporated into storage lipid, similar to the cis isomers, they are not further metabolized to eicosanoids. Nutritionally, trans isomers are in many ways like saturated fatty acids in that they are used for energy but cannot function as essential fatty acids.

temperature and fatty acid composition. A more unsaturated (increased number of double bonds) fatty acid makeup results in fats that have lower melting points compared with those of fats made from more saturated (decreased number or no double bonds) fatty acids. The length of the carbon chains in the fatty acids making up a fat also changes the melting point. Fats that contain fatty acids of shorter carbon chain length have lower melting points than do fats that contain longer fatty acids. Animals take advantage of these differences in physical characteristics to synthesize phospholipids containing appropriate classes of fatty acids that allow for membrane fluidity at physiologic temperatures.

Omega-3, Omega-6 and Omega-9 Fatty Acid Families

Fatty acids with the first double bond between the third and fourth carbon are in the omega-3 family, sixth and seventh carbon the omega-6 family and ninth and tenth carbon the

Box 5-9. Long-Chain vs. Medium-Chain Fatty Acid Metabolism.

Medium-chain fatty acids (mcFFA eight to 12 carbon lengths) are a minor component of natural compounds such as triglycerides from mother's milk or coconut milk. Triglycerides containing mcFFA are assigned the name medium-chain triglycerides (MCT). Even in foods "rich" with MCT, the overall contribution to the fat component of those foods is minor, compared with long-chain triglycerides. However, because MCT are subject to different metabolic regulation they may prove useful in certain disease states and have been included in some foods formulated for specific diseases (**Table 1**).

The Bibliography for **Box 5-9** can be found can be found at www.markmorris.org.

Table 1. Comparison between medium-chain triglycerides (MCT) and triglycerides.

Process	MCT	Triglycerides
Gut hydrolysis	Rapid, 5x triglycerides	Slower rate than MCT
Absorption	2x faster than triglycerides	Slower rate than MCT
Enterocyte reprocessing	Free fatty acid not reassembled in triglycerides	Free fatty acid reassembled in triglycerides
Transport	Portal vein, albumin bound	Chylomicrons, lymphatics and then general circulation
Hepatocyte		
Esterification	Not esterified to CoA	Esterified to CoA
Carnitine	Not bound to carnitine	Bound to carnitine
β-oxidation	Unregulated	Regulated

Table 5-18. Classification, structure and function of general lipids.

Classification	Structure	Function
Hydrocarbons	$-CH_3$, $-CH_2$, -CH	Building blocks
Nonesterified fatty acids	$CH_3(CH_2)n(CH_1)nCOOH$	
Saturated	Stearic, palmitic	Energy, membrane fluidity
Monounsaturated	Oleic, palmitoleic	Energy, membrane fluidity
Polyunsaturated	Omega-3, omega-6	Precursors of eicosanoids and prostaglandins
Simple lipids	Fatty acid + alcohol in ester bond	Energy storage, insulation
Triglycerides	Glycerol + three fatty acids	
Complex lipids		
Phospholipids	Diacyl glycerol 3' phosphate	Membrane lipids
Lecithin	3' phosphocholine	Emulsifying agent
Cephalin	3' phosphoserine/ethanolamine	CNS membrane
Inositol	Carbohydrate (3' phosphoinositol)	2nd messenger
Ceramide	Sphingosine + fatty acid	CNS membrane
Sphingomyelin	Ceramide + phosphocholine	Myelin
Glycolipids	Sphingomyelin + carbohydrate	CNS membrane/recognition
Cerebroside	Ceramide + monosaccharide	
Ganglioside	Ceramide + oligosaccharide	
Prostaglandins	20-carbon polyunsaturated fatty acids	Paracrine and autocrine action
Sterols and steroids	Four-ring hydrocarbon structures	Bile acids, hormones, membranes, lipoproteins, cholesterol, cholesterol esters
Fat-soluble vitamins	See vitamins	See vitamins

Box 5-10. Lipoprotein Lipase.

Lipoprotein lipase is an enzyme that hydrolyzes triglycerides into nonesterified fatty acids (NEFA) and glycerol. Lipoprotein lipase is located within the cell and is under hormonal control, specifically insulin. In its inactive state, lipoprotein lipase lies underneath the cell membranes that surround blood vessels. It is attached to the inner surface of the cell via a rope-like protein connection. Under the influence of insulin, this connection is loosened and the lipoprotein lipase is allowed to "float" to the cell surface where it can hydrolyze triglycerides in lipoproteins. Apo-CII is required as a coenzyme for lipoprotein lipase. The resulting NEFA diffuse into the cell for metabolism and glycerol is transported back to the liver for metabolism. Some lines of domestic cats have a genetic defect that results in absence of lipoprotein lipase activity.

Box 5-11. Good and Bad Cholesterol.

High-density lipoprotein (HDL) is the smallest of the lipoprotein molecules and is synthesized primarily in the liver and to a lesser degree in enterocytes. HDL is involved in reverse cholesterol transport. HDL transfers free cholesterol from cell membranes to the HDL molecule as cholesterol esters via an enzyme lecithin: cholesterol acyl transferase. The cholesterol esters may be transferred to very low-density lipoproteins (VLDL) by cholesterol ester transfer protein to eventually form low-density lipoprotein (LDL), which provides cholesterol to peripheral cells. Alternatively, the cholesterol esters may be delivered to the liver in HDL for excretion as bile salts. Because HDL is capable of transporting cholesterol from the periphery to the liver for disposal, it is said to contain "good cholesterol." LDL, on the other hand, is said to contain "bad cholesterol" because it transports cholesterol to the periphery where excess may result in arterial plaque and cardiovascular disease.

omega-9 family. The omega-3 and omega-6 fatty acid families are EFA because they cannot be synthesized de novo in mammals; lack of EFA in foods results in suboptimal physiologic activity (MacDonald et al, 1984a). Mammals are capable of de novo synthesis of saturated fatty acids and fatty acids of the omega-9 series up to 18 carbons (McGarry, 1986). Subsequently, mammals may elongate and desaturate de novo or dietary fatty acids of all classes via enzymes specific for certain carbons in the hydrocarbon chain (**Figure 5-19**). However, mammals cannot desaturate fatty acids between the n-1 carbon and the n-3, n-6 or n-9 double bond. Because of the specificity of these enzyme systems, unsaturated fatty acids cannot be converted between families (e.g., omega-6 or omega-9 to omega-3). Also, because of limitations and specificity in metabolism, monounsaturated and saturated fatty acids cannot be converted to EFA (e.g., omega-9 or stearate to omega-6).

Members of the omega-6 family include linoleic acid (18:2n-6), γ-linolenic acid (18:3n-6) and arachidonic acid (20:4n-6). Dogs, but not cats, are able to elongate and desaturate linoleic acid to form arachidonic acid (MacDonald et al, 1984b, 1984c; McLean and Monger, 1989). Thus, linoleic acid is usually listed as an EFA for dogs, whereas, both linoleic acid and arachidonic acid are EFAs for cats. The omega-6 fatty acid family is required for growth, reproduction and precursors of eicosanoid and prostaglandin synthesis.

Members of the omega-3 family include α-linolenic (18:3n-3), eicosapentaenoic (20:5n-3) (EPA) and docosahexaenoic (22:6n-3) acids (DHA). The omega-3 fatty acid family, especially 22:6n-3, is required for brain and retinal function (Neuringer et al, 1984; Arbuckle and Innis, 1992). Both fatty acid families contribute to cell membrane fluidity and skin health. Processing EFA in pet foods may affect their biologic activity (**Box 5-8**). **Table 5-19** summarizes the families, common names and biologic uses of several fatty acids found in nature.

Lipid Metabolism

GI Handling of Dietary Lipid

Lipids in foods include triglycerides, phospholipids, cholesterol, cholesteryl esters and fat-soluble vitamins. Long-chain NEFA make up a very small percentage of dietary lipids and will not be discussed here. Dogs and cats digest dietary lipids efficiently, with apparent lipid digestibility normally ranging between 80 and 95%. Increased levels of saturated and trans fatty acids reduce lipid digestibility (**Box 5-8**).

Fats and oils must undergo digestion via enzymatic and physical processes before they can be absorbed from the lumen of the gut. The following steps are involved in lipid digestion, absorption and initial metabolism (**Figure 5-19**) (Brody, 1994a):

- Gastric lipase in the stomach and duodenum degrades triglycerides of intact lipid micelles.
- Bile salts emulsify lipid micelles to form mixed micelles and coactivate pancreatic lipase.
- Pancreatic lipase and colipase hydrolyze triglycerides in mixed micelles.
- Gastric and pancreatic lipase activity results in 2-monoacylglyceride + two NEFA.
- NEFA and 2-monacylglyceride are absorbed into enterocytes.
- Triglycerides are reformed in enterocytes from long-chain NEFA and 2-monoacylglyceride.
- Apolipoproteins + triglycerides + cholesterol form chylomicrons in enterocytes and enter lymphatics.
- Chylomicrons in lymphatics enter the general circulation via the thoracic duct.
- Chylomicrons are partially metabolized and remnants attach to liver receptors.

Triglyceride-containing medium-chain fatty acids undergo similar processing until they enter the enterocyte at which point they are not re-esterified, but transported via albumin directly to the liver for metabolism (**Box-5-9**).

Short-chain fatty acids (particularly butyrate) resulting from fiber fermentation in the large intestine are an important source of fuel for colonocytes. Excess short-chain fatty acids enter the portal circulation for metabolism by the liver.

Hepatic Handling of Dietary Lipid

The liver determines the fate of dietary lipid under the direction of hormonal signals related to energy balance. The primary fuel source for hepatocytes is provided via β-oxidation of NEFA whether dietary or endogenous in origin (**Figure 5-8**). The fate of dietary lipid from chylomicron origin can be traced as follows (**Figure 5-19**) (Brody, 1994b):

- Chylomicron remnants attach to receptors on liver cells.
- Triglycerides are hydrolyzed to glycerol and CoA esterified fatty acids.
- CoA esterified fatty acids may be either shunted to β-oxidation in mitochondria or repackaged into triglycerides and then VLDL for use by peripheral tissues (storage or fuel). Their fate depends on the energy status of the animal.
- Glycerol is converted to 3-P-glycerol (only in liver) and enters the carbohydrate metabolic pathway.

Although fat storage is easily accomplished by de novo synthesis (production of fat from carbohydrate or protein), it is more energy efficient for animals to deposit dietary fat than to synthesize it. When fat is deposited from foods, the fatty acid profile tends to reflect the type of fat consumed. When fat is synthesized, stored fat composition reflects the fat synthetic enzyme activity of the animal.

Lipoprotein Metabolism

Lipoproteins are relatively large conglomerates of protein and lipid that are necessary to transport hydrophobic lipids effectively through the aqueous medium of physiologic solutions. **Table 5-20** gives a generic relative composition of the different lipoprotein classes observed in mammals (Chapter 28). As the protein component increases, the relative density of the lipoprotein increases reflecting dilution of the buoyant density of fat. Lipoproteins are made only in the liver (VLDL, HDL) and enterocytes (chylomicrons). The protein fraction, before it is integrated with the lipid component, is termed apolipoprotein.

Lipoprotein metabolism is very complex with species variation. However, a general introduction is necessary to understand lipoprotein metabolic disorders discussed in later chap-

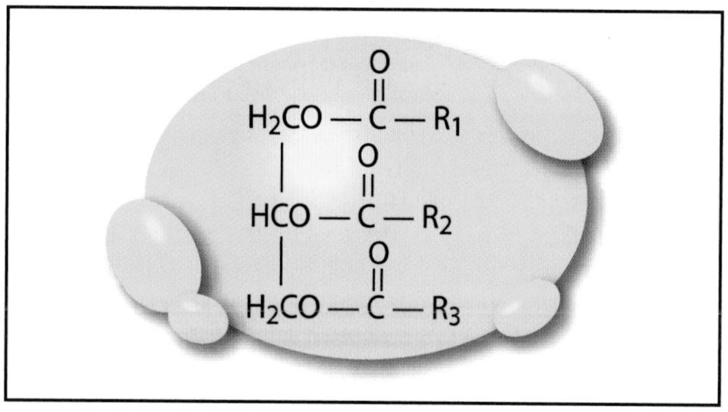

Figure 5-17. Triglycerides are the main storage forms of fatty acids, each molecule of which is composed of a three-carbon glycerol nucleus and three fatty acids (R_1, R_2, R_3).

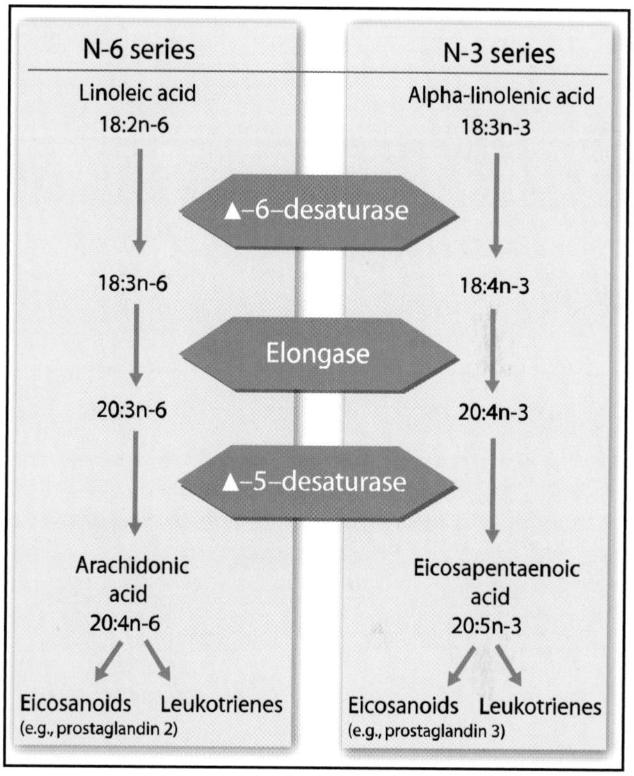

Figure 5-18. Diagram of metabolic pathways (elongation and desaturation) for essential fatty acids.

Table 5-19. Essentiality and biologic function of common fatty acids.

Structure	Common name	Essential	Biologic function
14:0	Myristic	No	Energy use and storage, acylation of proteins
16:0	Palmitic	No	Energy use and storage, acylation of proteins
16:1	Palmitoleic	No	Energy use and storage
18:0	Stearic	No	Energy use and storage, membrane fluidity
18:1n-9	Oleic	No	Energy use and storage, phospholipid structure
18:2n-6	Linoleic	Yes	Energy use and storage, arachidonic acid precursor (20:4n-6)
18:3n-3	Alpha-linolenic	Yes	Energy use and storage, eicosapentaenoic acid precursor (20:5n-3)
18:3n-6	Gamma-linolenic	Yes	Energy use and storage, arachidonic acid precursor
20:4n-6	Arachidonic	Yes (cat) No (dog)	Energy use and storage, synthesis of cytokines and eicosanoids, synthesis of steroid hormones, membrane fluidity, competitor of eicosapentaenoic acid (20:5n-3)
20:5n-3	Eicosapentaenoic	Probably	Energy use and storage, synthesis of cytokines and eicosanoids, retinal and nervous tissue development, membrane fluidity, competitor of arachidonic acid (20:4n-6)
22:6n-3	Docosahexaenoic	Probably	Energy use and storage, retinal and nervous tissue development, membrane fluidity, competitor of omega-6 fatty acids

Box 5-12. Hormone Sensitive Lipase.

Hormone sensitive lipase (HSL) catalyzes the reaction of triglycerides to nonesterified fatty acids (NEFA) and glycerol in adipocytes. Under the influence of insulin (following a meal), HSL is modified to a very low activity, which favors deposition of triglycerides in adipose tissue. Under the influence of glucagon (fasting) or epinephrine (flight or fight mechanism), HSL is highly active and the result is an efflux of NEFA and glycerol into the blood (bound to albumin) for transport to other tissues as an energy source. The NEFA that arrive back at the liver are catabolized or repackaged to triglycerides. In some pathologic conditions, triglycerides may accumulate in the liver (feline hepatic lipidosis) because the necessary repackaging materials for very low-density lipoprotein synthesis are not available in the liver.

Table 5-20. Composition of general lipoprotein classes in mammals.

Lipoprotein	Acronym	Protein:lipid (%)
Chylomicron	CM	1:99
Very low-density lipoprotein	VLDL	10:90
Low-density lipoprotein	LDL	25:75
High-density lipoprotein	HDL	50:50

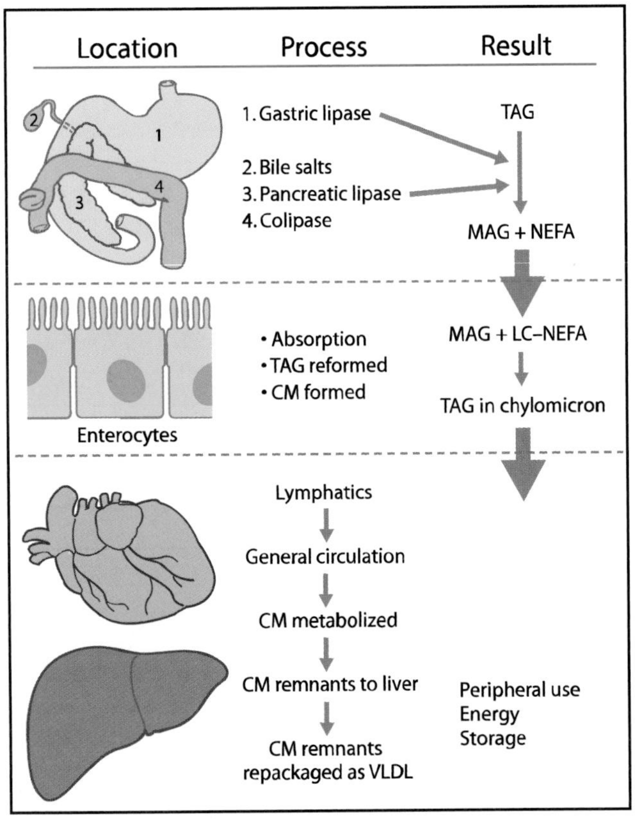

Figure 5-19. Digestion, absorption and fate of dietary triacylglycerides in mammals. See text for details. Key: TAG = triglyceride, MAG = monoacylglyceride, NEFA = nonesterified fatty acid, LC-NEFA = Long-chain NEFA, CM = chylomicron, VLDL = very low-density lipoprotein.

ters. An important point to remember is lipoprotein structure is not static and each class of lipoprotein has characteristics that may overlap with other classes. The following outline and **Figure 5-20** depict lipoprotein metabolism from the origin of lipoproteins in enterocytes or hepatocytes (Brody, 1994b):

- Chylomicrons are formed in enterocytes.
- HDL transfers apolipoprotein C-II and E (lipoprotein lipase cofactors) to chylomicrons and VLDL.
- Lipoprotein lipase in peripheral tissue hydrolyzes triglycerides in chylomicrons (**Box 5-10**).
- Chylomicron remnants bind to receptors in the liver.
- Liver hydrolyzes, reforms triglycerides and combines new apolipoproteins to form VLDL or HDL.
- VLDL triglycerides are hydrolyzed by lipoprotein lipase in the periphery to form VLDL remnants.
- VLDL remnants are taken up by the liver or converted to LDL for uptake by peripheral tissues.
- HDL made in the liver (major) and enterocytes (minor) transport excess cholesterol from the periphery to the liver for excretion in bile salts (**Box 5-11**).

Storage
Excess energy intake is stored in adipocytes as triglycerides. The triglycerides in adipocytes are formed directly from excess dietary fat or from de novo synthesis of fat in the liver under appropriate metabolic signals. The fat energy store in human adipocytes is capable of supporting life for one to two months. The key enzyme for release of energy from adipocytes is hormone sensitive lipase, which is under the control of hormonal signals (**Box 5-12**).

Lipid Function
Energy
Although providing dietary fat is an excellent way to meet an animal's energy requirement, this requirement can also be theoretically met by the protein and carbohydrate content of a food. On a per weight basis, the energy value of dietary fat is approximately 2.25 times that of protein or carbohydrate. Additionally, direct use of dietary fat for storage in adipocytes or use in functional lipid requires less energy for assimilation and storage when compared with de novo synthesis from protein or carbohydrate in food. In other words, fat stored directly from dietary fat has 10 to 15% more energy than fat made from excess dietary carbohydrate or protein because of the inherent loss of efficiency in de novo fat synthesis. This increased efficiency of fat use results in an increased energy value for dietary fat that animals may use to meet energy requirements or store as adipose tissue.

Essentiality
Fatty acids of the omega-6 family have functionally distinct effects compared with those of fatty acids of the omega-3 family. The addition of lipid-containing arachidonic acid to foods containing no arachidonic acid results in increased feed efficiency during growth and enhanced skin condition including reduced epidermal water loss. Arachidonic acid also allows processes requiring eicosanoids to occur such as reproduction

and platelet aggregation (MacDonald et al, 1984b, 1984c). Because dogs can convert linoleic acid (18:2n-6) to arachidonic acid (20:4n6), linoleic acid is usually listed as an EFA for dogs. A concentration of 1% of the food DM as linoleic acid is a safe and effective concentration for dogs (Wiese et al, 1962, 1965, 1966).

Because linoleic acid corrected many clinical signs of fatty acid deficiency in cats, it also is listed as an EFA for cats (McDonald et al, 1984a). Some of the signs of EFA deficiency in cats, however, were not ameliorated by linoleic acid but rather improvement depended on arachidonic acid supplementation. One group of investigators concluded that cats cannot convert linoleic acid to arachidonic acid in sufficient quantities for platelet aggregation and prevention of mild mineralization of the kidneys (McDonald et al, 1984b). Arachidonic acid supplementation allows normal reproduction in female cats (McDonald et al, 1984c). Male reproduction (spermatogenesis), unlike female reproduction, does not require dietary arachidonate because of the testes' ability to elongate and desaturate linoleate (McDonald et al, 1984c). These studies indicate that arachidonate is an EFA for cats. Foods for cats should contain at least 0.5% DM linoleic acid

Box 5-13. What's New in Fatty Acids: Resolvins, Protectins and Omega-3-Derived Mediators.

INTRODUCTION

Beneficial actions of polyunsaturated fatty acids were noted many years ago but the underlying mechanisms for these effects are poorly understood. It is clear that arachidonic acid is transformed into many potent bioactive compounds such as prostaglandins, leukotrienes and lipoxins. The departure of fatty acids from simply playing structural roles in cell membranes and/or as energy stores came largely from the recognition of the rapid transformation of arachidonic acid to these potent eicosanoids by both cyclooxygenase and lipoxygenase mechanisms. Many of the classic prostaglandins and leukotriene mediators are pro-inflammatory and play a decisive role in inflammation and/or in systems in which prostaglandins are key physiologic regulators. Inflammation is a vital reaction but it also plays a central role in many prevalent chronic diseases such as osteoarthritis, periodontal disease, inflammatory bowel disease, cancer, brain aging/dementia, allergic dermatitis and lower urinary tract disease.

In sharp contrast, it has become clear in recent years that counter-regulatory substances such as lipoxins are generated during resolution of acute inflammation, and that these serve as agonists for endogenous antiinflammatory mechanisms. This constitutes the first evidence that the resolution of inflammation, which was once thought to be a passive process, is actually an active process that involves up-regulating specific pro-resolution circuits. Thus, resolution of inflammation is an active endogenous process aimed at protecting the host from exacerbated inflammation.

THE OMEGA-3 FATTY ACID CONNECTION

The molecular mechanisms underlying the beneficial actions of polyunsaturated fatty acids remain an area of active research. Investigators have recently identified novel oxygenated products generated by enzymatic processes from the precursor omega-3 fatty acids eicosapentaenoic acid (EPA) and docosahexaenoic acid (DHA). These new compounds possess potent actions in the resolution of inflammation and may also have neuroprotective properties. The term resolvin (resolution phase interaction products) has been proposed for some of these compounds because they display potent antiinflammatory and immunoregulatory properties, reducing neutrophil traffic and the magnitude of the inflammatory response. The term protectin (or neuroprotectin) has been proposed given the protective actions of some of these compounds in neural and retinal tissues.

Resolvins are derived from EPA (E series) and DHA (D series). Both the D and E classes of resolvins appear as biosynthetic products involving cell-to-cell interaction with vascular endothelial cells and are potent regulators of leukocyte infiltration. Specifically, resolvin E1 (RvE1) dramatically reduces dermal inflammation, peritonitis, colitis, periodontitis, dendritic cell migration and interleukin (IL)-12 production. Resolvins of the D series block tumor necrosis factor-alpha activity and act as potent regulators to limit leukocyte infiltration into inflamed brain, skin and peritoneum.

Among the essential fatty acids, DHA is concentrated in the central nervous system, neurons and retina where it is thought to regulate membrane fluidity and ion fluxes. The term docosanoids has been proposed to describe products generated from DHA. DHA-derived docosatrienes have neuroprotective action in retinal cells and can improve the sequelae associated with stroke and dementia. The terms protectin or neuroprotectin describe these compounds, which are rapidly generated from DHA and released locally into tissues. There is emerging evidence that resolvins and docosanoid compounds may also have immunoregulatory actions by influencing antigen-presenting cells and T-cell traffic.

CONCLUSION AND CLINICAL IMPLICATIONS

Fatty acid supplementation has been used for many years to help manage patients with a variety of inflammatory diseases. The underlying mechanisms for the beneficial effects of fatty acid supplementation have been poorly understood. Recent research has identified novel oxygenated compounds termed resolvins and protectins, which are generated from EPA and DHA. These endogenous lipid/chemical mediators are "switched-on" in the resolution phase of an inflammatory response, thus acting as "braking-signals" in inflammation and reducing leukocyte-mediated injury in several different tissues. The discovery of resolvins and protectins offers molecular mechanisms that could underlie some of the beneficial actions of dietary fatty acid supplementation observed in many clinical settings.

Philip Roudebush, DVM, Dipl. ACVIM
(Small Animal Internal Medicine)
Hill's Scientific Affairs
Hill's Pet Nutrition, Topeka, KS, USA

The Bibliography for **Box 5-13** can be found can be found at www.markmorris.org.

Table 5-21. Fatty acid composition of commercial fats and oils.*

Fatty acid	Name	Butter**	Tallow**	Lard***	Chicken fat***	Fish oil***	Corn oil**	Sunflower oil**	Soybean oil**	Olive oil**
14:0	Myristic	8.4	2.6	1.4	0.5	4.2	<0.1	0.1	0.1	<0.1
16:0	Palmitic	21.3	7.4	24.1	20.4	16.2	9.9	6.3	10.1	11.4
16:1	Palmitoleic	1.1	1.9	3.5	7.6	11.6	0.1	0.1	<0.1	0.1
18:0	Stearic	8.9	24.2	12.2	4.4	2.4	2.1	3.8	1.4	2.4
18:1n-9	Oleic	18.8	13.8	42.8	37.6	10.9	25.6	20.9	20.4	65.5
18:2n-6	Linoleic	1.0	3.9	11.7	12.3	1.2	53.1	62.3	51.8	10.4
18:3n-3	Alpha-linolenic	0.4	0.5	0.5	0.5	1.2	1.0	0.1	7.3	0.5
18:3n-6	Gamma-linolenic	0.2	<0.1	0.1	0.2	0.4	<0.1	<0.1	<0.1	<0.1
20:4n-6	Arachidonic	0.7	0.6	0.1	0.2	0.4	<0.1	<0.1	<0.1	<0.1
20:5n-3	Eicosapentaenoic	<0.1	<0.1	<0.1	<0.1	14.1	<0.1	<0.1	<0.1	<0.1
22:6n-3	Docosahexaenoic	<0.1	<0.1	<0.1	<0.1	11.9	<0.1	<0.1	<0.1	<0.1

*All values are expressed as g/100 g.
**Adapted from Hyvonen L, Lampi AM, Varo P, et al. Fatty acid analysis, TAG equivalents as net fat value, and nutritional attributes of commercial fats and oils. Journal of Food Composition and Analysis 1993; 6: 24-40.
***Unpublished data, generally in agreement with published standards (Handbook 8, USDA, Washington, DC).

and at least 0.02% DM arachidonic acid.

Studies with primates have shown that 22:6n-3 (DHA) is essential for the normal development of nervous tissue and the retina (Neuringer et al, 1984). Studies with piglets have shown that dietary omega-3 fatty acids influence developing brain and retina (Arbuckle and Innis, 1992). The eicosanoids resulting from omega-3 fatty acid metabolism are less immunologically stimulating than those resulting from omega-6 fatty acids (**Figure 5-18**). Thus, feeding omega-3 fatty acids has been recommended in situations in which a reduced inflammatory response is desired such as: 1) before and after surgery, 2) after trauma, injury, burns and some types of cancer and 3) to assist in control of dermatitis, arthritis, inflammatory bowel disease and colitis (Hansen et al, 1995; Ogilvie et al, 1995; Kinsella et al, 1990).

Fatty acids of the omega-3 family, when compared with those in the omega-6 family, have been shown, in some cases, to decrease platelet aggregation and increase bleeding time (Leaf and Weber, 1988). Dietary omega-3 fatty acids slightly depressed platelet activity in rats and people; however, this finding is usually not a practical problem in healthy animals (Goodnight, 1989). Healthy adult dogs fed 7% of the food DM as omega-3 fatty acids from fish oil, over a period of two months, showed no problems with activated partial thromboplastin time, prothrombin time, buccal mucosal bleeding time clotting or platelet aggregation (Myers et al, 1996).

Although more research with omega-3 fatty acids in companion animals needs to be done, it is prudent to conclude that omega-3 fatty acids will be shown to be essential for normal function of the retina and brain as well as for physiologic homeostasis. At this time there are no conclusive data proving the optimal level or relationship of omega-3 fatty acids to omega-6 fatty acids for any species at any specific lifestage. The optimal relationship will likely depend on many individual parameters and differ depending on individual physiologic function (**Boxes 5-7** and **5-13**).

Neurologic Development

In children, during periods of early growth, DHA is needed to support retinal and auditory development (Pawlosky et al, 1997; Birch et al, 2002; Diau et al, 2003). DHA enhancement of visual and auditory development has also been demonstrated in other species. These enhancements reflect a general improvement in neurologic development overall, as a result of dietary supplementation of DHA during growth. Furthermore, brain development and learning ability are enhanced in infants supplemented with DHA (Birch et al, 2002; Hoffman et al, 2003). Because of these studies and others, it is now accepted that human infant formulas need supplemental DHA for proper brain development (Uauy and Mena, 2001; Birch et al, 2000).

Similar to findings in other species, inclusion of fish oil as a source of DHA in puppy foods improved trainability (Kelley et al, 2004). Conversion of short-chain polyunsaturated fatty acids to DHA is an inefficient process in mammals. Thus, there is a need to consider the essentiality of adding a source of DHA for growing puppies and kittens. The need for DHA supplementation during growth in kittens may be even more important than in puppies considering the cat's reduced ability to convert shorter chain fatty acids to DHA.

Osteoarthritis and Cartilage Health

Omega-3 fatty acids reduce inflammation associated with arthritis. Recent work suggests that incorporating EPA into canine cartilage models reduced the amount of glycosaminoglycan release when challenged with a stimulant compared to culturing with arachidonic acid (Chapter 34). Addition of EPA to dog food suppresses production of proinflammatory cytokines and cartilage degradative enzymes (Yamka et al, 2006a). Another study further demonstrated improved mobility and reduced cartilage degradation biomarkers. These data demonstrate the antiinflammatory effect of EPA in dogs, and the importance of omega-3 lipids for enhanced mobility.

Similarly, in cats, cartilage health can be enhanced by omega-3 fatty acid supplementation as in dogs (Yamka et al, 2006b).

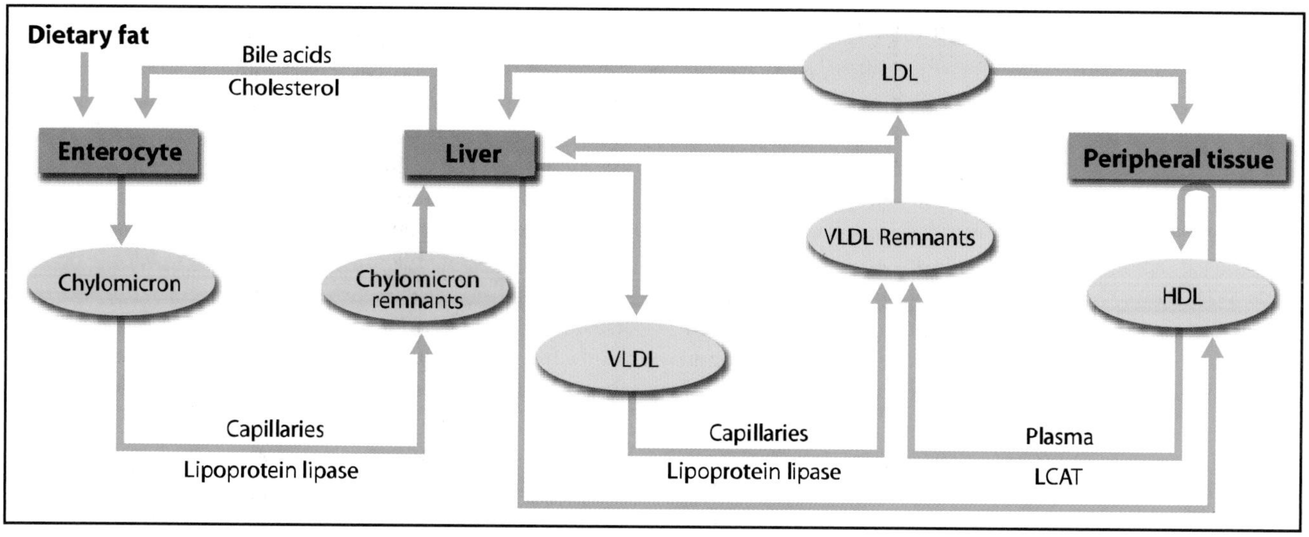

Figure 5-20. Lipoprotein metabolism. See text for details. Key: LDL = low-density lipoprotein, HDL = high-density lipoprotein, VLDL = very low-density lipoprotein, LCAT = lecithin cholesterol acyltransferase.

Addition of fish oil to cat foods reduced cartilage degradation and supported mobility. Geriatric cats (older than 12 years of age) fed foods supplemented with fish oil had reduced biomarkers of cartilage damage and enhanced mobility compared to cats fed food without fish oil.

Fat-Soluble Vitamin Absorption

Dogs and cats have a "requirement" for lipid to enhance absorption of the fat-soluble vitamins A, D, E and K. Dietary fat provides a physical environment in the gut that enhances absorption of fat-soluble vitamins. This requirement is in the range of 1 to 2% of the food and is not specific for any type of fat.

Lipid Requirements

Although not required for health, calories supplied by fat can be more beneficial than those provided by carbohydrate or protein. In cases of high-energy demand, the energy concentration of the food can limit total caloric intake. When the total bulk of the food is a limiting factor, increasing dietary fat allows for increased energy consumption. Increased aerobic capacity during exercise is supported by increased fat consumption because of the enhanced use of fat calories when compared with calories from carbohydrate (Chapter 18).

Lipid Deficiency

Deficiencies of fatty acids impair wound healing, cause a dry lusterless coat and scaly skin and change the lipid film on the skin, which may predispose the animal to pyoderma (Chapter 32). If deficiency persists, alopecia, edema and moist dermatitis may develop. Lesions of moist dermatitis, associated with EFA deficiency, are most common in the external ear canals and between the toes. However, lesions may develop anywhere on the body. Emaciation can result from severe, persistent EFA deficiency. An EFA deficiency can also impair reproductive performance (i.e., neonatal abnormalities and death may result if pregnancy occurs).

Lipid Excess

Increased dietary lipid is often associated with increased energy intake, because increasing the dietary lipid content of a food is nearly always associated with an increase in the food's caloric density. This relationship results from increased available energy. Changes in body composition result from changes in energy balance. Energy intake may be influenced by dietary fat; however, energy balance controls adiposity not the lipid intake.

Increasing the fat concentration of foods generally enhances palatability for dogs and cats. Fatty acid composition is an important aspect of palatability and influences acceptance through flavor and mouth feel. Dietary fat also influences subsequent food selection (Mullen and Martin, 1990), an effect mediated through serotonin, a neurotransmitter involved in control of food intake (Mullen and Martin, 1992).

Interactions with Other Nutrients

High dietary fat concentration requires increased antioxidant protection, such as added vitamin E. In the absence of adequate antioxidants, dietary lipids will become rancid (Chapter 8). Rancidity adversely affects the animal through reduced palatability, reduced vitamin activity and possibly subsequent oxidation of body fat. Because polyunsaturated omega-3 fatty acids are more susceptible to peroxidation than are most omega-6 fatty acids, increased amounts of antioxidants are needed in foods high in omega-3 fatty acids.

Excessive dietary unsaturated fat in conjunction with inadequate antioxidants may result in pansteatitis or "yellow fat disease." The end products of rancidification in adipose tissue cause a yellow, brown or orange discoloration of body fat. Affected animals are anorectic, depressed, febrile and lethargic. They move stiffly and generally show signs of cutaneous pain upon handling as the result of inflamed subcutaneous fat. Treatment involves dietary correction and oral vitamin E administration until clinical signs disappear (Cordy, 1954; Collins, 1983).

Lipid Sources

An array of animal and vegetable fats and oils in many combinations are currently used in commercial pet food production. Consumption of a specific fat results in a specific fatty acid profile that influences subsequent storage and metabolism. Because fatty acid intake strongly influences what type of fat is stored and which end products of fatty acid metabolism will occur, "you are what you eat" applies to fat more than any other macronutrient. **Table 5-21** shows the fatty acid compositions of different fat sources. Fatty acid composition of dietary fat within a single source varies for a number of reasons; therefore, the information in **Table 5-21** should be considered indicative of the fatty acid profiles possible within these specific types of fats and oils.

Fatty acid profiles in body fat change because of changes in fat consumption. For example, pigs consuming soybean oil had a 70% increase in linoleic (18:2n6) acid in depot lipid when compared with pigs fed diets containing tallow (Leszczynski et al, 1992). An equally large change in fatty acid composition can be found in plants due to changes in varieties within a species. An extreme example of this is safflower oil, which can vary from approximately 80% linoleic (18:2n6) to approximately 80% oleic (18:1n9), acid depending on the individual variety.

Fish oils have recently garnered the attention of nutritionists and veterinarians for their positive effects in managing a variety of disease processes. The oils most commonly associated with fish are those of the omega-3 and omega-6 families. The primary fish oil supplement is derived from menhaden and is very high in the omega-3/omega-6 families, compared with animal fat. The omega-3 family usually predominates over the omega-6 family in fish and shellfish, whereas polyunsaturated fatty acids from vegetable sources are usually higher in the omega-6 family. Threefold differences in fatty acid composition may occur in fish depending on season and geographic locale of the catch. Fish oil composition depends on dietary intake, type of fish (carnivore vs. plankton eater), warm vs. fresh water and season of catch. Unfortunately, data about specific variations based on the above factors are unavailable (Stansby et al, 1990).

REFERENCES

The References for **Chapter 5** can be found at www.markmorris.org.

CASE 5-1

Soft Feces in a Young Giant Schnauzer

Patient Assessment

A 10-month-old giant schnauzer weighing 44 kg was examined for persistently soft, mushy feces. An extensive diagnostic evaluation, including multiple fecal cultures, did not reveal a cause for the poor stool quality. The dog's body condition score was 3/5.

Assess the Food and Feeding Method

The owners had been feeding the dog a homemade food recommended by the breeder who sold them the dog. The food consisted of unspecified quantities of raw meat, liver, eggs, cooked brown rice, a few vegetables and approximately 100 g of various supplements.

The food was changed to a highly digestible commercial veterinary therapeutic food (Prescription Diet i/d Canine[a]). The dog was fed a mixture of moist and dry food that provided approximately 1,440 kcal (6.02 MJ) per day.

Feeding Plan

The dog's stool quality improved somewhat with the change from the homemade food to the veterinary therapeutic food, but its feces were still not formed. The owners continued to feed the dry form of the veterinary therapeutic food supplemented with a high-fiber cereal (Post All Bran[b] cereal [33% fiber]) to yield approximately a 10% fiber intake. (See Pearson square calculations in Chapter 1.) The final feeding recommendation was one cup of the cereal with 2.5 cups of dry Prescription Diet i/d Canine.

Two weeks later, the owner reported the dog's feces were normal. The food was subsequently changed to a veterinary therapeutic food that contained moderate levels of dietary fiber (Prescription Diet w/d Canine[a]).

Endnotes

a. Hill's Pet Nutrition, Inc., Topeka, KS, USA.
b. Kraft Foods, Inc., Rye Brook, NY, USA.

CASE 5-2

Lethargy and Weight Loss in a Mixed-Breed Dog

Patient Assessment

A five-year-old male dog of mixed breeding was admitted for lethargy, a dull coat and weight loss. The dog weighed 8 kg. Physical examination was normal except for a lusterless coat and a subnormal body condition score (2/5). Hypoproteinemia (total protein 4.1 g/dl, normal 5.0 to 7.5 g/dl) and hypoalbuminemia (albumin 1.2 g/dl, normal 2.2 to 3.5 g/dl) were noted on the serum biochemistry profile. The dog had several struvite urocystoliths surgically removed two years earlier.

Assess the Food and Feeding Method

For the past two years, the dog had been fed a veterinary therapeutic food (Prescription Diet s/d Canine[a]) that contained reduced levels of protein (7.9% dry matter), calcium, phosphorus and magnesium, and resulted in production of acidic urine. These nutritional characteristics have been shown to help dissolve struvite urocystoliths (Chapter 43). The dog had been fed one can (620 kcal [2.6 MJ]) daily.

Because of the low-protein content and other nutritional characteristics of this food, it is not recommended for long-term maintenance of adult dogs. The manufacturer recommends that Prescription Diet s/d Canine be fed for no more than six months. Because no other causes of hypoproteinemia and hypoalbuminemia were found, protein malnutrition was tentatively diagnosed.

Feeding Plan

The dog's food was changed to a different veterinary therapeutic food (Prescription Diet c/d Canine[a]). This food contains reduced levels of struvite precursor substances and produces an acidic urinary pH; however, it has a higher protein content (23.6% dry matter). This food is also nutritionally adequate for long-term maintenance of adult dogs. The dog was fed 1.5 cans (700 kcal [2.9 MJ]) daily until it reached optimal body condition.

Endnote

a. Hill's Pet Nutrition, Inc., Topeka, KS, USA.

Chapter 6

Micronutrients: Minerals and Vitamins

Karen J. Wedekind
Shiguang Yu
Lauren Kats
Inke Paetau-Robinson
Christopher S. Cowell

"Maybe my variety is due to bad absorption of vitamins."
Stephen Hawking

MINERALS

Introduction

Definition

The term "mineral" is generally used to denote all inorganic elements in a food. These inorganic elements constitute the majority of ash that remains after combustion of all organic matter. Ash analysis is of little value either for expressing mineral requirements or for indicating the useful mineral content of foods for two basic reasons: 1) body requirements are specific for certain inorganic elements (e.g., calcium, zinc, etc.) and 2) ash may not be a measure of total inorganic matter present, because some organic carbon may be bound as carbonate, and some inorganic elements (e.g., sulfur, selenium, iodine, fluorine and even sodium) may be lost during combustion.

The most important reason to determine total ash is to calculate the nitrogen-free extract by difference, as is required in the proximate analysis of foodstuffs. Specific minerals of interest can then be assayed (if not volatilized) from the ash component.

More than 18 mineral elements are believed to be essential for mammals (McDowell, 1992). By definition, macrominerals are required by the animal in the diet in percentage amounts, whereas microminerals or "trace" minerals are required at the mg/kg or parts per million (ppm). There are seven macrominerals: calcium, phosphorus, sodium, magnesium, potassium, chloride and sulfur. There are at least 11 trace elements or micronutrient minerals: iron, zinc, copper, iodine, selenium, manganese, cobalt, molybdenum, fluorine, boron and chromium. The last six are assumed to be essential for dogs and cats by analogy with other species. Calcium, phosphorus, magnesium, potassium, sodium and chloride are discussed below. Neither the Association of American Feed Control Officials (AAFCO) nor the National Research Council (NRC) lists a sulfur requirement for dogs or cats (AAFCO, 2007; NRC, 2006). Generally, there isn't a dietary need for sulfur per se, if a food is formulated to meet the sulfur-containing amino acid requirements of animals with simple stomachs.

Of the microminerals, only iron, zinc, copper, manganese, iodine and selenium will be discussed here. These trace minerals have been deemed essential for dogs and cats (although clinical cases of manganese deficiency have never been reported to occur in dogs or cats) (AAFCO, 2007). Cobalt and molybdenum are clearly important minerals in ruminant nutrition, but are not considered essential in monogastric species. Information about chromium and boron, two ultra-trace minerals, is included because of the potential importance these nutrients may have in companion animal nutrition. Other new trace elements discovered since 1970 include arsenic, lead, lithium, nickel, silicon, tin and vanadium. The essentiality of these minerals has not been elucidated in all species and under practical conditions may not be essential in the diet.

Function

Minerals are fundamental as: 1) structural components of body organs and tissues, such as calcium, phosphorus and magne-

Table 6-1. Mineral functions and effects of deficiencies and excesses.

Mineral	Function	Deficiency	Excess
Calcium	Constituent of bone and teeth, blood clotting, muscle function, nerve transmission, membrane permeability	Decreased growth, decreased appetite, decreased bone mineralization, lameness, spontaneous fractures, loose teeth, tetany, convulsions, rickets (osteomalacia in adults)	Decreased feed efficiency and feed intake, nephrosis, lameness, enlarged costochondral junctions. Increased calcium intake is a risk factor for calcium-containing urinary precipitates; however, moderate- to high-calcium levels may be protective against calcium oxalate precipitates. Calcium in meals may bind with oxalate in the gut decreasing the risk.
Phosphorus	Constituent of bone and teeth, muscle formation, fat, carbohydrate and protein metabolism, phospholipids and energy production, reproduction	Depraved appetite, pica, decreased feed efficiency, decreased growth, dull coat, decreased fertility, spontaneous fractures, rickets	Bone loss, uroliths, decreased weight gain, decreased feed intake, calcification of soft tissues, secondary hyperparathyroidism
Potassium	Muscle contraction, transmission of nerve impulses, acid-base balance, osmotic balance, enzyme cofactor (energy transfer)	Anorexia, decreased growth, lethargy, locomotive problems, hypokalemia, heart and kidney lesions, emaciation	Rare. Paresis, bradycardia
Sodium and chloride	Osmotic pressure, acid-base balance, transmission of nerve impulses, nutrient uptake, waste excretion, water metabolism	Inability to maintain water balance, decreased growth, anorexia, fatigue, exhaustion, hair loss	Occurs only if there is inadequate good-quality water available. Thirst, pruritus, constipation, seizures and death
Magnesium	Component of bone and intracellular fluids, neuromuscular transmission, active component of several enzymes, carbohydrate and lipid metabolism	Muscle weakness, hyperirritability, convulsions, anorexia, vomiting, decreased mineralization of bone, decreased body weight, calcification of aorta	Uroliths, flaccid paralysis
Iron	Enzyme constituent, activation of O_2 (oxidases and oxygenases), oxygen transport (hemoglobin, myoglobin)	Anemia, rough coat, listlessness, decreased growth	Anorexia, weight loss, decreased serum albumin concentrations, hepatic dysfunction, hemosiderosis
Zinc	Constituent or activator of 200 known enzymes (nucleic acid metabolism, protein synthesis, carbohydrate metabolism), skin and wound healing, immune response, fetal development, growth rate	Anorexia, decreased growth, alopecia, parakeratosis, impaired reproduction, vomiting, hair depigmentation, conjunctivitis	Relatively nontoxic. Reported cases of zinc toxicity from consumption of die-cast zinc nuts or pennies
Copper	Component of several enzymes (oxidases), catalyst in hemoglobin formation, cardiac function, cellular respiration, connective tissue development, pigmentation, bone formation, myelin formation, immune function	Anemia, decreased growth, hair depigmentation, bone lesions, neuromuscular disorders, reproductive failure	Hepatitis, increased liver enzyme activity
Manganese	Component and activator of enzymes (glycosyl transferases), lipid and carbohydrate metabolism, bone development (organic matrix), reproduction, cell membrane integrity (mitochondria)	Impaired reproduction, fatty liver, crooked legs, decreased growth	Relatively nontoxic
Selenium	Constituent of glutathione peroxidase and iodothyronine 5'-deiodinase, immune function, reproduction	Muscular dystrophy, reproductive failure, decreased feed intake, subcutaneous edema, renal mineralization	Vomiting, spasms, staggered gait, salivation, decreased appetite, dyspnea, oral malodor, nail loss
Iodine	Constituent of thyroxine and triiodothyronine	Goiter, fetal resorption, rough coat, enlarged thyroid glands, alopecia, apathy, myxedema, lethargy	Similar to those caused by deficiency. Decreased appetite, listlessness, rough coat, decreased immunity, decreased weight gain, goiter, fever
Boron	Regulates parathyroid hormone, influences metabolism of calcium, phosphorus, magnesium and cholecalciferol	Decreased growth, decreased hematocrit, hemoglobin and alkaline phosphatase values	Similar to those caused by deficiency
Chromium	Potentiates insulin action, therefore improves glucose tolerance	Impaired glucose tolerance, increased serum triglyceride and cholesterol concentrations	Trivalent form less toxic than hexavalent. Dermatitis, respiratory irritation, lung cancer

sium in bones and teeth, 2) constituents of body fluids and tissues such as electrolytes concerned with the maintenance of osmotic pressure, acid-base balance, muscle contraction, membrane permeability and tissue irritability (e.g., sodium, potassium, chloride, calcium and magnesium in blood, cerebrospinal fluid and gastric juice) and 3) catalysts/cofactors in enzyme and hormone systems, as integral and specific components of the structure of metalloenzymes, or as less specific activators within those systems. **Table 6-1** lists specific functions of each mineral.

Homeostasis

Specific concentrations and functional forms of minerals must be maintained within certain limits for optimal growth, health and fertility. Higher organisms possess homeostatic mechanisms that attempt to maintain concentrations of minerals at their active sites within narrow physiologic limits despite over- or under-ingestion. Such mechanisms include control of intestinal absorption or excretion, the availability of specific stores for individual elements and the use of "chemical sinks" such as metallothionein that can bind potentially toxic amounts of elements in an innocuous form (Underwood and Mertz, 1987).

The degree of homeostatic control varies from one element to another. Continued ingestion of diets or exposure to environments that are severely deficient, imbalanced or excessively high in a particular trace element, or in an interfering substance such as phytate or certain fibers, can induce changes in functioning forms, activities or concentrations of that element in body tissues and fluids so that they fall below or rise above the desired limits. Altered metabolism develops in these circumstances, which may affect physiologic function. Structural disorders may also arise in ways that differ with various elements, with the degree and duration of the dietary deficiency or toxicity and with the age, gender and species of the animal involved.

Deficiency/Adequacy/Toxicity

Traditionally, minerals were classified as "essential" or "toxic," but as more information was gathered, elements shifted from the latter to the former category (e.g., selenium). However, toxicity may occur with all elements. A "biologic dose-response curve" exists for each element (Underwood and Mertz, 1987). This curve (Figure 5-2) identifies a range of concentrations that spans three primary areas: 1) at low concentrations, physiologic function is consistently and reproducibly impaired (defined as deficiency), 2) at optimal concentrations, the nutrient is provided at levels necessary to meet the requirements of the animal and 3) at excessive concentrations, pharmaco-toxicologic effects occur. The intakes or dose levels at which these phases become evident and the width of the optimal plateau vary widely among minerals and can be markedly affected by the extent to which various other elements and compounds are present in the animal's body and in the food consumed (Box 6-1). Table 6-1 lists specific signs of mineral deficiencies and toxicities.

Several nutrients have specific therapeutic uses at high dosages (e.g., zinc is fed at growth-promoting levels in swine to prevent diarrhea). However, high doses may result in detrimental side effects after prolonged use. The pharmacologic actions of nutrients differ in several ways from their physiologic functions: 1) doses greatly exceeding the amount of a nutrient present in foods are usually needed to obtain a therapeutic response, 2) the specificity of the pharmacologic action is often different from the physiologic function and 3) chemical analogues of the nutrient that are often most effective pharmacologically may have little or no nutritional activity (RDA, 1989) (Box 5-7).

Claims of nutritional adequacy of pet foods are based on the current AAFCO nutrient allowances ("profiles"). These levels are neither minimal requirements nor necessarily optimal intake levels. It isn't possible to establish optimal levels without additional information about nutrient requirements for all lifestages and information concerning the availability of nutrients from pet food ingredients and complete diets. In some cases, insufficient margins of safety have been given to account for population variation, product diversity, processing effects and potentially low nutrient availabilities of certain pet food ingredients. In the case of trace minerals, the ratio between dietary allowance and absolute requirement can be as large as 100:1 (e.g., chromium) because of incomplete absorption, or can approach unity (e.g., iodine) when absorption is high (Underwood and Mertz, 1987). The nature of typical diets consumed strongly influences dietary allowances because numerous interactions among dietary components and different

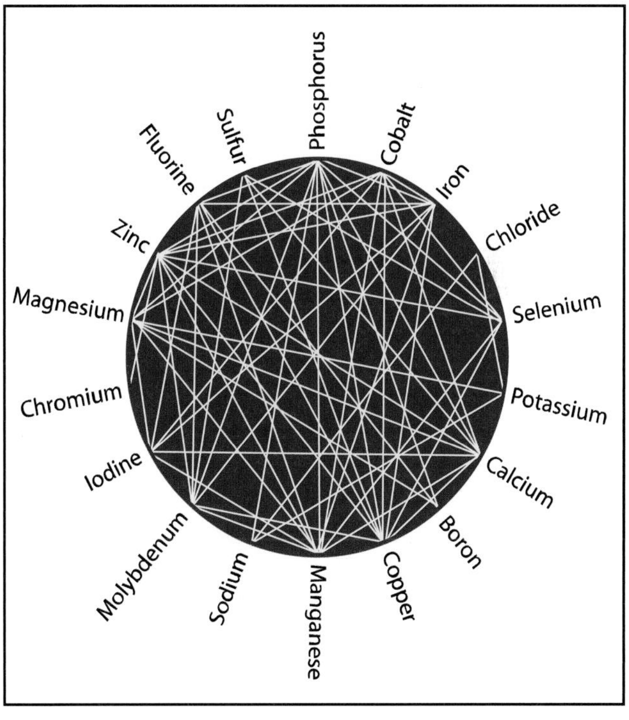

Figure 6-1. Mineral interrelationships. Minerals connected by a line clinically or experimentally interact with the other mineral. This interaction may be bidirectional (each mineral affects the use of the other) or unidirectional (one mineral affects the use of the second mineral but not vice versa). (Adapted from Puls R. Mineral Levels in Animal Health. Clearbrook, British Columbia: Diagnostic Data Sherpa International, 1990; 19.)

Box 6-1. Mineral Balance Studies.

The requirements for most nutrients are derived from experimental and clinical evidence of deficiency and the amount of nutrient needed to prevent signs of deficiency. When balance studies are used to estimate requirements, the requirement is defined as the intake at which zero balance is attained, or when intake is equal to excretion in urine and feces. However, the zero balance point will underestimate the requirement, if the measurement does not account for endogenous losses and losses in sweat.

Mineral balance studies have been criticized as inadequate and erroneous measures of body requirements. Small percentage errors in determining intakes and excretion can result in significant differences in balance calculations. One of the biggest problems in conducting balance studies is separating feces into time intervals that can be related to intake. Fecal markers aid in separation, but peristaltic reflux may still confound results. In addition, one animal's rate of passage can vary markedly. Adaptation to a different intake level may occur in a few days or weeks. Some adaptations, however, take several months or even years to occur. Thus, the adaptation period and collection period need to be sufficiently long to take into account animal adjustments to new foods, rates of passage and homeostatic adaptation.

Balance studies are probably more reliable when the mineral is excreted in the urine, rather than in the feces. This finding is true for sodium, potassium and selenium. When absorption of a nutrient is low, as is the case for a number of minerals, the amount of fecal mineral is large compared with the amount absorbed (e.g., the mineral concentration in feces is attributed to unabsorbed mineral and endogenous secretion). Failure to measure endogenous secretion may markedly underestimate the true amount of absorbed mineral. However, if radioisotopes or stable isotopes are used in conjunction with a balance study, the endogenous secretions can be distinguished from unabsorbed mineral and a measure of true absorption attained (as opposed to "apparent" absorption, which does not account for endogenous losses). Balance studies without the use of isotopes are fraught with inaccuracy and variability. Few analytical methods give a coefficient of variation as good as 5%, especially in complex matrices such as food, urine and feces. Thus, balance studies will not detect nutritionally important mineral differences when absorption efficiencies are low and radioisotopes or stable isotopes are not used.

Probably the biggest criticism of balance studies is that balance studies better reflect habitual intake than a requirement or zero balance. For example, an intake of 1 µg of selenium/kg body weight maintains a zero balance in Americans. Approximately one-tenth of that intake maintains a balance in people living in China; China is an area in which the risk of selenium deficiency is high and prevalence of Keshan disease is significant. Thus, zero balance does not necessarily indicate absence of disease. In New Zealand, selenium balance is maintained on an intake of one-third the amount required by Americans.

Analogous situations also exist worldwide for calcium balance. Widely different intakes of calcium result in zero balances in different countries. Thus, the previous dietary intake exerts a significant effect on the nutrient level that results in a zero balance and is more a reflection of the intake required to maintain an existing mineral pool size.

Balance studies should be evaluated with caution when attempting to determine requirements. A summary of their limitations follows:

- Prior long-term habitual intake influences whether positive, negative or equilibrium balance occurs at a particular intake.
- The duration of the study may not be long enough to allow for homeostatic adaptation.
- Cumulative errors occur from environmental contamination, individual variability and analytical methods. Thus, balance studies that demonstrate no treatment differences, may in fact be a result of the insensitivity and imprecision of the balance method.

The Bibliography for **Box 6-1** can be found at www.markmorris.org

chemical forms in individual foods determine biologic availability. Thus, it is important to understand the limitations of AAFCO nutrient profiles.

Mineral Interactions

A tremendous number of mineral-mineral interactions exist (**Figure 6-1**). In general, these interactions can be antagonistic (the presence of one mineral reduces the transport or biologic efficacy of the other) or synergistic (the two minerals act in a complementary fashion either by sparing or substituting for the other mineral or the two together enhance a biologic function). Most mineral interactions are antagonistic and can occur via a number of different mechanisms that include interactions (Solomons, 1988): 1) in the food during processing, before consumption, 2) in the digestive tract, where there is competition for uptake sites or intracellular-level mechanisms, 3) at the tissue level, either at storage sites or inhibition of enzyme activity, 4) at the time of transport and 5) in the excretory pathway.

The rigors of processing can affect the availability of minerals either positively or negatively via changes in solubility, pH, reduction potential and charge density and creation of complexes (Clydesdale, 1988). Charge density refers to the valence state and size of a metal. For example, the cations in the periodic table in groups 6B to 2B, with a relatively high ionic charge ($^+2$, $^+3$) and small size, form a large number of stable complex ions, whereas the large alkali metal cations, such as Na^+ and K^+, with a small charge are much less likely to form complexes with proteins or carbohydrate moieties via ionic, coordinate or covalent bonds. Furthermore, among the transition metals, which may form more than one cation, complexes formed by the $^+3$ valence state (e.g., Cr^{+3}, Co^{+3}) are more numerous and more stable than complexes formed by their respective $^+2$ ions. Charge is also involved with cell permeability and ion solubility before ions enter cells. Solubility varies tremendously depending on ion size and degree of polarity or charge.

Solubility is of obvious importance; a mineral must come in contact with the intestinal mucosa if it is to be absorbed. Charge density is less obvious but important for its effect on complex formation and membrane permeability. Solubility as it refers to mineral availability includes the solubility of an ion, salt, hydrate or complex, and to the type and strength of chemical bonds within these molecules. Inhibition of mineral absorption by a food can be overcome by the use of mineral enhancers, such as ascorbate, meat, citric acid and other ligands (e.g., ascorbate enhances iron absorption but negatively affects copper uptake; both effects are brought about by a change in pH and reduction in valence state).

Mineral-mineral interactions that occur in the digestive tract result from chemically similar minerals sharing "channels" for absorption. In this situation, simultaneous ingestion of two or more such minerals will result in competition for absorption (Solomons, 1988). In other words, when the dietary supply of a nutrient and/or the body reserves of a mineral are low, the intestine adapts to improve the efficiency of uptake and transfer. When the adaptation is nonspecific, other similar minerals have enhanced absorption. In iron deficiency, an up-regulation of iron also increases uptake of lead (Solomons, 1988). Other examples of interactions occurring in the digestive tract include the formation of insoluble mineral complexes (e.g., foods containing phytate and excessive calcium will form an insoluble calcium/phytate/zinc complex that reduces zinc availability).

Mineral-mineral interactions can also occur at the tissue storage level. High levels of dietary iron, for example, reduce hepatic copper stores. In studies, when ratios of iron to copper exceeded 20:1, hepatic copper levels were reduced to less than 50% of control values (Solomons, 1988). Likewise, trace minerals such as zinc can be mobilized when calcium is deficient because co-mobilization of both minerals takes place from the skeleton, making both available for use.

Mineral-mineral interactions can also occur at the time of transport. Transferrin is a serum transport protein for iron. Transferrin is generally less than 50% saturated with iron in its transit from site to site (Solomons, 1988). Transferrin can also transport chromium and manganese; therefore, these minerals may compete for binding sites contained in transferrin.

Finally, mineral-mineral interactions can also occur within pathways of excretion. For example, levels of circulating ionized calcium govern the release of parathyroid hormone (PTH) from the parathyroid gland. PTH status, in turn, influences renal tubular handling of filtered phosphate. Evidence also points to an interaction between calcium and magnesium at the level of renal excretion (Solomons, 1988).

Availability

Evaluation of feeds as sources of minerals depends not only on what the feed contains (i.e., the analyzed nutrient content), but also on how much of the mineral can be used by the animal. The adequacy of a food, as determined by its analytical mineral concentration, can be misleading because a number of factors can influence mineral availability. These include: 1) the chemical form (which influences solubility), 2) the amounts and proportions of other dietary components with which it interacts metabolically, 3) the age, gender and species of the animal, 4) intake of the mineral and the need (body stores) and 5) environmental factors (Underwood and Mertz, 1987) (**Box 6-2**).

Few studies have been completed in dogs and cats to evaluate the availability of minerals in foodstuffs used in commercial pet foods. Thus, there are many unknowns about the availability of nutrients in pet foods and whether a given food is truly adequate for a given lifestage. The availability of different forms of a mineral can vary widely even among inorganic mineral supplements. In general, different forms of trace minerals (iron, zinc, manganese and copper) differ in availability as follows: sulfate and chloride forms >carbonates >oxides (Aoyagi and Baker, 1993; Wedekind and Baker, 1990; McDowell, 1992a; Henry et al, 1986). The oxides of iron and copper are poorly available and should not be used as mineral supplements in pet food (McDowell, 1992a; Morris and Rogers, 1994).

In general, meat-derived foodstuffs are considered a more available source of certain minerals than plant-derived foodstuffs. The organic forms of minerals found in meats are often more available or as available as those from inorganic mineral supplements, whereas the minerals in plants are often less available (Aoyagi et al, 1993; Hortin et al, 1993). This finding applies more for iron, zinc and copper than for selenium.

Although the mechanism has not been fully delineated, one theory has been suggested to explain why organic forms of minerals are better used than inorganic forms. This theory postulates that chelates or complexes provide the mineral in a protected form (Kratzer and Vohra, 1986), analogous to the iron contained in heme, wherein the iron is complexed to a protoporphyrin ring. Because the metal is complexed or bound, it is protected from being sequestered by other dietary components (e.g., phytate, fiber and sugars) and is less likely to compete with mineral excesses.

Regardless of whether the molecular species is plant- or animal-derived, the complex must be able to be absorbed by mucosal cells or be cleaved to release the mineral in a soluble form or have stability constants that allow the mineral to be transferred to mucosal or serosal acceptors for availability (Clydesdale, 1988). Other explanations for why animal products are generally more available forms of certain minerals than plants include the "meat-factor" effect, wherein meat provides an available form of the mineral and enhances the absorption of the mineral supplied by the rest of the food (Kapsokefalou and Miller, 1993; Turnlund et al, 1983). In addition, meats, unlike plants, do not contain anti-nutritional factors, such as phytate, oxalate, goitrogens and fiber, which reduce mineral availability.

Not all fiber sources, however, negatively affect mineral availability. Research in chicks (Wedekind et al, 1995, 1996) and puppies (Wedekind et al, 1996a) indicated marked differences about how fiber sources affect mineral availability (Table 5-7). In these studies, beet pulp consistently reduced the availability of minerals (zinc, calcium, phosphorus and iron); however, cellulose, corn bran and sunflower hulls had negligible effects. Pea fiber, peanut hulls and soy hulls inhibited availability of some

Box 6-2. Organic vs. Inorganic Minerals.

There is some debate about whether organic forms of trace minerals are more available than inorganic forms. The answer depends on the specific mineral, the dietary conditions and the physiologic state of the animal. Clearly, the organic forms of certain minerals (e.g., selenium, chromium, iron) are better used than inorganic forms. (See the selenium, chromium and iron sections of this chapter.) Which form is better used is less clear for other minerals (e.g., zinc, copper). For example, there are as many studies that have failed to show increased availability with zinc/copper organic forms as there are studies demonstrating improved availability.

A number of factors influence the outcome of availability studies, including: 1) the presence of non-nutritional factors (e.g., phytate, fiber, goitrogens), 2) nutrient interactions (e.g., excesses of other minerals) and 3) physiologic state (e.g., demand for certain minerals increases with reproduction and growth compared to that of maintenance, thus in these situations, the differences in availability are magnified between organic and inorganic sources).

Results of studies in puppies showed that as calcium levels increased from 1.0 to 1.5%, zinc usage (as measured by changes in plasma zinc concentrations) decreased, irrespective of whether the source was organic (zinc propionate) or inorganic (zinc oxide). Zinc from zinc propionate was approximately 1.8 to 2 times more available than from zinc oxide.

Other investigators likewise noted increased zinc retention (as measured by zinc deposition in hair and fecal zinc excretion) for adult dogs fed a zinc-amino acid chelate compared with the same dogs fed zinc polysaccharide or zinc oxide. Increasing calcium from 1.2 to 3.2% reduced zinc retention when dogs were fed zinc polysaccharide or zinc oxide, but not the zinc-amino acid chelate.

Similarly, researchers have demonstrated in livestock and fish that growth rate and calcium and phytate levels are factors that significantly affect zinc use. Thus, these factors determine whether the use of organic zinc sources is beneficial. Together, these data suggest little or no benefit to using organic zinc in foods low in phytate and calcium (e.g., low calcium is defined as calcium levels approximating NRC recommendations for respective species). However, as phytate and/or calcium levels increase, or demand for zinc increases (e.g., rapid growth rate), there is greater zinc use from organic zinc sources (parameters used to assess zinc availability included bone zinc, immune response and/or growth rate). Furthermore, the more rapidly the animal grows, the greater the benefit demonstrated for organic zinc (e.g., fish >chicks [broiler breeds >leghorn-type] >puppies >pigs). The efficacy decreased as the animal matured, suggesting organic zinc sources in foods may be less beneficial for adult animals.

In summary, organic forms of minerals may be beneficial when dietary or physiologic conditions limit mineral availability. These conditions include: 1) mineral antagonisms caused by phytate, fiber and imbalances/excesses of other minerals and 2) increased metabolic demand such as rapid growth rate, reproduction and immune challenge.

The Bibliography for **Box 6-2** can be found at www.markmorris.org.

but not all of the minerals evaluated. Additional mineral supplementation is warranted for foods known to have reduced mineral availability.

Macrominerals

Calcium

Calcium serves two important functions: 1) as a structural component in bones and teeth and 2) as an intracellular second messenger that enables cells to respond to stimuli such as hormones and neurotransmitters. Calcium's two major physiologic functions in bone are to serve as a structural material and as an ion reservoir. When calcium in bone acts as an ion reservoir, it is in equilibrium with serum ionized calcium and under tight homeostatic control.

The mechanism of calcium homeostasis in blood is complex and involves several organs. Blood concentrations of ionized (or free) calcium are the major initiator of calcium regulatory mechanisms in the body. Calcium in blood is in equilibrium between a free or ionized state (~50%), a protein-bound state (~40 to 45%) and a complexed or chelated state (~5 to 10%). The effects of changing ionized calcium concentration in blood are highlighted below (**Figure 6-2**) (Nap and Hazewinkel, 1994). Low concentrations of ionized calcium:

- Stimulate PTH secretion, which stimulates conversion of 25-hydroxycholecalciferol (25-OH-D_3) to the biologically more potent 1,25-dihydroxycholecalciferol (1,25-$(OH)_2$-D_3) in the kidneys
- 1,25-$(OH)_2$-D_3 stimulates calcium uptake in the gut via receptor-mediated mechanisms
- 1,25-$(OH)_2$-D_3, in conjunction with PTH, stimulates bone resorption
- PTH induces phosphaturia.

High or normal concentrations of ionized calcium:

- Stimulate calcitonin secretion, which does not stimulate 1,25-$(OH)_2$-D_3 production
- 24,25-dihydroxycholecalciferol (24,25-$(OH)_2$-D_3) is now produced in the kidneys, which is considered biologically less active
- No stimulation of gut absorption or bone resorption occurs
- Increased renal calcium excretion results
- Calcitonin decreases osteoclastic activity.

PTH, calcitonin and 1,25-$(OH)_2$-D_3 act together to maintain calcium homeostasis in the face of variable dietary intakes and changing calcium requirements during growth, pregnancy and lactation.

The amount of true calcium absorption may range from 25 to 90%, depending upon calcium status, calcium form or intake (Nap and Hazewinkel, 1994). This exchangeable pool consists of the small amount of calcium in blood, lymph and other body fluids, and accounts for 1% of the total body calcium. The remaining 99% is located in bones and teeth. There are three routes of calcium absorption in the intestine. One is an active, saturable, transcellular process that occurs primarily in the duodenum and proximal jejunum. The process is regulated by vitamin D and involves a vitamin D-dependent, calcium-binding protein (CaBP or cal-bindin).

Active calcium absorption is affected by the physiology of the host (i.e., calcium and vitamin D status, age, pregnancy and lactation).

The other pathways of calcium absorption are facilitated and passive absorption, which are important in the distal gastrointestinal (GI) tract. Passive absorption is a nonsaturable, paracellular route that is independent of vitamin D regulation. The amount of calcium absorbed in this way depends primarily on quantity and availability of calcium in the food. No matter where absorption takes place, vitamin D is the most important regulator of calcium absorption (Birge and Avioli, 1990). Renal handling of calcium is also modulated by PTH and calcitonin but not as much by vitamin D.

Deficiencies and excesses of calcium, as well as calcium-phosphorus imbalances, should be avoided in dogs and cats (**Box 6-3**). A food grossly deficient in calcium, but adequate in phosphorus can cause secondary hyperparathyroidism. An all-meat diet devoid of bones, for example, is a very poor source of calcium. Inadequate calcium intake produces hypocalcemia, which stimulates release of PTH, which in turn stimulates production of 1,25-$(OH)_2$-D_3, resulting in a higher fractional absorption of calcium and phosphate, and lower calcium but higher phosphate concentration in urine. PTH acts with vitamin D to promote bone resorption and turnover, which may lead to pathologic fractures. Hypocalcemia is a common problem in diseased states (chronic or acute renal failure, pancreatitis, eclampsia, etc.), and parenteral supplementation of calcium and/or calcitriol (1,25-$(OH)_2$-D_3) is sometimes warranted (Chew and Carothers, 1995). Calcium excess is probably more detrimental in rapidly growing animals than in adults, especially large- and giant-breed puppies (Chapter 33). **Table 6-1** describes signs of calcium deficiency and excess.

Research suggests that the dietary requirement of calcium for growing puppies (especially large breeds) is higher at 1.2% dry matter (DM) (Hazewinkel et al, 1991; Schoenmakers et al, 1999; Nap et al, 1993) than the previous recommendation of 0.59% (NRC, 1985). The NRC (2006) recommended allowance for adult dogs and growing puppies after weaning is 0.40 and 0.59% DM calcium (both based on foods containing 4,000 kcal/kg), and for large- and giant-breed puppies at risk for developmental orthopedic disease, the recommendation is 0.7 to 1.2% DM calcium (based on foods containing 3,800 kcal/kg) (Chapter 33).

A balance study was conducted to determine the calcium requirement of adult cats (Pastoor et al, 1994). Four levels of calcium ($CaCO_3$) ranging from 0.27 to 1.62% DM were evaluated. The minimum level evaluated (0.27% calcium) resulted in positive mineral balance with no adverse effect on serum phosphorus, calcium, magnesium and alkaline phosphatase concentrations. This level is less than half that of current AAFCO (2007) recommendations (i.e., 0.6% calcium). Likewise, two groups of investigators conducting studies in kittens demonstrated lower calcium and phosphorus requirements than those currently recommended by AAFCO for growth (i.e., requirements for calcium and phosphorus were 0.5 and

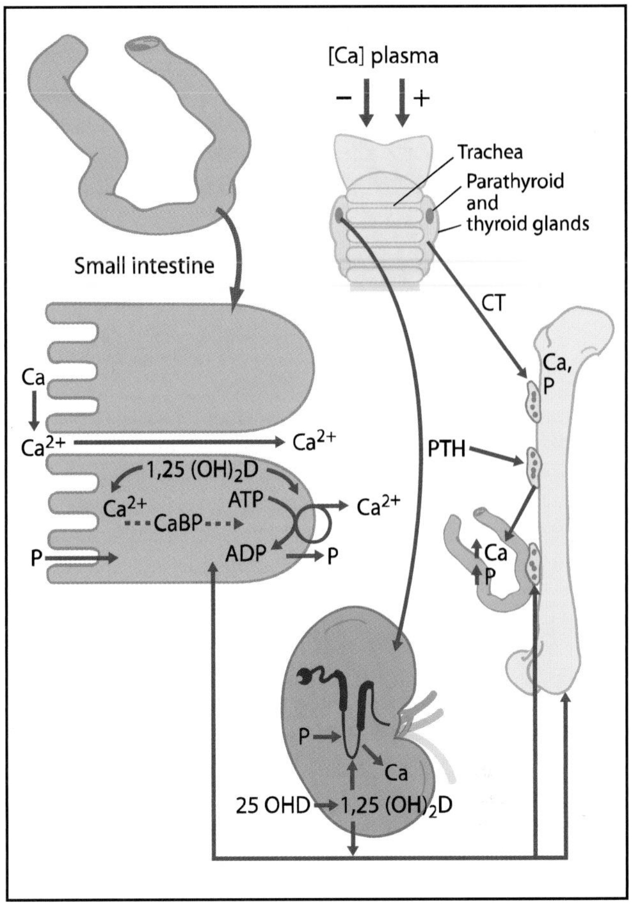

Figure 6-2. Calcium absorption by the intestine and bone resorption and reabsorption in the kidney are closely regulated by calcium-regulating hormones: parathyroid hormone, calcitonin and 1,25-$(OH)_2$-D_3. See text for details.

0.63% [Morris and Earle, 1996] and 0.36 and 0.28%, respectively [Pastoor, 1993]). These investigators concluded that the 1% DM calcium recommended by AAFCO (2007) for kittens is excessive and that the NRC recommendation (2006) of 0.8% DM calcium was a more defensible allowance for kittens fed typical moist foods. The current AAFCO (2007) canine and feline recommendations for calcium are 1.0% for growth/reproduction and 0.6% for adult maintenance (DM for both values). For dogs, this calcium requirement is based on an energy density of 3.5 kcal/g metabolizable energy (ME), whereas an energy density of 4.0 kcal/g ME is assumed for cats (AAFCO, 2007). Foods with increased energy densities should have a proportionally increased amount of calcium to account for decreased food consumption.

These meat meals are rich sources of calcium because of their bone content: poultry by-product meal, lamb meal and fish meal. Grains (corn, rice, etc.) are generally poor sources of calcium. Soybean meal and flaxseed have calcium contents between those of meat meals and grains. Meats without bone are poor sources of calcium. The most common calcium supplements used in pet foods are limestone (calcium carbonate), calcium sulfate, calcium chloride, calcium phosphate and bone meal, ranging in calcium from 16 to 39% (**Table 6-2**).

Box 6-3. Calcium-Phosphorus Ratios.

The "ideal" calcium-phosphorus ratio recommended for animals with simple stomachs is generally considered to be between 1:1 and 2:1. A number of factors, however, influence the importance of this ratio. Increasing levels of vitamin D reduce the significance of adverse calcium-phosphorus ratios. Furthermore, the ratio can differ markedly with the form and availability of the calcium and phosphorus supplied in the diet. For example, animals eating foods high in phytate phosphorus require greater phosphorus intake to meet their needs. Thus, the ideal calcium-phosphorus ratio would be lower when foods with these dietary characteristics are fed vs. foods composed of mostly meat ingredients.

Investigators sometimes debate whether the calcium-phosphorus ratio is more important than absolute calcium and phosphorus levels (**Table 1**). For all practical purposes, however, if a food were formulated to meet or slightly exceed an animal's requirement for calcium and phosphorus, it would by default provide an optimal calcium-phosphorus ratio. The more rapid the growth rate (e.g., large- and giant-breed puppies >small-breed puppies >adult dogs), the more critical it is to optimize calcium and phosphorus levels (Chapter 33). Increasing energy density increases the calcium and phosphorus requirement; the younger the animal the more critical it is that calcium and phosphorus be optimal.

Calcium-phosphorus ratios less than one have been evaluated in cats. Kealy et al compared the effects of feeding two foods with different calcium-phosphorus ratios to adult cats for 52 weeks. (The foods had 1:1 vs. 0.6:1 ratios; dry matter calcium and phosphorus levels were 1.27% calcium, 1.29% phosphorus and 0.75% calcium and 1.24% phosphorus, respectively.) Serum concentrations of total calcium, ionized calcium, phosphorus, PTH, alkaline phosphatase and vitamin D analogs did not differ between cats fed the two different foods at any sampling time and no signs of orthopedic diseases or bone loss developed during the study.

Likewise, Morris and Earle evaluated the effects of feeding foods containing calcium-phosphorus ratios as low as 0.65:1 to kittens and found no adverse effects, provided dry matter calcium and phosphorus levels exceeded 0.5 and 0.63%, respectively. Morris and Earle determined these calcium and phosphorus levels to be the calcium and phosphorus requirements for kittens. Results showed that this ratio (0.65:1) was well tolerated by kittens. Feed consumption, body weight gain, hematologic parameters and concentrations of plasma total and ionized calcium, total phosphorus, alkaline phosphatase, PTH, creatine phosphokinase, total plasma protein and albumin and plasma 25-OH-D did not differ from values in kittens fed foods with higher calcium-phosphorus ratios. Investigators noted significant changes in ionizable calcium concentrations; however, at 18 weeks in kittens fed foods with a calcium-phosphorus ratio of 0.38. These studies indicate that cats may tolerate wider dietary calcium-phosphorus ratios than the previously recommended ratios between 1:1 and 2:1.

The Bibliography for **Box 6-3** can be found at www.markmorris.org

Table 1. Examples of calcium-phosphorus percentages and ratios.

Examples	% calcium/% phosphorus (calcium-phosphorus ratio)
AAFCO adult allowance for calcium and phosphorus in dogs	0.6/0.5 (1.2:1)
AAFCO growth allowance for calcium and phosphorus in dogs	1.0/0.8 (1.25:1)
Example of why tuna is a poor source of calcium and has a poor calcium-phosphorus ratio	0.157/1.28 (0.12:1)
Example of a correct ratio, but excessive calcium and phosphorus levels	2/1.6 (1.2:1)

Phosphorus

Phosphorus is a vital participant in a number of tissues and functions. After calcium, phosphorus is the second largest constituent of bone and teeth. Phosphorus is a structural component of RNA and DNA, high-energy phosphate compounds such as ATP and cell membranes composed largely of phospholipids. As a component of nucleic acids, high-energy phosphate compounds and cell membranes, phosphorus is essential in cell growth and differentiation, energy use and transfer, fatty acid transport and amino acid and protein formation.

About 60 to 70% of phosphorus is absorbed from a typical diet (Allen and Wood, 1994). In general, phosphorus availability is greater from animal-based ingredients than from plant-based ingredients. Phosphorus in meat is found mainly in the organic form, whereas in plants, phosphorus is in the form of phytic acid. Phytate phosphorus is only about one-third available to monogastric animals but availability from different grains can vary markedly (McDowell, 1992). Intestinal phosphorus absorption represents the sum of a saturable, carrier-mediated component and a nonsaturable, concentration-dependent component. Regulation of total body phosphorus requires the coordinated efforts of the kidneys and intestine. Under conditions of low dietary phosphorus intake, the intestine increases its absorptive efficiency to maximize phosphorus absorption and the kidneys increase renal phosphorus transport or minimize urinary phosphorus losses. Hormonally, these adaptations result from changes in plasma levels of 1,25-$(OH)_2$-D_3 and PTH. Conversely, under conditions of dietary excess, the kidneys increase excretion of minerals. **Table 6-1** describes effects of deficiency and excess. Avoiding excess dietary phosphorus slows progression of kidney disease (Chapter 37).

There are few data to make a phosphorus recommendation; however, the most recent NRC (2006) suggests 1.0 and 0.30% DM for puppies and adult dogs, respectively.

Similar to the study design for calcium, investigators evaluated the minimum phosphorus requirement for adult cats (Pastoor et al, 1995). Four levels of phosphorus (provided as $NaH_2PO_4 \cdot 2H_2O$) ranging from 0.3 to 1.8% DM were evaluated. The minimum level evaluated (0.3% DM phosphorus) resulted in positive mineral balance with no adverse effect on serum phosphorus, calcium, magnesium and alkaline phos-

Table 6-2. Common mineral sources.*

Mineral	Source	Chemical formula	Mineral content (%)**			
Calcium	Calcium carbonate	$CaCo_4$	39 Ca	0.02 Na		
	Limestone	$CaCO_3$	38 Ca	0.05 Na	0.01 F	
	Calcium citrate		24 Ca			
	Calcium sulfate	$CaSO_4$	23 Ca			
	Calcium chloride	$CaCl_2$	35 Ca	64 Cl		
Calcium and phosphorus	Bone meal		24 Ca	12.6 P	0.37 Na	0.05 F
	Phosphate, curacao		36 Ca	14 P	0.3 Na	0.54 F
	Defluorinated		30-34 Ca	18 P	5.7 Na	0.16 F
	Dicalcium		18-24 Ca	18.5 P	0.6 Na	0.14 F
	Mono and dicalcium		16-19 Ca	21 P	0.6 Na	0.20 F
	Soft rock		17 Ca	9 P	0.1 Na	1.2 F
	Sodium tripolyphosphate		0 Ca	25 P	31 Na	0.03 F
Phosphorus	Phosphoric acid	H_3PO_4	0 Ca	23 P		
	Tricalcium phosphate	Ca_3PO_4	31-34 Ca	18 P		
Magnesium	Magnesium oxide	MgO	54 Mg			
	Magnesium sulfate	$MgSO_4$	9 Mg			
Potassium	Potassium citrate		36 K			
	Potassium chloride	KCl	50 K			
	Potassium sulfate	K_2SO_4	42 K			
Sodium and chloride	Sodium chloride	$NaCl$	39 Na	61 Cl		
	Sodium acetate		28 Na			
	Sodium tripolyphosphate		32 Na	25 P		
Iron	Ferrous sulfate	$FeSO_4 \bullet H_2O$	33 Fe			
	Ferrous sulfate	$FeSO_4 \bullet 7H_2O$	20 Fe			
	Ferric ammonium citrate		16.5-18.5 Fe			
	Ferrous fumarate	$FeC_4 \bullet H_2O_4$	32.9 Fe			
	Ferric chloride	$FeCl_3 \bullet 6H_2O$	20.7 Fe			
	Ferrous carbonate	$FeCO_3$	48.2 Fe			
	Ferric oxide	Fe_2O_3	69.9 Fe			
	Ferrous oxide	FeO	77.8 Fe			
Copper	Cupric carbonate	$CuCO_3 \bullet Cu(OH)_2$	57.5 Cu			
	Cupric chloride	$CuCl_2 \bullet 2H_2O$	37.3 Cu			
	Cupric hydroxide	$Cu(OH)_2$	65.1 Cu			
	Cupric oxide	CuO	79.9 Cu			
	Cupric sulfate	$CuSO_4 \bullet 5H_2O$	25.4 Cu			
Manganese	Manganese carbonate	$MnCO_3$	47.8 Mn			
	Manganous chloride	$MnCl_2 \bullet 4H_2O$	27.8 Mn			
	Manganous oxide	MnO	77.4 Mn			
	Manganese sulfate	$MnSO_4 \bullet 5H_2O$	22.7 Mn			
	Manganous sulfate	$MnSO_4 \bullet H_2O$	32.5 Mn			
Zinc	Zinc carbonate	$5ZnO \bullet 2CO_3 \bullet 4H_2O$	56.0 Zn			
	Zinc chloride	$ZnCl_2$	48.0 Zn			
	Zinc oxide	ZnO	72.0 Zn			
	Zinc sulfate	$ZnSO_4 \bullet 7H_2O$	22.7 Zn			
	Zinc sulfate	$ZnSO_4 \bullet H_2O$	36.4 Zn			
Iodine	Calcium iodate	$Ca(IO_3)_2$	65.1 I			
	Potassium iodide	KI	76.4 I			
	Cuprous iodide	CuI	66.6 I			
	Iodized salt		48.2 mg/kg I			
Selenium	Sodium selenite	Na_2SeO_3	45.6 Se	26.6 Na		
	Sodium selenate	Na_2SeO_4	41.8 Se	24.3 Na		

*Adapted from National Research Council. Nutrient Requirements of Cats. Washington, DC: National Academy of Sciences, 1986.
**Actual mineral levels in technical grade sources may vary.

phatase concentrations. Again, this is lower than the 0.5% DM phosphorus level currently recommended by AAFCO (2007). Levels of phosphorus exceeding 0.6% DM were associated with lower plasma phosphorus concentrations, reduced creatinine clearance and decreased magnesium absorption. Thus, the authors concluded continued feeding of high levels of dietary phosphorus might be detrimental to renal function. The AAFCO (2007) recommendation for phosphorus, for both dogs and cats, is 0.8% for growth and reproduction and 0.5% for adult maintenance (DM). These values (0.72 and 0.26% [DM] for kittens and adult cats, respectively) are higher than those listed in the current NRC (2006).

In general, meat tissue (poultry, lamb, fish, beef) is high in phosphorus. Eggs and milk products are also relatively rich in phosphorus. Oilseeds, protein supplements and grains likewise contribute significant amounts of phosphorus to pet foods, due more to their high inclusion rate than to high-phosphorus concentrations. A number of phosphorus supplements (**Table 6-2**) are used in pet foods, including calcium phosphate (monocalcium, dicalcium and tricalcium phosphate, defluorinated rock phosphate), sodium phosphates and phosphoric acid.

Magnesium

Magnesium is the third largest mineral constituent of bone, after calcium and phosphorus. Magnesium is involved in the metabolism of carbohydrates and lipids and acts as a catalyst for a wide array of enzymes. It is required for cellular oxidation (e.g., ATP production), it catalyzes most phosphate transfers (e.g., alkaline phosphatase, hexokinase and deoxyribonuclease) and it exerts a potent influence on neuromuscular activity. In light of these functions, it is not surprising that magnesium deficiency in animals is manifested clinically in a wide range of disorders, which include retarded growth, hyperirritability and tetany, peripheral vasodilatation, anorexia, muscle incoordination and convulsions. Other metabolic aberrations that may occur in magnesium-deficient animals include calcification of the kidneys and liver, decreased blood pressure and body temperature and decreased thiamin concentrations in tissues (Underwood and Mertz, 1987).

From 20 to 70% of dietary magnesium is absorbed (Brody, 1994). Intestinal magnesium absorption represents the sum of both a carrier-mediated system at low intraluminal concentrations, and simple diffusion at higher concentrations. A number of dietary and physiologic factors negatively influence magnesium absorption, including high levels of dietary phosphorus, calcium, potassium, fat and protein.

The kidneys play a critical role in magnesium homeostasis. Approximately 70% of serum magnesium is filtered by glomeruli; healthy kidneys reabsorb about 95% of the filtered magnesium (Shils, 1996). Several physiologic and metabolic factors, drugs and disease states influence magnesium reabsorption in nephrons. Certain drugs, such as diuretics, aminoglycosides, cisplatin, cyclosporin, amphotericin and methotrexate, can cause increased renal wasting of magnesium (Freeman, 1995).

Avoiding excess dietary magnesium is recommended for the prevention of struvite urinary precipitates in cats and dogs; however, magnesium deficiency is reported to increase the risk of calcium oxalate urolithiasis in rats (Driessens and Verbeeck, 1990). Furthermore, magnesium supplementation has been advocated to prevent calcium oxalate urolithiasis in people. However, this practice is very controversial because clinical trials have demonstrated mixed efficacy. The relationship of magnesium to feline and canine urinary calcium oxalate precipitates is unknown; however, ensuring magnesium concentrations above the minimum requirement is considered safe (Chapters 40, 43 and 46).

Conversely, increased magnesium supplementation may be warranted under certain clinical conditions in which magnesium stores are depleted. The GI tract and kidneys are the primary potential routes for magnesium excretion. Magnesium deficiencies may also result from renal losses secondary to renal tubular acidosis, hypercalcemia, hyperthyroidism, hypoparathyroidism and use of diuretics. Additionally, epidemiologic data and rat studies suggest that low urinary magnesium to calcium ratios may increase the risk for calcium oxalate formation (Driessens and Verbeeck, 1990). **Table 6-1** describes signs of deficiency and excess.

The minimum requirement for magnesium in adult cats has been evaluated (Pastoor, 1993). Four levels of magnesium ($MgCO_3$) were compared. Positive mineral balance was observed even at the lowest magnesium level (0.02% DM) and no adverse effects were noted in serum magnesium and alkaline phosphatase concentrations. This magnesium level is half of the current NRC (2006) and AAFCO recommendation (2007). Extrapolation of these results, which were obtained by feeding semi-purified diets, to commercial foods should be made cautiously because of the differences in ingredients used and the greater potential for mineral antagonisms and decreased availability that may occur in practical diets. AAFCO (2007) recommends 0.08% DM magnesium for growth and reproduction and 0.04% DM magnesium for adult maintenance for cats (AAFCO, 2007). The AAFCO (2007) magnesium recommendation for dogs is 0.04% DM for both lifestages, whereas the current NRC (2006) suggests 0.04% DM for puppies and 0.06% DM for adult dogs.

Ingredients containing bone (bone meal, lamb meal), oilseed/protein supplements (flaxseed, soybean meal and other legumes such as pea protein) and unrefined grains and fiber sources (wheat bran, oat bran, beet pulp, soymill run) are rich in magnesium. Common magnesium supplements include magnesium oxide and magnesium sulfate.

Potassium

Potassium is the most abundant intracellular cation and the third most abundant mineral in the body. Potassium is involved in a number of functions, including: 1) maintaining acid-base balance, 2) maintaining osmotic balance, 3) transmitting nerve impulses, 4) facilitating muscle contractility and 5) serving as a cofactor in several enzyme systems (energy transfer and use, protein synthesis and carbohydrate metabolism).

Potassium is absorbed primarily by simple diffusion from the upper small intestine, although some absorption also occurs in the lower small intestine and large intestine. Potassium availability is relatively high (95% or higher) for most foodstuffs (McDowell, 1992). Yet, in contrast to most minerals, potassium is not readily stored and must be supplied daily in the diet. Thus, it is important that foods for dogs and cats contain adequate potassium. Increased intake of potassium is unlikely to cause sustained hyperkalemia unless renal excretion of potassium is impaired. Administration of certain drugs predisposes patients to hyperkalemia (e.g., nonspecific β-adrenergic blockers and angiotensin-converting enzyme inhibitors).

Table 6-1 describes signs of deficiency and excess. Increasing protein, energy density or chloride, and other factors such as stress (heat, exercise, vomiting and diarrhea) and milk production increase the requirement for potassium. AAFCO (2007) recommends 0.6% DM potassium for both dogs and cats for all lifestages. These levels are higher than the current NRC (2006) DM potassium recommendation of 0.44% for puppies, 0.40% for adult dogs, 0.40% for kittens and 0.52% for adult cats.

Rich sources of potassium include soybean meal, unrefined grains and fiber sources (soymill run, sunflower hulls, rice bran, wheat bran) and yeast. Potassium supplements commonly added to pet foods include potassium citrate, potassium chloride and potassium sulfate.

Sodium and Chloride

Sodium and chloride, in addition to potassium, are important for maintaining osmotic pressure, regulating acid-base equilibrium and transmitting nerve impulses and muscle contractions via Na-K-ATPase (sodium pump). In addition, sodium and chloride control the passage of nutrients into cells. Sodium ions must be present in the lumen of the small intestine for absorption of sugars and amino acids. Insufficient sodium concentrations decrease the use of digested protein and energy. Sodium also influences calcium absorption and mobilization and may affect absorption of several water-soluble vitamins (e.g., riboflavin, thiamin and ascorbic acid) that are sodium coupled (McDowell, 1992).

Sodium and chloride are readily absorbed, principally from the upper small intestine, and excreted predominantly in the urine with smaller amounts in feces and perspiration. Marked losses of salt can occur through perspiration in some species, secretion in milk, vomiting and diarrhea. When sodium intake is inadequate, the body has a remarkable capacity for conserving sodium by excreting extremely low levels in the urine. Chloride metabolism is controlled in relation to sodium. For example, excess urinary excretion of sodium is accompanied by urinary excretion of chloride.

Hormones acting to maintain a constant sodium-potassium ratio in extracellular fluid regulate sodium concentrations in the body. Aldosterone, secreted from the adrenal cortex, regulates reabsorption of sodium from the renal tubules. Antidiuretic hormone from the posterior pituitary responds to osmotic pressure changes in the extracellular fluid. Both hormones maintain a constant sodium-potassium ratio.

A number of factors influence the sodium requirement. The requirement is increased during reproduction, lactation, rapid growth and heat stress and with high dietary potassium levels. In people, the average sodium intake exceeds the recommended requirement by 15-fold (Stamler, 1995). Likewise, the sodium content of certain pet foods exceeds the recommended level by four- to 15-fold (Chapter 36). Investigators determined the sodium requirement of kittens to be 0.16% (DM or 0.30 mg Na/kcal ME) based on aldosterone concentration in plasma (Yu and Morris, 1997). The same investigators determined the requirement for adult cats was 0.08% DM sodium or 0.15 mg Na/kcal ME (Yu and Morris, 1999). The AAFCO (2007) recommendation for sodium in cats is 0.2% DM for both lifestages, whereas in dogs, the recommendation is 0.3% DM for growth and reproduction and 0.06% DM for adult maintenance. The current NRC (2006) sodium recommendation is 0.14% DM for kittens and 0.068% DM for adult cats. The NRC (2006) suggests a 0.22% minimum DM sodium requirement for puppies and 0.08% DM for adult dogs.

High sodium intake has long been reported to increase the risk of hypertension in people and animals (Stamler, 1995). Pet populations with increased risk of hypertension include senior dogs and cats and those with renal disease, cardiac disease, hyperthyroid disease or obesity. Pet food manufacturers sometimes use dietary salt supplementation to increase water intake in cats with lower urinary tract disease. High sodium intake in the short term effectively increases water intake, urine output and urine dilution, thus lowering the risk of urolithiasis, but may have detrimental effects in the long term. Kirk (2002) showed that high-sodium intake (1.1% DM) over a three-month period, increased serum urea nitrogen, phosphorus and creatinine concentrations in cats with preexisting renal disease. In addition, the high-sodium food increased cardiac left ventricular fractional shortening and lowered plasma aldosterone levels, evidence suggesting that this sodium chloride load required both the heart and kidney to work harder. Similarly, both the NRC Mineral Tolerance of Animals (2005) and the NRC Nutrient Requirements of Dogs and Cats (2006) recommend a safe upper limit for sodium at 1.5% DM for adult dogs, and 1.0 and 1.5% DM for kittens and adult cats, respectively. At higher levels of sodium intake (≥2%), studies showed reduced food intake, negative potassium balance and vomiting.

In the absence of studies establishing chloride requirements for dogs or cats, the DM recommendation for chloride is 1.5 times that of sodium. This value is comparable to the Na:Cl requirement ratio for other species. **Table 6-1** describes signs of deficiency and excess (**Case 6-1**).

The effect of dietary sodium chloride on blood pressure has generally been attributed to the sodium ion. However, it is clear from a number of studies that both sodium and chloride are necessary to inhibit renin production (Kotchen et al, 1978; Kurtz et al, 1987). Salts such as sodium chloride, potassium chloride, lysine hydrochloride (but not lysine glutamate, sodium bicarbonate, potassium bicarbonate) inhibited renin production in sodium chloride-deprived rats and people.

Fish, eggs, dried whey, poultry by-product meal and soy isolate are ingredients high in sodium and chloride. Sodium and/or chloride supplements typically added to pet foods include salt, sodium phosphates, calcium chloride, choline chloride, potassium chloride and sodium acetate.

Microminerals

Iron

Iron is present in several enzymes and other proteins responsible for oxygen activation (oxidases and oxygenases), for electron transport (cytochromes) and for oxygen transport (hemoglobin, myoglobin). Because of the limited capacity of the body to excrete iron, iron homeostasis is maintained primarily by adjusting iron absorption. Iron in foods exists in two forms: 1) heme iron present in hemoglobin and myoglobin and 2) nonheme iron present in grains and plant sources.

Heme iron absorption is not greatly affected by iron status or other dietary factors. (Two exceptions are meat, which enhances heme iron absorption, and calcium, which inhibits heme and nonheme iron absorption.) In contrast to absorption of heme iron, absorption of nonheme iron is markedly influenced by iron status and by several dietary factors such as phytate, tannins and excesses of calcium, phosphorus, manganese, zinc, copper and ascorbic acid (Hallberg and Rossander-

Hulthen, 1993).

The amount of iron absorbed from food is thus determined by three factors: 1) iron status of the body, 2) availability of dietary iron (as affected by other ingredients and nutrients) and 3) amounts of heme and nonheme iron in food (Hallberg and Rossander-Hulthen, 1993).

Iron is transported by plasma and is taken up by the bone marrow for hemoglobin synthesis. Although a small amount of hemoglobin circulates in plasma, by far the greatest amount of plasma iron is complexed to the specific iron-binding β_1-globulin transferrin. The degree of saturation of transferrin affects deposition of iron in liver stores and the supply of iron to red blood cell precursors. At saturation levels above 60%, much of the iron is deposited in the liver. Under normal conditions, only 30 to 40% of the transferrin is saturated; the remaining 60 to 70% represents an unbound or latent reserve (Morris, 1987).

Iron is stored predominantly as ferritin and hemosiderin in liver, bone marrow and spleen. Normally, iron is stored primarily as ferritin. As tissue iron concentrations increase, however, the concentration of hemosiderin increases more than that of ferritin. Excretion of iron is limited. Only negligible amounts of iron appear in urine; the iron appearing in feces is predominantly unabsorbed iron. Iron is continuously lost in sweat, hair and nails.

Investigators determined that the iron requirement of kittens and puppies fed a phytate-free purified diet is 80 mg iron/kg of food (DM) (Chausow and Czarnecki-Maulden, 1987). This requirement is the AAFCO (2007) recommendation for iron for dogs and cats, for both growth/reproduction and adult maintenance lifestages. The new NRC (2006) recommends a minimum of 88 mg/kg DM iron for growth and 30 mg/kg DM iron for adult dogs. Similar to AAFCO allowances (2007), the minimum NRC (2006) iron recommendation for cats is 80 mg/kg DM for growth and adult lifestages. Most pet foods are high in iron because of the high iron concentrations found in meat ingredients, especially organ meats. Furthermore, studies have shown the availability of iron to be relatively high from liver, muscle and animal by-products (Elvehjem et al, 1933; Conrad et al, 1980). Consequently, iron deficiency is not of practical concern with most pet foods.

Although iron levels may be high in pet foods (levels sometimes exceed the requirement by 15-fold without supplementation), AAFCO has set a maximum level of 3,000 mg iron/kg of food for dogs (no maximum is established for cats), which clearly exceeds dietary concentrations of iron in most typical pet foods. Iron excesses should be avoided because of potential antagonism with other minerals (e.g., zinc and copper). **Table 6-1** lists signs of deficiency and excess.

Chronic blood loss eventually depletes iron reserves and causes a microcytic, hypochromic anemia. The most common chronic blood loss in dogs and cats occurs with blood-sucking intestinal (hookworms) and external (fleas, ticks) parasites. Young puppies and kittens are especially vulnerable because of the low-iron content of milk.

Iron concentrations are high in most meat ingredients, especially organ meats such as liver, spleen and lungs. Other ingredients rich in iron include dicalcium phosphate and fiber sources such as beet pulp, soymill run and peanut hulls. In fact, poultry studies have shown that the iron contained in dicalcium phosphate alone in a corn-soybean meal diet can meet a chick's requirement for iron (Deming and Czarnecki-Maulden, 1989).

Typical iron sources include ferrous sulfate, ferric chloride, ferrous fumarate, ferrous carbonate and iron oxide. The iron in iron oxide, however, is not biologically available. Iron oxide is often added to pet foods to impart a "meaty red" color. A relatively high level of iron oxide is added (up to 0.04%) when iron oxide is used as a pigment in pet foods. Analytically, a pet food containing iron oxide will appear to be high in iron, but may not be high in available iron. Thus, the contribution of iron from iron oxide should be considered when evaluating the iron adequacy of foods containing iron oxide (e.g., 0.04% DM iron oxide in a moist food contributes 933 mg iron/kg of food).

Zinc

Zinc is a constituent or activator of more than 200 enzymes, so it is involved in a number of diverse physiologic functions. Some of zinc's primary functions include: 1) nucleic acid metabolism, 2) protein synthesis, 3) carbohydrate metabolism, 4) immunocompetence, 5) skin and wound healing, 6) cell replication and differentiation, 7) growth and 8) reproduction. Zinc also interacts with hormone production, most notably testosterone, adrenal corticosteroids and insulin. Zinc homeostasis is controlled through absorption and excretion.

The mechanism and control of zinc absorption are still not fully understood. Zinc absorption occurs primarily in the duodenum, jejunum and ileum. Only small amounts are absorbed from the stomach. Zinc absorption is markedly affected by other dietary components. Phytate, for example, decreases zinc absorption, whereas low molecular weight binding ligands such as citrate, picolinate, ethylenediaminetetraacetic acid (EDTA) and amino acids such as histidine and glutamate enhance zinc absorption (Hambidge et al, 1986). The liver is the primary organ involved in zinc metabolism. When hepatic zinc content is increased above normal levels, additional zinc is associated with metallothionein, a metal-binding protein thought to have a role in storage and detoxification of zinc, copper, cadmium and other metals.

Zinc in plasma is bound to protein in two forms: 1) firmly bound zinc that appears to bind to globulin (approximately 33% of total plasma zinc) and 2) loosely bound zinc complexed with albumin (66% of total plasma zinc) (McDowell, 1992). Storage of zinc is limited except in bone; stores increase only slightly as dietary zinc increases. Zinc concentration in bone has been used as a measure of zinc absorption and/or zinc status in young growing animals, whereas plasma zinc is only a reliable index under controlled experimental conditions.

Zinc is excreted primarily in the feces as unabsorbed and endogenous zinc (pancreatic juice, bile, other digestive secretions). Excretion of endogenous zinc in feces varies according to the balance between true absorption and metabolic needs. Variable excretion is one of the primary mechanisms used to maintain zinc homeostasis. Thus, both absorption and excretion are important in regulating zinc balance.

Zinc deficiency is probably more of a practical concern with pet foods than is toxicity, because: 1) zinc is relatively nontoxic and 2) its availability is decreased by a number of factors (phytate, high dietary levels of calcium, phosphate, copper, iron, cadmium and chromium). The antagonistic effects of calcium are greatest when phytate is also present, resulting in the formation of a highly insoluble complex of calcium, phytate and zinc. Signs of zinc deficiency have been reported to occur in dogs fed cereal-based dry foods (e.g., grains may contain significant concentrations of phytate), even when the zinc content of the food exceeded NRC minimum requirements (NRC, 2006; Morris and Rogers, 1994).

AAFCO recommends 120 mg/kg DM zinc for dogs and 75 mg/kg DM zinc for cats (2007). For trace minerals, AAFCO makes the same recommendations for adult maintenance and growth/reproduction foods. In livestock, however, the requirement for zinc is greatly increased during growth and reproduction. NRC (2006) recommends a minimum of 100 mg/kg DM zinc for growth vs. 60 mg/kg DM zinc for adult dogs; NRC makes similar zinc recommendations for cats (i.e., 75 and 74 mg/kg DM zinc in foods for growth and adults, respectively).

Signs of zinc deficiency include anorexia, decreased growth rate, alopecia, parakeratosis, impaired reproduction, depressed immune function and growth disorders of the skeleton (Chapter 33). Naturally occurring zinc-responsive dermatoses have been described (Chapter 32).

Although relatively nontoxic, excess dietary zinc can interfere with other minerals (iron and copper), thus excesses should be avoided. The only reported cases of zinc toxicosis in dogs or cats have been due to dietary indiscretion (e.g., consumption of die-case nuts from animal carriers or pennies) (**Case 6-2**). **Table 6-1** describes effects of zinc deficiency and excess. Ingredients naturally high in zinc include most meats, fiber sources and dicalcium phosphate. Zinc supplements most commonly used in pet foods are zinc oxide, zinc sulfate, zinc chloride and zinc carbonate.

Copper

Of the many copper-containing proteins, four enzyme systems may play key roles in the clinical signs associated with copper deficiency: 1) the ferroxidase activity of ceruloplasmin explains in part the disturbances of hematopoiesis in copper deficiency, 2) the monoamine oxidase enzymes may account for the role of copper in pigmentation and control of neurotransmitters and neuropeptides, 3) lysyl oxidase is essential for maintaining the integrity of connective tissue, a function that explains disturbances in lungs, bones and the cardiovascular system and 4) the copper enzymes cytochrome C oxidase and superoxide dismutase (SOD) play a central role in the terminal steps of oxidative metabolism and the defense against superoxide radicals, respectively. These functions have been postulated to account for the disturbances of the nervous system as seen in neonatal ataxia in several animal species with copper deficiency (Davis and Mertz, 1987).

In most species, copper can be absorbed in all segments of the GI tract; however, the small intestine is the major site of absorption (Davis and Mertz, 1987). Although the biochemical mechanisms are not fully understood, there is good evidence that intestinal absorption of copper is regulated by the need of the animal and that metallothionein (a metal-binding protein) plays a key role in regulation. Copper appears to be absorbed by two mechanisms, one saturable, suggesting active transport at low dietary copper concentrations and the other unsaturable, suggesting simple diffusion at high dietary copper levels.

Most copper in plasma is bound to ceruloplasmin, a copper-binding protein. Newly absorbed copper, however, may be transported from the intestine loosely bound to albumin or certain amino acids. In this form, the element is readily available to the liver and other tissues, in contrast to the much more tightly regulated distribution of ceruloplasmin-bound copper. This difference in availability may explain the tissue damage caused by copper accumulation in hepatotoxicosis seen in Bedlington terriers and people with Wilson's disease, in which the ceruloplasmin transport protein is lacking.

The liver is the central organ for copper metabolism. Hepatic concentrations reflect an animal's intake and copper status. Copper is excreted primarily through the feces. Most fecal copper is unabsorbed, but active excretion also occurs via the bile. Copper homeostasis is maintained primarily through absorption.

Dietary copper deficiency has been reported to occur in dogs and cats and thus is of practical concern (Morris and Rogers, 1994) (**Case 6-3**) Availability of copper from different foods and supplements can vary greatly, so the requirement for copper is difficult to define. The requirement can vary several-fold depending on the source of copper in the food and the level of other ingredients/nutrients/non-nutrients (e.g., interactions with phytate, calcium, zinc and iron). The AAFCO (2007) recommendation for copper in dogs is 7.3 mg/kg DM.

Separate copper requirements are recommended for extruded cat foods (15 mg/kg DM) vs. moist cat foods (5 mg/kg DM) during growth/reproduction. The recommended AAFCO (2007) copper level for maintenance of adult cats is 5 mg/kg DM, regardless of the food form. The rationale for separate copper requirements for cats (extruded vs. canned) is unclear. Investigators demonstrated increased needs for copper during reproduction in queens fed extruded foods.[a] Separate requirements for extruded and canned foods were recommended in the absence of reproduction data for cats fed moist foods.

Researchers studied chicks to evaluate the availability of copper from feed ingredients typically used in pet foods (Aoyagi et al, 1993). Results showed that copper availability was essentially zero from copper oxide and pork liver. Beef, sheep and turkey liver, however, were highly available sources of copper. AAFCO (2007) has recommended that pet food companies discontinue the use of copper oxide as a copper source based on studies of swine, poultry, dogs and cats in which researchers have demonstrated the poor availability of copper from copper oxide (Aoyagi and Baker, 1993; Cromwell et al, 1989; Czarnecki-

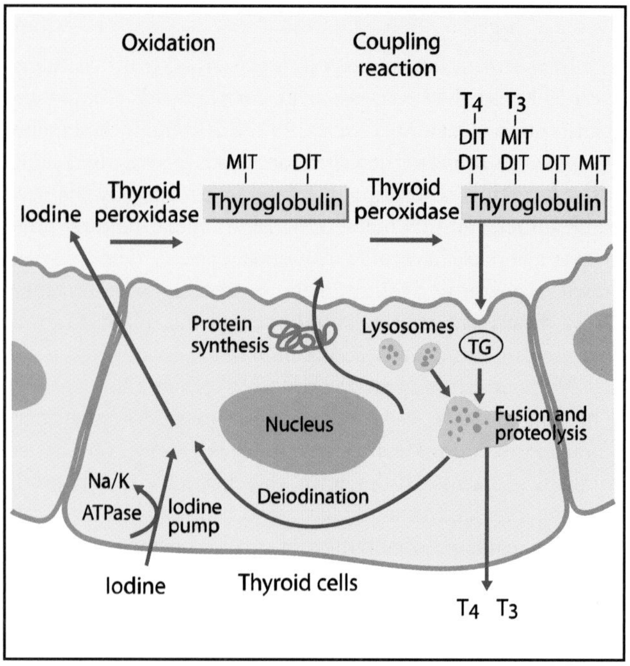

Figure 6-3. Diagram showing pathways of thyroid-hormone synthesis from iodine within the thyroid gland. (Adapted with permission from Hetzel BS, Maberly GF. Iodine. In: Mertz W, ed. Trace Elements in Human and Animal Nutrition, 5th ed. San Diego, CA: Academic Press Inc, 1986; 147.) See text for details.

Mauldin et al, 1993; Fascetti et al, 1998, 2000).

Signs of copper deficiency in cats include poor reproductive performance, early fetal loss, fetal deformities, cannibalism, coat hypopigmentation, kinked tails and inverted carpi.[a] Clinical signs in dogs include hair depigmentation and hyperextension of the distal forelimbs (Zentek and Meyer, 1991). **Table 6-1** lists signs of deficiency and excess.

Copper excess in dogs and cats with normal metabolism is of much less practical concern than copper deficiency, but can interfere with iron and zinc use. Bedlington, West Highland white and Skye terriers, however, are predisposed to hereditary autosomal recessive disease resulting in copper hepatoxicosis (Chapter 68). Anti-copper therapies such as zinc supplementation and orally administered tetrathiomolybdate have been used to treat dogs with this genetic disorder (NRC, 2006). AAFCO (2007) has set a safe upper limit of 250 mg/kg DM copper for dogs, but no safe upper limit for cats. NRC (2006) lists no safe upper limit of copper for either dogs or cats.

Most meat ingredients, especially organ meats, are rich in copper. Ruminant livers are extremely high in copper; concentrations are five to 10 times higher than in monogastric livers.[b] Typical copper supplements include cupric sulfate, cupric carbonate and cupric chloride.

Manganese

Manganese deficiency is of little practical relevance in dogs and cats, but is of practical relevance in birds. AAFCO (2007) recommends 5 mg/kg DM manganese for dogs and 7.5 mg/kg DM for cats, which is similar to NRC (2006) recommendations. The manganese requirement for birds is 10 to 12 times higher than that for people, pigs, dogs and cats (McDowell, 1992). Manganese functions as an enzyme activator or as a constituent of metalloenzymes. Although there are only a few manganese-containing metalloenzymes (e.g., arginase, pyruvate carboxylase and manganese-superoxide dismutase), many enzymes are activated by manganese, including hydrolases, kinases, decarboxylases and transferases. Other cations (especially magnesium), however, can partially substitute for manganese with little or no loss in enzymatic activity, thus manganese deficiency may not adversely affect physiologic or metabolic function (McDowell, 1992).

Manganese is also essential in bone and cartilage development because it activates glycosyltransferases (i.e., enzymes important for polysaccharide and glycoprotein synthesis). In addition, manganese is involved in reproduction and lipid metabolism (e.g., manganese is involved in the biosynthesis of choline and cholesterol).

Manganese homeostasis is maintained through regulation of absorption and excretion. Manganese is absorbed throughout the small intestine in a rapidly saturable process. Low molecular weight ligands, such as L-histidine and citrate, enhance absorption, whereas excessive concentrations of phosphorus, iron and cobalt can reduce absorption. Manganese is excreted via several routes that combine to provide an efficient homeostatic mechanism to regulate manganese levels in tissues. Bile flow is the primary route of excretion, but manganese is also excreted in pancreatic juice and in the small intestine.

Table 6-1 lists signs of manganese deficiency and excess. Ingredients rich in manganese include fiber sources, menhaden fish meal and dicalcium phosphate. Manganese supplements include manganese oxide, manganese sulfate, manganous chloride and manganese carbonate.

Iodine

Iodine is a constituent of the thyroid hormones 3,5,3',5'-tetraiodothyronine (thyroxine, T_4) and 3,5,3'-triiodothyronine (T_3). Thyroid hormones have an active role in thermoregulation, intermediary metabolism, reproduction, growth and development, circulation and muscle function. Thyroid hormones also: 1) influence physical and mental growth and differentiation and maturation of tissues, 2) affect other endocrine glands, especially the hypophysis and the gonads, 3) influence neuromuscular functioning and 4) have an effect on the integument, hair and fur (McDowell, 1992).

The thyroid glands actively trap iodine daily to ensure an adequate supply of thyroid hormone. This trapping mechanism regulates a more or less constant iodine supply to the thyroid glands over a wide range of plasma iodide levels. **Figure 6-3** outlines the steps of thyroid-hormone biosynthesis (Hetzel and Maberly, 1986). Iodine trapping is an active transport mechanism linked to Na^+/K^+-ATPase activity. Thyroid-stimulating hormone, which is released from the pituitary gland to regulate thyroid activity, also regulates this mechanism. A thyroid-peroxidase enzyme oxidizes iodide, which is released from thyroid cells into the colloid space. Iodine then combines with tyrosine residues associated with thyroglobulin protein to form monoiodotyrosine (MIT) and diiodotyrosine (DIT). The oxidation process proceeds further under the influence of the thyroid-peroxidase enzyme to couple MIT and DIT to form various iodothyronines (e.g., T_3 and T_4). Finally, iodinated thyroglobulin and thyroid hormones are reabsorbed into the thyroid cells and exposed to proteolytic enzymes. Much of the protein and iodinated tyrosines are lysed and returned as substrates to repeat the process. At the same time, some thyroid hormones are released into the circulation. Regulating the action of thyroid hormones is a complex process involving interaction among neurotransmitters, hormones and enzymes in the central nervous system, the pituitary gland, the thyroid glands, the circulation and peripheral tissues.

Investigators have estimated the iodine requirement for adult dogs to be 0.56 mg/kg DM (Belshaw et al, 1975). AAFCO (2007) recommends an iodine level of 1.5 mg/kg DM for dogs. This margin of safety is prudent in practical foods to overcome potential effects of goitrogens and negative mineral antagonisms.

A recent study (Wedekind et al, In press) estimated the iodine requirement for adult cats to be 0.46 mg/kg DM. This estimate was based upon three measurements of iodine status: regression of Tc 99m thyroid:salivary ratio (scintigraphy), iodine balance and urinary iodine excretion after iodine intake. These estimates agreed closely with the iodine requirement determined for dogs (Belshaw et al, 1975) and people (DRI, 2001). This estimate is higher than current AAFCO (2007) minimum iodine recommendations for adult cats (i.e., 0.35 mg/kg DM iodine), but is much lower than the NRC (2006) recommended iodine allowance (1.4 mg iodine/kg diet). Note that the NRC (2006) recommendation does not agree closely with current AAFCO recommendations and was based upon data derived from two studies (Scott et al, 1961; Ranz et al, 2002). Unfortunately, these studies should not have been used as a basis for establishing the iodine requirement of cats. The Scott (1961) study used a nutritionally incomplete or imbalanced diet (i.e., the diet used was an all meat diet [beef hearts], which was grossly deficient in calcium). The Ranz (2002) study was of short duration (i.e., 54 days total with only a seven-day period for each iodine level). In this study, the minimum iodine level evaluated, approximately 4.1 mg/kg iodine, was not low enough to yield a valid iodine requirement estimate. Interestingly, the previous NRC (1986) did not cite the Scott (1961) reference.

The iodine requirement is influenced by physiologic state and diet. Lactating animals require more dietary iodine because about 10% of the iodine intake is normally excreted in milk (McDowell, 1992). Likewise, the presence of goitrogenic substances and nutrient excesses of certain minerals (e.g., arsenic, bromide, fluoride, cobalt, manganese, calcium and potassium) may increase the need for iodine (NRC, 2005). Potential sources of goitrogens in pet foods include peas, peanuts, soybeans and flaxseed. Fish, eggs and iodized salt are rich sources of iodine, whereas most animal proteins are moderate sources of iodine. Iodine supplements typically used in pet foods include calcium iodate, potassium iodide and cuprous iodide.

Since the late 1970s, feline hyperthyroidism has become a more frequently diagnosed condition. However, much remains to be learned about this endocrinopathy (e.g., prevalence and cause). Hypothyroidism is a much more prevalent thyroid disorder in dogs. Both iodine excess and deficiency may result in subclinical or overt thyroid dysfunction.

Current AAFCO (2007) guidelines set a maximum safe level for iodine for dogs at 50 mg/kg, whereas NRC (2006) recommends 4 mg/kg as a safe upper limit. Neither NRC nor AAFCO sets a safe upper limit for iodine for cats. However, estimates for establishing safe upper limits and/or lowest observable adverse effect level for cats were determined in a recent study (Wedekind et al, In press). In people, guidelines have been established to define deficiency, adequacy and iodine excess (Laurberg et al, 2001) based upon urinary iodine concentrations. When these guidelines are applied to cats (corrected for metabolic equivalent basis; $BW^{0.67}$), dietary intakes between 0.46 and 3.5 mg/kg were considered optimal, whereas dietary intakes exceeding 3.5 mg/kg were defined as excessive. In addition, cats fed the highest dietary iodine intake (8.8 to 9.2 mg/kg iodine) for one year had significantly reduced FT_4 and numerically lowered TT_4 and TT_3 at 12 months. Thus, these findings suggest 3.5 mg/kg as a no observable adverse effect level or safe upper level and intakes of 8.8 mg/kg as a lowest observable adverse effect level. **Table 6-1** lists signs of iodine deficiency and excess. See Chapter 29 for more information about iodine.

Selenium

Selenium is an essential constituent of glutathione peroxidase, which helps protect cellular and subcellular membranes from oxidative damage. Glutathione peroxidase and vitamin E work synergistically to reduce the destructive effects of peroxidative reactions on living cells. Selenium spares vitamin E in at least three ways: 1) preserves the integrity of the pancreas, which allows normal fat digestion, and thus normal vitamin E absorption, 2) reduces the amount of vitamin E required to maintain integrity of lipid membranes via glutathione peroxidase and 3) aids retention of vitamin E in the blood plasma in some unknown way.

Vitamin E reduces the selenium requirement in at least two ways: 1) maintains body selenium in an active form, or prevents losses from the body and 2) prevents destruction of lipids within membranes, thereby inhibiting production of hydroperoxides and reducing the amount of the selenium-dependent enzyme needed to destroy peroxides formed in cells (Scott et al, 1982). Selenium also has a vital role in maintaining normal thyroid hormone and iodine metabolism, particularly through the control of deiodinase enzymes that regulate conversion of T_4 to T_3 (Arthur, 1993).

The duodenum is the main site of selenium absorption. There is no homeostatic control of selenium absorption regardless of the dietary selenium concentration. Likewise, selenium status also appears to have little effect on selenium uptake. Excretion of selenium, however, is homeostatically regulated. Urinary excretion of selenium is closely related to dietary intake in rats and people (Levander, 1986). A dietary threshold is reached at low-selenium intakes, wherein excretion is shut down, thus conserving selenium. Urinary selenium increases proportionally at higher selenium intakes. Fecal excretion, on the other hand, remains constant over a wide range of selenium intakes.

Although selenium deficiency has been observed experimentally in dogs (Van Vleet, 1975), the incidence of selenium deficiency has not been reported for dogs and cats. Likewise, selenium toxicity has not been noted in dogs and cats, despite high concentrations (>4 mg selenium/kg food) in seafood and fish-containing cat foods. AAFCO (2007) selenium recommendations are 0.11 mg/kg of food DM for dogs and 0.1 mg/kg of food DM for cats. The NRC (2006) recommended allowance is 0.35 and 0.30 mg DM selenium/kg diet for dogs and cats, respectively (growth and adult recommendations were not different). This increase in minimum recommendations, relative to previous NRC publications, takes into account potentially low availability of selenium in pet food ingredients.

Selenium availability is highly influenced by the chemical form of selenium (supplied as a supplement or from foodstuffs). Furthermore, the requirement for selenium can be partially replaced by vitamin E. Selenium in animal feeds is highly variable primarily due to the variable selenium status of soils. Studies with pigs demonstrated that inorganic selenium (sodium selenite) and organic selenium (selenium yeast) were equally effective in supporting glutathione peroxidase activity, but that selenium stores in tissues (liver and muscle) were greater when organic selenium was fed (Mahan, 1995). Selenium content in milk is also higher when selenium is supplied in the organic form.

Fish products are rich in selenium (1 to 6 mg selenium/kg), but selenium availability in these ingredients is low (Wedekind et al, 1997; Wedekind et al, 1998; Combs and Combs, 1986). Selenium levels exceeding 2 mg selenium/kg of food DM have not been reported to be toxic for cats. Cats may be able to tolerate higher selenium levels because the high-protein foods typically fed to cats are protective against high-selenium levels (Levander, 1986).

Current AAFCO (2007) guidelines set a maximum safe selenium level for dogs at 2 mg/kg; however, NRC (2006) does not list a safe upper limit for dogs. Neither NRC nor AAFCO has listed a safe upper limit for selenium for cats. Fish, eggs and liver are ingredients rich in selenium. **Table 6-1** lists signs of deficiency and excess (**Case 6-4**). Typical selenium supplements include sodium selenite and sodium selenite. See Chapter 29 for more information about selenium.

Ultra-Trace Minerals

The minimum dietary requirements for ultra-trace elements in dogs and cats have not been determined. Based on research in other species, it is probable that supplemental micronutrients, such as chromium and boron, may be beneficial under certain physiologic and dietary circumstances.

Chromium

In 1957, investigators identified a compound they called glucose tolerance factor (GTF) that restored impaired glucose tolerance in rats (Schwarz and Mertz, 1959). Chromium was identified as the active component. Chromium is ubiquitous in water, soil and living matter; however, tissue levels in animals are very low because of limited uptake by plants and absorption by animals. Furthermore, many forms of chromium are poorly available. Therefore, supplementation with an available form may be warranted. Chromium in an organically bound form (e.g., GTF) is absorbed better, has a different tissue distribution and is more available to fetuses than inorganic chromium (Mertz and Roginski, 1971).

Several studies in people and other animals have demonstrated beneficial effects of chromium supplementation (in chromium deficiency or diabetics) including: 1) improved glucose tolerance, 2) reversed hyperglycemia and glycosuria, 3) decreased circulating insulin concentrations, 4) decreased plasma lipid concentrations, 5) decreased body fat, 6) increased protein accretion, 7) improved immune response and 8) reduced cortisol production in response to heat and transport stress (Anderson, 1987; Page et al, 1993; Moonsie-Shageer and Mowat, 1993). Not all studies have shown improvements in these variables. This lack of consistent response may be accounted for by an adequate chromium nutriture for some individuals or some factor other than chromium deficiency that may have compromised the variable (impaired glucose tolerance, etc.). Few tests are available to specifically diagnose chromium status. The glucose tolerance test has been most commonly used to evaluate chromium deficiency. **Table 6-1** lists signs of deficiency and excess.

Boron

Boron indirectly influences PTH activity, thus it influences calcium, phosphorus, magnesium and cholecalciferol (vitamin D_3) metabolism. Investigators demonstrated that boron acts by at least three different mechanisms (Hunt et al, 1994): 1) it compensates for perturbations in energy substrate use induced by vitamin D deficiency, 2) it enhances macromineral content in normal bone and 3) it enhances some indices of growth and cartilage maturation, independent of vitamin D. Boron has a role in the control of urolithiasis. It decreases oxalate production in women fed magnesium-deficient diets (Hunt et al, 1994a). Boron also decreases calcium loss and bone demineralization in postmenopausal women (Nielsen et al, 1987). **Table 6-1** lists signs of deficiency and excess.

VITAMINS

Definition

The term "vitamine" was coined by Casmir Funk in 1912 when he described a class of nitrogen-containing compounds that were "vital-amines" (i.e., being vital to life). This term was later changed to vitamin when it was found that not all of these compounds contained nitrogen. The discovery, isolation and synthesis of vitamins have occurred in the last 100 years, although the effects of vitamin deficiency, specifically scurvy, have been recorded since about 1150 B.C. (Combs, 1998).

A vitamin can be defined by its physical and physiologic characteristics. For a substance to be classified as a vitamin, it must have five basic characteristics: 1) it must be an organic compound different from fat, protein and carbohydrate, 2) it must be a component of the diet, 3) it must be essential in minute amounts for normal physiologic function, 4) its absence must cause a deficiency syndrome and 5) it must not be synthesized in quantities sufficient to support normal physiologic function.

These definitions are important to note because not all vitamins are essential for every species. For example, vitamin C is essential for primates, guinea pigs and some species of fish, but not for most other animal species. Lack of the enzyme L-gulonolactone oxidase prevents those species from synthesizing vitamin C from glucose, thereby, making vitamin C a required vitamin. Under certain conditions of disease or increased metabolism, however, vitamin C may be "conditionally essential" in those species that have de novo synthesis.

Two other terms warrant definition: vitamers and provitamins. A vitamer is chemically the same compound as a vitamin, but may exert varying physiologic effects because it is an isomer. Vitamin E is a good example of vitamers, because of its many forms. α-tocopherol is the most biologically active form, whereas γ-tocopherol has little biologic function, but acts as an in vitro antioxidant. A provitamin is a compound that requires an activation step before it becomes biologically active. β-carotene, for example, is cleaved by enzymatic processes to release two molecules of retinol (vitamin A).

The two main categories of vitamins are distinguished by their miscibility in either lipids (fat soluble) or water (water soluble). There are four fat-soluble vitamins (A, D, E and K) and nine generally recognized water-soluble vitamins (thiamin [B_1], riboflavin [B_2], niacin, pyridoxine [B_6], pantothenic acid, folic acid, cobalamin [B_{12}], biotin and vitamin C). Though not a true vitamin in the classic sense, choline is generally added to commercial dog and cat foods and treated as a vitamin in this chapter. The AAFCO dog food nutrient profiles list three fat-soluble and eight water-soluble vitamins including choline (vitamin K, biotin and vitamin C are not listed). The AAFCO cat food nutrient profiles list four fat-soluble and nine water-soluble vitamins including choline (vitamin C is not listed) (2007). There are also a number of compounds that are classified as "vitamin-like compounds" or "quasi-vitamins," which will also be discussed later in this section.

Function

Vitamins have incredibly diverse physiologic functions. Vitamins act as potentiators or cofactors in enzymatic reactions (**Figure 6-4**). They also play a significant role in DNA synthesis, energy release from nutrient substrates, bone development, calcium homeostasis, normal eye function, cell membrane integrity, blood clotting, free radical scavenging, amino acid and protein metabolism and nerve impulse transduction (**Table 6-3**).

Because of the differences between fat and water solubility and in chemical structure, vitamins are absorbed in the body through a variety of means. Fat-soluble vitamins require bile salts and fat to form micelles for absorption. They are then passively absorbed, usually in the duodenum and ileum, and transported in conjunction with chylomicrons to the liver via the lymphatic system. In contrast, most of the water-soluble vitamins are absorbed via active transport. Some vitamins (e.g., cobalamin) require a carrier protein called "intrinsic factor" whereas others need a sodium-dependent, carrier-mediated absorption pump.

Deficiency/Adequacy/Toxicity

Similar to other essential trace or micronutrients, differences in ingestion levels of vitamins create deficiency, adequacy or toxicity. The biologic dose-response curve (Figure 5-2) is appropriate for vitamins (Box 5-5). A deficiency is a lack of the vitamin in quantities required for normal physiologic function. In general, fat-soluble vitamins are stored in the lipid depots of all tissues, making them more resistant to deficiency, but also more likely to cause toxicity. Conversely, water-soluble vitamins are depleted at a faster rate because of limited storage; therefore, they are less likely to cause toxicity and more likely to be acutely deficient.

Within the range of adequate intake, requirements are met for each lifestage and tissue stores are maximized. Consuming more vitamins than is required to maximize stores can, in many cases, lead to clinical signs of toxicity if the ingestion period is prolonged and the body cannot excrete excesses. It is, therefore, prudent to provide vitamins in the appropriate balance for each lifestage to meet requirements and build tissue stores, but not to over-supplement in the pharmaco-toxicologic range.

Factors Affecting Requirements

Different lifestages of animals affect vitamin requirements. Growing and reproducing animals accrete tissues and therefore require higher levels of vitamins, minerals, protein and energy for optimal performance. Over-supplementation, however, is still contraindicated because these animals are also more susceptible to toxicity. As animals age, metabolic and physiologic changes may increase the requirement for some vitamins.

Various disease conditions also affect vitamin status. Prolonged anorexia deprives animals of vitamins and other nutrients and depletes vitamin stores. Polyuric diseases such as diabetes mellitus and kidney disease may increase excretion of water-soluble vitamins. Kidney disease can also lead to a secondary vitamin D deficiency by reducing the final hydroxylation step converting 25-OH-D_3 to 1,25-$(OH)_2$-D_3, which occurs in the proximal tubules of the kidneys.

In addition, certain drugs (e.g., antibiotics) may decrease the intestinal microflora responsible for vitamin K synthesis. Also, diuretic therapy may increase excretion of water-soluble vitamins. Some vitamin requirements depend on other nutrient levels. The amount of cobalamin required is related to the amount of folic acid, choline and methionine present because these nutrients interact metabolically and are dependent on each other. In addition, the amount of tryptophan influences

Table 6-3. Summary of names, functions and clinical syndromes associated with deficiency and toxicity of vitamins.

Vitamin	Function	Deficiency	Toxicity
Vitamin A	Component of visual proteins, (rhodopsin, iodopsin), differentiation of epithelial cells, spermatogenesis, immune function, bone resorption	Anorexia, retarded growth, poor coat, weakness, xerophthalmia, nyctalopia, increased CSF pressure, aspermatogenesis, fetal resorption	Cervical spondylosis (cats), tooth loss (cats), retarded growth, anorexia, erythema, long-bone fractures
Vitamin D	Calcium and phosphorus homeostasis, bone mineralization, bone resorption, insulin synthesis, immune function	Rickets, enlarged costochondral junctions, osteomalacia, osteoporosis	Hypercalcemia, calcinosis, anorexia, lameness
Vitamin E	Biologic antioxidant, membrane integrity through free radical scavenging	Sterility (males), steatitis, dermatosis, immunodeficiency, anorexia, myopathy	Minimally toxic. Fat-soluble vitamin antagonism, increased clotting time (reversed with vitamin K)
Vitamin K	Carboxylation of clotting proteins II (prothrombin), VII, IX, X and other proteins, cofactor of the bone protein osteocalcin	Prolonged clotting time, hypoprothrombinemia, hemorrhage	Minimally toxic. Anemia (dogs)
Thiamin (B_1)	Component of thiamin pyrophosphate (TPP), cofactor in decarboxylase enzyme reactions in the TCA cycle, nervous system	Anorexia, weight loss, ataxia, polyneuritis, ventriflexion (cats), paresis (dogs), cardiac hypertrophy (dogs), bradycardia	Decreased blood pressure, bradycardia, respiratory arrhythmia
Riboflavin (B_2)	Component of flavin adenine dinucleotide (FAD) and flavin mononucleotide (FMN) coenzymes, electron transport in oxidase and dehydrogenase enzymes	Retarded growth, ataxia, collapse syndrome (dogs), dermatitis, purulent ocular discharge, vomition, conjunctivitis, coma, corneal vascularization, bradycardia, fatty liver (cats)	Minimally toxic
Niacin	Component of nicotinamide-adenine dinucleotide (NAD) and adenine dinucleotide phosphate (NADP) coenzymes, hydrogen donor/acceptor in energy-releasing dehydrogenase reactions	Anorexia, diarrhea, retarded growth, ulceration of soft palate and buccal mucosa, necrosis of the tongue (dogs), reddened ulcerated tongue (cats), cheilosis, uncontrolled drooling	Low toxicity. Bloody feces, convulsions
Pyridoxine (B_6)	Coenzyme in amino acid reactions (transaminases and decarboxylases), neurotransmitter synthesis, niacin synthesis from tryptophan, heme synthesis, taurine synthesis, carnitine synthesis	Anorexia, retarded growth, weight loss, microcytic hypochromic anemia, convulsions, renal tubular atrophy, calcium oxalate crystalluria	Low toxicity. Anorexia, ataxia (dogs)
Pantothenic acid	Precursor to coenzyme A (CoA), protein, fat and carbohydrate metabolism in the TCA cycle, cholesterol synthesis, triglyceride synthesis	Emaciation, fatty liver, depressed growth, decreased serum cholesterol and total lipids, tachycardia, coma, lowered antibody response	No toxicity established in dogs and cats
Folic acid (folate)	Methionine synthesis from homocysteine (vitamin B_{12} dependent), purine synthesis, DNA synthesis	Anorexia, weight loss, glossitis, leukopenia, hypochromic anemia, increased clotting time, elevated plasma iron, megaloblastic anemia (cats), sulfa drugs interfere with gut synthesis, cancer drugs (methotrexate) are antagonistic	Nontoxic
Biotin	Component of four carboxylase enzymes: pyruvate carboxylase, acetyl-CoA carboxylase, propionyl-CoA carboxylase and 3-methylcrotonyl CoA carboxylase	Hyperkeratosis, alopecia (cats), dry secretions around eyes, nose and mouth (cats), hypersalivation, anorexia, bloody diarrhea	No toxicity established in dogs and cats
Cobalamin (B_{12})	Coenzyme functions in propionate metabolism, aids tetrahydrofolate-containing enzymes in methionine synthesis, leucine synthesis/degradation	Cessation of growth (cats), methylmalonic aciduria, anemia	Altered reflexes (reduction in vascular conditioned reflexes and an exaggeration of unconditioned reflexes)
Vitamin C	Cofactor in hydroxylase enzyme reactions, synthesis of collagen proteins, synthesis of L-carnitine, enhances iron absorption, free radical scavenging, antioxidant/pro-oxidant functionality	Liver synthesis precludes dietary requirement, no signs of deficiency have been described in normal cats and dogs	No toxicity established in dogs and cats
Choline	Component of phosphatidylcholine found in membranes, neurotransmitter acetylcholine, methyl group donor	Fatty liver (puppies), increased blood prothrombin times, thymic atrophy, decreased growth rate, anorexia, perilobular infiltration of the liver (cats)	None described for cats and dogs
L-carnitine*	Transport long-chain fatty acids into the mitochondria for use in β-oxidation	Hyperlipidemia, cardiomyopathy, muscle asthenia	None described for cats and dogs

*L-carnitine is a vitamin-like substance.

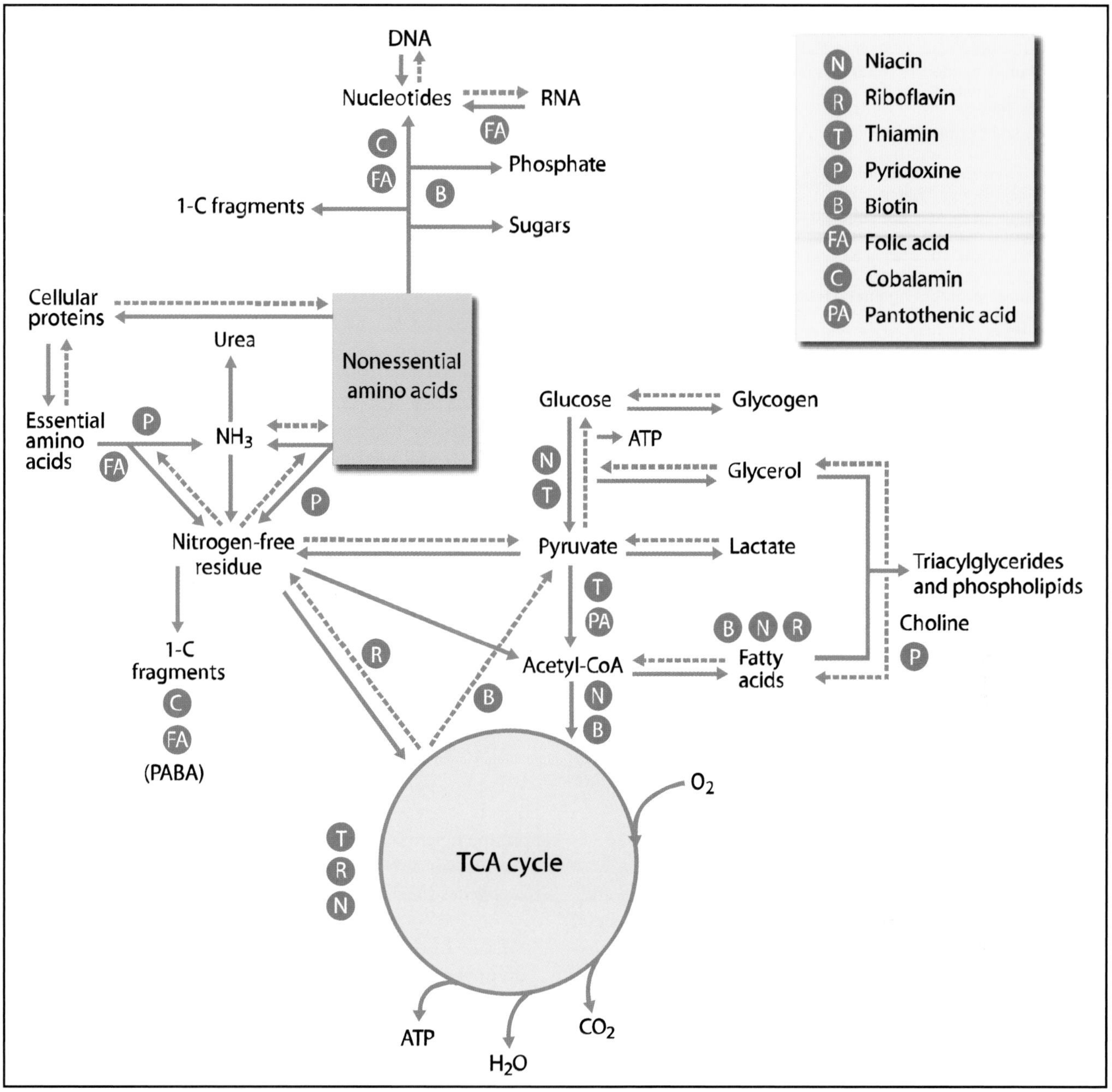

Figure 6-4. The role of B vitamins in intermediary metabolism.

niacin requirements because tryptophan is the precursor for that vitamin.

Finally, certain foods may contain antivitamin activity, for example, thiaminases in tissues of some fresh water fish may deactivate thiamin.

Feeding scientifically based formulas that specifically target the lifestage, nutrient interaction and disease condition will address changing vitamin requirements.

Vitamin Interactions

Much of the experimental work with vitamin deficiency disease has focused on the deficiency of a single vitamin. However, multiple deficiencies occur more frequently than a single-vitamin deficiency in patients. Pellagra is a classic example, in which deficiencies of niacin and tryptophan are usually accompanied by deficiencies of vitamin B_6 and riboflavin.

Many critical pathways require the concerted action of several B-complex vitamins (**Figure 6-4**). For example, one of the key reactions of metabolism is the conversion of pyruvate to acetyl-CoA. It is a key reaction because it occurs at the intersection of glycolysis and the TCA cycle. This pathway point is critical in the production of energy and the synthesis of fat and protein. Four different vitamins (niacin, thiamin, pantothenic acid and biotin) act as coenzymes in this one enzymatic conversion. Thus, a deficiency of any one of these four vitamins compromises the efficiency of the other three.

Table 6-4. Examples of vitamin-vitamin interactions.*

One vitamin needed for optimal absorption of another
Vitamin B_6 for vitamin B_{12}
Folate for thiamin
A high level of one vitamin may interfere with absorption or metabolism of another
Vitamin E interferes with vitamin K
Vitamin B_6 interferes with niacin
Thiamin interferes with riboflavin
One vitamin needed for metabolism of another
Riboflavin needed for vitamin B_6 and niacin
Vitamin B_6 needed for niacin
One vitamin protects against excess catabolism or urinary losses of another
Vitamin C spares vitamin B_6
One vitamin protects against oxidative destruction of another
Vitamin E spares vitamin A
Vitamin C spares vitamin E
A high level of one vitamin can obscure the diagnosis of deficiency of another
Folate deficiency obscures vitamin B_{12} deficiency

*Adapted from Machlin LJ, Langseth L. Vitamin-vitamin interactions. In: Bodwell LE, Erdman JW Jr, eds. Nutrient Interactions. New York, NY: Marcel Dekker Inc, 1988; 287-306.

The interactions between vitamins may involve the processes of absorption, metabolism, catabolism and excretion. Some vitamins may spare the requirements of others, whereas others may have potentially adverse effects. Even the marginal deficiency of one vitamin can exacerbate a deficiency or increase the requirement of another vitamin. Some examples of vitamin-vitamin interactions appear in **Table 6-4**.

Availability

Estimating the vitamin content of foods and foodstuffs and ultimately the adequacy of a given food is difficult at best because of cumulative errors made in estimating vitamin content and availability. These errors include: 1) analytical errors in sampling and determination of the vitamin, 2) variation in the actual amount of the vitamin (e.g., lot-to-lot variation, seasonal effects, demographics, different cultivars), 3) the presence of vitamins in bound forms in many foodstuffs and foods, 4) storage losses and 5) processing losses. All of these factors make it difficult to define what vitamin level is optimal for a given lifestage and food. To account for potential errors, references recommend that analytical values in databases be discounted by 10 to 25% (Combs, 1998).

Supplementation

Nearly all commercial pet foods contain added vitamins. Formulating a ration to meet vitamin requirements entirely from ingredient sources is extremely difficult and poses risks for the animal. The body uses synthetic and naturally formed vitamins in the same way, although they may have different availabilities. The effects of processing on vitamin stability and the availability in conjunction with disputed requirement levels in complex foods make fortification necessary (Chapter 8).

Commercial pet foods, therefore, are fortified to meet an animal's vitamin requirement for a given lifestage, overcome processing and storage losses and avoid toxicity. Because commercial pet foods are fortified with vitamins, it is usually unnecessary, and perhaps contraindicated, to concurrently give multipurpose vitamin-mineral supplements. Supplementation may be warranted in the management of diseases that affect vitamin metabolism, but should be monitored if long-term treatment is planned.

Fat-Soluble Vitamins

Vitamin A

Vitamin A is a general term describing a group of compounds with the biologic activity of retinol. Carotenoids are provitamin A. There are about 600 carotenoids known in nature, but only about 10% (e.g., α-carotene, β-carotene and β-cryptoxanthin) are provitamin A (Yeum and Russell, 2002). The international unit (IU) is still used by the pet food industry to measure the biologic activity of vitamin A. One IU of vitamin A activity can be provided by 0.3 µg of all-trans-retinol. In people, 12 µg β-carotene, 24 µg α-carotene or 24 µg β-cryptoxanthin is equal to one retinol activity equivalent (1 µg retinol) (DRI, 2001). Dogs, but not cats, can use provitamin A as a source of vitamin A. The retinol equivalent of β-carotene in dogs has not been defined. Most of the preformed vitamin A in food is in the form of retinyl esters, whereas the source of vitamin A from plants is in the form of provitamin A carotenoids.

FUNCTION

Vitamin A is essential for a number of distinct biologic functions. It is necessary for normal vision, growth, reproduction, immune function and maintenance of healthy epithelial tissue. Vitamin A is also involved in the expression and regulation of many genes (McClintick et al, 2005).

METABOLISM

Retinyl esters in food are hydrolyzed by hydrolases from the pancreas and the mucosal brush border to yield retinol. Retinyl esters and carotenoids are hydrophobic, thus their dispersion into the aqueous environment of the small intestinal lumen requires bile salts for micellar solubilization. This process allows access of hydrolytic enzymes to retinyl esters and exposes retinol to the mucosal surface, allowing free retinol and intact β-carotene to diffuse passively into mucosal epithelial cells. Absorption of vitamin A esters appears to be high (80 to 90%), but absorption may vary depending on the level and type of dietary fat and protein, which exert surfactant effects (Combs, 1998).

Dietary carotenoids are only absorbed half as well as preformed dietary vitamin A. As the amount of carotenoids in the food increases, however, the absorption efficiency decreases. Intestinal absorption of carotenoids is much more critically dependent on the presence of bile salts than is absorption of vitamin A. Cats can absorb β-carotene but are unable to convert it to retinol (Schweigert el al, 2002).

In the body, enzymes convert provitamin A carotenoids to retinols. β,β-carotene 15,15'-monooxygenase is a central cleavage enzyme that cleaves β,β-carotene into two molecules of retinol at the 15,15' double bond. The gene encoding for the enzyme has been cloned from several species including people, mice and chicks (Wyss, 2004). This central cleavage enzyme is found in the intestinal mucosa, liver, lungs, kidney, testes and brain. Recently, a second type of cleavage enzyme, β,β-carotene 9',10'-dioxygenase, was identified and cloned in mice (Kiefer et al, 2001). This enzyme exclusively catalyzes the asymmetric oxidative cleavage of β-carotene at the 9',10' double bond, resulting in the formation of β-apo-10'-carotenal and β-ionone.

Vitamin A is absorbed almost exclusively as the free alcohol retinol. Within mucosal cells, retinol is re-esterified mostly to palmitate and incorporated into the chylomicrons of the mucosa. Afterwards, it diffuses into lymph. A small amount of retinol may be oxidized first to retinal and then to retinoic acid, which may form a compound (glucuronide) that passes into the portal blood. Vitamin A is transported through the lymphatic system with low-density lipoprotein (LDL) to the liver, where it is deposited mainly in hepatocytes and stellate and parenchymal cells.

Some vitamin A derivatives are re-excreted into the intestinal lumen via the bile. This is true for much of retinoic acid and some retinol. The major vitamin A components of bile are vitamin A glucuronides, many of which are reabsorbed. Thus, enterohepatic circulation may provide an important means of conserving vitamin A. Although dogs and cats excrete vitamin A in urine, cats excrete a lesser amount.

When vitamin A is mobilized from the liver, stored vitamin A ester is hydrolyzed before it is released into the bloodstream. Vitamin A retinol is transported to tissues in the bloodstream by a specific transport protein called retinol-binding protein (RBP). RBP is synthesized and secreted by hepatic parenchymal cells.

In contrast to most other species, dogs and cats have a unique way of metabolizing vitamin A. Cats require preformed vitamin A because they lack the oxygenase enzyme necessary for β-carotene cleavage. In addition, studies have shown that cats and dogs do not depend on RBP to transport vitamin A in plasma (Schweigert, 1988; Wilson et al, 1987; Schweigert et al, 1990; Schweigert et al, 1990a). Cats and dogs transport vitamin A as retinyl esters (mostly retinyl stearate) bound to LDL and very low-density lipoprotein in amounts 10 to 50 times those of other mammals (Schweigert, 1988). This is of interest because free circulating retinyl esters are a sign of hypervitaminosis A in almost all other animal species, including people.

REQUIREMENTS

The AAFCO (2007) recommended allowance for vitamin A is 5,000 IU/kg DM for dogs for all lifestages (growth, reproduction and maintenance) and 9,000 IU/kg DM for cats for growth and reproduction and 5,000 IU/kg DM for maintenance. NRC (2006) recommends a vitamin A allowance of 1,515 RE (retinal equivalent) (5,050 IU)/kg DM for dogs for all lifestages, 1,000 RE (3,333 IU)/kg DM for cats for growth and maintenance and 2,000 RE (6,667 IU)/kg DM for cats during gestation and lactation. Unlike dogs, cats cannot meet their vitamin A requirement from carotenoids.

DEFICIENCY AND TOXICITY

The appreciable stores of vitamin A in the body are mobilized as needed to mitigate against the effects of low dietary intakes of the vitamin. The only unequivocal signs of vitamin A deficiency are the ocular lesions nyctalopia (night blindness) and xerophthalmia (extreme dryness of the conjunctiva). Other signs include anorexia, weight loss, ataxia, skin lesions, increased susceptibility to infection, retinal degeneration, poor coat, weakness, increased cerebrospinal fluid pressure, nephritis, skeletal defects (periosteal overgrowth and narrowing of foramina) and impaired reproduction (NRC, 2006).

Vitamin A toxicities have been encountered in numerous species. The most characteristic signs of hypervitaminosis A are skeletal malformation, spontaneous fractures and internal hemorrhage (**Case 6-5**). Other signs include anorexia, slow growth, weight loss, skin thickening, suppressed keratinization, increased blood clotting time, reduced erythrocyte count, enteritis, congenital abnormalities, conjunctivitis, fatty infiltration of the liver and reduced function of liver and kidneys. Queens fed a diet with 606,000 RE/kg food had an increased number of kittens born with defects such as cleft palate, cranioschisis, foreshortened mandible, stenotic colon, enlarged heart and agenesis of the spinal cord and small intestine (Freytag et al, 2003). Dogs seem less sensitive to excess dietary vitamin A than some other mammals (Cline et al, 1997).

The dietary maximum of vitamin A in the AAFCO (2007) dog and cat nutrient profiles is 250,000 IU/kg DM for dogs and 750,000 IU/kg DM for cats. NRC (2006) proposed a safe upper limit of 15,000 RE (50,000 IU)/kg DM for growing puppies and gestating and lactating bitches, and 64,000 RE (213,333 IU)/kg DM for adult dogs. The safe upper limit of vitamin A for cats is 80,000 RE (266,667 IU)/kg DM for growth and 100,000 RE (333,333 IU)/kg DM for maintenance, gestation and lactation.

SOURCES

Naturally rich sources of vitamin A include fish oil, liver, egg and dairy products. The most common vitamin A supplements used in pet foods include vitamin A esters (all trans retinyl palmitate, acetate or propionate) or vitamin A provided as fish oils. Because of stability issues, vitamin A sources are often coated, beaded, prilled or spray dried with antioxidants and emulsifying agents.

Concentrations of carotenoids in plants vary widely according to geographic location, maturity, method of harvest, amount and type of processing, length and conditions of storage and exposure to high temperature, sunlight and air. As a result, vitamin A is among the most variable nutrients in the diet. The vitamin A content in animal tissues can also be variable; concentrations can be very high in certain tissues such as liver. Levels of vitamin A in animal tissue vary depending on either the level of vitamin A or carotenoid present in the dog's or cat's diet.

Vitamin D

Two important forms of vitamin D are cholecalciferol (vitamin D_3), which occurs in animals and ergocalciferol (vitamin D_2), which occurs predominantly in plants. In pet food, vitamin D activity is typically expressed in IU. One IU of vitamin D can be provided by 0.025 µg of cholecalciferol or vitamin D_3. The skin of most mammals can produce cholecalciferol from the provitamin 7-dehydrocholesterol via activation with ultraviolet-B light. However, this photosynthesis pathway is inefficient in dogs (Hazewinkel et al, 1987) and cats (Morris, 1999) because of the higher activity of the enzyme 7-dehydrocholesterol- Δ^7 reductase that converts 7-dehydrocholesterol to cholesterol. Therefore, dogs and cats need dietary vitamin D.

FUNCTION

The primary function of vitamin D is to enhance intestinal absorption and mobilization, as well as retention and bone deposition of calcium and phosphorus. This function is manifested through its active form of 1,25-$(OH)_2$-D_3 as a hormone that binds to the nuclear 1,25-$(OH)_2$-D_3 receptor (VDR) in many types of cells. The active vitamin D_3 also has a direct effect on Ca^{2+} channels located on the plasma membrane (Norman et al, 1992).

METABOLISM

Vitamin D is absorbed from the small intestine by nonsaturable, passive diffusion, which depends on bile salts. Vitamin D then enters the lymphatic circulation primarily (~90%) in association with chylomicrons; the remainder of vitamin D is associated with an α-globulin fraction (Combs, 1998). Like other steroids, vitamin D is transported in association with proteins. In most species, the binding protein is vitamin D-binding protein (DBP) or "transcalciferin." The concentration of DBP greatly exceeds the concentration of vitamin D metabolites in blood. This concentration difference, in conjunction with the binding affinity, results in less than 5% of the available binding sites being occupied by vitamin D compounds. The distribution between bound and free vitamin D compounds greatly favors the bound form. In this fashion, DBP facilitates peripheral distribution of vitamin D from dietary origin and mobilizes endogenously produced vitamin D from the skin.

Vitamin D is distributed relatively evenly among the various tissues where it resides in lipid depots. Vitamin D can be found in adipose, kidneys, liver, lungs, aorta and heart. The primary circulating form of vitamin D is the parent vitamin D (~50%), with the next most abundant form (i.e., 25-OH-D_3 [also called calcidiol]) accounting for approximately 20% of the total (Combs, 1998).

In mammals, both vitamin D_2 and D_3 are not the active form of vitamin D. They are activated in the body by hydroxylation to 25-OH-D_3 first in the liver and again to 1,25-$(OH)_2$-D_3 (also called calcitriol) in the kidneys. Vitamin D_2 is less efficiently used than vitamin D_3 in cats (Morris, 2002). At normal plasma concentrations, only small amounts of 25-OH-D_3 are released from this pool to enter tissues. Thus, circulating levels of 1,25-$(OH)_2$-D_3 are a good indicator of vitamin D status.

Several factors tightly regulate the vitamin D endocrine system: 1,25-$(OH)_2$-D_3, PTH, calcitonin, several other hormones and circulating levels of calcium and phosphate. The vitamin D-dependent homeostatic system responds to perturbations in calcium concentration. For example, when serum calcium falls below a given level, PTH is secreted by the parathyroid glands, which function to detect hypocalcemia. The kidney responds to PTH, resulting in phosphate diuresis and stimulation of 25-OH-D_3 1-hydroxylase. The latter effect increases production of 1,25-$(OH)_2$-D_3, which acts to increase enteric absorption of calcium and phosphate. In addition, 1,25-$(OH)_2$-D_3 acts jointly with PTH in bone to promote mobilization of calcium and phosphate. The combined result of these responses is to increase plasma concentration of calcium and phosphate. Calcitonin is secreted by the thyroid gland ("C" cells) when circulating concentrations of calcium are increased. Calcitonin suppresses bone mobilization and may increase the renal excretion of calcium and phosphate. In that situation, 25-OH-D_3 1-hydroxylase may be inhibited by 1,25-$(OH)_2$-D_3, and may actually be converted to 24,25-$(OH)_2$-D_3, which may down-regulate the absorption of calcium in dogs (Tryfonidou et al, 2002).

These events tightly regulate hydroxylase activity and maintain nearly constant plasma concentrations of 1,25-$(OH)_2$-D_3, calcium and phosphorus. Once formed, 1,25-$(OH)_2$-D_3 binds to specific receptors on the enterocyte nucleus and initiates events that stimulate calcium and phosphorus absorption. In addition, 1,25-$(OH)_2$-D_3, acting with PTH, mediates resorption of bone with the release of calcium and phosphorus.

Many metabolites of vitamin D circulate in plasma other than 25-OH-D_3 and 1,25-$(OH)_2$-D_3. One metabolite, 24,25-$(OH)_2$-D_3, may also be biologically active, whereas other metabolites are generally considered physiologically inactive excretory forms (Combs, 1998).

REQUIREMENTS

The AAFCO (2007) dietary allowance for vitamin D is 500 IU/kg DM for dogs for all lifestages. For cats, the AAFCO (2007) allowance is 750 IU/kg DM for growth and reproduction and 500 IU/kg DM for maintenance. The vitamin D allowance recommended by NRC (2006) is 13.8 µg cholecalciferol (552 IU)/kg DM for dogs regardless of lifestage. The NRC recommended vitamin D allowance for cats is 5.6 µg cholecalciferol (250 IU)/kg DM for growth and 7 µg cholecalciferol (280 IU)/kg DM for maintenance and reproduction.

DEFICIENCY AND TOXICITY

Signs of vitamin D deficiency are frequently confounded by a simultaneous deficiency or imbalance of calcium and phosphorus. Clinical signs generally include rickets (young animals), enlarged costochondral junctions, osteomalacia (adult animals), osteoporosis (adult animals) and decreased serum calcium and inorganic phosphorus concentrations. Experimental vitamin D deficiency has been produced in cats, resulting in neurologic abnormalities associated with degeneration of the cervical spinal cord (Morris, 1996). Other signs included hypocalcemia, elevated PTH concentrations, posterior paralysis, ataxia and eventual quadriparesis.

Excessive intake of vitamin D is associated with increases in 25-OH-D_3, with the D_3 form being more toxic than the D_2 form. When circulating at very high concentrations, 25-OH-D_3 can compete effectively with 1,25-$(OH)_2$-D_3 for receptors in the intestine and bone. Therefore, during vitamin D toxicosis, 25-OH-D_3 can induce actions usually attributed to 1,25-$(OH)_2$-D_3. Thus, 25-OH-D_3 is believed to be the critical factor in vitamin D intoxication (NRC, 1987). Excessive vitamin D_3 supplementation below the toxic level decreases bone remodeling and causes focal enlargement of the growth plate in growing puppies (Tryfonidou et al, 2003). Excessive vitamin D concentrations may result in hypercalcemia, soft-tissue calcification and ultimately death (Morita et al, 1995; Nakamura et al, 2004) (**Case 6-6**).

The vitamin D maximum in the AAFCO (2007) dog and cat nutrient profiles is 5,000 IU/kg DM for dogs and 10,000 IU/kg DM for cats. The NRC (2006) proposed a safe upper limit of 80 μg cholecalciferol (3,200 IU)/kg DM for dogs and 750 μg cholecalciferol (30,000 IU)/kg DM for cats regardless of lifestages.

SOURCES

Marine fish and fish oils are the richest natural sources of vitamin D in foodstuffs but they may pose a risk for toxicity. One group of investigators found that moist foods generally contained higher levels of vitamin D than extruded foods and that some moist foods exceeded the AAFCO maximal recommended allowance of 10,000 IU/kg for cats (Morris, 1996). Other sources of vitamin D include fresh water fish and eggs (especially yolks). Beef, liver and dairy products contain smaller amounts of vitamin D. The most common synthetic sources of vitamin D in pet foods include cholecalciferol (D-activated animal sterol), vitamin D_3 supplement, ergocalciferol (D-activated plant sterol) and vitamin D_2 supplement.

Vitamin E

Vitamin E is a term for a group of compounds with the biologic activity of α-tocopherol. In nature, there are eight isomeric forms of vitamin E, four tocopherols (α, β, γ, δ) and four tocotrienols (α, β, γ, δ). Naturally occurring α-tocopherol (*d*-α-tocopherol) is now designated as RRR-α-tocopherol based on RS or CIP system of chiral configuration. Synthetic α-tocopherol (*dl*-α-tocopherol), a mixture of eight stereoisomers of α-tocopherol, is designated as all-*rac* (racemic)-α-tocopherol. Vitamin E activity in pet food is generally expressed in international units. One IU of vitamin E equals 1 mg of all-*rac*-α-tocopheryl acetate or 0.91 mg of all-*rac*-α-tocopherol. The most biopotent form of vitamin E is α-tocopherol. The relative biopotencies of vitamin E isomers are as follows: α >β >δ >γ (McDowell, 1989). Also, tocopherols are generally more available than tocotrienols (Combs, 1998). Because some forms of vitamin E have little biologic activity, total vitamin E analysis is not a reliable means of determining vitamin E activity.

FUNCTION

Vitamin E functions as an antioxidant in the body and in food. Of the vitamin E isomers, α-tocopherol is the most active biologic form in the body, whereas the γ-isomer is the most active form in food. Mixed tocopherols, including γ-tocopherols, are widely used to prevent lipid oxidation in pet food products (Chapter 8).

Vitamin E works in conjunction with glutathione peroxidase to protect cells against the adverse effects of reactive oxygen and other free radicals that initiate the oxidation of polyunsaturated membrane phospholipids. Vitamin E in cellular and subcellular membranes is the first line of defense against peroxidation of vital phospholipids. However, some peroxides are formed even when adequate levels of vitamin E are present.

Selenium, as part of the enzyme glutathione peroxidase, is a second line of defense that destroys peroxides before they damage membranes. Therefore, selenium, vitamin E and sulfur-containing amino acids, through different biochemical mechanisms, are capable of preventing some of the same nutritional diseases (McDowell, 1992). Vitamin E prevents fatty acid hydroperoxide formation, sulfur-containing amino acids are precursors of glutathione peroxidase and selenium is a component of glutathione peroxidase. In addition, vitamin E is important for normal reproduction and is involved in modulating cellular signaling, regulating gene transcription, modulating immune function and inducing apoptosis (Brigelius-Flohe et al, 2002).

METABOLISM

Vitamin E is absorbed from the small intestine by nonsaturable, passive diffusion, which depends on micellar solubilization. Whether presented as free alcohol or as esters, most vitamin E is absorbed as the alcohol. Esters are largely hydrolyzed in the gut wall before absorption, probably by a duodenal mucosal esterase. The free alcohol enters the intestinal lacteals and is transported via lymph to the general circulation.

The efficiency of vitamin E absorption is low and variable (35 to 50%); the absorption efficiency is much lower than that of vitamin A (Combs, 1998). Absorption of vitamin E is enhanced by the simultaneous digestion and absorption of dietary lipids. Transfer of vitamin E across epithelial cells may require several stages, most of them poorly understood. In mammals, vitamin E is transported from the intestine to lymphatic capillaries in association with chylomicrons. Conversely, in birds, tocopherol is transported via the portal vein directly to the liver. Unlike cholesterol or vitamin A, α-tocopherol is not re-esterified during the absorption process.

Vitamin E circulates in the lymph and blood bound to all of the lipoproteins. There is a very high correlation between tocopherol levels and the total lipid or cholesterol concentration in serum.

All tissues show linear increases in tocopherol concentrations with increases in tocopherol intake. This relationship differs from that of most other vitamins, which usually have distinct deposition thresholds in tissues other than the liver, and may provide an explanation for the pharmacologic effects of vitamin

E. Vitamin E levels in tissues vary markedly with no consistent relationship to lipid parameters. The vitamin is most concentrated in membrane-rich cell fractions such as mitochondria and microsomes.

Vitamin E undergoes very little metabolism. Usually less than 1% of orally ingested vitamin E is excreted in urine (Combs, 1998). The major route of excretion is fecal elimination.

The need for vitamin E in the diet is markedly influenced by dietary composition. The requirement increases with increasing levels of polyunsaturated fatty acids (PUFA), oxidizing agents, vitamin A, carotenoids and trace minerals and decreases with increasing levels of fat-soluble antioxidants, sulfur-containing amino acids and selenium. Various researchers have recommended up to 60 mg of α-tocopherol per g of PUFA; however, there is no consensus among experts about the quantitation of this relationship (Combs, 1998).

REQUIREMENTS

The AAFCO (2007) recommended allowance for vitamin E is 50 IU/kg DM for dogs and 30 IU/kg DM for cats, irrespective of the lifestage. For cat foods containing fish oils, AAFCO recommends an additional 10 IU vitamin E/g of fish oil/kg of food above the allowance. The vitamin E allowance recommended by NRC (2006) is 30 mg α-tocopherol (33 IU)/kg DM for dogs for all lifestages. For cats, the vitamin E allowance is 38 mg α-tocopherol (42 IU)/kg DM for growth and maintenance and 31 mg α-tocopherol (34 IU)/kg DM for gestation and lactation.

DEFICIENCY AND TOXICITY

The clinical manifestations of vitamin E deficiency vary markedly between species. In general, however, the neuromuscular, vascular and reproductive systems are affected most commonly. Signs of vitamin E deficiency are mostly attributed to membrane dysfunction as a result of the oxidative degradation of polyunsaturated membrane phospholipids and disruption of other critical cellular processes. Clinical findings of vitamin E deficiency in dogs include degenerative skeletal muscle disease associated with muscle weakness, degeneration of testicular germinal epithelium and impaired spermatogenesis, failure of gestation, brown pigmentation (lipofuscinosis) of intestinal smooth muscle and decreased plasma tocopherol concentrations. In cats, deficiency signs include steatitis, focal interstitial myocarditis, focal myositis of skeletal muscle and periportal mononuclear infiltration in the liver (**Case 6-7**).

Vitamin E is one of the least toxic fat-soluble vitamins. Animals and people apparently tolerate high levels without adverse effects. However, at very high doses, antagonism with other fat-soluble vitamins may occur, resulting in impaired bone mineralization, reduced hepatic storage of vitamin A and coagulopathies as a result of decreasing absorption of vitamins D, A and K, respectively. A maximum of 1,000 IU/kg DM was recommended by AAFCO for dogs; however, AAFCO (2007) set no maximum for cats. There is no evidence of vitamin E toxicity in dogs and very limited information when vitamin E is given orally to cats. In certain conditions, higher dietary vitamin E levels may be beneficial (Morris and Rogers, 1994). A number of inflammatory dermatoses in animals have been treated with oral vitamin (Chapter 32). People have been given much higher dietary concentrations of vitamin E without adverse clinical signs (Combs, 1998).

SOURCES

Only plants synthesize vitamin E. The richest sources of vitamin E are vegetable oils and, to a lesser extent, seeds and cereal grains. Tocopherol concentrations are highest in green leaves. Tocotrienols are not found in green leaves, but instead are found in the bran and germ fractions of certain plants. Animal tissues tend to be low in vitamin E, with the highest levels occurring in fatty tissues. Common vitamin E supplements used in pet foods include α-tocopherol and α-tocopherol acetate.

Vitamin K

Like other fat-soluble vitamins, vitamin K is a generic descriptor for a group of compounds exhibiting the antihemorrhagic activity of phylloquinone. Phylloquinone (vitamin K_1) and menaquinone (vitamin K_2) are the two major naturally occurring forms of vitamin K. Green leafy vegetables are the primary sources of vitamin K_1 whereas vitamin K_2 is produced from actinomycete bacteria found in normal intestinal microflora. Vitamin K_2 is now called menaquinone-7 (MK-7) in recognition of the seven-isoprenoid units. Menadione or vitamin K_3 (2-methyl-1,4-napthoquinone) is the parent compound of the vitamin K series. When used in pet food, it is usually added in a complex form such as menadione sodium bisulfate complex (MSBC) or menadione dimethylpyrimidinol bisulfate (MPB), as the bioactive form of vitamin K.

FUNCTION

Vitamin K plays a major role in the carboxylation of proteins (factors II, VII, IX, X and proteins C and S) to convert prothrombin to thrombin for normal blood clotting. Vitamin K is also involved in the synthesis of osteocalcin, a protein that regulates the incorporation of calcium phosphates in growing bone (Combs, 1998).

METABOLISM

The absorption of natural vitamin K in food is between 40 and 70% (Combs, 1998). Ingested phylloquinone is absorbed from the proximal small intestine into the lymphatic system by an energy-dependent process. Menaquinone is absorbed from the small intestine by a passive noncarrier-mediated process. Conditions that impair lipid absorption also adversely affect vitamin K absorption. Upon absorption, vitamin K is transported to the liver in chylomicrons. The vitamin is rapidly concentrated in the liver, but in contrast to other fat-soluble vitamins, vitamin K has a very rapid turnover in this organ. No specific carriers have been identified for any of the K vitamers.

Although phylloquinones and menaquinones are ingested, much of the vitamin K in tissues is from bacterial origin. Menadione is rapidly excreted in urine as the phosphate, sulfate or glucuronide form of menadiol. However, catabolism of phylloquinones and menaquinones is much slower than that of menadione and they are primarily excreted in feces as a glucuronide conjugate.

Because microbially synthesized K_2 is readily absorbed by passive diffusion in the colon in most mammalian species, dietary supplementation is unnecessary for most cats and dogs.

REQUIREMENTS

AAFCO (2007) does not have a recommended allowance for vitamin K for dogs, but recommends 0.1 mg/kg DM for cats when cat foods contain more than 25% fish. This recommendation is warranted because vitamin K deficiency has been observed in cats fed certain commercial foods containing high levels of salmon or tuna (**Case 6-8**). NRC (2006) recommends that the vitamin K allowance is 1 mg/kg DM for cats for all lifestages. For dogs, the recommended allowance of vitamin K is 1.64 mg/kg DM for growth, 1.63 mg/kg DM for maintenance and 1.6 mg/kg DM for gestation and lactation.

DEFICIENCY AND TOXICITY

Prolonged clotting times and excessive bleeding have been reported in vitamin K deficiency in cats and dogs under various conditions. Vitamin K deficiency usually occurs secondary to other conditions such as malabsorptive diseases (inflammatory bowel disease), ingestion of coagulant antagonists (coumarin, indanedione), destruction of gut microflora by antibiotic therapy (sulfonamides and broad-spectrum antibiotics) and congenital defects (γ-glutamyl carboxylase defect in Devon Rex breed of cats). Vitamin K_3 (menadione) has lower lipid solubility and is the most effective form of vitamin K for cases of malabsorption. Vitamin K_1 is the only form of vitamin K effective in anticoagulant antagonism (Edwards and Russell, 1987).

Phylloquinone produces no adverse effects when administered to animals in massive doses by any route (NRC, 1987). The menaquinones are similarly thought to have negligible toxicity. Menadione, however, can produce fatal anemia, hyperbilirubinemia and severe jaundice. The intoxicating doses appear to be at least three orders of magnitude above those levels required for normal physiologic function (Combs, 1998). Neither AAFCO nor NRC has set maximum or safe upper limits for dogs and cats.

SOURCES

Data for vitamin K content of foods are limited by the lack of good analytical methods. Nevertheless, because dietary needs for vitamin K are low, most foods contribute significantly to those needs. Rich sources of vitamin K include alfalfa meal, oilseed meals, liver and fish meals. Menadione sodium bisulfite complex and menadione dimethypyrimidinol bisulfate are commonly used as vitamin K sources in pet food because of their stability during manufacturing and storage.

Water-Soluble Vitamins

Deficiency of B vitamins occurs in veterinary medicine but may be difficult to specifically diagnose because analytical tests are not readily available. Therefore, diagnosis relies almost entirely upon clinical signs and nutrient intake history.

B vitamins are relatively nontoxic and may be supplied to veterinarians in individual or combination forms. Because many of the B-vitamin deficiencies present with overlapping clinical signs, it may be prudent to treat deficiency with vitamin-B complex. If signs are specific for a particular B-vitamin deficiency, and if the single preparation form of the vitamin is available, individual targeted treatment may be initiated. However, individual preparations of B vitamins are often more expensive, and the relative nontoxic levels of B vitamins warrant treatment with the combination form.

Thiamin

Thiamin or vitamin B_1 consists of one pyrimidine ring and one thiazole ring linked via a methylene group. Thiamin may exist as free thiamin or in the mono-, di-(pyro), or triphosphate configuration. Thiamin pyrophosphate (80%) is the major form found in tissues; the other three forms are found in lesser amounts (Rindi, 1996; Brody, 1994a). Thiamin is very labile, especially in wet foods, being susceptible to neutral and alkaline conditions, heat, oxidation and ionizing radiation.

FUNCTION

Thiamin pyrophosphate (TPP) is the major coenzymatic form of thiamin and is required for only a small number of enzymatic reactions. TPP is involved in the following general scheme of reactions: 1) nonoxidative decarboxylation of α-ketoacids, 2) oxidative decarboxylation of α-ketoacids and 3) transketolation reactions. Thiamin may also have a function unrelated to coenzyme activity. TPP is concentrated in neuronal cells and may affect chloride permeability by controlling the number of functional channels, possibly by phosphorylation.

METABOLISM

Dietary thiamin may be present in any of the four forms mentioned above or may be of synthetic origin. Whatever the form, thiamin is hydrolyzed to free thiamin by intestinal phosphatases before absorption by enterocytes. Absorption takes place primarily in the jejunum by an active, carrier-mediated transport that also phosphorylates the vitamin. Passive diffusion becomes an important mode of absorption when dietary thiamin intake is high.

Absorbed thiamin is transported in erythrocytes, which contain free thiamin and its phosphorylated forms, and in plasma, which only contains free thiamin and its monophosphate form. Tissues take up thiamin and may interconvert it between any of its four forms. The liver, heart and kidneys have the highest concentration of thiamin.

REQUIREMENTS

The AAFCO (2007) recommended allowance for thiamin is 1 mg/kg DM for dogs and 5 mg/kg DM for cats, irrespective of the lifestage. NRC (2006) recommends a thiamin allowance for dogs of 1.38 mg/kg DM for growth and 2.25 mg/kg DM for maintenance and reproduction. For cats, the NRC (2006)

Table 6-5. Blood levels, allowances and tests for B-complex vitamins in cats and dogs.

Cats

Vitamin	Blood level	AAFCO allowance*	NRC allowance*	Best test
Thiamin	20-90 ng/ml (WB)	5 mg/kg	5.6 mg/kg	Erythrocyte transketolase activity
Riboflavin	196-660 ng/ml (WB)	4 mg/kg	4 mg/kg	Erythrocyte glutathione reductase** Urine riboflavin
Niacin	1.8-5.8 μg/ml (WB)	60 mg/kg	40 mg/kg	Urine methyl nicotinamide or methyl-pyridones**
Pantothenic acid	104-270 ng/ml (WB)	5.0 mg/kg	5.75 mg/kg	Urinary excretion of pantothenate
Pyridoxine	86-350 ng/ml (P)	4.0 mg/kg	2.5 mg/kg	Blood levels of pyridoxine Urinary metabolites of pathway intermediates
Folic acid	3.2-34 ng/ml (P)	0.8 mg/kg	0.75 μg/kg	Serum folate
Vitamin B_{12}	120-1,200 pg/ml (WB)	20 μg/kg	22.5 μg/kg	Blood levels of cobalamin Serum and urine methylmalonic acid
Biotin	1,000-3,000 pg/ml (WB)	70 μg/kg	75 μg/kg	Urinary biotin Urinary organic acids
Choline	180-490 μg/ml (P)	2,400 mg/kg	2,550 mg/kg	Plasma choline and phosphatidylcholine

Dogs

Vitamin	Blood level	AAFCO allowance*	NRC allowance*	Best test
Thiamin	46-112 ng/ml (WB)	1.0 mg/kg	2.25 mg/kg	Erythrocyte transketolase activity
Riboflavin	185-420 ng/ml (WB)	2.2 mg/kg***	5.25 mg/kg	Erythrocyte glutathione reductase** Urine riboflavin
Niacin	2.7-12 μg/ml (WB)	11.4 mg/kg	17 mg/kg	Urine methyl nicotinamide or methyl-pyridones**
Pantothenic acid	120-380 ng/ml (WB)	10 mg/kg	15 mg/kg	Urinary excretion of pantothenate
Pyridoxine	40-270 ng/ml (P)	1 mg/kg	1.5 mg/kg	Blood levels of pyridoxine Urinary metabolites of pathway intermediates
Folic acid	4-26 ng/ml (P)	0.18 mg/kg	0.27 mg/kg	Serum folate
Vitamin B_{12}	135-950 pg/ml (WB)	22 μg/kg	35 μg/kg	Holotranscobalamin II**
Biotin	530-5,000 pg/ml (WB)	None established	0†	Urinary biotin Urinary organic acids
Choline	235-800 μg/ml (P)	1,200 mg/kg	1,700 mg/kg	Plasma choline and phosphatidylcholine

Key: WB = whole blood, P = plasma, AAFCO = Association of American Feed Control Officials, NRC = National Research Council.
*AAFCO allowances are similar for growth and adult maintenance and are expressed on dry matter basis (AAFCO Official Publication, 2007). NRC allowances are "recommended allowances" for adult maintenance and are also expressed on a dry matter basis (NRC. Nutrient Requirements of Dogs and Cats. Washington, DC: National Academies Press, 2006.
**Not currently available in veterinary medicine.
***Investigators have shown a riboflavin requirement approximately 20 to 33% higher than the AAFCO allowance listed here. (Cline JL, Odle J, Easter RA. The riboflavin requirement of adult dogs at maintenance is greater than previous estimates. Journal of Nutrition 1996; 126: 984-988.)
†For normal foods not containing raw egg whites, adequate biotin is probably provided by intestinal microbial synthesis (assuming the patient is not receiving antimicrobial therapy).

recommended allowance for thiamin is 5.5 mg/kg DM for growth, 5.6 mg/kg DM for maintenance and 6.3 mg/kg DM for gestation and lactation. **Table 6-5** lists AAFCO and NRC allowances for dogs and cats.

DEFICIENCY AND TOXICITY

Clinical thiamin deficiency is rarely observed in dogs and cats because most commercial pet foods have adequate supplementation. Signs of thiamin deficiency are often related to the nervous system and heart. They include anorexia, failure to grow, muscle weakness, paraparesis, convulsions, seizures, ventriflexion of the head, ataxia and cardiac hypertrophy (Read and Harrington, 1981; Jubb et al, 1956; Everett, 1944).

Thiamin deficiency may result from inadequate intake of thiamin, attributable to foods with low-thiamin content or processing losses, or high intake of thiamin antagonists. The processing conditions used to prepare commercial pet foods are destructive to thiamin. However, this anticipated loss is overcome by adding synthetic thiamin before processing (**Case 6-9**).

Thiamin antagonists may be synthetic or natural compounds that modify the thiamin structure rendering it inactive. The natural antagonists include thiaminases (enzymes that degrade thiamin), and polyhydroxyphenols (caffeic acid, chlorogenic acid, tannins), which inactivate thiamin by an oxyreductive process. Thiaminases are found in high concentrations in raw fish, shellfish, bacteria, yeast and fungi (**Table 6-6**). Cooking destroys thiaminases.

Thiamin deficiency may be diagnosed by measuring erythrocyte transketolase activity or thiamin metabolites in blood directly. **Table 6-5** lists concentrations of thiamin in blood for cats and dogs (Baker et al, 1986). Activity of erythrocyte transketolase is an excellent indicator of thiamin status, if determined in a laboratory familiar with the analysis. Thiamin toxicosis via the oral route is very rare.

SOURCES

Thiamin occurs in animal tissues almost entirely in phosphorylated forms, whereas it occurs mostly as free thiamin in plants. Thiamin is widely distributed in foods, but is mostly present at low concentrations. The richest sources are whole grains, yeast and liver (especially pork liver). Meat products may also supply significant amounts of thiamin. Up to 90% of thiamin in natural ingredients may be lost as a result of processing (Morris and Rogers, 1994). Therefore, thiamin supplementation is common in pet foods. Thiamin hydrochloride and thiamin mononitrate are the most commonly used supplements in commercial foods for dogs and cats.

Table 6-6. Thiaminase activity in fish products.*

Food	Thiaminase activity**
Marlin	0
Yellowfin tuna	265
Red snapper	265
Skipjack tuna	1,000
Dolphin (mahi mahi)	120
Ladyfish	35
Clam	2,640

*Adapted from Hilker DM, Peter OF. Anti-thiamin activity in Hawaii fish. Journal of Nutrition 1966; 89: 419-421.
**mg thiamin destroyed/100 g fish/hour.

Riboflavin

Riboflavin, or vitamin B_2 belongs to the class of isoalloxazines. Riboflavin has a planar structure and has limited solubility in water. This property has clinical significance because it is difficult to deliver massive doses of the vitamin via intravenous solutions. Riboflavin is heat stabile, but sensitive to light, and acidic and alkaline conditions.

FUNCTION

Riboflavin is the precursor to a group of enzymatic cofactors called flavins. Flavins linked to protein are called flavoproteins. The two major coenzymes derived from riboflavin are flavin mononucleotide (FMN) and flavin adenine dinucleotide (FAD). Flavins are used as coenzymes in about 50 enzymes in mammals. Flavins participate in intermediary energy metabolism and function mainly in oxidoreductase types of reactions (**Figure 6-4**).

METABOLISM

Most riboflavin found in food sources is in the form of free coenzyme derivatives that are not readily absorbed unless hydrolyzed, and covalently bound riboflavin that is not well used. The free flavin compounds are hydrolyzed before they are absorbed in the upper GI tract. A specialized transport system that is saturable and sodium dependent is necessary for absorption of flavins. After absorption, about 50% of the riboflavin in blood is bound to albumin and the other half to globulins (Brody, 1994a; Rivlin, 1996). Tissues requiring riboflavin convert it to FMN by phosphorylation catalyzed by flavokinase and subsequently to FAD catalyzed by FAD synthase. Excess riboflavin in the body is eliminated largely as riboflavin via the kidneys.

REQUIREMENTS

The AAFCO (2007) recomended allowance for riboflavin is 2.2 mg/kg DM for dogs and 4 mg/kg DM for cats for all lifestages. The NRC (2006) recommended allowance for riboflavin for dogs is 5.25 mg/kg DM for growth and maintenance and 5.3 mg/kg DM for gestation and lactation. For cats, the NRC (2006) recommended allowance for riboflavin is 4.0 mg/kg DM for all lifestages. **Table 6-5** lists AAFCO and NRC allowances for dogs and cats.

DEFICIENCY AND TOXICITY

Deficiency of riboflavin in dogs and cats is uncommon but may manifest as dermatitis, erythema, weight loss, cataracts, impaired reproduction, neurologic changes and anorexia (NRC, 1985; Street and Cowgill, 1939; Street et al, 1941). Measurement of erythrocyte glutathione reductase activity is commonly used to evaluate riboflavin status in people and animals. **Table 6-5** lists riboflavin blood values for dogs and cats. Most commercial pet foods are supplemented with synthetic riboflavin. Toxicity has not been reported to occur in dogs and cats.

SOURCES

Riboflavin is widely distributed in foods, primarily bound to proteins as FMN and FAD. Rich sources include dairy products, organ meats (e.g., liver, heart, kidney), muscle meats, eggs, green plants and yeast. Cereal grains are poor sources of vitamin B_2. The supplemental form for addition to foods is usually riboflavin.

Niacin

Niacin is the generic term used to describe compounds that exhibit biologic activity of nicotinamide. Two major forms of niacin are nicotinic acid and nicotinamide.

FUNCTION

Nicotinic acid and nicotinamide are substituted pyridine ring structures (pyridine 3-carboxylic acid and nicotinic acid amide). Niacin must be converted to either nicotinamide-adenine dinucleotide (NADH) or nicotinamide-adenine dinucleotide phosphate (NADPH) to participate in enzymatic reactions or protein modification.

Niacin, in its cofactor form, is essential to several physiologic reactions: 1) oxidoreductive reactions, 2) nonredox reactions, 3) cleavage of β-N-glycosidic bonds with transfer of ADP-ribose to proteins (post-translational modification) and 4) formation of cyclic ADP-ribose (mobilizes intracellular calcium).

Oxidoreductive reactions are the primary function, but the others are significant in proper cell function. Generally, NAD/NADH is involved in catabolic reactions and transfers the reducing power (electrons) acquired from intermediary metabolites to the electron transport chain to ultimately produce adenosine triphosphate. Alternatively, NADP/NADPH is generally involved in biosynthetic reactions that transfer reducing power (electrons) to macromolecules such as fat, protein and carbohydrate.

METABOLISM

Niacin in foods is found mainly as NADH and NADPH, which may be free or bound to other macromolecules. After ingestion, NADH and NADPH undergo hydrolysis by the intestinal mucosa to release free nicotinamide, which is readily absorbed (Brody, 1994a). Dietary niacin (nicotinic acid and nicotinamide) is absorbed readily through the gastric and small intestinal mucosa. Both free nicotinic acid and nicotinamide are found in blood. Tissues readily take up these compounds to synthesize required cofactors, which also trap the compound in cells. Excess niacin is methylated and excreted in urine.

Niacin may also be synthesized from tryptophan via the kynurenin pathway, which results in formation of nicotinic acid ribonucleotide. Some enzymes in this pathway require vitamin B_6 and iron as cofactors. In most mammals, foods high in tryptophan can alleviate signs of niacin deficiency. However, cats cannot efficiently use tryptophan to synthesize niacin because they have a very high enzymatic activity of picolinic carboxylase that decisively leads the metabolism of tryptophan to acetyl-CoA and CO_2 instead of NAD (Sudadolnik et al, 1957; Baker and Czarnecki-Maulden, 1991). Thus, cats have a strict dietary requirement for preformed niacin.

REQUIREMENTS

The AAFCO (2007) recommended allowance for niacin is 11.4 mg/kg DM for dogs and 60 mg/kg DM for cats for all lifestages. The NRC (2006) recommended allowance for niacin is 17 mg/kg DM for dogs and 40 mg/kg DM for cats for all lifestages. **Table 6-5** lists AAFCO and NRC allowances for dogs and cats.

DEFICIENCY AND TOXICITY

Deficiency of niacin results in pellagra with its classic 4D signs: dermatitis, diarrhea, dementia and death. Clinical deficiency is uncommon in dogs because most commercial pet foods are supplemented with niacin. Cats, however, are more likely to develop signs of deficiency because of their strict requirement for niacin. Niacin is a fairly stable vitamin. Processing conditions may release some bound niacin, which increases availability. Niacin deficiency may occur when foods with low quantities of niacin and tryptophan are ingested.

Measurement of methylated nicotinamide levels in urine best substantiates niacin deficiency. Niacin metabolites in whole blood have been reported for dogs and cats (**Table 6-5**), but these values generally have not been useful markers of deficiency in other species (Baker et al, 1986; Jacob and Swendseid, 1996). No niacin toxicity information in cats is available. However, excessive ingestion of nicotinic acid causes bloody stool, convulsions and even death (Chen et al, 1938).

SOURCES

Niacin is a very stable vitamin found in a variety of foodstuffs. The greatest amounts of niacin are found in yeast, animal/fish by-products, cereals, legumes and oilseeds. Niacin occurs in animal tissues as NAD and NADP and in plants mostly as protein-bound forms. Niacin is generally added to most pet foods as nicotinic acid or nicotinamide.

Pyridoxine

Pyridoxine is also generally called vitamin B_6. However, vitamin B_6 is a generic descriptor for all 3-hydroxy-2-methylpyridine derivatives exhibiting the biologic activity of pyridoxine. The three naturally occurring forms of vitamin B_6 are pyridoxal, pyridoxine and pyridoxamine.

FUNCTION

The biologically active forms of vitamin B_6 are the coenzymes pyridoxal phosphate (PLP) and pyridoxamine phosphate (PMP). PLP is involved in most reactions of amino acid metabolism, including transamination, decarboxylation, desulfhydration and nonoxidative deamination. PLP is also involved in the catabolism of glycogen and metabolism of lipids. As a coenzyme for decarboxylase enzymes, PLP functions in the synthesis of serotonin, epinephrine, norepinephrine and γ-aminobutyric acid (GABA). Pyridoxine is involved in vasodilatation through the production of histamine and is required in the pathway where niacin is produced from tryptophan. Pyridoxine helps catalyze the synthesis of taurine from cysteine and participates with ascorbic acid and NAD in the synthesis of carnitine from the amino acid lysine. Pyridoxine is also involved with the synthesis of the heme precursor porphyrin (as a coenzyme for δ-aminolevulinate synthase).

METABOLISM

The various forms of vitamin B_6 (pyridoxine, pyridoxal, pyridoxamine, PLP, PMP) are freely absorbed via passive diffusion in the small intestine. The glucuronide form is not absorbed.

The predominant form of vitamin B_6 in blood is PLP, which is tightly bound to proteins. Pyridoxal crosses cell membranes more readily than PLP does. After uptake by cells, the vitamin is again phosphorylated by pyridoxal kinase to yield the predominant tissue form, PLP, which is considered to be the most active vitamin B_6 form.

The vitamin B_6 forms are readily interconverted metabolically by reactions involving phosphorylation/dephosphorylation, oxidation/reduction and amination/deamination. Phosphorylation appears to be an important means of retaining the vitamin intracellularly. Only small quantities of vitamin B_6 are stored in the body. The products of vitamin B_6 metabolism are excreted in the urine; pyridoxic acid is the predominant metabolic product. Different from other species, cats excrete little pyridoxic acid in urine even after a large oral dose of pyridoxine hydrochloride (Coburn and Mahuren, 1987). The main metabolites of vitamin B_6 in cat urine are pyridoxine 3-sulfate, pyridoxal 3-sulfate and N-methylpyridoxine.

REQUIREMENTS

The AAFCO (2007) recommended allowance for pyridoxine is 1 mg/kg DM for dogs and 4 mg/kg DM for cats for all lifestages. The NRC (2006) recommended allowance for pyridoxine is 1.5 mg/kg DM for dogs and 2.5 mg/kg DM for cats for all lifestages. **Table 6-5** lists AAFCO and NRC allowances for dogs and cats.

DEFICIENCY AND TOXICITY

Signs of vitamin B_6 deficiency include anorexia, reduced growth, muscle weakness, neurologic signs, (e.g., hyperirritability and seizures), anemia, and irreversible kidney lesions. Oxalate crystalluria is also a notable sign in pyridoxine-deficient cats (NRC, 2006). **Table 6-5** lists normal plasma levels of pyridoxine for cats and dogs (Baker et al, 1986).

Because pyridoxic acid is not detected in the urine of vitamin B_6-deficient subjects, this metabolite is useful in the clinical assessment of vitamin B_6 status. Measurement of xanthurenic acid excretion after a tryptophan load, however, is a more sensitive indicator of vitamin B_6 status. When vitamin B6 is deficient, the conversion of tryptophan to niacin is impaired, resulting in increased production of xanthurenic acid. Other indices of vitamin B_6 status are plasma concentrations of PLP and erythrocyte transaminase.

The prevalence of vitamin B_6 toxicity appears to be low. Earliest detectable signs include ataxia and loss of small motor control. Many of the signs of toxicity resemble those of vitamin B_6 deficiency: ataxia, muscle weakness and loss of balance. Histologic examination of tissues from dogs fed more than 200 mg pyridoxine hydrochloride/kg body weight/day revealed bilateral loss of myelin and axons in the dorsal funiculi and loss of myelin in the dorsal nerve roots (Phillips et al, 1978). There is no information regarding vitamin B_6 toxicity in cats.

SOURCES

Vitamin B_6 is widely distributed in foods, occurring in greatest concentrations in meats, whole-grain products, vegetables and nuts. The chemical forms of vitamin B_6 tend to vary among foods of plant and animal origin; plant tissues contain mostly pyridoxine, whereas animal tissues contain mostly pyridoxal and pyridoxamine. Pyridoxine is far more stable than either pyridoxal or pyridoxamine, thus processing losses are greatest in foods containing animal products. Losses can be as high as 70% (average losses from 0 to 40%) (McDowell, 1989). Pyridoxine hydrochloride is most often used for supplementation because it is relatively stable.

Pantothenic Acid

Pantothenic acid is the trivial designation for dihydroxy-β, β-dimethylbutyryl-β-alanine. Only the dextrorotatory form of pantothenic acid has biologic activity. It occurs mainly in bound form, (i.e., coenzyme A [CoA] and acyl-carrier protein), in most foods and feedstuffs. Pantothenic acid in foods is fairly stable at cooking temperatures and during storage. However, appreciable losses (up to 50%) have been reported during canning and storage of some foods at pH values greater than 7 and less than 5 (Combs, 1998).

FUNCTION

CoA is found in all tissues and is one of the most important coenzymes for metabolism. CoA plays a critical role in the tricarboxylic acid cycle for production of ATP from fat (glycerol and fatty acids), glucose and amino acids. CoA is also involved in the synthesis of fatty acids, steroid hormones and cholesterol. CoA is necessary for oxidation of fatty acids, pyruvate and ketoglutarate (Machlin, 1991).

METABOLISM

CoA and acyl-carrier protein are the predominant forms of pantothenic acid in foods and foodstuffs. Thus, hydrolytic digestion of these protein complexes is the first step in metabolism of this vitamin. Both forms are degraded to pantothenic acid in the lumen of the intestine in a series of steps. Absorption occurs via a saturable, sodium-dependent, energy-requiring process. At high concentrations, simple diffusion occurs throughout the small intestine. In dogs, more than 80% of free pantothenate is absorbed from the gut (Taylor et al, 1974). Urinary β-glucuronide is the major form of excretion (Taylor et al, 1972). Pantothenic acid is transported in the free acid form in plasma. Erythrocytes contain predominantly acetyl-CoA.

REQUIREMENTS

The AAFCO (2007) recommended allowance for pantothenic acid is 10 mg/kg DM for dogs and 5 mg/kg DM for cats for all lifestages. Less pantothenic acid is apparently required to optimize growth when high-protein foods are fed, whereas high-fat diets may increase the requirement for pantothenic acid (McDowell, 1989). The NRC (2006) recommendation for pantothenic acid allowance is 15 mg/kg DM for dogs regardless of lifestage. For cats, the NRC (2006) allowance for pantothenic acid is 5.7 mg/kg DM for growth, and 5.75 mg/kg DM for maintenance and reproduction. **Table 6-5** lists AAFCO and NRC allowances for dogs and cats.

DEFICIENCY AND TOXICITY

Naturally occurring deficiency of pantothenic acid is rare. Dogs with pantothenic acid deficiency have erratic appetites, depressed growth, fatty livers, decreased antibody response, hypocholesterolemia and coma, in later stages. Pantothenic acid-deficient cats developed fatty livers and became emaciated (NRC, 2006). Normal whole blood concentrations of pantothenic acid for dogs and cats are listed in **Table 6-5** (Baker et al, 1986).

Pantothenic acid is generally regarded as nontoxic. No adverse reactions or clinical signs other than gastric upset have been observed in any species following ingestion of large doses.

SOURCES

"Pantothenic acid" is derived from the Greek word "pantos" meaning "found everywhere." Although this vitamin is found in practically all foodstuffs, the quantity present is generally insufficient for most monogastric species. The most important sources are meats (especially liver and heart), rice and wheat bran, alfalfa, peanut meal, yeast and fish solubles. Calcium pantothenate is the predominant form added to pet foods.

Folic Acid

Folic acid was first discovered in 1943 and was classified as vitamins B_{10} and B_{11}. The structure of folic acid may be subdivided into three functional components: the middle group is para-aminobenzoic acid (PABA), flanked on one side by a pteridine ring, and on the other side by a polyglutamic acid chain. Folate is the name commonly used to designate a family of compounds with the biologic activity of folic acid (Brody, 1994a; Selhub and Rosenberg, 1996).

FUNCTION

Folic acid functions as a one-carbon (methylene, methenyl, methyl) donor and acceptor molecule in intermediary metabolism. Specific pathways include nucleotide biosynthesis, phospholipid synthesis, amino acid metabolism, neurotransmitter production and creatinine formation. In addition, vitamin B_{12} is closely paired with folate in the production of methionine from homocysteine, which will be discussed later in this section.

METABOLISM

Natural sources of folic acid undergo hydrolysis by the intestinal enzyme γ-glutamyl hydrolase to form folylmonoglutamate, which is subsequently absorbed by enterocytes. Thus, the major form of folic acid in blood is the monoglutamate form. After target cells absorb folylmonoglutamate, additional glutamates are added to the tail, which trap the molecule within cells.

Folic acid must be in the reduced form (i.e., dihydro or tetrahydro) to participate in one-carbon metabolic reactions. The enzyme dihydrofolate reductase (DHFR) interconverts dihydrofolates to tetrahydrofolates. Inhibition of this enzyme interferes with intermediary pathways that require reduced folates for coenzymes. C677T mutation in the methylenetetrahydrofolate reductase (MTHFR) gene also affects folate metabolism and requirement (Golbahar et al, 2005).

REQUIREMENTS

The AAFCO (2007) recommended allowance for folic acid is 0.18 mg/kg DM for dogs and 0.8 mg/kg DM for cats for all lifestages, respectively. The NRC (2006) recommended allowance for folic acid is 270 μg/kg DM for dogs and 750 μg/kg DM for cats regardless of lifestage. **Table 6-5** lists AAFCO and NRC allowances for dogs and cats.

DEFICIENCY AND TOXICITY

Folate deficiency is characterized by poor weight gain, megaloblastic anemia, anorexia, leukopenia, glossitis and decreased immune function. In cats, folate deficiency is associated with hyperhomocysteinemia and greatly augmented urinary excretion of formiminoglutamic acid (Yu and Morris, 1998). Folate deficiency has been linked to the risk of neural tube defects in people (Mitchell, 2005). Folate levels in blood may be measured to confirm a deficiency suggested by clinical signs. **Table 6-5** lists plasma levels for healthy cats and dogs (Baker et al, 1986).

There have been no reported cases of folate toxicity. Neither NRC nor AAFCO has proposed a dietary maximum concentration for folic acid.

SOURCES

Folate is found in several foods, but is unstable in a variety of conditions. Liver, egg yolks and green vegetables are good sources of folate. The vitamin is destroyed by heating, prolonged freezing and during storage in water. Commercial pet foods are supplemented with folate to overcome the effects of processing and storage.

Biotin

Biotin consists of an imidazole ring fused to a tetrahydrothiophene ring with a valeric acid side chain. It has eight possible stereoisomers in nature but only d-(+)-biotin is physiologically active (NRC, 2006). Biotin is unstable to oxidation and heat.

FUNCTION

Biotin is an essential cofactor for four different carboxylase reactions in mammals. These carboxylases have important functions in the metabolism of lipids, glucose, some amino acids and energy.

METABOLISM

The majority of biotin in food sources is thought to be covalently bound to proteins. After ingestion, biotin must be hydrolyzed from protein by the enzyme biotinidase in pancreatic juice before absorption in the intestine (Brody, 1994a; Mock, 1996). After hydrolysis, free biotin is actively absorbed through a biotin transporter that requires both an intact ureide group and a free carboxyl group on valeric acid (NRC, 2006). Avidin in raw egg white can tightly bind biotin and is resistant to intestinal proteolysis and heat treatment, making biotin unavailable for absorption. After absorption from the intestine, biotin is transported in the free form in the plasma to the required tissues where it is linked to its target apoenzyme by the enzyme holocarboxylase synthetase. The kidneys eliminate excess biotin. Increasing urinary excretion of 3-hydroxyisovaleric acid, an indicator of reduced activity of the biotin-dependent enzyme methylcrotonyl-CoA carboxylase, and decreasing biotin in urine are early and sensitive indicators of biotin deficiency (Mock et al, 2002).

REQUIREMENTS

Neither AAFCO (2007) nor NRC (2006) has a recommendation for biotin for dogs. However, diets containing raw egg white and/or antibiotics may need biotin supplementation. The AAFCO (2007) biotin recommendation for cats is 0.07 mg/kg DM for all lifestages. The NRC (2006) recommended allowance for biotin for cats is 75 μg/kg DM regardless of lifestage. **Table 6-5** lists AAFCO and NRC allowances for dogs and cats.

DEFICIENCY AND TOXICITY

Naturally occurring biotin deficiency is very rare in dogs and cats (NRC, 2006). Feeding raw egg whites and administering oral antimicrobials are probably the two most common causes of biotin deficiency. Raw egg whites contain the glycoprotein avidin, which binds biotin rendering it unavailable for absorption. Feeding avidin to cats may result in signs of biotin deficiency that include dermatitis, alopecia and a dull coat (Pastoor et al, 1993). Because gut microbial synthesis may meet half the biotin requirement, antimicrobials that decrease the population of the intestinal microflora may also result in signs of biotin deficiency. Clinical signs include poor growth, dermatitis, lethargy and neurologic abnormalities (**Case 6-10**). **Table 6-5** lists biotin blood values for dogs and cats (Baker et al, 1986).

Biotin toxicity has not been reported. Neither AAFCO (2007) nor NRC (2006) has proposed a dietary maximum concentration for biotin.

SOURCES

Mammalian tissues are incapable of synthesizing biotin. The biotin requirement is probably met by two sources: diet and microbes (Brody, 1994a; Mock, 1996). Biotin is widely distributed in foods, but mostly in very low, highly variable concentrations. Oilseeds, egg yolks, alfalfa meal, liver and yeast are the most important natural sources of biotin. Marked losses of biotin may occur as a result of oxidation, canning, heat and solvent extraction of foodstuffs. Less than one-half of the biotin in various foodstuffs is biologically available (McDowell, 1989). Most commercial pet foods are supplemented with synthetic biotin.

Vitamin B_{12}

Vitamin B_{12} or cobalamin is the generic descriptor for all corrinoids exhibiting the biologic activity of cyanocobalamin. Vitamin B_{12} is the largest and most complex B vitamin and the only one to contain a metal ion, cobalt. The structure consists of four pyrrole rings linked to form a macrocyclic ring designated as corrin, which is similar to hemoglobin. Substitutions on the corrin ring account for the different recognized forms of vitamin B_{12}. The active forms of B_{12}, 5'deoxyadenosylcobalamin and methylcobalamin, are very unstable (Brody, 1994a; Herbert, 1996). Substituted forms of vitamin B_{12} are much more stable and may be used as pharmaceutical supplements (cyanocobalamin, hydroxocobalamin, nitritocobalamin).

FUNCTION

Vitamin B_{12} is important in one-carbon metabolism. In dogs and cats, methylcobalamin, which contains cobalt in the 1^+ state, is a coenzyme for methionine synthase and 5'deoxyadenosylmethionine, which contains cobalt in the 2^+ state is a coenzyme for methylmalonyl-CoA mutase. Vitamin B_{12} is required by the enzyme methionine synthase that removes a methyl group from methyl tetrahydrofolate (THF) to regenerate THF, which is needed for pyrimidine biosynthesis. This intimate relationship with folate may result in folate trapping in B_{12} deficiency and the resultant megaloblastic anemia of folate deficiency.

METABOLISM

Dietary vitamin B_{12} is freed from food peptides and proteins by hydrolysis (gastric acidification and pancreatic enzymes). Free vitamin B_{12} binds to intrinsic factor (IF), a glycoprotein secreted from gastric parietal cells. IF is essential for vitamin B_{12} absorption in people. In dogs, the pancreas is the major and the stomach a lesser source of IF. In cats, the pancreas appears to be the sole source of IF (NRC, 2006). The stable vitamin B_{12}-IF complex is absorbed in the ileum via cell surface specific receptors. Vitamin B_{12} may also be absorbed in the jejunum of dogs and cats (Gazet and McColl, 1967). After absorption, vitamin B_{12} is transported in blood by transcobalamin I and II. Transcobalamin I (haptocorrin) is a glycoprotein that carries almost all vitamin B_{12} in the blood of people. Transcobalamin II, a protein without a carbohydrate moiety, carries about 75% of vitamin B_{12} in the blood of dogs and cats. Cat and dog plasma do not contain transcobalamin I, but have another transport protein, transcobalamin O, which carries about 10 to 15% of vitamin B_{12} (Linnel et al, 1979). All DNA-synthesizing cells take up vitamin B_{12} from the blood via cell surface specific receptors.

REQUIREMENTS

The AAFCO (2007) recommended allowance for vitamin B_{12} is 0.022 mg/kg DM for dogs and 0.020 mg/kg cats for all lifestages. The NRC (2006) recommended allowance for vitamin B_{12} is 35 µg cobalamin/kg DM for dogs and 22.5 µg/kg DM for cats regardless of lifestages. **Table 6-5** lists AAFCO and NRC allowances for dogs and cats.

DEFICIENCY AND TOXICITY

Vitamin B_{12} deficiency is very rare but may result in poor growth and neuropathies in dogs (**Case 6-11**). Because vitamin B_{12} is only made by microbes and found in animal tissue, long-term feeding of vegetarian diets may lead to vitamin B_{12} deficiency.

Vitamin B_{12} may be directly assessed by determination of serum vitamin B_{12} levels or indirectly by determination of serum or urine methylmalonic acid (MMA) (Brody, 1994a). MMA levels in serum and urine increase with vitamin B_{12} deficiency. A newer test, serum holotranscobalamin II, may prove useful in the future to detect early vitamin B_{12} deficiency (Herbert, 1996). Whole blood levels of cobalamin for dogs and cats are listed in **Table 6-5** (Baker et al, 1986).

Oral toxicity of vitamin B_{12} has not been reported in dogs and cats. Neither AAFCO (2007) nor NRC (2006) has proposed a dietary maximum concentration for vitamin B_{12}.

SOURCES

Only certain microorganisms synthesize cobalamin. Microbes and yeast can make vitamin B_{12} for absorption by animals. Plants generally contain very small amounts of vitamin B_{12}. Meat and, to some degree, milk products are good sources of vitamin B_{12}. Most commercial pet foods are supplemented with stable vitamin B_{12}.

Choline

Choline is traditionally classified as one of the B-complex vitamins although it does not entirely satisfy the strict definition of a vitamin; many animals can synthesize choline in the liver. In addition, choline is required in the body in substantially greater amounts (>1,000 mg/kg) than the other B vitamins (<100 mg/kg). Furthermore, choline does not function as a coenzyme or cofactor as do most other B vitamins.

Choline, 2-hydroxy-N, N, N-trimethylethanaminium, has three methyl groups that enable choline to serve as a methyl donor in the body. It is an integral component of lecithin (phosphatidylcholine). Choline is a strong base and decomposes in alkaline solution.

FUNCTION

Choline plays several important roles in the body. It is an integrated component of phosphatidylcholine, a structural element of biologic membranes. Phosphatidylcholine also promotes lipid transport. Diminished synthesis of phosphatidylcholine in the liver due to choline deficiency results in accumulation of lipids in the liver. Choline, as acetylcholine, is a neurotransmitter. Choline, as a component of platelet-activating factor (1-O-alkyl-2acetyl-sm-glycero-3-phophocholine), is important in clotting and inflammation. After oxidation to betaine, choline is a source of labile methyl groups for transmethylation reactions (e.g., the formation of methionine from homocysteine and creatine from guanidoacetic acid).

METABOLISM

Choline is present in food predominantly as phosphatidylcholine; less than 10% is present as either the free base or sphingomyelin (Combs, 1998). Choline is released from phosphatidylcholine and sphingomyelin by digestive enzymes and absorbed from the jejunum and ileum mainly by a carrier-mediated process. Intestinal microorganisms metabolize most free choline ingested to trimethylamine, which is absorbed and excreted in urine. Phosphatidylcholine is not subject to such extensive microbial metabolism; therefore, metabolism of phosphatidylcholine results in less urinary trimethylamine. Once absorbed, choline is transported in the lymphatic circulation primarily in the form of phosphatidylcholine bound to chylomicrons.

Most species can synthesize choline, as phosphatidylcholine, by the sequential methylation of phosphatidylethanolamine. The activity is greatest in the liver, but is also found in many other tissues.

REQUIREMENTS

The requirement for choline is affected greatly by dietary factors such as methionine, betaine, myoinositol, folate and vitamin B_{12}, as well as the combination of different levels and composition of fat, carbohydrate and protein in the diet. In addition, age, gender, caloric intake and growth rate influence the lipotrophic action of choline and thereby its requirement.

Choline and methionine are the two principal methyl donors in transmethylation. Therefore, dietary adequacy of methionine and choline directly affects the requirement of the other. Methionine can completely replace choline as a methyl donor. For example, in cat foods, if dietary methionine exceeds 0.62% DM, 3.75 parts of methionine can be substituted for 1 part choline (AAFCO, 2007).

Vitamin B_{12} and folate are required for the synthesis of methyl groups and metabolism of the one-carbon unit. Biosynthesis of labile methyl from a formate carbon requires folate, whereas vitamin B_{12} plays a role in regulated transfer of the methyl group to tetrahydrofolic acid. Therefore, a deficiency of one or both of these vitamins increases the requirement for choline.

Excess dietary protein and/or high-fat foods increase the choline requirement. In most species, the choline requirement is greater for younger animals than for adults. Some adult species may not require choline.

The AAFCO (2007) recommended allowance for choline is 1,200 mg/kg DM for dogs and 2,400 mg/kg DM for cats for all lifestages. The NRC (2006) recommended allowance for choline is 1,700 mg/kg DM for dogs and 2,550 mg/kg DM for cats regardless of lifestage. **Table 6-5** lists AAFCO and NRC allowances for dogs and cats.

DEFICIENCY AND TOXICITY

Choline deficiency in most animal species is characterized by depressed growth, hepatic steatosis and hemorrhagic renal degeneration (Combs, 1998). Additional signs of choline deficiency in dogs include thymic atrophy and elevated plasma phosphatase values and increased blood prothrombin time. **Table 6-5** lists normal plasma levels of choline for cats and dogs (Baker et al, 1986). Choline and phosphatidylcholine levels in blood may be measured to confirm deficiency suggested by clinical signs.

Studies with dogs suggested a low tolerance to lecithin (phosphatidylcholine). Reduced erythrocytes resulted from daily oral administration of lecithin (equivalent to 150 mg of choline) (NRC, 1987). However, neither AAFCO (2007) nor NRC (2006) has recommended a maximum or safe upper limit for dietary choline for dogs and cats.

SOURCES

All natural fats contain some choline; therefore, choline is widely distributed in foods and foodstuffs. Lecithin has also been shown to be an effective emulsifying agent in foods and is the form of choline ingested in most foods. Egg yolks, glandular meals and fish are the richest animal sources and cereal germs, legumes and oilseed meals are the best plant sources. Choline is added to most pet foods as choline chloride and is added separately from the vitamin premix because of its hygroscopic nature and propensity to reduce the stability of other vitamins if added in the premix.

Vitamin C

Because of de novo synthesis, vitamin C is not technically a vitamin for healthy dogs and cats. (See vitamin definition.) However, it is included here because of its biochemical functions, including in vivo and in vitro antioxidant properties (Chapter 7).

FUNCTION

Vitamin C, ascorbic acid or specifically L-ascorbic acid, is a very labile compound that is readily oxidized to dehydroascorbic acid. It requires a reducing enzyme (dehydroascorbic acid reductase) to transform it back to the active form. Vitamin C primarily functions in the body as an antioxidant and free radical scavenger. Ascorbic acid is best known for its role in collagen synthesis, where it is involved in hydroxylation of prolyl and lysyl residues of procollagen (Combs, 1998). It is also involved in drug, steroid and tyrosine metabolism (McDowell, 1989) and electron transport. Ascorbic acid is also necessary for synthesis of L-carnitine, an important carrier of acyl groups across mitochondrial membranes. Normal circulating plasma levels are 4 µg/ml in dogs and 3 µg/ml in cats (Baker et al, 1986).

More recently, research into the role of ascorbic acid has shifted from prevention of deficiency to the treatment and prevention of disease. Because ascorbic acid protects against free-radical damage induced by the "oxidative burst" of neutrophils (Combs, 1998; Levine et al, 1994), and stimulates the phagocytic effect of leukocytes, it plays a role in immune function (McDowell, 1989). Larger doses may play a protective role against carcinogenesis. Ascorbic acid acts as a nitrate scavenger, thereby reducing nitrosamine-induced carcinogenesis. Vitamin C has been associated with a reduced risk for gastric cancer, oral cancer and perhaps lung cancer, but had no effect on cancer of the pancreas, colon and prostate gland (Sauberlich, 1991).

Vitamin C may even play a role in the prevention of gingival and periodontal disease. Studies with people have shown that 600 mg/day (10x the recommended dietary allowance) significantly reduced gingival bleeding upon probing (Leggott et al, 1986). Whether this effect can be demonstrated in species that synthesize their own ascorbate (i.e., cats and dogs) remains to be seen.

Ascorbic acid may have some benefit in exercise stress recovery (Kronfeld, 1983). However, megadose supplementation to prevent hip dysplasia has not proved effective (Richardson, 1992).

METABOLISM

Most higher animals can synthesize vitamin C from glucose via the glucuronic acid pathway. People and some animals such as guinea pigs, fish, fruit-eating bats, insects and some birds cannot synthesize vitamin C because they lack the key enzyme L-gulonolactone oxidase. In these species, vitamin C is absorbed by a saturable, carrier-mediated, active-transport mechanism that is sodium dependent. Species that can synthesize ascorbic acid absorb it strictly by passive diffusion. In either case, absorption efficiency of physiologic doses is more than 80% (Combs, 1998).

Vitamin C is transported in the plasma in association with albumin, mostly in a reduced form. Under physiologic conditions, vitamin C exists as ascorbate, which cannot cross most membranes readily. Cellular uptake of vitamin C involves dehydroascorbic acid in erythrocytes, lymphocytes and neutrophils. Once inside the cell, dehydroascorbic acid is quickly reduced to ascorbic acid by an intracellular enzyme (dehydroascorbic acid reductase), which uses reduced glutathione (GSH) as the source of reducing equivalents. Ascorbic acid is widely distributed throughout tissues, both in animals capable of synthesizing ascorbic acid and those that depend on dietary vitamin C. The pituitary and adrenal glands have the highest concentrations of vitamin C; high levels are also found in the liver, spleen, brain and pancreas. Ascorbic acid is excreted in urine, sweat and feces. Losses in feces and sweat are usually minimal.

Because vitamin C is not an essential nutrient for dogs and cats, neither AAFCO nor NRC lists recommendations.

DEFICIENCY AND TOXICITY

Acute vitamin C deficiency results in scurvy (in animals unable to synthesize the vitamin). In general, high intake of vitamin C is considered to be of low toxicity.

SOURCES

Fruits, vegetables and organ meats are generally the best sources of vitamin C. The vitamin C content of most foods decreases dramatically during storage and processing. Polyphosphorylated forms of vitamin C are available that can survive processing conditions.

Vitamin-Like Substances

Vitamin-like substances are substances that exhibit properties similar to those of vitamins, but do not fit the strict definition of a vitamin. They have physiologic functionality, but questionable essentiality. These compounds can be "conditionally essential" depending on the metabolic capacity of the animal.

L-carnitine

L-carnitine is one of the most well known vitamin-like substances. L-carnitine is a natural component of all animal cells (Bremer, 1983; Rebouche and Paulson, 1986). Its primary function is to transport long-chain fatty acids across the inner mitochondrial membrane into the mitochondrial matrix for β-oxidation (Bremer, 1983; Fritz, 1958). Skeletal and cardiac muscle contain 95 to 98% of the L-carnitine in the body and are significant storage sites (Rebouche and Engel, 1983).

The biosynthesis of L-carnitine requires five enzymatic steps that occur in many cells in the body (Bremer, 1983). The final step in which butyrobetaine is converted to L-carnitine is rate limiting and occurs primarily in the liver (Bremer, 1983). Lysine, methionine, ascorbic acid, ferrous ions, vitamin B_6 and niacin are important in L-carnitine metabolism; these nutrients are required substrates and cofactors for the enzymes involved in L-carnitine biosynthesis (Borum, 1986).

Clinical signs of L-carnitine deficiency include chronic muscle weakness, fasting hypoglycemia, cardiomyopathy, hepatomegaly and dicarboxylic aciduria (Stanley, 1987). In many cases of L-carnitine deficiency, no clinical signs are apparent (Borum, 1986).

Carotenoids

Carotenoids are a class of lipophilic natural pigments that are widely distributed throughout the plant and animal kingdom. Only plants, bacteria, fungi and algae synthesize carotenoids; however, animals can accumulate carotenoids in their tissues after oral ingestion. In plants, carotenoids play essential light-harvesting roles during photosynthetic events and protect membranes against photo-oxidative damage. More than 600 different compounds are classified as carotenoids, but fewer than 10% can be metabolized into vitamin A. In contrast to many other mammals, cats are unable to convert β-carotene to vitamin A; therefore, cats must rely solely on preformed vitamin A in their diet (Schweigert et al, 2002). The carotenoids found in greatest abundance in a variety of foodstuffs are β-carotene, α-carotene, lutein, lycopene, β-cryptoxanthin, zeaxanthin, canthaxanthin and astaxanthin. A primary characteristic of the carotenoids is their conjugated polyene structure.

ABSORPTION AND TRANSPORT

Because carotenoids are lipophilic compounds, concurrent ingestion of fat facilitates intestinal carotenoid absorption. Bile salts are necessary for absorption of ingested fat and carotenoids. The aggregation of bile salts into micelles, and the formation of mixed micelles with the products of lipid digestion and other lipid-soluble food constituents are essential in facilitating absorption of lipophilic compounds from the intestine. At the brush border, micelles interact with enterocytes where the lipophilic contents of micelles diffuse out of the micelles and across the cell membrane. It is believed that the uptake of carotenoids by enterocytes occurs passively and is not carrier-mediated. Enterocytes package carotenoids into chylomicrons, which migrate to the basal-lateral cell membrane where they are exocytosed into the intracellular space for passage to the lymphatic system. After transportation in chylomicrons via the lymphatic system, carotenoids are carried by lipoproteins and transported in the bloodstream.

FUNCTION

Although carotenoids do not strictly fit the definition of a vitamin for mammalian species, they have biologic activity beyond their provitamin A role. Carotenoids with nine or more double bonds function as antioxidants by quenching singlet oxygen and other reactive oxygen species such as hydroxyl radicals, superoxide anion radicals and hydrogen peroxide, which are produced in normal metabolism (Chew, 1995; Bendich, 1989). Carotenoids sacrifice highly reactive multiple double bonds to free radicals via hydrogen donation, thereby stabilizing reactive products. Carotenoids also protect cell membranes by stabilizing the oxygen radicals produced when phagocytic granulocytes undergo respiratory bursts that destroy intracellular pathogens (Bendich, 1989).

The immune-modulating properties of carotenoids have been studied in dogs and cats. Supplementation with β-carotene increases the CD4 T cell population in older dogs to levels found in young dogs and improves T-cell proliferation (Massimino et al, 2003). Supplementation with β-carotene or lutein, an oxycarotenoid found in corn and other vegetables, stimulates cell-mediated and humoral immune responses in dogs and cats (Chew et al, 2000; Kim et al, 2000; Kim et al, 2000a).

SOURCES

Carotenoids are responsible for the striking colors of many yellow, orange and red fruits and vegetables, plant leaves, as well as the colors in some species of fish, crustaceans and plumage of some birds.

Bioflavonoids

The flavonoids are a group of red, blue, yellow and colorless compounds that have vitamin-like activity. This class of compounds was originally mistaken for vitamin C because crude extracts of lemon juice and yellow peppers had antiscorbutic effects. Originally called citrin (mixture of eriodictyol and hesperidin), vitamin P or vitamin C_2, these compounds were reclassified as flavonoids in 1950 (Combs, 1998; Machlin, 1991; Harborne, 1994). More than 5,000 flavonoids have been identified (Harborne and Baxter, 1999). Flavonoids are classified in major and minor groups. Classes include flavonols, flavanols, flavones, isoflavones and anthocyanins. Flavonols, (e.g., kaempferol, quercetin and myricetin, are present in tea, apples and onions. Flavanols (also called catechins) are found in tea, apples and red wine. Isoflavones such as genistein and daidzein are constituents of soybeans. Anthocyanins provide the deep red color to fruits such as berries.

ABSORPTION AND TRANSPORT

The availability varies widely among flavonoids depending on the food source and the forms of flavonoids they contain. Flavonoids are usually found naturally as glycosides linked to sugars, except for catechins. The type of sugar moiety of the glycoside affects availability, (e.g., quercetin glucosides are more efficiently absorbed than quercetin rutinosides) (Hollman et al, 1999). Mammalian enzymatic systems are unable to hydrolyze flavonoid glycosides, but the necessary glycosidases are present in the gut microflora. After hydrolysis and absorption in the small intestine, flavonoids are bound in the liver as glucuronides or sulfate conjugates (Machlin, 1991). Recent studies with flavanols have shown that glycosides can be absorbed without previous hydrolysis by microorganisms (Hollman et al, 1995). Most of the flavonoids are further metabolized into phenolic compounds and rapidly excreted, usually within 24 hours.

FUNCTION

Although many different flavonoids exist with many different physiologic effects, this class of compounds shares some similar functions. The most notable is the sparing effect that flavonoids have on vitamin C. Flavonoids have the ability to perform similarly to vitamin C: reduce capillary fragility and permeability and chelate the divalent metal ions copper and iron (Combs, 1998). Flavonoids can act as antioxidants because they are very effective scavengers of free radicals. In fact, flavonoid assays in vitro often exhibit stronger antioxidant activity than vitamins E and C. Other non-antioxidant related beneficial effects include prevention of angiogenesis (Cao and Cao, 1999) and inhibition of cyclooxygenase and lipoxygenase (Laughton et al, 1991). Catechins, found in abundance in tea, have been shown to modulate signal transduction pathways, have antiinflammatory activities and decrease cell proliferation (Dong et al, 1997; McCarty, 1998). Data from studies using animal models have shown that green and black tea consistently decrease cancers of the skin, lung, stomach, liver, mammary gland and colon (Chung et al, 2003). Isoflavones present in soybeans have been associated with reduced risk of cardiovascular disease, certain cancers and other degenerative diseases.

SOURCES

Flavonoids are ubiquitous in the plant kingdom. Significant variation in the flavonoids present in leaf, petal, root, fruit and seed can occur within the same plant. Flavonoid concentration can vary within a given plant organ (i.e. in apples), flavonoids tend to concentrate in the skin (Harborne, 2000).

Other Vitamin-Like Substances

Some other substances with vitamin-like activity include lipoic acid, ubiquinones, orotic acid, inositol and p-aminobenzoic acid. Animals synthesize most of these compounds, which are important metabolic intermediates. They function: 1) in the metabolism of fatty acids, 2) in the electron transport chain, 3) as antioxidants and 4) as growth factors. Continued research in "conditionally essential" nutrients may lead to vitamin classification for many of these compounds.

ENDNOTES

a. Kirk CA. Hill's Science and Technology Center, Topeka, KS, USA. Personal communication, 1997.

b. Wedekind KJ. Hill's Science and Technology Center, Topeka, KS, USA. Unpublished data, 1997.

REFERENCES

The References for **Chapter 6** can be found at www.markmorris.org.

CASE 6-1

Seizures in an Airedale Terrier

Patient Assessment

A 20-kg, eight-year-old, neutered male Airedale terrier was admitted to an emergency clinic after a 45-minute episode of continuous seizure activity. The dog was moribund at presentation. Thirty-six hours before the onset of seizures, the dog had ingested a salt-flour figurine, weighing approximately 100 g. The dog vomited a clear fluid three times within 12 hours after ingesting the figurine and became progressively more polydipsic and polyuric. The dog then consumed an unknown additional volume of uncooked salt-flour dough. Within an hour after ingesting this mixture, the dog developed generalized, fine-muscular fasciculations, which rapidly progressed to clonic-tonic motor activity.

The moribund dog was unresponsive to painful stimuli, pyrectic (41.6°C [106.9°F]), tachypneic and had an irregular heart rhythm. A generalized seizure occurred during the examination. Serum electrolyte and blood gas analysis revealed severe hypernatremia (serum sodium 211 mEq/l, normal 145 to 158), hyperchloremia (serum chloride 180 mEq/l, normal 105 to 122) and metabolic acidosis (serum pH 7.135, normal 7.32 to 7.38).

Treatment Plan

Treatment was initiated with intravenous fluids (5% dextrose in water), sodium bicarbonate, diazepam, phenobarbital and furosemide. The dog was also cooled with ice-water wraps and electric fans. The dog suffered cardiopulmonary arrest five hours later and died.

Further Assessment

At postmortem examination, one liter of putty-like, grayish-white material and clear, watery fluid were found in the stomach. Hemorrhage was noted throughout the stomach and the proximal two-thirds of the small intestine. Acute renal and hepatic necrosis was found histopathologically. Sodium and chloride levels in tissues were higher than normal. The brain sodium level was 108 mEq/l (80 mEq/l is considered indicative of sodium salt toxicosis). Analysis of the liquid portion of the gastric contents showed that a minimum of 20 g of sodium chloride remained in the stomach.

Bibliography

Khanna C, Boermans HJ, Wilcock B. Fatal hypernatremia in a dog from salt ingestion. Journal of the American Animal Hospital Association 1997; 33: 113-117.

CASE 6-2

Vomiting and Diarrhea in a Yorkshire Terrier

Patient Assessment

A one-year-old, intact female Yorkshire terrier weighing 2.7 kg had a sudden onset of lethargy, watery diarrhea, vomiting, icterus and red-colored urine. Abnormal laboratory findings included hemolyzed plasma, anemia, azotemia, leukocytosis, hemoglobinuria and an elevated total bilirubin concentration. Abdominal radiographs revealed a metal object at the pylorus. The object was recognized by the owner as a nut that had been missing for two weeks from an airfreight kennel used to house the dog. Serum zinc concentration was 32 mg/kg, compared with 1.1 mg/kg in serum obtained from a clinically normal dog at the same time.

Assess the Food and Feeding Method

No dietary history was available. The manufacturer of the kennel indicated that the nut was made of pure zinc.

Treatment Plan

The nut was removed from the stomach using a fiberoptic endoscope. Additional therapy included intravenous fluids and a blood transfusion.

Reassessment

The dog stopped vomiting but remained depressed and continued to have profuse watery diarrhea. Semi-solid feces were passed on Day 5 after removal of the nut. The dog's appetite returned on Day 6 and the dog steadily improved until discharge seven days later. Serum zinc concentrations on Days 11 and 21 were 8.5 mg/kg and 1.0 mg/kg respectively (values for a clinically normal dog were 0.7 mg/kg). The owner reported that the dog seemed completely normal three months after discharge.

On analysis, the nut contained 97% zinc, 2% aluminum and other elements. The nut removed from the stomach was highly corroded and when its weight was compared with that of a new nut of the same design, it appeared that the dog received a total dose of 703 mg zinc/kg body weight.

Bibliography

Torrance AG, Fulton RB. Zinc-induced hemolytic anemia in a dog. Journal of the American Veterinary Medical Association 1987; 191: 443-444.

CASE 6-3

Reproductive Problems in a Group of Cats

Patient Assessment

A group of breeding domestic shorthair cats, ranging in age from two to five years and weighing from 3 to 4.5 kg, was presented for poor reproductive performance, including failure to conceive, fetal resorption, small weak kittens and cannibalism. Neonatal kittens from these queens had graying of hair, dry and curled coat texture and skeletal abnormalities including inverted carpi and metatarsi, "kinked" tails and fused digits.

Physical examinations of the unbred queens were unremarkable. Some pregnant queens appeared slightly underweight for their date of gestation but were otherwise normal when examined. Newborn litters contained several small kittens, weighing less than 70 g or kittens with gray-to-whitish coats over the caudal one-half to three-fourths of the body. The coat color over the head and feet was unaffected. The coat texture of kittens less than three days old was somewhat dry and had a slightly curled appearance. Several newborn kittens had kinked tails and inverted carpi. Kittens older than three weeks had normal coats and improvements in carpal and tarsal malformations, but normal function or structure did not return in many kittens. Kittens with kinked tails and fused toes did not improve with age.

Reproductive problems included a decline in conception rate from 100% to between 0 to 50% over an eight-month period. In utero monitoring of pregnant queens through biweekly ultrasound examinations showed that the fetal loss rate was 67% and occurred between 25 to 30 days of gestation. Food intake was only about two-thirds of that expected for the queens.

The initial evaluation included complete blood counts and serum biochemistry profiles for many of the queens and serum trace mineral analyses and heavy metal toxicity screens for queens and affected kittens. The hemogram results included normal hematocrit and hemoglobin values with low mean corpuscular hemoglobin concentrations (hypochromasia) in four of six queens evaluated. Heavy metal toxicity screens of affected kittens were unremarkable with the exception of high-hepatic zinc level in one kitten and a single low-hepatic iron value. Serum copper concentrations for queens were normal, but hepatic copper values were not determined because queens were in active reproduction. In one- to two-week-old affected kittens, hepatic copper concentrations ranged from 26.6 to 35.7 mg/kg and serum copper values from 0.3 to 0.4 mg/kg, which were deemed borderline low based on literature values.

Assess the Food and Feeding Method

A commercial dry cat food that had passed an AAFCO feeding trial for feline growth and maintenance had been fed for approximately eight months to cats in this colony before any abnormalities were noted. The food was plant-based; the first four ingredients were corn, corn gluten meal, soybean meal and poultry by-product meal. In addition to containing typical vitamin and mineral supplements, the food also included copper oxide as a copper source and iron oxide as a colorant.

Analysis of the food disclosed no deficiencies when compared with recommended levels established for growing kittens. However, high levels of zinc and iron were noted in the food. High levels of dietary phytates, which can reduce mineral absorption, were expected to be in the food because of the plant ingredients it contained.

Feeding Plan

A dietary copper deficiency was considered the most likely cause of the reproductive failure noted in these queens. Although food analysis revealed that dietary copper levels were more than adequate, the copper oxide used in the food is a completely unavailable copper source for animals. Additionally, factors that impair copper absorption by chelation (phytates in plants) or transport competition (zinc and iron) were found in high concentrations in the food and would further impair absorption of available copper.

The cat food was supplemented with 15 mg/kg copper from an available source (i.e., copper sulfate).

Reassessment

After the food was supplemented with copper sulfate, the conception rate increased to 80% of breedings and in utero fetal death rates decreased to 12.5%. Food intake increased to expected levels. Three months after feeding the supplemented food, coat pigmentation abnormalities and limb and tail deformities again became evident in newborn kittens. Serum samples were again collected from pregnant queens for copper analysis. Copper values were low in four of nine queens, indicating continuing copper deficiency. An additional 10 mg/kg of dietary copper as copper sulfate were added for a total of 25 mg/kg supplemental copper. No abnormal kittens were born during the next five months.

Some less severe clinical signs of copper deficiency in kittens not consuming copper-supplemented food (i.e., queen's milk only) were reversible. Pigmentation and coat texture returned to normal and improved carpal flexion was observed with skeletal maturation.

Bibliography

Morris JG, Rogers QR. Copper oxide is an ineffective source of copper in queen diets. In: Proceedings. Pet Food Forum, Chicago, IL, 1995: 107-108.

CASE 6-4

Sudden Death in a Chihuahua

Patient Assessment

A three-year-old female Chihuahua was found dead one hour after being given 1.5 ml of a vitamin E preparation by intramuscular injection. The owner routinely administered the vitamin preparation twice yearly to all dogs of breeding age in his kennel. One week earlier, a similar incident occurred with a two-year-old female Yorkshire terrier. The owner had purchased the vitamin E product from the same veterinarian for several years. The Chihuahua and the vitamin E preparation were delivered to a diagnostic laboratory for examination.

At necropsy, the lungs were wet, glistening and mottled pink. White foam was found in the trachea and bronchi. All other internal organs appeared normal. Histopathologic examination of the lungs showed congested capillaries, perivascular edema and abundant proteinaceous fluid in the alveolar lumina. Liver and kidney specimens from the dog contained 12.9 and 12.1 mg selenium/kg, respectively (normal values <3 mg/kg).

Assess the Food and Feeding Method

No food was available for evaluation. When contacted, the veterinarian suggested that the bottle of vitamin preparation might also contain selenium. Selenium had been added to a bottle of vitamin E intended for use in calves, but the mixture had not been dispensed. The veterinarian was concerned that the bottle might have been sold inadvertently to the owner of the dog.

Two liquid phases, one oily and the other watery, were visible in the vitamin preparation bottle. The water-base liquid from the bottle contained 5,317 mg selenium/l. Subcutaneous tissue at the injection site contained 129 mg of selenium/kg. The calculated dose of selenium that had been administered to the dog was 2.5 mg/kg. The minimal lethal dose of selenium administered by intramuscular injection in dogs is 2.0 mg/kg.

Comments

Selenium toxicosis in cattle, sheep, horses, swine and poultry has been documented and usually develops as a subacute to chronic disease resulting from ingestion of seleniferous plants or feeds that contain high concentrations of selenium because of errors in ration formulation. Lesions of subacute to chronic selenium toxicosis have also been produced in dogs by long-term parenteral selenium administration. Acute selenium toxicosis causes increased vascular permeability, which is manifested as hemorrhages and edema in many tissues.

Bibliography

Janke BH. Acute selenium toxicosis in a dog. Journal of the American Veterinary Medical Association 1989; 195: 1114-1115.

CASE 6-5

Cervical Rigidity in a Cat

Patient Assessment

A 10-year-old, castrated domestic shorthair cat weighing 7 kg was examined for lethargy, decreased appetite and weight loss of several months' duration. Weight loss of 2 kg over the preceding 12 months was evident from the medical record.

The cat appeared depressed, had a matted, unkempt coat and extended its cervical region and held its head low and directly in front of its body. The cat was afebrile, obese and dehydrated. On palpation, the cervical region was rigidly extended with tense musculature. A hard mass was palpable in the midcervical region. The rigidly extended neck was the only neurologic abnormality.

Evaluation included a complete blood count (mild leukocytosis with mature neutrophilia), serum biochemistry analysis (mild hyperglycemia and hypercholesterolemia), feline leukemia virus antigen test (negative) and cervical and thoracic radiographs. Radiography revealed a bone-dense, cervical mass ventral to the C_1-C_2 intervertebral space. Much of the normal vertebral architecture appeared to be obliterated and the trachea and soft tissues were deviated ventrally and laterally. Thoracic radiography revealed ventral, bony proliferations extending from thoracic vertebrae T_2 through T_7. Marked bony proliferation was evident along the sternum and several of the costal cartilages.

The cat's serum vitamin A concentration was markedly high (315 µg/dl, normal 20 to 80 µg/dl).

Assess the Food and Feeding Method

The cat was fed a commercial dry cat food ad libitum supplemented with fresh beef liver daily.

Treatment and Feeding Plan

A tentative diagnosis of hypervitaminosis A was made based on the dietary history, clinical signs and radiographic lesions. The daily liver supplementation was considered the source of the excess dietary vitamin A. The cat was given a single intramuscular injection of dexamethasone and an oral analgesic was prescribed. The owner was advised to discontinue feeding beef liver and to feed only a balanced commercial cat food. The owner was further advised to encourage the cat to eat with hand feeding.

Reassessment

Six months later, the cat was euthanatized for reasons unrelated to the hypervitaminosis A. The cat had been eating fairly well, although its stiff-necked posture remained.

Bibliography

Goldman AL. Hypervitaminosis A in a cat. Journal of the American Veterinary Medical Association 1992; 200: 1970-1972.

CASE 6-6

Vomiting and Anorexia in a German Shepherd Mixed-Breed Dog

Patient Assessment

A five-year-old, 10.6-kg, neutered female German shepherd mix was examined after three days of vomiting, anorexia and lethargy. The owners reported the dog was allowed free access to the neighborhood, which included a radiator machine shop where cholecalciferol-based rodenticides were used. The dog appeared depressed and moderately dehydrated.

Abnormal laboratory findings included moderate hypercalcemia, mild azotemia, proteinuria and isosthenuria. These results suggested vitamin D_3 toxicosis.

Assess the Food and Feeding Method

No dietary history was available.

Treatment and Feeding Plan

Treatment consisted of intravenous 0.9% saline solution, diuretics, salmon calcitonin and corticosteroids. Hypercalcemia persisted throughout hospitalization. Further diagnostic testing did not identify a cause for persistent hypercalcemia. After seven days of hospitalization, the dog improved markedly and was discharged to the owners' care. Oral prednisone (at tapering dosages) and a veterinary therapeutic food formulated for renal patients were given at home.

Reassessment

The dog was evaluated several times during the next four weeks and appeared normal despite persistent hypercalcemia. The dog became normocalcemic five weeks after discharge from the hospital and remained normocalcemic when examined at two and three months.

Bibliography

Livezey KL, Dorman DC, Hooser SB, et al. Hypercalcemia induced by vitamin D_3 toxicosis in two dogs. Canine Practice 1991; 16: 26-32.

CASE 6-7

Subcutaneous Nodules in a Young Cat

Patient Assessment

A five-month-old female domestic shorthair cat was examined for depression, anorexia, firm nodular subcutaneous fat in the groin region and abdominal hyperesthesia of one week's duration. The cat was normally docile and tractable but began to resist being handled and petted. Body condition was normal (3/5).

Hematologic abnormalities included a neutrophilic leukocytosis and a normocytic, normochromic, nonregenerative anemia. Urinalysis and fecal examination results were normal. Biopsy specimens were obtained from the affected subcutaneous tissue. The biopsy specimens were firm, nodular and brownish-orange when examined grossly. Serosanguineous fluid oozed from the biopsy sites. Histopathologic examination revealed pyogranulomatous panniculitis, ceroid pigment and multifocal areas of fat necrosis and mineralization.

Assess the Food and Feeding Method

Since weaning, the cat had only been fed sardines, anchovies and mackerel free choice.

Treatment and Feeding Plan

A diagnosis of pansteatitis was made based on the dietary history and histopathologic lesions. Treatment included α-tocopherol (50 mg/kg body weight) once daily per os for two months and prednisolone for 15 days in a decreasing dosage schedule. A fish-free, complete and balanced moist cat food was offered. Because the cat was anorectic and unaccustomed to commercial cat food, it was initially force-fed.

Reassessment
Marked clinical improvement occurred within one week and the cat appeared clinically normal within one month.

Comments
Vitamin E protects cells against lipid peroxidation. α-tocopherol appears to localize within cell membranes to prevent or inhibit initiation of lipid peroxidation. Animals fed oily fish and fish oils containing high levels of unsaturated fat require greater amounts of vitamin E to limit fat oxidation.

Bibliography
Koutinas AF, Miller WH, Kritsepi M, et al. Pansteatitis (steatitis, "yellow fat disease") in the cat: A review article and report of four spontaneous cases. Veterinary Dermatology 1993; 3: 101-106.

CASE 6-8

Hemorrhagic Diathesis in a Group of Kittens

Patient Assessment
A group of adult intact female cats and their kittens were involved in an AAFCO feeding trial to establish nutritional adequacy for gestation, lactation and growth. Necropsy of four kittens that died during the feeding trial revealed hepatic or GI hemorrhages. Fourteen of the surviving kittens were divided into two groups. Blood samples were taken on Days 1, 3, 4 and 6. After the Day 3 blood samples were taken, seven of the kittens were injected subcutaneously with a vitamin K preparation (200 mg K_1), and the other seven were left untreated. Clotting times were determined for each sample.

The mean clotting time for kittens not receiving vitamin K treatment was 50 ± 9 seconds (values for normal kittens 22 ± 0.1 seconds). Mean clotting times for kittens receiving treatment decreased significantly from 59 ± 10 seconds for Days 1 and 3 to 22 ± 0.4 seconds for Days 4 and 6.

Assess the Food and Feeding Method
Queens and kittens were fed a commercial feline food formulated primarily from tuna, free choice. Individual food intake measurements were not available for the kittens because they were group housed for the AAFCO feeding protocol.

Feeding Plan
Further studies using purified diets did not identify the specific cause of vitamin K deficiency in kittens eating this fish-based food. These studies led to a recommendation that pet food companies include a supplemental source of vitamin K in moist fish-based foods for cats.

Bibliography
Strieker MJ, Morris JG, Feldman BF, et al. Vitamin K deficiency in cats fed commercial fish-based diets. Journal of Small Animal Practice 1996; 37: 322-326.

CASE 6-9

Weight Loss in a Group of Cats

Patient Assessment
Twenty-eight cats in a humane shelter in England developed lethargy, a mild decrease in food consumption and weight loss. Analysis of blood samples taken from three of the cats revealed a normocytic, normochromic anemia.

Three days after the onset of clinical signs, 13 of the cats rapidly lost body condition and developed an uncoordinated gait. Within eight to 12 hours, these cats developed ventriflexion of the head and had fully dilated pupils with no light reflex. Five of the cats subsequently developed seizures and died despite treatment with anticonvulsant drugs. A diagnosis of thiamin deficiency was made based on necropsy results.

Assess the Food and Feeding Method

The cats were fed a commercial moist cat food for six months. The food was not a complete and balanced product but was designed as a "complementary" food to be mixed with other complete dry foods. Two different lots of the moist food contained 0.56 and 0.04 mg thiamin/kg food. Assuming the food contained 75% water and had a metabolizable energy content of 1.25 kcal/g as fed, the food should contain at least 1.25 mg/kg food of thiamin for kittens and 0.5 mg/kg food of thiamin for adult cats.

Treatment and Feeding Plan

The other severely affected cats were treated with intravenous fluids and intramuscular injections of vitamin B complex for five days. These cats responded to therapy within 12 hours and were clinically normal five days later. No other cases have occurred since the humane shelter switched to a complete and balanced moist cat food.

Bibliography

Davidson MG. Thiamin deficiency in a colony of cats. Veterinary Record 1992; 130: 94-97.
Finke MD. Alpo Viewpoints in Veterinary Medicine 1993; 3(1).

CASE 6-10

Skin and Hair Disorders in a Group of Kittens

Patient Assessment

Twenty female kittens were involved in a feeding trial to evaluate dietary phosphorus requirements. The kittens were eight weeks old at the beginning of the trial. After eating the experimental food for 11 weeks, most kittens developed dried secretions around the eyes, mouth, nose and feet, focal dermatitis of the lips near the canine teeth, alopecia along the back, neck and tail, achromotrichia, dull fur and a brownish appearance of the skin. Growth of the kittens was not impaired. Results of hemograms and urinalyses were normal.

Assess the Food and Feeding Method

The food was a purified diet that contained dried egg whites, fish meal, beef tallow, corn oil, glucose, cooked starch, cellulose, taurine, vitamins and minerals. Food and demineralized water were provided free choice.

Feeding Plan

A tentative diagnosis of biotin deficiency was made based on the dietary history and clinical signs. The biotin content of the food was increased from 0.066 mg/kg to 3.0 mg/kg of food.

Reassessment

The kittens were markedly improved after eating the biotin-supplemented food for 10 weeks. Serum biotin concentrations of kittens fed unsupplemented food was about one-fifth of that of adult female cats fed a commercial complete and balanced dry cat food. Serum biotin concentrations responded to increased biotin intake.

Comments

Biotin deficiency induced by avidin in raw egg whites is a classic example of vitamin deficiency in experimental nutrition. Avidin is a glycoprotein that irreversibly binds biotin and renders it unavailable. Biotin deficiency was an unwanted side effect in this group of research cats due to egg whites in the formulation. The researchers ordered ovalbumin expecting to receive a purified fraction of egg protein. However, they received dried total egg whites, which contained avidin.

Bibliography

Pastoor FJH, Van Herck H, Van't Klooster ATh, et al. Biotin deficiency in cats as induced by feeding a purified diet containing egg white (expanded abstract). Journal of Nutrition 1991; 121: S73-S74.

CASE 6-11

Cachexia in a Young Giant Schnauzer

Patient Assessment

A five-month-old female giant schnauzer was admitted for lethargy, depression and cachexia (body condition score 1/5). The dog weighed 7.8 kg and was 47 cm high at the shoulder. It had gained no weight in the previous eight weeks. The dog's four normal female littermates weighed 20.5 to 22.5 kg and were 48 to 52 cm high at the shoulder.

Hematologic abnormalities included chronic nonregenerative anemia and neutropenia. Peripheral blood smears revealed marked erythrocyte anisocytosis and poikilocytosis, occasional hypersegmented neutrophils and large platelets. Analysis of bone marrow aspirates revealed decreased to normal cellularity with adequate iron stores. Serum iron and total iron binding capacity were normal. Serum biochemistry analyses were within normal limits for age-matched controls.

Intestinal maldigestion and malabsorption were ruled out based on normal GI contrast radiography, normal absorption of starch and fat and normal serum trypsin-like immunoreactivity. Normal hepatic function was documented by ammonia tolerance and BSP retention tests.

A urine sample was submitted for metabolic screening. Analysis revealed methylmalonic aciduria, which is a sign of vitamin B_{12} deficiency. Two serum samples had vitamin B_{12} concentrations of 21 and 36 pg/ml (values for normal dogs 209 to 483 pg/ml). Results of a test to measure intestinal absorption of an orally administered dose of vitamin B_{12} were suboptimal.

Assess the Food and Feeding Method

The puppy was fed a variety of homemade and commercial dog foods free choice, supplemented with an oral liquid hematinic.

Treatment and Feeding Plan

Vitamin B_{12} (1 mg) was administered intramuscularly once daily for seven days. A complete and balanced commercial dry growth dog food was offered free choice.

Reassessment

Within 12 hours of the vitamin B_{12} injection, the puppy became bright and alert and developed a voracious appetite. Two weeks after treatment, the puppy had gained 7 kg; six weeks after treatment the puppy weighed 25 kg. Reticulocytosis occurred five days after parenteral vitamin B_{12} therapy was started. Neutrophil counts increased within 10 days and all hematologic abnormalities resolved within two months. The dog remained clinically normal when given 1 mg vitamin B_{12} intramuscularly every four to five months.

Subsequent testing of this puppy's mother documented an inborn error of vitamin B_{12} metabolism leading to selective vitamin B_{12} malabsorption. Inherited selective malabsorption of vitamin B_{12} has been described in other giant schnauzer puppies and in a cat.

Bibliography

Fyfe JC, Jezyk PF, Giger U, et al. Inherited selective malabsorption of vitamin B_{12} in giant schnauzers. Journal of the American Animal Hospital Association 1989; 25: 533-539.

Vaden SL, Wood PA, Ledley FD, et al. Cobalamin deficiency associated with methylmalonic acidemia in a cat. Journal of the American Veterinary Medical Association 1992; 200: 1101-1103.

Chapter 7

Antioxidants

Steven C. Zicker
Karen J. Wedekind

"Scientists now believe that free radicals are causal factors in nearly every known disease, from heart disease to arthritis to cancer to cataracts. In fact, radicals are a major culprit in the aging process itself."
Lester Packer

INTRODUCTION

Oxidation is characterized by the loss of electrons, which results in an increase in positive or a decrease in negative charges on an atom. Usually, in biologic systems this occurs by the loss of one or two electrons by transfer to another atom, which accepts the electron(s) into its orbit, resulting in a more stable state. Conversely, reduction of an atom is the gain of electrons. A substance that donates electrons (i.e., becomes oxidized) to another substance is a reducing agent and one that accepts electrons (i.e., becomes reduced) is an oxidizing agent. Oxidizing agents are always reduced in a reaction, whereas reducing agents are always oxidized. Redox reactions occur when oxidation and reduction take place in the same chemical equation between two substances. In general, the balance of this potential energy equation is a measure of the ease with which a molecule gives up an electron compared to its willingness to accept an electron in relation to the hydrogen half-cell equation developed by Nernst.

An antioxidant is any substance, that when present in low concentrations compared with those of an oxidizable substrate, significantly delays or prevents oxidation of that substrate (i.e., it prevents oxidation) (Halliwell, 2002). Thus, antioxidants may preserve the structural integrity and function of biologic molecules in cells. However, this concept may be too simplistic because some cellular signaling pathways appear to depend on redox chemistry to manifest "normal" biologic function.

Free radicals are unstable atoms (e.g., oxygen, nitrogen) with at least one unpaired electron in the outermost shell. Oxygen free radicals (also called reactive oxygen species or ROS) will be used as the prototypical molecule for this chapter (**Figure 7-1**).

An unpaired electron creates a thermodynamically unstable situation; therefore, the molecule will either attempt to gain (reduction) or lose (oxidation) an electron to achieve thermodynamic stability. Thus, a free radical may act as either an oxidizing or reducing agent depending on its thermodynamic propensity for stability. For example, superoxide (O_2^-) is a normal byproduct of cellular respiration. Thermodynamically, superoxide attempts to lose an electron to become oxygen and eventually water by a hydrogen peroxide intermediate. Alternatively, the hydroxyl radical (OH) strongly prefers to gain an electron (i.e., oxidize other molecules) to achieve its OH^- configuration. The chemistry of free radical reactions depends not only on which free radical species is generated in vivo but also where the molecule is generated within the cell. For example, a highly reactive free radical produced in mitochondria is unlikely to diffuse into the cytoplasm. A less reactive species, however, such as hydrogen peroxide may diffuse into the cytoplasm before it engages chemically in a redox reaction.

Redox and free radical chemistry reactions may occur directly or be catalyzed by other molecules, metals or proteins acting

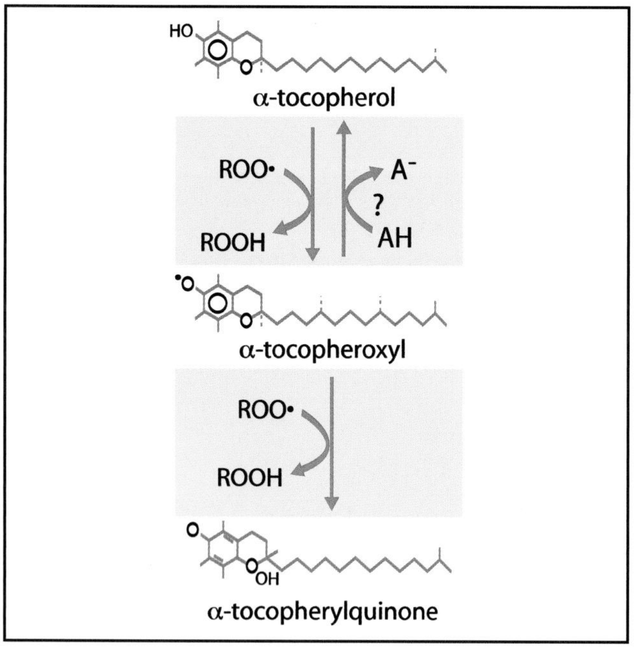

Figure 7-1. Oxidation of tocopherols by reaction with peroxyl radicals.

Reaction 1	$2O_2^{-\cdot} + 2H^+$	superoxide dismutase	$H_2O_2 + O_2$
Reaction 2	$2\ H_2O_2$	catalase	$2H_2O + O_2$
Reaction 3	$H_2O_2 + Fe^{2+}$		$OH + OH^- + Fe^{3+}$
Reaction 4	$O_2^- + Fe^{3+}$		$O_2 + Fe^{2+}$

Figure 7-2. An example of detoxifying free radicals.

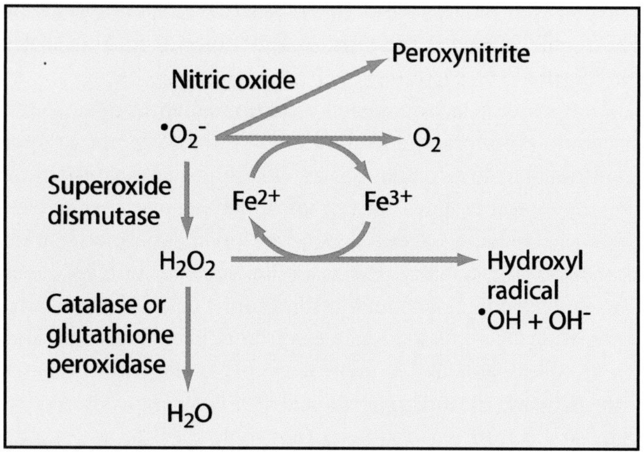

Figure 7-3. Metabolic schemes of superoxide anion.

as enzymes. Also, these systems may work in networks that depend on the proximity and species of redox coupling required. For example, mitochondria produce superoxide as a normal byproduct of cellular respiration. Normally, electrons "leak" from the electron transport chain, converting 1 to 3% of oxygen molecules into superoxide.

Cells can detoxify free radicals by several mechanisms; in the case of superoxide, cells use a two-step enzymatic method.

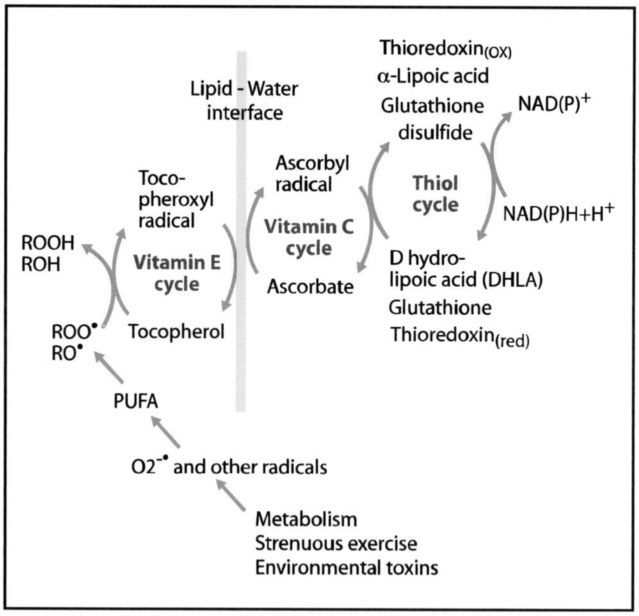

Figure 7-4. An antioxidant network to detoxify free radicals.

First, the superoxide free radical is simultaneously reduced and oxidized (dismutated) by superoxide dismutase to form hydrogen peroxide and oxygen (reaction 1) (**Figure 7-2**). Although hydrogen peroxide is a ROS, it is much less reactive than superoxide. As mentioned above, it may diffuse out of the mitochondria before reacting with another molecule. In the second step, catalase enzymes convert hydrogen peroxide into water and oxygen (reaction 2). Ironically, the hydroxyl (OH) free radical, the most mutagenic of the ROS, is generated when superoxide is converted to hydrogen peroxide. Peroxide readily reacts with ferrous iron (Fe^{2+}) or other transition metal ions (Fenton reaction) to produce hydroxyl radicals (reaction 3). Ferric iron (Fe^{3+}) can accept an electron from superoxide and cycle it back to the ferrous state where it is available to react with another peroxide molecule (reaction 4). Trace amounts of ionic iron can potentially catalyze formation of large quantities of hydroxyl free radicals.

A more dynamic metabolic picture of potential pathways emerges when these individual reactions are linked together in a biologic system (**Figure 7-3**). Thus, free radical production depends on multiple pathways and the availability of detoxification mechanisms vs. reactive materials. Overproduction of oxidative/reactive materials vs. detoxification mechanisms is called oxidative stress.

Hydroxyl radicals are highly reactive and oxidize most organic compounds at almost diffusion controlled rates (K >10/molar/sec.) (Dorfman and Adams, 1973). Due to their high reactivity, hydroxyl radicals are indiscriminate, reacting with the first substrate available. Therefore, hydroxyl radicals are highly destructive and have mutagenic potential. Mitochondrial membranes and DNA are particularly susceptible because ROS are formed in close proximity.

Redox reactions are complicated and involve multiple reactions for completion. As mentioned above, antioxidants may require several steps, cellular components or both to successfully detoxify oxidizing agents. **Figure 7-4** demonstrates the production and the stepwise detoxification of an oxidant.

NUTRITIONALLY EFFECTIVE ANTIOXIDANTS

Theoretically, adding antioxidants to a biologic system should positively affect the aging process (**Box 7-1**). However, many interventional studies designed to prove this hypothesis have produced limited or contradictory results.

Distribution and availability of antioxidants are important determinants of biologic outcome. For example, several plant flavonoids and other polyphenols have limited solubility and absorption in the gut compared to other water- or fat-soluble compounds (Carbonaro and Grant, 2005). Physiologic factors such as food intake and composition may markedly influence the effects of antioxidants considered to be easily absorbed and distributed (Hacquebard and Carpentier, 2005; Leonard et al, 2004). One study showed that vitamin E absorption was least effective from gel capsules given without a meal and variably effective when given with a meal. However, vitamin E adsorbed onto a cereal provided consistently higher rates of availability.

Metabolic transformation may alter biologic activity and distribution of orally administered antioxidants between species. Cats lack β-carotene 15,15'-dioxygenase that cleaves β-carotene (provitamin A) into two retinal molecules, whereas herbivores have relatively high activity of this enzyme (Combs, 1998). Thus, cats (and possibly other carnivores) are more likely to absorb carotenoids intact, whereas carotenoids serve relatively more of a pre-vitamin A function for herbivores.

Cats metabolize and eliminate α-lipoic acid at a much slower rate than other species (Hill et al, 2004). Age is another functional consideration. Although vitamin C is not considered essential for rats, as rats age the metabolic enzymes responsible for recycling and transporting vitamin C in hepatocytes become impaired which, if severe, may impart a conditionally essential status for vitamin C to older rats (Lykkesfeldt et al, 1998; Michels et al, 2003).

NON-CLASSIC ANTIOXIDANT MECHANISMS

Many "antioxidant" molecules have other important physiologic functions, including regulating second messengers, cell cycle signaling and controlling gene expression. These cellular redox functions are well regulated and coordinated and are probably inherent rather than random.

Resveratrol, a polyphenol from red grapes, activates sirtuin 2, a member of the sirtuin family of NAD^+ dependent de-acetylases, which mimics the effects of caloric restriction and prolongs cell life (Howitz et al, 2003). Hydrogen production mimics insulin signaling and is now recognized as a component of insulin signaling physiology (Goldstein et al, 2005). Nuclear factor kappaB (NF-κβ) signaling of apoptosis is activated by an alternative pathway via hydrogen. Furthermore, antioxidants that specifically target mitochondria alter this signaling pathway (Hughes et al, 2005; Kutuk and Basaga, 2003; Haddad, 2002). NF-κβ is not the only redox-sensitive transcription factor; several other factors have been characterized with these properties over the past several years (Azzi et al, 2004; Haddad, 2002). Antioxidant molecules are far reaching and go beyond the understanding of classic chemistry.

Box 7-1. Free Radical Theory of Aging.

Denham Harman first proposed the free radical theory of aging in 1956. His theory postulates that reactive oxygen species (ROS) damage cells with resulting age-dependent pathology. Today, it is generally accepted that mitochondria, through aerobic respiration byproducts, are the primary source of ROS in mammals. Accordingly, slowing or reversing the effects of ROS may slow aging.

The free radical theory of aging hypothesis has produced many strategies to mitigate the effects of ROS. One highly touted strategy is to suppress ROS effects with antioxidants or antioxidant defense mechanisms through nutritional supplementation. The effectiveness of this strategy depends on a wide range of different biologic factors.

The Bibliography for **Box 7-1** can be found at www.markmorris.org

MEASURING OUTCOMES OF ANTIOXIDANT STUDIES

Interpreting the vast number of studies involving antioxidant supplements is challenging. The biologic effects of antioxidants may occur by multiple divergent or convergent pathways, thus making interpretation difficult. The effects of ROS are considered insidious and temporally delayed, thus, predicting long-term outcomes from short-term experiments is another challenge to interpretation. Finally, determining the outcome event is also problematic because of the variety of endpoints that have been developed to measure the effects of antioxidants. Some outcomes discussed below highlight potential pitfalls of current methodologies.

Antioxidant Concentrations in Foods, Supplements and Tissues

Oral antioxidant administration as a supplement or in combination with food does not ensure absorption and distribution into tissues. Some antioxidants are more readily absorbed than others. Species differences may further affect absorption. Vitamin E is usually easier to absorb than water-insoluble plant phenols; however, variable absorption and distribution may occur depending on several factors. Vitamin E was more efficiently absorbed when administered with a meal (Leonard et al, 2004). Vitamin E depletion and repletion also appears to have different kinetic parameters depending on tissue type (Pillai et al, 1993, 1993a). Absorption and distribution of oral antioxidants must be relevant to the target tissue and the intended bio-

Table 7-1. Examples of biomolecules and specific markers.

Molecules	Markers
DNA	8-oxodeoxyguanosine
Lipids	Alkenals, malondialdehyde, thiobarbituric acid reaction substances
Prostaglandins	Isoprostanes
Protein	Nitrotyrosine, protein carbonyls
Advanced glycation end products	—

Table 7-2. Blood concentrations (µmol/l at seven days) of cats and dogs supplemented with β-carotene for at least seven days.

Species	Dose (mg/day)	Body weight (kg)	Peak plasma concentration
Cat	10	3 to 3.5 kg	0.95
Dog	25	7 to 9 kg	Approx. 0.02

logic outcome. Variabilities in bioavailability and distribution have not limited the number of studies attempting to link either increased ingestion or increased serum values of antioxidants to a variety of health outcomes in target tissues. If absorption and distribution fail to prove causality, what measurements are available for developing arguments about biologic efficacy?

Decreased Markers of ROS Damage

ROS are short-lived and difficult to measure as their native species. Several laboratory methods have been developed to measure biologically stable molecules as markers of ROS production in a biologic system. Presumably, if levels of these markers increase in serum or tissue, then more ROS are being produced and more damage results. If marker levels decrease, production of ROS has presumably also decreased. These markers are specific for different biomolecules (**Table 7-1**). The utility of these measurements has been debated because they indirectly measure presumed ROS reactions, sometimes in distant tissues. As such, they are responses to oxidative events, but do not provide direct mechanistic effects of antioxidant action in target tissues.

The next investigative modality is to look directly at target tissue effects of orally administered antioxidants. These studies can provide biochemical information about tissue mechanisms compared to indirect measures. Several interesting results have emerged with a variety of antioxidants. For example, aged rats, a vitamin C independent mammal, have decreased ability to recycle vitamin C in their hepatocytes, which may be restored by administration of lipoic acid and acetyl-carnitine (Lykkesfeldt et al, 1998). As mentioned above, aged rats had increased oxidative damage to hepatic proteins, which decreased enzymatic activity and increased susceptibility to protein degradation (Starke-Reed and Oliver, 1989). Finally, oxidative damage increases in the brains of aging beagles and rats; the damage was correlated with memory loss in rats (Head et al, 2002; Liu et al, 2002). Intervention with acetyl-carnitine and lipoic acid partially reversed the memory loss in older rats (Liu et al, 2002).

Biologic Outcomes of Antioxidant Interventions

Intervention studies are much more difficult to perform because of their greater expense, length of time required for intervention and the inability to control dietary intake of individuals. However, animals that have shorter lifespans are useful for developing strategies that may benefit people and other animals with longer lifespans. Models with shorter lifespans and/or accelerated aging, attributable to more rapid ROS damage, may; therefore, be more translucent to interventions and assessed more quickly for efficacy (Magwere et al, 2006). In addition, specific genetic models such as the senescent accelerated mouse, which overproduces free radicals, and transgenic models are becoming more available. These models may provide insight into efficacy and modes of action of supplemental dietary antioxidant regimens.

VETERINARY APPLICATIONS

The science of nutritional antioxidants has advanced over the past several years. Numerous studies have revealed biologic benefits to supplementing foods or dietary regimens with oral antioxidants in a variety of species. A review of mainstream antioxidants and their application to canine and feline nutrition follows.

Vitamin E

Dogs

Requirements for vitamin E in dogs and cats were suggested as early as 1939 and modified based on selenium and polyunsaturated fatty acid (PUFA) content of foods in the 1960s (Anderson et al, 1988; Harris and Embree, 1963; Hayes et al, 1969). From published research, the National Research Council (NRC) recommends that dogs receive 22 IU vitamin E per kg/food dry matter (DM) (based on a food containing 0.1 ppm selenium, not more than 1% linoleic acid and 3,670 kcal metabolizable energy/kg DM). This results in a range roughly equivalent to 0.4 to 1.4 IU/kg body weight for maintenance (lower number) up to pregnant/lactating dogs (upper number) (2006).

Effects of vitamin E on other biologic outcomes have been tested in dogs. Investigators found that levels higher than the requirement may confer targeted biologic benefits. Increasing dietary intake of vitamin E up to 2,010 mg/kg DM in geriatric beagles improved immune function (Hall et al, 2003; Meydani, 1998). Increased intake of vitamin E in food is related directly to increased vitamin E content of skin, which may provide health benefits for dermatologic disease processes (Jewell et al, 2002). Vitamin E concentrations in blood decrease with exercise, whereas higher levels have been associated with improved performance (Piercy et al, 2001; Scott et al, 2001). Finally, vitamin E protects from ischemic damage in a variety of tissues (Jorge et al, 1996; Sebbeg et al, 1994; Fujimoto et al, 1984).

There are no published toxicity data for vitamin E in dogs; however, concentrations exceeding 2,000 IU/kg DM of food have been fed for 17 weeks without observable negative reactions (Hall et al, 2003). Although an upper limit of toxicity has not been documented, a level of 1,000 IU/kg DM of food, or 45 IU/ kg of body weight, has been suggested (NRC, 2006).

Cats

Cat foods are often higher in fat and PUFAs than dog foods, which may provide a different matrix for determining requirements. Nonetheless, several studies have shown that the amount of vitamin E needed to support growth and reproduction in cats is approximately in the same general range as that for dogs, when accounting for adequate selenium and excessive PUFAs. Thus, a range of 0.5 to 1.7 mg of vitamin E/kg body weight has been suggested by NRC (2006) for maintenance and pregnancy/lactation, respectively.

Food supplemented with vitamin E at 272 and 552 IU/kg DM food improved immune function in aged cats (Hayek et al, 2000). Supplementation with 1,000 IU D-α-tocopherol enhanced neurologic recovery in a spinal cord compression model (Anderson et al, 1988). Vitamin E supplementation at 800 IU/day via gel caps did not protect better than placebo for preventing onion powder or propylene glycol induced Heinz body anemia in cats (Hill et al, 2001). Food supplemented with vitamin E and cysteine (2,200 IU vitamin E + 9.5 g cysteine/kg food DM) protected against acetaminophen-induced oxidative production of methemoglobinemia (Hill et al, 2005). Also, pretreatment of cats with vitamin E and selenium (200 IU vitamin E + 50 µg selenium) for five days delayed motor nerve degeneration in a model of axonal degeneration (Hall, 1987). A presumed safe upper level for oral administration has not been established; however, administration of vitamin E parenterally at 100 mg/kg body weight to kittens resulted in significant mortality (Phelps, 1981).

Vitamin C

Dog and Cats

Dogs and cats are capable of synthesizing required amounts of vitamin C by de novo mechanisms (Innes, 1931; Naismith, 1958). One group of investigators showed that hepatic in vitro synthesis of vitamin C in dogs and cats was much less (i.e., 10 to 25%) than in other mammals leading to speculation that ability to synthesize vitamin C may be limited in these species; however, no followup work has been performed (Chatterjee et al, 1975). In dogs, both ascorbic acid and ester-C are rapidly absorbed, possibly by use of an active transport mechanism in the gastrointestinal tract (Wang et al, 2001).

The subchronic intravenous toxicity (i.e., LD_{50}) dose for vitamin C has been reported to be greater than 500 mg/kg/day and 2,000 mg/kg/day for cats and dogs, respectively (Körner and Weber, 1972). Supplementation of vitamin C (0, 200, 400 or 1,000 mg/day) to cats resulted in a small progressive reduction in urinary pH (Kienzle and Maiwald, 1998). In people, intake of ascorbate at the upper recommended limit of 2,000 mg/day increased urine oxalate excretion and risk of kidney stone formation (Massey et al, 2005). However, moderate supplementation of vitamin C in healthy cats (i.e., up to 193 mg/kg DM food, approximately 2 mg/kg body weight), did not appear to increase the risk of oxalate stone formation (Yu and Gross, 2005). Supplementing rats with vitamin C at 1,500 mg/kg DM food may decrease erythrocyte fragility when vitamin E is near the requirement level in food (Chen, 1981). Additionally, oral vitamin C supplementation at 1 g/day may slow racing times in greyhounds (Chapter 18) (Marshall et al, 2002).

β-Carotene and Other Carotenoids

The carotenoids, predominately β-carotene, have been subjected to preliminary studies in canine and feline nutrition. β-carotene can serve as a precursor to vitamin A in dogs, but not cats. Although carotenoids possess antioxidant properties, most of the research in dogs and cats has focused on immunomodulatory benefits.

β-carotene supplementation increases concentrations of β-carotene in canine and feline plasma and white blood cells (Chew et al, 2000, 2000a). However, the concentrations reached in feline plasma are approximately 50-fold higher than those in canine plasma at the same approximate time and dose rate, indicating that most of the β-carotene administered to dogs is probably converted to vitamin A rather than absorbed directly as b-carotene. People convert approximately 60 to 75% of β-carotene into vitamin A and absorb approximately 15% intact. From this, the mean concentration of serum β-carotene in people is approximately 0.3 µmol/l, which is approximately 10-fold greater than concentrations found in dogs receiving supplements. Nevertheless, supplementation with β-carotene reportedly improves immune function in young and aged dogs (Kearns et al, 2000; Chew et al, 2000b).

Supplementation with the carotenoid lutein increases plasma and leukocyte concentrations in dogs and cats. Food supplemented with lutein improves immune function in both species (Kim et al, 2000, 2000a). A novel form of astaxanthin provides cardioprotection from vascular occlusion in dogs (Gross and Lockwood, 2005).

β-carotene has been evaluated in beagles at very high doses (i.e., 50 to 250 mg/kg/day as an oral dose in beadlets) (Heywood et al, 1985). Although coat discoloration and liver vacuolization were noted at all dose levels, no consistent findings of toxicity were found. Carotenoid safety is not well evaluated in cats; however, it may be presumed to be very safe based on wide margins of safety in other mammals and lack of conversion to vitamin A in this species. Canthaxanthine supplementation in cats for six months induced retinal pigment epithelial changes that included some vacuolization but no functional electroretinogram changes (Scallon et al, 1988).

Selenium

Selenium was first recognized as an essential nutrient in 1957 based on its ability to spare vitamin E in exudative diathesis in chicks (Schwarz et al, 1957). The metabolic basis for selenium's nutritional function remained unclear until it was discovered in

1973 (Rotruck et al, 1973) that selenium was a component of glutathione peroxidase. Subsequently, investigators discovered several selenium-dependent glutathione peroxidase isoforms (phospholipid, cytosolic, plasma and gastrointestinal). In addition, other selenoproteins were discovered including (three iodothyronine 5'-deiodinases [types I, II and III]); two thioredoxin reductases and four other selenoproteins (in plasma [P], muscle [W], liver and prostate) (Combs, 2001).

Glutathione peroxidase primarily defends against oxidative stress by catalyzing the reduction of hydrogen peroxide and organic hydroperoxides, which react with the selenol group of the active center of selenocysteine. As a constituent of 5'-deiodinases, types I to III, selenium combats oxidative stress by deactivating large amounts of hydrogen peroxide produced by the thyroid gland, which is used for iodination of thyronine residues. The activity of phospholipid and cytosolic glutathione peroxidase protects the thyroid gland from oxidative damage.

Glutathione peroxidase and thioredoxin reductase activities are involved in a variety of key enzymes, transcription factors and receptors. Thioredoxin reductase's involvement in the modulation of redox-regulated signaling including ribonucleotide reductase, prostaglandin and leukotriene synthesis, receptor-mediated phosphorylation cascades (i.e., activation of NF-κβ) and in apoptosis is of great interest (McKenzie et al, 1998; Neve, 2002).

The selenium requirement of most animals is similar and based on maximization of glutathione peroxidase in plasma and red blood cells. The estimated selenium requirement for kittens and adult cats is 0.15 and 0.13 mg selenium/kg food, respectively (Wedekind et al, 2003, 2003a) and 0.10 mg selenium/kg food for adult dogs (Wedekind et al, 2002). Recommended allowances of selenium in pet foods, which account for bioavailability, for dogs and cats are 0.35 and 0.30 mg selenium/kg food, respectively (NRC, 2006).

Animal studies and clinical intervention trials involving people have shown selenium to be anticarcinogenic at intakes 5- to 10-fold greater than recommended daily allowances or minimum requirements (Combs, 2001; Neve, 2002). Several mechanisms have been proposed to account for selenium's anticancer effects: 1) antioxidant activity through glutathione peroxidase and thioredoxin reductase, 2) enhanced immune function, 3) altered carcinogen metabolism, 4) inhibited tumor proliferation and enhanced apoptosis and 5) inhibited angiogenesis (Neve, 2002). Studies indicate antioxidant protective ranges for selenium would be approximately 0.50 to 1.3 mg selenium/kg food DM for dogs and cats. Interestingly, the complementary nature of antioxidants such as vitamins C and E and selenium suggests that one "spares" the need for the others in protecting against lipid peroxidation. In the case of all of these antioxidants, effective levels necessary to reduce disease risk are much higher than levels needed to merely prevent nutritional deficiency.

Safe upper limits for selenium for most species are similar (Koller and Exon, 1986), approximately 2 mg selenium/kg food, although neither the Association of American Feed Control Officials (AAFCO, 2007) nor NRC (2006) suggests a safe upper limit for cats (Wedekind et al, 2003). Cats have approximately fivefold higher serum selenium concentrations compared to other species (Foster et al, 2001). This is probably attributed to the fact that selenium intakes are higher for cats than for most other species. For example, fish and other seafood, which are highly concentrated sources of selenium, are fed much more widely to cats than dogs. However, studies show that even when dogs and cats are fed foods containing the same selenium concentration, serum selenium concentrations are 40 to 60% higher in cats. Cats have significantly higher selenium concentrations in blood even when fed similar dietary selenium intakes compared to most other species including dogs. It is unclear whether cats have a higher tolerance for selenium; however, the literature suggests that diets containing similar sources and levels of selenium were more toxic for swine (Kim and Mahan, 2001) than for cats (Wedekind et al, 2003). AAFCO (2007) suggests a safe upper limit of 2 mg selenium/kg diet for dogs (Wedekind et al, 2002).

Thiols: S-Adenosyl-L-Methionine, α-Lipoic Acid, N-Acetylcysteine

Thiol metabolism has gained research momentum as redox chemistry has matured. Thiols are capable of redox reactions similar to those of oxygen and have many metabolic correlates within cells. Glutathione, S-adenosyl-L-methionine (SAMe), thioredoxin and other sulfur-containing molecules have important roles in metabolism and antioxidant defenses.

SAMe has been used to successfully treat acetaminophen toxicity in cats and dogs (Wallace et al, 2002; Webb et al, 2003). Administration of SAMe to clinically healthy cats improved indices of redox status as indicated by decreased RBC thiobarbituric acid reaction substances and increased hepatic glutathione (Center et al, 2005).

α-Lipoic acid is another thiol that may influence reduced glutathione content of cells. As a food additive, α-lipoic acid resulted in increased ratios of reduced white blood cells to oxidized forms (GSH:GSSG) in dogs (Zicker et al, 2002). Administration to cats prolongs elimination of α-lipoic acid compared to that of other species; therefore, administration rates should be adjusted accordingly (Hill et al, 2004).

N-acetylcysteine increases reduced glutathione in cats challenged orally by onion powder compared to values in controls (Hill et al, 2001). N-acetylcysteine combined with ascorbic acid inhibits virus replication in cell lines infected with feline immunodeficiency virus (Mortola et al, 1998). Cysteine in combination with vitamin E also protects cats from acetaminophen-induced oxidative damage (Hill et al, 2005).

Fruits and Vegetables

Fruits and vegetables are often rich in flavonoid, polyphenol and anthocyanidin ingredients that may possess antioxidant properties. Exhaustive research of the effects of these ingredients in dogs and cats is unavailable; however, a few studies have tried to evaluate some potential benefits of adding fruits and vegetables to dietary regimens. Oral administration of a bioflavonoid complex reduced the extent of Heinz body anemia caused by acetaminophen administration to cats (Allison et al,

2000). A combination of fruits and vegetables in a supplemented food increased selected flavonoids in the blood of aged dogs (Zicker, 2005). Although effective doses and safety of fruits and vegetables are not well evaluated, administration of onion powder to cats can result in Heinz body anemia, perhaps through increased oxidation, although it has purported antioxidant benefits in some species (Robertson et al, 1998).

Combination Therapies

Because many antioxidants work in networks, several studies looked at complex mixtures of these compounds. Physiologic outcomes are variable, but generally, effects on immune function have been positive (Devlin et al, 2001) and markers of antioxidant status or damage from oxidative stress have been reduced (Baskin et al, 2000; Jewell et al, 2000; Piercy et al, 2000; Wedekind et al, 2002a; Yu and Paetau-Robinson, 2006). Long-term supplementation with a complex mixture of antioxidants slowed cognitive decline in aged dogs and resulted in improved behavioral correlates in an in-home study (Roudebush et al, 2005). The contribution to the final results of each individual compound is unknown in any of these studies; thus, this remains an area of future research.

REFERENCES

The references for **Chapter 7** can be found at www.markmorris.org.

Section 2

Pet Foods

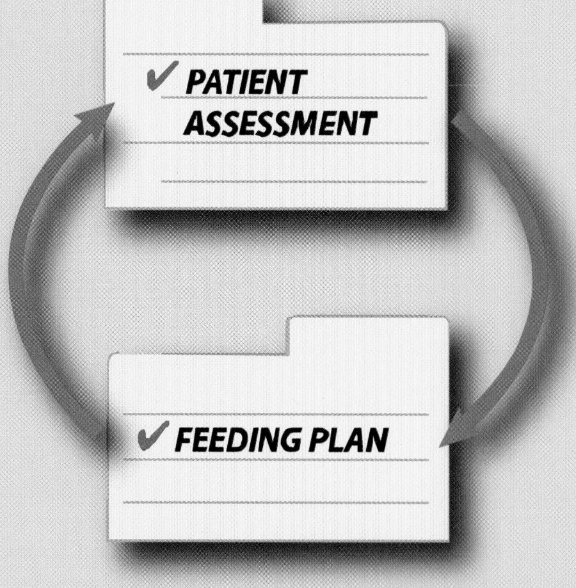

Chapter 8

Commercial Pet Foods

Stephen W. Crane
Christopher S. Cowell
Neil P. Stout
Edward A. Moser
Jerry Millican
Peter Romano, Jr.
Steven E. Crane

"The greatest obstacle to discovery is not ignorance-it is the illusion of knowledge."
Daniel J. Boorstin

INTRODUCTION

According to a 2005 report, there are 63.0 million dogs and 81.4 million cats in the United States (Euromonitor, 2006; United States Census Data, 2006). In 2005, 34.8% of households had at least one dog (Euromonitor, 2006), a small decline from 37.6% of households that had at least one dog in 1996 (Maxwell, 1996). In 2005, 33.9% of all households had at least one cat (Euromonitor, 2006), which reflects a small increase from 1996 when 32.9% had at least one cat (Maxwell, 1996).

Most pet owners in the United States feed commercially prepared pet foods daily (**Box 8-1**). In 2005, pet food sales in the United States reportedly increased from $9.3 billion in 1995 to $14.4 billion, up nearly 35% over a decade. In 1986, pet food sales in the United States were $5.1 billion (Enterline, 1986); thus, pet food sales have increased phenomenally in the United States during each of the past two decades.

European and Asian countries have followed this trend towards commercially prepared pet foods. North America is the largest market followed by Western Europe and Asia. In 2005, 62.3% of the total caloric needs of pets in the United Kingdom were met by commercial pet foods (Euromonitor, 2006). Pet food sales totaled $13.2 billion in Western Europe, $1.5 billion in Central and Eastern Europe and $2.8 billion in Japan during 2005 (Euromonitor, 2006).

Fulfilling the nutrient requirements of pet animals with commercially prepared pet foods has proved successful and economical for many years. Prepared pet foods account for 92.8% of calories consumed by cats and 78.1% of calories consumed by dogs in North America (Euromonitor, 2006). In Japan, 70.3% of caloric needs of cats and dogs combined and 58.8% of total caloric needs in Western Europe are being met by commercial foods (Euromonitor, 2006). In other parts of Europe, Latin America and the Pacific Rim, commercially prepared pet foods account for 35 to 50% of the calories consumed by dogs and cats (Corbin, 1995). In 2005, Central and Eastern Europe lagged behind with just over 9% of pets' caloric needs being met by commercially prepared pet foods (Euromonitor, 2006).

The popularity of commercial pet foods and their potential impact on pet wellness make understanding their features, benefits and applications highly relevant to companion animal veterinarians and their health care teams. In addition, foods formulated specifically for disease prevention and treatment are important adjuncts to medicine and surgery in daily veterinary practice.

Clients recognize veterinary practitioners and technicians as authorities on nutrition. Veterinarians have a strong influence on the foods clients choose to feed their pets. A 1995 study conducted by the American Animal Hospital Association found that 54% of pet owners interviewed sought veterinary advice about pet foods at least once, and 43% had received a recommendation from their veterinarian about which manufacturer's pet food to feed their puppies or kittens (AAHA,

Box 8-1. History of Pet Food Manufacturing in the United States.

Domestication of cats and dogs was probably influenced by the enticement of food. Formation of a mutually beneficial association between Egyptians who cultivated and stored grains and wild cats that found abundant rodent species in Egyptian homes and food storage areas likely affected feline domestication. In any case, feeding domestic cats and dogs with table scraps and supplemental scavenging was the method of feeding until the mid 1800s.

James Spratt, an American living in the United Kingdom, who was unimpressed with shipboard biscuits given to his dog on the passage across the Atlantic Ocean, created the first commercially available pet food in 1860. Spratt developed a dry "dog cake" or kibble that he sold to English huntsmen. Spratt's United States company continued to manufacture pet food until General Mills purchased it in the late 1950s. The next influential figure in the pet food industry was an Englishman named F. H. Bennett. In 1907, Bennett's company was formed in New York City and introduced Milk-Bone dog biscuits, which were marketed as a complete dog food.

Spratt and Bennett were the two primary manufacturers of commercial pet food until the early 1920s when the Chappel brothers of Rockford, IL, began canning horsemeat for dogs under the Ken-L-Ration brand name. By the mid 1920s, Clarence Gaines of Gaines Food Co., Sherburne, NY, began selling dog meal in 100-lb bags thus creating "Gaines Dog Meal."

In the 1930s, new dog food brands including Cadet and Snappy helped make canned pet food more popular than dry foods. In 1941, canned pet food represented 91% of the market. World War II changed that picture drastically as pet foods were classified as "nonessential" and the tin used to manufacture the cans was of great value to the war effort. By 1946, dry foods represented 85% of the market.

In Raritan, NJ, Dr. Mark Morris, Sr., began manufacturing small batches of specialized foods for dogs with kidney disease in his small animal hospital. In 1948, Dr. Morris signed a manufacturing agreement with Burton Hill of Hill's Packing Co., Topeka, KS, to manufacture Raritan Ration B, later known as Prescription Diet Canine k/d for sale in veterinary hospitals, thus creating a new category of pet foods designed to aid in the dietary management of disease.

The modern era of dry pet food manufacturing began in 1957 and continued through the 1960s when the Ralston Purina Company, St. Louis, MO, introduced the first extruded dog and cat foods called Dog Chow and Cat Chow. Moist cat foods, predominantly canned fish varieties in single-serving 6-oz. cans, were the top sellers of the day. During this time frame, General Foods created Gaines Burger, a new food that incorporated the convenience of dry food with the palatability of canned foods. It was the first semi-moist dog product. Tender Vittles, the first semi-moist cat food, was created by Ralston Purina in the early 1970s.

Originally produced as a consistent high-quality food for research kennels, Science Diet, manufactured by Hill's Pet Nutrition, Inc., Topeka, KS, became the first specialty product line designed for different lifestages and health maintenance in 1968.

Commercial pet food sales continued to grow from the 1970s to the present with many new product introductions every year including moist, semi-moist, soft-dry and dry pet foods, treats, beverages and edible toys.

1995). Seventy percent of the latter group fed the brand of food recommended by their veterinarian (AAHA, 1995). Clients frequently seek more detailed information than "feed any good commercial food" and also inquire about the relevance of new human nutritional information to their pets.

Notably, there exists a significant discrepancy in the perception of pet owners who desired a food recommendation from their veterinarian and the number of clients who believed they had received a recommendation from their veterinarian. About 90% of clients desire a food recommendation from their veterinarian and yet only 18 to 22% recall receiving veterinary advice in this critical area of pet health.[a]

This chapter provides general information about commercial pet food forms, pet food marketing concepts, pet food segments and manufacturing processes used to prepare commercial pet foods. It also includes common ingredients used in commercial pet foods, including their selection and nutritional and palatability contributions, quality manufacturing and ways of measuring features and benefits of pet foods. The content is necessarily general as there are more than 1,200 pet food manufacturers around the world (Mintel GNPD, 2006) and approximately 175 manufacturers in the United States alone (Research and Markets, Inc., 2006). Methods for assessing specific pet foods are described in Chapter 1.

PET FOOD FORMS

Commercial pet foods are available in three basic forms: dry, semi-moist and moist. As suggested by the category names, water content differs markedly among the three forms. Other differences include the typical nutrient profile and the advantages and disadvantages of each form. Pet food quality is independent of form; high-quality foods can be found in all three categories. Consumer preferences also vary. North Americans favor dry foods whereas Europeans feed a higher percentage of moist (usually canned) foods. The global trend is toward use of dry pet foods, especially for dogs.

Moist Foods

The moisture content of moist foods varies from 60 to more than 87%. The dry matter (DM) portion of the food contains all the nonwater nutrients: protein, fat, carbohydrate, vitamins and minerals (**Figure 8-1**). Small differences in moisture content greatly affect a moist food's DM content. For example, if the moisture content of Food A is 78% and Food B is 82%, the DM percentage differs significantly.

DM in Food A = (100 – 78) = 22%
DM in Food B = (100 – 82) = 18%

The % DM difference = (22 – 18) ÷ 18 = 4 ÷ 18 x 100 = 22% more nutrients in Food A than in Food B. Gums and gelling agents are often used to solidify the food and imbibe water in high-moisture foods to preclude "free" water in the container. Many moist pet foods contain high levels of meat and meat by-products. Higher levels of protein, phosphorus, sodium and fat than semi-moist or dry forms also characterize these foods. Some moist foods are promoted as "meaty" or having "meaty pieces" to fulfill the needs of "naturally carnivorous" pets. However, "meaty" is used as an adjective ("meat-like") and many meaty pieces are actually extruded soy or wheat flour (textured vegetable protein), starches, gum and meat meal combinations.

The high palatability of moist foods is a primary reason for the popularity of this form. The high preference that animals express for moist foods requires portion-controlled feeding to prevent over consumption.

Moist foods in North America are usually sold as "complete" with all nutrients present. A few moist foods are not complete and are usually intended as either treats or palatability enhancement modules for dry foods. In the United States, moist foods are rarely fed as the sole food source (<10%). Rather, moist foods are used to supplement the dry main meal as the pet owners' way to treat or pamper their pet. This behavior has fueled the growth of the "gourmet" moist food category, which is defined by its taste appeal and aesthetic attributes. The segment has seen a proliferation of flavor offerings as well as an increasing number of textures (pâté, ground, flaked, chunks, minced, stews, slices, etc.), and nontraditional packaging such as single serving, plasticized foil pouches for moist foods and other forms of single serving containers designed for consumer ease of use.

In some international markets, moist foods serve as primary protein and fat modules in complementary feeding systems. In complementary feeding systems, pet owners mix the protein-fat source of the moist module with a "mixer," which is a high-carbohydrate dry food. When mixing the complementary components, pet owners have the latitude to modify the recommended quantity of moist and dry feeding components. Whether mixing occurs for treatment purposes or as part of a complementary feeding system, the variation in nutrient intake may complicate obtaining an accurate dietary history.

Moist foods have a low caloric density as fed and typically yield 0.7 to 1.4 kcal (2.93 to 5.86 kJ) metabolizable energy (ME)/g food. The lower caloric density and higher packaging and shipping costs translate to a higher cost per calorie. Correspondingly, moist foods have the highest daily feeding cost.

Moist foods are preserved with heat sterilization and vacuum preservation in an anaerobic environment. An enamel liner insulates moist pet foods from their container. Nutrient stability is excellent. A shelf life of at least 18 months is anticipated, provided the mechanical integrity of the seams and lid seals is maintained. All moist foods are seriously damaged by even a single freeze-thaw cycle. Thus, care must be taken to store cans at nonfreezing temperatures.

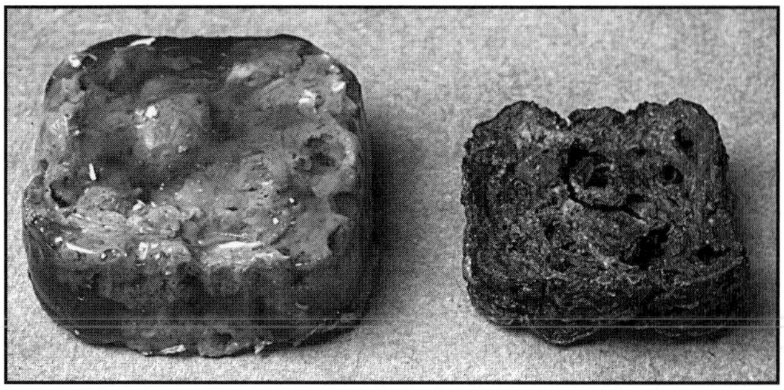

Figure 8-1. This cat food has a guaranteed analysis of 83% moisture. The food is shown after it has been removed from the package (left). Another specimen of the same food (right) was dried to constant weight in an oven. The dry matter portion of the food contains all the nonwater nutrients: protein, fat, carbohydrate, vitamins and minerals. Gums and other hydrocolloids are added to high-moisture pet foods to imbibe water, which helps maintain the product's shape. The low percentage of dry matter in this pet food means that feeding costs are high (**Box 8-4**).

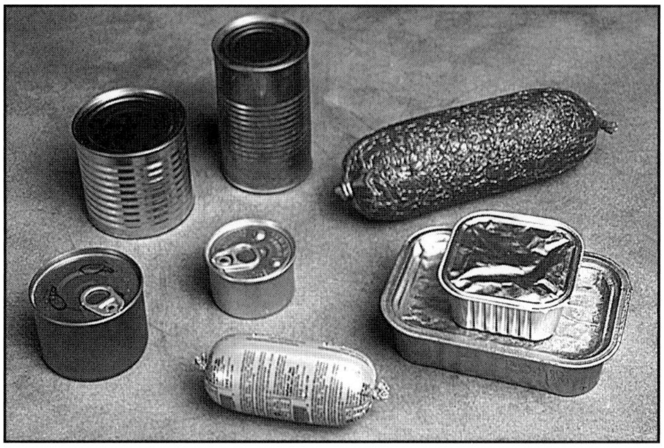

Figure 8-2. Moist pet foods are available in a variety of packages, including multiple sizes of traditional steel cans, aluminum and plastic trays, chubs and compressed tubes.

Moist foods are packaged in a variety of containers including paper trays, plastic pots and stuffed plastic tubes ("chubs"), in addition to the more popular steel cans and aluminum trays (**Figures 8-2** and **8-3**). The food in chubs often is incomplete, is unbalanced, contains excess mineral levels and does not have an extended shelf life (i.e., must be used within 48 hours after opening the package). Chub contents are often added to dry food or high-carbohydrate mixers, or are used as protein and fat modules in making homemade foods. In early 2006, in Australia where the chub form of food is commonly used, manufacturers of this form of pet food encountered problems with excessive levels of sulfur dioxide preservatives, which contributed to thiamin deficiencies in a number of dogs (Central Western Daily, 5/30/06).

Dry Foods

Dry pet foods contain 3 to 11% water. The high DM content of these foods allows the expression of different formulation concepts. Dry food has been produced with a caloric density of 2.7 to more than 7.1 kcal (11.3 to 29.7 kJ) ME/g food.

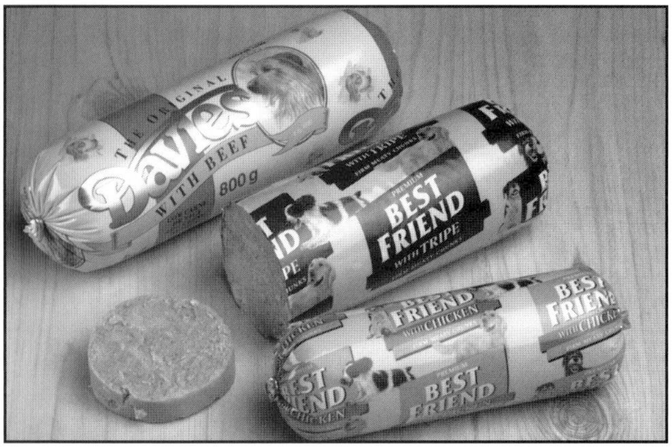

Figure 8-3. Chubs are plastic tubes used to package high-protein, high-fat moist foods. A chub's contents are usually mixed with dry pet food or high-carbohydrate modules.

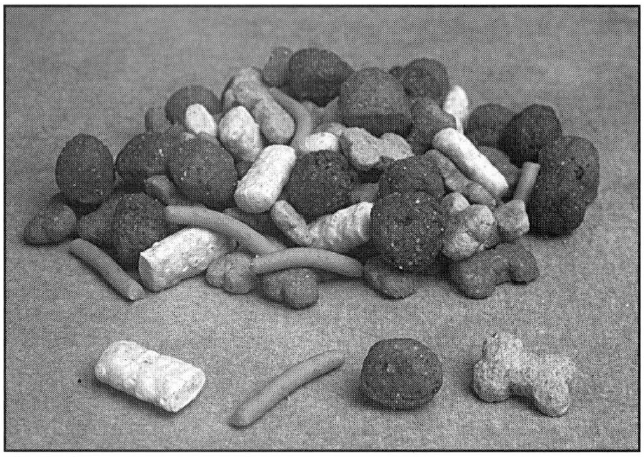

Figure 8-4. Semi-moist kibbles are frequently blended with dry kibbles to make soft-dry combinations. The soft-dry pet food shown here contains two different dry foods and two different semi-moist foods. The semi-moist food improves palatability and provides anthropomorphic appeal by simulating pieces of meat and cheese.

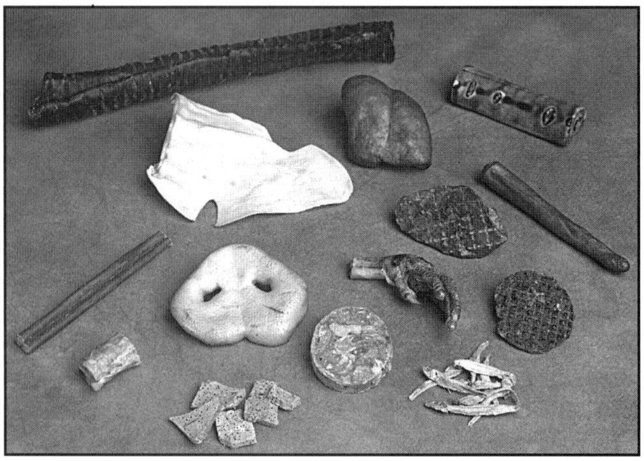

Figure 8-5. Dried animal tissues are popular pet treats. Examples shown here include bovine penis, porcine penis, porcine tail, ovine lung, beef kidney, porcine ear, bovine liver, porcine nose, bovine trachea, turkey feet, bovine chin tissue and whole fish.

Packaging and freight costs of dry pet foods are lower than those of moist products. Bags are cheaper than cans and it costs more to ship the additional water (60 to 87% water in moist foods). Thus, dry foods cost about one-third as much as moist foods on a cost-per-calorie basis. Dry food particles are usually formed through extrusion; however, baking, flaking, pelleting, crumbling and dry meals are other possible manufacturing methods.

Dry foods are usually acceptable to most pets, but generally have reduced average preference when compared with moist or semi-moist foods.

Dry foods are often perceived as providing dental benefits. However, the perception that dry foods are superior for dental health is a generalization. An epidemiologic study of progressive periodontitis in poodles found no correlation between food form and disease progression (Hoffman and Gaengler, 1996). Chapter 47 provides more details about the relationship between food and oral health.

Semi-Moist and Soft-Dry Foods

Semi-moist pet foods have an intermediate water content (25 to 35%), falling in between that of moist and dry pet foods. Semi-moist foods use humectants and acidification with simple organic acids to control water activity and inhibit mold growth. Semi-moist foods often contain meat meals and artificial flavors and provide a sweet, savory flavor to dogs and an acidic note for cats. This pet food form is highly palatable and has an average intermediate preference between moist and dry pet foods.

Semi-moist foods are often packed in pouches or wrappers. Although patients requiring weight control and management of diabetes mellitus benefit from a consistent food dose, the higher sugar content and lower fiber content of semi-moist foods make them ill-suited for these feeding applications. Once very popular, semi-moist pet foods experienced a greatly reduced market acceptance in the 1990s. However, this form continues to be important as the high-flavor "bits" component of some popular soft-dry pet food treats. In the soft-dry form, the semi-moist component may look like burger pieces, cheese, pasta or vegetables and provide anthropomorphic appeal to pet owners because of the appearance of ingredient variety (**Figure 8-4**).

Treats

Treats are small food rewards that owners use for reinforcement of their bonding with pets, as training aids and just for fun. Dog owners in the United States spent more than $1.7 billion on treats for their dogs, and nearly $234 million on treats for their cats in 2005 (Euromonitor, 2006). A survey of 1,000 United States households revealed that 80% of dog owners fed human foods or table scraps as treats and almost nine of 10 respondents had fed commercially prepared treats or snacks (BH&G, 1991). A second survey concluded that about 60% of dogs received treats in some form and 30% were also given meat or meat juice (Slater et al, 1995). Market research indicates that more than 90% of dog owners who purchase specialty dog food brands give their dogs treats.[a] Sixty-five percent purchase biscuits, 45% buy "bones" and 40% buy chews. About half of these dog owners give their dogs treats every day; on average, these respondents provide treats for their dogs five to six times per week. The pet typically receives two treats per treating occasion. Providing pets with treats continues to increase significantly; 88% of dog owners, 65% of cat owners and 73% of bird owners provide their pets with treats (PetPlace.com, 2006).

Pet owners and those taking and interpreting a dietary history can easily ignore the variable contribution of treats to the daily nutrient intake. As a generalization, dietary balance is maintained when less than 10% of the daily intake consists of table scraps or treats and the remainder is a prepared food that is complete and balanced. At low levels, treats can be considered nutritionally trivial except in certain medical conditions. Excessive feeding of treats interferes with normal appetite and dietary balance and can contribute to obesity. Inappropriate use of treats might include when: 1) the quantity consumed exceeds the manufacturer's recommendation, 2) the pet has a high intake of cream, meat, organ tissues and processed human foods and 3) up to 20% of the daily energy requirement is provided by treats used for dental benefits.

An increasingly popular treat form is dried animal tissues (e.g., bovine penis, tail, tendon or hoof and pig's ears) (**Figure 8-5**). Dried animal tissue treats are more than 85% protein, which often are characterized by a high-collagen content of low biologic value.

Treats can be part of the dietary management of obesity, diabetes mellitus, urolithiasis, cardiac failure, renal failure and adverse reactions to foods when used under medical supervision and when the nutrient profile of the treats is compatible with the appropriate veterinary therapeutic food.

Supplements

Supplements are different from treats, although the terms are sometimes used interchangeably. Treats are nutritionally trivial, but supplements are very concentrated nutrient modules. The proper role of a supplement is to correct a diagnosed nutrient deficiency. Unfortunately, many supplements are overused and present some risk for abuse and toxicosis.

The most common form of veterinary supplements is a wide variety of vitamin and vitamin-mineral combinations that are used by 10% of animal owners (Slater et al, 1995). Mineral and electrolyte supplements include calcium, phosphorus, sodium, potassium, magnesium, iron and zinc. Protein and amino acid supplements (including taurine) are also common but should only complement the base food in situations of repletion feeding.

Routine use of vitamin-mineral supplements is not needed when a dog or cat eats typical commercial pet food. One study evaluated the daily calcium and phosphorus intake of adult dogs and cats consuming an average dry commercial pet food compared with the daily-recommended allowances for these animals (**Table 8-1**) (Kallfelz and Dzanis, 1989). In dogs, average calcium and phosphorus intakes were almost three times the daily allowance, whereas in cats, intakes were 65 to 75% above the allowance. This finding suggests that supplementation of normal commercial foods with calcium and phosphorus is unnecessary. The study also found that dogs and cats consuming commercial dry rations were ingesting from two to five times the daily allowance of vitamins (**Table 8-1**). Thus, the need for routine supplemental vitamins is questionable at best when dogs and cats eat a typical commercial pet food. For pregnancy, lactation and growth, all-purpose or specific-purpose growth pet foods contain adequate nutrient levels; supplementation for these physiologic conditions is unnecessary.

Table 8-1. Daily intake of calcium, phosphorus, vitamin A and vitamin D by an adult dog or cat consuming a typical commercial dry pet food.*

Dog	MDR**	
Average intake		
Calcium (mg/kg/day)	25	74
Phosphorus (mg/kg/day)	19	54
Vitamin A (IU/kg/day)	23	67
Vitamin D (IU/kg/day)	2.3	11
Cat		
Calcium (mg/kg/day)	41	70
Phosphorus (mg/kg/day)	36	67
Vitamin A (IU/kg/day)	46	121
Vitamin D (IU/kg/day)	4.5	9.1

Key: MDR = minimum daily requirements.
*Adapted from Kallfelz FA, Dzanis DA. Overnutrition: An epidemic problem in pet animal practice? Veterinary Clinics of North America: Small Animal Practice 1989; 19: 433-446.
**From Nutrient Requirements of Dogs and Nutrient Requirements of Cats. National Academy of Sciences, Washington, DC: National Academy Press, 1985, 1986.

Fat supplements provide a concentrated source of calories and essential fatty acids. Corn, safflower, canola and sunflower oils mix easily with food and provide a cost-effective source of additional linoleic acid. Commercially available fatty acid supplements emphasize linoleic acid, gamma-linolenic acid and mixtures of various omega-3 fatty acids (eicosapentaenoic and docosahexaenoic acid). The usual objective for fat or fatty acid supplementation is to increase caloric intake or to improve a pet's coat. However, specific fatty acids are beneficial in certain disease conditions and are used in foods designed for those diseases.

Various herbs and yeasts have been advocated for flea control but these products have no demonstrated efficacy (Baker and Farver, 1983). Human health foods are also used to supplement pet foods. These items include sea salt, kelp, algae, lecithin, chelated minerals, enzymes and probiotic digestants of enteric microorganisms (Chapter 5). These items are sometimes used in homemade foods or provided by owners who take these supplements themselves.

The correct use of supplements is based on a diagnosis of a nutrient deficiency. Unfortunately, supplements are commonly used as "insurance" against suspected deficient intake. They may also be used when super-supplementation of a particular nutrient is perceived as a need. In the first case, a more effective, less costly and safer approach is to simply exchange the suspect food and its corrective supplement for a food that is nutritionally adequate. The super-supplementation approach creates risk for toxicosis or dietary imbalance and can violate the treatment principle of "Above All, Do No Harm."

PET FOOD MARKETING CONCEPTS

Marketing concepts identify how a product will be advertised and sold. Understanding basic marketing concepts helps veterinarians and their health care teams evaluate advertising and answer questions from pet owners who are influenced by the advertising. Most clients know little about their pet's nutritional needs and are susceptible to advertising claims (**Box 8-2**). Basic marketing concepts for pet food include: 1) specific-purpose foods, 2) all-purpose foods, 3) low price, 4) "people food," 5) flavors and varieties, 6) presence of an ingredient, 7) absence of an ingredient, 8) "more is better," 9) product name, 10) natural or "holistic" foods and 11) "organic" foods. There may be modifications, combinations and crossovers among these basic categories. Additionally, more than one concept may be used by the same company for different brands so that if one feature does not appeal to a pet owner, perhaps another will.

Specific-Purpose Foods

The objective of the specific-purpose concept is to provide a specialized nutrient profile for a particular feeding application. When owners select a specific-purpose product it is often because they have been educated to understand the points of difference between all-purpose and specific-purpose products.

Many specific-purpose foods are sold from value-added environments such as veterinary hospitals, where client-education opportunities often occur. Some grocery store brands also offer specific-purpose products and rely on advertising and packaging to communicate their purpose. Although a product is named or marketed as fulfilling a specific application, it may or may not actually deliver the expected benefit.

Specific-purpose foods can be divided into lifestage and special needs groups. Lifestage products are formulated to provide appropriate nutrition based on pet age or "lifestage." The primary lifestage types are: 1) growth or puppy/kitten foods, (many of which are also formulated to support gestation and lactation), 2) adult or maintenance foods and 3) senior/geriatric foods.

Special products provide specialized nutrition for individual pet needs. For example, rapidly growing puppies of the large and giant breeds have increased risk for developmental orthopedic disorders (Chapter 33). Therefore, these puppies may benefit from a growth-type food specially modified to control nutritional risk factors such as excess calcium and energy intake. Other examples are light products for obese-prone animals and active products for animals with higher caloric requirements, oral care foods, and hairball control foods.

All-Purpose Foods

The all-purpose marketing concept is based on the premise that one product satisfies all nutritional needs at all times. These products must provide adequate nutrients to support the most demanding lifestages, which are growth and lactation. The advantage of all-purpose pet foods is that they require little explanation for use. Thus, they are suited for a grocery store-type distribution. Many national-brand, regional-brand, private label and generic foods use the all-purpose approach.

It is often assumed that all-purpose foods are formulated for adult animals. This assumption is based on the fact they are not called puppy or kitten foods and have pictures of adult animals on the package. However, these foods must be balanced to support the nutritional requirements for growth and lactation, even if they are fed to adult or geriatric animals. Thus, all-purpose foods provide nutrients in excess of allowances for adult and geriatric pets.

Low Price

For many pet owners, low cost is an important criterion for selecting pet foods. The unit price (cost per weight) is the most obvious way for consumers to compare cost but may be a poor method of judging value. Value is best evaluated by actually measuring feeding costs (cost per calorie or cost per day or year). Actual feeding cost evaluation may reveal that there are only small price differences between pet foods perceived as "inexpensive" and those perceived as "expensive." Additionally, many manufacturers of low-priced foods base their claims of nutritional adequacy on nutrient profiles rather than on test feeding of dogs or cats. (See feeding cost discussion under Features and Benefits below.)

"People Food"

The concept behind "people-food" marketing is that a number of pet owners think their pets like and need the same foods people eat. Additionally, some people believe that human foods are inherently superior to pet foods. Some dogs and cats do like human foods, particularly meat-type foods. But, animals also voraciously eat items with no appeal to their owners (e.g., pet food, grass, vomitus, garbage and even feces). The concept of human food being superior to pet food is relative. First, people and pets have different nutrient requirements. Second, most pet foods are better balanced to meet the needs of dogs and cats than are typical human diets compared to the needs of people.

Indeed, there is widespread public-health concern for human nutritional health in affluent countries including inadequate intake of calcium, complex starches and fiber and excess intake of fat, saturated fat, cholesterol, salt and calories. Pet owners who use a similar approach to feeding their pets could be negatively affecting their pets' nutritional health as well. The desirability of feeding human food to pets is largely based on advertising themes designed to create anthropomorphic appeal. As a result, pet foods are often branded with recognizable human food names (chops, burgers, stews, pasta and gravy). This discussion is not intended to imply that pet foods that promote the people food concept are either good or bad, but simply to point out that the basis for the concept is not valid. Dogs and cats don't need to eat people food to be healthy.

Box 8-2. Product Claims.

A claim promotes the relationship between a product and a desired attribute or result. Claims are important because they help pet food manufacturers differentiate their products from those of competitors, and in some cases, demonstrate product superiority. In the process, companies spend thousands to millions of dollars substantiating claims.

Claims appear in several product sites and on promotional materials. A claim may appear as part of a product name (e.g., "light formula") or elsewhere as part of a product's labeling. "Labeling" is a broad term that includes the product's packaging or anything in association with the product at the point-of-sale (e.g., banners, brochures) (Chapter 9). Print or television advertising is not "labeling" under the law, but in many cases, websites are considered "labeling."

CLAIM REGULATION

In general, pet food labeling claims in the United States are regulated for legality, truthfulness, accuracy and fairness by the Center for Veterinary Medicine in the Food and Drug Administration (FDA) and by the individual states. In addition, the Federal Trade Commission has regulatory authority over media advertising (print, radio and television). Frequently, companies will choose to keep claims and/or advertising disputes out of the regulatory arena by mediating them with the National Advertising Division of the Better Business Bureau, a voluntary self-regulating industry body. When all else fails, these disputes enter the judicial system for final resolution. The Lanham Act is often the basis for these legal actions.

TYPES OF CLAIMS

Several types of claims exist: 1) general, 2) nutritional adequacy, 3) descriptive, 4) structure/function, 5) therapeutic foods, 6) health and 7) drug.

General Claims

General claims describe unique product attributes such as composition or ingredients, flavors and varieties, palatability and digestibility. These claims must be truthful and are often called "marketing" claims. Palatability claims are a frequently used type of general claim. Comparative claims have a lifespan of one year before they must be re-substantiated. "New" and "improved" claims are limited to six months production.

Nutritional Adequacy Claims

For all practical purposes, nutritional adequacy claims are primarily regulated in the United States using the procedures and protocols established by the Association of American Feed Control Officials (AAFCO). To make a "complete and balanced" nutritional adequacy claim, pet food manufacturers must either conduct a feeding test (AAFCO protocol) or meet the minimum AAFCO nutrient profile (Chapter 9). Lifestage claims are included as a subset of the nutritional adequacy claim.

Descriptive Claims

Descriptive claims must meet AAFCO requirements. Examples of descriptive claims include "light" or "low-calorie" foods. For example, dry canine and feline foods bearing a "low-calorie" claim must contain no more than 3,100 and 3,250 kcal/kg of food as fed, respectively. "Reduced" and "less calorie" pet foods do not have to meet specific maximum calorie content requirements. In those cases, though, the product of comparison and the percentage reduction must be specified. Similar AAFCO rules are in place for "low" and "reduced" fat products.

Structure/Function Claims

Because nutrition has an effect on the structure or function of the body, claims describing a food's role in maintaining health and well-being are generally allowed provided they relate to recognized nutrient effects. Acceptable structure/function claims include such things as, "Contains calcium for strong bones and teeth" and "Taurine is essential to the good health of your cat." Claims such as "for healthy skin and glossy coat" are also generally considered acceptable.

Therapeutic Food Claims

Therapeutic claims for veterinary medical foods are regulated at the discretion of FDA (**Box 8-3**). Generally, these claims are restricted to veterinarian-directed literature, but regulators may tolerate consumer information if the product is distributed under a valid veterinarian/client/patient relationship. Manufacturers who make therapeutic food claims formulate foods for the nutritional management of a condition or disease. Examples of therapeutic food claims include, "Helps control the clinical signs associated with sodium and fluid retention," "An aid in the dissolution of struvite uroliths" and "A nutritional aid for dogs with dental stain, plaque or calculus."

Health Claims

Health claims state or imply a relationship between food and disease. Technically, the health claim regulations only apply to human foods. However, FDA has allowed some health-related information on pet food labels provided certain conditions are met. For example, FDA allows "reduces urine pH to help maintain urinary tract health" on adult maintenance cat products based on controlled studies to demonstrate utility and long-term safety. Label claim wording must also meet FDA restrictions. A related claim on cat food labels is "low magnesium." Low-magnesium foods must contain less than 25 mg of magnesium/100 kcal of food and less than 0.12% magnesium on a dry matter basis.

FDA has also allowed "hairball control" claims for products after review of formulations and nutrient profiles, and "plaque/tartar control" claims for products provided the effect is achieved by mechanical means.

Drug Claims

Drug claims are highly regulated by the FDA under the authority of the Federal Food, Drug and Cosmetic Act (FFDCA). Basically, any expressed or implied intent to cure, treat, prevent, mitigate or diagnose disease is considered a drug claim. Such claims require pre-market approval by the FDA, and require extensive resources to document safety and efficacy. Such research takes years to conduct, but, if the research leads to FDA approval, the product usually has market exclusivity. A pet food whose labeling bears unapproved claims may be subject to regulatory action as an adulterated drug.

David A. Dzanis, DVM, PhD, Dipl. ACVN
Dzanis Consulting & Collaborations
Santa Clarita, CA, USA

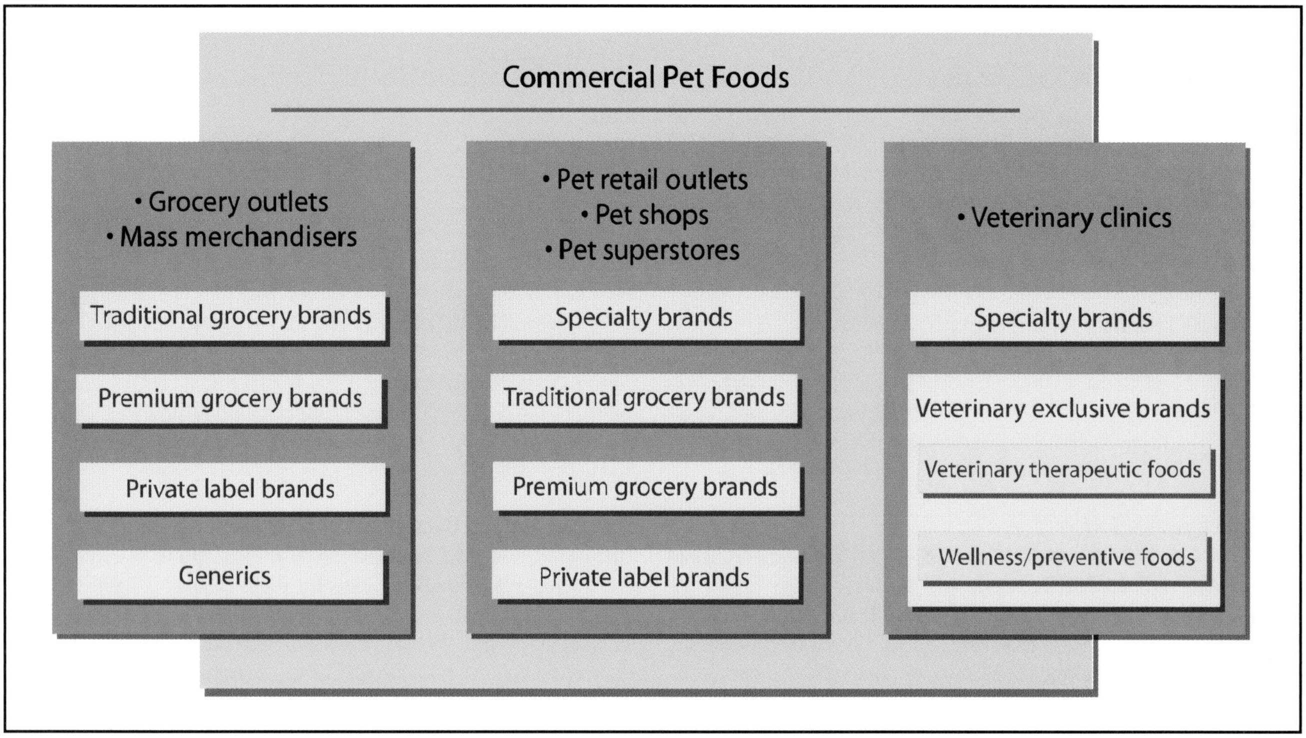

Figure 8-6. This diagram shows the market segments and usual distribution outlets of commercial pet foods.

Flavors and Varieties

Flavor and variety marketing concepts are also based on anthropomorphic appeal because they fulfill the pet owner's assumption of the need for variety. From a pet food manufacturer's standpoint, offering many flavors and varieties increases the brand's potential shelf presence and exposes the shopper to more opportunities for purchase. However, in the natural state, the diets of wild canids and particularly wild felids are somewhat monotonous.

Ingredients

Although flavor/variety descriptors often use ingredient names, ingredient-based marketing generally implies that the highlighted ingredients provide unique benefits to pets. However, fundamentally, ingredients and nutrients are not the same; the nutrient profile is important to animals and should be the primary focus rather than concern for specific ingredients.

In addition, products marketed on ingredient appeal usually contain other primary ingredients that may not be suggested by the ingredient name. If the veterinarian's objective is to restrict or exclude an antigen source, the ingredient list should be regarded as a better source of information than the product name. For example, most "lamb and rice" foods contain several protein sources in addition to lamb (Brown et al, 1995).

Two variations on the ingredient-based marketing concept are "presence" of an ingredient and "absence" of an ingredient.

Presence of an Ingredient

Promoting the presence of a particular component in a pet food is a common marketing concept. An ingredient frequently promoted as beneficial for dogs is meat. The implied corollary is that meat is a high-protein food that is natural and enhances performance. The theme of "meat as desirable" is extended to "meaty" and "animal-protein" advertising themes. Manufacturers of dry dog foods that make a "meat-based" claim imply the presence of a high meat content, which is not the case.

Likewise, fish is an excellent protein source for cats, but is not a natural food for most wild felids. Promotion of fish as desirable has historical roots in the low cost and availability of fish by-products from fish canning operations. Purported benefits have also been made for lecithin, wheat germ meal, mineral chelates, yucca extracts, herbs and probiotic bacterial cultures.

Absence of an Ingredient

Advertising the absence of a food component implies that a problem or danger may be associated with the ingredient. The marketplace example of "No Corn-Only Wheat!" or a competitor's reversed message, "Contains Corn-No Wheat!" creates consumer confusion and insecurity about both cereal sources. Although there are nutritional differences among grains, no specific grain commonly used in pet foods is harmful (Chapters 5 and 8). Other examples of negative marketing include denigration of the following ingredients: soy (purported to cause bloating and gastric dilatation-volvulus, but not proven), by-products ("inferior fillers"), "synthetics" (non-natural and therefore "harmful") and ethoxyquin ("poison" although proven safe at recommended levels).

In pet food advertising, "no fillers" is used by some manufacturers to take advantage of pet owner misconceptions. Some consumers consider pet food ingredients other than meat and vitamins "fillers," including grains, fiber sources and animal by-products, all of which can be excellent nutrient sources.

"More Is Better"

A variant on the presence of an ingredient theme is "more is better." For example, some pet owners believe a "high-protein" content in a pet food benefits exercise and is necessary for hard-working dogs. In reality, prolonged hard work only slightly increases the essential amino acid requirements of dogs. More energy-not more protein-is the primary need in athletics (Chapter 18). Therefore, specific-purpose foods for dogs with increased work levels should be energy dense and highly digestible and should contain adequate but not excessive levels of a high-quality protein. "Enough is best" is a better concept than "more is better."

Product Name

The product or brand name can become a marketing tool when it is amusing, easy to remember or authoritative. Brand names such as Happy Cat, Cycle 3, Bow-Wow, Eukanuba, Vet's, Vet's Choice, James Well-Beloved, Prescription Diet and Dr. Ballard's are examples. Product and brand names can also help identify and appropriately reinforce the food's application. Kitten Chow, and Science Diet Adult Feline are examples.

Natural/Organic/"Holistic" Foods

In 2000, the Association of American Feed Control Officials (AAFCO) defined "natural" as: "A food or ingredient derived solely from plant, animal or mined sources, either in its unprocessed state or having been subject to physical processing, heat processing, rendering, purification, extraction, hydrolysis, enzymolysis, or fermentation, but not having been produced by or subject to a chemically synthetic process and not containing any additives or processing aids that are chemically synthetic except in amounts which might occur unavoidably in good manufacturing practices" (AAFCO, 2007). This definition excludes the use of any synthetic preservatives, flavors and colors in products labeled as "natural." However, because most added trace nutrients such as vitamins, minerals and taurine are chemically synthetic, AAFCO guidelines do allow use of trace nutrients in "complete and balanced" pet foods with a disclaimer, e.g., "natural ingredients with added vitamins and minerals" (Box 9-1).

Research has identified several factors that consumers seek in natural pet foods. To pet owners, a natural pet food is nutritious and free of artificial preservatives and colors.[b] The absence of artificial preservatives appears to be the most important feature of natural pet foods to pet owners in the United States.[b]

"Organic" is not the same as "natural." Rather, the term characterizes the procedure by which the ingredients are grown, harvested and processed. For example, "organic beef" must be from cattle raised under certain conditions and without use of many drugs such as hormones and antibiotics. Sales of "organic" pet foods meeting the requirements of USDA Rule CFR part 205, which took effect October 21, 2002, are still very limited. As of June 2006, the USDA is still deliberating if and how the rules originally developed for human and livestock foods will apply to pet foods. At this time, pet foods meeting the human standard may display the USDA organic seal if the contents of the package meet the following:

1. 100% Organic-may carry new USDA Organic Seal.
2. Organic-at least 95% of content is organic by weight (excluding water and salt) and may carry the new USDA Organic Seal.
3. Made With Organic-at least 70% of content is organic and the front product panel may display the phrase "Made with Organic" followed by up to three specific ingredients or classes of ingredients. (These products may *not* display the new USDA Organic Seal.).
4. Less than 70% of content is organic and may list only those ingredients that are organic on the ingredient panel with no mention of organic elsewhere on the label. (These products may *not* display the new USDA Organic Seal.).

The term "holistic" has been applied to a wide range of pet foods with a variety of ingredients and characteristics. However, the term is not legally defined or regulated within applicable pet food regulations and is, therefore, essentially meaningless. In fact, some regulators consider the term misleading in that it may falsely imply therapeutic benefit.

PET FOOD SEGMENTS

Pet food brands have proliferated, each attempting to carve out a new "segment" in the market (**Figure 8-6**). The following discussion will provide a broad overview of the various segments, as well as, general definitions of the product types that fall into each segment.

Grocery Brands

Traditionally, pet foods were sold in grocery stores, and the brands sold there were called "grocery" brands. Grocery brands are national in scope. Many are well-recognized "household words" with high exposure levels due to large-scale advertising and wide distribution. Grocery outlets are the primary source of commercially prepared pet foods globally. Most grocery brands are "all-purpose" foods, balanced for growth/lactation. However, there has been a trend toward specific-purpose foods (lifestage and special needs) among traditional grocery dry brands.

The usual marketing theme for this segment combines a warm, friendly image with high palatability, flavor variety and moderate pricing. Palatability receives overwhelming attention in grocery brands through advertising that associates eating with gusto and rapid, voracious ingestion of food with pet satisfaction. In this context, pet owners feel that they are being "good" to their pets by providing a food that is enthusiastically consumed. "Gourmet" foods are a marketing sub-niche that further escalates the palatability message to accommodate "finicky" tastes.

"Premium" grocery brands are a relatively new set of brands sold in grocery outlets with a more nutritional focus. These foods are almost always specific-purpose foods with limited flavor offerings and a higher price.

Table 8-2. Examples of signs and disorders often managed with veterinary therapeutic foods.

Adverse reactions to food (food allergy or food intolerance)
Anemia
Anorexia
Ascites/edema
Cancer
Cardiovascular disease
Cognitive dysfunction
Colitis
Constipation
Convalescence
Dental plaque, calculus and stain
Diabetes mellitus
Diarrhea
Exocrine pancreatic insufficiency
Feline hepatic lipidosis
Feline lower urinary tract disease
Gastroenteritis
Gingivitis
Heart failure
Hepatic disease
Hyperlipidemia
Hypermetabolic states
Hypertension
Obesity
Oral malodor
Osteoarthritis
Pancreatitis
Renal failure
Surgical recovery
Urolithiasis

Private Label Brands
Private label or "store" brands are increasingly popular in larger national or regional supermarket chains and pet retail outlets. A third party usually manufacturers these foods according to specifications established by the customer (e.g., chain or pet retail outlet). Private label brands can be identified by the label, which will state "Distributed by ____" or "Manufactured for ____" instead of "Manufactured by ____." These brands may be formulated, packaged and priced similarly to traditional grocery and premium brands. Ingredient selection and quality varies from good to poor. Many private label brands use a least-cost formulation. Although private label brands lack advertising saturation, their higher profit margin provokes favorable in-store merchandising, making them increasingly competitive with other brands in their segment.

Generic Pet Foods
Generic pet foods are nonbranded products (package colors are often white or yellow with black lettering). Their primary selling point is low price, which is achieved through the use of the lowest cost ingredients, manufacturing and packaging. Generic pet foods are usually produced locally or regionally to reduce transportation costs. Poor growth performance and zinc deficiency have been described in dogs eating generic foods. A jargon expression of "generic pet food syndrome" has been used to describe some of the conditions that result from feeding certain generic pet foods (Chapter 32).

Specialty Brands
Specialty brands are also called "premium" and "super-premium" foods and, like premium grocery brands, are more likely to emphasize superior ingredients and nutrition as a guiding philosophy. Specialty brands are distinguished from premium grocery brands by the outlets from which they can be purchased. These outlets include pet stores, pet superstores, veterinary hospitals and some farm/feed stores and garden centers.

Most of these brands use the lifestage and special needs (specific purpose) approach. Specialty pet foods are likely to confirm ingredient and final product quality by regular analytical testing and nutritional adequacy through feeding trials. Although there are points of similarity between brands, manufacturers in this segment are also likely to maintain different nutritional philosophies for particular feeding applications.

The growth of the specialty pet food segment has been robust because many pet owners realize that daily feeding costs are reasonable despite higher unit costs. The distinction between premium and super-premium is ill defined, although ingredient choice and quality may be factors. Price is the primary differentiating factor.

Veterinary exclusive wellness brands are an additional subsegment within the specialty market. These products largely conform to the same descriptor as specialty brands except they are available only through veterinary hospitals.

Veterinary Therapeutic Foods
Although veterinary therapeutic foods represent a very small market segment of the overall pet food industry, they have disproportionate importance to veterinarians. These foods have unique nutrient profiles that provide therapeutic synergy with medical and surgical modalities for a wide variety of disease conditions (**Table 8-2**). These foods usually have a specific purpose, whereas some have contraindications, and should only be used under professional supervision (**Box 8-3**).

MEASURING PET FOOD FEATURES AND BENEFITS

Veterinarians are frequently asked by pet owners to recommend or compare various commercial pet foods. Palatability, digestibility, stool quantity and quality and feeding costs are often mentioned as important pet food features by pet owners and are often highlighted in advertising and promotional materials by pet food companies. It is important for veterinary health care teams to understand these pet food features and benefits in order to make informed recommendations to clients about advertising and other promotional materials. The following discussion explains how these commonly touted features and benefits are measured, what influences them and describes their actual value to pets and pet owners.

Box 8-3. FDA Perspective: Veterinary Medical Foods.

A "medical food" is defined by law as "a food that is formulated to be consumed or administered enterally under the supervision of a physician and is intended for the specific dietary management of a disease or condition for which distinctive nutritional requirements, based on sound scientific principles, are established by medical evaluation." Although the definition is only in reference to foods for human consumption, it could also be adapted to apply to "veterinary medical foods," which are generally intended to be offered as the sole source of nutrition to animals with specific medical conditions, and usually contain restricted amounts of certain nutrients to aid in the mitigation of some disease processes.

These products are often identified on the market by the label bearing the phrase "use under the direction of a veterinarian" or some similar wording. As foods, veterinary medical foods are subject to the same labeling requirements as are any other nonmedicated pet food. As such, labels generally may not bear drug claims. This restriction also applies to product names. Thus, these products are often given names that would not be easily recognized by the average consumer, such as initials or numbers. Also, veterinary medical food labels must meet the same criteria for substantiation of nutritional adequacy by meeting the AAFCO nutrient profile or passing an AAFCO feeding trial protocol or include the phrase "for intermittent or supplemental feeding only." Because directions for use are presumed to be given to the owner by the veterinarian, veterinary medical food labels are exempt from the requirement to include feeding directions.

Despite label restrictions, companies often establish the intended use of their veterinary medical food products as "drugs" through brochures, advertisements or other promotional materials. However, FDA recognizes that there are scientifically sound reasons for use of these products in some cases of disease in dogs and cats; thus these products serve a purpose for veterinarians, their clients and their patients. Also, veterinarians obviously must be informed of the indications, contraindications and directions for use of the products. Thus, FDA generally exercises regulatory discretion with respect to distribution of truthful information on diet and disease to veterinarians.

The same information distributed to pet owners; however, is of more concern. Proper use of these types of products requires adequate veterinary supervision. An owner who feeds a product for its desired therapeutic effect solely on the basis of labeling or advertising claims may cause harm resulting from improper diagnosis or treatment. However, FDA appears to grant some laxity in allowing claims on labels and consumer-directed information for products for which distribution is maintained under a valid veterinarian/client/patient relationship.

David A. Dzanis, DVM, PhD, Dipl. ACVN
Dzanis Consulting & Collaborations
Santa Clarita, CA, USA

Palatability

Pet Food Preference and Acceptability

Measuring the sensory aspects of eating evaluates the sum of the pleasant and unpleasant sensations that arise from the presentation and ingestion of food. Although "taste" is obviously important, the gustatory attributes of a food are only one of the variables involved. Olfaction, texture and eating experience also influence food intake.

PREFERENCE AND ACCEPTANCE TESTING

"Preference" and "acceptance" are specific measurement techniques to assist in the investigation of alleged pleasant or unpleasant sensations of food intake. Obviously, investigators must infer these sensations indirectly in nonverbal animals. The measurement methods used in such tests must be of sufficient statistical power to reduce bias errors. Testing should also incorporate controls for potentially confounding variables such as high or low caloric density, hunger, preference for a single-feeding pan position and environmental distractions.

The two primary assessment tools are the one-pan acceptance test (monadic test) and the two-pan preference test. The one-pan test measures acceptability; that is, it simply determines if a given food is palatable enough to be eaten in sufficient quantity to maintain the subject's body weight in a neutral state. The two-pan preference test measures "choice" between a pair of test foods that are fed simultaneously side by side. In application, the results of a two-pan preference test may indicate that animals distinctly prefer one of the foods, thus the preferred food would be termed more "palatable." However, the "losing" food could still be quite palatable and could be consumed in sufficient quantity to support body weight.

Preference Tests

Two-pan palatability tests are broadly used in the pet food industry to assess comparative food preferences. During the test, animals have simultaneous access to an excess quantity of the test foods. This allows the animal to eat all of one of the foods and none of the second, or some of each food and not become hungry. The total food consumed from each pan is measured after a timed interval. At each successive meal, the position of the food pans is alternated within the animal's enclosure to cancel any bias for a favored or habitual eating location.

The duration and number of animals required for a preference test depend on the animal days necessary to yield the statistical power requisite for test objectives. Sixty animal test days (30 animals for two days) provide a stable and repeatable assessment platform for screening purposes. However, 120 to 240 animal test days are commonly used for more statistically rigorous preference examinations.

Although there are several methods of quantifying and expressing preference results, the only bias-free method is based on the intake ratio (IR) (Griffin, 1995): $IR = A \div (A + B)$, where A and B are an individual animal's daily food consumption of each of two different foods. As an example, an animal ingests 200 g of Food A and 110 g of Food B. Using the equa-

Table 8-3. Taste chemosensory neural groups identified in dogs and cats.*

Neural group	Substances that stimulate the neural group
Dogs	
Group A	L-proline, L-cysteine, NaCl, fructose, sucrose
Group B	Malic acid, HCl, quinine hydrochloride
Group C	Nucleotides
Group D	Butyl chloride, phytic acid
Cats	
Group I	Malic acid, HCl
Group II	L-proline, L-cysteine, inorganic salts
Group III	Nucleotides

*Adapted from Boudreau JC, White TD. Flavor chemistry of carnivore taste systems. In: Bullard RW, ed. Flavor Chemistry of Animal Foods (ACS Symposium Series 67). Washington, DC: American Chemical Society, 1978; 102-128.

tion IR = 200 ÷ (200 + 110) = 200 ÷ 310 = 0.65. Thus, 65% of the food consumed by this animal was Food A. Ratios greater than 0.50 indicate the animal ate more Food A than Food B, ratios below 0.50 indicate more of Food B was consumed, and ratios equal to 0.50 mean equal amounts of Food A and Food B were consumed.

For groups of test animals, the ratio can be summarized in two ways. First, any animal with a ratio greater than 0.51 can be classified as preferring Food A, whereas animals with ratios less than 0.49 can be classified as preferring Food B. Those animals whose ratios fall between 0.49 and 0.51 would be classified as having no preference. The result for the group can then be expressed as the percentage of animals preferring Food A, preferring Food B or having no preference. Although this "percent preferring" measure tends to be statistically insensitive (e.g., either large sample sizes or large differences are required to achieve statistically significant results), it substantiates advertising claims that are "consumer friendly" (e.g., seven out of 10 dogs preferred Food A to Food B).

The ratio can also be summarized for a group of animals by simply reporting the average intake ratio. Average daily intake ratios should not be confused with average consumption ratios. Only the former ratio is free from measurement bias, is more statistically sensitive and is, therefore, recommended to guide product development.

Acceptance Tests

The one-pan or monadic test quantifies food acceptance. In most cases, this technique is less sensitive than the two-pan method. Although two-pan differences do not reliably produce one-pan differences, one-pan differences almost always produce two-pan differences.

Thirty animals (15 in each of the subgroups shown below) provide a reliable test platform as follows:

Group	Days 1-5	Days 6-7
A-B	Feed Food A	Feed Food B
B-A	Feed Food B	Feed Food A

Assuming consumption is stable after Day 3, the data collected across Days 4 to 7 are calculated and interpreted in the manner described above for two-pan preference tests.

SENSORY ASPECTS OF PREFERENCE

The primary sensory modalities for canine and feline food acceptance and preference are smell, taste and texture. The relative roles played by each modality in animals has been studied and debated.

Smell

The olfactory system of dogs and cats is very highly developed. People have about 3 to 4 cm^2 of olfactory epithelia. Cats have about 21 cm^2 and dogs have 18 to 150 cm^2, with a high density of central nervous system neurons related to olfaction (Dodd and Squirrell, 1980). This highly developed olfactory system gives some dogs their legendary ability to detect extremely low concentrations (1×10^{-11} molar) of some solutions and to discriminate between the scents of identical twins (Kalmus, 1955). Anosmic dogs have a greatly reduced ability to distinguish different foods. Despite the clear importance of olfaction to dogs and cats, foods must also provide taste for animals to show a sustained interest (Houpt et al, 1978).

Taste

In people, taste is confined to four basic groups: sweet, salty, bitter and acidic. Dogs and cats extend the range of taste sensitivity by detecting and responding to several amino acids that are only weakly bitter or acidic to people (**Table 8-3**). Some amino acids and peptides contribute to meaty and savory aromas. These effects can be intensified by complexing selected amino acids to selected sugars in Maillard ("browning") reactions.

Dogs and cats also respond to selected nucleotides and fatty acids that appear to increase the meaty taste perception. A nucleotide accumulates in decomposing animal tissue that cats dislike but not dogs, which may help explain the fascination of dogs with carrion (Houpt et al, 1978). Dogs respond to some simple monosaccharide and disaccharide sugars, whereas cats have a weak interest or no interest in sugar or sugar solutions (**Table 8-3**). However, foods acidified with phosphoric or citric acid appeal to cats. These acids have been used in some brands of dry and semi-moist cat foods for many years. However, an acid taste is less preferred in moist cat foods and the general effect of any pH change is less marked in dogs.

Texture/Mouth Feel

There is a significant oral-touch or mouth feel component to canine and feline food preferences. Neither cats nor dogs like sticky foods. The size of ground cereal particles in dry foods, and the particulates in wet foods affect preference. The size and shape of expanded particles can be important; some dogs prefer an identical formula as an extruded chunk to a loose burger presentation. Contrary to owner perceptions, dogs also like larger kibbles of the same formula. Some cats prefer one shape of an identical formula to another and may develop strong preferences for mouth feel and the surface-to-volume ratio of certain shapes of dry kibbles.

Vision

Vision is important to the hunting and prey-seeking behavior of wild animals. However, any relationship between the limited color vision of dogs and cats and their preference for a food's color is unknown. Thus, the degree to which visual stimuli influence food preference is speculative. Highly manipulated food colorings are common, but are probably more appealing to pet owners than to pets.

FACTORS AFFECTING FOOD PREFERENCES

Water Content

Dog and cat food preferences and moisture content correlate positively. On average, moist foods are preferred to semi-moist foods and semi-moist foods to dry foods. This effect is maintained but less clear-cut when intake is adjusted for caloric consumption. Adding water to dry food increases preference for some pets. Alternatively, some animals refuse to eat dry kibbles softened with water. Some dogs and cats strongly prefer or are "addicted" to one food form.

Making a self-originating "gravy" is another way of adding moisture to food. "Gravy making" occurs when water is added to kibbles that are coated with a combination of gums, carboxymethylcellulose and digest. Adding warm water rehydrates the coating and releases savory volatiles. The act of making a gravy adds anthropomorphic appeal for owners who desire an element of home cooking for their pet. However, food safety concerns may arise when water is added to dry pet food.

Nutrient Content and Ingredient Selection

In studies in which semi-purified foods were fed to cats, the food's protein content had little effect on preference levels (Morris, 1995). However, increasing protein levels in typical pet foods had a positive effect on preference for dogs and cats. Savory characteristics may be especially strong for cats; cats seem to prefer the inclusion of some liver in their foods. Cats prefer liver to muscle meats and muscle meats to lung tissue. Dogs prefer beef, pork and lamb to chicken and liver. Horsemeat is highly palatable to dogs (Heinicke, 1995). Both species prefer fish as a protein source in moist foods, but the quality of fish is critically important to preference. The type of fish (white vs. "oily" species), the season of the catch and the cut and freshness of the fish are important variables. Other animal-source proteins preferred by some pets include whey, cheese and egg.

Although dogs and cats prefer a high meat content to a high cereal content, cereal-based foods are acceptable to many animals. Dry foods must be cereal-based to facilitate the manufacturing process. The specific cereal grain(s) and quality and processing parameters affect the olfactory and gustatory characteristics of dry pet foods.

Gelling agents include alginates, carboxymethylcellulose, pectin and gum combinations. These agents imbibe water in the course of forming aspic and gravy loaves and increase a food's palatability through increased water content. Gels have a neutral taste unless they are hydrated with meat juices. Additionally, pets may prefer a gelled food to a non-gelled form of the same formula if gelling eliminates a sticky texture. Breaking a gelled loaf into chunks increases the anthropomorphic appeal for owners and provides positive oral-touch impressions for cats. The advertising theme of flesh tearing as "natural" for cats is prevalent in some markets.

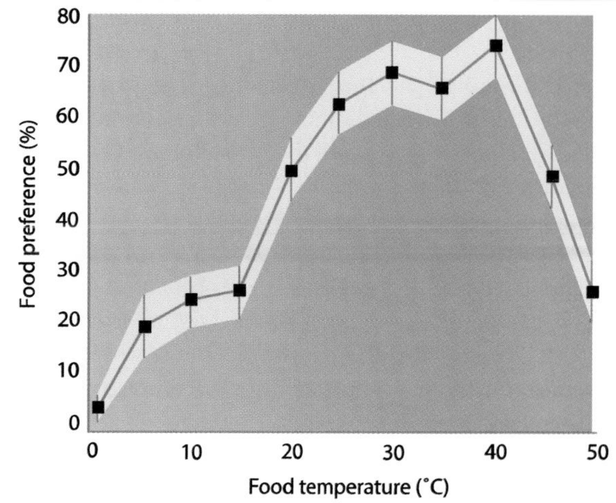

Figure 8-7. This graph demonstrates the influence of food temperature on food preference in cats. Data show the mean food preference of 23 cats fed moist food at various temperatures. Food preference was highest when food temperature approached the cats' body temperature. (Adapted from Sohail MA. The ingestive behavior of the domestic cat–A review. Nutritional Abstracts and Reviews–Series B, 1983; 53: 177-186.)

Dry foods have a lower total animal tissue content than moist foods, and the origin of animal source ingredients appears relatively less important than for moist foods. This effect may be due to the dilution effect of higher cereal content or the loss of savory volatiles during processing. Higher fat levels in foods increase energy density and usually increase preference. Both animal and vegetable fat sources are palatable. Dry pet food formulas often combine some of each. Fatty acid aldehydes indicate oxidation damage and rancidity. These negative palatability factors usually occur in food inadequately protected with antioxidants.

Cooking Effects and Food Temperature

Dogs and cats prefer cooked meats to fresh meats. However, overcooking decreases preference, which is especially important if a "burned" flavor permeates moist cat foods. The controlled cooking of cereal starches during extrusion of dry foods is important to starch digestibility and the pet's preference for the final food. The serving temperature of pet food modifies olfactory cues and mouth feel. Dogs and cats prefer food served at body temperature (**Figure 8-7**). Rewarming refrigerated moist foods in a microwave oven can produce "hot spots." Learned aversions to foods may occur following accidental mouth burning.

Palatability Enhancers

Most dry pet food particles are coated with flavor-enhancing agents such as "digests." Digests are animal tissues enzymatically altered by proteolytic enzymes. When the tissue digestive process produces a desired amino acid and peptide content, sterilization and acidification of the proteolyzed slurry stop the enzymatic action. The digest is then applied to kibbles as a topical liquid or a coating powder.

Other palatability enhancers include salt, topically or internally applied fats, L-lysine, L-cysteine, monosodium glutamate, sugar and soy sauce. Blood and feather meals, nucleotides, yeasts, whey, cheese powder, fermented meats and yeasts, meat slurries injected at extrusion, hydrolyzed vegetable protein, egg and onion and garlic powders have all been used by various manufacturers to enhance palatability. Artificial flavor technology is becoming increasingly evident; people may detect the odor of bacon, cheese and liquid hickory smoke in some pet foods and treats.

Effects of Past Feeding Patterns on Current Food Intake

Food experiences appear to influence canine and feline food acceptance and preference patterns. "Imprinting" is the preference for a familiar food as influenced by an animal's early ingestion experiences (Thorne, 1995). While puppies and kittens imprint on the inherent flavor cues found in mother's milk and preweaning solids delivered by their mother, they learn these flavors are "safe." Imprinting may be one way puppies and kittens learn what is to be hunted in addition to what is safe and nutritious (Thorne, 1995).

Aversion to new and unfamiliar foods and flavors occurs most commonly when animals receive a single food from an early age. "Novelty" is the behavior of enjoying new foods and flavors. In studies, dogs preferred novel foods and flavor changes when exposed to food rotation from weaning to two years of age (Corbin, 1995; Thorne, 1995). Experience-based ingestive imprinting, aversion and novelty behaviors may help wild animals survive by allowing them to adapt to foods they are unaccustomed to when their typical food becomes scarce.

The surroundings in which a pet eats may also influence conditioned ingestive behaviors. Cats preferred a novel food when fed in their normal housing, but became aversive when the same food was presented in an unfamiliar environment (Boudreau et al, 1985). Additionally, preference tests can differ between a laboratory setting and a home-feeding environment (Griffin, 1995). One effect of presenting a new food is a measurable, transitory increase in food intake (Mugford, 1977). This novelty response may occur even if the old flavor is preferred to the new one. The pet owner's anthropomorphic inference is that flavor boredom is a problem and the experience prompts more frequent flavor rotations. These events may set the stage for pets becoming "finicky."

Finicky Behavior

Finickiness is defined as excessively particular or fastidious behavior. This behavior is commonly described as a human-caused problem resulting from a pet's conditioned expectations for frequent changes in food variety or flavor. Supermarket shelves contain a proliferating number of varieties and flavors. Some pet owners take advantage of this phenomenon and rotate the flavor they feed daily. Clearly, the emphasis given by many owners to satisfying the food preference(s) of their pets is a strong indication of how much pets are viewed as human surrogates.

Finicky can also be an intermittent, slow or "picky" eating pattern. In these circumstances, pet health care providers should consider the possibility that the pet is simply being overfed or the owner is confusing an appropriate autoregulation of food consumption with food refusal or flavor boredom. In either case, pet owners may be concerned when their pet's consumption doesn't match the high consumption/gusto portrayed by television advertising.

The pets' body condition score (Chapter 1) will need to be evaluated when helping clients deal with finicky pets. If the body condition score is normal (3/5) or the pet is overweight (4/5 to 5/5), the finicky behavior was probably acquired from excessive flavor rotation. Behavior modification, or gradually weaning the pet from a high-frequency flavor rotation to a more stable platform of less frequent changes, may correct the problem. Ritualizing the feeding routine to the same time, place, quantity and brand of food may also help.

Food Addictions

Single-ingredient food addictions almost always cause an imbalance in nutrient intake, leading to nutritional deficiency, or excess or both. Progressive counter-conditioning (adding dilute pepper sauce to the addicting ingredient) while concurrently offering a complete and balanced pet food of the same general flavor as the addicting substance can be successful. In 14 separate single-food addiction cases, this technique worked in all but three cats and one dog.[c]

Digestibility

Digestion is the sum of the various mechanical, chemical and bacteriologic degradation processes that occur when food passes through the digestive tract. Digestion reduces complex food substances into absorbable entities such as amino acids, peptides, fatty acids and disaccharide and monosaccharide sugars. Digestibility is an important pet food feature. Although simple in concept, the integrated physiologic aspects of digestion are highly complex with numerous neuroendocrine control mechanisms operating at systemic and local levels.

Two measurable aspects are "apparent" and "true" digestibility. Apparent digestibility is quantified by measuring the difference between the DM content of an individual nutrient in the food and the quantity in the feces (Lewis et al, 1987). As an example, the % apparent protein digestibility is calculated:

$$\frac{\text{Protein food} - \text{Protein feces}}{\text{Protein food}} \times 100$$

Nondietary factors may influence fecal nutrient levels. An

example would be the contribution of sloughing intestinal cells, bacteria, mucus, blood, ammonia and urea to protein and other nitrogen sources in the feces. Nondietary factors that increase the fecal protein level reduce apparent digestibility.

True digestibility is a calculated value that must be established by first measuring the baseline value of endogenous output when a food devoid of a given nutrient is fed (Kendall et al, 1982). As an example, the % true protein digestibility is calculated as follows:

$$\frac{\text{Protein food} - (\text{Protein feces} - \text{Endogenous fecal protein}) \times 100}{\text{Protein food}}$$

High digestibility yields more available nutrients for passive or active transport in intestinal absorption. Another benefit of increased digestibility is less food is needed to meet a pet's energy and nutrient requirements. Accordingly, high digestibility reduces food costs such that a pet food that appears more expensive to purchase on a unit price basis may actually be a better value than less expensive foods with lower digestibility and caloric density.

The primary determinants of digestibility are differences in ingredient selection and processing. For example, undercooked carbohydrates markedly reduce digestibility. The undigested residue can also alter the pH of intestinal chyme and may produce osmotic effects expressed as decreased stool quality and diarrhea (Schunemann et al, 1989). Additionally, interbreed anatomic differences influence food digestibility in some dogs. In one study, Great Dane dogs had reduced relative gastrointestinal (GI) tract mass (weight) when compared with beagles. Giant-breed dogs also had more rapid oral-colon transit times, more voluminous feces and a higher content of fecal water and electrolytes. These effects were independent of food composition and form (Schunemann et al, 1989; Meyer et al, 1993; Zentek and Meyer, 1995). These findings suggest that, compared with smaller dogs, some large dog breeds are more prone to loose stools and may benefit more from highly digestible foods.

The results of testing for apparent digestibility are commonly used in pet food marketing as a measure of quality. This is often advertised under the "More is Better" concept. However, digestibility trial protocols permit either free choice or meal feeding of food quantities to maintain a neutral weight. If free choice feeding is chosen to test a more palatable food against a less palatable one, the more palatable food will probably be over consumed and apparent digestibility will decline. Thus, the less palatable brand would appear more digestible.

Digestibility is one feature that can be altered to support specific applications in veterinary therapeutic foods.

Stool Quantity and Quality

Fecal volume and consistency are of concern to many pet owners. In normal animals, fecal volume correlates with overall DM digestibility of the food, whereas the consistency of feces is affected by overall GI motility and colonic function. Higher digestibility influences the quantity (**Figure 8-8**) and

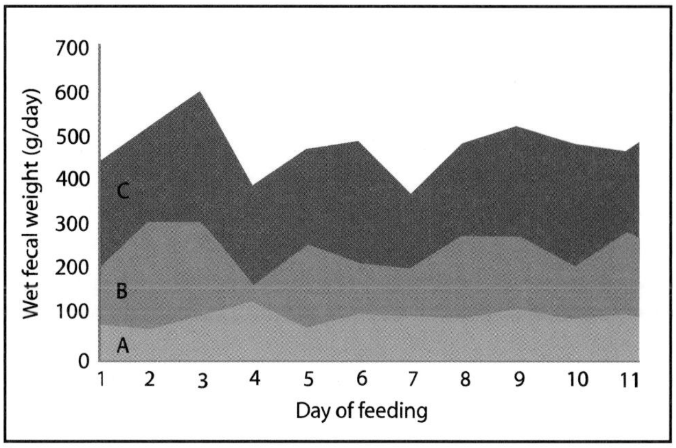

Figure 8-8. This graph shows the volume of feces (wet stool weight; grams per day) produced by the same group of laboratory beagles fed three different foods at quantities to maintain body weight. Food A is a commercial dry product formulated to provide concentrated calories and high digestibility for dogs with high-caloric requirements and those that have difficulty maintaining optimal body weight. Food A has a caloric density of 4.2 kcal/g (17.57 kJ/g) of food and energy digestibility of 88.5%. Foods B and C are commercial products. Food B was formulated with a caloric density of 4.0 kcal/g (16.74 kJ/g) and an energy digestibility of 85%. Food C has a caloric density of 3.5 kcal/g (14.64 kJ/g) and an energy digestibility of 80%.

quality of feces. Reduced DM intake reduces stool volume and may also improve the form and texture attributes relating to easy "clean-up". Fecal volume, water content and firmness are especially important to owners of urban dogs who must pick up their pet's feces. These fecal attributes are also important to animal caretakers who care for dogs and cats in kennels and colonies where sanitation may be facilitated by washing fecal elimination areas with high-pressure water sprayers. House-training puppies is easier if fecal volume is small and bowel movements are infrequent.

Feeding Costs

The energy content and digestibility of a pet food directly affect feeding costs. The methods by which energy content can be determined and stated are regulated to ensure standardized reporting, which supports fairness to consumers. In the United States, any label statement for energy content must be limited to kcal of ME/kg food and familiar measuring units (per can or measuring cup).

Feeding costs are directly related to the energy provided by a given volume of food and the cost of that food volume. True costs of feeding are best reflected by the cost of the food per day or year or the cost per calorie (**Box 8-4**).

COMMON PET FOOD INGREDIENTS

Ingredients available for use in the pet food industry range from human non-edible pet food grade by-products to human grade ingredients found in grocery stores. In the United States, ingredients are legally defined in the Association of American Feed Control Officials (AAFCO) Official Handbook and are listed

Box 8-4. True Cost of Feeding.

Pet owners usually compare the cost of pet foods on the price per unit (price per bag or price per can) rather than the true cost of feeding (cost per day or cost per year). It is easy to compare the price per unit when evaluating two different pet foods, but more difficult to compare the true cost of feeding. The following example demonstrates that veterinarians and their health care team need to discuss the true cost of feeding with pet owners when clients are concerned about the price of a particular food.

MOIST CAT FOOD

A 5-kg, three-year-old neutered male cat is diagnosed with lower urinary tract disease due to struvite urolithiasis. A moist veterinary therapeutic food is recommended to help prevent further episodes of struvite urolithiasis. The cat's owner is concerned about the cost of the veterinary therapeutic food. She now feeds her cat more than two small cans/day of a gourmet grocery brand. This calculation shows that the veterinary therapeutic food costs less to feed than the cat's current food.

	Veterinary therapeutic food	Current food
a) Cost/can ($)	1.52	0.69
b) Weight of contents of container (g) (from label)	404	85
c) Cost/g ($) (a ÷ b = c)	0.004	0.008
d) Feeding amount (g) (300 kcal/1,255 kJ)*/**	285***	185
e) Cost/day ($) (c x d = e)	1.07	1.50
f) Cost/year ($) (e x 365 = f)	391.38	547.68

*The amount of energy currently being fed was obtained from the label (in this example it was 138 kcal or 418 kJ/can). Manufacturer's recommended feeding equals 2.17 cans/day; therefore, 2.17 cans x 138 kcal/can = 300 kcal/day.

**To feed the same amount of energy in the form of the veterinary therapeutic food, first the amount of energy/can is determined from the label (424 kcal or 1,773 kJ). Then the amount of energy currently being fed is divided by the energy/can of the veterinary therapeutic food: 300 kcal/day ÷ 424 kcal/can = 0.70 cans/day.

***To obtain the grams of the veterinary therapeutic food to feed, multiply 0.70 x 404 g/can = 285 g/day.

on the label in order of predominance (Chapter 9). This section will discuss the benefits and characteristics of ingredients available to pet food manufacturers.

Carbohydrate Ingredients

Grains are typically classified as carbohydrate ingredients. These ingredients are composed primarily of starch (>60%) with protein, fat and fiber fractions making up most of the balance. The amount of starch, as a percentage of the whole ingredient, will vary depending on the degree of milling, as in the case of whole corn vs. cornstarch. Examples of carbohydrate ingredients used in pet foods are found in **Table 8-4** (**Box 8-5**).

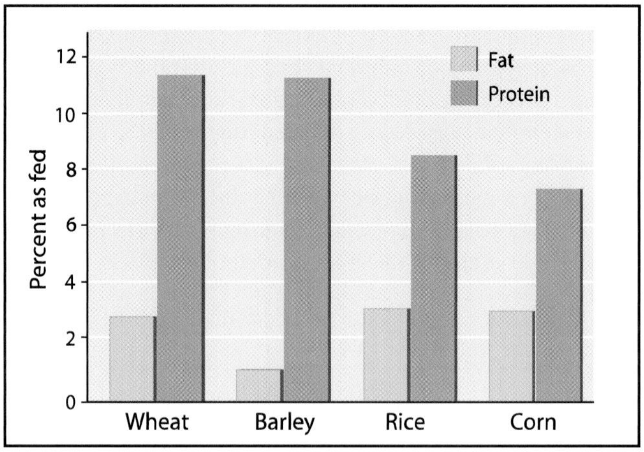

Figure 8-9. Typical fat and protein concentrations (% as fed) of common grains used in commercial pet foods.

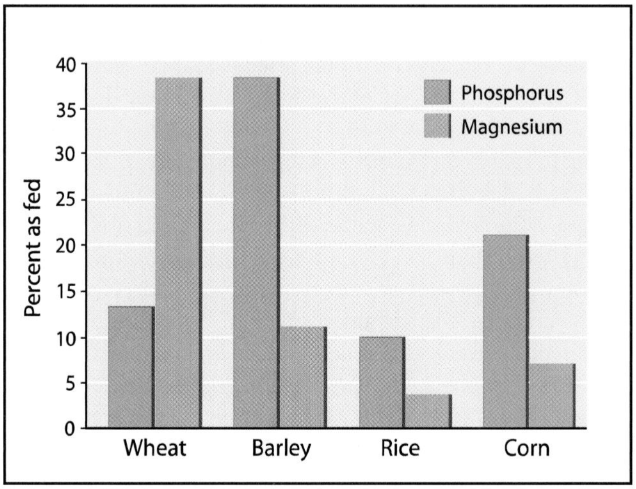

Figure 8-10. Typical phosphorus and magnesium concentrations (% as fed) of common grains used in commercial pet foods.

Nutritional Characteristics

Grains primarily provide energy to the food, but are also a source of many different nutrients (protein, fat, fiber, minerals, vitamins) at various proportions. For example, corn contains average levels of protein, but is a good source of linoleic acid. By comparison, rice is lower in fat, phosphorus and magnesium. Barley and rice bran are higher in protein, but also higher in phosphorus. Wheat middlings are higher in protein, but also higher in fiber, and higher in nutrient variability (**Figures 8-9** and **8-10**). Grains differ analytically and in nutrient availability. Although corn, rice, barley and oats have nearly identical ileal and total tract carbohydrate digestibility (all >98%), whole grains have differing DM digestibility (rice >corn >barley >oats). Varying fiber levels between the grains account for this difference (Walker et al, 1994).

Awareness of nutrient composition and availability differences is important when formulating foods in order to select ingredients with nutrient compositions that agree with the overall design of the food being formulated. For example, if a product were being formulated to maximize energy and linoleic acid content, then corn would be the prime choice as the car-

Box 8-5. Ingredient Myths and Facts.

Sometimes pet foods are marketed based on ingredient stories that have consumer appeal. Ingredient stories are simple and believable but sometimes mislead consumers. Animals require nutrients, not ingredients. Ingredients are the means to achieve the nutritional and palatability goals of a product. What are some of the myths and facts surrounding ingredients commonly used in pet foods?

MYTH NO. 1: Corn is a filler, is poorly digested and causes allergies.
FACT: Fillers are ingredients that serve no nutritional purpose, and corn does not fit that description. Corn is a nutritionally superior grain compared with others used in pet foods because it contains a balance of nutrients not found in other grains. Corn provides a highly available source of complex carbohydrates and substantial quantities of linoleic acid, an essential fatty acid important for healthy skin. Corn also provides essential amino acids and fiber. In a survey of veterinary dermatologists, corn was not listed among the ingredients most often suspected to cause food allergies. A review of 15 different studies representing 278 dogs described primary cutaneous lesions associated with adverse reactions to specific foods or ingredients: beef, dairy products and wheat represented 69% of reported cases; lamb, chicken egg, chicken and soy represented an additional 25% of the cases (Chapter 31).

MYTH NO. 2: Soybean meal causes bloat in dogs.
FACT: Bloat, or gastric dilatation/volvulus, is a condition usually seen in large, deep-chested dogs. Research has shown that food ingredients do not affect gastric motility and emptying (moist meat-based vs. dry cereal-based food) (Chapter 53).

MYTH NO. 3: Chicken meal is superior to poultry by-product meal.
FACT: Both chicken meal and poultry by-product meal contain quality protein that is digestible and palatable. Chicken meal, however, contains mostly rendered chicken necks and backs, which means it provides more ash per unit protein (**Table 8-6**) than poultry by-product meal. This may make it less desirable for use in formulations in which controlling the mineral content of the product is indicated. Poultry by-product meal is a slightly more concentrated protein source (**Table 8-5**).

MYTH NO. 4: By-products are of lesser quality than meat.
FACT: Pet food ingredients including muscle meat are by nature by-products. Some of the by-products used in pet foods are ingredients that are considered human grade both domestically and internationally. Examples of these are pork and beef liver, tripe and spleen. Many by-products such as liver offer superior palatability compared to muscle meats when used in dog and cat foods.

MYTH NO. 5: There is one best fiber source.
FACT: Various fiber types can be used to provide distinct functions in pet foods. Though fiber does not serve as a major energy source for dogs or cats, it can help promote normal bowel function, maintain the health of the intestinal tract and aid in the nutritional management of certain diseases. No single fiber source or type can optimally deliver all the benefits fiber can provide in pet nutrition. Insoluble fiber is preferred in weight-loss regimens. Soluble fiber is more appropriate in the maintenance of intestinal tract health. It is important to use the fiber source or sources that achieve the nutritional goals of the product (Chapter 5).

MYTH NO. 6: Cellulose fiber binds minerals and decreases the digestibility of other nutrients.
FACT: As with other fibers, dry matter digestibility decreases with increasing cellulose levels. However, research has shown that fiber type does not affect protein digestibility in dogs. In addition, purified cellulose does not decrease protein digestibility in cats. Purified cellulose is inert when it comes to mineral binding and has no effect on calcium or zinc availability in chicks or iron in dogs. More soluble fibers such as beet pulp bind calcium and zinc in chicks and iron in growing puppies (Chapter 5).

MYTH NO. 7: Holistic foods are superior.
FACT: There is no legal definition of the term "holistic" for pet foods. Any manufacturer can make claims of "holistic" in literature and brochures regardless of the ingredients used in its foods.

MYTH NO. 8: A product contains or is made from human grade ingredients.
FACT: Claims that a product contains or is made from ingredients that are "human grade," "human quality," "people foods," "ingredients you (the purchaser) would eat," "foods that you (the purchaser) would feed your family" or similar claims are false and misleading unless the entire product, itself, meets the USDA and FDA standards for food edible by people. At this time, the use of the descriptors "human grade" or "human quality" for pet foods is not allowed (AAFCO, 2007).

Myth No. 9: "BARF" diets (Bones and Raw Foods) better meet the archetypical needs of dogs that cannot digest grains commonly used in commercial pet foods.
FACT: The BARF philosophy appears to be a decision primarily driven by emotion. Currently there are no published peer-reviewed clinical papers or scientific support for BARF diets (Chapter 11).

bohydrate source. If the design is to minimize phosphorus or magnesium, rice is a good candidate (**Figure 8-10**). No single carbohydrate is best for every situation. Each has its own strengths and weaknesses, and combinations are often used to achieve the desired nutrient profile.

Process Characteristics

The principal function of carbohydrates in the process of manufacturing dry pet foods is to provide structural integrity to kibbles. The starch works like a "cement" that holds kibbles together, preventing crumbling throughout the manufacturing process. It is unusual for a dry pet food to be formulated with fewer than 40% carbohydrate ingredients because of the minimum requirement for extrusion. Formulations designed for obesity management, however, often contain less than 40% carbohydrate and higher levels of fiber.

Table 8-4. Common grain ingredients and their carbohydrate or nitrogen-free extract (NFE) concentrations (as fed).

Grain	NFE (%)*
Barley	76
Corn	81
Corn flour	85
Cornstarch	88
Grain sorghum	80
Oat groats	70
Rice	90
Rice bran	46
Rice flour	90
Wheat	78
Wheat flour	82
Wheat middlings	66

*NFE is the nonfiber carbohydrate fraction and is calculated as follows: % NFE = 100% – % moisture – % crude protein – % crude fat – % crude fiber – % ash.

Table 8-5. Dry protein sources used in commercial pet foods and their typical protein ranges (as fed).

Ingredient	Protein (%)
Poultry by-product meal	65-70
Meat and bone meal	50-55
Chicken meal	63-67
Lamb meal	48-55
Fish meal	60-65
Soybean meal	46-50
Corn gluten meal	60-64
Rice gluten meal	40-50
Dried egg product	43-48

Table 8-6. Protein-to-ash ratios of dry protein sources used in commercial pet foods.

Ingredient	Protein:ash
Poultry by-product meal	6:1
Meat and bone meal	2:1
Chicken meal	4:1
Lamb meal	2.5:1
Fish meal	3:1
Soybean meal	10:1
Corn gluten meal	25:1
Rice gluten meal	20:1
Dried egg product	8:1

The choice of a carbohydrate in a moist formulation can markedly affect processing characteristics. The starch will gelatinize in moist products and combine with the denaturing protein to give the loaf structure. This structure will maintain even distribution of the formulation. However, the textural characteristics of the structure will vary widely among carbohydrates, especially if the starch is in purified form, because each reacts uniquely to cook temperature and time.

Dry Protein Ingredients

Protein ingredients contain higher levels of protein (>20%). Protein ingredients typically used in dry pet foods and their protein contents are listed in **Table 8-5** (**Box 8-6**). Protein ingredients vary widely in the levels of protein and other nutrients they deliver to a formulation. For example, ash represents the total mineral element of the formula (the sum of calcium, phosphorus, magnesium, potassium, sodium, etc.). Ash is the material that remains after combustion or hydrolysis of the organic material. The protein-to-ash ratio is a good indicator of an ingredient's efficiency in providing protein and the ingredient's DM digestibility. The higher an ingredient's ash content, the lower its digestibility.

The ratios of total protein content to total ash content described in **Table 8-6** are critical to formulating dry pet foods. This is especially true for cats, which require a higher proportion of protein from animal tissue and which have higher protein requirements than dogs. A protein ingredient choice that has a low protein-to-ash ratio will make it difficult to meet a cat's protein requirement without delivering excessive levels of magnesium and phosphorus. Dogs and cats readily accept poultry by-product meal. Because it contains viscera, it provides an excellent source of protein with lower mineral levels than chicken meal, which is composed primarily of rendered chicken necks and backs. Thus, poultry by-product meal is an excellent choice for feline foods to avoid excess mineral levels.

Nutritional Characteristics

Dogs are omnivorous and have lower protein requirements than cats. Therefore, formulations for dogs are more flexible and may include more vegetable proteins. Vegetable proteins typically have higher protein-to-ash ratios and contain some fiber. Soybean meal is an excellent source of the amino acids lysine and tryptophan. However, because dogs prefer animal tissues to vegetable meals, it is advantageous to add animal source proteins to the formulation. A blend of animal tissue meals and vegetable meals is appropriate and often optimal.

Wet Protein Ingredients

Wet protein ingredients are classified as fresh or frozen meats and meat by-products. These ingredients generally have moisture contents above 60%. **Table 8-7** lists the typical protein ingredients used in canned pet foods. Controlling excess minerals in moist foods is easier because the protein-to-ash ratio for fresh meat ingredients is higher overall (i.e., they contain less bone) than that of rendered meat meals used in dry pet foods.

Process Characteristics

Protein ingredients provide structural integrity to kibbles, but not nearly as much as that provided by carbohydrates. The exception to this is textured vegetable protein (TVP), which is made from wheat or soy flour. Sulfur is usually added to give the matrix more structure by increasing the disulfide bonding between protein strands. TVP absorbs moisture readily and has a texture similar to that of meat when hydrated. The meat tissues used in moist pet foods contribute greatly to the firmness and structure of the finished product. Overheating or adding strong acids will cause the structure to degenerate, affecting the finished product.

Fiber Ingredients

Fiber ingredients contain levels of crude fiber between 18 and 80%. **Table 8-8** lists fiber ingredients typically used in pet foods and the usual amount of fiber in each ingredient.

Nutritional Characteristics

Fiber may be classified as soluble or insoluble based on solubility in water. Soluble fiber is easily fermented in the gut by intestinal flora and provides energy and substrates for colonocyte health (Chapter 5). Examples of soluble fiber include pectin, gum and hemicellulose. Beet pulp, citrus pulp and soymill run are good sources of soluble fiber. These types of fibers improve stool consistency without compromising total digestibility.

Insoluble fiber, which is found in cellulose and peanut hulls, improves stool quality (e.g., adds bulk and holds water) and modulates GI motility. Insoluble fiber is also useful in obesity management because it dilutes calories, maintains satiety and can be used at higher levels without causing flatulence. The efficiency of the fiber source is critical for formulation. For example, a product formulated for obesity management with a crude fiber content of 20% would need much greater amounts of fiber ingredients such as beet pulp to achieve the same result as cellulose (**Figure 8-11**).

Cellulose and peanut hulls are more efficient for diluting calories than beet pulp or soymill run. This advantage is critical when space is needed in the formula to provide protein in moist and dry products, and starch necessary for kibble integrity in dry products. As is the case for carbohydrate and protein ingredients, the choice of a fiber ingredient should be dictated by the overall formulation strategy and food purpose.

Process Characteristics

Fiber ingredients typically contribute an anti-caking effect to the flow of materials in the manufacturing process. However, they also cause high degrees of friction in an extruder and may require fat for lubrication, which may negate fiber's caloric dilution purpose.

Fat Ingredients

Fat ingredients contain more than 50% fat. Fat ingredients typically used in pet foods are animal fat (pork fat, beef tallow, poultry fat) and various types of vegetable oil (soybean, sunflower, corn). Each type of fat has several different grades of quality, as measured by peroxide values and free fatty acid levels, which are indicators of rancidity. Selection of high-quality fat ensures a low oxidative potential and increases the palatability of the finished product.

Nutritional Characteristics

Fat ingredients are extremely efficient in delivering energy to a food. Fats contribute calories at 2.25 times the rate of carbohydrates or proteins. Use of fat ingredients is the most efficient method of increasing the energy density of a food to limit a pet's consumption of other nutrients. However, preventing or managing obesity in sedentary pets limits the broad application of this approach.

Table 8-7. Wet protein sources used in commercial pet foods and their typical protein ranges (as fed).

Ingredient	Protein (%)
Liver (pork, beef, turkey, sheep)	17-22
Meat by-products (lungs, spleens, kidneys)	15-20
Beef (carcass)	18-22
Chicken (whole, backs, necks)	10-12
Fish (freshwater)	12-15
Fish (ocean)	20-27

Table 8-8. Common fiber ingredients used in commercial pet foods and their typical crude fiber ranges (as fed).

Ingredient	Crude fiber (%)
Cellulose	72-78
Soymill run	32-36
Wheat bran	13-16
Beet pulp	17-20
Peanut hulls	52-58

Box 8-6. Incorporating Fresh or Frozen Meat Into Dry Extruded Pet Foods.

Until the late 1980s, the only animal source proteins used in dry commercial pet foods were dry rendered meat, chicken or poultry meals. Extrusion technology advanced during that time allowed the addition of fresh or frozen meat or poultry to dry pet foods.

A slurry composed of animal tissues, fat and water, containing about 25 to 35% of the formula, is ground and mixed in a separate tank. It is then pumped into the preconditioner where it replaces some of the process water. The product is then extruded in the same way as when dry meat meals are used.

Because labeling regulations in the United States stipulate that ingredients must be listed in order of predominance by weight, the wet weight of the meat or poultry can be within the top three ingredients. The water in the meat (60 to 70%), however, must be dried off to make a dry product. Therefore, the actual meat or poultry ingredient would be listed much farther down on the label if it were added as a dry meat meal.

Process Characteristics

Fats that have low melting points can be added to the inside or sprayed on the outside of a kibble. Hard fat ingredients (tallow, grease) must be heated before they can be applied to the exterior of kibbles. Antioxidants are necessary to help prevent rancidity during prolonged heating of fats, and to extend the shelf life of dry products. Because fats are lubricants, they are extremely useful for managing product expansion and density in the extrusion process. Adding large amounts of fat, especially hard fat ingredients, to moist products without proper mixing results in fat separation.

Table 8-9. Common pet food additives.*

Antioxidant preservatives
Butylated hydroxyanisole (BHA)
Butylated hydroxytoluene (BHT)
Ethoxyquin
Propyl gallate
Rosemaric acid/rosmarequinone
Tocopherols
Antimicrobial preservatives
Calcium propionate
Citric acid
Fumaric acid
Hydrochloric acid
Phosphoric acid
Potassium sorbate
Propionic acid
Pyroligneous acid
Sodium nitrite
Sodium propionate
Sorbic acid
Humectants
Cane molasses
Corn syrups
Propylene glycol
Sorbitol
Sucrose/dextrose
Coloring agents/preservatives
Aluminum potassium sulfate
Artificial color(s)
Azo dyes (tartrazine [FD&C yellow No. 5], sunset yellow [FD&C yellow No. 6], allura red [FD&C red No. 40])
Caramel color
Iron oxide
Natural color(s)
Nonazo dyes (brilliant blue [FD&C blue No. 1], indigotin [FD&C blue No. 2])
Sodium erythrobate
Sodium metabisulfite
Sodium nitrite
Titanium dioxide
Flavors/flavor enhancers
Artificial flavors
Citrus bioflavonoids
Dehydrated cheese/dried cheese powder
Digests
Liver meal
Monosodium glutamate
Natural flavors
Natural smoke flavor
Palatability enhancers
Acidified yeast
Digests
Garlic powder/oil
Hydrochloric acid
L-lysine
Meat extracts (beef, chicken, turkey)
Onion powder/oil
Phosphoric acid
Spices
Sucrose, dextrose, cane molasses
Water (moisture)
Whey
Emulsifying agents, stabilizers and thickeners
Diglycerides (of edible fats and oils)
Glycerin
Glyceryl monostearate
Gums (hydrocolloids)
Seaweed extracts (carrageenan, alginates)
Seed gums (guar gum)
Microbial gums (xanthan gum)
Chemically modified plant materials
Modified starch
Monoglycerides (of edible fats and oils)
Miscellaneous
Charcoal
Mineral oil (reduces dust)
Polyphosphates (dental calculus prevention)
Sodium tripolyphosphate (dough conditioner)
Disodium phosphate
Tetrasodium pyrophosphate
Yucca schidigera extract (flavor, odor control)

*Adapted from Roudebush P. Pet food additives. Journal of the American Veterinary Medical Association 1993; 203: 1667-1670.

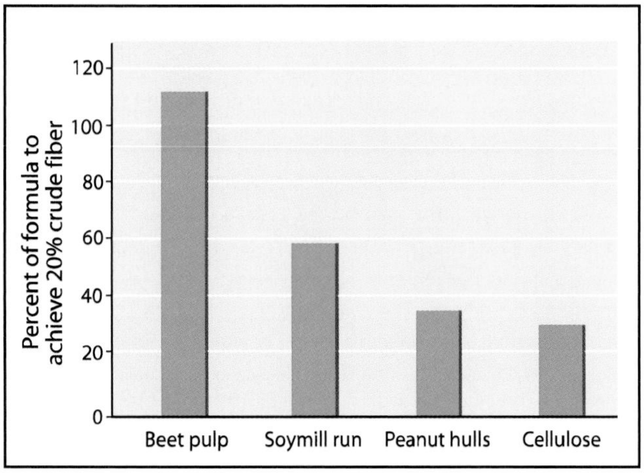

Figure 8-11. The amount (% of formula) of a particular fiber ingredient necessary to produce a product containing 20% crude fiber. Note that it is impossible to achieve 20% crude fiber in the finished food using beet pulp because the percentage exceeds 100.

Additives

Since 1920, legally sanctioned food additives have been used commonly in human and animal foods. Pet food manufacturers use various additives to generate products with visual appeal, prolonged nutritional quality, palatability and a long shelf life.

Because most commercial pet foods are designed as complete foods, nutrient enrichment with vitamins and minerals is the most important and beneficial use of pet food additives. Most ingredients with unfamiliar, chemical-sounding names are, in fact, nutrients. In general, additives other than vitamins and minerals are found least often or in smallest amounts in moist foods, and most commonly or in largest amounts in dry foods, semi-moist foods, treats and snacks.

The term "additive" is inclusive for anything imparting increased nutritional, gustatory or cosmetic appeal. Additives commonly used in prepared human and pet foods include colors, flavors, flavor enhancers, emulsifying agents, gelling substances, stabilizers, thickeners and processing aids. The terms preservative and additive are often used synonymously, but they are distinctly different. Preservatives are substances added to foods to protect or retard decay, discoloration or spoilage under normal use or storage conditions. Thus, all preservatives are additives, but not all additives serve a preservative function.

Many additives have multiple purposes in pet foods as outlined in **Table 8-9**. A few additive categories are described here in more detail.

Antioxidant Preservatives

See the shelf life and antioxidant sections in this chapter.

Antimicrobial Preservatives

Because semi-moist pet foods and treats have a high moisture content and are not maintained in a sterile environment, they often contain antimicrobial preservatives. These compounds inhibit bacterial putrefaction, mold formation or both. Examples include acids, propylene glycol and propionate and sorbate salts.

Humectants
Humectants reduce water activity and prevent loss of water after processing. See the soft-moist manufacturing section in this chapter for more details.

Coloring Agents/Preservatives
Natural and synthetic colors are often added to pet food products to enhance consumer appeal. Examples of natural colors include the carotenoids. Synthetic colors used in pet foods include iron oxide; coal tar derivatives (azo dyes) such as tartrazine (Food, Drug & Cosmetic [FD&C] yellow No. 5), sunset yellow (FD&C yellow No. 6) and allura red (FD&C red dye No. 40) and none-azo dyes such as brilliant blue (FD&C blue No. 1) and indigotin (FD&C blue No. 2). An artificial color may only be used in a pet food in the United States if it is listed as safe in the United States Food and Drug Regulations (21 CFR 73 and 74). Several additives are not colors themselves but are used to prevent discoloration of products. Examples of color enhancers or preservatives are the nitrites and bisulfites.

Emulsifying Agents and Stabilizers/Thickeners
Gums (hydrocolloids), glycerin, glycerides and modified starch are used to prevent separation of ingredients and create the gravy, sauce or jelly portion of moist pet foods. These additives allow manufacture of high-moisture foods that are highly palatable to pets, but that do not have an excess of free water.

Gums are long-chain, high molecular weight polysaccharides that dissolve or disperse in water to build viscosity in or thicken products. Gums also are used for secondary effects that include stabilization of emulsions, suspension of particulates, inhibition of syneresis (release of water from fabricated foods) and formation of films or gels. Gums frequently used in pet foods include seaweed extracts such as alginates (brown seaweed) and carrageenan (red seaweed), seed gums such a guar gum (ground endosperm of guar plants), microbial gums such as xanthan gum (bacteria originally isolated from the rutabaga plant cultured on carbohydrate media) and chemically modified plant materials such as sodium carboxymethylcellulose (cellulose chemically modified to become water soluble). Modified celluloses and vegetable gums are frequently sprayed on the surface of commercial dry foods with digests. Water mixed with these dry foods creates a gravy.

Miscellaneous Additives
Polyphosphates are frequently used as additives in baked treats and moist pet foods. These additives serve as dough conditioners and help to improve texture, retain natural moisture and protein in meat ingredients, reduce oxidation and allow better color development.

Extracts of *Yucca schidigera* are marketed in pet foods as a means of reducing fecal odor. Yucca extracts, in higher concentrations, reduce atmospheric ammonia in livestock and poultry confinement units. Saponins or other active compounds in the extract appear to reduce levels of free ammonia by binding ammonia or converting ammonia to other products. Some yucca extracts may also inhibit urease enzymes. Whether binding or preventing free ammonia is an effective way of reducing pet fecal odor has not been proved. Yucca extract is not officially approved for odor reduction use in pet food, although it is approved as a flavoring agent for pet and human foods.

Palatability Enhancers
Pet food companies have done a great deal of work in the area of palatability enhancement. In general, dogs like fats, sugars, meat ingredients and digests, which are animal tissues that have been chemically or enzymatically altered. The digestion process from which digests are made releases amino acids, such as lysine, and dipeptide combinations that enhance palatability for dogs. Cats strongly prefer meat ingredients and inorganic acids such as phosphoric acid to fats and sweet ingredients such as whey and sugar. Cats also strongly prefer the amino acids cystine and glycine. Feline digests generally have a low pH, which also aids in preservation. Digests are available in dry and liquid forms to best accommodate the manufacturer's application process.

Formulating dry pet foods with wet meat ingredients combined with fat (up to about 25% of the product) also improves palatability (**Box 8-6**). In this process, a liquid mixture of meat, water and fat is pumped into the extruder raising the overall moisture, which is then driven off during the drying process. The palatability of the finished product is enhanced because the wet meat ingredient is cooked once in the extruder, as opposed to meat meals, which are rendered first then extruded.

Palatability enhancers are less effective in a canned matrix because of the high-moisture environment and deactivation from high processing temperatures. Therefore, meat selection becomes the most important factor in improving the palatability of a moist product. In addition, a higher moisture content can increase the palatability of moist foods. **Table 8-9** lists some palatability enhancers commonly used in the pet food industry.

COMMERCIAL PET FOOD MANUFACTURING

Principles of Extrusion/Dry Manufacturing
Most commercially prepared dry pet food is manufactured using a batch system (**Figure 8-12**). This system grinds and blends raw ingredients in predetermined amounts ranging from 1,000 to 5,000 kg, depending on capacity, then transports the resulting matrix to an extruder where it is cooked and formed into kibbles. After extrusion, the kibbles are transported to a dryer where they are dried to target moisture, and then transported again by air or vibratory or conveyor belts to sites where fat and flavor enhancers are sprayed or dusted on the surface. The kibbles may or may not be sent through a cooler. The finished product is then transported to packaging machines that place it in containers for shipment and distribution. The entire process is usually automated and computer controlled.

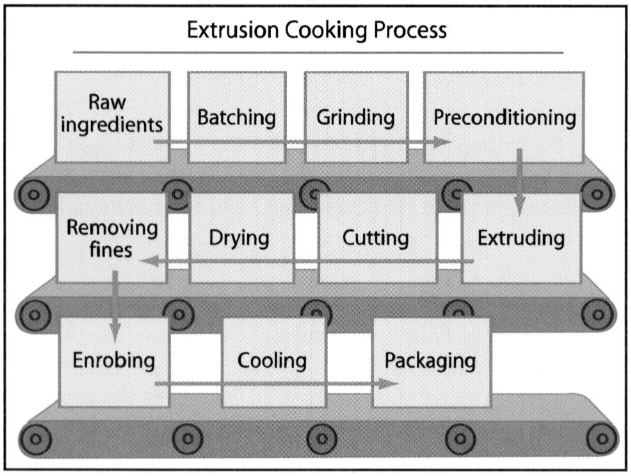

Figure 8-12. Process flow diagram for dry commercial pet food production.

Raw Materials

Ingredients used to manufacture pet foods often are received in bulk (90,000 kg by train cars; 25,000 kg by truckload) as in the case of grains or meat meals, which are the primary ingredients of any dry product, or in 25- to 50-kg bags for ingredients used in small proportions (e.g., trace minerals, crystalline amino acids and vitamins). Ingredients received in bulk are usually stored in silos until needed. Generally, the form in which a manufacturer receives ingredients depends on the physical makeup of the manufacturing plant and how much and what kind of storage units are available. Most ingredient suppliers offer multiple shipment options to best suit the needs of the manufacturer.

Grinding

Ingredients supplied as large particles may need to be ground before mixing (pregrinding) to enhance their nutritional and process characteristics. Generally, the larger the particle size, the more likely that pregrinding is necessary. A good example of this type of ingredient is whole yellow corn. A milling device known as a hammer mill is most often used to grind raw materials and the final dry mix. The hammer mill is a large capacity-milling machine that contains multiple free-swinging steel hammers and a sieve or screen that can be changed to create the desired particle size. Centrifugal force spins the hammers against the screen, pulverizing whole grains to 1,000 microns or less (Rokey, 1995).

The entire dry mix is usually ground to achieve the desired uniform particle size (e.g., usually the consistency of coarse flour). A uniform size is critical for proper water absorption, optimal passage through the extruder and thorough cooking by the extruder (Rokey, 1995). Large uncooked particles may clog the extruder die and may reduce palatability, product appearance and digestibility.

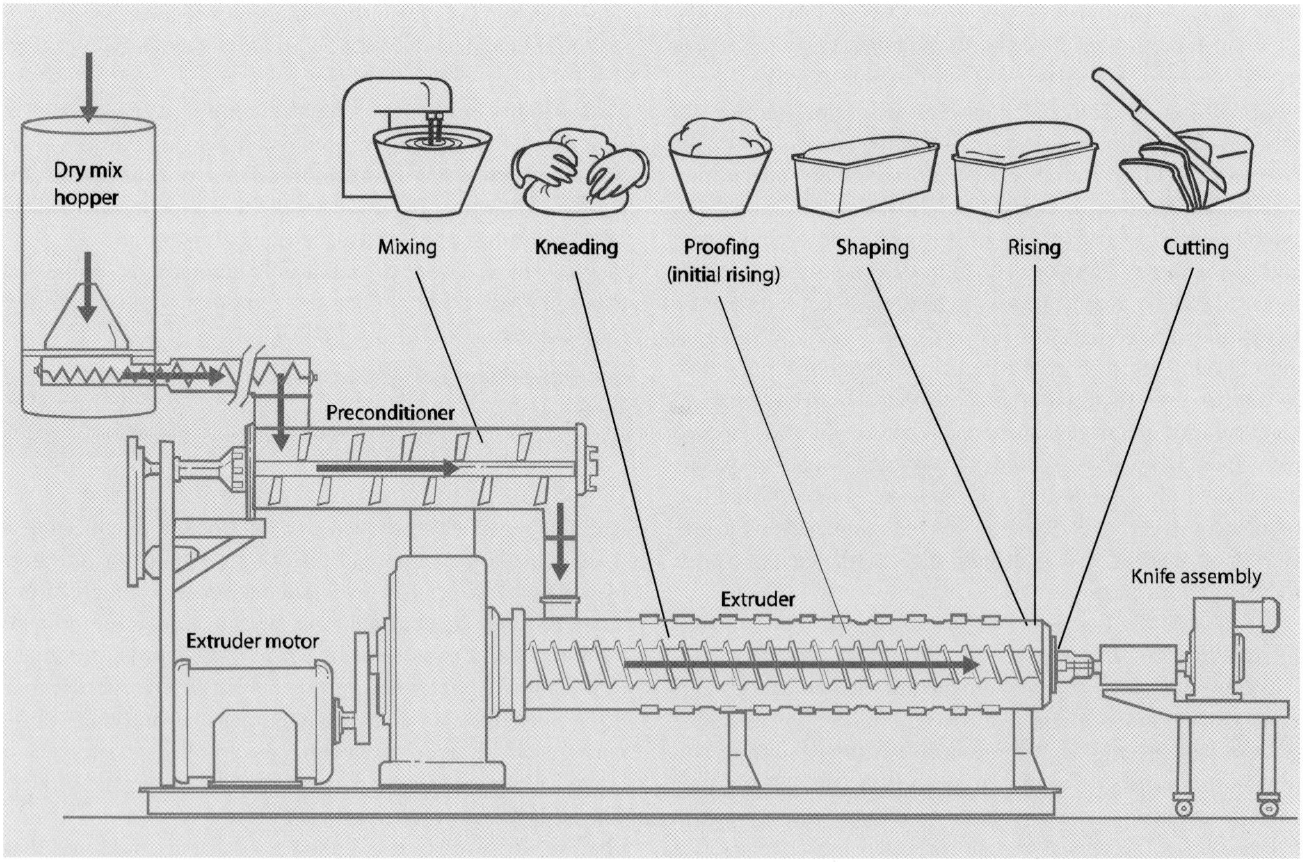

Figure 8-13. The same steps are used in bread baking and extrusion cooking: 1) mixing (preconditioner), 2) kneading (extruder barrel), 3) proofing (extruder barrel), 4) shaping (die plate), 5) rising (die plate) and cutting (rotating knives).

Compounding and Mixing

Good compounding (physically combining all of the dry mix ingredients) and mixing are essential to delivering a consistent, nutritionally adequate product. Improper compounding will result in unequal distribution of essential nutrients or lack of key ingredients in a product.

Ground bulk ingredients are usually stored in large bins. From here, they are blown, via negative airflow, into mixing hoppers. Ingredients that form a smaller percentage of the product can be added by hand and combined with bulk ingredients. Computer-controlled scales weigh dry mix ingredients to ensure they are present in desired quantities.

After a "batch" of dry mix is compounded it must be properly mixed. Mixer types and times are carefully selected based on the flow characteristics of the ingredients that compose the mixture. Because particle size, density and shape influence flow characteristics, a ribbon blender is often used for thorough mixing (Harnby, 1993). A ribbon blender is a horizontal blending machine that has a shaft running through the middle of the mixer. A ribbon of steel attached to the shaft is the mixing element. A ribbon blender is able to thoroughly mix large quantities of dry ingredients (up to 5,000 kg) and is the most commonly used mixing device. After the finished dry mix is ground for the last time, it is transferred to the extrusion process area and stored in a bin.

Extrusion

Extrusion is the primary processing method for commercially prepared dry and semi-moist pet foods. The process itself can be thought of in terms of bread making: mixing, kneading, proofing (rising of the dough), shaping, rising and slicing (**Figure 8-13**). The first step in extrusion cooking is proper preconditioning of the dry mix to start gelatinization of the starches.

The dry mix is fed into the preconditioner by a weighing system that accurately maintains a constant feed rate. The preconditioner contains mixing/conveying paddles (**Figure 8-14**) that mix the dry mix and liquid additions (fat, meat slurries, etc.), along with water and steam to increase the moisture content and prepare the mixture for cooking and forming. Generally, the dry mix and any liquid additions are retained in the preconditioner for about 45 seconds. The preconditioner achieves a 20 to 25% cook of the starch (a measure of the completeness of extrusion cooking). Extrusion provides much more flexibility in processing different formulations than do pelleting or baking technologies (**Box 8-7**).

SINGLE-SCREW EXTRUDERS

Single-screw extruders were originally used in the plastics industry and later converted to all types of food applications and are used by approximately 90% of pet food manufacturers (Rokey, 1995). Extruders come in a variety of sizes from pilot plant prototype machines to large volume machines capable of extruding 12 to 15 tons of food per hour. Single-screw extruders consist of a cylindrical multi-segmented barrel with a single screw that propels, mixes and cooks the material and forces it

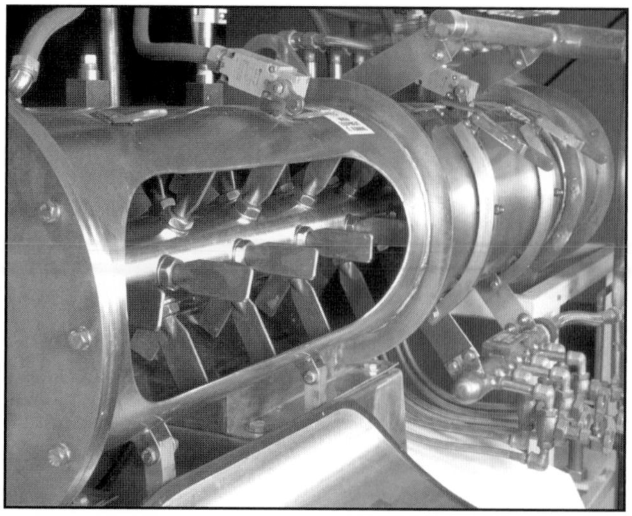

Figure 8-14. Extruder preconditioner used in commercial pet food production. The mixing and conveying paddles shown here initiate starch gelatinization and move the dry mix toward the extruder for cooking.

through a multi-holed die where it is cut to the desired length by a rotating knife (**Figures 8-15** through **8-17**). This type of extruder operates on the principle of friction. The desired cooking of the dough is achieved when the material comes in contact with the barrel wall (Johnson, 1993). The most common type of single-screw extruder used in the pet food industry is called a high shear cooker extruder (Dziezak, 1989).

The process conditions of the single-screw extruder can be adjusted to produce different types of products. For example, a high-fiber, low-fat formula produces significantly more friction, and is therefore more prone to overcooking than more conventional formulas. Reducing the screw speed, screw profile, feed rate or amount of preconditioning, increasing the fat, which helps lubricate the extruder barrel or a combination of these factors will compensate for this processing challenge by reducing the cook time (residence time). Residence times can be varied from 10 to 270 seconds with temperatures ranging from 80 to 200°C (Dziezak, 1989). Because of the ingredient matrix used in pet foods, a high-temperature, short residence time (HTST) approach is used. The benefits of HTST extrusion include: 1) complete cooking, 2) destruction of microorganisms and 3) denaturing of anti-nutritional factors such as trypsin inhibitor and hydrolytic enzymes that lead to rancidity (Dziezak, 1989). Nutrient losses, however, are also incurred because of the high temperatures and shear forces (**Box 8-8**). Vitamin A and E losses of 21 to 26% and thiamin losses of 12% may occur (Frye, 1995). Adding higher levels of these vitamins compensates for losses during extrusion.

TWIN-SCREW EXTRUDERS

Similar to the single-screw extruder, the twin-screw extruder was borrowed from the plastics industry and introduced to the food industry in the early 1970s (Dziezak, 1989). As their name implies, twin-screw extruders have components similar to those of single-screw extruders, except there are two screws. These

Box 8-7. Baking and Pelleting Technology.

The first commercial pet foods were produced using baking technology. Currently, the baking process is used primarily for the manufacture of treats. The baking process uses equipment similar to that used for extrusion in the initial phases. Raw materials need to be finely ground and mixed before they are combined with water to form a "dough." Rollers then flatten the dough as it proceeds to the forming stage called a rotary molding. The dough flows along a conveyor belt where it passes underneath a cylindrical rotor that contains the desired product shape outlines, similar to a large multi-shape cookie cutter. As the dough is "molded" into shapes, the rotor turns and releases the product now cut into shapes. An oven then bakes the product and in the final stages cools it so that it can be packaged.

Shape and product definition in baking are almost always superior to that of extrusion. Because the rotor can be tooled to make any detailed outline with little product expansion, the baked treat can have detail that extruded foods cannot achieve. The baking process, however, is less flexible than extrusion. High-wheat formulations (and, therefore high gluten) are necessary to provide product shape and rigidity. Fat levels must be contained in a relatively small range. Too much fat will inhibit the molding process and too little will cause the newly formed pieces to stick in the rotor. Leavening agents must be used to expand the product and maintain texture.

The pelleting process, which is mainly used to make livestock feeds, is similar to extrusion, but has notable differences. The dry mix must be even more finely ground because the pellet mill has less flexibility in particle size than an extruder. The preconditioning phase is also longer in pelleting because most of the starch gelatinization must occur before product enters the pellet mill. Pressure from pressing the dry mix into the multi-hole die translates to cooking the mix and forming pellets.

The pelleting process is markedly slower and has lower output than extrusion. Ingredient selection and process flexibility are limited in pelleting; the extruder can generate much more cooking energy, thereby allowing addition of internal fat and liquid that is incompatible with pelleting. Because pelleting uses less cooking time than extrusion (two to 16 seconds at 71 to 82°C vs. 10 to 270 seconds at 80 to 200°C), there is a greater risk for microbial growth and production of a non-commercially sterile product. In addition, extruded products are more digestible than pelleted products. The benefit of the pelleting process is its lower cost.

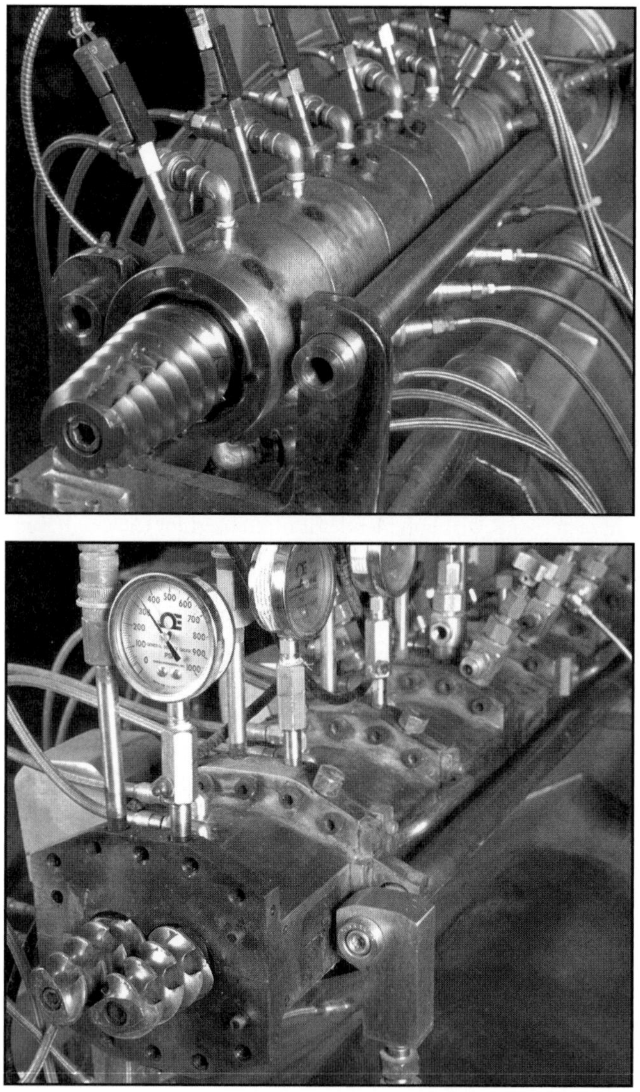

Figure 8-15. Pictures of single- (top) and twin-screw (bottom) extruders. The head of the extruder barrel has been removed showing the screw assemblies. Steam and liquid can be injected directly into the extruder barrel to modify the cooking process.

screws may be co-rotating or counter-rotating, intermeshing or non-intermeshing. The most common twin-screw extruder is the co-rotating, intermesh design (**Figure 8-15**).

The twin-screw design offers benefits over the single-screw extruder because its intermeshing screws mix more thoroughly, transfer more frictional energy and convey the dough forward more effectively. This allows a shorter residence time distribution (i.e., the amount of time the dough is in the extruder barrel) and more uniform cooking. Certain product formulations benefit from twin-screw extrusion. Products that contain a large percentage of internal fat (25%) can be made in the twin-screw extruder, but not in the single-screw extruder because of the lubricating effects of fat. Other products that are difficult to extrude, such as very sticky mixtures or formulas containing fresh meat, are more readily processed in twin-screw extruders because of their increased pumping action and increased cooking ability.

DIE AND KNIFE

The final stage in the extrusion process occurs when the gelatinized dough-like material is forced through the openings of the die. The die is a removable plate with one or more holes of the desired shape that is bolted to the head of the extruder barrel. Die configuration is an important piece of the process because the shape of the openings in the die contributes to the shape of the finished product (**Figure 8-16**). In addition, the die provides the backpressure required for developing shear. The

Box 8-8. Vitamin Losses During Processing and Storage.

In a study conducted by a major supplier of vitamins to the human and pet food industries, investigators analyzed vitamin-fortified extruded and canned pet foods for vitamin levels. The purpose of the study was to examine the processing losses of vitamins and the recommended supplementation guidelines to offset those losses. The foods were sampled before processing, after processing and after three, six, 12 and 18 months of storage. The results are shown in **Tables 1** and **2**.

In the high-moisture environment of moist pet foods, ascorbic acid (vitamin C) was completely unstable even when bound in the protective polyphosphate form. Typically stable vitamins (e.g., riboflavin, niacin, pantothenic acid, choline, vitamin B_{12} and biotin) had good processing resistance with the exception of biotin in moist dog foods. Heat- and moisture-labile vitamins (e.g., thiamin, folic acid and β-carotene) showed losses during the canning process. The fat-soluble vitamins benefit from research into protective coatings that make them much more resistant to processing losses. Storage losses were minimal due to the protective environment of the can.

Polyphosphate-bound ascorbic acid and the water-soluble B vitamins were more resistant during extrusion than in canning. Thiamin and vitamin B_{12} were lost during storage. The fat-soluble vitamins A and E had processing losses, but vitamin A remained stable, unlike vitamin E, through 18 months of storage.

Pet food manufacturers are aware of processing and storage losses of vitamins and overcome these predictable losses by supplementation. Principles of vitamin supplementation of pet foods include: 1) considering the lifestage of the animals to be fed, 2) understanding that vitamins from natural ingredients may be variable or unavailable, 3) meeting the animal's requirements with the supplemented level, 4) considering total levels from supplementation and natural sources to prevent toxicity, 5) considering the energy density of the product and 6) compensating for processing, storage and compounding losses.

Table 1. Vitamin losses (%) incurred during processing and storage of moist dog and cat foods.

	Moist cat food		**Moist dog food**	
Vitamin	**Processing**	**Storage***	**Processing**	**Storage***
Vitamin A	0.0	0.0	10.0	0.0
Vitamin E	0.0	9.2	4.3	10.7
Vitamin B_{12}	5.7	11.3	0.0	0.0
Riboflavin	0.0	38.0	0.0	0.0
Niacin	0.0	31.7	15.1	18.3
Pantothenic acid	0.0	0.0	0.0	0.0
Choline	0.0	-	-	-
Folic acid	0.0	20.0	0.0	14.5
Thiamin	51.7	0.0	52.7	0.0
Pyridoxine	18.5	0.0	88.9	0.0
Biotin	0.0	0.0	55.4	0.0
Vitamin C	100.0	-	100.0	-
β-carotene	43.7	-	57.7	-

*Additional amount of vitamin loss during 18 months of storage.

Table 2. Vitamin losses (%) incurred during processing and storage of dry dog and cat foods.

	Dry cat food		**Dry dog food**	
Vitamin	**Processing**	**Storage***	**Processing**	**Storage***
Vitamin A	16.3	0.0	9.5	0.0
Vitamin E	20.6	31.6	15.4	29.1
Vitamin B_{12}	0.0	38.0	0.0	34.2
Riboflavin	0.0	21.2	0.0	32.0
Niacin	3.3	20.0	0.0	33.6
Pantothenic acid	0.0	4.8	0.0	0.0
Choline	5.5	-	-	-
Folic acid	9.6	23.1	8.5	0.0
Thiamin	11.8	34.2	4.0	57.5
Pyridoxine	11.5	10.0	0.0	0.8
Biotin	0.0	0.0	0.0	0.0
Vitamin C	0.0	12.4	11.1	14.3
β-carotene	19.7	-	34.2	-

*Additional amount of vitamin lost during 18 months of storage.

die is also the final cooking point in the extruder. The number of holes in the die, the shape of the holes and the thickness of the die all contribute to the density, texture and shape of the extrudate (i.e., the material in the extruder). Generally, several die holes will cause less expansion than a single die hole and thicker dies will produce smoother kibbles.

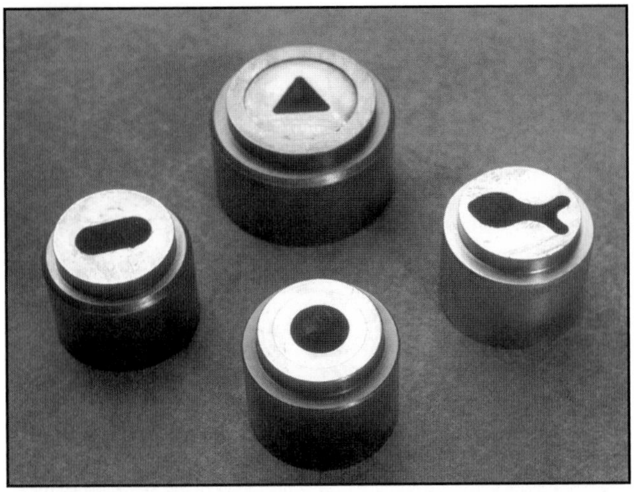

Figure 8-16. Various die inserts can be fitted into the plate at the end of the extruder barrel. The shape of the die will determine the shape of the dry kibble pieces. The dies shown here will produce oval, round, triangular or fish-shaped pieces.

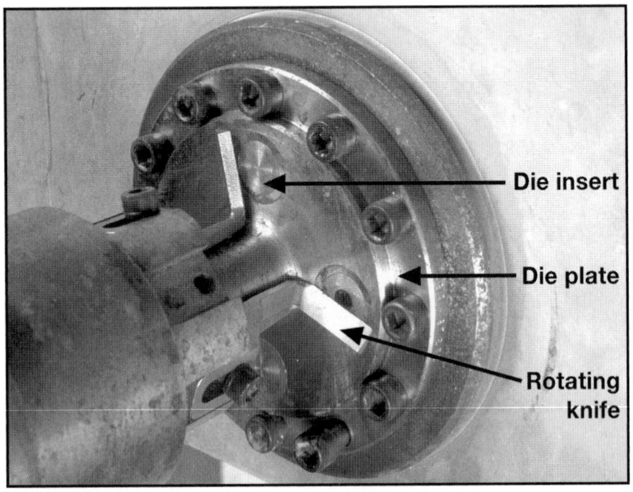

Figure 8-17. Rotating knives fit flush onto the plate at the end of the extruder barrel. The speed of rotation determines the length of the individual food pieces.

The temperature of the extrudate is between 100 to 200°C. It contains approximately 25 to 27% moisture and is under tremendous pressure (i.e., 34 to 37 atmospheres) (Dziezak, 1989). When the extrudate encounters ambient pressure and temperature at the die, moisture is flashed off, expanding the product (i.e., at least 50% greater than the die diameter) and creating the characteristic porous texture of dry pet food. The loss of between 3 to 5% moisture markedly cools the product and helps retain its shape (Colonna et al, 1989).

The extrudate resembles a rope as it leaves the die. A knife assembly on the face of the die is used to cut the extrudate to the desired size (**Figure 8-17**). The design and sharpness of the knife are critical to product appearance and size. The multi-bladed knife assembly rotates at high speed shearing off the "rope," creating kibbles. The speed the knife assembly rotates determines the length of the kibbles.

Drying/Cooling

The high-moisture, soft, spongy kibbles are conveyed by air to the dryer. During this conveyance, the kibbles lose another 2 to 3% moisture. The primary purpose of the dryer is to remove another 10 to 15% moisture from the kibbles. Heated air draws moisture out of the center of the kibble through the external surface where the moisture evaporates into the atmosphere. Reducing product moisture to between 8 and 10% inhibits mold and bacterial growth, thereby improving product shelf life.

Two types of dryers are commonly used in the production of pet foods: horizontal bed dryers and vertical bed dryers. Horizontal bed dryers are usually long rectangular machines that contain an inlet with a swing feeder, a slow-moving conveyor belt and an exit (**Figure 8-18**). Horizontal bed dryers can be single or multiple pass, meaning that the product makes one pass through or, in the case of a double-pass dryer, the product tumbles from one level and doubles back before exiting.

Vertical dryers are typically tall box-shaped machines that contain several levels or "decks" to support the newly extruded pet food as it cascades from the top to the bottom of the unit. These decks separate the product so that the drying profile can be varied to meet the needs of a specific product. Each deck uses a controlled discharge grid that can be cycled to allow all or part of the product on that deck to flow down to the next level using gravity.

Various zones of either type of dryer can be heated to different temperatures to optimize drying. The first zones are usually heated to about 80 to 100°C where the product is warmed and then moved into primary drying zones with temperatures of 120 to 150°C. Finally, the kibbles are cooled to 80 to 100°C before they exit the dryer. The typical retention time in a double-pass dryer with a cooling zone is 15 minutes for drying and seven minutes for cooling (Colonna et al, 1989).

Bed depth (height of the product on the conveyor belt or dryer deck), zone temperature, retention time and humidity all influence drying of pet food products. If the initial zones are too hot, the external surface of the kibble will dry too quickly sealing in moisture, which is known as "case-hardening." As the moisture migrates through the external surface, microfissures can form that will make the kibble more fragile, leading to breakage and excess fine particles (fines) during and after packaging. If the product is too hot as it exits the dryer and is packaged without proper cooling, condensation will occur, creating an environment that encourages mold and bacterial growth.

Enrobing

Enrobing is the process by which coatings, either liquid or dry, are applied to the kibbles in the final step before packaging. For example, coatings may be applied in a rotating drum (**Figure 8-19**) to which liquids (usually fat, flavor enhancers or both) are added in predetermined amounts. Fat is usually added in the enrobing step because it disrupts starch gelatinization and adversely affects expansion of the product. Flavor enhancers have their greatest effect upon palatability when they are applied topically. Three to four times the amount of enhancer may be needed if applied internally to achieve the same effect if applied topically. As the drum turns, the product tumbles upon itself further coating each kibble. When dry coatings are used, a fat coating is applied first to help the dry mixture adhere to the kibbles, which are then tumbled similarly.

Packaging

Dry pet food packaging increases shelf life, protects the food from infestation and provides product information. Classically, the package of choice for dry pet foods is the bag, which can contain as little as 100 g of product for use as samples or up to 20 kg or more of product for sale in mass merchandising outlets and warehouses. Filling machines come in a variety of sizes and capacities to handle various package sizes and shapes. The process is usually automated and calibrated to ensure that the fill weight matches the guaranteed weight on the package label. An overage of 0.5 to 2% is not uncommon to ensure weight compliance.

An important consideration in choosing packaging is the type and amount of fat in the product to be packaged. As the fat percentage increases, protection from "grease out" must also increase. Grease out is caused by fat leaching out of the kibble through the bag, leaving grease stains on the bag surface. It is, therefore, of cosmetic concern and an indication of packaging integrity, and doesn't necessarily indicate rancidity or compromised product quality. The lamination of a polyethylene, or polypropylene, inner liner at a thickness proportional to the amount of fat, a natural paper middle liner and a clay-coated outer liner protect against grease out. Another consideration is the saturation of the fat used. Vegetable oils, because of their high degree of unsaturation, are liquid even at low temperatures and tend to migrate out of the kibble into the surrounding packaging. This process is accelerated if the kibble has rough or sharp edges that puncture the bag liner. Grease out may also occur more readily in conditions of high temperature during storage and distribution. Failure to compensate for these effects will lead to grease out and unsightly, stained packages.

Dry pet food products are increasingly found in nontraditional packaging. Milk cartons, buckets and jugs are just a few examples seen in retail outlets. A consideration when using alternative packaging is the effect the material has on the flavor or odor of the food. Some plastics used in packaging materials impart "off" flavors that decrease palatability.

Modified atmosphere packaging can be used to limit oxidation of fats in pet foods. Such packaging materials have a polymer with barrier properties that preclude diffusion of air including oxygen through to the kibbles. The significant reduction in gas exchange also allows for the use of nitrogen as a flushing agent, just before sealing the package, to remove oxygen from the bag, which further reduces product oxidation. This is particularly helpful with dietary fats (e.g., eicosapentaenoic acid and docosahexaenoic acid), which are highly susceptible to oxidation.

Principles of Semi-Moist Manufacturing

Extrusion

The pre-extrusion equipment used to manufacture semi-moist pet foods is very similar to that used in dry product manufacturing. Because of the higher moisture levels and humectants in semi-moist foods, extruders are generally configured to produce lower cooking temperatures and lower die pressures than found in dry product processing. These requirements are ideal for the twin-screw design, but single-screw extruders may be used. Post-extrusion equipment differs because the product does not go through the drying step, but rather goes through low agitation coating drums where water, humectants and acids are added, then through a cooler (refrigerated air) to set the product's structure and retain the high moisture content and spongy texture.

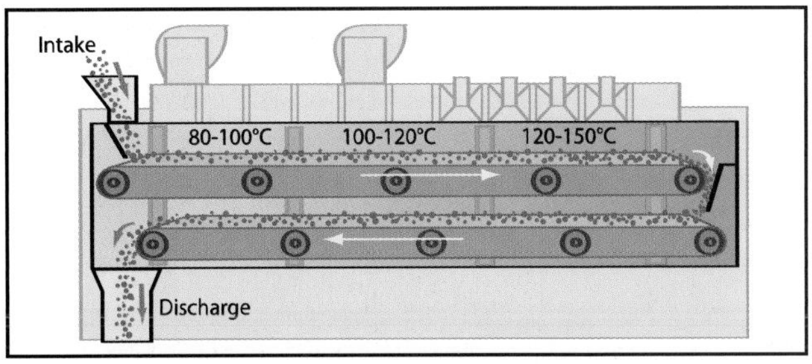

Figure 8-18. Diagram depicting pet food dryer components. Freshly extruded kibbles enter the dryer and pass through heating zones on the upper conveyor, tumble to the next conveyer, pass through the cooler zones and finally exit the dryer. (Adapted with permission, Aeroglide Corporation, Raleigh, North Carolina.)

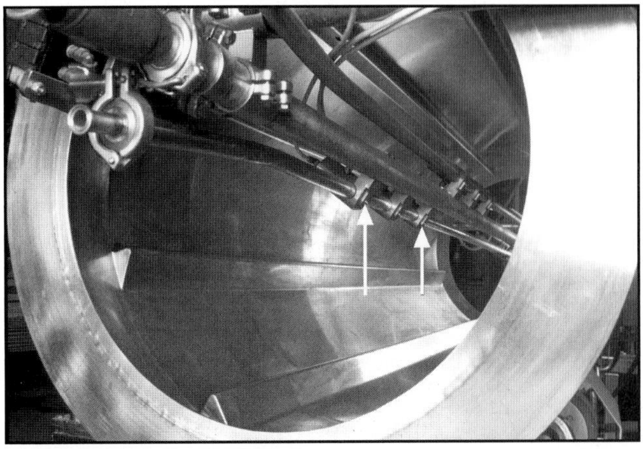

Figure 8-19. Rotating coating drum used for applying fat and flavor enhancers to dry food. Nozzles (arrows) spray the appropriate ingredient while the product tumbles upon itself further coating each kibble.

Mold Inhibition

Semi-moist pet foods are high in moisture (25 to 35%) and, as such, are more prone to spoilage from mold and bacteria. In addition, semi-moist foods are susceptible to moisture loss leading to loss of product integrity and texture. Semi-moist products are formulated with mold and bacterial inhibitors and humectants to retain moisture and packaged in moisture-proof barrier packaging.

The measurement of how susceptible a product is to mold growth is called a_w, or water activity. It is defined as the amount of moisture available for microbial growth and is calculated

Table 8-10. Relationship between water activity and microbial growth.*

Water activity (a_w)	Phenomenon
0.90	Lower limit for general growth of bacteria (e.g., *Salmonella, Clostridium and Lactobacillus* species)
0.80	Lower limit for most enzymatic activity and growth of most fungi
0.60	Lower limit for osmophilic/xerophilic yeast and fungi
0.55	DNA becomes disordered, no growth possible

*Adapted from Bush A. Encyclopaedia of Food Science, Food Technology and Nutrition, vol. 3. London, UK: Academic Press Ltd, 1993; 1490.

Box 8-9. Maillard Reactions.

The Maillard reactions (nonenzymatic browning reaction) between protein and reducing sugars can deteriorate the nutritional quality of foods during processing or storage by affecting the availability of some amino acids. The reaction occurs when reducing sugars, such as glucose, fructose, lactose or maltose, combine with free amino groups found on amino acids such as lysine. Heat accelerates the reaction. Digestive enzymes cannot cleave the peptide bonds adjacent to an amino acid that has a sugar attached to it. Lysine typically can be made unavailable through Maillard reactions with the reducing sugars found in most pet foods. Maillard products may also increase microbial degradation of taurine in the large intestine. Amino acid and sugar Maillard reaction products are generally not absorbed or if they are absorbed they are typically excreted in the urine and are of no nutritional value to the animal. On the other hand, controlled Maillard reactions can be used during the cooking process to produce desirable flavors, colors or aromas.

In addition to Maillard reactions, heat and alkaline pH may result in unusual cross-linking of certain amino acids and peptides that are not normally found naturally. Examples such as lysinoalanine (lysine linked with alanine), lanthionine (cysteine linked with alanine) or ornithoalanine (ornithine linked with alanine) may be formed. These compounds are not used well by animals, thus they reduce the protein quality of the food. This type of amino acid cross-linking may occur during the processing of dried meat meals, ingredients often used in pet foods. However, Maillard binding of amino acids only becomes a practical nutritional problem when the amino acid is limiting. When lysine is abundant, the protein quality is not significantly degraded.

using the following formula:

a_w = % Equilibrium Relative Humidity ÷ 100.

The value for a_w is a number between 0.0 and 1.0 and is obtained using a glass jar containing the product and a humidity probe. The product is allowed to equilibrate in varying levels of humidity, which are then measured and the a_w calculated. Each strain of mold or bacteria has an a_w value at which growth is no longer possible (Bush, 1993). **Table 8-10** describes the effect of a_w upon microbial growth.

Water activity, not moisture content, becomes more important in semi-moist pet foods. Most semi-moist pet foods have high moisture contents (>30%), but relatively low a_w values because added humectants bind free water making it unavailable for microbial growth. Early preservation techniques such as salting or adding sugar lowered the a_w value of meats and, therefore, increased the shelf life stability of those foods. Common pet food humectants include: 1) high-fructose corn syrup, 2) salt, 3) propylene glycol, 4) glycerol, 5) sorbitol and 6) other polyols. Adding large amounts of humectants results in an a_w value of around 0.70, which will inhibit most microbial growth. In the United States, the Food and Drug Administration has removed propylene glycol from GRAS (generally recognized as safe) status for use in cats (Christopher et al, 1989) because of its potential toxic effects. Manufacturers in the United States have responded by removing propylene glycol in favor of glycerin or polyols. To add a margin of safety, antimycotic agents (e.g., sorbate, propionate salts or both) are added in small amounts to inhibit growth of resistant organisms. In addition, acids (phosphoric, hydrochloric, etc.) may be added to lower a food's pH to maximize antimycotic effects.

Semi-Moist Packaging

Exposure to ambient air markedly increases moisture loss in semi-moist foods. About 50% loss occurs over a 24-hour period and much of that in the first four hours. Moisture loss affects product plasticity, and therefore palatability, creating a hard, crystalline structure considerably tougher than that of dry products. Barrier packaging retains moisture that is critical to maintaining shelf life.

Most feline semi-moist products are packaged in a polypropylene inner layer bound to an aluminum foil layer that inhibits diffusion of water molecules. Most manufacturers use this type of inner layer regardless of the type of outer packaging (pouch, canister, etc.). Canine products usually contain less moisture (around 25%) but contain large amounts of sugars to control the water activity. Because the a_w value and moisture are lower in these products, the packaging can be less stringent. Nonpermeable polypropylene pouches without the foil membrane are often used.

Principles of Canning

The Frenchman Nicholas Appert invented canning as a method of food preservation in 1810 in response to the French government's need for preserved foods to support its military campaigns (Lopez, 1987). Later work by Louis Pasteur showed the relationship between processing and the reduction of food spoilage. In the 1920s, the toxic effects of mesophilic bacteria such as *Clostridium botulinum* (anaerobic spore-former) were documented and the importance of controlling these species with heat and pH was first understood.

Canning is a time/temperature-dependent process that can be adjusted to create different textural results with the ultimate goal being to achieve commercial sterility. Lower temperatures will require more time to attain proper core temperatures; conversely, higher temperatures require less time to achieve sterilization. Because of high process temperatures and vacuum conditions in cans, canning destroys aerobic and anaerobic bacteria, making it the best method to preserve high-moisture foods for extended periods.

One newer method is the increasing use of foil pouches that most often contain a single serving of food. Products packaged in pouches usually contain increased moisture levels compared to that of loaf style cans. The high moisture content allows foods to be poured from the package into the feeding bowl. Pouches meet the needs of consumers who desire easy to store foods and single serving freshness. However, pouches increase the cost of feeding compared to dry or conventionally canned foods.

Product Form

Several types of moist pet food products and various sizes and shapes of packaging materials exist. Early canned dog foods were composed primarily of ground offal and horsemeat as by-products of the human food industry. These products were high in protein, fat and moisture and were similar in appearance to pâté. More contemporary forms include chunk and gravy, flaked, ground meat and shredded, all of which mimic foods consumed by people.

"Loaf" products contain some carbohydrate sources (corn, rice, etc.) that balance the amount of protein and fat. These products are usually lower in moisture, and because of the structural properties that starch imparts, are found in finely formed loaves. Vegetable gums and other hydrocolloid thickeners are used to create a firmer texture in canned products that contain little carbohydrate. A popular form for moist dog and cat foods is pieces of meat or fish in jelly. These products may range in form from a finely ground pâté in jelly to large chunks of meat suspended in aspic (e.g., jelly mold). A hygroscopic medium is used to create a two-phase food texture: a "piece" suspended in a medium. The viscosity of the suspension medium can vary from a semi-liquid gravy, to a jellied, savory coating to a solid, suspending jelly.

In manufacturing, the viscosity of the suspension medium is selectively regulated by using different combinations and ratios of hygroscopic sucroglycerides, starches, gums, pectins and alginates. (See Additives.) Many gums and starches are functional food "thickeners" for binding free water into semi-liquid gravies or soft jellies at room temperature. Carrageenan, carboxymethylcellulose, agar, carob, guar, acacia and xanthan gums are examples of thickeners. Pectin and alginates (seaweed derivatives) create more "solid" jellies, suspend pieces and conform to the container to form a loaf. Jellies are often golden and translucent to reveal the internally embedded pieces. Gravies are frequently opaque due to the inclusion of animal tissue meals, caramel coloring or both.

In addition to the water-binding capacity of the jellying agents, the viscosity and specific gravity of the suspension medium should approximate the density of the pieces at processing temperatures. Parity in density will help prevent separating during processing, so the pieces remain suspended.

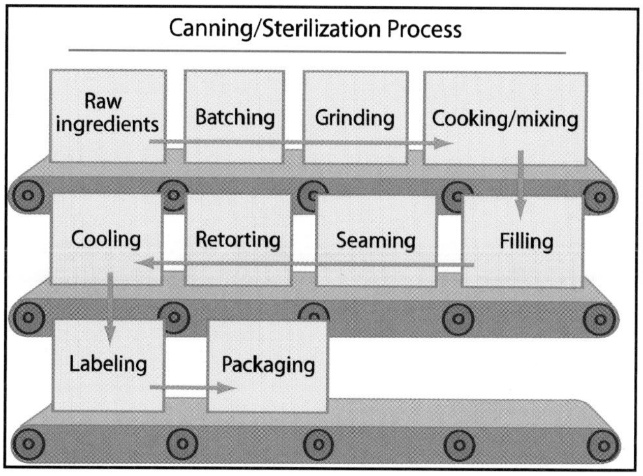

Figure 8-20. Process flow diagram for moist commercial pet food production.

The food pieces may be natural tissues or extruded vegetable and meat proteins. In some pet food markets, intact vegetable matter such as peas and carrots have consumer appeal. These elements can be natural or made from textured vegetable protein. Diced pieces can originate from large, flat cakes made from dough premix.

Canning Process

The canning process is usually continuous flow, highly automated and carefully controlled. Fresh and/or frozen meats are: 1) ground, 2) may or may not be mixed with grains, 3) subjected to steam and water, 4) filled into cans, 5) sealed and sterilized with a pressure cooking device, 6) cooled, 7) labeled and 8) put in cases (**Figure 8-20**).

MEATS/ANIMAL PROTEIN GRINDING

One of the major ingredients of any moist pet food is the animal protein component. Fresh meats and meat by-products require frequent shipments, a large refrigerated area for storage and a system of "just-in-time" manufacturing that uses the ingredients quickly to reduce waste and spoilage and assure freshness. Frozen meats require a very large freezer storage capacity and specialized grinding equipment, but offer the manufacturer flexibility in ingredient use.

Generally, meats, whether fresh or frozen, require grinding before canning and sterilization. In a continuous canning process using frozen ingredients, a predetermined sequence and amount of meat is fed into a machine that chips the frozen blocks of meat into smaller portions. The chipped meat is then conveyed to the final grinding step where it is forced through a plate that contains many one-fourth- to three-fourth-inch openings. The mechanical shear grinds the frozen meats and begins the thawing process. If multiple meat sources are used, meats may require mixing to create a homogeneous blend. The meat mixture then proceeds to a cooking step that increases the temperature of the product to a level appropriate for processing.

In a batch process, the ingredients are measured by weight, ground and placed into a cooker/mixer in one large batch. The

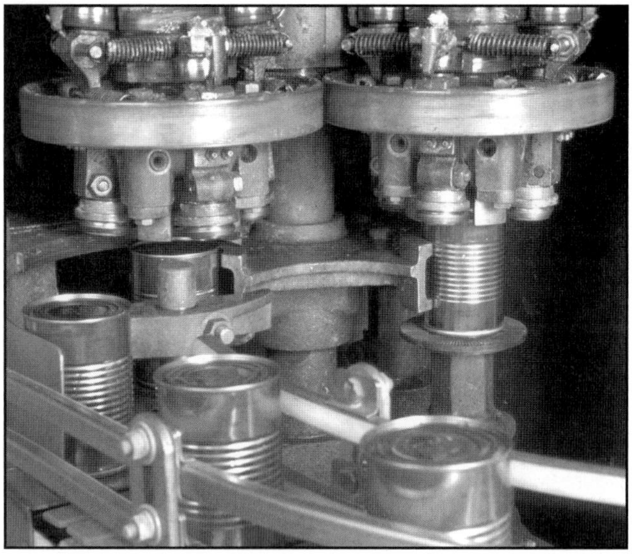

Figure 8-21. As individual cans rotate, the filler/seamer fills the can and then places and seams the lid.

process is repeated as necessary to achieve the desired amount for the manufacturing run.

COOKER/MIXER

The cooker/mixer plays a critical role in the processibility, texture and flavor of the final product. In this step, the meat mixture can be blended with pre-ground or blanched grains, starches, gums, vitamin and mineral premixes and water to complete the formulation. In addition, the entire mixture is heated to specific temperatures (25 to 85°C) to gelatinize starches and begin protein denaturation, which affects the texture, flowability and flavor of the product (**Box 8-9**). The ingredients are mixed and propelled forward in the cooker/mixer by a screw that controls the speed at which the mixture travels, and therefore, the degree of cooking.

In general, high-carbohydrate moist products will require higher processing temperatures (>70°C) to fully hydrate the starch component and maintain viscosity. When the mixture does not attain appropriate viscosity, a condition known as "spin-out" occurs. As the cans are sealed the machine rotates the cans at high speeds developing centrifugal forces. If the viscosity is low, the mixture cannot "hold" ingredients like cracked corn or rice and they will migrate to the edge of the can's contents creating a product with a tough exterior and a soft interior.

Lower temperatures (<55°C) are needed to create the proper viscosity for processing formulations high in animal tissue. Excessive cooker/mixer temperature will ruin the texture of the product after sterilization.

FILLER/SEALER

The hot mixture is usually transported to a heated storage reservoir above the filler/seamer machine. The filler/seamer is a high capacity machine (300 to 1,000 cans/min.) that fills the cans, places a lid on each can and seams the lid (**Figure 8-21**). To create the vacuum necessary for commercial sterility, steam is injected over the product just before sealing. Steam effectively displaces air and after the can is sterilized and cooled, water vapor condenses and contracts, creating a relative vacuum. The steam injection step is not required if the product is hot enough to generate water vapor to displace the air in the can.

The filling/sealing process is precisely controlled to prevent potentially hazardous conditions. The closure step on any moist pet food container is critical to ensure the product's stability. Underfilled cans will be underweight and subject to regulatory action. In addition, vacuum difficulties may lead to increased oxidation resulting in fat and vitamin destruction and product discoloration. Overfilled cans lack sufficient headspace to create a vacuum, thus the lid may improperly seal resulting in product spoilage and distended cans. Cases are stamped with a date code that identifies the year, month, day and time of production. This information may be coded or in "open" form that is easily recognized. Reputable manufacturers will provide decoding information for those who call their toll-free numbers.

STERILIZATION/RETORTING

After filling and sealing is completed, the cans are sterilized in a machine called a retort. The main objectives in retorting products are to preserve the food and achieve commercial sterility. Commercial sterility is defined as the conditions in which heat processing frees a product of microorganisms of public health significance (i.e., pathogens) (Lopez, 1987). This is not to be confused with complete sterility in which all pathogenic and nonpathogenic microorganisms are killed. The main pathogen of concern is *C. botulinum*, a rod-shaped, spore-forming, mesophilic anaerobe that produces a neuroparalytic exotoxin that causes botulism. *C. botulinum* is destroyed by temperatures above 116°C and will not grow in acidic conditions (pH <4.6). In general, process temperatures should be at least 121°C for a minimum of three minutes to kill pathogenic bacteria.

Manufacturers must document process times and temperatures for each formula produced. This time/temperature relationship can be established by process testing using cans of the formula that have thermocouples attached so that internal temperature at the coldest spot can be measured. More time is needed at lower temperatures to kill the same organism. As an example, process temperatures of 121°C for three minutes are equivalent to 100°C for six hours. The relationship is established when the temperature at the coldest spot is greater than 116°C for the required time.

Various pressure-cooking devices (retorts) are available. All retorts follow the same basic process steps, or "phases," that ensure commercial sterility: 1) bring-up phase, 2) sterilization phase and 3) cooling phase. The bring-up phase uses hot water or steam to gradually heat the can contents to 80 to 100°C. In the sterilization phase, pressurized steam or water at temperatures between 116 and 129°C raise and maintain the temperature of the can above 116°C, long enough (60 to 90 min.) to kill all pathogenic bacteria. The cool-down phase (80 to 100°C) starts the cooling process. The cooling phase uses water at a temperature of 18 to 25°C, depending on the retort used. The cans are cooled to between 32 and 40°C to allow non-mechanical drying of the outside of the can and to prevent rusting.

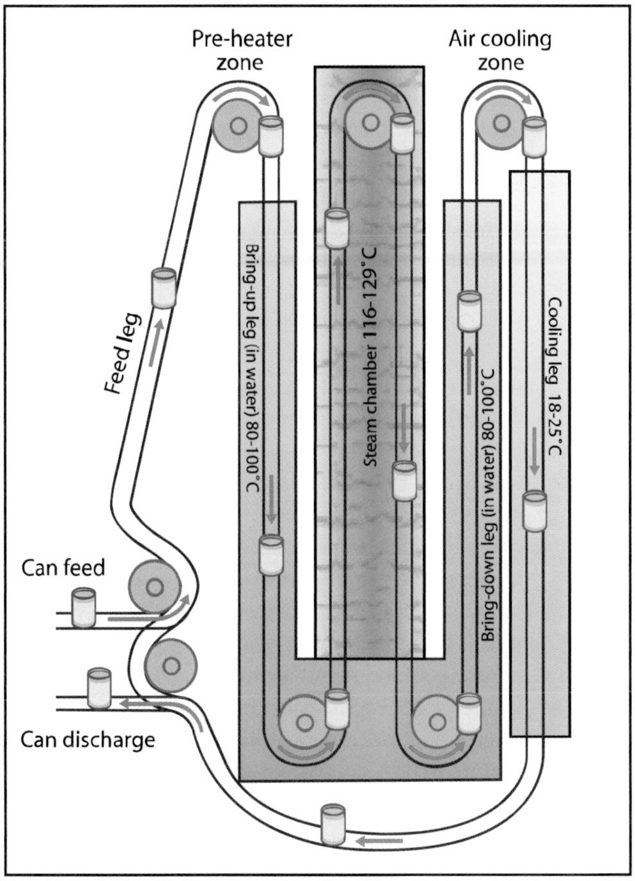

Figure 8-22. A diagram of the continuous process flow of the hydrostatic retort. Cans enter the feed leg and are brought up to temperature in the bring-up leg, then enter the sterilization leg (steam chamber) where the product is sterilized and finally enter the bring-down leg and cooling leg where the cooling process is completed.

These temperatures are not hot enough to continue cooking the cans' contents.

RETORTS

Retorts have been designed to process all types of packages from baby food jars to cans that hold more than 3 kg of fruit or vegetables. Several types of retorts are used by the pet food industry, but hydrostatic and batch retorts are most common.

The hydrostatic retort is a continuous process machine that conveys the cans on carriers that are connected to a chain drive in a tower layout. The cans advance through the various legs of the process in a continuous loop transitioning from water to steam and back to water again (**Figure 8-22**). This type of sterilization method is called hydrostatic because the steam pressure, and therefore temperature, is controlled by water pressure in the water legs. Because the cans slowly rotate on their sides throughout the process, the gas bubble is evenly distributed on the outside surface as the cans' contents. This is evident by the uniform appearance of pâté and loaf-type products produced in this manner.

Batch retort sterilizers, as the name implies, are loaded, processed and cooled in a batch-type manner. These sterilizers can be configured vertically or horizontally; the vertical configuration is used most commonly in the pet food industry (**Figure 8-23**). Some batch retorts have three to four baskets that are filled and lowered into the retort for processing. The baskets must then be lifted out of the retort, the cans cooled and sent for labeling. The benefit to this system is that the headspace is kept constant because the cans are oriented vertically without agitation, resulting in a uniform appearance. The disadvantages are that the system is labor intensive and has a low production capacity. This system works well for test batches and pilot work.

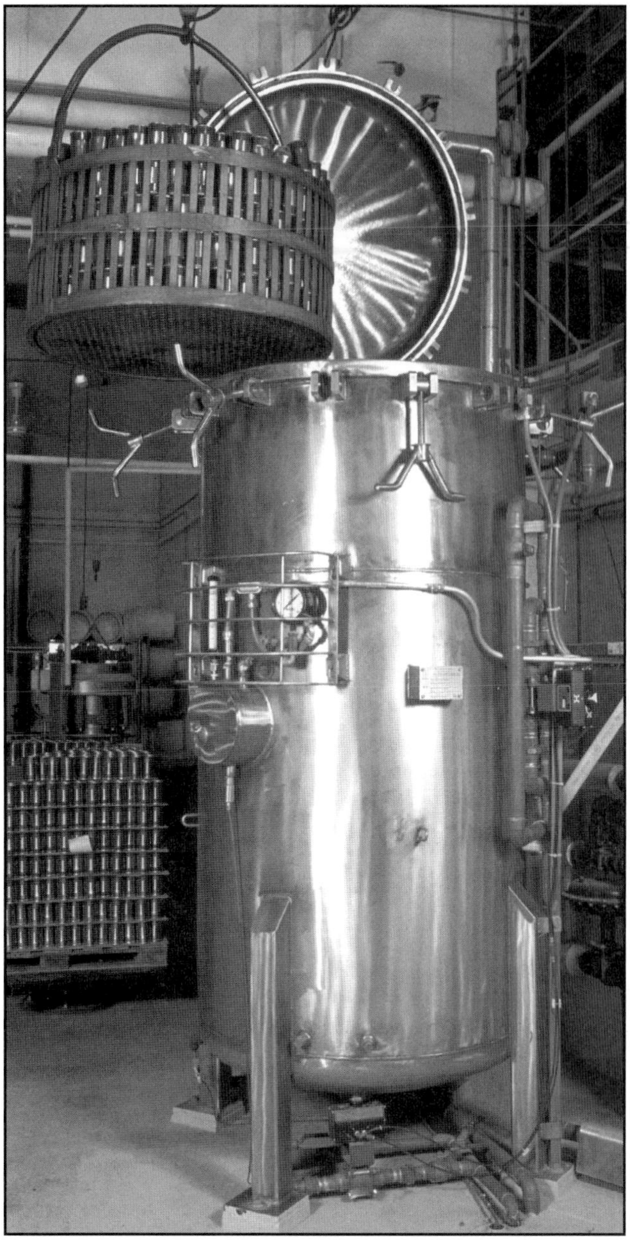

Figure 8-23. In a batch retort sterilizer, cans are loaded, processed and cooled in baskets (batch-type manner) rather than in a continuous process as occurs in hydrostatic retorts.

The automated crateless system is a newer batch retort. In

Table 8-11. Standard accelerated stability tests and their conditions.*

Test	Conditions	Comments
Ambient storage	Room temperature Atmospheric pressure	Too slow
Light	Room temperature Atmospheric pressure	Different mechanism
Metal catalysts	Room temperature Atmospheric pressure	More decomposition
Weight-gain method	30 to 80°C Atmospheric pressure	Endpoint questionable
Schaal oven	60 to 70°C Atmospheric pressure	Fewest problems
Oxygen uptake	80 to 100°C Atmospheric pressure	Different mechanism
Oxygen bomb	99°C 65 to 115 psi O_2	Different mechanism
Active oxygen (AOM)	98°C Air bubbling	Different mechanism
Rancimat	100 to 140°C	Endpoint questionable

*Frankel EN. Trends in Food Science & Technology 1993; 4: 220-225.

this system, cans from the sealer are conveyed to a bank of vertical retorts filled with water and situated over a cooling canal filled with cold water. The first retort loads cans from the top, where they tumble to the bottom and are cushioned by water. When the first retort is filled, the conveyor moves to the next sterilizer and the process is repeated. After the retort is filled with cans, the cushion water removed, the retort vented, the cans sterilized by steam, an unloading valve at the bottom allows the cans to tumble into the cooling canal. The cans are cooled and conveyed forward for labeling and casing. This system has four to five times the capacity of the crate retort system. Product appearance, however, may be inconsistent because the headspace bubble will settle to the top regardless of the can's orientation.

LABELING/CASING

The temperature of cans coming out of the cooling leg will be between 32 and 40°C, which causes rapid evaporation of exterior moisture. The vacuum in the can is a critical quality component that assures seal integrity. Can vacuum is determined with a sensor that scans the tops of the cans just before labeling. If the can lid is convex, the can will be rejected automatically.

The dry cans then proceed to the labeling system, which automatically applies adhesive and the appropriate label at a rate of about 450 to 500 cans per minute.

After labeling, the cans proceed to casing, which is an automated process that orients the cans, prepares the cardboard or paper case from flat stock, loads the appropriate number of cans per case and then seals the case with adhesive at a rate of about 1,000 to 1,300 cases per hour. Date code information is ink-jetted on the case for rapid identification, and the cases are loaded onto pallets for transportation.

QUALITY CONTROL PROCEDURES

Because pet owners depend on people at the distribution outlet (veterinary hospital, pet store, etc.) or word of mouth (breeder, veterinarian, other pet owners) for information about a company or its products, endorsements and company reputation are direct or indirect statements about quality. Quality is a relative term meaning different things to different people.

Quality procedures for manufacture of pet foods are neither required nor regulated. Implementation of a quality program is the sole responsibility of individual pet food manufacturers. Some companies go to the expense of studying and implementing world-class manufacturing processes (benchmarking); others do very little. Some companies use high-quality human and pet food grade ingredients; others purchase the least costly ones. Some companies conduct multiple tests to evaluate the quality of raw ingredients and finished products; others do what is minimally necessary. Some companies submit to voluntary plant inspections; others avoid such evaluations.

The rest of this chapter describes quality-manufacturing procedures that some pet food manufacturers follow in the continuous pursuit of product excellence. The information discussed below should give the reader examples of a quality manufacturing program employed by companies whose reputation is built upon the products and services they provide.

Ingredients and Process

Understanding and controlling raw ingredients and the manufacturing process are the keys to manufacturing a high-quality pet food. A good quality program to ensure raw ingredient integrity is essential. The key elements of such a program include: 1) ingredient specifications, 2) ingredient receiving and testing procedures and 3) ingredient handling procedures at the plant.

The contractual agreement with suppliers should list ingredient specifications including nutrient composition, purity requirements, key analytical criteria and shipping conditions. Receiving procedures at the manufacturing site should include analytical testing of ingredients, physical inspections and checks to ensure raw ingredients are segregated appropriately and maintained properly. Handling procedures after receiving and initial bulk storage are designed to ensure ingredients are not damaged in any fashion. Proper conveyance mechanisms, rodent and insect control procedures and appropriate design of holding vessels to ensure first-in, first-out ingredient flow help eliminate damage and help ensure freshness. Good quality control practices include internal audits of these procedures and systems and audits by a third party, such as the American Institute of Baking.

Attention to the use of high-quality raw ingredients and high-quality processing will ensure a high-quality product. The essential element of a good quality program for the processing of pet foods is a complete understanding of each manufacturing unit's operation and its effect on the attributes of the finished product. Once these effects are understood, critical control points can be established around unit operations and quality systems set up to monitor and ensure conformance. The manufacturing process of pet foods primarily involves proper compounding of raw ingredients and then working this mixture for moist or dry extruded products. Therefore, quality programs must include: 1) calibration procedures for conveying the individual ingredients, 2) proper time and temperature measuring and 3) calibration procedures for the cooking process. For moist products, the sterilization program must be documented and recorded. Detailed records should be kept for each lot of product manufactured, clearly detailing the processing conditions. Routine, clearly documented calibration and correlation programs must be established for each process variable (i.e., weighing or scaling, temperatures, flow rates, etc.). Analytical and physical testing of finished product is another essential element of a good quality program.

Vendors

Pet foods contain numerous raw materials from many suppliers. A vendor quality control program is critical to ensuring receipt of high-quality raw ingredients.

A good quality vendor control program begins with: 1) testing methods for nutrient levels, 2) microbiologic evaluation and 3) toxicity testing. Defining these test methods ensures that multiple vendors of raw ingredients deliver against the same purchasing specification. A routine calibration and correlation program should be established to minimize method and operator variations. A vendor quality program should establish the frequency of analytical testing; however, each lot of an ingredient must be tested initially for moisture, protein and fat, at a minimum, to see if it adheres to ingredient specifications and for accurate compounding. Ingredients should also be routinely analyzed for other nutrients of concern (e.g., calcium, phosphorus, magnesium and sodium).

Beyond the testing required in a purchasing specification, further quality assurance can be attained through programs the food industry calls vendor self-certification. The objective of these programs is to shift the focus from final ingredient shipment testing to building of quality control procedures upstream in the vendors' process. For example, purchasing specifications for cereal grains would include a target value for percent moisture of the grain. Most certification programs require vendors to keep detailed records on the lots of material they purchase. The intent is to encourage vendors to define, understand and control their raw materials and processes so that they manufacture and supply ingredients that will fall within the pet food manufacturer's specifications.

Product Quality

The quality of the finished pet food product is quantified by how well the product meets the formulated nutrient content as well as other critical parameters, such as: 1) consistent appearance, 2) physical integrity, 3) package integrity, 4) adequacy of sterilization and 5) freedom from toxins and microbiologic concerns.

Sampling frequency should be established to ensure that any nonconforming product is identified and removed. This frequency depends on batch sizes, length of storage and normal ingredient variation history. Sampling every 30 minutes for moisture, protein, fat, calcium, phosphorus, sodium, potassium and magnesium to determine variation in the process is a good starting point. Samples can be analyzed either separately or as a composite sample collected over time if the manufacturing process is well controlled.

For dry pet foods, sampling should include: 1) each lot of raw ingredients received, 2) the mix of raw ingredients once compounded (weighed and mixed), 3) the product leaving the extruder, 4) the product leaving the dryer, 5) after any topical enrobing and 6) finished product in the package. For moist pet foods, samples should be taken from: 1) raw materials, 2) product in the cooker/mixer and 3) sterilized product.

Statistical Process Control

To ensure the most consistent quality of the finished product, modern factories use statistical process control in the manufacturing process. Statistical process control determines normal variation through chemical analysis of the product at various points in the process compared with nutrient specifications of the finished product. It also establishes control limits based on this variation.

Variables analyzed can be moisture, protein, fat or any other nutrient of concern for a particular product where consistency is required. Usually, two to three standard deviations from the mean represent the control limits. Adjustments to the manufacturing process are made only when finished product attributes are outside these control limits.

Analytical Tests

Finished products are analyzed to ensure conformity to formulated nutrient content and freedom from toxins and microbiologic concerns. At a minimum, a good quality program should include routine testing to determine percentages of moisture, protein, fat, ash, calcium, phosphorus, sodium, magnesium, potassium and crude fiber. Additionally, incoming raw ingredients and finished products should be tested for *Salmonella* and *Clostridium* species, aflatoxin and vomitoxin.

Each manufacturing facility should have an in-house laboratory that can run the above analyses as the product is produced. The results help operators adjust the process controls to ensure the finished product meets specifications. Faster analytical methods (e.g., near infrared) that can analyze several nutrients simultaneously with speed and accuracy help operators control the process. In addition to chemical analysis, the physical size, density and color should be part of the finished product specifications. In the case of canned pet foods, can seal, product texture and vacuum should be recorded in addition to chemical analysis results.

Shelf Life

Shelf life is the amount of time a product maintains nutritional, microbial, physical and organoleptic (sensory) integrity. The main cause of diminished shelf life in dry products is oxidation.

Fat, either bound in the ingredient matrix or applied to the surface of dry products is subject to the second law of thermodynamics, which states that a system follows an irreversible cascade toward entropy, or disorder. The double bonds of polyunsaturated fatty acids are particularly susceptible to attack by oxygen molecules to form fatty acid radicals and peroxide byproducts. This process is initiated by oxygen and catalyzed by iron, copper, light and warm temperatures to create a series of chemical reactions called auto-oxidation (Robey, 1994; Pappas, 1991; Halliwell, 1994). Unless checked, auto-oxidation will decrease palatability and destroy fat and fat-soluble vitamins. Oxidation does not occur in an environment lacking oxygen; therefore, moist products have a longer shelf life.

There are no recognized industry standards for shelf life. However, reasonable estimates include up to 36 months for moist foods, nine to 12 months for semi-moist foods and 12 to 18 months for dry foods. Although improved packaging technology and development of natural antioxidants (e.g., vitamins E and C, rosemary and citric acid) have increased effectiveness compared to early methods, they still do not preserve dry foods as effectively as synthetic antioxidants. Dry pet foods preserved with natural antioxidants therefore may have a shelf life markedly shorter than 12 to 18 months. Shelf-life information for products should be available from manufacturers, and can be commonly found on product bags or cans.

Antioxidants

Antioxidants are a class of compounds that function as one or more of the following: 1) electron donors, 2) oxygen scavengers, 3) free radical scavengers or 4) hydrogen donors (Pappas, 1991; Hilton, 1989). **Table 8-9** lists common antioxidants used in pet foods. Antioxidants can be synthetic or natural, used in combination with other antioxidants or alone. They also gain synergism with mineral chelators (e.g., citric and ascorbic acid), and emulsifiers (e.g., lecithin, propyl gallate) and have vastly different potencies depending on the matrix being modified and the antioxidant used. Antioxidants bind with free radicals breaking the cascade of auto-oxidation. Synthetic antioxidants (e.g., ethoxyquin and butylated hydroxyanisole [BHA]) are much more effective than the same quantities of natural antioxidants, such as mixed tocopherols or ascorbic acid. Synthetic antioxidants better resist processing losses and are effective longer, thereby extending shelf life.

Shelf-Life Determination

Shelf life in the pet food industry is usually determined through chemical analysis of oxidation products and by sensory evaluation (palatability testing and olfaction). Some of the chemical methods used for oxidation analysis include oxygen uptake, oxygen bomb, Schaal oven technique, active oxygen method and the Rancimat test (**Table 8-11**).

The methods used must be compatible with the types of fat in the food because different fats will give different results when similar analytical methods are used. In addition, most tests for oxidation rely on high temperatures (80 to 140°C), catalysts or oxygen exposure to simulate the oxidation process. These accelerated methods may produce different results than lower temperature, long-term storage tests because the process of oxidation changes dramatically at temperatures above 100°C, but at lower temperatures the results are less confounded (Frankel, 1993). Many of these tests, however, still have practical value to estimate the antioxidant potential of a given product because they can be conducted rapidly and produce results that correlate reasonably well with ambient storage conditions.

Although there is no standard format for shelf-life evaluation, one study incorporated peroxide value analysis and palatability trials in their assessment of different antioxidant systems in dog foods (Gross et al, 1994). Their design used accelerated storage (16 weeks at 48.8 ± 2.2°C) and ambient storage (12 months at 22.2 ± 1.2°C) methodologies. Peroxide values and proximate analyses were determined monthly, and feeding trials were conducted initially and after 16 weeks of accelerated storage and after five months and 12 months of ambient storage. This method of shelf-life determination was sensitive enough to detect oxidation products (rancidity) through both chemical means and reduced palatability scores.

Nutrient Stability

The oxidation cascade not only creates rancidity with its objectionable odors and flavors, but also destroys the functionality of nutrients. Pet foods contain fat, which provides essential fatty acids and the fat-soluble vitamins A, D, E and sometimes K. These compounds can be markedly reduced by oxidation, possibly leading to a food with vitamin deficiencies.

ENDNOTES

a. Data on file. Hill's Pet Nutrition, Inc., Topeka, KS.
b. Laurie D. Hill's Pet Nutrition Inc., Topeka, KS, USA. Personal communication. October 1996.
c. Crane SW. Personal observation. April 1996.

REFERENCES

The References for **Chapter 8** can be found at www.markmorris.org

Chapter 9

Pet Foods Labels

Philip Roudebush
David A. Dzanis
Jacques Debraekeleer
Hilary Watson

"Tell me what you eat and I will tell you what you are."
Anthelme Brillat-Savarin, 1825

INTRODUCTION

The pet food label is an important means by which specific product information is communicated between a manufacturer or distributor and consumers, veterinarians and regulatory officials. Commercial pet foods differ from human food products in that the final consumer, the animal, is not the purchaser. Thus, there are two different "customers" with regards to safety, nutritional balance and palatability. Pet food label information is not directed to the final consumer, but to the owner or veterinarian who decides what the animal will be fed.

Implementation of the Nutrition Labeling and Education Act of 1990 and the Dietary Supplement Health and Education Act of 1994 in the United States has led to increased consumer awareness of the contents and effects of various human foods. Consumer interest in human food label information has increased awareness of information available on pet food labels. The regulations governing pet food labeling are similar to human food labeling rules in many respects, but deviate significantly in some important ways. Thus, veterinarians and pet owners need to understand the rules specific to pet food labeling to obtain and best interpret information about a pet food.

The Label as a Legal Document

The pet food label is more than an attractive package cover designed to sell the product; the pet food label is also a legal document. A number of agencies and organizations regulate the production, marketing and sales of commercial pet foods in different countries. Each agency or organization has different responsibilities with varying degrees of authority (**Table 9-1**). Some of these agencies and organizations regulate the information found on pet food labels whereas others influence the regulatory process.

Pet foods are regulated at their point of sale. As an example, pet food manufactured in the United States for sale outside the United States must meet the labeling requirements established by the country in which the food is sold. Conversely, pet foods manufactured outside the United States must conform to Food and Drug Administration (FDA) and state pet food labeling requirements when sold in the United States.

PET FOOD LABELS IN THE UNITED STATES

Regulation in the United States

Association of American Feed Control Officials

Early regulators recognized the need for uniform and consistent regulation of animal feeds by forming the Association of American Feed Control Officials (AAFCO) in 1909. AAFCO is a private organization, not a regulatory body per se. However, all AAFCO members must be state or federal government officials. Members include animal feed control officials from individual U.S. states and territories, federal agencies such as FDA and government representatives from Canada and Costa Rica.

Table 9-1. Major governing agencies and organizations for commercial pet food manufacturers.

Agency	Key functions
Association of American Feed Control Officials (AAFCO)	Sets nutrient standards for substantiation of claims Provides model regulations for the states Provides ingredient definitions
U.S. Food and Drug Administration (FDA)	Specifies some label requirements Regulates health claims Ensures food safety Approves food additives
U.S. Department of Agriculture (USDA)	Regulates some pet food ingredients Inspects animal research facilities
State Department of Agriculture (or similar agency)	Adopts and enforces animal food regulations
National Research Council (NRC)	Evaluates and compiles nutrition research Makes nutrient recommendations
Pet Food Institute (PFI)	Trade organization that represents major pet food manufacturers in the United States
Canadian Veterinary Medical Association (CVMA)	Administers voluntary product certification in Canada
European Commission	The main legislative body in the European Union responsible for creating new directives and regulations
European Council of Ministers	Approves directives and regulations Creates basic laws
National Government (Ministry of Agriculture)	Implements European legislation and controls its application Houses national experts
European Federation of the Pet Food Industry (FEDIAF = Fédération Européenne de l'Industrie des Aliments pour Aminaux Familiers)	Trade organization that represents major pet food manufacturers in Europe
Confederation of the Food and Drink Industries of the EU (CIAA = Confédération des Industries Agro-Alimentaires de l'UE)	Trade organization that represents human food manufacturers in Europe Works closely with FEDIAF on matters of mutual interest

Representatives from pet food trade associations such as the Pet Food Institute (PFI) and the American Pet Products Manufacturers Association and professional organizations such as the American Veterinary Medical Association, Canadian Veterinary Medical Association and American College of Veterinary Nutrition cannot be members of AAFCO, but do attend AAFCO meetings and often serve as advisors to various AAFCO committees and investigators.

AAFCO provides a forum for local, state and federal feed regulatory officials to discuss and develop uniform and equitable laws, regulations and policies. In that capacity, AAFCO has developed model laws and regulations, which although are not directly enforceable (because AAFCO is not a government agency), have become the foundation for most state laws and regulations for all animal feeds. AAFCO addressed the need for information about pet nutrition and pet food regulations by forming a permanent Pet Food Committee in 1959. Model regulations applying specifically to pet foods were adopted in 1967. Amendments to the AAFCO Model Pet Food Regulations occur frequently as needed to address new information and issues relating to pet foods and nutrition. They have been adopted in various degrees by approximately two-thirds of the states. Today, individual members look to AAFCO for guidance when establishing and revising state laws and regulations.

In addition, AAFCO remains the recognized information source for pet food labeling, ingredient definitions, official terms and standardized feed testing methodology. The Model Pet Food Regulations include calorie content statement guidelines and definition of the pet food descriptive terms "light," "lean" and "reduced calorie." The Pet Food Committee has also developed criteria for the official definition of product "families" whose lead member has been tested via the AAFCO feeding trial protocol.

Many pet owners recognize the need to feed their animals nutritionally balanced pet foods. As a consequence, consumers usually purchase pet foods that are labeled "complete and balanced." One means of ensuring nutritional adequacy of a food requires that the food be formulated so essential nutrients meet specified levels. Nutrient minimums before the early 1990s were based on the recommendations of the National Research Council (NRC). In 1990 and 1991, AAFCO established the Canine Nutrition Expert (CNE) and Feline Nutrition Expert (FNE) Subcommittees to establish updated practical profiles based on commonly used ingredients. The CNE and FNE Subcommittee reports formed the basis for new dog and cat food nutrient profiles to be used as minimum standards for the formulation of dog and cat foods (AAFCO, 2007). Two separate AAFCO profiles exist for each species: one for growth and reproduction, and one for adult maintenance. Lower amounts of some nutrients were established for adult dogs and cats, eliminating unnecessary excesses. In addition, maximum levels were established for some nutrients in dog foods, including calcium, phosphorus, magnesium, fat-soluble vitamins and many trace minerals. Maximum methionine, zinc and vitamin A and D levels were established for cat foods. The AAFCO Dog and Cat Food Nutrient Profiles have replaced NRC recommendations as the basis for the substantiation of label claims.

AAFCO (2007) also publishes minimum feeding protocols

for dog and cat foods. These are minimum testing protocols used by manufacturers for substantiating the nutritional adequacy of pet foods via feeding trials and determining metabolizable energy of dog and cat foods.

Food and Drug Administration

Under the Federal Food, Drug, and Cosmetic Act, the FDA has broad responsibilities, including authority over pet foods. Today, the Center for Veterinary Medicine (CVM), in FDA, regulates pet foods in cooperation with the individual states. FDA is responsible for: 1) establishing certain animal food labeling regulations, 2) specifying certain permitted ingredients such as drugs and additives, 3) enforcing regulations about chemical and microbiologic contamination and 4) describing acceptable manufacturing procedures. Feed control officials within each state inspect facilities and enforce these regulations. Health claims on pet food labels or literature accompanying the product are subject to regulation by CVM. A health claim is defined as the assertion or implication that consumption of a food will treat, prevent or otherwise affect a disease or condition (Dzanis, 1994).

United States Department of Agriculture

The United States Department of Agriculture (USDA) is responsible for ensuring that pet foods are labeled so they are not mistaken for human foods. The USDA inspects animal ingredients used in pet foods to ensure proper handling and to guarantee that such ingredients are not used in human foods. The USDA also inspects and regulates animal research facilities. All animal research facilities owned and operated in the United States by pet food companies must fulfill USDA requirements for: 1) record keeping, 2) physical structure, housing and care of animals, 3) food and water quality and 4) sanitation. Research facilities are subject to unannounced inspections by USDA officials at least annually.

National Research Council

The NRC is a private, nonprofit organization that evaluates and compiles research conducted by others. The NRC functions as the working arm of the National Academy of Sciences, the National Academy of Engineers and the Institute of Medicine (Phillips, 1992). The National Academy of Sciences was created in 1863 to advise the United States federal government about scientific and technological matters (Phillips, 1992). The NRC was created in 1916 in response to the increased need for scientific and technical services during World War I (Phillips, 1992). The NRC is not part of the United States government, is not an enforcement agency and is not a basic research organization with laboratories of its own.

The NRC includes a Board on Agriculture and Natural Resources. One of the major activities of the Board has been the development of nutrient requirement recommendations for domestic animals. Numerous ad hoc committees have assisted in developing the series, *Nutrient Requirements of Domestic Animals*. As part of that series, a new edition of *Nutrient Requirements of Dogs and Cats* was published in 2006 (NRC, 2006). Before that, the most current NRC recommendations for dogs and cats were published in 1985 and 1986, respectively (1985, 1986). Before the development and acceptance of AAFCO's Dog and Cat Food Nutrient Profiles, the NRC publications on nutrient requirements for normal dogs and cats were the recognized authority for substantiation of label claims on commercial pet foods. The AAFCO Dog and Cat Food Nutrient Profiles have replaced the NRC recommendations as the standard to be used by pet food manufacturers in the United States for formulating foods for normal dogs and cats.

Currently, pet food labels in the United States that make reference to NRC nutritional recommendations are considered to be misbranded. The NRC recommendations are still used by some pet food manufacturers in countries other than the United States and reference to NRC is still found on some pet food labels. With the most recent NRC edition, it is anticipated that AAFCO will reconvene its expert panel to review and update the AAFCO Dog and Cat Food Nutrient Profiles in light of the new NRC recommendations. AAFCO is not expected to reinstate the NRC recommendations as the authority cited on pet food labels.

Pet Food Institute

The PFI was organized in 1958 as the national trade association of dog and cat food manufacturers in the United States. Active members of PFI produce 95% of the total dog and cat food tonnage in the United States (PFI, 1994). Affiliate members of PFI include the leading suppliers of equipment, ingredients, packaging and services to the United States pet food industry.

PFI works closely with veterinarians, humane groups and local animal control officers to sponsor public affairs and owner education programs that encourage responsible dog and cat ownership. It also represents the industry before legislative and regulatory bodies at the federal and state levels. In the past 20 years, PFI has sponsored research on amino acid requirements of dogs and cats, as well as research on the benefits of pet ownership and the beneficial role of pets in society.

Individual States

Each individual state is responsible for adopting and enforcing pet food regulations. Many, but not all, states have adopted pet food regulations that follow the model bill and model regulations established by AAFCO. The State Department of Agriculture, Regulatory Protection Division or State Chemist administers pet food regulation and enforcement in most states.

Label Design

A pet food label is divided into two main parts: 1) the principal display panel and 2) the information panel (**Figure 9-1**). The principal display panel is defined by FDA as "the part of a label that is most likely to be displayed, presented, shown or examined under customary conditions of display for retail sale." The principal display panel is the primary means of attracting the consumer's attention to a product and should immediately communicate the product identity. The information panel is defined as "that part of the label immediately contiguous

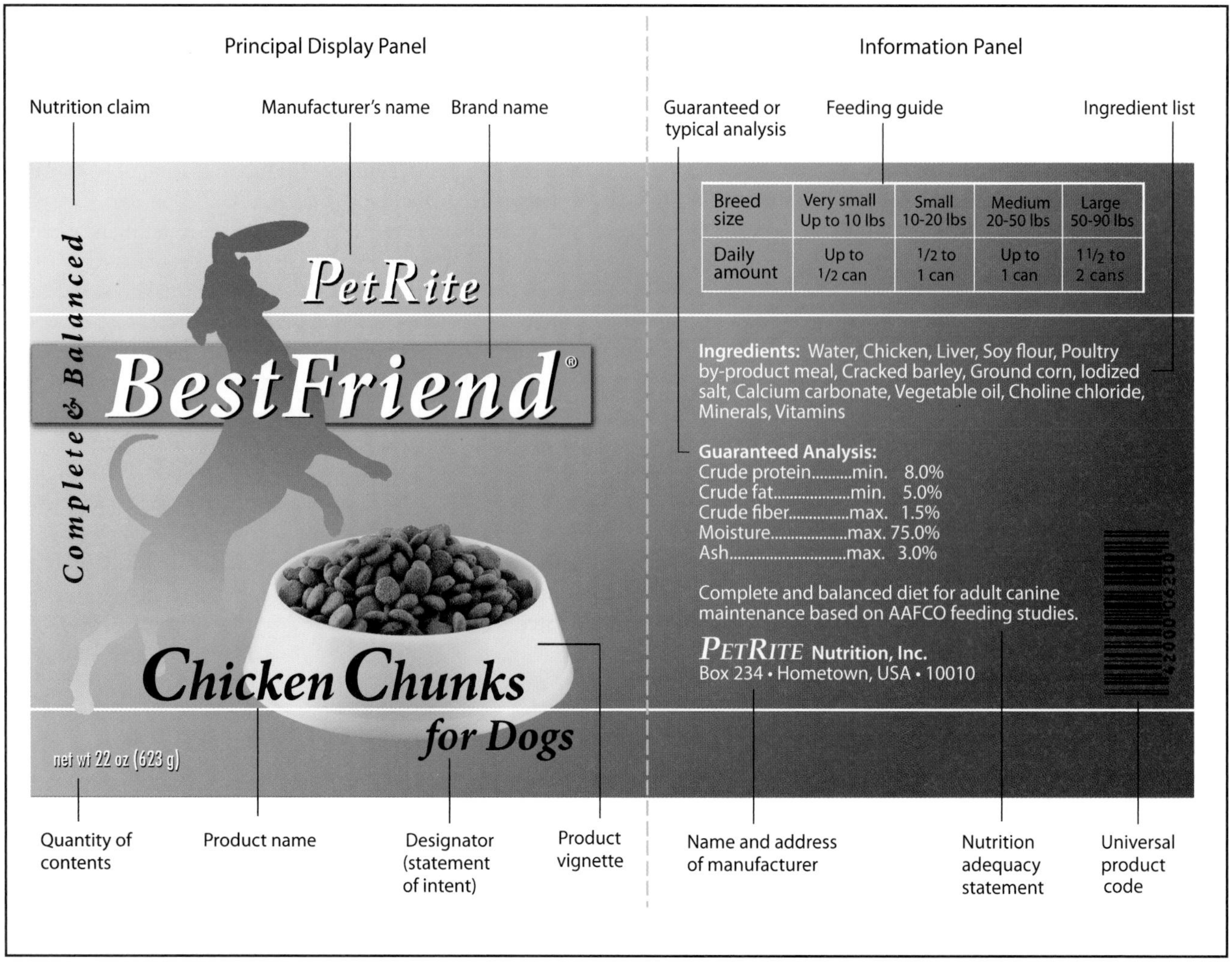

Figure 9-1. Typical pet food label with all elements.

Table 9-2. Key elements found on pet food labels in the United States and Canada.

Principal display panel	Information panel
Product identity	Ingredient statement*
Manufacturer's name	Guaranteed analysis*
Brand name	Nutritional adequacy or nutritional purpose statement (product description)*
Product name*	
Designator (intended species)*	Feeding guidelines*
Net weight*	Statement of calorie content
Product vignette	Manufacturer or distributor*
Nutrition claim	Universal product code
Bursts and flags	Batch information
	Freshness date

*Elements required on pet food labels in the United States, on labels certified by the CVMA Program and in some other countries.

and to the right of the principal display panel" (FDA) and usually contains important information about the product. In the United States and some other countries, several items are required by law to be included on the principal display and information panels (**Table 9-2**). The following discussion will focus on the major features found on these two portions of the pet food label.

Principal Display Panel

PRODUCT IDENTITY

The product identity is the primary means by which a specific pet food is identified by consumers. In the United States, the product identity must legally include a product name but may also include a manufacturer's name, a brand name or both. The brand name is the name by which pet food products of a given company are identified and usually conveys the overall image of the product. The product name provides information about the individual identity of the particular product within the brand. The manufacturer or distributor is not required to include its name as part of the product identity on the principal display panel, but must include its name and address on the label.

Initial assessment of pet foods is best determined by looking at the product name on the principal display panel. The product name is usually descriptive of the food and in the United States is subject to AAFCO regulations about composition of ingredients. Percentage rules are important; beef ingredients

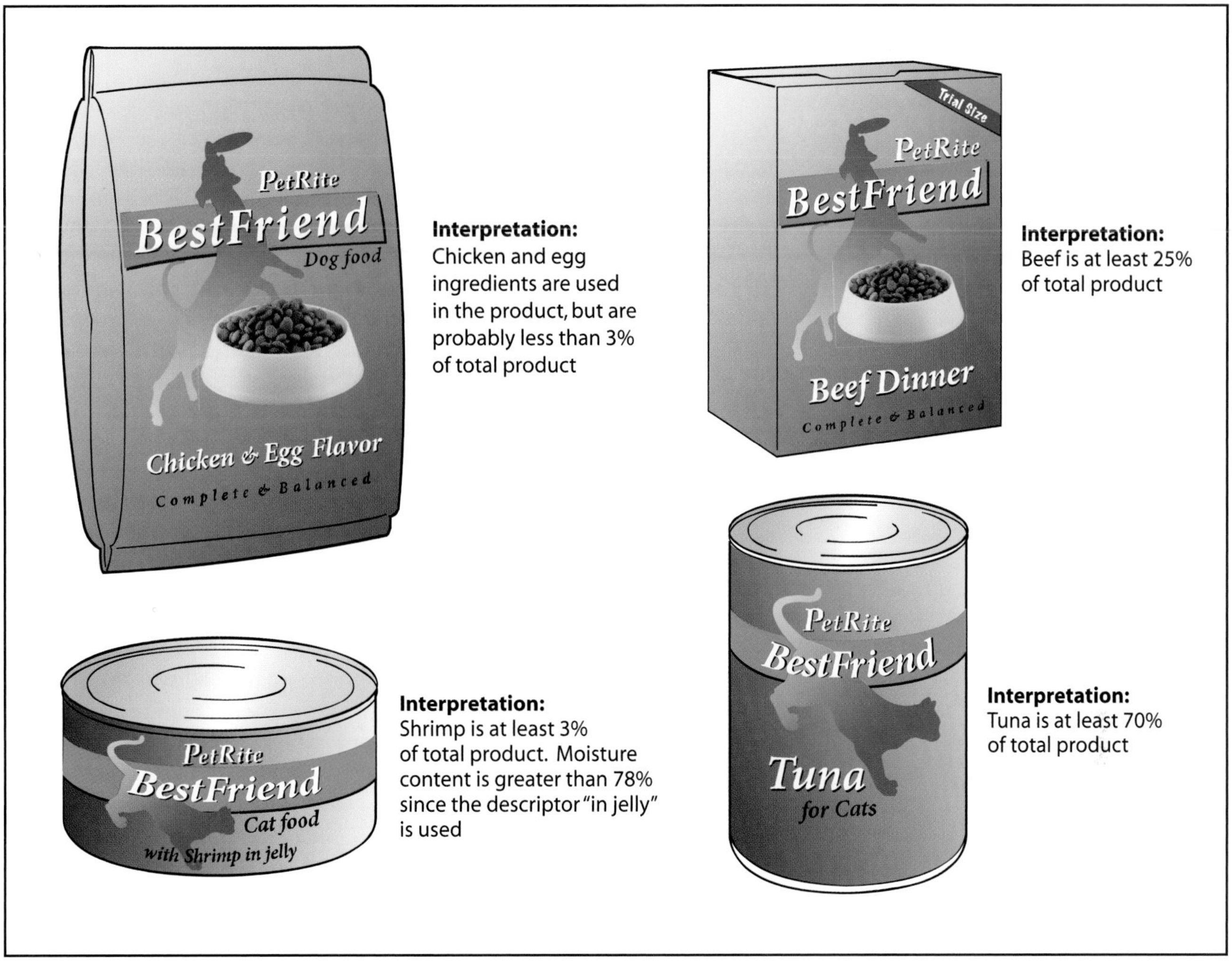
PetRite
BestFriend
Dog food
Chicken & Egg Flavor
Complete & Balanced
Interpretation:
Chicken and egg ingredients are used in the product, but are probably less than 3% of total product
Trial Size
PetRite
BestFriend
Beef Dinner
Complete & Balanced
Interpretation:
Beef is at least 25% of total product
PetRite
BestFriend
Cat food
with Shrimp in jelly
Interpretation:
Shrimp is at least 3% of total product. Moisture content is greater than 78% since the descriptor "in jelly" is used
PetRite
BestFriend
Tuna
for Cats
Interpretation:
Tuna is at least 70% of total product

Figure 9-2. Examples of pet food descriptor terms.

will be used as an example (**Figure 9-2**): 1) unqualified use of the term "Beef" in a product name requires that beef ingredients be at least 95% or more of the total weight of all ingredients exclusive of water used in processing, but in no case less than 70% of the total product, 2) use of the term "Beef" with a qualifier such as "Beef dinner," "Beef platter," "Beef entree," "Beef formula," or any similar designation requires that beef ingredients be at least 25% of the total weight of all ingredients exclusive of water used in processing, but in no case less than 10% of the total product, 3) the term "With Beef" is intended to highlight minor ingredients and this example requires that beef ingredients be at least 3% of the total product and 4) the term "Beef flavor" does not stipulate a minimum percentage. The beef flavor designation usually indicates that beef is less than 3% of the total product. An ingredient that gives the characterizing flavor (e.g., beef digest, beef by-products) can be used instead of the actual named flavor, beef. In fact, some ingredients may be less than 1% of the total product and still appear in the product name as a flavor. This type of regulation is also found in human foods in which the product names cranberry juice, cranberry juice cocktail and cranberry drink indicate different levels of actual juice in the product.

Percentage rules also apply to product names and moisture content of foods. In the United States, the maximum moisture content in all pet foods should not exceed 78%. However, pet foods can have moisture contents higher than 78% if they are labeled as a stew, gravy, broth, juice or milk replacer. High-moisture pet foods in cans, pouches or tins will contain terms such as "in sauce," "in aspic," "in gravy" or some similar designation in the product name.

DESIGNATOR

The words "dog food," "for cats" or some similar terminology must appear conspicuously on the principal display panel of pet foods sold in the United States. These terms clearly identify the animal for which the product is intended and that the product is not for human consumption.

NET WEIGHT

FDA regulations state that the principal display panel shall bear a declaration of the net quantity of contents. The term "Net Weight" is used most often and must be displayed in conspicuous and easily legible print. Most often, "dual declarations" are made, so that the net weight is stated in avoirdu-

Box 9-1. AAFCO Guidelines for "Natural" Claims.

"Natural" ingredients must be from animal or plant origin or a mined product (e.g., salt). Processes such as extraction, hydrolysis and fermentation are permitted.

Any chemical synthetic process, such as addition of a chemical moiety to a vitamin, is not "natural" under AAFCO definitions.

A pet food bearing an unqualified "natural" claim may not contain ANY ingredients that do not meet the AAFCO definition for "natural."

"Natural" pet foods may contain synthetic nutrients provided a qualifying disclaimer is added, e.g., "Natural ingredients with added vitamins, minerals and taurine," but not other synthetic substances such as artificial preservatives or colors.

The term "natural" may also be used to characterize a single ingredient, e.g., "natural cheese flavor," provided it does not imply that the product itself is "natural."

Table 9-3. Examples of words used on bursts and flags on pet food labels.

5 pounds more
Even fewer calories than ____
Freshness guaranteed
Great new taste
Great taste
More delicious taste than ____
New
New & improved
New flavor
New formula
New pâté style
New recipe
New taste
No artificial colors and flavors
Pleasant aroma
Soy free
Taste preferred 4 to 1 over leading national brand
Taste preferred over leading dog biscuit

pois (pounds and ounces) and metric (kilograms or grams) units. The regulation of net weight declarations is complex. Net weight descriptions must be placed on the principal display panel within the bottom 30% of the panel in lines generally parallel to the base of the package, and they must be separated from all other text above, below and to each side by minimum specifications. The regulations also specify minimum type sizes depending on the square inch area of the principal display panel.

PRODUCT VIGNETTE

The term product vignette refers to a vignette, graphic or pictorial representation of a product on a pet food label. This representation should not misrepresent the contents of the package. This means that a picture or other depiction of the product or ingredients on the label should not look better than the actual product or ingredients.

NUTRITION CLAIM

Nutrition statements appearing on the principal display panel are usually brief. Examples include the terms "complete and nutritious," "100% nutritious," "100% complete nutrition" or some similar designation. A nutritional adequacy statement on the information panel must substantiate nutrition claims on the principal display panel. If the nutritional adequacy statement on the information panel is for a limited lifestage (e.g., for maintenance only), the principal display panel claim must be suitably qualified, such as "100% complete nutrition for adult dogs." Manufacturers can substantiate these nutrition claims by meeting the appropriate AAFCO nutrient profile or successfully completing a protocol feeding trial. Nutrition claims substantiation for "natural" foods is discussed in more detail below (**Box 9-1**).

BURSTS AND FLAGS

Bursts and flags (**Figure 9-3**) are areas of the principal display panel that are designed to highlight information or provide specific information with visual impact. **Table 9-3** lists the type of information often included in bursts and flags. New products, formula or ingredient changes and improvements in taste are most often highlighted. The time allowed for a burst or flag to be on the label varies with the type of information. "New" or "New & Improved" can only appear on the label for six months, whereas a comparison such as "Preferred 4 to 1 over the leading national brand" can remain on the label for one year, unless resubstantiated.

Information Panel

INGREDIENT STATEMENT

Pet foods sold in the United States must list each ingredient of the food in the ingredient statement. Ingredients are listed in descending order by their predominance by weight according to the product's formula. AAFCO has established the name and definition of a wide variety of ingredients. The ingredient names must conform to the AAFCO name (e.g., poultry by-product meal, corn gluten meal, powdered cellulose) or when a suitable AAFCO name does not exist, should be identified by the common or usual name (e.g., beef, lamb, chicken). Ingredients listed as "meat" or "meat by-products" must designate the mammal from which the ingredients are derived unless the meat or meat by-products are derived from cattle, swine, sheep or goats. For example, ingredients derived from deer would be listed as venison or venison by-products. Brand or trade names cannot be used in the ingredient statement and no reference to quality or grade of ingredients can be made. Collective terms (e.g., "animal protein products"), allowed for use on livestock and poultry feed labels, are not allowed on pet food labels in the United States (**Table 9-4**).

The list of ingredients may be helpful, although it has some shortcomings that limit its usefulness for evaluating pet foods. The nutritive value of ingredients can be estimated, but not definitively determined, from the ingredient statement alone. A consumer must rely on the reputation or word of the manufacturer to assess the nutritive value of the ingredients appearing on the list. A serious limitation of the ingredient statement is that terms such as "meat by-products" are difficult to evaluate. The nutritive value of various meat by-products varies widely. As an example, meat by-products such as liver, kidney and lungs have excellent nutritive value whereas other meat by-products such as udder, bone and connective tissue have poor nutrient availability.

Because individual ingredients are listed in descending order by weight for the product as a whole, careful reading of the ingredient list may be needed to fully understand the true relative proportions of ingredients in the product. A pet food that lists several related ingredients or different forms of the same ingredient separately (e.g., wheat germ meal, wheat middlings, wheat bran, wheat flour) could make wheat-based ingredients appear to be a lower portion of the food than is the fact. Also, because an ingredient's position on the list includes its inherent water content, this allows dry ingredients to appear lower on the list than ingredients that are naturally high in moisture.

This basic principle is commonly used in moist meat-type dog foods in which textured vegetable protein (TVP) is a major portion of the product. The ingredient list may look like this for a food named a "beef dinner:" Water sufficient for processing, meat by-products, beef, soy flour, cornstarch.... In this kind of food, water is typically combined with soy flour to produce TVP. The TVP makes up a predominant portion of the food, but soy flour appears lower on the ingredient statement because it is a "dry" ingredient whereas other components of the food are added as "wet" ingredients. The consumer thinks he or she is purchasing a beef-based food when in fact, there is more soy flour than beef when the two are compared on an equal moisture ("dry matter") basis.

This same principle is used in dry pet foods in which "fresh" meats are highlighted. The ingredient list may look like this for a lamb and rice dog food that claims to provide "real lamb meat:" Lamb, brewers rice, ground yellow corn, corn gluten meal, oat groats, poultry by-product meal, beef tallow.... Lamb appears first on the ingredient list because its moisture content is higher than that of the other dry ingredients. The predominant portion of the food contains a mixture of grains (rice, corn, oats) rather than "real meat."

Pet food additives such as vitamins, minerals, antioxidant preservatives, antimicrobial preservatives, humectants, coloring agents, flavors, palatability enhancers and emulsifying agents that are added by the manufacturer must be listed in the ingredient statement. Pet food additives must conform to the requirements of the applicable regulations in the United States Code of Federal Regulations as food additives (21 CFR 573) or as ingredients generally recognized as safe (GRAS) (21 CFR 582). Some additives are listed only in the sections for human direct food additives or for GRAS substances, but are allowed in pet foods by informal review. With FDA review and concurrence, AAFCO has also established definitions for some additives that are not formally codified in the federal regulations.

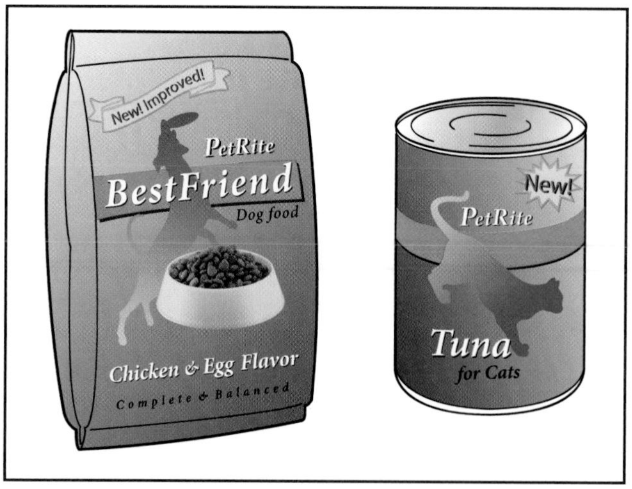

Figure 9-3. One label with a flag and one label with a burst.

Table 9-4. Ingredient statement from the same dry dog food as it would appear on pet food labels from selected countries.

United States
Ingredients: Corn Meal, Chicken Meal, Soybean Meal, Animal Fat (Preserved With Mixed Tocopherols And Citric Acid), Natural Chicken Liver Flavor, Vegetable Oil, Dried Egg Product, Flaxseed, Salt, Calcium Carbonate, Minerals (Ferrous Sulfate, Zinc Oxide, Copper Sulfate, Manganous Oxide, Calcium Iodate, Sodium Selenite), Vitamins (Choline Chloride, Vitamin A Supplement, Vitamin D_3 Supplement, Vitamin E Supplement, L-Ascorbyl-2-Polyphosphate [A Source Of Vitamin C], Niacin, Thiamine Mononitrate, Calcium Pantothenate, Pyridoxine Hydrochloride, Riboflavin, Folic Acid, Biotin, Vitamin B_{12} Supplement), Beta-Carotene.

Canada
Ingredients: Grain Products, Poultry Products, Soybean Meal, Stabilized Poultry and/or Animal Fat, Vitamins and Minerals.
CVMA-Certified Product
Ingredients: Corn Meal, Chicken Meal, Soybean Meal, Animal Fat, Dried Whole Egg, Vegetable Oil, Salt, Plus All Necessary Vitamins and Minerals.

Europe*
In Europe there are two options:
1) Ingredient groupings
Ingredients: Cereals, Meat and Animal Derivatives, Vegetable Protein Extracts, Oils and Fats, Eggs and Egg Derivatives, Minerals.
2) Individual ingredient listing
Ingredients: Ground Corn, Chicken Meal, Soybean Meal, Animal Fat, Dried Egg Product, Brewers Rice, Vegetable Oil, Iodized Salt, Calcium Carbonate, Magnesium Oxide.
*Antioxidants, preservatives, vitamins and coloring agents are not listed under ingredients because they are considered additives and are declared elsewhere on the label.

GUARANTEED ANALYSIS

In the United States, pet food manufacturers are required to include minimum percentages for crude protein and crude fat and maximum percentages for crude fiber and moisture (**Table 9-5**). Guarantees for other nutrients may follow moisture, but a nutrient need not be listed unless its presence is highlighted elsewhere on the label (e.g., "contains taurine," "calcium enriched"). Guarantees for substances not listed in the AAFCO Dog or Cat Nutrient Profiles (e.g., vitamin C, L-carnitine, glucosamine, chondroitin sulfate) should immediately

Table 9-5. Guaranteed or typical analysis from the same dry cat food as it would appear on pet food labels from selected countries.

United States (guaranteed analysis)		
Crude protein	Minimum	30.0%
Crude fat	Minimum	18.0%
Crude fiber	Maximum	2.0%
Moisture	Maximum	10.0%
Vitamin E	Minimum	275 IU/kg
Ascorbic acid (vitamin C)*	Minimum	50 mg/kg
Canada (guaranteed analysis)		
Protein	-	30.0%
Fat	-	18.0%
Moisture	-	10%
CVMA-Certified Food in Canada (guaranteed analysis)		
Crude protein	Minimum	30.0%
Crude fat	Minimum	18.0%
Crude fibre	Maximum	2.0%
Moisture	Maximum	10.0%
Ash	Maximum	5.0%
Europe (typical analysis)		
Crude protein	-	31.3%
Crude oils and fats	-	21.3%
Crude fibre	-	2.0%
Crude ash	-	4.7%
Moisture	-	7.5%
Additives (per kg)		
Vitamin A	-	17,100 IU
Vitamin D_3	-	1,710 IU
Vitamin E	-	290 mg
Copper (copper chloride)	-	21 mg
Contains EU permitted antioxidant		
Contains EU permitted colorant		

*Not recognized as an essential nutrient by the AAFCO Cat Food Nutrient Profiles.

follow the listing of recognized nutrients and be accompanied by an asterisk referring to the disclaimer "Not recognized as an essential nutrient by the AAFCO Dog (or Cat) Food Nutrient Profiles." The sliding scale method of listing guarantees as percentage ranges (e.g., minimum 15 to 18%) is not allowed. It is important to recognize that these percentages generally indicate the "worst case" levels for these nutrients in the food and do not reflect the exact or typical amounts of these nutrients. This differs from pet food labels in Europe where "typical" percentages are used.

The term crude protein refers to a specific analytical procedure that estimates protein content by measuring nitrogen. Crude protein is an index of protein quantity but does not indicate protein quality (amino acid profile) or digestibility (Chapter 5).

Crude fat refers to a specific analytical procedure that estimates the lipid content of a food obtained through either ether extraction or acid hydrolysis. In addition to lipids, this procedure also isolates certain organic acids, oils, pigments, alcohols and fat-soluble vitamins. Because fats have more than twice the energy density of proteins and carbohydrates, crude fat can be used to estimate the energy density of the food. If the moisture and crude fiber content of two foods are somewhat similar, the food with the higher crude fat guarantee will usually have the higher energy density.

Crude fiber represents the organic residue that remains after plant material has been treated with dilute acid and alkali solutions. It is determined by a specific analytical procedure that was originally developed for the wood pulp industry and then applied to animal foods. Although crude fiber is used to report the fiber content of commercial pet foods, it usually underestimates the true level of fiber in the product. Crude fiber is an estimate of the indigestible portion of the food for dogs and cats (Chapter 5). The crude fiber method typically recovers a large percentage of cellulose and lignin in a sample, and a variable percentage of hemicellulose and even ash.

Moisture is determined by drying a sample of the product to a constant weight. The drying procedure measures water in the product as a whole, but does not distinguish between added water and water in the ingredients. Subtle differences in moisture content of moist products can result in marked differences in dry matter content and therefore the economics of feeding a given pet food. Remember, the dry matter content of the food contains all of the nutrients except water. For example, compare the dry matter content of three different moist cat foods: 1) Food A contains 72% moisture, 2) Food B contains 78% moisture and 3) Food C contains 82% moisture.

Food A 100 - 72% water = 28% dry matter
Food B* 100 - 78% water = 22% dry matter
Food C** 100 - 82% water = 18% dry matter

*28 - 22 ÷ 22 x 100 = 27% more dry matter in Food A (72% moisture) vs. Food B (78% moisture)

**28 - 18 ÷ 18 x 100 = 55% more dry matter in Food A (72% moisture) vs. Food C (82% moisture)

Therefore, what appears to be a small difference in water content of a food produces a marked difference in dry matter content. Guarantees are expressed on an "as is" or "as fed" basis. It is important to remember to convert these guarantees to a dry matter basis when comparing foods with differing moisture content (e.g., moist vs. dry foods).

Although a maximum ash guarantee is not required in the United States, many pet food manufacturers include one on the labels of their foods. In the United States, "low ash" claims are not allowed because "ash" per se is of no true significance. "Low magnesium" claims on cat food labels are allowed if the food meets certain FDA criteria. In such cases, a maximum magnesium guarantee is required. To be labeled as a "low magnesium" food, the product must contain less than 0.12% magnesium, on a dry matter basis, and less than 25 mg per 100 kcal metabolizable energy. Actual analytical values must show that the product consistently meets these levels. The estimation of magnesium content based on calculation from the guaranteed analyses must meet these criteria as well. The only exception occurs when the label bears an AAFCO calorie content statement that is higher than would be estimated from the guaranteed analysis.

Ash consists of all noncombustible materials in the food, usually salt and other minerals. A high ash content in dry and soft-moist foods generally indicates a high magnesium content. However, the ash content of moist cat foods usually correlates poorly with the magnesium content. Excessive magnesium intake may be one risk factor for feline struvite urolithiasis (Chapter 43).

Table 9-6. How to interpret label claims of nutritional adequacy.*

Claim 1: "Good Things Beef Flavor Dog Food is formulated to meet the nutritional levels established by the AAFCO (Association of American Feed Control Officials) Dog Food Nutrient Profiles for maintenance of adult dogs."
Interpretation: This food has been formulated to meet the nutrient levels in the AAFCO Dog Food Nutrient Profile for adult maintenance. This product does not meet the nutrient profile for growth/lactation and has probably not undergone AAFCO feeding tests.

Claim 2: "Good Things Chicken Recipe Cat Food meets the nutrient requirements established by the AAFCO Nutrient Profile for all stages of a cat's life."
Interpretation: This food has been formulated to meet the nutrient levels in the AAFCO Cat Food Nutrient Profile for growth/lactation and adult maintenance. This product has probably not undergone AAFCO feeding tests. The language of the statement is not in compliance with AAFCO regulations.

Claim 3: "Animal feeding tests using the AAFCO procedures substantiate that Good Things Lamb Meal and Rice Formula Dog Food provides complete and balanced nutrition for the growth of puppies and maintenance of adult dogs."
Interpretation: This food has successfully completed an AAFCO minimum protocol feeding trial for growing puppies (10 weeks of feeding) or is a family member of a tested product. It probably, but not necessarily, is formulated to meet the AAFCO Dog Food Nutrient Profiles for maintenance and growth/reproduction.

Claim 4: "Good Things Cat Food with Tuna provides complete and balanced nutrition for kittens and adult reproducing queens as substantiated by feeding tests performed in accordance with procedures established by the Association of American Feed Control Officials (AAFCO)."
Interpretation: This cat food (or a family member) has undergone AAFCO minimum protocol feeding studies for gestation/lactation and growth. This food would be nutritionally adequate for adult cats but is not recommended by this manufacturer for long-term maintenance of adult cats. The language of the statement is not in compliance with AAFCO regulations.

Claim 5: "Complete and balanced nutrition for adult maintenance based on AAFCO protocol feeding studies conducted at the Good Things Nutrition Center."
Interpretation: This food (or a family member) has undergone AAFCO minimum protocol feeding studies for adult maintenance only and has not been tested for gestation/lactation or growth. The language of the statement is not in compliance with AAFCO regulations.

Claim 6: "Complete and balanced nutrition for all lifestages of the dog, substantiated by testing performed in accordance with feeding protocols established by AAFCO."
Interpretation: This dog food (or a family member) has undergone AAFCO minimum protocol feeding trials for gestation/lactation and growth. The language of the statement is not in compliance with AAFCO regulations.

Claim 7: "Meets or exceeds the nutritional levels established by the National Research Council recommendations for all stages of a cat's life."
Interpretation: This cat food has been formulated to meet or exceed the nutrient levels established for growth, gestation/lactation and adult maintenance by the National Research Council (NRC) in the United States. This product has probably not undergone feeding tests. This nutrition statement would be considered misbranded in the United States because the NRC nutrient recommendations have been replaced by AAFCO Cat Food Nutrient Profiles. However, references to NRC are still made on pet foods sold in countries other than the United States.

Claim 8: "Good Things for Dogs: CVMA Certified; Certified by the Canadian Veterinary Medical Association to meet its nutritional standards on the basis of comprehensive feeding trials, chemical analysis and on-going monitoring."
Interpretation: This dog food meets or exceeds the standards established by the CVMA Pet Food Certification Program for adult maintenance. The food meets or exceeds the CVMA standards for nutrient content, digestibility and labeling requirements. Nutrient digestibility is the only feeding test performed after the product is initially certified.

*Claims 2, 4, 5 and 6 appear on pet food labels in the United States market, but Claim 3 is the preferred wording for products that have passed an AAFCO protocol feeding trial, and Claim 1 is the preferred wording for products that meet the profiles.

NUTRITIONAL ADEQUACY STATEMENT

Since 1984, regulations in the United States have required that all pet food labels, with the exception of products clearly labeled as "treats" and "snacks" (and more recently as "supplements") contain a statement and validation of nutritional adequacy. When a claim of "complete and balanced," "100% nutritious" or some similar designation is used, manufacturers must indicate the method and lifestage that was used to substantiate this claim (**Table 9-6**).

AAFCO (2007) regulations allow three basic methods to substantiate claims. The formulation method requires that the manufacturer formulate the food to meet the AAFCO Dog or Cat Food Nutrient Profiles. The feeding trial (protocol) method requires that the manufacturer perform an AAFCO-protocol feeding trial using the food as the sole source of nutrition. The family method allows product analyses to ensure that the pet food is a member of a product family in which the lead member has successfully passed a feeding trial.

AAFCO (2007) nutrient profiles are published for two categories: 1) growth and reproduction and 2) adult maintenance. The formulation method allows the manufacturer to substantiate a "complete and balanced" claim by calculating the nutrient content of a food using standard nutrient information about ingredients or by chemical analysis of the final product. **Table 9-6** lists some of the wording that connotes this type of claim, but the only statement that is acceptable in states that follow AAFCO Model Pet Food Regulations is "(Complete name of product) is formulated to meet the nutritional levels established by the AAFCO Dog (or Cat) Food Nutrient Profiles for (lifestage)." The formulation method is less expensive and time-consuming, but has been criticized because it does not account for acceptability of the food or nutrient availability. A report in 1991 documented that some commercial pet foods that made "complete and balanced" claims by formulation methods alone did not provide adequate growth of normal animals because of poor availability of nutrients in the food (Huber et al, 1991). However, that study was based on the older

NRC recommendations, not the AAFCO Dog Food Nutrient Profiles, which had additional safety considerations built in to help mitigate the potential for these types of deficiencies.

The feeding trial (protocol) method is generally considered the preferred method for substantiating a claim. Feeding tests can be used to support a nutritional adequacy claim for one or more of the following categories: 1) gestation and lactation, 2) growth, 3) maintenance and 4) all lifestages. AAFCO has published minimum testing protocols for adult maintenance, growth and gestation/lactation. A food that successfully completes a gestation/lactation trial followed by a growth trial using the offspring from the gestation/lactation trial can make a claim for all lifestages. The required terminology for labels of pet foods that have passed these tests is: "Animal feeding tests using AAFCO procedures substantiate that (complete product name) provides complete and balanced nutrition for (lifestage)." The wording must appear verbatim. Deviations from the above statement, while occasionally observed on some pet food labels, are currently considered misbranded in the United States (**Table 9-6**).

AAFCO feeding trials are minimum protocols. As an example, the adult maintenance protocol uses eight animals that are fed the food as the sole source of nutrition for six months. A veterinarian examines the animals at the beginning of the study and at the end of 26 weeks for clinical signs of nutritional deficiency or excess. Body weight is recorded weekly and minimal laboratory evaluations (total erythrocyte count, hemoglobin, packed cell volume, serum alkaline phosphatase, serum albumin and whole blood taurine in cats) are performed. This type of protocol will usually detect the vast majority of nutrient deficiencies but might not detect some nutrient excesses that may be harmful when fed over a longer period. In this respect, the AAFCO profiles are better because maximum levels of some nutrients are also established. Growth protocols include feeding the food for a minimum of 10 weeks. Because this test is conducted during the most critical stage of the puppy's or kitten's development, it is very sensitive in detecting deviations from normal growth. The gestation/lactation trial considers factors such as litter size and survivability and health of the dam.

The family method of nutritional substantiation is a combination of the formulation and feeding trial methods. An individual product can be a member of a product family and be nutritionally similar to a lead product that has undergone AAFCO feeding tests. AAFCO (2007) has established clear procedures for establishing pet food product families. To qualify, the family member must be the same processing type as the tested product, sufficiently close to the tested product in metabolizable energy content, analyzed and shown to meet the levels of the tested product for crude protein, calcium, phosphorus, zinc, lysine and thiamin (plus potassium and taurine for cat foods), meet either the tested product or the AAFCO Dog or Cat Food Nutrient Profiles minimums for all other nutrients and meet all established AAFCO Dog or Cat Food Nutrient Profiles maximums. When the calorie content of both the tested product and family members are determined by an AAFCO-sanctioned metabolizable energy feeding trial, the nutritional adequacy statement as used for the tested product may also be used for the family members. Although infrequently observed in the market, labels of family members whose calorie content was determined by calculation methods must state,"(complete product name) provides complete and balanced nutrition for (lifestage), and is comparable in nutritional adequacy to a product which has been substantiated using AAFCO feeding tests."

Pet foods that are clearly labeled as snacks, treats or supplements may make a nutritional adequacy claim but are not required to do so. Pet foods that fail to meet AAFCO requirements by any of the standard methods and are not clearly labeled as snacks, treats or supplements are required to have the nutritional statement: "This product is intended for intermittent or supplemental feeding only."

Veterinary therapeutic/wellness foods are those products that are intended for use by or under the supervision or direction of a veterinarian. These foods may contain the nutritional statement "use only as directed by your veterinarian." In addition to this statement, the label must include the appropriate lifestage AAFCO nutritional adequacy claim or an "intermittent or supplemental" feeding statement.

FEEDING GUIDELINES

In the United States, dog and cat foods labeled as complete and balanced (including snacks and treats) for any or all lifestages must list feeding directions on the product label for all lifestages for which the product is intended. These directions must be expressed in common terms and must appear prominently on the label. Feeding directions should, at a minimum, state, "Feed (weight/unit of product) per (weight unit) of dog (or cat)" and frequency of feeding. These feeding statements are general guidelines at best. Because of individual variation, many animals will require more or less food than that recommended on the label to maintain optimal body condition and health.

There is an exception to this rule for products that bear the "use only as directed by your veterinarian" statement. Because the veterinarian will presumably provide proper instruction about feeding of the product, explicit feeding directions are not required. Many veterinary therapeutic/wellness products, however, may still provide specific directions either on the label or in accompanying product literature.

STATEMENT OF CALORIE CONTENT

The label of a dog or cat food in the United States may bear a statement of calorie content provided the statement is separate from the guaranteed analysis and appear under the heading "calorie content." At this time, it is required for "light" and "less calorie" pet foods, but is voluntary on others. The statement is based on kilocalories of metabolizable energy (ME) on an as fed basis and must be expressed as kilocalories per kilogram (kcal/kg) of product. The statement may also be expressed as kilocalories per familiar household measure (e.g., kcal/cup, kcal/can), in addition to, but in lieu of, the kcal/kg value.

There are two methods for determining calorie content. The

first is the "calculation method," wherein analytical values for the calorie-containing nutrients in the food (protein, fat and carbohydrates) are used to estimate metabolizable energy by the "modified Atwater" formula. This formula is based on average digestibility of these nutrients in commonly used pet food ingredients. As such, it tends to underestimate the true calorie content of very highly digestible foods and overestimate the calorie content of poorly digestible foods.

Calorie content may also be determined by conducting AAFCO-sanctioned feeding trials to obtain a more accurate measurement of digestibility. The most common method is to feed animals the pet food in question for five days, then to very carefully measure food intake and fecal excretion for an additional five days. Comparing "what goes in" to "what comes out," with some additional estimates for nitrogen loss in urine, is a more reliable method for determining metabolizable energy.

To differentiate the two methods on a pet food label, a calorie content statement determined by the calculation method must include the word "calculated."

GENERAL INFORMATION

In the United States, the name and address of the manufacturer, distributor or dealer must be found on the label, usually on the information panel. The phrases "Distributed by...." or "Manufactured for...." or "Imported by...." indicate that a company other than the one selling the product has manufactured the pet food. This is a common practice with private label brand pet foods. The manufacturer in this case is called a co-packer. Regulations require that if the product is manufactured in a country other than where it is sold, the manufacturer's information be accompanied by "Product of (country of origin)."

Although not a legal requirement, most manufacturers include the universal product code (UPC) or bar code on the label. Other information such as batch numbers and date of manufacture are also frequently found on pet food containers or labels. This information is important to know when communicating with a manufacturer about product in a specific container. Some manufacturers will use a freshness date such as "Best before (date)" or list other guarantee policies.

PET FOOD LABELS IN CANADA

Regulation in Canada

The Canadian government has few pet food labeling regulations. The *Consumer Packaging and Labelling Act* specifies that three basic mandatory statements must appear in English and French languages on a pet food label for food sold in Canada: 1) product identity, 2) product net quantity (metric units first) 3) and the dealer's name and principal place of business.

The Canadian government's Competition Bureau has published a "Guide for the Labeling and Advertising of Pet Foods" (2001). This guide provides a voluntary code of conduct setting out best practices for the labeling and advertising of Canadian-produced pet foods. Although these guidelines are not law, the guide is used by the Competition Bureau in evaluating possible violations of Canadian labeling legislation and in assessing complaints about false or misleading pet food labels or advertising. For this reason, most reputable Canadian pet food companies adhere to the Competition Bureau guidelines.

CVMA Pet Food Certification

The Canadian Veterinary Medical Association (CVMA) Pet Food Certification Program was established in 1976 as a voluntary, third-party, quality assurance program for pet foods sold in Canada. The CVMA Program establishes nutrient standards, lifestage feeding protocols and digestibility feeding protocols for dogs and cats (CVMA, 1999; Allard, 1988). Similar to PFI and NRC, the CVMA is not a regulatory agency but provides a method of voluntary enforcement of certain standards for pet foods. Involvement in the CVMA Pet Food Certification Program is not mandatory.

The mission of the CVMA Pet Food Certification Program is:

> "To improve the health and well-being of pets by: 1) providing a nutritional standard for pet foods for manufacturers to meet in order to satisfy the nutritional requirements of a normal pet throughout its life, 2) certifying pet foods that meet the CVMA nutritional standards and monitoring continuously those foods to ensure that they continue to meet the standards of composition, digestibility and palatability, 3) providing the consumer with a quality assurance program and a means of identifying a nutritionally sound pet food in the marketplace, 4) ensuring the CVMA Seal of Certification becomes synonymous in the Canadian public's mind with quality and integrity by assuring that all advertising statements are fairly presented and can be supported by the advertiser and 5) helping pet owners understand the importance of proper nutrition in preventive health care and 6) encouraging the funding of small animal nutrition research" (1999).

All CVMA-certified pet foods are allowed to display the CVMA Seal of Certification on their labels for products sold in Canada. Because of AAFCO restrictions, pet food containers sold in the United States cannot display the CVMA Seal.

Principal Display Panels

Principal display panels on Canadian pet food containers may vary. The Canadian government requires that product identity and net quantity (net weight) be listed on all principal display panels of pet foods sold in Canada. Other elements of the principal display panel described under United States regulations may appear on the container depending on several factors.

The CVMA Pet Food Certification Program requires more extensive labeling requirements than does the Canadian law (Allard, 1988). The CVMA Program labeling requirements include product identity, designator and net quantity, which are usually found on the principal display panel (Allard, 1988). Nutritional claims can be stated but must be substantiated. Product names can contain ingredients (Beef stew, Beef flavor, etc.) as described earlier for United States' labels and follow roughly the same percentage rules. Pet foods that meet the requirements can display the CVMA Seal of Certification on the principal display panel (**Figure 9-4**) (CVMA, 1999). Requirements dictate the maximum size of the logo for different sizes of containers (CVMA, 1999).

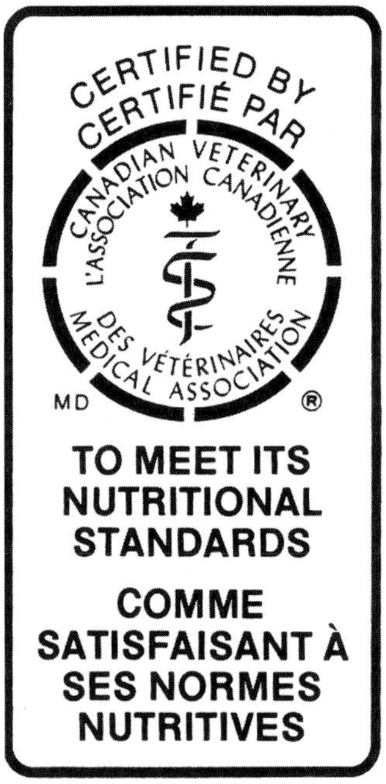
CERTIFIED BY
CERTIFIÉ PAR
CANADIAN VETERINARY MEDICAL ASSOCIATION
L'ASSOCIATION CANADIENNE DES VÉTÉRINAIRES
MD
®
TO MEET ITS NUTRITIONAL STANDARDS
COMME SATISFAISANT À SES NORMES NUTRITIVES

Figure 9-4. The CVMA seal.

The Competition Bureau voluntary guidelines regarding the principal display panel are similar to those for the United States and the CVMA Certification Program. These guidelines require the substantiation of any nutritional claims, and provide definitions for ingredients referenced in the product name (i.e., Beef dog food, Beef dinner etc). The Competition Bureau's guidelines follow similar percentage rules to those of the United States.

Commercial pet foods produced in the United States for sale in Canada will usually contain the elements of the principal display panel legally required in the United States; namely, 1) a product name, 2) designator and 3) net weight. Pet foods produced in Canada that are not CVMA certified are not legally required to conform to the stricter labeling requirements of the United States or CVMA Program, but most Canadian pet foods do follow the comparable guidelines published by the Competition Bureau. Other elements of the principal display panel such as the manufacturer's name, brand name, product vignette and bursts/flags are also found on Canadian labels.

Information Panels

Ingredient Statements

Ingredient statements on pet food containers in Canada also vary. Canadian government regulations do not require an ingredient statement. However, the Competition Bureau guidelines state that ingredients must be listed on the label, that manufacturers should follow the AAFCO feed ingredient definitions and ingredients should be listed in descending order by percentage of weight. The CVMA Program states that ingredients should be listed on the label in decreasing order of concentration in the product. Pet foods produced in the United States and sold in Canada will usually meet the United States regulations for ingredient lists. Pet foods produced in Canada that are not CVMA certified generally follow the Competition Bureau's guidelines even though they are not required to by law (**Table 9-4**).

Guaranteed Analysis

Canadian law does not require guarantees on pet food labels. The voluntary Competition Bureau Guidelines state that a guaranteed analysis must be shown on the label and must include the following on an "as fed" basis: crude protein (minimum %), crude fat (minimum %), crude fibre (maximum %) and moisture (maximum %). Pet foods certified by the CVMA Program must also include the above guarantees. Ash maximums (not more than 6% dry matter) are required for cat foods certified by the CVMA Program, and magnesium maximums (not more than 0.1% dry matter) are required for cat foods that make a "low ash" claim.

Nutritional Adequacy Statements

The CVMA Pet Food Certification Program has published nutrient standards and protocols for digestibility feeding trials for dogs and cats (1989). Nutrient, digestibility, feeding protocol and feeding guideline standards have also been published for "special foods" including light (lite) foods, calorie-reduced foods, geriatric foods, growth foods, gestation/lactation foods and low-ash, low-magnesium cat foods. Feeding trials are incorporated into the standards for geriatric foods (three-month period) and growth foods (weaning to six months). Products that meet these standards can display the CVMA Seal of Certification and use the following words as a nutritional statement: "This product meets nutritional standards established by the Canadian Veterinary Medical Association (CVMA)." In addition to the CVMA certification logo, products certified as special foods may carry language to the effect that: "This product is formulated to provide (claim for level of nutrients)" or "This product meets the CVMA standard for a (type of special food)."

The Competition Bureau Guidelines state that nutritional adequacy claims can be made if they are based on animal feeding protocols and nutrient profile programs such as those administered by the Pet Food Association of Canada, the CVMA or AAFCO. The guidelines further state that products that are formulated for or suitable for only a limited purpose, such as supplemental feedings or that are limited to specific lifestages, must contain a statement to that effect. If a product is intended to be used under the supervision of a veterinarian, the following claim must be included on the product label: "Use only as directed by your veterinarian." The guidelines specifically forbid drug claims (i.e., the words "diagnose," "cure," "mitigate," "treat" or "prevent" disease must not be used on a pet food label).

Some products in Canada will reference the NRC for complete and balanced nutrition claims, although this reference is no longer legal in the United States. Based on published NRC nutrient standards, these claims refer to the formulation/analysis method. **Table 9-6** includes nutritional claims that appear on pet foods sold in Canada.

Other Items on Information Panels

In Canada, pet foods certified by the CVMA must provide feeding instructions on the label if they are sold as light, calorie-reduced or geriatric foods. Pet foods certified by the CVMA Program as light, calorie-reduced or geriatric foods have energy density (kcal/gram of dry matter gross energy) standards, but caloric density is not required on the label.

Competition Bureau guidelines also require that feeding instructions appear on the product label. The guidelines also cover misrepresentations with respect to business claims (i.e., rank of the company in the industry, length of time in business, etc.) as well as deceptive endorsements or testimonials.

PET FOOD LABELS IN EUROPE

Regulation in Europe

The regulations about pet food labeling for Europe, as discussed in this chapter, apply primarily to the 25 member states of the European Union (EU) and Switzerland. Legislation controlling pet food labels originates in EU institutions and is then implemented into national law. Outside the EU, individual countries have different structures and rules.

European Union

COUNCIL

The Council of the EU is the EU's main decision-making institution. The Council of the European Union is the forum within which the ministers of the EU meet. Depending on the subject on the agenda, each country is represented by the minister responsible for that particular subject (e.g., agriculture, public health etc.) There are nine different Council "configurations."

The Council passes laws, usually in cooperation with the EU Parliament. In principle, the EU Commission proposes laws for the Council, which examines and adopts them or proposes modifications.

EUROPEAN COMMISSION

The Commission acts with complete political independence, and must not take instructions from any member state government. The Commission has the right to propose new EU legislation and ensures that the regulations and directives adopted by the Council and Parliament are implemented. A civil service made up of 36 "Directorates-General" (DGs) and services, based mainly in Brussels and Luxembourg, assists the Commission. Each DG deals with specific matters; DG Sanco (Health and Consumer Protection Directorate General) largely regulates pet food and labeling issues. DG Sanco's work is divided into three main areas: public health, food safety and consumer protection.

In most cases, the various DGs of the European Commission prepare an initial text for adoption as a Commission Proposal. During this preparation phase, national civil servants, the industry, consumers and other interest groups and outside professionals may be consulted.

EUROPEAN PARLIAMENT

The European Parliament is the only supranational institution whose 732 members are directly elected by the citizens of the 25 member states. The European Parliament is involved in legislative activity through its 20 parliamentary committees.

Table 9-7. National member organizations of FEDIAF.

Austria: ÖHTV	Italy: ASSALCO
Belgium: BKVH/CPAF	Netherlands: VKH
Denmark, Norway & Sweden: NPFA	Poland: Polikarma
Finland: Lemmikkieläinruokayhdistys	Portugal: ALIAN
France: FACCO	Slovenia: GIZ_PHMZ
Germany: IVH	Spain: ANFAAC
Greece: GPFMA	Switzerland: VHN
Hungary: HPFA	United Kingdom: PFMA
Ireland: PFAI	

These Committees draw up legislative proposals, and amend and adopt Commission and Council proposals. Two Committees can be involved in pet food legislation: "the Committee responsible for environment, public health and food safety" and "the Committee responsible for agriculture and rural development."

LEGISLATIVE PROCESS

Two kinds of legislative pieces can come forth: a directive or a regulation. A directive must be implemented into national law within a period stipulated in the directive. The national law can be more restrictive than the European directive but must always be within the scope and spirit of the directive. A regulation must be adopted by national law without changes and is applicable almost immediately after publication. The directives for feeding stuffs contain strict provisions and stipulate definitions for ingredients, for methods of sampling and analysis and for types and maximum levels of permitted additives.

NATIONAL AUTHORITIES

The national, regional or local governments in EU countries apply the EU's health and consumer protection laws. Their job is to ensure traders, manufacturers and food producers in their country observe the rules. After a piece of legislation has been published in the Official European Journal, the national government must implement it immediately (regulation) or, in the case of a directive, translate the legislation into national law within the specified time (Borchardt, 1994). The individual countries through their Ministries of Agriculture are responsible for controlling the application of the law by checking labels and taking samples for analysis. National experts, who work closely with the European Commission on legislation, reside under the Ministries of Agriculture of the different member states.

FÉDÉRATION EUROPÉENNE DE L'INDUSTRIE DES ALIMENTS POUR AMINAUX FAMILIERS

Established in 1970, the Fédération Européenne de l'Industrie des Aliments pour Aminaux Familiers (FEDIAF) represents the pet food industry in Europe and unites the national professional organizations of 19 countries, whether they belong to the EU or not (**Table 9-7**) (FEDIAF, 1993; PFMA, 1993). FEDIAF represents approximately 450 compa-

Table 9-8. Product descriptors used in Europe.

Claim/description	Level of the named ingredient
With beef flavor Beef flavor	Greater than 0 but less than 4% of the named flavor should be present
With rabbit Contains rabbit	At least 4% of the named species should be present
High in chicken With extra chicken Extra chicken	At least 14% of the named species should be present
Beef variety Beef dinner Beef recipe Beef menu Beef with cereal	At least 26% of the named species should be present
Brand name rabbit	All contents are of the named origin with no other ingredients present except gravy, jelly, sauce, permitted additives and nutrient supplements

Table 9-9. Information found in the statutory statements of European pet food labels.

Additives
Address of person (company) responsible for the accuracy of declarations
Complete/complementary food
Expiration date and reference to manufacturing date
Ingredient list
Instructions for use
Net weight and/or volume
Reference (batch) number
Registration number of the plant
Species/category
Typical analysis

nies responsible for producing more than 90% of European pet food. The national organizations represent manufacturers, packers and importers of prepared pet food, including foods for dogs, cats, birds and other pets.

FEDIAF's main role is to represent the European pet food industry in all external forums (FEDIAF, Website 2006). FEDIAF cooperates with the European authorities to implement pet food law designed to ensure the manufacture and distribution of healthy, balanced and quality products. New legislation is translated by FEDIAF into labeling guidelines, which in some countries is then implemented into a "Code of Practice" for the members.

Through the nutrition working party, FEDIAF publishes nutrition guidelines as a policy paper for members. To develop these guidelines the group uses NRC recommendations, AAFCO guidelines and studies published by internationally recognized nutritionists, veterinarians and other researchers. These guidelines are updated yearly.

Through their national organizations, FEDIAF also collaborates with local and national authorities to make pet owners more aware of their responsibilities toward their pets and society.

CONFÉDÉRATION DES INDUSTRIES AGRO-ALIMENTAIRES DE L'UE

The Confédération des Industries Agro-Alimentaires de l'UE (CIAA), also known as the Confederation of the Food and Drink Industries, is analogous to FEDIAF for human foodstuffs. Both federations work closely together in matters of common interest that are regulated by the same legislation. Advertising, claims and environmental matters are regulated for human and animal foods by the same law.

Label Design

Pet food labels in Europe are divided into a Principal Display Panel and the Statutory Statement, although the distinction may be less visible than that for pet food labels in the United States. The Council Directive on the circulation of compound feeding stuffs (79/373/EEC, April 1979) regulates the statutory statement. This directive has been updated several times with a major update (Council Directive 90/44/EEC), which has been in force since January 1992. The pet food industry is also protected by Directive 2002/32/EC and amendments, which regulate maximum residue levels of undesirable substances such as heavy metals, mycotoxins and dioxins in feeding stuffs for animals and ingredients for commercial foods/feeds.

Principal Display Panel

As in the United States, this part of the label gives information about product identity, shows graphics and pictures, includes marketing claims to promote the product and contains descriptions of meat types and other information that companies may choose to convey outside of the statutory statements.

No specific rules apply to the principal display panel other than general legislation concerning misleading claims that applies to all advertising (Council Directive 84/450/EEC and amendments). Labels should not mislead the purchaser; the label must not suggest that the product possesses properties that it does not have, nor should the label imply that the product is special when similar properties are found in other products. A pet food label must not claim that the product will prevent, treat or cure disease.

Directive 90/44/EEC, Art. 5.c.4 is the only text directly referring to claims on pet food labels. It allows pet food manufacturers to claim a low or high level of a specific ingredient on the condition that the percentage is specified and that the claim reflects an essential aspect of that particular food. In the absence of more specific legislation and to protect the consumer against unsubstantiated claims, a policy for claiming meat and flavor varieties has been proposed within the FEDIAF (**Table 9-8**). These guidelines serve an advisory role and are currently under discussion. Although they are not official law with force of application, in some countries (e.g., France) the authorities use those guidelines to judge labels for misleading claims.

Statutory Statement

GENERAL

The mandatory and optional declarations are encapsulated in a space provided for that purpose and called "The Statutory

Statement" (United Kingdom) or "Cadre Réservé" (France) (Art. 5 of 90/44/EEC). In addition to being visible, legible and indelible, the statutory statement must be separate from all other information on the label (**Table 9-9**).

Some of this information may be outside the statutory statement, but the statutory statement must indicate where to find the information. Such information as the "best before" date, net weight and the name and address of the company responsible for the product are often found elsewhere on the label.

A pet food label must indicate whether the food is a complete or a complementary pet food (in other words, whether the food can satisfy all nutritional demands without an additional ration [complete] or whether it must be fed with another product [complementary]). For complementary foods, the other food or supplement should be stated (Burger, 1993). The description "complete" or "complementary" must be considered in relation to the intended purpose of the food or to the particular lifestage for which it is defined (e.g., adult, growth or all lifestages).

The species or category of animals must be stated with the indication complete or complementary (e.g., Brand X is a complete food for adult dogs). This statement of intent is often communicated on the principal display panel, but is repeated in the statutory statement.

INGREDIENT LIST

In Europe, ingredients are declared by the individual name or grouped under various categories (**Table 9-4**). These categories are designed to provide consumers with some indication of the source of raw materials used, while allowing the manufacturer some flexibility in the selection of the ingredients within a specific category (Burger, 1993). These categories are well defined and names and descriptions are officially published (**Table 9-10**). Ingredients should be listed in descending order by weight of each individual ingredient or category.

Vitamins are considered additives and are not listed under ingredients. Water does not have to be declared as an ingredient even if added during processing.

TYPICAL ANALYSIS

Contrary to pet food labels in the United States, where minimum and maximum guarantees are stated, the EU regulations dictate that the typical analysis must be declared for: 1) crude protein, 2) crude fat, 3) crude fiber and 4) ash (**Table 9-5**). Moisture must be declared if it exceeds 14%. Typical analysis (percentage) is the average of the nutrient level calculated from several samples and should correspond with the target level of each nutrient for which precise limits of variation are defined.

The typical analysis gives the percentages found in the actual food. Declaration of nutrients such as calcium, phosphorus, sodium, potassium and magnesium is optional. Energy declaration is forbidden in the EU except for some veterinary dietetic pet foods. Other nutrients must be declared if a manufacturer wants to draw attention to them by saying a food is "high in" or "low in" a particular nutrient.

Table 9-10. Common ingredient categories found on European pet food labels.

Cereals
All types of cereals, regardless of their presentation, or ingredients made from the starchy endosperm
Derivatives of vegetable origin
Derivatives resulting from the treatment of vegetable products in particular cereals, vegetables, legumes and oilseeds
Egg and egg derivatives
All egg products, fresh or preserved by appropriate treatment, and derivatives from the processing thereof
Fish and fish derivatives
Fish or parts of fish, fresh or preserved by appropriate treatment, and derivatives from the processing thereof
Meat and animal derivatives
All fleshy parts of slaughtered warm-blooded land animals, fresh or preserved by appropriate treatment, and all products and derivatives of the processing of the carcass
Milk and milk derivatives
All milk products, fresh or preserved by appropriate treatment, and derivatives from the processing thereof
Minerals
All inorganic substances suitable for animal feed
Oils and fats
All animal and vegetable oils and fats
Various sugars
All types of sugars
Vegetable protein extracts
All products of vegetable origin in which the proteins have been concentrated by an adequate process to contain at least 50% crude protein, as related to the dry matter, and which may be restructured or textured
Vegetables
All types of vegetables and legumes, fresh or preserved by appropriate treatment
Yeasts
All yeasts, the cells of which have been killed and dried

ADDITIVES

Five types of substances are commonly declared as additives: 1) vitamins, 2) copper, 3) preservatives, 4) antioxidants and 5) coloring agents (**Table 9-5**).

Vitamins A, D and E must be declared when added by the manufacturer. The added amount should be declared although some countries ask the manufacturer to declare the total amount of the vitamins found in the food. Vitamins are declared in IU or in milligrams per kilogram (mg/kg) of food.

Pet foods are regulated by the same legislation that regulates livestock feed. Although clear exceptions are made for companion animal foods, situations arise in which an unusual nutrient must be declared. This is the case for copper because sheep are much more sensitive to copper toxicity. If a copper salt is added to a pet food, the name of the salt and the total copper content must be declared.

If a container has a net weight of up to 10 kg, the manufacturer can use the following statements: "Contains European Economic Community (EEC) permitted antioxidant(s)," "contains EEC permitted preservative(s)" or "contains EEC permitted colorant(s)." However, if a container has a net weight of more than 10 kg, the name of the additive must be stated in the following way: "With antioxidant X," "with preservative Y," or "preserved with Y" and "with colorant Z," or "colored with Z."

Table 9-11. Indications permitted for dietetic pet foods in Europe.

Support of renal function in case of chronic renal insufficiency
Dissolution of struvite uroliths
Reduction of struvite urolith recurrence
Reduction of urate urolith formation
Reduction of oxalate urolith formation
Reduction of cystine urolith formation
Reduction of ingredient and nutrient intolerances
Reduction of acute intestinal absorptive disorders
Compensation for maldigestion (including exocrine pancreatic insufficiency)
Support of heart function in case of chronic cardiac insufficiency
Regulation of glucose supply (diabetes mellitus)
Support of liver function in case of chronic liver insufficiency
Regulation of lipid metabolism in case of hyperlipidemia
Reduction of copper in the liver
Support of skin function in case of dermatosis and excessive loss of hair
Reduction of excessive body weight
Nutritional restoration, convalescence

Table 9-12. Required information on labels of dietetic pet foods in Europe.

Particular nutritional purpose (**Table 9-11**)
Essential nutritional characteristics
Species or category of animals
Labeling declarations
Recommended length of time for use
Other provisions

Only those additives are declared that have been added during production of the food. Additives (e.g., preservatives or antioxidants) added during rendering to preserve raw materials (e.g., meat or fish meals) do not have to be declared on the label.

Maximum permitted levels of additives are strictly regulated. Additives are only permitted after European authorities accept a dossier that documents efficacy and safety.

BEST BEFORE DATE

The Best Before Date is listed as a day, month and year. The date itself can be found outside of the statutory statement in a place in which it may be more convenient for printing on the container (e.g., the can lid or top of the bag). In this case the statement "Best before..." must appear within the statutory statement with instructions of where to find the date.

FEEDING INSTRUCTIONS

Feeding instructions are compulsory on European pet food labels but are not as strictly regulated as in the United States. The manufacturer will usually list the weight of the food to feed per body weight of the animal.

NET WEIGHT

The "net weight" declaration is regulated by packaged goods regulations. The "e" often seen after the net weight is not specific for pet foods, but indicates that the net weight is an average. Strict rules regulate the limits of variation permitted under or above the declared net weight statement to ensure that the consumer receives the full amount purchased. The net weight declaration is often mentioned on the front of the label but some countries require that the statutory statement declare where the net weight can be found.

OTHER DECLARATIONS

Regulations now incorporate the batch number into the obligatory declarations for pet foods as well as the plant-specific registration number. The name and address of the company responsible for the product must also appear.

Dietetic Pet Foods in Europe

In July 1995, labeling of dietetic pet foods for dogs and cats became strictly regulated. Definitions and scope of the legislation are published in Council Directive 93/74/EC, whereas Commission Directives (i.e., 94/39/EC and 95/9/EC) give the applications (Council Directive 93/74/EC; Commission Directive 93/39/EC; Commission Directive 95/9/EC). Consequently, a number of statements have appeared on the labels of dietetic pet foods. The Commission Directives publish lists (**Table 9-11**) with the permitted indications for dietetic foods ("Particular Nutritional Purposes"), the characteristics of the corresponding foods and specific label declarations (**Table 9-12**). The objective of the legislation is to prevent unsubstantiated and misleading claims on pet food labels.

The term "dietetic pet food," and its official translations, is the only term to be used to indicate that a product falls under this legislation. The new label declarations apply without prejudice to the Council Directive on the circulation of compound feeding stuffs and other provisions regulating nonveterinary medical pet foods.

The legislation considers most indications for nutritional management as "temporary situations" making it mandatory to publish a defined length of use on the labels. This period of time has been determined by the commission and its experts, and does not always reflect the manufacturer's recommendations.

Energy declaration is not permitted on pet food labels other than dietetic foods marketed for obesity and convalescence. The energy density is a calculated value expressed in megajoules per kilogram (MJ/kg) of product.

New nutritional purposes may be accepted when new products are marketed and the manufacturer has introduced a dossier showing sufficient data to support the claims.

REFERENCES

The References for **Chapter 9** can be found at www.markmorris.org.

Chapter 10

Making Pet Foods at Home

Rebecca L. Remillard
Stephen W. Crane

"Teach thy tongue to say 'I don't know' and thou shall progress."
Anonymous

CLINICAL IMPORTANCE

Clients are increasingly interested in their own nutrition and that of their pets. Feeding commercially prepared pet foods offers several advantages over feeding homemade foods, including convenience, cost, consistency and better nutritional balance. Nevertheless, a growing number of pet owners prefer to prepare homemade foods. In doing so, they have less guilt, and feel like they are preparing a "real meal" that is "more natural" and "more traditional" (Wolter, 1988).

According to pet owners, veterinarians are the best source of pet health care (Practice Health, 1993); advice about good nutrition is a reasonable extension of this role. Therefore, veterinarians and their health care teams should be able to provide sound and practical advice about home-cooked pet foods. The first part of this chapter gives practitioners more insight into why some pet owners prefer homemade foods, and covers some pet owner concerns about commercially prepared foods because it is possible to provide a balanced homemade food. Veterinarians should not routinely discourage owners who wish to feed such foods. The second part gives practical recommendations for assessing homemade foods. The tables and boxes describe ingredients and methods for formulating homemade foods and resources to correct imbalanced foods.

Nearly all dogs and cats in the United States consume table food at some time in their lives (PFI, 1997). Many dogs fed commercial foods "exclusively" have learned about the availability of table scraps after a meal, garbage on trash day and food from children and generous neighbors. The vast majority of dogs and cats in the United States, however, receive 90% or more of their nutrition from complete and balanced commercially prepared foods (Lund et al, 1996). In one survey, 20% of pet owners answered that they feed their pet candy or table foods every day (AAHA, 1995). The occasional feeding of table foods should not be of concern for healthy pets unless the food composes more than 10% of the daily dry matter intake (Lewis et al, 1987). However, for various reasons, some clients prefer to feed their pets a homemade food exclusively. In the United States, these clients are probably more prevalent in urban areas. Some veterinarians who practice holistic medicine strongly recommend that their clients feed only a home-prepared food. The number of websites offering nutritional consultations about homemade foods by veterinary nutritionists is increasing.

In the United Kingdom and northern European countries, pet owners provide a high proportion of their pets' diets in the form of commercial pet foods. In countries with a longstanding tradition of gourmet cooking, such as France, Italy, Spain and Belgium, many pets receive a portion of the family meal as the cultural norm. In 1987, about 13% of the dog and cat owners in France fed table foods exclusively to their dogs and cats, and another 15% purchased traditional food for home cooking (Pibot, 1989). In 1987, 62% of French dog owners and 79% of cat owners professed to feed commercial pet foods regularly (Bonnavaud, 1989). However, this does not mean pet owners

Table 10-1. Common Reasons Pet Owners and Veterinarians Want to Use a Homemade Food.

They want to use ingredients that are fresh, wild-grown, organic or natural.
They want to avoid additives that are present in some commercial pet foods.
They want to avoid contaminants thought to be present in prepared foods.
They are concerned that the ingredient list is an indecipherable list of chemicals.
They fear an ingredient in a commercial food such as a "by-product."
They wish to maintain adequate food intake in a finicky pet through exceptional palatability.
They desire to personally cook for the pet.
The pet is addicted to table foods or a single grocery item.
They wish to feed major quantities of an ingredient not found in commercial pet foods.
They hope to construct a nutritional profile for dietary management of a disease for which no commercial food is available.
They hope to restrict the allergens/causative substances during an elimination trial or for long-term feeding of animals with adverse reactions to food.
They wish to support a sick or terminally ill animal through home cooking and hand feeding.
They wish to provide food variety as a defense against malnutrition, or because of the popular idea that pets need variety.
They wish to lower feeding costs by using significant quantities of table food and leftovers.
They wish to feed a pet according to human nutritional guidelines (e.g., low fat, low cholesterol, etc.).

feed commercial pet foods "exclusively." One survey estimated that commercial dog foods only provided 27% of the dogs' nutrient needs (Bonnavaud, 1989). In the same period, pet owners spent about one-third of their pet food budget for commercial pet foods and two-thirds for homemade foods (Kieffer, 1989).

In Europe, moist pet foods often are considered a meat source (protein source), rather than a complete pet food. Consequently, some pet food companies have developed a concept that is intermediate between homemade and commercially prepared foods: moist foods, high in protein and fat. To balance the diet, the food's feeding guide recommends supplementing with a specific amount of rice or pasta. A cereal-based mixer is often sold as an alternative to rice and pasta. These latter modules contain carbohydrate and fiber ingredients that are often fortified with calcium, vitamins and trace minerals. When proper ratios are used, the meal provides adequate mineral balance and appropriate protein-to-energy ratios. This may not be the case, however, when the mixer is combined with fresh meat instead of the complementary moist food. Combining, mixing, cooking and serving the modular components fulfills the owner's expectation of "proper" feeding.

RATIONALE FOR CHOOSING HOMEMADE FOODS

When a client wants to prepare pet foods at home, it is important for veterinarians to understand the client's reasons and motivation (**Table 10-1**). In many cases it is possible to address their concerns and to recommend an appropriate commercial food. In one survey, at least 25% of pet owners said they would be influenced to purchase a specific brand of pet food based on a recommendation by their veterinarian (AAHA, 1995). However, when owners strongly prefer to cook for their pet, it is better to provide them with a well-designed homemade recipe, rather than allow them to prepare food according to their own or other well-intentioned pet owner's recipes that may have deficiencies and excesses (Donoghue and Kronfeld, 1994).

Appeal of "Natural" and "Organic" Foods

Independent health food stores in the United States sold $25 million of pet foods marketed as "organic" or "natural" pet foods in 1990, which increased to $29.4 million in 2001. Sales of natural pet food in 2005 reached $520 million, and estimated sales for 2010 are $1.042 billion, with the organic segment approaching $100 million (Kvamme, 2007). These sales figures may well represent the value some pet owners place on natural or organic labeled foods. The United States Department of Agriculture (USDA) has developed national standards for organically produced agricultural products to assure consumers that products marketed as organic meet consistent uniform standards (Jones, 2006). In general, all natural (non-synthetic) substances are allowed in organic production and all synthetic substances are prohibited. Under current definitions, it is not possible to formulate a complete and balanced organic pet food because it is not possible to meet the nutritionally complete and balanced claim without adding inorganic trace minerals and vitamins (Dzanis, 2007). Likewise, it is not possible to formulate a complete and balanced homemade food without using inorganic supplements; therefore, it is only possible to offer a homemade food "made with" organic ingredients. It is important to understand that the definition of organic relates only to how a food product is made and does not relate to the quality or safety of the product.

Appeal of Vegetarian and Vegan Foods

Pet owners who want to feed a vegetarian food to their dog or cat may assume they must prepare the food at home. Commercially prepared vegetarian foods exist for dogs, and can be well-balanced using egg and milk products. Vegan foods (no animal products) should be carefully checked because they may be deficient in arginine, lysine, methionine, tryptophan, taurine, iron, calcium, zinc, vitamin A and some B vitamins (Dwyer, 1991; McDonald et al, 1995). People should be discouraged from preparing vegetarian or vegan foods at home for cats, because cats are strict carnivores. Without adequate supplementation using synthetic ingredients, cats fed vegetarian and vegan diets are at high risk for taurine, arginine, tryptophan, lysine and vitamin A deficiencies.

Concerns about Additives, Preservatives and Contaminants

Additives

In one survey that studied consumer understanding of the word "natural," most respondents mentioned freedom from various types of additives (Miller, 1991). In surveys, additives are always high on the list of food items that consumers feel may damage their health, or are a sufficient reason not to buy a food (Miller, 1991). However, when ranking the known risks of food hazards in people, the relative risk of food-borne disease (microbial contamination) is highest, about 100,000 times the risk associated with additives (Miller, 1991).

Because food technology and additives are a difficult and confusing matter for non-experts, additives often evoke emotional responses from the misinformed (Potter, 1986). For example, minerals and vitamins added to a pet food to complete the nutritional balance are considered additives. In addition, the issue is not always presented correctly; consumer associations and some so-called experts often accuse additives of causing all kinds of disorders in pets. Advertising occasionally abuses the negative image of synthetic additives to promote "natural" or "additive-free" products. However, evidence linking a particular food or food constituent with a particular disease is often circumstantial and great care must be exercised in assessing its significance (Aruoma et al, 1991). Veterinarians do not always have the answers when owners are alarmed by nutrition gossip, but should become more knowledgeable about pet food additives so they can accurately address client concerns.

Additives (e.g., flavorings, colorings, binders and emulsifiers) in pet foods are the same or very similar to those approved for use in human foods. In the United States, no additive may be legally used in foods unless the Food and Drug Administration (FDA) recognizes that the additive is safe at the intended level of use in the intended food. The FDA usually requires at least two-year feeding tests in two species of animals to reveal short- and long-term effects. Additives currently used in human and pet foods are generally regarded as safe (GRAS; 21 CFR 582) and must be removed from human and/or pet foods if there is an indication of harmful effects (Roudebush, 1993). For example, propylene glycol has been removed from the GRAS list for cats.

Clients who want to avoid "additives" as a generic group are often poorly informed about pet food additives and the possible negative consequences of not adding these compounds to foods. Veterinarians should be able to explain the positive aspects of additives to give clients a sufficient comfort level to feed a commercial product instead of a homemade food (Chapter 8).

In general, additives provide three benefits: 1) organoleptic-to provide structure, texture and color, 2) technologic-to serve as binding and gelling agents and 3) nutritional-to serve as vitamins and antioxidants. Clients interested in additive-free products must first specifically identify which additive (intentional vs. unintentional) they wish to avoid. Some commercially available products do not contain artificial colors, flavors and synthetic preservatives. After a pet owner's specific concerns have been identified and discussed, it is likely that an acceptable commercially prepared complete and balanced product can be located.

Preservatives

Consumer research has identified several factors that pet owners associate with natural pet food including freedom from artificial preservatives (Potter, 1986). Veterinarians and their health care teams should become knowledgeable about pet food preservatives so they can accurately address client concerns. A preservative may be defined as "any substance that is capable of inhibiting or retarding the growth of microorganisms or of masking the evidence of such deterioration" (Aruoma et al, 1991). Protection against microbial attack may be achieved by several methods: chemical treatment (semi-moist and some dry foods), dehydration (dry foods), heat (moist and dry foods), irradiation or storage at a low temperature. Preservatives are very important to prevent molding or bacterial deterioration of semi-moist foods. Many preservatives are organic acids and their salts, such as sorbates, and are the same as those used in many human foods and dressings.

ANTIOXIDANTS

Antioxidants function to stabilize fats and fat-soluble vitamins against oxidation. There are two types of antioxidants: natural and synthetic (Hilton, 1989).

Natural Antioxidants

Commonly used natural antioxidants include tocopherols, ascorbic acid (vitamin C) and rosemary. Tocopherols are often referred to as vitamin E. Although vitamin E (alpha-tocopherol) is the biologically active form in the body, it does not effectively stabilize fats in food. The gamma- and delta-tocopherols exert the best antioxidant activity in food, but have very low vitamin E activity. Thus, the term "Preserved with vitamin E" is technically inaccurate, but it is commonly used to assuage client concerns. Instead, the label should indicate whether gamma- or delta-tocopherol was added.

Ascorbic acid and its salts and esters are most effective when combined with other antioxidants. Salts (L-calcium ascorbate) and esters (ascorbyl-5,6-diacetate) of ascorbic acid are synthesized compounds, but may be perceived as acceptable natural alternatives to a "more chemical sounding" antioxidant.

Rosemary has been investigated for use in pet foods. Although always considered a natural antioxidant, rosemary is not used in its original form, but as a refined extract to avoid influence on taste and odor (Löliger, 1991).

Synthetic Antioxidants

The more commonly used synthetic antioxidants are butylated hydroxytoluene (BHT), butylated hydroxyanisole (BHA) and ethoxyquin. BHT and BHA have been used in human foods since 1954 and are most effective when combined. Ethoxyquin has been approved for use in animal feeds and pet foods in the United States for more than 30 years. All three antioxidants are considered safe at their recommended levels in the United States and Europe (AAFCO, 2007; Dzanis, 1991; Council Directive 70/524/EEC, 1970; Council Directive 91/248/EEC, 1991).

Synthetic antioxidants are more effective than natural antioxidants and better withstand the heat, pressure and moisture during food processing. In doing so, they also preserve the fat-soluble vitamins A, D and E for activity in the body. Clients

Box 10-1. AAFCO Definitions for Meat Ingredients Commonly Used in Commercial Pet Foods.

MEAT
Meat is the clean flesh derived from slaughtered mammals and is limited to that part of the striate muscle which is skeletal or that which is found in the tongue, in the diaphragm, in the heart, or in the esophagus; with or without the accompanying and overlying fat and the portions of the skin, sinew, nerve and blood vessels which normally accompany the flesh. It shall be suitable for use in animal foods (IFN 5-00-394).

MEAT BY-PRODUCTS
Meat by-products are the non-rendered, clean parts, other than meat, derived from slaughtered mammals. It includes, but is not limited to lungs, spleen, kidneys, brain, livers, blood, bone, partially defatted low temperature fatty tissue and stomachs and intestines freed of their contents. It does not include hair, horns, teeth and hooves. It shall be suitable for use in animal food (IFN 5-00-395).

MEAT MEAL
Meat meal is the rendered product from mammalian tissues, exclusive of any added blood, hair, hoof, horn, hide trimmings, manure, stomach and rumen contents except in such amounts as may occur unavoidably in good processing practices. It shall not contain added extraneous materials not provided for by this definition. The calcium level shall not exceed the actual phosphorus level by more than 2.2 times. It shall not contain more than 12% pepsin indigestible residue, and not more than 9% of the crude protein in the product shall be pepsin indigestible (IFN 5-00-385).

MEAT AND BONE MEAL
Meat and bone meal is the rendered product from mammal tissues, including bone, exclusive of any added blood, hair, hoof, horn, hide trimmings, manure, stomach and rumen contents except in such amounts as may occur unavoidably in good processing practices. It shall not contain added extraneous materials not provided for by this definition. It shall contain a minimum of 4.0% phosphorus, and the calcium level shall not be more than 2.2 times the actual phosphorus level. It shall not contain more than 12% pepsin indigestible residue, and not more than 9% of the crude protein in the product shall be pepsin indigestible (IFN 5-00-388).

should be aware that most canned foods do not contain antioxidants, and that many commercially prepared dry pet foods use vitamin antioxidants. Awareness of these facts may help clients choose a more appropriate commercially prepared food.

Contaminants

Some clients are concerned about compounds that may be present unintentionally or accidentally in pet foods (pesticides, drug residues and heavy metals) (Chapter 11). Analyses have shown that contamination of pet foods with pesticides, polychlorinated biphenyls (PCBs) and heavy metals is insignificant (Mumma et al, 1986). In the late 1990s, the FDA Center for Veterinary Medicine (CVM) developed and used a sophisticated process to detect and quantify minute amounts of pentobarbital in dog food (2002). Upon finding pentobarbital residues in some samples of dry dog food, CVM scientists conducted further tests that led them to conclude that dogs eating dry dog food are unlikely to have any adverse health effects from the low levels of pentobarbital found in the dog food samples tested. CVM scientists also developed a test to detect dog and cat DNA in the protein of dog food. Because pentobarbital is used to euthanize dogs and cats at animal shelters, finding pentobarbital could suggest that pets were rendered and used in pet food. Test results indicated a complete absence of protein derived from euthanized dogs or cats (Bren, 2002). As a result, CVM scientists assumed the source of pentobarbital in dog food was euthanized farm livestock.

Clients may elect to feed a homemade food to avoid all types of contaminants. However, ingredients in homemade foods may also contain contaminants. Therefore, making a food at home does not ensure against unintentional contaminants. For example, mercury may be found in fish-based pet foods, but the same concern is real for pets fed fresh fish (Mumma et al, 1986; Ferrando, 1989).

Inability to Understand Pet Food Labels

The ingredient list on a pet food label often uses language unfamiliar to most pet owners; however, each term has a specific definition. Pet owners can easily be confused by terms such as meat, meat meal, meat and bone meal and meat by-products (**Box 10-1**).

Furthermore, pet owners may be alarmed about what they read in the popular press and on the Internet about ingredients commonly used in commercial pet foods (Stein, 1993; Pitcairn and Pitcairn, 1995; Martin, 1997, 2002, 2007), which are often undocumented material presented as "investigative research." Consequently, pet owners often assume the worst possible composition of pet food ingredients (Phillips, 1990; Remillard, 1994). Veterinarians should encourage pet owners to identify ingredient terms of concern and provide more accurate information about the composition of these ingredients. Regulatory agency descriptions exist for all ingredients commonly used in commercial pet foods; one source is the Official Publication of the Association of American Feed Control Officials (AAFCO). For example, a pet owner who has read that meat by-products include hair and fecal material (Stein, 1993; Pitcairn and Pitcairn, 2005; Martin, 1997, 2002, 2007), should be informed that it is illegal for meat by-products to contain such materials (AAFCO, 2007).

Some pet owners may still find meat by-products objectionable after learning the AAFCO definition. However, they may be comfortable with the definition of meat as an ingredient and feed a commercially prepared product containing meat instead of a homemade food.

Some pet owners consider the last half of the ingredient list to be nothing more than a list of chemicals and cannot identify the nutrients provided by synthetic sources. Veterinarians should ask pet owners to identify bothersome ingredient terms and then explain to them which essential nutrients are provided by those ingredients. As examples, calcium carbonate provides calcium, zinc oxide provides zinc and sodium selenite provides sodium and selenium. Some vitamin examples are: thiamin mononitrate provides vitamin B_1, calcium pantothenate provides pantothenic acid and D-activated animal sterol provides vitamin D_3. Pet owners may have fewer objections to feeding commercially made products after biochemical names have been translated into more commonly recognized vitamins and minerals.

Other points of concern include whether the ingredients are available to the pet (i.e., whether the animal is able to digest and absorb the nutrients they contain). In the United States, the pet owner's attention should be directed to the AAFCO statement required on every product that claims to be complete and balanced (Chapter 9). The AAFCO statement provides valuable information (i.e., the testing procedures used and the lifestage for which the food has been substantiated). If the complete and balanced claim was not substantiated by feeding tests for the specific lifestage of the pet (i.e., growth, maintenance, reproduction), another more appropriate product should be recommended.

"My dog eats what I eat" is an expression often heard from people who prefer to cook for their pet. Preparing elaborate meals at home gives the owner the feeling of "being involved" and can be an integral part of the human-animal bond. This may be particularly important for elderly, solitary persons who benefit from feeling responsible for somebody and are motivated to remain active. Other people choose to cook simply because they feel guilty, as if they don't care enough. The latter circumstance is a minor concern in the United States, but is more important in countries such as France (AAHA, 1995; Pibot, 1989).

Quite often, the pet that receives home-cooked meals is a geriatric animal with a diminishing appetite, body weight and condition due to a slowly progressive disease (e.g., chronic renal failure, hepatic disease, cancer). Meal preparation and hand-feeding allow the owner to participate in the pet's supportive care. Formulating a simple homemade recipe that is approximately balanced for the animal with a chronic, progressive fatal disease is a reasonable, compassionate gesture on the part of veterinarians.

Table 10-2. Balanced reduced-protein/low-phosphorus homemade formulas for adult dogs and cats with kidney disease.*/**/***

Daily food formulation for an 18-kg (40-lb) dog (as fed)

Ingredients	Grams	Nutrient content (% dry matter)†††	
Rice, white, cooked†	237	Dry matter	41.0
Beef, regular, cooked††	78	*Protein*	21.1
Egg, large, boiled	20	Fat	13.7
Bread, white	50	Linoleic acid	1.8
Oil, vegetable	3	Crude fiber	1.4
Calcium carbonate	1.5	Calcium	0.43
Salt, iodized	0.5	*Phosphorus*	0.22
Total	390	*Potassium*	0.26
		Sodium	0.33
		Magnesium	0.09
		Energy (kcal/100 g)	445

Daily food formulation for a 4.5-kg (10-lb) cat (as fed)

Ingredients	Grams	Nutrient content (% dry matter)†††	
Liver, chicken, cooked	21	Dry matter	37.8
Rice, white, cooked†	98	*Protein*	24.4
Chicken, white, cooked	21	Fat	17.5
Oil, vegetable	7	Linoleic acid	7.9
Calcium carbonate	0.7	Crude fiber	0.85
Salt, iodized	0.5	Calcium	0.54
Salt, substitute (KCl)	0.5	*Phosphorus*	0.29
Total	149	*Potassium*	0.66
		Sodium	0.42
		Magnesium	0.09
		Energy (kcal/100 g)	458

*Also feed one human adult vitamin-mineral tablet (1 g) daily to dogs and 0.5 g tablet to cats to ensure all vitamins and trace minerals are included. Cats should be given one-half to one taurine tablet (500 mg/tablet) daily.

**ESHA Research. Diet Analysis Software. Food Processor Plus, version 5.03, 1990 Salem, OR. Agricultural Software Consultants, Inc. Mixit 2+, version 3.0, 1991, Kingsville, TX.

***__Disclaimer for all homemade food recipes:__ These are computer-formulated homemade foods that meet current recommended nutrient minimums without exceeding the known maximums for dogs and cats. These foods have never been analyzed for actual nutrient content, nor have they been tested in animals (e.g., AAFCO feeding trial) as are some approved, commercially prepared, pet foods. Likewise, the urinary pH produced by these recipes is unknown, but should be adjusted using appropriate oral medications when indicated in certain medical conditions.

†May substitute rice baby cereal and flavor either selection with meat broth during cooking.

††Retain the fat.

†††Nutrients of concern are italicized.

Table Foods Have Become a Bad Habit

Pet owners may begin feeding a young or sick dog or cat from the table only to realize that later the pet will not eat commercially prepared food. Therefore, table food is 100% of the animal's daily intake. There are several methods of weaning pets off one particular food and onto another. However, if the animal is persistent, the owner reluctant to make a change or both, formulating a diet from table foods commonly used in the household may be the only way to ensure the pet receives balanced nutrition. In addition, these animals may have very selective eating habits. In such cases, the veterinarian should inform the owner to thoroughly mix all ingredients of the homemade food to ensure balanced nutrient intake.

A Veterinary Therapeutic Food is Unavailable or Unacceptable

Specific types or forms of nutritional management required by the pet are not always available commercially, or one pet food

Table 10-3. Balanced low-fat homemade formulas for overweight adult dogs and cats.*/**/***

Daily food formulation for an 18-kg (40-lb) dog (as fed)

Ingredients	**Grams**	**Nutrient content (% dry matter)††**	
Chicken, white meat	65	Dry matter	36.5
Egg, large, boiled	81	Protein	22.6
Rice, white, cooked†	325	*Fat*	8.0
Cereal, All Bran	26	Linoleic acid	1.1
Calcium carbonate	2	*Fiber*	5.8
Salt, iodized	1	Calcium	0.50
Salt substitute (KCl)	1	Phosphorus	0.37
Total	501	Potassium	0.63
		Sodium	0.45
		Magnesium	0.14
		Energy (kcal/100 g)	398

Daily food formulation for a 4.5-kg (10-lb) cat (as fed)

Ingredients	**Grams**	**Nutrient content (% dry matter)††**	
Liver, chicken, cooked	125	Dry matter (%)	33.8
Rice, white, cooked†	46	Protein	52.7
Cereal, All Bran	8	*Fat*	11.4
Calcium carbonate	1.2	Linoleic acid	1.2
Salt, iodized	0.3	*Fiber*	5.2
Salt, substitute (KCl)	0.3	Calcium	0.85
Total	180	Phosphorus	0.77
		Potassium	0.67
		Sodium	0.44
		Magnesium	0.11
		Energy (kcal/100 g)	420

*Also feed one human adult vitamin-mineral tablet (1 g) daily to dogs and 0.5 g tablet to cats to ensure all vitamins and trace minerals are included. Cats should be given one-half to one taurine tablet (500 mg/tablet) daily.

**ESHA Research. Diet Analysis Software. Food Processor Plus, version 5.03, 1990 Salem, OR. Agricultural Software Consultants, Inc. Mixit 2+, version 3.0, 1991, Kingsville, TX.

***Disclaimer for all homemade food recipes:** These are computer-formulated homemade foods that meet current recommended nutrient minimums without exceeding the known maximums for dogs and cats. These foods have never been analyzed for actual nutrient content, nor have they been tested in animals (e.g., AAFCO feeding trial) as are some approved, commercially prepared, pet foods. Likewise, the urinary pH produced by these recipes is unknown, but should be adjusted using appropriate oral medications when indicated in certain medical conditions.

†May substitute rice baby cereal and flavor either selection with meat broth during cooking.

††Nutrients of concern are italicized.

may not address a patient's multiple medical problems. Some patients' medical problems may require apparently contradictory dietary management. For example, a patient with little or no pancreatic tissue may require: 1) a highly digestible food because of a deficiency in digestive enzymes but also 2) a food with moderate fiber levels to help manage diabetes mellitus.

A veterinary therapeutic food may be commercially available for a patient with a particular medical problem, but the product may be unacceptable to the patient or owner. Although some veterinary therapeutic foods are even more palatable than many specialty and grocery brands, most commercial veterinary therapeutic foods are not available in a variety of flavors, and the ingredient formulation is usually fixed. If a pet is finicky, the one flavor or formulation may be unacceptable and, the patient may not consume adequate quantities of the food to support body weight and condition.

However, it should be noted that in general, homemade formulas won't be as effective as commercially prepared veterinary therapeutic foods. Also, not all veterinary therapeutic foods can be formulated at home (**Tables 10-2** through **10-6**).

Dietary Elimination Trials

The prevalence of adverse reactions to food (including food intolerances and food allergies) has been roughly estimated at 1% of all hospital cases, or 10 to 20% of cases with allergic dermatoses presented to specialists (Brown et al, 1995; Carlotti et al, 1990). Although adverse reactions to food are a small segment of practice, there is strong evidence that they do occur in pets. Homemade foods may be fed to companion animals as a diagnostic or therapeutic measure in cases in which adverse food reactions are suspected. Veterinarians should investigate possible food reactions in cases in which gastrointestinal or dermatologic signs do not fully resolve with standard therapy (Chapter 31).

A dietary history is required to identify ingredients that must be eliminated from the patient's food; however, examining pet food labels rarely ensures that a particular protein is not in the product. For example, the words meat and liver do not specify the species of origin (i.e., cattle, swine, sheep or goats). In Europe, most pet food labels do not list individual ingredients, which makes the dietary history even less accurate. Thus, some sources of protein (and species) cannot be adequately identified from the ingredient list, and so cannot be effectively eliminated from the food. Veterinarians should not hesitate to contact pet food manufacturers for more detailed information.

The recommended protocol for demonstrating a food allergy requires feeding a food composed of protein ingredients not previously fed to the pet or a pet food product containing hydrolyzed protein sources. All protein and carbohydrate sources in a novel food must be changed (i.e., the meat and grain sources). Game meats (venison, bison, elk), rabbit, ostrich and duck are relatively novel meat sources, whereas potato, barley and pea are novel carbohydrate sources in North America. All other possible dietary sources of protein and carbohydrate should be discontinued including treats, snacks, table foods, vitamin-mineral supplements and chewable medications. Patients not successfully managed with a commercially prepared novel food or a food containing protein hydrolysates are often fed a homemade food for four to 12 weeks. Homemade foods may have an advantage because they can be better tailored to the patient's specific needs, but many have been shown to be deficient in essential nutrients (Roudebush and Cowell, 1992).

Homemade foods used in dietary elimination trials can easily be supplemented with calcium, vitamins and microminerals. Most veterinary and children's vitamin-mineral supplements and chewable/flavored medications contain proteins not derived from novel sources. Adult vitamin-mineral supplements without additives are available from health food stores and pharmacies. Supplements are also available that contain no proteins but complete the nutritional balance for dogs and cats with a variety of concurrent medical conditions (www.balanceit.com).[a] These products are a line of all-in-one patent pending supplements specifically designed to make the preparation of foods for healthy and sick dogs and cats easier and less expensive. Any supplement should be added individually to the homemade food on a trial basis (i.e., one per week) because it may contain an item to which the pet is allergic or intolerant.

COMMON PROBLEMS WITH HOMEMADE FOODS

It is possible to achieve the same nutrient balance with a homemade food as with a commercially prepared food. However, this largely depends on the accuracy and competence of the veterinarian or animal nutritionist formulating the food, and on the compliance and discipline of the owner. Unfortunately, some homemade recipes are flawed even when followed exactly and consistently. In one survey, 90% of the homemade elimination foods prescribed by 116 veterinarians in North America were not nutritionally adequate for adult canine or feline maintenance (Roudebush and Cowell, 1992). Unlike most commercial foods, many published homemade recipes are not complete or balanced to fulfill animal requirements (Roudebush and Cowell, 1992; Kallfez, 1996; Donoghue et al, 1987). Few of the numerous published homemade food recipes for dogs and cats have been tested to document performance over sustained periods (Donoghue and Kronfeld, 1994; Kelly and Willis, 1996). Additionally, making homemade foods requires knowledge, motivation, additional financial resources and careful, consistent attention to recipe detail to ensure a consistent, balanced intake of nutrients.

Very few pet food products sold in the United States are designed to be mixed with another food at home. Some prepared meatless products are available, but the manufacturer clearly instructs the pet owner to feed the food for a limited time or to add a protein source when feeding the product long-term. In North America, homemade foods are more likely to be made "from scratch" than from modules, as in Europe.

Formulations for homemade foods should not be assumed to be complete or balanced for any canine or feline lifestage until sufficiently tested (feeding tests, nutrient analysis, etc.). Most recipes have been crudely balanced using the average nutrient content of specific foods and computer assimilation. The palatability, digestibility and safety of these recipes have not been adequately or scientifically tested (Donoghue and Kronfeld, 1994; Stein, 1993; Pitcairn and Pitcairn, 2005; Martin, 1997, 2002, 2007). Even formulations that are initially complete and balanced put pets at risk when pet owners make their own food substitutions, omit ingredients because of personal preferences or convenience or make preparation errors. Therefore, veterinarians and their health care teams should encourage regular dietary histories and patient monitoring for pets fed homemade foods.

Table 10-4. Balanced low-sodium and low-mineral homemade formulas for adult dogs and cats with heart disease.*/**/***

Daily food formulation for an 18-kg (40-lb) dog (as fed)

Ingredients	Grams	Nutrient content (% dry matter)†††	
Beef, regular cooked†	94	Dry matter	38.7
Rice, white, cooked††	330	Protein	20.8
Cereal, All Bran	9.0	Fat	12.4
Oil, vegetable	2.0	Linoleic acid	1.0
Calcium carbonate	2.0	Fiber	2.9
Salt, substitute (KCl)	1.0	*Calcium*	0.49
Total	438	Phosphorus	0.26
		Potassium	0.59
		Sodium	0.12
		Magnesium	0.11
		Energy (kcal/100 g)	431

Daily food formulation for a 4.5-kg (10-lb) cat (as fed)

Ingredients	Grams	Nutrient content (% dry matter)†††	
Beef, lean, cooked†	67	Dry matter	37.9
Rice, white, cooked††	67	Protein	36.4
Calcium carbonate	0.7	Fat	21.5
Salt, iodized	0.1	Linoleic acid	0.73
Salt, substitute (KCl)	0.1	Fiber	0.65
Total	135	*Calcium*	0.55
		Phosphorus	0.28
		Potassium	0.54
		Sodium	0.17
		Magnesium	0.07
		Energy (kcal/100 g)	500

*Also feed one human adult vitamin-mineral tablet (1 g) daily to dogs and 0.5 g tablet daily to cats to ensure all vitamins and trace minerals are included. Cats should be given one-half to one taurine tablet (500 mg/tablet) daily.

**ESHA Research. Diet Analysis Software. Food Processor Plus, version 5.03, 1990 Salem, OR. Agricultural Software Consultants, Inc. Mixit 2+, version 3.0, 1991, Kingsville, TX.

***Disclaimer for all homemade food recipes:** These are computer-formulated homemade foods that meet current recommended nutrient minimums without exceeding the known maximums for dogs and cats. These foods have never been analyzed for actual nutrient content, nor have they been tested in animals (e.g., AAFCO feeding trial) as are some approved, commercially prepared, pet foods. Likewise, the urinary pH produced by these recipes is unknown, but should be adjusted using appropriate oral medications when indicated in certain medical conditions.

†Retain the fat.

††May substitute rice baby cereal and flavor either selection with meat broth during cooking.

†††Nutrients of concern are italicized.

Common Nutrient Problems in Homemade Foods

It is difficult to characterize homemade foods designed by owners because each food and patient is unique. However, many formulations contain excessive protein, but are deficient in calories, calcium, vitamins and microminerals. Commonly used meat and carbohydrate sources contain more phosphorus than calcium; therefore, homemade foods may have inverse calcium to phosphorus ratios as high as 1:10. Most homemade foods for dogs contain excessive quantities of meat, often providing excessive phosphorus and far exceeding the animal's protein requirements.

Table 10-5. Balanced low-protein/low-purine homemade formula for adult dogs with urate urinary calculi (daily food formulation for an 18-kg (40-lb) dog, as fed).*/**/***

Ingredients	Grams	Nutrient content (% dry matter)†	
Rice, white, cooked	431	Dry matter	29.5
Egg, large, boiled	49	*Protein*	9.8
Oil, vegetable	27	Fat	21.8
Calcium carbonate	1.2	Fiber	2.2
Salt, substitute (KCl)	1.2	Calcium	0.38
Total	509	*Phosphorus*	0.10
		Energy (kcal/100 g)	483

*Also feed one human adult vitamin-mineral tablet (1 g) daily.
**ESHA Research. Diet Analysis Software. Food Processor Plus, version 5.03, 1990 Salem, OR. Agricultural Software Consultants, Inc. Mixit 2+, version 3.0, 1991, Kingsville, TX.
***__Disclaimer for all homemade food recipes:__ These are computer-formulated homemade foods that meet current recommended nutrient minimums without exceeding the known maximums for dogs and cats. These foods have never been analyzed for actual nutrient content, nor have they been tested in animals (e.g., AAFCO feeding trial) as are some approved, commercially prepared, pet foods. Likewise, the urinary pH produced by these recipes is unknown, but should be adjusted using appropriate oral medications when indicated in certain medical conditions.
†Nutrients of concern are italicized.

Table 10-6. A balanced low-residue homemade formula for adult dogs with gastrointestinal disease (daily food formulation for an 18-kg (40-lb) dog, as fed).*/**/***

Ingredients	Grams	Nutrient content (% dry matter)†	
Rice, white, cooked	232	Dry matter	27.7
Cottage cheese	232	Protein	30.4
Egg, large, boiled	116	Fat	15.6
Oil, vegetable	2.0	*Fiber*	0.71
Salt, substitute (KCl)	1.0	Calcium	0.42
Calcium carbonate	1.0	Phosphorus	0.39
Total	585	Energy (kcal/100 g)	450

*Also feed one human adult vitamin-mineral tablet (1 g) daily to dogs to ensure all vitamins and trace minerals are included.
**ESHA Research. Diet Analysis Software. Food Processor Plus, version 5.03, 1990 Salem, OR. Agricultural Software Consultants, Inc. Mixit 2+, version 3.0, 1991, Kingsville, TX.
***__Disclaimer for all homemade food recipes:__ These are computer-formulated homemade foods that meet current recommended nutrient minimums without exceeding the known maximums for dogs and cats. These foods have never been analyzed for actual nutrient content, nor have they been tested in animals (e.g., AAFCO feeding trial) as are some approved, commercially prepared, pet foods. Likewise, the urinary pH produced by these recipes is unknown, but should be adjusted using appropriate oral medications when indicated in certain medical conditions.
†Nutrients of concern are italicized.

Feline foods designed by clients are commonly deficient in fat and energy density or contain an unpalatable fat source (vegetable oil). Homemade foods are rarely balanced for microminerals and vitamins because over-the-counter veterinary vitamin-mineral supplements are neither complete nor are the nutrients well-balanced within the product. In the United States, there is an all-in-one vitamin-mineral supplement specifically designed to balance homemade foods;[a] this supplement is available to pet owners through veterinarians and nutritionists.

Common Ingredient Problems in Homemade Foods

People are taught that eating a variety of foods is nutritionally sound. Clients often extend this principle to their pet's nutrition. As an example, owners who purchase commercial pet foods may not be brand loyal and often change brands "just in case" one brand is really not complete and balanced. Other pet owners will feed both moist and dry versions of complete and balanced products (of the same or different brands) "just in case there's something in one that's not in the other." Pet owners perceive that feeding a variety of foods is their best defense against malnutrition. Many times pet owners feed a variety of foods because they perceive the pet enjoys the frequent dietary changes.

Likewise, some owners feel a homemade food better meets their pet's nutritional requirements because they use a variety of ingredients. Nutritionally, this may or may not be accurate depending on ingredient substitutions. Inappropriate substitutions are a common error made by owners who design homemade pet foods.

Some owners choose the meat and carbohydrate ingredients for the pet's food based on their own preferences, product availability or affordability. Other pets are fed a variety of "leftover" ingredients such as fat trimmings, bones, vegetable skins, crusts and condiments. Pet food composed of table "leftovers" rarely represents the owner's food and is not complete and balanced for the pet.

On the other hand, some owners mistakenly feed their pet according to current and popular human nutritional guidelines such as avoiding fat, cholesterol and sodium. Such practices do not lead to consumption of a complete and balanced food for the pet. Many owners, who make their pet's food according to published canine or feline recipes, over time, make their own ingredient substitutions that may or may not be correct. Foods made at home, therefore, are typically designed from a variety of table foods, and generally have no consistent ingredient composition. Inconsistency is the rule.

The second most common error made by pet owners who cook for their pets is to eliminate the vitamin-mineral supplement because of its inconvenience, expense or a failure to understand its importance. Foods made from recipes that were once crudely balanced become grossly unbalanced when owners eliminate supplements. Regular veterinary checkups are necessary to monitor the patient's progress and response to the food and to monitor the owner's level of compliance.

Some owners and breeders encourage the use of uncooked meat, liver and eggs in their homemade pet food recipes. This practice can be dangerous because uncooked animal ingredients can harbor pathogenic bacteria that normally would be killed during cooking (Chapter 11).

RECOMMENDING HOMEMADE FOODS

Veterinarians should be willing to: 1) assess an existing recipe, 2) offer nutritionally adequate recipes for healthy pets, if the client insists on cooking for the pet (**Tables 10-7** and **10-8**) or 3) if necessary, make appropriate formula substitutions for the client when the pet is diagnosed with a medical problem (**Tables 10-2** through **10-6**).

Assessing Recipes

Veterinarians encounter a wide variety of pet food recipes from breeders, chat rooms and the popular press. Improving the ingredients in such recipes is not a simple task. It requires knowledge and good formulation skills, and an up-to-date database of locally available ingredients. The ingredients should be selected on the basis of nutrient content, tolerance, availability and cost. Information about the nutrient composition of commonly available homemade ingredients can be obtained from readily available sources; however, the information is usually presented in an obscure format such as amounts of "nutrient per serving" on an as fed basis (Watt and Merrill, 1975; Carper, 1975; Pennington, 1994; Pitcairn and Pitcairn, 2005). Information in human food tables is not readily converted to common forms used to compare pet food formulations (e.g., percent as fed or dry matter basis). A simpler method to correct an inadequate homemade formulation is to adjust the proportions or change the ingredients in the recipe. Homemade formulations can be checked for nutritional adequacy and adjusted using the "quick check" guidelines below.

1. Do Five Food Groups Appear in the Recipe?

- A carbohydrate/fiber source from a cooked cereal grain.
- A protein source, preferably of animal origin, or if more than one protein source is used, one source should be of animal origin.
- A fat source.
- A source of minerals, particularly calcium.
- A multivitamin and trace mineral source.

2. Is the Carbohydrate Source a Cooked Cereal and Present in a Higher or Equal Quantity than the Meat Source?

The carbohydrate source to protein source ratio should be at least 1:1 to 2:1 for cat foods and 2:1 to 3:1 for dog foods. Carbohydrate sources for dog and cat foods are used for energy and are usually a cereal such as cooked corn, rice, wheat, potato or barley. These carbohydrate sources have similar caloric contributions, but some carbohydrate sources also contribute a significant amount of protein, fiber and fat (**Table 10-9**). A specific carbohydrate may be chosen based on specific changes in the patient's protein, fat and fiber requirements. For example, soybean may be substituted for corn if more protein is needed, or peas may be substituted if more fiber is needed.

3. What is the Type and Quantity of the Primary Protein Source?

The overall protein quality in a homemade food can be improved by substituting an animal-source protein for a vegetable-source protein. Skeletal muscle protein from different animal species has very similar amino acid profiles. The protein content of various mammalian and avian skeletal muscle tissues is generally equivalent on a water-free basis. Thus, there is no great advantage to feeding one meat source over another. Any cooked animal protein source should provide the majority of a dog's or cat's essential amino acids.

The final food should contain 25 to 30% cooked meat for dogs, (one part meat to two or three parts carbohydrate, respectively) and 35 to 50% cooked meat for cats (one part meat to one to two parts carbohydrate).

Providing some liver in the meat portion is recommended once a week or no more than half of the meat portion regularly. Liver corrects most potential amino acid deficiencies in homemade foods for dogs and cats. Liver not only improves the amino acid profile over that provided by vegetable and skeletal meat sources, but also contributes essential fatty acids, choles-

Table 10-7. Balanced generic homemade daily formulation for a healthy 18-kg (40-lb) adult dog that meets AAFCO allowances.*

Ingredients	Grams	Percent
Carbohydrate, cooked**	240	58
Meat, cooked***	120	29
Fat†	10	2
Fiber††	30	7
Bone meal†††	4.0	-
Potassium chloride∫	1.0	-

***Disclaimer for all homemade food recipes:** These are computer-formulated homemade foods that meet current recommended nutrient minimums without exceeding the known maximums for dogs and cats. These foods have never been analyzed for actual nutrient content, nor have they been tested in animals (e.g., AAFCO feeding trial) as are some approved, commercially prepared, pet foods. Likewise, the urinary pH produced by these recipes is unknown, but should be adjusted using appropriate oral medications when indicated in certain medical conditions.
**Examples include rice, cornmeal, oatmeal, potato, pasta and various infant cereals.
***Examples include all typical meats, poultry, fish and liver.
†Chicken fat, beef fat, vegetable oil or fish oil.
††Prepared high-fiber cereals (All Bran, Fiber One) or vegetables (raw or cooked).
†††Dicalcium phosphate can be used instead of bone meal.
∫Readily available as a salt substitute in grocery stores.
Human adult vitamin-mineral tablet (1 g/tablet, give 1 tablet/day)

Nutrient content (% dry matter)	
Protein	21
Fat	20
Crude fiber	6.5
Calcium	0.66
Phosphorus	0.59
Magnesium	0.1
Sodium	0.2
Potassium	0.6
kcal (as fed)	820

Directions: Bake or microwave meat component and cook starch component separately. Grind or finely chop meat if necessary. Pulverize the bone meal or dicalcium phosphate. Mix with other components except the vitamin-mineral supplement. Mix well and serve immediately or cover and refrigerate. Feed the vitamin-mineral supplement with the meal; give as a pill or pulverize and thoroughly mix in food before feeding.

Table 10-8. Balanced generic homemade daily formulation for a healthy 4.5-kg (10-lb) adult cat that meets AAFCO allowances.*

Ingredients	Grams	Percent
Carbohydrate, cooked**	60	50
Meat, cooked***	40	34
Fat†	10	8
Bone meal††	1.2	-
Salts (NaCl/KCl)†††	1.0	-
Taurine	0.5	-

***Disclaimer for all homemade food recipes:** These are computer-formulated homemade foods that meet current recommended nutrient minimums without exceeding the known maximums for dogs and cats. These foods have never been analyzed for actual nutrient content, nor have they been tested in animals (e.g., AAFCO feeding trial) as are some approved, commercially prepared, pet foods. Likewise, the urinary pH produced by these recipes is unknown, but should be adjusted using appropriate oral medications when indicated in certain medical conditions.
**Examples include rice, cornmeal, oatmeal, potato, pasta and various infant cereals.
***Examples include all typical meats, poultry, fish and liver.
†Chicken fat, beef fat, vegetable oil or fish oil.
††Dicalcium phosphate can be used in place of bone meal.
†††Readily available as a lite salt in grocery stores.
Human adult vitamin-mineral tablet (1 g/tablet, give 0.5 tablet/day).

Nutrient content (% dry matter)	
Protein	31
Fat	28
Crude fiber	2.0
Calcium	0.69
Phosphorus	0.58
Magnesium	0.1
Sodium	0.4
Potassium	0.75
kcal (as fed)	250

Directions: Bake or microwave meat component and cook starch component separately. Grind or finely chop meat if necessary. Pulverize the bone meal or dicalcium phosphate. Mix with other components except the vitamin-mineral supplement. Mix well and serve immediately or cover and refrigerate. Feed the vitamin-mineral supplement with the meal; give as a pill or pulverize and thoroughly mix in food before feeding.

terol, energy, vitamins and microminerals. If a pet owner requests an ovo-lacto vegetarian food, eggs are the best ingredient. If a vegan food is requested, soybeans provide the next best, but incomplete, amino acid profile.

4. Is the Primary Protein Source Lean or Fatty?

The fat content of different cuts of meat varies. When the specified protein source is "lean," an additional animal, vegetable or fish fat source should compose at least 2% of the formula weight for dogs, and 5% of the formula for cats to ensure adequate energy density and essential fatty acids. If a homemade food lacks sufficient caloric density (fat), the addition of cooked beef or chicken fat, poultry skins, vegetable or fish oils (tuna, mackerel, sardine) can increase the caloric density without adding other nutrients. Changing the cut of meat can also markedly increase the fat content of a food (**Box 10-2**).

5. Is a Source of Calcium and Other Minerals Provided?

A homemade food is almost never spontaneously balanced in minerals; an absolute calcium deficiency is common. Unfortunately, pet owners erroneously assume cottage cheese, cheese or milk added in small quantities to homemade pet foods provides adequate calcium. Most foods require a specific calcium supplement. When the protein fraction equals or is greater than the carbohydrate fraction, usually only calcium carbonate is added to the food (0.5 g/4.5-kg cat/day and at least 2.0 g/15-kg dog/day). Calcium carbonate, containing 40% calcium and less than 1% phosphorus, is available in various size tablets from most pharmacies, health food and grocery stores.

Calcium and phosphorus supplementation may be necessary when the protein fraction is less than the carbohydrate fraction. Steamed bone meal, dicalcium phosphate and certain proprietary mineral supplements contain approximately 27% calcium and 16% phosphorus (about 2:1) and microminerals. These supplements, fed at the same dose as calcium carbonate, usually correct the calcium and phosphorus content.

6. Is a Source of Vitamins and Other Nutrients Provided?

Supplements providing vitamins, microminerals, fatty acids and specific nutrients of concern for cats and dogs can be obtained, but they may be cumbersome to feed and greatly increase the cost of the food. An adult over-the-counter vitamin-mineral tablet that contains no more than 200% of the recommended daily allowances for people works well for both dogs and cats at one-half to one tablet per day. One tablet per day of a human adult product will not oversupplement pets with calcium, phosphorus, magnesium, vitamins A, D and E, iron, copper, zinc, iodine and selenium, according to AAFCO maximum allowances for canine and feline foods (2007). In general, veterinary supplements contribute between 0 and 300% of the vitamin-mineral requirements of dogs and cats.

Specific nutrients of concern for cats-such as arginine, arachidonic acid, L-carnitine and choline-can be purchased as individual nutrient products. However, levels in homemade cat foods are usually adequate when a combination of animal proteins is used. Cats fed a homemade formula exclusively should receive 200 to 500 mg taurine daily, depending on the calculated taurine content of the food. Iodized salt should be used whenever salt is added to the food. It is difficult to meet the iodine requirement without using the iodized form (400 µg of iodine/6 g [1 tsp] sodium chloride). The alternative is to prescribe the canine or feline supplement designed for homemade foods.[a]

Making Ingredient Substitutions

When formulating a homemade recipe, proportions of carbohydrate, protein, fat and fiber must be maintained. **Table 10-10** suggests starch, meat, fat and fiber ingredient substitutions and their relative nutrient values. When substituting one ingredient for another, determine the relative nutrient value of the old ingredient and that of the replacement ingredient. If the old

Table 10-9. Nutrient profiles of cooked grains and vegetables for homemade foods.

Cereal	Calories*	Total carbohydrate**	Sugar**/***	Protein**	Dietary fiber**	Fat**
Corn	352	81	12.2	9.0	6.1	4.3
Chickpeas	412	68	3.0	22.0	12.3	6.5
Barley	388	85	2.0	10.6	20	3.2
Peas	383	72	19.5	24.6	25.9	2.0
Potato	374	87	2.0	7.4	6.5	<1.0
Rice, brown	411	85	1.5	9.6	6.3	3.3
Rice, white	406	87	<1.0	8.4	1.6	<1.0
Rice, instant	408	88	1.4	8.6	3.3	<1.0
Soybean	467	27	8.1	44.9	17.0	24.3
Wheat (pasta)	422	80	<1.0	16.7	6.5	3.2

*Expressed on a kcal/100 g dry matter.
**Expressed on a percent dry matter basis.
***Readily available sugars (e.g., mono- and disaccharides).

recipe recommended 75 g of rice, and the owner would like to use pumpkin instead of rice, 200 g of pumpkin will be needed to supply the same amount (15 g) of carbohydrate as 75 g of rice (**Table 10-10**). As fed weights of foods can be found at the USDA National Nutrient Database (www.nal.usda.gov/fnic/foodcomp/search).

Several methods can be used to formulate homemade foods. Veterinary nutritionists in North America commonly use nutrition software programs such as those listed in Chapter 1. Most practicing veterinarians in North America either contact a veterinary nutritionist directly or use one of these software programs. A third method is to hand calculate the formulation using these steps: 1) determine the ingredients to be used from each food category (**Table 10-10**) and 2) determine the appropriate amount of each ingredient that will supply the needed amount of nutrient for the dog or cat. Each ingredient supplies more than just one nutrient (e.g., rice supplies carbohydrates and some protein). However, this simplified method of formulating a homemade food minimizes nutrient deficiencies by providing overlapping sources of nutrients.

Nutritionally Adequate Recipes

Tables 10-7 and **10-8** are homemade food recipes for healthy adult dogs and cats, respectively. These recipes should be considered all-purpose foods. It should be noted that all-purpose foods do not provide the ideal nutrient profile for most dogs and cats. All-purpose foods, however, provide excess nutrients to adult and older cats and dogs (Chapters 13, 14, 20 and 21).

There are also homemade food recipes for clinical patients. **Table 10-2** contains recipes for reduced protein/low-phosphorus foods for dogs and cats with kidney disease. **Table 10-3** contains recipes for low-fat/high-fiber foods for overweight dogs and cats. **Table 10-4** contains recipes for low-sodium/low-mineral foods for dogs and cats with heart disease. **Table 10-5** is a recipe for a low-protein/low-purine food for dogs with urinary calculi. **Table 10-6** is a recipe for a low-residue food for dogs with gastrointestinal disease.

Because these foods are for clinical patients, it is imperative that clients follow these recipes meticulously. Well-intentioned but ill-informed substitutions or other modifications could result in ineffective, or even counterproductive, nutritional therapy. Furthermore, it is unlikely that these recipes will be as effective as commercial foods in managing clinical patients, even when followed closely.

Box 10-2. Effect of Meat Substitutions on Fat and Energy Levels in Homemade Recipes.

The fat content of the animal protein source in homemade pet food recipes can greatly affect the energy density of the food. In general, animal protein sources such as fish, beef, turkey, chicken and mutton or lamb have similar protein and amino acid contents (**Table 1**). As a result, they can usually be substituted for one another on an as fed basis in most typical homemade food recipes. On the other hand, the fat content and therefore the energy density can increase greatly depending on whether the cut of meat is regular (typical), lean or extra lean (**Table 2**). See **Table 10-10** for more information about ingredient substitutions.

Table 1. Protein and energy content of interchangeable protein sources for a homemade cat food recipe (as fed).

Protein/energy	Lean beef	Chicken	Tuna
Protein	28	28	29
kcal ME/g	4.5	4.4	4.4
kJ ME/g	18.7	18.5	18.2

Table 2. Protein, fat and energy density of ground beef (30 g) with varying fat levels (as fed).

Protein/ fat/energy	Extra lean (>90%)	Lean (>80%)	Regular (<80%)
Protein (g)	7	7	7
Fat (g)	3	5	8
Energy (kcal)	55	73	100
Energy (kJ)	230	305	418

The Bibliography for **Box 10-2** can be found at www.markmorris.org.

Table 10-10. Cooked ingredient substitution lists.

Ingredients	Major nutrient	18-kg (40-lb) dog	4.5-kg (10-lb) cat
Starch, cooked	Carbohydrate	60 g	12 g
Meat, cooked	Protein	28 g	9 g
Fat	Fat	10 g	10 g
Fiber	Dietary fiber	10 g (max)	5 g (max)

Starch: These foods in these amounts yield 15 g carbohydrate with 3 g protein, trace fat and 80 kcal

Bread	25 g	Breadsticks, raisin, rye, whole wheat, white
	30 g	Bagel, English muffins, buns, rolls, pita, tortilla
Cereal	20 g	Ready to eat cereals
	25 g	Bran cereals, shredded wheat
	30 g	Bran flakes, Chex
	100 g	Cooked cereals and grits
Grains	20 g	Cornmeal, flour, cornstarch, popcorn, tapioca
	75 g	Rice
	100 g	Barley, pasta
Vegetables	50 g	Baked beans, sweet potato
	75 g	Beans, peas, lentils, plantain
	80 g	Corn
	100 g	Corn on the cob, lima beans, green peas, potato, yam
	150 g	Squash, parsnips
	200 g	Pumpkin

Protein: Should be weighed after cooking and after bone, skin and excess fat have been removed

Low fat: These foods in these amounts yield 7 g protein with 3 g fat and 55 kcal

Beef	30 g	Baby beef, chipped beef, flank tenderloin, plate ribs, round (bottom, top), all rump cuts, lean spareribs, tripe, ground beef (>90% lean) and USDA good and choice
Dairy	30 g	Cottage cheese
	45 g	Cheeses (low fat 3 g or less/oz.)
Fish	30 g	Any fresh or frozen, tuna or mackerel canned in water
Mixed meats	30 g	Low-fat luncheon meats with 3 g fat or less /oz., >90% lean
Pork	30 g	Leg, tenderloin, ham, Canadian bacon
Poultry	30 g	Chicken or turkey meat without skin
	90 g	Egg whites
Seafood	30 g	Clams, crab, lobster
	50 g	Scallops
	60 g	Shrimp
	90 g	Oysters
Veal	30 g	Leg, loin, rib, shank, shoulder
Wild game	30 g	Venison, rabbit, squirrel, pheasant, goose without skin

Medium fat: These foods in these amounts yield 7 g protein with 5 g fat and 73 kcal

Beef	30 g	Ground beef (>80% lean), corned beef, ribeye
Dairy	30 g	Cheese: mozzarella, ricotta, farmer
Fish	30 g	Tuna, salmon canned in oil, drained
Lamb	30 g	Leg, rib, sirloin, loin, shank, shoulder
Mixed meats	30 g	Low-fat luncheon meats with 3-5 g fat/oz., 85-90% lean
Organ meats	30 g	Liver, kidney, heart, sweetbreads
Pork	30 g	Loin, shoulder arm and blade, butt
Poultry	30 g	Chicken or turkey meat with skin, duck and goose well-drained of fat
	50 g	Egg whole
Veal	30 g	Cutlet
Vegetable	120 g	Tofu

High fat: These foods in these amounts yield 7 g protein with 8 g fat and 100 kcal

Beef	30 g	Ground beef (<80% lean), brisket, chuck, ribs, USDA prime
Dairy	30 g	Cheese spreads, all regular American, blue, cheddar, Monterey, Swiss
Lamb	30 g	Breast, ground
Mixed meats	30 g	Cold cuts, sausages
	45 g	Frankfurter
Pork	30 g	Spareribs, back ribs, ground, country style and deviled ham, sausage
Veal	30 g	Breast
Vegetable	30 g	Peanut butter

Fats: These foods in these amounts yield 5 g fat with 45 kcal

Monounsaturated	5 g	Margarine with soybean, cottonseed, partially hydrogenated oils, peanut oil, olive oil
Polyunsaturated	5 g	Soft tub margarine, oil (safflower, corn, sunflower, cottonseed, sesame)
	15 g	Diet margarine with safflower, corn, sun–flower oil
Saturated	5 g	Chicken fat, beef fat, bacon fat, lard, butter, shortening
	15 g	Heavy cream, cream cheese
	30 g	Sour cream, nondairy substitutes, gravy
	45 g	Light cream, half & half

Fiber: Grams of dietary fiber per 100 g of these foods

Low (0-2 g)	Asparagus, cucumber, lettuce, zucchini, alfalfa sprouts, eggplant, mushrooms, celery, green pepper, tomatoes
Medium (2-4 g)	Bamboo shoots, carrots, peas, string beans, bean sprouts, chickpea, pinto beans, summer squash, broccoli, cauliflower, pumpkin, turnips, cabbage, kidney beans, spinach, watercress
High (5 g or more)	Beans (white, red, lima, black, broad, soy)

Additional Instructions

Specific instructions for preparing, storing and feeding of homemade foods should be given to pet owners. Explaining the importance of a balanced food and providing practical recommendations about how to mix and cook the food will increase compliance. Some owners may even prefer a commercially prepared food when they realize what is involved in preparing a balanced homemade recipe.

Some owners and breeders encourage the use of uncooked meat and eggs in their homemade pet food recipes. Pet owners should be informed that uncooked meat and eggs can harbor pathogenic bacteria that are normally killed during cooking (Chapter 11). Animal ingredients (meat and eggs) should be cooked for at least 10 minutes at 82°C (180°F). Vegetable ingredients should be washed or rinsed and cooked if increased digestibility is desired. Owners can make homemade foods that lack preservatives and antioxidants in three- to seven-day batches but must refrigerate the food in airtight containers between meals (0 to 4°C [32 to 40°F]). Larger quantities of food can be frozen (-20°C [<0°F]). Because homemade foods are relatively high in moisture and lack a preservative system, they are highly susceptible to bacterial and fungal growth when left at room temperatures for more than a few hours. Pet owners who feed homemade foods must also check the food daily for color and odor changes that may indicate spoilage or deterioration. Clients should be advised of these food safety issues when feeding homemade foods (Chapter 11).

Pet owners should be encouraged to use a dietary gram scale to weigh ingredients. Later, they can convert weights to volumes for easier compounding. Ingredient compositions are published in different ways. For example, some recipes specify cooked rice, whereas others specify rice to be weighed as purchased. Formulation must take this variability into account, and the owner should be informed about it.

Cooking is necessary to improve the digestibility of starch in carbohydrate sources (Walker et al, 1994; Wolter, 1982). Cooking also destroys anti-nutrient factors that may be present (e.g., anti-trypsin in soybeans, thiaminase in some fish). However, carbohydrate and animal protein sources should be cooked separately. Carbohydrate sources need a longer cooking time to increase digestibility, due to swelling and gelatinizing of starch granules. Meat and liver, on the other hand, should not be overcooked to avoid protein denaturation. Cooking vegetables may increase starch digestibility, but does not decrease the value of vegetables as a source of fiber. Longer cooking times, however, may increase vitamin losses (Meyer, 1990).

After cooking, all ingredients should be thoroughly mixed in a blender to prevent the animal from picking out single food items. An unbalanced intake of nutrients may occur if ingredients of a nutritionally balanced homemade food are allowed to separate and the animal does not consume the entire mixture. Be sure the owner understands the dietary formulation only approximates the recommended nutrient intake of the pet at a given weight for a certain number of days.

Owners should be warned that although vitamins and minerals are present in only small quantities, they are very important and are not optional. Vitamin-mineral supplements should not be cooked or heated or stored with the food. Vitamins may be destroyed by heat or oxidation. The vitamin-mineral supplement should be kept separate from the food, and administered just before, during or after a meal to ensure proper dosing. Overall digestibility and availability of vitamin-mineral supplements are improved when using USP labeled products and when these nutrients are present in the small intestine with a meal composed of proteins, fats and carbohydrates.

The food should be warmed to just below body temperature before feeding. Clients should be advised to carefully check for "hot spots" that could burn a pet's mouth after food has been rewarmed in a microwave oven. Wetting the food may improve palatability. Moisture content of homemade foods is approximately 70%, which is more similar to that of moist than dry commercial foods. Animals that favor dry forms of commercial foods may reject homemade foods.

When stored too long, the food mixture may separate and dry out, becoming less palatable. Therefore, it is best not to prepare large amounts of food that cannot be eaten in a few days. Mixing the food before warming will improve palatability.

When choosing the ingredients for specific foods, keep in mind that some ingredients are acceptable for one species, but may markedly decrease the palatability for another. For example, dogs like sugar but cats do not. When formulating a food for patients with diabetes mellitus or colitis, for example, beans and peas may be a suitable carbohydrate and protein source for dogs, but increasing the amount of these ingredients may make a food unacceptable to cats.

Vegetable and meat sources may be substituted for similar ingredients in a recipe (**Table 10-10**). Owners who feed a variety of foods decrease the risk that a particular nutrient might be below requirement long enough to cause clinical signs of deficiency. Clients should receive a list of possible substitutes, and be informed that inappropriate substitutions may jeopardize nutritional balance.

If the patient has a history of food rejection or gastrointestinal upset with food changes, advise the client to feed the homemade food without supplements for a week or so, and then add the supplements one at a time (one per week) to avoid the problem or better identify the source of the problem.

In practices where homemade foods are regularly recommended, the staff should have experience preparing the recipes to become familiar with the preparation of homemade foods. Furthermore, it is worthwhile and probably cost effective to send the most commonly recommended formulas to a food analytical laboratory to confirm the calculated analysis. In the United States, AAFCO provides valuable guidelines for minimum and maximum nutrient allowances within which a food for healthy dogs and cats should be formulated if no feeding tests are done. These guidelines may be a useful target for formulating homemade foods as well.

PATIENT ASSESSMENT/MONITORING

Patients that eat homemade foods should be brought in for regular veterinary examinations (two to three visits per year). Because the nutritional profile of homemade foods is quite variable, a nutritional review is recommended at least twice a year. If a dog or cat eats a homemade food exclusively for more than six months, the veterinarian should ask the client to record and submit a three- to five-day food history so that the nutrient profile and ingredient substitutions can be reevaluated.

The effectiveness of a food can be grossly evaluated by noting the patient's body weight, body condition and activity level. Laboratory data such as albumin level, red blood cell number and size and hemoglobin concentration are gross estimations of the animal's nutritional status and can be used with other clinical observations to evaluate homemade foods.

More specifically, the skin and hair should be examined closely and an ophthalmic examination, including evaluation of the lens and retina, should be performed. These tissues are more sensitive than others to nutritional status (Remillard et al, 1993; Glaze and Blanchard, 1983; Sousa et al, 1988; Harvey, 1994). Stool quality should also be assessed.

Veterinarians should always: 1) offer to have a homemade recipe evaluated by a nutritionist and 2) recommend the feeding of a consistent complete and balanced commercial product as often as possible. This is especially true if the pet has a medical condition for which dietary management depends on the highest level of diet consistency and quality assurance.

ACKNOWLEDGMENTS

The authors and editors acknowledge the contributions of Drs. Bernard-Marie Paragon and Jacques Debraekeleer and Mr. Christopher Cowell in the previous edition of Small Animal Clinical Nutrition.

ENDNOTE

a. Balance IT Supplements, DVM Consulting Prof. Corp., Davis, CA, USA.

REFERENCES

The references for **Chapter 10** can be found at www.markmorris.org.

CASE 10-1

Lethargy and Vomiting in Three Cats

Rebecca L. Remillard, PhD, DVM, Dipl. ACVN
MSPCA Angell Animal Medical Center
Boston, Massachusetts, USA

Patient Assessment

Three cats were examined for lethargy and occasional vomiting. Two cats were at their optimal body weight and condition (weight = 4.5 kg, body condition score = 3/5); one cat weighed 5.5 kg and had a body condition score of 4/5. All three cats were icteric, had elevated hepatic enzyme levels and were diagnosed as having hepatic lipidosis.

Assess the Food and Feeding Method

The owners read about pet food manufacturing in a popular cat publication and decided they no longer wanted to feed a commercially produced food to their three cats. They discarded all pet food products in the house, chose a recipe suggested in the text that suited them and began feeding the homemade food exclusively for two weeks. Two cats reluctantly ate a little food almost every day, whereas one cat refused food completely.

Questions

1. How should the veterinarian advise these clients about making food changes in the future?
2. These owners did not want to feed a commercially produced cat food because they were convinced the ingredients used were making their cats subclinically but progressively ill. What food recommendations should be made for these cats?

Answers and Discussion

1. When making food changes for cats, a gradual transition schedule that decreases the old food and increases the proportion of new food is highly recommended (Chapter 1). Generally, cats should eat daily and should not go more than three days without eating a sufficient quantity of food to meet their resting energy requirement. Hepatic lipidosis can occur in normal and overweight cats. The condition occurs more commonly when cats are completely anorectic, but can also occur in cats that have been partially anorectic for weeks to months.
2. Because the owners are convinced they should feed a homemade food, they should be offered a nutritionally adequate generic recipe or should be referred to a nutritionist who could formulate a recipe that takes into consideration their particular concerns.

Progress Notes

The three cats were fed a complete and balanced liquid feline formula for three days (30 ml every three hours) by nasogastric tube. Moist kitten food was offered free choice. Two cats began eating on Days 4 and 5 and were discharged. The third cat progressively deteriorated and was euthanized on Day 5.

CASE 10-2

Weight Loss in an Older Cat

Rebecca L. Remillard, PhD, DVM, Dipl. ACVN
MSPCA Angell Animal Medical Center
Boston, Massachusetts, USA

Patient Assessment

The owner of a 17-year-old, neutered female domestic shorthair cat with chronic renal failure requested a recipe so she could cook for her cat at home. The owner thought the cat's poor appetite would improve if the cat were fed a food that contained chicken, the cat's favorite ingredient. She asked the veterinarian to review a homemade recipe she obtained from a cat breeder. The cat weighed 3.2 kg (7 lb) and had a body condition score of 2/5.

Assess the Food and Feeding Method

The recipe's nutrient content follows:

Ingredient	(g)	(%)
Meat (chicken, white)	25	25
Rice or pasta	55	55
Vitamin-mineral supplement	13	13
Brewer's yeast	5	5
Spirulina (blue green algae)	2	2

Question

Using the quick check guidelines for homemade foods (See chapter text.), what suggestions should be made about nutrients, ingredient levels and food preparation?

Answer and Discussion

The meat source should constitute at least 30% of the as fed homemade food and contain more fat. The recipe as presented contains virtually no fat. This cat is underweight and has a less than optimal body condition score; it needs a more energy dense food. If the cat prefers white meat then approximately 10 to 20 g of fat is necessary. Chicken skin, beef fat or vegetable or fish oils may be used to constitute at least 10% of the as fed weight of the food.

The food needs a calcium source, such as 0.3 g of calcium carbonate per day. Review the vitamin-mineral supplement label to ensure the supplement contains trace minerals (copper, zinc, manganese, iron, iodine and selenium), B vitamins, vitamin A and taurine. Encourage the owner to use a dietary gram scale to weigh and blend all ingredients to prevent the cat from picking out the chicken, but administer the vitamin-mineral supplement with the meal. The revised recipe follows:

Ingredient	(g)	(%)
Meat (chicken, white)	35	31
Rice or pasta	60	52
Fat (chicken skin)	15	13
Vitamin-mineral supplement	4	3
Calcium carbonate	0.3	0.25

The client was advised to feed chicken liver once a week in place of the chicken meat. The vitamin-mineral supplement recommended was one-half of an adult vitamin-mineral tablet. Brewer's yeast adds magnesium, B vitamins, microminerals and fiber; however, nutritional yeast is fortified and has a better nutritional profile of B vitamins and microminerals. The *Spirulina* is of questionable nutritional value, but probably causes no harm.

CASE 10-3

Understanding Pet Food Labels

Rebecca L. Remillard, PhD, DVM, Dipl. ACVN
MSPCA Angell Animal Medical Center
Boston, Massachusetts, USA

Patient Assessment

A dog owner recently went to a local kennel club meeting and heard that synthetic preservatives in pet foods should be avoided. She was especially concerned about a preservative with a long name that begins with an "e." Because she didn't know which pet foods in the grocery store contained the compound, she preferred to make her dog's food at home. She asked her veterinarian to review the ingredient list and specifically asked if the ingredient called "ethylenediamine dihydroiodide" is the preservative she should avoid.

Questions

1. What is ethylenediamine dihydroiodide?
2. Where or how can this information be found?
3. What should be the recommendation to the dog owner?

Answers and Discussion

1. Ethylenediamine dihydroiodide is a source of iodine in pet foods in the United States. It is not the preservative ethoxyquin.
2. The Association of American Feed Control Officials (AAFCO) manual provides this information. Alternatively, the pet food company could be contacted directly.
3. The owner need not be concerned about feeding ethoxyquin; however, if she wishes to avoid this preservative, she could choose a commercial pet food product preserved with other antioxidants (e.g., a natural preservative). A commercially prepared complete and balanced pet food is preferable to a homemade food.

CASE 10-4

Back Pain and Weakness in a Springer Spaniel

Rebecca L. Remillard, PhD, DVM, Dipl. ACVN
MSPCA Angell Animal Medical Center
Boston, Massachusetts, USA

Patient Assessment

A 13-month-old female English springer spaniel was examined for chronic small bowel diarrhea of seven months' duration. The dog weighed 5.5 kg and had a body condition score of 2/5.

Assess the Food and Feeding Method

The owner was unwilling to feed any commercially produced dog food because "he had tried them all and none of them ever worked." According to the client, the dog does well and had normal stools when fed a homemade food containing only one part boiled white chicken and two parts instant rice. The pet owner would like for the veterinarian to balance this food.

The veterinarian gave the client the following recipe:

Ingredient	(g)	(%)
Chicken, dark meat with skin	80	24
White rice, cooked	250	74
Calcium carbonate	0.6	0.2
Vitamin-mineral supplement	8	2
Salt (NaCl), iodized	0.4	0.1

The owner was also given a printed complete set of instructions and cautions.

Reassessment
Six months later the dog presented with severe back pain, rear leg weakness, inappetence, depression and lethargy. The dog ate the homemade food exclusively for six months and had few episodes of diarrhea. The dog's serum calcium concentration was 8.9 mg/dl (reference range = 9 to 11 mg/dl). The dog's serum albumin concentration was normal.

Questions
1. What additional information would be important to obtain about feeding the homemade food?
2. What is the most likely food-related problem given the clinical signs of generalized muscle weakness and lethargy?
3. What common omission do clients who feed a homemade food often make?

Answers and Discussion
1. The recipe should be checked item by item to ascertain whether the owner is following the recipe and then the instructions for mixing and feeding the food should be reviewed with the client.
2. Long-term feeding of a calcium-deficient food can result in marked muscle weakness, lethargy and osteoporosis.
3. Omitting the vitamin-mineral supplement is a common error made by owners who feed a homemade food.

Progress Notes
After reviewing the food formulation with the owner, he admitted that he had not been giving calcium carbonate supplementation because it was inconvenient to give the dog one (0.5 g calcium carbonate) tablet per day. Ten percent calcium gluconate solution was administered intravenously at 15 mg/kg slowly over one hour. Within hours the dog's attitude improved and the dog was able to stand. The dog was apparently difficult to medicate, so liquid or powdered supplements mixed in the food were suggested.

Chapter 11

Food Safety

E. Phillip Miller
Neil W. Ahle
Mary C. DeBey

*"Do not eat any detestable thing . . .
Do not eat anything you find already dead."
Deuteronomy 14: 3, 21*

INTRODUCTION

Each year more than 24 million Americans are affected by foodborne illnesses such as salmonellosis, botulism and staphylococcal food poisoning (Ensminger et al, 1995). In people, both identified and undocumented pathogens likely cause 76 million cases of foodborne illness, 323,000 hospitalizations and 5,200 deaths annually (Mead et al, 1999). Luckily, the typically affected person often improves in 24 hours and has little more than an upset stomach. Likewise, domesticated pets can become ill from ingesting contaminated food. Most animal feedstuffs including spoiled foods such as garbage and carrion are rich in the nutrients needed to support rapid microbial colonization (Coppock and Mostrom, 1986). This phenomenon occurs quickly because most bacteria have the ability to double their number every 30 minutes under favorable moisture and temperature conditions.

Microbes of all shapes and sizes are everywhere in our environment. Foods can be contaminated at any stage of production, starting in the field and ending with storage in the home. The time between the harvesting of pet food ingredients, food handling and preparation in the home and consumption of the final product provides multiple opportunities for microbial populations to proliferate. Microbial growth can result in either food spoilage or risk of foodborne illness. The current methods of food processing and preservation simply forestall the final outcome: spoilage. The earlier in the food production cycle the contamination occurs, the more widespread the outbreak.

Foodborne diseases (**Figure 11-1**) can be divided into two types: 1) food infections (usually bacterial) and 2) food intoxication (microbial toxicoses) (Ensminger et al, 1995). Food infections such as salmonellosis and salmon disease (*Neorickettsia helminthoeca*) result from ingestion of infectious microbial cells that invade the host's tissues, and after an appropriate incubation period, produce the disease. Because it takes time for these cells to replicate to pathogenic numbers, clinical disease in food infections does not become evident until at least 12 to 24 hours after ingestion.

Food intoxications do not depend on the ingestion of viable cells, but result from ingestion of a food that already contains a microbial toxin. Because cell replication is not required, the signs of food poisoning appear rapidly, sometimes in less than one hour after ingestion. The term "food poisoning" is often incorrectly used as a synonym for foodborne illness or any illness thought to be food related.

CLINICAL IMPORTANCE

When a pet exhibits signs of gastrointestinal (GI) disease, the owner often concludes that food must be the culprit. In the past, when pets relied on table foods, carrion, garbage and improperly cooked pet foods for sustenance, this conclusion would have been credible (Galton, 1955; Thornton, 1972).

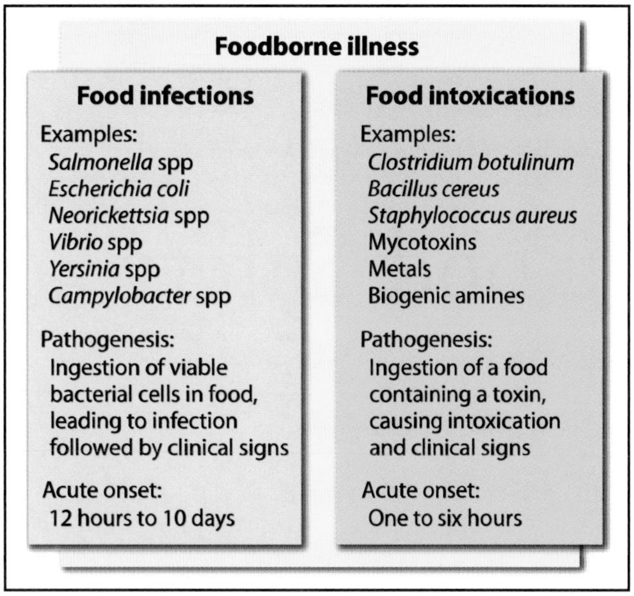
Foodborne illness
Food infections
Examples:
Salmonella spp
Escherichia coli
Neorickettsia spp
Vibrio spp
Yersinia spp
Campylobacter spp
Pathogenesis:
Ingestion of viable bacterial cells in food, leading to infection followed by clinical signs
Acute onset:
12 hours to 10 days
Food intoxications
Examples:
Clostridium botulinum
Bacillus cereus
Staphylococcus aureus
Mycotoxins
Metals
Biogenic amines
Pathogenesis:
Ingestion of a food containing a toxin, causing intoxication and clinical signs
Acute onset:
One to six hours

Figure 11-1. Classification of foodborne illnesses.

Table 11-1. Causes of poisonings in dogs and cats.*

Substance	Total cases (%)
Drugs	25.0
Insecticides	19.6
Plants	12.1
Miscellaneous/unknown	8.9
Rodenticides	8.4
Cleaning products	5.9
Cosmetics	2.9
Hydrocarbons	2.9
Foreign bodies	2.8
Chemicals	2.7
Fertilizers	2.2
Food	1.7
Herbicides	1.6
Paints	1.6
Bites/stings	1.2
Heavy metals	0.5

*Adapted from Hornfeldt CS, Murphy MJ. 1990 Report of the American Association of Poison Control Centers: Poisonings in Animals. Journal of the American Veterinary Medical Association 1992; 200: 1077-1080.

Today, foodborne disease in household pets is rare (Dillon, 1986). The 1993-1994 report of the American Association of Poison Control Centers (AAPCC) indicated that of the 116,432 dog and 19,489 cat poisoning cases reported, foodborne illnesses accounted for only 0.11 and 0.13%, respectively (**Table 11-1**) (Hornfeldt and Murphy, 1998). However, foodborne illness is still a common disease in the United States racing greyhound industry (Fenwick, 1996).

The low incidence of foodborne illnesses in domestic pets can be attributed to two primary changes in feeding practices. First, most pets in developed countries depend totally on commercial pet foods to meet their nutritional needs. More than 90% of the pet owners in the United States purchase commercial pet foods for their pets (Lund et al, 1996). Although these figures are lower for the United Kingdom and Europe, the majority of pet owners in those geographic regions also feed commercial pet foods (Pet Food Manufacturers Association, 1994).

Second, present-day commercial pet foods are much safer than in the past. Modern pet foods are not composed of a single ingredient, but are formulated from multiple ingredients including grains, meats, meat by-products, vegetables, eggs, dairy products, fish and other added nutrients. The use of many and varied ingredients tends to dilute any contamination that might occur in a particular commodity or ingredient. Commercial pet food manufacturers commonly use manufacturing techniques such as extrusion and retorting to produce heat levels sufficient to destroy many pathogens and heat-labile toxins (Dziezak, 1989; Lopez, 1987). Improved packaging materials and a better knowledge of proper warehousing also help to protect raw materials and finished products from moist conditions and possible contamination during storage. Furthermore, manufacturers use sensitive analytical techniques to verify that ingredients and final products are high quality and free of contaminants. The value of these efforts is supported by a study in which researchers analyzed 35 dog and 17 cat foods and found that most were remarkably free of toxic contaminants (Mumma et al, 1986).

REGULATION OF COMMERCIAL PET FOOD

To ensure safety, pet foods and individual pet food ingredients are regulated by several governmental agencies in addition to meeting manufacturer's quality control and storage standards. In the United States, the Food and Drug Administration (FDA) regulates foods and ingredients that are shipped across state or international boundaries under the authority of the Federal Food, Drug and Cosmetic Act (FFDCA) (Superintendent of Documents, 2004; Van Houweling et al, 1977; Price et al, 1993). Section 402 of the FFDCA states that foods, including pet foods, shall be considered adulterated when they contain an added substance that may render the food injurious to health. Section 406 of the FFDCA empowers the Secretary of Health and Human Services to promulgate regulations and tolerances that limit the quantity of contaminants, such as mycotoxins. Additionally, sections 501, 505 and 512 of the FFDCA authorize the FDA control over the use of veterinary drugs. As part of the drug approval process, the FDA can set the conditions of drug use in animal feeds. The use levels established for veterinary drugs prevent excessive drug residues in meat, milk and other by-products from food-producing animals that may be used as ingredients in pet foods. The FDA and the Association of American Feed Control Officials (AAFCO) publish annually the approved animal drug levels in feeds along with the species for which the drug is approved (Superintendent of Documents, 2005; AAFCO, 2007).

The threat of terrorism to the nation's food supply has also prompted expansion of the federal role. The Federal

Government has the authority under the Public Health Security and Bioterrorism Preparedness and Response Act of 2002 (i.e., the Bioterrorism Act) to administratively detain food items that may present a threat of serious adverse health consequences or death to people or animals. The Act also authorizes enforcement actions that may be taken against perishable foods subject to a detention order.

A tolerance is a codified legal regulation whereas action and advisory levels constitute nonbinding FDA guidelines that the agency uses in exercising its enforcement discretion. Instead of a tolerance, the FDA may choose to issue either an action or an advisory level for some unnatural additives. All three are considered maximum allowable levels, but an action level is generally supported by more definitive safety data than is an advisory level. Therefore, some circumstances may elicit enforcement action at levels below an action or advisory level whereas others may not, even when an action or advisory level has been exceeded.

The FDA does not set tolerances for pesticides; instead these fall under the jurisdiction of the United States Environmental Protection Agency (EPA) by the authority of the FFDCA and the Federal Insecticide, Fungicide and Rodenticide Act (Superintendent of Documents, 1995). The EPA establishes and publishes pesticide tolerances for the various plant and animal commodities in 40 CFR 180. These tolerances are developed by combining the results of field trials and laboratory animal toxicity testing (NRC, 1993). The United States Department of Agriculture (USDA) and FDA are then jointly responsible for enforcing the pesticide tolerances.

For contaminants not covered by a tolerance, an action level or advisory level, the limit remains theoretically at zero. However, present day analytical methods have become so sensitive that minuscule amounts can be detected. Fortunately, the FDA has discretionary power when a contaminant is detected at a low level not considered to be a safety concern.

In Europe, the regulation of intentional additives (e.g., vitamins and minerals) and unintentional additives (e.g., pesticides, drug residues and metals) falls under the authority of the European Union (EU) (Ministry of Agriculture, Fisheries and Food, 1995). Control measures are implemented on a national basis and can be stricter but never more permissive than the EU legislation. Non-EU foreign countries regulate pet food safety with a variety of internal regulations and policies.

Most regulatory agencies, both domestic and international, use monitoring programs to maintain surveillance over pet food products. Specifically, in the United States, the FDA monitors pet food and individual pet food ingredients for pesticides, mycotoxins and heavy metals as part of its Feed Contaminants Program (Van Houweling et al, 1977).

Intrastate pet foods are under less federal scrutiny, with primary regulation left to state and local officials. This relationship has created concern that unsuitable food components, most notably mycotoxin-contaminated grains, may be used inadvertently (Nicholson, 1986). In addition, such products are often pelleted instead of extruded; therefore, processing temperatures may not be sufficient to kill bacteria and inactivate heat-labile toxins. Both factors tend to increase the risk of foodborne disease in locally produced foods.

The risk of litigation also encourages pet food manufacturers to be diligent in maintaining high product quality standards. Under tort claims law, all products offered for sale to the public contain an implied warranty (The American Law Institute, 1965). The law specifically provides "that a person who sells a product in a defective condition unreasonably dangerous to the user or consumer or his property is liable for the physical harm the product causes . . ." News programs frequently report large verdicts against manufacturers of human food products because of the harm allegedly caused by their products (Taylor, 1996). Animal feed and pet food manufacturers have also been caught up in this trend. Procedural breakdowns or oversights during production or storage can have a catastrophic effect on profits or even company viability. Mycotoxin litigation alone cost the pet food industry an estimated $7 million in the early 1990s (McCoy, 1996). Recent problems with mycotoxin contamination had financial repercussions and severely damaged the reputation of companies involved (Industry News, 1995; Anonymous. FDA Recall, 2005). Such experiences have made it necessary for manufacturers to devote extensive resources to documenting product quality.

HOME-PREPARED FOODS

The use of home-prepared pet foods also has clinical relevance to foodborne disease. Meat and eggs produced for human consumption and used to prepare homemade pet foods are contaminated with microbes (Notermans et al, 1995; Fenlon et al, 1996; Remillard, 2005). Research indicates that many people are careless about cross-contamination during food preparation at home (Patil et al, 2005). If breeders and pet owners use grocery store ingredients that have been stored properly, heat foods to temperatures sufficient to destroy pathogens and prepare amounts that are readily consumed, the potential for foodborne illness in the pet is expected to be similar to that for people in the same household. Some health-conscious pet owners forgo commercial foods and, instead, prepare foods for their pets daily. These owners must be fastidious and very careful about preparing and storing their pets' food, and truly be committed to the long-term maintenance of proper hygiene and preparation methods. Otherwise, the best method to lessen the risk of foodborne illness is to feed the pet a high-quality commercial pet food manufactured by a company that uses state of the art quality control procedures. There are no such requirements or regulations for pet food manufacturers to do so and most do not; however, there are a few world-wide manufacturers that maintain self-imposed rigorous product quality control procedures.

RAW INGREDIENT DIETS

Feeding raw ingredient diets (commercially available or homemade) to household pets has become increasingly popular.

Some advocates of raw food claim that dogs should be fed raw meat because their wild canine ancestors survived and present day relatives survive on uncooked food. There is no evidence to support dogs evolved from jackals, foxes or coyotes (Wayne, 1993). Comparisons of mitochondrial DNA indicate that dogs most likely descended from wolves. However, the mitochondrial DNA patterns of modern dogs and wolves are distinctly different, and there is no single wolf ancestor that is common to all dogs (Semyenova et al, 2002). No compelling scientific evidence based on evolution supports statements that dogs should eat uncooked food as did wild canids. Claims that dogs are carnivores, rather than omnivores, are likely due to confusion of taxonomy (*Carnivora*) with feeding behavior (carnivore). Dogs belong to the order *Carnivora*, but their eating habits are those of an omnivore (Chapter 12). Panda bears, for example, are herbivores in their feeding behavior, but are included in the order *Carnivora* taxonomically.

Advocates of raw food emphasize the importance of ingredients (Billinghurst, 1993; Schultze, 1998; Volhard and Brown, 2000) with less emphasis on nutrient balance. Advocates claim the nutrients from commercial moist or extruded pet foods are less or not available or even absent (Pottenger, 1939; Billinghurst, 1993; Schultze, 1998; Volhard and Brown, 2000) when compared with feeding raw ingredients. Although no digestibility studies of a complete raw diet have been published to date, average apparent digestibilities of nutrients in commercial pet food have been published. Opponents to feeding raw food point out that some nutrients actually are more readily available from cooked ingredients (Zia-ur-Rehman and Salariya, 2005), and that overall nutrient availability and balance are more significant than for certain individual ingredients.[a]

Advocates of feeding raw food report coat and/or dental benefits (Pottenger and Simonson, 1939; Billinghurst, 1993; Schultze, 1998; Volhard and Brown, 2000) based upon empirical and anecdotal evidence (Billinghurst, 1993; Schultze, 1998; Volhard and Brown, 2000); however, some who recommend raw meat recognize the limits of using such evidence (Silver, 2004). The high fat content (>50%) of raw food diets compared to that found in most dry kibble (<30%) often can account for owners' reports of improvement in the appearance of their pet's coat (Dunn, 1999). The incidence of periodontitis and fractured teeth, however, increased with age in 67 dogs eating raw animal carcasses with bones in a dental health study (Robinson and Gorrel, 1997). None of the homemade and commercially available raw food diets analyzed were appropriate for long-term feeding (Freeman and Michel, 2001, 2001a), which is consistent with the clinical experience of one editor of this textbook (RLR). To date, no scientific evidence exists that demonstrates raw food diets provide additional or exceptionally unique nutrients that cannot be obtained from cooked food.

Professionals at zoos and racing greyhound kennels, who have historically fed raw meat, recognize the potential for contamination and attempt to decrease risks of foodborne illness. Raw meat may make up 50 to 75% of the food consumed by racing greyhounds in the United States (Chengappa et al, 1993). Sporadic fatalities and contamination of the environment with *Salmonella enterica* have occurred in greyhound facilities in which raw meat was fed (Morley et al, 2006). Unlike raw food advocates in the dog-racing industry, pet owners share their household and food-preparation area with their pet. The FDA "does not believe raw meat foods for animals are consistent with the goal of protecting the public from significant health risks, particularly when such products are brought into the home and/or used to feed domestic pets." Thus, the FDA has drafted guidelines for companies selling raw meat diets to pet owners (2000).

Often, pet owners will refer to the quality of their raw homemade diet ingredients as "all natural," "whole food" "or organic," none of which decreases the potential for microbial contamination. Numerous studies have demonstrated the presence of bacterial pathogens in retail meat for human consumption (Sinell H-J et al, 1984; Fenlon et al, 1996; Tamplin et al, 2001; Duffy et al, 2001; Whyte et al, 2001; Zhao et al, 2001; White et al, 2001; Villani et al, 2005; O'Keefe, 2005). Raw meat diets prepared by pet owners fed to dogs and cats have been documented to contain pathogenic *Yersinia enterocolitica* 4/O:3, *Salmonella* spp. and *Escherichia coli* O157:H7 (Fredriksson-Ahoma et al, 2001; Joffe and Schlesinger, 2002; Freeman and Michel, 2001; Chengappa et al, 1993). Commercially available raw meat diets (beef, lamb, chicken and turkey), sampled over a two-month period, cultured positive for non-type specific *E.coli* and *S. enterica* (Strohmeyer et al, 2006). Of 25 commercial raw meat diets (beef, lamb, quail, chicken and ostrich), 64% were positive for *E. coli* and 20% were positive for *Salmonella* spp. In addition, 20% were contaminated with *Clostridium perfringens* and a toxigenic strain of *C. difficile* was isolated from one food (Weese et al, 2005). Any claims that a finished pet food is "human grade," or any connotation that a pet food is derived from raw ingredients "like, or similar to, what your own human family members eat" is considered false and misleading under current AAFCO rules and regulations.[a]

Advocates of feeding raw meat, bone and eggs claim that pathogenic organisms in raw meat do not affect dogs and cats due to the lower stomach pH and shorter GI transit times in these species. Stomach pH and GI transit times are in fact similar among people, dogs and cats and do not lower the risk to pets. Dogs and cats succumb to foodborne pathogens and exhibit clinical signs similar to those in people (Fredriksson-Ahomaa et al, 2001; Gayle, 2003; Remillard and Wynn, 2005). Neither freezing raw meat before feeding nor purchasing freeze-dried commercial foods eliminates pathogens; freezing and freeze-drying are ineffective means for killing bacteria. In fact, both methods are used for long-term preservation of valuable stock bacterial cultures in laboratories. Grape seed extract itself does not kill microorganisms and does not render meat safer. The antimicrobial activity attributed to grapefruit seed extract is merely due to the synthetic preservative agents added to the product. Natural grape seed appears not to have antimicrobial activity (von Woedtke et al, 1999).

Opponents to feeding raw food point out that meat and egg supplies for people are contaminated with microorganisms and that feeding raw meat increases the likelihood of exposure of owners and pets to foodborne bacterial diseases (LeJeune and Hancock, 2001). Advocates of raw food do not deny its potential health risks to pets (Volhard and Brown, 2000; Hofve and Smith, 2001; Silver, 2004). Pet owners may not realize that infected dogs shed bacteria capable of infecting people. Dogs may be excreting *Salmonella* spp., *Campylobacter* spp. or *Y. enterocolitica* in their feces, yet remain clinically normal (LeJeune and Hancock, 2001). Pets fed homemade raw meat diets shed viable organisms in their feces. In one study, *Salmonella* spp. were isolated from 80% of the raw meat and bone diets sampled and in 30% of the stool samples from dogs consuming those diets (Joffe and Schlesinger, 2002). Greyhounds fed raw meats diets shed the same subspecies of *Salmonella* in their feces as that found in their diets (Stone et al, 1993). Sled dogs were subclinical shedders of *Salmonella* spp. when fed a contaminated diet (Cantor et al, 1997). Dogs infected with *Campylobacter* spp. excrete organisms in their feces, but may remain clinically normal (Hald and Madsen, 1997). However, serovars of *Campylobacter* isolated from diarrheic dogs were the same as those isolated from poultry carcasses fed to the dogs (Varga et al, 1990). Therefore, pets fed contaminated raw meat diets are a source of contamination to people and other pets in the same household. Transmission of *Salmonella* infection from pets to people in the same household has been documented (Morse et al, 1976; Sato et al, 2000; Tauni and Osterlund, 2000). Pet owners feeding raw chicken necks and backs or other raw meat are putting themselves, their family and their pet at increased risk for exposure to *Salmonella* spp. Household transmission of foodborne *Y. entercolitica* from dogs to people has been documented (Gutman et al, 1973). Exposure may occur either by direct contact with food/utensils, or by contact with the contaminated environment shared between people and pets (Sanchez et al, 2002).

A recent meta-analysis demonstrated that consumers engage in risky behaviors regarding food handling. High-income individuals were less knowledgeable about food hygiene and performed higher risk, cross-contamination practices more often than other groups studied (Patil et al, 2005). Exposure to foodborne illness due to ingestion of pathogens from undercooked hamburger or eggs, raw chicken and work surfaces used to slice raw vegetables is a continuous threat to people who prepare raw foods for their pets (Hedberg, 2001). Safe handling of food and feeding containers is of paramount importance for pet owners who feed raw meat. Some people are unaware of any food safety issues because the raw meat used to feed their pet is sometimes derived from the same source as meats they use for their own consumption. However, USDA product labels on meat sold in grocery stores give clear warnings and cooking instructions to reduce the risk of foodborne illnesses. Foodborne pathogenic organisms may infect people handling contaminated meat and egg products and products intended for pets (bones, pig ears and treats) (Grimsrud, 1999).

Even advocates of feeding raw foods or ingredients admit that people "extremely susceptible to infectious disease" should not feed raw meat (Hofve and Smith, 2001). Individuals who clean the cat's litter box or pick up their dog's stool should consider the feces contaminated with viable pathogenic microbes. Households with elderly persons who may be immunocompromised should avoid raw food and soiled environments. Extra precautions should be taken when persons (or other pets) in the household have immunosuppressive (human immunodeficiency virus, feline leukemia virus or feline immunodeficiency virus) infections, are undergoing chemotherapy or being treated with antiinflammatory medications. Additional caution should be emphasized when young children are in the household and pet food-oral or fecal-oral contamination is possible. Because children are more susceptible than healthy adults, families with children who crawl and those with children who play with the family pet may decide to feed commercially prepared moist or extruded foods to prevent foodborne illness in the child (Trevejo et al, 2003). Veterinarians recommending commercial or homemade foods containing raw meat or eggs have an ethical responsibility to fully inform pet owners of the increased potential risk of foodborne pathogens not only to the pet but the entire household (LeJeune and Hancock, 2001; Remillard, 2005).

PATIENT ASSESSMENT

The most important goal in dealing with a case of suspected foodborne illness is to obtain an accurate diagnosis. However, this may be difficult because many factors, including the pet owner, can mislead the veterinarian. One must adhere stubbornly to the principles of a proper toxicologic investigation, including the careful evaluation of information supplied by: 1) the history, 2) clinical signs, 3) postmortem findings, 4) chemical analyses and 5) laboratory animal tests (Osweiler et al, 1985). For live patients, an accurate diagnosis will aid in the initiation of specific treatments and preventive measures. The veterinarian should also use preliminary information and clinical signs to guide the history-taking process.

History

Although an adequate history is important in all clinical cases, it is especially important when foodborne illness is suspected because some of the critical facts in the case may be lacking. For example, it may not be possible to obtain a sample of garbage or a carrion source. Pet owners who often express the opinion that food is to blame also complicate the history-taking process. In such cases, veterinarians must be methodical if they are to reach an unbiased and accurate diagnosis.

The natural starting place is the discussion with the pet owner. First, ascertain when and what clinical signs first appeared. From here, veterinarians can annotate the sequence and relevant facts about the events that transpired before the patient's presentation. Aspects of the history that seem vague or incomplete should be probed further. Facts that seem unrelated should be noted for later consideration. For example, it is important to know what day the neighborhood trash is left out for pickup, especially if it was the day before the illness occurred. The recent application of a pesticide to the premises or yard, coupled with signs typical of pesticide toxicity, would

Table 11-2. Clinical signs of selected foodborne illnesses.

Clinical signs	Agents causing the foodborne illness
Vomiting/diarrhea	*S. aureus, Salmonella* spp., *Neorickettsia* spp., *E. coli, B. cereus, Yersinia* spp., *Campylobacter* spp., biogenic amines, aflatoxins, vomitoxin, cyclopiazonic acid, lead, arsenic, zinc, cadmium
Liver disorders, jaundice	Aflatoxins, fumonisins, lead, arsenic, rubratoxin, *Yersinia* spp.
Blood disorders, e.g., anemia, hemorrhages	Aflatoxins, *Neorickettsia* spp., lead, onions, garlic, rubratoxin, cyclopiazonic acid, mycotoxins
CNS/nervous disturbances	*C. botulinum*, fumonisins, penitrem A, lead, arsenic, mercury, chocolate
Kidney pathology	Ochratoxin, cyclopiazonic acid, *E. coli*, lead, arsenic, mercury, cadmium, chocolate, grapes/raisins
Skin lesions	*E. coli*, garlic, arsenic, cyclopiazonic acid

be important, particularly if the pet owner, instead of a professional exterminator, had applied the pesticide. Exposure to other toxicants in the pet's environment, such as recent use of certain cleaning chemicals, is always a distinct possibility and should be thoroughly investigated. A run or hike in the woods may allow the pet access to contaminated material containing bacteria or mycotoxins that induce foodborne illness. The AAPCC reported that home exposures are responsible for 91.6% of canine and 93.3% of feline poisonings (Hornfeldt and Murphy, 1998). If pets are allowed to roam freely outdoors, the scope of investigation must be expanded. Free-roaming animals have access to pesticides, other toxic chemicals, poisoned bait, trash, garbage and spoiled foods. Pets on farms and ranches have an increased exposure to pesticides and agricultural chemicals. They also have the freedom to ingest animal feeds intended for other species that may contain feed additives such as ionophores and organic arsenicals, which are toxic to pets.

These examples lend credence to the fact that one cannot achieve an adequate history by allowing the pet owner to simply describe the events that preceded the illness. Instead, it is imperative that the veterinarian take the initiative to tactfully probe and query the pet owner for every piece of key information. Most pet owners feel that such facts are irrelevant, and others may refuse to admit that their pet would scavenge garbage cans. Still others may even give incorrect information to conceal their own negligence. All family members should be included in these discussions if possible. This is a good time to request that the pet owner bring the food in its container to the hospital for testing. It is important that the entire food container be brought, not just a sample selected by the pet owner (to be discussed later in the chapter).

Contamination of a commercial pet food will usually produce an epizootic of sick pets within a wide geographic area, as exemplified by events in Europe and recently in the United States. A popular brand of cat food was inadvertently contaminated with the food animal drug salinomycin, causing paralysis and death in several hundred cats (Spillers Petfoods, 1996). Toxic levels of aflatoxin in a commercial food led to numerous reports of affected dogs (Derezynski et al, 2006; Stenske et al, 2006). Therefore, knowledge of this information can be used in the diagnostic process. If other animals in the same household are eating food from the same bag or container and remain asymptomatic, then implication of the food is diminished, and other possible causes should be investigated. Date codes on bags or cans of food may be used by the manufacturer to link illness of multiple pets in widely separated geographic areas. The food is not a likely suspect if pets consuming food with the same date code are not experiencing similar clinical signs.

However, even if it appears that the commercial food has been exonerated in a wide geographic area, one should not end the commercial food investigation because the pet owner may have compromised the product's integrity by improper storage or usage. The veterinarian should contact the manufacturer to determine if similar cases have been reported. Company technical personnel can also help the differential diagnostic process by supplying key information about product testing, additional areas of investigation and beneficial laboratory tests. Major pet food companies frequently check raw ingredients for mycotoxins, mineral levels, heavy metals, pesticides, spoilage indicators, peroxides and other substances as part of their quality control and specifications for incoming raw materials.

Physical Examination

The physical examination of patients suspected to have a foodborne illness should be thorough, just as for other diseases. Although signs of GI disease may be obvious, one should also be alert for other clinical signs such as cutaneous lesions or signs that might signify central nervous system or hepatic disease (**Table 11-2**). If possible, samples of vomitus and feces should be obtained for laboratory testing. Veterinarians should also use their own olfactory senses. Many toxicities impart unique odors to the patient. For example, fishy breath emanating from a dog known to be consuming a cereal-based dry dog food with no added fish oil or fish meal would be noteworthy. Likewise, a pesticide odor on a cat's coat would be a significant observation. Again, one cannot overemphasize the investigative prowess that must be exercised in foodborne illness cases.

Another important reason for conducting a routine physical examination is to evaluate the need for symptomatic treatment. Patients may have signs such as dehydration, seizures or high fever that require symptomatic or supportive treatment before a final diagnosis is made. This determination is best made during the physical examination. If emergency treatment is warranted, consultation with a local veterinary school, state veterinary diagnostic laboratory, hospital poison control center or the American Society for Prevention of Cruelty to Animals may be useful. The National Animal Poison Control Center (888-426-4435) may also prove helpful.

Clinical Laboratory Testing

Clinical laboratory testing should be performed routinely in all suspected foodborne illness cases. Many such illnesses are short-lived so hematologic and serum biochemistry values may be within normal limits. However, clinical biochemistry values may be invaluable in establishing the diagnosis and prognosis in serious illnesses such as mycotoxicosis.

Vomitus, feces and urine should be collected, labeled, frozen and tested for bacteria, viruses, biotoxins, metals, pesticides or chemicals as deemed appropriate by discussions between the veterinarian and laboratory testing personnel. The collection and analysis of a urine sample is also important because many toxic compounds are concentrated in urine. In fatal cases, organ tissue samples, bile, urine and stomach and intestinal contents should be collected during the postmortem examination.

Risk Factors

Individual factors such as age, species and state of health influence susceptibility to foodborne illness. Young and old animals are most susceptible. Debilitated and immunocompromised animals are more prone to foodborne illness. Dogs are at higher risk than cats because they are more likely to forage spoiled foods (e.g., trash, garbage and carrion). The AAPCC reported that dogs account for 75% of all animal poisonings (Hornfeldt and Murphy, 1998). Historically, the risk of foodborne illnesses in pets is increased when raw ingredient diets are fed, during warm weather, during hunting seasons, and around two holidays: Thanksgiving and Christmas (Coppock and Mostrom, 1986).

Cats tend to be more discerning and fastidious in their eating habits. Cats may vomit because of subtle variations between different batches of the same food. Slight changes in moisture content or application of palatability enhancers can lead to vomiting in cats. If a cat vomits after eating a recently opened can or bag of a commercial product, but is otherwise healthy, you may choose to try a food with a different date code before concluding that the food is adulterated. If the cat is truly ill, and you suspect the food, call the company to check for other reports of illness in cats eating that product or a product with the same date code. Reputable companies will want to know about any problems.

The most important factors to consider in establishing risk are the food source and the environment. Knowledge of these factors will help quantify the patient's exposure to other sources of toxicants and microbial agents. If the pet owner feeds a commercial pet food and follows label directions and proper storage recommendations, the likelihood of foodborne illness is low. However, if the same pet is allowed to roam freely outdoors, then the risk of exposure to foodborne disease agents is increased greatly. Home-prepared foods are riskier if owners do not follow proper preparation and storage procedures. Animals fed foods containing uncooked meat, eggs or offal are at much greater risk for foodborne agents. In general, the risk of contracting foodborne illness from various food sources increases as follows (from least to greatest risk):

- Federally regulated canned pet foods
- Federally regulated dry pet foods
- Federally regulated semi-moist pet foods
- Individual homemade fresh foods
- Locally prepared commercial dry pet foods
- Mass-produced kennel foods
- Free access to garbage, trash and carrion.

The risk of contracting a foodborne agent from any of these food sources can be markedly increased by improper storage of the food. All of the effort that goes into selection of raw ingredients, product manufacturing and choice of food or home preparation is wasted if the pet owner fails to properly store the food. Proper storage depends on control of three factors: 1) temperature, 2) moisture and 3) availability of oxygen (Ensminger et al, 1995). If these factors are controlled, commercial canned products will have a shelf life of well over a year and dry foods of at least six months. Therefore, risk is also influenced by proper food storage.

Consumers should store dry food in the closed bag, at room temperature if possible, and away from moisture (Chapter 8). If the consumer puts the food in a plastic container, the bag itself should be placed in the container to retain integrity of the product and preserve the date code (Chapter 8). Opened cans of food should be covered and immediately refrigerated for no longer than specified by the manufacturer, usually three to five days.

Etiopathogenesis

The bacteria of major concern as potential causes of foodborne illnesses in people include: *C. perfringens, C. botulinum, Staphylococcus aureus, Bacillus cereus, Salmonella* spp., *Listeria* spp., *Yersinia* spp., *Aeromonas* spp., *C. jejuni, E. coli, Vibrio* spp., *Enterococcus faecalis, E. cloacae* and *Klebsiella ozaenae* (Potter, 1992; Council for Agricultural Science and Technology, 1994). These organisms also have the potential to cause disease in pets. However, as stated previously, the prevalence of foodborne disease is low in dogs and cats. The following discussion involves the etiopathogenesis of bacteria and other agents that can cause foodborne disease in pets.

Bacteria and Rickettsia

SALMONELLA SPECIES

Salmonellae are gram-negative, aerobic bacilli that are normally present in the intestinal tracts of many mammals, birds and reptiles. Healthy adult dogs and cats are fairly resistant to the pathogenic effects of salmonellae but serve as important sources of infection for people and weak, debilitated animals. It has been estimated that 36% of healthy dogs and 17% of healthy cats harbor these organisms in their GI tracts (Green, 1995; Morse and Duncan, 1975).

The most common route of exposure is through ingestion of fecal-contaminated food and water. The presence of salmonellae in food or water indicates inadequate hygiene and improper cooking. Racing greyhounds are frequently infected when they consume foods largely composed of contaminated raw meat and offal from rendering plants. Researchers who sampled and cultured raw meat used in greyhound foods found that 45% of the meat samples were contaminated with salmonellae. *S. typhimurium* was the most commonly isolated serotype (Chengappa et al, 1993). When racing greyhounds ingest raw meat containing large numbers of cells, a clinical enteritis syndrome termed "kennel sickness" or "blowout" results (Fenwick, 1996).

Salmonellae produce a heat-labile endotoxin, which is responsible for their pathologic effects. Clinical syndromes can be divided into gastroenteritis, bacteremia/toxemia and organ localization. Infections can usually be treated successfully with a combination of appropriate antibacterial drugs and supportive treatment. Persistent carriers are common and can be a source of human exposure. Proper cooking of foods and boiling water will kill vegetative bacterial cells and inactivate the endotoxin.

CLOSTRIDIUM BOTULINUM

The heat-labile toxin of the gram-positive, anaerobic, spore-forming bacterium *C. botulinum* causes botulism. These saprophytic bacilli are commonly found in soil and as contaminants in raw meat, carrion and vegetables. They are not considered dangerous to man or animals unless allowed to grow under anaerobic conditions in uncooked meats, improperly canned foods and the carcasses of dead animals. Under anaerobic conditions, *C. botulinum* produces the most potent biotoxin known (Klassen and Eaton, 1993). This powerful exotoxin blocks the release of the neurotransmitter acetylcholine. Dogs are less susceptible to the effects of the toxin than people, but naturally occurring botulism has occurred in dogs (Green, 1995; Barsanti, 1984; Barsanti et al, 1978). Cats, previously thought to be resistant to botulinum toxin, have also been found to be susceptible. Eight cats fed pelican carrion contracted the disease, and four died during the course of the illness. Toxigenic *C. botulinum* type C bacteria were found in the stomach of one cat and in the pelican muscle (Elad et al, 2004). Clinical signs can occur as early as 12 hours or as late as five to six days after the exotoxin is ingested. The primary clinical sign is generalized paralysis that starts in the posterior limbs and progresses to quadriplegia.

Primary care consists of supportive treatment. Spontaneous recovery will occur provided the dose of toxin ingested was insufficient to severely affect vital functions, such as respiration. Prevention can be achieved by heating foods before consumption to either 80°C (176°F) for 30 minutes or 100°C (212°F) for 10 minutes (Ensminger et al, 1995). These heating protocols are sufficient to destroy the heat-labile toxin of *C. botulinum*; however, any bacterial spores present will survive this procedure.

STAPHYLOCOCCUS AUREUS

The ubiquitous staphylococci are common inhabitants of the skin and mucous membranes of man and other animals (Jawetz et al, 1980). *S. aureus* is the most common cause of foodborne illness in people. The typical GI signs result from a potent *S. aureus* enterotoxin. Although *S. aureus* organisms are easily killed by heat, their enterotoxin can withstand typical cooking temperatures and even the canning process (Tatini, 1976). Ingestion of about 25 µg of enterotoxin will produce nausea and vomiting within two to four hours in people. Spontaneous recovery occurs in 24 to 48 hours. Dogs and cats are reported to be tolerant to staphylococcal enterotoxin and have remained asymptomatic after administration of oral doses as high as 100 µg/kg body weight (Freer and Arbuthnott, 1986).[b]

ESCHERICHIA COLI

E. coli is a well-known pathogen of people. However, the role of *E. coli* as a pathogen of dogs and cats has been unclear (Burrows et al, 1995; Olson et al, 1985). *E. coli*, strain O157:H7 has been involved in a number of outbreaks of foodborne illnesses stemming from improperly cooked meat purchased from fast-food restaurants (Potter, 1992). The same strain has been incriminated in an unusual clinical syndrome in racing greyhounds termed "Alabama rot" or "Greenetrack disease" (Fenwick et al, 1995). This disease is characterized by erythema, ulceration of the extremities and renal glomerular pathology (Fenwick, 1996; Fenwick et al, 1995; Hertzke et al, 1995). No particular treatment has proved effective, but many animals will recover with symptomatic treatment and good nursing care.

BACILLUS CEREUS

B. cereus causes vomiting and diarrhea in people, but it is not thought to pose a significant danger for foodborne illness in animals (Turnbull and Kramer, 1991). At room temperature, *B. cereus* flourishes, producing a potent endotoxin. The organism is a ubiquitous, spore-forming aerobic saprophyte found in soil, grains, cereal products and other foods (van Netten and Kramer, 1992). As an example, it is commonly found in uncooked rice (Ensminger et al, 1995). *B. cereus* has been found as a common isolate in samples of dry pet food.[c] It has also been isolated from food packaging paper and materials (Vaisanen et al, 1992).

The standard heat used to manufacture pet foods is not likely to destroy the spores of this organism. However, the number of organisms isolated from pet food samples ($<10^5$ cells/g of food) is unlikely to cause foodborne disease in pets unless the food is exposed to moisture and heat conditions conducive to bacterial proliferation (van Netten and Kramer, 1992; Claus and Berkeley, 1986; Drobniewski, 1993). Therefore, pet owners should be warned not to add water to dry pet foods and leave them exposed to high ambient temperatures for prolonged periods.

NEORICKETTSIA SPECIES

In dogs, *Neorickettsia helminthoeca* and *N. elokominica,* cause a serious systemic infection known as salmon poisoning (Breitschwerdt, 1995; Gorham and Foreyt, 1984). The disease is transmitted by ingestion of raw salmon containing the vector, a fluke named *Nanophyetus salmincola.* The fluke matures in five to seven days and then attaches to the intestinal mucosa of the host animal. The rickettsiae leave the fluke, invade the intestinal mucosa and enter the bloodstream to produce an acute systemic infection.

Clinical signs include vomiting, hemorrhagic diarrhea, high fever, dehydration and peripheral lymphadenopathy. Tetracycline therapy is the treatment of choice. Supportive treatment with parenteral fluids is also indicated. The anthelmintic preferred for elimination of the fluke is fenbendazole. If timely treatment is not instituted, mortality can reach 50 to 90% (Burrows et al, 1995).

Mycotoxins

Estimates suggest that one-quarter of the world's annual food crop is affected by mold metabolites called mycotoxins (Mannon and Johnson, 1985). Produced by a wide variety of saprophytic and pathologic fungi, they can be highly toxic (Council for Agricultural Science and Technology, 1989). Toxic syndromes range from mild GI discomfort and vomiting to an acute fulminating episode with death. Long-term, low-level exposure can produce vague signs such as chronic organ damage (e.g., hepatic cirrhosis), immunosuppression and decreased production or performance. Mycotoxins interfere with absorption of antioxidant compounds from food, and modulate activity of antioxidant enzyme systems in cells. Combinations of mycotoxins may be more toxic than single mycotoxins (Surai and Dvorska, 2005). Although cereal grains are most commonly associated with mycotoxins, a wide variety of foodstuffs including cheeses, nuts, forages, fruits and even beer can be contaminated (Council for Agricultural Science and Technology, 1989).

Mycotoxin production occurs in the field and during harvesting, processing, transportation and storage. Stressors, such as drought and insect damage, predispose crops to infestation and mycotoxin production. Warm ambient temperatures and high humidity also favor mycotoxin production. Some molds thrive in cooler, wet conditions. Presence of mold, however, does not necessarily mean mycotoxin production. The conditions under which mycotoxins are formed are relatively narrow when compared to conditions favorable to mold growth (Pitt, 2001). Some degree of mycotoxin production is unavoidable. Mycotoxin content may be controlled through identification, quantification and regulation. The genera of the three major mycotoxin-producing fungi are *Aspergillus, Fusarium* and *Penicillium.* Dietary supplementation with antioxidants proved protective against the toxic effects of mycotoxins in various animal species (Surai and Dvorska, 2005).

AFLATOXINS

Aflatoxin, a mycotoxin produced by *Aspergillus flavus* or *A. parasiticus*, can produce varying degrees of toxicity in birds and mammals. Corn, peanuts, cottonseed and grains are potential sources of aflatoxins in pet foods. Dogs and cats are among the species most sensitive to the effects of aflatoxin, with LD_{50} values ranging from 0.5 to 1.0 mg/kg (Newberne and Butler, 1969; Edds, 1973). Aflatoxin B_1 is metabolized in the liver to highly reactive intermediates that bind to DNA, disrupt transcription and lead to abnormal cell proliferation, mutagenesis and carcinogenesis. Aflatoxins also inhibit various enzymes (Hocking, 2001). The net effect is decreased protein synthesis, leading to hypoalbuminemia and a shortage of clotting factors.

The onset and severity of the clinical syndrome depend on the dose and duration of exposure. In 1955, the canine disease known as hepatitis X was successfully reproduced by feeding dogs a brand of dog food previously incriminated in cases of the same disease (Seibold and Bailey, 1952; Newberne et al, 1955). Later, researchers discovered that the identical disease syndrome could be elicited in dogs fed purified aflatoxin B_1 (Newberne et al, 1966). Cases of canine aflatoxicosis resulting from contaminated food have been reported in South America and Africa (Coppock and Mostrom, 1986; Hagiwara et al, 1990). Consumption of an aflatoxin-contaminated commercial pet food was reported to result in the deaths of more than 100 dogs in the United States in 2006 (Stenske et al, 2006).

The principal target organ in all species is the liver. Clinical signs, such as anorexia, severe GI disturbances, jaundice and hemorrhage, with a corresponding increase in hepatic enzyme activities and a decrease in serum protein values, are typical (Newberne and Butler, 1969; Edds, 1973; Neal, 1973; Stenske et al, 2006). The most frequently observed hepatic lesions are centrilobular necrosis, fibrosis and bile duct proliferation (Puschner, 2002). Intravascular coagulation can also be a complication of chronic aflatoxicosis (Green, 1977). Marked cytoplasmic vacuolar degeneration consistent with accumulation of hepatocellular lipids was noted in dogs with confirmed aflatoxicosis. Progression of clinical signs corresponded with increases in alanine aminotransaminase (ALT) and aspartate aminotransaminase activities, hyperbilirubinemia, hypoalbuminemia, hypocholesterolemia and coagulopathy (Stenske et al, 2006). Hematemesis or melena was associated with a grave prognosis. In another report, dogs that died were significantly younger, had lower total protein and higher total bilirubin, ALT and alkaline phosphatase values when compared to the same parameters in survivors. The authors concluded that hypocholesterolemia and reduced protein C values were biomarkers for aflatoxicosis (Dereszynski et al, 2006).

Today, manufacturers and governmental regulatory agencies strive to minimize exposure to aflatoxins by using low-level detection methods. Aflatoxins are heat stable and not destroyed by boiling, autoclaving or food manufacturing methods. The FDA has established an action level of 20 ppb for total aflatoxins in pet food (Office of Enforcement, 1994). Therefore, prevention strategies involve identification of raw materials with unacceptable levels (>20 ppb), maintenance of proper storage conditions and assay of final feeds.

VOMITOXIN

Vomitoxin, chemically known as deoxynivalenol, is a mycotoxin produced by members of the genus *Fusarium* (Council for Agricultural Science and Technology, 1989). Vomitoxin can be found in any grain but most commonly affects wheat and barley. Like most other mycotoxins, it is heat stable and survives extrusion and drying (Hughes et al, 1999).

Dogs and swine, the species most susceptible to the effects of vomitoxin, are affected at relatively low concentrations. The mechanism of action is inhibition of protein synthesis (Bohm and Razzazi-Fazeli, 2005). Experimentally, acute toxicity affects rapidly dividing cells in lymph nodes, spleen, thymus and intestinal mucosa, and may be immunosuppressive (Bondy and Pestka, 2000). Clinical signs include feed refusal, vomiting and diarrhea. Vomiting and feed refusal are apparently due to neurochemical changes in the brain, rather than taste (Riley and Pestka, 2005). In a study using 0 to 10 mg deoxynivalenol/kg pet food, individual dogs and cats were highly variable in their response to vomitoxin. Some animals vomited immediately after eating, whereas others exhibited food refusal or decreased food intake without vomiting. Compared to dogs, cats tolerate higher levels of deoxynivalenol. Cats consumed small, frequent meals, whereas dogs ate one large meal when the food was presented. Feeding behavior of cats may have influenced their ability to tolerate higher levels of deoxynivalenol (Hughes et al, 1999).

In 1993, the FDA advisory level for deoxynivalenol in grains and grain by-products used in pet foods was 5 ppm with the added recommendation that these ingredients not exceed 40% of the food (i.e., 2 ppm deoxynivalenol in the complete pet food) (Chesemore, 1993). However, feed refusal in dogs has been reported in levels approaching 2 ppm (Maune, 1995). Therefore, a more practical maximum level is 1 ppm. In 1995, vomitoxin levels in winter wheat were reportedly as high as 32 ppm. One major pet food company recalled 16,000 tons of products due to deoxynivalenol contamination at a cost of about $20 million (Industry News, 1995).

FUMONISINS

The fumonisins are a group of recently described mycotoxins produced by *Fusarium moniliforme*, a common field fungus found in grains, beans and fruit (Gelderblom et al, 1988; Haschek and Haliburton, 1986). Although *F. moniliforme* reportedly infects 80 to 100% of all corn harvested in the United States, little information is available about the toxicity of fumonisins in dogs and cats. However, these potent mycotoxins cause leukoencephalomalacia in horses and liver disease in a number of other species. Fumonisin-contaminated pet foods have not been a problem to date.

OTHER MYCOTOXINS

The mycotoxins produced by *Penicillium* can be roughly categorized into those that cause kidney or liver lesions, such as ochratoxin A, and those that are neurotoxins, called tremorgens. The tremorgens are mold metabolites that act as neurotoxins. Mortality resulting from tremorgens is difficult to diagnose postmortem because they cause no visible lesions (Pitt, 2001). The toxic effects of penitrem A have been reported (Arp and Richard, 1979; Hayes et al, 1976). Penetrim A toxicity led to life-threatening tremors in dogs that ingested moldy cream cheese or unidentified materials in a compost pile (Boysen et al, 2002; Young et al, 2003). Affected animals recover with no residual effects if the tremors are addressed with anesthesia and dehydration is prevented (Richard, 2000).

Ochratoxin A primarily affects the kidney, but can affect the liver if levels are high. Toxicity in dogs has been reported (Szczech et al, 1973). The toxin is not rapidly removed from the body and may accumulate. High levels of ochratoxin have been detected in house dust (Richard, 2000).

Canine and feline toxicity data for many of the other food-borne mycotoxins are scant in the scientific literature. The toxic effects of rubratoxin B and cyclopiazonic acid have been described and documented (Hayes and Williams, 1977; Nuehring et al, 1985).

Biogenic Amines

"Cadaveric alkaloids" isolated from putrefied bodies have been known to forensic toxicologists for more than 100 years (Blanke and Poklis, 1993). Modern chemistry has now established that these decomposition products are not alkaloids but instead are "biogenic amines." They are produced when bacteria decarboxylate amino acids in animal tissue. Examples of biogenic amines include histamine, putrescine and cadaverine.

Detection of histamine in the tissues of fish indicates decomposition or spoilage. Normal commercially canned fish contain histamine levels less than 5 to 6 ppm (Dykstra, 1995). As the level of histamine approaches 20 ppm, spoilage becomes organoleptically and physically evident.

Excessive levels of histamine (around 500 ppm) in the flesh of spoiled fish in combination with a toxin called saurine are thought to be involved in the pathogenesis of a human food-borne illness called "scombroid fish poisoning" (Dykstra, 1995; Russell and Dart, 1993; Morrow et al, 1991). This common seafood-related illness is named for its association with consumption of scombroid fishes, such as tuna, wahoo, mackerel and sardines, although other fishes and cheese have been implicated (Morrow et al, 1991; Taylor, 1986). The disease produces clinical signs of an allergic nature, i.e., flushing, sweating, nausea, diarrhea, rash, dizziness, facial swelling, respiratory distress and occasionally vasodilatory shock, but the disease is rarely fatal (Morrow et al, 1991; Taylor, 1986). The FDA has recognized histamine's role in scombroid poisoning by setting a maximum action level of 500 ppm histamine in canned fish (Dykstra, 1995).

Histamine and other biogenic amines such as putrescine and cadaverine have also been detected in pet foods. Their presence has been attributed to the use of poultry, fish and meat by-products as raw ingredients. The levels of histamine in pet foods reported in each of two different studies ranged from 3.8 to 88.8 ppm and 16 to 65.5 ppm, respectively (Guilford et al, 1994; Guraya and Koehler, 1991). Dogs and cats are tolerant to much higher levels of histamine (2,500 ppm), but research is needed to determine whether certain hypersensitive animals may be at risk (Blonz and Olcott, 1978).

Metals

Metals are probably the oldest toxic agents known to man (Goyer, 1993). They are unique in that they are never destroyed nor created, just redistributed in the environment. Food is the most common source of metal toxicity in people and other animals. Pets frequently serve as sentinels for human exposure.

Pet foods can become contaminated in several ways. First, metals tend to accumulate in plant and animal matter, creating the possibility of toxic levels in food ingredients. Foods can also become contaminated during commercial manufacturing and home preparation by the inadvertent addition of metal shavings, grease, oils and other chemicals. Acidic foods can leach paint, soldered joints or plating agents from food containers. Young animals may ingest lead by chewing on painted wood, linoleum, metal toys, golf balls, roofing materials, drapery weights and ornaments (Osweiler et al, 1985).

Most foodborne metal toxicities in dogs and cats involve lead, zinc, cadmium and arsenic. These agents cause a variety of clinical syndromes depending on age, dose ingested and length of exposure. The specifics of metal toxicities are well described in several veterinary toxicology textbooks and are beyond the scope of this chapter.

The tendency of metals to accumulate in plants and animals has ramifications for the manufacture of commercial pet foods. Several studies have been conducted to quantify such accumulations. In one study, researchers analyzed 28 brands of commercial dog food and seven brands of cat food and found that average levels of lead, arsenic and cadmium were 1.26, 0.37 and 0.22 ppm, respectively (Edwards et al, 1979). A later study of 35 dog foods and 13 cat foods found the average levels of lead, cadmium and zinc were 0.88, 0.80 and 122.0 ppm, respectively (Mumma et al, 1986). These studies confirm that nontoxic levels of metals may be present in some pet foods; however, their presence at these levels would not support a diagnosis of metal toxicity. Instead, a definite diagnosis must be based upon finding toxic levels in the food that correspond to elevated levels in the patient's tissues, such as blood, liver and kidney.

Other Sources

SUPPLEMENTS

Many people supplement their own food with vitamins, herbal remedies and other items purchased at health food stores. Well-meaning pet owners likewise think that what is good for them is also good for their pets. Unfortunately, this practice fails to consider species and dose differences. Cats, in particular, may be adversely affected by medications considered safe for people. Certainly, vitamin A and D toxicity is well documented. It is also known that many herbal remedies cause adverse effects in people and animals (Poppenga, 1995; Remillard and Wynn, 2005). Therefore, the safety of other "natural" supplements such as aloe, ginseng root, eucalyptus, ginger and oil of wintergreen has yet to be established for dogs and cats. As the investigation of the clinical case proceeds, the veterinarian should ask the owner how and why the animal's food is being supplemented with these substances.

ONIONS AND GARLIC

Owners may also supplement a pet's food with onions or garlic. Onions derive part of their flavor from n-propyl disulfide, which is toxic to the erythrocytes of several species (Jain, 1993). In 1990, a phenolic compound was extracted from onions that increased methemoglobin concentrations and caused the formation of Heinz bodies in canine erythrocytes (Miyata, 1990).

Onions may injure the lipid membranes of erythrocytes and irreversibly denature hemoglobin (Jain, 1993). These changes result in Heinz body formation, hemolytic anemia and hemoglobinuria. The most common cause of Heinz body hemolysis in dogs is related to ingestion of onions. Although the toxicity has been known for more than 50 years, animal owners still unknowingly feed onions to dogs as part of table food or intentionally as a supplement. The hemolytic episode may be difficult to correlate with onion ingestion because it occurs several days postingestion. Clinical signs related to moderate Heinz body anemia have occurred in dogs consuming relatively small amounts (5 to 10 g of onions/kg body weight) of raw, cooked or dehydrated onions (Harvey and Rackear, 1985; Ogawa et al, 1986). In one study, consumption of approximately 30 g of raw onions/kg body weight for three consecutive days produced severe anemia, erythrocyte Heinz bodies and hemoglobinuria in all dogs fed onions (Ogawa et al, 1986). One animal developed severe icterus and died on Day 5.

Cats are prone to developing erythrocyte Heinz bodies after exposure to many chemicals in food (Jain, 1993; Hickman et al, 1990; Christopher et al, 1989). Likewise, Heinz body anemia has occurred in cats after consumption of onions (Kobayashi, 1981). Baby food or other foods containing similar amounts of onion powder should not be fed to cats because of Heinz body formation and the potential for development of anemia, especially with high food intake. Cats with concurrent oxidative diseases may develop additive hemoglobin damage when fed baby food containing onion powder (Robertson et al, 1998).

Garlic (*Allium sativum*) is also a member of the onion family. Long-term exposure to garlic and garlic extracts caused anemia, contact dermatitis and asthmatic attacks in dogs (Poppenga, 1995). Eccentrocytosis appears to be a major diagnostic feature of garlic-induced hemolysis in dogs. The constituents of garlic have the potential to oxidize erythrocyte membranes and hemoglobin, inducing hemolysis associated with the appearance of eccentrocytes in dogs. Thus, foods containing garlic should not be fed to dogs (Lee et al, 2000).

CHOCOLATE

Pets today are often fed "people" food. One delicacy that has potential to cause toxicity is chocolate. Chocolate products contain variable amounts of theobromine, a potent cardiovascular and central nervous system stimulant (Clark et al, 1981). Although pet owners might believe that chocolate is innocuous, one poison control center documented six cases of chocolate poisoning in dogs during a single year (Hornfeldt, 1987). Signs such as vomiting, diarrhea, panting, nervousness, excitement, tremors, tachycardia, cardiac dysrhythmias, coma, convulsions and sudden death may appear in four to 15 hours after ingestion (Hornfeldt, 1987; Gauberg and Blumenthal, 1983; Hooser, 1984; Sutton, 1981). Renal damage may occur in severe cases.

The toxic dose of theobromine has been reported to be greater than 200 mg/kg body weight (Hornfeldt, 1987). However, a springer spaniel died after ingestion of two lb of milk chocolate, corresponding to a dose of only 92 mg of theobromine/kg body weight (Gauberg and Blumenthal, 1983). Based on this case, consumption of one typical 1.55-oz. milk chocolate bar (93 mg theobromine)/kg body weight could produce clinical signs and possibly death (Hooser, 1984). Unsweetened baking chocolate also contains high levels of theobromine (450 mg/oz.) and has been implicated in cases of toxicity (Hooser, 1984). Finally, dogs have also been poisoned by ingesting cocoa powder (1 to 3% theobromine) (Sutton, 1981).

Theobromine is eliminated very slowly in dogs. This metabolic peculiarity prolongs the clinical syndrome and increases the risk of toxicity from repeated ingestion of small doses of theobromine. Because there is no available antidote for theobromine toxicity, symptomatic treatments such as administration of emetics, activated charcoal, tranquilizers, sedatives and lidocaine should be used in clinical cases of chocolate toxicity.

GRAPES AND RAISINS

Acute renal failure has been associated with ingestion of variable amounts of grapes or raisins by dogs; as little as 0.41 oz./kg in one case (Gwaltney-Brant et al, 2001). Vomiting and azotemia are the most consistent findings, occurring in 100% of the cases in a retrospective review (Eubig et al, 2005). Varying degrees of renal tubular degeneration and proximal necrosis also occur (Morrow et al, 2005). A number of etiologies have been proposed, including heavy metals, mycotoxins and pesticide residues, but given the lack of a dose-response relationship, no clear toxic principle has been identified. Suggested therapy includes gastric decontamination protocols to induce emesis followed by activated charcoal administration and fluid diuresis (Mazzaferro et al, 2004).

FEEDING PLAN

If a diagnosis of foodborne illness seems feasible, then the pet owner should be questioned extensively about the animal's food. First, the veterinarian should identify all possible food sources (including commercial foods, home-prepared foods and table scraps) and determine the feeding amounts and the availability of unintentional food sources. Common questions concerning commercial foods should include: 1) brand name, 2) manufacturer, 3) lot or date code, 4) form of food (i.e., dry, semi-moist, moist), 5) feeding method (i.e., meal fed, free choice), 6) the length of time the pet has been consuming the brand of food, 7) the length of time the pet has been fed from the present container of food (i.e., bag or can), 8) whether water is mixed with the food, 9) how long the food is left in the food bowl, 10) the ambient temperature at feeding, 11) the method of storing the food and 12) whether other pets in the household consume the same food.

Questions about home-prepared foods should include: 1) the source of ingredients, 2) storage methods for the ingredients and the food, 3) method of preparation, 4) preparation temperatures, 5) method of measuring temperatures and 6) feeding method. Any recent change in either the food ingredients or preparation methods should be investigated further.

The amount of food consumed should be compared with the calculated amount typically consumed by an animal of similar size. If the amount consumed is markedly less than the calculated amount, it could mean that the animal does not like the food and may be foraging other food sources or garbage. Decreased intake may also indicate food refusal typical of vomitoxin contamination.

Sampling Procedures

Most veterinary diagnostic laboratories can perform the tests necessary to facilitate a diagnosis of foodborne illness. Many investigative tests and techniques are available to the diagnostic laboratory to help assess the case. In fact, the number is so overwhelming that only a few can be used on a particular sample. It is essential that the veterinarian discuss the likely diagnoses with laboratory personnel before test initiation to ensure the tests most critical to a correct diagnosis are performed. Veterinarians also need to determine the laboratory's preferred specimens and methods of specimen preservation.

Sample/specimen collection should follow the rules of physical evidence even if the possibility of litigation seems remote or nonexistent to ensure results are admissible in court if circumstances change. The admissibility of this information in a trial depends on whether: 1) all specimens and/or samples were properly identified, 2) the "chain of custody" (**Table 11-3**) is documented by a specific and detailed description of all events and changes of possession starting at the time of collection, through transportation and transferal to final sample analysis at the laboratory and 3) the evidence is relevant to the case (Grau, 1993). Therefore, it is also important to inform laboratory personnel if there is any possibility of litigation.

The best sources of samples for assessment of the food for possible etiologic agents are: 1) the actual food source, 2) food ingredients (homemade foods), 3) stomach contents, 4) intestinal contents and 5) feces. The following procedures and methods relate primarily to assessment of the food but also could be used to evaluate any previously described specimens (e.g., urine, blood, tissues, etc.).

The pet owner should bring the entire container of food or containers of food ingredients to the veterinarian to ensure that sample collection follows aseptic technique and the rules of evidence collection (Grau, 1993; Edwards, 1989). Sample collection techniques are described in detail in **Table 11-4**. Label all sample containers as space allows with a sample number and a description of the contents, submitter's name, pet owner's name, date, product label information and lot number. Supporting information and descriptions that cannot be written on the sample label because of space constraints should be numbered identically to the sample and submitted with the sample (Osweiler et al, 1985; Edwards, 1989; Galey, 1992).

Detection Methods

Bacterial Isolation and Identification

Pet food ingredients, like most other foods, contain a diverse microbial flora. Therefore, no single growth medium will satisfy the requirements of all organisms that may be present in a sample. The veterinarian should discuss likely pathogens with laboratory personnel so that the best methods, enrichment techniques and selective media can be used (Galey, 1992; Quinn et al, 1994).

Most laboratories will use a variety of direct examination and culture techniques to attempt a successful identification (Quinn et al, 1994). First, smears of the specimens collected by either the veterinarian or laboratory personnel will be stained and examined. Then growth and colony characteristics of bacterial isolates will be determined using a variety of media. The presence or absence of certain bacterial biochemical characteristics and atmospheric growth conditions will also be explored. Finally, a variety of other tests and techniques will be used to facilitate the identification process (e.g., API 20E strips and Staph-Trac).[d]

Analytical Chemistry

Metal assays are usually performed using some type of atomic spectroscopy, e.g., atomic absorption spectroscopy and inductively coupled plasma emission spectroscopy (Galey, 1992). Organic compounds such as pesticides and solvents are usually detected by chromatography, e.g., gas chromatography, high-pressure liquid chromatography, thin-layer chromatography. After a compound has been identified preliminarily by chromatography, results are often confirmed using mass spectrometry.

Mycotoxins can be detected by chromatography methods, radioimmunoassay (RIA) and enzyme-linked immunosorbent assay (ELISA) (Quinn et al, 1994). Staphylococcal enterotoxins can be identified using ELISA, RIA, serologic, precipitin and gel diffusion techniques (Freer and Arbuthnott, 1986). ELISA can also be used to detect the exotoxins and endotoxins of other bacterial species. *C. botulinum* exotoxins can be identified by serum neutralization using commercially available antisera followed by assay in laboratory animals (Quinn et al, 1994).

Significant Pathogen Levels in Food

Commercial foods are not sterile and may contain species of organisms associated with foodborne illnesses in people. However, the infective dose of each foodborne pathogen can vary greatly depending on the food substrate, the immunologic status of the host and the resistance of the normal intestinal flora (Council for Agricultural Science and Technology, 1994).

The same factors apply to foodborne illness in animals with the exception that the animal species can also influence the infective or toxic dose. Therefore, the relationship between microbial populations and the quality of foods can only be estimated and must be viewed with caution, especially when one considers that most sampling and microbial counting procedures possess inherent inaccuracies. Also, many organisms have fastidious growth and unique colonization requirements (i.e., medium, temperature and atmosphere). Although laboratory personnel will try various permutations, it is not always possible to find the correct combination given the limitations of sample size. In addition, the specimen may contain a microorganism that produces antimicrobial peptides that inhibit the growth of other species. Finally, the various counting procedures will also kill some of the bacteria present in the sample.

The scientific literature contains few data establishing the relative risk of foodborne illness and the microbial content of pet foods. Measuring the microbial content of pet foods is difficult but interpreting the results with respect to wholesomeness or food safety is even more difficult because risk quantification also depends on other factors, such as storage conditions.

Table 11-3. Procedures for the collection, transfer and preservation of physical evidence.*

- Collect, package and identify all samples according to the procedures listed in **Table 11-4.**
- Maintain a record of every person who had custody of any sample(s) or other evidence from the time that it was collected until presented in court ("chain of custody") by keeping a written log or diary of all relevant facts and sample transfers.
- Write notes documenting the time, place, description and circumstances of all samples entered in the log. Describe in detail how the samples were identified (numbered), processed, packaged, stored and shipped.
- If possible, photograph any apparent pathologic lesions, mold growth, foreign matter in the food, etc. Number the photographs consecutively and describe each photograph in the written notes.
- Write notes about all telephone conversations related to the case in the log, including the date, time and content of the conversation.
- Date all new entries in the log and have the person writing in the log initial the entry.
- Retain and store all relevant product labels in a safe place.
- Use a shipping method that expedites delivery of the samples to the laboratory. Keep copies of all shipping records. Hand carry the samples to the laboratory if possible. Obtain written proof of delivery (e.g., receipt).

*Adapted from Grau JJ. Criminal and Civil Investigation Handbook, 2nd ed., New York, NY: McGraw-Hill, Inc, 1993.

However, measurement of microbial populations may yield valuable information when used to compare one sample of a pet food with another sample of the same product. For example, it would be valuable to know whether bacterial numbers had increased dramatically while the food was in the pet's bowl. This information helps establish the level of hygiene and timeliness of the pet's feeding schedule. In summary, the presence of an organism in a food does not alone establish the diagnosis but must be considered as one piece of the diagnostic "puzzle."

Control and Prevention

Methods for control and prevention of foodborne illness in pets apply to commercial (after purchase) and home-prepared foods. Following the practices described in **Table 11-5** can best prevent foodborne illnesses in pet foods.

Food storage is an important preventive measure. Proper storage depends on control of: 1) temperature, 2) moisture and 3) availability of oxygen. First, high temperatures markedly decrease the shelf life of both canned and dry foods, especially when temperatures exceed 20°C (68°F) (Emsminger et al, 1995; Containers, 1968). Therefore, all commercial pet foods should be stored in the 4.4 to 15.6°C (40 to 60°F) temperature range. Fresh, home-prepared foods should be refrigerated at –1.6 to 15.5°C (29 to 60°F) before feeding. (Most household refrigerators hold foods at 4.4 to 7.2°C [40 to 45°F].) The length of time that a food can be kept refrigerated depends on its type and age. Fresh meats, fish and poultry can be kept for two to 10 days whereas fruits and vegetables will remain wholesome for weeks when refrigerated.

Moist products are sealed and therefore not affected by moisture or air; control of these factors applies only to storage of

Table 11-4. Sampling procedures for foodborne illnesses.

- Collect samples for toxicologic and microbiologic studies as separate samples and label them accordingly.
- Collect several samples from the same source, e.g., different areas of the food bag, stool specimen.
- Treat samples as though they were being prepared for a legal case by following the rules of evidence.
- Collect duplicate samples or split samples so that the veterinarian can retain one sample and the other can be submitted to the laboratory.
- Collect samples for microbiologic testing aseptically using sterile gloves, instruments and containers.
- Use watertight sample containers, preferably with screw-type lids.
- Label all sample containers with an accurate and complete description of the contents, e.g., submitter's name, client's name, date and time collected, product name, etc. Submit other sample information and any supporting descriptions with the samples.

Table 11-5. Prevention of foodborne illness in animals.

Commercial pet foods (moist or dry kibble)
Discard foods from bulging or leaking cans and damaged bags.
Discard all foods with an abnormal color, foreign materials, odor or moldy appearance.
Discard dry foods 30 minutes after adding water.
Avoid frozen raw diets.
Homemade diets
Use raw ingredients appropriate for human consumption.
Cook ground meat thoroughly to the center.
Sear the surface of whole meat cuts.
Cook all eggs: whole, yolks, whites and shells if used as calcium supplement.
Wash all raw fruits and vegetables.
Control food contamination
Use stainless steel utensils, feeding bowls, etc. whenever possible.
Keep food preparation areas, cooking utensils and food bowls spotlessly clean. Wash and disinfect bowls and utensils daily.
Store dry, commercial foods in a cool, dry environment, free from insects and rodents.
Empty the feeding bowl of moist or moistened foods not consumed within two to four hours if the ambient temperature is above 10°C (50°F).
Clean, wash and disinfect food utensils and food bowls after each feeding.
If feeding free choice, check food daily for mold and spoilage.
Control microorganisms in food using physical means
Cook all home-prepared foods at 82°C (180°F) for at least 10 minutes.
Verify cooking temperatures with a cooking thermometer and internal meat temperatures with a meat thermometer.
Validate thermometer accuracy periodically with boiling water.
Cover all perishable foods and opened cans of pet food and store in the refrigerator at 4°C (40°F) when not being prepared, cooked or consumed.
Control the pet's access to unintentional foods
Minimize roaming on trash pick up days.
Monitor closely when off leash.

bulk dry commercial foods. Spoilage bacteria require at least 30% moisture for growth whereas molds require 5 to 15%. Dry pet foods have moisture content in the range of 6 to 9%. Therefore, dry commercial pet foods will have a satisfactory shelf life if stored in a cool dry place with the top of the bag or container closed. These precautions limit the availability of moisture and air needed for oxidative chemical degradation and microbial growth. Placing the food still in its sack in a canister or other closed container will extend the shelf life by further reducing the availability of moisture and oxygen. This method of storage has the added advantage of preventing rodent and insect damage and maintaining palatability. In addition, storing the product in the original bag will preserve the date code information stamped on the bag and enhance investigation of a problem if one occurs.

REASSESSMENT

The type and duration of therapy will be dictated by the diagnosis and the physical condition of the patient. Therapy typically will consist of supportive, symptomatic treatment because most foodborne illnesses are self-limiting. With illnesses such as metal poisoning or mycotoxicoses that produce characteristic blood or biochemical changes, those specific parameters should be monitored routinely for evidence of recovery. In those cases in which the patient does not recover, veterinarians should first reassess the patient to ascertain whether exposure to the foodborne agent has been discontinued. If so, then an inaccurate diagnosis or other pathologic factors may have complicated the case. Continued monitoring of laboratory parameters is warranted. Animals that recover only to suffer another bout of foodborne illness at a later date are obviously being exposed to unsafe foods. Therefore, the veterinarian should counsel the pet owner to prevent further recurrences (**Table 11-5**).

ACKNOWLEDGMENT

The authors and editors acknowledge the contribution of Dr. James Cullor in the previous edition of Small Animal Clinical Nutrition.

ENDNOTES

a. Crane S. Feeding raw diet mythology. Personal communication. 2006.
b. Miller EP. Unpublished data. September 1996.
c. Cullor JS. Unpublished data. May 1995.
d. Analytab Products, Inc, Plainview, NY, USA.

REFERENCES

The references for **Chapter 11** can be found at www.markmorris.org.

CASE 11-1

Ulcerative Dermatitis in a Greyhound

Laine Cowan, DVM, Dipl. ACVIM (Internal Medicine)
College of Veterinary Medicine
Kansas State University
Manhattan, Kansas, USA

Patient Assessment

A two-year-old female greyhound that had been in training at a racetrack in Arkansas was examined for depression, swelling of the distal limbs and feet and skin ulceration. Other dogs from the same racing kennel had been affected with similar problems in the past.

Results of physical examination included depression, vomiting, subcutaneous edema involving both rear limbs, primarily distal to the stifle, and skin lesions. The skin lesions were focal, reddened areas that became dark red or black on the surface after a few hours. Several small ulcers were present on the distal extremities (**Figure 1**) and a large, well-demarcated ulcer was present on the left medial thigh (**Figure 2**). A large area of bruising and ecchymoses was evident on the ventral abdomen.

Clinical pathologic abnormalities included leukocytosis with neutrophilia, thrombocytopenia (29,000 platelets/µl; reference range = 200,000 to 500,000/µl), and severe azotemia (urea nitrogen = 240 mg/dl [10 to 20 mg/dl]; serum creatinine = 5.6 mg/dl [0.6 to 1.2 mg/dl]).

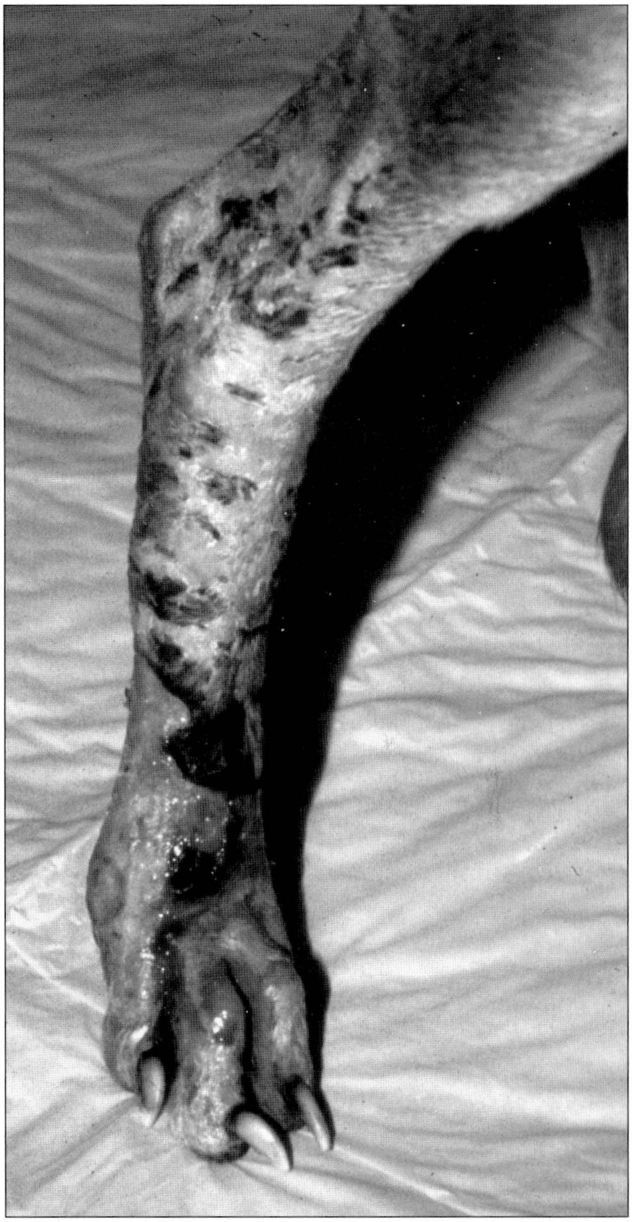

Figure 1. Right distal limb of a two-year-old female greyhound. Note the numerous small, well-demarcated ulcers.

Assess the Food and Feeding Method

All dogs in the kennel were fed a mixture of raw ground beef, dry commercial dog food and a powdered vitamin-mineral supplement. The beef was obtained from a commercial vendor in frozen packages and thawed before it was mixed with the dry food and supplement. The dogs were fed a portion of this mixture once daily.

Questions

1. What foodborne illnesses might be responsible for the clinical signs in this patient?
2. What specific diagnostic tests should be performed to investigate causes of foodborne illness in this patient?
3. What measures should be instituted to prevent outbreaks of foodborne illness in this kennel?

Answers and Discussion

1. Outbreaks of *Salmonella* enteritis ("kennel sickness," "blowout") and systemic salmonellosis are common among greyhounds in kennels. The clinical signs are usually mild to severe diarrhea that typically resolves in a few days. Occasional systemic infections occur with high morbidity rates, especially in puppies and young dogs. Racing greyhounds contract salmonellosis primarily by eating contaminated raw meat. Other foodborne bacterial diseases that result in gastrointestinal or systemic signs include campylobacteriosis, shigellosis and listeriosis.

   A syndrome of cutaneous multifocal ulceration, often accompanied by limb edema or acute renal failure, has been recognized in young, adult greyhound dogs. The syndrome has been referred to as "Alabama rot" and described as idiopathic cutaneous

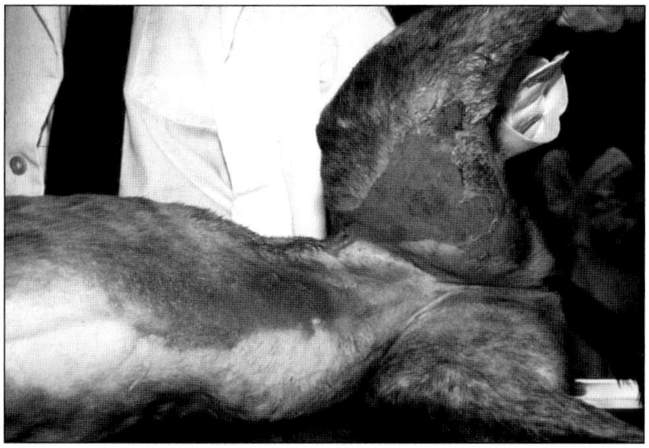

Figure 2. View of the ventral abdomen and left medial thigh of the same dog. Note the extensive contusions on the ventral abdomen and large, well-demarcated ulcer involving a large portion of the medial thigh

and renal glomerular vasculopathy. Reports of this syndrome have been limited to the greyhound breed. Clinical signs include acute erythema and edema progressing rapidly to well-demarcated cutaneous ulcers of the distal extremities, especially the hind limbs. Some dogs develop acute renal failure, which is usually fatal. Significant microscopic lesions are limited to the skin and kidney. Cutaneous lesions are characterized by vascular necrosis of arterioles, with ischemic necrosis and ulceration of the epidermis. Renal lesions are predominantly glomerular, including thrombi in glomerular capillaries and glomerular endothelial necrosis.

This syndrome in greyhound dogs resembles hemolytic uremic syndrome in people and edema disease in swine, which are thought to involve a Shiga-like toxin binding to and damaging vascular endothelium. Platelet aggregation contributes to thrombosis. Shiga-like toxins can be produced by a variety of bacteria, but *Escherichia coli* strain O157:H7 is incriminated most often. Because most racing greyhounds are fed raw meat, there is the potential for them to be exposed to Shiga-like toxin-producing *E. coli*

2. Bacterial organisms can be recovered by culturing the raw meat and commercial dry food and the patient's feces and blood. Large numbers of toxin-producing *E. coli* have been found in meat samples fed to greyhounds and in fecal samples from clinical cases.
3. The occurrence of disease related to contaminated meat is closely related to how the meat is handled on the farm or track before feeding. Preventive measures should include proper cooking and storage of meat whenever possible. Of primary importance is the temperature of the meat once it has thawed. When large blocks of frozen meat are thawed at room temperature, the outermost surface of the meat can reach unacceptably high temperatures before the center has thawed. Thawing meat slowly at refrigerator temperatures or in a camp cooler will markedly reduce surface bacterial growth.

   Many foodborne pathogens persist in the environment for extended periods. In some cases, the occurrence of food poisoning is associated with inadequate hygiene and failure to isolate dogs with diarrhea that are shedding large numbers of organisms. All facilities and equipment should be frequently cleaned with soap and then disinfected with bleach or phenolic compounds.

Progress Notes

The dog was treated with intravenous fluids, parenteral antibiotics and whirlpool baths in dilute povidone-iodine solution. Cimetidine and antiemetics were given to help control vomiting. Despite these efforts, the dog died 48 hours later of acute renal failure.

Necropsy findings included slightly pale, swollen kidneys with prominent, congested glomeruli and capsular petechiae. Mural edema of the stomach and black tarry colonic contents were also evident. Microscopic renal lesions included glomerular thrombotic microangiopathy; hyalin thrombi were present in glomerular capillaries and afferent arterioles. Glomerular capillary walls were thickened.

Bibliography

Chengappa MM, Staats J, Oberst RD, et al. Prevalence of *Salmonella* in raw meat used in diets of racing greyhounds. Journal of Veterinary Diagnostic Investigation 1993; 5: 372-377.

Cowan LA, Hertzke DM, Fenwick BW, et al. Clinical and clinicopathologic abnormalities in greyhounds with cutaneous and renal glomerular vasculopathy; 18 cases (1992-1994). Journal of the American Veterinary Medical Association 1997; 210: 789-793.

Fenwick BW, Hertzke D, Cowan LA. Alabama rot: Almost the complete story. In: Proceedings. Eleventh Annual International Canine Sports Medicine Symposium. Orlando, FL, 1995: 15-21.

Hertzke DM, Cowan LA, Schoning P, et al. Glomerular ultrastructural lesions of idiopathic cutaneous and renal glomerulopathy of greyhounds. Veterinary Pathology 1995; 32: 451-459.

CASE 11-2

Food Poisoning in Two Dogs

Lawrence H. Arp, DVM, PhD, Dipl. ACVP
Nutley, New Jersey, USA

Patient Assessment

A three-month-old male Australian shepherd dog was examined for severe muscle tremors, polypnea, hyperkinesias and ataxia, with intermittent opisthotonos and generalized seizures. The dog was anesthetized with sodium pentobarbital to control motor activity. Intravenous fluids were administered. After recovery from anesthesia, the dog was still atactic but less hyperkinetic.

On the same day, a one-year-old male Irish setter from the same neighborhood was admitted for treatment of muscle tremors and clonic seizures. The dog vomited 30 minutes before clinical signs were observed. It was treated in a similar manner to the first dog. Both dogs were clinically normal 12 hours later except for slight incoordination.

Assess the Food and Feeding Method

The owner of the first dog reported finding a partly eaten package of moldy cream cheese in his yard. The cream cheese had been purchased about one month earlier, had been partially used and then refrigerated until it was found covered with mold. The owner had thrown it out the previous day. Both dogs had access to the cream cheese but were not seen eating it. The cream cheese was covered with a dark blue-green fungal mat. Both dogs were of normal weight for their age and had normal body condition scores (3/5). No other nutritional history was available.

Questions

1. What potential foodborne diseases might cause the clinical signs in these dogs?
2. What diagnostic tests could be performed to confirm a foodborne illness?

Answers and Discussion

1. Members of the genera *Penicillium* and *Aspergillus* produce penitrem A and aflatoxin, respectively, two potent mycotoxins. These fungi are isolated most frequently from refrigerators and moldy foodstuffs in the home. These fungal genera also may be isolated from stored feeds and cereal grains that may eventually enter the pet food chain.

   Penitrem A causes acute muscle tremors, seizures and prostration in several animal species. The severity of clinical and pathologic features is dose dependent. Mildly affected dogs have transitory muscle tremors and ataxia lasting two to four hours, whereas larger doses may cause seizures and death. Normal neurologic function progressively returns after one or two days in animals that recover. Visceral petechiae, hepatic necrosis and hyperthermia may occur in dogs with mycotoxicosis.

   Ingestion or topical exposure to a variety of other compounds may also cause neurologic signs. Examples include various insecticides (pyrethrins, pyrethroids, organophosphates, carbamates), methylxanthines (chocolate), metaldehyde, various ornamental plants (Chinaberry, English ivy, jimson weed, tulip, yellow iris), illicit drugs (marijuana, cocaine, amphetamines), strychnine and lead.
2. The moldy cream cheese could be sent to a laboratory for identification of fungal elements and further toxicologic testing. Establishing a diagnosis of plant or illicit drug poisoning is difficult without specific evidence of ingestion. Whole blood cholinesterase activity will be depressed in organophosphate and carbamate toxicosis.

Progress Notes

Because both dogs recovered rapidly there was no need to change the foods or the feeding methods. The owners were instructed to limit access to spoiled food by proper disposal.

Examination of the moldy cream cheese by light microscopy revealed fungal elements typical of the genus *Penicillium*. The organism was later identified as *P. crustaceum*, a common contaminant of refrigerated foodstuffs. *P. crustaceum* produces large quantities of penitrem A at 4°C.

Three mice were given a moldy cheese emulsion by mouth and developed hyperkinesia, irritability, generalized muscle tremors and tonic-clonic seizures within two hours. Penitrem A was identified by thin-layer chromatography from a sample of the moldy cream cheese; therefore, this mycotoxin was considered the cause of the clinical signs in both dogs.

Bibliography

Arp LH, Richard JL. Intoxication of dogs with the mycotoxin penitrem A. Journal of the American Veterinary Medical Association 1979; 175: 565-566.

CASE 11-3

Vomiting and Diarrhea in a Puppy

James S. Cullor, DVM, PhD
School of Veterinary Medicine
University of California, Davis
Davis, California, USA

Patient Assessment

A nine-week-old male German shepherd puppy was examined for evaluation of vomiting and diarrhea. There had been no problems until six days earlier when the puppy's feces became liquid and bowel movements more frequent. The puppy vomited twice several hours after the diarrhea was first noticed. The vomitus contained undigested food, but no evidence of foreign material, blood or parasites. The dog was confined to the house or a fenced outdoor enclosure. The puppy was vaccinated a week before the clinical problems began. When examined the puppy was mildly lethargic, about 5% dehydrated, but otherwise healthy.

Assess the Food and Feeding Method

The dog was fed a commercial dry grocery brand food formulated for puppies. Fresh water and the dry food were offered free choice. The food had been purchased from a large retail outlet one week before the onset of clinical signs. The puppy was eating the dry food with no obvious problems. Three days before the onset of clinical signs, the owner began mixing the dry food with water. The moistened food remained at room temperature or outside where temperatures reached 32.2°C (90°F) for several days. The puppy became ill several hours after eating most of the moistened food.

Questions

1. What potential foodborne illnesses could be causing the clinical signs in this dog?
2. What techniques could be used to diagnose whether foodborne illness is causing the vomiting and diarrhea in this patient?

Answers and Discussion

1. A variety of foodborne illnesses can cause vomiting and diarrhea. These include contamination of food with bacterial organisms or their toxins (*Staphylococcus aureus, Salmonella* spp., *Neorickettsia* spp., *Escherichia coli, Bacillus cereus, Yersinia* spp., *Campylobacter* spp.), biogenic amines, aflatoxins, vomitoxin and heavy metals (lead, arsenic, zinc, cadmium). The fact that the dry food was moistened with water and left at high ambient temperatures makes bacterial proliferation a likely cause of clinical signs.
2. Most veterinary diagnostic laboratories can perform the tests necessary to facilitate a diagnosis of foodborne illness. It is important to determine the laboratory's preferred specimens and method of specimen preservation. Bacterial isolation techniques can often be performed on the food, vomitus and feces. Heavy metal, pesticide, biogenic amine and toxin assays can be performed on food, serum, feces and other biological samples.

Progress Notes

There was no history that the puppy had access to illicit drugs, heavy metals, pesticides, toxic ornamental plants and garbage. Results of a hemogram were normal, which made a diagnosis of viral enteritis unlikely. Three samples from the dry commercial puppy food and three from the moistened food were cultured and grown aerobically. Feces were also cultured daily over the next three days. Cultures revealed 1 x 10^2 colony forming units (cfu) of *Bacillus cereus*/g dry food and 1 x 10^7 cfu of *B. cereus*/g moistened food. These results confirmed that bacteria had proliferated after the food was moistened and left at warm to hot ambient temperatures. *B. cereus* was also cultured once from diarrheic feces. No other bacterial pathogens were recovered from the food or feces.

The puppy was treated with subcutaneous fluids and was fed a complete, balanced homemade food consisting of boiled lean ground beef and rice, offered in small, frequent meals. The puppy's feces gradually became firmer. After two days of therapy with the homemade food, the original commercial dry puppy food was offered, without added moisture. The puppy was feeling well, eating normal amounts of food and had normal stools by Day 7 after the onset of clinical signs. The pet owner was advised to not add water to dry pet foods and leave them exposed to ambient temperatures for more than a few hours.

A tentative diagnosis of *B. cereus* enterotoxemia was made. *B. cereus* is known to cause vomiting and diarrhea in people; however, it is not thought to pose a significant danger for foodborne illness in animals. *B. cereus* flourishes at room temperature, and certain isolates possess the genetic capability to produce a potent enterotoxin. The organism is a ubiquitous, spore-forming aerobic saprophyte found in soil, grains, cereal grain products and other foods. As an example, it is commonly found in uncooked rice. *B. cereus* has been found as a common isolate in samples of dry pet food. It has also been isolated from food packaging paper and materials.

The standard heat treatments used in pet food manufacturing are not likely to kill the spores of this organism. However, the number of organisms isolated from the pet food (<10^5 cells/g of food) is unlikely to cause foodborne disease in pets unless the food is exposed to moisture and heat conditions conducive to bacterial proliferation.

Bibliography

Claus D, Berkeley RCW. Genus *Bacillus.* In: Sneath PHA, Mair NS, Sharpe ME, et al, eds. Bergey's Manual of Systematic Bacteriology. Baltimore, MD: Williams and Wilkins, 1986; 1105-1139.

Drobniewski FA. *Bacillus cereus* and related species. Clinical Microbiology Reviews 1993; 6: 324-328.

Turnbull PCB, Kramer JM. *Bacillus.* In: Balows A, Hausler WJ, Herrmann KL, et al, eds. Manual of Clinical Microbiology, 5th ed. Washington, DC: American Society for Microbiology, 1991: 296-303.

Vaisanen OM, Mentu J, Salkinoja-Salnen MS. Bacteria in food packaging paper and board. Journal of Food Microbiology 1992; 71: 130-133.

CASE 11-4

Acute Renal Failure in a Yorkshire Terrier

Kenneth R. Harkin, DVM, Dipl. ACVIM (Small Animal Internal Medicine)
College of Veterinary Medicine
Kansas State University
Manhattan, Kansas, USA

Patient Assessment

A 10-year-old, spayed female Yorkshire terrier was presented for evaluation of vomiting after consuming 1/2 to 3/4 cup of raisins (organic flame variety), either in the overnight hours before or in the early morning hours of the day of presentation. The dog vomited a large quantity of raisins in the late morning and also had a bout of diarrhea that contained raisins. The dog vomited foam and bile four to five more times throughout the day. Although the dog wasn't anorectic, it would vomit shortly after eating.

Physical examination revealed an alert patient with a normal body temperature, a heart rate of 140 beats/min. and a normal body condition score (3/5; body weight was 7.2 kg). The patient was minimally dehydrated (5%) and had a full, but non-painful abdomen.

Abnormalities noted on the complete blood count and serum biochemistry profile included hemoconcentration (hematocrit 58% [reference range 37 to 55%]), azotemia (urea nitrogen 49 mg/dl [reference range 8 to 30 mg/dl], creatinine 4.0 mg/dl [reference range 0.5 to 1.4 mg/dl], hyperphosphatemia (8.6 mg/dl [reference range 2.3 to 6.5 mg/dl]), hyperkalemia (6.6 mmol/l [reference range 3.8 to 5.5 mmol/l]), hypercalcemia (15.6 mg/dl [reference range 7.2 to 12.8 mg/dl]) and elevated alanine transaminase (220 U/l [reference range 13 to 79 U/l]) and alkaline phosphatase (913 U/l [reference range 12 to 122 U/l]) activities. The total protein was 6.4 g/dl (reference range 5.6 to 7.9 g/dl) and the albumin was 3.7 g/dl (reference range 3 to 4.5 g/dl). A stress leukogram was also noted. The serum was moderately hemolyzed and moderately lipemic. There was no urine in the urinary bladder.

Problems identified included azotemia with hyperkalemia, hypercalcemia, elevated liver enzymes, vomiting, historical idiopathic hyperlipidemia and unknown urine production.

Assess the Food and Feeding Method

The dog had been diagnosed with idiopathic hyperlipidemia three years earlier and was being fed a low-fat, high-fiber veterinary therapeutic food (Prescription Diet r/d Canine,[a] dry). No additional medications were necessary to control the hyperlipidemia. The dog was meal fed twice daily and fresh water was always available.

Questions

1. What is the likely cause of the azotemia?
2. What is the likely cause of the hyperkalemia and hypercalcemia?
3. What parameters need to be closely monitored?
4. What treatment options need to be considered for this patient?

Answers and Discussion

1. The historical ingestion of raisins makes acute renal failure from raisin toxicity the most likely differential diagnosis for this dog. The clinical course and laboratory abnormalities identified are characteristic of raisin toxicity. (See chapter text.) Without a urine specific gravity, however, the possibility that this dog has pre-renal azotemia cannot be dismissed. The disproportionately high

creatinine to urea nitrogen would be less supportive of prerenal azotemia. Possible differential diagnoses to consider for this constellation of clinical signs and laboratory findings could include: 1) diseases that cause hypercalcemia (neoplasia such as lymphoma, anal sac adenocarcinoma, parathyroid adenoma), however, the chronic nature of these diseases and the lack of previously recognized polydipsia/polyuria would make them seem unlikely, 2) hypoadrenocorticism, although the sodium concentration was normal and the dog had a stress leukogram, 3) acute pancreatitis, however, hypocalcemia is more common than hypercalcemia in this disorder and the dog had a non-painful abdomen when palpated and 4) vitamin D toxicity (e.g., rodenticides, dermatologic creams) would present with all of the changes seen in this dog; however, there was no historical evidence for this toxicity.

2. The hyperkalemia in this patient is caused by a combination of decreased glomerular filtration rate from the intrinsic damage to the renal tubules and dehydration. Aldosterone deficiency (i.e., hypoadrenocorticism) is unlikely given the lack of other supportive evidence for that disease.

   Hypercalcemia is a commonly recognized laboratory abnormality with raisin toxicity. The etiology is unknown. Other differential diagnoses for hypercalcemia include hypercalcemia of malignancy, primary hyperparathyroidism, granulomatous disease, vitamin D toxicosis and hypoadrenocorticism. The serum calcium concentration in this dog decreased to 13.9 mg/dl 12 hours later and to 11.3 mg/dl 36 hours later. The patient's ionized calcium, performed when the serum calcium was 13.9 mg/dl was normal.
3. The most critical parameters to monitor in this dog include urine production and serum potassium concentration. Urine production can be monitored directly with placement of a urinary catheter and closed collection bag. Indirect measures of urine production include frequent weighing of the dog and weighing of the pads in the kennel before and after urination. Placement of a central venous catheter for measurement of central venous pressure is critical if the patient becomes oliguric or anuric to prevent potentially life-threatening overhydration. In anuric and severely oliguric patients, serum potassium values can rise precipitously, resulting in cardiac arrhythmias and death. Avoiding potassium-containing fluids for rehydration is important as an initial step in an attempt to lower the serum potassium concentration. If necessary, emergency measures can be implemented including administration of calcium gluconate, sodium bicarbonate and insulin:dextrose infusions.
4. For this patient, the first steps should be rehydration and establishing whether the dog is anuric, oliguric or polyuric. If the dog is anuric, the best options include hemodialysis and peritoneal dialysis. If the dog is oliguric, furosemide, mannitol and dopamine may increase urine production. Patients in polyuric renal failure are easily managed as long as fluid losses are met with intravenous fluid replacement and electrolytes are monitored to prevent hypokalemia.

Progress Notes

On the night of admission, a catheter was placed in the cephalic vein and the dog was administered 0.9% sodium chloride at 11 ml/kg/hour. The following morning the dog was still alert; however, urine production was minimal; the patient had gained 0.45 kg (6.25%) after receiving approximately 700 ml of fluids. A serum biochemistry profile performed that morning showed that the azotemia had worsened (urea nitrogen 68 mg/dl, creatinine 5.3 mg/dl, phosphorous 9.0 mg/dl), the hypercalcemia had improved (13.4 mg/dl) and the hyperkalemia was essentially unchanged (6.5 mmol/l). A jugular catheter was placed that morning to monitor central venous pressure. The initial pressure was measured at 5 to 6 cmH_2O; however, this value increased to 10 cmH_2O approximately eight hours later. A urinary catheter was also placed that morning; no urine was produced over the next eight hours. The dog became progressively depressed over that time period. A serum chemistry profile was repeated that afternoon: the urea nitrogen was 84 mg/dl, creatinine 6.5 mg/dl, phosphorous 12.4 mg/dl and potassium was 8.6 mmol/l.

Cardiotoxicity from the hyperkalemia was now evident, as the heart rate had decreased from 120 beats/min. to 60 beats/min. The respiratory rate had increased to more than 80 breaths/min. and breathing was becoming more labored. The decision was made to place catheters for peritoneal dialysis. The dog was given butorphanol (1.4 mg IV) as a preanesthetic agent and anesthesia was induced and maintained with sevoflurane inhalation. The dog developed atrial standstill on induction and was given intravenous sodium bicarbonate (3 ml), which temporarily resolved the cardiac dysrhythmia. Three Jackson-Pratt tubes were placed through 2-cm incisions made in the right ventral abdomen, left ventral abdomen and along the ventral midline for use as peritoneal dialysis catheters. No attempt was made to remove the omentum because the dog's critical state necessitated minimal anesthesia time. Atrial standstill developed again during the procedure; the dog was administered sodium bicarbonate (3 ml IV), 50% dextrose (5 ml IV) and two doses of calcium gluconate (10% solution, 1.5 ml IV).

Peritoneal dialysis was initiated immediately after the dog recovered from anesthesia. A dialysate was made by placing 25 ml of 50% dextrose in 500 ml of lactated Ringer's solution. A total of 125 ml of dialysate was infused into the abdomen every hour for 15 exchanges and allowed to remain for 40 minutes, after which it was allowed to drain for 20 minutes. The amount of dialysate was then increased to 210 ml and was allowed a dwell time of 100 minutes. This process was repeated for the next four days, at which time the dwell time was increased to six hours and the volume of dialysate was left at 210 ml.

A constant infusion rate of furosemide (0.1 mg/kg/hour) was started at the time of dialysis to stimulate urine production; however, the dog remained markedly oliguric (<1 ml/kg/hour) for the following three days. Urine production began to increase from Days 4 through 6, although the dog was still considered oliguric (2 to 3 ml/kg/hour). On Day 7, the dog became markedly polyuric, with hourly urine production of approximately 10 ml/kg/hour.

The dog was hospitalized for 20 days. Additional therapies administered included famotidine (0.5 mg/kg IV q12hours) to minimize gastric hyperacidity, cefazolin (22 mg/kg IV q8hours) for prophylaxis to prevent infection from the peritoneal dialysis catheters and total parenteral nutrition, which was administered for seven days, at which time the dog began to eat on its own. A biochemistry profile performed at the time of discharge revealed these values: urea nitrogen 52 mg/dl, creatinine 3.0 mg/dl and phosphorous 11.5 mg/dl.

Because of the previously diagnosed idiopathic hyperlipidemia, a diet change was not initiated in this dog. A chitin-based phosphate binder (Epakitin[b]) was added to the food to control hyperphosphatemia. The higher protein content of the food (vs. foods formulated for renal failure) necessitated three to four times the standard dose of phosphate binder to control hyperphosphatemia. There was also a concern that the increased protein in the food would increase intraglomerular pressure; therefore, the dog was given enalapril (0.25 mg/kg PO q24hours). At four months from discharge, the dog had a stable creatinine at 3.7 mg/dl, phosphorous of 6.0 mg/dl and was reported to be active and eating well.

Endnotes

a. Hill's Pet Nutrition, Inc., Topeka, KS, USA.
b. Vetoquinol, Buena, NJ, USA.

CASE 11-5

Acute Vomiting in a German Shepherd Dog

Kiko Bracker, DVM, Dipl. ACVECC
Angell Animal Medical Center
Boston, Massachusetts, USA

Patient Assessment

A nine-year-old, neutered male, German shepherd dog was examined for a three-day history of occasional vomiting and progressive lethargy. The dog was uninterested in food for the past few days and was drinking excessively. Before the onset of these signs, the dog had been healthy and no medications had been administered.

Physical examination revealed a 46-kg dog with a normal body condition score (5/9 [BCS]). Vital signs were within normal limits. The dog was lethargic, but responsive and able to walk around the exam room. The abdomen was not painful and abdominal palpation was normal. The mucous membranes were tacky and faintly icteric, as were the sclera. Thoracic auscultation was normal.

Diagnostic evaluation included a complete blood count, which showed hemoconcentration (hematocrit = 55%), and a serum biochemistry panel, which revealed hyperbilirubinemia and increased liver enzyme activities (**Table 1**). A coagulogram showed that the prothrombin time (PT) and activated partial thromboplastin time (aPTT) were prolonged (**Table 1**). Results of a urinalysis were normal except for bilirubinuria.

Abdominal radiography showed no significant abnormalities. An abdominal ultrasound found the gallbladder to be full, but showed no dilatation of the bile ducts. The liver appeared structurally normal although a small amount of fluid was noted between the liver lobes that could not be sampled due to its location. Because of the prolonged clotting times and concern of bleeding, no liver biopsy or aspirates were taken. The tentative diagnosis was an acute hepatic insult of unknown cause.

Assess the Food and Feeding Method

The dog had been eating the same brand of dry dog food for several years. The exact daily caloric intake was unknown because the dog was fed free choice. Upon further questioning, the owner admitted the dog had been eating a food that was identified as being contaminated with aflatoxin. Based on national recall information, a primary rule out of aflatoxin toxicosis was established.

Questions

1. What method of delivering nutrition to this patient is most appropriate during its hospitalization?
2. How can a diagnosis of aflatoxicosis be confirmed?
3. Is there a specific antidote for this toxin?

Answers and Discussion

1. For patients that are not vomiting, enteral feeding is the method of choice because it increases mucosal blood flow, preserves enterocyte function and decreases bacterial translocation from the intestinal tract. This dog was vomiting; therefore, enteral feeding would likely worsen its nausea. Additionally, placement of a feeding tube (nasoesophageal tube, esophagostomy tube, gastrostomy tube, etc.) carries the risk of hemorrhage because the patient was found to be hypocoagulable. Administration of parenteral nutrition (PN) is the most appropriate method of providing nutrition to this patient.
2. A sample of the contaminated food can be submitted to a diagnostic lab for analysis. Alternatively, a fresh or frozen sample of hepatic tissue may be used to identify the presence of aflatoxin by thin-layer chromatography or high-performance liquid chromatography; however, the toxin may be eliminated from the body in 24 hours; therefore, these tests are often negative. Formalin preserved liver tissue can be submitted for histologic evaluation because the histologic changes (diffuse lipidosis and hepatocellular necrosis) are fairly unique to this toxin in dogs.
3. There is no antidote for aflatoxin toxicosis. Aggressive treatment to support the liver and treat signs of liver failure are recommended.

Progress Notes

The dog was treated in two hospitals for five days. Although the specific treatments at both hospitals differed slightly, the goals were the same: 1) intravenous fluid support, 2) replacement of clotting factors with fresh frozen plasma and supplementation with vitamin K_1, 3) use of gastroprotectants to minimize gastrointestinal ulceration (omeprazole, famotidine), 4) antiemetic therapy (metoclopramide, dolasetron), 5) nutritional support, 6) antioxidants and antioxidant precursors to minimize damage to the liver (N-acetylcysteine, Denosyl,[a] vitamins E and C) and 7) prophylactic antibiotics (ampicillin) to minimize the chance of infection due to intestinal bacterial translocation and incompetent hepatic immune function.

Occasional hematemesis occurred during the first two days of hospitalization. Although the patient was offered several different types of dog food, it refused to eat. Therefore, it was occasionally syringe fed 100 ml of a highly palatable, homogenized veterinary therapeutic food (Prescription Diet a/d Canine/Feline [b]). Although this food is relatively calorie dense (1.4 kcal/ml), the dog's resting energy requirement (RER) was much higher (70 x (46 kg)$^{0.75}$ = RER = 1,236 kcal/day). Furthermore, the dog's vomiting made enteral feeding impractical.

On the third day of hospitalization, PN was started through a peripheral catheter. A central line was not used due to concerns about hemorrhage. The PN was formulated to contain a minimum of amino acids (1.0 g/100 kcal), due to the liver's inability to process ammonia derived from deamination of amino acids.

In several separate infusions, the dog received 1,170 ml of fresh frozen plasma (24 ml/kg) to replace clotting factors. This treatment improved the dog's clotting times. Nonetheless, the patient's clinical condition deteriorated; the dog became weaker, vomited more often and began to have bloody diarrhea. Hepatic encephalopathy was suspected on the fifth day of hospitalization. Within two hours the patient underwent cardiac arrest and died.

Table 1. Biochemistry and clotting values for a nine-year-old German shepherd dog.

Test	Day 1	Day 5	Reference values
ALP (IU/l)	124	221	71-120
AST (IU/l)	ND	502	13-50
ALT (IU/l)	194	885	21-97
Bilirubin (mg/dl)	8.2	23.2	0.1-0.3
Albumin (g/dl)	2.7	2.2	3.1-4.2
PT (seconds)	70	24.5	7.3-11.8
aPTT (seconds)	>100	28.4	10.6-14.8

Key: ALP = alkaline phosphatase, AST = aspartate aminotransferase, ND = not done, ALT = alanine aminotransferase, PT = prothrombin time, aPTT = activated partial thromboplastin time.

Endnotes

a. Nutramax Laboratories, Inc., Edgewood, MD, USA.
b. Hill's Pet Nutrition Inc., Topeka, KS, USA.

Bibliography

Hooser SB, Talcott PA. In: Peterson ME, Talcott PA, eds. Small Animal Toxicology, 2nd ed. St. Louis, MO: Elsevier Inc, 2006; 889-892.

Marik PE, Zaloga GP. Early enteral nutrition in acutely ill patients: A systematic review. Critical Care Medicine 2001; 29: 2264-2270.

Proulx J. Nutrition in critically ill animals. In: Raffe MR, Wingfield WE, eds. The Veterinary ICU Book, 1st ed. Jackson, WY: Teton NewMedia, 2002; 202-217.

CASE 11-6

Azotemia in a Cat

Candace Berkshire, DVM
Washington State University
Pullman, Washington, USA

Patient Assessment

A 10-year-old, castrated male domestic shorthair cat was enrolled in a cohort of blood donor cats. Initial diagnostics at enrollment included testing for feline leukemia virus, feline immunodeficiency virus, heartworm, toxoplasmosis, haemobartonellosis, bartonellosis and ehrlichiosis. Prior medical history included mild periodontal disease, constipation that resolved with lactulose treatment and, recently, forelimb lameness.

The patient was fed a high-protein therapeutic food for more than a year. When the food was listed as a product recalled due to contaminated wheat gluten, the cat was examined for possible adverse effects. Physical examination findings were within normal limits, although the cat was less active than usual. Results from a serum biochemistry profile indicated that the patient was azotemic, with blood urea nitrogen (BUN) and creatinine values of 66 mg/dl and 3.3 mg/dl, respectively. Urine collected by cystocentesis had a specific gravity of 1.018, with many crystals, originally thought to be ammonium urate (**Figure 1**). An abdominal ultrasound was performed; pathologic changes included hydronephrosis of the left kidney, bilateral nephrocalcinosis, fluid surrounding the left kidney and a large amount of gravity-dependent sediment in the urinary bladder. A peripheral intravenous catheter was placed and fluid therapy was initiated. Therapy included intravenous fluids, a histamine receptor antagonist (famotidine[a]) and lactulose.

The patient was transitioned to a therapeutic food targeted for management of renal disease (Prescription Diet k/d Feline[b]). Despite therapy, lethargy, anorexia and the degree of azotemia continued to progress for several days (**Figures 2** and **3**). A central intravenous catheter was placed for delivery of fluids and measurement of central venous pressure. Urine output was monitored by routinely weighing litter box contents. Urine volume was large and dilute; therefore, the patient was classified as polyuric. Following four days of fluid and drug therapy, BUN and creatinine values decreased markedly. Renal panels were repeated daily; the azotemia continued to improve over the following five days. After 10 days of treatment for acute renal failure (ARF), the cat was transitioned to subcutaneous fluids, therapy with famotidine was discontinued; however, the renal therapeutic food was continued. After the acute crisis, azotemia resolved in three weeks.

Assess the Food and Feeding Method

When enrolled in the blood donor program, the cat was fed an adult feline maintenance food. Approximately one year before the pet food recall, the patient and its cohorts were transitioned to a high-protein, low-carbohydrate food (Prescription Diet m/d Feline[b]). Food was administered in measured amounts by kennel staff twice daily. As mentioned above, the cat was fed Prescription Diet k/d Feline when it was affected with ARF.

Questions

1. Could ARF be related to contamination of pet food with a toxic agent?
2. How can ARF be differentiated from chronic renal failure?
3. What treatment plan(s) should be considered for suspected cases of ARF?
4. What are some risks following successful treatment of ARF?

Answers and Discussion

1. In March 2007, a massive recall of pet food was instituted following reports of renal failure in animals following a palatability trial. Over several weeks, many contaminants were considered. Melamine was isolated from pet food ingredients, pet food and renal and urine samples from affected patients. In vitro studies demonstrated that melamine, when combined with a similar moiety (i.e., cyanuric acid), would form crystals in cat or dog urine. ARF was thought to result from severe crystalluria, similar to ARF in ethylene glycol cases.

   In December 2005, a pet food manufacturing company issued a similar recall because aflatoxin was identified as the cause of severe hepatic necrosis and cirrhosis in dogs. Ten years earlier, in 1995, pet food was recalled for excessive levels of vomitoxin in pet food.

   Product contamination should be considered in unexplained acute disease, particularly if the incidence of that disease process increases dramatically and other causes have been ruled out. Reputable pet food manufacturers conduct multiple tests on raw ingredients and finished products and can provide immediate information about calls involving products to their toll-free numbers. When the pet food recall was instituted, renal failure caused by melamine ingestion was undocumented, and the agent was considered relatively nontoxic. In cases of unexplained acute illness, exposures to toxins, whether environmental or in pet food

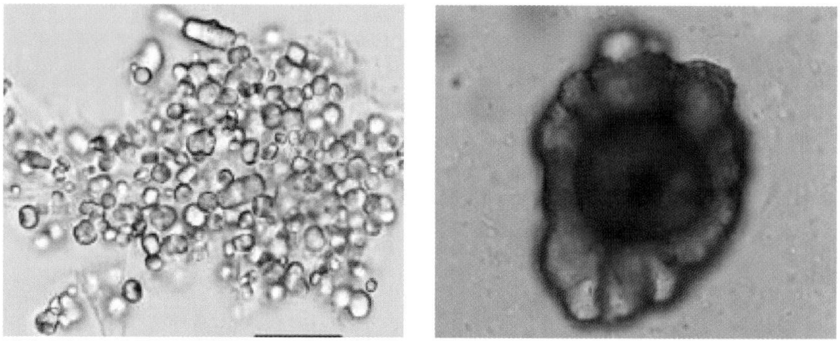

Figure 1. Melamine/cyanuric crystals produced in vitro (left). Crystal from the urine of an affected cat (Magnification 1,000x) (right).

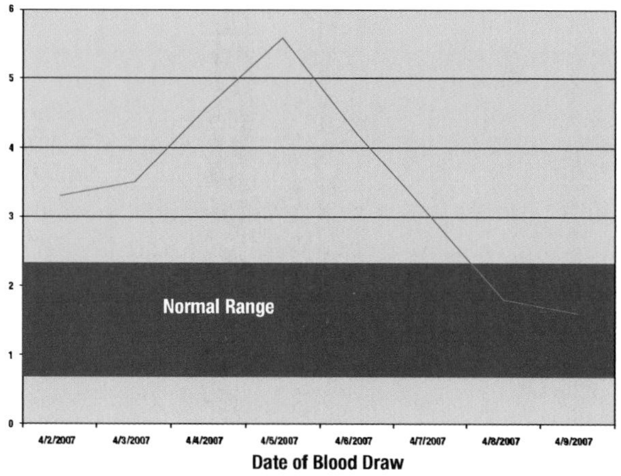

Figure 2. Creatinine changes during ARF.

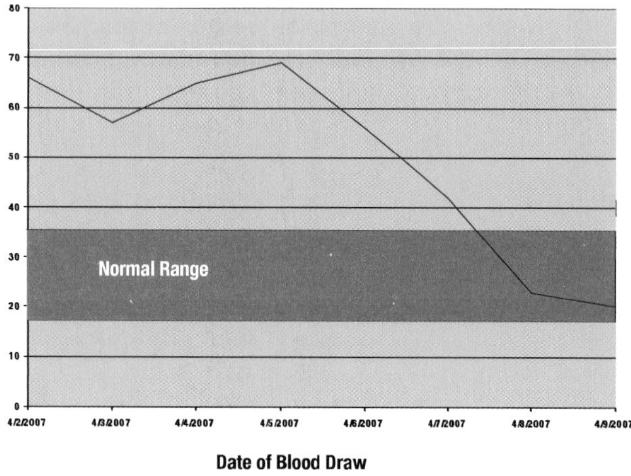

Figure 3. BUN changes during ARF.

should be documented.

2. The most obvious differences between acute and chronic renal failure are the speed of onset and duration of signs. In ARF, signs appear rapidly with illness usually lasting less than one week. ARF patients are oliguric or anuric, whereas animals with chronic renal failure are usually polyuric. However, normal or increased urine production should not be used to rule out ARF. In cases of acute uremia, mucous membranes remain pink, as opposed to pale mucous membranes and anemia often noted in chronic renal failure. Mineral and electrolyte imbalances may also be more apparent in cases of ARF, and may include hypocalcemia and hyperphosphatemia. Patients with chronic renal disease also show outward signs of chronic disease including poor body condition and coat, whereas patients with ARF generally present with good body condition and a normal coat.
3. Management of ARF is multifactorial. Immediate actions should include removing the inciting source, in this case, discontinuing use of the contaminated food. Fluid therapy should be instituted to correct extracellular fluid imbalances and deficits. After replacement fluids have been administered and adequate hydration achieved, fluid therapy should continue with respect to maintenance and continued fluid loss. Diuresis is the optimal method of preventing medullary tubule blockage by crystals. To prevent further acid-base derangements, gastric protectants should be administered, and continued for two to three weeks, until uremic gastritis has been effectively controlled. Caloric intake should be carefully monitored. Uremia and metabolic acidosis can induce protein catabolism, which is compounded by anorexia and vomiting. Patients should be routinely weighed to evaluate weight loss, although this measure can be confounded by changes in hydration status and lean body mass. A low-protein, low-phosphorus food is typically recommended for uremic patients. The protein should be highly digestible, and the food should have increased amounts of fat to increase caloric density. Whenever possible, enteral feeding methods should be employed to promote gastrointestinal health.
4. Risks associated with acute uremia include derangements of fluid balance, electrolyte imbalances and cardiovascular and pulmonary complications. If morphologic changes are not treated and reversed during the recovery phase, acute uremia can progress to chronic renal failure. Overaggressive fluid therapy can potentially result in volume overload, leading to hypertension and pulmonary edema. Care should be taken to continually assess the hydration status of the patient.

Progress Notes

The patient was assessed and diagnostic studies were conducted to detect ARF before the onset of clinical signs. Due to aggressive treatment, the patient recovered fully within three weeks. The patient was discharged from the blood donor program and given to a private owner. At the time of discharge, the cat's BUN and creatinine concentrations had decreased to normal limits, and no signs of renal disease were present. The cat was bright, alert and responsive and fully recovered. Recommendations were made to continue feeding the therapeutic kidney food, due to the patient's increased risk for developing chronic renal disease at a later date. Lactulose treatment was continued, and considered unrelated to the ARF episode.

Acknowledgement

The author thanks Dr. Amy Tamulevicus of the Veterinary Teaching Hospital, Kansas State University, Manhattan, for providing clinical information about this patient.

Endnotes

a. Pepcid. Merck & Co., West Point, Pennsylvania, USA.
b. Hill's Pet Nutrition, Inc., Topeka, KS, USA.

Bibliography

Cowgill LD, Francey T. Acute uremia. In: Ettinger SJ, Feldman EC. Textbook of Veterinary Internal Medicine: Diseases of the Dog and Cat, 6th ed. St. Louis, MO: Elsevier Saunders, 2005; 1731-1751.

Grauer G. Early detection of renal damage and disease in dogs and cats. Veterinary Clinics of North America: Small Animal Practice 2005; 35: 581-596.

Interim melamine and analogues safety/risk assessment. U.S. Food and Drug Administration Center for Food Safety and Applied Nutrition. www.cfsan.fda.gov/~dms/melamra.html.

Lees G. Early diagnosis of renal disease and renal failure. Veterinary Clinics of North America: Small Animal Practice 2004; 34: 867-885.

Section 3

Nutritional Management of Healthy Dogs

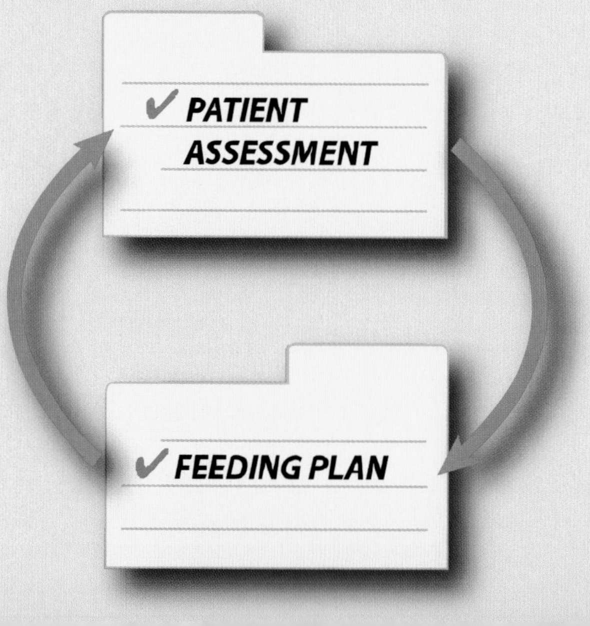

Chapter 12

Introduction to Feeding Normal Dogs

Jacques Debraekeleer

Kathy L. Gross

Steven C. Zicker

"What dogs? These are my children, little people with fur who make my heart open a little wider."
Oprah Winfrey

CLINICAL IMPORTANCE

Much has changed in our perception and use of dogs over the past half century. Our society has moved from an agrarian phase into a postindustrial phase with a concomitant shift of the human population into urban settings. Dogs have, by necessity, made the shift to urban living along with us and in doing so we have discovered their remarkable adaptability and versatility.

Dogs have found a job in virtually every niche of society. Dogs have been useful in law enforcement, as nursing home companions, in the military, in drug enforcement, as paraplegic assistants and in search and rescue. The human-animal bond has become a commonly taught subject in veterinary schools, which testifies to the importance of animals, including dogs, for our mental and physical well-being. The Centers for Disease Control and Prevention (CDC) describe some of the health benefits of pet ownership, including decreased blood pressure, cholesterol levels, triglyceride levels and feelings of loneliness and increased opportunities for exercise, outdoor activities and socialization (2006). Many organizations support the health benefits of pet ownership including the American Veterinary Medical Association, The Delta Society and the National Institutes of Health; these organizations and others have issued statements or provided information supporting the health benefits of pet ownership. According to this national poll of working Americans 18 years of age and over, nearly one in five U.S. companies allow pets at work. A majority of those polled believe pets at work provide benefits such as relieving stress, improving relationships with coworkers, making for a happier workforce and creating a happier work environment (CDC, 2006). Another health benefit for both dogs and people is related to exercise and weight loss. When overweight people and overweight pets exercise together, they both have lower dropout rates from their weight-loss programs (Jewell et al, 2004).

The emphasis on dogs as valued members of society (**Box 12-1**) has driven the development of canine nutrition towards the same goals we strive for in human nutrition: long life, high quality life and enhanced performance.

Demographics

Globally, pet ownership has increased, possibly due to reduced human birth rates, changing family structure and aging populations (Anonymous, 1997). Regardless of a pet's size or species, pet owners consider their pet to be a family member. One survey indicated that 63% of the U.S. population own pets. There are nearly 75 million dogs in the U.S. Furthermore, 45% of U.S. households own dogs; this equates to approximately 1.7 dogs per household (AAMA, 2007). **Table 12-1** lists countries with the most prevalent dog ownership. Breed popularity varies from year to year and from region to region; however, some breeds always appear to be more desired than others (**Table 12-2**). Worldwide, mixed-breed and crossbred dogs are most popular.

Box 12-1. People Treat their Dogs like Family Members.

A majority of American households (62%) own at least one pet, but virtually everyone, more than nine in 10, considers his or her pet a member of the family. Here are some other interesting facts about dog ownership.

- 70% of owners said they give their dogs presents at Christmas.
- 22% of owners celebrate their dogs' birthday by giving a special treat, making a special meal, giving their dog a cake, ice cream, a new toy, a new bone, singing happy birthday, throwing a birthday party with other dogs, taking their dog to a favorite place or taking photographs.
- More than 50% of American dog owners are more attached to their pets than to at least one other person; 36% say they are more attached to their dog than their best friend and 12% say they are more attached to their dog than their spouse.
- 25% of owners let their dog sleep either on top of or in their bed.

The Bibliography for **Box 12-1** can be found at www.markmorris.org.

Table 12-1. Comparisons of dog populations in selected countries.*

Country	Pet dog population
USA	61,080,000
Brazil	30,051,000
China	22,908,000
Japan	9,600,000
Russia	9,600,000
South Africa	9,100,000
France	8,150,000
Italy	7,600,000
Poland	7,520,000
Thailand	6,900,000

*Source: Infobase Pvt. Ltd.

Table 12-2. Ten most popular dog breeds registered by the American Kennel Club in 1996 compared with their popularity in 2005.

	1996*		2005**	
Breed	Rank	Number	Rank	Number
Labrador retriever	1	149,505	1	137,867
Rottweiler	2	89,867	16	15,916
German shepherd dog	3	79,076	4	45,014
Golden retriever	4	68,993	2	48,509
Beagle	5	56,946	5	42,592
Poodle	6	56,803	8	31,638
Dachshund	7	48,426	6	38,566
Cocker spaniel	8	45,305	15	16,343
Yorkshire terrier	9	40,216	3	47,238
Pomeranian	10	39,712	14	19,511

*Adapted from U.S. Pet Ownership & Demographics Sourcebook. Schaumburg, IL: Center for Information Management, American Veterinary Medical Association, 1997; 32-35.
**American Kennel Club Registration Statistics, 2005.

The terms "mixed breed" and "crossbred" have slightly different meanings. Mixed-breed dogs' ancestry might not be discernable, whereas breeders often plan crossbreeding by mating two different purebred dogs.

Coinciding with increasing numbers of pets, from 2001 to 2006, sales of commercial pet foods increased 5.4% in the U.S. and more than 10% worldwide. In the U.S., the trend is for less pet food to be sold through grocery stores and more through specialty and mass merchandisers. Packaged dry dog foods are almost universally fed by dog owners (95% of dog owners) compared to canned food use (34% of dog owners) (Packaged Facts, 2006). This highly competitive market and increased demand, coupled with the importance of nutrition to the health and performance of dogs, make it necessary for practicing veterinarians to understand not only the basics, but also the subtleties of canine nutrition to make knowledgeable recommendations to clients about optimal feeding programs.

Species Diversity

The modern domestic canine species encompasses a vast number of breeds each with its own genetic idiosyncrasies (Fogle, 1997). Using genomic techniques (microsatellite genotyping), the genetic similarities of 85 modern breeds were organized into four distinct groups. The breeds in each of the four groups had similar geographic origins, morphology or role in human activities (Parker et al, 2004). The variety of dog breeds has arisen out of selection efforts by people to produce animals with specific traits that may enhance performance, show or behavioral characteristics (**Table 12-3**). The result is a species that displays a wide variety of morphology; head shape, size, coat characteristics (color, length, etc.) and musculoskeletal structure. By selecting for these traits, we have probably unknowingly selected for variations in metabolism and nutrient usage as has been evidenced in other species. Our knowledge about breed variation in metabolism and nutrient requirements is growing. Furthermore, nutrigenomic technologies create a potential for an even better understanding of breed-specific nutrition (Chapter 4). Nutrigenomics is currently applied to many species including people (Swanson et al, 2003). Because dogs are good models for certain human diseases, the outcome will be an increasing body of knowledge about metabolism and nutrition of the diverse canid species. A common unifying theme is dogs are omnivores.

DOGS AS OMNIVORES

The word carnivore can be used to indicate either a taxonomic classification or a type of feeding behavior. The order Carnivora is quite diverse (**Table 12-4**) and consists of 12 families containing more than 260 species. Omnivorous and carnivorous feeding behaviors are most common among members of the order Carnivora; however, the order also includes species that are herbivores (e.g., pandas) (Corbet and Hill, 1986; Morris and Rogers, 1983, 1989).

Eating Behavior

Several researchers have examined the eating habits of wolves (*Canis lupus*), the nearest ancestors of our domestic dogs, and close relatives such as coyotes (*Canis latrans*). Both are opportunistic predators and scavengers, hunting and eating what is available regionally (Sheldon, 1992). Coyotes eat carrion and hunt rodents, other small mammals, birds, amphibians and other species (Sheldon, 1992; Landry and Van Kruiningen, 1979). Additionally, they have been reported to consume droppings of herbivorous prey; domestic dogs also will readily consume herbivore feces (Lewis et al, 1987). Regional ungulates such as buffalo, deer, elk, moose, wildebeest, antelope and zebra are the natural prey of wolves (Sheldon, 1992; Landry and Van Kruiningen, 1979). Viscera are typically consumed; therefore, partially digested vegetable material is a normal part of the wolf's diet (Beaver, 1981). Both coyotes and wolves also eat plant matter such as fruits, berries, persimmons, mushrooms and melons (Sheldon, 1992; Landry and Van Kruiningen, 1979; Röhrs, 1987). Similarly, dogs are opportunistic eaters and have developed anatomic and physiologic characteristics that permit digestion and usage of a varied diet.

Anatomy and Physiology

Oral Cavity

The oral cavity functions to decrease the physical size of food for introduction into the rest of the alimentary tract. Decreasing the physical size of food creates particles small enough to pass through the esophagus and increases the surface area of the food, which enhances enzymatic digestion in the stomach and small intestine. Dogs have cutting canine teeth for ripping and tearing and molar teeth with large occlusal tables for crushing, which are associated teleologically with the capacity to use plant material (**Figure 12-1**) (Morris and Rogers, 1989). Dogs may fix large pieces of food with their paws to tear off small pieces with their cutting canine teeth, after which the food particle is advanced to the back of the oral cavity where it may be crushed by the molar teeth and mixed with saliva before being swallowed (Meyer, 1990).

Stomach

Wild canids typically eat large meals, usually infrequently, due to intermittent food availability. Dogs may consume their daily energy requirement in one or two large rapidly ingested meals (Ruckebusch et al, 1991). This eating pattern means that the stomach must be able to expand markedly. On average, a medium-sized, adult domestic dog has the capacity to ingest 30 to 35 g of dry matter per kg body weight per day (Meyer, 1990a; Meyer et al, 1980). However, the canine stomach can adjust, within limits, to accommodate the amount of food ingested and can hold 1 to 9 liters depending on the breed (Schummer and Nickel, 1960).

Small and Large Intestine

The characteristics of the canine small intestine are consistent with those of animals that digest an omnivorous diet (Morris and Rogers, 1989). The small intestine composes approximately 23% of the total gastrointestinal (GI) volume of dogs (Ruckebusch et al, 1991) vs. 15% for cats (Wolter, 1982). The ratio of GI tract length to total body length is 6:1 for dogs, 4:1 for cats, 10:1 for rabbits and as high as 20:1 for some herbivores (Morris and Rogers, 1989; Meyer, 1990; Wolter, 1982). This anatomic relationship is consistent with ingestion of an omnivorous diet with intermediate digestibility (i.e., between low digestible herbaceous forages and highly digestible animal flesh). Dogs digest starch effectively via pancreatic enzymes and mucosal disaccharidases.

Table 12-3. Examples of various functions dogs perform in society.

Assisting hearing or physically impaired persons
Entertainment
Guiding blind persons
Herding
Hunting
Military and law enforcement
Pets
Racing (sprint or endurance)
Rescue operations
Show and breeding
Social interactions

Nutrient Requirements and Metabolism

Much can be learned about an animal's nutritional requirements simply by analyzing its natural food source. True carnivores, such as cats, are limited to what is available from prey tissues such as skeletal muscle and liver to provide energy and nutrients, including protein, taurine, arginine, arachidonic acid and niacin. Consequently, carnivorous animals (e.g., cats) developed more efficient pathways to use these nutrients, and have lost the ability or have a decreased ability to synthesize them from precursors (Chapter 19). Being omnivorous and feeding on a varied diet of plant and animal tissue, dogs maintained or improved the ability to synthesize nutrients from precursors. These differences lend more evidence to early evolutionary divergence (Martin, 1989) and further support the premise that dogs are omnivores.

Table 12-5 compares the recommendations for daily nutrient intake of adult dogs to the nutrient content of meat (ground beef). This comparison confirms that an all-meat food would be unbalanced for dogs. Specific aspects of nutritional requirements of dogs are discussed in Chapters 5 and 6 and Chapters 13 through 18.

LIFESTAGE NUTRITION

Lifestage nutrition is the practice of feeding animals foods designed to meet their optimal nutritional needs at a specific age or physiologic state (e.g., maintenance, reproduction, growth or senior). The concept of lifestage nutrition recognizes that feeding either below or above an optimal nutrient range can negatively affect biologic performance or health (Chapters

Table 12-4. Taxonomy and natural feeding behavior of the order Carnivora.*

Family	Canidae	Ursidae	Procyonidae	Ailuropodidae	Mustelidae	Viverridae
Feeding behavior	Omnivores	Omnivores Carnivores	Omnivores	Herbivores	Carnivores Omnivores	Omnivores
No. of species	35	7	13	2	63	35
Examples	Dogs Jackals Coyotes Foxes Wolves	Bears	Raccoons Coatis Kinkajou Olingos	Pandas	Weasels Polecats Mink Ferrets Martens Wolverine Badgers Skunks Otters	Genets Civets Linsangs
Family	**Herpestidae**	**Hyaenidae**	**Felidae**	**Otariidae**	**Odobenidae**	**Phocidae**
Feeding behavior	Carnivores Omnivores	Carnivores	Carnivores	Carnivores	Carnivores	Carnivores
No. of species	37	4	36	14	1	19
Examples	Mongooses Meerkats	Hyenas	Leopards Pumas Cats Ocelots Serval Jaguars Lynxes Bobcats Lions Tigers Cheetahs	Eared seals Sea lions	Walrus	Earless seals

*Adapted from Corbet GB, Hill JE. A World List of Mammalian Species. New York, NY: Facts on File Publications, 1986; 105-121. Nowak RM, Paradiso JL. Walker's Mammals of the World, 4th ed. Baltimore, MD: The Johns Hopkins University Press, 1983. Ridgway SH, Harrison RJ. Handbook of Marine Mammals. New York, NY: Academic Press Inc, 1981.

Table 12-5. Comparison between the recommended daily allowances of selected nutrients for a 10-kg adult dog and the nutrient content of meat (beef).*

	RDA	Regular ground beef	Amount meeting the DER of a 10-kg dog		
Nutrient	**10-kg dog**	**per 100 g**	**482 g**	**% of RDA**	**Adequacy**
Metabolizable energy (kcal)	650	135	650	100	Yes
Moisture (ml)	650	60	289	44	na
Protein (g)	24	17	82	341	No
Fat (g)	≥8	20	96	1,204	No
Calcium (mg)	1,000	10	48	5	No
Phosphorus (mg)	750	200	963	128	Maybe
Ca/P ratio	1:1-2:1	1:20	1:20	na	No
Sodium (mg)	250-500	70	337	100	Yes
Potassium (mg)	550	325	1,565	285	No
Magnesium (mg)	150	25	120	80	Maybe
Iron (mg)	14	3.25	16	112	Yes
Copper (mg)	1	0.05	0.2	24	No
Zinc (mg)	10	1.5	7	70	No
Iodine (mg)	0.15	0.003	0.014	10	No

Key: RDA = recommended daily allowance, DER = daily energy requirement, na = not applicable, Yes = meets the optimal recommendations, Maybe = does not meet the optimal recommendations, but is neither deficient nor excessive, No = deficient or excessive.
*Adapted from Gesellschaft für Ernährungsphysiologie Ausschuß für Bedarfsnormen. Energie-und Nährstoffbedarf Nr. 5 Hunde. Frankfurt, Germany: DLG Verlag, 1989. Meyer H, Heckötter E. Futterwerttabellen für Hunde und Katzen. Hannover, Germany: Schlütersche Verlaganstalt und Druckerei, 1986. National Research Council. Nutrient Requirements of Dogs. Washington, DC: National Academy Press, 1985. Randoin L, Le Gallic P, Dupuis Y, et al. Tables de composition des aliments. Institut Scientifique d'Hygiène Alimentaire, 6th ed. Malakoff, France: LT Editions J. Lanore, 1990. Watt BK, Merrill AL. Composition of Foods-Raw, Processed, Prepared. Agriculture Handbook No 8.Washington, DC: Agricultural Research Service, USDA, 1975.

5 and 6). This concept differs markedly from feeding a single product for "all lifestages" (all-purpose foods) in which nutrients are added at levels to meet the highest potential need (usually growth and reproduction). Adult animals at maintenance are always provided nutrients well in excess of their biologic needs when fed all-purpose foods. Because the goals in nutrition are to feed for optimal health, performance and longevity, feeding foods designed to more closely meet individual needs is

preferred. This philosophy is the central tenant to lifestage nutrition and preventive medicine. In addition to providing advice about basic nutritional requirements of their patients, veterinarians should assess and minimize the nutrition-related health risks at each lifestage. For maximal benefit, risk assessment and prevention plans should begin well before the onset of disease.

The value of lifestage feeding is enhanced if risk factor management is incorporated into the feeding practice. In many instances, when the nutritional needs associated with a dog's age and physiologic state are combined with the nutritional goals of disease risk factor reduction, a more narrow, but optimal, range of nutrient recommendations results. For example, essentially all commercial dog foods sold in the U.S. meet or exceed the Association of American Feed Control Officials (AAFCO) minimum nutrient requirements for dog foods. Regulatory agencies such as AAFCO ensure ingredient safety and nutritional adequacy. However, even foods that are nutritionally adequate may have levels of certain nutrients outside a desired range for disease risk factor reduction or optimal performance (these nutrients are nutrients of concern). As mentioned in Chapter 1, besides nutrients of concern, specific food factors such as digestibility and texture can also affect health and modify disease risk. Together, nutrients of concern and specific food factors are referred to as key nutritional factors. The key nutritional factors for commercial foods for different lifestages of healthy dogs will be discussed in Chapters 13 through 18, including those associated with reducing the risk of specific diseases and those involved with optimizing performance during different physiologic states.

Homemade foods, unlike commercial foods, are not regulated. Thus, unless experts in canine nutrition have formulated the recipes from which they are made, there are no assurances that homemade foods will provide adequate nutrition or that the ingredients used to make them are safe for dogs (Chapter 10). However, even if the recipes for homemade foods ensure nutritional adequacy and ingredient safety, key nutritional factors should also be considered, depending on the lifestage of the dog being fed.

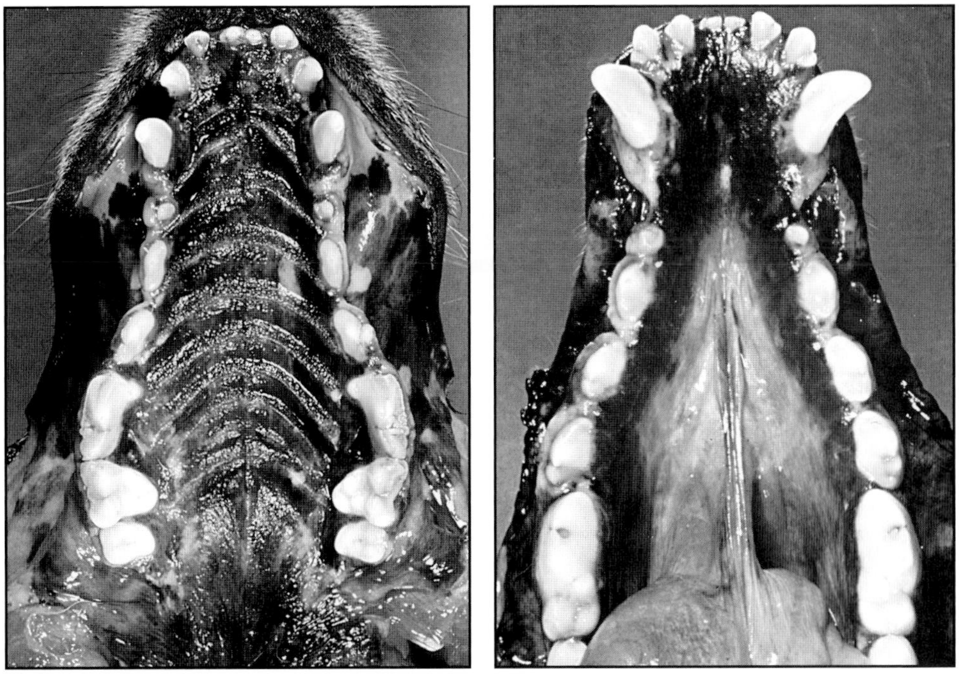

Figure 12-1. Maxillary dentition and palate of a dog (left). Mandibular dentition and sublingual mucosa of the same dog (right). These photographs demonstrate tooth anatomy associated with an omnivorous eating behavior. The cuspid (canine) teeth are long and cutting and are used for capturing and puncturing prey. The maxillary and mandibular premolar teeth interdigitate and provide a shearing action. The carnassial teeth (upper fourth premolar and lower first molar) have broad occlusal surfaces and are used for grinding and chewing. (Adapted with permission from Harvey CE, Emily PP. Function, formation, and anatomy of oral structures in carnivores. Small Animal Dentistry. St. Louis, MO: Mosby-Year Book Inc, 1993.)

In sequence, the chapters that follow cover Feeding Young Adult Dogs: Before Middle Age, Feeding Mature Adult Dogs: Middle Aged and Older, Feeding Reproducing Dogs, Feeding Nursing and Orphaned Puppies from Birth to Weaning and Feeding Growing Puppies: Postweaning to Adulthood. The next chapter begins with feeding young adult dogs because most dogs are adults, and the nutrient needs of adult dogs serve as a good basis for comparing nutrient needs for other lifestages. Chapter 18 covers recommendations for feeding adult working and sporting dogs for optimal physical and olfactory performance.

REFERENCES

The references for **Chapter 12** can be found at www.markmorris.org.

Chapter 13

Feeding Young Adult Dogs: Before Middle Age

Jacques Debraekeleer
Kathy L. Gross
Steven C. Zicker

"If you get to thinking you're a person of some influence, try ordering somebody else's dog around."
Will Rogers

INTRODUCTION

Depending on breed, dogs one through five to seven years of age are generally considered young adults. They are usually fully grown (about 12 months old for most breeds) but are not yet middle aged. In people, middle age is often considered to coincide with the third quarter of the average lifespan. Other than obesity and periodontal disease, this age range represents a relatively healthy period in a dog's life. Generally, many of the more common mortal diseases are more often diagnosed in middle-aged or older dogs.

The goals of nutritional management for young adult dogs are to maximize longevity and quality of life (disease prevention). A basic premise is that the foods fed should be nutritious; they should provide the recommended allowances of all known required nutrients. Most regulated commercial foods provide all the necessary nutrients in amounts that avoid deficiencies (Chapter 9). However, to meet the feeding goals described above, nutritional recommendations must exceed simply preventing diseases associated with nutrient deficiencies.

Nutritional recommendations for people living in affluent countries include nutrient and food recommendations that help prevent important diseases such as obesity, diabetes mellitus, cardiovascular disease, cancer, Alzheimer's disease and others. Thus, as in people, optimal feeding plans for pet dogs should include recommendations for specific nutrients and non-nutrient food ingredients (key nutritional factors) that influence important canine diseases. **Table 13-1** lists the important health concerns that may be positively affected by proper nutritional management in this age group of dogs. To achieve these feeding goals, besides selecting the best food, the food needs to be properly fed (amounts and methods).

PATIENT ASSESSMENT

Patient assessment should be a structured process that includes: 1) obtaining accurate and detailed medical and nutritional histories, 2) reviewing the medical record, 3) conducting a physical examination and 4) evaluating results of laboratory and other diagnostic tests. During assessment, the feeding goals should be established and explained, risk factors for nutrition-related diseases considered and key nutritional factors identified.

History and Physical Examination

Often, in a typical busy clinical setting, the time available to obtain a dietary history and conduct a physical examination is limited. However, a minimum dietary database for all canine patients should be obtained and include: 1) the type of food fed (homemade, commercial, dry, moist, semi-moist, etc.), 2) recipes if homemade food represents the majority of the diet, 3) brand names of commercial foods, if known, 4) names of supplements, treats and snacks and 5) method of feeding (free

Table 13-1. Important diseases for adult dogs that have nutritional associations.*

Disease/ health concern	Incidence/prevalence/ mortality/pet owner concern
Dental disease	Most prevalent disease; numerous associated health risks (e.g.kidney disease)
Obesity	Approximate 30% prevalence; associated health risks (e.g., diabetes mellitus, musculoskeletal disease); major concern
Kidney disease	Second leading cause of non-accidental death; major concern
Arthritis	6% prevalence; primary concern
Cancer	Primary cause of death; primary concern
Skin/coat problems	Second most common cause of disease (26% prevalence); second most common health concern

*Adapted from DeBowes LJ, Mosier D, Logan EI. Association of periodontal disease and histologic lesions in multiple organs from 45 dogs. Journal of Veterinary Dentistry 1996; 13: 57-60. Egenvall A, Bonnet BN, Hedhammar A, et al. Mortality in over 350,000 insured Swedish dogs from 1995-2000: II. Breed-specific age and survival patterns and relative risk for causes of death. Acta Veterinaria Scandinavica 2005; 46(3): 121-136. Lund EM, Armstrong PJ, Kirk CA, et al. Health status and population characteristics of dogs and cats examined at private veterinary practices in the United States. Journal of the American Veterinary Medical Association 1999; 214: 1336-1341. Morris Animal Foundation Survey Results, August 12, 2005. Morris Animal Foundation Survey Results, 1998.

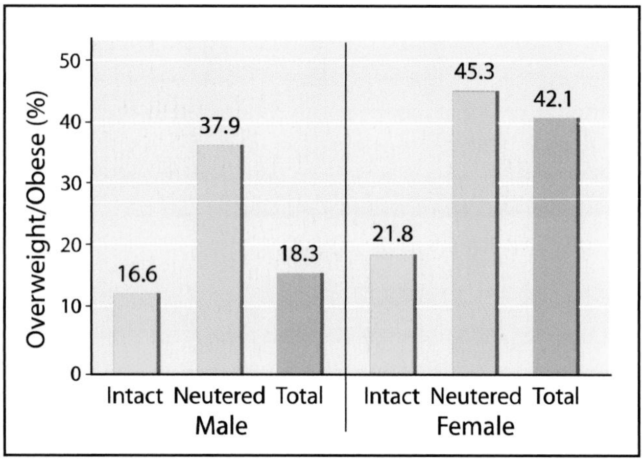

Figure 13-1. Percentage of overweight and obese dogs in intact, neutered and total female (3,828) and male (4,109) populations. (Adapted from Edney ATB, Smith PM. Study of obesity in dogs visiting veterinary practices in the United Kingdom. Veterinary Record 1986; 118: 391-396.)

choice, meal feeding, etc.). An extended dietary database includes: 6) quantities fed, 7) recent changes in food type, intake and preferences, 8) access to food for other pets or livestock, 9) who in the family buys food for the pet, 10) who in the family feeds the pet and 11) appetite changes with estimates of magnitude and duration. The general type and level of activity (e.g., house pet, confined to kennel, working dog, etc.) and neuter status should be noted because these factors are important determinants of energy requirements. The dietary history should be expanded if nutrition-related problems such as obesity are identified in the initial evaluation of the patient.

Body weight, body condition score (BCS) (Chapter 1), oral health and overall appearance of the skin and coat of all adult dogs should be assessed and recorded in the medical record. These parameters are general indicators of nutritional adequacy. An otherwise healthy young adult dog with normal body weight, skin and coat and BCS (2.5/5 to 3.5/5) and no evidence of significant dental disease is unlikely to need further nutritional assessment. However, for purposes of disease prevention, nutritional intervention, such as switching to a food that matches the recommended levels of key nutritional factors, may be warranted. The health concerns listed in **Table 13-1** are discussed in the risk factor review that follows.

Gender and Neuter Status

No controlled studies have been performed to delineate differences in nutritional requirements of intact male vs. intact female dogs. It may be presumed that, like other mammals, intact females require less caloric intake than intact males. If this assumption is true it is probably because of gender-related differences in lean body mass. Lean body mass accounts for nearly all of an animal's resting energy requirement (RER) (Blaxter, 1989). Women require fewer calories than men because of a lower relative amount of lean body mass than men (Pellett, 1990). One study showed that female dogs had an average of 16% more body fat than male dogs (Meyer and Stadtfeld, 1980). Surveys have found a much higher prevalence of overweight and obese conditions in female than male dogs (**Figure 13-1**) (Edney and Smith, 1986; Mason, 1970). These findings suggest that intact female dogs may need fewer calories than intact males.

Obesity occurs twice as often in neutered dogs than in reproductively intact dogs (**Figure 13-1**) (Edney and Smith, 1986). Very little is known, however, about the pathophysiology of this phenomenon. Neutering does not appear to have a marked impact on the resting energy expenditure of female dogs (Anantharaman-Barr, 1990); however, it may significantly increase food intake (Houpt et al, 1979). The increased food intake in neutered bitches is thought to be a consequence of a reduction of appetite-suppressing estrogen activity (Houpt et al, 1979; O'Farrell and Peachey, 1990). A decrease in physical activity is also assumed to occur in many dogs after neutering and may play a more important role in male dogs because of decreased roaming (Hopkins et al, 1976; Lewis, 1978). The daily energy intake should be limited to prevent rapid weight gain in neutered dogs; 1.6 x RER is a good starting point. For some breeds and individual dogs, it may be necessary to lower the energy intake of neutered dogs to 1.2 to 1.4 x RER (Chapters 1 and 5).

Breed

The breed classification should be determined in the initial assessment. Different breeds may be at risk for specific diseases or metabolic alterations that require nutritional management. As an example, certain canine breeds appear to be predisposed to obesity (Chapter 27). In addition, daily energy requirement (DER) differences have been delineated among different breeds, possibly because of differences in lean body mass, temperament and activity level. As examples, Newfoundland dogs have energy requirements about 20% less than average (Kienzle and Rainbird, 1991), whereas Great Danes and Dalmatians may have energy requirements up to 60% higher than average (Rainbird and Kienzle, 1990; Kienzle and Rainbird, 1991; Zentek and Meyer, 1992; Männer, 1990). Careful attention to specific local lineage and personal clinical impressions of breed differences may prove useful in food recommendations.

Activity Level

Activity significantly influences the energy requirements of individual dogs and should be taken into account when estimating energy requirements. For example, standing requires 40% more energy than lying down (Meyer, 1983). DER may range from RER for sedentary dogs to almost 15 x RER for endurance athletes under extreme conditions (Hinchcliff et al, 1997). A consistently higher level of physical activity probably would result in a relative increase in lean body mass, which would result in an increase in energy use, even at rest (Blaxter, 1989). However, because the activity of individual dogs often cannot be defined precisely, feeding recommendations should initially be conservative to avoid overfeeding and the risk of obesity. Food intake should be adapted as needed to maintain optimal body weight. Chapter 18 presents more information about the influence of specific nutrients on athletic performance (**Box 13-1**).

SEDENTARY DOGS

Estimations for DER include enough energy to support spontaneous activity, such as eating, sleeping, going outside and up to three hours of play and exercise per day. However, most pet dogs are minimally active (NRC, 2006). Approximately 19% of owners never play with their dogs and 22% take their

Box 13-1. Special Nutritional Considerations for Stressed Dogs.

STRESS

Police dogs, sentry dogs and other working dogs may refuse to eat, lose weight, develop diarrhea or become reluctant to work for inapparent reasons. Physiologically induced weight loss is most common in sentry dogs, in which a combination of mental stress, weather extremes and activity may result in loss of up to 10% of body weight during a six-hour tour of duty. Stress stimulates release of cortisol and induces a discharge of catecholamines. Besides stimulating alertness, catecholamines may depress food intake in stressed animals by activating the β-adrenergic and dopaminergic receptors in the lateral hypothalamus. This is obvious in highly stressed sentry dogs that may be reluctant to eat the volume of food they need to meet energy requirements. Dogs in various stressful situations demonstrate the same behavior. Some show dogs and racing greyhounds eat sparingly when the owner/handler prepares to depart to a show or a competition. A decrease in food intake, a slight increase in energy requirement and the catabolic effect of cortisol justify feeding a food with increased fat content (at least about 15% dry matter [DM]) and a protein level of about 25% DM. This recommendation does not compensate for energy spent for activity in addition to the stress (e.g., long-distance performances in which fat must be further increased to meet additional energy requirements).

Changing environments such as boarding or hospitalization may influence food intake due to stress. Dogs may develop diarrhea or refuse to eat when boarded. Practitioners commonly see dogs that refuse to eat in the hospital, but readily eat at home.

EFFECTS OF THE SHOW CIRCUIT

The success of a show dog is determined by genetics, general health, socialization, training and nutrition. Therefore, the preparation of a show dog starts with the correct choice of parents, sound breeding practices and correct rearing of puppies. Good nutrition allows for optimal expression of inherited qualities of a dog. Nutrition of a show dog involves feeding for correct development of skeleton and dentition, and maintenance of long-term health. More specific to show dogs are the nutritional needs for optimal condition of skin and coat, and the support of stress.

Preparation for the show may require particular attention. Skin health and correct color, length and glossiness of hair are important for adult show dogs. The first requirement for a shiny coat is good overall health and nutrition throughout the year. See Chapter 32 for more information about the nutritional effects on skin and coat.

Some show dogs may be finicky eaters, so they may need to be fed a more concentrated, palatable food, containing 25 to 30% DM protein and ≥15% DM fat. During a show, dogs don't spend much energy for physical activity; the primary increase is probably due to stress. Generally, a food that supports the health of skin and coat will provide all the nutrients needed to counteract stress.

EFFECTS OF MULTI-DOG HOUSEHOLDS

Individually housed dogs with limited exercise may have daily energy requirements (DER) as low as 90 to 95 kcal (375 to 400 kJ) metabolizable energy (ME)/$BW_{kg}^{0.75}$, or 1.3 x resting energy requirement (RER). When housed in kennels with other dogs in situations where much mutual interaction occurs, DER may increase to 130 to 140 kcal (545 to 585 kJ) ME/$BW_{kg}^{0.75}$, or 1.9 to 2.0 x RER or more.

In the U.S., more than a third of dog-owning families have more than one dog and many families own more than one species. Some dogs may increase their interest in food when a new pet is introduced to a household, whereas others may refuse to eat for a day or two. Jealousy may arise over food, bones or toys, or over space in the bed. Dogs may defend their food bowl and raise the hair on their crest, withers and back or growl. Free-choice feeding may have a quieting effect in kennels or multiple-dog households, and less dominant dogs may have a better chance to get their share of the food provided. In some cases, dogs need to be fed in separate places. However, those situations are often created by the owner's intervention in the pecking order.

The Bibliography for **Box 13-1** can be found at www.markmorris.org.

Table 13-2. Influence of age on daily energy requirements of active pet dogs.*

Age (years)	Typical DER ranges** kcal ME/$BW_{kg}^{0.75}$	kJ ME/$BW_{kg}^{0.75}$	x RER
1-2	120-140	500-585	1.7-2.0
3-7	100-130	420-550	1.4-1.9
>7	80-120	335-500	1.1-1.7

Key: DER = daily energy requirement, ME = metabolizable energy, RER = resting energy requirement, kcal = kilocalories, kJ = kilojoules.

*Most pet dogs are minimally active and have a DER of approximately 95 kcal/$BW_{kg}^{0.75}$ or 1.2 to 1.4 x RER.

**The energy requirements indicated in this table are only starting points and should be adapted for individual dogs.

dogs out for exercise fewer than three hours per week (Slater et al, 1995). Solitary dogs are less active than dogs housed as a group (Hubrecht et al, 1992). In one study, large dogs (Labrador retrievers) were active for half as many hours per day as small dogs (Manchester terriers) (Patil and Bisby, 2002). An association was also reported between increasing age and declining activity; older dogs spent less time running and more time walking (Head et al, 1997; Siwak et al, 2002).

ACTIVE AND SPORTING DOGS

Dogs and horses are often regarded as the elite athletes of domesticated mammals (Rose and Bloomberg, 1989). Greyhounds are sprint athletes and can reach average speeds of 56 to 60 km/hour (35 to 37.5 miles/hour) over typical race distances (Tompkins and Heasman, 1988). Sled dogs are endurance athletes and can maintain a trot of about 16 km/hour (10 miles/hour) for 10 to 14 hours per day for several consecutive days (Grandjean and Paragon, 1992). Energy requirements of dogs performing work between the two extremes (i.e., sedentary and sled dogs) need to be tailored to the individual. Chapter 18 describes how to feed active working and sporting dogs.

Age

Age-related changes occur between the onset of adulthood and five to seven years of age. The prevalence of dental disease, obesity, cancer, arthritis and kidney disease generally increases over this time span (Chapters 27, 30, 34, 37, 47). The cumulative effects of oxidative damage can result in beta-amyloid deposition in the brain as early as five to seven years of age, predisposing to cognitive dysfunction (Chapter 35). Furthermore, apart from reproduction and imposed activity during work or sport, age may be the single most important factor that influences the DER of most adult dogs (**Table 13-2**) (Finke, 1994).

Environment

The influence of the environment should not be neglected when evaluating energy and nutrient requirements. Temperature, humidity, type of housing, level of stress and the degree of acclimatization should be considered with respect to breed and lifestage nutrient requirements of dogs (**Box 13-1**). Animal factors including insulative characteristics of skin and coat (i.e., subcutaneous fat, hair length and coat density) and differences in stature, behavior and activity interact and affect DER.

Dogs can tolerate extreme cold. Adult dogs can maintain normal body temperature in ambient temperatures as low as -46 to -50°C (-51 to -58°F) for four to 27 hours and six out of seven dogs maintained normal body temperatures at -75 to -79°C (-103 to -110°F) for three to five hours (Hume and Egdahl, 1959). One study found that an ambient temperature of -160°C (-256°F) was necessary to make a dog hypothermic after one hour (Giaja, 1938). When kept outside in cold weather, dogs may need 10 to 90% more energy than during optimal weather conditions (Meyer, 1983; Durrer and Hannon, 1962). Heat losses are minimal at a temperature called the lower critical temperature (Blaxter, 1989a). This is the environmental temperature at which dogs reach their minimum metabolic rate. It is breed specific and is lower when the thermic insulation (i.e., coat density and length) is greater (Zentek and Meyer, 1992; Meyer, 1983, 1990; Männer, 1991; Kleiber, 1975). The lower critical temperature is estimated at 15 to 20°C (59 to 68°F) for longhaired breeds, 20 to 25°C (68 to 77°F) for shorthaired breeds and may be as low as 10 to 15°C (50 to 59°F) for arctic breeds (Männer, 1990, 1991; Kleiber, 1975; Meyer, 1990).

Energy use by dogs in cold environments is similar to energy use during endurance exercise (Minaire et al, 1973). In part, skeletal muscle is involved in shivering and non-shivering thermogenesis (NRC, 2006). As with endurance exercise, muscle glycogen stores may limit the ability to withstand cold (Minaire et al, 1973). Thus, high-fat foods are probably well suited for cold-acclimatized dogs in a cold environment. No published studies currently exist about the influence of changing the relative proportions of the nutrient composition of a food for improved resistance to cold in dogs. But for long-term exposure to cold, the amount of food fed should be increased to ensure increased energy availability.

Compared to cold ambient temperatures, a relatively smaller amount of energy is expended to dissipate heat at temperatures above the thermoneutral zone; however, increased amounts of water are required (**Box 13-2**). Adult dogs tolerated high ambient temperatures up to 56°C (133°F) for three hours or more in dry air (Adolph, 1947) but became poikilothermic at 33°C (91°F) or higher in moist air after one hour (Lozinsky, 1924). The metabolic rate increased by 10% in adult dogs when ambient temperatures were 35°C (95°F) (Minaire et al, 1973).

Housing conditions may influence energy and water requirements by modifying the immediate environment. Many housing options are possible; however, any shelter with temperatures closer to the thermoneutral zone will decrease energy requirements in cold environments and water requirements in hot environments (i.e., protection from wind chill, excess sun, etc.). Conversely, housing that moves dogs farther away from the thermoneutral zone will have the opposite effects (e.g., closed spaces in hot humid conditions, damp shady shelters in cold weather). The number of dogs in a shel-

Box 13-2. Nutrients Used for Body Cooling.

When ambient temperature exceeds a dog's thermoneutral zone, water and energy are used for heat loss. The ability of dogs (and people) to withstand extremely high ambient temperatures is well demonstrated by a study conducted in 1775 by Blagden. It was reported that Blagden, and a dog in a basket (to protect its feet from being burned), entered a room kept at a 126°C (259°F) and remained there for 45 minutes. A steak he took with him was cooked; however, he and the dog were unaffected.

Bodies cool by radiation, conduction, convection and vaporization of water. As the ambient temperature increases, the conditions for heat loss by radiation, conduction and convection become increasingly unfavorable. When the ambient temperature exceeds the dog's body temperature, the dog's entire metabolic heat production and the heat received from the environment by conduction, convection and radiation must be removed by evaporation of water to maintain normal body temperature.

Vaporization of water can occur via insensible perspiration, respiration, panting and sweating. Dogs have few sweat glands and thus must pant to evaporate additional water for cooling. Panting is facilitated by the elastic properties of the thorax and respiratory system. Depending on the size of the dog, the respiratory apparatus oscillates to a natural frequency (the resonant frequency of the chest is proportional to the square root of the body mass). The amount of cooling is regulated by the duration of panting. If not for resonant elasticity, the increased muscular effort of breathing would generate more heat than the total heat that could be dissipated by panting. As a result of these elastic properties, however, panting requires only a small amount of energy.

The amount of heat lost via vaporization of water is approximately 580 kcal (2,426 kJ)/kg water. In hot desert-like conditions, in which the heat gained from the environment can be 10 times the metabolic heat production, the water required for cooling a 15-kg dog may equal 2.5% of its body mass per hour. At this rate, if uncompensated for evaporative water loss, a dog could experience a 10% reduction of its total body water within 2.5 hours. Thus, from a nutritional perspective, dogs in hot environments may have a significant increase in water requirement with only a small increase in energy needs to maintain normal body temperature.

The Bibliography for **Box 13-2** can be found at www.markmorris.org.

ter may also affect the adequacy of the housing; increased numbers of dogs will increase the temperature in the local environment (Blaxter, 1989a; Kleiber, 1975).

Regarding environmental factors, and unrelated to the nutritional needs of dogs, pet food manufacturers develop products to address owner conveniences and concerns. This practice led to the development of specific pet food flavor varieties, kibble shapes, colors and sizes and packaging improvements. In the U.S., products have been introduced for pets that spend the majority of their lives indoors or in high population density urban settings. As an example, these products address the desire by pet owners for a very small stool volume, which makes cleanup easier. In addition, pets fed highly digestible, calorically dense foods eat less, resulting in less food carried home by the owner. Such trends, however, are not new to urban high population density countries such as Japan.

Laboratory and Other Clinical Information

Healthy young adult dogs require few laboratory and other diagnostic tests as part of routine assessment. The most common extended database includes a fecal examination for intestinal parasites, tests for heartworm infection and fundic examination. For dogs older than five years, a urinalysis performed on a fresh urine specimen collected after an all-night fast is added. A complete blood count, serum biochemistry profile and urinalysis should be obtained for ill dogs and those with suspected abnormal nutrition.

Key Nutritional Factors

Table 13-3 summarizes key nutritional factors for young adult dogs. The following section describes these key nutritional factors in more detail. Calcium is also a nutrient of concern for young adult dogs, especially when they are fed homemade foods (**Box 13-3**).

Table 13-3. Key nutritional factors for foods for young adult dogs.

Factors	Recommended food levels* Normal weight and body condition	Inactive/obese prone
Water	Free access	Free access
Energy density (kcal ME/g)	3.5-4.5	3.0-3.5
Energy density (kJ ME/g)	14.6-18.8	12.5-14.6
Fat and essential fatty acids (%)	10-20	7-10
Crude fiber (%)**	≤5	≥10
Protein (%)	15-30	15-30
Phosphorus (%)	0.4-0.8	0.4-0.8
Sodium (%)	0.2-0.4	0.2-0.4
Chloride (%)	1.5 x Na	1.5 x Na
Antioxidants (amount/kg food)		
Vitamin E (IU)	≥400	≥400
Vitamin C (mg)	≥100	≥100
Selenium (mg)	0.5-1.3	0.5-1.3
Food texture (VOHC Seal of Acceptance)	Plaque	Plaque

Key: DM = dry matter, kcal = kilocalories, kJ = kilojoules, ME = metabolizable energy, VOHC = Veterinary Oral Health Council Seal of Acceptance (Chapter 47).

*Dry matter basis. Concentrations presume an energy density of 4.0 kcal/g. Levels should be corrected for foods with higher energy densities.

**Crude fiber measurements underestimate total dietary fiber levels in food.

Box 13-3. Nutritional Factors of Concern for Homemade Foods Intended for Adult Dogs.

In addition to the key nutritional factors for commercial foods for adult dogs (See Key Nutritional Factors discussion.), calcium is also a nutritional factor of concern for homemade foods for adult dogs.

Commercial foods may contain inadequate, adequate and sometimes excessive amounts of calcium and/or phosphorus and; therefore, should not be supplemented. However, calcium is often deficient and phosphorus may be excessive in homemade foods, especially when most of the diet comes from meat and leftovers from the table (Table 12-5). Existing commercial multiple vitamin-mineral mixes (powders, tablets, etc.) are seldom designed to correct imbalances encountered in homemade foods. When formulating homemade foods, it is better to correct calcium-phosphorus imbalances by adding mineral sources such as calcium carbonate or dicalcium phosphate, both of which are usually available from drug stores (Chapter 10).

Water

Water accounts for approximately 56% of an adult dog's body weight (73% of lean body mass) (Stadtfeld, 1978). The body has a limited capacity to store water, and although healthy dogs can replenish a water deficit of up to 8% of body weight in a few minutes (Anderson, 1982), water deprivation will result in death more quickly than withholding any other nutrient (NRC, 1985). Therefore, it can be argued that water is the most important nutrient.

Total water intake (i.e., drinking and water from food) is influenced by several factors such as environment, physiologic state, activity, disease processes and food composition. Total water intake increases almost linearly with increasing salt levels in food (Anderson, 1982; Burger et al, 1980). Switching from a moist to a dry food and vice versa markedly affects the amount of water taken with the food; however, dogs compensate well for this difference by changing the quantity of water they drink, thus keeping their total daily water intake constant (Burger et al, 1980). Generally, dogs self-regulate water intake according to physiologic need. Healthy adult dogs need roughly the equivalent of their energy requirement in kcal metabolizable energy (ME)/day, expressed in ml/day (Lewis et al, 1987). Dogs should be offered free access to water at rest and before, during and after exercise (NRC, 2006). During warm weather, enough water should be available to compensate for evaporation by panting (Anderson, 1982) **Box 13-2**.

Energy

Domestic canids are the most diverse mammalian species in body weight and size. Therefore, energy requirements are not linearly correlated with kg body weight, but are more closely related to metabolic weight ($BW_{kg}^{0.75}$) (Meyer, 1986; NRC, 2006). DER recommendations of adult, non-athletic, non-reproducing dogs have varied from 85 kcal (355 kJ) ME/$BW_{kg}^{0.75}$ to more than 220 kcal (920 kJ) ME/$BW_{kg}^{0.75}$ (Zentek and Meyer, 1992; Männer et al, 1987; Heusner, 1991). This range may confuse dog owners, but it is not surprising considering that breed, neuter status, age, daily activity, environmental temperature and insulative characteristics of the integument markedly influence the DER of a particular dog (Rainbird and Kienzle, 1990; Kienzle and Rainbird, 1991; Männer, 1990, 1991; Meyer, 1983; NRC, 2006; Gesellschaft, 1989; Burger, 1994; Finke, 1991). Graphically, the DER for a population of dogs results in a bell-shaped curve; therefore, the energy intake of individual dogs may vary by about 50% above or below the average requirements, even within the same age group (Chapter 1). The RER, however, is not markedly influenced by these factors, and is similar for all dogs, independent of breed or age. RER is approximately 70 kcal (293 kJ)/$BW_{kg}^{0.75}$ (NRC, 2006; Kleiber, 1975) (Chapter 1). A simple linear formula can also be used to estimate RER for dogs weighing more than two kg: RER_{kcal} is approximately (30 x BW_{kg}) + 70 (Lewis et al, 1987). To convert from kcal to kJ, multiply kcal by 4.184. Table 5-2 provides RER values for dogs with body weights from 1.5 to 70 kg.

Because DER is the sum of RER plus all the above influences, it is better to use RER as the basis for calculating energy requirements of adult dogs and to assign different multipliers to account for differences in activity, age and environmental influences. When assigning multipliers to RER, it is important to account for neuter status because this variable can be an important factor in determining DER of household dogs. Neutered dogs may have a lower DER than intact counterparts. Surveys have shown that the prevalence of obesity increases progressively and peaks in middle-aged dogs (Armstrong and Lund, 1996; Kronfeld et al, 1991). Thus, prevention of obesity should be an important goal of feeding programs for young adult dogs. Animals benefit more from an appropriate weight-maintenance program than treatment for obesity (Chapter 27).

Three groups of adult dogs can be distinguished based on DER: 1) one to two years old, 2) three to seven years old and 3) more than seven years old (**Table 13-2**) (Rainbird and Kienzle, 1990; Kienzle and Rainbird, 1991; Finke, 1991, 1994). The differences in DER probably reflect an age-related decrease in activity and lean body mass.

Most pet dogs are minimally active and may have a DER that approaches their RER. Such dogs fed caloric intakes recommended for maintenance (1.6 x RER) will be overfed and are likely to become overweight. A recommendation of 1.2 to 1.4 x RER (85 to 98 kcal [355 to 410 kJ] ME/$BW_{kg}^{0.75}$/day) is a good starting point for feeding sedentary dogs (Männer, 1990, 1991; Männer et al, 1987; Heusner, 1991; NRC, 2006).

A good starting point for estimating the DER of more active adult dogs would be 1.6 x RER (115 kcal [480 kJ] ME/$BW_{kg}^{0.75}$). Such dogs between two and seven years of age would probably have a DER between 1.4 to 1.9 x RER (100 to 130 kcal [420 to 550 kJ] ME/$BW_{kg}^{0.75}$) with the higher number used in the lower age group and the lower number applied to the higher age group (**Table 13-2**). All initial estimates of energy needs must subsequently be evaluated by body condition assessment and adjusted as needed for individual dogs. It has been estimated that sled dogs may require more than 10,000 kcal/day (41.8 MJ/day) (up to 15 x RER) to maintain body weight under racing conditions (Hinchcliff et al, 1997). Active young adult dogs should be fed a food with an energy density range of 3.5 to 4.5 kcal/g dry matter (DM). The energy density range of foods for inactive/obese prone dogs should be lower (3.0 to 3.5 kcal/g DM).

Fat and Essential Fatty Acids

Fats are an excellent source of energy, but the real requirement for fat is to supply essential fatty acids (EFAs). In addition, fat serves as a carrier for the absorption of fat-soluble vitamins (i.e., A, D, E and K). Linoleic and α-linolenic acids are considered essential because dogs lack the enzymes to synthesize them (Watkins, 1997). Linoleic acid (18:22n-6) is the parent fatty acid of the omega-6 (n-6 series), as is α-linolenic acid for the omega-3 (n-3) series. EFAs have structural functions in cell membranes and are precursors of eicosanoids such as prostaglandins, thromboxanes and leukotrienes (NRC, 1985a; Lands, 1991). Linoleic acid deficiency results in two primary skin defects: hyperproliferation and increased permeability to water (Ziboh and Miller, 1990). The epidermal water barrier consists of lamellae of lipids (sphingolipids) in the stratum corneum of the epidermis. Linoleic acid is incorporated into the ceramide-portion of sphingolipids where it provides the specific characteristics needed for barrier function (Ziboh and Miller, 1990). Additionally, linoleic acid plays a role in fertility (Lands, 1991). Ensuring an adequate intake of EFAs is key to maintaining normal skin and coat quality.

Whether omega-3 fatty acids are essential is less certain because of the inability of omega-3 fatty acids to support all of the physiologic functions that are supported by omega-6 fatty acids (Lands, 1991). Nevertheless, a source of dietary omega-3 fatty acids is recommended (Watkins, 1997). The minimum recommended allowance for dietary eicosapentaenoic plus docosahexaenoic acids is 0.044% DM (NRC, 2006). Omega-3 fatty acids may moderate excessively vigorous actions of omega-6-derived eicosanoids (Lands, 1991) and are of value in the management of certain diseases (Chapters 30, 32, 34, 37). The minimum recommended allowance for dietary fat in foods for normal, healthy adult dogs is 8.5%, with at least 1% of the food as linoleic acid (DM) (NRC, 2006). Depending on the type/source of fat, increasing the amount of fat in foods increases palatability and EFA levels; however, energy content also increases. The recommended range of fat for foods intended for young adult dogs is 10 to 20% (DM). Lower levels of dietary fat are recommended for obese-prone adult dogs (7 to 10% DM).

Fiber

The levels of dietary fat and fiber are important determinants of a food's energy density. Fat provides more than twice as much energy on a weight basis than carbohydrate or protein. High-fat foods have increased energy density; conversely, low-fat foods have decreased energy density. Fiber is a poor source of energy for dogs; thus, as the fiber content of foods increases, energy density decreases. Dietary fiber reduces the energy density of the food and helps promote satiety (Chapters 5 and 27). Inclusion of fiber in foods may therefore help maintain ideal body weight in dogs fed free choice. In pet foods, fiber is listed as crude fiber, which is an imprecise measure because most soluble fiber is omitted. A better measure would be total dietary fiber; however, regulations only permit declaration of crude fiber because no method for determination of total dietary fiber is yet officially recognized for pet foods. It is difficult to determine the optimal concentration of crude fiber in a complete food for dogs; however, up to 5% DM seems adequate. Obese-prone dogs may benefit from at least 10% DM crude fiber and DM fat should be restricted to between 7 to 10%. Foods that are low in fat and high in fiber tend to have the lowest energy density and are recommended for obese-prone dogs.

Protein

The amount of protein in commercial foods for healthy dogs varies widely (15 to 60% DM). After the amino acid requirements are met for an individual animal, addition of more protein provides no known physiologic benefit. This fact often runs contrary to the popular belief that more protein is better. Also, the addition of extra protein in commercial dog foods is sometimes marketed as necessary for carnivores and misrepresents the fact that dogs are omnivores. Excess dietary protein, above the amino acid requirement, is not stored as protein, but rather is deaminated by the liver. Subsequently, the kidneys excrete the by-products of protein catabolism and the remaining keto acid analogues are used for energy or stored as fat, or as glycogen in some cases.

The subject of whether excess dietary protein contributes to the progression of subclinical kidney disease has yet to be resolved (Chapter 37). Studies in people suggest that protein restriction may help slow progression of kidney disease (Mitch et al, 1998; NKF, 1998). In addition to any potential aggravating effects excess dietary protein may have on subclinical kidney disease, foods high in protein also tend to contain high levels of phosphorus. As mentioned above, excess dietary phosphorus accelerates the progression of kidney disease in dogs. Minimum protein requirements for healthy adult dogs eating high-quality protein have been determined using nitrogen balance and endogenous nitrogen excretion. A more reliable estimate based on endogenous nitrogen excretion equates to a minimum requirement of 1.7 g metabolizable protein/$BW_{kg}^{0.75}$ for an ideal protein (NRC, 1985a; Kendall et al, 1982; Schaeffer et al, 1989). When protein of average quality is used (biologic value of about 70), the minimum requirements are increased to 2.1 to 2.5 g digestible protein/$BW_{kg}^{0.75}$ (Gesellschaft, 1989b).

The minimum crude protein content of food depends on digestibility and quality. For example, if the digestibility of an average quality protein is 75%, then about 12% DM crude protein is adequate. Foods containing less than 12% DM crude protein must be of higher biologic value. Biologic value becomes less important for healthy adult dogs if foods contain crude protein levels greater than 12%. A daily protein intake for adult maintenance of 4.3 to 5.0 g digestible protein/$BW_{kg}^{0.75}$ (biologic value = 70) or 4.0 to 6.5 g digestible protein/100 kcal ME is recommended (Gesellschaft, 1989b). The minimum recommended allowance for DM crude protein is 10% for a commercial food with an energy density of 4 kcal/g DM (NRC, 2006). Foods formulated to meet the lower limits in crude protein must also have the recommended allowances for essential amino acids. Thus, the recommended range of DM crude protein for foods for young adult dogs is between 15 to 30%.

Phosphorus

Minimum requirements for phosphorus for adult dogs are not very different from those established for other mammals. Commercial foods contain adequate and sometimes excessive amounts of phosphorus and, therefore, should not be supplemented.

Based on endogenous losses, a daily intake of 75 mg phosphorus/kg body weight is adequate (Gesellschaft, 1989a). At an energy density of 3.5 kcal (14.6 kJ)/g DM this corresponds to an average content of about 0.4 to 0.6% DM phosphorus. These levels are adequate, but not excessive; daily intakes 20 to 30% less are still sufficient (Gesellschaft, 1989a). Therefore, it is unnecessary to feed foods with higher levels of phosphorus, or to add calcium-phosphorus supplements to commercial foods. Moreover, higher phosphorus levels are contraindicated for a substantial part of the dog population; up to 25% of the young adult dog population may already be affected by subclinical kidney disease (Oehlert and Oehlert, 1976; Rouse and Lewis, 1975; Shirota et al, 1979). One clinical study revealed that 22.4% of all dogs over five years of age examined at a European veterinary teaching hospital for a variety of reasons had abnormally elevated kidney function tests (Leibetseder and Neufeld, 1991). Excess dietary phosphorus can accelerate progression of chronic renal disease (Brown et al, 1991), whereas phosphorus restriction may slow the progression of chronic renal disease and improve long-term survival (Brown et al, 1991; Finco et al, 1992). It is therefore prudent to feed foods that contain adequate but not excessive amounts of phosphorus (Chapter 37 contains more information about how excess dietary phosphorus affects progression of kidney disease).

The minimum recommended allowance for phosphorus in foods for adult dogs is 0.3% (DM); this recommendation is appropriate for foods with an energy density of 4 kcal/g (DM) (NRC, 2006). The recommended range of phosphorus for foods intended for young adult dogs is 0.4 to 0.8% (DM) when the energy density ranges from 3.5 to 4.5 kcal/g DM.

Sodium and Chloride

Essential hypertension is not considered a common problem in dogs; therefore, higher intakes of dietary sodium and chloride have not been considered harmful in young, healthy dogs (Bodey and Mitchell, 1996; Bovée, 1990). However, one study suggested that up to 10% of apparently healthy dogs may have high blood pressure (Remillard et al, 1991).

High sodium and chloride intake is contraindicated in dogs with certain diseases that may have a hypertensive component such as obesity, renal disease and some endocrinopathies (Anderson and Fisher, 1968; Cowgill and Kallet, 1986; Rocchini et al, 1987; Littman, 1990; Ross, 1992). Uncontrolled high blood pressure may lead to kidney, brain, eye, heart and cardiovascular damage (Cowgill and Kallet, 1986; Littman, 1990). Dietary sodium chloride restriction is the first step in, and an important part of, antihypertensive therapy (Cowgill and Kallet, 1986; Littman, 1990; Ross, 1992).

It is prudent to meet but not greatly exceed sodium and chloride requirements when selecting foods for adult dogs. The best estimate for a minimum requirement of sodium is about 4 mg/kg body weight/day (Morris et al, 1976). Generally, 25 to 50 mg/kg body weight/day (Gesellschaft, 1989a) is recommended for adult maintenance; these levels are six to 12 times more than the minimum. The minimum recommended allowance for sodium content of commercial foods is 0.08% (DM); this allowance is for foods with an energy density of 4 kcal/g (DM) (NRC, 2006). For risk factor management, the recommended range for dietary sodium is 0.2 to 0.4% (DM), which is more than adequate. Sodium levels in commercial foods for adult dogs range from 0.11 to 2.2% DM and are higher in moist foods than in dry foods. In the absence of studies establishing chloride requirements in dogs, a value 1.5 times the sodium requirement is recommended.

Antioxidants

The consequences of prolonged oxidative stress (i.e., free radical damage) to cell membranes, proteins and DNA may contribute to and/or exacerbate a wide variety of degenerative diseases. A partial list includes cancer, diabetes mellitus, kidney/urinary tract disease, heart disease, liver disease, inflammatory bowel disease and cognitive dysfunction (Ames et al, 1993; Kesavulu et al, 2000; Ha and Le, 2000; Thamilselvan et al, 2000; Freeman et al, 1999; Cheng et al, 1999; Center, 1999; Knight, 1999). The consequences of free radical damage to cells and tissues have also been associated with the effects of aging (Harman, 1956).

The body synthesizes many antioxidant enzyme systems and compounds but relies on food for others. Commonly supplemented food-source antioxidants include vitamins E and C, β-carotene and other carotenoids, selenium and thiols. Fruits and vegetables are good sources of flavonoids, polyphenols and anthocyanidins. The following discussion focuses on vitamins E and C and selenium as antioxidant key nutritional factors because: 1) they are biologically important, 2) they act synergistically (e.g., vitamin C regenerates vitamin E after it has reacted with a free radical), 3) they are safe and 4) information about inclusion levels in pet foods is usually available. For improved antioxidant performance, foods for mature dogs should contain at least 400 IU vitamin E/kg (DM) (Jewell et al, 2000), at least 100 mg vitamin C/kg (DM) and 0.5 to 1.3 mg selenium/kg (DM).

VITAMIN E

Vitamin E is the main lipid-soluble antioxidant present in

plasma, erythrocytes and tissues (NRC, 2006). It is transported in plasma proteins and partitions into membranes and fat storage sites where it is one of the most effective antioxidants for protecting polyunsaturated fatty acids from oxidation. It functions as a chain-breaking antioxidant that prevents propagation of free radical damage of biologic membranes. Vitamin E inhibits lipid peroxidation by scavenging lipid peroxyl radicals much faster than these radicals can react with adjacent fatty acids or with membrane proteins (Gutteridge and Halliwell, 1994). Vitamin E plays a dominant role in defending against oxidative damage in cells.

The requirement for vitamin E for foods (DM) for adult dogs is 30 mg/kg (NRC, 2006). Research indicates that a level of vitamin E much higher than the requirement confers specific biologic benefits. One antioxidant biomarker study in dogs indicated that for improved antioxidant performance, dog foods should contain at least 500 IU vitamin E/kg (DM) (Jewell et al, 2000). Besides helping to prevent chronic diseases associated with oxidative stress, increasing dietary intake of vitamin E up to 2,010 mg/kg food (DM) in older dogs improved immune function (Hayes et al, 1969; Hall et al, 2003; Meydani et al, 1998). Furthermore, increased vitamin E intake is also directly related to increased vitamin E content of skin in dogs (Jewell et al, 2002). The skin is uniquely challenged by oxidants due to its role as a barrier. It is exposed to air pollutants, ultraviolet radiation and oxidants released as a result of normal metabolism, parasites and aerobic microbes. An upper limit of 1,000 to 2,000 IU/kg food (DM) has been suggested for dogs (AAFCO, 2007; NRC, 1985). In one study that demonstrated improved immune function associated with ingestion of 2,010 IU vitamin E/kg food (DM) (Hall et al, 2003), dogs had no safety issues at this intake level for one year.[a] A prudent recommendation is that foods for young adult dogs should contain at least 400 IU vitamin E/kg (DM).

VITAMIN C

Vitamin C is the most powerful reducing agent available to cells. As such, it is important for regenerating oxidized vitamin E. Besides regenerating vitamin E, vitamin C: 1) regenerates glutathione and flavonoids, 2) quenches free radicals both intra- and extracellularly, 3) protects against free radical-mediated protein inactivation associated with oxidative bursts of neutrophils, 4) maintains transition metals in reduced form and 5) may quench free radical intermediates of carcinogen metabolism.

Dogs can synthesize required amounts of vitamin C (Innes, 1931; Naismith, 1958; Chatterjee et al, 1975) and they can rapidly absorb supplemental vitamin C (Wang et al, 2001). However, in vitro studies indicated that dogs (and cats) have from one-quarter to one-tenth the ability to synthesize vitamin C as other mammals (Chatterjee et al, 1975). Whether or not this translates to a reduced ability in vivo is unknown. In conjunction with the recommended levels of vitamin E, above, for improved antioxidant performance, foods for adult dogs should contain at least 100 mg of vitamin C/kg (DM).

Excessive supplementation of vitamin C should be avoided. In people, high levels of oral vitamin C increased urine oxalate excretion and stone risk (Massey et al, 2005). Vitamin C supplementation to cats resulted in a small, progressive reduction of urinary pH (Kienzel and Maiwald, 1998). However, moderate supplementation of foods for healthy adult cats with vitamin C (193 mg/kg of food, DM) did not increase the risk of oxalate production in urine (Yu and Gross, 2005).

SELENIUM

Glutathione peroxidase is a selenium-containing antioxidant enzyme that defends tissues against oxidative stress by catalyzing the reduction of H_2O_2 and organic hydroperoxides and by sparing vitamin E. The minimum requirements for selenium in foods for dogs and cats are 0.10 and 0.13 mg/kg (DM), respectively (Wedekind et al, 2002, 2003, 2003a). Animal studies and clinical intervention trials in people have shown selenium to be anticarcinogenic at levels much higher (five to 10 times) than human recommended allowances or minimal requirements (Combs, 2001; Neve, 2002). Several mechanisms have been proposed for this effect, including enhanced antioxidant activity via glutathione peroxidase (Neve, 2002). Therefore, for increased antioxidant benefits, the recommended range of selenium for adult dog foods is 0.5 to 1.3 mg/kg (DM). There are no data to base a safe upper limit of selenium for dogs, but for regulatory purposes, a maximum standard of 2.0 mg/kg (DM) has been set for dog foods in the U.S. (AAFCO, 2007).

Food Texture

Periodontal disease is the most common health problem of adult dogs (Harvey et al, 1994) and may predispose affected animals to systemic complications (DeBowes et al, 1996). Periodontal disease can be prevented in many dogs with routine veterinary care and frequent plaque control at home. Feeding recommendations for oral health commonly include feeding a dry pet food (Golden et al, 1982). However, typical dry dog foods contribute little dental cleansing and the general statement that dry foods provide significant oral cleansing should be regarded with skepticism. Research has demonstrated that maintenance dog foods with specific textural properties and processing techniques can significantly reduce plaque accumulation and maintain gingival health. If the labels of such foods carry the Veterinary Oral Health Council (VOHC) seal, they have been successfully tested according to specific protocols and shown to be clinically effective in reducing accumulation of plaque (Chapter 47).

FEEDING PLAN

Assess and Select the Food

After the nutritional status of the dog has been assessed and the key nutritional factors and their target levels determined, the adequacy of the food is assessed. The steps for assessing foods for normal adult dogs are to: 1) ensure that the nutritional adequacy of the food has been assured by a credible regulatory agency such as the Association of American Feed Control Officials (AAFCO) for foods sold in the U.S., 2) compare the

Table 13-4. Selected commercial foods for young to middle-aged adult dogs compared to recommended levels of key nutritional factors.*

Dry foods	**Energy density (kcal/cup)****	**Energy density (kcal ME/g)**	**Fat (%)**	**Fiber (%)**	**Protein (%)**	**P (%)**	**Na (%)**	**Vit E (IU/kg)**	**Vit C (mg/kg)**	**Se (mg/kg)**	**VOHC plaque (Yes/No)**
Recommended levels (normal body condition)	**-**	**3.5-4.5**	**10-20**	**≤5**	**15-30**	**0.4-0.8**	**0.2-0.4**	**≥400**	**≥100**	**0.5-1.3**	**-**
Hill's Science Diet Lamb Meal & Rice Recipe	364	4.0	16.0	2.5	23.0	0.67	0.29	582	174	0.54	No
Hill's Science Diet Oral Care Adult	273	3.8	15.5	10.1	25.1	0.65	0.24	564	175	0.62	Yes
Iams Adult Lamb Meal & Rice Formula	330	4.0	14.2	4.2	25.1	1.6	0.65	123	52	0.37	No
Iams Chunks	381	4.4	17.8	2.9	29.8	1.1	0.6	103	43	0.27	No
Iams Eukanuba Medium Breed Adult	404	4.7	17.9	2.1	27.8	1.16	0.55	na	na	na	No
Iams ProActive Health Chunks	374	4.0	17.0	1.9	28.9	1.21	0.58	na	na	na	No
Medi-Cal Dental Formula	290	na	12.7	5.3	19.7	0.9	0.4	na	na	na	No
Medi-Cal Preventive Formula	340	na	16.3	2.7	23.9	0.8	0.4	na	na	na	No
Nutro Natural Choice Dental Care Lamb Meal and Rice	287	3.7	15.4	4.4	23.6	1.54	0.22	275	71	1.65	No
Nutro Natural Choice Lamb Meal and Rice	342	3.8	14.3	2.2	24.2	1.54	0.33	220	66	0.77	No
Purina Dog Chow	430	4.2	11.4	5.1	23.9	0.91	0.42	144	na	0.64	No
Purina ONE Total Nutrition Lamb & Rice Formula	451	4.7	20.1	1.8	30.5	1.09	0.52	na	na	na	No
Purina Pro Plan Chicken & Rice Formula	489	4.8	16.9	3.4	33.8	1.22	0.46	na	na	na	No
Royal Canin MINI Adult 27	352	4.3	17.4	1.6	29.3	0.87	0.43	717	326	0.22	No
Royal Canin MINI Dental Hygiene 24	320	4.2	15.4	1.8	26.4	0.77	0.33	659	330	0.21	No
Waltham Pedigree Small Crunchy Bites	290	3.8	13.7	2.0	26.0	1.55	0.65	256	80	na	No
Moist foods	**Energy density (kcal/can)****	**Energy density (kcal ME/g)**	**Fat (%)**	**Fiber (%)**	**Protein (%)**	**P (%)**	**Na (%)**	**Vit E (IU/kg)**	**Vit C (mg/kg)**	**Se (mg/kg)**	**VOHC plaque (Yes/No)**
Recommended levels (normal body condition)	**-**	**3.5-4.5**	**10-20**	**≤5**	**15-30**	**0.4-0.8**	**0.2-0.4**	**≥400**	**≥100**	**0.5-1.3**	**-**
Hill's Science Diet Adult Advanced Savory Chicken Entrée	345/13 oz.	3.9	17.1	1.3	26.7	0.67	0.25	200	na	1.00	No
Medi-Cal Preventive Formula	435/396 g	na	20.1	3.3	23.8	0.7	0.3	na	na	na	No
Purina Pro Plan Adult Chicken & Rice Entrée Classic	426/13 oz.	4.9	36.6	0.9	40.4	1.36	0.47	na	na	na	No

food's key nutritional factor content with the recommended levels (**Tables 13-3** and **13-4**).

Whether or not commercial foods for healthy pets have been AAFCO approved can usually be determined from the nutritional adequacy statement on the product's label (Chapter 9). Although it is important to ensure nutritional adequacy, AAFCO approval does not ensure the food will be effective in preventing long-term health problems. Thus, in addition to having AAFCO approval, the food should be evaluated to ensure the key nutritional factors are at appropriate levels for delivering the feeding goal of promoting long-term health.

Table 13-4 compares the key nutritional factor recommendations for foods for young adult dogs to the key nutritional factor profiles of selected commercial foods sold in the U.S. and Canada. The manufacturer should be contacted if the food in question cannot be found in **Table 13-4.** Manufacturers' addresses, websites and toll-free phone numbers are listed on pet food labels.

Comparing a food's key nutritional factor content with the key nutritional factor target levels will help identify any significant discrepancies in the food being fed. This comparison is fundamental to determining whether or not to feed a different food. The current food should be changed if significant differences are seen between the recommended key nutritional factor levels and those in the food currently fed.

Commercial treats, snacks and table food should also be included in the food assessment step because they are part of the total food intake of an animal and, if misused, may create

Table 13-4 (cont.) Selected commercial foods for young to middle-aged adult dogs compared to recommended levels of key nutritional factors.*

Dry foods	Energy density (kcal/cup)**	Energy density (kcal ME/g)	Fat (%)	Fiber (%)	Protein (%)	P (%)	Na (%)	Vit E (IU/kg)	Vit C (mg/kg)	Se (mg/kg)	VOHC plaque (Yes/No)
Recommended levels (inactive/obese prone)	**-**	**3.0-3.5**	**7-10**	**≥10**	**15-30**	**0.4-0.8**	**0.2-0.4**	**≥400**	**≥100**	**0.5-1.3**	**-**
Hill's Science Diet Light Adult	295	3.3	8.8	14.6	24.5	0.58	0.23	586	276	0.45	No
Iams Eukanuba Medium Breed Weight Control	275	4.2	10.5	1.9	21.3	0.76	0.50	206	42	0.34	No
Iams Weight Control	328	4.2	12.5	2.8	22.2	0.85	0.37	103	44	0.35	No
Medi-Cal Weight Control/Mature	320	na	8.5	4.0	19.5	0.8	0.2	na	na	na	No
Nutro Natural Choice Lite	244	3.4	7.2	4.4	16.7	1.22	0.33	161	67	0.44	No
Purina Pro Plan Chicken & Rice Weight Management	337	3.7	10.2	2.7	30.5	1.06	0.27	503	na	0.33	No
Royal Canin MINI Weight Care 30	326	3.8	12.0	6.2	32.6	0.82	0.33	652	326	0.16	No
Moist foods	**Energy density (kcal/can)****	**Energy density (kcal ME/g)**	**Fat (%)**	**Fiber (%)**	**Protein (%)**	**P (%)**	**Na (%)**	**Vit E (IU/kg)**	**Vit C (mg/kg)**	**Se (mg/kg)**	**VOHC plaque (Yes/No)**
Recommended levels (inactive/obese prone)	**-**	**3.0-3.5**	**7-10**	**≥10**	**15-30**	**0.4-0.8**	**0.2-0.4**	**≥400**	**≥100**	**0.5-1.3**	**-**
Hill's Science Diet Light Adult	322 kcal/13 oz.	3.4	8.6	9.7	19.5	0.51	0.31	385	na	0.78	No
Medi-Cal Weight Control/Mature	370 kcal/396 g	na	10	5.5	21.5	0.6	0.3	na	na	na	No

Key: ME = metabolizable energy, Fiber = crude fiber, P = phosphorus, Na = sodium, Se = selenium, VOHC = Veterinary Oral Health Council, na = information not available from manufacturer, g = grams.
*From manufacturers' published information or calculated from manufacturers' published as-fed values; all values are on a dry matter basis unless otherwise stated.
**Energy density values are listed on an as fed basis and are useful for determining the amount to feed; cup = 8-oz. measuring cup. To convert to kJ, multiply kcal by 4.184.

an imbalance in an otherwise balanced feeding plan. Excessive feeding of treats and snacks may markedly affect the cumulative nutritional profile (**Box 13-4**). The impact of snacks on daily nutrient intake depends on two factors: 1) the nutrient profile of the snack and 2) the number provided daily. Thus, if snacks are fed, it is prudent to recommend those that best match the nutritional profile recommended for a particular lifestage. However, meeting nutrient requirements is not the primary goal of feeding treats; consequently, many commercial treats are not complete and balanced. A few treats are complete and balanced and are approved by AAFCO, or some other credible regulatory agency. Similarly, most table foods are not nutritionally complete and balanced and may contain high levels of fat or minerals. If snacks are fed, it is simplest to recommend that they be commercial treats that, if possible, match the nutritional profile recommended for a particular lifestage (see product label). Generally, any snacks should not be fed excessively (<10% of the total diet on a volume, weight or calorie basis). Otherwise, the nutritional composition of the snack and food should be combined and assessed as the entire diet.

Assess and Determine the Feeding Method

The feeding method includes the amount fed and how it is fed (free choice vs. some type of restricted feeding). It may not always be necessary to change the feeding method when managing healthy adult dogs in optimal body condition. However, a thorough evaluation includes verification that an appropriate feeding method is being used. In addition, current or future risk factors such as obesity should be considered when evaluating the current method. Current feeding methods should have been obtained when the history was taken.

Nutrient requirements of dogs and intake of appropriate levels of key nutritional factors are met, not only by the amount of nutrients in the food, but also by how much food is fed. If the dog in question has an ideal BCS (2.5/5 to 3.5/5), the amount being fed is probably appropriate. The amount fed can be estimated either by calculation (Chapter 1) or by referring to feeding guides on product labels. Such calculated amounts and feeding guides represent population averages and, likely, may need to be adjusted for individual dogs. If possible, owners should check the dog's body weight and/or be taught to regularly evaluate their dog's BCS. If these measurements indicate a trend of increasing or decreasing body weight or BCS, pet owners should be counseled to change the amount fed by 10% increments.

Besides establishing how much food is being fed, another part of feeding method assessment is to determine how the food is offered (i.e., when, where, by whom and how often). An

Box 13-4. Impact of Treats on Daily Nutrient Intake.

From 60 to 86% of owners regularly give their dogs commercial treats. If table foods are considered, 90% or more of dogs receive treats, snacks and biscuits as a supplement to their regular food. People like to give treats and snacks for emotional reasons, to change their pet's behavior or to improve and maintain oral health. Because several daily treats will have a marked effect on a dog's cumulative nutritional intake, specific questions about treats should be asked when taking the dietary history. Specific recommendations about treats should be provided when prescribing a food regimen for diseased or healthy dogs. This information is critical when managing specific problems such as developmental orthopedic disease in growing large- and giant-breed dogs, adverse reactions to food, obesity, urolithiasis, diabetes mellitus, heart failure and renal disease.

The impact of snacks on a dog's daily nutrient intake depends on two factors: 1) the nutrient profile of the treat and 2) the number of treats provided daily. It is best to recommend a treat that matches the nutritional profile preferred for a given lifestage or disease. Snacks provide energy; a handful of dog snacks, for example, can easily be equivalent to 40% of a small dog's daily energy requirement (DER) or 10% of a large-breed dog's DER. Therefore, the owner must compensate for the additional energy by feeding less of the dog's usual food. This recommendation is especially important for dogs in which a small snack can have a marked impact (i.e., toy- and small-breed dogs). The following two examples illustrate the impact of treats on daily nutrient intake.

A six-year-old, neutered male miniature pinscher weighing 4.5 kg is fed two commercial biscuit treats per day, in addition to its regular food. Each biscuit provides 15 kcal (62.8 kJ), so the dog receives a total of 30 kcal (125.5 kJ) per day from the treats. The dog's DER is about 330 kcal (1,381 kJ). Therefore, the treats provide almost 10% of the dog's DER. If the dog's DER is being met with the regular food, then the treats may contribute to long-term excess energy intake and obesity.

A five-month-old, 20-kg, female German shepherd dog is given a commercial treat marketed as a snack with "real marrow bone." Calcium is not declared on the guaranteed or typical analysis of the treat label. The owner gives the dog 10 treats daily as part of a training program. This number of treats is within the feeding guidelines on the label. However, analysis shows that each treat contains 426 mg of calcium. Consuming 10 treats daily increases the dog's daily calcium intake by more than 80% compared with feeding a commercial food formulated for large-breed puppies. This feeding practice increases the risk of developmental orthopedic disease (Chapter 33). To facilitate learning, dogs do not need to receive edible reinforcement every time and the pieces can be very small. If praise is paired with treats, praise alone will rapidly become sufficient reinforcement for the desired behavior.

The Bibliography for **Box 13-4** can be found at www.markmorris.org.

Table 13-5. Advantages and disadvantages of various feeding methods for dogs.

Method	Advantages	Disadvantages
Free-choice feeding	Less labor intensive Less knowledge required Quieting effect in a kennel Less dominant dogs have a better chance to get their share	Less control over food intake Predisposes to obesity Less monitoring of individual changes in food intake
Meal-restricted feeding	Better control of food dose Early detection of altered appetite Better control of body weight	Intermediate labor intensive Most knowledge required for food dose calculation
Time-restricted feeding	Intermediate control of food dose Some monitoring of appetite possible	Inaccurate control of food intake Risk of obesity similar to free choice Most labor intensive

important determinant of food intake in domestic dogs is the owner's and other family members' involvement because these factors usually control the amounts and types of food fed (Rabot, 1993; Mugford and Thorne, 1980; Houpt and Smith, 1981; Houpt, 1991). Studies show that owners typically feed their dogs one (26 to 77% of owners) to two (19 to 50% of owners) meals per day (Slater et al, 1995; Mugford and Thorne, 1980; Campbell, 1986). Often, pet owners overestimate needs and feed too much (Rabot, 1993). Furthermore, despite widespread concern about obesity among pet owners, most people do not recognize overweight/obesity in their own dog (Singh et al, 2002). Pet dogs may eat several small meals daily when fed a commercial dry food free choice and still maintain an ideal body weight (Mugford and Thorne, 1980). However, relatively inactive dogs fed a highly palatable, energy-dense food free choice are at increased risk for obesity (Houpt, 1991). Most pet dogs are relatively inactive (NRC, 2006).

Both free choice and restricted feeding methods (time restricted or food restricted) have advantages and disadvantages. Although free-choice feeding is most popular, it can lead to the most problems. As an alternative, meal-restricted feeding is simple and more precise in delivering the required

Box 13-5. Alternative Eating Behaviors.

RESPONSE TO FOOD VARIETY

Dogs may display preferences for specific types of foods according to taste and texture. However, the notion that dogs require a variety of flavors or taste in their meals is incorrect and may be detrimental in some instances. Dogs prefer novel foods or flavors to familiar foods; therefore, feeding a variety of novel foods free choice may lead to overeating and obesity. Dogs may correct for excessive energy intake by decreasing or refusing food intake the next day(s). Reduction of food intake to maintain weight following engorgement may erroneously be interpreted as a dislike of the current food instead of an auto-regulatory mechanism to achieve the previous set-point weight.

GARBAGE EATING

Garbage eating is probably normal behavior. Many dogs prefer food in an advanced stage of decomposition. However, garbage eating is oftentimes unhealthy. Ingestion of garbage may cause brief, mild gastroenteritis or more serious intoxication (Chapter 11). Because the etiology is complex and may involve bacterial toxins, mycotoxins and by-products from putrefaction or decomposition, the clinical signs vary widely from vomiting, diarrhea, abdominal pain, weakness, incoordination and dyspnea, to shock, coma and death. Scavenging dogs may eat less of their regular meal; therefore, garbage eating may be mistaken for anorexia at home.

Spraying garbage bags with a dog repellent usually will not stop the problem. Preventing access to garbage is the obvious best solution.

GRASS EATING

Owners often ask why dogs eat grass. Plant and grass eating is normal behavior. Herbivores are the natural prey for wolves and most other canids. The viscera of prey are often eaten first and contain partially digested vegetable material. Because dogs' ancestors and close relatives in the wild regularly ingest plant material, some investigators have suggested that domestic dogs must also eat grass. Probably the better explanation is that, to date, no one knows for sure why dogs eat plants or grass, but they may simply like the way plants taste or prefer the texture. Plant chlorophyll can bind mycotoxins, such as those found in moldy grains, decreasing their absorption.

BEGGING FOR FOOD

Begging for food may be fun when dogs sit up or perform other tricks; however, the behavior can become annoying when whining, barking, persistent nudging and scratching take over. Begging for food was one of the most common complaints addressed in a study involving more than 1,400 owners and was perceived as a problem in one-third of the dogs. Additionally, begging may encourage owners to feed more of the dog's regular food. Begging tends to increase with age and may indicate that most owners don't realize that they reinforce begging by continuing to offer tidbits to their begging pet. Treats reinforce begging. Also, the fact that begging for food is directly proportional to the number of people in the family may be related to an increase in the number of tidbits fed.

Treatment consists of ignoring behaviors such as begging, barking and whining. Owners should be prepared for a prolonged period of such behaviors before begging subsides completely. Intermittent reinforcement of begging when these behaviors become problematic can be more powerful than continuous rewarding, even though the owner may have refused to provide snacks in the interim. It may also help to keep the dog out of the kitchen and dining areas when preparing and eating food and to feed the dog before or after the family has eaten.

PICA

Pica is defined as perverted appetite with craving for and ingestion of non-food items. The etiology of true pica is unknown. Suggested causes include mineral deficiencies, permanent anxiety and psychological disturbances. A few cases of pica have been noted in relation to zinc intoxication and hepatic encephalopathy. Pica is common in dogs with exocrine pancreatic insufficiency, probably as a manifestation of polyphagia, and perhaps as a consequence of some specific nutritional deficiency. Sometimes, coprophagy and garbage eating are mistakenly considered forms of pica.

Pica can be treated with aversion therapy by offering a counter attraction at the moment the dog begins to eat foreign material and by punishment if there is no response. Outdoors, the dog should be kept on a leash or even muzzled. Most treatments for pica are unrewarding. Physically preventing the animal from engaging in pica is sometimes the only solution.

COPROPHAGY

Coprophagy is defined as eating feces and may involve consumption of the animal's own stools or the feces of other animals. Coprophagy is probably widespread among pet dogs and is probably more disturbing to owners than it is harmful to dogs. Bitches normally eat the feces of their puppies during the first three weeks of lactation. Feral dogs and dogs in rural areas have access to and consume large-animal feces, which is considered normal behavior. In many cases, however, coprophagy is a behavioral problem and the etiology is unknown. Coprophagy can also be related to certain diseases.

Table 1 lists behavioral and metabolic disorders that may be associated with coprophagy. The risk of transmitting parasitic diseases is probably the most important health reason for managing coprophagy; however, the associated halitosis is of primary concern to owners. The dog's motivation must be reduced to correct coprophagy. Several measures have been proposed.

Punishment may deter the dog's behavior, but may violate the confidence between owner and pet. Punishment may also aggravate the coprophagic behavior. Thus, a good balance has to be found. Walking the dog on a leash and keeping it away from feces after the dog defecates is helpful.

Box 13-5 continued

Repulsive substances can be used to create aversion for feces. Many different products have been recommended including spices (e.g., pepper, sambal, hot pepper sauce), quinine, strong perfumes and specific products such as cythioate, meat tenderizers and For-Bid.[a] Adding repulsive substances to feces can be time-consuming and has questionable efficacy.

Food changes to deter coprophagy have been recommended; however, most of these recommendations lack substantiation. Using foods with increased fiber levels has been reported to help. Free-choice feeding has also been recommended, whereas a strict schedule of two meals per day and avoiding all tidbits or table foods has worked for others.

ENDNOTE

a. Alpar Laboratories Inc., La Grange, IL, USA.

The Bibliography for **Box 13-5** can be found at www.markmorris.org.

Table 1. Factors associated with coprophagy.

Behavior
Confinement in a kennel leading to stress or competitive behavior
Confinement leading to boredom with all exploratory effort focused on feces
Reaction to punishment during housetraining
Strong dominance or extreme submissive attitude towards the owner
To attract the owner's attention
Young animals with a natural interest in feces

Gastrointestinal disorders
Malassimilation
Parasitic infections
Polyphagia due to diabetes mellitus or Cushing's syndrome

Food
Overfeeding
Poorly digestible food

Table 13-6. Feeding plan summary for young adult dogs.

1. Select a food or foods with the best levels of key nutritional factors (**Table 13-4**); for foods not in **Table 13-4**, contact the manufacturer for key nutritional factor content.
2. The selected food should also be approved or meet requirements established by a credible regulatory agency (e.g., AAFCO).
3. Determine the preferred feeding method (**Table 13-5**); when the correct amount of food is fed, meal-restricted feeding is least likely to result in obesity.
4. For food-restricted meal feeding, estimate the initial quantity of food based on DER calculation (DER ÷ food energy density).
5. Body condition and other assessment criteria will determine the DER. DER is calculated by multiplying RER by an appropriate factor (Table 5-2). Remember, DER calculations should be used as guidelines, starting points and estimates for individual dogs and not as absolute requirements.
   - Neutered adult = 1.6 x RER
   - Intact adult = 1.8 x RER
   - Inactive/obese-prone adult = 1.2 to 1.4 x RER (Most pet dogs are relatively inactive)
   - Working adult = 2.0 to 8.0 x RER (Chapter 18)
6. Monitor body weight, body condition and general health. These parameters are used to refine the amount to feed.

Key: AAFCO = Association of American Feed Control Officials, DER = daily energy requirement, RER = resting energy requirement.

amount of food. Time-restricted feeding is less effective for controlling the amount of food consumed and is more labor intensive. **Table 13-5** provides a brief review of these feeding methods. See Chapter 1 for a more in-depth discussion of feeding methods.

If a food change is in order and/or the amount fed needs to be modified, knowledge of the presence of other pets in the home, which family member is responsible for selecting and purchasing the dog's food and who feeds the dog regularly are helpful for evaluating the feasibility of new dietary recommendations and improving compliance. Most healthy adult dogs adapt well to new foods. However, it is good practice to allow for a transition period to avoid digestive upsets. This is particularly true when switching from lower fat foods to higher fat foods or when changing forms of food (e.g., changing from dry to moist food). The new food should be increased and old food decreased in progressive amounts over a three- to seven-day period until the changeover is completed (Nott et al, 1993) (Chapter 1).

Dogs may eat an insufficient amount or completely refuse new food, especially if the new food is lower in palatability as may be required for health concerns (e.g., lower fat content). Investigation of food refusal may reveal problems with owner compliance rather than a finicky appetite. The following guidelines may be useful when a food change must be made: 1) Explain clearly to the owners why a change in food is necessary or preferable. 2) Justify your recommendation to the owners (i.e., food profile vs. specific needs of the dog). 3) As a general rule, start with one or two meals per day, always presented at the same time. Uneaten food should be removed after 15 to 20 minutes. 4) Don't give treats or table foods between meals for the first few days. If a small snack is given, it should be given immediately (i.e., within seconds) after the new food is eaten. Most dogs will accept the new food within a few days. **Table 13-6** summarizes the feeding plan recommendations discussed above.

Finally, owners are often concerned about alternative eating behaviors displayed by their dogs. In fact, these behaviors may be more offensive to the owner than detrimental to the dog. Alternative eating behaviors may be of nutritional or non-nutritional origin, and some may indicate underlying disease (**Box 13-5**).

REASSESSMENT

Owners should be encouraged to weigh their dog every month, and should be trained to observe their dog and adapt the food intake according to its needs. Dogs whose nutrition is well managed are usually alert, have an ideal BCS (2.5/5 to 3.5/5) with a stable, normal body weight and a healthy coat. Stools should be firm, well formed and medium to dark brown.

Reassessment by a veterinarian should take place regularly. Healthy dogs should be reassessed every six to 12 months. Because few if any homemade recipes have been tested according to prescribed feeding protocols, dogs should be reassessed more frequently if homemade food is a significant part of their caloric intake. Reassessment should take place immediately if clinical signs arise indicating that the current feeding regimen is inappropriate, or if the dog's needs change (e.g., reproduction or change in activity).

If expected results are not obtained, the owner should also be questioned in detail about compliance with the feeding regimen or the possibility that the dog has access to other food sources.

ENDNOTE

a. Jewell DE. Hill's Science and Technology Center, Topeka, KS. Personal communication (data on file). March 30, 2007.

REFERENCES

The references for **Chapter 13** can be found at www.markmorris.org.

CASE 13-1

Feeding a Young Basset Hound after an Ovariohysterectomy

Philip Roudebush, DVM, Dipl. ACVIM (Internal Medicine)
Hill's Scientific Affairs
Topeka, Kansas, USA

Patient Assessment

A 12-month-old female basset hound was admitted for an ovariohysterectomy. The owners had observed no problems since purchasing the dog from a pet store eight months before. Physical examination revealed a normal 20-kg dog (body condition score [BCS] 3/5) except for excessive accumulation of waxy debris in both ears. Results of preanesthetic blood work were normal. The ovariohysterectomy was performed with no complications. The owners returned to pick up the dog the next day.

Assess the Food and Feeding Method

The dog was fed a commercial specialty brand growth formula (Science Diet Lamb Meal & Rice Formula Canine Growth[a]) that the owners purchased from the pet store where they obtained the dog. The owners had been following the feeding directions on the pet food label. They were currently feeding one can of the growth formula in the morning (520 kcal, 2.18 MJ) and two cups (200 g) of the dry formulation of the same brand in the evening (780 kcal, 3.26 MJ). The dog's appetite had been good. The owners also gave the dog two commercial treats each day (Science Diet Canine Growth Treats[a]) (19 kcal [79 kJ] per treat).

Questions

1. What are the key nutritional factors to consider in developing a feeding plan for this young neutered adult dog?
2. What response should be given when the owners ask whether the ovariohysterectomy will change the feeding recommendations for their dog?
3. Outline a specific feeding plan for this patient including an appropriate food and feeding method.

Answers and Discussion

1. Key nutritional factors for young adult dogs include water, energy, phosphorus, calcium, protein, sodium, chloride, fat and essential fatty acids, antioxidants and food texture. In general, water requirements are met by allowing free access to a source of potable water. Energy, fat and fiber are important because prevention of obesity is an important goal of feeding adult dogs. Phosphorus, calcium, sodium and chloride requirements should be met but not greatly exceeded. Essential fatty acids are important for maintenance of normal skin and coat, a primary concern of many dog owners. Food texture is important in controlling periodontal disease, the most common health problem of adult dogs. Antioxidants may help prevent certain diseases.
2. Gonadectomy increases the risk of obesity in dogs. Neutered female dogs are about twice as likely to be overweight as intact female dogs. A similar trend occurs in castrated male dogs. Gonadectomy predisposes dogs to weight gain and eventual obesity

for several reasons. Daily energy requirement (DER) may decrease because of metabolic changes associated with gonadectomy. Furthermore, studies have demonstrated that neutered female dogs eat more food and gain more weight than sham-operated females fed identical food. Thus, removal of the metabolic effects of estrogens and androgens by gonadectomy may lead to increased food consumption when the animal's energy requirement is simultaneously lower due to decreased metabolic rate and physical activity. These are important considerations when creating a feeding plan for young neutered adult dogs.

3. Basset hounds are predisposed to obesity. Gonadectomy and the breed predisposition to obesity make obesity prevention a primary goal in developing a feeding plan for this patient. This dog has also reached adulthood; therefore, the levels of nutrients found in growth-type formulas are unnecessary.

   The food should be changed from a growth formula to an adult maintenance formula. In general, adult maintenance formulas of the same brand contain less energy, fat, phosphorus, calcium, sodium and chloride than growth formulas. These lower levels of nutrients exceed the minimum nutrient requirements of adult dogs while avoiding the higher nutrient levels found in growth or all-purpose type formulas. This dog's optimal BCS suggests that it is eating an appropriate amount of food. However, gonadectomy and other metabolic changes associated with maturity will probably decrease the DER. The estimated DER would be 1.4 to 1.6 x resting energy requirement (RER) (940 to 1,070 kcal, 3.93 to 4.48 MJ). The dog is currently consuming 1,300 kcal (5.44 MJ) or 2 x RER. The feeding method will be dictated somewhat by whether moist, dry, semi-moist or homemade foods are fed. The owners are currently meal feeding a combination of moist and dry foods; this feeding method can be continued with the new food.

Progress Notes

The dog was discharged to the owners' care with instructions to limit exercise for several days, examine the suture line daily for signs of swelling or inflammation and return for suture removal in 10 to 14 days. The owners were shown how to clean the ears and an otic cleaning solution was dispensed.

The owners were interested in continuing to feed a combination of moist and dry food. They were instructed to purchase the same brand adult maintenance food (Science Diet Lamb Meal & Rice Formula Canine Maintenance[a]) and gradually mix the new food with the old food until the moist and dry growth formulas were completely gone. A combination of the adult maintenance food consisting of one large (418 g) can of moist food in the morning (420 kcal, 1.76 MJ) and 1 2/3 cups (165 g) of dry food in the evening (610 kcal, 2.59 MJ) would provide approximately 1.6 x RER for the dog's current weight of 20 kg. Two treats per day were also continued; however, the owners were encouraged to use the adult maintenance formula of the same treat (18 kcal [75 kJ] per treat).

Prevention of obesity was emphasized to the owners because of the risk factors discussed earlier. They were given an instruction sheet that outlined how to score the dog's body condition and encouraged to weigh the dog monthly. They were instructed to call the practice if the dog appeared to be gaining weight or if the dog's BCS increased. Periodontal disease, veterinary oral care and routine home oral care were also discussed.

Endnote

a. Hill's Pet Nutrition, Inc., Topeka, KS, USA. Science Diet Lamb Meal & Rice Formula Canine Growth and Science Diet Lamb Meal & Rice Formula Canine Maintenance are currently marketed as Science Diet Lamb Meal & Rice Recipe Puppy and Science Diet Lamb Meal & Rice Recipe Adult.

Bibliography

Anantharaman-Barr G. The effect of ovariohysterectomy on energy metabolism in dogs (research abstract). Friskies Veterinary International 1990; 2: 19-20.

Feeding Mature Adult Dogs: Middle Aged and Older

Jacques Debraekeleer
Kathy L. Gross
Steven C. Zicker

"Old dogs, like old shoes, are comfortable. They might be a bit out of shape and a little worn around the edges, but they fit well."
Bonnie Wilcox 'Old Dogs, Old Friends'

INTRODUCTION

For a number of reasons, the mature segment (six to eight years of age and older) of the pet dog population is growing. More than 35% of dogs in the U.S. are at least seven years old and, in Europe, the number of dogs older than seven years increased by about 50% from 1983 to 1995 (Lund et al, 1999; Kraft, 1998). In this chapter, mature dogs include dogs that are middle aged and older. In people, middle age is often considered as being approximately the third quarter of the average lifespan.

Aging increases vulnerability (Mosier, 1989; Hayflick, 1994). Aging isn't a disease; however, morbidity increases with age because normal changes make animals more vulnerable to diseases (Hayflick, 1994). The influence of nutrition on vulnerability to chronic or acute disease is difficult to evaluate, and has not been explored thoroughly in dogs. In people and companion animals, nutrition may be one of the more important aspects of geriatric care because delay or elimination of the two or three leading causes of death would profoundly affect life expectancy (Hayflick, 1994a). In dogs, the three leading non-accidental causes of death are cancer, kidney disease and heart disease (Bronson, 1982; MacDougall and Barker, 1984; MAF, 1991, 1998). Other diseases and disorders are also common (Table 13-1). Moreover, older animals seldom suffer from a single disease and one problem may markedly influence the course of another (Mosier, 1990).

The overall feeding goals for mature adult dogs are to optimize quality and longevity of life and minimize disease. To understand the specific nutritional needs of mature dogs, it is necessary to know the major effects of aging on canine body systems (**Box 14-1**). Aging is characterized by progressive and, usually, irreversible change (Mosier, 1988), and its rate and manifestations are determined by intrinsic and extrinsic factors, one of which is nutrition. Because aging is progressive, the point in time at which a food change should be made is arbitrary, and in a way philosophical. Dogs often are considered mature or likely to start having diseases associated with aging between seven and one-half and 13.5 years (Goldston, 1989). Smaller dogs tend to live longer than large dogs (**Table 14-1**). The life expectancy of smaller dogs may be more than 20 years. Because dogs are often considered older when they reach half of their life expectancy (Grandjean and Paragon, 1990), a food change should be considered around the age of five years for large- and giant-breed dogs and around seven years for small dogs (Markham and Hodgkins, 1989).

At these ages, dogs may gradually start to gain weight and develop age-related physical and behavioral changes (Armstrong and Lund, 1996; Markham and Hodgkins, 1989; Landsberg and Ruhl, 1997). Clinical signs of cognitive dysfunction and brain pathology associated with aging begin at about seven to eight years of age (Head et al, 2000).[a]

However, veterinarians should not accept the tenant that poor health and old age are synonymous (Goldston, 1989). There is a real opportunity to improve the quality and possibly

Box 14-1. The Mature Dog.

Aging is the progressive change that occurs after maturity in various organs and leads to decreased ability of an organism to meet environmental demands. This definition underscores two primary aspects of aging. First, aging occurs "after maturity." Although nutrition in young animals will have an affect on longevity and health, changes occurring during growth should not be considered aging. Second, aging results in a "decreased ability to meet the demands of the environment." Although young organisms adapt easily to fluctuations in nutrient intake and quality, mature animals may no longer be able to cope with excesses, borderline deficiencies or changes in nutrient intake and quality. Therefore, foods for mature dogs should meet allowances more rigorously and consistently because of lack of reserve capacity to handle large excesses and deficiencies.

An important feature of aging is that, compared with a group of younger adults, the mature dog population has a "large variation in health status" between individuals. In addition, diseases may be subclinical and not apparent by results of a physical examination; more in depth assessments are necessary, including diagnostic evaluations. Mature animals, therefore, must be evaluated individually rather than as a group and their nutritional needs determined accordingly.

The Bibliography for **Box 14-1** can be found at www.markmorris.org.

Table 14-1. Percent survival rates of mature dogs.*

Age	10 years	15 years
Small-breed dogs	38%	7.0%
Large-breed dogs	13%	0.1%

*Adapted from Deeb BJ, Wolf NS. Studying longevity and morbidity in giant and small breed dogs. Veterinary Medicine 1994; 89 (Suppl.7): 702-713.

the length of life of mature dogs through nutritional management. An important example is cognitive dysfunction (Chapter 35). Nutritional intervention in combination with mental stimulation can halt and even reverse its progression.

There is considerable interest in the potential benefits of pet nutrition on the part of pet owners. In one survey, 51% of respondents indicated that they were interested in learning about clinical signs and treatments for older pets and 47% were interested in pet nutrition (MAF, 2005).

PATIENT ASSESSMENT

History and Physical Examination

A thorough history should be taken and a physical examination performed to identify potential areas of nutritional concern. All of the considerations discussed for young adult dogs in Chapter 13 (i.e., breed, gender and health status) should be considered when developing key nutritional factors for mature dogs. Special attention should be directed to physiologic changes associated with aging and diseases that are more prevalent in mature animals such as renal disease, cancer, degenerative joint disease, cardiac disease, endocrine disorders, periodontal disease, cognitive dysfunction and obesity (Harvey et al, 1994; Alexander and Wood, 1984; Hoskins, 1995; Goldston, 1995; Landsberg and Ruhl, 1997). Many diseases may be subclinical, emphasizing the importance of a thorough evaluation.

This chapter builds on many of the recommendations in Chapter 13 for feeding young adult dogs. The minimum nutrient requirements of mature dogs are similar to those of young adult dogs. The few studies evaluating the effect of aging on the nutritional needs of dogs have shown minimal changes in nutrient requirements. Therefore, nutritional recommendations for mature dogs are based on risk factor management, extension of learning from other species and prudence. For several of the key nutritional factors for mature dogs, this results in reducing the recommended upper range of some nutrients, compared to that for young adult dogs. The only nutritional modification known to slow aging and increase the lifespan consistently in multiple species is caloric restriction. Reducing caloric intake by 20 to 30% of normal, while meeting essential nutrient needs, slows the aging process and reduces the risk for cancer, renal disease, arthritis and immune-mediated diseases in several animal models (Sheffy and Williams, 1981; Kealy et al, 2002). This level of restriction seems difficult to achieve in the long term but should be considered for incorporation into mainstream nutritional advice. Carefully monitoring food intake and body condition in mature dogs is important because these parameters may indicate underlying disease processes.

Laboratory and Other Clinical Information

Laboratory analyses become more important in health screening of dogs older than five years. All mature dogs should be screened for renal disease and hypertension. Chronic renal disease is best diagnosed with a urinalysis (i.e., urine specific gravity, urine protein, urine sediment examination) and a serum biochemistry profile, including urea nitrogen, creatinine, electrolyte, calcium and phosphorus measurements (DiBartola, 1995). Additional blood parameters should be evaluated based on historical and physical examination findings. Generally, indirect blood pressure measurements obtained routinely during hospital visits are reasonable estimates of a dog's true blood pressure (Remillard et al, 1991). However, uncooperative, anxious dogs may have elevated blood pressure values in the hospital setting that do not reflect normal values (Littman and Drobatz, 1995). Fundic examination may also detect changes associated with hypertension and other systemic diseases (Littman and Drobatz, 1995). Thoracic radiographs and echocardiography should be performed if a cardiac murmur is detected or if there is a history of coughing or an abnormal respiratory pattern.

Key Nutritional Factors

Veterinarians should appreciate the diversity in health status of mature dogs and adapt care and nutrition to the specific needs of each patient (MacDougall and Barker, 1984; Knapp, 1964; Kronfeld, 1983). **Table 14-2** summarizes key nutritional factors for mature dogs. The following section describes these key nutritional factors in more detail. Most of these are the same as for young adult dogs. A more thorough discussion of the overlapping key nutritional factors can be found in the key nutritional factors section in Chapter 13.

Water

Mature dogs are more prone to dehydration due to possible osmoregulatory disturbances, medications (diuretics) and chronic renal disease, with compromised urine concentrating ability. Therefore, continuous access to a fresh, clean water supply is very important and water intake should be routinely monitored.

Energy

With increasing age, lean body mass decreases, subcutaneous fat increases, basal metabolic rate gradually declines and body temperature may decrease. As dogs age, they become slower and less active, and their thyroid function may be impaired (Siwak et al, 2000; Armstrong and Lund, 1996; Finke, 1991; MacDougall and Barker, 1984; Mosier, 1990; Meyer, 1990; Sheffy et al, 1985). All these changes result in a 12 to 13% decrease in daily energy requirement by around seven years of age (Chapter 13, Table 13-2) (Kienzle and Rainbird, 1991). For mature dogs, a daily energy intake of 1.4 x resting energy requirement (100 kcal [418 kJ] metabolizable energy/$BW_{kg}^{0.75}$) is a good starting point (Leibetseder, 1989). This amount should be modified if a dog tends to lose or gain weight when fed at the recommended level. Very old dogs are often underweight and may have inadequate energy intake (Armstrong and Lund, 1996; Kronfeld, 1991; Donoghue et al, 1991). Underweight, very elderly people increase body weight when a food of higher caloric density is provided (Olin et al, 1996). Thus, it may be appropriate to feed a more energy-dense food to very old dogs. Because of the potential for mature dogs to have different energy needs, energy densities in foods recommended for this age group may vary from 3.0 to 4.0 kcal (12.6 to 16.7 kJ)/g dry matter (DM).

Fat

A relatively low fat intake helps prevent obesity in healthy mature dogs. However, some dogs may need different foods at seven years of age than they will at 13 years of age. Very old dogs may have a tendency to lose weight (Armstrong and Lund, 1996; Kronfeld et al, 1991). For these dogs, increasing the fat content of the food increases energy intake, improves palatability and improves protein efficiency (NRC, 1985; Schaeffer et al, 1989).

Research in people has indicated that increased energy intake can correct immunosenescence due to mild protein-energy malnutrition (Morley, 1994). The general condition of elderly people improved significantly by increasing the energy density of the food (Olin et al, 1996). Thus, a good balance should be maintained between preventing obesity and providing sufficient caloric intake.

Generally, fat levels between 7 and 15% DM are recommended for most mature dogs. Fat levels for obese-prone dogs should be between seven to 10%. The fat level should be selected as needed to meet the desired energy density to achieve ideal body weight and condition (body condition score 2.5/5 to 3.5/5). Essential fatty acid requirements should also be met as outlined for young adult dogs.

Table 14-2. Key nutritional factors for foods for mature dogs.

Factors	Recommended food levels* Normal weight and body condition	Inactive/ obese prone
Water	Free access	Free access
Energy density (kcal ME/g)	3.0-4.0	3.0-3.5
Energy density (kJ ME/g)	12.5-16.7	12.5-14.6
Crude fat (%)	10-15	7-10
Crude fiber (%)**	≥2	≥10
Protein (%)	15-23	15-23
Phosphorus (%)	0.3-0.7	0.3-0.7
Sodium (%)	0.15-0.4	0.15-0.4
Chloride (%)	1.5 x Na	1.5 x Na
Antioxidants (amount/kg food)		
Vitamin E (IU)	≥400	≥400
Vitamin C (mg)	≥100	≥100
Selenium (mg)	0.5-1.3	0.5-1.3
Food texture (VOHC Seal of Acceptance)	Reduced plaque accumulation	Reduced plaque accumulation

Key: kcal = kilocalories, kJ = kilojoules, ME = metabolizable energy, VOHC = Veterinary Oral Health Council Seal of Acceptance (Chapter 47).
*All foods expressed on a dry matter basis unless otherwise noted. If the caloric density of the food is different, the nutrient content in the dry matter must be adapted accordingly (Chapter 1).
**Crude fiber measurements underestimate total dietary fiber levels in food.

Fiber

Mature dogs are prone to develop constipation (Twedt, 1993), which may justify increased fiber intake. Additionally, fiber added to foods for obese-prone mature dogs dilutes calories. Fiber also decreases postprandial glycemic effects in diabetic dogs (Nelson, 1989). Very old dogs that tend to lose weight, however, should be offered a food with increased caloric density. The recommended levels of crude fiber in foods intended for mature dogs are at least 2% (DM).

Protein

Recommendations for protein intake in mature dogs are controversial, which parallels the debate in people (Pellet, 1990). The decrease in lean body mass, seen with age, together with alterations in protein synthesis and turnover have been the basis for the argument that protein intake in mature dogs should be higher than for younger adults (Grandjean and Paragon, 1990; Kronfeld, 1983; Wannemacher and McCoy, 1966). In contrast, other investigators have recommended reduced protein intake because of the increased prevalence of renal pathology in dogs older than five years of age (Leibetseder and Neufeld, 1991; Lewis et al, 1987).

As with all lifestages, healthy mature dogs should receive enough protein and energy to avoid protein-energy malnutrition. Improving protein quality, rather than increasing its intake, can provide sufficient protein (Sheffy et al, 1985; Leibetseder, 1989; Mundt, 1989). Additionally, data suggest that mild protein-energy undernutrition in older people plays a role in immunosenescence; however, supplementation with calories returned helper T cells and suppressor cells to values seen in younger people (Morley, 1994). Serum protein concentrations, lymphocyte counts and muscle protein-to-DNA ratios have indicated that foods with 18% DM protein are adequate to maintain immunocompetence in older dogs (Finco et al, 1994). These findings confirmed earlier observations that foods with 16 to 20% DM protein are sufficient to maintain nitrogen balance and protein stores in older dogs (Wannemacher and McCoy, 1966). In addition, alterations in protein metabolism and plasma protein concentrations seen in healthy elderly people are unrelated to daily protein intake, suggesting that other factors play a role (Munro et al, 1987).

High protein intake has not been shown to contribute to the development of kidney disease in healthy animals. However, after kidney function is impaired, protein may play a role in progression of renal disease. In a four-year study with uninephrectomized healthy dogs, investigators recognized no difference in kidney function between dogs receiving a food with 34% DM protein and a food with 18% DM protein (Finco et al, 1994). However, histologic examination revealed an increase in mesangial matrix scores and fibrosis in the high-protein group (Finco et al, 1994). Mesangial proliferation has been described in glomerulonephritis and chronic interstitial nephritis in dogs (Müller-Peddinghaus and Trautwein, 1977a; Spencer and Wright, 1981) and may indicate more rapid renal impairment at a higher protein intake (Finco et al, 1994). Moderately reduced protein intake during early stages of canine renal disease improved the subjects' general condition (Leibetseder and Neufeld, 1991). In conclusion, commercial foods containing 15 to 23% DM protein provide sufficient protein for apparently healthy mature dogs.

Phosphorus

Some degree of clinical or subclinical renal disease is often present in mature dogs; as many as 25% of all dogs may be affected (Oehlert and Oehlert, 1976; Rouse and Lewis, 1975; Shirota et al, 1979; Leibetseder and Neufeld, 1991; Bloom, 1954; Crowell and Finco, 1975; Müller-Peddinghaus and Trautwein, 1977). Excessive phosphorus intake should therefore be avoided (Finco et al, 1992). Researchers have observed that dogs with advanced renal disease had slowed progression and reduced severity of renal disease when phosphorus levels in foods were decreased, thereby improving survival time (Brown et al, 1991; Finco et al, 1992; Lopez-Hilker et al, 1990). The minimum recommended DM allowance of phosphorus for foods for adult dogs is 0.3% (NRC, 2006). Therefore, foods for mature dogs should contain 0.3 to 0.7% DM phosphorus.

Sodium and Chloride

There is no nutritional need for the higher levels of sodium and chloride found in some commercial dog foods, especially considering the increased prevalence of heart and renal disease in mature dogs (Detweiler and Patterson, 1965; Whitney, 1974). High sodium chloride intake may be harmful in diseases that have a hypertensive component. Secondary hypertension is associated with obesity, chronic renal disease and some endocrinopathies, which are frequently seen in mature dogs (Anderson and Fisher, 1968; Cowgill and Kallet, 1986; Rocchini et al, 1987; Littman, 1990; Ross, 1992). Mature dogs with heart disease have decreased ability for eliminating excess dietary sodium (Chapter 36). Kidney disease and certain other diseases with a hypertensive component may be subclinical in their early phases. The minimum recommended allowance for sodium in foods for healthy adult dogs is 0.08 % DM; this recommendation is based on foods with a DM energy density of 4 kcal/g (NRC, 2006). For purposes of risk factor management, the recommended range for dietary sodium in foods for mature dogs is 0.15 to 0.4% DM, which is more than adequate. Some commercial all-purpose foods contain more than 2% DM sodium. Although the chloride requirement of dogs has not been established, a chloride level 1.5 times the sodium requirement is a reasonable recommendation.

Antioxidants

The consequences of prolonged oxidative stress (i.e., free radical damage) to cell membranes, proteins and DNA contribute to and/or exacerbate a wide variety of degenerative diseases including those listed in Table 13-1. In addition to these diseases, cognitive dysfunction was shown to affect 28% of dogs between 11 and 12 years of age and 68% of dogs 15 to 16 years old. Cognitive dysfunction is responsive to certain combinations of antioxidants (Chapter 35).

The consequences of free radical damage to cells and tissues have also been associated with the effects of aging. Although aging is a complex, multifactorial process, one explanation for many of the degenerative changes associated with aging is the free radical theory of aging (Harman, 1956). This theory proposes that free radicals produce cell damage and that age-dependent pathologic alterations may, at least in part, be the cumulative result of these changes.

Many phenomena initiate free radical formation within the body. Although environmental pollutants and radiation are direct and indirect sources of free radicals, the primary source is endogenous from normal oxidative metabolism. However, the body defends itself against the effects of free radicals through a complex network of protective antioxidant compounds.

Antioxidants protect biomolecules by scavenging free radical compounds, minimizing free radical production and binding metal ions that might increase the reactivity of poorly reactive compounds. In addition, many antioxidants exhibit second messenger regulatory function, cell cycle signaling and control of gene expression (Chapter 7). Also, combinations of antioxidants are more effective in relieving oxidative stress than are individual antioxidants.

The following key nutritional factor recommendations focus on the antioxidant vitamins E and C and on selenium as an essential component of the antioxidant enzyme, glutathione peroxidase. These compounds make up the list of antioxidant key nutritional factors because: 1) they are biologically important, 2) they act synergistically (e.g., vitamin C regenerates vitamin E after it has reacted with a free radical), 3) they are safe and 4) information regarding inclusion levels in pet foods is usually available. For improved antioxidant performance, foods for mature dogs should contain at least 400 IU vitamin E/kg (DM) (Jewell et al, 2000), at least 100 mg vitamin C/kg (DM) and 0.5 to 1.3 mg selenium/kg (DM).

Food Texture

Oral disease is the most common health problem in mature dogs and may predispose affected patients to systemic complications (DeBowes et al, 1996). Both veterinary care and home care are important in the treatment and prevention of periodontal disease. Foods designed to reduce the accumulation of dental substrates (e.g., plaque) and help control gingivitis and malodor are an important part of an oral home-care program for mature dogs (Chapter 47). If the labels of such foods carry the Veterinary Oral Health Council (VOHC) seal for plaque control, they have been successfully tested according to specific protocols and shown to be clinically effective in reducing accumulation of plaque. However, with older dogs, it is best if an adequate periodontal management program is in place (veterinarian/client/patient) so that there is sufficient periodontal health to ensure that the patient can chew the product (Chapter 47).

Other Nutritional Factor

Calcium

Osteoporosis occurs frequently in older people but is not a clinical problem in mature dogs (Weigel and Alexander, 1981). This finding is probably due, in part, to lifetime feeding of calcium-replete commercial foods to most dogs. There should be little concern about calcium deficiency in mature dogs unless unbalanced homemade foods are fed. Foods with 0.4 to 0.8% DM calcium are recommended for mature dogs. The calcium-phosphorus ratio should not be less than 1:1.

FEEDING PLAN

Mature dogs are more prone to obesity, degenerative joint disease, cardiac disease, renal disease, cognitive dysfunction and metabolic aberrations. They also are usually less active than young adult dogs. The feeding plan should be based on potential risk factors and information attained in the assessment. Because of the larger variation in health among mature dogs, more attention should be paid to individual needs. Nutritional surveillance is more important for mature dogs than for young adult dogs; therefore, the number of veterinary assessments per year should be increased. Goals remain the same as listed in the introduction; however, each patient should be evaluated individually.

Assess and Select the Food

Assessment of the food for mature dogs is similar to those procedures outlined for young adult dogs in Chapter 13. Compare the current food's key nutritional factor levels with the key nutritional factors reviewed above, identify discrepancies between key nutritional factor levels and current intake and decide whether food changes are required. **Table 14-3** compares key nutritional factor levels in selected commercial foods formulated for mature dogs to the key nutritional factor recommendations. Check with manufacturers for key nutritional factor content of foods not found in **Table 14-3**. Contact information can be found on pet food labels, websites or published information. Also, as with young adult dogs, the pet food label should indicate that the product has been approved by a regulatory agency such as the Association of American Feed Control Officials (AAFCO) (Chapter 9).

Commercial treats, snacks and table food should also be included in the food assessment step. Excessive feeding of treats and snacks may markedly affect the cumulative nutritional profile (Chapter 13, Box 13-4). The impact of snacks on daily nutrient intake depends on two factors: 1) the nutrient profile of the snack and 2) the number provided. Thus, if snacks are fed, it is prudent to recommend those that best match the key nutritional profile recommended for mature dogs. Because meeting nutrient requirements is not the primary goal of feeding treats, many commercial treats are not complete and balanced. However, a few treats are complete and balanced and are approved by AAFCO, or some other credible regulatory agency. Most table foods are not nutritionally complete and balanced and may contain high levels of fat or sodium and other minerals. If snacks are fed, it is simplest to recommend that they be commercial treats that, if possible, match the nutritional profile recommended for a particular lifestage (see product label). Generally, snacks should not be fed in excessive amounts (<10% of the total diet on a volume, weight or calorie basis). Otherwise, the nutritional composition of the snack and food should be combined and assessed.

Assess and Determine the Feeding Method

It may not be necessary to change the feeding method when managing healthy mature dogs. However, a thorough evaluation includes verification that an appropriate feeding method is being used.

The feeding method should be monitored more closely in mature than in younger dogs. Free-choice feeding should not be used for obese or overweight patients; however, this method may be preferred for thinner, very old animals to allow increased food intake. It is very important to measure food intake of mature dogs; this measurement may be more accurate when dogs are meal fed. Measures to stimulate food intake may be necessary for some very old dogs. Most mature adult dogs adapt well to new foods, but some patients may have difficulty. It is always good practice to allow for a transition period to avoid digestive upsets. This is particularly true when switching from lower to higher fat foods. The new food should be increased and the old food decreased in progressive amounts

Table 14-3. Comparison of recommended levels of key nutritional factors for foods for mature adult dogs with levels in selected commercial foods.*

Dry foods	**Energy density (kcal/cup)****	**Energy density (kcal ME/g)**	**Fat (%)**	**Fiber (%)**	**Protein (%)**	**P (%)**	**Na (%)**	**Vit E (IU/kg)**	**Vit C (mg/kg)**	**Se (mg/kg)**	**VOHC plaque*** (Yes/No)**
Recommended levels (normal body condition)	**-**	**3.0-4.0**	**10-15**	**≥2**	**15-23**	**0.3-0.7**	**0.15-0.4**	**≥400**	**≥100**	**0.5-1.3**	**-**
Hill's Science Diet Mature Adult 7+ Original	363	4.0	15.8	4.2	19.3	0.58	0.18	700	271	0.41	No
Hill's Science Diet Oral Care Adult	273	3.8	15.5	10.1	25.1	0.65	0.24	564	175	0.62	Yes
Iams Eukanuba Medium Breed Senior	350	4.6	12.8	2.2	29.3	0.95	0.40	236	83	na	No
Medi-Cal Dental Formula	280	na	12.7	5.3	19.7	0.9	0.4	na	na	na	No
Nutro Natural Choice Senior	267	3.8	12.1	2.2	23.1	1.21	0.27	275	99	0.49	No
Purina ONE Senior Protection Formula	375	4.1	14.0	3.4	32.3	1.12	0.30	1,012	na	0.99	No
Purina Pro Plan Chicken & Rice Senior	408	4.2	15.6	2.3	30.4	1.14	0.44	na	na	na	No
Royal Canin MINI Aging Care 27	378	4.3	17.4	1.7	29.3	0.71	0.33	717	326	0.22	No
Moist foods	**Energy density (kcal/can)****	**Energy density (kcal ME/g)**	**Fat (%)**	**Fiber (%)**	**Protein (%)**	**P (%)**	**Na (%)**	**Vit E (IU/kg)**	**Vit C (mg/kg)**	**Se (mg/kg)**	**VOHC plaque*** (Yes/No)**
Recommended levels (normal body condition)	**-**	**3.0-4.0**	**10-15**	**≥2**	**15-23**	**0.3-0.7**	**0.15-0.4**	**≥400**	**≥100**	**0.5-1.3**	**-**
Hill's Science Diet Gourmet Beef Entrée Mature Adult 7+	164/5.8 oz. 368/13 oz.	4.0	14.4	1.6	18.8	0.52	0.16	316	na	0.70	No
Hill's Science Diet Gourmet Turkey Entrée Mature Adult 7+	369/13 oz.	4.1	12.8	2.1	19.4	0.62	0.17	426	na	0.83	No
Hill's Science Diet Savory Chicken Entrée Mature Adult 7+	155/5.8 oz. 347/13 oz.	3.8	13.1	1.6	18.4	0.57	0.16	520	na	0.82	No
Dry foods†	**Energy density (kcal/cup)****	**Energy density (kcal ME/g)**	**Fat (%)**	**Fiber (%)**	**Protein (%)**	**P (%)**	**Na (%)**	**Vit E (IU/kg)**	**Vit C (mg/kg)**	**Se (mg/kg)**	**VOHC plaque*** (Yes/No)**
Recommended levels (inactive/obese prone)	**-**	**3.0-3.5**	**7-10**	**≥10**	**15-23**	**0.3-0.7**	**0.15-0.4**	**≥400**	**≥100**	**0.5-1.3**	**-**
Hill's Science Diet Light Adult	295	3.3	8.8	14.6	24.5	0.58	0.23	586	276	0.45	No
Iams Eukanuba Medium Breed Weight Control	275	4.2	10.5	1.9	21.3	0.76	0.50	206	42	0.34	No
Iams Weight Control	328	4.2	12.5	2.8	22.2	0.85	0.37	103	44	0.35	No
Medi-Cal Weight Control/Mature	320	na	8.5	4.0	19.5	0.8	0.2	na	na	na	No
Nutro Natural Choice Lite	244	3.4	7.2	4.4	16.7	1.22	0.33	161	67	0.44	No
Purina Pro Plan Chicken & Rice Weight Management	337	3.7	10.2	2.7	30.5	1.06	0.27	503	na	0.33	No
Royal Canin MINI Weight Care 30	326	3.8	12.0	6.2	32.6	0.82	0.33	652	326	0.16	No
Moist foods†	**Energy density (kcal/can)****	**Energy density (kcal ME/g)**	**Fat (%)**	**Fiber (%)**	**Protein (%)**	**P (%)**	**Na (%)**	**Vit E (IU/kg)**	**Vit C (mg/kg)**	**Se (mg/kg)**	**VOHC plaque*** (Yes/No)**
Recommended levels (inactive/obese prone)	**-**	**3.0-3.5**	**7-10**	**≥10**	**15-23**	**0.3-0.7**	**0.15-0.4**	**≥400**	**≥100**	**0.5-1.3**	**-**
Hill's Science Diet Light Adult	322/13 oz.	3.4	8.6	9.7	19.5	0.51	0.31	385	na	0.78	No
Medi-Cal Weight Control/Mature	370/396 g	na	10.0	5.5	21.5	0.6	0.3	na	na	na	No

Key: ME = metabolizable energy, na = information not published by manufacturer, Fiber = crude fiber, Se = selenium, P = phosphorus, Na = sodium, VOHC = Veterinary Oral Health Council, na = information not available from manufacturer, g = grams.

*From manufacturers' published information or calculated from manufacturers' published as-fed values; all values are on a dry matter basis unless otherwise stated.

**Energy density values are listed on an as fed basis and are useful for determining the amount to feed; cup = 8-oz. measuring cup. To convert to kJ, multiply kcal by 4.184.

***An adequate periodontal management program should be in place (veterinarian/client/patient) to ensure that there is sufficient periodontal health to enable the patient to chew these products.

†The manufacturers of most of the foods listed for inactive/obese-prone dogs recommend these foods for young adults.

over a three- to seven-day period until the changeover is completed (Nott et al, 1993) (Chapter 1). **Table 14-4** summarizes feeding recommendations for mature adult dogs.

REASSESSMENT

Nutritional status for healthy mature dogs should be assessed at least every six to 12 months. Immediate reassessment should take place if clinical signs arise that indicate the current nutritional regimen is inappropriate or if the dog's needs change due to altered use.

ENDNOTE

a. Zicker SC. Hill's Pet Nutrition, Inc., Topeka, KS. U.S. Marketing Research Summary: Omnibus Study on Aging Pets. Data on file. November 2000.

REFERENCES

The references for **Chapter 14** can be found at www.markmorris.org.

Table 14-4. Feeding plan summary for mature dogs.

1. Select a food or foods with levels of key nutritional factors listed in **Table 14-3**; for foods not in this table, contact the manufacturer for levels of key nutritional factors in the food in question.
2. The selected food should also be approved or meet requirements established by a credible regulatory agency (e.g., AAFCO).
3. Body condition and other assessment criteria will determine the DER. DER is calculated by multiplying RER by an appropriate factor (Table 5-2). Remember, DER calculations should be used as guidelines, starting points and estimates for individual dogs and not as absolute requirements.
   Dogs in ideal body condition =
   3.0 to 4.0 kcal (12.5 to 16.7 kJ) ME/g DM
   Inactive/obese-prone dogs =
   3.0 to 3.5 kcal (12.5 to 14.6 kJ) ME/g DM
4. Determine the preferred feeding method (Table 13-5); when the correct amount of food is fed; meal-restricted feeding is least likely to result in obesity.
5. For food-restricted meal feeding, estimate the initial quantity of food based on DER calculation (DER ÷ food energy density). Food energy density can be obtained from **Table 14-3** or from the manufacturer.
6. Monitor body weight, body condition and general health. These parameters are used to refine the amount to feed.

Key: AAFCO = Association of American Feed Control Officials, DER = daily energy requirement, RER = resting energy requirement, ME = metabolizable energy, DM = dry matter.

CASE 14-1

Feeding a Mature Miniature Pinscher

Jacques Debraekeleer, DVM
Hill's Science and Technology Center
Etten Leur, The Netherlands

Kathy L. Gross, PhD
Hill's Science and Technology Center
Topeka, Kansas, USA

Patient Assessment

An eight-year-old intact male miniature pinscher was examined as part of a routine health maintenance program. The owners saw a magazine article recently promoting preventive health programs for mature dogs. They realized that their dog was aging but had not noticed any specific problems.

The dog weighed 4.5 kg and had an optimal body condition score (BCS 3/5). Physical examination was normal except for a slightly enlarged prostate gland, mild periodontal disease and a grade II/VI holosystolic cardiac murmur loudest over the mitral valve. Results of a complete blood count, serum biochemistry profile, urinalysis and ocular fundic examination were normal. Thoracic radiographs were normal with no evidence of cardiomegaly or pulmonary disease.

Assess the Food and Feeding Method

The dog was fed several different kinds of commercial moist grocery brand dog foods and commercial jerky-type dog treats. Ice cream was also fed regularly. The owners were somewhat concerned because the dog did not seem to be eating as much as it did previously.

Questions

1. What are the key nutritional factors that should be considered in this patient?
2. Outline a feeding plan (foods and feeding method) for this dog.
3. How should the owner's concern about the reduction in appetite be addressed?

Answers and Discussion

1. Key nutritional factors for mature dogs include water, energy, fat, fiber, protein, phosphorus, sodium, chloride, antioxidants and food texture. Chronic progressive renal disease is a leading cause of morbidity and mortality in mature dogs. However, classic diagnostic tests such as the serum biochemistry profile and urinalysis that were performed for this dog will not detect renal disease until it is advanced. Although not definitively proven, dogs with subclinical renal disease may benefit from foods that avoid excess levels of phosphorus, protein, sodium and chloride. Clean water should also be available at all times. In general, fat levels between 7 and 15% dry matter (DM) are recommended for most mature dogs. Fat levels and energy density of the food should be adjusted based on the body condition of the patient. Obese-prone mature dogs may benefit from lower fat, less energy-dense foods whereas very old dogs often lose weight and need higher fat, more energy-dense foods. Increased levels of dietary fiber may be important for obese-prone mature dogs and those with constipation. Oral disease is the most common health problem of mature dogs; more than two-thirds of mature dogs suffer from significant periodontal disease. Both veterinary care and home care are important in treatment and prevention of periodontal disease. Foods formulated to decrease the accumulation of dental plaque and help control gingivitis and malodor are an important part of the oral home-care program for mature dogs.
2. Commercial moist grocery brand dog foods may contain excessive levels of phosphorus, fat, energy, protein, sodium and chloride. Jerky-type commercial treats also contain excessive levels of protein, fat, sodium and chloride. Mature healthy dogs may benefit from commercial foods for "senior" or "geriatric" dogs and treats that contain lower yet adequate levels of these nutrients. Excessive levels of dietary sodium and chloride should also be avoided in mature dogs with evidence of cardiac disease. Ice cream should also be discontinued as a regular treat or offered in smaller amounts. Moist foods do not provide textural characteristics that prevent the accumulation of dental plaque. Dental foods formulated to improve oral health are available and would be appropriate for this patient. The dog's body condition suggests that the current caloric intake is appropriate and should be maintained if a new food is selected. The estimated daily energy requirement (DER) should be 1.6 to 1.8 x resting energy requirement (RER) (330 to 370 kcal, 1,390 to 1,550 kJ). The feeding method will be dictated somewhat by whether a moist, dry, semi-moist or homemade food is fed. Moist and homemade foods should be fed once or twice daily as discrete meals, whereas dry or semi-moist food may be fed free choice and left out for prolonged periods.
3. The optimal BCS suggests that the dog is eating an appropriate amount of food. There may be several reasons why the owners expressed concern about the amount of moist food eaten by the dog. The moist foods currently fed are probably high in fat and energy dense; as little as one-half to two-thirds of a standard 400- to 450-g can will meet this dog's DER. The addition of jerky-type treats and ice cream would also decrease the amount of food the dog needed. Mature dogs may not be as active as they were earlier in life, which decreases their energy requirements. Periodontal disease was recognized during the physical examination and significant oral pain will discourage eating in some patients. Finally, an underlying disease may be contributing to partial anorexia despite the normal diagnostic results. All these factors should be explained to the owners and they should be encouraged to monitor food intake and body condition closely.

Progress Notes

The food was changed to a commercial moist specialty brand food formulated for mature dogs (Science Diet Mature Adult 7+ Canine[a]). The dog was fed three-fourths of a large can per day. The commercial jerky-type treats and ice cream were discontinued and replaced with a dry treat formulated for mature dogs. The dog was given two treats per day. A thorough oral examination including dental prophylaxis and polishing was recommended.

Endnote

a. Hill's Pet Nutrition, Inc., Topeka, KS, USA.

Chapter 15

Feeding Reproducing Dogs

Jacques Debraekeleer

Kathy L. Gross

Steven C. Zicker

"Acquiring a dog may be the only opportunity a human ever has to choose a relative."
Mordecai Siegal

INTRODUCTION

The objectives of a good reproductive feeding program are to optimize: 1) conception, 2) number of puppies per litter, 3) the ability of the bitch to deliver and 4) viability of prenatal and neonatal puppies (Grandjean and Paragon, 1986). Appropriate feeding and management will increase the likelihood of successful reproductive performance, whereas improper or inadequate nutrition can negatively affect reproductive performance in bitches (**Table 15-1**).

Females undergo the greatest extremes in nutrient requirements when the entire reproductive cycle is considered. Estrus, pregnancy and lactation are each associated with specific nutrient concerns that must be addressed. The concerns change with intrinsic physiologic alterations and may be influenced by environmental and other extrinsic factors. Males also need adequate nutrition to achieve optimal performance and conception rates.

Experienced breeders seem to have knowledge about nutritional programs for reproducing dogs based primarily on personal experience, augmented to varying degrees by scientific information. To be effective, veterinarians and their health care teams should have a good understanding of appropriate and practical nutritional programs for reproduction and the neonatal period. These programs should be based on up-to-date, science-based information about the nutritional demands of estrus, gestation and lactation.

PATIENT ASSESSMENT

Estrus and Mating

Optimal nutrition for reproducing animals should precede mating and conception (Sheffy, 1978). As a rule, only healthy dogs in a good nutritional state (body condition score [BCS] 2.5/5 to 3.5/5) should be used for breeding because effects of malnutrition before breeding are often unnoticed until puppies are born (**Table 15-1**). A BCS of 2/5 may be acceptable for a house pet that is only bred for an exceptional occasion (Donoghue, 1992). Obese bitches may have a lower ovulation rate, smaller litter size and insufficient milk production (Meyer, 1990). Obesity may also cause silent heat, prolonged interestrous intervals and anestrus. Therefore, to optimize fertility, overweight bitches should lose weight before breeding (Grandjean and Paragon, 1986). A good history and general physical examination should precede breeding to document and correct problems that may interfere with successful breeding.

Pregnancy

Gestation in dogs averages 63 days and is typically divided into 21-day trimesters. Assessment includes a detailed dietary history, a physical examination and pertinent laboratory analyses. During the physical examination, particular attention should be given to body weight, body condition and vaginal discharges. Ultrasound of the abdomen can provide additional information. Adequately fed bitches gain about 15 to 25% more than

Table 15-1. Effects of improper nutrition on reproductive performance and health in bitches.*

Factors	Reproductive and health consequences
Underfeeding	Small litter size
	Low birth weight
	Increased neonatal morbidity and mortality
	Decreased milk yield
	Decreased immunity and decreased response to vaccination
	Decreased fertility later
	Hair loss and weight loss in bitches
Obesity	Decreased ovulation
	Decreased fertility
	Silent heat
	Prolonged interestrous interval
	Anestrus
	Smaller litters
Malnutrition*	
Protein deficiency	Low birth weight
	Increased neonatal morbidity and mortality
	Decreased neonatal immunity
Carbohydrate-free food	Low birth weight
	Increased neonatal morbidity and mortality
	Increased numbers of stillbirths
Zinc deficiency	Fetal resorption
	Smaller litters
Iron deficiency	Decreased immunity and response to vaccination
Pyridoxine and biotin deficiency	Decreased immunity and response to vaccination
Hypervitaminosis A	Congenital abnormalities
	Smaller litters
Hypervitaminosis D	Soft-tissue calcification

*Malnutrition is uncommon when balanced commercial foods are fed, but may occur if homemade foods are not properly formulated.

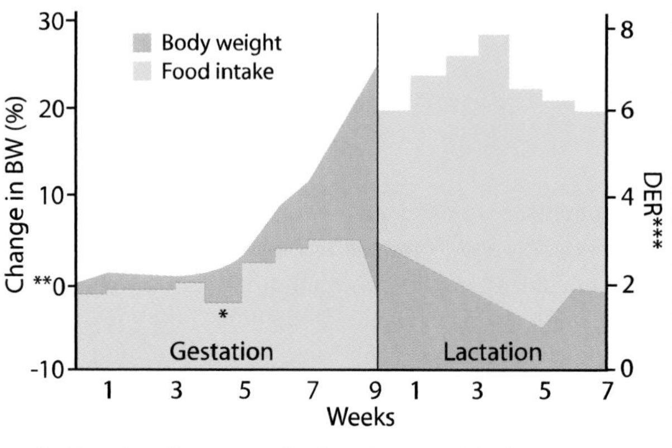

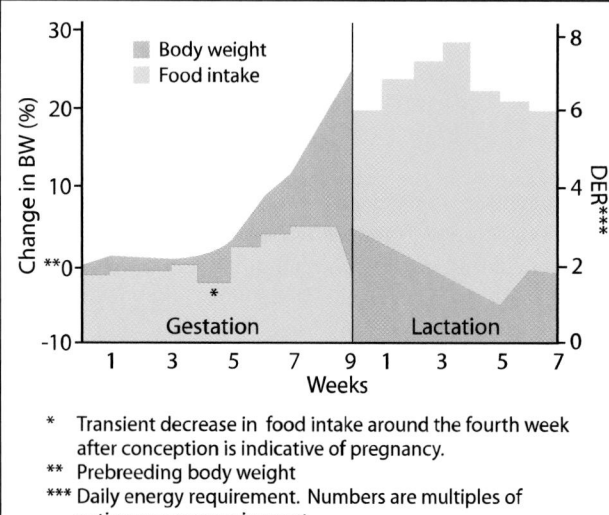

* Transient decrease in food intake around the fourth week after conception is indicative of pregnancy.
** Prebreeding body weight
*** Daily energy requirement. Numbers are multiples of resting energy requirement.

Figure 15-1. Typical changes in body weight and food intake of a bitch during gestation and lactation. A bitch only weighs 5 to 10% above pre-breeding weight after parturition, and should not lose more than 5% of its body weight during the first month of lactation. Food intake may drop precipitously during the last days of gestation.

their pre-breeding weight before whelping (**Table 15-2** and **Figure 15-1**) (Meyer, 1990; Gesellshaft, 1989; Leibetseder, 1989). After parturition, bitches should weigh about 5 to 10% more than their pre-breeding weight. This weight gain corresponds with development of mammary tissue, extracellular water and some gain in extragenital tissue (Meyer, 1990; Gesellshaft, 1989; Leibetseder, 1989; Mosier, 1978). Retention of more than 10% above pre-breeding weight may adversely affect whelping. Furthermore, unlike cats, dogs do not need to maintain a body fat reserve to provide energy for the subsequent lactation because they can increase their food intake during lactation (Meyer, 1990; Grandjean and Paragon, 1986).

Laboratory analyses can include a complete blood count, serum protein, glucose, calcium, phosphorus and potassium concentrations and culture of vaginal discharges, if present. During pregnancy, red blood cell counts, hematocrit values and red cell volume may decrease because of plasma volume expansion, and may reach their lowest level during the second week of lactation (Concannon et al, 1989; Wallace and Davidson, 1995; Meyer et al, 1985). In most bitches, serum albumin and calcium concentrations also decrease during gestation (Meyer et al, 1985; Kaneko, 1989). Urea nitrogen concentrations may be below the normal range just before parturition; however, this finding should not be alarming, because levels return to normal during the first weeks of lactation (Meyer et al, 1985).

Malnutrition, due to inadequate and/or excessive intake of nutrients, may affect pregnancy and lactation (**Table 15-1**). Fertilized eggs may die at an early stage resulting in embryo loss. Alternatively, fetuses may develop incorrectly, die and be resorbed, expelled before term (abortion) or carried to full term (stillbirth) (McDonald et al, 1995). Embryo loss and in utero resorption are manifested by smaller litter size. Malnutrition during pregnancy is also a cause of low birth weight puppies that are particularly prone to hypoglycemia, sepsis, pneumonia and hemorrhage and have reduced survival (Mosier, 1978, 1978a; Schroeder and Smith, 1994).

Obesity at the end of pregnancy may increase dystocia, prolong labor and therefore predispose puppies to hypoxia and hypoglycemia. Studies indicate that obesity in pregnant women is the most important factor predisposing to preterm parturition and increases perinatal mortality sixfold (Prentice and Goldberg, 1996). Obesity in pregnant women increases the risk of congenital central nervous system defects (e.g., neural tube defects) and low birth weight infants (Prentice and Goldberg, 1996). Rats that were obese during gestation and lactation had inadequate milk production and were unable to maintain their litters. Surviving pups were significantly smaller than normal. These findings occurred irrespective of whether rats were underfed or overfed during lactation (Rasmussen, 1992).

Lactation

Successful lactation depends on body condition before breeding, and adequate nutrition throughout gestation and lactation. During lactation, nutrient requirements are directly related to milk production, which in turn depends primarily on the number of suckling puppies. A bitch's nutrient requirement during lactation is greater than at any other adult lifestage and equal to or higher, in some cases, than for growth. Only extreme exercise (Chapter 18) is more energy demanding. The superior ability of bitches to produce milk is illustrated by the following examples. A German shepherd bitch, with six puppies, may produce about 1.7 liters of milk/day during the third and fourth week of lactation (Rüsse, 1961). Beagles with five to seven puppies are able to produce an average of 964 ml of milk/day (7.6% of body weight) at three weeks postpartum, and 1,054 ml/day (8.3% of body weight) at four weeks (Oftedal, 1984). In contrast, a woman produces about 750 ml/day during a three-month lactation (Pellet, 1990). Peak milk production of bitches equates to that of dairy cows, which produce about 7.3% of body weight during peak lactation (exceptional cows can peak at 11% or higher) (Rothbauer, 1994). Additionally, bitch's milk contains more than twice the protein and fat of cow's milk (**Table 15-3**) and more protein than goat's milk. More nutrient-dense milk is necessary to support the more rapid growth rate (as a percent of birth weight) of puppies vs. that of calves, kids and children (**Table 15-4**). A physical examination and anamnesis should be performed as described for gestation, above.

During the first week of lactation, milk production is approximately 2.7% of body weight. Thereafter, milk production steadily increases and peaks during the third and fourth week of lactation and has been estimated to be as much as 8% of a bitch's body weight (Ontko and Phillips, 1958; Rüsse, 1961; Oftedal, 1984; Meyer et al, 1985; Zentek and Meyer, 1992; Scantlebury et al, 2000; NRC, 2006).

After the first two to five days of lactation, the composition of the milk is stable and the bitch's nutrient requirements are primarily determined by the quantity of milk produced (Meyer et al, 1985; Rüsse, 1961; Oftedal, 1984; Mundt et al, 1981). During peak lactation, the quantity of milk produced depends primarily on the number of nursing puppies (Meyer et al, 1985; Ontko and Phillips, 1958). The puppies' intake of solid food begins to increase around the fifth week, after which milk production progressively declines (Gesellshaft, 1989). Therefore, the stage of lactation and the number of nursing puppies primarily determine the bitch's protein and energy requirements for lactation.

Urea nitrogen levels may be decreased just before parturition; however, values normalize during the first few weeks of lactation. Serum total protein concentrations should be within the normal physiologic range (6.0 to 6.5 g/dl) and remain stable during lactation (Meyer et al, 1985). A decrease in total protein may indicate undernutrition. Serum calcium concentrations may temporarily decrease during Weeks 3 and 4 of lactation, whereas inorganic phosphorus concentrations should be normal or slightly increased (Meyer et al, 1985).

Key Nutritional Factors

Compared with maintenance for young adult dogs, there are no special nutritional requirements for bitches during estrus (Grandjean and Paragon, 1986). As for maintenance, breeding bitches should be fed to be in ideal body condition (2.5/5 to

Table 15-2. Distribution of the accretion of the bitch's body weight (BW) at the end of gestation.*

Tissues	% of pre-breeding BW
Fetal mass	12
Placenta	3
Growth of uterus, mammary tissue and amniotic fluid	3
Extragenital accretion of tissue and extracellular water	7
Total accretion	25

*Adapted from Meyer H. Praktische Fütterung. In: Ernährung des Hundes, 2nd ed. Stuttgart, Germany: E Ulmer Verlag, 1990; 162-223. Gesellschaft für Ernährungsphysiologie. Grunddaten für die Berechnung des Energie- und Nährstoffbedarfs. Ausschuß für Bedarfsnormen der Gesellschaft für Ernährungsphysiologie Energie- Nährstoffbedarf/Energy and Nutrient Requirements, No. 5 Hunde/Dogs. Frankfurt/Main, Germany: DLG Verlag, 1989; 9-31.

Table 15-3. Nutrient comparison (% as fed) between bitch's milk and cow's milk.*

Nutrients	Canine milk	Bovine milk
Total protein	7.5	3.3
Arginine	0.42	0.13
Isoleucine	0.38	0.21
Leucine	0.98	0.36
Lysine	0.37	0.27
Valine	0.46	0.18
Total fat	9.5	3.5
Linoleic acid (C18:2)	11.7	2.5
Lactose	3.4	5.0
Gross energy (kcal/100 g)	146	74

*Adapted from Meyer H, Kienzle E, Dammers C. Milchmenge und Milchzusammensetzung bei und Hündin sowie Futteraufnahme und Gewichtsenwicklung ante und post partum. Fortschritte in der Tierphysiologie und Tierernährung (Advances in Animal Physiology and Animal Nutrition) 1985; Suppl. No. 16: 51-72. Swaisgood HE. Protein and amino acid composition of bovine milk. In: Jensen RG, ed. Handbook of Milk Composition. San Diego, CA: Academic Press Inc, 1995; 464-468.

Table 15-4. Composition of mammals' milk as related to growth rate of young mammals.*

Species	Days required to double birth weight	Protein (%)	Fat (%)	Calcium (%)	Phosphorus (%)
Man	180	1.6	3.75	0.03	0.014
Horse	60	2.0	1.4	0.10	0.07
Cow	47	3.3	3.7	0.12	0.10
Goat	22	2.9	3.8	na	na
Sheep	15	4.1	7.3	0.19	0.10
Pig	14	6.0	8.0	0.21	0.15
Cat	9.5	7.5	8.6	0.18	0.16
Dog	9	7.5	9.5	0.24	0.18
Rabbit	6	11.5	15.0	0.61	0.38

Key: na = not available.
*As-fed basis.

Table 15-5. Key nutritional factors for reproducing dogs.

Factors	Recommended levels in food (DM) Mating*	Gestation/lactation
Water	Fresh water should always be available	Fresh water should always be available
Energy density	3.5-4.5 (kcal ME/g)**	≥4.0
Energy density	14.6-18.8 (kJ ME/g)**	≥16.7
Crude protein (%)	15-30	25-35
Crude fat (%)	10-20	≥20
DHA (%)	-	≥0.02
Digestible Carbohydrate (%)	≥23	≥23
Calcium (%)	0.5-1.0	1.0-1.7
Phosphorus (%)	0.4-0.7	0.7-1.3
Ca:P ratio	1:1-1.5:1	1:1-2:1
Digestibility	Foods with higher energy density are more likely to have higher digestiblity	Foods with higher energy density are more likely to have higher digestibility

Key: DM = dry matter, ME = metabolizable energy, kcal = kilocalories, kJ = kilojoules, DHA = docosahexaenoic acid.
*Foods for most breeding males and females are usually similar to those for young and middle-aged adults (Table 13-4).
**If the caloric density of the food is different, the nutrient content in the DM must be adapted accordingly.

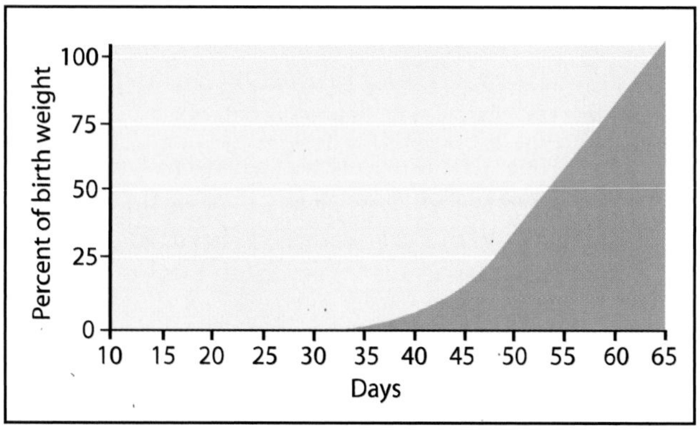

Figure 15-2. The development of fetal mass during pregnancy in beagle dogs. Only 2% of total fetal mass is developed at 35 days of pregnancy and 5.5% at 40 days. After Day 40, fetal tissue growth becomes exponential. (Adapted from Gesellschaft für Ernährungsphysiologie. Empfehlungen für die Versorgung mit Energie. Ausschuß für Bedarfsnormen der Gesellschaft für Ernährungsphysiologie Energieund Nährstoffbedarf/Energy and Nutrient Requirements, No. 5 Hunde/Dogs. Frankfurt/Main, Germany: DLG Verlag, 1989; 32-44. Leibetseder J. Ernährung der Zuchthündin und der Junghunde. Der Praktischer Tierarzt 1989; 70: 12-20.)

3.5/5). Like breeding females, most sires do not have special nutritional needs beyond maintenance requirements for young adults and do well when fed foods for young adult dogs (Chapter 13). However, intact males and females may require more energy than their neutered counterparts to maintain ideal body condition (BCS 2.5/5 to 3.5/5).

Table 15-5 summarizes key nutritional factors for breeding males and females and for pregnant and lactating bitches. The following section describes these key nutritional factors in more detail.

Water

Although often overlooked, water is the first nutrient needed for lactation. Water is needed in large quantities to produce milk and aids in thermoregulation. Water requirements in ml are roughly equal to energy requirements in kcal. A 35-kg bitch nursing a large litter may require five to six liters of water per day at peak lactation. Therefore, it is critical that clean, fresh water be available at all times during gestation and lactation.

Energy

Only 2% of total fetal mass is developed at 35 days of pregnancy and 5.5% at 40 days (**Figure 15-2**). Therefore, during the first two-thirds of gestation, energy requirements are not different from those of young adult dogs (Gesellshaft, 1989a; Ontko and Phillips, 1958). However, during this period bitches should be adequately fed and not allowed to lose weight or body condition. After Day 40, fetal tissue grows exponentially (Gesellshaft, 1989a; Leibetseder, 1989); energy needs correspondingly increase markedly during Week 5 and peak between Weeks 6 and 8 of gestation (Meyer, 1990; Ontko and Phillips, 1958; Romsos et al, 1981). Energy requirements for gestation peak at about 30% above adult maintenance for bitches with smaller litters, whereas energy needs for bitches with larger litters can increase by 50 to 60% (**Table 15-6**) (Meyer, 1990; Romsos et al, 1981; Meyer et al, 1985a).

Although energy needs are highest during Weeks 6 to 8 of gestation, food intake is limited by abdominal fullness as a result of the gravid uterus. Giant breeds may have difficulty ingesting enough food and maintaining body weight even before the last week of gestation (Zentek and Meyer, 1992). Food intake may decrease precipitously just before whelping with some bitches becoming completely anorectic (Romsos et al, 1981; Meyer et al, 1985). Enough energy should be provided to bitches during the earlier weeks of gestation, otherwise bitches may be underweight during mid and late gestation and have difficulty maintaining body condition and milk production after whelping (Bebiak et al, 1987). As mentioned above, bitches should not be allowed to lose body condition during the earlier weeks of gestation. Thus, during gestation, particularly during the last few weeks, the food should be high in energy density (≥4.0 kcal/g [≥16.7 kJ/g]) to provide adequate energy, especially for large-breed bitches.

After whelping, the bitch's energy requirement steadily increases and peaks between three and five weeks (Leibetseder, 1989; Ontko and Phillips, 1958) at a level two to four times higher than the daily energy requirement (DER) for non-lactating adults (Grandjean and Paragon, 1986; Bebiak et al, 1987; Meyer et al, 1985). The energy requirement returns to maintenance levels about eight weeks after whelping (Ontko and Phillips, 1958). Bitches are capable of increasing food intake during lactation (Meyer et al, 1980, 1985); however, the energy density of the food is usually the limiting factor for meeting DER of lactating dogs (Lewis et al, 1987). If foods with low energy density are fed (<3.5 kcal [<14.6 kJ]/g), the bitch may not be physically able to consume enough food and may lose weight, have decreased milk production and display signs of severe exhaustion (Meyer et al, 1985). These signs are most pronounced in giant-breed dogs with large litters (Zentek and Meyer, 1992). Therefore, for these bitches, foods should provide at least 4 kcal metabolizable energy [ME] (16.7 kJ)/g dry matter (DM).

Energy requirements for lactating bitches can be subdivided into energy for maintenance and energy used for milk production. The DER for lactating bitches, without allotment for milk production, is slightly higher than that for average adults because of stress and increased activity associated with caring for puppies. Energy requirements have been estimated to be approximately 145 kcal (600 kJ) digestible energy/$BW_{kg}^{0.75}$ or about 2.1 x resting energy requirement (RER) (Meyer et al, 1985). This is compared to 132 kcal (550 kJ) ME/$BW_{kg}^{0.75}$ for maintenance of active dogs (NRC, 2006) or about 1.9 x RER. The energy used for milk production, by week of lactation, can be estimated using the method described in **Table 15-7. Table 15-8** provides a method for calculating milk production.

Other methods for determining energy requirements of lactating bitches have also been reported but each has limitations (Debraekeleer et al, 2000). Regardless, the body condition of bitches should be evaluated and food adjustments made as necessary to maintain a BCS on the high end of the ideal range

Table 15-6. Practical recommendations for energy intake during gestation.*

Week of gestation	Total DER	
-	**kcal ME/day****	**kJ ME/day****
1-4	DER***	DER***
5	DER + 18 kcal ME/kg BW	DER + 75 kJ ME/kg BW
6-8	DER + 36 kcal ME/kg BW	DER + 150 kJ ME/kg BW
9	DER + 18 kcal ME/kg BW	DER + 75 kJ ME/kg BW

Key: DER = daily energy requirement, kcal = kilocalories, kJ = kilojoules, ME = metabolizable energy, BW = body weight, RER = resting energy requirement.

*Adapted from Gesellschaft für Ernährungsphysiologie. Empfehlungen für die Versorgung mit Energie. Ausschuß für Bedarfsnormen der Gesellschaft für Ernährungsphysiologie Energie- und Nährstoffbedarf/Energy and Nutrient Requirements, No. 5 Hunde/Dogs. Frankfurt/Main, Germany: DLG Verlag, 1989; 32-44.

**Energy requirements during gestation are the sum of the energy needed for normal adult maintenance of a non-pregnant dog plus what is needed for accretion of fetal and maternal tissue. Because accretion of fetal and maternal tissue is minimal during the first 35 days of gestation, the increase in energy requirement only becomes significant after Week 6. However, it is better to increase the food intake progressively during Week 5. This allows the bitch to build reserves for the last week of gestation, when food intake is compromised by abdominal fill.

***During gestation DER is estimated as 1.9 x RER (DER = 132 kcal ME/$BW_{kg}^{0.75}$ or 550 kJ ME/$BW_{kg}^{0.75}$).

Table 15-7. Two methods for calculating the total daily energy requirements for lactating bitches.

Method 1*

The total energy for lactation consists of the bitch's daily energy required for maintenance and the energy required for lactation and uses the formula: ME (kcal) = DER + (BW_{kg} x [24n + 12m] x L), where DER equals the DER for maintenance.

The calculation requires the DER for lactating bitches, without allotment for milk production, which is 145 kcal x $BW_{kg}^{0.75}$ (DER for maintenance of lactating bitches is thought to be higher than for bitches not lactating [see text]).

The calculation also requires the energy needed for lactation, which is based on the bitch's body weight in kg, the week of lactation and the number of puppies in the litter. The week of lactation (L) uses correction factors: Week 1 = 0.75; Week 2 = 0.95; Week 3 = 1.1; Week 4 = 1.2. The number of puppies in the litter is represented by "n" if one to four puppies are in the litter and "m" if the number of puppies in the litter is between five and eight; for fewer than five puppies, m = 0.

These values are inserted into the formula to determine the energy requirement for a lactating bitch:
ME (kcal) = DER + (BW_{kg} x [24n + 12m] x L) where DER is the daily maintenance energy requirement without lactation and BW_{kg} x [24n + 12m] x L represents the energy requirement for lactation.

For example, what would be the total energy requirement for a 20-kg bitch, in the second week of lactation, with a litter of six puppies?

DER (without lactation) = 145 kcal x $20^{0.75}$ = 145 kcal x 9.5 = 1,378 kcal
Number of puppies = 6: n = 4, m = 2
Week of lactation = L = 0.95 (correction factor for Week 2)
Requirement for lactation = 20 x (24 x 4 + 12 x 2) x 0.95 kcal = 2,280 kcal
Total requirement for maintenance and lactation = 1,378 + 2,280 = 3,658 kcal

Method 2

A simplified approach exists to determine DER for peak lactation; however, this method does not allow variation due to week of lactation as does Method 1. It uses the $ME_{peak\ lactation}$ (kcal) = 2.1 x RER_{bitch} plus 25% per puppy.

Using the same example, what would be the total energy requirement for a 20-kg bitch, in the second week of lactation, with a litter of six puppies?

DER = 2.1 x 70($20^{0.75}$) = 1,390 kcal
Requirement for lactation = 25%/puppy or 348 kcal x 6 = 2,088 kcal.

*Adapted from NRC, 2006.

Table 15-8. Calculation of milk production in bitches.*

TP (liters) = (BW_{kg} x k) + [(n–4) x (0.1 x BW_{kg})]
Peak milk production (Weeks 3 to 4) = TP x 0.04.
Example = 30-kg bitch with 8 puppies
TP = (30 x 2) + [(8–4) x (0.1 x 30)] = 60 + (4 x 3) = 72 liters milk
Peak milk production (Weeks 3 to 4) = 72 x 0.04 = 2.9 liters/day
Key: TP = total milk production through Day 45 of lactation, n = number of puppies, k = 1.6 for bitches ≤8 kg BW, 1.8 for bitches >8 to <25 kg BW and 2.0 for bitches ≥25 kg BW, BW = bitch's body weight.
*Adapted from Grandjean D, Paragon B-M, Grandjean R. Rationnement alimentaire et prévention chez le chien 1. Le Point Vétérinaire 1986; 18: 519-524.

(BCS 3.5/5). Foods for lactation should provide at least 4.0 kcal ME (16.7 kJ)/g DM (Leibetseder, 1989; Meyer et al, 1985; Grandjean et al, 1987).

Protein

Protein needs during mating are the same as for maintenance for young adult dogs (i.e., 15 to 30% DM) and do not increase substantially during the first two trimesters of gestation. During late gestation, the protein requirement increases from 40 to 70% above maintenance (Gesellshaft, 1989b; Leibetseder, 1989; Meyer et al, 1985a), and follows the increase in energy requirement. Thus, foods for dogs in late gestation should also have increased levels of protein to meet nutrient requirements at the same time that DM intake is limited. The increased protein requirement can be met by providing about 7 g of digestible protein/$BW_{kg}^{0.75}$ (an increase of 30 to 50% vs. recommendations for young adults) (Gesellshaft, 1989b; Meyer et al, 1985a). The food should contain about 4 g digestible protein/100 kcal ME (about 10 g of digestible protein/MJ) (Gesellshaft, 1989b; Meyer and Heckötter, 1986). A food containing 20 to 25% DM crude protein and 4.0 kcal/g DM (16.7 kJ/g) provides this level of protein. The quality of the protein should also be higher to improve vigor of newborn puppies and minimize neonatal mortality (Ontko and Phillips, 1958). Protein deficiency during pregnancy may decrease birth weight, increase mortality during the first 48 hours of life and decrease immunocompetence of offspring (**Table 15-1**) (Ontko and Phillips, 1958).

The requirement for protein appears to increase more than the requirement for energy during lactation (Meyer et al, 1985). Therefore, the protein-energy ratio must be higher in foods for lactation than in foods for adult maintenance. Ratios of 4.8 to 6.8 g digestible protein/100 kcal ME (10.5 to 15 g/MJ digestible energy) have been recommended (Leibetseder, 1989; Meyer et al, 1985; Meyer and Heckötter, 1986). This recommendation corresponds to about 19 to 27% DM digestible protein of an energy-dense food (4.0 kcal [16.7 kJ] ME/g).

The minimum recommended crude protein allowance for foods for gestation and lactation in bitches ranges from 20% (NRC, 2006) to 22% (AAFCO, 2007). For optimal reproductive performance, foods for gestation and lactation should contain between 25 to 35% DM crude protein.

Fat and Fatty Acids

Fat provides essential fatty acids and enhances absorption of fat-soluble vitamins. Increasing fat levels in foods improves digestibility and provides energy, which in turn improves nitrogen retention (Schaeffer et al, 1989). Although young adult maintenance-type foods are appropriate for the first two-thirds of pregnancy in most breeds, a food with an energy density of approximately 4.0 kcal (16.7 kJ) ME/g is recommended for the last third of gestation. Feeding a food containing slightly more than 19% DM fat usually achieves this recommendation; however, this level may need to be altered depending on litter size, body condition of the bitch, food intake of the bitch and other extraneous factors as discussed previously. The minimum recommended allowance for fat in foods intended for late gestation and peak lactation is 8.5% DM (NRC, 2006). The Association of American Feed Control Officials (AAFCO) recommends at least 8% DM fat (2007). However, to ensure optimal reproductive performance, particularly for late gestation and for lactating bitches with fewer than four puppies, at least 20% DM crude fat is recommended. At least 20% DM fat is also recommended for giant-breed bitches throughout gestation and lactation.

Increased fat intake results in better food efficiency during lactation (Siedler and Schweigert, 1954). One study showed that increasing the fat content in the food from 12 to 20% DM might increase the fat content in the milk by 30% (Gross, 1993). Because puppies are born with a very low energy reserve (Stadtfeld, 1978; Meyer et al, 1985a), sufficient energy should always be available via the milk. Increasing concentrations of fat also increase the caloric density of foods and help meet the high energy requirements of bitches during lactation. An increase in fat should be balanced by increasing other nutrients proportionally to match the increased energy density.

Milk fat and fatty acid composition are highly variable components of milk. Perhaps because of the type of food typically consumed by dogs and cattle, fat in bitch's milk contains a high percentage of unsaturated fatty acids and is rich in linoleic acid compared to cow's milk (**Table 15-3**). The type of fat fed and the fatty acid profiles of endogenous fat deposits may affect the fatty acid composition of milk. In one study, the fatty acid composition of bitch's milk reflected that of foods fed during gestation and lactation. Furthermore, the milk of bitches fed foods enriched with α-linolenic acid (ALA) but not docosahexaenoic acid (DHA) was high in ALA. Puppies fed this milk accumulated more plasma phospholipid DHA than the control group (but not as much as puppies fed preformed DHA) (Heinemann et al, 2005). In children, during early growth, DHA supports retinal and auditory development (Pawlosky et al, 1997; Birch et al, 2002; Diau et al, 2003). Furthermore, brain development and learning ability were enhanced in infants supplemented with DHA (Birch et al, 2002; Hoffman et al, 2003). Similar to findings in other species, including fish oil as a source of DHA in puppy foods improved trainability (Kelley et al, 2004). Foods containing long-chain omega-3 (n-3) polyunsaturated fatty acids fed during gestation and lactation improve retinal func-

Table 15-9. Comparison of key nutritional factors in selected commercial foods for reproducing (gestation and lactation) bitches to recommended levels.*

Dry foods	Energy density (kcal/cup)**	Energy density (kcal ME/g)	Protein (%)	Fat (%)	DHA (%)	Carbohydrate (%)	Ca (%)	P (%)	Ca:P
Recommended levels	**-**	**≥4.0**	**25-35**	**≥20**	**≥0.02**	**≥23**	**1.0-1.7**	**0.7-1.3**	**1:1-2:1**
Hill's Science Diet Nature's Best Chicken & Brown Rice Dinner Puppy	445	4.3	30.2	22.1	0.20	37.7	1.43	1.05	1.4:1
Hill's Science Diet Nature's Best Lamb & Brown Rice Dinner Puppy	442	4.2	30.1	22.1	0.17	36.5	1.5	1.1	1.4:1
Hill's Science Diet Puppy Healthy Development Original	384	4.2	31.8	22.9	0.22	33.2	1.59	1.21	1.3:1
Hill's Science Diet Puppy Lamb Meal & Rice Recipe	377	4.2	31.7	21.7	0.22	35.3	1.58	1.1	1.4:1
Iams Smart Puppy	428	4.7	32.1	19.9	na	38.7	1.37	1.04	1.3:1
Medi-Cal Development Formula	425	na	28.4	17.5	0.09	na	1.2	1.1	1.1:1
Purina ONE Healthy Puppy Formula	465	4.6	31.7	20.6	na	38.4	1.61	1.11	1.5:1
Purina Pro Plan Chicken & Rice Formula Puppy Food	473	4.6	31.6	20.7	na	36.6	1.23	1.04	1.2:1
Purina Puppy Chow	416	4.2	30.7	13.6	na	41.7	1.25	1.02	1.2:1
Royal Canin Veterinary Diet Development Formula	322	4.3	28.4	17.0	na	45.0	1.32	0.99	1.3:1
Moist foods	**Energy density (kcal/can)****	**Energy density (kcal ME/g)**	**Protein (%)**	**Fat (%)**	**DHA (%)**	**Carbohydrate (%)**	**Ca (%)**	**P (%)**	**Ca:P**
Recommended levels	**-**	**≥4.0**	**25-35**	**≥20**	**≥0.02**	**≥23**	**1.0-1.7**	**0.7-1.3**	**1:1-2:1**
Hill's Science Diet Puppy Healthy Development Savory Chicken Entrée	205/5.8 oz. 459/13 oz.	4.1	28.2	23.6	na	39.2	1.33	0.96	1.4:1
Medi-Cal Development Formula	445/396 g	na	32.2	14.1	0.02	na	1.3	0.9	1.4:1
Royal Canin Veterinary Diet Development Formula	430/396 g	4.6	31.8	19.6	na	40.4	1.45	1.2	1.2:1

Key: ME = metabolizable energy, Ca = calcium, P = phosphorus, Ca:P = calcium-phosphorus ratio, na = information not available from manufacturer, g = grams, DHA = docosahexaenoic acid.

*From manufacturers' published information or calculated from manufacturers' published as-fed values; all values are on a dry matter basis unless otherwise stated. Digestibility: Foods with higher energy density are more likely to have higher digestibility. Foods for most breeding males and females are usually similar to those for young and middle-aged adults (Table 13-4).

**Energy density values are listed on an as fed basis and are useful for determining the amount to feed; cup = 8-oz. measuring cup. To convert to kJ, multiply kcal by 4.184.

tion of young dogs (Bauer et al, 2006, 2006a). Because milk concentrations of DHA parallel dietary intake, it seems prudent to include DHA in foods fed to lactating bitches. Common ingredients such as fish and poultry meal are sources of DHA in foods for reproducing bitches. Foods for late gestation and peak lactation should contain the minimum recommended allowance of DHA plus eicosapentaenoic acid (EPA) of at least 0.05% (DM) (NRC, 2006). Therefore, DHA needs to be at least 40% of the total DHA plus EPA, or 0.02% DM.

Carbohydrate

Technically the term "carbohydrate" includes digestible (soluble) carbohydrates (mono-, di- and polysaccharides such as starch and glycogen) and dietary fiber. This chapter refers to digestible carbohydrates. Feeding a carbohydrate-free food to pregnant bitches may result in weight loss, decreased food intake, reduced birth weight and neonatal survival of the puppies and may increase the risk of stillbirth (**Table 15-1**) (Romsos et al, 1981; Kienzle et al, 1985; Kienzle and Meyer, 1989). Because more than 50% of the energy for fetal development is supplied by glucose (Romsos et al, 1981), bitches have a high metabolic requirement for glucose during the last weeks of gestation. Feeding a carbohydrate-free food to pregnant bitches increases the risk of hypoglycemia and ketosis during late pregnancy. Furthermore, the lactose concentration in the milk may decrease by 40% during peak lactation (Romsos et al, 1981; Kienzle et al, 1985; Kienzle and Meyer, 1989) (**Box 15-1**).

Providing approximately 20% of the energy from carbohydrate is sufficient to prevent the negative side effects of a carbohydrate-free diet (Kienzle et al, 1985; Kienzle and Meyer,

Box 15-1. Periparturient Hypoglycemia.

Clinical hypoglycemia (i.e., glucose values <45 mg/dl or 2.5 mmol/l) occurs infrequently in bitches, but when it develops it is usually observed during the last two to three weeks of gestation. Neurologic signs of hypoglycemia predominate, and differentiation from eclampsia is not always easy. Elevated levels of serum ketones (mainly β-hydroxybutyrate) are characteristic in bitches with clinical disease; however, ketonemia may be missed when strips or tablets containing nitroprusside are used to detect ketones. Nitroprusside primarily detects acetone and acetoacetate.

Risk factors that may predispose bitches to this syndrome include: 1) poor body condition during pregnancy, 2) malnutrition and 3) feeding a high-fat, carbohydrate-free food. If a carbohydrate-free food is fed, gluconeogenic precursors such as protein should be increased by at least 50% when energy requirements are moderate and may have to be doubled if the energy requirement of the dam is high.

Treatment of clinical hypoglycemia during pregnancy should consist of intravenous administration of a bolus of 20 to 50% glucose solution, which can be followed by intravenous infusion of a 5% glucose solution at a rate of 2 ml/kg body weight/hour. During or soon after the infusion, a palatable food should be provided that has adequate carbohydrate, protein and calories (**Table 15-5**) and has above average digestibility (**Table 15-9**).

The Bibliography for **Box 15-1** can be found at www.markmorris.org.

1989). If no carbohydrate is given, protein intake must almost be doubled; the food must provide at least 12 to 13 g digestible protein/$BW_{kg}^{0.75}$ (Gesellshaft, 1989b; Kienzle et al, 1985; Kienzle and Meyer, 1989). In a study in which a food that had about 50% DM protein was fed, no problems with hypoglycemia or ketosis resulted and puppies were born healthy (Blaza et al, 1989). These protein levels are very high and may cause soft, foul-smelling stools (Paquin, 1979). Providing approximately 20% of the energy from carbohydrate translates to about 23% DM carbohydrate. Foods for gestation should contain at least 23% DM digestible carbohydrate.

When lactating bitches are fed foods without digestible carbohydrates, the lactose level in the milk may decrease to about 2% vs. the normal range of 3 to 3.5% (Romsos et al, 1981; Kienzle et al, 1985). In one study, increasing the digestible carbohydrate level in the food corrected low lactose levels; however, the same effect was not achieved by increasing protein levels (Kienzle et al, 1985). Therefore, these and other investigators recommend that foods for lactation provide at least 10 to 20% of the energy intake in the form of digestible carbohydrate to support normal lactose production (Leibetseder, 1989; Kienzle et al, 1985). Foods for bitches during lactation should also contain at least 23% DM digestible carbohydrate.

Calcium and Phosphorus

For most breeds, during the first two trimesters of gestation, calcium and phosphorus needs are similar to those for maintenance of young adults (0.5 to 1.0% DM calcium and 0.4 to 0.7% DM phosphorus: Ca-P ratio 1:1 to 1.5:1). During the last part of gestation, requirements for calcium and phosphorus roughly increase by 60% because of rapid skeletal growth of the fetuses (Gesellshaft, 1989c; Meyer et al, 1985a). The minimum recommended allowance for calcium in foods intended for late gestation and peak lactation is 0.8% (DM) (NRC, 2006). The AAFCO minimum allowance is 1% (2007). As occurs with some dairy cows, excessive calcium intake during pregnancy may decrease activity of the parathyroid glands and predispose the bitch to eclampsia during lactation (Smith, 1986; Drazner, 1987). Therefore, it has been recommended for most breeds to feed a food during pregnancy that avoids large excesses of calcium (1.0 to 1.7% DM) and has a calcium-phosphorus ratio of 1.1:1 to 2:1 (**Box 15-2**). The range for phosphorus should be from 0.7 to 1.3% (DM). These amounts are also recommended for giant-breed bitches.

Mineral requirements during lactation are determined by mineral excretion in milk (Meyer, 1982) and thus by the number of nursing puppies. A definite increase in calcium content is seen over the course of lactation; however, the calcium-phosphorus ratio is consistently maintained around 1.3:1 (Meyer et al, 1985). This is reflected by the fact that even without clinical eclampsia, plasma calcium levels tend to decrease during the third and fourth week of lactation (Meyer et al, 1985a). Bitches need two to five times more calcium during peak lactation than for adult maintenance (Meyer, 1982, 1990a) (**Box 15-2**). Depending on the number of puppies, bitches need 250 to 500 mg calcium and 175 to 335 mg of phosphorus/kg body weight per day (Gesellschaft, 1989c). One investigator recommended that a food for lactation contain at least 0.8 to 1.1% calcium and 0.6 to 0.8% phosphorus (Leibetseder, 1989); however, reducing these needs by 10 to 20% will not necessarily lead to disturbances in milk mineral content. The recommended range for calcium during gestation and lactation is 1.0 to 1.7% and the corresponding recommended range for phosphorus is 0.7 to 1.3% (DM), respectively. The calcium-phosphorus ratio should be 1.1:1 to 2:1. Calcium supplementation is not recommended during gestation or lactation when appropriately balanced commercial foods are fed.

Digestibility

Nutrients in foods should be highly available due to the considerable nutritional demands associated with late gestation and lactation. Apparent digestibility is the difference between the amount of food ingested and that excreted in feces. During late gestation, the ability to ingest adequate amounts of food may exceed food intake capacity, especially if the food is poorly digestible. Therefore, it is important to assess digestibility and recommend foods with above average digestibility for the reproductive process.

Digestibility information for commercial foods marketed for reproduction is not readily available. However, energy density is an indirect indicator of digestibility. Foods that have an energy

Box 15-2. Eclampsia in the Bitch.

Eclampsia is an acute, life-threatening condition due to a sudden decrease in extracellular calcium concentration. Bitches are at highest risk for developing eclampsia (puerperal tetany) during Weeks 2 and 3 of lactation when calcium losses via secretion in milk are highest. Eclampsia is less common during Weeks 1 and 4 of lactation, and is seen rarely in the last two weeks of gestation. Occasionally, bitches may be affected at or just before whelping.

The number of nursing puppies is the most important stimulus for milk production; therefore, it is not surprising that eclampsia is seen commonly in bitches nursing large litters. Typically, affected bitches are primipara, are less than four years of age, are toy-breed dogs and have low body weight-to-litter size ratio. Investigators have suggested that toy breeds may be more predisposed to developing eclampsia than large breeds because toy breeds tend to receive more meat-based homemade foods, which are low in calcium. Serum total calcium and ionized calcium concentrations usually are decreased. Serum total calcium concentration is an insensitive measure of ionized calcium concentration. Ionized calcium is the biologically active form. In-hospital serum chemistry analyzers and point-of-care analyzers allow veterinarians to obtain serum total calcium and ionized calcium concentrations rapidly. Diagnosis of hypocalcemia is based on low serum ionized calcium concentrations. Serum ionized calcium concentrations were <0.8 mmol/l (reference range, 1.13 to 1.33 mmol/l) in a retrospective study of eclampsia in the bitch. Other causes of clinical signs typical of hypocalcemia should be considered if the serum ionized calcium concentration is >0.8 mmol/l.

Although most bitches with eclampsia are hypocalcemic, some may be normocalcemic. Some bitches with hypocalcemia, on the other hand, may not exhibit clinical signs. Typical clinical signs are anxiety, panting, whining, hypersalivation, vomiting, ataxia, stiff gait, muscle tremors, tetany and seizures. Other signs include hyperthermia, tachycardia and death, if the condition is untreated. However, clinical signs vary, based on the degree of hypocalcemia and the time over which it develops.

Lack of clinical signs may indicate that factors other than hypocalcemia determine whether tetany manifests clinically or not. The bitch may have additional serum biochemical abnormalities. Blood glucose should be measured, because hypoglycemia may be present concurrently. Magnesium levels in bitches with eclampsia may be low or normal. The ratio of serum total magnesium to total calcium may be significantly lower in affected bitches than in normal bitches. Hyperkalemia has been reported and some bitches may have abnormal serum phosphorus concentrations (either hypophosphatemia or hyperphosphatemia). Further study is needed about the role of other serum biochemical abnormalities in the clinical signs of eclampsia. The incorporation of magnesium into the treatment and prevention of the disorder should be evaluated.

Hypocalcemia leads to increased neuromuscular irritability resulting in restlessness and whining, stiffness of gait, ataxia and tonic-clonic seizures. Decrease in extracellular calcium ion levels leads to increased permeability of nerve cells (primarily of peripheral nerves) to sodium ions. Neuromuscular irritability is directly proportional to:

$$[Na^+] \times [K^+] \div [Ca^{++}] \times [Mg^{++}] \times [H^+]$$

Suggested causes of hypocalcemia during the periparturient period include calcium supplementation during pregnancy, poor dietary calcium and loss of calcium through fetal skeletal ossification and lactation. High calcium intake may down-regulate parathyroid gland secretion and impair normal mobilization of calcium from skeletal stores. As demand for calcium increases during late gestation and lactation, calcium homeostasis is unable to maintain critical serum levels.

Slow intravenous infusion (over five to 10 minutes) of 10% calcium gluconate, administered to effect (1 to 2 mg calcium/kg body weight), results in rapid clinical improvement. Heart monitoring (e.g., auscultation, electrocardiography) should be performed during intravenous calcium gluconate infusion. If bradycardia or dysrhythmias develop, the infusion must be slowed or discontinued. In addition, body temperature should be monitored because hypothermia may occur following calcium gluconate administration. To lessen the risk of relapse, calcium may be injected subcutaneously or intramuscularly, in addition to the immediate intravenous infusion. However, subcutaneous injections may cause skin necrosis and should be administered only when other routes are inaccessible. Following correction of acute signs, the bitch should be provided with oral vitamin D and calcium supplementation (e.g., calcium carbonate, 100 mg/kg/day, divided with meals) throughout lactation.

If possible, puppies should be separated from the bitch for the first 24 hours of treatment and fed canine milk replacer by bottle or orogastric tube feeding. If tetany recurs during the same lactation, the puppies should be weaned. Administration of corticosteroids is contraindicated because they may further decrease plasma calcium levels.

Prevention of eclampsia starts during pregnancy by feeding a balanced food, without excess calcium and with a balanced calcium-phosphorus ratio. Foods with a calcium-phosphorus ratio close to 1:1 have been recommended during pregnancy. Vitamin D therapy (10,000 to 25,000 IU daily) during the last week of gestation has been proposed, just as cows are treated to prevent postparturient paresis. This approach may not be valid for bitches because eclampsia and the highest calcium losses generally do not occur immediately after whelping.

The Bibliography for **Box 15-2** can be found at www.markmorris.org.

density of 4 kcal ME/g (16.7 kJ/g) or higher have more fat and less fiber. Fat is typically highly digestible; fiber is poorly digestible. Thus, high-fat, low-fiber foods are usually more digestible.

Other Nutritional Factors

In addition to the key nutritional factors for commercial foods discussed above, the following nutritional factors are highlighted because they are of particular concern for homemade foods intended for reproducing dogs (Chapter 10).

Essential Fatty Acids

Homemade foods with rice and meat as the main ingredients may not provide enough essential fatty acids for lactation, and may need to be supplemented with vegetable oil (Meyer, 1990b).

Iron, Zinc and Copper

Requirements for most trace elements depend on litter size. Hematocrit, hemoglobin and plasma iron values often decrease in bitches near the end of gestation (Meyer et al, 1985a). Iron requirements are particularly high during the last week of gestation, when large quantities are stored in the liver of the fetuses, and mobilized from the bitch's body for colostrum (Meyer et al, 1985a). Colostrum is very rich in iron; however, levels decrease within 48 hours (Meyer et al, 1985a). Iron concentrations are low in mature milk. Because of this, iron requirements increase only slightly during lactation when compared with adult maintenance requirements (Gesellshaft, 1989d). Therefore, neonates must have an iron reserve to overcome the initial three-week nursing period, when milk is the only source of food (Meyer et al, 1985a). Latent iron deficiency may impair neutrophil phagocytic function and cell-mediated immunity, increasing susceptibility to infections (Bhaskaram, 1988). The minimum recommended allowance for iron is 70 mg/kg (DM) (NRC, 2006). Oxides of iron should not be used as an iron source because they are poorly available (NRC, 2006).

During periods when requirements for tissue synthesis are greater than normal (e.g., pregnancy, lactation and growth), animals are particularly susceptible to zinc deficiency. Most commercial foods provide adequate zinc. However, if zinc deficiency does occur during pregnancy, it may lead to fetal resorption or fewer, less viable offspring (Fletcher et al, 1988). The minimum recommended allowance for zinc during gestation/lactation is 96 mg/kg (DM) (NRC, 2006).

Copper is an integral constituent of enzymes that catalyze oxidation reactions and plays an important role in connective tissue formation via lysyl oxidase. It is involved in hematopoiesis because it is a constituent of ferroxidases. It is also a cofactor of superoxide dismutase and thus helps protect against oxidative stress. There are numerous sources of copper but oxides of copper should not be used because they are poorly available (NRC, 2006). The minimum recommended allowance for copper is 12.4 mg/kg DM (NRC, 2006). Copper needs during gestation/lactation increase disproportionately to increased energy needs (Gesellshaft, 1989d).

Phenylalanine and Tyrosine

Tyrosine is not an essential amino acid but is made from phenylalanine. However, tyrosine in adequate amounts spares about half of the need for phenylalanine. Therefore, it is appropriate to consider the amount of phenylalanine required as the sum of phenylalanine plus tyrosine. Although phenylalanine and tyrosine are not thought to be the most limiting amino acids for growth in commercial foods, at least twice as much phenylalanine, or phenylalanine plus tyrosine, is required for maximal black hair color as for growth (NRC, 2006; Biourge and Serheraert, 2002). Other metabolic needs for phenylalanine and tyrosine include protein, thyroid hormone and catecholamine synthesis (NRC, 2006). The minimal recommended DM phenylalanine allowance for foods for bitches during late gestation/peak lactation is 0.83% and 1.23% DM for phenylalanine plus tyrosine (NRC, 2006). About one and one-half to two times this much tyrosine is required to maximize black hair color (NRC, 2006).

FEEDING PLAN

Generally, recommendations are based on information from populations of dogs at similar stages of reproduction. However, the feeding plan should be tailored to meet the needs of individual dogs based on unique variations in genetics, environment, litter size and health status. Information gleaned from the assessment step (i.e., patient, food and feeding method) sets the stage for developing the feeding plan; specifically which foods to feed and which feeding methods to use in providing the food.

Assess and Select the Food

Food assessment includes a comparison of the current food's levels of key nutritional factors with those recommended in **Table 15-5.** For convenience, **Table 15-9** compares the key nutritional factor content of selected commercial foods marketed for dogs during reproduction to the key nutritional factor targets determined above. Pet food labels usually lack information about carbohydrate content (other than crude fiber), digestibility, energy density and specific vitamins and minerals. If the food in question is not listed in **Table 15-9**, it may be necessary to contact the manufacturer for information.

The food should also be approved by a credible regulatory agency to ensure it will support gestation and lactation (i.e., AAFCO or equivalent). This information should be listed on the product label. The food assessment step determines the appropriateness of the current food. Food selection involves choosing the food that most closely fits the key nutritional factor recommendations. If a food change is warranted, gradually transition the bitch to the new food over several days as described in Chapter 1.

Oftentimes foods marketed for gestation/lactation are also growth-type foods. Thus, they can be referred to as growth/reproduction-type foods. Generally, foods for non-reproducing sexually intact adult dogs (Table 13-4) will suffice for the first four weeks of gestation (Gesellshaft, 1989a). However, it is probably best to feed a growth/reproduction food throughout gestation, particularly for giant breeds. This recommendation also negates the need for a food change during mid- to late-gestation. Lactation represents an extreme test of a food's nutritional adequacy, because no other physiologic endeavor, other than extreme exercise, requires such a marked increase in energy density and nutrient content (Lewis et al,

1987). The nutrient demands are directly related to the dam's ability to produce milk. Because nutritional requirements for lactation increase markedly over a relatively short period of time, it is very important to provide the correct food. A more appropriate food should be selected if food assessment indicates inadequacies or if lactation performance is suboptimal. Lactating bitches are best fed commercial foods.

Dry foods are more nutrient dense, as fed, and have higher levels of carbohydrates than moist foods. These foods may benefit bitches experiencing weight loss and those spending little time eating. Conversely, moist foods are often higher in fat and provide additional water to support lactation. The added water also improves palatability so bitches may be more likely to eat. Because both food types have advantages, many breeders choose to feed both forms during gestation and lactation.

Assess and Determine the Feeding Method

Breeding Males

Some males in heavy service may have decreased food consumption and lose weight. If weight loss is a problem in reproducing males, the amount of food provided should be increased or a more energy-dense food should be fed to help maintain body condition, provided other causes of weight loss have been ruled out.

Bitches

For females, it has been recommended to increase food intake by 5 to 10% above maintenance levels at the time of proestrus, and to reduce the amount back to maintenance levels after mating; a practice known as flushing (Sheffy, 1978). The purpose of flushing is to optimize conception and litter size. However, flushing is unnecessary for a bitch in good body condition (Nguyen and Dumon, 1988). Because no specific nutritional differences exist for this particular stage of reproduction, feeding methods recommended for young adult dogs are adequate during estrus (Chapter 13).

If a bitch is underfed before breeding and in poor body condition (BCS <2/5), it may be prudent to postpone mating and bring the bitch into good body condition for the next breeding. If breeding cannot be postponed, the bitch should be fed a growth/reproduction-type food, such as those listed in **Table 15-9**, in sufficient quantities to improve body condition throughout gestation (Meyer, 1990). During estrus, bitches tend to have a depressed appetite; therefore, a 17% decrease in food intake can be expected during peak estrus (Houpt et al, 1979; Bebiak et al, 1987). Occasional vomiting may occur in bitches due to hormonal changes, nervousness, travel and environmental changes associated with mating. To reduce these problems, it may be better to feed small meals or not to feed the bitch at all immediately before or after mating (Bebiak et al, 1987).

During the first two-thirds of gestation, bitches are usually fed the same amount of energy as intact adult dogs (approximately 1.8 x RER). This amount is increased to approximately 3.0 x RER during the last three weeks of gestation. Energy intake may need to be increased further to maintain normal body condition in some dogs, especially larger breeds.

During the third or fourth week of gestation, bitches commonly experience a decrease in appetite that may result in up to a 30% reduction in food intake (Lewis et al, 1987; Bebiak et al, 1987; Schroeder and Smith, 1995). This decrease may be due to the effect of embryo implantation, which starts around 20 days of pregnancy (**Figure 15-1**) (Schroeder and Smith, 1995).

Because overfeeding during gestation may have similar negative effects as underfeeding, it is recommended that small- and medium-sized bitches be meal fed. One or two meals per day will suffice for most bitches during the first half of pregnancy. At least two meals per day should be provided in the last half of pregnancy (Meyer, 1990). Giant breeds may need to be fed free choice (Zentek and Meyer, 1992). Bitches pregnant with a large litter may also need to be fed free choice because of abdominal fill. Restriction of food during gestation may lead to smaller litter size, lower birth weights and may compromise the subsequent lactation (Mosier, 1977).

As with gestation, a lactating bitch's nutrient needs are met by a combination of the nutrient levels in the food and the amount fed. Even if the food has an appropriate nutrient profile, significant undernutrition may result if the bitch is fed an insufficient amount. If the bitch maintains normal body condition (BCS 2.5/5 to 3.5/5) and the puppies are growing at a normal rate, then the amount being fed is probably appropriate. The amount to feed can be estimated either by calculation (Chapter 1) or by referring to feeding guides on product labels. As a rough estimate, bitches should ingest their DER + 25% of their DER for each nursing puppy. During peak lactation, a bitch's energy needs may be three to four times greater than its requirements for adult maintenance.

The amount fed during lactation is usually offered either three times per day or free choice. In practice, it is best to feed bitches free choice during lactation (Lewis et al, 1987), except when the bitch has only one puppy and may have a tendency to gain weight. Free-choice feeding is especially important for lactating bitches with more than four puppies (Meyer et al, 1985). Some bitches are nervous throughout lactation and free-choice feeding will allow them to eat on their schedule. Meal-fed lactating bitches should receive at least three meals daily (Lewis et al, 1987; Leibetseder, 1989). Puppies may begin to eat the bitch's food at three weeks of age; therefore, it is important to allow them access to the food. **Table 15-10** summarizes the feeding plan discussed above for reproducing dogs.

Before and during weaning, restricting the food intake of the bitch may help prevent excessive mammary gland distention and discomfort associated with abrupt weaning. Reducing the amount of food fed to the bitch will help decrease lactation. On Day 1 of the weaning process, separate the bitch from the puppies and withhold food but allow the puppies to eat their weaning food. Reunite the bitch and puppies that night and remove all food. Take the puppies away from the bitch again on Day 2. However, this time they are not returned at the end of the day; and at this point they are considered weaned. Also on Day 2, feed the bitch about one-fourth of the amount fed before breeding. Over the next three to four days, gradually increase

Table 15-10. Feeding plan summary for reproducing dogs.

1. For gestating and lactating bitches, use **Table 15-9** to select a food with the appropriate levels of key nutritional factors; for breeding males, use Table 13-4. For foods in neither table, contact manufacturers for key nutritional factor content.
2. The selected food should be approved by a credible regulatory agency (e.g., Association of American Feed Control Officials).
3. Determine an appropriate feeding method (Table 13-5). Free-choice feeding is the preferred method for feeding bitches during late gestation and lactation; food-restricted meal feeding may be best for breeding males.
4. For food-restricted meal feeding, estimate the initial quantity of food based on daily energy requirement (DER) calculation (DER ÷ food energy density).
5. DER is calculated by multiplying resting energy requirement (RER) (Table 5-2) by an appropriate factor. Remember, DER calculations are estimates and should be used as guidelines or starting points for amounts to feed individual dogs and not as absolute requirements; the amount fed should be refined by monitoring body condition score and weight.
   Gestation = 1.8 to 2.0 x RER for the first four weeks, then 2.2 to 3.5 x RER for the last five weeks
   Lactation = 4.0 to 8.0 x RER (peak lactation: 2.1 x RER + 25% per puppy) or use Method 1 (**Table 15-7**)
6. At the end of lactation, bitches should be fed for weaning as described in Box 16-5.
7. Monitor body condition, body weight, general health, reproductive performance and puppy growth rates to adjust the feeding plan.

the amount fed to the bitch until by Day 5 or so, the prebreeding amount (maintenance) is fed. Leaving one or two puppies to nurse will not alleviate mammary gland engorgement in bitches that are still producing a large amount of milk at weaning. This practice continues to stimulate milk production, and therefore prolongs the problem. When it is decided to completely separate the puppies from the bitch, all puppies should be taken away at once. Chapter 16 provides more information regarding weaning.

REASSESSMENT

In general, breeding dogs should be reassessed before every estrous cycle in which a pregnancy is planned. Breeders should be encouraged to present reproducing bitches for a checkup at least a month before the upcoming estrus. Problems detected by the assessment still may be corrected before breeding. See the young adult section for assessment methods (Chapter 13).

There are two occasions during pregnancy when owners should present a bitch for assessment by a veterinarian. The first time is to confirm pregnancy with ultrasonography between 17 to 20 days after breeding, or by palpation between 25 to 36 days after breeding (Wallace and Davidson, 1995; Yeager and Concannon, 1995). A thorough physical examination should be conducted at the first visit. The owner should be encouraged to present the bitch again one week before parturition, or earlier if an abnormality is found during the first checkup. In addition to another physical examination, the following parameters should be assessed at the second checkup: a complete blood count and serum glucose, calcium and total protein concentrations.

The bitch should receive a veterinary checkup around the third or fourth week of lactation. This evaluation should include a physical examination with special attention given to mammary glands and body condition.

During lactation, owners should be advised to carefully observe the bitch and litter. Although experienced breeders usually are good observers, they still should be reminded to look for signs of impending problems. Owners should consult their veterinarian if the bitch's food intake decreases or an abnormal vaginal discharge develops. Other signs that should prompt veterinary care include hypersalivation, muscle contractions, seizures and/or weakness. Poor quality maternal care is another reason for owners to consult their veterinarian. Rectal temperature and mammary gland health should be evaluated regularly (Wallace and Davidson, 1995).

Body weight gain by puppies during early lactation provides an indication of milk production by the bitch (quantity and quality) and milk intake by puppies. Failure to gain weight for more than one day or continuous vocalization may indicate that the quantity or quality of milk production is insufficient due to mastitis, agalactia or inadequate nutrition.

Body condition scoring is an important tool to assess nutritional adequacy. Breeders can easily be taught how to assess and score body condition. A bitch should not lose more than 5% of body weight during the first month of lactation, and optimal body weight should again be reached within a month after lactation ceases (Grandjean and Paragon, 1986; Wolter, 1982). BCS should be maintained around 3/5 throughout lactation, otherwise adjustments should be made in the food or feeding method, assuming other potential causes of weight loss are ruled out.

REFERENCES

The references for **Chapter 15** can be found at www.markmorris.org.

CASE 15-1

Weight Loss in a Lactating Great Dane Bitch

Jacques Debraekeleer, DVM
Hill's Science and Technology Center
Etten Leur, The Netherlands

Kathy L. Gross, PhD
Hill's Science and Technology Center
Topeka, Kansas, USA

Patient Assessment

A five-year-old Great Dane bitch was examined for weight loss. The dog was in its fourth week of lactation and was nursing 11 puppies. Although most of the puppies grew according to breed expectations, three had slightly lower body weights. Delivery had been uneventful.

Physical examination revealed an underweight dog (body condition score 2/5) with no vaginal discharge or other abnormalities. The bitch currently weighed 59 kg but weighed 65 kg before the pregnancy. The mammary glands were well developed with no signs of inflammation.

A complete blood count and serum biochemistry profile were performed. Serum albumin (2.5 g/dl, normal 2.4 to 3.5 g/dl) and serum calcium (9.0 mg/dl, normal 9 to 11.8 mg/dl) concentrations were low normal. The other biochemical parameters were within normal ranges. The hemoglobin concentration (11.8 g/dl, normal 12 to 18 g/dl), packed cell volume (32%, normal 37 to 55%) and total erythrocyte count (5.13 million/ml, normal 5.5 to 8.5 million/µl) were slightly below normal.

Assess the Food and Feeding Method

The owners reported that the bitch's appetite was voracious. The dog was fed twice daily; early in the morning before the owners went to work and in the evening when they returned home. The bitch received a commercial grocery brand dry food that the owners had fed for several years. The owners were feeding 15 cups (90 g/cup) twice daily; they commented that this seemed like a large amount of food. One cup of low-fat (2%) milk was poured over the food at each meal.

The manufacturer was contacted and provided the following information about the dry matter (DM) nutrient content of the food: crude protein 19.6%, crude fat 11.4%, carbohydrate (nitrogen-free extract [NFE]) 58.0%, crude fiber 3.45%, ash 7.6%, calcium 1.65%, phosphorus 1.23% and sodium 0.48%. The energy density was 3.4 kcal metabolizable energy (ME) (15.5 kJ)/g of food, as fed.

Questions

1. How should this patient's laboratory results be interpreted?
2. What are the key nutritional factors for a lactating bitch with a large litter?
3. What are the caloric requirements of the patient?
4. What feeding method should be recommended for this dog?
5. What other management techniques should be used with this bitch and its puppies?

Answers and Discussion

1. Normal pregnancy and lactation can affect canine hematologic values. Mild decreases in hemoglobin concentration, packed cell volume and total erythrocyte count occur during late gestation and lactation. These values should return to normal within several weeks after lactation ceases. Profound changes in hematologic values in pregnant and lactating bitches signal serious malnutrition and/or concurrent disease. The low normal serum albumin and calcium concentrations in this Great Dane bitch are not of immediate concern but may indicate marginal protein and calcium intake. Serum albumin has a long half-life in dogs (approximately eight days); therefore, serum albumin concentrations may not reflect changes over the last one to two weeks. Bitches with large litters secrete large quantities of calcium into the milk during peak lactation (Weeks 3 and 4 of lactation). Thus, serum calcium concentrations may be low normal to mildly decreased.
2. Key nutritional factors for lactating bitches include water, energy, protein, carbohydrate, fat, calcium, phosphorus and food digestibility. Water is needed in large quantities to produce milk. A 60-kg bitch nursing a large litter may require 10 to 11 liters of water per day during peak lactation. Energy requirements steadily increase after whelping and peak between three and five weeks at levels two to four times higher than the daily energy requirement (DER) of non-lactating young adult dogs. Foods for lactating large-breed dogs should provide at least 18% DM fat and 4.0 to 5.0 kcal ME (16.7 to 21 kJ)/g DM. During lactation, the requirements for calcium and protein increase more rapidly than the energy requirements. Generally, foods containing 25 to

35% DM crude protein and 1.0 to 1.6% DM calcium are adequate. Lactose concentrations in milk decrease when lactating bitches are fed foods without digestible carbohydrates. Food should provide at least 10 to 20% of energy intake in the form of carbohydrate to support normal milk lactose production. Because of the considerable nutritional demands associated with lactation, nutrients in the food should be highly available. Foods with above average digestibility are recommended for lactating dogs.

3. Energy requirements for lactating dogs can be subdivided into energy for maintenance and energy used for milk production. The DER, without allotment for milk production, may be slightly higher than that for average young adult dogs because of stress and increased activity associated with caring for puppies. The maintenance portion of the DER for lactating dogs has been estimated to be approximately 1.9 x resting energy requirement (RER). As a rough estimate, at peak lactation the bitch will need an additional 25% of this amount for each puppy. This amount should be adjusted based on body weight changes and body condition assessment. For this bitch, energy for maintenance at ideal body weight would be approximately 1.9 x RER (65 kg body weight) = 3,000 kcal (12.6 MJ). Energy for peak milk production (11 puppies) would be an additional 8,250 kcal (34.7 MJ). The total DER = 11,250 kcal (47.3 MJ). The bitch was currently being fed approximately 9,180 kcal (38.6 MJ) from the food plus 240 kcal (1 MJ) from the supplemental milk for a total of 9,420 kcal (39.6 MJ) per day. The estimated daily deficit is 1,830 kcal (7.7 MJ) vs. the calculated DER.
4. In general, lactating dogs should be offered food free choice. Meal feeding several times a day may be sufficient for smaller dogs or dogs with small litters.
5. The puppies should be introduced to food as soon as possible. A warm gruel prepared from moist or blended dry commercial foods formulated for canine growth should be used and can be offered several times daily to the puppies. This feeding plan will relieve the physical and nutritional stress on the bitch and begin the transition to solid food for the puppies.

Progress Notes

The bitch's food was changed to a commercial, dry specialty brand product (Science Diet Puppy Healthy Development Original[a]) that was higher in energy density (3.94 kcal [16.48 kJ]/g as fed) than the current food. This food also had appropriate levels of other key nutritional factors. The food and fresh, clean water were offered free choice and the milk was discontinued. Approximately 24 cups of the growth/lactation food would provide the estimated DER for peak lactation. The owners were also instructed to prepare a warm gruel for the puppies using the moist formulation of the product several times daily.

Three weeks later the owners returned with the bitch and six puppies that had not yet been sold. The puppies had been completely weaned the previous week and were now eating the dry growth formula for large-breed puppies. The bitch weighed 63.5 kg and appeared normal. The owners were encouraged to slowly change the bitch's food back to the original dry food for maintenance of young adult dogs over the next week. The DER was estimated to be 1.8 x RER at an ideal weight of 65 kg, which equals 2,850 kcal (12 MJ) or nine to 10 cups of food per day.

Endnote

a. Hill's Pet Nutrition, Inc., Topeka, KS, USA.

Bibliography

Gesellschaft für Ernährungsphysiologie. Empfehlungen für die Versorgung mit Mengenelementen. In: Ausschuß für Bedarfsnormen der Gesellschaft für Ernährungsphysiologie Energie- und Nährstoffbedarf/Energy and Nutrient Requirements, No. 5 Hunde/Dogs. Frankfurt/Main, Germany: DLG Verlag, 1989; 56-72.

Kaneko JJ. Appendices. In: Clinical Biochemistry of Domestic Animals, 4th ed. San Diego, CA: Academic Press Inc, 1989; 877-901.

Chapter 16

Feeding Nursing and Orphaned Puppies from Birth to Weaning

Jacques Debraekeleer
Kathy L. Gross
Steven C. Zicker

"Happiness is a warm puppy."
Charles M. Schulz

INTRODUCTION

Compared with the young of other species, newborn puppies are relatively immature at birth. For example, their skeletons have a low degree of mineralization (Meyer and Stadtfeld, 1980; Meyer et al, 1985). Large-breed puppies are less mature than small-breed puppies, which may be one of the reasons why they are more susceptible to malnutrition and developmental orthopedic diseases during the rapid growth phase.

Growing puppies progress through three critical phases in the first 12 months of life, during which nutrition is essential for survival and healthy development.

- A nursing period during which the transition is made from in utero nutrition to postpartum nutrition. This period is largely influenced by the nutrition of the bitch during gestation and early lactation. This chapter focuses on feeding nursing and orphaned puppies.
- A weaning period, which is very stressful due to changes in food and environment. The transition from bitch's milk to solid food for further growth must therefore be handled properly. Because weaning overlaps with the nursing period, it is also covered in this chapter.
- A postweaning period that occurs from two to 12 months of age and is a critical time for development. Proper feeding during this period is especially critical for large- and giant-breed puppies because nutrition has proved to be the most important non-genetic factor for healthy bone development. Chapter 17 covers postweaning feeding of growing puppies.

Before weaning, mortality may be as high as 10 to 30%, with two-thirds of the deaths occurring during the first week of life (Pibot and Jean-Blain, 1989; Lawler and Evans, 1989). Three factors are critical to successful transition from fetal life to the nursing period: 1) the bitch's nutrition during gestation and early lactation, 2) the bitch's behavior and physical health and 3) provision of good neonatal care (husbandry practices) by the owner.

Puppies are considered orphaned if they lack sufficient maternal care for survival from birth to weaning. Several physiologic needs normally provided by the bitch must be met to ensure survival of neonates: heat, humidity, nutrition, immunity, elimination, sanitation, security and social stimulation. A foster bitch or the caregiver must meet these needs for orphaned puppies. Most orphans can be raised successfully with proper care and nutrition.

Box 16-1. Puppy Behavior from Birth to 12 Weeks of Age.

Three phases of puppy behavior are described during the first 12 weeks of life:
- Neonatal period: From whelping to when the eyes open at about 13 days of age.
- Transition period: From when the eyes open to three weeks of age.
- Socialization period: From three weeks of age to weaning.

NEONATAL PERIOD

A newborn puppy has two basic activities: sleeping and nursing. Puppies quickly learn to find the bitch's teats when the bitch lies down for nursing. Nursing should be vigorous and active, and after nursing, the puppy's abdomen should be enlarged. Following nursing, puppies usually return to sleep. Neonates spend more than 80% of their time sleeping. However, a healthy puppy never sleeps deeply and quietly. Involuntary muscle contractions such as jerks and twitches (especially of the facial muscles) and irregular respiration are common. This pattern of activity is called "activated sleep" and should not be mistaken for shivering, a reflex that is not operant until about seven days of age. A puppy sleeping without these movements may be ill and should be observed closely. Puppies start crying when hungry or away from the litter; however, healthy puppies will stop crying soon and sleep again, even without nursing. Weak puppies may also have an enlarged abdomen but are restless and continue to vocalize. Such vocalizing is a constant high-pitched crying and is different from the crying of healthy puppies when they are hungry.

TRANSITION PERIOD

Puppies become more responsive to their environment as they become older. They no longer cry consistently when hungry or separated from littermates, but will cry when placed in an unfamiliar environment, even if warm and fed. Puppies begin to respond to visual stimuli when their eyes open. Puppies first start to play fight, clumsily pawing and mouthing at one another during this period. Tail wagging also occurs.

The first teeth may begin to erupt during the third week of life. Puppies lose the need for perineal stimulation to eliminate. Sucking on objects other than the bitch's nipples progressively decreases. By the end of the transition period puppies begin to lap liquids. A gruel or milk replacer should be presented in a bowl or saucer at this time; ground meat or thick gruels can be handfed.

SOCIALIZATION PERIOD

After a puppy can see and hear, it begins more active social interactions with its dam, littermates and people. Social bonds are formed and social hierarchies are begun. The critical period for socialization lasts until about 12 weeks, and exposure to people and other dogs is essential. Puppies achieve the full-grown dog form of locomotion, although they are still clumsy and have little endurance. Play fighting among puppies becomes a predominant behavior during this period. Eruption of deciduous teeth is complete by the first half of this period. Puppies no longer eliminate reflexively when the perineum is stimulated and they leave the nest box to do so. During the socialization period, puppies develop the ability to lap liquids well and are able to eat solid foods. The dam becomes less tolerant to nursing.

The Bibliography for **Box 16-1** can be found at www.markmorris.org.

PATIENT ASSESSMENT

History

When raising puppies, owners should be encouraged to maintain a logbook that may provide important information about the health and nutritional status of the puppies and dam. Owners should record birth weights of the puppies followed by their body weights every one to two days for the first four weeks of life, which also helps with socialization. Changes in behavior and other indicators of health such as opening of eyes, eruption of teeth, consistency of feces and food intake should also be recorded. **Box 16-1** provides a brief review of normal behavior for nursing puppies. **Table 16-1** lists normal physiologic values for neonatal puppies. Puppies should be identified in some manner (e.g., with a colored collar, nail polish, etc.) to facilitate easy recognition (**Box 16-2**).

Physical Examination

The goal of a physical examination is to assess indicators of impaired health that may reveal serious metabolic perturbations such as hypoglycemia, hypothermia and dehydration. Special attention should be paid to assessing puppy behavior, environmental conditions and hygiene. These parameters are important markers/risk factors for potential health problems. However, because puppies depend on bitch's milk during the neonatal period, assessment must always include a thorough evaluation of the health and maternal behavior of the bitch.

The most important areas of evaluation of nursing puppies are assessment of body weight and condition (especially with respect to temporal changes), body temperature and other physical parameters.

Orphaned puppies should be thoroughly evaluated when first seen. A careful physical examination of neonates and the bitch, if available, should be performed to detect the potential cause for abandonment. Particular attention should be given to detect common problems such as hypothermia, hypoglycemia, dehydration and congenital defects. The nutritional and hydration status should also be noted.

Body Weight

Low birth weight is highly correlated to neonatal mortality. Low birth weight puppies are particularly prone to hypoglycemia and sepsis, and are less likely to survive without special care. **Table 16-2** provides birth weights for selected dog breeds. Nursing puppies should be weighed daily or every other day on a gram scale. Monitoring the puppies' weight is a good way to evaluate the quality and quantity of milk the bitch is producing and the milk intake and health status of the puppies

Table 16-1. Normal physiologic values for neonatal puppies and data for neonatal care.

Birth weight	Individual	1-6.5% of mother's weight
	Total litter	12-14% of mother's weight
	BW at 8-10 days	2 x birth weight
Daily weight gain	Week 1	8% (5-10%)
	Weeks 2-4	5% (3.5-6%)
	Weeks 5-10	2 g/kg adult BW
	>10 weeks	2-4 g/kg adult BW
Body temperature	24 hr after birth	35.5 ± 0.8°C (96 ± 1.4°F)
	Weeks 1-2	34.5-37.2°C (94-99°F)
	Weeks 2-4	36.0-37.8°C (97-100°F)
	>4 weeks	37.8-38.3°C (97-101°F)
Heart rate	Weeks 1-2	230-240 beats/min.
	Weeks 3-4	210-220 beats/min.
	Weeks 5-6	195 beats/min.
	Week 7	185 beats/min.
	Weeks 8-12	165-175 beats/min.
Respiratory rate	At birth	15-35 breaths/min.
Shivering reflex develops	-	6-8 days
Eyes	Eyes open	10-14 days
	Visual following of moving objects	3-4 weeks
	Recognition of owner and mother	4-5 weeks
Ears	Open	12-17 days
	Reaction to auditory stimuli	3-4 weeks
Locomotion	Stepping movements with forelimbs	5-6 days
	Stepping movements with pelvic limbs	7-10 days
	Ability to stand	10 days
	Steady gait	3 weeks
	Walking and running	4 weeks
Micturition and defecation	Voluntary control	16-21 days
Activated sleep	Muscle tic disappears	4 weeks
Descent of testes	-	18-45 days
Urine specific gravity	-	1.006-1.007
Water requirement	-	180 (130-220) $ml/BW_{kg}/day$
Eating solid food	-	4-5 weeks
Deciduous teeth eruption	Incisors	3-4 weeks
	Canines	3 weeks
	Premolars	4-12 weeks
Permanent teeth eruption	Incisors	3-5 months
	Canines	4-6 months
	Premolars	4-6 months
	Molars	5-7 months
Body water	At birth	80%
Fat reserves	At birth	1-2%
	At 2 weeks	10%
	At 1 month	17%
	Non-obese adult dogs	22-23%

Key: BW = body weight, C = centigrade, F = Fahrenheit.

(**Box 16-3**). Puppies should neither lose weight nor fail to gain weight for more than one day. Loss or failure to gain weight in an individual puppy or the entire litter may indicate disease in the puppies or bitch, inadequate milk production or inability to suckle. It is essential to evaluate puppies' growth rate in relation to changes in behavior such as restlessness and continuous vocalization.

Body Temperature

When examining a puppy, the clinician should determine whether the puppy is warm. Neonates show a certain degree of poikilothermy during the first two weeks of life (Mosier, 1978), and have an extremely low amount of body fat (Rauchfuss, 1978). Therefore, it is vital for newborn puppies to eat and be kept in a warm environment. During the first week, the immediate environment of the puppies should be kept between 29 and 32°C (84 to 90°F). This means that the temperature in the room with the bitch and its litter should be maintained between 24 and 27°C (75 to 81°F). **Table 16-3** lists optimal environmental temperatures for orphaned puppies. Marginal hypothermia can often be detected by palpation of the lower limbs (**Box 16-4**). The behavior of the bitch may indicate whether a puppy is hypothermic or ill. A bitch may push a puppy away and neglect its cries when the puppy's skin temperature drops below a certain level (Mosier, 1978).

Box 16-2. General Husbandry Practices for Neonates.

Puppies should be housed in warm draft-free enclosures. Incubators are ideal, particularly for newborns. Pet carriers, shoeboxes or cardboard boxes are suitable substitutes. The bedding should be soft, absorbent and warm. Thread-free cloth, fleece and wood shavings are appropriate materials and help puppies feel secure as they snuggle into them.

Neonates demonstrate a certain degree of poikilothermy and are unable to regulate body temperature well during the first four weeks of life. Puppies huddle together close to the bitch, which generates an optimal microclimate, protects them against changes in environmental temperature and decreases the rate of heat loss. Orphans cannot seek protection near the bitch and are more sensitive to suboptimal environmental conditions.

Without the bitch, puppies can quickly become hypothermic, which leads to circulatory failure and death. Artificial heat should provide age-optimal environmental temperatures (**Table 16-3**). It is best to set the heating source to establish a gradation of heat in the nest box. A gradation of environmental temperatures allows neonates to move toward or away from the heat source as needed to avoid hyperthermia, which can be as detrimental as hypothermia. Puppies can rapidly become dehydrated secondary to overheating. Maintaining humidity near 50% helps reduce water loss and maintains the moisture and health of mucous membranes.

To fulfill non-nutritive nursing needs, hand-reared puppies often nurse other littermates in the nest box. To avoid skin trauma related to excessive nursing, puppies can be housed individually or separated by dividers. Although beneficial for alleviating problems due to non-nutritive nursing, separation of the litter reduces temperature and humidity in the immediate environment and social stimulation by littermates. Brief, but regular handling, provides social stimulation. The stress associated with regular handling may increase neural development and improve weight gain in puppies. Neonates raised without social stimulation develop abnormal behavior patterns (i.e., reduced normal exploratory behavior and neonates become more suspicious and aggressive as adults). Peer contact can compensate for maternal deprivation. Therefore, benefits of separating neonates must be weighed against the potential for development of abnormal behavior and increased risk for hypothermia. Puppies should interact with littermates as much as possible until weaning.

Puppies obtain passive systemic immunity from colostrum and passive local immunity from continued ingestion of bitch's milk. If possible, neonates should receive colostrum or bitch's milk within the first 12 to 16 hours of birth. This is particularly critical for puppies fed only milk replacers because they lack systemic and local immune protection.

Normally the bitch will sever the umbilical cord. If not, it should be cut to 1.5 in. (3.5 to 4 cm) and an appropriate topical antiseptic applied. Orphaned puppies are at greater risk for infectious diseases; thus, sanitary husbandry practices are important. To reduce risk for diseases, puppies should not be exposed to older animals or grouped within multiple litters. Feeding equipment and bedding should be kept clean and sanitized frequently. Caretakers should wash their hands before handling neonates and after stimulating elimination.

Puppies cannot voluntarily urinate or defecate until about three weeks of age. Until that time, they rely on the bitch to stimulate the urogenital reflex to initiate elimination. Caretakers should stimulate puppies after feeding by gently swabbing the perineal region with a warm moistened cotton ball or cloth.

Often, puppies within a litter look similar; therefore, it may be difficult to tell them apart when hand rearing, especially in large litters. Different colored nail polish can be applied to the claws to help differentiate individuals; owners can paint a different paw for each puppy (e.g., blue front left paw, blue right rear paw, pink right front paw, etc.).

Other Physical Parameters

When evaluating neonates, the clinician should hold each puppy to assess alertness, muscle tone and response to handling. Attentive, experienced breeders often are good observers and make these evaluations routinely. Gastric fullness should be evaluated and the owner asked if the puppies are nursing. Healthy puppies, if hungry, might start crying but in a short time they generally stop crying and sleep, even without nursing (**Box 16-1**). Small and weak puppies may appear to nurse and develop abdominal fullness, yet fail to thrive. Weak puppies may also have an enlarged abdomen but are often restless and vocalize, which should alert the owner. This distention may result from aerophagia (Bebiak et al, 1987); however, more often it is caused by malnutrition or illness of the bitch or puppy. Weak puppies cannot reach the bitch's nipples and stimulate milk release, which is usually achieved by kneading the mammary glands with their forelimbs.

Key Nutritional Factors

Colostrum and Milk

The liquid secretions from the mammary glands during the first few days postwhelping are known as colostrum. The composition of the milk changes rapidly to become normal or "mature" milk between 24 hours postpartum and the end of the first week of lactation. Colostrum transfers immunoglobulins, provides a concentrated source of energy and selected nutrients and produces a laxative effect.

The immune system of neonatal puppies is immature, which is offset by passive transfer of immunoglobulins from the bitch across the placenta and in the colostrum (Banks, 1981; Tizard, 1992). Investigators estimate that puppies receive only 5 to 10% of IgG from transplacental transfer; therefore, they depend primarily on immunity derived from the intake of colostrum (Tizard, 1992). Colostrum contains about twice as much protein as mature milk; globulin proteins make up the entire difference (Meyer et al, 1985a; Rüsse, 1971). Colostrum is particularly rich in IgG, as opposed to mature milk, which is richer in IgA (Banks, 1981).

Colostrum has a very different composition than mature milk. Due to its high dry matter (DM) content, colostrum is sticky and viscous (Meyer et al, 1985a), which makes nursing more difficult, especially for weaker puppies. The DM content of colostrum decreases within 12 to 24 hours after whelping, primarily reflecting a decrease in protein.

The lactose concentration of colostrum is very low compared with that of mature milk (i.e., 1.0 vs. 3.4%) (Meyer et al, 1985a). Levels of calcium, phosphorus and magnesium are very high in colostrum and decrease after two to three days to levels that are lower than in mature milk (Meyer et al, 1985a).

Just after whelping, colostrum contains high levels of iron, copper and zinc, which decrease within 48 hours postpartum (Meyer et al, 1985a). Colostrum is high in vitamin A (Meyer et al, 1985; Ferrando et al, 1975); colostrum levels increase the liver reserve of vitamin A in puppies by 25% within a week (Meyer et al, 1985).

Milk is assumed to be a complete food for neonates. The composition of milk (i.e., water, protein, fat, lactose, minerals and vitamins) is designed to support the normal growth rate of neonates. Thus, the nutrient content of bitch's milk in **Table 16-4** summarizes the key nutritional factors for nursing puppies. For nutrients in which the concentration in mature milk is unknown, values recommended by the Association of American Feed Control Officials for growth should suffice (2007). In lieu of other information, the key nutritional factor discussion for weaning and postweaning puppy growth provides information that could be extrapolated to neonates (Chapter 17).

Milk from different mammalian species contains the same components but in different proportions. One reason for the difference in milk composition may be the relative growth rates of each species (Johnson, 1974). The faster the rate of growth, the more concentrated the milk nutrients to support growth (Table 15-4). Bitch's milk is higher in energy, protein and minerals than cow's milk (Table 15-3). As with other species, the nutrient concentration in bitch's milk changes with duration of lactation (Adkins et al, 2001).

Water

Water is one of the most important nutrients in orphan feeding. The normal water intake of puppies is relatively high. A normal puppy needs about 60 to 100 ml of fluid/lb body weight per day (130 to 220 ml/kg body weight per day) (Lawler, 1991; Mosier, 1977). On average, orphaned puppies should receive about 180 ml of water/kg body weight to make orphan feeding successful. Water should be given until 180 ml/kg body weight is reached if the milk replacer doesn't provide this much water at the recommended dilution.

Energy

Data from two studies show that bitch's milk is extremely digestible (Mundt et al, 1981; Kienzle et al, 1985). The energy intake of suckling puppies can be expressed in terms of gross energy (GE) because the energy digestibility is greater than 95%. The high digestibility of milk maximizes its usage and helps puppies survive the critical first weeks. Bitch's milk is high in energy and provides about 146 kcal GE (610 kJ)/100 g of milk.

Total milk intake per puppy is lowest during the first week of

Table 16-2. Average litter size and birth weight of dogs.*

Breed	Litter size	Birth weight (g)
Airedale terrier	9	300
Appenzell mountain dog	10	465
Australian silky terrier	3	-
Bernese mountain dog	5	445
Borzoi	9	450
Boxer	8	440
Cavalier King Charles spaniel	4	230
Chihuahua	2-3	140
Chow chow	6	460
Dachshund	4	215
Dalmatian	5-6	-
Doberman pinscher	7	410
English bulldog	7	295
English cocker spaniel	6	230
English springer spaniel	11	375
Fox terrier	3	260
French bulldog	5	215
German shepherd dog	6	445
German shorthaired pointer	7-8	415
Great Pyrenees	≥5	705
Hovawart	11	435
Irish terrier	6	270
Labrador retriever	5	450
Maltese	3	155
Miniature dachshund	3	210
Miniature pinscher	3	-
Miniature poodle	2-3	165
Miniature schnauzer	4	155
Newfoundland	7	595
Norwich terrier	5	225
Papillon	3	120
Pekingese	2-3	-
Pomeranian	2	-
Pug	3	-
Rottweiler	7	-
Saint Bernard	7	640
Scottish terrier	5	240
Shetland sheepdog	4-5	260
Shih Tzu	2-3	-
Sloughi	3	670
Standard schnauzer	6	285
Yorkshire terrier	5	95

*Because of the very large variation in adult body weight (BW) and number of puppies per litter, there is no direct relationship between the birth weight of a puppy and the BW of the mother. Puppies from largest breeds are approximately 1% of the bitch's BW, whereas a Chihuahua puppy averages 6.4% of its mother's BW. However, there is a strong relationship between the weight of the total litter and the bitch's BW. On average, the total litter weight is about 12 to 14% of the bitch's BW. This relationship and the values in this table may be helpful to determine if individual puppies are far below the average expected birth weight, and to assess the bitch's nutritional status during pregnancy.

Table 16-3. Optimal environmental temperatures for orphaned puppies.

Age	°Centigrade	°Fahrenheit
	Immediate environment/ incubator for orphans	
Week 1	29-32	84-90
Week 2	26-29	79-84
Week 3	23-26	73-79
Week 4	23	73
	Environment around litter	
Week 1	24-27	75-81

Box 16-3. Body Weight Gain in Puppies.

Birth weight of puppies is the single most important measure of their chances of survival, and reflects, among other factors, the adequacy of the bitch's nutrition during pregnancy. The evolution of a puppy's body weight gives useful information about food intake and general health. Body weight should be recorded within 24 hours after parturition, and then daily or every other day for the first four weeks of life, using an accurate gram scale.

BIRTH WEIGHT

Due to variation in breed size, an exact optimal birth weight is difficult to estimate for individual puppies. Body weight at birth correlates primarily with the weight of the mother; birth weights range from 1% for some large and giant breeds to about 6.5% in Chihuahuas. Interestingly, investigators found a consistent ratio between the weight of the total litter and the body weight of the dam. Birth weight of the entire litter averages about 12 to 14% of adult body weight. The ratio can be slightly smaller in large breeds. Given the number of puppies and the ratio of litter to adult body weight, the birth weight of individual puppies can be evaluated in relation to the expected total number of puppies per litter.

BODY WEIGHT GAIN

Daily weight gain averages about 5% of the puppy's current body weight during the first four weeks after parturition. The absolute daily weight gain is lowest during the first week of life; however, the relative increase is largest (average 7.7% of body weight), and can reach 10% of body weight (**Table 1**). In the first 48 hours, the increase in body weight is not related to the puppy's body weight, because healthy smaller puppies eat relatively more in an effort to replete body reserves.

The puppy's body weight often doubles by eight to 10 days after parturition and it may triple by the third week. Although the relative weight gain gradually decreases, weight gain in g/day varies little from the second to the fourth week of life.

Daily gain can vary markedly. Although puppies should be weighed every day or every other day, a more precise evaluation should be based on the average weekly weight gain.

Between one and two months of age, daily weight gain may average 3 g/kg adult body weight, and between 2 and 4 g/kg adult body weight through weaning. These numbers may be used to help assess growth rates. However, dogs do not grow linearly; the growth curve has a sigmoid shape, with a fast exponential growth component first followed by slower growth. The exact timing of these phases differs from breed to breed. As a rule, small- and medium-sized dogs (up to 25 kg) reach about 50% of their adult weight around four months of age, whereas dogs with adult weights above 25 kg reach the 50% point at about five months of age.

Table 1. Average daily weight gain of puppies.*

Week	% of current body weight
1	8 (5-10)
2	6
3	4
4	3.5

*Adapted from Kienzle E, Meyer H, Dammers C, et al. Milchaufnahme, Gewichtentwicklung, Milchverdaulichkeit, sowie Energie- und Nährstoffretention bei Saugwelpen. Fortschritte in der Tierphysiologie und Tierernährung (Advances in Animal Physiology and Animal Nutrition) 1985; Suppl. No. 16: 27-50. Mundt H-C, Thomée A, Meyer H. Zur Energieund Eiweißversorgung von Saugwelpen über die Muttermilch. Kleintierpraxis 1981; 26: 353-360.

The Bibliography for **Box 16-3** can be found at www.markmorris.org.

life. However, expressed per kg body weight, puppies' milk intake is highest during the first week and decreases progressively (Kienzle et al, 1985). Puppies born with a lower body weight ingest an amount of milk similar to that of their larger littermates during the first 48 hours of life (Oftedal, 1984; Kienzle et al, 1985).

The energy requirement of a puppy is the sum of energy needed for maintenance and the requirement for growth. Because puppies sleep more than 80% of the time, and huddle together in a warm whelping box, they are able to decrease their energy requirements for maintenance to a level that approaches resting energy requirement (70 kcal/$BW_{kg}^{0.75}$) (Mundt et al, 1981) during the first week of life. Therefore, all additional ingested energy can be used for growth. Their energy intake averages about 240 kcal (1 MJ)/kg body weight/day during the first four weeks of life. Averages, however, may vary from as high as 287 kcal GE (1.2 MJ)/kg body weight during the first week of life to as low as 190 kcal GE (0.8 MJ)/kg body weight by Week 4 (Oftedal, 1984; Mundt et al, 1981; Kienzle et al, 1985).

This information can also be generally applied to orphaned puppies. A very common mistake is to underestimate the energy requirements of neonates. In the beginning, however, it is better not to over feed orphaned puppies to avoid diarrhea. **Table 16-5** summarizes the estimated energy requirements of orphans to transition them to milk replacers. The initial amounts in **Table 16-5** are lower than the amounts discussed above. These lower levels are intended to help orphaned puppies adapt to orphan formulas. When using commercial milk replacers, it is usually best to follow the label recommendations.

Protein

Protein digestibility of bitch's milk is very high (up to 99%), and nitrogen retention is about 90% during the first week (Mundt et al, 1981). Compared with cow's milk, bitch's milk contains more than twice as much protein per 100 ml (7.5 vs. 3.3%) (Table 15-3). Bitch's milk also provides high levels of arginine, lysine and branched-chain amino acids (Meyer et al, 1985a; Swaisgood, 1995). This nutrient profile is important when assessing and formulating milk replacers, and reflects the enormous anabolic activity of puppies at this young age. Protein requirements should be met if puppies ingest adequate amounts of energy as that contained in bitch's milk.

Commercial milk and homemade replacer formulas should have adequate protein and essential amino acid content and appropriate ratios of these constituents. The arginine and histidine levels in a formula are particularly important. Deficiency of these amino acids can cause cataract development in neonates and contribute to anorexia and poor growth. The minimum recommended levels of these two amino acids for growth in puppies after weaning are 0.79 and 0.39% (DM), respectively (NRC, 2006). These recommendations are based on a food with 22.5% DM crude protein. For four- to 14-week-old puppies, 0.01 g of arginine should be added for every 1% of crude protein in excess of 22.5% (NRC, 2006). The amount of arginine in milk is 420 mg/kg (as fed) or 1.85% (DM) (**Table 16-4**).

Fat

Approximately 1.5% of a puppy's total body mass at birth is fat, which is very low compared to the 22% body fat of non-obese adult dogs (Stadtfeld, 1978; Rauchfuss, 1978). Puppies increase body fat during the first month of lactation; accretion of body fat is about 50% of total weight gain (Kienzle et al, 1985). Fat increases to about 10% of body weight by two weeks of age (Meyer and Stadtfeld, 1980) and to 17% after one month (Kienzle et al, 1985). The dam's milk, therefore, must contain enough energy (fat) to support development of these reserves. Milk fat and fatty acid composition are two of the most variable components of milk. The fat content and fat quality of milk depend on the food the bitch receives during lactation (Gross, 1993). Bitch's milk should contain 9 g or more fat/100 g of milk. Fat in bitch's milk contains a high percentage of unsaturated fatty acids and is rich in linoleic acid compared with cow's milk (Table 15-3).

Milk fat and fatty acid composition are highly variable components of milk and often reflect dietary intake of the bitch. The type of dietary fat fed in conjunction with the fatty acid profile of endogenous fat deposits may affect the fatty acid composition of milk. In one study, the fatty acid composition of bitch's milk reflected the foods fed during gestation and lactation. Furthermore, the milk of bitches fed foods enriched with α-linolenic acid (ALA) but not docosahexaenoic acid (DHA) was high in ALA. Puppies fed this milk accumulated more plasma phospholipid DHA than the control group (but not as much as puppies fed preformed DHA) during suckling (Heinemann et al, 2005). In children, during periods of early growth, DHA may be needed to support retinal and auditory

Box 16-4. Hypoglycemia, Hypothermia and Dehydration in Neonates.

Before weaning, mortality of puppies can be as high as 10 to 30%, with 65% of the deaths occurring during the first week of life. Healthy puppies sleep and nurse; when a puppy continues to vocalize it is probably ill, malnourished, cold or dehydrated.

The syndrome of hypoglycemia, hypothermia and dehydration is by far the most common nutrition-related condition seen in neonates. Orphaned puppies are at a much higher risk than nursing puppies, especially when deprived of colostrum. Low fat stores and the degree of poikilothermy make puppies dependent on effective nursing and optimal environmental temperature during the first two weeks of life. The first three days of life, however, are the most critical. Rectal temperatures of newborn puppies may decrease up to 4 to 5°C (7 to 8°F) immediately after parturition. Furthermore, healthy puppies may lose about 0.5 g of body weight every 30 minutes that they sleep without being fed.

When food intake is inadequate or when the environmental temperature is too low, newborn puppies rapidly deplete glycogen and fat stores and soon chill and become hypoglycemic, weak and dehydrated. Etiology includes inadequate milk production by the bitch (qualitative or quantitative), and all the causes of anorexia and reasons why a puppy refuses or is unable to nurse, including early maternal rejection, prematurity and low birth weight.

Infections, parasites and other illnesses lead to anorexia and may cause hypoglycemia, dehydration and hypothermia. Diarrhea rapidly causes dehydration in young puppies.

Hypoxia is an important cause of anorexia and hypoglycemia. Hypoxia may result from dystocia, prolonged birth or trauma caused by the bitch. Neonates have significantly lower blood glucose levels during the first day of life when their dam refused food during the last days of pregnancy.

Hypoglycemia, hypothermia and dehydration are interrelated; one can cause or worsen the others, starting a vicious cycle (**Figure 1**).

HYPOTHERMIA

After a puppy's rectal temperature drops below 34.5°C (94°F) the puppy becomes less active and nurses ineffectually, bowel movements stop and digestion no longer occurs. When a puppy's skin feels cold, the dam will push the puppy away and ignore its cries. The puppy then becomes hypoglycemic and is too weak to nurse, initiating a vicious cycle from which the puppy will not survive without help. Tissue hypoxia and metabolic acidosis may reach profound proportions. After the body temperature reaches the critical level of 32°C (90°F), hypothermia becomes severe and the puppy lies motionless, with a very slow respiratory rate and an occasional air hunger response. It has been reported that healthy newborn puppies can survive up to 12 hours of deep hypothermia and recover if warmed slowly. In practice, however, hypothermic puppies can be rescued only when the problem is detected early and treated correctly.

Hypothermia that develops in puppies kept at the correct environmental temperature may indicate insufficient milk intake by the puppy due to disease or weakness, inability to reach the bitch's nipples, insufficient milk production and/or inadequate maternal behavior and poor milk quality or quantity due to insufficient nutrition of the dam, disease of the dam and/or inherited factors.

Orphaned puppies are at greater risk because they are more sensitive to suboptimal temperatures without the dam. Additionally, the milk replacer formula or feeding schedule may be inadequate.

HYPOGLYCEMIA

Fetuses receive continuous infusion of glucose from the placenta, so they do not depend on their own gluconeogenesis. Because they have very low fat and glycogen reserves at birth, canine neonates may develop hypoglycemia after only 12 hours of fasting. In contrast, adult dogs can undergo weeks of starvation without developing hypoglycemia. During starvation, gluconeogenesis becomes the

Box 16-4 continued

sole means of glucose homeostasis. The neonate's small muscle mass, decreased use of free fatty acids as an alternate energy source and a possible lack or decreased levels of gluconeogenic enzymes limit the neonate's capacity to maintain normal glucose levels. Dietary carbohydrate and protein levels can also affect activities of gluconeogenic enzymes in puppies. Transient hypoglycemia is sometimes seen in toy-breed puppies between two and three months of age; however, transient hypoglycemia is different from this syndrome.

DEHYDRATION

Dehydration is characterized by wrinkled skin and dry, sticky mucous membranes, which may appear deep pink or red.

TREATMENT

The three treatment goals for hypoglycemia, hypothermia and dehydration are to: 1) achieve optimal core body temperature, 2) maintain glucose within physiologically normal levels and 3) achieve adequate hydration status.

Chilled puppies should receive a mixture of equal amounts of physiologic saline solution (or lactated Ringer's solution) and a 5% glucose solution by subcutaneous injection before rewarming. Glucose is necessary to meet the sudden increase in energy requirements during warming.

Hypothermic puppies should first be warmed to 34.5°C (94°F), a temperature that allows digestive enzymes to become active again. If they are not warmed before being fed, hypothermic puppies will develop diarrhea, resulting in further dehydration and hypothermia, because of nonfunctioning digestive enzymes.

Hypothermic puppies should be warmed slowly and progressively over one to three hours to prevent oxygen and energy requirements of tissues from increasing faster than the puppy can supply. Aggressive, rapid warming can compromise vascular integrity and aggravate fluid loss and dehydration, resulting in hyperthermia, hypovolemia, shock and death. Slow warming is best accomplished by using body heat. A simple method such as placing a chilled puppy in an inside pocket of a loose-fitting garment will result in slow warming and gentle massage. Warm water (36.5°C [98°F]) or a warm-water heating blanket is a good alternative. If a closed incubator is used, humidity should be around 60%. Because their normal body temperature is lower than that of adult dogs, newborn puppies should not be warmed to adult body temperature, but to about 36 to 36.7°C (97 to 98°F). Hypothermic animals are susceptible to infections, so administration of antibiotics may be lifesaving.

Dehydration should not be treated orally in markedly hypothermic puppies because of their depressed gastrointestinal motility. Parenteral fluid solutions, warmed to body temperature, can be given subcutaneously, at the dose of 1 ml/30 g body weight, and repeated as needed. After body temperature is restored, oral solutions can be administered by stomach tube. Nursing should recommence as soon as possible, although hand rearing will be necessary if the bitch is incapable of feeding the puppies.

Tube feeding with an appropriate milk replacer, parenteral fluid administration and other supportive therapy should be implemented at once each time a young puppy becomes weak and before hypothermia and dehydration are a problem.

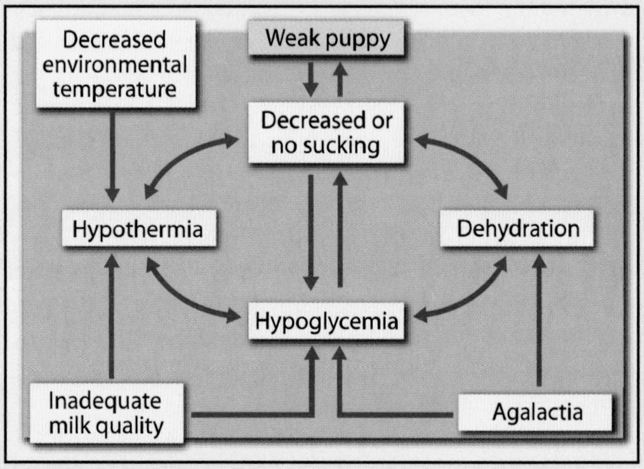

Figure 1. This figure shows how hypothermia, hypoglycemia and dehydration interrelate, creating a cycle that often results in neonatal death.

The Bibliography for **Box 16-4** can be found at www.markmorris.org.

development (Pawlosky et al, 1997; Birch et al, 2002; Diau et al, 2003). In addition, infants supplemented with DHA had enhanced brain development and learning ability (Birch et al, 2002; Huffman et al, 2003). As in other species, including fish oil as a source of DHA in puppy foods improved trainability (Kelley et al, 2004). Retinal function of young dogs improved when foods containing long-chain omega-3 (n-3) polyunsaturated fatty acids were fed during gestation and lactation (Bauer et al, 2006). The recommended level of DHA plus eicosapentaenoic acid (EPA) for puppies after weaning is 0.05% (DM). At this level, EPA should not exceed 60% of the total amount of DHA plus EPA (NRC, 2006). These levels probably also apply to orphan formulas. Thus, DHA needs to be at least 40% of the total DHA plus EPA, or 0.02%.

Linoleic acid is an essential fatty acid and is required for normal growth. The DM linoleic acid content of bitch's milk is 4.9% (**Table 16-4**). Bitch's milk has an energy density of 6.43 kcal/g (DM). Converting this amount of linoleic acid to a 4 kcal/g basis results in a linoleic acid equivalent of 3.0% (DM). This is greater than the minimum recommended allowance of 1.3% for foods for puppies after weaning (NRC, 2006) and probably reflects the more rapid growth rate and subsequently higher requirement of neonates.

Carbohydrate

Lactose is the primary carbohydrate in milk. Lactose levels in bitch's milk vary between 3.0 and 3.5%, which are about 30% lower than those in cow's milk (Table 15-3). Although the lactose content of milk varies widely among animal species, it is very consistent and maintained within narrow limits within a species. Lactose and minerals in milk primarily contribute to osmolarity. Any increase or decrease in lactose content is offset by changes in the content of other soluble components (Johnson, 1974).

Lactose, a disaccharide, is absorbed after digestion into its constituent monosaccharides. Lactose is unique in that its glucose and galactose molecules are linked with a β-1,4 bond instead of the α-1,4 linkage commonly found in other soluble glucose polymers (Stryer, 1988; Newberg and Neubauer, 1995). This linkage makes lactose a less suitable substrate for microbes that may infect the mammary gland or the neonate's gastrointestinal tract. Furthermore, large amounts of lactose may favor colonization of the intestine by more beneficial microflora, which compete with and exclude many potential pathogens (Newberg and Neubauer, 1995). To avoid diarrhea, lactose should be the main carbohydrate source during the first weeks of life. Pancreatic amylase activity is insignificant at four weeks of age and low at eight weeks, whereas intestinal lactase activity is enhanced until about four months of age (Kienzle, 1988; Meyer, 1992).

Calcium and Phosphorus

Calcium levels are very high in colostrum; however, after two to three days, levels decrease to less than those found in mature milk (Meyer et al, 1985a). Calcium content increases over the course of lactation; however, the calcium-phosphorus ratio remains consistent around 1.3:1 (Meyer et al, 1985a). Calcium and phosphorus levels in milk are similar among canine breeds. Canine milk is rich in calcium and phosphorus; the amounts of these minerals in bitch's milk could be regarded as recommendations for daily intake by growing puppies, despite the fact that skeletal calcification does not keep pace with the increase in body size until after weaning (Gesellshaft, 1989; Baines, 1981).

Potassium, Sodium, Magnesium and Copper

Potassium helps maintain acid-base and osmotic balance, transmit nerve impulses, facilitate muscle contractility and serves as a cofactor in several key enzyme systems. Sodium is also important for maintaining acid-base and osmotic balance, and transmitting nerve impulses and muscle contractions. Sodium controls passage of nutrients into cells, including absorption of sugars and amino acids from the intestinal lumen. Sodium is involved in calcium absorption and the absorption of several water-soluble vitamins. Magnesium is involved in carbohydrate and lipid metabolism and is a catalyst for a wide variety of enzymes. It is required for ATP production, catalyzes most phosphate transfers and has a potent influence on neuromuscular activity. Numerous copper-containing enzyme systems exist including those involved in hematopoiesis, control of neurotransmitters, connective tissue integrity, oxidative metabolism and protection against superoxide radicals. Thus, it is important that these minerals be present in adequate amounts and correct proportions. **Table 16-4** lists the levels of these minerals in milk.

Iron

Deficiency may occur if iron stores are not accumulated during the last week of pregnancy, or if excessive blood loss occurs due to severe hookworm infection or severe flea infestation. During the first three to four weeks of life, body iron stores and hematocrit and hemoglobin values decrease below levels at birth. Decreasing hematocrit and hemoglobin values might also be due to a relative increase in total body water over this time period. The decrease is more pronounced in fast-growing, large-breed puppies (Gesellshaft, 1989a).

Milk is a poor source of iron and puppy requirements are usually higher than intake (Kienzle et al, 1985). Iron reserves increase when puppies receive food at weaning; body iron stores normalize around four months of age (Kienzle et al, 1985).

Table 16-4. Key nutritional factors for foods for nursing puppies (the nutritional content of bitch's milk).*

Nutrient	Per 100 g milk, as fed	DM basis**
Moisture (g)	77.3	0
Dry matter (g)	22.7	100
Crude protein (g)	7.5	33
Arginine (mg)	420	1.85
Fat (g)	9.5	41.8
Linoleic acid (g)	1.11	4.9
Lactose (g)	3.3	14.5
Calcium (mg)	240	1.06
Phosphorus (mg)	180	0.79
Sodium (mg)	80	0.35
Potassium (mg)	120	0.53
Magnesium (mg)	11	0.05
Copper (mg)	0.33	0.0015
Iron (mg)	0.7	0.003
ME (kcal)	146 (610 kJ)	6.43 kcal/g (26.9 kJ/g)
Osmolarity (mOsm/kg)	569	Not applicable
DM digestibility	>95%	>95%

Key: DM = dry matter, ME = metabolizable energy.

*Adapted from Anderson RS, Carlos GM, Robinson IP, et al. Zinc, copper, iron and calcium concentrations in bitch milk. Journal of Nutrition 1991; 121:S81-S82. Gesellschaft für Ernährungsphysiologie. Grunddaten für die Berechnung des Energie- und Nährstoffbedarfs. In: Ausschuß für Bedarfsnormen der Gesellschaft für Ernährungs-physiologie Energie-Nährstoffbedarf/Energy and Nutrient Requirements, No. 5 Hunde/Dogs. Frankfurt/Main, Germany: DLG Verlag, 1989; 9-31. Kienzle E, Meyer H, Dammers C, et al. Milchaufnahme, Gewichtentwicklung, Milchverdaulichkeit, sowie Energie- und Nährstoffretention bei Saugwelpen. Fortschritte in der Tierphysiologie und Tierernährung (Advances in Animal Physiology and Animal Nutrition) 1985; Suppl. 16: 27-50. Meyer H, Kienzle E, Dammers C. Milchmenge und Milchzusammensetzung bei der Hundin sowie Futteraufnahme und Gewichtsenwicklung ante und post partum. Fortschritte in der Tierphysiologie und Tierenahrung (Advances in Animal Physiology and Animal Nutrition) 1985; 16:27-50. Mundt H-C, Thomée A, Meyer H. Zur Energie- und Eiweißversorgung von Saugwelpen über die Muttermilch. Kleintierpraxis 1981; 26: 353-360. Oftedal OT. Lactation in the dog: Milk composition and intake by puppies. Journal of Nutrition 1984; 114: 803-812. Rüsse I. Die Laktation der Hündin. Zentralblatt für Veterinär Medizin 1961; 8: 252-281.

**Units are expressed in percentages unless otherwise indicated.

Table 16-5. Recommendations for energy intake of orphaned puppies as a basis for determining orphan formula dose.*

Feeding period	kcal ME/100 g BW	kJ ME/100 g BW
Days 1-3	15	60
Days 4-6	20	85
>6 days	20-25	85-105

Key: ME = metabolizable energy, BW = body weight.

*Do not over feed orphan formulas initially. The feeding amount for the first six days intentionally provides less energy than would normally be provided, which is gradually increased so that the orphaned puppies' energy requirements are being met after about one week.

Table 16-6. Feeding plan summary for nursing puppies.

1. Ensure good husbandry practices are understood and in place (Box 17-2).
2. Ensure colostrum intake by the puppies within the first 24 hours.
3. Provide bitch's milk until three to four weeks of age; then gradually initiate the weaning process by introducing small amounts of semisolid to solid food, which augments nursing of bitch's milk (**Box 16-5**).
4. The weaning food should be a good quality growth/reproduction type commercial food (Tables 15-9 and 17-4).
5. Assess nursing puppies daily, including recording of body weight and tracking weight gain for the first month of age (**Box 16-3**); then weekly. Recommend weekly veterinary checks for the first month.
6. Puppies failing to thrive on bitch's milk should be fed via partial or total orphan feeding techniques; check bitch, including bitch's food, to ensure no health or nutrition issues are affecting lactation.
7. Wean at six to seven weeks (**Box 16-5**) and feed according to recommendations in Chapter 17 (growing puppies).

Table 16-7. Feeding plan summary for orphaned puppies.

1. Ensure good husbandry practices are understood and in place (**Box 16-2**); have owner(s) attempt to provide as much total care as the bitch would have.
2. Puppies should have colostrum within the first 24 hours of birth; if not, administer frozen colostrum or consider colostrum from other species, commercial colostrum sources or serum from vaccinated dogs given subcutaneously.
3. Use foster bitch if possible; partial orphan feeding is next best and bottle feeding is the best of hand-feeding techniques (**Figures 16-1** through **16-3**).
4. **Table 16-9** provides three homemade formulas and **Table 16-10** compares them to bitch's milk. Commercial milk replacers are best.
5. To determine the initial amount to feed, use **Table 16-5** to estimate the puppies' daily energy requirement (DER); divide the DER by the energy density of the milk replacer to determine the daily amount to feed. Besides energy and other nutrients, orphaned puppies should receive about 180 ml of water/kg body weight/day; if necessary, add additional water to the milk replacer if the recommended dilution doesn't provide this amount of total fluid intake.
6. Milk replacers should be heated to 38°C (100°F) and the daily amount divided and fed ≥4 times/day at equal intervals.
7. Good hygiene is critical and includes washing/boiling feeding utensils before each feeding, preparing no more than the amount of milk replacer that can be fed in 24 hours (keep refrigerated) and carefully washing puppies with a moist, soft cloth twice weekly.
8. Have owners gradually initiate the weaning process by introducing small amounts of semisolid to solid food, which augments the milk replacer (**Box 16-5**).
9. The weaning food should be a good quality growth/reproduction type commercial food (Table 17-4).
10. Assess nursing puppies daily, including recording of body weight and tracking weight gain for the first month of age (**Box 16-3**); then weekly. Recommend weekly veterinary checks for the first month.
11. For puppies not thriving on milk replacer, review milk replacer quality (**Table 16-8**), dilution calculations and feeding amounts; switch to a different milk replacer if necessary.
12. Wean at six to seven weeks (**Box 16-5**) and feed according to recommendations in Chapter 17 (growing puppies).

Therefore, puppies should receive solid food as soon as possible (around three weeks of age).

Milk replacers are often fortified with iron at concentrations higher than those found in bitch's milk. Orphaned puppies, especially low birth weight neonates born with low iron reserves, may benefit from iron intakes higher than those normally found in milk. The additional iron supports hematopoiesis and helps avoid anemia sometimes observed in three- to four-week-old neonates.

Digestibility

DM digestibility of bitch's milk is very high (>95%) (Mundt et al, 1981; Kienzle et al, 1985). Digestibility of milk replacer formulas should also be high (>90%) to allow for smaller quantities to be fed and avoid diarrhea.

Osmolality

The osmolality of bitch's milk is approximately 569 mOsm/kg. Milk replacers with osmolality values considerably higher than these concentrations should be avoided because they may cause hyperosmolar diarrhea and potentiate dehydration. High osmolality may delay gastric emptying and predispose to regurgitation, vomiting and aspiration during the next meal, if the stomach is not completely empty.

FEEDING PLAN

The feeding plan includes determining the best food and feeding method. **Tables 16-6** and **16-7** provide feeding plan summaries for nursing and orphaned puppies, respectively.

Assess and Select the Food

Puppies should receive colostrum within the first 12 to 24 hours after birth to ensure adequate intake of immunoglobulins. If bitch colostrum is unavailable, colostrum from a different species may be used. Although antibody protection may be limited, providing nonspecific defense substances such as lactoferrin, oligosaccharides, lactoperoxidases and lysozymes may be beneficial. Alternatively, sterile serum from vaccinated dogs administered subcutaneously has been recommended (England, 2005).

Direct assessment of milk quality is difficult; therefore, indirect parameters should be evaluated, including failure to grow, weakness, an enlarged abdomen and abnormal behavior such as restlessness and continuous vocalization. After illness is ruled out, these signs may indicate insufficient milk production by the bitch and/or deficient milk quality.

Milk intake can be estimated by weighing puppies before and after they nurse. The ratio of weight gain to milk intake may indicate milk quality. However, weight gains range from about one g/two g of milk intake to one g/to almost five g of milk intake during the first weeks of life (Oftedal, 1984; Mundt et al, 1981; Jean-Blain, 1973). This wide range results primarily from differences in ability to estimate milk intake. Also, an underweight bitch (body condition score 1/5 or 2/5) may be at risk for producing inadequate or poor quality milk. Therefore,

Box 16-5. Weaning.

Weaning is a gradual process with two phases. The first phase begins when puppies start eating solid food between three and four weeks of age. This phase should be encouraged, especially if the bitch has a large litter. Additionally, nursing is an important stimulus for milk production. Therefore, milk production will progressively decline as the puppies' intake of solid food increases, making complete weaning (second phase) less stressful. However, some bitches may continue to produce large quantities of milk and are at risk for development of mammary congestion when the puppies are completely separated. The feeding schedule in **Table 1** may be helpful, particularly in cases of early weaning (around the fifth week of age).

Limiting food intake for a day or two while weaning reduces nutrients available for milk production, thereby reducing mammary gland engorgement. Leaving one or two puppies to nurse will not alleviate mammary gland engorgement in bitches that are still producing a large amount of milk at weaning. This practice continues to stimulate milk production, and therefore prolongs the problem. When it is decided to completely separate the puppies from the mother, all puppies should be taken away at once.

Puppies should be encouraged to start eating solid food as soon as possible. This practice will reduce reliance on the bitch, reduce the nutritional burden on the bitch and make complete weaning less stressful. Most puppies will start eating solid food between three and four weeks of age, the time when deciduous teeth begin to erupt. Oftentimes, during play, puppies will come in contact with the bitch's food and progressively start eating small amounts.

Puppies can be offered gruel to stimulate food intake at three weeks of age. Gruels are made by blending a moist growth/reproduction-type food with an equal volume of warm water. Alternatively, one part of dry food can be ground and mixed with three parts of warm water (volume basis). Puppies should be encouraged to lap the gruel; owners can dip their fingertips in the gruel and then into the puppies' mouth. Ideally, the food used to make the gruel should be highly digestible, contain at least 25 to 30% protein and have an energy content of at least 4.0 kcal (16.7 kJ) metabolizable energy/g (dry matter). A good quality growth/reproduction-type food such as the bitch is eating should be appropriate (Chapters 15 and 17). Puppies are very prone to vomiting and diarrhea during this period. If gastrointestinal disturbances occur, gruel can be made from a highly digestible moist food intended for dietary management of diarrhea with a minimum of about 25% dry matter protein.

As the puppies' interest in solid food increases, the water content of the gruel can be reduced progressively. Puppies should be eating sufficient quantities of solid food at five weeks of age because the bitch's milk production will probably start declining.

From three weeks of age on, puppies can be separated from their mother for short periods of time. The time away from the dam can be progressively increased to about four hours a day by around six weeks of age. Weaning should be effectively completed between six and seven weeks of age and puppies can be removed from the dam. After weaning, the puppies should be fed the same food to minimize stress and the risk of diarrhea.

Table 1. Recommended feeding schedule for reducing mammary congestion in bitches during weaning of puppies.*

Day of weaning	No food
First day after weaning	One-fourth of DER for adult maintenance (0.5 x RER)
Second day after weaning	One-half of DER for adult maintenance (RER)
Third day after weaning	Three-fourths of DER for adult maintenance (1.4 x RER)

Key: DER = daily energy requirement, RER = resting energy requirement.
*Adapted from Meyer H. Praktische Fütterung. In: Ernährung des Hundes, 2nd ed. Stuttgart, Germany: E Ulmer Verlag, 1990; 162-223.

The Bibliography for **Box 16-5** can be found at www.markmorris.org.

the bitch's food and feeding method should also be assessed. Most lactating bitches should be fed free choice (Chapter 15).

Foods used to feed orphans may consist of bitch's milk, commercial milk replacer or homemade replacer formulas. Milk from a healthy bitch is the food of choice and is assumed to provide nutrients in the proper levels for nursing puppies. Bitch's milk is rarely available in sufficient quantities to hand raise orphans. Of the alternatives, commercial milk replacers are preferred although several homemade formulas have proved sufficient. **Table 16-8** lists commercial milk replacers and compares their nutrient profiles (key nutritional factors) with bitch's milk. **Table 16-9** provides three homemade milk replacer recipes and **Table 16-10** compares these recipes' nutrient profiles with that of bitch's milk. Commercial and homemade milk replacers should closely mimic the profile of bitch's milk. Unsupplemented ruminant milk may be used as a base for homemade formulas but doesn't meet the nutritional needs of puppies. For puppies, goat's milk provides no nutritional benefit over cow's milk.

Foods should be liquid until nursing puppies and orphans are three to four weeks old, then semisolid to solid foods should be introduced. This transition marks the beginning of weaning (**Box 16-5**).

Assess and Determine the Feeding Method

Puppies should be encouraged to nurse often during the first week of life (eight to 12 times per day); after Week 1, they should be encouraged to nurse at least three to four times daily. Inexperienced bitches should be carefully observed to ensure that all puppies receive sufficient amounts of colostrum within 24 hours of birth, when puppies are able to absorb intact proteins such as immunoglobulins. This involvement may include positioning the puppies on the bitch's nipples at feeding time or encouraging a nervous bitch to lie quietly as the puppies nurse. Handling the dam and puppies facilitates monitoring the progress of the litter.

Table 16-8. Nutrient content of milk replacers compared with that of bitch's milk/100 grams of milk, as fed*

Nutrients**	Bitch's milk	Esbilac Liquid	Esbilac Reconstituted Powder	Nurturall C Puppy Liquid†	Nurturall-C Reconstituted Powder†	Just Born Puppy Liquid†	Just Born Reconstituted Powder†	Goat's Milk Esbilac Liquid	Goat's Milk Esbilac Reconstituted Powder
Manufacturer	-	**PetAg**	**PetAg**	**VPL**	**VPL**	**Farnam**	**Farnam**	**PetAg**	**PetAg**
Dilution***	na	na	1+2	na	1+2	na	1+2	na	1+2
Moisture (g)	77.3	84.9	na	80.1	85.7	80.1	85.7	84.2	-
Dry matter (g)	22.7	15.1	na	19.9	14.3	19.9	14.3	15.9	-
Crude protein (g)	7.5	5.1	6.2	7.6	4.5	7.6	4.5	4.7	6.12
Arginine (mg)	420	290	390	200	102	200	102	210	390
Lysine (mg)	380	370	470	na	na	na	na	360	470
Fat (g)	9.5	6.4	7.5	4.3	4.4	4.3	4.4	6.2	7.5
Linoleic acid (g)	1.1	na	0.4	na	na	na	na	-	0.86
Carbohydrate									
NFE (g)	3.8	2.9	2.7	6.4	4.3	6.4	4.3	2.9	2.7
Lactose (g)	3.3	na	-	na	na	na	na	-	-
Crude fiber (g)	na	0	0	<0.1	<0.1	<0.1	<0.1	0	0
Minerals									
Total ash (g)	1.2	0.8	1.3	1.5	1.1	1.5	1.1	1.2	1.3
Calcium (mg)	240	145	220	254	215	254	215	150	207
Phosphorus (mg)	180	110	178	221	186	221	186	-	149
Sodium (mg)	80	65	53	na	na	na	na	110	94
Potassium (mg)	120	130	194	113	186	113	186	250	142
Magnesium (mg)	11	12	12.6	6.5	7.0	6.5	7.0	18	14.2
Copper (mg)	0.33	0.18	0.23	0.2	0.16	0.2	0.16	0.22	0.46
Iron (mg)	0.70	0.60	0.82	2.70	2.17	2.7	2.17	1.90	0.83
Energy									
ME (kcal)	146	82	95	86	68	86	68	82	94.7
ME (kJ)	610	343	396	358	285	358	285	343	396
Osmolarity (mOsm/kg, H_20±SD)	568.7±41.2	na	-	na	na	na	na	na	-
Nutrient content of milk replacers compared with that of bitch's milk/100 kcal metabolizable energy††									
Protein (g)	5.20	6.21	6.56	8.89	6.63	8.89	6.63	5.70	6.46
Arginine (mg)	288	354	411	234	149	234	149	256	412
Lysine (mg)	260	451	495	na	na	na	na	439	496
Fat (g)	6.40	7.78	7.92	5.03	6.41	5.03	6.41	7.55	7.94
Linoleic acid (g)	0.76	na	0.43	na	na	na	na	na	0.91
Carbohydrate									
NFE (g)	2.60	3.51	2.80	7.49	6.29	7.49	6.29	3.51	2.81
Lactose (g)	2.3	na	na	na	na	na	na	na	na
Crude fiber (g)	na	0	0	<0.1	<0.1	<0.1	<0.1	0	0
Minerals									
Total ash (g)	0.82	0.98	1.32	1.75	1.62	1.75	1.62	1.46	1.38
Calcium (mg)	164	177	232	297	314	297	314	183	219
Phosphorus (mg)	123	134	187	258	272	258	272	0	157
Sodium (mg)	55	79	56	na	na	na	na	134	99
Potassium (mg)	82	159	204	132	272	132	272	305	150
Magnesium (mg)	7.5	14.6	13.3	7.6	10.2	7.6	10.2	22.0	15.0
Copper (mg)	0.23	0.22	0.24	0.23	0.24	0.23	0.24	0.27	0.49
Iron (mg)	0.48	0.73	0.86	3.16	3.18	3.16	3.18	2.32	0.88

Key: na = not applicable/available, NFE = nitrogen-free extract, ME = metabolizable energy, mOsm = milliosmoles.
*Manufacturers' data; nutrient content for reconstituted powdered products are manufacturers' calculations based on the recommended dilution. Nutrient data per 100 ml would be reduced slightly (between 1 to 2%) because the specific gravity of milk is greater than that of water.
**g/100 g = %.
***The first number is the milk powder, the second the water (e.g., 1+2 = one part of powder plus two parts of water).
†Nutrients in liquid and powder forms are averages from the yearly laboratory analyses of composite samples from 2004 to date.
††The nutrient levels per 100 kcal ME were calculated from the nutrient and energy levels in the top portion of the table.

Competition in large litters may prevent smaller, weaker puppies from nursing and predispose them to dehydration and hypoglycemia. Partial orphan rearing of the entire litter should be done in these cases (see below). Partial orphan rearing allows the puppies to stay with the dam in their normal environment and permits proper socialization.

Puppies that fail to thrive when receiving bitch's milk should be fed immediately via partial or total orphan feeding techniques (see below) to avoid the risk of hypoglycemia, hypothermia and dehydration.

It may be necessary to alter the feeding method when managing orphaned puppies, especially if they are hand reared. Evaluation of the current feeding method with knowledge of growth demands will facilitate this part of feeding plan development. Orphaned puppies and those too weak to nurse are candidates for fostering, partial orphan rearing or hand feeding. The caregiver for orphans should provide the level of care provided by the bitch; good husbandry is essential.

Fostering

The optimal means of feeding orphaned or rejected puppies is to foster them to another lactating bitch. In general, fostering is the least labor intensive, provides optimal nutrition, reduces mortality, improves immune status, usually provides an optimal physical environment and promotes normal social development of puppies. Unlike large animals, bitches readily accept additional puppies during lactation. If several foster mothers are available, it is best to place orphans in litters with fewer than 14 days age difference. Larger puppies often crowd out smaller individuals if the age discrepancy is too large. This situation can be managed by supervised feeding until the orphans can fend for themselves. Unfortunately, foster mothers are not normally available and alternative techniques must be used. Foster mothers should be well fed.

Puppies fostered onto another bitch should be supervised initially to detect any behavioral problems between the foster parent, its young and the orphans. Puppies should be accepted immediately and allowed to nurse. Encourage owners to watch for signs of rejection or impending cannibalism by the mother.

Table 16-9. Homemade milk replacers for puppies.

Recipe 1		Recipe 2		Recipe 1 (modified)	
Skim milk	43.8 g	Cow's milk**	800 ml	Skim milk	64 g
Low-fat curd*	40 g	Half cream***	200 ml	Low-fat curd*	15 g
Egg yolk (2/3)	10 g	Bone meal	6 g	One egg yolk	15 g
Vegetable oil	6 g	Citric acid	4 g	Vegetable oil	3 g
Vitamin-mineral mix	0.2 g	One egg yolk	15 g	Vitamin-mineral mix	2.5 g
-	-	Vitamin A	2,000 IU	$CaCO_3$	0.5

*Do not use cottage cheese because it may increase the risk of clotting in the neonate's stomach.
**3% fat.
***12% fat (i.e., half cream in the UK).

Table 16-10. Comparisons between bitch's milk and homemade milk replacers for puppies (See **Table 16-9**).

Nutrients*	Bitch's milk	Homemade milk replacers		
	-	Recipe 1**	Recipe 2**	Recipe 1 (modified)***
Moisture (g)	77.3	76.6	85.3	79.9
Dry matter (g)	22.7	23.4	14.7	20.1
Crude protein (g)	7.5	9.9	3.5	7.5
Fat (g)	9.5	9.5	5.5	8.1
NFE (g)	3.8	3.3	4.6	3.5
Ash (g)	1.2	0.8	0.7	1.3
Calcium (mg)	240	92.6	290	287
Phosphorus (mg)	180	177	200	186
Sodium (mg)	80	32	50	34
Potassium (mg)	127	96	150	110
Copper (mg)	0.33	0.03	na	0.05
Iron (mg)	0.7	0.68	na	0.95
Zinc (mg)	0.95	0.79	na	1.01
Energy				
ME (kcal)†	146	130	80	110
ME (kJ)†	610	544	335	460

Key: NFE = nitrogen-free extract, ME = metabolizable energy.
*g/100 ml or g/100 g = %.
**Calculated before addition of the vitamin-mineral mix.
***Calculated based on the addition of 2.5 g Pecutrin (Bayer).
†Calculated except for bitch's milk, for which the actual energy density was known from the literature.

Partial Orphan Rearing

Puppies that cannot be successfully raised by the bitch for reasons such as poor health, poor lactation performance or too large of a litter may be left with the mother but given supplemental feeding to support nutritional needs. Supplemental food may be given by hand feedings or timed feedings using a surrogate bitch. Puppies may also be reared in a communal situation. Partial orphan rearing can be accomplished by dividing the litter into two groups of equal number and size. One group remains with the mother while the other is removed and fed milk replacer. The groups are exchanged three to four times daily. It is important to feed the separated group before it is returned to the mother. As a result, the group just placed with the dam will be less inclined to nurse immediately (Björck, 1984). It is better to supplement all the puppies in the litter rather than just a few. The advantages of partial orphan rearing are similar to those of fostering. In addition, continued access to the mother can help stimulate milk production and mothering behaviors. When using foster or surrogate mothers, clients should monitor for signs of rejection and cannibalism. Partial orphan rearing may be necessary to assist the efforts of foster mothers. Unfortunately, foster and surrogate mothers are rarely available.

Hand Feeding

The most common method of raising orphaned puppies is hand feeding. Eyedroppers, syringes, bottles and stomach tubes are typically used to feed orphans.

BOTTLE FEEDING

Bottle feeding is the preferred method for vigorous puppies with good nursing reflexes (**Figures 16-1** and **16-2**). Bottle feeding has the advantage that neonates will nurse until they are satiated and reject the milk or formula when full. However, bottle feeding can be time consuming, especially with large litters.

Most puppies will readily suckle small pet nursers, which are available in pet stores (**Figure 16-3**). Feeding bottles for dolls or bottles with nipples for premature human infants are alternatives. The nipple opening should only allow one drop at a time to fall from the nipple when the bottle is inverted. A horizontal slit made with a razor blade instead of a round hole may make it easier for neonates to obtain milk or formula. Milk should be sucked-never squeezed-from the bottle. A rapid flow rate may lead to aspiration of milk and pneumonia and/or death.

Puppies should normally be held horizontally with the head in a natural position (**Figure 16-1**). This position reduces the risk of aspiration. Although some puppies may prefer a different position during feeding (**Figure 16-2**), careful observation is necessary because the risk of aspiration is increased.

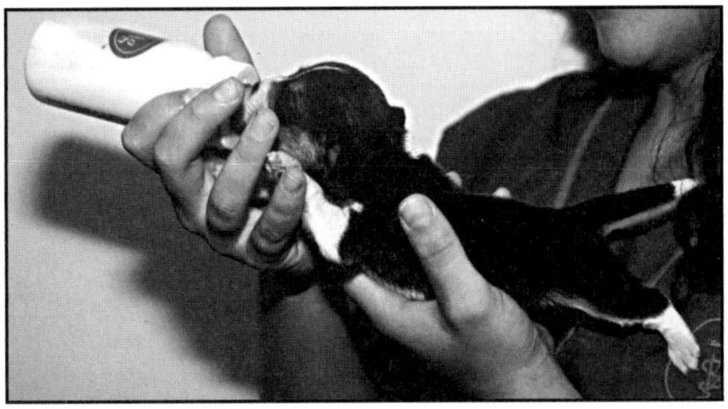

Figure 16-1. This is the preferred position for bottle feeding puppies. This position mimics the normal nursing position and decreases the likelihood of aspiration.

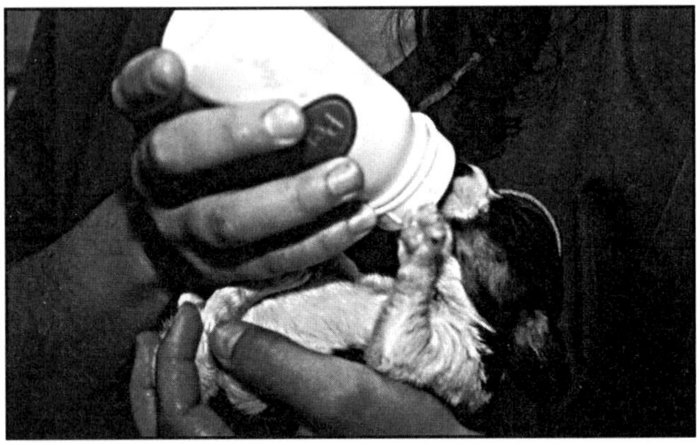

Figure 16-2. Some neonates prefer different positions for bottle feeding. This puppy prefers nursing in dorsal recumbency. Close observation is required because this position may predispose to aspiration.

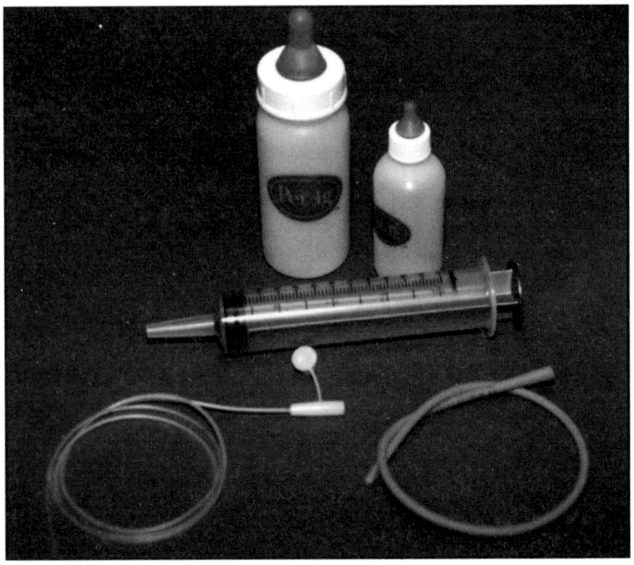

Figure 16-3. Various bottles and feeding tubes can be used for hand feeding orphaned puppies.

TUBE FEEDING

Puppies that are weak or suckle poorly may need to be tube fed. Tube feeding is quicker than bottle feeding and is often used when the same person must care for several orphans. Bottle feeding allows puppies to control the amount of food intake, whereas tube feeding bypasses this control mechanism. Infant feeding tubes (5 to 8 Fr.) or soft urethral or intravenous catheters may be used (**Figure 16-3**).

The tube should be lubricated and placed in the lower esophagus, which is approximately 75% of the distance from the nose to the last rib. Measure and mark the tube with an indelible marker or a piece of tape before insertion. Recheck measurements every few days to account for growth. The orphan should normally be placed horizontally in the palm of the hand with its head in a natural position.

The mouth can be opened using the same hand that steadies the head. Gently advance the tube to the premeasured mark. If resistance is encountered or the puppy suddenly struggles, the tube may be in the trachea. It should be removed and repositioned into the esophagus. Do not feed until proper placement is ensured. After the tube is placed, attach the feeding syringe and slowly administer the warmed formula (over about one to two minutes). The stomach may be palpated to determine the degree of distention. Administration should be stopped if the stomach becomes taut or resists formula flow. Continuation of feeding may result in overdistention and regurgitation. If regurgitation occurs, withdraw the tube and discontinue feeding until the next meal.

Feeding Schedule: Amount, Rate and Formula Temperature

An important part of successful hand feeding is adhering to a strict feeding schedule. Orphans should be fed at least four times daily. Very young neonates and weak puppies should preferably be fed every two to four hours. Older puppies should be fed every four to six hours. Normally, one- to two-week-old puppies will obtain more than 90% of their normal daily intake in four to five meals.

To determine the initial daily amount to feed, first use **Table 16-5** to estimate a puppy's daily energy requirement (DER). Then divide the DER by the energy density of the milk replacer to determine the daily amount to feed. When properly diluted, most milk replacers will provide approximately one kcal/ml. Besides energy and other nutrients, on average, orphaned puppies should receive about 180 ml of diluted milk replacer/kg body weight/day; if necessary, add additional water to the milk replacer if the recommended dilution doesn't provide for this amount of total fluid intake. This amount might underfeed energy but is less likely to cause diarrhea. During the first week of life, the capacity of milk intake by smaller breeds may be limited to about 10 to 15 ml per feeding.

Milk replacers should be warmed to 38°C (100°F) and delivered slowly. Cold foods, rapid feeding rates and over feeding may result in regurgitation, aspiration, bloating and diarrhea. Review and correct the feeding methods if untoward signs develop. If diarrhea is observed, food volume should be reduced or the food should be diluted with water, then gradually returned to levels to meet caloric requirements over successive feedings. It is better to underfeed than over feed neonatal puppies.

Hygiene

Success of hand feeding orphans also depends on how well the caregiver fulfills the daily routine of hygienic measures. Hygienic measures must be more stringent for orphaned puppies because they may have received less colostrum and be more susceptible to infections than other neonates.

- Feeding materials (e.g., bottles and nipples) should be cleaned thoroughly and boiled in water between uses.
- Ingredients for homemade milk replacers should be fresh and refrigerated until used.
- Never prepare more milk replacer than can be used in 24 hours and refrigerate.
- Formulas should be discarded after one hour at room temperature.
- At least twice a week, orphans should be washed gently with a soft moistened cloth to simulate cleaning by the dam's tongue.

REASSESSMENT

Nursing puppies should be reassessed daily. Puppy body weights should be obtained at birth, daily or every other day for the first four weeks and then weekly. Adequacy of the bitch's milk production can be assessed by the growth rate of the puppies, puppy contentment and mammary gland distention. To determine whether an individual mammary gland is producing milk, gently express milk from the nipple while the bitch is relaxed. Most breeders are experienced enough to do this without help. Less experienced owners may need to be taught how to do this; weekly veterinary checkups during the first month may be helpful.

Orphaned puppies should be evaluated daily for the first two weeks of life. They should remain normally hydrated, sleep quietly between feedings and gain weight at a rate similar to bitch raised neonates. Alertness, eagerness to suckle, general behavior, body temperature (i.e., temperature of skin and lower limbs), body weight and stool character should be recorded daily or more often if neonates appear weak or listless.

Orphan rearing requires precise measurement of food intake. Nursing puppies should gain from one g body weight/two to five g of milk intake during the first weeks of life. It is realistic to expect orphaned puppies to gain somewhat less because they are fed at a lower energy intake and milk replacers are not the same as bitch's milk. However, if orphaned puppies do not thrive when fed a commercial milk replacer or homemade replacer, the nutrient content should be compared with mother's milk (**Tables 16-8** through **16-10**). The dilution recommended by the manufacturer should also be checked. In some cases, it may be necessary to switch to another formula.

Puppies with rectal temperatures less than 35°C (95°F) should not be fed milk formula. At this temperature, the sucking reflex is usually absent and normal gut motility has ceased. Neonates should first be warmed slowly after receiving a warm solution of 2.5% glucose by subcutaneous injection (1 ml/30 g body weight).

Weaning is an important event and is integral to successful feeding of nursing and orphaned puppies (**Box 16-5**).

REFERENCES

The references for **Chapter 16** can be found at www.markmorris.org.

Chapter 17

Feeding Growing Puppies: Postweaning to Adulthood

Jacques Debraekeleer
Kathy L. Gross
Steven C. Zicker

"Whoever said you can't buy happiness forgot little puppies."
Gene Hill

INTRODUCTION

This chapter covers puppy growth from immediately post-weaning to adulthood, which generally occurs between 10 to 12 months of age, depending on breed. The goal of a feeding plan for puppies is to create a healthy adult. The specific objectives of a good puppy feeding plan are to achieve healthy growth, optimize trainability and immune function and minimize obesity and developmental orthopedic disease. Growth is a complex process involving interactions between genetics, nutrition and other environmental influences. Nutrition plays a role in the health and development of growing dogs and directly affects the immune system (Sheffy, 1985), body composition (Meyer and Zentek, 1992; Toll et al, 1993), growth rate (Meyer and Zentek, 1992) and skeletal development (Hazewinkel, 1985; Hedhammar et al, 1974; Kealy et al, 1992). Chapter 33 provides in-depth recommendations for feeding large- and giant-breed puppies (>25 kg adult weight) to avoid developmental orthopedic disease.

PATIENT ASSESSMENT

Puppies should be assessed for risk factors before weaning to allow implementation of recommendations for appropriate nutrition. A thorough history and physical evaluation are necessary. Special attention should be paid to large- and giant-breed puppies (Chapter 33) and breeds and sexes (intact and neutered) at risk for obesity (Chapter 27). In addition, growth rates and body condition scores (BCS) provide valuable information about nutritional risks.

Besides being breed dependent, growth rates of young dogs are affected by the nutrient density of the food and the amount of food fed (Meyer and Zentek, 1992). Puppies should be fed to grow at an optimal rate for bone development and body condition rather than at a maximal rate. Growing animals reach a similar adult weight and size whether growth rate is rapid or slow. Feeding for maximum growth increases the risk for skeletal deformities (Hedhammar et al, 1974; Kealy et al, 1992) and decreases longevity in other species (Chipalkatti et al, 1983). In Labrador retrievers, even moderate overfeeding resulted in overweight adults and decreased longevity (Kealy et al, 2002).

The most practical indicator of whether or not a puppy's growth rate is healthy is its BCS. All puppies should have their body condition evaluated and reassessed at least every two weeks to allow for adjustments in amounts fed and, thus, growth rates (Chapter 1). Owners can be trained to assess body condition and are likely to become more aware of the appearance of a healthy growing puppy. A markedly less effective option is to compare the puppy's weight to breed standards for

Table 17-1. Key nutritional factors for foods for growing puppies.*

	Recommended levels in food (DM)	
Factors	Puppies with an adult BW <25 kg	Puppies with an adult BW >25 kg
Energy density (kcal ME/g)	3.5-4.5	3.5-4.5
Energy density (kJ ME/g)	14.6-18.8	14.6-18.8
Crude protein (%)	22-32	22-32
Crude fat (%)	10-25	10-25
DHA (%)	≥0.02	≥0.02
Calcium (%)	0.7-1.7	0.7-1.2
Phosphorus (%)	0.6-1.3	0.6-1.1
Ca:P ratio	1:1-1.8:1	1:1-1.5:1
Digestibility	See energy density recommendations, above; foods with higher energy density values tend to be more digestible	See energy density recommendations, above; foods with higher energy density values tend to be more digestible

Key: DM = dry matter, BW = body weight, kcal = kilocalories, kJ = kilojoules, ME = metabolizable energy, DHA = docosahexaenoic acid.
*For large- and giant-breed dogs (adult BW >25 kg), also see Table 33-5.

Table 17-2. Recommendations for initial estimate of energy intake of growing dogs.

Time frame	x RER	kcal/$BW_{kg}^{0.75}$	kJ/$BW_{kg}^{0.75}$
Weaning to 50% of adult BW*	3	210	880
50 to 80% of adult BW	2.5	175	735
≥80% of adult BW	1.8-2.0	125-140	525-585

Key: RER = resting energy requirement, kcal = kilocalories, kJ = kilojoules, BW = body weight. RER can be obtained from Table 5-2 or calculated. If calculating RER, use one of these two formulas: for puppies of all body weights, $RER_{kcal} = 70(BW_{kg}^{0.75})$; or for puppies weighing more than 2 kg, $RER_{kcal} = 30(BW_{kg}) + 70$. To convert kcal to kJ, multiply by 4.184.
*Great Dane puppies may need 25% more energy during the first two months after weaning = 250 kcal or 1,050 kJ/$BW_{kg}^{0.75}$. See text.

various months of age based on its estimated mature weight. Furthermore, regularly assessing body condition provides more immediate feedback about optimal nutritional status than using body weights based on estimated adult size.

Key Nutritional Factors

The requirements for all nutrients are increased during growth compared with requirements for adult dogs. Most nutrients supplied in excess of that needed for growth cause little to no harm. However, excess energy and calcium are of special concern; these concerns include energy for puppies of small and medium breeds (for obesity prevention) and energy and calcium for puppies of large and giant breeds (for skeletal health). Also, essential fatty acids can affect neural development and trainability of puppies.

Table 17-1 summarizes the key nutritional factors for growing puppies. The following sections describe these key nutritional factors in more detail. The concept of key nutritional factors is based on the assumption that commercial foods are fed.

Energy

Energy requirements for growing puppies consist of energy needed for maintenance and growth. During the first weeks after weaning when body weight is relatively small and the growth rate is high, puppies use about 50% of their total energy intake for maintenance and 50% for growth (Gesellshaft, 1989; Sheffy, 1978). Gradually, the growth curves reach a plateau, as puppies become young adults (**Figure 17-1**). The proportion of energy needed for maintenance increases progressively, whereas the part for growth decreases. Energy needed for growth decreases to about 8 to 10% of the total energy requirement when puppies reach 80% or more of adult body weight. Because of the shift in energy usage, total food intake of a typical German shepherd puppy (adult body weight ~35 kg), based on energy needs, may no longer increase after about four months of age.

A puppy's daily energy requirement (DER) should be about 3 x its resting energy requirement (RER) until it reaches about 50% of its adult body weight (**Table 17-2**). Thereafter, energy intake should be about 2.5 x RER and can be reduced progressively to 2 x RER. When approximately 80% of adult size is reached, 1.8 to 2 x RER is usually sufficient. Great Dane puppies may have energy requirements 25% higher than those of other breeds. Young Great Dane puppies may not grow when daily energy intake is less than 175 kcal (735 kJ) metabolizable energy (ME)/$BW_{kg}^{0.75}$ (2.5 x RER) (Meyer and Zentek, 1992; Meyer and Zentek, 1991). However, this finding should not be extrapolated to other giant-breed puppies (Rainbird and Kienzle, 1990). These factors are general recommendations or starting points to estimate energy needs. Body condition scoring should be used to adjust these energy estimates to individual puppies.

Prevention of obesity is essential and should start at weaning. As in people, after puppies become overweight, it is very difficult to return to, and maintain, normal weight. Excessive food intake during growth may contribute to skeletal disorders in large- and giant-breed puppies (Chapter 33) (Kealy et al, 1992). If overweight and obesity are carried into adulthood, the risk for several important diseases is increased (Chapter 27). These include hypertension, heart disease, diabetes mellitus, dyslipidemias, osteoarthritis, heat and exercise intolerance and decreased immune function. Obesity also increases cellular oxidative stress. Long-term oxidative stress has its own serious health implications (Chapter 7). Studies show that moderate energy and food restriction during the postweaning growth period reduces the prevalence of hip dysplasia in large-breed (Labrador retriever) puppies and increases longevity in rats without retarding adult size (Kealy et al, 1992; Chipalkatti et al, 1983; Nolen, 1972; Ross and Bras, 1973; Ross, 1972). However, feeding a food with a very low energy density and low digestibility may not supply enough energy and nutrients to support optimal growth. This approach can lead to intake of large quantities of the food, which can overload the gastrointestinal (GI) tract resulting in vomiting and diarrhea. Together, these factors make for a prudent argument to initiate monitoring of energy and food intake and body condition at an early age. Recommended energy density requirements for growing dogs are listed under the key nutritional factor "Fat" below.

Protein

Protein requirements of growing dogs differ quantitatively and qualitatively from those of adults. Quantitatively, at this stage of growth, protein requirements are highest at weaning and decrease progressively (Meyer, 1990; Burns et al, 1982; Case and Czarnecki-Maulden, 1990). For example, the level of crude protein in bitch's milk is 33% dry matter (DM). Bitch's milk is a highly digestible food with an energy density of 6.4 kcal/g DM. This level is equivalent to 21% highly digestible protein in a commercial food with 4 kcal/g DM. In one study, beagle puppies needed a food with a minimum of 15% DM protein of high biologic value and 90% digestibility to achieve optimal growth immediately after weaning. Only 11.7% (DM) of the same high-quality protein was needed at three months of age (Burns et al, 1982).

For puppies 14 weeks and older, the minimum recommended allowance for crude protein is 17.5% DM (NRC, 2006). The recommended protein range in foods intended for growth in all puppies (small, medium and large breed) is 22 to 32% DM (**Table 17-1**). Most dry commercial foods marketed for puppy growth provide protein levels within this range.

Protein levels above the upper end of this range have not been shown to be detrimental but are well above the level in bitch's milk. Earlier work suggested that excessive protein intake might play a role in the development of skeletal deformities in giant-breed dogs (Hedhammar et al, 1974). Since then, it has been shown that foods containing 23 to 31% crude protein (6.4 to 8.8 g/100 kcal ME) do not have a deleterious effect on skeletal development. Furthermore, these levels support optimal growth, provided calcium and energy levels are appropriate (Nap et al, 1991; Nap, 1993). Most commercial foods for puppy growth contain more protein than is needed.

Protein requirements of growing dogs differ quantitatively and qualitatively from those of adults. An important difference is that arginine is an essential amino acid for puppies, whereas it is only conditionally essential for adult dogs (Young et al, 1978) (Arginine is present in ample amounts in essentially all pet foods and thus is not considered a key nutritional factor for commercial foods).

Foods formulated for adult dogs should not be fed to puppies. Although protein levels may be adequate, energy levels and other nutrients may not be balanced for growth.

Fat

Dietary fat serves three primary functions: 1) a source of essential fatty acids, 2) a carrier for fat-soluble vitamins and 3) a concentrated source of energy. Growing dogs have an estimated daily requirement for essential fatty acids (linoleic acid) of about 250 mg/kg body weight (Meyer, 1990b), which can be provided by a food containing between 5 to 10% DM fat (Meyer, 1990). The fat source must be carefully chosen when low-fat foods (<10% DM fat) are fed to ensure that sufficient amounts of linoleic acid are provided.

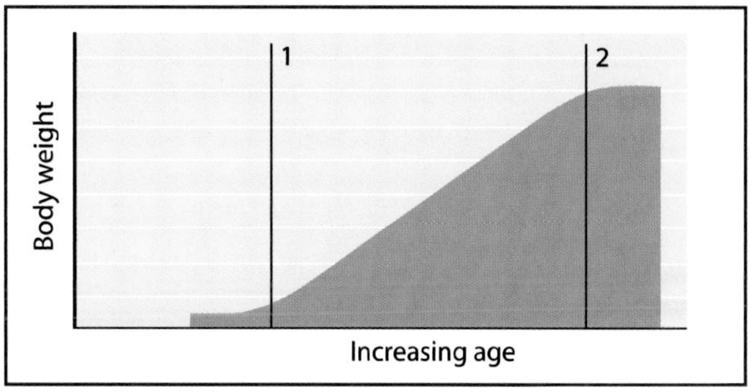

Figure 17-1. Typical sigmoidal growth curve of puppies. Growing puppies' energy needs may be subdivided into two components: the energy needed for maintenance and the energy required for accretion of body tissue. During the first weeks after weaning, when body weight is relatively small and growth rate exponential, puppies use about 50% of the energy for maintenance and 50% for growth. Gradually, the growth curve reaches a plateau. As body weight increases, the share of energy needed for maintenance increases progressively, whereas the part for growth becomes proportionately less important. The starting (line 1) and endpoint (line 2) of exponential growth can shift depending on the breed and individual variation. (See text and references.)

Studies indicate that docosahexaenoic acid (DHA) is essential for normal neural, retinal and auditory development in puppies (Pawlosky et al, 1997). Similar results have been found in other species (Pawlosky et al, 1997; Birch et al, 2002; Diau et al, 2003; Hoffman et al, 2003). Inclusion of fish oil as a source of DHA in puppy foods improves trainability (Kelley et al, 2004). Conversion of short-chain polyunsaturated fatty acids to DHA is an inefficient process in puppies (Bauer et al, 2006). Thus, adding a source of DHA should be considered essential for growth. The minimum recommended allowance for DHA plus eicosapentaenoic acid (EPA) is 0.05% DM; EPA should not exceed 60% of the total (NRC, 2006). Thus, DHA needs to be at least 40% of the total DHA plus EPA, or 0.02% DM.

Fat contributes greatly to the energy density of a food; however, excessive energy intake can cause overweight/obesity and developmental orthopedic disease, as discussed above. The minimum recommended allowance of dietary fat for growth (8.5% DM) is much less than that needed for nursing, but more than is needed for adult maintenance (5.5% DM) (NRC, 2006). To provide a DM energy density between 3.5 to 4.5 kcal/g, between 10 and 25% DM fat is required; this range of dietary fat is recommended from postweaning to adulthood.

Calcium and Phosphorus

Although growing dogs need more calcium and phosphorus than adult dogs, the minimum requirements are relatively low. Puppies have been successfully raised when fed foods contain-

Table 17-3. Feeding plan summary for growing puppies.

1. Estimate adult body weight for determination of the recommended calcium range (>25 kg adult weight, use large-/giant-breed recommendation).
2. Using **Table 17-4** (or manufacturer's information), select a food with the recommended levels of key nutritional factors; ensure the selected food has been approved for puppy growth by a credible regulatory agency (e.g., AAFCO).
3. Avoid free-choice feeding; use food-restricted meal feeding, dividing the amount fed into two to four daily feedings.
4. Estimate the initial amount to feed from recommendations on product package or by calculation (**Table 17-5**). Remember, such recommendations and calculations should be used as guidelines or starting points and not as absolute requirements.
5. Teach owners to perform body condition scoring and have them monitor body condition at least every two weeks and adjust the amount fed by 10% increments to maintain a BCS of 2.5/5 to 3/5.
6. Veterinarians should assess body condition and weight of puppies in conjunction with routine vaccinations and more frequently if any indication of under- or overnutrition is detected. The feeding plan, including food dosage, should be modified as necessary.
7. Underfeeding through the growth phase is healthier than overfeeding and results in the same mature size.

Key: AAFCO = Association of American Feed Control Officials, BCS = body condition score.

Box 17-1. Digestible Carbohydrates in Foods for Growing Puppies.

No specific recommendations for digestible (soluble) carbohydrate levels are available for growing dogs. It has been suggested that foods contain about 20% digestible carbohydrate until puppies are four months of age to ensure optimal health. In one study, feeding young puppies a food high in protein and fat without carbohydrate resulted in lethargy, poor appetite, diarrhea and mortality, which were attributed to fatty liver syndrome. However, another study failed to confirm these results. Body fat is higher when puppies are fed a very high-fat, low-carbohydrate food during growth.

The Bibliography for **Box 17-1** can be found at www.markmorris.org.

ing 0.37 to 0.6% DM calcium and 0.33% DM phosphorus (Jenkins and Phillips, 1960; Jenkins and Phillips, 1960a). Intestinal absorption of calcium can vary from almost 0 to 90% (Hazewinkel, 1985; Nap, 1993), and phosphorus absorption can increase to almost 80% to adapt to intake (Gesellshaft, 1989a; Jenkins and Phillips, 1960). Generally, calcium absorption depends on requirements and calcium intake (Meyer, 1990a). Calcium homeostatic mechanisms may be less precise in young puppies. In puppies between two and six months of age, intestinal absorption of calcium never decreases below approximately 40%, even if they receive high levels of calcium in foods (Hazewinkel, 1985; Hedhammar et al, 1974; Nap, 1993; Jenkins and Phillips, 1960). Retention of calcium, therefore, increases when young dogs receive high levels of calcium, either in the food or as a supplement (Hazewinkel, 1985; Nap, 1993). Absorption of calcium gradually is more regulated after puppies are about 10 months old (Hedhammar et al, 1974).

Foods for large- and giant-breed puppies should contain 0.7 to 1.2% DM calcium (0.6 to 1.1% phosphorus) (Chapter 33). Foods with a calcium content of 1.1% DM provide more calcium to puppies just after weaning than if bitch's milk is fed exclusively (Resnick, 1978). Because small- to medium-sized breeds are less sensitive to slightly overfeeding or underfeeding calcium (Nap, 1993), the level of calcium in foods for these puppies can range from 0.7 to 1.7% DM, (0.6 to 1.3% phosphorus) without risk. The phosphorus intake is less critical than the calcium intake, provided the minimum requirements of 0.35% DM are met and the calcium-phosphorus ratio is between 1:1 and 1.8:1 (Jenkins and Phillips, 1960; Jenkins and Phillips, 1960a). For large- and giant-breed dogs, the calcium-phosphorus ratio should be between 1:1 and 1.5:1.

Digestibility

The ability of 11-week-old puppies to digest foods was less than at 60 weeks of age (Weber et al, 2003). Also, puppies fed foods low in energy density and digestibility need to eat larger quantities of food to achieve growth, increasing the risk of flatulence, vomiting, diarrhea and the development of a "pot-bellied" appearance. Therefore, foods recommended for puppies should be more digestible than typical adult foods. Most pet food companies, however, do not provide digestibility data. An indirect indicator of digestibility is energy density. Foods with a higher energy density are likely to be more digestible.

Other Nutritional Factors

Copper

Most commercial pet foods should contain adequate levels of copper unless the availability is low (e.g., when sources such as copper oxide are used) (Aoyagi and Baker, 1993). Puppies with copper deficiency may have loss of hair pigmentation, with graying of black and dark brown hair (Zentek, 1991; Zentek et al, 1991). Hyperextension of the distal phalanges and splayed toes on the front feet and normochromic, normocytic anemia may develop in more extreme cases (Zentek, 1991; Zentek et al, 1991). The recommended minimum allowance for copper in growing puppies is 1.1% DM (NRC, 2006).

Phenylalanine and Tyrosine

Tyrosine is not an essential amino acid but is made from phenylalanine. Also, tyrosine spares about half of the need for phenylalanine. Therefore, it is appropriate to consider the amount of phenylalanine required as the sum of phenylalanine plus tyrosine. Although phenylalanine and tyrosine have not been shown to be the most limiting amino acids for growth in commercial food, at least twice as much phenylalanine, or phenylalanine plus tyrosine, is required for maximal black hair color as for growth (Biourge and Sergheraert, 2002). Other metabolic needs for phenylalanine and tyrosine include protein, thyroid hormone and catecholamine synthesis (NRC, 2006). The recommended minimum allowance for phenylalanine plus tyrosine in foods for puppy growth is 1.0% DM.

Carbohydrates

Although no specific level of digestible (soluble) carbohydrates exists for growing puppies, inclusion of about 20% (DM) may optimize health (**Box 17-1**).

FEEDING PLAN

The feeding plan consists of choosing the best food and the best feeding method. Reassessment at appropriate intervals is another key to a successful feeding plan. **Table 17-3** summarizes the feeding plan.

Assess and Select the Food

The food assessment phase will help determine the best food to feed or whether it is necessary to change foods if a food has already been selected. If a change is indicated, select a food that has been approved by a credible regulatory agency such as the Association of American Feed Control Officials (AAFCO). However, AAFCO feeding trials only last 10 weeks. During this time, potential problems related to excess calcium and energy consumption, especially in large- and giant-breed puppies may not have had time to manifest. Therefore, foods selected for growth should have key nutrients in the ranges provided in **Table 17-1.**

If the appropriate food was selected for reproduction, puppies of small- to medium-sized breeds (<25 kg anticipated adult weight) may continue to receive the same food as the bitch received during lactation. These puppies were probably transitioned to this food during weaning. Large- and giant-breed puppies should be fed a food that contains less calcium and energy to decrease the risk of developmental orthopedic disease. If possible, such foods should be fed during early weaning. Chapter 33 contains more detailed information about feeding large- and giant-breed puppies. The greatest nutritional influence on the incidence of phenotypic hip dysplasia occurs when energy is restricted very early in life (Lust et al, 1973).

Besides selecting an AAFCO (or a food approved by another credible organization) approved food, the food assessment/selection process includes comparing the nutrient profile of the current food, or the food under consideration, with the key nutritional factors in the amounts discussed above. **Table 17-4** lists levels of key nutritional factors in selected commercial foods marketed for healthy puppy growth and compares them to the recommended levels. If the food in question is not listed in **Table 17-4**, contact pet food manufacturers for this or other missing information. The guaranteed or typical analysis on pet food labels is of limited use and will not contain information about digestibility. Information about digestibility and energy density should be obtained from the manufacturer; digestibility must be sufficiently high to avoid GI problems. Also, foods with similar label declarations can have markedly different nutrient availabilities and growth performance (Huber et al, 1986; Huber et al, 1991).

Growing dogs should not receive vitamin-mineral supplements when fed complete, balanced commercial foods. Supplements may be justified to balance homemade foods. Because it is very difficult for breeders to exactly balance a homemade food, large- and giant-breed puppies should only receive a commercially prepared food specifically designed for such breeds. If an owner insists on using homemade foods, it is best to consult with a qualified veterinary nutritionist to ensure a homemade recipe is balanced (Chapter 10).

The calcium and energy content of treats should be similar to that recommended for the food (**Table 17-4**). If not, the number of treats fed should be limited to no more than 10% of the total amount of food fed. Treats given in large amounts may almost double a puppy's calcium intake (Box 33-5). Most treats are not complete and balanced for puppy growth. Check the product label for this information.

Assess and Determine the Feeding Method

Feeding method assessment is critical to successful management of growing puppies, especially those of large and giant breeds. The feeding method includes how much food is fed and how it is offered. Food can be offered three ways: free choice, time-restricted meal feeding and food-restricted meal feeding. Free-choice and time-restricted feeding should be avoided during rapid growth.

Free-choice feeding may increase body fat, predispose the dog to obesity and, in large breeds, induce skeletal deformities at a young age. Breeders who want to maximize growth of large- and giant-breed puppies should be informed that overfeeding predisposes to developmental orthopedic disease. Even under these circumstances, rate of weight gain and body condition should be monitored closely (at least every two weeks).

Previously, time-restricted meal feeding was recommended (feeding a puppy all it can eat in 20 minutes, twice daily) (Lewis et al, 1987). However, more recent research showed that puppies fed using this method had increased body weight, more body fat and increased bone mineral accretion than puppies receiving the same food free choice (Toll et al, 1993).

During periods of rapid growth, puppies should be fed a measured amount of food (food-restricted meal feeding) every day based on body condition and age. The allotted amount of food can be offered in one or two meals per day. This recommendation includes thin puppies owned by clients who are tempted to feed more food so their puppies can "catch up."

Feeding puppies an allotted amount of food is best for most puppies because it allows for better control of body condition and rate of growth. Using this feeding method for growing puppies is complicated because the amount fed per unit body weight needs to be adjusted regularly. Initially the amount fed needs to be greater per unit body weight and then is reduced as the growth rate and energy requirements per unit body weight decline (**Figure 17-1** and **Table 17-2**). Also, the initial amount fed needs to be determined.

The initial daily food dose can be estimated by dividing the puppy's DER by the energy density of the food. From a practi-

Table 17-4. Comparison of recommended levels of key nutritional factors for small- to medium-breed puppies (adult BW <25 kg) to the key nutritional factor content of selected commercial foods marketed for healthy puppy growth.* For large- to giant-breed puppies (>25 kg), see foods and recommended levels in Table 33-6.

Dry foods	Energy density (kcal/cup)**	Energy density (kcal ME/g)***	Protein (%)	Fat (%)	DHA (%)	Ca (%)	P (%)	Ca:P
Recommended levels	**-**	**3.5-4.5**	**22-32**	**10-25**	**≥0.02**	**0.7-1.7**	**0.6-1.3**	**1:1-1.8:1**
Hill's Science Diet Puppy Healthy Development Original	384	4.2	31.8	22.9	0.22	1.59	1.21	1.3:1
Hill's Science Diet Puppy Lamb Meal & Rice Recipe	377	4.2	31.7	21.7	0.22	1.58	1.10	1.4:1
Hill's Science Diet Nature's Best Chicken & Brown Rice Dinner Puppy	445	4.3	30.2	22.1	0.20	1.43	1.05	1.4:1
Hill's Science Diet Nature's Best Lamb & Brown Rice Dinner Puppy	442	4.2	30.1	22.1	0.17	1.50	1.10	1.4:1
Iams Eukanuba Medium Breed Puppy	463	4.1	31.7	19.2	na	1.50	1.07	1.4:1
Iams ProActive Health Smart Puppy	432	4.2	30.8	18.9	na	1.30	1.10	1.2:1
Medi-Cal Veterinary Diet Development Formula	425	na	28.4	17.5	na	1.20	1.10	1.1:1
Nutro Natural Choice Puppy Lamb Meal and Rice	333	3.8	29.7	14.3	na	1.98	1.54	1.3:1
Purina ONE Healthy Puppy Formula	465	4.6	31.7	20.6	na	1.61	1.11	1.5:1
Purina Puppy Chow	416	4.2	29.8	15.6	na	1.31	1.01	1.3:1
Purina Pro Plan Chicken & Rice Formula Puppy	473	4.6	31.6	20.7	na	1.23	1.04	1.2:1
Royal Canin Medium Puppy 32	402	4.6	35.6	20.0	na	1.12	0.88	1.3:1
Moist foods	**Energy density (kcal/can)****	**Energy density (kcal ME/g)*****	**Protein (%)**	**Fat (%)**	**DHA (%)**	**Ca (%)**	**P (%)**	**Ca:P**
Recommended levels	**-**	**3.5-4.5**	**22-32**	**10-25**	**≥0.02**	**0.7-1.7**	**0.6-1.3**	**1:1-1.8:1**
Hill's Science Diet Puppy Healthy Development Savory Chicken Entrée	205/5.8 oz. 459/13 oz.	4.1	28.2	23.6	na	1.33	0.96	1.4 : 1
Purina Pro Plan Puppy Chicken & Rice Entrée Classic	459/13 oz.	4.9	42.4	38.4	na	1.92	1.48	1.3:1

Key: BW = body weight, ME = metabolizable energy, DHA = docosahexaenoic acid, Ca = calcium, P = phosphorus, na = not available from manufacturer.
*From manufacturers' published information or calculated from manufacturers' published as-fed values; all values are on a dry matter basis unless otherwise stated.
**Energy density values are listed on an as fed basis and are useful for determining the amount to feed; cup = 8-oz. measuring cup.
***Energy density also reflects digestibility; foods with higher energy density are likely to have better digestibility than foods with lower energy density; for kJ/g, multiply kcal/g by 4.184.

cal standpoint, the energy requirement can be estimated but not determined precisely. Estimates of a puppy's DER can be obtained from **Table 17-2** (i.e., this phase of growth can be divided into three periods). The DER can also be calculated. DER calculations are simple and are based on the puppy's RER; **Table 17-2** lists RER factors. RER can be calculated (**Table 17-5**) or obtained directly from Table 5-2 or the food manufacturer.

The initial daily food dose estimate is merely a starting point. Body condition scoring (Figure 1-2) should be used to adjust the food dose estimate to individual puppies and will need to be readjusted regularly (10% increments) to allow for changes in growth rate. This amount can be fed in two to four meals per day. Note that Great Dane puppies may have energy requirements 25% higher than those of other breeds. As mentioned above, young Great Dane puppies may not grow when daily energy intake is less than 175 kcal (735 kJ) ME/$BW_{kg}^{0.75}$ (2.5 x RER) (Meyer and Zentek, 1992; Meyer and Zentek, 1991).

However, this finding should not be extrapolated to other giant-breed puppies (Rainbird and Kienzle, 1990).

REASSESSMENT

Owners should weigh growing puppies weekly and record body weights and food intake (including snacks and treats). Veterinarians, or members of their health care team, can instruct owners about how to BCS their own puppies. A BCS should be obtained at least every two weeks. During office calls for routine vaccinations, veterinarians can compare the owners' scores with their own. This level of attention to BCS can be important to the development of a healthy puppy. The owner is then prepared to continue to make these observations throughout the life of the dog. Such dogs, as adults, should be less likely to experience skeletal diseases (large and giant breeds) and overweight or obesity and the myriad of related problems (most breeds).

Veterinarians should reassess puppies at the time of routine vaccinations and more frequently if any indication of under- or overnutrition is detected. Reassessment should include body weight and body condition assessment, food assessment and determination of correct food dosage (**Table 17-5**).

Table 17-5. Example of a food dosage calculation for a growing puppy.

Problem: what is the estimated amount of a growth food (375 kcal/cup) that should be fed to a five-month-old male Labrador retriever puppy weighing 18 kg?

1) Determine RER by using the linear formula: RER_{kcal} = 30(BW_{kg}) + 70; RER_{kcal} = 30(18) + 70 = 610 kcal/day or from Table 5-2.
2) Determine DER by using the RER factors in **Table 17-2**, based on age: 2.5 x RER = 2.5 x 610 kcal = 1,525 kcal/day.
3) Divide the DER by the energy density of the food (**Table 17-4**), to obtain the estimated daily amount to feed: 1,525 kcal ÷ 375 kcal/cup = 4 cups/day.
4) Divide the daily amount to feed into two to four individual meals.
5) This amount is only an estimate and is intended to be used as a starting point. The puppy's body condition should be monitored regularly (at least every two weeks) and the amount fed should be increased or decreased by 10%, depending on body condition score.

Key: cup = 8 volume oz. measuring cup (240 cc), RER = resting energy requirement, DER = daily energy requirement.

REFERENCES

The references for **Chapter 17** can be found at www.markmorris.org.

CASE 17-1

Initial Health Care for a Welsh Corgi Puppy

Jacques Debraekeleer, DVM
Hill's Science and Technology Center
Etten Leur, The Netherlands

Kathy L. Gross, PhD
Hill's Science and Technology Center
Topeka, Kansas, USA

Patient Assessment

A 10-week-old, female Welsh corgi puppy was examined as part of a routine health maintenance program. The owners had recently purchased the puppy from a local breeder and had never owned a dog before. They were interested in vaccinations and any other information about caring for puppies. They had had the puppy for two days and indicated that everything appeared normal.

Physical examination revealed an alert and active puppy with no obvious problems. The puppy weighed 6.5 kg and had a normal body condition (body condition score [BCS] 3/5). The estimated adult weight was about 17 kg. Results of a fecal flotation test were negative for intestinal parasites. Routine vaccinations were given.

Assess the Food and Feeding Method

The breeder provided a small amount of an unknown dry food in a plastic bag. The owners had offered small amounts of this food three times per day, and the puppy ate the food very well. They were also given a bottle of chewable vitamin-mineral tablets by the breeder and instructed to give the puppy one tablet per day.

Questions

1. What are the key nutritional factors to consider in developing a feeding plan for this puppy?
2. Outline a specific feeding plan for this patient including an appropriate food and feeding method.
3. Should the owners continue to provide the chewable vitamin-mineral supplement?

4. Besides nutrition, what other health care topics for puppies should be discussed with these owners?

Answers and Discussion

1. Key nutritional factors for growing dogs include energy, protein, fat, calcium, phosphorus and digestibility. Energy is required to support rapid accretion of new tissue; however, excessive energy intake increases the risk of obesity and, in some breeds, developmental orthopedic disease. Foods for puppies should contain 3.5 to 4.5 kcal (14.6 to 18.8 kJ) metabolizable energy (ME)/g dry matter (DM). Fat makes the greatest contribution to the energy density of food and should be 10 to 25% DM in growth-type foods. Puppies also have higher protein requirements than adult dogs to support tissue growth. Protein levels of 22 to 32% DM are recommended for puppies. Adequate calcium is important in foods for growing dogs to support skeletal development. Known calcium deficiency is rarely a concern in growing dogs fed commercial foods, but it may be a problem for dogs fed homemade foods. Excess calcium intake is a risk factor for developmental orthopedic disease and may occur in growing dogs eating some commercial foods and/or receiving mineral supplements. Calcium levels of 0.7 to 1.7% DM are generally recommended for growing dogs. Phosphorus is less critical than calcium provided minimum requirements of 0.35% DM are met and the calcium-phosphorus ratio is between 1:1 and 1.8:1. No specific recommendations for dietary carbohydrate are available for growing dogs; however, puppies appear to do better if growth-type foods contain more than 20% complex carbohydrate DM. Gastrointestinal (GI) distention ("pot-bellied" appearance) and GI disturbances (i.e., flatulence, vomiting, diarrhea) are less common in puppies fed highly digestible foods.
2. A food specifically formulated for growing dogs that addresses the key nutritional factors described above should be recommended. A number of commercial products meet these objectives. Homemade foods can also be fed to growing dogs; however, recipes should be used that contain adequate protein, fat, calcium, vitamins and trace minerals to support growth.Feeding methods for growing dogs include free-choice (ad libitum) feeding, time-limited feeding and food-limited feeding. Free-choice feeding is relatively effortless and may reduce abnormal behavior such as barking at feeding time. In addition, frequent trips to the food bowl may help reduce boredom and coprophagy, and timid or unthrifty dogs experience less competition when eating. Disadvantages of free-choice feeding include food wastage, only dry or semi-moist forms of pet food can be fed and competition or boredom may stimulate overeating. The most serious disadvantage in young growing dogs is increased risk for obesity and developmental orthopedic disease due to over consumption of even a properly balanced food.

   Time-limited feeding is a method in which dogs are allowed free access to food for a defined period, usually 10 to 15 minutes, once or twice daily. This feeding method may result in less overall food consumption when compared with puppies fed free choice. Time-limited feeding may also help in disciplining and housetraining young puppies. The owner interacts with the puppy during this time and is able to observe its general condition and behavior, which may lead to earlier detection of problems. A routine of feeding a puppy and then taking it outdoors can reinforce housetraining by taking advantage of the gastrocolic reflex. Advocates of this feeding method suggest that when some dogs fed in this manner reach adulthood they may voluntarily limit their feeding to once or twice a day and thus avoid overeating. However, research has shown that some dogs may eat as much in 15 minutes as when fed free choice. In this study, dogs fed by a time-limited method had higher weight gain, more body fat and increased bone mineral accretion than dogs receiving the same food free choice. This method is also less convenient for the owner than free-choice feeding.

   Food-limited feeding (feeding a measured amount of food every day) requires knowing how much to feed. This is best obtained by estimating the amount to feed based on the puppy's calculated daily energy requirement or as recommended by the manufacturer, and then adjusting the amount as necessary to maintain a BCS between 2.5/5 to 3.5/5. This amount is divided into two to four meals per day. This is the method of choice for feeding all puppies to reduce the risk of obesity and developmental orthopedic disease because it limits food intake to maintain optimal growth rate and body condition. This method is also less convenient and more time consuming than free-choice feeding because food amounts must be increased as growth occurs.
3. Routine vitamin-mineral supplementation is not necessary for healthy puppies eating balanced commercial growth foods. Supplementation is important if homemade foods are used.
4. In addition to vaccination, intestinal parasite control and nutritional counseling, the following health maintenance procedures should be discussed with puppy owners: 1) external parasites and appropriate control programs, 2) heartworm preventive programs, in endemic areas, 3) the pet's behavior and socialization, 4) specific breed characteristics, 5) routine grooming procedures, 6) basic obedience training and reputable obedience schools, 7) recommendations for neutering, 8) housetraining and 9) manipulation of the mouth to accustom the puppy to toothbrushing later on. All of these topics should be discussed with these clients, especially because they are novice dog owners.

Progress Notes

All of the health maintenance procedures mentioned above were discussed with the owners by the veterinarian or veterinary technician. A commercial specialty brand dry food formulated for canine growth (Science Diet Puppy Healthy Development Original[a]) was recommended. The quantity of food to be fed was based on the feeding instructions on the pet food bag. This amount was divided into three equal daily meals. The owners were instructed to discontinue the vitamin-mineral supplement and were given an instruction sheet that outlined how to assess the body condition of puppies. The food amount was to be adjusted as the puppy grew according to the feeding guidelines on the bag. The owners were asked to weigh and assign a BCS for the puppy every other week and adjust the food amount as needed to maintain optimal body condition. The veterinary technician would also assess the body weight and condition during subsequent office visits when the puppy was 14 to 16 and 20 to 22 weeks of age.

Endnote

a. Hill's Pet Nutrition, Inc., Topeka, KS, USA.

Bibliography

Toll PW, Richardson DC, Jewell DE, et al. The effect of feeding method on growth and body composition in young puppies (abstract). In: Abstract Book. Waltham Symposium on the Nutrition of Companion Animals. Adelaide, Australia, September 23-25, 1993: 33.

Section 4

Feeding Working and Sporting Dogs

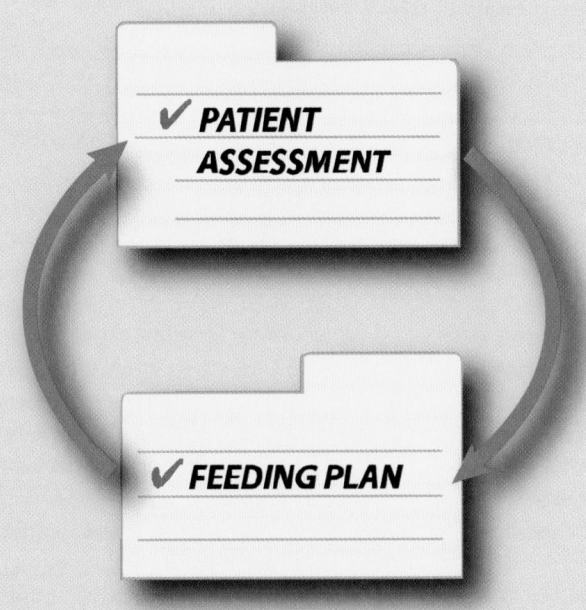

Chapter 18

Feeding Working and Sporting Dogs

Philip W. Toll
Robert L. Gillette
Michael S. Hand

"We derive immeasurable good, uncounted pleasures, enormous security, and many critical lessons about life by owning dogs."
Roger Caras, A Celebration of Dogs

INTRODUCTION

Working and sporting dogs undertake a wide range of activities (**Table 18-1**). Depending on the activity, there is a need for athletic performance, scent detection or both. Athletic performance and scent detection depend on genetics, training and nutrition. All three must be optimal for maximal performance. A deficiency in any one of these factors limits performance; therefore, each factor must be assessed in light of the activity performed by an individual dog.

Genetics

The genetic characteristics of the dog must be appropriate for the type of activity it does. Mental, physical and metabolic characteristics all play a role. As an example, rat terriers are bred to have the physical and mental characteristics that make them effective in the pursuit and capture of rats and other burrowing animals. Also, as a result of genetic selection, sight hounds excel at pursuing and capturing prey in open fields. Physical characteristics such as conformation, heart size and muscle fiber type dictate the limits of athletic performance. Genetics likely also play a role in a dog's desire to perform. Certainly, it is desirable that sporting or working dogs be willing, or even eager, to perform the tasks asked of them. For example, if a Labrador retriever has no desire to enter the water or a sheepdog has no desire to herd, or a sled dog no desire to pull, whether or not physical characteristics are ideal becomes irrelevant. Thus the basis of a dog's performance depends on its innate physical and mental potential. This generalization assumes that any lack of desire that may be present is not due to injury, illness, improper training or malnutrition. But, if a working or sporting dog has the desired physical, metabolic and mental characteristics, its performance can be optimized by appropriate training and nutrition.

Training

Assessment of training should ensure that the intensity, duration and frequency match the desired level of performance. Many canine athletes are poorly trained. This is especially true for intermittent athletes such as hunting dogs that spend much of the year in a run or small yard but are expected to hunt for many hours at the onset of hunting season. This also applies to other "weekend athletes" (i.e., dogs that compete or participate in weekend activities with their owners). It seems the trend is for more dogs to participate as workout companions with their owners.

Table 18-1. Working and sporting dog activities listed by exercise type.

Exercise type	Activity
Sprint (high-intensity physical activity that can be sustained less than two minutes)	Coursing (sight hounds) Racing (greyhounds, whippets) Weight pulling
Intermediate (physical activity lasting a few minutes to a few hours)	Agility Border patrol, customs Drug detection Exercise with people (running, bicycling) Field trials Frisbee trials Guarding Hunting (game birds, rabbits) Livestock management (cattle, sheep, hogs) Military Police work Pursuit (raccoon, coyote, fox, deer, wild boar) Search and rescue Service work (guide dogs, assistance dogs) Tracking
Endurance (physical activity that last many hours)	Sled pulling (racing, expedition)

Table 18-2. Popular books about training scent-detection dogs.

Pearsall MD, Verbuggen H. Scent. Training to Track, Search and Rescue, 1982. Alpine Publications, Inc. PO Box 7027, Loveland, CO 80537.
Tweedie J. On the Trail! A Practical Guide to the Working Bloodhound and Other Search and Rescue Dogs, 1998. Alpine Publications, Inc. PO Box 7027, Loveland, CO 80537.
Syrotuck WG. Scent and the Scenting Dog, 1972. Barkleigh Productions, Inc. 6 State Road #113, Mechanicsburg, PA 17050.
Johnson GR. Tracking Dog. Theory and Methods, 1975. Barkleigh Productions, Inc. 6 State Road #113, Mechanicsburg, PA 17050.

Exercise training is simply the consistent performance of some type of exercise over an extended period of time. Although genetics dictate the mental, anatomic and metabolic characteristics of an individual dog, training can alter some of these characteristics and enhance exercise and scent-detection performance. **Table 18-2** lists four popular books that include methods for training scent-detection dogs.

Exercise training means subjecting a dog to a workload of sufficient intensity, duration and frequency to produce a measurable adaptation of the systems being trained. The types of adaptations produced by training are specific; that is, physiologic changes occur that favor the type of activity performed. To improve aerobic power, exercise intensity should be greater than 50% of maximum oxygen consumption (VO_2 max) for sedentary individuals. As the level of training or fitness improves, intensity and duration must be increased to produce further improvement. The general principle is that intensity and duration must be increased until a level of overload is reached for the systems being trained to induce adaptation. Furthermore, training adaptations are specific to the type of exercise performed.

Examples of training-induced changes include increased bone mass, muscle hypertrophy, increased mitochondrial density in muscle and plasma volume expansion. All of these changes support enhanced performance. Muscle hypertrophy is a well-known phenomenon. Muscle size and strength increase with use. Changes in content of various muscle enzymes and numbers of mitochondria can occur depending on the type of activity performed. Bones, ligaments and tendons also hypertrophy in response to increasing stresses but at a slower rate than muscle.

Cardiovascular function increases to meet increased needs of muscle for substrates and waste removal. Plasma volume expansion is a well-known result of long-term exercise training that supports increased cardiac output (McKeever et al, 1985; Convertino et al, 1980). Heart rates of trained animals are lower for a given workload because of greater cardiovascular efficiency. Training also influences the type and amount of substrate that can be used to support exercise.

Nutrition

Nutrition cannot overcome deficits in genetics and training. However, matching the food and feeding methods to the type of activity (i.e., intensity, duration and frequency) allows a sporting or working dog to perform to its genetic potential and level of training. The feeding goals for sporting and working dogs are to provide appropriate nutrition to optimize exercise and olfactory performance and long-term health.

Because many successful working and sporting dogs rely on both athletic and scent-detection abilities, this section of the chapter reviews exercise and olfactory physiology, followed by a discussion of how to assess the nutritional needs of individual sporting and working dogs. The key nutritional factors are developed as the basis for ensuring that the best food is selected to help achieve the goals of optimizing performance and long-term health.

The second section covers the feeding plan and how well the feeding plan meets the feeding goals (reassessment). The feeding plan includes food selection and how the food should be fed including amount, how it is offered and the timing of feeding. Depending on the results of the reassessment process, changes to the original feeding plan may be required to ensure delivery of the feeding goals.

CLINICAL IMPORTANCE

Canids represent one of the most diverse mammalian species. The wide range of athletic ability and types of sporting and working dogs come as no surprise in light of this diversity. In regards to athleticism, at one extreme is the racing greyhound, which is capable of sprinting a quarter mile in less than 26 seconds and reaching maximum speeds in excess of 40 mph (64 km/hr). At the other extreme is the sled dog, which is capable of running vast distances, day after day, in arctic conditions. In between these extremes is a plethora of different kinds of working, hunting and sporting dogs that participate in a wide range of athletic activities (**Table 18-1**).

The American Kennel Club lists 26 sporting breeds, 18 herding breeds and 25 breeds of working dogs; however, it is difficult to quantify how many of these dogs actually participate in athletic events (American Kennel Club, 2007). Eighty different breeds of hounds are found worldwide and all these breeds were originally hunting dogs. In addition, there are 13 sight hound breeds, 49 herding or shepherd dogs and 31 recognized terrier breeds (Palmer, 1994; van Lier, 1995; van Leeuwen, 1995). Another classification system lists 91 hounds, 43 working breeds, 44 herding dogs, 49 gun dogs and 31 terriers (Palmer, 1994).

Scent-detection type working dogs are employed by many government agencies including those involved in national defense, customs service and border patrol. Additionally, in the United States, more than 28,000 dogs work for state and local law enforcement agencies. Numbers of active scent-detection type sporting dogs are difficult to document. In the United States, survey results from one publisher estimate that readers of their hunting magazines own more than 700,000 active hunting dogs.[a] These same readers spend 150 to 200 hours per year training their dogs and 40 days per year hunting in the field with their dogs. In the United States, the National Greyhound Association registered about 26,000 greyhound puppies per year in 2004 and 2005 and about 22,900 in 2006 (National Greyhound Association, 2007). There are 37 dog tracks in 14 states.[b]

Because dogs participate in a wide variety of working and sporting activities, and the level of participation varies from full-time athlete to intermittent activity, it is difficult to assess how much of the canine population participates in sporting and working events. It is clear, however, that large numbers of dogs participate in these activities.

OLFACTORY PHYSIOLOGY

Olfaction is a very important special sense for dogs. Besides the obvious value of facilitating obtaining prey, olfaction is significant in the overall communication process of canids. For dogs, communication is fundamental to maintaining affiliations, reducing competition and identifying individuals (Simpson, 1997). Urine scent marking by dogs is one example. It is thought that a dog can identify the sex and even specific individuals from the odor of another dog's urine (Houpt, 1998). Urine is not the only olfactory cue for dog-to-dog communication. Anal gland and ear secretions are also thought to function in individual identification. Common greeting behaviors for dogs include sniffing under each other's tails and investigating odors of each other's ears (Houpt, 1998; Fox and Bekoff, 1975). Also, as writing is to people, dogs can use olfaction-based communication to send a message that can be transmitted and received in their absence. The sender must be present for visual or auditory signals to be sent, but an odor persists for minutes to many days after the sender has gone (Houpt, 1998). Olfactory cues may help newborn puppies locate their mother and its teats (Houpt, 1998a) and later might confer survival advantages by promoting the acquisition of information about safety of different foods (Hepper and Wells, 2005).

Table 18-3. Various scent-detection activities conducted by working and sporting dogs.

Brown tree snake detection
Cadaver detection
Conservation work
Drug detection
Explosives detection
Fire accelerant detection
Game hunting
Identification of individuals
Pipeline leak detection
Search and rescue
Termite detection
Tracking for work or sport
War dogs

Scent-detection ability is important to the function of many classes of sporting and working dogs. Based on tomb evidence, the use of dogs as chemical detectors dates back to their use as hunting dogs 12,000 years ago (Furton and Meyers, 2001). Today many scent-detection dogs do potentially life-saving work including detecting explosives, leading search and rescue teams, finding and detaining potentially dangerous criminals or alerting to the presence of enemies. Interestingly, with minimal training, dogs are reportedly able to closely match biopsy results in distinguishing between normal controls and lung and breast cancer patients by sniffing breath samples (McCulloch et al, 2006). Dogs can also distinguish patients with bladder cancer on the basis of urine odor. Apparently tumor-related volatile compounds are present in the urine, imparting a characteristic odor signature (Willis et al, 2004). **Table 18-3** includes various activities in which scent-detection dogs are used.

A review of the physical and chemical aspects of scent and the functioning of the olfactory system under different conditions sets the stage for understanding how exercise training and proper nutrition can affect olfactory performance and scent detection.

Physics and Mechanics of Scent

The following discussion pertains primarily to scent trails from animals or people. However, much of the information also applies to odors from inanimate and/or stationary objects. There are thought to be two general types of odors that are left on a scent trail: individual odor and contact/disturbance odor. Sources of individual odors could be skin cells, glandular secretory products (sebaceous, apocrine and eccrine secretions) and, in the case of people, the smell of their clothes, deodorants, soap, etc. Contact/disturbance odors are generated as an animal or person walks over the ground. In the process, their footsteps disrupt the surface, crushing vegetation, soil and other materi-

Box 18-1. Genes and Olfaction: People vs. Dogs.

Olfactory receptors constitute the largest gene family in vertebrates. Species that have highly developed olfactory senses are referred to as macrosmatic (e.g., dogs), whereas species with a weak sense of smell are termed microsmatic (e.g., people). There are likely several reasons dogs are much better at odor detection than people. The surface area of the canine olfactory epithelium is as much as 20 times greater than that of people. The density of neuronal cells and the number of olfactory receptors that are expressed on their surface as well as the size of the olfactory bulb have to be taken into consideration when comparing the olfactory capabilities of different species. The canine olfactory epithelium can express up to 20 times more olfactory receptors than that of people. This contributes to the ability of dogs to detect odorant molecules at a much lower concentration. The binding affinity of odorant molecules for their related olfactory receptor is also likely to be an important variable that could explain differences in sensing abilities between people and dogs. The range of types of olfactory receptors of dogs is around 30% larger than for people, which could contribute to the wider range of odorant molecules that dogs can detect.

The Bibliography for **Box 18-1** can be found at www.markmorris.org.

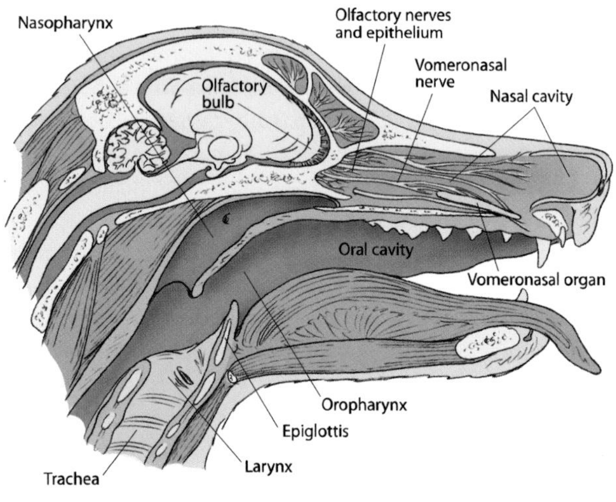

Figure 18-1. Drawing of a mid-sagittal section of a canine head showing olfactory and upper respiratory anatomy.

als, and as a result, these materials release odors. When following scent, dogs may be detecting airborne odors arising directly from air moving past an animal or person, from contact/disturbance odors that become airborne if such odors are volatile or from the ground, which could include both individual odors and contact/disturbance odors (Hepper and Wells, 2005).

Scents tend to be concentrated at their source. Odors spread and become less concentrated, forming a scent cone. When air is stagnant around the source of an odor, scent pools can form. Factors such as wind, terrain, air temperature, humidity and soil temperature can affect the scent cone or scent pool, including where and how far it is dispersed (Jones et al, 2004). Hunters using dogs generally agree that the best scent conditions include moderate humidity and moderate ambient temperatures (early morning and late afternoon on warm sunny days) (Holloway, 1961). Wind can be channeled by obstructions or terrain and can rapidly disperse scent in unexpected directions (Jones et al, 2004). Thus, odors do not disperse in a linear continuous gradient but result in odor fragments or patches. These pockets of odors vary in concentration and are separated by areas of clean air where no odor is present. Thus, dogs are often exposed to variable and intermittent odor signals. In the face of this complexity, dogs and many other animals are able to determine the direction of a trail and find the source of an odor. Furthermore, they can be trained to identify specific odors (Hepper and Wells, 2005). Human handlers who are aware of factors affecting odor dynamics can improve detection success by directing the activity of a scent-detection dog accordingly (**Table 18-2**).

Olfactory System

The olfactory system consists primarily of the nose, nasopharynx (including the vomeronasal organ and olfactory epithelium), olfactory and vomeronasal nerves and the olfactory bulb (**Figure 18-1**). The pulmonary system and oro- and nasopharynx facilitate olfaction by moving and directing air over the olfactory epithelium.

The olfactory epithelium contains the olfactory receptors. This is where odor molecules interact to stimulate an olfactory sensation. Chemicals that are best detected by the olfactory system are volatile and both water and lipid soluble. Such molecules are readily made airborne and dissolve in the mucus that covers the olfactory epithelium. After this occurs, they bind to specific substances called G-protein-coupled-receptors, which are on the cilia of the olfactory receptor neurons. As a result, a signal transduction of smell is initiated (Jones et al, 2004). **Box 18-1** discusses gene-based differences between the olfactory capabilities of people and dogs.

For olfaction to occur, odorants need to contact the olfactory receptors in the olfactory epithelium. Thus, air from the environment must pass into the nasal cavity to reach the olfactory epithelium. The course taken by air as it passes through the nasal cavity is difficult to predict because of the complex anatomy of the nasal cavity. There are distinctly different routes of airflow during normal inspiration and during sniffing. Sniffing draws considerably more air over the olfactory epithelium as opposed to normal inspiration. During normal inspiration, air tends to route below the olfactory epithelium, a more efficient route for pulmonary function (Becker and King, 1957).

Sniffing occurs at 160 to 240 breaths/min. compared to 40 to 44 breaths/min. in typical bird dogs while ranging. When bird dogs are pointing, their mouth is slightly open, their nasal openings move in accordance with sniffing and the head is stretched forward. These postures and movements might be optimizing airflow over the olfactory epithelium (Steen et al, 1996).

Dogs exhibit three types of scenting behavior: 1) air scenting, 2) trailing and 3) tracking. While air scenting, dogs are thought to be following the airborne scents emanating directly from the source of the odor and being carried away by air currents. These dogs are nearly always working upwind. When trailing, dogs follow the trail with their head up while moving upwind and head down while following the scent downwind. They usually do not follow directly on the trail path and may overrun a path if it turns. The assumption is that when dogs are trailing they are following the individual's scent deposited by contact with the ground surface. When tracking, dogs follow the trail with their head down and nose on the path and very closely follow the footsteps of the subject being tracked. It is assumed that while tracking, dogs are following odor deposited on the ground and contact/ground disturbance odor. It should be noted that these three characterizations are based on observations (Hepper and Wells, 2005). Also, dogs can be trained to do primarily one type of these three scent-detection behaviors (Jones et al, 2004).

In addition to the general scent-detection behaviors characterized above, dogs seem to display three different phases when ground tracking. During a searching phase, they move quickly and sniff intermittently, supposedly trying to find a track. After they find a track they usually stop for a moment. Then they enter a deciding phase, characterized by moving slower and by more frequent sniffing episodes. The deciding phase can be as short as following two to five human footprints while they determine the direction of the track. After the direction of the track is decided upon, the tracking phase follows. During this phase they move more quickly, suggesting that following the track is a simpler task than determining its direction. Apparently the deciding phase is based on decay/dilution of the odorants as a result of time. In the case of human footsteps, this time frame can be as short as three to five seconds (Thesen et al, 1993).

Hunting dogs often air scent while running at top speed. During these periods they are usually mouth breathing. One question is how they mouth breath and detect scents at the same time because scent detection requires ambient airflow inward through the nasal cavity. One explanation is based on the Bernoulli principle as follows. Because the oropharynx has a larger cross sectional area it offers less aerodynamic resistance than the nasopharynx. If the mouth is open during heavy breathing, air moves more easily back and forth via the oropharyngeal route. The more restrictive anatomy of the nasal airway suggests that air moving through this passage would do so at a lower speed. Thus (based on the Bernoulli principal), during heavy breathing, air velocity in the oropharynx would likely be high, and the pressure would be low compared to the air velocity and pressure in the nasal cavity. Thus, air would flow into and through the nasal cavity and then into the oropharynx. This would allow ventilating the nasal cavity and the olfactory mucosa while performing open-mouthed breathing during inhalation and exhalation (Steen et al, 1996). However, this phenomenon would not allow simultaneous sniffing and panting. Sniffing improves olfactory acuity, apparently by exposing the olfactory epithelium to more ambient air and thus more odors (Laing, 1983).

Effect of Physical Fitness on Olfaction

The rate a dog is panting and the quality of its olfactory work are inversely related. As mentioned above, dogs cannot pant and sniff at the same time. Panting results from a need to cool and dogs cool primarily by panting (Box 13-2). This can pose a dilemma for detection dogs in hot, humid environments. It is exacerbated if physical exercise is imposed and/or if the dog is neither physically fit nor properly fed. There is a direct correlation between rate of sniffing and efficiency of olfaction and an inverse relationship between the rate of panting and ability to detect scents. The searching phase is prolonged in dogs that have exercised and are panting. Dogs that are panting also have difficulty in determining the direction of a track (Gazit and Terkel, 2002). In a treadmill exercise-based study, physically trained dogs did not experience a decline in olfactory acuity following moderate physical stress compared to untrained stressed dogs. In this study, the olfactory acuity of the untrained dogs declined by 67% (Altom et al, 2003). Many bird-hunting dogs are pets, or kept in kennels, and hunt only a few weekends each year. They are asked to perform seasonal, intermittent endurance exercise coupled with scent detection. Their ability to hunt successfully could be enhanced by increasing their physical training before and through the hunting season.

A dog's ability to perform physically can also be improved through proper nutrition, which, as discussed above, could indirectly improve olfaction. Separately, a dog's olfactory ability can be improved directly through proper nutrition. The nutritional approaches to improved performance are discussed later in the chapter.

EXERCISE PHYSIOLOGY

Exercise requires increased function of several organ systems and energy metabolic pathways. Dramatic changes take place within dogs to support exercise, and as a result, of exercise. Certainly, nutritional needs are affected by exercise. An understanding of exercise physiology is fundamental to assessing and developing a feeding plan for canine athletes.

The following review of exercise physiology relates particularly to nutrition of canine athletes. This discussion includes: 1) a review of muscle metabolism that outlines the energy needs of working muscles, substrate requirements and the by-products of energy metabolism, 2) exercise type and intensity, which determine the preferred metabolic substrates and therefore the nutrient profile, 3) some of the physiologic changes that occur

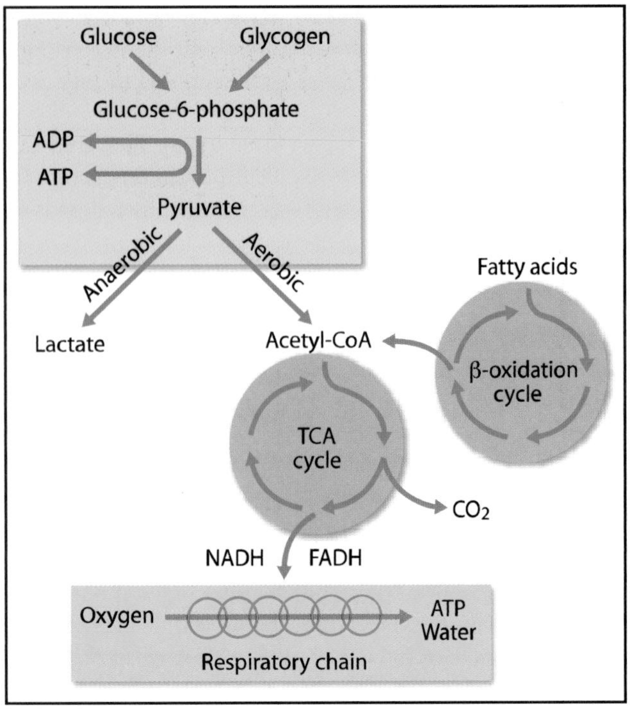

Figure 18-2. Summary of major energy-generating pathways used during exercise. Key: ADP = adenosine diphosphate, ATP = adenosine triphosphate, TCA = tricarboxylic acid, NADH = reduced form of nicotinamide dinucleotide, FADH = reduced form of flavin-adenine dinucleotide.

during exercise and how they may affect nutrient needs and 4) the energy cost of running, which dictates dietary energy needs. All of these factors are important to nutritional assessment of canine athletes and form the basis for a good feeding plan.

Muscle Metabolism

Muscle Fiber Types

Muscles are not homogeneous. They are composed of fibers with different contractile and metabolic characteristics. Muscle fibers are classified into two groups based on contractile properties and histochemical staining: Type I or slow twitch and Type II or fast twitch. Type I fibers have high oxidative capacity and endurance. These fibers are smaller than Type II fibers and have high capillary density and high numbers of mitochondria. They are low in glycolytic ability and low in staining for myofibrillar ATPase, an enzyme associated with fast contraction and relaxation. Conversely, Type II fibers are high in myofibrillar ATPase, larger, contain more glycolytic enzymes and have greater strength. In most species, Type II fibers can be further subdivided into Type IIa and Type IIb. Contraction characteristics are similar for Type IIa and Type IIb fibers, but Type IIa fibers have greater oxidative capacity than Type IIb fibers; the latter are more fatigable. However, dogs and perhaps other members of their genus and subfamily, appear not to have classic Type IIb fibers but, instead, two other kinds of Type II fibers that are more oxidative (called Type IIDog and Type IIC). This fits with the general observation that dogs are tireless runners (Snow et al, 1982; Latorre et al, 1993; Rivero et al, 1994).

The fiber composition varies between muscles and between individuals. High-power athletes such as racing greyhounds have a higher proportion of Type II fibers, whereas endurance athletes have a higher proportion of Type I fibers (**Table 18-4**). Because the work performed by most intermediate athletes resembles that done by endurance athletes, but is of shorter duration, the muscle fiber-type profile of intermediate athletes should resemble that of endurance athletes more than that of sprint athletes. Muscle fiber type is a function of genetics and dictates the type of exercise for which an individual is best suited. However, some modification is possible through training. Endurance training increases the number and volume of mitochondria and increases capillary density in all fiber types (Åstrand, 1986).

Muscle Energetics

Exercise requires the transfer of chemical energy into physical work. Chemical energy stored in high-energy phosphate bonds of adenosine triphosphate (ATP) is the sole source of energy for muscle contraction. ATP is cleaved to ADP during contraction. The amount of ATP used is proportional to the amount of work performed (i.e., Fenn effect). ATP is vital not only for the events of contraction but also for relaxation and maintenance of important ion gradients (**Box 18-2**). Normal excitability of nerve and muscle is due to an electrochemical gradient maintained by the sodium-potassium pump at the expense of ATP. The calcium pump uses ATP to maintain a low concentration of calcium in the muscle cell in the relaxed state. An estimated one-third of the basal energy requirement is used to maintain electrolyte concentration gradients across cellular membranes (Blaxter, 1989; Pivarnik, 1994).

Although ATP is the high-energy compound that cells use as fuel to perform work, the energy required for exercise can ultimately come from a variety of sources. Because the concentration of ATP in muscle cells is relatively low in comparison to the cell's need during exercise, ATP must be replenished from other fuel sources. These metabolic fuels are stored in muscle (endogenous) and at other body sites (exogenous). The metabolism of these fuels occurs either with oxygen (aerobic) or without oxygen (anaerobic). The anaerobic pathways (i.e., the creatine phosphate shuttle and glycolysis) occur in the cytoplasm, whereas the aerobic pathways (i.e., complete oxidation of glucose, fatty acids and amino acids) take place in mitochondria. **Figure 18-2** shows an overview of these pathways. The proportion of each pathway used is determined by the duration and intensity of the task performed and by the conditioning and nutritional status of the animal (Blaxter, 1989; Nadel, 1985; Williams, 1985; Kronfeld and Downey, 1981; Kronfeld et al, 1977; Hammel et al, 1977). **Table 18-5** lists metabolic fuels, their uses and storage sites.

The concentration of ATP is tightly regulated, although it is rapidly consumed during exercise (Blaxter, 1989; Nadel, 1985; Stryer, 1988; Rusko et al, 1986). Resting muscle cells have only enough ATP to fuel muscle contraction for a few seconds. If work continues beyond this point, ATP must be regenerated from other metabolic fuels at a rate comparable to that at which

Box 18-2. The Events of Muscle Contraction.

Muscle contraction occurs when a nerve excites a muscle fiber resulting in a muscle action potential (loss of the normal -90 millivolt resting membrane potential). The action potential travels throughout the muscle fiber causing calcium to be released into the cytoplasm from the sarcoplasmic reticulum. This flood of calcium around the contractile proteins elicits a conformational change that allows the contractile proteins (actin and myosin) to bind together (**Figure 1**). This attachment allows the energy stored in the "pre-cocked" head of the myosin filament to be discharged in a "power stroke" that causes muscle shortening. The two filaments are released when ATP binds to the myosin active site. The head of the myosin filament is re-cocked when this ATP molecule is cleaved. When the calcium concentration remains high, the head of the myosin filament binds to another site on the actin filament and the sequence is repeated. This sequence of events continues until either minimum fiber length (maximum shortening) or maximum load is exceeded. Relaxation occurs when the calcium concentration drops to pre-contraction levels because of the action of the calcium pump.

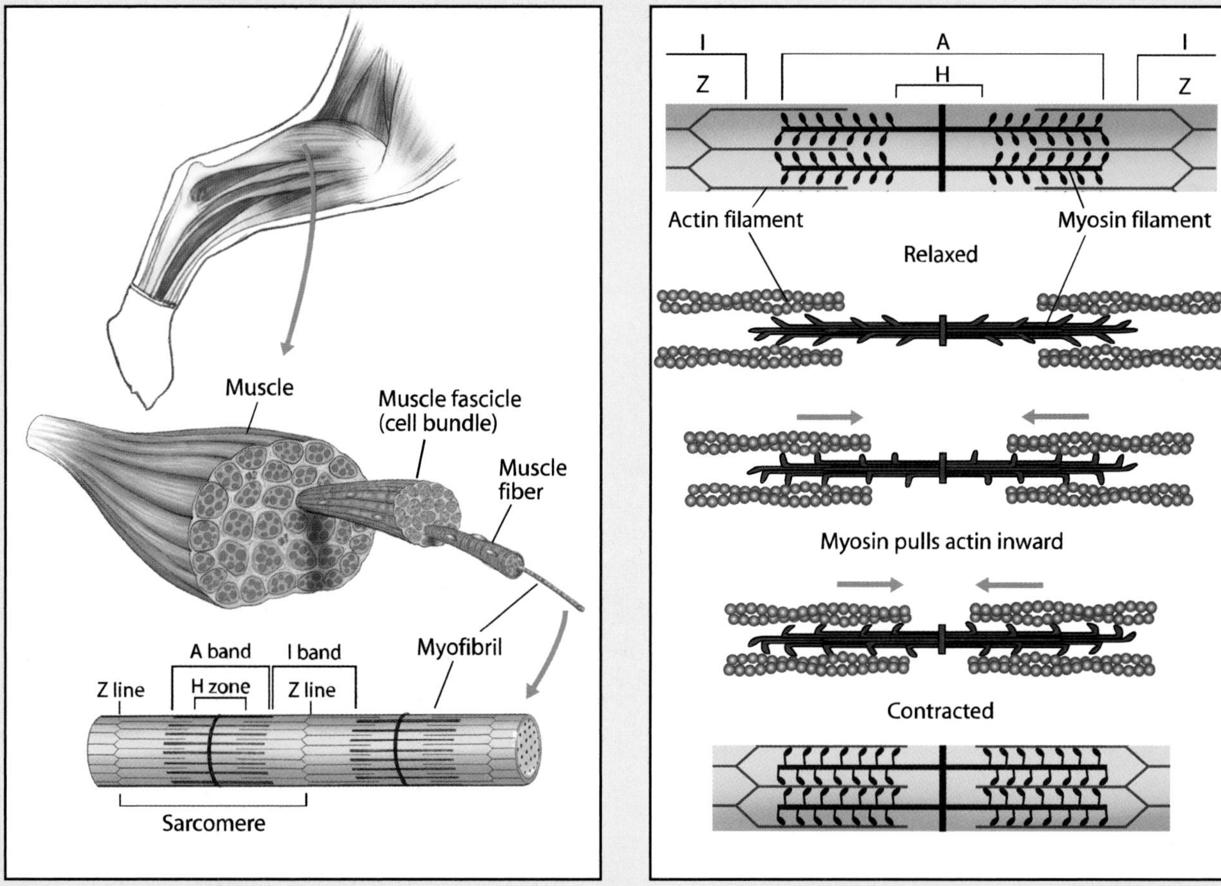

Figure 1. Components of striated muscle cells. Each striated muscle cell or fiber contains hundreds to thousands of myofibrils. Each myofibril contains a series of interlocking myofilaments (i.e., actin and myosin filaments). The **H band** is the center of the myosin filaments, the **A band** is the entire length of the myosin filaments, the **Z disk or plate** is the center and attachment site of the actin filaments, the **I band** encompasses the entire length of the actin filaments except for the portions that overlap the myosin filaments. The compartments between the Z plates are called **sarcomeres.** During contraction, the Z plates are pulled towards one another as the degree of overlap of thick and thin filaments increases; I band and H bands shorten. Maximum contraction is attained when the ends of the thick filaments butt against Z plates.

it is being consumed (Blaxter, 1989; Nadel, 1985; Williams, 1985; Rusko et al, 1986; Pate and Brunn, 1989). Creatine phosphate (Cr-P) is an endogenously stored fuel that muscles can rapidly convert to ATP. The Cr-P shuttle permits the maximum rate of ATP synthesis possible; however, this pathway can only support maximal efforts for five to 15 seconds (**Figure 18-3**) because muscle Cr-P stores are very limited (Williams, 1985; Pate and Brunn, 1989; Newsholme, 1986).

Glucose is a versatile metabolic fuel that is stored endogenously as muscle glycogen and exogenously as glycogen in the liver and to a much smaller extent as free glucose in the blood. Glucose can be metabolized to regenerate ATP by both anaerobic and aerobic pathways. Anaerobic metabolism of glucose (glycolysis) results in very rapid ATP production (**Figure 18-3**) or high metabolic power (**Box 18-3**), but only yields two ATP per molecule of glucose. Aerobic metabolism, the complete oxi-

Table 18-4. Percent fast twitch fibers (Type II) by selected canine breeds.*

Muscle	Greyhound	Crossbred	Foxhound
Biceps femoris	88.6	67.2	63.0
Semitendinosus	98.9	85.3	69.6
Triceps (long head)	94.2	77.2	64.9
Vastus lateralis	96.6	61.4	80.7

*Adapted from Guy PS, Snow DH. Skeletal muscle fibre composition in the dog and its relationship to athletic ability. Research in Veterinary Science 1981; 31: 244-248.

Table 18-5. Metabolism, use and storage sites of metabolic fuels.

Fuel	Metabolism	Use	Storage sites
ATP	Anaerobic	Primary fuel for synthetic processes, ion pumps and muscle contraction	Muscle cells (concentration is low and highly regulated)
Cr-P	Anaerobic	Regenerate ATP	Muscle cells (low concentration)
Glucose	Anaerobic (glycolysis) and aerobic (TCA cycle)	Rapidly available energy source	Muscle and liver glycogen (1 to 2% of body weight)
Fatty acids	Aerobic (β-oxidation and TCA cycle)	Long-lasting energy source	Adipose tissue (2 to 20% of body weight)
Amino acids	Aerobic (TCA cycle)	Small contribution to energy (may contribute up to 5 to 15%)	Structural proteins

Key: ATP = adenosine triphosphate, Cr-P = creatine phosphate, TCA = tricarboxylic acid.

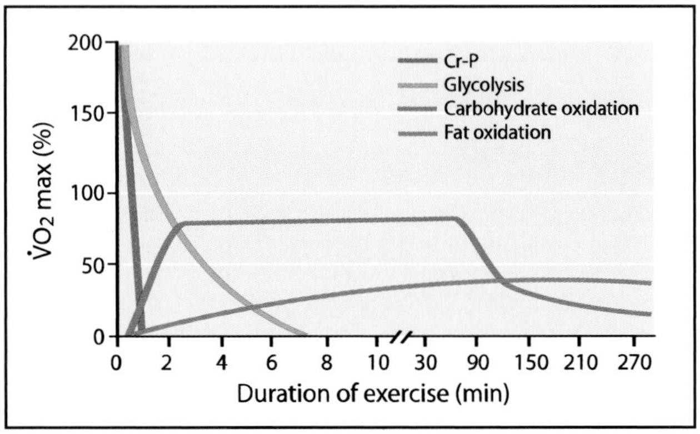

Figure 18-3. Relative contributions of the four energy-generating pathways, depending on exercise intensity and duration. Key: Cr-P = creatine phosphate.

dation of glucose to CO_2 and water, regenerates ATP less rapidly (**Box 18-3**), but results in a much greater yield (36 ATP per molecule of glucose). Because total body glucose stores (glycogen) are relatively small (1 to 2% of body weight), even aerobic metabolism of glucose cannot sustain exercise for extended periods of time. Fatty acids are stored in ample supply in adipose tissue and within muscle. They are the primary energy source for long-lasting exercise. Although small amounts of fatty acids are stored in muscle, this source may contribute up to 60% of the fatty acids oxidized during the first two to three hours of exercise (Weber et al, 1993).

Amino acids are usually not a primary energy source for exercise. Oxidation of amino acids may contribute up to 5 to 15% of the energy used during exercise, depending on the intensity and duration of the task (Young et al, 1962; Zackin, 1990; Hickson and Wolinsky, 1989). Most of this energy comes from the oxidation of the branched-chain amino acids leucine, isoleucine and valine (Miller and Massaro, 1989; Blomstrand et al, 1988). Most amino acids are structural or functional components of proteins and the size of the labile amino acid pool is very small, making amino acids a less significant fuel source for exercise in most circumstances.

The proportion of energy substrates and metabolic pathways used during exercise depends on the intensity and duration of the exercise. As exercise intensity increases, the power output and the rate of energy metabolism must also increase. As exercise duration increases, total substrate availability and energy yield become more important (**Box 18-3**). High-power activities (e.g., sprinting) rely heavily on anaerobic metabolism, whereas more prolonged activities require the higher energy yield provided by oxidation of glucose and fatty acids. As the duration of exercise increases, oxidation of fatty acids becomes more important (**Figure 18-3**).

By-Products of Muscular Work

Heat is the primary by-product of muscle contraction; 75 to 80% of the energy used during muscular work is converted to heat. A 10-fold increase in metabolism results in a 10-fold increase in heat production. Unless the animal is working in a very cold environment, this heat is a by-product that must be removed (even some sled dogs overheat). In dogs, the respiratory tract is responsible for dissipating most of this heat. Normal body temperatures of dogs doing physical work are higher than their normal resting temperatures. During very intense exercise or exercise in hot environmental temperatures, heat production exceeds the ability of the respiratory tract to lose heat, increasing body temperature. The body temperature of racing greyhounds may increase more than 1°C (1.8°F) after a 30-second race (Rose and Bloomber, 1989). Pointing breeds can have normal working temperatures up to 41.1°C (106°F) (Gillette, 2002). Labrador retrievers can have normal working temperatures up to 41.6°C (107°F) (Matwichuk et al, 1999). Because evaporative heat loss is the primary way dogs dissipate heat, ensuring adequate hydration is crucial for maintenance of normal body temperature.

Metabolic acid is another by-product of energy metabolism that must be eliminated during and after exercise. Aerobic metabolism generates ATP by combustion of carbohydrates and fats to CO_2 and water. Lactate is the endpoint of anaerobic metabolism. Either way, acid is produced that must be eliminated in some way for exercise to continue. Muscle enzyme

Box 18-3. Metabolic Power and Yield.

Metabolic power is the speed with which energy substrates can be converted to ATP, whereas metabolic yield is the amount of ATP that can be made from energy substrates. High-intensity exercise (e.g., sprinting) requires rapid mobilization of stored energy for a very short time; therefore, metabolic power is very important. Because duration of exercise is very short for sprinters, metabolic yield is less important. Conversely, endurance activities are longer in duration and lower in intensity. For these activities, the rapidity with which ATP is made from substrates (power) is less important than the amount of ATP made (yield). **Tables 1** and **2** show maximum power and yield from various substrates using aerobic and anaerobic pathways.

Clinically, canine sprint athletes rely heavily on anaerobic metabolism of carbohydrates whereas canine endurance athletes rely more on oxidation of fats.

CLINICAL EXAMPLE

Compare a 30-kg racing greyhound with a 30-kg sled dog. Assume the racing greyhound runs an 800-m race in about 48 seconds. The total energy needed for the race is about 24 kcal, whereas the energy use rate or metabolic power is about 30 kcal per minute (an increase of more than 25 times resting). Total daily energy requirement (DER) is about 1,600 kcal. In contrast, consider a sled dog that runs 80 km pulling a sled (its share is about 15 kg) for five hours. The sled dog needs about 3,600 additional kcal for the event and uses them at a rate of 12 kcal per minute. Total DER is about 5,000 kcal (more than 5 x resting energy requirement). To convert to kJ, multiply kcal x 4.184.

Table 1. Estimated maximum metabolic power output for human skeletal muscle using different substrates and metabolic profiles.*

Process	Metabolic power output (μmole of ATP/g of muscle/min.)
Aerobic metabolism	
Fatty acid oxidation	20.4
Glycogen oxidation	30
Anaerobic metabolism	
Glycogen glycolysis	60
Creatine phosphate and ATP hydrolysis	96-360

*Adapted from Hochachka PW. Design of energy metabolism. In: Prosser CL, ed. Environmental and Metabolic Animal Physiology, 4th ed. New York, NY: Wiley-Liss, 1991; 332.

Table 2. Energy yield using different substrates and metabolic pathways.*

Process	Energy yield (moles of ATP/moles of substrate)
Aerobic metabolism	
Triglyceride oxidation (glycerol + 3 palmitate)	403
Fatty acid oxidation (palmitate)	129
Glycogen oxidation	38
Glucose oxidation	36
Proline oxidation	21
Lactate oxidation	18
Anaerobic metabolism	
Glycolysis (glycogen)	3
Glycolysis (glucose)	2
Creatine phosphate hydrolysis	1

*Adapted from Hochachka PW. Design of energy metabolism. In: Prosser CL, ed. Environmental and Metabolic Animal Physiology, 4th ed. New York, NY: Wiley-Liss, 1991; 327-329.

The Bibliography for **Box 18-3** can be found at www.markmorris.org.

activity is highly pH sensitive. Therefore, if energy metabolism and muscle contraction are to proceed optimally, muscle pH must be tightly regulated. Intracellular buffers can blunt some of the acute effects of increased concentrations of CO_2 and lactate. However, elimination of organic acids from muscle cells is the primary strategy for avoiding deleterious decreases in muscle pH. Because it is a weak electrolyte, CO_2 has less effect on pH than lactate (a strong salt of lactic acid) and is handled differently by the body.

Assuming no other primary acid-base changes, CO_2 and bicarbonate (HCO_3^-) increase in parallel because of the following relationship:

$$CO_2 + H_2O \leftrightarrow HCO_3^- + H^+$$

The CO_2 load produced during exercise can be eliminated via two routes: 1) respiratory loss of CO_2 (acute) and 2) renal excretion of HCO_3^- (long-term). The ability of the kidneys to respond acutely may be impaired because of decreased plasma volume and renal blood flow during exercise. The respiratory

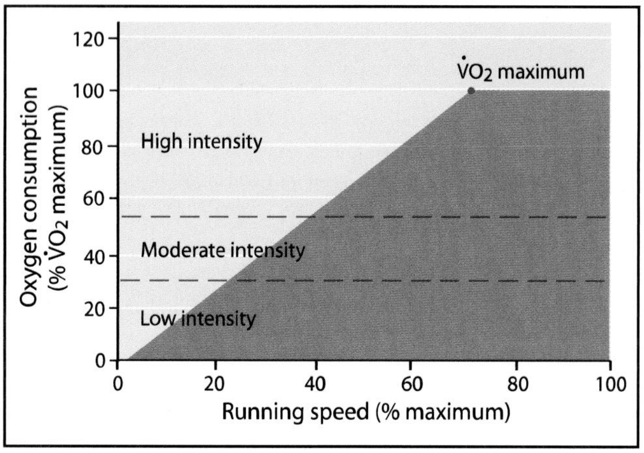

Figure 18-4. Relationship between energy consumption (VO_2) and running speed (workload). VO_2 max is the point at which VO_2 no longer increases with increasing workload.

system responds very quickly by increasing ventilation to excrete excess CO_2 (and excess heat). Aerobic exercise generally does not produce large acid-base changes, because the respiratory system can excrete CO_2 as fast as it is produced.

The acid-base consequences of anaerobic metabolism are more severe and less easily handled by the body. Lactate is the anionic form of a strong organic acid and does not participate in any dissociation equilibria. This means that lactate has a greater effect on pH than CO_2 and its acid-base effects must be ameliorated by other compensatory changes until it is metabolized. Lactate is oxidized for energy by muscle or converted back to glucose in the liver (Cori cycle).

Exercise Intensity and Duration

Energy and other nutrient requirements for canine athletes are determined by the intensity and duration of exercise. Exercise intensity can be described in a variety of ways depending on body weight and type of activity. Exercise intensity is a measure of work done per unit time. For dogs, the type of work done is usually running and the amount of work done depends on body weight, distance traveled and changes in elevation. The amount of work done is directly proportional to the amount of energy used. Therefore, energy use describes work done.

For example, a 30-kg dog expends about 30 kcal to cover 1 km on a flat surface, regardless of how fast it walks or runs (minor differences may occur due to differences in efficiency of various gaits for running at a specific speed). Running speed (distance/time) is a measure of exercise intensity (work/time) or power (energy/time). A direct relationship exists between running speed (km/hr) and energy use rate (kcal/hr or kJ/hr) for an individual of a given size. However, individuals of different sizes expend different amounts of energy to run the same speed, making running speed a poor measure for comparison of workload between individuals of different sizes.

Exercise physiologists have traditionally used oxygen consumption (VO_2) as a measure of workload. The body only uses oxygen for combustion of substrates to produce energy. Each liter of oxygen consumed represents an energy expenditure of about 4.8 kcal or 20.1 kJ. Therefore, the VO_2 indicates the rate of energy use, at least at submaximal exercise levels. At very high workloads, exercise intensity can be increased without a further increase in VO_2 (**Figure 18-4**). The workload at which this occurs is called maximal oxygen consumption (VO_2 max).

Exercise intensity is frequently expressed as a percentage of VO_2 max in order to compare different types of activities for individuals of different size within a species and between species. Exercise intensity dictates the severity and types of physiologic changes associated with exercise, including substrate use, metabolic pathways and waste production. Low-intensity exercise is up to 30% of VO_2 max and is completely aerobic, using mostly fatty acids. Exercise intensities from 30 to 50% of VO_2 max (moderate intensity) are still completely aerobic, but carbohydrates become an important energy substrate (carbohydrate threshold). At high-intensity exercise (75 to 100% of VO_2 max), anaerobic metabolism becomes important and lactate begins to accumulate in the blood. The anaerobic threshold is the workload at which lactate concentrations in the blood increase to 4 mmol/l or more (Hollman, 1985). When working at exercise intensities at or above the anaerobic threshold, lactate in the blood begins to accumulate at an exponential rate, potentially limiting the duration of the exercise. Workloads above VO_2 max are called either maximal or supramaximal, are highly dependent on anaerobic metabolism and result in large increases in blood lactate concentrations.

Exercise intensity dictates metabolic pathways and substrate use. High-intensity activities (sprinting) depend on anaerobic metabolism of carbohydrate (glucose and glycogen), which is supported by high-carbohydrate foods. The severe acidemia produced by high-intensity activities underscores the need for adequate electrolyte and water intake. Endurance events that take place at low to moderate intensity for long periods are completely aerobic and rely mostly on oxidation of fatty acids. Thus, as exercise duration increases, the fat fraction of the food becomes more important to supply energy needs. Intermediate exercise (as performed by most canine athletes) is usually of low to moderate intensity, but may include some short periods of high-intensity work. Both fats and carbohydrates are important fuel sources in intermediate exercise.

Physiologic Changes Due to Activity Anticipation

Anticipation to perform work can affect metabolism in dogs. Foxhounds, Labrador retrievers and sled dogs have significant blood parameter changes as a result of anticipation to perform specific tasks. Labrador retrievers had a significant increase in serum calcium and total bilirubin and a significant decrease in serum glucose, total protein, cholesterol and insulin associated with anticipation (Gillette et al, 2001). A regimen of physical conditioning had a significant affect on the anticipatory changes in foxhounds and sled dogs (Gillette et al, 2006). The effects of anticipation can play a role in a dog's ability to perform selected activities.

Physiologic Changes Due to Exercise

The hallmark of exercise is increased metabolism. Many organ systems increase their activity, some by several-fold, whereas some systems decrease their function. The systemic changes that occur during exercise seem to be driven by the muscles' need for substrates and removal of metabolic waste. Working muscle metabolizes substrates (mostly fatty acids and glucose) to release energy stored in chemical bonds for contraction. The products of muscle metabolism are contraction, heat, CO_2, NH_3/NH_4^+, water, and in some cases, lactate.

Muscle metabolism can increase more than 20-fold in dogs, depending on the intensity of the exercise. Likewise, cardiac output increases proportionally with the workload. Both stroke volume and heart rate increase. Blood is the transport medium that carries oxygen and other substrates to the working muscle and removes by-products such as heat, CO_2 and lactate. Increased function of the respiratory system (both increased rate and depth) supplies more oxygen and disposes of more CO_2. Dogs and other mammals with contractile spleens can increase effective circulating blood volume and hematocrit by expelling red blood cells from the spleen before or during exercise. For example, racing greyhounds increase blood volume as much as 24% before racing, even in the face of a 10% shift of plasma volume to other fluid compartments. Probably as a result of both the plasma shift and splenic contraction, hematocrit can increase as much as 29% (Toll et al, 1995) (**Box 18-4**). Plasma volume decreases during exercise because of hydrostatic and osmotic forces. Increases in blood pressure during exercise cause a shift of fluid from the intravascular space to the interstitial compartment (Harrison et al, 1975). Muscle activity tends to increase intracellular osmotic pressure, encouraging fluid movement from the interstitial to the intracellular spaces (Pivarnik, 1994). The kidneys conserve plasma volume losses during exercise. Decreases in plasma volume that decrease central venous pressure cause renal vasoconstriction and diminish glomerular filtration rate (GFR) (Pivarnik, 1994; Houpt, 1984). Decreasing GFR will normally decrease urine output and thus diminish plasma volume losses. Increases in plasma osmotic concentration that occur during prolonged exercise also stimulate secretion of antidiuretic hormone (ADH), which conserves plasma volume by stimulating production of a more concentrated urine (Pivarnik, 1994; Houpt, 1984).

Exercise affects plasma volume and composition. Loss of fluid to the intracellular compartment increases the concentrations of plasma proteins, electrolytes and all other solutes in the extravascular compartment. Other primary plasma changes that are needed to support increased muscle activity are a direct result of that activity. Glucose concentration may increase or decrease depending on the intensity and duration of exercise. The concentration of free fatty acids increases during prolonged exercise. At very high workloads, the partial pressure of oxygen may fall dramatically. Acidemia is also common with maximum intensity exercise because of anaero-

Box 18-4. Acute Physiologic Changes in Racing Greyhounds.

Because racing greyhounds exercise at a very high intensity, they exhibit very dramatic physical and biochemical changes during and after racing. Packed cell volume (PCV) may increase to 68%, jugular venous pH values may decrease to 6.95 and plasma lactate concentrations may increase to 32 mEq/l (normal 1 to 2 mEq/l). Hyperventilation after a race can result in jugular venous pCO_2 values as low as 14 torr (normal = 40 torr) and rectal temperatures can increase more than 1°C (1.8°F) during a 30-second race. After the race, plasma sodium concentrations may reach 171 mEq/l (an 18 mEq/l increase from rest) and potassium concentrations may increase to 7.8 mEq/l (normal = 4 mEq/l). Plasma protein concentrations also increase after racing, implying a fluid shift out of the plasma compartment.

A study examined the effect of excitement before racing on these variables and quantified the effects of fluid shift on plasma volume, blood volume and PCV before and after racing. Arterial blood samples were obtained at rest, just before and five minutes after a 704-m race to quantify changes in hematologic variables, plasma electrolyte and protein concentrations, osmolality and acid-base variables. Changes in plasma volume were estimated from the change in plasma protein concentration. Immediately before the race, plasma volume decreased by 10% from rest and total circulating red blood cell (RBC) volume increased by 60% attributable to increased RBC numbers rather than size. Increases in blood volume (BV) by 24% and PCV by 29% also were detected before the race. Five minutes after the race, plasma volume was 21% below the resting value and total circulating RBC volume had increased 73% above the resting value, resulting in a 40% increase in PCV. Contraction of the spleen appeared responsible for the increased PCV and BV before the race and maintenance of BV after the race.

Plasma chloride concentration was the same before and after the race, meaning it decreased by the same fraction (22%) as the plasma volume, indicating Cl^- loss from the plasma. Plasma Na^+ content decreased by a smaller fraction (13%), causing Na^+ concentration to increase from 151 mEq/l at rest to 167 mEq/l after the race. Assuming that Na^+ concentration was the same throughout the extracellular fluid, water likely moved into the intracellular compartment. As a consequence of these changes, the inorganic strong ion difference in plasma increased by about 16 mEq/l, which tended to minimize the acid-base disturbance induced by the 33 mEq/l increase in lactate concentration.

These results indicate that the physiologic changes taking effect during strenuous sprint exercise in racing greyhounds enhance blood volume and aid in acid-base homeostasis, both of which are adaptive for this type of exercise.

The Bibliography for **Box 18-4** can be found at www.markmorris.org.

Table 18-6. Caloric cost of running 1 km for dogs of varying size.

Body weight (kg)	Cost of running (kcal) 1 km/kg body weight*	Cost of running 1 km (kcal)**
5	1.77	9
10	1.41	14
15	1.23	19
20	1.13	23
25	1.05	26
30	0.99	30
35	0.94	33
40	0.90	36
45	0.87	39
50	0.84	42
70	0.76	53

*Formula: $Energy_{(kcal)}/BW_{(kg)} = 1.77 \times distance_{(km)} \times BW_{(kg)}^{-0.4} + 1.25 \times BW_{(kg)}^{-0.25}$.
**To convert to kJ, multiply kcal x 4.184.

bic metabolism and accumulation of lactate in the blood.

The important points from the above discussion are: 1) exercise increases metabolism and therefore increases the need for energy, 2) cardiovascular function increases and fluid shifts/losses occur during exercise-adequate water intake is important to support these needs and 3) transient changes also occur in the composition of blood that can influence the interpretation of results from blood samples drawn soon after exercise.

Energy Cost of Running

The energy cost of running depends on body size and distance traveled. **Table 18-6** shows the caloric cost of running 1 km for dogs of various sizes. This table also illustrates an important principle about the mass-specific caloric cost of running as size changes. As body size increases, the efficiency of running increases (i.e., larger animals use fewer kcal/kg to run the same distance). By using the data in **Table 18-6**, it is possible to estimate the energy requirement for a dog of a known size to run a given distance (**Box 18-5**).

PATIENT ASSESSMENT

History

In addition to the normal historical information that is usually obtained about a patient, the following information should be gathered from owners: environmental/housing data, medications, dietary history and exercise type, amount, frequency and performance. Detailed information should be gathered about how the dog is housed, including: indoors or outdoors, size and type of housing, opportunity for spontaneous exercise, type of surfaces, number of dogs housed together and access to food and water. All medications used should be recorded, including drugs used to suppress estrus and drugs used to enhance performance.

The dietary history should include all foods and supplements used. The amount fed, nutrient profile and timing of feeding in relation to exercise should be noted. The amount eaten should also be assessed (i.e., Does the dog have a normal appetite and is it actually consuming a reasonable amount?). In some cases, the composition of the overall diet (food plus supplements) may be complex and individual meals may vary in composition. It is also important to ascertain the duration of a particular feeding plan. Abrupt or frequent changes in food or feeding method may affect performance.

Exercise Type

Functionally, exercise can be divided into three types (**Table 18-1**) based on intensity and duration: 1) sprint-high-intensity physical activity that can be sustained less than two minutes, 2) intermediate-physical activity lasting a few minutes to a few hours and 3) endurance-physical activity that lasts many hours. These definitions are arbitrary and vague, but are useful for assessing and developing feeding plans.

Most canine sprinters are sight hounds, racing greyhounds being the most notable example. Metabolically, weight-pull dogs might also fit into this category. Some racing sled dogs that participate in shorter, high-speed events are referred to as "sprinters." However, they fit better in the intermediate or endurance categories from a metabolic and nutritional standpoint because their events may last several hours. Other breeds that engage in activities such as agility, fly ball and lure coursing also do considerable sprinting. However, because they compete multiple times per day, they too fit better in the intermediate category.

Based on energy needs, most canine athletes participate in intermediate exercise activities. Most of these activities are of low to moderate intensity and last only a few hours. Intensity and duration of exercise vary widely within this category. For example, most guide dogs work at a low level of physical exertion for variable lengths of time throughout the day, whereas a search and rescue dog may work at a much higher level for many consecutive hours. Other dogs at the upper end of the intermediate exercise range can include foxhounds, coonhounds and other hunting dogs in the field. At times, they work at levels that are near the lower end of the energy requirement range for endurance dogs. Dogs that work at a relatively high intensity level for many hours, such as racing sled dogs, have much greater energy requirements and are true endurance athletes.

Exercise amount can be quantified as hours per day or week. Frequency is how often the animal exercises: daily, weekly, weekends only or seasonally. Many hunting dogs only work hard on weekends during hunting season, whereas some livestock dogs may work several hours daily. Canine athletes should be categorized as either "full-time" or "part-time" athletes.

Environmental Influences on Exercise

Ambient temperature and humidity, psychological stress and geography are environmental factors that may influence performance and nutritional needs of working and sporting dogs. Of these, ambient temperature and humidity exert the greatest effect. Hot temperatures result in increased work and water loss (i.e., to excrete metabolic heat and maintain body temperature

Box 18-5. The Energy Cost of Running.

Daily energy requirement (DER) for canine athletes is highly variable and is directly related to the amount of work done in a day. Work for canine athletes is usually running. A racing greyhound that usually only runs a fraction of a mile in a race has a DER very similar to that of a house pet (1.6 to 1.8 x resting energy requirement [RER]). At the other extreme is the sled dog that runs many miles a day pulling a load and has a very high DER (up to 11 x RER). Understanding the energy cost of running and being able to quantify it in kcal is central to the correct feeding of canine athletes.

The following discussion and calculations are based on experimental data and on running on a flat surface. However, these data show good agreement with data from food consumption records. These calculations are essential for assessing feeding methods (food dose) and making feeding recommendations for canine athletes.

RUNNING

Running is the predominant type of work done by canine athletes. Force generation in the muscle is transmitted through the skeleton to move the dog's mass through a distance. The physics and biomechanics of running are complicated and are described elsewhere. The rate of energy use (power) is proportional to running speed. However, the amount of energy used to cover a given distance is independent of velocity. For running on a flat surface, energy use is a function of body size and distance. One study described the effect of size on the energy cost of running for a variety of mammals; the study used an equation to relate VO_2 to velocity and body weight. The following equation, which was derived from the research equation, relates the energy cost of running to body weight and distance, assuming an energy yield of 4.8 kcal (20.1 kJ)/l of oxygen consumed.

$$ERR = 1.77d \times BW^{-0.40} + 1.25BW^{-0.25}$$

Where ERR is the energy requirement for running in kcal/kg, d is distance in km, and BW is body weight in kg. Larger animals have a biomechanical advantage resulting in greater efficiency of running and lower mass specific cost of running (kcal/kg) for a given distance. The negative exponents in the equation make calculations difficult. Therefore, **Table 18-6** summarizes the caloric cost of running for dogs of various sizes.

RUNNING WITH WEIGHTS

The caloric cost of running with weights is the sum of the cost of running without added weight and the incremental cost of carrying that weight. When carrying added weight, VO_2 increases the same percentage as gross weight. In other words, the percentage increase in the cost of running is equal to the percentage increase in gross weight. This is not the same as simply increasing the dog's size. Efficiency of running changes with body size whereas simply adding weight increases workload without affecting efficiency (increased gross weight with no change in body size). The total cost of running (ERR_{tot}) is calculated by adding the cost of running (ERR) and the incremental cost of running with added weight (ERR_{incr}). The incremental cost of running is the product of ERR and the percent increase in gross weight.

$$ERR_{incr} = ERR \times \% \text{ increase in gross weight}$$
$$ERR_{tot} = ERR + ERR_{incr} \text{ or}$$
$$ERR_{tot} = ERR \times \text{gross weight} \div \text{body weight}$$

Clinical Example

What is the caloric requirement of 30-kg dog carrying a 3-kg pack on a 15-mile (25-km) hike with its owner? The energy requirement of running for a 30-kg dog is 30 kcal/km (**Table 18-6**) or 750 kcal for 25 km. The incremental energy required for carrying the 3-kg pack is 750 kcal x 3 kg ÷ 30 kg or 75 kcal. The total energy required for exercise is 750 kcal + 75 kcal or 825 kcal. The DER for an average dog this size is 1.6 x RER or 1,435 kcal/day. With the added activity of carrying extra weight, the DER becomes 2,260 kcal/day (2.5 x RER). To convert to kJ, multiply kcal x 4.184.

PULLING WEIGHT

The kinematics of running and center of mass seem to be unaffected with added weight, at least up to 30% of body weight (i.e., the biomechanics do not change with added weight). This finding is unlikely to be true for dogs pulling weight such as sleds. However, it seems reasonable to assume that the cost of pulling a weight on a flat surface is similar to that of carrying the same weight. When applied to sled dogs, the calculations used above agree well with food record data. The incremental cost of running for a sled dog is based on the fraction of sled weight pulled by that dog.

Clinical Example

What is the caloric requirement for a 25-kg racing-sled dog that runs 167 km (100 miles) per day pulling a sled and driver with a combined weight of 180 kg in a team of 12 dogs? The cost of running (ERR) for this 25-kg dog is 4,342 kcal, based on an efficiency of a 25-kg dog of 26 kcal/km (**Table 18-6**) and a distance of 167 km. Assuming all dogs pull equally, the weight pulled by this dog is 15 kg (total sled weight ÷ number of dogs) or 60% of the dog's body weight. The incremental cost of running (ERR_{incr}) is 60% of ERR or 2,605 kcal. The total cost of running (ERR_{tot}) for this dog is 6,947 kcal. Note that RER for a 25-kg dog is 783 kcal (3.28 MJ). The energy needed for exercise is almost 9 x RER. The DER for this dog is 10 x RER, assuming no additional energy is needed for thermogenesis. To convert to kJ, multiply kcal x 4.184.

The Bibliography for **Box 18-5** can be found at www.markmorris.org.

Table 18-7. Disorders affecting olfaction in people.*

Disorder	Effect on olfaction
Adrenal cortical insufficiency	Increased detection
Allergic rhinitis	Absent or diminished
Bronchial asthma	Absent or diminished
Chronic kidney failure	Absent or diminished
Cobalamin deficiency	Absent or diminished
Cushing's syndrome	Absent or diminished
Diabetes mellitus	Absent or diminished
Head trauma	Absent or diminished
Hepatic cirrhosis	Absent or diminished
Hypothyroidism	Absent, diminished or distorted
Nasal polyposis	Absent or diminished
Upper respiratory infections	Absent, diminished or distorted
Viral hepatitis (acute)	Absent, diminished or distorted

*Many of these diseases would also be expected to cause similar problems in dogs. Adapted from: Schiffman SS. Taste and smell in disease. New England Journal of Medicine 1983; 308: 1275-1279.

Table 18-8. Drugs that can cause changes in the sense of smell in dogs and people.*

Drug	Effect on olfaction
Amiodarone	Abnormal sense of smell reported in 1 to 3% of human patients
Amlodipine	Disturbance of smell reported rarely in human patients; resolves after drug withdrawal
Bromocriptine	Olfactory hallucination in 9% of human patients receiving 0.5 to 5 mg/day
Cimetidine	Decrease in olfactory acuity in human patients; reported rarely
Dexamethasone	Reduced olfactory acuity in dogs after only one week
Doxycycline	Loss or distortion of sense of smell in a small number of human patients
Nifedipine	Disturbance of sense of smell in human patients; rare and symptoms resolve after drug withdrawal
Phenylephrine	Decreased ability to smell in 1% of human patients

*Adapted from: Bleasel AF, McLeod JG, Brown ML. Anosmia after doxycycline use. Medical Journal of Australia 1990; 152: 440. Ezeh PI, Myers LJ, Hanrahan LA, et al. Effects of steroids on olfactory function of the dog. Physiology and Behavior 1992; 51: 1183-1187. Henkin RL. Drug induced taste and smell disorders: Incidence, mechanisms and management related primarily to treatment of sensory receptor dysfunction. Drug Safety 1994; 11: 318-377. Levenson JL, Kennedy K. Dysosmia, dysgeusia and nifedipine. Annals of Internal Medicine 1985; 1102: 135-136. Product Information: Amiodarone, 2004.

homeostasis). High humidity impairs evaporative cooling thus adding to the work of heat excretion. Cold temperatures without exercise increase the energy requirement for thermogenesis. For working dogs, cold environmental temperatures aid in heat dissipation during exercise. Excitement or stress associated with some activities increases body temperature and respiration, leading to greater requirements for energy, water and perhaps electrolytes. Stress may also negatively affect food intake. Geographic factors such as high elevation, changing elevation (running up and down hills), bodies of water (swimming) and the presence of sand or tall grass underfoot can increase workload. These factors are important to consider for their potential effects on exercise and olfactory performance. Dogs that are out of breath and are panting excessively have reduced ability to detect scent (Gazit and Terkel, 2002).

Physical Examination

During the physical examination, the veterinarian should evaluate the dog's general health, musculoskeletal soundness, hydration, upper respiratory function, cardiopulmonary function and body condition. A complete physical examination is crucial because disease affecting any body system can impair performance. For example, severe periodontal disease can cause sufficient pain to affect food intake, thus causing a retriever to retrieve poorly or a greyhound to run poorly. Likewise any injury or deterioration of the musculoskeletal system affects performance. All major muscle groups and joints should be palpated and moved through a complete range of motion during the routine physical examination of canine athletes.

Certain infectious, traumatic, endocrine and metabolic diseases can affect olfaction. **Table 18-7** summarizes diseases that modify olfaction in people. Many of these diseases would be expected to cause similar problems in dogs. For example, viral upper respiratory infections (e.g., canine distemper), including intranasal inoculation with modified-live virus distemper vaccine will cause dysosmia (Myers, 1990). In a survey of field trial participants requesting information about the prevalence of anosmia in their hunting dogs, 85% of owners reported that they currently owned or had owned a dog with some loss of its sense of smell (Holloway, 1961). In another report, only 40% of canine patients presenting with complaints of dysosmia actually had dysosmia. In the remaining 60%, other disorders were interfering with the dogs' ability to hunt, including one dog with hip dysplasia (Myers, 1990).

Drugs can also negatively affect olfaction (**Table 18-8**). For example, corticosteroids reduce olfaction in dogs. The combination of hydrocortisone plus desoxycorticosterone acetate resulted in a reduction of olfactory acuity after 18 days of administration. Dexamethasone administration reduced olfactory acuity in dogs after only one week (Ezeh et al, 1992). These results are not surprising because Cushing's disease results in reduced olfactory acuity and adrenal cortical insufficiency results in increased olfaction (**Table 18-7**). Many hunting dogs receive corticosteroid therapy for skin or musculoskeletal disorders. On the other hand, zinc supplementation is effective in some olfactory disorders (Henkin et al, 1999). In lieu of zinc deficiency, supplemental zinc is not warranted and could be toxic when given at high levels (NRC, 2006).

Cardiopulmonary function is best assessed during routine physical examination by thorough auscultation of the heart and lung fields in a quiet environment. Energy balance can be evaluated by body condition scoring. The body condition score (BCS) is an indication of fat mass. If dietary energy intake is less than energy needs, fat mass declines and BCS decreases. Conversely, if intake exceeds requirement, fat mass and BCS increase. Chapter 1 describes body condition scoring in detail. A BCS of 2.5/5 to 3.5/5 is normal for most pets and for many canine athletes. However, a much leaner body composition is desirable for some canine athletes (e.g., racing greyhounds and sled dogs). Even small excesses of body fat may represent an unnecessary handicap for racing dogs.

The ability of any athlete to excel at a given event depends on that athlete's physical and metabolic characteristics, level of training and drive or desire. Some dogs are not well suited to some activities. Greyhounds make poor sled dogs and sled dogs make poor retrievers. Assessing how well an individual is suited to a particular type of exercise is partly common sense and partly experience; the fine points may take years of careful observation.

It is possible, however, to make some generalizations about characteristics that favor athletic performance. Sprinters tend to be very lean and fine-boned. A study comparing racing greyhounds to other breeds of dogs noted that as a percent of total body mass, greyhounds have more muscle (58% of body mass), the same amount of bone and less fat than other breeds (Gunn, 1978). Maximal muscle mass with no extra weight in the form of fat or excess bone is an obvious advantage for a sprinter. These characteristics benefit greyhounds in oval track racing. Different body types allow other breeds to perform well in various sprint sports. The smaller body of whippets allows for higher performance in the tight turns of lure coursing fields. The body conformation of Border collies allows for high levels of performance in agility competition and herding livestock. Endurance athletes may require more body fat to meet energy needs during long trips.

Laboratory and Other Clinical Information

Laboratory tests are not usually required for the routine assessment of healthy dogs. However, a few factors should be kept in mind when performing laboratory tests. Laboratory tests should address the two major factors of activity or work: anticipation to work and work itself. Anticipation to perform transiently affects the metabolism of dogs bred and trained for specific activities. Exercise can cause transient changes in blood and serum parameters. Concentrations of blood-borne substrates such as glucose and fatty acids may increase or decrease in relation to exercise. Total protein and electrolyte concentrations may increase simply due to fluid shift. As discussed above, contraction of the spleen and fluid shifts may dramatically increase packed cell volume. Lactate may accumulate in the plasma and blood pH may decrease with very intense exercise.

Excitement and conditioning of dogs bred and trained for working and sporting activities produce metabolic states that need to be addressed when performing nutritional studies (Gillette et al, 2006). Anticipation can initiate metabolic changes that result in exercise-related disease processes. An example is exercise-induced collapse in Labrador retrievers, a two-part problem in which event anticipation leads to medical problems.

Changes related to normal exercise physiology may be present to variable degrees up to two hours following exercise. Persistence of these changes may indicate a problem and should be investigated further. Small, persistent increases in concentration of the muscle isoenzyme of creatine phosphokinase (CPK) may occur in response to continuous exercise training. However, grossly elevated values indicate major muscle injury or rhabdomyolysis.

Key Nutritional Factors

The key nutritional factors for foods for working and sporting dogs are summarized in **Table 18-9**. The following section discusses the bases for these key nutritional factors and their recommended levels in foods.

Water

Water is arguably the most essential of all nutrients. It is the solvent for nearly all biologic solutes and a transport medium for nutrients, wastes and heat. Water also absorbs physical shock and lubricates various internal and external body surfaces. Approximately two-thirds of the body's weight is composed of water (Pivarnik, 1994; Houpt, 1984; Swenson, 1984). Total body water is divided into four major compartments. Approximately 62 to 64% of water is located within cells, 22% within interstitial spaces and 7% within the intravascular space in plasma (Wolter, 1985; Ivy et al, 1988). The remaining 7% is present as transcellular fluids such as vitreous and aqueous humor, cerebral spinal fluid, joint fluid and digestive secretions (Pivarnik, 1994; Houpt, 1984). Osmotic, oncotic and hydrostatic pressures as well as the permeability characteristics of individual membranes direct fluid balance between compartments. Dietary water intake and metabolic water production (10 to 16 ml/100 kcal and 3 to 4 ml/g glycogen) on one hand and evaporative, urinary and fecal losses on the other maintain total body water balance (Pivarnik, 1994; Houpt, 1984).

The fluid content of individual tissues and compartments changes with the onset of muscular activity. Cardiac output, partially a function of plasma volume, increases during exercise to meet the muscle's heightened demand for nutrient delivery and waste removal. The increase in blood flow also helps dissipate the heat produced by working muscles. Only about 20 to 30% of the energy consumed within muscle cells during exercise produces work; the remaining 70 to 80% is converted into heat. This is about the same efficiency as a gasoline engine (Serway, 1984). This heat must be dissipated to prevent performance impairments and perhaps life-threatening increases in body temperature (Pivarnik, 1994; Kozlowski et al, 1985; Kruk et al, 1985).

During prolonged periods of exercise in warm and humid environments, heat dissipation leads to a decrease in total body water and plasma volume. Approximately 60% of the heat dissipated during exercise is lost through fluid evaporation from the upper respiratory tract (Young et al, 1959). Water requirements essentially double in dogs when the ambient temperature reaches 45°C (113°F) (NRC, 2006). Exercise in very cold, dry environments also increases evaporative fluid losses. Significant fluid loss during exercise may impair performance. Even mild dehydration can limit exercise performance (Swenson, 1984) and probably negatively affects olfactory performance. Several studies indicate that hydration status is the single most impor-

Table 18-9. Key nutritional factors for foods for working and sporting dogs.

Factors	Sprint activity	Intermediate activity (low/moderate duration and frequency)	Intermediate activity (high duration and frequency)	Endurance activity
Water	Unlimited access except just before a race	Unlimited access	Unlimited access	Unlimited access
Energy density	Use food with 3.5 to 4.0 kcal ME/g DM	Use food with 4.0 to 5.0 kcal ME/g DM	Use food with 4.5 to 5.5 kcal ME/g DM	Use food with >6.0 kcal ME/g DM
Fat	Use food with 8 to 10% DM fat or 20 to 24% of calories from fat	Use food with 15 to 30% DM fat or 30 to 55% of calories from fat	Use food with 25 to 40% DM fat or 45 to 65% of calories from fat	Use food with >50% DM fat or >75% of calories from fat
Unsaturated fatty acids	-	>60% unsaturated fatty acids to optimize olfaction	>60% unsaturated fatty acids to optimize olfaction	-
Digestible carbohydrate	Use food with 55 to 65% DM NFE or 50 to 60% of calories from NFE	Use food with 30 to 55% DM NFE or 20 to 50% of calories from NFE	Use food with 30 to 35% DM NFE or 15 to 30% of calories from NFE	Use food with <15% DM NFE or <10% of calories from NFE
Protein	Use food with 22 to 28% DM protein or 20 to 25% of kcal (ME) from protein	Use food with 22 to 32% DM protein or 20 to 25% of kcal (ME) from protein	Use food with 22 to 32% DM protein or 18 to 25% of kcal (ME) from protein	Use food with 28 to 34% DM protein or 18 to 22% of kcal (ME) from protein
Digestibility	DM digestibility >80%	DM digestibility >80%	DM digestibility >80%	DM digestibility >80%
Antioxidants				
Vitamin E	≥500 IU vitamin E/kg food (DM)	≥500 IU vitamin E/kg food (DM)	≥500 IU vitamin E/kg food (DM)	≥500 IU vitamin E/kg food (DM)
Vitamin C	150 to 250 mg vitamin C/kg food (DM)	150 to 250 mg vitamin C/kg food (DM)	150 to 250 mg vitamin C/kg food (DM)	150 to 250 mg vitamin C/kg food (DM)
Selenium	0.5 to 1.3 mg/kg food (DM)	0.5 to 1.3 mg/kg food (DM)	0.5 to 1.3 mg/kg food (DM)	0.5 to 1.3 mg/kg food (DM)

Key: ME = metabolizable energy, DM = dry matter, NFE = nitrogen-free extract (represents digestible [soluble] carbohydrate fraction).

tant determinant of endurance capacity (Kronfeld and Downey, 1981; Downey et al, 1980; Young et al, 1959a).

There is currently much debate over the best strategy to maintain fluid and electrolyte balance in working dogs. Under most exercise situations, these athletes lose more water than electrolytes, causing a decrease in plasma volume and an increase in plasma osmolality. Efforts to return electrolyte values to normal should thus concentrate on water replacement. Ideally, fresh clean water should be available at all times. There are occasions when such accommodations cannot be made due to the nature of the athletic event or the environmental conditions. Under these conditions, water should be offered at least three times a day and more often if possible. "Baiting" the water with a flavor enhancer such as meat juice can encourage water intake.

Energy

Providing the right amount of energy from the right sources is central to feeding working and sporting dogs. Providing the correct amount of energy is determined by the food's energy density and the amount fed. The energy density can limit the maximum possible caloric intake and a food's overall digestibility. Additionally, the preferred source of energy (fat vs. carbohydrate) depends on exercise type. Energy for exercise comes from three nutrients: fat, carbohydrate and protein. Fats and carbohydrates are the primary energy substrates for exercise. Fat is the preferred substrate for longer duration exercise, whereas sprinters depend more on carbohydrate. Under most conditions, the energy contribution of protein during exercise is small (Hickson and Wolinsky, 1989); however, its contribution will increase in fatigued dogs.

Energy required depends on the intensity, duration and frequency of exercise. The amount of energy required for exercise depends on total work done (intensity x duration x frequency). The preferred source of energy depends mostly on intensity. Greyhounds, even though they work at a very high intensity, have relatively low energy requirements because the duration of their events is so short and frequency is usually only a few times each week. Generally, 1.6 to 2 x resting energy requirement (RER) is adequate for most sprint athletes. Note the daily energy requirement (DER) for most pet dogs is 1.2 to 1.4 x RER. Most pet dogs are minimally active.

For activities of very short duration and high intensity, the energy substrate source is the main determinant of the nutrient profile. Foods for sprint athletes should be high in carbohydrate and lower in fat, with a resulting energy density lower than that of many dog foods. Intensity, duration and frequency of exercise are variable for intermediate athletes; therefore, the energy requirement is highly variable. DER for these athletes ranges from 2 to 5 x RER. Foods with a higher fat content are typically fed to provide adequate dietary energy density. Endurance athletes require more than 5 x RER. For activities of long duration, providing adequate energy is a major determinant in the choice of a nutrient profile for exercising dogs. Foods that are very high in fat are required.

Table 18-9 lists target energy density levels for foods for working and sporting dogs, depending on the type, level and duration of physical activity.

Fat

Fat provides approximately 8.5 kcal (36 kJ) of metabolizable energy (ME) per gram of dry matter (DM) or more than twice the amount provided by protein and carbohydrate. Because of these differences in caloric density, the only practical means of significantly increasing the energy density of a food is to increase its fat concentration. Reasonable increases in fat usually also increase palatability. Energy density and palatability make dietary fat levels an important consideration in the formulation of foods for working and sporting dogs. Increasing dietary fat generally also increases a food's digestibility because fat tends to be more digestible than protein or carbohydrate. Also, when a greater quantity of a lower energy density food is eaten in an attempt to provide adequate calories, there is a more rapid rate of passage through the gastrointestinal (GI) tract, further reducing digestibility and energy intake (Davenport et al, 2001).

Ingesting adequate calories to meet daily energy expenditure is often a serious challenge for working dogs. In extreme cases, sled dogs in long-distance races expend from 6,000 to 10,000 kcal/day (25 to 42 MJ/day), in which case DM intake becomes a performance-limiting factor. Because the total daily DM intake is limited to about 3.5% of body weight,[c] the energy density of a food should be maximized. Under these circumstances, each nonessential gram of protein and carbohydrate ingested potentially robs the dog of 5 kcal (21 kJ). The calorie deficit is paid through mobilization of body fat stores. Overreliance on these depots may lead to catabolism of more functionally crucial energy sources, such as muscle and plasma proteins. In addition to its role as an energy store, adipose tissue also functions as an insulator. Excessive adipose depletion may increase a dog's cost of maintaining its body temperature, especially at rest in cold environments.

Even under the less severe conditions of intermediate exercise, increased dietary fat levels provide needed energy and other valuable benefits. Fatigue and dehydration may decrease appetite. Increasing dietary fat concentration increases energy intake and encourages stressed dogs to ingest more food because the higher fat content improves palatability.

Feeding high levels of fat can positively affect endurance. Training may elevate the carbohydrate threshold, thus increasing the proportion of energy supplied by free fatty acid (FFA) oxidation at all but the highest intensities of exercise. Increasing dietary fat concentration may augment this process by enhancing FFA availability (Kronfeld and Downey, 1981; Kronfeld et al, 1977; Reynolds et al, 1994). Working dogs fed high-fat foods have higher circulating levels of FFA at rest and respond to exercise stimuli by releasing more FFA than those fed isocaloric amounts of a high-carbohydrate food (Kronfeld and Downey, 1981; Kronfeld et al, 1977; Young et al, 1962). This difference in FFA availability may be related to the decreased resting plasma concentration of insulin in animals fed high-fat foods, and the induction of key lipolytic enzymes.

Table 18-10. Effect of nutrient profile on stamina.*

	Food A	Food B	Food C
Nutrient (DM)			
Energy density (kcal/g)	4.7	5.9	6.0
Fat (%)	12.8	28.3	33.1
Protein (%)	22.9	48.7	30.5
Performance			
Time (minutes)	103.7	136.1	137.6
Distance (miles)	15.5	20.4	20.6

Key: DM = dry matter, Food A = grocery brand dry food, Food B = grocery brand moist food, Food C = specialty brand dry food.
*Adapted from: Downey RL, Kronfeld DS, Banta CA. Diet of beagles affects stamina. Journal of the American Animal Hospital Association 1980; 6: 273-277.

The effect of food on insulin levels has also been demonstrated in well-trained human athletes (Gleeson et al, 1986; Martin et al, 1978; Coyle et al, 1985; Yoshida, 1986; Brouns et al, 1989). People eating high-fat foods had significantly lower resting insulin concentrations than those eating high-carbohydrate foods (Maughan et al, 1987). Insulin decreases the release of FFA from peripheral adipose stores through its inhibitory effects on the activity of hormone-sensitive lipase. Dogs rely more heavily on FFA for energy generation at all exercise intensities than people do; therefore, the effect of food on resting insulin levels is a matter of even greater concern for working and sporting dogs (Reynolds et al, 1997). Increased dietary fat (from 25 to 65% of kcal) increases VO_2 max and the maximal rate of fat oxidation by 20 to 30% in well-trained dogs (Reynolds et al, 1995). These increases were associated with a 25 to 30% increase in mitochondrial volume, possibly accounting for the increased oxidative capacity. Protein and total caloric intake were identical between groups. Also, event anticipation can suppress insulin concentrations before and during an event activity (Gillette et al, 2006).

The relationship between fat intake and canine endurance is well established. The time to exhaustion for well-conditioned beagles running on a treadmill was directly related to energy density, digestibility and digestible fat intake (**Table 18-10**) (Downey et al, 1980). Practical applications of this concept are evident in the performance foods currently fed to many successful working and sporting dogs. As the duration of the event performed by a dog increases, so should the dietary fat intake.

Dogs can tolerate high levels of dietary fat if fat is gradually introduced and an adequate intake of non-fat nutrients is maintained. Steatorrhea and a decrease in food palatability are indicators that the fat content of a food has exceeded a dog's fat tolerance. Under conditions of extreme training, sled dogs may ingest up to 60% of their energy as fat. During ultra-endurance events, such as the Iditarod or the Yukon Quest, fat intake may compose 80% of the calories ingested.[d] This "super fat loading" should be attempted only during the most strenuous periods of such events, when it is difficult or impossible for dogs to ingest as much energy as they are expending.

Anemia has been associated with impaired performance in dog teams fed very high-fat foods (i.e., 80% kcal from fat) for prolonged periods (i.e., weeks to months) (Reynolds, 1997).

Table 18-11. Saturated and unsaturated fatty acid content of selected fat sources used in commercial pet foods.*

Ingredient	Saturated fatty acids (%)	Unsaturated fatty acids (%)**
Beef tallow	47.4	52.6
Choice white grease	38.7	61.3
Lard (swine fat)	28.6	71.4
Poultry fat	28.6	71.4
Fish oil (menhaden)	20.2	79.8
Corn oil	12.7	87.3
Flax oil (linseed)	9.4	90.6
Safflower oil	8.6	91.4
Soybean oil	14.2	85.8
Sunflower oil	8.9	91.1

*National Research Council. Nutrient Requirements of Dogs and Cats. Washington, DC: National Academies Press, 2006; 328-329.
**Includes both polyunsaturated and monounsaturated fatty acids; derived by subtracting % saturated fatty acid values from 100.

However, during several long expeditions (including the trans-Antarctica expedition of 1991), Will Steger observed no decrement of performance when dogs were fed food containing 80% fat kcal and 17% protein kcal.[e] Other factors such as environment, training and dietary intake of non-fat nutrients (e.g., protein) may play a role in the development of anemia.

The type of fat used must also be considered in the formulation of foods for working and sporting dogs. Essential fatty acids should make up at least 2% of the DM of a food (Chapter 5). The remainder of the fat may come from any of a number of plant or animal sources. Many greyhound and sled-dog trainers believe that dogs run "hotter" when fed saturated rather than unsaturated fats. No objective evidence supports this theory. However, there is evidence that foods containing high levels of saturated fat (60% of the fatty acids saturated) will reduce olfactory performance in dogs, particularly if they are not physically conditioned (Altom et al, 2003). This may be due to effects of dietary fatty acids on brain function. Membrane composition of the central nervous system can be affected by the dietary fat source. Rats fed food high in saturated fat (beef tallow) showed a deficiency of 18:3 fatty acids in the brain vs. rats fed a food with unsaturated fat (corn oil) (MacDonald et al, 1996). The fatty acid composition of membrane phospholipids dictates membrane fluidity and permeability (Coutre and Hulbert, 1995). Changes in membrane fluidity can affect the functions of membrane enzymes. Sodium-potassium ATPase is one of several major components of the pathway that mediates molecular events of olfaction. Dietary fat can affect brain synaptic membrane sodium-potassium ATPase activity (Gerbi et al, 1994; Altom et al, 2003). In the study above that noted a decrease in olfaction when 60% of the fatty acids were saturated (37% unsaturated), another group of dogs fed a food with only 24.5% saturated fatty acids (72% unsaturated) maintained olfactory performance over time, even if the dogs were not physically fit. Thus, higher levels of unsaturated fatty acids in a food appear to protect against decline of olfaction over time in untrained dogs. Anecdotal reports support the use of supplemental unsaturated fatty acids (corn oil) to improve olfactory performance.[f] If corn oil is added to dry commercial foods to increase the fat and/or unsaturated fatty acid content, 1 tablespoon of corn oil for approximately each pound of dry food will increase the overall fat content by about three percentage points. For example, if two tablespoons of corn oil are added to one pound of dry food that contains 20% fat, the resultant mixture of food and corn oil will contain about 26% fat and would have increased levels of unsaturated fatty acids. However, if commercial foods are properly formulated for active dogs, supplementation with fat sources such as corn oil should not be necessary.

Alternatively, large intakes of unsaturated fatty acids may increase the risk of oxidative damage to membrane lipids (NRC, 1985; Van Vleet, 1980), which can severely damage cell membrane function with potentially disastrous implications for working dogs. Relative to their sedentary colleagues, dogs participating in endurance events are at particular risk for developing oxidative membrane damage because they consume more fat and metabolize more oxygen per unit body weight per day. Feeding only well-stabilized (preserved) unsaturated fatty acids reduces the risk of oxidative damage to tissues. Increasing intake of vitamins E and C and selenium to bolster cellular antioxidant capacity has also been recommended (Kronfeld, 1989) and is discussed below in the Antioxidants section.

Unsaturated fatty acids are an important component in a well-balanced food. As mentioned above, they are largely responsible for membrane fluidity, a property critical to the function of all cell membranes. Unsaturated fatty acids are also required for biosynthesis of many regulatory molecules and maintenance of epidermal integrity. All essential fatty acids are unsaturated. In weighing the biologic significance of unsaturated fatty acids with the possible health risks associated with their overconsumption, balanced amounts of saturated and unsaturated fatty acids may be the best solution. **Table 18-11** shows the percentage of saturated and unsaturated fatty acids in various ingredients used as fat sources for pet foods. For commercial foods, product labels will include ingredient listings in descending order of predominance by weight. By reviewing a product's ingredient list, one can obtain an approximate idea of the levels of saturated and unsaturated fatty acids in the food. If additional unsaturated fat sources are added to a commercial food, adequate vitamin E should be provided. (See Antioxidants discussion, below.)

Certain fatty acids are purported to have ergogenic effects. The omega-3 (n-3) family of fatty acids contained in fish oils has been reported to enhance oxygen uptake (Brilla and Landerholm, 1990). The results reported in this study lacked statistical significance, prompting the need for further investigations. Medium-chain triglyceride (MCT) supplementation reportedly enhances performance (Grandjean and Paragon, 1987; Wolter, 1985). These intermediate length (eight to 12 carbon) fatty acids do not rely on L-carnitine for transport across the inner mitochondrial membrane. Because they bypass this rate-limiting step in fatty acid oxidation, some investigators have theorized that increasing the dietary MCT level may increase the maximal rate of fatty acid oxidation. A study of the effects of MCT supplementation failed to demonstrate an increase in oxygen consumption or FFA oxidation in human athletes (Brilla and Landerholm, 1990). Further research is needed to determine the consequences of MCT supplementation in working dogs.

Sprint exercise depends almost entirely on carbohydrate; therefore, the fat requirement for sprinters is not different than that for other dogs. Total fat content should be 8 to 10% of DM or 20 to 24% of kcal. Dietary fat needs for intermediate athletes are directly proportional to the amount of work done. Part-time athletes during off-season should be fed as other dogs (Chapter 13). Dietary fat content should be increased as the amount of work increases: 15 to 30% DM (30 to 55% fat kcal) for moderate amounts of work and 25 to 40% DM (45 to 65% fat kcal) for large amounts of work. Endurance athletes require very high levels of dietary fat to meet their energy needs, in excess of 50% DM and 75% fat kcal. A balance of saturated and unsaturated fat sources is recommended. **Table 18-9** summarizes recommendations for fat and other nutrients by exercise type. Currently, it is recommended that working and sporting dogs not be fed high-fat meals immediately before or during intense exercise (NRC, 2006).

Digestible Carbohydrate

Provided sufficient gluconeogenic precursors are available, dogs have no dietary requirement for carbohydrates except during gestation and neonatal development (Chapters 15 and 16). Dogs are quite capable of maintaining normal blood glucose and tissue glycogen levels when fed carbohydrate-free foods (Kronfeld et al, 1977; Hammel et al, 1977). Compared with people, dogs are less likely to develop ketosis during long periods of exercise or starvation (Kronfeld et al, 1977; Crandall, 1941). Despite these facts, dogs have great ability to use carbohydrate.

Canine athletes requiring less than twice maintenance levels of energy may derive a significant portion of their kcal from carbohydrate sources. This is an advantage for high-power athletes, such as racing greyhounds that are highly dependent on anaerobic metabolism. Because carbohydrates contain only about 3.5 kcal (15 kJ) ME/g, they cannot be used to increase the energy density of a food. This limitation is an important consideration for endurance athletes that have difficulty ingesting a sufficient volume of food to meet caloric requirements.

Racing greyhounds are highly dependent on carbohydrate stored in muscles as glycogen because they must mobilize energy quickly to run a race. Studies have shown that greyhounds use significant amounts of glycogen during a race; up to 70% of available glycogen in some muscles for an 800-meter race (Dobson et al, 1988; Rose and Bloomberg, 1989). Furthermore, evidence suggests that the rate of glycogen use (and, therefore, energy production) depends on the concentration of glycogen in muscle (Richter and Glabo, 1986). It is logical; therefore, to hypothesize that increasing muscle glycogen will enhance sprint performance. Muscle glycogen content can be increased through a combination of dietary and training protocol changes in some animals (rats, people [Conlee, 1987], horses [Oldham et al, 1989]); these techniques have been used as a means of improving endurance performance (Conlee, 1987; Bergstrom et al, 1967). The possible benefits of increased muscle glycogen on sprint exercise performance of dogs have not been established. It is also unclear if continuous feeding of high-carbohydrate foods to dogs will increase muscle glycogen. For sled dogs, it may be more advantageous to promote glycogen sparing by feeding a high-fat food than increasing pre-exercise glycogen concentrations via ingestion of a high-carbohydrate food. Studies have demonstrated an increase in the amount of muscle glycogen stored and a greater rate of glycogen use in sled dogs fed a high-carbohydrate food (65% of kcal) (Reynolds et al, 1997). When isocaloric amounts of a high-fat food were fed, glycogen was used at a much slower rate, promoting better endurance at all submaximal exercise intensities. In sled dogs, carbohydrate sparing appears to be a more successful strategy than carbohydrate loading.

Two studies have reported the effect of different fat and carbohydrate levels on race time in greyhounds (Toll et al, 1992; Hill et al, 1996). Both studies used seven adult racing greyhounds in a crossover design and used race time in a 5/16-mile (502-m) race as the measure of performance. Investigators in the first study used two foods similar in composition except for fat and carbohydrate content (Toll et al, 1992). The high-carbohydrate food contained 16% DM fat (34% of kcal) and 52% DM carbohydrate (44% of kcal), whereas the low-carbohydrate food contained 56% fat (80% of kcal) and 8% carbohydrate (5% of kcal). No significant difference in race times between the two food groups was detected for the first four weekly measurements. At the end of the fifth week, the dogs fed the high-carbohydrate food ran faster (33.08 ± 0.05 sec) than when they were fed the low-carbohydrate food (33.34 ± 0.05 sec). The results were statistically significant ($p < 0.05$). In this study, dogs performed better when fed a high-carbohydrate/low-fat food than they did when fed a high-fat/low-carbohydrate food. The delay before differences occurred may indicate that some time may be required to adapt to a new food before performance is affected.

The second study compared results of feeding a "high-fat" food (38.2% energy from fat, 23% energy from protein, 38.8% energy from carbohydrate) with those of feeding a "moderate-fat" food (27.6% energy from fat, 20.4% energy from protein, 52.1% energy from carbohydrate) (Hill et al, 1996). Dogs were fed each food for eight weeks. Race times were faster when the dogs were fed the high-fat food than when they were fed the medium-fat food (32.9 ± 0.7 vs. 33.1 ± 0.6 sec at $\alpha = 0.1$, $\beta = 0.2$).

Neither of these studies evaluated a truly high-carbohydrate level (60 to 70% of dietary kcal) as is now recommended for glycogen loading in people (Goodyear et al, 1990). Furthermore, although the results of these two studies are mixed, physiologic principles suggest that carbohydrate supplementation should benefit racing greyhounds.

Even endurance athletes may benefit from a low level of dietary carbohydrate. Studies involving sled dogs fed 0 or 17% of their kcal as carbohydrate showed that dogs were more susceptible to developing "stress" diarrhea when fed foods devoid of carbohydrate (Kronfeld, 1973). There are other advantages associated with feeding carbohydrates to sprint athletes. Because these dogs derive more of their energy for exercise from glucose/glycogen, glycogen depletion may play a role in the onset of fatigue for athletes working at or above their anaerobic threshold (Pate and Brunn, 1989; Miller and Massaro, 1989; Keizer et al, 1986; Issekutz, 1981; Burke and Read, 1987).

Carbohydrate availability to working muscles is a limiting factor for prolonged exercise in people and other species. This finding has led to development of strategies for carbohydrate loading or glycogen super-compensation. The classic method (Åstrand method) uses a combination of exhaustive exercise and low-carbohydrate foods (≤10% kcal from carbohydrate) to deplete muscle glycogen. Glycogen depletion is followed by consumption of high-carbohydrate foods (80 to 90% kcal from carbohydrate) and little activity. This method dramatically increases muscle glycogen in people (Bucci, 1993). An alternative carbohydrate-loading method (Sherman/Costill method) simply requires consumption of 60 to 70% of kcal from carbohydrate consistently over time. In people, this method produces results similar to those achieved by the classic method (Bucci, 1993).

Glycogen loading is probably not as beneficial for canine endurance athletes as continuous feeding of foods with high-fat levels. However, high-power athletes (e.g., racing greyhounds) should benefit from glycogen loading. Because racing greyhounds do not have dramatically increased energy needs and cannot use fatty acids effectively during a race lasting less than 60 seconds, there is no benefit to feeding high levels of fat. Additionally, glycogen stores are rapidly mobilized during racing. In one study, greyhounds running an 800-m race in 48 seconds mobilized 50 to 70% of their glycogen stores in specific running muscles (Dobson et al, 1988).

Studies in people have shown that feeding moderate amounts of carbohydrate (2 g glucose/kg body weight) during a brief postexercise time window permits very rapid rates of glycogen resynthesis (Goodyear et al, 1990; Keizer et al, 1986; Ivy et al, 1988). This period begins about 30 minutes postexercise (Kronfeld, 1973). Glucose administered during this window permits up to four times the rate of glycogen resynthesis supported by the same amount of glucose administered after this two-hour window. The form of the glucose (i.e., polymer or simple sugar) does not seem to affect the rate of glycogen repletion (Keizer et al, 1986). Severely hypertonic solutions should be avoided to prevent excessive osmotic movement of fluid into the gut, which may lead to cramping and GI distress (Williams, 1985; Buskirk and Puhl, 1989). This strategy for glycogen repletion is effective in human athletes and dogs. Glucose solutions (from 1.5 to 3 g glucose/kg body weight) given before, during or after exercise have been shown to minimize the exercise-associated decline in blood glucose, promote more rapid repletion of muscle glycogen postexercise and improve thermoregulation (Kruk et al, 1987; Reynolds et al, 1997; Wakschlage et al, 2002). Although only speculation, resultant improvements in exercise performance and thermoregulation might also protect against a reduction in olfactory performance by precluding excessive panting. The carbohydrates used in foods for canine athletes should be highly digestible to limit fecal bulk. Excessive amounts of undigested carbohydrates reaching the colon may increase water loss via the stool, increase colonic gas production and increase overall fecal bulk. These changes in fecal consistency have been proposed to increase an athlete's risk of developing "stress diarrhea," further increasing fecal water losses (Kronfeld, 1973). Bulky stools have also been associated with rectal bleeding during exercise-induced colonic evacuation (Kronfeld, 1973). Excessive fecal bulk is also extra weight that must be carried by the athlete. One study estimated that 150 g of extra stool generated by a racing-sled dog was equal to a 7-kg handicap for a thoroughbred horse (Kronfeld and Downey, 1981).

Metabolic power or a high rate of ATP generation is required for sprint performance. Consequently, anaerobic metabolism of glucose and glycogen is the dominant energy generation pathway. High-carbohydrate foods should be fed to maximize muscle glycogen. Dietary carbohydrates should compose 50 to 70% of total kcal to maximize muscle glycogen levels (based on research done with people).

The dietary carbohydrate recommendation for intermediate athletes is highly variable, depending on the intensity and duration of work. Dogs that perform relatively long bouts of low to moderate intensity work require more dietary energy (higher fat) and relatively low carbohydrate levels (as low as 15% of kcal). Dogs that perform short bursts of higher intensity work should be fed more carbohydrate, up to 50% of kcal.

Endurance athletes require very little carbohydrate. Endurance rations should contain less than 15% of kcal from carbohydrate to achieve the energy density required for the amount of work done by these dogs. Some carbohydrate and/or soluble fiber should be included in the food to avoid loose stools.

Technically, the total carbohydrate portion of a food includes fiber. The digestible (soluble) carbohydrate portion of total carbohydrate consists of starches and sugars, typically referred to simply as "carbohydrate." The digestible carbohydrate fraction of a food is also called the nitrogen-free extract (NFE). The percent digestible carbohydrate is usually not stated on the guaranteed analysis listing of a commercial product's label. Such information should be available from product literature supplied by the manufacturer (e.g., product "keys," websites, etc.). However, percent digestible carbohydrate can also be estimated from the guaranteed analysis listing by subtracting the percent crude protein, fat, crude fiber and ash (mineral) from 100. If fiber and ash are not listed, assume 3% fiber and 9% ash in dry foods and 1% fiber and 6% ash in moist (canned) foods. Another, perhaps simpler means of estimating digestible carbohydrate content is to check if the protein and fat recommendations in **Table 18-9** are close to what is listed on the guaranteed analysis portion of the label of the food in question, if they are, its digestible carbohydrate content should also be close to what is recommended.

Table 18-9 summarizes carbohydrate recommendations for canine athletes by exercise type.

Soluble fiber and resistant starches may provide some benefit to racing dogs, particularly if they are fed raw meat. Rapid fermentation of oligosaccharides may decrease colonic pH and inhibit clostridial growth (Amtsbert et al, 1989). Fructo-oligosaccharides inhibit cecal colonization by *Salmonella* species in chickens and could conceivably do so in dogs (Baily et al, 1991).

Protein

Dietary protein is used to fulfill structural, biochemical and, to a lesser extent, energy requirements. Work increases the requirement for protein. The magnitude of this increase and the best strategy for meeting it are subjects of much debate in canine performance nutrition.

The work-induced elevation in protein requirement is most pronounced when the intensity and/or duration of exercise performed is rapidly increased above an animal's present level of conditioning. These circumstances are encountered at the onset of a training program, when the duration or intensity of training bouts is increased and especially during performances (Zackin, 1990; Hickson and Wolinsky, 1989). A common example would be when a bird dog that is also a minimally active pet is hunted the first time during hunting season with little or no exercise training. The increase in protein demand is due to combined increases in the rates of tissue protein synthesis and catabolism.

Several anabolic processes contribute to the exercise-induced increment in protein requirement. Protein demand is elevated due to an increase in the synthesis of structural and functional proteins. Training induces synthesis of many enzymes and transport proteins in each of the energy-generating pathways (Nadel, 1985; Williams, 1985; Costill et al, 1979, 1979a). Blood volume also expands during aerobic training (Nadel, 1985; Williams, 1985; Zackin, 1990; Hickson and Wolinsky, 1989). Such expansion necessitates an increase in plasma protein synthesis to maintain oncotic and osmotic balance between plasma and interstitial fluids (Pivarnik, 1994). The increase in hematocrit sometimes observed during endurance conditioning programs may reflect an increase in tissue protein synthesis (Nadel, 1985; Williams, 1985; Kronfeld and Downey, 1981). Anaerobic training regimens may also induce muscle hypertrophy (Hickson and Wolinsky, 1989). Amino acids are used in the formation of new muscle tissue and in the repair of damage that may occur to muscle and connective tissue during intensive conditioning programs. In addition to enhancing the rate of tissue protein synthesis, exercise increases the rate of amino acid catabolism. Amino acids may provide between 5 and 15% of the energy used during exercise, depending on the intensity and duration of the task (Young et al, 1962; Zackin, 1990; Hickson and Wolinsky, 1989). Most of this energy comes from the oxidation of branched-chain amino acids (Miller and Massaro, 1989; Blomstrand et al, 1988). All three amino acids belonging to this group (leucine, isoleucine, valine) are "essential" and thus cannot be synthesized from other amino acids in sufficient quantities to meet requirements. The branched-chain amino acids lost through exercise must be replaced through dietary intake.

The proportion of energy supplied by amino acids may be even greater in underfed athletes and those participating in ultra-endurance events in which there is a high risk for depletion of endogenous carbohydrate stores (Zackin, 1990; Miller and Massaro, 1989). In these instances, gluconeogenesis becomes the major pathway for maintaining blood glucose levels (Zackin, 1990; Miller and Massaro, 1989). Because amino acids are the predominant substrate used by the gluconeogenic pathway, their rate of catabolism is increased whenever this pathway is accelerated (Hickson and Wolinsky, 1989; Cahill et al, 1970).

This concept raises an important point: it is disadvantageous for an athlete to rely heavily on endogenous sources of protein for energy. There are no known labile stores of protein in the canine body. All protein sources serve a structural or functional purpose (Cahill et al, 1970). Interestingly, skeletal muscle is readily mobilized. Overuse of this source would have an obvious negative impact on performance. Because the small pool of circulating amino acids is insufficient to meet the amino acid requirements of the anabolic and catabolic processes described above, dietary protein intake must supply the deficit if nitrogen balance is to be maintained (Zackin, 1990).

For endurance athletes, there may be some disadvantages inherent to exploiting dietary protein sources for energy. Protein has only about 3.5 kcal (15 kJ) ME/g DM. Thus, increasing the proportion of protein in the formulation cannot increase the energy density of a ration. The energy density of the food is one of the major determinants of endurance capacity when working dogs have difficulty ingesting as many kcal as they expend (Downey et al, 1980).

Excessive protein intake may predispose an animal to increased amino acid catabolism because dietary amino acids are not stored in labile protein depots, but are deaminated (Hickson and Wolinsky, 1989). The resulting ketoacids are either oxidized for energy directly or converted into fatty acids and/or glucose and then stored as adipose tissue or glycogen. The urea produced from amino acid breakdown is excreted from the body in urine. In healthy animals, the amount of water lost increases with increased urea production.

An optimal food for a working or sporting dog should contain enough high-quality protein to meet the dog's anabolic requirements and enough non-protein energy nutrients to meet its energy requirements. Such a food encourages the use of ingested protein in synthetic rather than energy-generating processes. As non-protein caloric intake increases, less dietary protein is used for energy and more is available for use in anabolic processes. Energy requirements should be met by fat and carbohydrate, leaving the majority of amino acids available for synthetic purposes. During long-duration exercise, DER may increase several-fold whereas protein requirement increases only a few percent. To meet the energy needs of hard-working dogs, either more food must be consumed (increasing both energy and protein intake equally) or a higher energy, lower protein food must be fed (increasing energy intake more than protein intake). Providing sufficient dietary energy by increasing fat content should limit the use of amino acids for energy production. Because the protein requirement is actually a requirement for available amino acids, the digestibility and essential amino acid content of ingested protein will also determine how efficiently amino acids are incorporated into tissue proteins.

Research attempts that define the optimal dietary protein intake for working dogs have been inconclusive. Several field studies performed on racing-sled dogs in the 1970s and early 1980s found that well-conditioned dogs fed a high-fat, high-protein food maintained higher packed cell volumes and serum albumin concentrations than those fed a relatively high-carbohydrate, low-protein food (Kronfeld et al, 1977; Kronfeld, 1977; Adkins and Kronfeld, 1982). The investigators concluded that the high-fat, high-protein food might offer a performance advantage by maintaining better blood volume and oxygen carrying capacity than the other foods tested. These investigators recommended that 30 to 40% of kcal of a performance ration should come from protein.

Another study examined the effects of feeding isocaloric foods (4.5 kcal [19 kJ] ME/g) containing 16, 24, 32 or 40% of their energy as protein on performance and biochemical parameters (Reynolds et al, 1999). During training and racing, dogs fed only 16% of ME as protein suffered significantly more injuries and had a significant decline in VO_2 max when compared with age-, gender- and ability-matched sled dogs fed 24, 32 or 40% of ME as protein. Additionally in people, long-duration exercise leading to glycogen depletion increases protein requirement more than weight lifting. There were no noticeable differences in performance between the dogs fed 24, 32 or 40% of ME as protein, although the dogs fed 40% of ME as protein maintained a significantly higher packed cell volume and total plasma volume. This study indicated that 16% of ME as protein may be insufficient to meet the needs of extremely hard-working dogs and that such animals should ingest a minimum of 24% of their energy requirement as protein.

Work in greyhounds shows a different response to food protein levels. When raced for 500 m twice/week, dogs ran 0.3 km/hr faster and their hematocrits were higher when fed a lower protein (63 g/1,000 kcal, 24% ME), higher carbohydrate (106 g/1,000 kcal, 43% ME) food vs. a higher protein (96 g/1,000 kcal, 37% ME), lower carbohydrate (75 g/1,000 kcal, 30% ME) food (Hill et al, 2001a). The fat content of the foods was similar. Thus, for sprint athletes, a lower level of food protein appears desirable.

The protein requirement for exercise is only mildly increased (5 to 15%) regardless of exercise type. Protein is used for muscle hypertrophy and muscle maintenance/repair. Furthermore, the branched-chain amino acids can contribute to energy production. Dietary protein should be at least 24% of kcal. Because the energy requirement of some endurance athletes is so high (up to 11 x RER), it may not be feasible to feed even this level of protein and provide adequate kcal. For these dogs, 16% of the ME as protein should be viewed as an absolute minimum. Note that for endurance exercise, energy requirement increases up to 11-fold, whereas protein requirements increase much less (5 to 15%). For a given food, as intake increases to meet energy requirements, protein intake increases proportionally. Because of the disparity between the increase in need for energy and protein for exercise, as total dietary energy requirement increases, the percent of the ME as protein of the food can decrease. **Table 18-9** summarizes protein recommendations by exercise type.

Digestibility

DM digestibility of food is important to canine athletes for two reasons. First, exercise may be limited by a dog's ability to obtain sufficient amounts of nutrients (usually energy). Enhanced digestibility increases the maximum possible delivery of nutrients to tissues. Second, lower digestibility means greater fecal bulk, and therefore a greater handicap. Although increased animal size results in greater running efficiency, increased fecal weight creates a greater energetic cost of running with no benefit. Total DM digestibility of any food for canine athletes should exceed 80% (Downey et al, 1980; Lewis et al, 1987). Foods having a higher energy density are likely to have increased DM digestibility.

Antioxidants

There are at least two questions to consider when discussing antioxidants for working and sporting dogs: 1) do supplemental antioxidants provide a health benefit and 2) do they influence performance.

Exercise is associated with an increase in the rate of oxygen consumption. The extent of the increase depends on the intensity of the exercise. Even normal oxidative metabolism results in the production of highly reactive free radical molecules. Proportionate increases in free radical production appear to accompany exercise-associated increases in oxygen consumption (Hinchcliff et al, 2000). Aerobic, anaerobic and mixed exercise cause varying degrees of free radical production. Besides mitochondrial production of free radicals, such as with endurance exercise, anaerobic and mixed exercise result in ischemia reperfusion, acidosis and catecholamine oxidation that further contribute to oxidative stress. The body's typical adaptive response is increased mobilization of a variety of enzymatic and non-enzymatic antioxidant systems. However, with exercise these innate antioxidant capabilities are oftentimes overwhelmed, which leads to oxidative stress. The consequences of prolonged oxidative stress may contribute to and/or exacerbate a wide variety of degenerative diseases (Chapter 7). In human athletes, unchecked oxidative stress seems to be involved in chronic muscular fatigue and may lead to a condition called "overtraining" (Finaud et al, 2006). It is possible that canine athletes experience a similar phenomenon.

Considerable research into the use of supplemental antioxidants to augment the body's antioxidant capacity during exercise has been done in a variety of species. However, because of the complexity of the associated variables, many of the research results are equivocal making it challenging to apply the knowledge to practice (Finaud et al, 2006). These complexities include degree of training, positive effects of free radicals, doses of antioxidant supplements and the number of different antioxidant supplements used.

Oxidative stress can be mitigated to a degree through training. In marathon runners, free radicals generated during exercise up-regulated the expression of antioxidant enzyme systems (Gomez-Cabrera et al, 2006). Also, in other studies, endurance, anaerobic and mixed exercise training programs reduced post-exercise oxidative stress. The positive effects of training are seen in antioxidant enzyme systems in muscle, fat, plasma, liver and heart (Finaud et al, 2006; Aksoy et al, 2006). In one study in minimally trained dogs, the antioxidant mechanisms were insufficient to meet the antioxidant needs associated with repetitive endurance exercise (Hinchcliff et al, 2000). Not surprisingly, training matters. Many hunting dogs have a leisurely lifestyle for most of the year, associated with being the family pet. However, on the opening day of hunting season, they are expected to function at peak athletic and olfactory performance. Such dogs should have adequate levels of antioxidants in their food. Better yet, combine that recommendation with a preseason exercise-training program. It should be noted that free radicals appear to also have a physiologic function and total mitigation of reactive oxygen molecules can negatively affect certain types of exercise performance. In human subjects, free radicals have been shown to have a regulatory function at the vascular level, causing vasodilatation (Richardson et al, 2006). Excessive doses of antioxidants have been shown to impair muscle force production (Stone and Yang, 2006). When racing greyhounds were supplemented with high doses (1 g/day) of vitamin C, they ran slower (Marshall et al, 2002). Racing greyhounds also ran slower when supplemented with high doses of vitamin E (1,000 IU/day) but not lower doses (100 IU/day) (Hill et al, 2001).

Besides interfering with normal redox signaling, high doses of antioxidants, particularly of individual antioxidant supplements, can be counterproductive in a different way. Single antioxidant supplementation can have a pro-oxidant effect. For example, as part of its antioxidant function, vitamin E temporarily becomes a radical species known as the α-tocopherol radical. Normally, co-antioxidants, such as vitamin C, reduce the α-tocopherol radical back to α-tocopherol. If co-antioxidants are absent or decreased, the α-tocopherol radical can exhibit pro-oxidant activity (McNaulty et al, 2005). Antioxidant balance is important because supplementation with large amounts of a single antioxidant may change the balance to one of a pro-oxidative state. High doses of vitamin C and selenium may act as pro-oxidants (Atalay et al, 2006). Multi-nutrient antioxidant supplementation using lower doses is a better approach.

Commonly supplemented food-source antioxidants include vitamins E and C, β-carotene and other carotenoids, selenium and thiols. Fruits and vegetables are good sources of flavonoids, polyphenols and anthocyanidins. The following recommendations, however, will focus on vitamins E and C and selenium as antioxidant key nutritional factors because: 1) they are biologically important, 2) they act synergistically and 3) there is published information regarding safety and inclusion levels.

VITAMIN E

Vitamin E is the primary lipid-soluble antioxidant in plasma, erythrocytes and tissues (NRC, 2006). It is transported in plasma proteins and partitions into membranes and fat storage sites where it is one of the most effective antioxidants for protecting polyunsaturated fatty acids from oxidation. The minimum DM requirement for vitamin E for foods for adult dogs is 30 mg/kg (NRC, 2006). Research indicates that a higher level of vitamin E confers specific biologic benefits. In minimally trained sled dogs, 136 IU of vitamin E/kg was not enough to maintain normal vitamin E levels in plasma after three successive 58-km exercise runs (Hinchcliff et al, 2000). In another sled dog study, 400 IU vitamin E/day in conjunction with β-carotene and lutein resulted in increased plasma concentrations of antioxidants and decreased DNA and lipoprotein oxidation (Baskin et al, 2000). In a study that measured plasma vitamin E concentrations in racing-sled dogs during the 1998 Iditarod Race, dogs that had high pre-race vitamin E concentrations were almost twice as likely to finish the race (Piercy et al, 2000). These results could reflect a higher vitamin E intake and/or better fitness and a resultant higher anaerobic threshold. As noted above, unchecked oxidative stress can result in muscle fatigue. Endurance exercise in sled dogs results in considerable oxidative stress (Hinchcliff et al, 2000). Trained subjects present a higher vitamin E status whereas overreaching seems to decrease it (Finaud et al, 2006).

Based on antioxidant biomarker studies in non-exercising dogs, for improved antioxidant performance, dog foods should contain at least 500 IU/kg of DM vitamin E (Jewell et al, 2000). For a 25-kg dog engaged in moderate exercise for several hours/day, this would amount to approximately 250 IU/day. Compared to the amounts in the studies mentioned above, this is not an excessive amount.

VITAMIN C

Vitamin C is the most powerful reducing agent available to cells. As mentioned above, it is an important co-antioxidant because it regenerates oxidized vitamin E. Besides regenerating vitamin E, vitamin C also: 1) regenerates glutathione and flavonoids, 2) quenches free radicals both intra- and extracellularly, 3) protects against free radical-mediated protein inactivation associated with oxidative bursts of neutrophils, 4) maintains transition metals in reduced form and 5) may quench free radical intermediates of carcinogen metabolism.

Dogs can synthesize amounts of vitamin C required for maintenance (Innes, 1931; Naismith, 1958; Chatterjee et al, 1975) and they can rapidly absorb supplemental vitamin C (Wang et al, 2001). However, in-vitro studies indicated that dogs (and cats) have from one-quarter to one-tenth the ability to synthesize vitamin C as other mammals (Chatterjee et al, 1975). Whether or not this translates to a reduced ability in vivo is unknown.

Studies in exercising people and horses have shown improvements in indicators of oxidative stress associated with exercise

Box 18-6. Vitamins, Minerals and Exercise.

Although vitamins and minerals are obviously important for exercise, it is unclear if exercise alters the requirements for these nutrients. Additionally, some vitamins and minerals are believed to be beneficial as ergogenic aids. Unfortunately, little well controlled research has been conducted in this area and current results are conflicting.

Exercise-induced increases in demand have been suggested for nearly all of the B-complex vitamins. Many of these compounds are used as cofactors in key enzymes of energy-generating pathways; others function in tissue synthesis and repair initiated by exercise. Likewise, the demand for vitamin C has been postulated to increase due to its role in L-carnitine and collagen synthesis and its antioxidant functions. Exercise may also hasten the excretion of water-soluble vitamins because exercise increases total body water turnover. Five to 10 times maintenance levels of the water-soluble vitamins have been safely fed to working dogs.

High consumption of polyunsaturated fatty acids (PUFA) and increased oxygen metabolism may also increase a working or sporting dog's risk for oxidative damage of cell membranes. Such damage may induce myodystrophy and decrease endurance. Increased intake of antioxidants is recommended for prophylaxis. At present, there is no evidence to indicate that exercise increases dietary requirements for vitamins D and K.

Metabolic acidosis induced by lactic acidosis associated with strenuous work may increase excretion of calcium, magnesium and potassium. Foods containing low levels of magnesium (but at levels above the minimum Association of American Feed Control Official's allowance) resulted in clinical signs of magnesium deficiency in greyhound dogs. These signs were alleviated when foods containing magnesium at 0.12% of the dry matter (DM) were fed.

Canine athletes fed high-fat foods or those whose food is supplemented with meat (as is common with greyhounds and sled dogs) may require additional calcium. The high level of fat in performance foods enhances the formation of insoluble calcium soaps, thus rendering a portion of the ingested calcium unavailable. Additionally, red meat is rich in phosphorus and nearly devoid of calcium. Meat supplementation may thus require calcium supplementation to maintain a normal calcium content and calcium-phosphorus ratio in the diet. Dietary calcium levels of 1.2 to 2.0% of a food's DM have been successfully fed to working dogs. Very high-fat foods with lower calcium concentrations may be deficient in available calcium. Excessive calcium supplementation may also predispose a dog to zinc deficiency by inhibiting absorption of this nutrient (Chapter 32).

The requirement for iron is also thought to increase with exercise. Commercial performance foods and foods supplemented with substantial quantities of red meat should easily meet this increased demand. In such instances, iron supplementation is contraindicated because it may irritate the lower gastrointestinal tract and predispose canine athletes to develop bloody diarrhea.

Large doses of vitamins and minerals individually or in combination have not been demonstrated to increase the physical capabilities of human or canine athletes. Dietary intake of these nutrients should be aimed at meeting increased physiologic requirements rather than attempting to produce an unproved pharmacologic enhancement of performance.

Several considerations must be weighed when determining the optimal vitamin and mineral content of a performance food. One must estimate the availability and the tolerance levels of these nutrients as well as possible nutrient interactions. For example, iron and zinc must be present in proper proportions; an excess of one may lead to a relative deficiency of the other because they share a common mechanism of absorption. Similarly, a disproportionate supplementation of one fat-soluble vitamin may inhibit absorption of the others. The concentrations and types of energy-producing nutrients in the food can also influence vitamin and mineral requirements. As mentioned, PUFA intake can alter the demand for vitamin E and selenium.

Although dogs have no known dietary vitamin C and L-carnitine requirement, some researchers argue that canine athletes may be unable to synthesize adequate quantities of these nutrients to meet the metabolic demands of extremely hard work. It is also unclear whether requirements for vitamins and minerals increase in proportion to caloric intake or whether they approach an asymptote. Further research is needed to resolve these issues.

Those wishing to supplement with vitamins and minerals are advised to do so carefully. Such supplementation should only be undertaken with knowledge of nutrient availability, interactions and tolerance levels because dietary overcompensation of these nutrients may be as detrimental to performance as dietary deficiencies. One report noted that a mineral mixture solution containing potassium, phosphorus, sodium, magnesium, copper and iron given free-choice to exercising dogs caused diarrhea.

The Bibliography for **Box 18-6** can be found at www.markmorris.org.

as a result of vitamin C supplementation (Goldfarb et al, 2005; White et al, 2001). However, as mentioned above, a study in greyhounds that were supplemented with high doses of vitamin C resulted in slower racing times. As mentioned previously, multi-nutrient antioxidant supplementation using lower doses is a better approach than using high doses of a single antioxidant supplement. To augment antioxidant protection, in conjunction with recommended levels of vitamin E above, improved antioxidant performance foods for working and sporting dogs should contain between 150 to 250 mg of vitamin C/kg (DM). The upper end of this range would be about 70 to 100 mg/day for a 30-kg dog. This is about 7 to 10% of the amount (1 g/day) that slowed race times in the greyhound study described above.

SELENIUM

Glutathione-peroxidase is a selenium-containing antioxidant enzyme that defends tissues against oxidative stress by catalyzing the reduction of H_2O_2 and organic hydroperoxides and by sparing vitamin E. In people, following eccentric exercise-

Box 18-7. Electrolytes and Exercise.

Electrolytes are integral components of nearly all chemical reactions and transmembrane transport systems. About one-third of basal energy requirement is expended to maintain electrolyte concentration gradients across cellular membranes. The narrow range within which these concentrations are regulated and the high cost of achieving this regulation is evidence of their biologic significance. The electrolytes sodium, potassium and chloride are involved in control of fluid balance, maintenance of normal muscle and nerve excitability and acid-base status.

The electrolytes (primarily sodium) play a major role in regulation of total body water. Hyperosmolality stimulates thirst and causes the kidneys to conserve water. In cases of electrolyte depletion, aldosterone may reduce renal losses by stimulating tubular reabsorption of sodium and water. Sodium depletion occurs commonly in horses, people and other mammals that sweat; however, exercise-related loss of sodium may also be significant in canine athletes. The amount of sodium lost via saliva in exercising dogs depends on salivary flow rate. As salivary flow increases, the osmotic concentration of the initially hypotonic saliva increases; saliva approaches isotonicity with plasma at maximum flow rates. Warm or humid conditions that elicit increased salivary flow rates during exercise may also significantly increase sodium, bicarbonate and chloride losses.

Abnormal electrolyte concentrations impair physical performance by altering membrane potentials across muscle and nerve cells, and altering the functions of catalytic and contractile proteins. These changes hinder performance by diminishing the rate of energy and force generation. They also interfere with heat dissipation, which is particularly impaired by increases in plasma osmolarity.

Either water or an electrolyte solution may be used to maintain or replace fluid-electrolyte losses during and after exercise. Electrolyte solutions, while popular, are of limited value for most dogs eating a balanced food. Additionally, there is much debate about the proper concentration of these solutions. Hypertonic and even isotonic solutions administered orally may not return postexercise plasma osmolarity to normal. These solutions may encourage water transfer into cells if they are more hypertonic than the fluid of the interstitial spaces. Such fluids may lead to gastrointestinal cramping, vomiting and diarrhea and thus exacerbate dehydration. Anecdotally, even isotonic solutions administered before exercise have been associated with snow "dipping" or ingesting snow during sled-dog races. This phenomenon may be caused by the effect of the electrolyte solution on plasma osmolarity and thus thirst. Snow dipping is considered undesirable in racing dogs because it disturbs the rhythm and speed of the team.

Proponents of electrolyte supplementation note that in proper concentrations, such solutions increase fluid palatability and the rate of fluid absorption from the gut. Some argue these solutions may help maintain plasma volume during exercise and may aid in its restoration in the postexercise period. Because diarrhea is a common disorder among working dogs, the use of electrolyte replacement solutions may play a role in the clinical management of these cases.

Clearly, more research is needed before recommendations can confidently be given about the administration of electrolyte solutions to canine athletes before, during and after exercise. Under nearly all conditions, it is more important to replace water losses. Under conditions where electrolyte administration is deemed beneficial, it is safer to err on the side of hypotonic rather than hypertonic oral supplementation.

The Bibliography for **Box 18-7** can be found at www.markmorris.org.

induced muscle injury, suboptimal selenium status worsens muscle functional decrements (Milias et al, 2006). The minimum requirement for selenium in foods for dogs is 0.10 mg/kg (DM) (Wedekind et al, 2002). Animal studies and clinical intervention trials in people have shown selenium to be anticarcinogenic at much higher levels (five to 10 times) than the human recommended allowance or minimal requirement (Combs, 2001; Neve, 2002). Several mechanisms have been proposed for this effect, including enhanced antioxidant activity via glutathione peroxidase (Neve, 2002). Therefore, for increased antioxidant benefits, the recommended range of selenium for dog foods is 0.5 to 1.3 mg/kg (DM). There are no data to base a safe upper limit of selenium for dogs or cats, but for regulatory purposes, a maximum standard of 2.0 mg/kg (DM) has been set for dog foods in the United States (AAFCO, 2007).

Other Nutritional Factors

Vitamins, minerals and electrolytes play important roles in maintaining homeostasis and chemical reactions during exercise (**Boxes 18-6** and **18-7**). However, they are of secondary concern when feeding canine athletes and are found in adequate amounts in most commercial foods. Likewise, the acid-base composition of the food and base loading may also affect performance (**Box 18-8**); however, these effects are poorly understood in canine athletes. Deficiencies of vitamin A, iodine and zinc have been associated with disturbances of smell in people (Mattes, 1999) but are not of practical concern in dogs being fed commercial foods.

FEEDING PLAN

The feeding plan should be formulated based on realistic and quantifiable nutritional objectives after the patient, food and feeding method have been assessed. The feeding plan guides the selection of foods and feeding methods.

Assess and Select the Food

Although the working or sporting dog's nutritional needs could conceivably be met by many different dietary approaches, all foods for canine athletes (performance foods) should share a few important characteristics. First, the food should be calori-

Box 18-8. Acid-Base Balance and Exercise.

Muscle contraction produces metabolic acid (CO_2 and/or lactate), which decreases the intracellular pH of muscles. Changes in intracellular pH can affect the function of muscle enzymes responsible for ATP generation and contraction. The mechanisms that act to blunt the detrimental effects of acid production within muscles include: 1) intracellular buffering and 2) removal of acids by the bloodstream.

In equine athletes, two approaches have been used to help counteract exercise-induced acidosis to improve athletic performance. The first is to base load the horse via stomach tube several hours before exercise. Sodium bicarbonate in water is the base used most often. This solution is frequently called a "milkshake" due to its milky white appearance. This approach can effectively alter resting acid-base status, but hasn't been proven to alter performance. The second approach is to alter the ionic composition of food to change the acid-base status of the animal. Investigators have been able to alter resting acid-base status by altering the dietary cation-anion balance of the food, but again it is unclear if this alteration affects performance. Alteration of acid-base status by dietary or supplementation means has not been investigated extensively in dogs; however, the basic principles investigated in horses should apply to dogs.

The Bibliography for **Box 18-8** can be found at www.markmorris.org.

cally dense so that canine athletes can consume enough food to meet their energy requirements. Second, the food must be acceptable and highly digestible. DM digestibility should exceed 80% (Downey et al, 1980; Lewis et al, 1987). High digestibility reduces fecal bulk and fecal water loss and may decrease the risk of developing stress diarrhea (Houpt, 1984; Downey et al, 1980). Finally, the food should be practical. Factors such as the cost of the food, the form of the food, the environment in which the food is stored and fed and the number of dogs being fed are all important considerations. What is practical for a single hunting dog at home may not be practical for a team of sled dogs hundreds of miles from civilization, agility dogs at an out-of-town competition or racing greyhounds at a track.

Because the greatest nutritional demand of exercise is for energy, foods for canine athletes must provide sufficient kcal from the right sources. Increasing the fat content of the food usually enhances energy density. The appropriate fat content is dictated by energy need and exercise intensity. Dogs participating in short-duration, maximal exercise may benefit from lower fat, higher carbohydrate foods.

Assessment of the food includes: 1) physical evaluation of the food, 2) evaluation of the product label for commercial foods and 3) evaluation of the food's nutritional content relative to the animal's needs (key nutritional factors) (Chapter 1).

Working and sporting dogs are fed a wide variety of foods and supplements. When assessing the overall ration, it is important to assess all foods and supplements fed. The nutrient profile of the total daily ration should be evaluated for the key nutritional factors based on the type and amount of exercise performed by each dog.

Most intermediate athletes are fed commercial foods, whereas many elite sprint and endurance athletes (racing dogs) are fed homemade foods or more commonly a mixture of commercial food and other ingredients. The use of supplements is prevalent with working and sporting dogs of all types.

Comparing the nutritional content of the current food to the key nutritional factors allows decisions to be made about the adequacy of the food for individual dogs. If the current food is appropriate (key nutritional factors in balance with the dog's needs) then that food can continue to be fed. If discrepancies exist between the key nutritional factors for the dog and the content of the food, the food should be changed or "balanced" to meet the dog's needs.

Commercial Foods

Table 18-12 lists the key nutritional factors for working and sporting dogs and compares them to the key nutritional factor content of selected commercial foods formulated for these dogs. For those commercial foods not found in **Table 18-12**, minimum fat and protein levels are listed in the guaranteed or typical analysis on the pet food label. (See Chapter 1 for limitations of this information.) The carbohydrate portion of a food can also be estimated as described above under "Carbohydrates" in the "Key Nutritional Factors" section or in Chapter 5. Digestibility information is usually only available from the manufacturer. The energy density of most commercial foods is not high enough for dogs engaged in true endurance activity. **Table 18-12** provides energy density information for commercial foods supplemented with vegetable oil in order to meet the energy density needs for endurance athletes.

Homemade Foods

Homemade foods can be very complicated mixtures of many ingredients. Chapter 10 discusses assessment of homemade foods in detail. Fortunately, most recipes for homemade foods for working and sporting dogs use a commercial dry dog food as a base. Many racing greyhound food regimens contain dry dog food mixed with either raw or cooked meat, water, vitamin-mineral supplements and a variety of other ingredients. Likewise, many sled-dog mushers mix animal fat or both meat and fat with dry dog food and other ingredients. If the commercial dry food constitutes 50 to 75% of the mixture on a weight basis and most of the added ingredients are wet ingredients or fat, it is unlikely that vitamin and mineral deficiencies will occur.

Because many elite canine athletes (racing greyhounds and sled dogs) are fed homemade foods containing meat and animal by-products of variable quality, the safety of these foods should always be evaluated. Some raw meat sources contain abundant bacteria and bacterial toxins (Case 11-1). Raw foods may pose a health hazard for people who care for these dogs and for the dogs themselves. Chapter 11 discusses food safety.

Supplements

Feeding glucose solutions minimizes the exercise-associated decline in blood glucose, promotes more rapid repletion of muscle glycogen postexercise and improves thermoregulation. However, when such solutions are fed is important. Glucose solutions (from 1.5- to as much as 5-g glucose/kg body weight) have been used (Kruk et al, 1987; Reynolds et al, 1997; Wakshlag et al, 2002; NRC, 2006). As an option to a glucose solution, an anecdotal report recommends using up to one 8-oz. measuring cup of sucrose per quart of water (~240 g/l).[f] To receive an amount of sucrose equal to the upper end of the previously recommended range for glucose (5 g/kg body weight), a 35-kg dog would have to ingest approximately three-fourths of a quart of the sucrose-water solution.

Several commercial products are available to support energy levels during exercise. These products are available as powders to be added to drinking water (so called "canine sports drinks") or dry snacks. They can be found online or at pet or sporting goods stores. Small amounts of a high-carbohydrate low-fat commercial dog food could also be used for this purpose.

Vegetable oils (plant-source edible oils, e.g., corn oil and soybean oil) can be used to increase the unsaturated fatty acid content of a commercial food for improving olfaction (see "Fat" under Key Nutritional Factors discussion) and for increasing the energy density of a commercial food. If corn oil is added to dry commercial foods to increase the fat and/or unsaturated fatty acid content, 1 tablespoon of corn oil for approximately each pound of dry food will increase the overall fat content by about three to four percentage points. For example, if two tablespoons of corn oil are added to one pound of dry food that contains 20% fat, the resultant mixture of food and corn oil will contain about 27% fat and would have increased levels of unsaturated fatty acids. Corn and vegetable oils provide about 125 kcal ME/tablespoon (14 g). **Table 18-12** provides energy density information for commercial foods. The foods listed would need to be supplemented with vegetable oil to increase energy density to a level to support needs for dogs engaged in endurance activity. Dogs can tolerate high levels of dietary fat if the fat is gradually introduced and an adequate intake of non-fat nutrients is maintained. Steatorrhea and a decrease in food palatability are indicators that the fat intake of a food has exceeded an individual dog's fat tolerance.

Assess and Determine the Feeding Method

Performance can be influenced by the composition of the food and how it is fed. It is possible to feed the right food in the wrong way and vice versa. Items to be assessed should include amount fed, frequency of feeding and timing of meals in relation to exercise, food adaptation, access to water and the use of supplements. All of these factors should be matched to the individual athlete and the type of exercise performed (intensity, duration, frequency and season). If the current feeding method matches the individual's needs based on the assessment, no changes are necessary. Changes should be made if the assessment reveals discrepancies in the feeding method. If the animal is in appropriate body condition and hydration status, it is likely that the amount of food and water consumed is appropriate.

The amount of a new food to feed can be estimated several ways. Feeding guidelines from the manufacturer and those on pet food labels are seldom correct for active working and sporting dogs. Energy needs and food doses usually must be calculated. If the amount of the previous food was correct (i.e., appropriate body condition was maintained) and the energy density of the food is known, simply feed the same amount of the new food to supply the same energy intake. If this method isn't feasible, the food dose should be calculated based on the dog's needs as shown above. In all cases, the dog should be assessed frequently and adjustments should be made to maintain correct body condition.

Timing of feeding and timing of food changes are important for working and sporting dogs. Timing of feeding in relation to exercise influences hormonal status, substrate availability and performance. When changing foods, adequate time must be allowed for the dog to adapt to the new food type to take full advantage of its nutrient profile.

Amount to Feed

An increase in energy requirement is the hallmark of exercise. The wide variation in the intensity and duration of exercise and therefore energy requirement of different types of working and sporting dogs emphasizes the need for food dose calculations. The basics of energy requirement and food dose calculation are covered in Chapter 1.

The dog's DER is the product of its RER and a factor that accounts for activity. For the average neutered, minimally active adult dog, DER is 1.2 to 1.4 RER (Chapters 1 and 13). DER for exercising dogs has a wide range of values from 1.6 x RER to 11 x RER, depending on the intensity and duration of exercise. The DER range for sprint dogs is 1.6 to 2 x RER, for intermediate (mixed) type activity the DER range is 2 to 5 x RER, for endurance-type activity the DER is more than 5 x RER. As discussed earlier, the caloric cost of running is determined by the size of the animal (body weight), weight carried or pulled and distance traveled.

Energy is also used to maintain body temperature. Extreme arctic and tropical temperatures increase a dog's RER (Lewis et al, 1987; Young et al, 1959). Dogs working in cold climates may require less energy than the sum of those determined for work and thermoregulation because exercise generates significant quantities of heat. RER for nonworking dogs in hot environments increases only marginally as a result of increased work of the respiratory muscles (panting) (Chapter 13). Working dogs already have increased respiratory rates, thus, additional energy for thermoregulation during exercise in hot climates should be negligible. Total DER is the sum of the needs for rest (RER), exercise (EER) and thermoregulation (ET) (i.e., DER for canine athletes = RER + EER + ET).

Most working dogs expending fewer kcal than 3 x RER can adequately fulfill their energy needs by eating a commercial

Table 18-12. Levels of key nutritional factors (DM) in selected dry commercial foods used for working and sporting dogs compared to recommended key nutritional factor values.*

Recommended levels for sprint activity

Foods	Energy density (kcal/cup)**	Energy density (kcal ME/g)***	Fat (%)	Carbohydrate (%)	Protein (%)	Vitamin E (IU/kg)	Vitamin C (mg/kg)	Selenium (mg/kg)
	-	3.5-4.0	8-10	55-65	22-28	≥500	150-250	0.5-1.3
Hill's Science Diet Adult Lamb Meal & Rice Recipe	364	4.0	16.0	52.9	23.0	582	174	0.54
Hill's Science Diet Adult Active	560	5.0	27.2	35.4	29.8	556	152	0.54
Iams Eukanuba Premium Performance Sporting Dog Food	431	4.8	22.2	33.8	33.3	na	na	na
Iams Proactive Health Lamb Meal & Rice Formula	330	4.0	14.2	46.3	25.1	123	52	0.37
Nutro Natural Choice High Energy	396	4.3	23.1	32.4	34.1	na	66	0.33
Nutro Natural Choice Lamb Meal & Rice Formula	342	3.8	14.3	50.0	24.2	220	66	0.77
Pedigree Small Crunchy Bites Dog Food	290	3.8	13.7	48.1	26.0	256	80	na
Purina Dog Chow	430	4.2	11.4	51.9	23.9	144	na	0.64
Purina Pro Plan Performance Formula	493	4.8	23.2	31.3	35.0	na	na	na
Royal Canin Energy 4800	591	5.2	33.3	15.8	35.6	856	389	0.28
Royal Canin Maxi German Shepherd 24	314	4.5	21.2	37.0	26.8	670	na	0.22
Royal Canin Maxi Golden Retriever 25	412	4.1	14.7	38.7	27.5	769	na	0.20
Royal Canin Maxi Labrador Retriever 30	321	4.1	14.3	35.3	33.0	659	na	0.18
Royal Canin Medium Active Special 25	349	4.6	18.9	na	27.8	667	333	0.16

Recommended levels for intermediate activity (low/moderate duration and frequency)

Foods	Energy density (kcal/cup)**	Energy density (kcal ME/g)***	Fat (%)	Carbohydrate (%)	Protein (%)	Vitamin E (IU/kg)	Vitamin C (mg/kg)	Selenium (mg/kg)
	-	4.0-5.0	15-30 (>60% unsaturated)†	30-55	22-32	≥500	150-250	0.5-1.3
Hill's Science Diet Adult Lamb Meal & Rice Recipe	364	4.0	16.0 (na)	52.9	23.0	582	174	0.54
Hill's Science Diet Adult Active	560	5.0	27.2 (64% unsaturated)	35.4	29.8	556	152	0.54
Iams Eukanuba Premium Performance Sporting Dog Food	431	4.8	22.2 (na)	33.8	33.3	na	na	na
Iams Proactive Health Lamb Meal & Rice Formula	330	4.0	14.2 (na)	46.3	25.1	123	52	0.37
Nutro Natural Choice High Energy	396	4.3	23.1 (na)	32.4	34.1	na	66	0.33
Nutro Natural Choice Lamb Meal & Rice Formula	342	3.8	14.3 (na)	50.0	24.2	220	66	0.77
Pedigree Small Crunchy Bites Dog Food	290	3.8	13.7 (na)	48.1	26.0	256	80	na
Purina Dog Chow	430	4.2	11.4 (na)	51.9	23.9	144	na	0.64
Purina Pro Plan Performance Formula	493	4.8	23.2 (na)	31.3	35.0	na	na	na
Royal Canin Energy 4800	591	5.2	33.3 (na)	15.8	35.6	856	389	0.28
Royal Canin Maxi German Shepherd 24	314	4.5	21.2 (na)	37.0	26.8	670	na	0.22
Royal Canin Maxi Golden Retriever 25	412	4.1	14.7 (na)	38.7	27.5	769	na	0.20
Royal Canin Maxi Labrador Retriever 30	321	4.1	14.3 (na)	35.3	33.0	659	na	0.18
Royal Canin Medium Active Special 25	349	4.6	18.9 (na)	na	27.8	667	333	0.16

food formulated for performance (**Table 18-12**). These foods are palatable, complete/balanced and convenient in most situations. Working and sporting dogs exercising in extremely warm or extremely cold environments or those working for several hours a day for several consecutive days may expend more calories than 3 x RER. DM intake is limited to about 3.5% of body weight under most physiologic conditions.[C] A performance food containing these amounts (30% DM protein, 20% DM

Recommended levels for intermediate activity (high duration and frequency)

Foods	Energy density (kcal/cup)**	Energy density (kcal ME/g)***	Fat (%)	Carbohydrate (%)	Protein (%)	Vitamin E (IU/kg)	Vitamin C (mg/kg)	Selenium (mg/kg)
Recommended	**-**	**4.5-5.5**	**25-40 (>60% unsaturated)†**	**30-35**	**22-32**	**≥500**	**150-250**	**0.5-1.3**
Hill's Science Diet Adult Active	560	5.0	27.2 (64% unsaturated)	35.4	29.8	556	152	0.54
Iams Eukanuba Premium Performance Sporting Dog Food	431	4.8	22.2 (na)	33.8	33.3	na	na	na
Iams Proactive Health Lamb Meal & Rice Formula	330	4.0	14.2 (na)	46.3	25.1	123	52	0.37
Nutro Natural Choice High Energy	396	4.3	23.1 (na)	32.4	34.1	na	66	0.33
Nutro Natural Choice Lamb Meal & Rice Formula	342	3.8	14.3 (na)	50.0	24.2	220	66	0.77
Pedigree Small Crunchy Bites Dog Food	290	3.8	13.7 (na)	48.1	26.0	256	80	na
Purina Dog Chow	430	4.2	11.4 (na)	51.9	23.9	144	na	0.64
Purina Pro Plan Performance Formula	493	4.8	23.2 (na)	31.3	35.0	na	na	na
Royal Canin Energy 4800	591	5.2	33.3 (na)	15.8	35.6	856	389	0.28
Royal Canin Maxi German Shepherd 24	314	4.5	21.2 (na)	37.0	26.8	670	na	0.22
Royal Canin Maxi Golden Retriever 25	412	4.1	14.7 (na)	38.7	27.5	769	na	0.20
Royal Canin Maxi Labrador Retriever 30	321	4.1	14.3 (na)	35.3	33.0	659	na	0.18
Royal Canin Medium Active Special 25	349	4.6	18.9 (na)	na	27.8	667	333	0.16

Recommended levels for endurance activity

Foods	Energy density (kcal/cup)**	Energy density (kcal ME/g)***	Fat (%)	Carbohydrate (%)	Protein (%)	Vitamin E (IU/kg)	Vitamin C (mg/kg)	Selenium (mg/kg)
Recommended	**-**	**>6**	**>50††**	**<15**	**28-34**	**≥500**	**150-250**	**0.5-1.3**
Hill's Science Diet Adult Active	560	5.0	27.2	35.4	29.8	556	152	0.54
Iams Eukanuba Premium Performance Sporting Dog Food	431	4.8	22.2	33.8	33.3	na	na	na
Nutro Natural Choice High Energy	396	4.3	23.1	32.4	34.1	na	66	0.33
Purina Pro Plan Performance Formula	493	4.8	23.2	31.3	35	na	na	na
Royal Canin Energy 4800	591	5.2	33.3	15.8	35.6	856	389	0.28

Key: DM = dry matter, ME = metabolizable energy, na = not available from manufacturer.
*This table lists selected products for which manufacturers' published information is available. **Table 18-1** provides examples of types of activities conducted by working and sporting dogs.
**Energy density values are listed on an as-fed basis and are useful for determining the amount to feed; cup = 8-oz. measuring cup. To convert to kJ, multiply kcal x 4.184.
***Foods higher in energy density are generally more digestible.
†For improved olfaction, fat sources should provide >60% total unsaturated fatty acids (**Table 18-11**).
††To increase fat content and energy density, adding two tablespoons of vegetable oil per pound (454 g) of food would increase fat content by approximately 6 percentage points; one tablespoonful of vegetable oil = 125 kcal ME; adding vegetable oil to dry commercial foods intended to support endurance activity is recommended.

fat, 40% DM carbohydrate and >80% DM digestibility) provides a maximum of 5 x RER for a 25-kg dog.

Because true endurance athletes have a DER greater than 5 x RER, providing sufficient dietary energy becomes the focus of feeding these athletes. Long-distance sled-dog drivers frequently encounter situations in which their 25- to 30-kg dogs require 6,000 to 10,000 kcal/day (25 to 42 MJ/day) (7 to 11 x RER). Under these extreme circumstances, dogs are fed 1,500

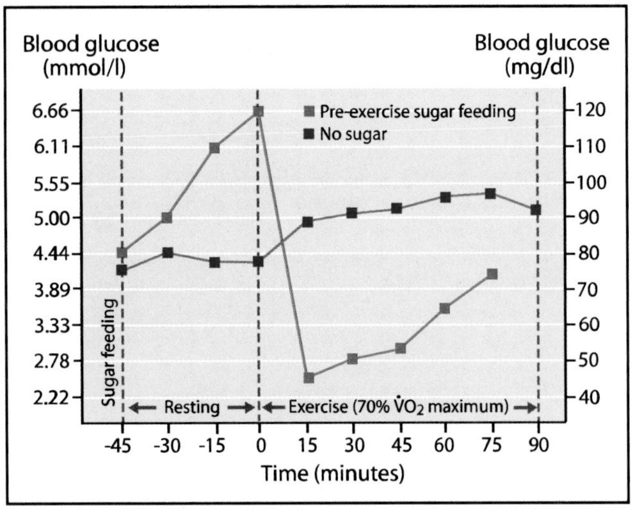

Figure 18-5. Differences in blood glucose concentrations between people exercising on a bicycle ergometer following administration of a glucose drink or placebo. (Adapted from Costill DL, Miller JM. Nutrition for endurance sport: Carbohydrate and fluid balance. International Journal of Sports Medicine 1980; 1: 2-14.)

to 2,500 kcal (6 to 11 MJ) of a dry commercial food in an attempt to fulfill protein, carbohydrate, vitamin and mineral requirements. Fulfilling the rest of the dog's DM intake with fat or fatty meat then maximizes energy intake. Strategies that maximize fat intake have been successfully used in virtually all of the recent Iditarod, Quest and Alpirod victories and in sled-dog expeditions to both poles.[d,e,g,h] These extremely high-fat foods, which derive up to 80% of their kcal from lipid sources, should be fed only to dogs previously acclimated to high-fat intake (i.e., 30 to 60% fat kcal), through feeding and training. Also, there may be a limited amount of time that dogs can be maintained on such a food or at such a level of stress.

Another strategy used by sled-dog mushers is to feed their dogs so they begin a long-distance race with 1.36 to 2.3 kg of extra adipose tissue. This gives the dogs a reserve to draw upon when caloric intake cannot meet energy expenditure. The additional insulation may also help dogs reduce heat loss during rest periods.

Feeding to Maintain Proper Body Condition

Food-dose calculations are based on average energy needs for a population of dogs and therefore will not be accurate for all dogs in various circumstances. Variation in individual metabolic rate, environmental temperature and exercise affect energy requirement and food dose. Repeated or continual body condition assessment is clearly the best clinical measure of energy balance. Body condition scoring is primarily a measure of body fat. Increasing body fat indicates positive energy balance; therefore, food dosage should be decreased. If body fat falls below optimal, energy balance is negative and food dosage should be increased to ensure adequate energy for maximal performance. One method of body condition scoring is presented in Chapter 1. A BCS of 2/5 to 3/5 is normal for most working and sporting dogs, with a bias towards the lean side of this range. Hunting dogs' BCS should be in the range of 2.5/5 to 3.5/5. Unfortunately, some of these dogs will have BCS greater than 3.5/5 because they are pet dogs and thus are more prone to being overweight.

Because fat in excess of what is needed for energy reserves during racing adds weight and may affect performance, many sight hounds are kept very lean (BCS 1/5 to 2/5). Most racing greyhounds normally have a BCS of 1/5. Being very lean may be an important physical characteristic for maximal sprint performance plus the fact that greyhounds have a very limited ability to use fat as an energy source for sprinting. Racing sled dogs should have a BCS of 2.5/5 (Reynolds et al, 1999).

When to Feed

To gain maximum benefit from a specific food, meals must be fed at the right time in relation to exercise and ample time must be allowed for metabolism to adapt to a new food type when changing foods.

After the amount to feed has been determined, an appropriate feeding schedule should be used. The temporal relationship between food intake and exercise greatly affects nutrient use. In one study, dogs fed within six hours of exercise developed a higher working body temperature than those fed 17 hours before exercise (Young et al, 1962). The elevated body temperatures in dogs fed closer to the onset of exercise may have been caused by heat released by the digestive process (specific dynamic action of food), and by vasodilatation of the splanchnic vessels. Such shunting may decrease cutaneous circulation and thus diminish heat dissipation. In performing the same task, dogs fed within six hours of exercise used more glucose and less fat than postabsorptive dogs (Young et al, 1962, 1959a; Young, 1959). Higher circulating insulin levels in the more recently fed dogs may cause this alteration in substrate use (Pate and Brunn, 1989). Because insulin tends to decrease free fatty acid mobilization from peripheral adipose depots, feeding too close to exercise may impair endurance by encouraging use and thus depletion of limited carbohydrate (glycogen) stores (Pate and Brunn, 1989).

The importance of the temporal relationship between feeding and exercise is seen in the poorly documented syndrome known as hunting dog hypoglycemia. The exact etiology of this syndrome is unknown. It is often associated with hyperactive, under-conditioned hunting dogs. Elevated ambient temperature has also been implicated as a risk factor (Lewis et al, 1987). Dogs experiencing this syndrome begin working normally and then develop signs of weakness and tremors that may progress to seizures and even death. Their purported inability to maintain normoglycemia has been attributed to inadequate glycogen mobilization (due to a lack of a glycogen debranching enzyme), excessive rates of glycogen mobilization or a combination of the two (Lewis et al, 1987). Feeding these dogs several hours (≥4) before the onset of exercise may help decrease insulin levels at the onset of exercise. Exercise also dampens the insulin response to ingested carbohydrate (Pate and Brunn, 1989). Providing exogenous carbohydrate via small amounts of food offered at the onset of, and periodically during, exercise may aid blood glucose homeostasis in these dogs (Lewis et al, 1987). It is best if this food is not high in fat (NRC, 2006). As mentioned above (Supplements), glucose or sucrose solutions can also be used (Kruk et al, 1987; Reynolds et al, 1997; Wakshlag et al, 2002; NRC, 2006). Such solutions can be given immediately before, during or after exercise and have been shown to minimize the exercise-associated decline in blood glucose, promote more rapid repletion of muscle glycogen postexercise and improve thermoregulation. The same timing of feeding is recommended for the several commercial products that are marketed to support energy levels during exercise (specific-purpose hydratable powders and dry snacks).

Figure 18-5 shows blood glucose results from a study that examined the effect of feeding time on blood glucose concentration during exercise in people riding a stationary bicycle (Costill and Miller, 1980). One group was given a drink containing glucose 45 minutes before the onset of exercise, whereas the other group received a placebo drink. Blood glucose levels remained constant in the non-fed group, whereas people ingesting the glucose drink had a normal postprandial increase in blood glucose followed by a severe drop at the onset of exercise.

Feeding long before exercise (more than four hours) may also aid endurance by allowing the dog to evacuate its bowels before it begins work. This decreases the weight carried by the dog and may decrease its risk of developing stress diarrhea. Although the cause of loose stools postexercise has not been determined, some researchers have attributed it to the presence of stool in the colon at the onset of exercise.[h] As with pre-exercise feedings, the timing of postexercise meals also influences nutrient use. Glycogen synthesis postexercise occurs much more rapidly in human athletes given exogenous substrates within 30 minutes to two hours postexercise. Feeding within this time frame may aid repletion of glycogen stores in athletes who must perform strenuous exercise on several consecutive days.

The practical application of the above information is feed: 1) more than four hours before exercise, 2) within two hours after exercise and 3) small amounts of food during exercise. Feeding must be done during exercise or during short breaks. Feeding a hunting dog that has hypoglycemic tendencies at the beginning of a 45-minute lunch break may contribute to exercise-induced hypoglycemia (**Figure 18-5**).

Because large volumes of urine represent additional weight and a possible time handicap for racing dogs, many handlers will not water an animal closer than two hours before a competition. The dog is then confined for one and one-half to two hours after drinking and will usually empty its bladder upon being released from the cage. Water should be offered as soon as is practicably possible after exercise. Cooler fluids seem to be absorbed most rapidly (Bucci, 1993). Canine athletes may become significantly dehydrated after prolonged exercise and under relatively warm or humid conditions. Attempts should not be made to replace the entire fluid deficit orally or at once. Gradual oral replacement can be supplemented with subcutaneous (or in severe cases intravenous) isotonic solutions. Body temperature should be monitored because dehydrated animals are less capable of regulating this parameter (Greenleaf et al, 1976).

Table 18-13. Feeding plan summary for working and sporting dogs.

Sprint activity
1. Feed a food with the appropriate amounts of key nutritional factors for this type of activity (**Table 18-12**).
2. Feed the right amount of food (DER = 1.6 to 2 x RER).
3. Check body condition frequently to assess energy balance and food dose.
4. Time meals and snacks correctly. Provide food or snack >four hours before activity; offer high-carbohydrate snack within 30 minutes after racing to enhance glycogen repletion.
5. Allow free access to water except just before racing.
6. Monitor hydration status frequently.

Intermediate activity (working/hunting)
1. Feed a food with the appropriate amounts of key nutritional factors for this type of activity (**Table 18-12**).
2. Feed the right amount of food. The food dose will be highly variable depending on duration and frequency of exercise (DER = 2 to 5 x RER) and should be calculated after assessing the amount of exercise performed.
3. Check body condition frequently to assess energy balance and food dose.
4. Time meals and snacks correctly. Feed after exercise or >four hours before exercise. Snacks should be given during exercise or at the end of breaks <15 minutes before resuming exercise.
5. Allow free access to water.
6. Monitor hydration status frequently.

Intermediate athletes (training)
1. Feed the same as for work (See above).
2. Allow adequate time to adapt to new food (>six weeks) before seasonal work.
3. Begin training and new food at least six weeks before seasonal work begins.
4. Allow free access to water.

Intermediate athletes (idle)
1. Feed as typical adult dog (Chapter 13).
2. Feed a performance food (smaller amount) or typical adult maintenance food as needed to maintain optimal body condition.
3. Allow free access to water.

Endurance athletes
1. Feed a food with the appropriate amounts of key nutritional factors for this type of activity (**Table 18-12**).
2. Feed the right amount of food. The food dose will be highly variable depending on duration and frequency of exercise (DER = 5 to 11 x RER) and should be calculated after assessing amount of exercise performed.
3. Check body condition frequently to assess energy balance and food dose.
4. Time meals and snacks correctly. Feed after exercise or >four hours before exercise. If snacks are used they should be given during or after exercise.
5. Allow free access to water.
6. Monitor hydration status frequently.

Key: DER = daily energy requirement, RER = resting energy requirement.

Table 18-13 summarizes the feeding plans for sprint-, intermediate- and endurance-type activities.

Food Adaptation

Dogs require some time to adapt to a new food whenever a dietary change is made. When dramatic changes in proportion of fat and carbohydrate are made, GI and metabolic adaptations occur. The GI adjustments usually happen in a few days provided the transition to the new food is gradual. The metabolic changes generally take more time. Muscle glycogen responds to feeding a high-carbohydrate food in a few days to a few weeks (Reynolds et al, 1995). Changes in muscle enzymes and oxidative capacity occur in response to high-fat rations in six to eight weeks. Allowing appropriate time for these adaptations to occur is especially important for seasonal athletes that may be fed a high-fat performance food only part of the year and a maintenance food the remainder of the year (Reynolds et al, 1994). Both training and dietary change should occur six weeks before exercise season (e.g., hunting season).

REASSESSMENT

After the feeding plan has been implemented, the dog should be monitored to evaluate the appropriateness of the feeding plan. This process is identical to the original assessment of the dog. Frequent physical examinations are important for early detection of injuries or illnesses. Daily monitoring of food consumption is an early indicator of problems. Frequent evaluation of stool quality may indicate how well the dog is tolerating the food. Weekly measurements of body condition and weight allow assessment of energy balance (i.e., whether food intake matches energy expenditure). Appropriate body condition is also important for optimal performance. Excess fat represents an unneeded handicap, whereas excessively lean dogs may not have sufficient energy stores.

Hydration status should be monitored frequently. Water plays a vital role in supporting cardiovascular function, transport of metabolic substrates and wastes and thermoregulation. Respiratory water losses can be large, particularly during lengthy exercise or under hot or cold environmental conditions.

Ultimately, assessing both exercise and olfactory performance is the best means of monitoring the feeding plan for working and sporting dogs. Generally, what is good for exercise performance is good for olfaction.

ACKNOWLEDGMENT

The authors and editors thank Dr. Arleigh J. Reynolds for his contribution to this chapter in the previous edition.

ENDNOTES

a. Publisher. Gun Dog Magazine, Stover Publishing Co, Des Moines, IA, USA. Personal communication. Summer 1997.
b. National Greyhound Association. Abilene, KS, USA. Personal communication. Summer 2007.
c. Burrows C. University of Florida, Gainesville, USA. Personal communication. Summer 1991.
d. Runyan J. Fairbanks, AK, USA. Alaska Dog Racing Association Annual Meeting. Personal communication. October 1994.
e. Steger W. International Arctic Project, Minneapolis, MN, USA. Personal communication. Summer 1994.
f. Gillette RL, Director, Veterinary Sports Medicine Program, College of Veterinary Medicine, Auburn University, Auburn AL, USA. Personal clinical and field work.
g. Champaigne C, Champaigne-Wright R. Fairbanks, AK, USA. Personal communication. October 1994.
h. Kronfeld D. University of Pennsylvania, Philadelphia, USA. Personal communication. Spring 1991.

REFERENCES

The references for **Chapter 18** can be found at www.markmorris.org.

CASE 18-1

Poor Performance in Racing Greyhounds

Philip W. Toll, DVM, MS
Hill's Science and Technology Center
Topeka, Kansas, USA

Patient Assessment

A litter of 14-month-old greyhound dogs (four males, two females) was examined for poor performance. The dogs were owned by a rural mail carrier who recently started a small greyhound farm. This litter of dogs was currently in training and was to begin racing within 60 days. The dogs were being schooled by racing 3/16 mile twice a week at a local training track; however, their performance was not up to the owner's expectations.

The physical examination of all dogs was normal except for a profound overbite (brachygnathia) in two males and one female. All dogs had body condition scores (BCS) of 1/5 and weighed approximately 30 kg each. Fecal examination (composite sample) was negative for parasites. Results of complete blood counts and serum biochemistry profiles from samples obtained from two of the dogs were normal.

Assess the Food and Feeding Method

The dogs were fed individually once daily. They received a ration composed of the following:

2 cups dry puppy food
1 lb raw meat (90% lean)
1 tbs bone meal
1 tbs dry vitamin supplement
1 cup milk

A trainer at a neighboring greyhound farm suggested feeding more meat and adding one-fourth cup vinegar to the ration.

Questions

1. What are the key nutritional factors and dietary recommendations for sprint athletes?
2. What additional information is necessary to fully assess the food and feeding method for these dogs?
3. What recommendations should be made about the food recipe for these dogs?
4. What is an appropriate feeding method?

Answers and Discussion

1. The key nutritional factors for sprint athletes include energy density, fat, digestible carbohydrate, protein, water and food digestibility. The ideal food or ration for sprint athletes should have an energy density between 3.5 to 4.0 kcal (15 to 17 kJ) metabolizable energy (ME)/g dry matter (DM) and contain these levels of nutrients: fat 8 to 10% DM, digestible carbohydrate 55 to 65% DM, protein 22 to 28% DM and DM digestibility greater than 80%. Water should be available at all times except just before a race.
2. Further assessment should include the following: 1) Nutrient levels in the final ration are needed. **Table 1** estimates the key nutrient levels for the current ration. 2) Amount of food fed to each dog and the timing of feeding in relationship to exercise (training). 3) Food safety issues must be addressed for animals that are fed a homemade ration containing raw meat. Greyhounds are frequently fed raw meat that may contain large numbers of bacteria and toxins. Information is needed about how the meat is stored, thawed and handled.
3. The current ration is a typical food for racing greyhounds. The recommendation from the other trainer to increase the meat fraction will increase the protein and fat content of the ration. Although most greyhound trainers believe that meat is essential for optimal performance, the protein and fat content of this recipe is already more than adequate. The appropriate recommendation is to increase the carbohydrate content of the ration by increasing the amount of a balanced commercial dry dog food. This food should be a commercial dry food formulated for adult dogs (lower in fat and protein and higher in carbohydrate than the puppy food). Vitamin and micronutrient deficiencies are unlikely to occur if a balanced commercial dry food makes up at least 50% of the recipe on an as fed weight basis. Cooking raw meat is recommended for homemade dog foods although many greyhound trainers believe that raw meat is vital for optimal performance. Therefore, efforts should focus on meat quality, storage, handling and sanitation (Chapter 11). Food storage and preparation should emphasize sanitation and minimize the opportunity for bacterial growth in the food mixture. Meat should be kept frozen until near the time of use and be cooked to kill bacteria and decrease quantities of heat-labile toxins. Greyhound trainers often use and recommend a wide variety of unusual dietary supplements. However, most of these supplements are unnecessary and no data exist to support their use. Because greyhounds produce large amounts of metabolic acid when racing, adding an acid such as vinegar to the ration is inappropriate.
4. Meals should be fed more than four hours before training or racing. Water should be available at all times except just before racing. Food dose should be adjusted to maintain proper body condition (usually 1/5 or 2/5 for racing greyhounds).

Progress Notes

The recipe was changed to the following:

3 cups dry adult food
0.5 lb meat
1 cup milk
1 tbs vitamin supplement

The recommendations decreased the protein and fat levels and increased the digestible carbohydrate levels of the ration while not markedly changing the overall feeding regimen. Nutritionally speaking, this was not an ideal ration, but rather a compromise between the need to improve the nutrient profile, while maintaining the owner's desire to continue feeding raw meat. **Table 2** lists the key nutrient levels. The owner was pleased with these suggestions and they were implemented as part of the training program.

Table 1. Nutrient levels in the current ration for greyhounds during training.

	Dry puppy food (as fed)	Meat (as fed)	Milk (as fed)	Total ration (as fed)	Total ration (DM)
Moisture (%)	8	68	87	58.3	0
Energy (kcal/g)*	3.95	1.79	0.65	1.87	4.44
Protein (%)	27	21	3.5	17.9	42.8
Fat (%)	18	10	3.5	10.2	24.6
NFE (%)	39	0	4.9	10.9	26
Amount (g)	226	454	244	924	na

Key: DM = dry matter, NFE = nitrogen-free extract (digestible carbohydrate), na = not applicable.
*To calculate kJ, multiply kcal x 4.184.

Table 2. Nutrient levels in the recommended ration for greyhounds during training.

	Dry adult food (as fed)	Meat (as fed)	Milk (as fed)	Total ration (as fed)	Total ration (DM)
Moisture (%)	8	68	87	48.6	0
Energy (kcal/g)*	3.4	1.79	0.65	1.72	3.37
Protein (%)	23	21	3.5	16.6	32.2
Fat (%)	14	10	3.5	9.7	18.9
NFE (%)	49	0	4.9	22	42.8
Amount (g)	340	227	244	811	na

Key: DM = dry matter, NFE = nitrogen-free extract (digestible carbohydrate), na = not applicable.
*To calculate kJ, multiply kcal x 4.184.

Bibliography

Hill RC, Butterwick R. New developments in the nutrition of racing greyhounds. In: Proceedings. Fourteenth International Sports Medicine Symposium, Orlando, FL, 1998: 12-14.

Toll PW. Racing greyhound nutrition: Metabolic considerations. In: Proceedings. Eighth International Racing Greyhound Symposium, Orlando, FL, 1992: 19-21.

CASE 18-2

Weight Loss in a Cattle Dog

Philip W. Toll, DVM, MS
Hill's Science and Technology Center
Topeka, Kansas, USA

Patient Assessment

A 14-month-old, intact male Australian cattle dog cross that weighed 20 kg was examined for weight loss. A cowboy who worked on a 10,000-acre ranch in the western United States owned the dog. According to the owner, the dog had always been thin but had recently lost weight and was having trouble keeping up when the owner checked cattle on horseback. The owner estimated that the daily ride was about 15 to 20 miles. The dog had been kicked by horses several times in the past and was treated for rattlesnake envenomation three months earlier. There were no apparent long-term health effects from these problems.

The results of a physical examination were unremarkable except for one testicle in the scrotum and a body condition score (BCS) of 1/5. Ideal body weight was estimated to be 25 kg. Fecal examination and heartworm test results were negative. Complete blood count, serum biochemistry profile and urinalysis results were normal.

Assess the Food and Feeding Method

The dog was fed a generic, "high-protein" dry dog food produced at a local feed mill. The food was offered free choice, but the dog usually ate in the morning and evening. The guaranteed analysis on the food bag was as follows: Crude protein, not less than 32%; Crude fat, not less than 11%; Crude fiber, not more than 4%; Moisture, not more than 12%; Calcium, not less than 1.2%; Phosphorus, not less than 0.9%. The ingredient list was as follows: corn, corn gluten meal, rice, meat and bone meal, soybean meal, animal fat, wheat, vitamins and minerals. The nutritional adequacy statement read "provides complete and balanced nutrition for adult dogs as established by the AAFCO Dog Food Nutrient Profiles."

Questions

1. What additional dietary history would be important to obtain for this patient?
2. Outline an appropriate feeding plan (food and feeding method) for this dog, assuming there are no underlying metabolic or medical problems contributing to the weight loss.
3. What client education is appropriate about the feeding plan?

Answers and Discussion

1. The normal physical examination and laboratory database in an otherwise healthy young dog rules out many causes of chronic weight loss. The weight loss could be due to insufficient food intake in the face of strenuous exercise. The actual amount of food that is being offered free choice and the actual amount being consumed by the dog should be documented. This result can be compared with the daily energy requirement (DER) calculated in Answer 2 below.
2. The food for this dog should provide the nutrient levels outlined for intermediate athletic dogs (high duration and frequency) in **Table 18-9**. In general, the food should have moderate protein and carbohydrate levels, high fat levels, high energy density and above average digestibility.

   The estimated DER should include energy for maintenance of young, intact adult dogs (1.8 x resting energy requirement [RER]) plus energy for additional running. RER at an ideal weight of 25 kg = 820 kcal x 1.8 = 1,476 kcal/day (3.4 MJ x 1.8 = 6.2 MJ) for adult maintenance activities. Energy required for a 25-kg dog running 20 miles (33 km)/day = 33 km x 30 kcal/km = 990 kcal/day (4.1 MJ). The added energy cost of running increases the DER to 2,460 kcal (10.3 MJ) (3 x RER). The amount of food to achieve the estimated DER should be divided into two to three meals.
3. The owner should be told that hard work dramatically increases the requirement for calories. By comparison, the need for protein and other nutrients increases only slightly with increasing workload. The idea that athletic dogs require markedly more protein than nonworking dogs is inaccurate. The energy density of the current food is probably less than 3.5 kcal metabolizable energy (ME)/g dry matter (DM), which will not provide enough kcal in the amount of food the dog normally consumes. Using a food with higher fat levels will ensure a higher energy density. A food with 25 to 30% DM fat is recommended. The current food has 12 to 13% DM fat (estimated from the guaranteed analysis).

   The food should also have above average digestibility to ensure that the energy and nutrients are readily available to the dog. The nutritional adequacy statement shows that the food has not undergone feeding trials, which suggests that the digestibility of the food is unknown.

   Routine body condition scoring is the best way to assess whether the appropriate food is being fed in the correct amounts. A food with a higher fat content and higher energy density should be fed free choice until the dog achieves an ideal body condition (BCS 3/5). Then the amount should be adjusted to maintain that weight and body condition.

Progress Notes

The dog was eating 5 cups of the current food per day, which was estimated to provide 1,700 kcal/day (7.1 MJ/day). This caloric intake was clearly inadequate to provide the estimated DER with the added cost of running. The food was changed to a dry commercial specialty brand food (Science Diet Canine Active[a]) with 30.5% DM protein, 26.2% DM fat, 4.4 kcal ME/g DM and DM digestibility exceeding 85%. The new food was gradually exchanged for the old food over several days. The new food was offered free choice until a BCS of 3/5 was achieved, and the daily amount was then stabilized at 2,500 kcal (10.5 MJ) (5 cups) when the dog was working cattle. The amount was decreased to approximately 1,500 kcal (6.3 MJ) (3 cups) on days the dog was not working.

Endnote

a. Hill's Pet Nutrition, Inc., Topeka, KS, USA. This product is currently available as Hill's Science Diet Canine Adult Active Formula.

CASE 18-3

Poor Performance in a Hunting Dog

Philip W. Toll, DVM, MS
Hill's Science and Technology Center
Topeka, Kansas, USA

Patient Assessment

A five-year-old neutered female golden retriever was examined for collapsing during a game bird hunting trip. The dog was a sedentary house pet for most of the year, but was used as a retriever for game bird hunting each fall. The dog's general health had always been good but its retrieving ability was considered only fair. The dog had received routine heartworm preventive medication since it was a puppy.

On the opening day of hunting season, the dog was fed at 5:30 a.m., loaded in the truck about 6:00 a.m. and began hunting at 7:00 a.m. The dog worked hard through the morning and covered about 10 miles. The weather was unseasonably warm (23.8°C; 75°F) for the fall season in the upper Great Plains region of the United States. The hunters and dog took a lunch break from 11:00 a.m. to noon. The dog was given 1 cup of food and water at 11:00 a.m. and snacked on a small bag of potato chips around 11:30 a.m. The dog rested peacefully until noon when hunting resumed. Half an hour after hunting resumed, the dog began to falter, became ataxic and then collapsed. The dog never appeared to lose consciousness or develop seizures.

The dog was carried back to the truck and taken immediately to a veterinary hospital. During the trip to the hospital the dog seemed to improve. The physical examination was normal. The dog weighed 30 kg and had a body condition score of 3/5. Heart rate and heart sounds were normal with no pulse deficits. Hydration status was normal. Packed cell volume and serum glucose concentration were normal. A heartworm test was negative.

Assess the Food and Feeding Method

The dog was fed a commercial private label brand dry food formulated for adult dogs. The owners fed the dog one meal daily (1,500 kcal [6.3 MJ]; 4.5 cups) at 7:00 a.m. before they went to work. The dog received several biscuit treats in the evening and occasionally leftover food from family meals.

Questions

1. What are possible causes of the dog's collapse during the hunting trip?
2. What education should be provided to the owner about management of the dog?
3. What food should be recommended for this dog during the hunting season?
4. What feeding methods should be used during the hunting season?

Answers and Discussion

1. Causes of sudden collapse of a healthy appearing dog while hunting include hyperthermia, dehydration, hypoglycemia, heartworm disease, cardiac dysrhythmia and/or muscle cramping. Heartworm disease is unlikely based on the history of a good preventive medication program and negative heartworm test. A cardiac dysrhythmia may have occurred in the field and spontaneously resolved during travel to the veterinarian. Dehydration is unlikely because the dog received water during the lunch break and no clinical evidence of dehydration was found. Hyperthermia may have occurred due to excessive work in a warm environment, but the dog's rectal temperature was not elevated at the hospital. Transient hypoglycemia may have occurred. Muscle cramping may accompany electrolyte abnormalities, dehydration and poor training and conditioning.
2. The dog was poorly trained and went from being a sedentary house pet to working dog very abruptly. Physical training should begin about six weeks before hunting season for part-time athletes such as this dog. One hour of brisk walking each day is a good starting point. The dog should work for several hours at an intensity level similar to what is expected in the field during the last two weeks of training. Besides improving exercise tolerance, such a training program would likely improve olfactory ability. Preseason exercise is also recommended to prepare the dog's footpads for the work in the field.
3. A performance-type food (**Table 18-12**) should be recommended if the dog is to be used frequently for long periods of time during the hunting season. Performance foods are usually higher in fat, the preferred muscle fuel for longer lasting exercise and improved olfaction. Olfaction is further enhanced if the fat contains a significant amount of unsaturated fatty acids. Also, higher fat levels increase a food's energy density, which is needed for additional work in the field. A 30-kg dog traveling 10 miles requires 480 kcal (2.0 MJ). The food should be changed well before hunting season (preferably six weeks before) to allow for metabolic adaptation. Adaptation allows a dog to take full advantage of the higher dietary fat content.
4. Timing of feeding is also important. Working dogs should be fed four or more hours before exercise to allow some time for food assimilation and for blood glucose and insulin concentrations to return to normal. Snacks during exercise are helpful. However,

they should be spaced throughout the day and each snack should compose no more than 10% of the normal daily food amount. Feeding at the end of a break will cause less blood glucose disturbance.

Progress Notes

The food was changed to a commercial specialty brand dry food that was higher in fat, energy density and digestibility (Science Diet Canine Active[a]) than the previous food. The owner reported that the dog performed well through the rest of the hunting season with no further collapsing episodes. In addition to the change in feeding plan, the dog now runs four to five miles several times weekly with the owner's daughter.

Endnote

a. Hill's Pet Nutrition, Inc., Topeka, KS, USA. This product is currently available as Hill's Science Diet Canine Adult Active Formula.

CASE 18-4

Diarrhea in a Team of Sled Dogs

Arleigh J. Reynolds, DVM, PhD, Dipl. ACVN
Cornell University
Ithaca, New York, USA

Patient Assessment

A team of Alaskan husky-type dogs was examined for recurrent bouts of hemorrhagic diarrhea during exercise. The owner was a neophyte musher from upstate New York and noted that the dogs were eating well and eager to work. However, they would defecate loose feces during and immediately after each training run. Sometimes the feces were flecked with bright red blood. At other times during the day, the feces were of normal consistency without blood. At the time they were examined, the dogs were running four 10-mile training sessions each week.

Physical examination revealed a group of bright, alert, well-hydrated dogs with an average body weight of 20 kg. Muscle tone and mass were slightly greater than is usual for sedentary dogs. Their body condition score (BCS) was 2/5. Their overall condition was judged to be normal for this breed at this stage of training. The only abnormality noted on physical examination was mild brown staining of the hair on the ventral aspects of the tail and caudal aspects of both hind limbs.

The results from fecal smears and flotation tests for parasite ova, blood and abnormal bacteria were negative. Manual rectal palpation results, hematocrit and total solids measurement were normal.

Assess the Food and Feeding Method

The owner was feeding a dry commercial dog food with the following guaranteed analysis: Crude protein, not less than 26%; Crude fat, not less than 12%; Crude fiber, not more than 9%; Moisture, not more than 10%; Ash, not more than 8%. The dogs did quite well on this food during the summer and early fall training. By November, with the cold, wet climate and increased training mileage, the owner was feeding twice the volume of food he fed during the summer. Each 20-kg dog was receiving 800 g of food per day to maintain body weight. The dogs were fed half that amount in the morning (8:00 a.m.) and half in the evening (8:00 p.m.). The training runs usually occurred around noon.

Questions

1. What is the most likely cause of the diarrhea observed in these dogs?
2. What characteristics of the food and feeding method might have contributed to the diarrhea?
3. What recommendations should be made to the owner to prevent this problem from continuing?

Answers and Discussion

1. The observation that the dogs had normal feces except during and immediately after running suggests that stress or physiologic diarrhea is the most likely diagnosis. This problem is usually observed when exercise takes place while feces remain in the lower gastrointestinal tract.
2. The food is relatively low in fat and energy density for a performance ration; therefore, a large volume of food must be fed to meet the increased energy requirements associated with intense training and cold environmental temperatures. Feeding a large volume of food and feeding close to the time of exercise increases the fecal volume present during exercise. One theory is that the constant concussion between feces and colonic mucosa, termed "cecal slap," may irritate the colonic mucosa and alter colonic

motility, thereby inducing diarrhea during and immediately after exercise.

3. The musher should switch to a commercial food with a higher fat content and energy density so that a smaller volume can be fed (**Table 18-12**). For sled dogs exercising once a day, a single meal given within two hours after exercise will give maximal time for ingesta to pass completely through the gastrointestinal tract before the next exercise session.

Progress Notes

The dogs' food was changed to commercial performance ration (Eukanuba Original[a]) containing 32% protein and 20% fat (as fed). Each day, the dogs were fed approximately 500 g of the commercial food and 2 oz. of a fat supplement (poultry fat, beef tallow or corn oil) within two hours postexercise. Within two weeks, the problem had resolved in all dogs and defecation during performance was nearly eliminated.

Endnote

a. The Iams Co., Dayton, OH, USA.

Section 5

Nutritional Management of Healthy Cats

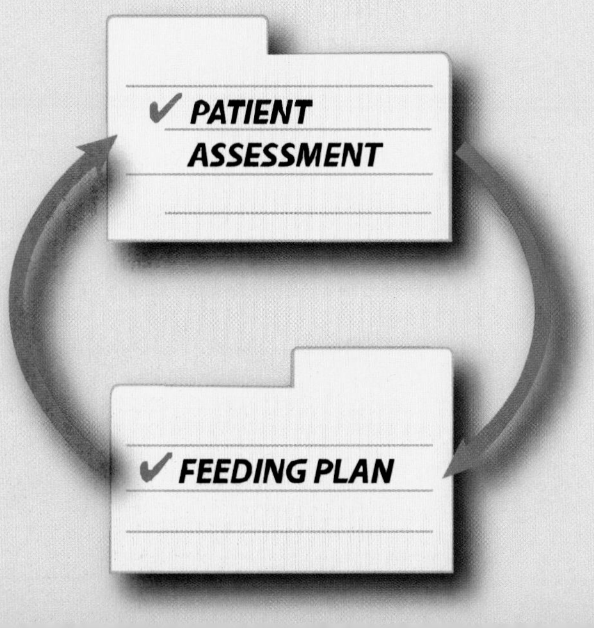

Chapter 19

Introduction to Feeding Normal Cats

P. Jane Armstrong
Kathy L. Gross
Iveta Becvarova
Jacques Debraekeleer

"The smallest feline is a masterpiece."
Leonardo da Vinci

INTRODUCTION

Cats were probably domesticated between 1600 and 1500 BC. Early Egyptians considered cats sacred and valued them for their natural hunting and predatory behavior, which helped control rodent populations. Little consideration for the nutritional needs of cats was required during the early days of domestication. As domestic cats evolved from mouse catcher to household companion, the need to understand their unique nutritional requirements also increased. Today, it is well accepted that proper nutrition and care throughout life maximizes health, longevity and quality of life. Providing proper guidance about the nutritional management of cats requires an understanding of: 1) the basic principles of nutrition (Chapters 5 and 6), 2) the foods and nutrients commonly fed to cats, 3) how to assess nutrient availability and quality of various foodstuffs and foods, 4) foods and feeding practices that may positively or negatively affect health and 5) the unique nutritional needs of cats throughout the lifecycle.

Demographics

Cats are the most popular pets in the United States, totaling approximately 77 million (APPMA, 2003). More than one-third of the households in the U.S. own cats with an average of 2.1 cats per cat-owning household. In 1996, the ratio of male to female cats was roughly equal and nearly 80% of pet cats in the U.S. were neutered (**Table 19-1**) (Lund et al, 1999). **Table 19-2** lists the 10 countries with the largest pet cat populations. Mixed-breed cats, domestic shorthairs and longhairs, make up an estimated 95% of the world's domestic cat population. They result from random rather than selective breeding. Domestic shorthair and longhair cats display a wide variety of sizes, and coat colors, patterns and lengths. Although most cats in the U.S. are non-pedigreed, the Cat Fanciers Association registered 41 different breeds in 2005. The four most common breeds were Persians, Maine coons, Siamese and Abyssinians (CFA, 2005).

Compared with dogs, cats make up a smaller proportion of the pets seen by veterinarians, but that proportion is increasing. Now, nearly 68% of cat owners in the U.S. regularly use veterinary services. In 2001, cats visited veterinary clinics once per year compared with 0.79 visits per year in 1987 (Center for Information Management, 2002). In 2001, cat owners spent $6.3 billion toward the health and well being of their cats. Cat food sales followed the upward trend in cat ownership and health care with almost $4.3 billion of sales in the U.S. in 1997

Table 19-1. Age and gender distribution of cats in the United States (1996).*

	Status	% of population
Gender	Male	9.7
	Neutered male	41.2
	Female	11.7
	Spayed female	34.4
Age (years)	0-1	25.7
	1-4	27
	4-7	17.6
	7-10	12
	10-15	13.4
	15+	4.4

*Adapted from Lund EM, Armstrong PJ, Kirk CA, et al. Health status and population characteristics of dogs and cats examined at private veterinary practices in the United States. Journal of the American Veterinary Medical Association 1999; 214: 1336-1341.

Table 19-2. Comparisons of cat populations in the 10 countries with the highest numbers of cats.*

Country	Pet cat population (millions)
USA	76.43
China	53.10
Russia	12.70
Brazil	12.47
France	9.60
Italy	9.40
UK	7.70
Germany	7.70
Ukraine	7.35
Japan	7.30

*Source: Infobase Pvt. Ltd.

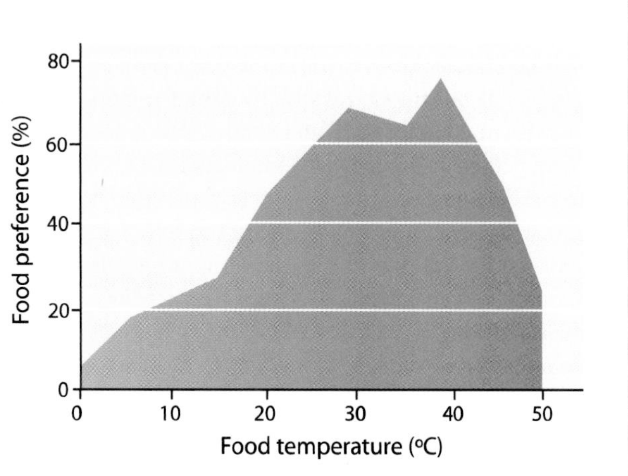

Figure 19-1. Influence of food temperature on food preference in cats (mean food preference demonstrated by 23 cats fed moist food at various temperatures vs. the same food at 20°C [68°F]). Note how preference increases for food served at body temperature but decreases when food is served at temperature extremes. (Adapted from Sohail MA. The ingestive behavior of the domestic cat–A review. Nutritional Abstracts and Reviews Series B 1983; 53: 177-186.)

(Maxwell, 1998). The greatest growth occurred in dry cat foods and treats, whereas sales of moist foods were static, and sales of semi-moist products decreased. Pet owners are very interested in nutritional information. In one pet owner survey, interest in obtaining nutritional information equaled obtaining information about diseases. Furthermore, the pet owners' top two preferred sources of pet health information were the Internet and veterinarians (MAF, 2005).

CATS AS CARNIVORES

Taxonomically, cats and dogs are members of the order Carnivora and are therefore classified as carnivores (Table 12-4). From a dietary perspective, however, dogs are omnivores (Chapter 12) and domestic cats and other members of the superfamily *Feloidea* are strict or true carnivores, along with raptors, mosquitoes and some coldwater fish. This basic difference is supported by specific behavioral, anatomic, physiologic and metabolic adaptations of cats to a strictly carnivorous diet.

Adaptations in Feline Feeding Behavior

Domestic cats share several feeding behaviors with their wild counterparts. Unlike most mammals, cats do not display a regular daily rhythmicity in sleep-wake cycles, activity, feeding and drinking. Cats typically eat 10 to 20 small meals throughout the day and night (Kane et al, 1981; MacDonald et al, 1984). This eating pattern probably reflects the evolutionary relationship of cats and their prey. With the exception of African lions, cats are solitary hunters. Small rodents (e.g., voles and mice) make up 40% or more of feral domestic-type cats' food source; however, young rabbits and hares may compose a large portion of their natural diet (Fitzgerald, 1988). A variety of other prey (e.g., birds, reptiles, frogs and insects) is also eaten, but in smaller amounts. The average mouse provides approximately 30 kcal (125 kJ) of metabolizable energy (ME) (Mugford, 1977). This amount is about 12 to 13% of a feral cat's daily energy requirement. Repeated cycles of hunting throughout the day and night are required to provide sufficient food for an average cat. Thus, meal feeding cats once per day is in conflict with their natural feeding behavior.

The predatory drive is so strong in cats that they will stop eating to make a kill (Adamec, 1976). This behavior may frustrate owners who confuse predatory behavior with hunger (**Box 19-1**). Many owners reason that a fed cat will not hunt and are disappointed when their housecat kills songbirds. Supplemental feeding may reduce hunting time, but otherwise does not alter hunting behavior (Turner and Meister, 1988).

Cats are very sensitive to the physical form, odor and taste of foods. Oral tactile sensation is important to normal feeding behavior and should be considered when feeding novel foods. Unless accustomed to foods with different textures such as dry foods, cats generally prefer solid, moist foods and reluctantly accept food with powdery, sticky and very greasy textures (NRC, 2006, 1986; Kane et al, 1981a). The flavor and texture preferences of individual cats are often influenced by early experience

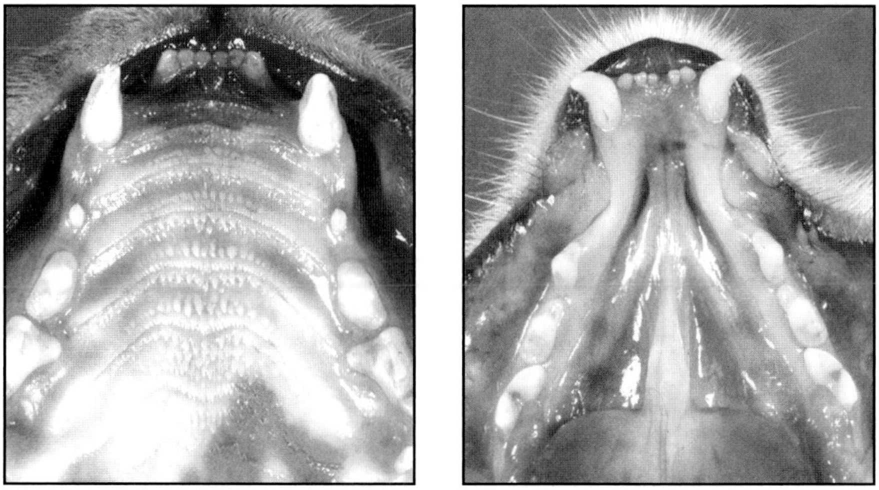

Figure 19-2. Maxillary dentition and hard palate of a cat (Left). Mandibular dentition and sublingual mucosa of the same cat (Right). These photographs demonstrate tooth anatomy associated with a carnivorous eating behavior. The canine teeth are slightly curved and taper to a pointed tip suitable for grasping and puncturing prey. The premolar and molar teeth are conical and sharply pointed, making them suitable for shearing and tearing flesh. There are no grinding (flat, table) surfaces present. (Adapted with permission from Harvey CE, Emily PP, eds. Function, formation, and anatomy of oral structures in carnivores. In: Small Animal Dentistry. St. Louis, MO: Mosby-Year Book, 1993.)

that can affect preferences throughout life. Cats accustomed to a specific texture or type of food (i.e., moist, dry, semi-moist) may refuse foods with different textures. This becomes an important consideration when feeding cats novel foods.

Cats find certain flavors very attractive, which seems to reflect the nutritional characteristics of their natural foods. Cats prefer the tastes of animal fat, protein hydrolysates (digests), meat extracts and certain free amino acids abundant in muscle tissue (i.e., alanine, proline, lysine, histidine and leucine). Cats search out wild prey more often when meat is not in their diet (Robertson, 1998). Even the feeding behaviors of cats in the wild reflect their preference for animal tissues. When ingesting prey, wild cats avoid consuming plant materials contained in the entrails. African lions have been observed to first empty the digesta from the entrails by expressing the contents with their tongues (Leyhausen, 1979). This behavior contrasts with that of a pack of wild dogs or wolves eating similar game. Wolves often first consume the viscera of prey (Mech, 1970). Herbivores are common prey; therefore, the gastrointestinal contents are generally of plant origin and have a high carbohydrate content. Unlike dogs and other omnivores, cats are not attracted to the taste of sugars and are averse to flavors derived from plant products (e.g., glutamic acid and medium-chain triglycerides) (MacDonald et al, 1984). Cats are also sensitive to bitter tastes when compared to tastes of other species (Carpenter, 1956). A great deal of variation in preference is apparent in the cat population; owners often report that cats have an appetite for cantaloupe, pumpkin, bananas or celery.

Food temperature also influences food acceptance by cats (**Figure 19-1**). Cats prefer that moist foods be offered at, or near, body temperature (38.5°C [101.5°F]). This preference is logical considering that in the wild, a cat's food typically consists of freshly killed prey.

Anatomic and Physiologic Adaptations

Sensory Structures

Cat eyes are well adapted to hunting. Their visual acuity is greater than that of dogs because of their larger optic cortex. A cat's ears are upright, face forward and have 20 associated muscles to provide the fine control needed to precisely locate sound. Cats also respond to high-pitched sounds, which represent the range of sound frequencies emitted by typical prey (Tabor, 1983). Finally, the highly sensitive facial whiskers and tactile hairs are thought to help cats hunt in dim light and to protect their eyes.

Limbs

The retractable claws of cats are a unique adaptation to hunting. The sharp tips of the claws with hook-like curves and needle features are ideal for capturing and securing prey, yet they are easily retracted so they do not make noise when cats stalk prey. In contrast, the claws of dogs play only a secondary role in capturing prey.

Oral Cavity

Cats and dogs have the same number of incisor, canine and carnassial teeth (i.e., the enlarged upper premolar and lower molar teeth specialized for shearing flesh); however, cats have fewer premolar and molar teeth, and they do not possess fissured crowns, which are a hallmark of omnivorous animals (**Figure 19-2**). The jaws of cats have limited lateromedial and craniocaudal movement, thereby limiting grinding ability. The scissors-like action of the carnassial teeth is ideal for delivering the cervical bite used to transect the spinal cord and immobilize or kill prey. Cats lack salivary amylase used to initiate digestion of dietary starches. This adaptation reflects the nutritional composition of the typical prey (i.e., low starch content).

Stomach

Because cats evolved to eat small frequent meals, the stomach is less important as a storage reservoir compared with the stomach of dogs. Thus, the stomach of domestic cats is simpler than that of dogs (i.e., relatively smaller with a smaller glandular fundus).

Small and Large Intestine

Intestinal length, as determined by the ratio of intestine to body length, is markedly shorter in cats than in omnivores and herbivores (**Table 19-3**). A greater villus height in cats increases the absorptive surface area. Overall, however, the absorptive capacity is estimated to be 10% less than that of dogs (Kendall et al,

Box 19-1. Alternative Eating Behaviors.

Although there are such things as aberrant eating behaviors, many of the behaviors observed are normal behaviors that owners happen to find objectionable.

COPROPHAGIA
Coprophagia, or consumption of excreta, is normal behavior for queens with kittens less than 30 days of age. The queen stimulates the kittens' elimination reflexes by grooming the kittens' perineal areas and then consumes the products of elimination. This process is important as an aid to elimination in young kittens. In addition, coprophagia maintains sanitation and reduces odors in the nest area. Thus, coprophagia has important survival value in wild or feral cats by reducing factors that could attract predators to the nest site. It is very uncommon for cats to continue coprophagia after the kittens are weaned.

CANNIBALISM/INFANTICIDE
Cannibalism or infanticide is often normal behavior in male and female cats. Queens typically cannibalize aborted, dead and weak kittens. This behavior may serve to reduce the spread of disease to healthy kittens, conserve maternal resources and optimize survival of the fittest kittens and help keep the nest box clean. In addition, the queen derives nutritional benefits from consuming dead kittens. Occasionally, queens will kill an apparently healthy litter. Environmental factors that cause kittens to mimic early signs of illness (e.g., inactivity, hyperthermia or hypothermia) may trigger infanticide and cannibalism. Maternal stress, malnourishment and hormonal insufficiency may contribute to unexplained cannibalism as well. Maternal experience or parity does not appear to play a role.

Tomcats may indiscriminately kill unrelated kittens. This behavior usually occurs when a strange male enters a new territory and encounters a lactating queen and kittens. A queen rapidly returns to estrus after the loss of its kittens. Thus, infanticide optimizes a male's genetic potential because it now has an opportunity to sire subsequent litters. Infanticide is an uncommon behavior by resident male cats.

The health status, dietary management and husbandry practices should be reviewed in queens or catteries experiencing persistent problems with cannibalism. Males should not have access to young kittens to reduce the chance of infanticide. Although resident male cats rarely pose a problem, it is prudent to err on the side of safety. Factors contributing to maternal stress should be evaluated and, if possible, reduced.

PLANT AND GRASS EATING
Plant and grass eating is a natural behavior of both cats and dogs. A variety of explanations have been advanced for grass eating. Because grass is not digested within the cat's gastrointestinal (GI) tract, it acts as a local irritant and sometimes stimulates vomiting. Thus, grass eating may serve as a purgative to eliminate hair or other indigestible material. However, many cats readily seek out grass to eat, appear to enjoy eating it and do not vomit. Other explanations for the behavior include a response to nutritional deficiencies, boredom or a taste preference. In contrast to eating grass, eating other plants, including many indoor ornamental plants, carries risk of toxicity (e.g., lily toxicity).

RESPONSE TO CATNIP
The smell or ingestion of catnip (*Nepeta cataria*) can invoke unusual behavioral changes for five to 15 minutes after exposure. The active ingredient, cis-trans-nepetalactone, is thought to act as a hallucinogen although stimulation of neurologic centers associated with estrous behaviors has also been suggested. Cats may respond to catnip by head rubbing and shaking, salivating, gazing, skin twitching, rolling and animated leaping. Only 50 to 70% of cats exhibit a behavioral response, which may have a genetic basis. Prolonged exposure may lead to a chronic state of partial unawareness. Cats may become refractory for an hour or more after cessation of the initial response.

WOOL SUCKING
A commonly reported behavioral abnormality in cats is wool sucking. The behavior first appears near puberty when cats begin to lick, suck, chew or eat wool or other clothing articles. Although the cause is poorly understood, nutritional deficiencies are unlikely. Affected cats may be seeking the odor of lanolin or human sweat or the behavior may be a manifestation of prolonged nursing. Siamese, Siamese-cross and Burmese cats are primarily affected, suggesting a genetic link. Wool sucking is managed by limiting access to attractive items and through behavior modification. Feeding a high-fiber food or providing a continuous supply of dry food reduces the behavior in some cats.

PROLONGED NURSING
Prolonged nursing may occur in kittens that strive to satisfy a desire for non-nutritional sucking. Non-nutritional sucking normally subsides near weaning. Kittens may develop nursing vices when nursing fails to take place because they were orphaned, prematurely weaned or required bottle feeding. Within the litter, kittens will often nurse tails, ears, skin folds and/or the genitalia of their littermates. After a kitten is separated from its litter, it may transfer sucking vices to people, stuffed toys, clothing or other pets.

1982; Morris and Rogers, 1989). Therefore, dogs can more efficiently use a variety of foods, some of which may require more digestion than animal tissues.

Unlike in omnivores, the sugar transport systems of the small intestine of cats are not adaptive to varying levels of dietary carbohydrate (Buddington and Diamond, 1992). Cats do not waste energy or protein by turning over carriers or enzyme systems of little value because free sugars and complex carbohydrates normally make up a negligible percentage of their food (**Table 19-4**). This lack of adaptability has been noted in other strict carnivores, such as raptors and coldwater fish. Also, cats have low activities of intestinal disaccharidases (i.e., sucrase, maltase and isomaltase) (Kienzle, 1993). This reflects adaptation to foods limited in simple sugars and other carbohydrates. In cats, pancreatic amylase production is about 5% of that in dogs (Kienzle, 1987, 1993a). Pancreatic amylase production is relatively nonadaptive in cats, as would be expected in a species unaccustomed to significant changes in dietary carbohydrate levels. Cats have higher concentrations of bacteria in their small intestine than dogs and other omnivores studied (Johnston et al, 1993, 2001; Gruffydd-Jones et al, 1998). Interestingly, the numbers typical for cats would be diagnostic for small intestin-

ANOREXIA
Although a few days of inappetence is not particularly detrimental to an otherwise healthy cat, prolonged inadequate calorie intake results in malnutrition, reduced immune function and increased risk for hepatic lipidosis. Anorexia may be caused by stress, unacceptable foods or concurrent disease. Most commonly, cats presented to veterinarians for anorexia have a concurrent disease. Cats may endure prolonged starvation rather than eat an unpalatable food. Therefore, advising owners that a cat will "eat when it gets hungry enough" can have deadly results. Anorexia of more than three days duration, even in an otherwise healthy-appearing cat, warrants investigation by a veterinarian.

A thorough history is useful for differentiating potential causes of anorexia. To determine if inadequate food acceptance is the cause, offer a small selection of highly palatable foods along with the typical food. Because improperly stored foods may develop off flavors, bacterial contamination or fungal growth, confirm that the product is fresh and wholesome. Environmental or emotional factors reported to result in stress-mediated anorexia include hospitalization, boarding, travel, introduction of new people or pets to the household, loss of a companion, overcrowding, high temperatures and excessive handling. Stress-mediated anorexia is usually diagnosed from the history and by ruling out other diseases. Providing a quiet secluded area will often allow a cat to relax sufficiently enough to begin eating. Often, increasing the food's palatability will improve food intake. Warming food, changing the food form, adding water or choosing foods high in animal protein and fat can enhance food palatability. If cats are highly stressed or appropriate feeding sites are unavailable, mild tranquilizers or appetite stimulants (e.g., mirtazapine, oxazepam or cyproheptadine) may be beneficial (Chapter 25). Force feeding may be accepted by some cats but others find the process so stressful that any benefit is far outweighed by the additional stress.

FIXED-FOOD PREFERENCES
The food type fed by the owner during a kitten's first six months influences the pattern of food preferences throughout life. Although uncommon, kittens exposed to a very limited number of foods may develop a food fixation, refusing to eat anything but a single food. Adult cats fed highly palatable, single-item foods have been reported to develop fixed-food preferences as well.

Cats with food fixations can be particularly troublesome if dietary modifications are necessary. Cats with strong food preferences should be transitioned to the new food over a prolonged period. Convert to the desired food by replacing 10 to 20% of the old food with an equal amount of the new food on Day 1, then gradually increase the ratio of new to old over the next 14 days. A more gradual transition may be required if food intake drops below 70% of maintenance levels. Cats should be monitored to ensure they are not selecting the preferred food from the food dish and that food intake remains adequate. Feeding kittens and cats a variety of foods (both different forms of food and different brands) and not feeding single-item foods can avoid food fixations. This approach is strongly recommended as disease management later in life often requires a dietary change.

LEARNED TASTE AVERSIONS
Cats may develop learned aversions to certain foods when feeding is paired with a negative GI experience. The negative experience can be physical, emotional or physiologic. Typically, aversions occur when cats consume a food immediately before an episode of nausea or vomiting. Foods that were readily consumed before the negative incident will be avoided subsequently. Clinically, aversions may develop when GI upset is induced by various diseases, drugs or treatment protocols. Foods with high salience (i.e., strong odors or high protein levels) are more likely to become aversive and should not be fed within 24 hours of anticipated GI upsets. Aversions have been documented to last up to 40 days in cats. Learned aversions are considered an adaptive response. By avoiding foods that previously caused gastric distress, cats will avoid eating foods likely to be spoiled or tainted. From a clinical perspective, consideration of food aversions often equates to delaying introduction of a therapeutic food, such as a diet for chronic kidney disease, until the cat's GI signs have been controlled with other medical management.

POLYPHAGIA
Various diseases, drugs and psychological stresses can mediate excessive food consumption. Rarely, polyphagia (hyperphagia) may occur with diseases involving the central nervous system, particularly with lesions of the ventromedial hypothalamus. Presence of weight loss or gain is of key diagnostic importance. Polyphagia with weight loss is almost always associated with an underlying disease process or simple underfeeding. Caloric intake should always be calculated because underfeeding can result in a ravenous appetite that may be misinterpreted as abnormal. Nutritional management of polyphagia requires an accurate diagnosis because treatment is aimed at the primary disease.

The Bibliography for **Box 19-1** can be found at www.markmorris.org.

al bacterial overgrowth in dogs (NRC, 2006). Although the reason for this finding is unclear, their relatively short small intestine and carnivorous physiology have been suggested as possibilities. Increased numbers of small intestinal bacteria might enhance protein and fat digestion (Zoran, 2002).

Certain amino acid transporters in the small intestines of cats are highly adaptable, particularly the transporter responsible for arginine uptake. This finding underscores the importance of the amount of protein and specific amino acids in foods for cats. Unlike omnivores, cats are unable to synthesize significant quantities of ornithine or citrulline within the intestine. Both are precursors to arginine synthesis. This inability results in the absolute requirement for arginine in cat foods, which is discussed below.

Cats have a vestigial cecum and a relatively short colon (0.4 m). These anatomic features would appear to limit cats' capability to use poorly digestible starches and fiber by microbial fermentation in the large bowel (Morris and Rogers, 1989). The primary end products of bacterial fermentation (i.e., short-chain fatty acids: acetate, propionate and butyrate), however, are present in relatively high concentrations in the large bowel of cats (Brosey et al, 2000). Large intestinal fermentation may be

Table 19-3. Comparison of small intestinal length to body length in selected species.

Species	Ratio
Cat	4:1
Dog	6:1
Rabbit	10:1
Pig	14:1

Table 19-4. Nutrient levels in rat carcass.

Nutrients*	Rat carcass**
Moisture (%)	63.6
Protein (%)	55
Fat (%)	38.1
Linoleic acid (%)	9.1
Carbohydrate (%)	1.2
Fiber (%)	0.55
Ash (%)	5.22
Calculated ME (kcal/g)***	5.7
Calcium (%)	1.15
Phosphorus (%)	0.98
Potassium (%)	0.79
Magnesium (%)	0.08
Sodium (%)	0.25
Zinc (mg/kg)	71.4
Copper (mg/kg)	12.4
Iron (mg/kg)	288
Vitamin A (IU/kg)	84,800
Vitamin E (IU/kg)	33
Thiamin (mg/kg)	5.8
Riboflavin (mg/kg)	10.7
Niacin (mg/kg)	156.6
Folic acid (mg/kg)	2.8
Pantothenic acid (mg/kg)	54.9
Pyridoxine (mg/kg)	5.2
Vitamin B_{12} (µg/kg)	22.5
Choline (mg/kg)	3,242

Key: ME = metabolizable energy.
*All nutrients expressed on a dry matter basis except moisture.
**Fresh intact rat carcasses. Adapted from Vondruska JF. The effect of a rat carcass diet on the urinary pH of the cat. Companion Animal Practice 1987; 1 (August): 5-9.
***To convert from kcal to kJ multiply kcal by 4.184.

more important to cats than previously thought.

Feline Nutrient Requirements and Metabolic Adaptations

Energy Metabolism

The liver of most animals has two enzyme systems for converting glucose to glucose-6-phosphate: hexokinase and glucokinase. This conversion is necessary before the liver can use glucose. The glucokinase system operates only when the liver receives a large amount of glucose from the portal vein. Because the typical food source of wild cats is primarily animal not plant tissue, it contains only small amounts of digestible (soluble) carbohydrate and the portal system delivers very little absorbed glucose to the liver. Thus, adult cats have very low hepatic glucokinase activity and a limited ability to metabolize large amounts of simple carbohydrates. Omnivores (e.g., people, dogs and rats) have higher hepatic glucokinase activity (MacDonald et al, 1984).

Kittens ingest digestible carbohydrates (i.e., lactose or milk sugar) before weaning. Adult cats must rely primarily on gluconeogenesis from glucogenic amino acids (ketoacids), lactic acid and glycerol for maintenance of blood glucose concentration. In omnivores, maximal gluconeogenesis occurs in the post-absorptive state when the direct contribution of dietary glucose is absent. In cats, gluconeogenesis is maximal in the absorptive phase immediately after a meal.

Feline liver apparently lacks fructokinase. This finding is compatible with the observations by Kienzle that cats consuming high-sucrose diets (>25%) have significant fructosuria. The fact that cats, unlike many mammals, have no taste preference for sucrose further supports adaptation to a diet devoid of simple carbohydrates (Kienzle, 1993b).

Protein Metabolism

Protein metabolism is unique in cats and is manifested by an unusually high maintenance requirement for protein as compared with canine requirements (**Table 19-5**) and a special need for four amino acids: arginine, taurine, methionine and cystine. The protein requirement for growth in kittens is only 50% higher than that of puppies, whereas the protein requirement for feline maintenance is twice that of adult dogs. The higher protein requirement of cats is not due to an exceptionally high requirement for any specific amino acid (**Table 19-6**); instead, it is caused by a high activity of hepatic enzymes (i.e., transaminases and deaminases) that remove amino groups from amino acids so the resulting ketoacids can be used for energy or glucose production. Unlike omnivores and herbivores, cats have a limited ability to decrease the activity of these enzymes when fed low-protein foods. The cat's strict adherence to a diet of animal tissue likely resulted in a lack of evolutionary pressure to accommodate lower protein food sources. Hepatic enzyme systems are constantly active; therefore, a fixed amount of dietary protein is always catabolized for energy (MacDonald et al, 1984). The gluconeogenic enzymes in feline liver appear to be continuously active, unlike the situation in most other species, including dogs (MacDonald et al, 1984). In addition, an alternate hepatic gluconeogenic pathway common in flesh-eating animals is active in cats (Beliveau and Freedland, 1982). This pathway uses serine as a glucose precursor. Serine is a nonessential amino acid found in large amounts in muscle, milk and egg.

ARGININE

Arginine deficiency in cats causes one of the most dramatic responses of any nutrient deficiency. Cats cannot synthesize sufficient ornithine or citrulline for conversion to arginine, which is needed for the urea cycle. After a cat eats a meal, the highly active protein catabolic enzymes in its liver produce ammonia, which is absorbed from the colon.

Without arginine, the urea cycle cannot convert ammonia to urea and ammonia toxicity occurs (MacDonald et al, 1984). Eating a single meal devoid of arginine may result in hyperammonemia in less than one hour. Affected cats exhibit severe signs of ammonia toxicity (i.e., vocalization, emesis, ptyalism, hyperactivity, hyperesthesia, ataxia, tetanic spasms, extended limbs with exposed claws, apnea and cyanosis) and may die within two to five hours (MacDonald et al, 1984). Because the diet of wild cats is high in animal protein (that contains arginine), cats have apparently lost the flexibility in protein metabolism seen in other animal species that eat foods with more limited amino acid composition. Arginine deficiency, however, has only been reported to occur in cats fed experimental foods specifically formulated to be arginine deficient or in cats fed certain casein-based human enteral products (Diehl and Wheeler, 1992). Although not necessarily supporting the argument that cats are carnivores, excess dietary lysine does not cause arginine antagonism in cats, as it can in dogs (Fascetti et al, 2004).

TAURINE

Taurine is a β-amino sulfonic acid, abundant as a free amino acid in the natural food of cats, such as small rodents, birds and fish. Taurine is found at lower concentrations in large animal species such as cattle. In cats, dietary taurine is essential and clinical disease results if insufficient amounts are present. Many species can use either glycine or taurine to conjugate bile acids into bile salts before they are secreted into bile. Cats can only conjugate bile acids with taurine. The loss of taurine in bile coupled with a low rate of taurine synthesis contributes to the obligatory taurine requirement of cats (**Box 19-2**).

METHIONINE AND CYSTINE

The sulfur-containing amino acids methionine and cystine are required in higher amounts by cats than most other species, especially during growth. Cystine is the amino acid formed when a pair of cysteine molecules are joined by a disulfide bond. Methionine and cystine are considered together because cystine can replace up to half of the methionine requirement of cats (NRC, 2006). Methionine serves as a precursor to cysteine; therefore, cysteine is not an essential amino acid. Cysteine cannot be converted to methionine; however, a minimal requirement for methionine must be met with methionine. Although these amino acids are present in high amounts in animal flesh, methionine tends to be the first limiting amino acid in many food ingredients. Nutritional deficiencies are possible, especially in cats fed home-prepared or vegetable-based foods. Clinical signs of methionine deficiency include poor growth and a crusting dermatitis at the mucocutaneous junctions of the mouth and nose. Approximately 19% of a food must be composed of animal protein to meet the methionine requirement of kittens (MacDonald et al, 1984). Foods high in plant proteins require additional methionine, which can be supplied as DL-methionine, a crystalline form of the amino acid. Cats appear to prefer foods with added methionine compared to foods deficient in methionine (Rogers et al, 2004).

Numerous theories have been advanced to explain the high methionine and cystine requirement of cats. Methionine needs may be increased because of an increased S-adenosyl methionine requirement, cysteine synthesis, taurine synthesis or because of a high rate of methionine catabolism. Additional cystine may be required for the synthesis of the antioxidant glutathione and the amino acid felinine. Felinine is a branched-chain, sulfur-containing α-amino acid found in the urine of domestic cats. Its biologic function has not been fully elucidated. The most widely accepted possible role for felinine, or its breakdown product in urine, is as a pheromone, which is of importance in territorial marking. Sexually immature kittens have been reported not to excrete felinine and adult males excrete more

Table 19-5. Comparison of dietary protein requirements during maintenance and growth in selected mammals.

Classification	Species	Growth (%)*	Maintenance (%)*	G:M ratio**
Omnivore***	Dog	12	4	3
Omnivore†	Dog	18	8	2.25
Omnivore***	Rat	12	4.2	2.9
Carnivore†	Cat	18	16	1.1
Carnivore***	Cat	29	19	1.5
Carnivore†	Mink	31	20	1.6
Carnivore†	Fox	24	16	1.5

*Percent of diet (dry matter basis).
**G:M ratio = ratio of growth to maintenance requirements.
***Ideal protein (i.e., meets all known essential amino acid requirements).
Adapted from MacDonald ML, Rogers QR, Morris JG. Nutrition of the domestic cat, a mammalian carnivore. Annual Review in Nutrition 1984; 4: 521-562.
†NRC minimal requirements. Adapted from National Research Council. Nutrient Requirements of Dogs and Cats. Washington, DC: National Academies Press, 2006.

Table 19-6. Comparison of minimal protein and amino acid requirements for growth in kittens and puppies.*

Nutrients	Recommended allowance for kittens** % DM	Recommended allowance for puppies** % DM
Crude protein	22.5	17.5
EAA	-	-
Amino acids		
Arginine***	0.96	0.66
Histidine	0.33	0.25
Isoleucine	0.54	0.50
Leucine	1.28	0.82
Lysine	0.85	0.70
Methionine (met + cys)	0.44 (0.88)	0.26 (0.53)
Phenylalanine (phe + tyr)	0.5 (1.91)	0.50 (1.00)
Threonine	0.65	0.63
Tryptophan	0.16	0.18
Valine	0.64	0.56
Taurine (extruded)	0.1	–
Taurine (canned)	0.17	–

Key: EAA = essential amino acids, DM = dry matter.
*Adapted from Rogers QR, Morris JG. Optimizing protein and amino acid nutrition for cats and dogs. In: Proceedings. Roche Technical Symposium and 1997 Petfood Institute Conference and Trade Show, Chicago, IL: 19-32.
**National Research Council. Nutrient Requirements of Dogs and Cats. Washington, DC: National Academies Press, 2006. Based on a dietary energy content of 4.0 kcal/g dry matter.
***Arginine requirement increases in kittens with increased dietary protein; approximately 2 g/kg should be added for each 10% increase in crude protein above the minimum allowance (22.5%).

Box 19-2. Taurine.

As a β-amino acid, taurine is neither incorporated into proteins nor degraded by mammalian tissues. However, taurine has important functions in virtually all body systems. In addition to its importance in normal bile salt function, taurine is essential for normal retinal, cardiac, neurologic, reproductive, immune and platelet function. Taurine is needed for normal fetal development and may function as an antioxidant, osmolyte and neuromodulator. Most animal tissues, particularly skeletal muscle, heart, viscera and brain, contain high levels of taurine; plants contain none. Taurine is essential in foods for cats because of two factors.

- The feline liver has a limited capacity to synthesize taurine. The rate-limiting enzymes responsible for conversion of methionine and cysteine to taurine (i.e., cysteine dioxygenase and cysteine sulfinic acid decarboxylase) are minimally active.
- Cats have an obligate loss of taurine via the enterohepatic circulation of bile acids. Taurine is important in the conjugation and secretion of bile acids. Many animals conserve taurine by switching to glycine conjugation when dietary taurine becomes scarce. Feline hepatic enzymes do not use glycine, but conjugate bile acids mostly to taurine. Most bile salts secreted into the intestinal lumen are returned to the liver after intestinal uptake. However, once deconjugated, taurine is available for intestinal uptake, fecal excretion or degradation by intestinal microbes. Microbial degradation appears to account for deconjugation and substantial wasting of free taurine. This process also results in an obligate taurine loss.

The requirement for taurine is influenced by dietary factors and the metabolic needs of cats. The protein source, commercial processing, sulfur-containing amino acid content and dietary fiber levels alter taurine requirements. In general, taurine is abundant in animal tissues and absent in plants; thus, homemade vegetarian diets and cereal-based dog foods have long been known to cause taurine deficiency when fed to cats. However, in 1987, taurine deficiency was reported to occur in cats fed commercial foods containing the National Research Council's recommended levels of taurine (400 mg taurine/kg food). This finding underscored the food-dependent nature of the taurine requirement and prompted an increase in taurine recommendations by the Association of American Feed Control Officials to 1,000 mg/kg and 2,000 mg/kg (ppm) food in commercial dry and moist foods, respectively. However, taurine levels of 2,500 ppm are often recommended for moist products. Taurine adequacy is best established through feeding trials.

Because taurine functions throughout the body, signs of deficiency have been demonstrated in virtually all body systems. Three syndromes of taurine deficiency in cats have been well established: 1) feline central retinal degeneration (FCRD), 2) reproductive failure and impaired fetal development and 3) feline dilated cardiomyopathy (DCM). Hearing loss, platelet hyperaggregation and impaired immune function have also been demonstrated although specific clinical disorders have not been recognized.

CLINICAL SIGNS

Clinical signs of taurine deficiency occur only after prolonged periods of depletion (i.e., five months to two years). Typically in nonreproducing adults, taurine deficiency may manifest as FCRD, DCM or both, with only about 40% of taurine-deficient cats exhibiting clinical signs.[a,b]

Clinical signs of FCRD are inapparent until significant visual impairment has occurred. Then, owners may notice their cat bumping into objects or "miscalculating" jumps. Early disease may be detected during ophthalmic examination. Changes in retinal function can be demonstrated by electroretinograms before retinal lesions appear. The development of FCRD apparently requires three or more months of taurine depletion. Initially, lesions appear as dark granular focal defects in the area centralis, slightly temporal to the optic disk. As degeneration progresses, the lesion becomes hyperreflective and extends in a band across the tapetum. Complete blindness ensues with full degeneration of the retina and attenuation of retinal vessels. Structural changes within the retina are permanent. Therefore, a diagnosis of FCRD does not reflect the current taurine status of a cat, but indicates a period of prolonged taurine deficiency has occurred.

Cats with DCM may be clinically normal or present acutely with signs of heart failure. Clinical signs may include lethargy, anorexia and dyspnea. Physical findings may include pleural effusion, pulmonary edema, gallop heart rhythms, systolic murmurs and ventricular dysrhythmias. Cats in severe heart failure are hypothermic, have pale mucous membranes, poor pulse quality and are often too weak to stand. Only about one-third of cats with DCM have concurrent FCRD. DCM is confirmed by echocardiography. Findings most often include dilatation of the left atrium and ventricle and decreased left ventricle contractility.

REPRODUCTION AND FETAL DEVELOPMENT

Reproduction and fetal development are severely impaired in taurine-deficient queens. Conception and implantation appear normal; however, fetal death is frequently observed near 25 days of gestation, followed by abortion or resorption. In a group of taurine-deficient queens, only 38% of 33 matings resulted in term deliveries, with an average of 2.1 live births.

Developmental abnormalities reported to occur in kittens born to taurine-deficient queens include poor survival, cerebellar dysgenesis, abnormal hind-limb development and thoracic kyphosis, which appears as a dorsoventral flattening of the thoracic cavity. Severe hydrocephalus and anencephaly may be present in aborted fetuses. Surviving kittens are often small and weak. Growth is depressed up to 40% in the immediate postnatal period.

DIAGNOSIS

The diagnosis of taurine deficiency is based on clinical signs and low plasma and whole blood taurine concentrations. Care must be used when evaluating plasma taurine concentrations because levels may be altered by sample handling errors and feeding. Fasting may reduce plasma taurine concentrations, whereas poor handling may allow taurine contamination from platelets and white blood cells. Although plasma taurine concentrations reflect the labile taurine pool, whole blood taurine concentrations better reflect tissue taurine status. Normal plasma taurine levels in cats may vary up to fivefold (50 to 250 nmol/ml). Plasma taurine values less than 40 nmol/ml may suggest taurine deficiency. Cats with clinical signs of deficiency typically have plasma taurine values less than 10 nmol/ml. Therefore, taurine deficiency is best evaluated using whole blood taurine concentrations. Whole blood taurine levels are normally greater than 300 nmol/ml, and values less than 160 nmol/ml are considered deficient, whereas values less than 50 nmol/ml are common. Samples should be collected and submitted according to protocols recommended by the individual clinical laboratory. Care should be used when collecting blood and plasma for taurine analysis. Falsely elevated plasma taurine levels may result from even small amounts of clotting, hemolysis or inclusion of platelets and white cells in the plasma sample. Use of serum for determining taurine status is not recommended because the quantity of taurine in serum varies with the procedure and the time allotted for coagulation and retraction of the clot.

PATHOPHYSIOLOGY

A central uniform mechanism of taurine action has not been determined, and may not exist. FCRD represents a disruption and loss of the photoreceptor outer segment. Within the retina, taurine may stabilize cell membranes, possibly acting as an antioxidant. In DCM, taurine is thought to regulate myocardial calcium flux through ionic channels, thereby regulating myocardial contractility and/or mitochondrial energy production. Taurine may act as a neuromodulator or neurotransmitter in fetal development. Finally, taurine appears to influence reproduction at the level of the uterus and placenta by unknown mechanisms.

TREATMENT

Cats with taurine deficiency should be supplemented with 250 to 500 mg of taurine twice daily to rapidly replete tissue stores. Cats with DCM may show clinical improvement within one to three weeks, whereas FCRD and developmental defects are irreversible.

PREVENTION

The taurine requirement of cats depends on diet composition. Poor-quality protein, Maillard reaction products or other factors that enhance bacterial overgrowth in the intestinal tract may increase the requirement two- to sixfold. Cats require approximately 50 mg of available taurine per day, which can be supplied by high-quality animal tissues or as a crystalline amino acid supplement. Commercial foods are typically supplemented with taurine in addition to the taurine provided naturally by ingredients. Animal feeding trials are essential to ensure dietary taurine adequacy.

ENDNOTES

a. Pion PD. University of California, Davis, USA. Personal communication. 1994.
b. Rogers QR. University of California, Davis, USA. Personal communication. 1990.

The Bibliography for **Box 19-2** can be found at www.markmorris.org.

than adult females (NRC, 2006). Felinine excretion rates of 95 mg/day have been recorded in intact male cats and may significantly increase the daily sulfur amino acid requirement (Hendriks et al, 1995).

Fat Metabolism

Cats have the ability to digest and use high levels of dietary fat (as is present in animal tissue). Like other true carnivores, cats have a special need for arachidonic acid (AA) (20:4n6) because they have a limited ability to synthesize it from linoleic acid (18:2n6), unlike dogs and other omnivores (MacDonald et al, 1984, 1984a). An exogenous source of AA is especially important for more demanding lifestages, such as gestation, lactation and growth. The basis for this additional requirement is the low hepatic delta-6 desaturase activity in cats (Sinclair et al, 1979). Delta-6 desaturase is the rate-limiting factor in the conversion of linoleic acid to γ-linolenic acid, which is further elongated and desaturated to form AA. AA is abundant in animal tissues, particularly in organ meats and neural tissues, but absent in plants. Thus, the dietary requirement for AA has little consequence if cats consume animal tissues (MacDonald et al, 1984).

Vitamin Metabolism

The vitamin needs of cats differ from those of dogs in several ways. Cats do not convert sufficient amounts of tryptophan to niacin (DaSilva et al, 1952). An animal tissue-based diet is well supplied with niacin from NAD and NADP (nicotinamide-adenine dinucleotide phosphate) coenzymes; therefore, cats don't need to produce niacin from tryptophan. Although cats possess all the enzymes needed for niacin synthesis, the high activity of enzymes in the catabolic pathway (picolinic carboxylase) far exceeds the rate of niacin synthesis (Morris and Rogers, 1983). As a result, the niacin requirement of cats is 2.4 times higher than that of dogs (NRC, 2006).

The prosthetic group of all transaminases is pyridoxine (vitamin B_6) (Stryer, 1975). Cats have high transaminase activities, consistent with consuming a diet from which considerable energy is derived from dietary protein. Therefore, it is logical to expect that their pyridoxine turnover and requirement would be higher than that of omnivores. The pyridoxine requirement of cats is estimated to be 1.7 times higher than that of dogs (NRC, 2006).

Vitamin A occurs naturally only in animal tissue. Plants synthesize vitamin A precursors (e.g., β-carotene). Omnivorous and herbivorous animals can convert β-carotene to vitamin A; cats cannot because they lack intestinal dioxygenase that cleaves β-carotene to retinol. In addition, cats have insufficient 7-dehydrocholesterol in the skin to meet the metabolic need for vitamin D photosynthesis; therefore, they require a dietary source of vitamin D (How et al, 1994, 1994a; Morris, 1996). Vitamin D is relatively abundant in animal liver; therefore, the need for dermal production is minimal and alternate pathways rapidly metabolize 7-dehydrocholesterol. Vitamin D is fairly ubiquitous in animal fats and primary vitamin D deficiency has been identified only in cats fed experimental diets.

Water

Water needs of cats also differ from those of dogs, not because of feline feeding behaviors (i.e., carnivorous vs. omnivorous) but because of their ancestors' adaptation to environmental extremes. Domestic cats are thought to have descended from the African wildcat (*Felis silvestris libyca*), a desert dweller. Several unique features of water balance in cats may be explained by adaptation to a dry environment. Cats are able to survive on less water than dogs and may fail to increase water intake at minor levels of dehydration, up to 4% of body weight (Anderson, 1982). Cats compensate for reduced water intake, in part, by forming highly concentrated urine. Unfortunately, this strong concentrating ability coupled with a weak thirst drive may result in highly saturated urine, increasing the risk of crystalluria or urolithiasis, both components of the feline lower urinary tract disease complex.

Cats consume 1.5 to 2 ml of water/g of dry matter (DM). This 2:1 ratio of water to DM is similar to that of typical prey. This ratio represents approximately 0.5 ml water/kcal ME intake. Practical recommendations for water provision are somewhat higher at 1 ml water/kcal ME. Water ingested from moist foods containing 78 to 82% moisture will result in diuresis.

LIFESTAGE NUTRITION

Lifestage nutrition is the practice of feeding foods designed to meet an animal's optimal nutritional needs at a specific age or physiologic state (e.g., maintenance, reproduction or growth). The concept of lifestage nutrition recognizes that feeding either below or above an optimal nutrient level can negatively affect biologic performance and health (Figure 5-2). This concept differs markedly from feeding a single product for all lifestages (i.e., all-purpose foods), whereby nutrients are added at levels to meet the highest potential need (i.e., usually growth and reproduction). For maximum benefit, risk assessment and preventive plans should begin well before the onset of disease. The value of lifestage nutrition is greater if risk factor management is also incorporated into the feeding practice. A narrower range of nutrient recommendations often emerges when age and physiologic needs are reviewed in conjunction with reducing nutritional risk factors for disease.

Box 19-3. Commercial Treats and Table Foods.

An estimated 41 to 60% of cats are regularly fed table foods and 34% of cats are fed commercial treats.[a] Feeding treats and table food allows more social interaction with the owner, increases diet variety and provides additional caloric intake. Some commercial treats claim dental benefits either by mechanical cleansing or through use of an active ingredient (Chapter 47). When fed in excess, treats and table foods may negatively affect a well-balanced food. Because most commercial cat foods contain vitamins and minerals well above the nutritional needs of cats, table foods and treats fed at less than 10% of the total daily intake should be safe. Providing high-calorie treats or table foods can also contribute to obesity and must be considered in the calculation of total calories for a cat.

MILK

One of the most common human foods offered to cats is milk. Milk is highly palatable and small quantities are well tolerated by most healthy cats. However, after weaning, intestinal lactase activity declines unless milk is a regular part of the diet. Undigested lactose is subject to bacterial fermentation and promotes osmotic diarrhea. Feeding milk to cats unaccustomed to receiving it may overwhelm digestive capacity resulting in diarrhea, flatulence or gastrointestinal distress. Although commercial lactase supplements may alleviate signs of lactose intolerance, lactose avoidance is more prudent for affected cats.

NUTRITIONAL SUPPLEMENTS

Although many supplements are legitimate sources of essential nutrients, others represent food fads that reflect current trends in human nutrition. Poor-quality foods are rarely "fixed" by adding a supplement. Changing to a higher quality food is a more appropriate recommendation and often less expensive.

Calcium

Breeders sometimes provide supplemental calcium during pregnancy, lactation or growth. Additional calcium is rarely necessary, except for cats fed a homemade food or queens with eclampsia, and may lead to nutritional excess or nutrient imbalances in cats fed complete and balanced commercial cat foods.

Chromium

Chromium has been called a "glucose tolerance factor" for its role in normal glucose homeostasis and insulin action in experimental animals. Chromium supplementation promotes lean tissue accretion in growing livestock. Thus, health food stores now stock chromium as an "anti-diabetic" nutrient and "fat-burner" for people. Little information exists about the effect of chromium supplementation in cats. Some caution may be warranted given excess chromium has been associated with chromosomal damage.

Brewer's Yeast/Thiamin

Brewer's yeast and thiamin have been promoted as coat conditioners and flea preventives for dogs and cats. Although brewer's yeast is a good source of B vitamins, particularly thiamin, research has not proven its efficacy as a flea repellent.

RAW MEATS

Breeders and owners commonly feed raw meats to cats. Raw muscle and organ meats are highly palatable, digestible and generally nutritious when supplemented with appropriate vitamins and minerals. Cooking destroys some nutrients and increases the availability of others. A benefit to feeding raw meat to cats has not been documented, and the disadvantages far outweigh any advantages. Raw meat, even when "flash frozen," may contain harmful bacteria (e.g., *Salmonella* spp. and *Escherichia coli*) and parasites (e.g., *Toxoplasma*

Nearly all commercial cat foods meet or exceed the minimum nutrient requirements; however, certain nutrients may still be outside of the desired nutrient range for optimal health. For cats fed commercial foods, these nutrients require particular consideration and, thus, are referred to as nutrients of concern. Specific food factors (e.g., digestibility, texture and effect on urinary pH) can also affect health and risk of disease (Chapter 1). Together, nutrients of concern and specific food factors are called key nutritional factors. Cats eating homemade foods are at greater risk for nutrient deficiencies (e.g., calcium) and excesses (e.g., phosphorus) than those eating commercial foods. Therefore, these cats have a longer list of key nutritional factors, which are discussed in Chapter 10. **Box 19-3** includes information about a variety of popular topics regarding foods for cats including commercial treats, table foods, vegetarian foods and dog foods. The key nutritional factors for different lifestages of healthy cats will be discussed in the following chapters, including those factors associated with reducing the risk of specific diseases and those involved with optimizing performance during different physiologic states. In sequence, these chapters cover Feeding Young Adult Cats: Before Middle Age, Feeding Mature Adult Cats: Middle Aged and Older, Feeding Reproducing Cats, Feeding Nursing and Orphaned Kittens from Birth to Weaning and Feeding Growing Kittens: Postweaning to Adulthood. The chapter about feeding young adult cats is presented first because most pet cats are adults and the nutrient needs of adults serve as a good basis for comparing nutrient needs for reproduction, lactation and growth.

ACKNOWLEDGMENT

The authors and editors acknowledge the contributions of Dr. Claudia A. Kirk in the previous edition of Small Animal Clinical Nutrition.

REFERENCES

The references for **Chapter 19** can be found at www.markmorris.org.

gondii, Cryptosporidium parvum) (Chapter 11). Some of these microbes can also be a health risk for people. Unless supplemented with vitamins and minerals, raw meat is nutritionally incomplete and can lead to nutritional secondary hyperparathyroidism, iodine deficiency or both. Meat mixes composed of large percentages of organ meats may provide excessive levels of vitamin A. Finally, cats fed raw meat diets sometimes develop fixed-food preferences, making subsequent food changes difficult.

FEEDING BONES

Bones are a concentrated source of calcium, phosphorus and magnesium. Steamed bone meal is a very good choice for supplying calcium in homemade or all-meat diets. However, feeding whole bones to cats should be discouraged. Bones with jagged or sharp points are often to blame for oral trauma and can become esophageal foreign bodies. Bone feeding is also associated with colitis and constipation in small animals. Commercial foods approved by the Association of American Feed Control Officials (AAFCO) are replete in calcium, phosphorus and magnesium and should not be supplemented.

VEGETARIAN AND VEGAN DIETS

Although the nutritional needs of cats are best met by a carnivorous diet, vegetarian diets can be designed to provide adequate nutrition. Vegetarian formulas are commercially available and several commercial supplements are available to provide nutrients normally missing, inadequate or poorly available in plant-based diets. The commonly reported pitfalls of commercially available feline vegan diets include taurine, arachidonic acid and vitamin A deficiencies. Several nutrients (below) require special attention in vegetarian formulations.

Protein

Plants are typically low in protein relative to the dietary needs of cats. Additionally, the quality of protein, in many cases, is much lower than protein from animal sources. Concentrated sources of plant protein available to supplement feline foods include isolated soybean protein and corn gluten meal. Care must be taken to feed sufficient protein both to meet the overall nitrogen needs and the minimum requirements of available individual amino acids.

Amino Acids

Taurine is not present in plant ingredients. Therefore, cats fed plant-based foods require taurine supplementation. Chemically synthesized sources of taurine are available from pharmacies and health food stores. Similarly, only animal tissues synthesize carnitine, a vitamin-like amino acid. Although healthy cats do not require dietary carnitine, a dietary source may be conditionally essential during growth or under disease conditions. Synthetic supplements are available. The common limiting amino acids in plants are methionine, lysine and tryptophan. Diets must be closely evaluated to ensure the availability of sufficient quantities of these amino acids. Plant proteins contain large amounts of glutamate. Cats may poorly tolerate high-glutamate foods.

Vitamins

Because cats cannot use β-carotene, pre-formed vitamin A must be supplied in the food. Also, many vitamin A supplements contain vitamin D. All sources of vitamin D should be considered to avoid excess. Vegetarian diets also require supplementation with vitamin B_{12}, which is not supplied by plant ingredients. Vitamin B_{12}-enriched yeast and synthetic supplements are commercially available. Finally, the niacin content of vegetarian diets should be closely evaluated. Although niacin is present in high amounts in many plant ingredients, the availability is often poor and additional supplementation may be required.

Box 19-3 continued

Minerals
Providing adequate calcium is a concern in any homemade food. A variety of calcium supplements are available from health food stores and pharmacies. Many plant ingredients contain components (e.g., fibers or phytates) that severely compromise the availability of certain trace elements. The availability of iron, zinc and copper is of particular concern in high-phytate and high-fiber foods (Chapter 5). These minerals should be provided as a highly available source.

Fat
Of the nutrients required by cats, arachidonic acid is the one not commercially available. To provide arachidonate directly, cats must be given animal fat or tissue as a nutritional source. However, cats can convert γ-linolenic acid (18:3n6) to arachidonic acid (20:4n6) via delta 5-desaturase. γ-linolenic acid is available from plant oils (e.g., borage and evening primrose oils). Prolonged feeding and reproductive trials using γ-linolenic acid have not been reported; thus, the suitability of these oils as long-term arachidonic acid supplements is unknown. Because cats fed foods high in polyunsaturated fatty acids may develop steatitis, cats fed vegetarian foods with large quantities of plant oils should be protected with added vitamin E.

DOG FOOD
Most dog foods are not nutritionally adequate for the maintenance, growth and reproduction of cats. Nutrients most likely to be deficient are protein, taurine, niacin, vitamin B_6, methionine and choline. Clinical signs of deficiency depend on which nutrients are deficient and to what degree.

FOOD TOXINS
Food toxicities are relatively infrequent in cats. Most notable is hemolytic anemia caused by onion toxicity. Certain disulfides found in onions promote oxidative damage to cat hemoglobin, resulting in Heinz body production and red cell removal. The toxic compound appears to be highly stable, because it remains active in cooked onion-based broth and onion powder. Hemolytic anemia has been described in a cat fed commercial baby food containing onion powder. Onion toxicity was not proved but the anemia resolved with a diet change. Subsequent studies have demonstrated toxic effects at levels of 2.5% dry matter. Therefore, it is prudent to avoid feeding food or seasonings containing onion powder or onions. Chapter 11 provides more information about foodborne toxins.

Theobromine
Theobromine is a toxic methylxanthine found in chocolate. The clinical signs of toxicity include vomiting, diarrhea, vascular collapse and death. The oral LD_{50} of theobromine is 200 mg/kg body weight. Approximately 40 to 50 g of cocoa would need to be consumed to provide this dose of theobromine, which is undoubtedly why clinical reports of chocolate toxicoses in cats are rare.

Histamine
Histamine is a primary amine arising from the decarboxylation of histidine. Histamine toxicosis has been reported to occur in cats after ingestion of certain species of spoiled fish. Affected cats developed salivation, vomiting and diarrhea about 30 minutes after eating uncooked anchovies. Myosis, lacrimation, tachypnea and tachycardia were evident upon physical examination. A survey detailing the histamine content of North American cat foods found foods were well below the 500 mg/g (wet/weight) level considered hazardous in people. Thus, histamine toxicosis is most likely to occur in cats fed improperly handled fish that has undergone spoilage.

ENDNOTE
a. Kirk CA. Unpublished data. 1992.

The Bibliography for **Box 19-3** can be found at www.markmorris.org.

Chapter 20

Feeding Young Adult Cats: Before Middle Age

Kathy L. Gross
Iveta Becvarova
P. Jane Armstrong
Jacques Debraekeleer

"In a cat's eyes, all things belong to cats."
English Proverb

INTRODUCTION

Cats generally reach adulthood between 10 to 12 months of age and, not uncommonly, live up to 20 years or more. The span of time from 12 months to death represents the total adult life of cats. After approximately six to eight years of age, however, there is an increasing prevalence of age-related diseases and onset of mild behavioral, physical and metabolic changes related to aging. In this chapter, the term "young adult" refers to non-reproducing cats one to six or seven years of age. The term "mature adult" (Chapter 21) refers to cats seven or eight years of age (beginning of middle age) and older.

The feeding goals for young adult pet cats include ensuring that the food fed and the feeding methods used will help maximize health, longevity and quality of life (disease prevention). Nutritional requirements for young adult cats tend to be the most broadly defined of any lifestage. This is partly because healthy young adult cats have the greatest ability to tolerate or compensate for metabolic and physiologic perturbations. Most regulated commercial foods provide all the necessary nutrients in amounts that avoid deficiencies (Chapters 5 and 6). To achieve the feeding goals described above, however, nutritional recommendations must go beyond simple prevention of nutrient deficiencies.

Nutritional recommendations for people who live in affluent societies include advice about nutrients, non-nutrient food ingredients and caloric intake guidelines for the prevention of important diseases such as obesity, diabetes mellitus, cardiovascular diseases, cancer, Alzheimer's disease and others. Although much remains to be learned in terms of the role of nutrients in feline disease prevention, optimal nutrient recommendations for young adult cats should also include recommendations based on our current understanding of nutrient and non-nutrient ingredients and feeding guidelines to help prevent important diseases of cats. **Table 20-1** lists relevant health issues for young adult cats that have a known nutritional association and which may be positively influenced by feeding for disease prevention.

PATIENT ASSESSMENT

The purpose of assessing the patient is to confirm the feeding goals, recognize risk factors for diseases (**Table 20-1**) and become acquainted with the associated key nutritional factors.

Table 20-1. Important diseases for adult cats that have nutritional associations.

Disease/health concern	Incidence/prevalence/mortality/pet owner concern	References*
Dental disease	Most prevalent disease; numerous associated health issues	Lund et al, 1999
Obesity	Approximate 30% prevalence; numerous associated health issues; neutered and indoor cats are at increased risk	Lund et al, 1999
FLUTD	0.85 to 1.5% per year incidence; 3% prevalence; most common reason cat owners seek veterinary care; kidney/urinary diseases are the most common cat owner concerns	Lawler et al, 1985; Lund et al, 1999; Willeberg, 1984; Westropp et al, 2005; Hostutler et al, 2005; Anon, Vet Economics, 2005; MAF, 2005
Kidney disease	Second leading cause of non-accidental death; kidney/urinary diseases are the most common cat owner concerns	Polzin et al, 2005; Ross et al, 2006; MAF, 1998, 2005
Cancer	Leading cause of non-accidental death	MAF, 1998
Arthritis	Incidence in general population unknown, but 22% in cats over one year of age in one study; overweight cats are three times likelier to have arthritis	Godfrey, 2005; Scarlett and Donoghue, 1998

Key: FLUTD = feline lower urinary tract disease.

*The references for **Table 20-1** can be found at www.markmorris.org.

Table 20-2. Factors to consider during nutritional assessment.

Signalment	Dietary history	Weight history	Physical examination	Diagnostic studies
Activity level	Adverse food reactions	Current weight	Body condition	Albumin
Age	Amount eaten	Ideal weight	Bone structure	Creatine kinase
Breed	Amount offered	Percent weight change	Coat condition	Hematocrit
Disease status	Appetite (interest)	Rate of change	Eyes	Hemoglobin
Environment	Brand fed	Usual weight	Hydration	Lymphocyte count
Gender	Feeding method		Muscle mass	Potassium
Reproductive status	Feeding schedule		Oral health	Prothrombin time
Use	Food aversions		Skin condition	Serum urea nitrogen
	Food storage		Strength/activity	Sodium
	Food form (e.g., dry, moist)			
	Nutritional losses			
	Previous foods			
	Supplements			
	Treats			
	Water availability			

(See below.) Assessment includes the complete evaluation of the patient and its environment (**Table 20-2**). Information from the signalment (age, breed, gender and neuter status), history and physical examination should be incorporated into nutritional recommendations.

History and Physical Examination

Key features from the signalment and history include the age, gender, activity level, weight history, environment (indoor vs. outdoor) and hunting history. Differences in these factors influence energy requirements and risks for certain diseases. The initial dietary history for healthy young adult cats should establish the brand, type and amount of foods fed regularly, including treats, table foods and nutritional supplements. The feeding method (including the amount fed) and appetite should be noted as well as any recent changes in body weight and stool quality. The extent of the evaluation depends on preliminary findings. A more detailed dietary history may be required if significant abnormalities are uncovered during the history or physical examination (e.g., anorexia, unexplained weight loss, poor diet, etc.). A detailed dietary history should evaluate the factors listed in **Table 20-2**.

If the dietary history is perceived to be incomplete, it may prove useful to have owners continue to feed and medicate their cat as usual and record amounts, types and brands of all foods and supplements given for one to two weeks. Such dietary records help better define nutrient intake, nutritional problems and errors in feeding management.

A thorough physical examination should include a systematic evaluation of each body system. Special attention should be given to the oral cavity, hydration status, skin and coat condition, body weight and body condition score (BCS) (Chapter 1). Careful observation is needed to assess lean body mass, muscle tone and body composition. Apparent loss of lean body mass may indicate recent weight loss, nutritional deficiency or disease, even in obese cats. For example, a study of 57 cats with neoplasia documented that fat mass was reduced in 60% of the patients and muscle mass was reduced in 91% (Baez et al, 2007). Any physical abnormalities should be correlated to the signalment and history to pinpoint issues that require further exploration. Important diseases or health issues that have either a direct or indirect nutritional association include the conditions listed in **Table 20-1**. Some of these data come from epidemiologic studies. Unfortunately, this type of study can only show an association and cannot prove causality. Most of the time these conditions won't be present and the focus will be on their prevention.

Age
Aging in healthy cats is associated with metabolic changes that affect nutritional recommendations. Overlaid on these changes are the concerns of age-associated diseases. There are specific nutrient and/or ingredient considerations for foods intended for young adult cats, especially with respect to weight control, lower urinary tract health, dental health, cancer, arthritis and subclinical kidney disease (VPI Pet Insurance, 2007; Ross et al, 2006; Lund et al, 2005, 1999; Godfrey, 2005; Polzin et al, 2005) (**Table 20-1**).

Breed
Although different breeds of cats may have varying nutritional requirements, the variation is less pronounced than that of dog breeds. Certain feline breeds (e.g., Abyssinians) are noted for their lively, rambunctious disposition, whereas others (e.g., Persians or ragdolls) tend to be quiet and tranquil (Pugnetti, 1983). Thus, disposition affects energy requirements among breeds. In the future, it is possible that other nutritional variances may be elucidated with continued research into specific requirements of different cat breeds. Currently, some commercial foods are marketed for various cat breeds, but no published data exist to support specific nutrient requirements by breed.

Gender/Neuter Status
Small differences in body composition and energy intake between male and female adult cats have been reported (Jewell et al, 1996). The differences in energy intake appear to be due to gender-related differences in lean body mass (Jewell et al, 1996; Klausen et al, 1997). Risk factors for certain diseases vary by gender; however, these differences are less than the individual variation between cats and rarely warrant a gender-specific nutritional plan. Exceptions include reproducing (Chapter 22) and neutered cats.

Neutering increases the risk of overweight and obesity. Neutered cats are more likely to be overweight than intact cats of either sex (Lund et al, 2005; Scarlett et al, 1994; Root, 1995; Flynn et al, 1996). Chapter 27 reviews probable mechanisms.

Nutritional counseling should be provided to owners at the time that cats are brought to the veterinarian for neutering. Although most cats are apparently able to maintain a healthy BCS (2.5/5 to 3.5/5) after neutering, feeding controlled amounts of low-energy foods reduces the risk for obesity (Scarlett et al, 1994) and should be a routine postneutering recommendation (Laflamme, 2006). Kittens neutered at less than six months of age should be fed foods designed for growth until they reach skeletal maturity (between eight and 10 months of age). Many foods designed for growing kittens are energy dense; therefore, portion control and regular monitoring of body condition is recommended.

Environment/Activity Level
The daily energy requirement (DER) for cats may be markedly altered when ambient temperatures deviate significantly from their thermoneutral zone (NRC, 2006). Behavioral responses usually compensate for minor deviations in temperature with little effect on a cat's water or energy needs. Temperatures low enough to cause shivering (5 to 8°C [41 to 46.4°F]), however, can increase a cat's DER to 2 to 5 x resting energy requirement (RER) (Hensel and Banet, 1982; Precht et al, 1973).

Cats kept in hot environments (>38°C [>100.4°F]) may initially reduce food intake by 15 to 40%; however, as respiratory rate and grooming behavior increase and panting begins, the requirements for calories and water increase. Water is critically important to prevent heat stress in hot environments. Heat-stressed cats pant and wet their coats with saliva to maximize cooling via evaporative water loss. Dehydrated cats have a 50% reduction in ability to use evaporative water loss for thermoregulation (Doris and Baker, 1981). Significant elevations of core body temperature may occur with loss of evaporative cooling. Owners should be advised to monitor body condition and adjust feeding protocols as needed to meet these changing demands.

Cats thrive in ambient conditions of low humidity and warm temperatures (Pedersen, 1991). National Institutes of Health (NIH) and United States Department of Agriculture (USDA) guidelines for feline housing recommend humidity between 30 to 70%, room temperatures between 18 to 29°C (64.4 to 84.2°F) and 10 to 15 air exchanges/hour (ventilation) (Guide for the Care and Use of Laboratory Animals, 1996; APHIS, 1985). Practical options to the NIH and USDA recommendations are temperatures between 10 to 29.5°C (50 to 85°F) and humidity levels between 10 to 50% (Pedersen and Wastlhuber, 1991). Energy requirements change very little within these ranges.

Multi-cat environments refer to individual households with two or more cats; however, the definition also includes catteries, shelters and research institutions. Cats are solitary animals; therefore, multi-cat environments can lead to social and psychological stress, particularly if there is overcrowding (Hart and Pedersen, 1991). Households with more than five cats appear to be at increased risk for problems typically associated with multi-cat households including changes in food intake, behavioral problems and infectious diseases such as feline leukemia (Beaver, 1992).

The combination of chronic stress, overcrowding, poor ventilation and inadequate nutrition makes infectious diseases very difficult to control. Unsanitary litter boxes can result in elevated environmental ammonia concentrations that impair health (Pedersen and Wastlhuber, 1991). Stress levels in multi-cat environments may be reduced by modifying the environment to include safe outdoor areas (See Box 27-8 for cat-proof fencing.), multilevel indoor and outdoor resting areas, visual barriers and quiet hiding spots where cats can retreat from unwanted social interactions.

Stressed cats may exhibit partial or complete anorexia. Less

Table 20-3. Key nutritional factors for foods for young adult cats.

Factors	Recommended food levels* Normal weight	Inactive/ obese prone
Energy density (kcal ME/g)	4.0-5.0	3.3-3.8
Energy density (kJ ME/g)	16.7-20.9	13.8-15.9
Fat (%)	10-30	9-17
Fiber (%)	<5	5-15
Protein (%)	30-45	30-45
Phosphorus (%)	0.5-0.8	0.5-0.8
Sodium (%)	0.2-0.6	0.2-0.6
Chloride (%)	1.5 x Na	1.5 x Na
Magnesium (%)	0.04-0.1	0.04-0.1
Average urinary pH	6.2-6.4	6.2-6.4
Antioxidants		
Vitamin E (IU/kg)	≥500	≥500
Vitamin C (mg/kg)	100-200	100-200
Selenium (mg/kg)	0.5-1.3	0.5-1.3
VOHC Seal of Acceptance	Plaque control	Plaque control

Key: ME = metabolizable energy, VOHC = Veterinary Oral Health Council (Chapter 47).
*Dry matter basis. Concentrations presume an energy density of 4.0 kcal/g. Levels should be corrected for foods with higher energy densities. Adjustment is unnecessary for foods with lower energy densities.

commonly, overeating and resultant weight gains are reported consequences of stress (Beaver, 1992). Short-term bouts of anorexia (i.e., one to three days) have little overall effect on otherwise healthy young adult cats, although metabolic changes are evident by the third day of fasting (Biourge et al, 1994; Pazak, 1997). A prolonged reduction in food intake in healthy cats or short-term food deprivation in sick cats can lead to undernourishment and increased risk of hepatic lipidosis.

Challenges associated with feeding cats in a multi-cat environment include difficulty in monitoring food and water intake, ensuring all cats have unfettered access to food and providing specialized foods to individual cats. Obtaining accurate dietary histories and achieving good dietary compliance for cats from multi-cat households can be challenging for veterinarians and owners. However, modification of feeding and management practices can alleviate many problems.

Activity level is one of the key determinants of DER. By nature, cats do not participate in heavy work or endurance-type activities, thus the variation in energy requirement between active and sedentary cats is small compared with that of dogs. Nevertheless, twofold differences in energy requirement have been observed between active and sedentary cats (Earle and Smith, 1991; Finke and Lutschaunig, 1995).

Most, but not all cats confined indoors are minimally active. Although most indoor cats have "run of the house," some indoor housing includes confinement to small areas (e.g., caging in hospitals, kennels, animal shelters or catteries). Activity is markedly limited under these circumstances as reflected by lower energy requirements. Thus, sedentary, inactive and caged cats often have DERs very near or even below the average RER (0.8 to 1.2 x RER) or 40 to 60 kcal/kg body weight/day (167 to 251 kJ/kg body weight/day) (Flynn et al, 1996; Earle and Smith, 1991) and may be as low as 24 kcal/kg body weight/day (100 kJ/kg body weight/day) (Hoenig et al, 2007). Therefore, indoor cats have an increased prevalence of overweight and obesity. They also are more likely to have hairballs and calcium oxalate urolithiasis (Lund et al, 1999).

Cats housed outdoors have less protection from the environment and temperature fluctuations and are presumably more active than indoor cats. As a result, the optimal food and feeding methods may differ for outdoor cats. Cats allowed unlimited activity may have energy needs 10 to 15% above average (Miller and Allison, 1958). Very active cats may expend markedly more energy than other cats. For example, the energy requirement of Abyssinian cats has been reported as 79 kcal/kg body weight/day (330 kJ/kg body weight/day), or 1.6 x RER, which is 30% greater than that required by the average adult housecat (Finke and Lutschaunig, 1995).

Both food selection (i.e., energy content) and amount fed should match activity levels and are important to prevent overweight or obesity.

Laboratory and Other Clinical Information

Laboratory analyses provide limited insight into nutritional status but can be very helpful in excluding disease processes. Special diagnostic tests (e.g., plasma aminograms, clotting profiles, urinary clearance ratios and hormone assays) may help assess specific disease processes or specific deficiencies such as Vitamin K deficiency. Fecal analysis for intestinal parasites is routinely performed for healthy young adult cats, although malnutrition from intestinal parasitism occurs rarely.

Key Nutritional Factors

Table 20-3 summarizes key nutritional factors for young adult cats. The sections that follow review key nutritional factors in more detail.

Water

Although water is the most important nutrient for cats, a definitive water requirement has been not established because: 1) cats adjust water intake to the dry matter (DM) content of the food and 2) the water requirement of cats varies with physiologic and environmental conditions. Generally, cats need 1 ml water/kcal metabolizable energy (ME) requirement. In practice, adult cats should have unlimited access to fresh water. Although cats conserve total body water by forming highly concentrated urine, such concentrated urine is undesirable in the prevention and treatment of feline lower urinary tract disease (FLUTD). Increased water intake is useful for managing urolithiasis by reducing the urinary concentration of urolith-forming minerals. To date, of all treatments evaluated, feeding moist food (>60% of calories) was the only one associated with a statistically significant decrease in recurrence of clinical signs in cats with feline idiopathic cystitis (FIC). Currently, FIC is the most common cause of FLUTD (Lekcharoensuk et al, 2001; Gerber et al, 2005) (Chapter 46). Feeding moist foods (vs. dry foods) increases water intake and urine volume in most cats (Gaskell, 1989), but unlike dogs, cats do not fully compensate for differences in food moisture content by altering free water intake. When allowed free access to water, the total water intake of cats eating dry food is only half that of cats eating moist food (Burger et al, 1980; Seefeldt and Chapman, 1979).

Energy

Determination of DER for a population of cats results in a bell-shaped curve (Figure 1-5). Individual cats may have energy requirements 50% or more above or below the average requirement. This range is not surprising considering that the DER of a particular cat is influenced by differences in lean body mass, gender, neuter status, environmental temperature, genetic traits, housing and activity level. Despite the relative uniformity of size within the domestic cat population, there are size-associated differences in energy requirements. Generally, smaller cats consume more calories per kg body weight than larger cats (Earle and Smith, 1991; Finke and Lutschaunig, 1995). Thus, it is important to remember that calculated energy requirements are only estimates for individual cats. The true caloric requirement for an individual cat is what is needed to maintain an ideal body condition (BCS 2.5/5 to 3.5/5) and stable weight.

Data in the literature indicate that, under a variety of conditions, the DER of young adult cats ranges widely from 31 to 100 kcal/kg body weight/day (129 to 418 kJ/kg body weight/day) (NRC, 2006). However, the DER of average young adult pet cats is more likely to range between 40 to 75 kcal/kg body weight/day (167 to 314 kJ/kg body weight/day) or approximately 1.0 to 1.6 x RER, where RER in kcal = $70(BW_{kg})^{0.75}$ or RER in kJ = $293(BW_{kg})^{0.75}$. A simple linear formula can also be used to estimate RER for cats weighing more than 2 kg: RER is approximately 70 kcal + 30 kcal x BW_{kg} (293 kJ + 125.5 kJ x BW_{kg}) (Lewis et al, 1987). Table 5-2 lists RER values for body weights greater than 1.5 kg. Caloric requirements for active neutered cats are calculated using the lower end of the range (1.2 x RER), whereas the upper end of the range (1.4 to 1.6 x RER) is used for active and sexually intact cats. Most housecats are neutered and are minimally active (NRC, 2006) and, therefore, are more prone to overweight and obesity. Thus, it is prudent to use 1.0 x RER or 39 to 66 kcal/kg body weight/day [163 to 276 kJ/kg body weight/day]) (Earle and Smith, 1991) as a starting point for most housecats and increasing their energy intake, if necessary, to maintain ideal body condition. This same starting point, 1.0 x RER, is recommended when calculating the energy needed for maintenance at ideal body weight for an obese cat. Obese cats may require as few as 0.8 x RER or 44 to 54 kcal/kg ideal body weight (184 to 226 kJ/kg ideal body weight/day) to achieve an average weight loss of 1% of body weight per week (LaFlamme and Jackson, 1995) (Chapter 27). After obese cats have returned to their original lean weight, as few as 24 kcal/kg body weight (100 kJ/kg body weight) may be needed for maintenance (Hoenig et al, 2007). Controlling energy intake is important for managing and preventing obesity. Approximately 35% of adult cats seen by veterinarians in the United States are overweight or obese (Lund et al, 2005). The prevalence is highest in seven- to eight-year-old cats; nearly 50% of this age group are overweight or obese (BCS 4/5 or 5/5) (Scarlett et al, 1994; Lund et al, 1999). Obesity increases the risk of death in young to middle-aged cats 2.7 times above that of lean cats (Scarlett and Donoghue, 1997); thus, preventing obesity has important consequences for long-term health (Chapter 27). Risk factors associated with obesity include: 1) middle age, 2) male gender, 3) neutering, 4) low activity/indoor/apartment dwelling and 4) feeding high-fat, high-calorie foods free choice (Lund et al, 2005; Scarlett et al, 1994). Food digestibility and energy density may influence the risk for FLUTD. Energy-dense foods reduce overall DM intake. Lower DM intake decreases stool volume, which subsequently reduces fecal water loss. Both features reduce total magnesium intake and increase urine volume. Food intake should be controlled when feeding high-calorie foods. Excessive intake of calorically-dense foods coupled with free-choice feeding can induce obesity, also a risk factor for urolithiasis.

The recommended range of energy density in foods for inactive/obese-prone young adult cats is 3.3 to 3.8 kcal/g (13.8 to 15.9 kJ/g) (DM). The recommended range for foods for normal weight young adult cats is 4.0 to 5.0 kcal/g (16.7 to 20.9 kJ/g).

Fat

Cats use dietary fat for energy, as a source of essential fatty acids and to facilitate absorption of fat-soluble vitamins. A minimum requirement for fat has not been established for cats although foods containing less than 5% DM fat have been fed successfully to hyperlipidemic cats. The minimum recommended DM allowance of fat in adult cat foods is 9% (NRC, 2006). Fat levels above 9.0% DM are recommended for most cats. Fat enhances the palatability of food; cats prefer foods with levels near 25% DM fat vs. foods containing 10 or 50% DM fat (Kane et al, 1981). High-fat foods have been associated with an increased incidence of obesity in cats (Scarlett et al, 1994). Most cats do well when fed foods containing 10 to 30% DM fat. Cats prone to obesity, however, should be fed foods with lower levels of dietary fat (9 to 17% DM).

Current AAFCO allowances for the essential fatty acids, linoleic acid and arachidonic acid (AA), are appropriate for adult cats (2007). Therefore, commercial foods that have AAFCO label statements acknowledging that a food is appropriate for adult maintenance should provide adequate amounts of linoleic acid and AA. **Box 20-1** discusses the role of omega-3 (n-3) fatty acids in foods for adult cats.

Fiber

Although cats do not require dietary fiber, small amounts in commercial foods enhance stool quality and promote normal gastrointestinal (GI) function. The natural foods of cats typically contain less than 1% dietary fiber although much higher levels are well tolerated (Vondruska, 1987; Dimski and Buffington, 1991). Fiber concentrations less than 5% DM are recommended for normal young adult cats. Because increased levels of dietary fiber reduce energy density and can induce satiety, obese-prone cats may benefit from foods that contain from 5 to 15% DM crude fiber (Chapter 27). Fiber supplementation may also benefit cats that are prone to develop hairballs.

Box 20-1. The Emerging Role of Omega-3 Fatty Acids in Feline Nutrition.

Fatty acids of the omega-3 (n-3) series (linolenic acid, 18:3n-3) are probably required in the food of all animals. However, studies establishing requirements for omega-3 fatty acids in adult cats have not been performed. Cats would normally consume omega-3 fatty acids when eating the neural tissues of their prey. The role of omega-3 fatty acids in companion animal medicine has focused mostly on their pharmacologic-like properties and ability to modulate the immune response and inflammation associated with dermatitis, arthritis, cancer and obesity. Although these effects may benefit some animals, untoward effects are possible. In one study, cats developed increased bleeding times and decreased platelet function when fed foods supplemented with high levels of omega-3 fatty acids. However, no adverse effects were found in similar studies. The current understanding of omega-3 fatty acid metabolism in cats is limited; thus, aggressive omega-3 fatty acid supplementation should be used judiciously. The recommended dry matter allowance for omega-3 fatty acids in foods for healthy adult cats is 0.01% (total eicosapentaenoic and docosahexaenoic acids).

The Bibliography for **Box 20-1** can be found at www.markmorris.org.

Clinical evidence and field trials have demonstrated a reduction in the frequency of hairball vomiting with fiber supplementation (Hoffman and Tetrick, 2003; Dann et al, 2004).

Protein

The protein requirements of adult cats have generally been established using experimental foods containing essential amino acids at or above the minimum requirement for growth. From these studies, the National Research Council (2006) suggested the minimum protein requirement for adult cats is 16% and the minimum recommended allowance is 20% (DM, food energy content of 4 kcal/g [16.7 kJ/g]). Commercial foods prepared from natural ingredients and processed may have lower protein digestibility than the experimental foods used to establish these minimums. To provide a margin of safety and account for differences in protein quality, the Association of American Feed Control Officials (AAFCO) has suggested a minimum dietary protein level of 26% DM for adult maintenance (2007). Protein and amino acid requirements vary with the energy content of a food. The minimum protein allowance suggested by AAFCO is based on foods containing 4.0 kcal/g (16.7 kJ/g) DM and should be corrected for foods with energy densities greater than 4.5 kcal/g (18.8 kJ/g). (See Chapter 1 for the correction method.)

Meeting the minimum protein needs of cats is critical because they have minimal capacity to adapt to low levels of dietary protein. Protein in excess of the requirement is rapidly catabolized and used to provide energy and maintain blood glucose levels. Any excess energy will be stored as fat; therefore, there appears to be little benefit to feeding large excesses of protein to cats. Furthermore, dietary protein excess may increase proteinuria and the progression of subclinical renal disease (Adams et al, 1994; Brown et al, 1997; Ross, 1992). Similar to findings in people and dogs, the role of protein in the progression of renal disease in cats is controversial. There is, however, strong (Grade 1, [See Chapter 2]) evidence to support the recommendation to feed a veterinary therapeutic food designed for kidney disease to cats with serum creatinine concentrations in excess of 2 mg/dl (stage mid-II through IV chronic kidney disease [CKD]) (Polzin et al, 2008; Ross et al, 2006; Elliot et al, 2000). The point being that, among other things, these foods are typically lower in protein.

Although cats can be fed vegetable-based foods, most protein in the food should be derived from animal tissues. The amino acid profile of most animal tissues better reflects the nutritional requirements of cats. Moist products should list animal-based ingredients within the first two ingredients (excluding water), whereas dry products should list animal-based ingredients in the first three ingredients. The recommended DM protein allowance for both normal weight and inactive/obese-prone young adult cats is 30 to 45%. Current AAFCO allowances for taurine are appropriate for adult cats (2007). Foods that have AAFCO label statements acknowledging that a food is appropriate for adult maintenance should provide adequate amounts. Therefore, taurine, although a very important nutrient for cats, is considered an "other" nutritional factor and is discussed under that heading below.

Phosphorus

Dietary phosphorus levels of 0.5 to 0.8% DM are recommended for young adult cats. The minimum recommended allowance for phosphorus in foods for adult cats is 0.26% DM (NRC, 2006). Deficiencies of phosphorus are rare in cats fed commercial foods. Phosphorus excess appears to be of greater concern. Dietary phosphorus is a key nutrient in the management of two common feline diseases: struvite-mediated FLUTD and CKD. The mineral constituents of struvite are magnesium, ammonium and phosphate. Although the primary objectives for preventing FLUTD due to struvite precipitates are to increase urine volume, reduce urinary pH and, to a lesser extent, restrict dietary magnesium, limiting dietary phosphorus may be beneficial (Chapter 46). The kidneys excrete excess dietary phosphorus. The risk of clinically apparent struvite crystalluria and urolithiasis is highest in cats from two to five years of age. Controlling phosphorus intake in combination with appropriate reductions in dietary magnesium concentrations and urinary pH, and increasing water intake, if possible, should help reduce the risk of struvite-associated FLUTD in cats of this age group.

Excess dietary phosphorus is not considered a cause of renal damage but may accelerate the progression of renal disease towards failure and death (Ross et al, 1982). High levels of dietary phosphorus (1.2 to 1.8% DM) reduce creatinine clearance values and possibly reduce renal function in young, healthy cats (Pastoor et al, 1995). Excess phosphorus should be avoided in the early nutritional management of renal disease in cats to decrease the renal excretory workload and avoid phosphorus retention (Chapter 37). The evidence for recommending a phosphorus-restricted food for cats with CKD, however, is weak. Studies in dogs on the specific effect of phosphorus intake on clinical outcome in induced CKD have shown that dietary phosphorus restriction slows progression and improves survival. Similar studies have not been reported in cats. Phosphorus restriction has been shown, however, to reduce renal mineralization in cats with induced CKD (Polzin et al, 2008). Dietary phosphorus may be reduced as low as 0.3% DM in cats with overt renal disease.

Sodium and Chloride

The minimum sodium requirement for adult cats is 0.065% DM; the minimum recommended allowance is not much greater (0.068%) (NRC, 2006). The average sodium content of prey is relatively low (i.e., approximately 0.25% DM in whole rat carcasses) (Vondruska, 1987). Sodium concentrations from 0.2 to 0.6% DM satisfy the needs of healthy young adult cats without providing excessive levels. In people, limiting sodium intake to levels that meet the requirement without significant excess reduces the risk of hypertension and is considered important to long-term health (Stamler, 1995). This same nutritional practice has been advocated for cats. In a study involving feline hypertension, nearly 50% of hypertensive cats fed a low-sodium food had a significant reduction in blood pressure (Littman, 1994). This response is similar to that seen in people in that not all people are "salt-sensitive." In cats, hypertension is commonly associated with diseases such as renal failure, hyperthyroidism and cardiac disease (Cowgill and Kallet, 1986; Kobayashi et al, 1990). High blood pressure has been associated with significant end-organ damage in hypertensive cats. Blindness, retinal hemorrhage, stroke, cardiac dilatation and murmurs and renal damage were common findings among cats studied (Littman, 1994). Thus, as it relates to cats with hypertension, avoiding excess sodium chloride seems prudent because: 1) hypertension has significant deleterious health effects, 2) diagnostics to detect hypertension are not commonly performed and 3) the medical conditions associated with hypertension are common in cats.

Dietary sodium chloride supplementation is used in commercial cat foods to reduce the occurrence of FLUTD by increasing water intake. Sodium chloride added at concentrations of 4% DM or greater markedly enhanced water intake and increased urine volume (Burger et al, 1980). Short-term studies have shown adult cats tolerate a wide range of dietary sodium intakes (i.e., 0.04 to 2.0%) (MacDonald et al, 1984; NRC, 2006; Burger et al, 1980). A longer-term study (three months) evaluated the safety of salt supplementation (0.35% vs. 1.1% sodium and 0.7% vs. 2.06% chloride, DM) in normal, obese, aged cats and cats with pre-existing CKD. In this study, none of the cats were hypertensive at the beginning of the study and blood pressure was unaffected when they were fed the high-salt food. Cats with pre-existing kidney disease fed the salt-supplemented food, however, experienced increased serum urea nitrogen, phosphorus and creatinine concentrations, suggesting progressive deterioration of renal function. Because apparently healthy cats can have a significant degree of undetected renal dysfunction when screened routinely with biochemistry profiles, it would follow that the risks associated with feeding high-sodium chloride foods to reduce the occurrence of FLUTD outweigh the benefits (Kirk et al, 2006).

Furthermore, in addition to possibly exacerbating hypertensive disorders and contributing to the progression of pre-existing renal disease, high dietary sodium levels reportedly enhance urinary calcium excretion (Osborne et al, 1992), particularly in cats with impaired renal function (Kirk et al, 2006). This may explain the common occurrence of calcium oxalate uroliths in cats with kidney disease. Thus, sodium excess, particularly in the form of sodium chloride, should be avoided in adult cats.

Chloride has been implicated more recently as a major determinant in the development of hypertension in salt-sensitive people. The interaction of sodium with chloride appears to cause the greatest increase in blood pressure compared with sodium combined with other anions (Kurtz et al, 1987) (Chapter 36). The minimum chloride requirement has been determined for kittens but not adult cats. The NRC recommended allowance for adult cats (0.096% DM) is based on kitten data (2006). Typically, dietary chloride recommendations are 1.5 times dietary sodium recommendations.

Magnesium

The minimum magnesium requirement for adult cats is 4.1 mg/100 kcal (9.7 mg/MJ or 0.016% DM) (Pastoor, 1993). The NRC minimum requirement is 0.02% (DM, 4 kcal/g) and the minimum recommended allowance is 0.04% (DM, 4 kcal ME/g [16.7 kJ/g]) (2006). Excessive magnesium restriction may be associated with the prevalence of calcium oxalate uroliths in cats (Thumchai et al, 1996). Therefore, excessive restriction of magnesium (i.e., $<0.04\%$ DM) is not recommended. For practical purposes, a magnesium content between 0.04 to 0.1% DM is recommended in foods for young adult cats (**Table 20-3**). These levels are similar to those found in the natural food of cats. Magnesium concentrations of 0.08% DM were measured in whole rat carcasses (Vondruska, 1987). Magnesium is an essential nutrient, but is also a major constituent of struvite crystals. To reduce the risk of FLUTD due to struvite, dietary magnesium concentrations should be less than 20 mg/100 kcal of food ($<0.10\%$ DM) and the food should be formulated to produce the appropriate urinary pH (Chapter 46).

Urinary pH

Food ingredients and feeding methods contribute to the urinary pH produced by cats. The normal urinary pH of cats eating mice and rats is 6.2 to 6.4 (Hand et al, 1988). Thus, 6.2 to 6.4 is considered the "normal acidic urinary pH" of cats fed a wild-type food and the recommended range for healthy young adult cats.

The risk of struvite precipitation and FLUTD is greatly reduced at urinary pH values less than 6.5 (Buffington, 1991). Many cats develop metabolic acidosis when the urinary pH

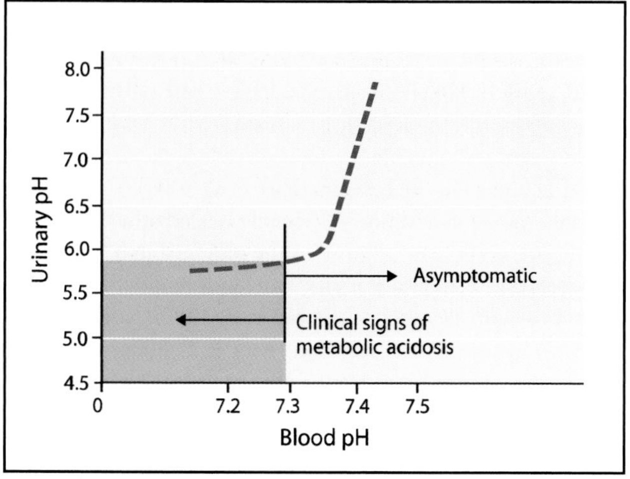

Figure 20-1. Correlation between urinary and blood pH in cats. Many cats develop metabolic acidosis when urinary pH is consistently less than 6.0. (Adapted from Allen TA, Bartges JW, Cowgill LD, et al. Colloquium on Urology. Feline Practice 1997; 25: 32.)

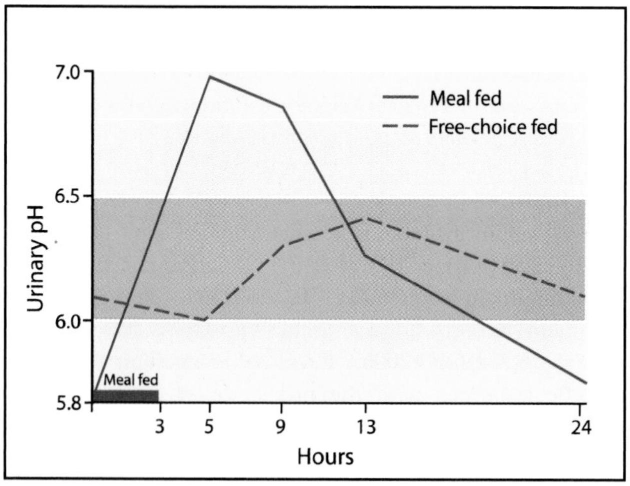

Figure 20-2. Effect of feeding method on urinary pH in cats. Note the significant increase in urinary pH after a single meal (meal fed). This effect is termed "postprandial alkaline tide." Food provided free choice modulates urinary pH by dampening the postprandial alkaline tide that occurs three to six hours following ingestion of larger meals. The shaded area represents the acceptable urinary pH range for adult cats. (Adapted from Taton GF, Hamar D, Lewis LD. Evaluation of ammonium chloride as a urinary acidifier in the cat. Journal of the American Veterinary Medical Association 1984; 184: 433-436.)

is less than 6.0 (**Figure 20-1**) (Dow et al, 1990). Metabolic acidosis may promote bone demineralization, urinary calcium and potassium loss (Ching et al, 1989, 1990) and increase the risk of calcium oxalate urolithiasis (Thumchai et al, 1996; Kirk et al, 1995). Free-choice food intake modulates urinary pH by dampening the postprandial alkaline tide that occurs three to six hours following larger meals. Meal feeding promotes a much greater alkaline tide and higher average urinary pH (**Figure 20-2**). Commercial foods commonly balance dietary cations and anions to achieve an appropriate urinary pH. Animal proteins, corn gluten meal, certain mineral salts, methionine and phosphoric acid are common ingredients that reduce urinary pH when added to feline foods (Hand et al, 1988).

Foods that produce average urinary pH values of 6.2 to 6.4 when fed free choice reduce the risk of struvite-mediated FLUTD, avoid metabolic acidosis and reduce the risk of calcium oxalate urolithiasis in most young adult cats.

Antioxidants

The body synthesizes many antioxidants (e.g., superoxide dismutase) but relies on food for others (e.g., vitamin E). Common food-source antioxidants include vitamins E and C, β-carotene and other carotenoids, selenium and thiols. Fruits and vegetables are good sources of flavonoids, polyphenols and anthocyanidins. The following discussion will focus on vitamins E and C and selenium as antioxidant key nutritional factors in foods for young adult cats because: 1) they are biologically important, 2) they act synergistically (e.g., vitamin C and selenium-containing glutathione peroxidase regenerate vitamin E after it has reacted with a free radical), 3) of safety concerns and 4) information regarding inclusion levels in pet foods is usually readily available.

The consequences of prolonged oxidative stress (i.e., free radical damage) to cell membranes, proteins and DNA contribute to and/or exacerbate a wide variety of degenerative diseases. A partial list includes cancer, diabetes mellitus, kidney and urinary tract disease, heart disease, liver disease, inflammatory bowel disease and cognitive dysfunction (Ames et al, 1993; Kesavulu et al, 2000; Ha and Le, 2000; Thamilselvan et al, 2000; Freeman et al, 1999; Cheng et al, 1999; Center, 1999; Knight, 1999).

The consequences of free radical damage to cells and tissues have also been associated with the effects of aging. Although aging is a complex, multifactorial process, one possible explanation for many of the degenerative changes is the free radical theory of aging (Harman, 1956). This theory proposes that free radicals produce cell damage and that age-dependent pathologic alterations may, at least in part, be the cumulative result of these changes. Examples of research supporting this theory include invertebrate studies that found the normal endogenous production of reactive oxygen species limits lifespan (Melov et al, 2000) and studies involving superoxide dismutase-deficient mice that died within the first week of life (Melov, 2000).

Many phenomena initiate free radical formation within the body. Although such things as environmental pollutants and radiation are direct and indirect sources of free radicals, the primary source is endogenous from normal oxidative metabolism in mitochondria. The body defends itself against the effects of free radicals through a complex of protective antioxidant compounds. These compounds protect biomolecules by scavenging free radical compounds, minimizing free radical production and binding metal ions that might increase the reactivity of poorly reactive compounds. Besides these classic mechanisms, many antioxidants exhibit second messenger regulatory function, cell cycle signaling and control of gene expression (Chapter 7 covers antioxidants in detail).

VITAMIN E

Vitamin E (α-tocopherol) is the main lipid-soluble antioxidant present in plasma, erythrocytes and tissues (NRC, 2006). It is transported in plasma proteins and partitions into membranes and fat storage sites where it is one of the most effective antioxidants for protecting polyunsaturated fatty acids (PUFAs) from oxidation. It functions as a chain-breaking antioxidant that prevents propagation of free radical damage in biologic membranes. Vitamin E inhibits lipid peroxidation by scavenging lipid peroxyl radicals much faster than these radicals can react with adjacent fatty acids or with membrane proteins (Gutteridge and Halliwell, 1994).

Research indicates that a level of vitamin E higher than the requirement confers specific biologic benefits. The minimum recommended allowance of vitamin E in foods (DM) for adult cats is 38 mg/kg (NRC, 2006). The concentration of vitamin E in a food necessary to protect against lipid peroxidation of PUFAs in cell membranes depends on the concentration of PUFAs in the food. Foods high in PUFAs, such as foods containing fish oils, may require four or more times increased vitamin E concentration to prevent steatitis (NRC, 2006). Besides helping to prevent chronic diseases associated with oxidative stress, increasing dietary intake of vitamin E to 272 and 552 IU/kg of food (DM) in aged cats improved immune function (Hayes et al, 1969; Hall et al, 2003; Meydani et al, 1998). Furthermore, increased vitamin E intake is also directly related to increased vitamin E content of skin in cats (and dogs), which may help prevent certain skin diseases (Jewell et al, 2002). No safe upper limit has been established for cats. One antioxidant biomarker study suggested that cat foods should contain 600 IU/kg DM for improved antioxidant function (Jewell et al, 2000). Based on these data, foods for young adult cats should contain at least 500 IU/kg DM.

VITAMIN C

Vitamin C (ascorbic acid) is the most powerful reducing agent available to cells. As such, it is important for regenerating oxidized vitamin E. Ascorbic acid also: 1) regenerates glutathione and flavonoids, 2) quenches free radicals intra- and extracellularly, 3) protects against free radical-mediated protein inactivation associated with oxidative bursts of neutrophils, 4) maintains transition metals in reduced form and 5) may quench free radical intermediates of carcinogen metabolism (Chapter 7). Dogs and cats can synthesize required amounts of vitamin C (Innes, 1931; Naismith, 1958) and, while not shown in cats, dogs can rapidly absorb supplemental vitamin C (Wang et al, 2001). In vitro studies, however, indicated that cats (and dogs) have from one-fourth to one-tenth the ability to synthesize vitamin C as other mammals (Chatterjee et al, 1975). Whether or not this finding translates to a reduced ability in vivo is unknown.

Excessive vitamin C supplementation can be a problem. In people, high vitamin C intake increased urine oxalate excretion and risk for urolithiasis (Massey et al, 2005). Vitamin C supplementation resulted in a small progressive reduction of urinary pH in cats and 1,000 mg vitamin C per day induced diarrhea in some cats (Kienzle and Maiwald, 1998). Moderate supplementation of foods with vitamin C (193 mg/kg of food, DM) did not appear to increase the risk of urinary oxalate production in healthy adult cats (Yu and Gross, 2005).

Foods for young adult cats should contain 100 to 200 mg vitamin C/kg DM. This is based on the recommendation for vitamin E and data that show that vitamin C regenerates vitamin E at about a 1:1 molar ratio (Barclay et al, 1985). Also, this range is not a risk for urinary oxalate production (Yu and Gross, 2005).

SELENIUM

Glutathione peroxidase is a selenium-containing antioxidant enzyme that defends tissues against oxidative stress by catalyzing the reduction of H_2O_2 and organic hydroperoxides and by regenerating vitamin E. The minimum recommended allowance for selenium in foods for adult cats is 0.3 mg/kg DM (NRC, 2006). The minimum requirement for selenium in foods for cats is 0.13 mg/kg DM (Wedekind et al, 2003, 2003a). Animal studies and clinical intervention trials in people have shown selenium to be anticarcinogenic at much higher levels (five to 10 times) than the recommended allowances for people or the minimum requirements for animals (Combs, 2001; Neve, 2002). Several mechanisms have been proposed for this effect, including enhanced antioxidant activity via glutathione peroxidase (Neve, 2002). Therefore, for increased antioxidant benefits, the recommended range of selenium for cat foods is 0.5 to 1.3 mg/kg DM. There are no data on which to base a safe upper limit of selenium for cats, but for regulatory purposes, a maximum of 2 mg/kg DM has been set for dog foods in the United States (AAFCO, 2007). In the absence of cat data, the safe upper limit for dogs may provide a working guideline for cat foods.

Texture

Food texture influences oral health (Chapter 47). Dry foods specifically designed to promote oral health can help reduce accumulation of dental plaque and calculus and the severity of gingivitis. If the labels of such foods carry the Veterinary Oral Health Council (VOHC) Seal of Acceptance, they have been successfully tested, according to specific protocols, to clinically reduce plaque (Chapter 47).

Generally, dry foods result in less plaque accumulation in cats than do moist and semi-moist foods (Logan, 1996; Studer and Stapley, 1973). This effect appears not to be clinically important because most cats eat dry foods and dental disease is the most prevalent disease of adult cats (Lund et al, 1999). Food texture also influences the palatability and acceptability of foods for cats. A sudden change in texture may result in reduced food intake or food refusal. Cats accustomed to eating only dry foods may refuse moist foods and vice versa.

Other Nutritional Factors

In addition to the key nutritional factors for commercial foods for young adult cats discussed above, the following nutritional

Table 20-4. Selected commercial foods for young adult cats (normal and inactive/obese prone) compared to recommended levels of key nutritional factors.*

Dry foods	Energy density (kcal/cup)**	Energy density (kcal ME/g)	Fat (%)	Fiber (%)	Protein (%)	P (%)	Na (%)
Recommended levels (normal body condition)	**–**	**4.0-5.0**	**10-30**	**<5**	**30-45**	**0.5-0.8**	**0.2-0.6**
Hill's Science Diet Adult Hairball Control Feline	339	4.1	22.1	8.1	34	0.69	0.31
Hill's Science Diet Adult Optimal Care Ocean Fish & Rice Recipe	488	4.3	22.7	1.2	34	0.72	0.27
Hill's Science Diet Adult Oral Care Feline	337	4.2	22.0	7.5	34.1	0.75	0.37
Hill's Science Diet Nature's Best Ocean Fish & Brown Rice Dinner Adult	470	4.3	20.6	1.2	33.9	0.74	0.33
Iams Eukanuba Adult Chicken Formula	436	4.4	23.6	1.4	38.5	0.99	0.55
Iams Original with Chicken Cat Food	368	4.1	17.3	1.8	37.3	1.06	0.50
Nutro Max Cat Adult Roasted Chicken Flavor	421	4.2	20.9	2.2	36.3	1.1	0.44
Nutro Natural Choice Complete Care Adult	452	4.3	22.0	2.7	37.4	1.1	0.44
Purina ONE Natural Blends Chicken & Oat Meal Formula	450	4.4	17.9	1.9	37.9	1.44	0.60
Purina ONE Total Nutrition Salmon & Tuna Flavor	430	4.4	15.7	1.8	37.9	1.29	0.52
Purina Pro Plan Indoor Care Turkey & Rice Formula	433	4.2	15.2	5.3	46.0	1.28	0.48
Royal Canin Adult Fit 32	351	4.2	16.5	8.1	35.2	1.12	0.66

Moist foods	Energy density (kcal/can)**	Energy density (kcal ME/g)	Fat (%)	Fiber (%)	Protein (%)	P (%)	Na (%)
Recommended levels (normal body condition)	**–**	**4.0-5.0**	**10-30**	**<5**	**30-45**	**0.5-0.8**	**0.2-0.6**
Hill's Science Diet Adult Hairball Control Savory Chicken Entrée Minced	91/3 oz. 168/5.5 oz.	4.4	23.3	9.8	35.9	0.65	0.49
Hill's Science Diet Adult Indoor Cat Savory Chicken Entrée Minced	91/3 oz. 168/5.5 oz.	4.4	23.3	9.8	35.5	0.65	0.49
Hill's Science Diet Adult Optimal Care Gourmet Beef Entrée Minced	93/3 oz. 171/5.5 oz.	4.4	22	4.8	37.6	0.72	0.32
Nutro MAX Cat Gourmet Classics Adult Chicken & Liver Formula	169/5.5 oz.	4.6	29.8	2.1	42.6	1.28	0.64
Nutro Natural Choice Complete Care Adult Chicken & Liver Entrée	167/5.5 oz.	4.7	30.4	1.7	47.8	1.30	0.65
Purina Pro Plan Adult Cat Chicken & Rice Entrée in Gravy	78/3 oz.	3.9	15.1	0.4	59.1	0.95	1.38

Dry foods	Energy density (kcal/cup)**	Energy density (kcal ME/g)	Fat (%)	Fiber (%)	Protein (%)	P (%)	Na (%)
Recommended levels (inactive/obese prone)	**–**	**3.3-3.8**	**9-17**	**5-15**	**30-45**	**0.5-0.8**	**0.2-0.6**
Hill's Science Diet Adult Hairball Control Light Feline	283	3.5	9.1	8.3	36	0.72	0.33
Hill's Science Diet Adult Indoor Cat	281	3.5	9.1	8.3	36	0.72	0.33
Hill's Science Diet Adult Light Feline	316	3.5	9.5	6.9	35.1	0.73	0.4
Hill's Science Diet Oral Care Adult Feline	337	4.2	22	7.5	34.1	0.75	0.37
Iams Eukanuba Adult Weight Control	315	3.9	14.4	1.8	34.7	0.99	0.54
Nutro Natural Choice Complete Care Indoor Weight Management	359	3.8	13.2	2.7	36.3	0.82	0.22
Nutro Natural Choice Complete Care Weight Management	308	3.8	13.2	3.3	37.4	1.10	0.44
Purina ONE Indoor Advantage Hairball & Healthy Weight Formula	416	4.1	11.7	3.8	42.9	1.42	0.45
Purina ONE Special Care Healthy Weight Formula	362	3.7	12.2	3.7	46.1	1.41	0.40
Purina Pro Plan Weight Management Formula	413	4.2	12.0	3.4	50.5	1.08	0.54
Royal Canin Indoor 27	324	4.0	14.3	7.5	29.7	1.08	0.70
Royal Canin Indoor Light 37	285	3.5	9.9	10.2	40.7	1.07	0.80

Moist foods	Energy density (kcal/can)**	Energy density (kcal ME/g)	Fat (%)	Fiber (%)	Protein (%)	P (%)	Na (%)
Recommended levels (inactive/obese prone)	**–**	**3.3-3.8**	**9-17**	**5-15**	**30-45**	**0.5-0.8**	**0.2-0.6**
Hill's Science Diet Adult Indoor Cat Savory Seafood Entrée Minced	90/3 oz. 165/5.5 oz.	4.1	23	9.4	37.9	0.7	0.43
Hill's Science Diet Adult Light Liver & Chicken Entrée Minced	75/3 oz. 138/5.5 oz.	3.6	14.2	10.1	35.6	0.69	0.32
Nutro MAX Cat Gourmet Classics Lite with Chicken & Lamb	140/5.5 oz.	3.9	15.2	1.7	41.3	1.3	1.09

Key: ME = metabolizable energy, P = phosphorus, Na = sodium, Mg = magnesium, Se = selenium, VOHC = Veterinary Oral Health Council Seal of Acceptance (Chapter 47), na = information not available from manufacturer, g = grams.

*From manufacturers' published information or calculated from manufacturers' published as fed values; all values are on a dry matter basis unless otherwise stated.

**Energy density values are listed on an as fed basis and are useful for determining the amount to feed; cup = 8-oz. measuring cup. To convert to kJ, multiply kcal by 4.184.

Mg (%)	Urinary pH	Vit. E (IU/kg)	Vit. C (mg/kg)	Se (mg/kg)	VOHC plaque (Yes/No)
0.04-0.1	**6.2-6.4**	**≥500**	**100-200**	**0.5-1.3**	**Yes**
0.053	6.3	705	119	0.79	No
0.065	6.3	1,042	197	0.86	No
0.058	6.3	670	171	0.55	Yes
0.088	6.2	739	270	0.83	No
na	na	na	na	na	No
0.109	na	na	na	na	No
0.082	na	132	38	0.49	No
0.088	na	330	88	0.77	No
na	na	na	na	na	No
na	na	na	na	na	No
0.110	na	na	na	na	No
0.121	na	604	220	0.49	No
Mg (%)	**Urinary pH**	**Vit. E (IU/kg)**	**Vit. C (mg/kg)**	**Se (mg/kg)**	**VOHC plaque (Yes/No)**
0.04-0.1	**6.2-6.4**	**≥500**	**100-200**	**0.5-1.3**	**Yes**
0.069	6.4	694	241	1.1	No
0.082	6.4	816	257	1.06	No
0.072	6.4	396	80	1.2	No
0.106	na	170	106	0.43	No
0.10	na	174	261	0.43	No
0.04	na	na	na	na	No
Mg (%)	**Urinary pH**	**Vit. E (IU/kg)**	**Vit. C (mg/kg)**	**Se (mg/kg)**	**VOHC plaque (Yes/No)**
0.04-0.1	**6.2-6.4**	**≥500**	**100-200**	**0.5-1.3**	**Yes**
0.071	6.2-6.4	689	176	0.68	No
0.071	6.2	689	176	0.68	No
0.068	6.2	693	189	0.67	No
0.058	6.3	670	171	0.55	Yes
na	na	na	na	na	No
0.088	na	330	110	0.71	No
0.093	na	330	88	0.60	No
na	na	na	na	na	No
na	na	na	na	na	No
0.84	na	na	na	na	No
0.11	na	604	220	0.49	No
0.11	na	604	220	0.49	No
Mg (%)	**Urinary pH**	**Vit. E (IU/kg)**	**Vit. C (mg/kg)**	**Se (mg/kg)**	**VOHC plaque (Yes/No)**
0.04-0.1	**6.2-6.4**	**≥500**	**100-200**	**0.5-1.3**	**Yes**
0.094	6.4	961	195	1.72	No
0.077	6.2	401	na	1.46	No
0.104	na	174	87	0.43	No

factors are of concern for young adult cats fed homemade foods (Chapter 10). Occasionally, these factors also become important for cats that are intentionally, or unintentionally, fed commercial dog foods.

Taurine

The AAFCO allowances for taurine are appropriate for adult cats (2007). Therefore, commercial cat foods that have AAFCO label statements acknowledging that a food is appropriate for adult maintenance should provide adequate amounts. However, sporadic cases of taurine depletion continue to be diagnosed. Therefore, dietary taurine concentrations should be evaluated in cats with signs of deficiency or disease (Chapter 19). The minimum recommended allowance for taurine in foods depends on the form of the food. Dry and moist foods should provide 0.1 and 0.17% DM taurine, respectively (NRC, 2006). Taurine is not required in commercial dog foods and is usually not added, yet another reason cats should not be fed dog foods.

Essential Fatty Acids

Signs of essential fatty acid deficiency in cats include fatty degeneration of the liver, kidneys and adrenal glands. Scaly skin, mild hyperkeratosis and hair loss have also been noted. Linoleic acid and α-linolenic acid are essential for normal membrane structure and function, including growth, lipid transport, maintenance of the epidermal permeability barrier and normal skin and coat (MacDonald et al, 1984a). Definitive studies about the essentiality of α-linolenic acid have not been conducted in cats. AA, on the other hand, is important for functions that rely on eicosanoid synthesis. In cats, AA deficiency is associated with impaired platelet aggregation, inflammatory skin lesions and reproductive failure in queens (MacDonald et al, 1984b, 1984c). Male cats are capable of converting linoleic acid to AA within the testes, resulting in normal spermatogenesis (MacDonald et al, 1984c). The minimum DM recommended allowances for linoleic acid and AA are 0.55 and 0.006%, respectively (NRC, 2006). The AAFCO allowances for linoleic acid and AA, however, are appropriate for adult cats (2007). Thus, provision of adequate amounts of these essential fatty acids via commercial foods is usually not a problem.

Calcium

Calcium deficiencies are uncommon in cats fed commercial foods. Most cases of calcium deficiency occur in cats fed only meats, in which the calcium concentration is excessively low, particularly relative to the moderately high phosphorus concentration. The recommended DM allowance for calcium in foods for growing kittens is 0.8% of the diet (NRC, 2006). Adult needs are typically less than those for growth. The recommended DM allowance for calcium in foods for adult cats is 0.29% (NRC, 2006). Typical commercial foods contain calcium levels well in excess of these guidelines.

Daily calcium intakes of 200 to 400 mg result when adult cats are fed foods with a calcium-phosphorus ratio of 0.9:1 to 1.1:1 (Scott and Scott, 1967). Although foods with much broader ratios of calcium to phosphorus have been fed successfully, ratios near 1:1 calcium to phosphorus optimize the availability of phosphorus (Kienzle et al, 1998). When the calcium-phosphorus ratio is increased to 2:1, phosphorus availability declines by 41%. Calcium-phosphorus ratios between 0.9:1 to 1.5:1 appear optimal for most cat foods.

Potassium

The potassium requirement of cats varies with the dietary protein concentration and the effect of the food on urinary pH. High-protein foods and foods that result in an acidic urinary pH increase the potassium requirement (Hills et al, 1982; Ching et al, 1989, 1990; Dow et al, 1990; DiBartola et al, 1993). Previously recommended levels of 0.4% DM potassium (NRC, 1986) resulted in hypokalemia in adult cats and kittens when combined with dietary acidification. Dietary potassium levels in foods for adult cats should be at least 0.52% DM (NRC, 2006) and ideally between 0.6 to 1.0% DM to prevent hypokalemia. The current AAFCO allowance for potassium is 0.6% DM (2007). Therefore, foods that have AAFCO label statements acknowledging that a food is appropriate for adult maintenance should provide adequate amounts of potassium.

Negative potassium balance may occur in cats with certain metabolic abnormalities (e.g., renal insufficiency, renal tubular acidosis, diabetes mellitus and enteritis). Supplementation may be necessary to maintain normal potassium balance in cats with these conditions, even when they are fed a food containing 0.6% DM potassium.

FEEDING PLAN

Assess and Select the Food

After the nutritional status of the cat has been assessed and the key nutritional factors and their target levels have been determined, the adequacy of the food being fed can be assessed. The steps to assessing foods include: 1) determining if the nutritional adequacy of the food has been assured by a credible regulatory agency such as AAFCO and 2) comparing the food's key nutritional factors with recommended levels.

In the U.S., commercial foods approved by AAFCO will usually have a nutritional adequacy statement on the label (Chapter 9). Commercial cat foods that have received AAFCO or other credible regulatory approval provide reasonable assurance of nutritional adequacy. Few homemade recipes have been formulated according to such protocols. Even foods bearing nutritional adequacy statements, however, are not infallible. Nutritional adequacy statements do not assure the food will be effective in preventing certain important long-term health problems (**Table 20-1**). Therefore, in addition to having passed nutritional adequacy protocols, the food should be evaluated to ensure that the key nutritional factors are at levels appropriate for delivering the feeding goal of promoting long-term health through disease prevention. Besides providing recommended levels of key nutritional factors for young adult cats, **Table 20-4** lists key nutritional factor profiles for selected commercial foods. The manufacturer should be contacted if the food in question cannot be found in this table. Manufacturers' addresses, websites and toll-free customer service numbers are listed on pet food labels. If the manufacturer cannot provide the necessary information, consider switching to a food for which this information is available. Because of the propensity for developing food fixations, feeding a combination of food forms (dry and moist) is sometimes recommended. It is unnecessary to change foods if the food currently fed supplies the correct amounts of the key nutritional factors and the food has a nutritional adequacy statement appropriate for adult cats. However, a new food should be selected if discrepancies were determined. The new food should, as closely as possible, provide the recommended levels of the key nutritional factors.

Snacks are either human foods (table foods) or commercial treats and are offered to cats for a variety of reasons. Small amounts of snacks will not have an important effect on the overall food regimen. Excessive feeding of treats, however, can markedly affect the cumulative nutritional profile. Therefore, it is important to assess the impact of treats with respect to the dietary needs of individual cats. The impact of treats on daily nutrient intake depends on three factors: 1) the nutrient profile of the treat, 2) the number of treats provided daily and 3) the nutrient composition of the cat's regular food. Meeting nutrient requirements is not the primary goal of feeding treats; consequently, many commercial treats are not complete and balanced. Similarly, most table foods are not nutritionally complete and balanced and may contain high levels of fat or minerals. If snacks are fed, it is simplest to recommend commercial treats that best match the nutritional profile recommended for young adult cats. Generally, snacks should not be fed in excessive amounts (<10% of the total dietary regimen on a volume, weight or calorie basis). Otherwise, the nutritional composition of the snack and food should be combined and assessed as the total food regimen.

Assess and Determine the Feeding Method

Veterinarians should evaluate the feeding method, including how the food is fed, the feeding frequency and the amount of food offered. It is also useful to know how the food is prepared (e.g., heated, water added, etc.) and by whom and where the cat is fed. This information may help explain any apparent discrepancies between the dietary history and the physical findings and help identify risk factors associated with various feeding methods. For example, a thorough evaluation of an obese cat includes verification that an appropriate feeding method is being used (Chapters 1 and 27).

No single feeding method is optimal for all cats. The preferred method of feeding an individual cat is often determined by non-nutritional factors (i.e., food type, owner preference, owner schedule and feeding environment including whether there are other pets [cats, dogs] in the household). Nutritional considerations for selecting an appropriate feeding regimen include the cat's body condition, health status/disease risk factors and the food's energy density and palatability.

There are basically two ways to feed cats: 1) free choice in

Table 20-5. Advantages and disadvantages of various feeding methods for cats.

Methods	Advantages	Disadvantages	Food types
Free choice	Convenient Ensures adequate food availability Mimics natural feeding behavior Dampens postprandial alkaline tide (lower mean urinary pH)	Overconsumption leads to weight gain or obesity, unless a specific amount is fed Difficult to monitor appetite and food intake Moist food may spoil Less owner contact	Dry Semi moist
Meal fed*	Enhances human-animal bond Facilitates monitoring of appetite and food intake Enhanced control of food intake	Enhanced postprandial alkaline tide (higher mean urinary pH) Large meals may result in vomiting Less convenient Three or more meals for pregnant or nursing queens, kittens or debilitated cats	Dry Semi moist Moist
Combination**	Enhances human-animal bond (vs. free choice) Variable effect on urinary pH	Poor monitoring of appetite and food intake unless a specific amount is fed Poor control of food intake Less convenient than free choice Variable effect on urinary pH	Dry Semi moist Moist

*One or more individual feedings per day, one to two hour availability per feeding.
**Dry foods available free choice, moist foods meal fed one or more times daily.

which the food is continuously available and the cat eats as much as it wants whenever it wants and 2) meal feeding in which a specific amount of food is offered one or more times per day. Most cats tolerate once daily feeding with no problems; however, meal feeding at least twice daily is preferred. Cats should be allowed one to two hours to complete a measured meal; many cats will return for several small feedings before finishing the entire offering. Many owners use a combination of free-choice and meal-feeding methods. Usually, dry food is available throughout the day and supplemented with one or more meals of moist food. Free-choice or combination feeding accommodates the normal feeding behavior of cats by allowing them to eat several small meals spaced irregularly throughout the day and night (Kane et al, 1981a). Each feeding method has advantages and disadvantages that should be considered when making recommendations (**Table 20-5**).

Unless a specific amount of food is fed, the major disadvantage to combination feeding is the inability to accurately monitor and control food intake. Most obese-prone cats should be fed a measured quantity of food; however, some obese-prone cats can be fed low-calorie foods free choice. Food should be available at all times for underweight cats to encourage sufficient food intake.

Clean drinking water should always be available. Water intake can be encouraged by providing a source of fresh flowing water, such as from a water fountain, which many cats seem to enjoy and can be an important aid in reducing the risk for FLUTD. Chapter 46 provides other tips for increasing water intake in cats.

The amount fed is important because nutrient requirements are met, or exceeded, by a combination of nutrient levels in the food and the amount of food fed. Even if a food has an appropriate profile of key nutritional factors, significant malnutrition could result from feeding excessive or insufficient amounts. The amount fed is appropriate if the cat has an optimal BCS (2.5/5 to 3.5/5) (Chapter 1) and body weight is stable. The amount fed can be estimated by calculation (Table 5-2) or by referring to feeding guides on product labels or product information. These guides, however, usually represent population averages and thus may not be optimal for individual cats. **Table 20-6** summarizes the feeding plan for young adult cats.

Table 20-6. Feeding plan summary for young adult cats.

1. Select a food from **Table 20-4** that most closely matches the recommended levels of key nutritional factors; for foods not listed in **Table 20-4**, contact the manufacturer for key nutritional factor content.
2. The selected food should be approved by a credible regulatory agency (e.g., AAFCO).
3. Determine the preferred feeding method (**Table 20-5**); when the correct amount of food is fed, food-restricted feeding is least likely to result in obesity.
4. For food-restricted meal feeding, first, estimate the cat's DER by multiplying RER (Table 5-2) by an appropriate factor.
    - Neutered adult = 1.2 to 1.4 x RER
    - Intact adult = 1.4 to 1.6 x RER
    - Inactive/obese-prone adult = 1.0 x RER (Most pet cats are minimally active)
5. Second, divide the cat's DER estimate by the food energy density (as fed) from **Table 20-4** or manufacturer's information. This calculation will determine the number of cups (dry food) or cans (moist food) to feed each day.
6. Remember, these DER calculations are estimates and should be used as guidelines or starting points for individual cats and not as absolute requirements. Body condition and body weight are used to refine the amount to feed.
7. Regularly monitor body condition, body weight and general health.

Key: AAFCO = Association of American Feed Control Officials, DER = daily energy requirement, RER = resting energy requirement, cup = 8-oz. measuring cup.

A reduction in the amount of food fed is usually necessary in normally active cats that are temporarily confined, such as during boarding, or if their environment changes permanently. These cats may become overweight if food intake is not adjusted accordingly. A normal decline in food intake should not be confused with inappetence due to stress or disease. Domestic cats display a variety of feeding behaviors that may have nutritional or non-nutritional bases (Box 19-1). Some of these behaviors are worrisome to owners and considered abnormal, when in fact they are normal. Other behaviors may indicate an underlying disease.

Cats do not typically develop digestive problems associated with food changes; furthermore, food variety stimulates increased food intake (Mugford, 1977). Unfortunately, rapid changes in the food or feeding method can cause GI upsets or food refusal for some cats. Transitioning to a new food over four to seven days may be necessary to avoid food intolerances. To change to a new food, replace 25% of the old food with the new food on Day 1 and continue this incremental change daily until the change is complete on Day 4. A slower transition may be required for cats that have been historically sensitive to dietary changes, those with GI diseases and when the new food differs markedly from the old (e.g., low fat vs. high fat or raw meat vs. dry food).

Food and water bowls should be cleaned regularly with warm soapy water and rinsed well. Water fountains should be cleaned weekly and refilled with fresh water. Dishes used for moist foods need daily cleaning, whereas dry food feeders should be cleaned at least weekly. Many cats prefer shallow dishes, especially breeds with less prominent faces such as Persians. For multi-cat households, multiple feeding stations and individual feeding dishes, particularly if placed at different levels, allow timid and low-status cats to eat alone or away from dominant cats. These practices also benefit dominant cats by reducing tension and allowing time for dominant cats to eat quietly instead of defending food or constantly harassing cats of lower social status.

REASSESSMENT

Cats provided proper nutritional management are healthy and alert and have ideal body condition, stable weight and a clean, well-groomed, glossy coat. The owner should evaluate body condition every two to four weeks. Owners should monitor daily food and water intake and observe the cat's interest in its food and its appetite. Stools should be evaluated regularly because changes in frequency or character may signify nutritional problems or disease. Normal stools should be firm, well-formed and medium to dark brown. Any abnormalities should be investigated. The veterinarian should also conduct a nutritional assessment as part of the annual wellness visit.

ACKNOWLEDGMENT

The authors and editors acknowledge the contributions of Dr. Claudia A. Kirk in the previous edition of Small Animal Clinical Nutrition.

REFERENCES

The references for **Chapter 20** can be found at www.markmorris.org.

CASE 20-1

Elective Surgery in a Young Siamese Cat

Claudia A. Kirk, DVM, PhD, Dipl. ACVN and ACVIM (Internal Medicine)
College of Veterinary Medicine
University of Tennessee
Knoxville, Tennessee, USA

Patient Assessment

An 11-month-old female Siamese cat was presented for routine ovariohysterectomy. The owner obtained the cat from a friend as a young kitten. The cat had been healthy except for one episode of upper respiratory infection, flea infestation and tapeworm infection. The cat lived with the owner in an apartment and rarely went outdoors.

Physical examination revealed a normal young adult cat. Body weight was 3.2 kg with ideal body condition (body condition score [BCS] 3/5). A packed cell volume (normal), feline leukemia virus test (negative) and fecal flotation test (negative) were performed before surgery. The ovariohysterectomy was uneventfully and the cat was released to the owner's care the next day.

Assess the Food and Feeding Method

The cat was fed a dry commercial grocery brand food formulated for growing kittens (Purina Kitten Chow Dairy Flavor[a]) and several varieties of moist commercial grocery brand foods. The dry food was available free choice and a small portion of moist food was fed each evening when the owner returned from work. Tuna flavor cat treats were also offered daily. Dairy products were fed intermittently; the cat was allowed to lick bowls used for cereal and ice cream.

Questions

1. When should the owner stop feeding kitten food?
2. Will the ovariohysterectomy change the nutrient requirements for this young cat?
3. What are the key nutritional factors for a cat entering adulthood?
4. Outline an appropriate feeding plan.

Answers and Discussion

1. An 11-month-old cat has reached its adult size and is finishing the maturation process. Foods specifically formulated for growing cats are usually fed until approximately one year of age. At that time, the food can be slowly changed to one formulated for young adult cats.
2. Neutering markedly alters a cat's metabolism. Changes occur within three months of neutering and include decreased resting energy requirement (RER) (basal metabolic rate; approximate decline 27 to 33%) and less ability to regulate food intake. These changes make gonadectomy a risk factor for obesity. Neutered cats are more likely to become overweight than are intact cats of either gender. Therefore, neutered cats should be fed less energy than intact cats to reduce the risk for obesity.
3. Key nutritional factors for young adult cats include water, energy, protein, fat, minerals (phosphorus, sodium, chloride, magnesium), urinary pH, antioxidants and food texture. Foods that produce average urinary pH values of 6.2 to 6.4 when fed free choice reduce the risk of struvite urolithiasis and avoid metabolic acidosis in most adult cats. Food texture influences oral health. Dental disease is the most prevalent disease in cats one year old and older. Dry foods specifically designed to promote oral health are beneficial in reducing plaque and calculus accumulation and controlling gingivitis.
4. A food specifically formulated for young adult cats should be chosen based on appropriate levels of key nutritional factors. A commercial dry adult cat food or a combination of dry and moist adult cat foods can be used. The form(s) of food chosen will dictate the feeding method used; meal feeding rather than free-choice feeding helps control obesity. The owner should be informed that neutering might markedly decrease the energy requirements of the cat. An estimated daily energy requirement (DER) can be calculated as a target for the owner. The DER of average young adult cats is approximately 1.4 x RER (70 kcal/kg body weight/day [293 kJ/kg body weight/day]). Caloric requirements for neutered or inactive cats may be less than this amount, whereas active intact cats may require a higher energy intake. Treats should be eliminated or used sparingly. The owner should monitor body weight and condition every two to three months to determine if DER should be adjusted. Free-choice access to potable water is important.

Progress Notes

The veterinary technician discussed the metabolic and behavioral changes that result from ovariohysterectomy with the owner when the cat was discharged. Dry and moist formulations of a commercial food formulated for adult cats (Science Diet Feline Maintenance[b]) were sent home with the owner. The owner was instructed to mix the dry adult food with the remaining growth food. The moist adult food was dispensed to replace the other moist foods after they were fed. The estimated DER was 1.4 x RER = 230 kcal (962 kJ). Offering one-fourth cup dry food in the morning and giving two-thirds of a 5.5-oz. can of food in the evening would meet this DER. The owner was given a body condition scoring chart for cats, and she indicated her willingness to evaluate the cat regularly.

Endnotes

a. Ralston Purina Co., St. Louis, MO, USA.
b. Hill's Pet Nutrition, Inc., Topeka, KS, USA. This product is currently available as Science Diet Adult Original.

Bibliography

Buffington CA, Rogers QR, Morris JG. Effects of age and food deprivation on urine pH of cats. Veterinary Clinical Nutrition 1994; 1: 12-17.

Flynn MF, Hardie EM, Armstrong PJ. Effect of ovariohysterectomy on maintenance energy requirement in cats. Journal of the American Veterinary Medical Association 1996; 209: 1572-1581.

Lund EM, Armstrong PJ, Kirk CA et al. Prevalence and risk factors for obesity in adult cats from private U.S. veterinary practices. International Journal of Applied Research in Veterinary Medicine 2005; 3(2): 88-96.

Munday HS, Earle KE, Anderson P. Changes in the body composition of the domestic shorthaired cat during growth and development. Journal of Nutrition 1994; 124: 2622S-2623S.

NRC. (National Research Council). Nutrient Requirements of Cats. Washington, DC: National Academy Press, 1986.

Root MV. Early spay and neuter in the cat: Effect on development of obesity and metabolic rate. Veterinary Clinical Nutrition 1995; 2: 132-134.

Scarlett JM, Donoghue S, Saidla J, et al. Overweight cats: Prevalence and risk factors. International Journal of Obesity 1994; 18: S22-S28.

Chapter 21

Feeding Mature Adult Cats: Middle Aged and Older

Kathy L. Gross
Iveta Becvarova
Jacques Debraekeleer

"Every life should have nine cats."
Anonymous

CLINICAL IMPORTANCE

More pet cats are getting older. Thirty-five percent of cats in the United States are at least seven years of age (Lund et al, 1999). The number of pet cats older than six years in the U.S. nearly doubled (from 24 to 47%) over a recent decade (Stratton-Phelps, 1999). Similarly, in Europe, the number of cats older than seven years increased by 100% between 1983 and 1995 (Kraft, 1998). For the purposes of this chapter, the term "mature" indicates cats that are seven to eight years old and older. It includes cats that could be considered "middle-aged," "senior" and "geriatric."

Age-related diseases begin to increase in prevalence around seven or eight years of age; this prevalence is coupled with the gradual onset of behavioral, physical and metabolic changes related to aging (Lund et al, 1999). Instituting appropriate changes in nutritional management and preventive care at this point are important to reduce risk factors for common age-associated diseases (Table 20-1), thereby helping to maintain good health and maximize longevity. Furthermore, a cat's chronologic age may not accurately reflect its physiologic age (e.g., an eight-year-old cat with kidney disease and poor nutritional status is likely to be "physiologically older" than a healthy 11-year-old cat).

This chapter builds on many of the recommendations in Chapter 20 for feeding young adult cats. The minimum nutrient requirements of mature adult cats are similar to those of young adult cats. The few studies evaluating the effects of aging on the nutritional needs of cats have shown minimal changes in nutrient requirements. Therefore, nutritional recommendations for mature adult cats are based on risk factor management, extension of learning from other species and prudence. Several key nutritional factors for mature adult cats, however, are lower than the recommended upper range for young adults. To date, the only nutritional modification proven to slow aging and increase the lifespan is caloric restriction. Reducing caloric intake by 20 to 30% of normal, while meeting essential nutrient needs, slows the aging process and decreases susceptibility to cancer, renal disease, arthritis and immune-mediated diseases in animal models studied (Sheffy and Williams, 1981; Kealy et al, 2002). This level of caloric restriction is difficult to achieve in the long term and has not been incorporated into mainstream nutritional advice.

Older mature cats become less active and have reduced lean body mass. Together, these changes reduce their basal metabol-

Table 21-1. Common physiologic changes and diseases associated with aging in cats.*

Body systems/functions	Age-related changes	Associated conditions and diseases
Metabolism	Decreased thirst sensitivity	Dehydration
	Decreased thermoregulation	Hypothermia or hyperthermia
	Decreased immunocompetence	Susceptibility to infections, disease and cancer
	Decreased rate of drug metabolism	Drug intolerance
	Increased sleep	Irritability
	Decreased activity and metabolic rate	Loss of body mass, reduced BMR and obesity
Special senses	Decreased olfaction	Reduced food intake and weight loss
	Decreased taste perception	Reduced food intake and weight loss
	Decreased hearing	
	Decreased visual acuity	
Oral cavity	Decreased salivary secretion	Increased oral disease
	Increased tooth loss, dental calculus	Painful or difficult prehension
	Increased periodontal disease	Reduced food intake and weight loss
		Susceptibility to sepsis and end-organ damage
Gastrointestinal	Decreased liver function	Reduced nutrient assimilation
	Increased cellular infiltrates	
	Decreased digestive function	Reduced nutrient digestibility
	Decreased colonic motility	Constipation
	Decreased pancreatic function	Reduced nutrient digestibility
Endocrine	Decreased pancreatic function	Glucose intolerance and diabetes mellitus
	Decreased adrenal function	Reduced ability to respond to stress
	Alterations in thyroid structure and function	Hyperthyroidism
Integumentary	Loss of elasticity, dry, thin coat, hyperplasia of sebaceous glands with decreased sebum and increased waxy secretions	Dermatitis Intradermal cysts Dry, flaky coat
Urinary	Decreased total renal function	Chronic renal failure
		Hypokalemia
	Alterations in acid excretion	Decreased acid-base regulation
		Metabolic acidosis
Reproductive	Testicular tumors and atrophy, mammary gland nodules	Reproductive gland neoplasia
	Irregular estrous cycles	Reproductive failure
	Decreased conception rates	Pyometra
	Cystic endometrial hyperplasia	
Musculoskeletal	Decreased lean mass and tone	Decreased BMR, weakness, decreased activity
	Decreased bone mass	Osteoarthritis, spondylosis
	Degenerative joint changes	
Cardiovascular	Decreased cardiac output, increased peripheral resistance, hypertension	Cardiomyopathy, valvular regurgitation Hypertension and end-organ damage
	Valvular thickening	
Respiratory	Reduced vital capacity and compliance	Chronic respiratory disease
	Increased respiratory rate and residual air capacity	
Nervous	Alterations in neurotransmitter levels	Senility
	Progressive decline in cellularity of nervous tissues	Decline in special senses
	Decreased reactivity to stimuli and cognition decline	Behavioral changes

Key: BMR = basal metabolic rate.
*As in any biologic system there is much individual variation. An individual aging animal may have few to many of these changes. Also, the age at which changes occur, and their severity, is quite variable.

ic rate. Additionally, changes occur in virtually all body systems. Age-associated changes in physiologic function include reduced digestive function, immune response, glucose tolerance, renal function, smell, taste perception and numerous other changes (**Table 21-1**) (Harper, 1996; Markham and Hodgkins, 1989; Cowan et al, 1998). Not all cats develop all age-associated changes nor will the changes that develop necessarily occur in any predictable sequence. Aging cats become less adaptable and have reduced physiologic reserve to withstand perturbations in their health and environment, including changes in their food. Older cats age at different rates; thus, greater diversity exists in individual needs than at any other lifestage. Individualization of nutritional management becomes even more important because of the reduced adaptability of older mature adult cats. The goals for nutritional management of mature adult cats are:

- Maintenance of optimal nutrition (i.e., maintenance of ideal body condition and weight, adequate intake of a nutritious food and good hydration).
- Risk factor management (i.e., minimization of associated disease risks [Table 20-1]).
- Disease management (i.e., amelioration of clinical signs of common diseases, slowing progression of certain chronic diseases).

• Improvement in the quality and length of life.

This chapter describes how to assess mature adult cats and how to determine and meet their nutritional needs.

PATIENT ASSESSMENT

History and Physical Examination

A complete history should be taken and physical examination performed as described for young adult cats (Chapter 20). Physiologic changes associated with aging and age-related diseases are of particular interest. Note any changes in appetite, food or water intake, activity, oral health and body condition. Abnormalities in these parameters are often early indicators of underlying disease. Oral disease is the most prevalent disease in adult cats; however, weight loss, cancer, renal disease, cardiac disorders, diabetes mellitus and hyperthyroidism are frequently diagnosed in this age category. Kidney disease may affect nearly 30% of older mature adult cats and is a major cause of death (MAF, 1998; Lulich et al, 1992). Physical evaluation of renal size, shape and firmness may uncover kidney abnormalities, whereas thoracic auscultation may expose cardiac disease. Hyperthyroidism may be detected by palpating enlarged thyroid glands or may be suspected based on the history and other physical findings. A fundic examination may help detect hypertension, which is often secondary to renal, cardiac or thyroid disease in older mature adult cats. Retinal hemorrhage was a common finding in a group of older hypertensive cats (Littman, 1994).

Laboratory and Other Clinical Information

Specific abnormalities in the physical and historical examination should be pursued further using appropriate diagnostic procedures. A geriatric-type blood panel to screen for common age-associated diseases should be performed at least annually. The minimum database should include a complete blood count, urine specific gravity and sediment examination and a serum biochemistry profile. The biochemistry panel should include measurements of albumin, globulin, urea nitrogen, creatinine, glucose, alkaline phosphatase, alanine aminotransferase, calcium, potassium, phosphorus, sodium, chloride and bicarbonate. Serum total thyroxine (T_4) concentrations should be assessed if clinical or biochemical abnormalities suggest hyperthyroidism. Feline leukemia and feline immunodeficiency virus testing should be current and repeated if potential exposure has occurred or suspicious clinical signs are present. Specialized diagnostics may be indicated by physical and/or biochemical findings (e.g., electrocardiography, ultrasonography, radiography, blood pressure monitoring).

Key Nutritional Factors

The recommended range of nutrient allowances can be optimized to support changes in physiologic function and reduce risk factors for common age-related diseases. **Table 21-2** summarizes key nutritional factors for mature adult cats.

Table 21-2. Key nutritional factors for foods for older cats.

Factors	Recommended food levels* Normal and underweight	Inactive/ obese prone
Energy density (kcal ME/g)	4.0-4.5	3.5-4.0
Energy density (kJ ME/g)	16.7-18.8	14.6-16.7
Fat (%)	18-25	10-18
Fiber (%)	≤5	5-15
Protein (%)	30-45	30-45
Calcium (%)	0.6-1.0	0.6-1.0
Phosphorus (%)	0.5-0.7	0.5-0.7
Sodium (%)	0.2-0.4	0.2-0.4
Potassium (%)	≥0.6	≥0.6
Magnesium (%)	0.05-0.1	0.05-0.1
Average urinary pH	6.4-6.6	6.4-6.6
Antioxidants		
Vitamin E (IU/kg)	≥500	≥500
Vitamin C (mg/kg)	100-200	100-200
Selenium (mg/kg)	0.5-1.3	0.5-1.3
VOHC Seal of Acceptance	Plaque control	Plaque control

Key: ME = metabolizable energy, VOHC = Veterinary Oral Health Council (Chapter 47).

*Dry matter basis. Concentrations presume an energy density of 4.0 kcal/g. Levels should be corrected for foods with higher energy densities. Adjustment is unnecessary for foods with lower energy densities.

Water

Water is an often overlooked but critical nutrient in the health of mature adult cats. Aging impairs thirst sensitivity, which is already low in cats compared with other species (MacDonald et al, 1984; Markham and Hodgkins, 1989). Additionally, the decline in renal function observed in many mature adult cats may increase water losses due to impaired urine concentrating ability. Together, these characteristics predispose older cats to dehydration. Chronic dehydration can impair normal metabolic processes and exacerbate subclinical disease. Dehydration also reduces a cat's ability to thermoregulate. Water intake in healthy cats without increased losses is 200 to 250 ml per day (Burger and Smith, 1987). This intake comes from a combination of free water, metabolic water and water contained in food. Changing to a moist food or adding water to the food (moist or dry) can increase water intake. Offering low-salt broth, meat juices and "pet drinks" have been advocated to enhance water consumption; however, the long-term effectiveness of these strategies is unknown. Clean fresh water should be available at all times and readily accessible to further encourage water intake.

Energy

Reductions in lean body mass, basal metabolic rate and physical activity decrease energy requirements as animals age (Sheffy and Williams, 1981; Taylor et al, 1995). In many species, the decrease in lean body mass is counterbalanced by an increase in total body fat such that obesity becomes more prevalent with age (Armstrong and Lund, 1996; Sheffy and Williams, 1981). However, studies reveal the prevalence of obesity plateaus and then declines in cats after seven years of age, whereas the preva-

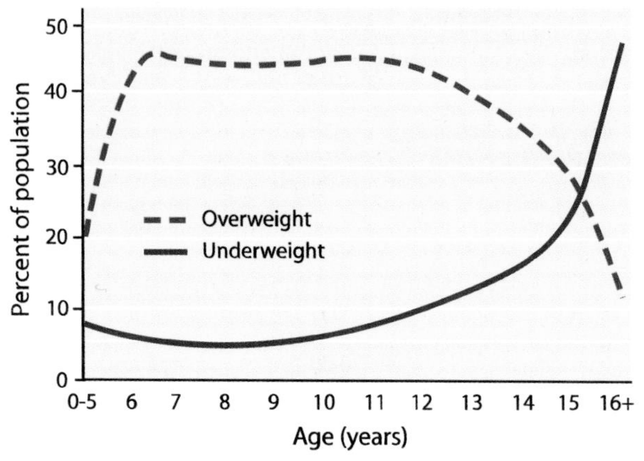

Figure 21-1. Proportion of overweight (body condition score [BCS] 4/5 or 5/5) and underweight (BCS 1/5 or 2/5) cats. Note that six- to 12-year-old cats are commonly overweight, whereas cats over 12 years old are at greater risk of being underweight. (Adapted from Armstrong PJ, Lund EM. Changes in body composition and energy balance with aging. Veterinary Clinical Nutrition 1996; 3: 83-96.)

lence of underweight cats increases dramatically after 11 years of age (**Figure 21-1**) (Scarlett et al, 1994; Armstrong and Lund, 1996). This observation may be explained by the high occurrence of disease in this age group, reduced food intake due to impaired appetite or sensory function, an age-related decline in food digestion or assimilation or a combination of these factors. Although the prevalence of obesity declines after seven years, a significant proportion of mature adult cats remain overweight (**Figure 21-1**). Both obesity and cachexia significantly increase the risk of mortality in cats over eight years of age, with obese cats nearly three times as likely to die as cats of optimal weight (Scarlett and Donoghue, 1997). Therefore, it is critical to recommend foods and feeding methods that will achieve optimal weight and body condition in individual mature cats.

In a study of healthy cats, energy intake declined slightly until approximately 10 years of age. However, a sharp increase in food intake was observed in cats 12 years and older (Taylor et al, 1995). In another study, the energy requirement of cats also decreased with age through approximately 11 years; likewise, the energy needs of these cats increased at approximately 12 years onward (Laflamme and Ballam, 2002). A 10% reduction in fat digestibility was responsible for a similar reduction in total food digestibility in the cats 12 years and older mentioned in the first study (Taylor et al, 1995). The digestibility of dietary fat declined significantly with age, whereas protein and carbohydrate digestibility remained unchanged. Thus, reduced fat digestibility in these mature cats was offset by increased food intake; as a result, digestible energy intake was not different between age groups (Harper, 1996). A later study also found an age-related decrease in ability to digest fat that involved about one-third of cats over 12 years of age (Perez-Camargo, 2004). From these studies, it is unclear if changes in the metabolic rate of older cats are compensated for by a reduction in fat digestion, or if older cats simply compensate for impaired digestion by consuming more food. The latter seems more likely based on observations that weight loss is more prevalent than obesity in very old cats. A decline in pancreatic enzyme secretion is a common physiologic change associated with aging in many species and could be expected to reduce digestibility of dietary fat. In addition, hepatic changes seen in older mature cats may influence nutrient assimilation (Armstrong and Lund, 1996). Based on these studies, the energy density of foods formulated for mature cats should be between 3.5 to 4.5 kcal/g (14.6 to 18.8 kJ/g) dry matter (DM), depending on their predisposition to be overweight and caloric intake may have to be restricted. Inactive/obese-prone cats should be fed foods with lower energy density (3.5 to 4.0 kcal/g [14.6 to 16.7 kJ/g] DM). Normal and underweight cats should be fed energy-dense foods (4.0 to 4.5 kcal/g [16.7 to 18.8 kJ/g] DM) and caloric intake should not be restricted, except to prevent or treat obesity.

Reasonable estimates of caloric needs in mature adult cats are 1.1 to 1.4 x resting energy requirement (RER) (55 to 70 kcal/kg body weight [230 to 293 kJ/kg body weight]), with more active or underweight cats needing up to 1.6 x RER (80 kcal/kg body weight [344 kJ/kg body weight]) (Taylor et al, 1995). Obese cats can be managed with standard weight-control programs appropriate for adult maintenance (Chapter 27).

Fat

Although weight loss is prevalent in very old cats, obesity still affects a large portion of the mature adult cat population (**Figure 21-1**) (Armstrong and Lund, 1996; Lund et al, 2005). Certain diseases associated with obesity are also common in these cats (e.g., diabetes mellitus, hypertension and heart disease). Additionally, the risk of death increases nearly threefold in older obese cats (i.e., eight to 12 years) (Scarlett and Donoghue, 1997; Markham and Hodgkins, 1989; Kirk and Toll, 1996). Moderate to low levels of fat are indicated to reduce the risk of obesity (Scarlett et al, 1994; Hand et al, 1989). However, very old cats need energy-dense foods and ample levels of essential fatty acids. Essential fatty acids (i.e., linoleic, arachidonic and possibly linolenic) help maintain normal skin and coat condition. As animals age, they tend to lose skin elasticity, develop epidermal and follicular atrophy and have reduced sebum secretion (Markham and Hodgkins, 1989). Markedly reducing dietary fat (i.e., calorie-restricted or "light" foods) is not recommended for older mature adult cats unless they are obese prone. Fat should be highly digestible in foods intended for older cats. As discussed above, fat digestion declines with age, which may account for the weight decline noted in very old cats (Taylor et al, 1995). Dietary fat improves food palatability and contributes significantly to energy density. Therefore, maintaining moderate fat concentrations improves food and caloric intake in older mature adult cats and enhances absorption of fat-soluble vitamins (Kane et al, 1981). The recommended range for fat content in foods for mature adult cats is 10 to 25% DM, depending on whether or not they are prone to obesity. Foods for cats that are inactive or prone to obesity should contain 10 to 18% DM fat and foods for cats that are normal or underweight should contain 18 to 25% DM fat. Foods with lower fat levels are recommended for obese-prone cats, and foods with higher fat levels should be fed to thin cats (body condition score <2.5/5) and cats with poor appetites. Essential fatty acids should be provided at levels at or above those recommended for young adult cats (Chapter 20).

Fiber

Fiber facilitates gastrointestinal health by a variety of mechanisms. Dietary fiber promotes normal intestinal motility and provides nutrition (i.e., volatile fatty acids) for colonocytes due to fermentation by colonic microbes. Feeding small amounts (i.e., <5%) of soluble and insoluble fiber can attain these desirable effects. Promoting intestinal motility may benefit cats with constipation (Markham and Hodgkins, 1989). Constipation is common in older cats due to reduced water intake, limited activity and reduced colonic motility. Although fiber should not be the sole factor for managing constipation, it is beneficial when provided regularly. Dietary fiber also benefits the management of obesity, diabetes mellitus and hyperlipidemia (Hand et al, 1989; Nelson and Lewis, 1990; Nelson et al, 1994; Bauer, 1992) (Chapters 27 through 29).

Increased levels of dietary fiber (5 to 15%, DM) reduce food DM digestibility and dilute caloric density; such levels are recommended for foods for inactive cats and cats that are prone to obesity. Normal and underweight cats should receive foods with increased energy density; thus, lower levels (≤5% DM) of dietary fiber are recommended.

Protein

Dietary protein should not be restricted in apparently healthy mature adult cats. Adequate protein and energy intake are needed to sustain lean body mass, protein synthesis and immune function. Besides increasing protein intake, another approach to influencing body composition (i.e., preventing loss of lean body mass in older cats), is increasing the dietary lysine-calorie ratio (**Box 21-1**). Although controversial, the protein needs of older patients may be somewhat greater than those of young adults (Wannemacher and McCoy, 1966; Carter, 1991). The recommended daily protein allowance for elderly people is increased by 25% above that for adult maintenance. The minimum recommended allowance for DM protein for adult cats is 20% (NRC, 2006). The equivalent increase in the minimum protein allowance for cats results in 25% DM protein. The minimum recommended protein allowance for healthy older cats fed commercial foods is further increased to 30% of the food DM to allow for variable digestibility and protein quality of food ingredients. An additional benefit to maintaining this moderate protein concentration in foods for older mature adult cats is the palatability-enhancing effect of animal protein, which may conceivably improve food intake and weight maintenance in very old cats. However, the long-term effects of feeding foods with high dietary protein levels to healthy cats are still largely unknown. High-protein foods have been associated with increased bone loss and increased formation of urinary calcium oxalate crystals in people (Barzel and Massey, 1998; Reddy et al, 2002). In cats, high-protein foods have been implicated in the progression of renal failure (Polzin et al, 1996). Protein restriction in foods for older cats has been advocated because of the high prevalence of renal disease in this age group (Taylor et al, 1995; Lulich et al, 1992) and the knowledge that renal failure is rarely diagnosed until at least three-fourths of renal function is lost. The potential benefits of this restriction include a delay in age-related renal impairment and slowed progression of subclinical renal disease. In one study, investigators examining the effect of protein-calorie restriction in cats following five-sixths nephrectomy observed a reduction in proteinuria and glomerular injury in cats fed reduced-protein foods (27.6% DM) compared with high-protein foods (51.7% DM) (Adams et al, 1993). A secondary finding was an increased occurrence of hypokalemia in cats fed the high-protein food (Adams et al, 1993). However, a subsequent study demonstrated no change in renal pathology following protein restriction and a slight benefit (i.e., reduced cellular infiltrates and tubular lesions) to caloric restriction (i.e., 56 kcal/kg body weight [low-calorie group] vs. 75 kcal/kg body weight [high-calorie group]) (Finco et al, 1998). Unfortunately, these studies may not be directly comparable because the dietary protein sources were markedly different. Thus, there is no clear consensus about the role of protein reduction in slowing progression of clinical or subclinical feline renal disease (Polzin et al, 2005). Healthy older cats should receive sufficient protein to adequately meet protein needs and avoid protein-calorie malnutrition. Improving protein quality without increasing protein intake can fulfill any additional protein needs of older cats. Until further research defines an optimal range of dietary protein for older cats, moderate levels of dietary protein (30 to 45% DM) are recommended.

Box 21-1. The Dietary Lysine-Calorie Ratio and Lean Body Mass of Geriatric Cats.

Besides increasing protein intake, another approach to influencing body composition (i.e., preventing loss of lean body mass) in older cats is the dietary lysine-calorie ratio. The lysine-calorie ratio affects body composition in swine and appears to do so in older cats. In a study involving older mature adult cats (>12 years old), increasing the dietary lysine-calorie ratio was correlated with variation in lean body mass. As the lysine-calorie ratio increased, loss of lean body mass was reduced. Cats fed a food with 36% dry matter (DM) protein and a lysine-calorie ratio of 6.30:1 maintained body weight and lean mass similar to that seen with a higher protein food (45% DM) that had a lower lysine-calorie ratio (4.38:1). Such nutritional technologies might hold promise for foods for older mature adult cats.

The Bibliography for **Box 21-1** can be found at www.markmorris.org.

Calcium and Phosphorus

After skeletal growth is complete, the nutritional requirement for calcium and phosphorus declines to levels needed by adult

Table 21-3. Most common causes of mortality in cats.*

Cause of death	Proportion of deaths (%)
Cancer	35
Kidney disease	24.9
Heart disease	10.7
Diabetes mellitus	7.6

*MAF (Morris Animal Foundation). Animal health survey: Top four causes of death as reported by owners. Denver, CO. 1998.

cats and is thought to remain relatively constant for life. Unlike the situation in people, osteoporosis is not commonly diagnosed in old cats. Nevertheless, the bone mass of adult cats remains stable until seven years of age and then declines (Jewell et al, 1996). The reason for the decline has not been elucidated but is presumably related to the loss of lean and total body mass that occurs with aging. With loss of body mass, less bone mass is required for structural support. Alternatively, bone loss resulting from buffering chronic elevations of metabolic acids cannot be ruled out. Older cats have been reported to maintain a greater metabolic acid load and a significantly lower urinary pH compared with young adult cats (Lawler and Ballam, 1996; Smith et al, 1997). Interestingly, a lower urinary pH (i.e., higher metabolic acid load) is also a risk factor for development of calcium oxalate urolithiasis, which is most prevalent in older cats (Thumchai et al, 1996; Kirk et al, 1995). Mature adult cats should receive foods with moderate levels of available dietary calcium (0.6 to 1.0%, DM) to help maintain bone mass and possibly reduce the risk of calcium oxalate urolithiasis.

In contrast to the moderate calcium needs during aging, reduction of dietary phosphorus is commonly recommended in foods designed for mature adult cats. The recommendation is predicated on the fact that nearly 30% of older cats may have kidney disease (Lulich et al, 1992). Furthermore, in a survey of pet owners, kidney disease was the second leading cause of non-accidental death in cats (**Table 21-3**) (MAF, 1998). Renal insufficiency is rarely diagnosed until significant loss of renal function has occurred. Thus, large proportions of older cats have subclinical renal damage and may benefit from reduced dietary phosphorus. It is commonly accepted that phosphorus restriction slows the progression of renal disease in cats (Chapter 37). Phosphorus reduction helps decrease: 1) the renal excretory workload, 2) phosphorus retention, 3) renal secondary hyperparathyroidism and 4) the subsequent renal mineralization in cats with chronic renal insufficiency (Ross et al, 1982; Polzin et al, 1996). Therefore, in the early nutritional management of renal disease in cats, phosphorus levels should be reduced from those typically found in commercial foods (Brown et al, 1997). Slowing progression of early renal disease in affected older cats should increase longevity (Ross et al, 2006). Phosphorus may be reduced to as low as 0.3% of the food DM for cats with overt renal disease, otherwise the general population of mature adult cats should be fed foods containing 0.5 to 0.7% DM phosphorus. Although adult cats appear to be remarkably tolerant to perturbations in dietary calcium-phosphorus ratios (Kealy et al, 1996), a ratio between 0.9:1 to 1.1:1 maximizes availability (Scott and Scott, 1967) and ratios between 0.9:1 to 1.5:1 are recommended.

Sodium and Chloride

Avoiding excessive sodium intake to reduce risk factors appears even more important in older cats than in young adult cats. Although the sodium and chloride requirements of older cats are not likely to be different from those of young adults, the prevalence of chronic diseases associated with hypertension (e.g., renal disease, hyperthyroidism, cardiac disease) increases with age. The exact prevalence of secondary hypertension in the feline population is unknown, but it appears highest in older cats. In one study, systolic arterial pressures were significantly higher in older cats (Lawler et al, 1996). Furthermore, hypertension affects 60 to 65% of cats with renal disease and 23% of cats with hyperthyroidism (Ross, 1992; Kobayashi et al, 1990; Stiles et al, 1994). Chronic hypertension results in end-organ damage and progression of renal and cardiac disease; therefore, control of risk factors for "salt-sensitive" individuals is desirable. Unfortunately, accurate monitoring of blood pressure in all feline patients is uncommon and hypertension is rarely diagnosed until clinical signs are evident. Therefore, nutritional needs for sodium and chloride should be met, but excesses should be avoided.

Supplemental sodium chloride is used in commercial foods to reduce the occurrence of feline lower urinary tract disease (FLUTD) by increasing water intake. A long-term study (three months) evaluated the safety of salt supplementation (1.1 vs. 0.35% sodium and 0.7 vs. 2.06% chloride, DM) in normal, obese, aged cats and cats with preexisting kidney disease. In this study, none of the cats were hypertensive and blood pressure was unaffected when they were fed the high sodium chloride food. However, cats with preexisting kidney disease fed the salt-supplemented food had increased serum urea nitrogen, phosphorus and creatinine concentrations, suggesting progressive deterioration of renal function. Because many apparently healthy cats can have undetected renal dysfunction based on results of routine serum biochemistry screening, the risks associated with feeding high-salt foods to reduce the occurrence of FLUTD outweigh the benefits (Kirk et al, 2006).

Furthermore, in addition to possibly exacerbating hypertensive disorders and contributing to the progression of preexisting renal disease, high dietary sodium reportedly enhances urinary calcium excretion (Osborne et al, 1992), particularly in cats with impaired renal function (Kirk et al, 2006). This may explain the common occurrence of calcium oxalate uroliths in cats with kidney disease. Thus, sodium excess, particularly in the form of sodium chloride, should be avoided.

Regulation of acid-base homeostasis and normal plasma osmolality depends, in part, on adequate sodium and chloride intake. Deficiencies of sodium and chloride can have deleterious effects in older cats; therefore, over restriction should be avoided. The minimum dietary allowance of sodium for adult cats is 0.068% DM (NRC, 2006). The Association of American Feed Control Officials (AAFCO) recommends an intake of 0.2% of the food DM, or almost threefold the minimum recommended allowance (2007). Some commercial moist foods exceed 1.0% DM sodium or almost 15 times the minimum recommended allowance. Sodium intake at this level is markedly above that needed for optimal health. The recommended range for dietary sodium for mature adult cats is 0.2 to 0.4% DM.

Chloride is now recognized as a co-determinant in salt-sensitive hypertension; thus, control of dietary excess is also important (Kurtz et al, 1987; Kotchen et al, 1987) (Chapter 36). Unfortunately, little information is available about the chloride requirement of cats. The minimum recommended allowance for dietary chloride is 0.096% DM (NRC, 2006); however, more typically, chloride values are approximately 1.5 times the concentration of sodium.

Potassium

The potassium requirement for older cats is thought to be greater than that for young adult cats. This impression comes from anecdotal reports of low serum potassium levels and improved attitude, appetite, muscle strength and renal function following oral potassium supplementation in older cats. However, the potassium requirement of healthy older cats has not been determined and an increased need remains speculative. Nevertheless, factors common in mature adult cats that support the need for increased dietary potassium include: 1) kaliuresis as a result of kidney disease, high dietary protein or high metabolic and/or dietary acid load, 2) reduced food intake and 3) increased intestinal loss. Mature adult cats with normal appetite and renal function probably do not benefit significantly from increased dietary potassium levels. However, hypokalemia can cause signs ranging from mild lethargy to marked polymyopathy and nephropathy. Thus, increasing dietary potassium to support moderate losses may benefit some older cats. Levels as low as 0.3% resulted in hypokalemia when provided in high-protein or acidified foods (DiBartola et al, 1993). The minimum recommended allowance for potassium in foods for adult cats is 0.52% DM (NRC, 2006). Dietary potassium levels for foods for mature adult cats should be at least 0.6% DM.

Magnesium

Increased losses of magnesium, similar to those seen with potassium, may affect magnesium balance in older cats. Hypomagnesemia has also been associated with refractory hypokalemia, particularly in cats with diabetes mellitus (Dhupa, 1995). The benefit of limiting dietary magnesium in cats is a reduced risk of struvite-mediated lower urinary tract disease. However, the risk of struvite-mediated disease is low in older cats (**Figure 21-2**) (Bartges, 1996). Furthermore, foods containing very low levels of magnesium have been associated with the development of calcium oxalate uroliths in an epidemiologic survey of cats (Thumchai et al, 1996) and deficiency increases risk of urolith formation in rats (Su et al, 1991). Therefore, magnesium should be provided at moderate levels (0.05 to 0.1% DM) and severe magnesium restriction should be avoided (<0.04% DM). The minimum recommended allowance for foods for adult cats is 0.04% DM (NRC, 2006).

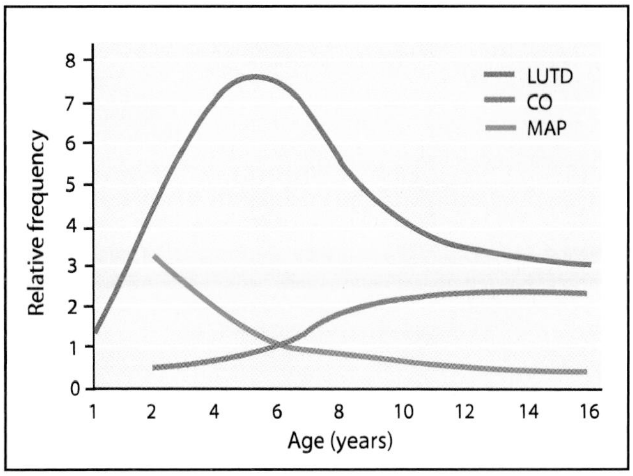

Figure 21-2. Relative frequency of feline lower urinary tract disease (LUTD), struvite (magnesium ammonium phosphate, MAP) urolithiasis and calcium oxalate (CO) urolithiasis in cats of varying age. Note that LUTD is most common in adult cats, struvite urolithiasis is most common in adult cats less than six years old and calcium oxalate urolithiasis is most common in cats over six years old. (Adapted from Bartges JW. Lower urinary tract disease in older cats: What's common, what's not. Veterinary Clinical Nutrition 1996; 3: 57-62. Thumchai R, Lulich JP, Osborne CA, et al. Epizootiologic evaluation of urolithiasis in cats: 3498 cases (1982-1992). Journal of the American Veterinary Medical Association 1996; 208: 547-551.)

Urinary pH

Older cats frequently have clinical or subclinical renal disease that may impair their ability to compensate for acid-base alterations resulting from metabolic and dietary influences. In a study in which cats were fed a food with higher urinary acidifying potential (pH 6.39 vs. 6.6 in the control food), older cats lost more weight, had lower red cell counts and had greater systemic acid loads than younger cats (Lawler and Ballam, 1995). This observation, combined with the reduced risk of struvite urolithiasis, increased risk of calcium oxalate urolithiasis and high frequency of kidney disease in older cats, supports the theory that foods fed to older cats should have a lower urine acidifying potential (i.e., higher published urinary pH averages) than foods for young adult cats. A safe range of measured urinary pH values in mature adult cats is between 6.4 and 6.6.

The acidifying potential of commercial foods for older cats is not typically tested despite the fact that older cats generate a significantly lower urinary pH than younger cats fed the same foods (Smith et al, 1997). To achieve a normal urinary pH, the acidifying potential of foods for mature adult cats should be lower than that of foods for young adult cats. Published urinary pH averages should be greater for foods for older cats than for foods for young adults, unless the foods have been specifically tested in old or very old cats and found to be safe. Providing food with less acidifying potential helps avoid metabolic acidosis and its complications in older cats (Thumchai et al, 1996; Kirk et al, 1995).

Table 21-4. Comparison of recommended levels of key nutritional factors for foods for mature adult cats (normal/underweight and inactive/obese prone) with levels in selected commercial foods.*

Dry foods	**Energy density (kcal/cup)****	**Energy density (kcal ME/g)**	**Fat (%)**	**Fiber (%)**	**Protein (%)**	**Ca (%)**	**P (%)**	**Na (%)**	**K (%)**
Recommended levels (normal/underweight)	**–**	**4.0-4.5**	**18-25**	**≤5**	**30-45**	**0.6-1.0**	**0.5-0.7**	**0.2-0.4**	**≥0.6**
Hill's Science Diet Adult Oral Care	337	4.2	22	7.5	34.1	0.82	0.75	0.37	0.69
Hill's Science Diet Mature Adult Hairball Control	326	4.0	20	8	34	0.86	0.70	0.39	0.80
Hill's Science Diet Mature Adult Indoor	326	4.0	20.1	8	34	0.86	0.71	0.39	0.81
Iams Eukanuba Senior Mature Care	414	4.1	19.0	2.0	39.5	1.39	1.12	0.43	0.85
Nutro MAX Cat Senior Roasted Chicken Flavor	359	3.9	14.3	2.2	31.9	1.10	0.99	0.38	0.66
Nutro Natural Choice Complete Care Senior Cat Food	329	4.0	16.5	2.7	34.1	1.10	1.04	0.44	0.66
Purina Cat Chow Vitality 7+ Formula	397	4.1	13.7	5.4	37.6	1.49	1.32	0.40	0.71
Purina ONE Vibrant Maturity 7+ Senior Formula	437	4.4	16.0	1.7	42.0	1.65	1.39	0.48	0.90
Purina Pro Plan Senior 11+ Indoor Care Turkey & Rice Formula Cat Food	513	4.8	19.8	3.1	50.2	1.45	1.25	0.47	0.78
Royal Canin Mature 27	282	4.2	16.5	7.1	29.7	0.86	0.69	0.34	0.92
Moist foods	**Energy density (kcal/can)****	**Energy density (kcal ME/g)**	**Fat (%)**	**Fiber (%)**	**Protein (%)**	**Ca (%)**	**P (%)**	**Na (%)**	**K (%)**
Recommended levels (normal/underweight)	**–**	**4.0-4.5**	**18-25**	**≤5**	**30-45**	**0.6-1.0**	**0.5-0.7**	**0.2-0.4**	**≥0.6**
Hill's Science Diet Mature Adult Active Longevity Gourmet Turkey Entrée Minced	87/3 oz. 160/5.5 oz.	4.1	20.1	4.8	34.5	0.96	0.64	0.28	0.84
Hill's Science Diet Mature Adult Active Longevity Savory Chicken Entrée Minced	91/3 oz. 168/5.5 oz.	4.4	23.3	3.7	39.2	1.02	0.69	0.49	0.82
Nutro Natural Choice Complete Care Indoor Senior Chicken & Lamb Formula	169/5.5 oz.	4.5	27.1	1.3	39.6	1.25	1.04	0.29	na
Dry foods	**Energy density (kcal/cup)****	**Energy density (kcal ME/g)**	**Fat (%)**	**Fiber (%)**	**Protein (%)**	**Ca (%)**	**P (%)**	**Na (%)**	**K (%)**
Recommended levels (inactive/obese prone)	**–**	**3.5-4.0**	**10-18**	**5-15**	**30-45**	**0.6-1.0**	**0.5-0.7**	**0.2-0.4**	**≥0.6**
Hill's Science Diet Mature Adult Hairball Control	326	4.0	20	8	34	0.86	0.70	0.39	0.80
Hill's Science Diet Mature Adult Indoor Cat	326	4.0	20.1	8	34	0.86	0.71	0.39	0.81
Hill's Science Diet Adult Light	316	3.5	9.5	6.9	35.1	1.00	0.73	0.4	0.67
Iams Eukanuba Senior Mature Care	414	4.1	19.0	2.0	39.5	1.39	1.12	0.43	0.85
Nutro Natural Choice Complete Care Indoor Senior	364	4.0	16.5	2.7	34.1	1.32	0.88	0.38	0.71
Purina ONE Special Care Healthy Weight Formula	362	3.7	12.2	3.7	46.1	1.42	1.41	0.40	1.15
Purina Pro Plan Senior 11+ Indoor Care Turkey & Rice Formula	513	4.8	19.8	3.1	50.2	1.45	1.25	0.47	0.78
Purina Pro Plan Weight Management Formula	413	4.2	12.0	3.4	50.5	1.19	1.08	0.54	0.82
Royal Canin Indoor Light 37	285	3.5	9.9	10.2	40.7	1.16	1.07	0.80	0.68
Moist foods	**Energy density (kcal/can)****	**Energy density (kcal ME/g)**	**Fat (%)**	**Fiber (%)**	**Protein (%)**	**Ca (%)**	**P (%)**	**Na (%)**	**K (%)**
Recommended levels (inactive/obese prone)	**–**	**3.5-4.0**	**10-18**	**5-15**	**30-45**	**0.6-1.0**	**0.5-0.7**	**0.2-0.4**	**≥0.6**
Hill's Science Diet Adult Light Liver & Chicken Entrée Minced	75/3 oz. 138/5.5 oz.	3.6	14.2	10.1	35.6	0.85	0.69	0.32	0.77
Nutro MAX Cat Gourmet Classics Lite with Chicken & Lamb	140/5.5 oz.	3.9	15.2	1.7	41.3	1.74	1.30	1.09	1.09
Nutro Natural Choice Complete Care Indoor Senior Chicken & Lamb Formula	169/5.5 oz.	4.5	27.1	1.3	39.6	1.25	1.04	0.29	na

Key: ME = metabolizable energy, g = grams, Ca = calcium, P = phosphorus, Na = sodium, K = potassium, Mg = magnesium, VOHC = Veterinary Oral Health Council Seal of Acceptance (plaque control, Chapter 47), na = information not available from the manufacturer.
*From manufacturers' published information or calculated from manufacturers' published as fed values; all values are on a dry matter basis unless otherwise stated.
**Energy density values are listed on an as fed basis and are useful for determining the amount to feed; cup = 8-oz. measuring cup. To convert to kJ, multiply kcal by 4.184.

Antioxidants

The consequences of prolonged oxidative stress (e.g., free radical damage) to cell membranes, proteins and DNA contribute to and/or exacerbate a wide variety of degenerative diseases including several of those listed in Table 20-1. The consequences of free radical damage to cells and tissues have also been associated with the effects of aging. Although aging is a complex, multifactorial process, the free radical theory of aging may account for many of associated degenerative changes (Harman, 1956). This theory proposes that free radicals produce cell damage and age-dependent pathologic alterations may be the cumulative result of some of these changes.

Many phenomena initiate free radical formation. Although environmental pollutants and radiation are direct and indirect sources of free radicals, the primary source is normal oxidative metabolism (McMichael, 2007). The body defends itself

Mg (%) 0.05-0.1	Urinary pH 6.4-6.6	Vit. E (IU/kg) ≥500	Vit. C (mg/kg) 100-200	Se (mg/kg) 0.5-1.3	VOHC plaque (Yes/No) Yes
0.06	6.3	670	171	0.7	Yes
0.06	6.6	940	133	0.8	No
0.07	6.6	940	193	0.6	No
na	na	na	na	na	No
0.088	na	330	88	0.9	No
0.088	na	330	99	0.6	No
0.12	na	na	na	na	No
na	na	na	na	na	No
0.09	na	na	na	na	No
0.12	na	725	330	0.4	No
Mg (%) 0.05-0.1	**Urinary pH 6.4-6.6**	**Vit. E (IU/kg) ≥500**	**Vit. C (mg/kg) 100-200**	**Se (mg/kg) 0.5-1.3**	**VOHC plaque (Yes/No) Yes**
0.07	6.5	217	na	1.0	No
0.07	6.5	241	na	1.2	No
na	na	na	na	na	No
Mg (%) 0.05-0.1	**Urinary pH 6.4-6.6**	**Vit. E (IU/kg) ≥500**	**Vit. C (mg/kg) 100-200**	**Se (mg/kg) 0.5-1.3**	**VOHC plaque (Yes/No) Yes**
0.06	6.6	940	133	0.8	No
0.07	6.6	940	193	0.6	No
0.07	6.2	693	189	0.7	No
na	na	na	na	na	No
0.09	na	330	104	0.9	No
na	na	na	na	na	No
0.09	na	na	na	na	No
0.84	na	na	na	na	No
0.11	na	604	220	0.5	No
Mg (%) 0.05-0.1	**Urinary pH 6.4-6.6**	**Vit. E (IU/kg) ≥500**	**Vit. C (mg/kg) 100-200**	**Se (mg/kg) 0.5-1.3**	**VOHC plaque (Yes/No) Yes**
0.08	6.2	401	na	1.5	No
0.10	na	174	87	0.5	No
na	na	na	na	na	No

against the effects of free radicals through a complex network of protective antioxidants. Antioxidants protect biomolecules by scavenging free radical compounds, minimizing free radical production and binding metal ions that might increase the reactivity of poorly reactive compounds. Besides these classic mechanisms, many antioxidants exhibit second messenger regulatory function, cell cycle signaling and control of gene expression (Chapter 7). Combinations of antioxidants work synergistically to reduce oxidative stress and are more effective than individual antioxidants.

The following key nutritional factor recommendations focus on vitamins E and C and selenium. Selenium is an essential component of the antioxidant enzyme glutathione peroxidase. These antioxidants are key nutritional factors because: 1) they are biologically important, 2) they act synergistically (e.g., vitamin C regenerates vitamin E after it has reacted with a free radical), 3) of safety and 4) information regarding inclusion levels in pet foods is usually available. Animal studies and clinical intervention trials in people have shown selenium to be anticarcinogenic at much higher levels (five to 10 times) than the recommended allowances for people or the minimum requirements for animals (Combs, 2001; Neve, 2002). For improved antioxidant performance, foods for older cats should contain at least 500 IU vitamin E/kg DM, 100 to 200 mg vitamin C/kg DM and 0.5 to 1.3 mg selenium/kg DM. The antioxidants discussion in Chapter 20 reviews the basis for these recommendations.

Palatability and Digestibility

Reduced smell or taste, oral disease or metabolic disturbances, medication use or a combination of factors can impair appetite and food intake in older cats (**Table 21-1**). Foods for very old cats should be highly palatable and highly digestible to lessen concerns about weight loss and inadequate food intake. Foods with an energy density greater than 4 kcal/g (16.7 kJ/g) DM are more likely to be highly digestible because they are likely to be lower in fiber and higher in fat.

Texture

Oral disease is the most common disease of mature adult cats (Lund et al, 1999). Age-related changes include an increased prevalence of dental calculus, periodontal disease, loss of teeth and oral neoplasia (Guilford, 1996). Cats with poor oral health have more difficulty eating, and pathologic lesions may act as a portal for bacteria into the body. Additionally, decreased salivary secretions and immune function may exacerbate oral infection and disease (Hefferren et al, 1996). Food texture can play an important role in the well-being of older cats. As in young adult cats, the texture of dry foods fed to older cats may result in less calculus and plaque accumulation than if moist foods are fed (Logan, 1996; Studer and Stapley, 1973). However, the dental efficacy afforded by most commercial dry foods appears not to be clinically important and such claims should generally be regarded with skepticism. Dry foods designed with dental cleansing benefit improve oral health by reducing accumulation of dental plaque and the severity of gingivitis (Logan, 1996; Logan et al, 1997). If the labels of such foods carry the Veterinary Oral Health Council (VOHC) Seal of Acceptance, they have been successfully tested, according to specific protocols, to clinically reduce plaque (Chapter 47). Conversely, hard dry foods (e.g., bones) may cause oral pain if fed to cats with gingivitis or periodontitis. Dry foods with softer texture, semi-moist foods or moist foods may be easier to chew. The optimal texture depends on

Table 21-5. Feeding plan summary for mature adult cats.

1. Select a food from **Table 21-4** that most closely matches the recommended levels of key nutritional factors; for foods not in **Table 21-4**, contact the manufacturer for key nutritional factor content.
2. Select a food with an appropriate energy density. Inactive/obese-prone mature adult = 3.5 to 4.0 kcal (14.6 to 16.7 kJ) ME/g dry matter. Underweight/low body condition mature adult = 4.0 to 4.5 kcal (16.7 to 18.8 kJ) ME/g dry matter.
3. The selected food should be approved by a credible regulatory agency (e.g., AAFCO).
4. Determine the preferred feeding method (Table 20-5); food-restricted meal feeding is best for obese-prone cats.
5. For food-restricted meal feeding, estimate the initial quantity of food based on DER calculation (DER ÷ food energy density, as fed); food energy density as fed (the amount/8-oz. measuring cup or can may be obtained from **Table 21-4** or from the manufacturer's information).
6. Body condition and other assessment criteria will determine DER. DER estimate is calculated by multiplying RER by an appropriate factor (Table 5-2). Remember, DER calculations are estimates and should be used as guidelines or starting points for individual cats and not as absolute requirements. Body condition and other assessment criteria are used to refine the amount to feed.
7. RER can be calculated from Table 5-2. Inactive/obese-prone mature adult (eight to 11 years) = 1.1 to 1.4 x RER. Normal or underweight mature adult (≥12 years) = 1.1 to 1.6 x RER
8. Regularly monitor body condition, body weight and general health.

Key: ME = metabolizable energy, AAFCO = Association of American Feed Control Officials, DER = daily energy requirement, RER = resting energy requirement.

the oral health and food texture preference of individual mature adult cats.

FEEDING PLAN

Older cats are more prone to weight loss, cardiac disease, renal disease, cancer and metabolic aberrations and usually have a decreased activity level than younger cats. The feeding plan should be based on the information obtained in the assessment and any detected risk factors. Nutritional surveillance and therefore the number of contacts per year should be increased for older cats. Although general feeding goals remain the same as those listed in Chapter 20 for young adult cats (maximize health, longevity and quality of life), each patient should be evaluated individually. The feeding plan includes assessing and selecting the best food and feeding method for the individual patient as described for young adult cats.

Assess and Select the Food

Foods currently being fed should be evaluated to:

- Ensure the food was formulated according to the guidelines of a competent regulatory agency (e.g., AAFCO). Review product labels for nutritional adequacy statements (Chapter 9).
- Compare the key nutritional factor levels of the current food with key nutritional factor targets. **Table 21-4** lists selected foods for mature adult cats and key nutritional factor levels for those foods and compares them to the key nutritional factor recommended levels.
- Identify discrepancies between the key nutritional factor targets and those in the food currently fed. A different food should be selected if important discrepancies are found between the recommended levels of key nutritional factors and those in the current food.

It may not always be necessary to change the food and feeding method when managing healthy mature adult cats. However, a thorough evaluation includes verification that an appropriate food and feeding method are being used. Older cats should be reevaluated at each examination because nutrition and health needs change with disease status, risk factors and overall health.

An important goal when managing the nutrition of mature adult cats is to ensure adequate food intake. There is little need to change the form of food a cat eats well because of age. In fact, some cats will refuse to eat a new food with a different form or texture. However, cats with inadequate food intake may benefit from changing food forms if the new food is more palatable and easier to chew.

Assess and Determine the Feeding Method

The feeding method includes how much to feed and how it is fed. Healthy mature cats may be fed free choice, meal fed or fed by a combination of methods. Overweight cats should be offered measured amounts of food. The measured quantity may be fed in meals or dispensed at one time to allow continuous access throughout the day. Underweight cats should be allowed to eat free choice. Only dry and semi-moist foods may be fed free choice and these foods are generally less palatable than moist foods. Table 20-5 summarizes advantages and disadvantages of feeding methods. Older cats may have reduced olfaction and taste perception; therefore, it may be preferable to feed moist and warm foods to encourage food intake. Providing dry foods free choice and several moist food meals throughout the day may optimize food intake. Adding broth or canned meat juices to dry foods may enhance food and water intake in older cats. However, when considering broths or meat juices to improve palatability, evaluate the product for excessive sodium chloride content. (See Key Nutritional Factor discussion, above.) **Table 21-5** summarizes a feeding plan for mature adult cats.

Although most cats do not experience digestive upsets with typical food changes, a gradual transition to a new food may benefit mature adult cats. Progressively exchanging the new food for the usual food over four to seven days will minimize untoward effects and food refusal (Chapters 1 and 20 provide exact details).

REASSESSMENT

Veterinarians should examine older cats and conduct a nutritional assessment regularly. The frequency of monitoring depends on the overall health of the cat and the presence or absence of chronic diseases. Annual veterinary examinations are usually recommended for mature adult cats, whereas biannual checkups are recommended for very old cats.

The owner should evaluate body condition every two to four weeks. Although lean body mass tends to decline as cats reach 16 years or so, significant loss of muscle mass or body weight warrants immediate evaluation by a veterinarian. Owners should also monitor daily food and water intake and stools and urination. Any persistent change, whether increased or decreased, should prompt the owner to seek veterinary advice. The veterinarian should assess the cat and perform diagnostics as indicated.

Dental disease is the most frequent diagnosis made in older cats (Lund et al, 1999). Therefore, a dental health program should be a part of every mature adult cat's preventive health care plan (Chapter 47).

ACKNOWLEDGMENTS

The authors and editors acknowledge the contributions of Drs. Claudia A. Kirk and P. Jane Armstrong in the previous edition of Small Animal Clinical Nutrition.

REFERENCES

The references for **Chapter 21** can be found at www.markmorris.org.

CASE 21-1

Weight Loss in a Mature Adult Cat

Claudia A. Kirk, DVM, PhD, Dipl. ACVN and ACVIM (Internal Medicine)
College of Veterinary Medicine
University of Tennessee
Knoxville, Tennessee, USA

Patient Assessment

A 14-year-old neutered male domestic shorthair cat was examined as part of a routine geriatric health maintenance program. The owner reported no major illnesses except for one episode of urethral obstruction four years earlier. The diagnosis at that time was bacterial cystitis. The cat spends most of its time sleeping on the couch interspersed by brief forays into a pasture to catch voles, field mice and crickets. The owner mentioned that the cat seemed to be losing weight although its appetite had not changed.

Physical examination revealed a bright, alert, 3.5-kg cat with slight loss of body fat and muscle (body condition score [BCS] 2/5). The cat weighed 4.4 kg and had a BCS of 4/5 when last examined 18 months earlier. Oral examination revealed moderate dental disease with several missing teeth and odontoclastic resorptive lesions involving the left upper 4th premolar and both 1st molar teeth. The lesions on the upper 4th premolar were so severe that the crown had fractured leaving a small portion of the tooth root exposed. Moderately severe gingivitis was present. No other abnormalities were noted.

The hospital at which this cat was seen had a health maintenance program for mature adult cats that included a complete blood count, serum biochemistry profile, urinalysis, fecal flotation test, thoracic radiographs, thyroxine (T_4) measurement, ocular fundic examination and tests for feline leukemia and feline immunodeficiency virus infection. Results of the complete blood count, fundic examination, T_4 measurement, thoracic radiographs and urinalysis were normal. The fecal flotation test and tests for viral infection were also negative. The serum biochemistry profile was normal except for a slightly elevated serum urea nitrogen concentration (28 mg/dl, normal 10 to 25 mg/dl) and slightly decreased serum potassium concentration (3.5 mEq/l, normal 3.7 to 5.2 mEq/l). The urinalysis was normal; the urinary pH was 6.0 and the urine specific gravity was 1.030.

Assess the Food and Feeding Method

The cat ate commercial dry and moist specialty brand foods (Science Diet Feline Maintenance[a]). The dry food was offered free choice, and a variety of moist products (beef formula, seafood formula or turkey formula) were offered once daily. The owner was unsure how much dry food was consumed daily. The bowl was filled with dry food as needed. The cat also caught one to two voles or mice per week and ate only the head, leaving the body on the porch. Water was available at all times. The cat often drank from the faucet when allowed.

Questions

1. Has the assessment found any reason for the cat's weight loss?
2. What key nutritional factors are important for this patient?
3. Outline a treatment and feeding plan (food and feeding method) for this cat.
4. How should this patient be monitored?

Answers and Discussion

1. The only abnormalities noted on the assessment are dental disease and laboratory results consistent with possible early chronic renal disease. The extensive dental disease may contribute to weight loss if food intake is reduced because of oral pain. Renal insufficiency would not be expected to cause weight loss at this time. Hyperthyroidism is a common cause of weight loss in older cats, but is less likely in this patient because no cervical mass was found and the serum T_4 concentration was normal. However, hyperthyroidism may occur in cats without these abnormal findings. Repeating the resting T_4 concentration test or performing a T_3 suppression test should be considered for this patient. Many older cats have reduced lean body mass due to: 1) the high occurrence of disease in this age group, 2) reduced food intake because of impaired appetite or sensory function and 3) an age-related decline in food assimilation.
2. Key nutritional factors in older cats include water, energy, protein, fat, minerals (phosphorus, calcium, magnesium, potassium, sodium, chloride), urinary pH, palatability, digestibility and food texture. Water intake is important in older cats because chronic renal disease is very common in this age group. Fat and energy intake are also important in older cats that are susceptible to weight loss. Cats over 12 years of age should be fed energy-dense foods (4.0 to 4.5 kcal metabolizable energy [ME]/g dry matter [16.7 to 18.8 kJ ME/g]) and caloric intake should not be restricted, except as necessary to treat or prevent obesity. Excessive dietary phosphorus, protein, sodium and chloride should be avoided to help control progression of renal disease and hypertension. Hypokalemia is a potential complication of chronic renal disease and has also been reported to occur in older cats. Therefore, potassium-replete foods should be used. The reduced risk of struvite urolithiasis, increased risk of calcium oxalate urolithiasis and decline in renal function observed in older cats support the use of foods with a lower urine acidifying potential (higher published urinary pH values) compared with foods for young adult cats. Because weight loss and inadequate food intake are concerns for many very old cats, their foods should be highly palatable and digestible to ensure optimal intake and nutrient usage. The optimal food texture for older cats depends on the individual's oral health and food texture preference.
3. The cat should be anesthetized for a thorough dental examination and appropriate treatment (i.e., cleaning, extractions, etc.). Commercial foods formulated for older cats are appropriate for this patient. Many of these products have appropriate nutrient levels as discussed above. Many cats and their owners favor the concurrent use of dry and moist foods. The use of more than one form of food and the current feeding method are appropriate and can be continued. An estimated daily energy requirement (DER) should be calculated and the owner encouraged to monitor whether the cat is eating enough food to meet this requirement.
4. Monitoring should include an oral examination and complete physical examination every six months, including a complete blood count, serum biochemistry profile and urinalysis to assess renal function and measurement of potassium and resting T_4 concentrations. Feeding a veterinary therapeutic food formulated for cats with renal failure may be indicated if renal function deteriorates. Adding a potassium supplement will be necessary if serum potassium concentrations remain low.

Progress Notes

An oral antibiotic (clindamycin[b]) was dispensed for administration at home for one week before anesthesia was planned for dental examination and treatment. Tooth scaling, polishing and extractions were performed and the cat recovered uneventfully. The antibiotic was continued for another week. The food was changed to a formula for older cats (Science Diet Feline Senior[a]). The DER was estimated to be 1.2 to 1.4 x resting energy requirement for an ideal body weight of 4.0 kg (230 to 270 kcal [962 to 1,130 kJ]). This energy requirement would be met by feeding one 5.5-oz. can (165 kcal [690 kJ]) and one-fourth to one-third cup of dry food per day. The owner agreed to monitor the cat's daily food intake and to weigh the cat weekly. An appointment was made to reassess the cat in six months.

Endnotes

a. Hill's Pet Nutrition, Inc., Topeka, KS, USA. These products are currently available as Science Diet Adult Original and Science Diet Mature Adult 7+ Original.

b. Antirobe. The Upjohn Company (Animal Health Division), Kalamazoo, MI, USA.

Bibliography

Armstrong PJ, Lund EM. Changes in body composition and energy balance with aging. Veterinary Clinical Nutrition 1996; 3: 83-96.

Bartges JW. Lower urinary tract disease in older cats: What's common, what's not. Veterinary Clinical Nutrition 1996; 3: 57-62.

Bodey AR, Sansom J. Epidemiological study of blood pressure in domestic cats. Journal of Small Animal Practice 1998; 39: 567-573.

Graves TK, Peterson ME. Diagnostic tests for feline hyperthyroidism. Veterinary Clinics of North America: Small Animal Practice 1994; 24: 567-576.

Hefferren JJ, Boyce E, Bresnahan J. Aging and oral health. Veterinary Clinical Nutrition 1996; 3: 97-100.

Markham RW, Hodgkins EM. Geriatric nutrition. Veterinary Clinics of North America: Small Animal Practice 1989; 19: 165-185.

Chapter 22

Feeding Reproducing Cats

Kathy L. Gross
Iveta Becvarova
Jacques Debraekeleer

"The greatness of a nation and its moral progress can be judged by the way its animals are treated."
Mahatma Gandhi

INTRODUCTION

Domestic cats generally reach puberty by six to nine months of age. However, the best age for breeding is between one and one-half to seven years of age (Feldman and Nelson, 1996). Queens 10 to 12 months of age are still growing and must meet nutritional demands for their own growth as well as for their fetuses. Queens older than seven years should not be bred due to reproductive complications, irregular estrous cycles and reduced litter size (Feldman and Nelson, 1996). The reproductive stage of the queen can be divided into four periods: 1) estrus and mating, 2) gestation, 3) lactation and 4) weaning. In general, reproducing queens have increased nutritional needs compared with maintenance requirements, especially during late pregnancy and lactation. During reproduction, energy requirements increase and the minimum requirements for certain nutrients exceed even those required for growth.

The objectives of a good feeding program for reproduction are to optimize: 1) the health and body condition of the queen throughout the various reproductive periods, 2) reproductive performance and 3) kitten health and development through the weaning period. Key indicators of optimal reproduction are ease of conception, a low rate of fetal and neonatal deaths, normal parturition, maximum litter size, adequate lactation and an optimal growth rate of healthy kittens. Providing adequate nutrition throughout reproduction has long-range health implications for the offspring. Immune function is impaired for life in animals born to nutritionally deficient dams (Burkholder and Swecker, 1990). Meeting the nutritional needs of reproducing queens is critical to successful conception, delivery and weaning of healthy kittens.

Lactation begins at parturition and lasts six to 12 weeks depending on breed, kitten growth rates and management practices. Most kittens are sufficiently mature at eight weeks of age to maintain adequate food intake for optimal development. Purebred kittens are typically weaned later than domestic shorthair kittens. Lactation is the most demanding stage of reproduction. The queen must maintain its own nutritional needs and provide nutritionally complete, nutrient-dense milk to support the needs of growing kittens. Consequently, queens should enter lactation with sufficient energy stores to support needs above those supplied by daily food intake. Poor lactation performance is common without these reserves. Thus, successful lactation depends on appropriate nutritional management during the pre-breeding period, gestation and lactation.

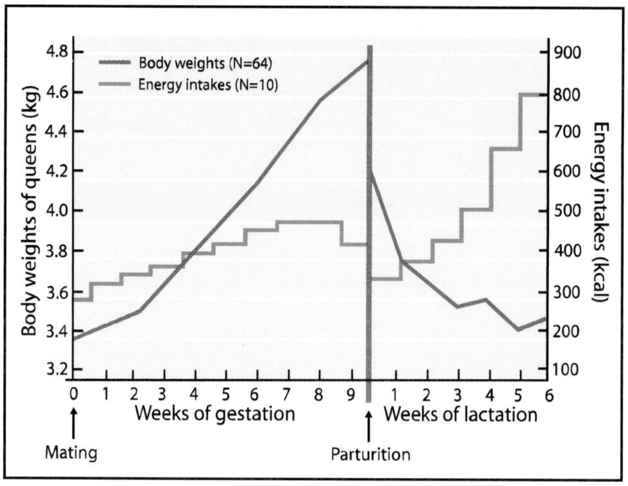

Figure 22-1. Body weight and energy intake during gestation and lactation in queens. Unlike bitches, which have a dramatic increase in energy intake and body weight during the last trimester, queens have a regular linear increase in both body weight and energy intake throughout gestation. Mobilized stores of body fat provide needed energy during lactation, which accounts for weight loss during this period. Food intake parallels lactation and peaks during the sixth to seventh week. (Adapted from Loveridge GG. Body weight changes and energy intake of cats during gestation and lactation. Animal Technology 1985; 37: 7-15.)

PATIENT ASSESSMENT

Estrus and Mating

Optimal nutrition for reproducing cats should precede mating and conception, and ideally start when the animal is a kitten. Female cats are seasonally polyestrous. Repeated estrous cycles occur throughout the breeding season, which typically occur from January through September in the northern hemisphere. Light duration and intensity are major determinants for the estrous period. Therefore, artificial lighting and latitude variation alter the breeding period for individual cats. Vocalizing, rolling, rubbing and treading characterize estrus in the queen; these behaviors culminate in acceptance of the male. Behavioral estrus averages seven to nine days (range one to 21). Cats are induced ovulators (i.e., coital contact is typically required for a luteinizing hormone surge and ovulation).

Queens should have a current vaccination history and be treated for internal and external parasites before breeding. A history and physical examination should precede breeding to assess problems that may interfere with conception, parturition and lactation. Queens should be at ideal body weight at mating (body condition score [BCS] 3/5). Small variations in body condition can be corrected during pregnancy; however, cats that are significantly under- or overweight (BCS <2/5 or >4/5) should not be bred. Both obesity and undernourishment can be detrimental to reproductive performance. Malnourished queens may fail to conceive, abort or bear small, underweight kittens and have a markedly reduced lactation. Lactating queens normally lose weight, but their body weight should return to normal before the next breeding. Obese cats reportedly have a greater incidence of dystocia (Lawler and Monti, 1984). Historical or physical evidence of a narrow pelvic canal, whether due to trauma, genetics or nutritional deficiency warrants careful assessment. Mammary tissue and teat development should be evaluated. Although congenital defects (e.g., multiple teats or teat malformation) rarely prevent queens from raising normal-sized litters, genetic selection away from such traits is advisable. Only cats in excellent health should be considered for breeding.

Tomcats should also be healthy and in optimal body condition (BCS 3/5); however, decreased reproductive performance associated with moderate deviations from ideal (BCS <2/5 to >4/5) have not been reported. In addition to a standard physical examination, the penis, prepuce and testes should be evaluated for anatomic defects. Previous reproductive performance including a weight history should be reviewed. The level of activity required during the breeding period should be ascertained. Single matings result in minimal changes in energy needs, whereas multiple matings may require an increase in the amount of food provided, based on body condition.

Pregnancy

The first assessment step is to diagnose pregnancy. Abdominal palpation is used most commonly to diagnose pregnancy in cats. The fetal vesicles can be reliably palpated from 14 to 25 days of gestation (Feldman and Nelson, 1996). An enlarged uterus is palpable from Day 25 to parturition. Ultrasound can detect pregnancy by Day 11 of gestation and fetal heartbeats are typically heard at 22 days (Davidson et al, 1986). Radiographic diagnosis requires calcification of the fetal skeleton and is most reliable after Day 45 of gestation. Gestation usually lasts 63 to 65 days (range 58 to 70 days) in queens, thus radiography is not useful for early pregnancy diagnosis, but is useful for determining litter size. In addition to the diagnosis of pregnancy, an assessment should include a dietary history, physical examination and any indicated laboratory analyses. Evaluations of body condition, weight gain and food intake are most important. Minimal diagnostics are usually required if the pelvic structures and mammary glands were evaluated and parasite, feline leukemia virus/feline immunodeficiency virus and vaccination status were determined before breeding.

One of the early indicators of successful breeding and conception is a steady gain in body weight. Weight gain increases linearly from conception to parturition in queens (**Figure 22-1**). This pattern is different from that of most other species, which experience small increases in body weight until the last third of gestation when weight gain and energy intake greatly increase. Weight gain in early pregnancy is not associated with significant growth of reproductive tissues or conceptuses but appears to be stored in energy depots (presumably as fat) to support lactation (Loveridge and Rivers, 1989). Mean weight gain during gestation is approximately 40% of the pre-mating weight (900 to 1,200 g for a litter of average size) and has been described by the equation (Loveridge and Rivers, 1989):

Weight gain (g) = 888.9 + (106.5)n (where n = number of neonates).

At parturition, only 40% of the weight gained by queens during gestation will be lost (Loveridge and Rivers, 1989), whereas bitches should return to pre-breeding weight (Feldman and Nelson, 1996a). The remaining 60% of prepartum weight gain will be used during lactation to sustain milk production. Poor nutrition may lead to failure to conceive, fetal death, fetal malformations and underweight kittens. Queens underweight at parturition may subsequently experience poor lactation performance and inability to maintain body condition. Poor maternal nutrition may impair the kittens' immunocompetence for life.

Overnutrition or obesity (BCS 5/5) has an equally negative effect on pregnancy outcome. Stillbirths, dystocia and cesarean sections occur more frequently in obese queens than in cats at ideal body condition (Lawler and Monti, 1984; Bilkei, 1990). Ensuring the queen is at ideal weight (BCS 3/5) before breeding is preferable to limiting food intake during gestation. Therefore, good nutritional management is important to optimal reproductive performance.

If queens are listless or have a poor appetite, the physical examination should closely evaluate uterine size and shape and any vaginal discharges. Laboratory evaluation should include a complete blood count and measurement of serum concentrations of glucose, calcium, protein, urea nitrogen, creatinine, phosphorus and potassium. The abdomen and uterus should be evaluated by ultrasound to evaluate fetal viability or if pyometra is suspected.

Lactation

Unless difficulties arise during parturition or lactation, a veterinarian will not examine most queens. Thus, pre-lactation counseling of the breeder or owner is important because most of the assessment will be performed without veterinary supervision. The queen and kittens should be weighed within 24 hours after parturition. The queen should weigh 700 to 900 g above the pre-breeding weight and each kitten should weigh approximately 100 g. The queen should be evaluated for vaginal discharges, body temperature and maternal behavioral characteristics. A dark reddish vaginal discharge is normal. Bright red discharges indicate hemorrhage, whereas foul-smelling, greenish, gray or brown discharges may indicate a retained fetus, retained placenta or infection. The queen's appetite, which is reduced 24 to 48 hours before parturition, should return to normal or to an increased level within 24 hours of parturition (Lawler and Bebiak, 1986). All kittens should nurse soon after parturition and within the first six to eight hours to ensure transfer of colostral antibodies. Neonatal kittens may not absorb immunoglobulins after 12 hours postpartum. This window of absorption is much shorter in kittens than in puppies and livestock (Casal et al, 1996).

Milk production should begin at parturition. Colostrum is produced during the first 24 to 72 hours of lactation. Milk yield depends on litter size and stage of lactation, with peak lactation occurring at three to four weeks. Investigators measured average milk yields of 1 to 3% of the queen's body weight/day during Week 1 (Dobenecker et al, 1998). Yields increase to 1.3 to 5.9% of the queen's body weight/day at peak lactation then decline slightly until weaning. Although mammary glands should be closely evaluated to ensure health and ready access for the kittens, expressing milk from each gland does not ensure adequate milk production. Continuous weight gain by the kittens is the best indicator of the queen's lactation performance. Neonatal kittens should gain between 10 to 15 g daily. Gains less than 7 g/day are inadequate (Lawler and Bebiak, 1986).

A veterinarian should immediately evaluate the queen and litter if health problems arise during lactation or kitten growth rates are suboptimal. A complete physical evaluation, anamnesis and review of the reproduction records and the nutritional plan should be performed. Blood and urine should be collected from the queen; a minimum database should include a complete blood count, urinalysis and serum biochemistry analysis including electrolytes. Ancillary tests should be performed as indicated.

Table 22-1. Key nutritional factors for foods for reproducing cats.

Factors (units)*	Mating**	Gestation/lactation
Energy density (kcal ME/g)	4.0-5.0	4.0-5.0
Energy density (kJ ME/g)	16.7-20.9	16.7-20.9
Protein (%)	30-45	35-50
Fat (%)	10-30	18-35
DHA (%)	-	≥0.004
Digestible carbohydrate (%)***	-	≥10
Calcium (%)	-	1.1-1.6
Phosphorus (%)	0.5-0.7	0.8-1.4
Ca:P ratio	-	1:1-1.5:1
Sodium (%)	0.2-0.5	0.3-0.6
Average urinary pH	6.2-6.4	6.2-6.5

Key: ME = metabolizable energy, DHA = docosahexaenoic acid.
*Units expressed on a dry matter basis. Concentrations presume an energy density of 4.0 kcal/g. Levels should be corrected for foods with higher energy densities. Adjustment is unnecessary for foods with lower energy densities.
**Foods for most breeding males and females are usually similar to those for young adult cats (Chapter 20).
***Important for lactation.

Key Nutritional Factors

Few studies establish the minimum nutritional requirements for reproducing queens and breeding male cats. Most nutrient recommendations are extrapolated from growth studies, results from other species and clinical experience. Although most commercial foods appropriate for growing kittens are deemed adequate for female reproduction, ideally, complete and balanced foods specifically designed to support gestation/lactation should be fed. Key nutritional factors for tomcats and queens during mating do not appear to be significantly different from those of young adults (Chapter 20). Exceptions will be noted below. **Table 22-1** summarizes key nutritional factors for reproducing cats eating commercial foods. The following section describes these key nutritional factors in more detail.

Water

Water is important for normal reproduction. Expansion of extracellular fluid compartments and maternal and fetal tissues

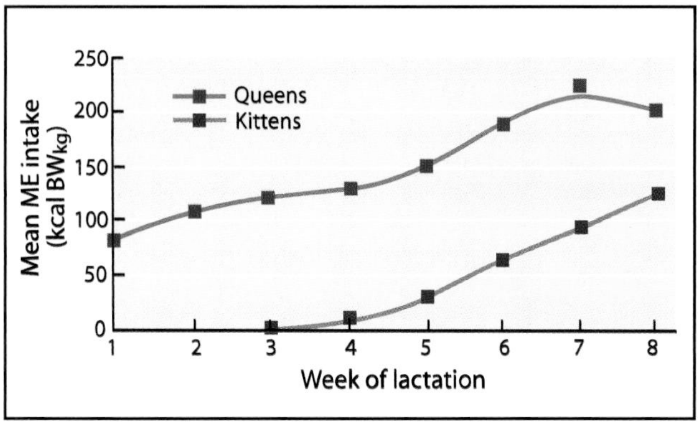

Figure 22-2. Food energy intake during lactation of queens and their kittens. Kittens begin eating the queen's food in increasing amounts from about four weeks of age until weaning. Energy intake peaks for queens at seven weeks and then decreases as kittens consume a larger percentage of their energy from food rather than milk. (Adapted from Munday HS, Earle KE. The energy requirements of the queen during lactation and kittens from birth to 12 weeks. Journal of Nutrition 1991; 121: S43-S44.)

during pregnancy increases the need for water. Water is particularly important for milk production during lactation. Water needs for lactating queens vary according to maintenance needs, type of food (moist vs. dry) and the rate of milk production. Although specific levels of water intake have not been established, reproducing queens should be provided with ample potable water at all times. Some queens are reluctant to leave the nest box during the first few days after parturition. Water intake should be encouraged by placing water very near the enclosure to allow easy access. Feeding moist foods or adding water to food can improve water intake.

Energy

ENERGY NEEDS DURING ESTRUS AND MATING

The energy requirements of most queens during mating do not appear to be significantly different from those of young adults (Chapter 20). The recommendation for energy density for foods for normal weight young adult cats is 4.0 to 5.0 kcal/g (dry matter [DM]) (16.7 to 20.9 kJ/g [DM]). However, during behavioral estrus, queens typically reduce food intake and body weight may decline. Food intake and body weight rebound upon cessation of estrus. In some queens, it may be advisable to feed a highly palatable food with an energy density at the upper end of the recommended range (4.5 to 5.0 kcal/g food [18.8 to 20.9 kJ/g food]) before mating to ensure optimal body condition at conception. Intact female cats typically require more calories than neutered housecats. The daily energy requirement (DER) for sexually intact cats is 1.4 to 1.6 x resting energy requirement (RER).

Breeding male cats that are used infrequently or in small catteries have energy needs similar to those of intact young adult cats (4.0 to 5.0 kcal/g or 16.7 to 20.9 kJ/g [DM]) (1.4 to 1.6 x RER). Tomcats that are used extensively for breeding may have difficulty maintaining proper body condition due to increased energy expenditure or, more often, reduced food intake. The stress of travel, new environments, social interactions and preoccupation with breeding may contribute to inappetence. These tomcats should be managed similarly to cats that are very active or under stress. Foods at the upper end of the recommended range of energy density for young adult cats (4.5 to 5.0 kcal/g food [18.8 to 20.9 kJ/g food]) with above average palatability should help these cats maintain ideal body condition (BCS 3/5) and activity.

ENERGY NEEDS DURING PREGNANCY

One of the most important changes in nutrient requirements of gestating cats is an increase in energy requirement. Although many essential nutrients are required at increased levels during gestation, dietary energy is often the most limiting "nutrient."

As mentioned previously, energy intake and weight gain increase linearly from conception to parturition in queens (**Figure 22-1**). However, food intake normally fluctuates slightly throughout gestation. Reduced food intake occurs approximately two weeks after mating and is thought to occur in association with fetal implantation at about Day 15 postconception (Feldman and Nelson, 1996). Energy intake increases then peaks between six to seven weeks of gestation. A second decline in food intake occurs during the last week of gestation. These transient declines in food intake do not appear harmful. However, inadequate food intake over the course of gestation may impair weight gain, the subsequent lactation and kitten health. The recommended energy allowance for gestation is 25 to 50% above maintenance levels or approximately 90 to 110 kcal/kg body weight/day (376 to 460 kJ/kg body weight/day), although total caloric intake may increase as much as 70% above maintenance (NRC, 1986; Loveridge and Rivers, 1989). The increased need for energy can be met by providing 1.6 x RER at breeding with a gradual increase to 2 x RER at parturition. Energy requirements sometimes exceed the recommended energy allowance due to individual cat variation and increased energy needs of queens with large litters. Therefore, free-choice feeding allows queens to adjust food intake as needed to meet the energy requirement for gestation. **Table 22-2** lists energy requirements of gestating queens at various body weights.

Feeding energy-dense foods (metabolizable energy [ME] = 4.0 to 5.0 kcal/g DM [16.74 to 20.9 kJ/g DM]) helps meet the energy needs of pregnant queens, especially during late gestation when the gravid uterus reduces stomach capacity.

ENERGY NEEDS DURING LACTATION

Lactation is the most energy-demanding stage of a cat's life. Peak milk production typically occurs at three to four weeks of lactation and, theoretically, peak energy demand should occur concurrently. However, actual peak energy demand occurs at six to seven weeks postpartum when energy requirements may exceed 250 kcal/kg body weight/day (1.05 MJ/kg body weight/day) or 2 to 6 x RER (**Table 22-3**). Observed energy intakes of queens and their litters during lactation increase from 90 kcal/kg body weight/day (376 kJ/kg body weight/day) at parturition to 270 kcal/kg body weight/day (1.13 MJ/kg body weight/day) at Week 7 (Loveridge, 1985). The discrepancy in the timing of peak lactation and peak energy demand is due to combined food consumption by kittens and the queen. Kittens begin eating the queen's food in increasing amounts from three weeks of age until weaning. Therefore, the above estimates of energy requirement for the lactating queen include energy consumed by the queen and its kittens (**Figure 22-2**). When energy intake was measured for the queen alone, the energy requirement at Week 6 of lactation was 229 kcal/kg body weight/day (962 kJ/kg body weight/day) (Munday and Earle, 1991). Within large litters, up to 50% of the total energy was consumed by kittens, increasing the total energy consumption (i.e., kittens and queens) to as high as 306 kcal/kg body weight/day (1.28 MJ/kg body weight/day). Even with these large increases in energy intake, queens will continue to lose weight during lactation and return to pre-mating weight by weaning. Queens that lose excessive weight are prone to lactation failure. **Table 22-3** estimates the energy requirements of lactating queens. However, it is preferable to feed lactating queens free choice because the wide variation in energy needs makes accurate prediction difficult.

The high-energy demands during lactation require a marked increase in total food intake. Feeding an energy-dense food (4.0 to 5.0 kcal ME/g DM, [16.7 to 20.9 kJ ME/g]) helps meet these demands without overwhelming gastric capacity.

If kittens are encouraged to eat a solid food beginning at three weeks of age, the energy demands placed on the lactating queen will decline as kittens increasingly obtain nutrition from solid food. Maintenance energy levels are sufficient for queens at ideal body condition after the kittens are weaned. Queens that have lost excess body weight during lactation should be provided additional food to restore body condition.

Table 22-2. Energy requirements of pregnant queens.*

Body weight		kcal ME per day		kJ ME per day	
		At 90 kcal/kg BW	At 100 kcal/kg BW	At 375 kJ/kg BW	At 420 kJ/kg BW
kg	lb				
2	4.4	180	200	750	840
3	6.6	270	300	1,125	1,260
4	8.8	360	400	1,500	1,680
5	11.0	450	500	1,875	2,100
6	13.2	540	600	2,250	2,520
7	15.4	630	700	2,625	2,940
8	17.6	720	800	3,000	3,360

Key: ME = metabolizable energy, BW = body weight.
*Adapted from the National Research Council. Nutrient Requirements of Cats. Washington, DC: National Academy Press, 1986.

Table 22-3. Daily energy requirements of lactating queens over the lactation period.*

Weeks of lactation	Daily energy requirements		
-	Factor x RER	kcal/kg BW**	kJ/kg BW
1	2.3	115	481
2	2.5	125	523
3	3.0	150	628
4	3.5	175	732
5	4.0	200	837
6	5.0	250	1,046

Key: RER = resting energy requirement, $70(BW_{kg})^{0.75}$ or $30(BW_{kg}) + 70$, BW = body weight.
*Based on average queen at parturition (3.8 kg) nursing four to five kittens. These values represent average energy requirements for lactating queens. Individual animal variation and litter size may alter total daily energy needs.
**Adapted from the National Research Council. Nutrient Requirements of Cats. Washington, DC: National Academy Press, 1986.

Protein

Protein synthesis in the queen is greatly increased during gestation. Additionally, protein quality and quantity are important to provide essential amino acids for healthy fetal growth and development. Protein levels of 20% DM have sustained adequate gestation in gestating queens fed energy-dense (4.8 kcal/g [20 kJ/g]) purified foods. The minimum recommended allowance is 21.3% DM (NRC, 2006). However, 30% DM dietary protein results in near optimal weight gain in queens during gestation and kittens during lactation (Piechota et al, 1995). Considering the varying nutrient availability in typical pet food ingredients compared with purified foods, protein levels at or above 35% DM are recommended for gestating queens (range of 35 to 50%, DM). Animal-based proteins are preferred as the major source of dietary protein because they are usually more digestible and have more desirable amino-acid profiles. Protein deficiency during pregnancy may result in lower birth weights, higher neonatal mortality and impaired immunocompetency in kittens (Burkholder and Swecker, 1990). Additionally, when queens are fed protein-restricted foods during late gestation and lactation, their kittens can have delayed home orientation (i.e., ability to orient to and return to the nest), aberrant locomotor development and decreased emotional responsiveness (Gallo et al, 1984).

During lactation, queens increase protein synthesis to provide milk with adequate protein content for kitten growth (i.e., approximately 36% DM milk protein). Milk protein output for a 4-kg queen nursing a large litter may reach 19 g crude protein/day (Dobenecker et al, 1998). Thus, it is not surprising that protein needs during lactation exceed even gestational requirements.

The minimum recommended allowance for protein for peak lactation is 30% DM (NRC, 2006). Inadequate protein concentrations result in poor lactation and kitten growth. Queens fed foods containing 20% DM protein had lower hematocrit values at Week 6 of lactation compared with queens fed foods with higher protein levels (Piechota et al, 1995). Providing 25% DM crude protein to lactating queens results in satisfactory reproductive performance (Piechota et al, 1995). However, near optimal performance is achieved with foods containing 30% DM crude protein. Queens fed foods with 30% protein lose less body weight than those fed foods with levels of 20 or 25% DM protein. Additionally, food intake and kitten growth rates are higher at dietary protein levels of 30% DM (Piechota et al, 1995). Because of variations in food digestibility and ingredient quality and the goal to promote optimal reproductive performance, the recommended crude protein allowance for lactation is at least 35% DM (range of 35 to 50%, DM). The protein sources in commercial foods should be highly digestible and have high biologic value. Animal-based protein ingredients should provide the major source of amino acids and protein for lactating queens.

For breeding males, the range recommended for young adult non-breeding cats is adequate (30 to 45%, DM).

Fats and Essential Fatty Acids

Fat delivers 2.25 times the number of calories as the same amount of protein or digestible (soluble) carbohydrate; therefore, increasing dietary fat increases a food's energy density. Thus, smaller amounts of food can be consumed to meet the queen's energy demands. The minimum recommended allowance for queens for late gestation and peak lactation is 9% DM (NRC, 2006). However, as discussed above, higher-energy foods are beneficial because of the increased energy demand during gestation and lactation and because such foods improve reproductive performance. For example, in one study, increasing dietary fat from 15 to 27% of the food DM: 1) increased the number of kittens per litter, 2) decreased kitten mortality from more than 20 to 9% and 3) improved reproductive efficiency in queens (more litters per year) (Olovson, 1986). For optimal reproductive performance, foods for gestating and lactating queens should contain at least 18% DM fat (range of 18 to 35%, DM), although foods with lower levels of fat have been successfully fed during gestation. Nutrients in the food should be balanced to the higher energy content of energy-dense foods (>4.5 kcal/g DM [18.8 kJ/g DM]). The fat content in foods for mating cats is typically between 10 to 30% DM.

Minimum essential fatty acid requirements for lactation do not differ significantly from those of gestation. However, a dietary source of docosahexaenoic acid (DHA, 22:6n-3) is required for normal development of retinal function in nursing kittens (Pawlosky et al, 1997). In children, during periods of early growth, DHA is needed to support retinal and auditory development (Pawlosky et al, 1997; Birch et al, 2002; Diau et al, 2003). Furthermore, brain development and learning ability were enhanced in infants supplemented with DHA (Birch et al, 2002; Hoffman et al, 2003). Similar to findings in other species, the inclusion of fish oil as a source of DHA in puppy foods improved trainability (Kelley et al, 2004). The need for DHA during growth in foods for kittens may be even more important than in foods for puppies considering the cat's reduced ability to convert shorter chain fatty acids to DHA. Milk concentrations of DHA parallel dietary intake. Therefore, DHA should be included in foods fed to lactating queens. Common ingredients such as fish and poultry meal represent a source of DHA in the food of queens. For foods for queens in late gestation and peak lactation, the minimum recommended allowance of DHA plus eicosapentaenoic acid (EPA) is at least 0.01% DM (NRC, 2006). Thus, DHA needs to be at least 40% of the total DHA plus EPA, or ≥0.004% DM.

Long-term deficiency of dietary arachidonic acid (AA) results in reproductive failure in cats (MacDonald et al, 1984). However, Association of American Feed Control Officials (AAFCO) allowances for AA are appropriate for gestating cats (AAFCO, 2007). Therefore, foods with AAFCO label statements acknowledging that a food is appropriate for growth or reproduction should provide adequate amounts (See the Essential Fatty Acid discussion in Other Nutritional Factors, below).

Digestible Carbohydrate

Although a true digestible carbohydrate requirement for cats has not been demonstrated, digestible carbohydrates apparently protect against weight loss in queens during lactation (Piechota et al, 1995). Digestible carbohydrates spare protein necessary to sustain blood glucose concentrations in queens and provide a substrate for lactose during milk production. Providing some digestible carbohydrate improves lactation performance even with an abundant supply of dietary protein (Piechota et al, 1995). Until further studies define optimal levels of digestible carbohydrates for lactation, at least 10% DM digestible carbohydrate should be included in foods for lactating queens.

Calcium and Phosphorus

Calcium and phosphorus are required at levels greater than maintenance to support fetal skeletal development and lactation. The minimal recommended DM allowances for dietary calcium and phosphorus for queens in late gestation and peak lactation are 1.08 and 0.76%, respectively (NRC, 2006). Recommended levels for foods for feline gestation and lactation should be within the ranges of 1.1 to 1.6 for calcium and 0.8 to 1.4 for phosphorus DM. Levels at, or greater, than these recommendations are typically found in commercial cat foods. The calcium-phosphorus ratio should be between 1:1 to 1.5:1. Although eclampsia is uncommon in cats, it does occur pre- and postparturiently (**Box 22-1**). The calcium and phosphorus recommendations for mating cats are the same as for young adult cats (Chapter 20).

Sodium

Reproducing queens, particularly during lactation, consume increased quantities of food to meet their energy and protein needs. In doing so, they consume considerably more sodium than in the non-reproducing state. Some women are predisposed to hypertension during pregnancy, but it is unknown whether or not there is a population of queens predisposed to hypertension during gestation.

There is no direct information to support a minimum recommended allowance for dietary sodium for gestation in queens but it is estimated to be about four times the amount recommended for adult maintenance (NRC, 2006). The minimal recommended DM allowance for foods for late gestation and peak lactation (0.27%) (NRC, 2006) is six to seven times the amount recommended for maintenance. Thus, an upper limit of 0.6%

Box 22-1. Eclampsia in the Queen.

Eclampsia, or periparturient hypocalcemia, is uncommon in cats. Clinical signs result from severe hypocalcemia, with or without other biochemical abnormalities. Predisposing factors may include improper perinatal nutrition, inappropriate calcium supplementation and heavy lactation demands. Whereas dogs typically present within the first four weeks of lactation, cats more commonly are presented during the last three weeks of pregnancy. Affected cats exhibit nonspecific clinical signs of lethargy, depression, weakness, tachypnea and mild muscle tremors. Additional signs may include vomiting, anorexia, and hypothermia, flaccid paralysis, hyperexcitability and other signs of malaise. Eclampsia should be considered as a diagnostic rule-out in queens with vague signs of illness late in gestation.

The pathophysiology of periparturient hypocalcemia in cats is not well understood. Some investigators have implicated excessive prenatal calcium intake. High calcium intake may down-regulate parathyroid gland secretion and impair normal mobilization of calcium from skeletal stores. As demand for calcium increases during late gestation and lactation, calcium homeostasis is unable to maintain critical serum levels. Although high calcium intake is an accepted cause of periparturient tetany in cattle, it remains speculative as the cause of the disease in cats.

Serum total calcium and ionized calcium concentrations usually are decreased. Ionized calcium is the biologically active form. In-hospital serum chemistry and point-of-care analyzers allow veterinarians to obtain serum total calcium and ionized calcium concentrations rapidly. Diagnosis of hypocalcemia is based on low serum ionized calcium concentrations. Blood glucose should be measured as well, because hypoglycemia may be present concurrently.

Treatment is aimed at immediate correction of hypocalcemia with a slow intravenous infusion of 10% calcium gluconate (1.0 to 1.5 ml/kg body weight over 10 to 30 minutes), given to effect. Heart monitoring (e.g., auscultation, electrocardiography) should be performed during intravenous calcium gluconate infusion. If bradycardia or dysrhythmias develop, the infusion must be slowed or discontinued. Dextrose may be administered by intravenous bolus (50% solution) or intravenous infusion (5% dextrose in saline solution) to correct hypoglycemia, if present. After acute signs are corrected, oral supplementation of calcium carbonate (10 to 30 mg/kg body weight every eight hours) is begun and continued throughout gestation and lactation.

If eclampsia is diagnosed following queening, the litter should be removed from the queen for 24 hours, during which time, the kittens should be fed kitten milk replacer by bottle or orogastric tube feeding. In contrast to dogs, it is rarely necessary to wean kittens early. Recurrence of periparturient hypocalcemia has not been reported in cats.

The Bibliography for **Box 22-1** can be found at www.markmorris.org.

DM is recommended for foods for queens in late gestation/peak lactation. The recommendation for sodium in foods for mating cats is the same as for young adult cats (Chapter 20).

Urinary pH
Highly acidified foods should be avoided during gestation because metabolic acidosis may impair bone mineralization in adult cats and kittens, which can be especially detrimental to developing fetuses (Ching et al, 1989, 1990; Dow et al, 1990; Buffington, 1988; Hardardottir et al, 1997). Foods designed to produce average urinary pH values between 6.2 to 6.5 appear to be safe (Allen et al, 1997). Foods for mating cats should produce average urinary pH values between 6.2 to 6.4, as for young adult cats.

Digestibility
For reproducing queens, foods with above average DM digestibility are better suited than less digestible foods because: 1) nutrient needs increase as pregnancy progresses 2) increased abdominal fullness as the pregnancy progresses may impair the queen's ability to ingest adequate amounts of nutrients, especially if the food is poorly digestible and 3) the nutritional demands of lactation are even greater than for gestation.

DM digestibility information for commercial foods marketed for reproduction is not readily available. However, energy density indirectly indicates digestibility. Foods with an energy density of 4 kcal ME/g (16.7 kJ/g) or higher have more fat and less fiber. Fat is typically highly digestible and fiber is poorly digestible. Thus, high-fat, low-fiber foods are usually more digestible.

Other Nutritional Factors
In addition to the key nutritional factors for commercial foods discussed above, the following nutritional factors may be important in some instances, especially when homemade foods are fed (Chapter 10).

Phenylalanine and Tyrosine
Tyrosine is not an essential amino acid but is made from phenylalanine. Also, tyrosine spares about half of the need for phenylalanine. Therefore, it is appropriate to consider the amount of phenylalanine required as the sum of phenylalanine plus tyrosine. Although phenylalanine and tyrosine are not the most limiting amino acids in commercial food, at least twice as much phenylalanine, or phenylalanine plus tyrosine, are required for maximal black hair color as for growth (Yu et al, 2001; Anderson et al, 2002). Other metabolic needs for phenylalanine and tyrosine include protein synthesis and synthesis of thyroid hormones and catecholamines (NRC, 2006). The minimal recommended DM allowance for foods for queens during late gestation/peak lactation for phenylalanine plus tyrosine is 1.91%. To maximize black hair color, 50% or more of this amount must be from phenylalanine (NRC, 2006).

Taurine
Taurine is required for normal reproduction and fetal development (Chapter 19). Taurine deficiency in gestating queens may result in fetal death near the 25th day of gestation, abortions throughout gestation, fetal deformities and delayed growth and development (Sturman, 1991). However, the taurine requirement for gestation is similar to that for other lifestages (i.e., a minimum of 0.1% DM taurine in dry foods and 0.17% DM in moist foods) (NRC, 2006; Kirk et al, 1995). Current AAFCO allowances for taurine are appropriate for reproducing cats (2007). Therefore, foods that have AAFCO label statements acknowledging appropriateness for growth or reproduction should provide adequate amounts.

Essential Fatty Acids
Linoleic and AA and possibly α-linolenic acid are required in foods for cats. Signs of linoleic acid deficiency in cats are similar to those in other animals (Chapter 32). However, the long-term deficiency of dietary AA also results in reproductive failure. Queens with an AA deficiency appear unable to bear live kittens (MacDonald et al, 1984). In contrast to queens, male cats do not appear to require AA for reproduction. Spermatogenesis remains normal in males with an AA deficiency possibly because testes convert linoleic acid to AA. AA at 0.04% of the dietary energy supports normal reproduction in queens. However, lower levels have been used when interference from omega-3 fatty acids is avoided (MacDonald et al, 1984). Current AAFCO allowances for linoleic and AA are appropriate for gestating cats (2007). Therefore, foods that have AAFCO label statements acknowledging that a food is appropriate for growth or reproduction should provide adequate amounts.

Magnesium
Magnesium should not be overly restricted in foods for reproducing queens. Most cat foods intended for prevention of struvite urolithiasis have magnesium levels above the minimum recommended allowance for late gestation and peak lactation (0.05%, DM) (NRC, 2006). Dietary magnesium levels of 0.08 to 0.15% DM are recommended in foods for reproducing queens.

Copper
Copper is required for normal iron metabolism and as an enzyme cofactor in several key metabolic pathways, including those responsible for myelin, melanin and connective tissue production. Copper requirements for growth and reproduction are thought to be approximately 5 mg/kg food (Doong et al, 1983). However, copper deficiency has been reported to occur in queens fed a food containing 15 mg copper/kg food, supplied, in part, by copper oxide (Morris and Rogers, 1994). Copper from copper oxide is poorly available. The combination of poorly available copper from food and competition from high levels of dietary zinc, iron, calcium and phytate significantly impair copper availability. Clinical signs of copper deficiency include fetal death and abortions, achromotrichia, arthrogryposis, fusion of digits, craniofacial deformities and cerebral dysgenesis.[a] For this reason, DM copper levels of 15 mg/kg food from an available source have been recommended for queens eating dry foods (AAFCO, 2007). The minimum recommended DM allowance for foods for late gestation and peak lactation in queens is 8.8 mg/kg (NRC, 2006).

A previous report of experimental copper deficiency cited histochemical defects of the aorta (Doong et al, 1983). Hematologic abnormalities are not a typical feature of copper deficiency in cats, as in other species. Supplemental copper in feline foods should be highly available. Copper sulfate and copper chelates appear to be good dietary sources.

FEEDING PLAN

Generally, feeding plan recommendations are based on information from populations of cats at similar lifestages. However, the feeding plan for reproducing cats should be tailored to meet the needs of the individual cat based on unique variations in genetics, environment, litter size and health status. The feeding plan includes the food to be fed and the feeding method (how much food is fed and how it is offered).

Assess and Select the Food
The process of food assessment includes comparing the current food's key nutritional factor content with the key nutritional factor recommendations for reproduction. **Table 22-4** lists the key nutritional factors in selected commercial foods and compares them to the recommended levels. For foods not listed, the same information can usually be obtained from pet food manufacturers (see pet food labels for toll-free numbers or websites). The comparison discloses potential discrepancies between the key nutritional factors and the cat's current food. Also, the food should be shown to be appropriate for reproduction based on AAFCO or other credible regulatory agency guidelines or feeding trials. Generally speaking, commercial growth-type foods are also intended for feeding to queens for gestation/lactation.

Food assessment during lactation also includes assessment of lactation performance. Evaluation of kitten growth rate and rate of weight loss in the queen can point to nutritional inadequacies in the queen during late gestation and lactation. Nursing kittens should gain approximately 100 g/week or 10 to 15 g/day. Weight gains less than 7 g/day require immediate evaluation of the food, the queen and the kittens. Queens normally lose some weight during lactation but should return to within 2% of their pre-breeding body weight by weaning (**Figure 22-1**). Weight loss is also related to litter size. The anticipated weight loss of queens from Week 0 to 3 can be approximated by the following equation (Loveridge and Rivers, 1989):

Total queen's body weight loss (g) = 339.2 + (58.8)n (where n = number of kittens).

If either the queen's rate of weight loss is excessive, or the kittens' growth rate is inadequate, the food and feeding method

Table 22-4. Comparison of recommended key nutritional factor levels in selected commercial foods for reproducing (gestation and lactation) queens to recommended levels.*

Dry foods	**Energy density (kcal/cup)****	**Energy density (kcal ME/g)**	**Protein (%)**	**Fat (%)**	**DHA (%)**	**Carbohydrate (%)*****	**Ca (%)**	**P (%)**	**Ca:P ratio**	**Na (%)**	**Urinary pH**
Recommended levels	**–**	**4.0-5.0**	**35-50**	**18-35**	**≥0.004**	**≥10**	**1.1-1.6**	**0.8-1.4**	**1:1-1.5:1**	**0.3-0.6**	**6.2-6.5**
Hill's Science Diet Kitten Healthy Development Original	510	4.5	42.3	26.1	0.24	22.2	1.3	1.1	1.1:1	0.39	6.4
Hill's Science Diet Kitten Indoor	510	4.5	42.2	26.1	0.24	22.3	1.3	1.1	1.1:1	0.39	6.4
Hill's Science Diet Nature's Best Chicken & Brown Rice Dinner Kitten	487	4.4	37.6	26.0	0.26	27.6	1.45	1.2	1.2:1	0.46	6.4
Hill's Science Diet Nature's Best Ocean Fish & Brown Rice Dinner Kitten	487	4.4	38.0	26.3	0.23	26.6	1.4	1.1	1.2:1	0.59	6.4
Iams Eukanuba Chicken Formula Kitten	469	4.5	40.0	25.7	na	25.4	1.3	1.1	1.2:1	0.43	na
Iams Kitten	470	5.0	37.8	24.6	na	28.4	1.15	0.9	1.2:1	0.54	na
Nutro Natural Choice Complete Care Kitten	463	4.4	40.7	24.2	0.077	25.3	1.3	1.2	1.1:1	0.44	na
Purina Kitten Chow	457	4.5	44.8	15.6	na	30.8	1.4	1.42	1:1	0.56	na
Purina ONE Healthy Kitten Formula	512	4.8	45.5	21.1	na	24.8	1.3	1.2	1.1:1	0.40	na
Purina Pro Plan Kitten Chicken & Rice Formula	472	4.3	46.0	20.1	na	26.6	1.3	1.2	1.1:1	0.42	na
Royal Canin Babycat 34 Formula	531	4.8	37.4	27.5	na	21.6	1.3	1.1	1.1:1	0.64	na
Royal Canin Kitten 34 Formula	393	4.6	37.4	22.0	na	26.5	1.25	1.1	1.1:1	0.67	na
Moist foods	**Energy density (kcal/can)****	**Energy density (kcal ME/g)**	**Protein (%)**	**Fat (%)**	**DHA (%)**	**Carbohydrate (%)*****	**Ca (%)**	**P (%)**	**Ca:P ratio**	**Na (%)**	**Urinary pH**
Recommended levels	**–**	**4.0-5.0**	**35-50**	**18-35**	**≥0.004**	**≥10**	**1.1-1.6**	**0.8-1.4**	**1:1-1.5:1**	**0.3-0.6**	**6.2-6.5**
Hill's Science Diet Kitten Healthy Development Liver & Chicken Entrée Minced	114/3 oz. 210/5.5 oz.	4.7	49.3	23.9	0.243	16.2	1.3	1.0	1.4:1	0.32	6.4
Hill's Science Diet Tender Chunks in Gravy Real Chicken Dinner Kitten	84/3 oz. (pouch)	4.3	47.8	22.6	0.087	19.5	1.2	1.1	1.1:1	0.43	6.3

Key: ME = metabolizable energy, DHA = docosahexaenoic acid, Ca = calcium, P = phosphorus, Na = sodium, na = not available from manufacturer.

*From manufacturers' published information or calculated from manufacturers' published as fed values; all values are on a dry matter basis unless otherwise stated. Digestibility: Foods with higher energy density are more likely to have higher digestibility. Foods for most breeding males and females are usually similar to those for young and middle-aged adults (Chapter 20).

**Energy density values are listed on an as fed basis and are useful for determining the amount to feed; cup = 8-oz. measuring cup. To convert to kJ, multiply kcal by 4.184.

***Important for lactation.

should be carefully reviewed. If inadequacies exist, a more appropriate food should be selected. Supplements should not have to be given to improve lactation performance. Supplements, unless carefully balanced to the nutrients in the food, can unbalance a food or impair availability of other nutrients.

Queens should be fed a food appropriate for gestation and lactation at or before mating. Although, nutritional demands are greatest in the last one-half to one-third of pregnancy, conception rate and in utero fetal viability are markedly impaired in queens fed foods with marginal nutrient content and avail-

Table 22-5. Feeding plan summary for reproducing cats.

1. For gestating and lactating queens, use **Table 22-4** to select a food with the appropriate levels of key nutritional factors; for breeding males, use Table 20-4. For foods in neither table, contact manufacturers for key nutritional factor content.
2. Food should be approved by a credible regulatory agency (e.g., the Association of American Feed Control Officials).
3. Determine an appropriate feeding method (Table 20-6). Free-choice feeding is the preferred method for feeding gestating/lactating queens; food-restricted meal feeding may be best for breeding males.
4. For food-restricted meal feeding, estimate the initial quantity of food based on daily energy requirement (DER) calculation (DER ÷ food energy density).
5. DER is calculated by multiplying resting energy requirement (RER) (Table 5-2) by an appropriate factor. Remember, DER calculations are estimates and should be used as guidelines or starting points for amounts to feed individual cats and not as absolute requirements; the amount fed should be refined by monitoring body condition score and body weight.
   Breeding male = 1.4 to 1.6 x RER
   Breeding female = 1.6 x RER
   Gestation = 1.6 to 2.0 x RER
   Lactation = 2.0 to 6.0 x RER
6. At the end of lactation, queens should be fed for weaning as described in Box 23-2.
7. Monitor body condition, body weight, general health, reproductive performance and kitten growth rates.

ability at breeding and early gestation. Changing to a new food more suitable for gestation and lactation before conception: 1) avoids any reduction in food intake or gastrointestinal upsets during the critical time of conception and implantation, 2) improves any marginal nutrient stores and 3) typically increases energy intake.

The food form selected for reproducing queens also warrants consideration. Many semi-moist foods produce urinary pH values below desired levels for reproducing queens. Dry foods are more nutrient dense on an as fed basis and have higher carbohydrate levels than moist foods. Dry foods may benefit queens undergoing rapid weight loss and those spending little time eating. Conversely, moist foods often have higher fat levels and provide additional water to support lactation. The added water also improves palatability; therefore, queens may spend more time eating. Dry and moist food types each have advantages; therefore, many breeders choose to feed both forms during reproduction. If both dry and moist foods are fed, it may be desirable to feed dry foods free choice and provide multiple moist food meals daily. Only fresh moist food should be offered.

Intact male cats in heavy service and those stressed during breeding (e.g., stress of travel, preoccupation with breeding, etc.) should be fed foods with high energy density (4.5 to 5.0 kcal/g DM [18.8 to 20.9 kJ/g DM]). Otherwise, foods appropriate for young adult cats are adequate (Chapter 20). Male cats used in harem-breeding programs are typically fed the same foods as the queens. Although the vitamin and mineral levels of these foods are typically well in excess of the male cat's needs, the high energy density may be beneficial.

Assess and Determine the Feeding Method

It may be necessary to alter the feeding method when managing reproducing cats. This is especially true for queens in late-term pregnancy, those carrying large litters and during lactation. Evaluation of current feeding methods with foreknowledge of reproductive demands will allow for development of a good feeding plan.

Reproducing queens have an increased need for energy and therefore, food. The increased need can be met by providing food on a calorie basis at the daily rate of 1.6 x RER at breeding with a gradual increase to 2 x RER at parturition. The queen's energy needs may increase fourfold over maintenance requirements during peak lactation. However, energy needs sometimes exceed the recommended energy allowances due to individual cat variation and increased energy requirements of queens with large litters. Free-choice feeding is the preferred method for reproducing queens. Note that meal size and therefore calorie intake may be limited as the uterus and fetal mass occupy much of the abdominal cavity and limit gastrointestinal capacity. Providing food free choice allows reproducing queens to consume sufficient calories in multiple small feedings. Queens may also be fed multiple meals (three to four/day) using the recommended energy allowances in **Table 22-1.** However, food intake should not be limited unless obesity becomes a problem. **Table 22-3** lists estimates of average energy intake during lactation. **Table 22-5** provides a feeding plan summary for reproducing cats.

Obesity increases the risk of dystocia and kitten mortality. Thus, careful weight management before breeding and weight monitoring during gestation are important (Lawler and Monti, 1984). Obese-prone queens should be fed three to four meals per day in controlled portions. Obese queens (i.e., those with heavy fat accumulations over the ribs and bony prominences [BCS ≥4/5]) should be fed controlled amounts of food during gestation; however, they should not be fed to lose weight.

The practice of flushing, that is, increasing food intake by 5 to 15% from proestrus through breeding, has been not been evaluated in cats. Even if flushing were proven to be of value, it would be difficult to do because proestrus is rarely observed in cats because they are induced ovulators.

Clean water should be available at all times. Food and water should be placed within easy reach for the queen. Food should be placed directly in or very near the box during the first few days after parturition, when many queens refuse to leave the nest box. Some people have advocated removing the kittens from the nest box for 30 to 60 minutes at a time to encourage queens to eat (Lawler and Bebiak, 1986). This recommendation is effective for some queens, but makes others so frantic it becomes counterproductive. Other methods to improve food intake include adding water or moist food to dry food to enhance palatability and increase water intake.

Kittens should be allowed access to the queen's food, which they typically begin eating at three weeks of age. Kittens may need to be fed away from the queen if the queen is fed portion-controlled amounts of food.

Some queens with strong maternal instincts are reluctant to

leave the nest box. When this occurs, their food and water should be placed in the immediate vicinity. Advise clients to use care when placing water bowls near neonates to avoid accidental drowning. If the queen's food intake does not improve, the kittens may be removed from the queen for short periods three to four times a day.

At the end of lactation, queens should be fed for weaning. On Day 1 of weaning, the kittens and food are withheld from the queen; during this time the kittens are allowed free access to their weaning food. At the end of Day 1 they are returned to the queen and allowed to nurse. On Day 2 the kittens are removed and allowed free access to their weaning food but not returned to the queen; they are weaned. Also on Day 2, the queen is given one-fourth of the amount it was fed for maintenance (pre-breeding ration). Over the next three days, food amounts for the queen are gradually increased to pre-breeding levels. The kittens should continue to be housed and fed separately. To minimize mammary gland engorgement in queens that are abruptly removed from their kittens and/or those that are heavy milk producers, restrict their food intake a day or two before the weaning process, just described.

REASSESSMENT

Breeding queens and tomcats should be reassessed before every reproductive cycle. Females should have returned to optimal body weight and condition (BCS 3/5) before the next breeding. Oral health should be optimal and vaccinations and parasite control should be completed before the next reproductive cycle. The last reproductive performance should be evaluated and compared with previous performance and the cattery average. If performance was suboptimal, a detailed review of genetic selection, husbandry and nutritional management should be completed to identify deficiencies. Modifications can be then be incorporated to improve subsequent reproductive outcomes.

Monitoring the queen during gestation should include weekly assessment of food intake and body weight. Body condition scoring is particularly important in assessing weight gain during gestation. Inadequate nutrition and poor weight gain may be overlooked if total body weight and the queen's expanding abdomen are the only criteria used to monitor weight gain. If underfed, the queen may continue to gain weight as the kittens grow but fail to develop the energy reserves needed for lactation. Body condition scoring during gestation should ignore the abdominal component of the scoring process and allow for slight increases in body fat (Figure 1-3). When assigning body condition scores to pregnant queens, the areas of focus include muscle mass and fat covering the ribs and bony prominences. Body weight and food intake should change gradually in a pattern similar to that depicted in **Figure 22-1**. The queen and each kitten should be thoroughly evaluated at parturition. Average weight loss of the queen at parturition is 6 to 14% (254 to 638 g) of the prepartum weight, depending on litter size (Loveridge, 1985). The remaining 700 to 850 g of gain will be used to sustain normal lactation. Evaluation of gestational performance should include: 1) the queen's weight record, 2) litter size, 3) kitten birth weights, 4) kitten growth rates, 5) kitten vigor, 6) mortality rates and 7) congenital defects. Although stools may normally vary from soft to firm during reproduction, stool quality should be monitored. Constipation and diarrhea are always considered abnormal and should be evaluated and treated as needed.

Reassessment of lactating queens is similar to that of pregnant queens. Most observations will be made by the owner/breeder. The queen should be regularly evaluated for vaginal discharge, mammary gland engorgement or mastitis and matted abdominal hair that interferes with nursing. Body weight and condition should be evaluated after parturition and weekly thereafter. Kittens should exhibit steady weight gain, have good muscle tone and suckle vigorously. Young kittens are quiet between feedings. Kittens are often restless and cry excessively if milk production is inadequate. Gastric distention is not a good indicator of adequate nursing. Aerophagia can give the appearance of gastric fullness in kittens, despite inadequate milk intake.

Kitten mortality reportedly varies from 9 to 63% depending on the source of cats and the cattery (Pedersen, 1991). Breeders should compare reproductive performance of each queen to the cattery standard. Several genetic, husbandry and nutritional factors may cause high kitten mortality. If kitten death or cannibalism rates are high, all three areas should be investigated thoroughly.

ACKNOWLEDGMENTS

The authors and editors acknowledge the contributions of Drs. Claudia A. Kirk and P. Jane Armstrong in the previous edition of Small Animal Clinical Nutrition.

ENDNOTE

a. Kirk CA. Unpublished data. 1994.

REFERENCES

The references for **Chapter 22** can be found at www.markmorris.org.

CASE 22-1

Alopecia in a Lactating Cat

Claudia A. Kirk, DVM, PhD, Dipl. ACVN and ACVIM (Internal Medicine)
College of Veterinary Medicine
University of Tennessee
Knoxville, Tennessee, USA

Patient Assessment

A five-year-old intact female domestic longhair cat was examined for hair loss. The alopecia was generalized and patchy with no evidence of pruritus, excoriations, crusts or primary lesions (e.g., papules or pustules). There was no evidence of flea or other external parasite infestation. The coat was dull, dry and unkempt. The cat appeared thin (body condition score [BCS] 2/5) and weighed 3.0 kg. The remainder of the physical examination was normal.

The queen had delivered five kittens four weeks earlier. The kittens were apparently healthy but had become restless and cried constantly during the previous five days. The kittens had attempted to nurse, but the owner did not know if they were actually obtaining milk. The owner also commented that the kittens had not grown during the past week. The queen's mammary glands did not appear adequately distended for the stage of lactation.

Multiple skin scrapings and a tape preparation were negative for ectoparasites. The hairs appeared somewhat brittle and were easily epilated. Results of a packed cell volume (PCV) were slightly below normal (28%, normal 30 to 52%).

Assess the Food and Feeding Method

The cat was fed a commercial private label dry cat food purchased from a local farm and feed store. The nutritional adequacy statement on the bag indicated that the product "meets the nutritional levels established by the Association of American Feed Control Officials (AAFCO) nutrient profiles for all stages of a cat's life." One cup of dry food mixed with chicken broth was offered twice daily.

Questions

1. What is the most likely cause of this patient's alopecia?
2. Is there a connection between the alopecia and restless, crying kittens?
3. Are there any other diagnostic tests that should be performed?
4. Outline a more appropriate feeding plan for this queen.

Answers and Discussion

1. The integument is a metabolically active organ that is affected by the nutritional status of the animal. Protein and energy are required for development of new hair and skin. Developing hair requires sulfur-containing and other amino acids. Therefore, the animal's food should provide optimal protein quantity, quality (i.e., appropriate levels of essential amino acids) and digestibility for normal skin and hair. Animals have increased protein and energy requirements during growth, gestation, lactation and some illnesses. Abnormal skin and hair will often be noted if nutritionally inadequate foods are fed during these stages and conditions. Telogen defluxion is usually recognized as hair loss associated with a stressful event (e.g., pregnancy, severe illness, surgery) that causes the abrupt, premature cessation of growth of many anagen hair follicles and the synchronization of these hair follicles in catagen, then in telogen. Short-term deficiency of protein, energy or other nutrients during growth, gestation, lactation and illness may cause telogen defluxion if appropriate dietary changes are not instituted. Bitches and queens in late gestation and lactation and growing puppies and kittens are at risk unless they are fed nutritionally balanced, highly digestible foods that meet their increased nutritional requirements.
2. Excessive crying, restless behavior and poor weight gain of kittens are clinical signs associated with lactation failure in queens. Lactation failure can result from inadequate intake of energy and protein to support proper lactation and can thus be linked to the same cause of telogen defluxion.
3. A complete blood count and serum biochemistry profile should be considered to rule out systemic disease as the cause of alopecia and lactation failure. Plucking hairs from the skin and examining them microscopically is termed trichography. This technique is helpful in diagnosing a number of conditions affecting the skin and coat including nutritional diseases. Estimating the ratio of anagen to telogen hair bulbs can be useful. All the hair of normal animals should not be in telogen. A diagnosis of telogen defluxion or follicular arrest is suggested when all the hair is in telogen. Inappropriate numbers of telogen hairs (e.g., mostly telogen hairs during the summer when the ratio should be approximately 50:50) suggest a diagnosis of nutritional, endocrine or metabolic disease. In people, the ratio of telogen to anagen hair increases with prolonged protein deficiency. Unfortunately, well-established normal values are not available for trichograms, which somewhat limits their usefulness in veterinary medicine.

The use of site-, age-, breed- and climate-matched controls, if possible, may increase the usefulness of this diagnostic technique.

4. The commercial dry food fed currently does not appear adequate to support normal lactation, body condition or coat quality in this lactating queen. A commercial food specifically formulated for feline growth and lactation should be recommended. The label of the new product should indicate that the food has undergone AAFCO or similar feeding trials in gestating and lactating cats. This documentation ensures that the nutrient levels and availability are adequate to support normal lactation. The food and water should be offered free choice. If a dry food is chosen, chicken broth or moist foods can also be offered to encourage food intake by the queen.

Progress Notes

The results of a complete blood count and serum biochemistry profile were normal. Plucked hairs had bulbs that exhibited changes consistent with only telogen hairs. The food was changed to a commercial dry specialty brand food specifically formulated for feline growth and reproduction (Science Diet Feline Growth[a]). The dry food and water were offered free choice. The queen's daily energy requirement (DER) was estimated to be 4 to 6 x resting energy requirement (RER) for an ideal weight of 3.5 kg (DER = 700 to 1,000 kcal [2.9 to 4.2 MJ]). Approximately one-fourth of the estimated DER (200 kcal [837 kJ]) was offered as dry food mixed with a highly palatable, gravy-style flavor enhancer (Science Diet Canine & Feline Mixit[b]). This combination of dry food with gravy mixer was offered twice daily in addition to dry food offered free choice.

The kittens were allowed to remain with the queen but were offered a supplemental gruel made from equal parts commercial milk replacer (KMR Liquid[c]) and moist Science Diet Feline Growth four times per day. The queen and kittens were separated during these feedings. The kittens readily consumed the food mixture. The amount of milk replacer was gradually decreased over the following week until the kittens were eating moist food three times daily without milk replacer. The kittens also consumed increasing amounts of the dry growth formula that was available for the queen. The kittens' crying and excessive activity declined with supplemental feeding. The kittens were weaned at six weeks of age when they all weighed at least 500 g.

The owner reported that the queen ate both the dry food and dry food mixed with flavor enhancer very well. The cat gained a small amount of weight during the next month, seemed to produce more milk and stopped losing hair. The queen was fed the growth food for six weeks after the kittens were weaned to improve its body condition and coat. At that point, the food was changed to a similar brand food for adult maintenance.

Endnotes

a. Hill's Pet Nutrition, Inc., Topeka, KS, USA. This product is currently available as Science Diet Kitten Healthy Development Original.

b. Hill's Pet Nutrition, Inc., Topeka, KS, USA.

c. Pet-Ag Inc., Elgin, IL, USA.

Bibliography

Hoskins JD. Clinical evaluation of the kitten: From birth to eight weeks of age. Compendium on Continuing Education for the Practicing Veterinarian 1990; 12: 1215-1225.

Lawler DF, Bebiak DM. Nutrition and management of reproduction in the cat. Veterinary Clinics of North America: Small Animal Practice 1986; 16: 495-519.

Morris JG, Rogers QR. Assessment of the nutritional adequacy of pet foods through the life cycle. Journal of Nutrition 1994; 124: 2520S-2534S.

National Research Council. Nutrient Requirements of Cats. Washington, DC: National Academy Press, 1986.

Piechota TR, Rogers QR, Morris JG. Nitrogen requirements of cats during gestation and lactation. Nutrition Research 1995; 15: 1535-1546.

Scott DW, Miller WH, Griffin CE. Small Animal Dermatology, 5th ed. Philadelphia, PA: WB Saunders Co, 1995.

Chapter 23

Feeding Nursing and Orphaned Kittens from Birth to Weaning

Kathy L. Gross
Iveta Becvarova
Jacques Debraekeleer

"Kittens are angels with whiskers."
Author Unknown

INTRODUCTION

Kittens usually depend on the queen to provide food during the neonatal or nursing period. Proper nutrition of the queen during gestation and lactation, the behavior and health of the queen and good neonatal care are important to achieving a successful transition from fetal life to the nursing period. The transition from queen's milk to solid food (weaning) is a gradual process and is an integral part of the nursing period. This chapter includes feeding normal nursing kittens, feeding orphaned kittens and integrating the weaning process.

Kittens are considered orphaned if they lack sufficient maternal care for survival from birth to weaning. Several physiologic needs normally provided by the queen must be met to ensure survival of neonates: heat, humidity, nutrition, immunity, elimination, sanitation, security and social stimulation. A foster queen or the caregiver must meet these needs for orphaned kittens (**Box 23-1**).

PATIENT ASSESSMENT

History

Clients should be encouraged to keep logbooks of all data that may provide information about the health and nutritional status of kittens (i.e., orphaned, fostered and normal) and the reproductive performance of the queen. Records should include food intake, body weight, body temperature and stool characteristics, especially during the first two weeks postpartum. Changes in kitten behavior, activity and other indicators of normal development (e.g., opening of eyes, eruption of teeth and coat quality) may prove useful as well (**Table 23-1**). In some instances, it may be helpful to differentiate individual kittens (**Box 23-1**).

It is particularly important that good records be maintained for orphaned and foster kittens. Orphaned kittens are hand-raised kittens, whereas foster kittens are those raised by a queen other than their mother. Successful management of these kittens depends on the quick recognition and correction of health and management problems. Parameters such as weight gain, daily food intake, stool characteristics and kitten vigor (i.e., muscle tone, activity and alertness) should be recorded. Kittens should be observed for suckling activity in addition to the above parameters.

Orphaned kittens should have consistent weight gains similar to those of suckling kittens (**Figure 23-1**) (Remillard et al, 1993). Orphans, in particular, should be examined for common problems such as hypothermia, hypoglycemia, dehydration and congenital defects. The current nutritional and hydration status

Box 23-1. General Good Husbandry Practices for Neonatal Kittens.

Kittens should be housed in warm draft-free enclosures. Incubators are ideal, particularly for newborn kittens. Pet carriers, shoeboxes or cardboard boxes are suitable substitutes. The bedding should be soft, absorbent and warm. Thread-free cloth, fleece and shavings are appropriate materials and help kittens feel secure as they snuggle into them.

Neonates demonstrate a certain degree of poikilothermy and are unable to regulate body temperature well during the first four weeks of life. Kittens huddle together close to the queen, which generates an optimal microclimate, protects them against changes in environmental temperature and decreases the rate of heat loss. Orphans cannot seek protection near the queen and are more sensitive to suboptimal environmental conditions.

Without the queen, neonates can quickly become hypothermic, which leads to circulatory failure and death. Artificial heat should provide age-optimal environmental temperatures (**Table 23-2**). It is best to set the heating source to establish a gradation of heat in the nest box. A gradation of environmental temperatures allows neonates to move toward or away from the heat source as needed to avoid hyperthermia, which can be as detrimental as hypothermia. Kittens can rapidly become dehydrated secondary to overheating. Maintaining humidity near 50% helps reduce water loss and maintains the moisture and health of mucous membranes.

To fulfill non-nutritive nursing needs, hand-reared kittens often nurse other littermates in the nest box. To avoid skin trauma related to excessive nursing, kittens can be housed individually or separated by dividers. Although beneficial for alleviating problems due to non-nutritive nursing, separation of the litter reduces temperature and humidity in the immediate environment and social stimulation by littermates. Brief, but regular handling, provides social stimulation. The stress associated with regular handling increases neural development and improves weight gain in kittens. Kittens raised without social stimulation develop abnormal behavior patterns (i.e., kittens reduce normal exploratory behavior and become more suspicious and aggressive as adults). Peer contact can compensate for maternal deprivation. Therefore, benefits of separating neonates must be weighed against the potential for development of abnormal behavior and increased risk for hypothermia. Kittens should interact with littermates as much as possible until weaning.

Kittens obtain passive systemic immunity from colostrum and passive local immunity from continued ingestion of queen's milk. If possible, neonates should receive colostrum or queen's milk within the first 12 hours of birth. This is particularly critical for kittens fed only milk replacers because they lack systemic and local immune protection.

Normally the queen will sever the umbilical cord. If not, it should be cut to 1.5 in. (3.5 to 4 cm) and an appropriate topical antiseptic applied. Orphaned kittens are at greater risk for infectious disease; thus, sanitary husbandry practices are important. To reduce risk for diseases, kittens should not be exposed to older animals or grouped within multiple litters. Feeding equipment and bedding should be kept clean and sanitized frequently. Caretakers should wash their hands before handling neonates and after stimulating elimination.

Kittens cannot voluntarily urinate or defecate until about three weeks of age. Until that time, they rely on the queen to stimulate the urogenital reflex to initiate elimination. Caretakers should stimulate kittens after feeding by gently swabbing the perineal region with a warm moistened cotton ball or cloth.

Often, kittens within a litter look similar; therefore, it may be difficult to tell them apart when hand rearing, especially in large litters. Different colored nail polish can be applied to the claws to help differentiate individuals; ask clients to paint a different paw for each kitten (e.g., blue front left paw, blue right rear paw, pink right front paw, etc.).

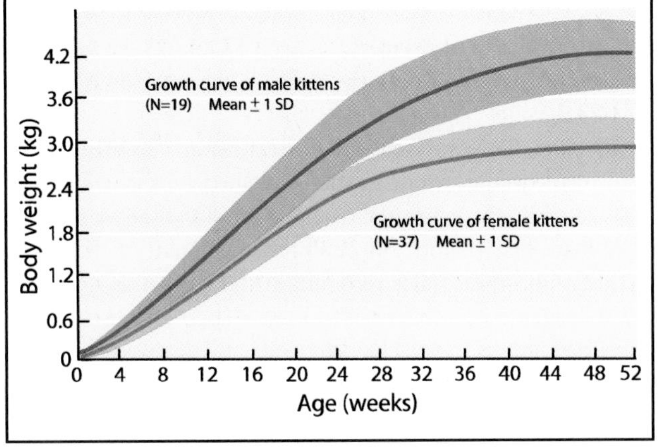

Figure 23-1. Growth curve for female and male kittens. Note after four weeks of age there are significant gender differences in growth rates; female kittens grow at a slower rate and are normally smaller than males. (Adapted from National Research Council. Nutrient Requirements of Cats. Washington, DC: National Academy Press, 1986; 2.)

should also be noted. Kittens fostered onto another queen should be supervised initially to detect any behavioral problems between the foster parent, its young and the orphans. Ideally, kittens should be accepted immediately and allowed to nurse. Ask clients to watch for signs of rejection or impending cannibalism by the foster queen.

Queens should also be monitored for signs of impending cannibalism (e.g., extreme nervousness, aggressiveness toward the kitten(s) and kitten rejection). Unfortunately, cannibalism often occurs without warning. In the case of orphans, the queen, if available, should be examined to detect the potential cause for abandonment.

Additionally, housing and environmental hygiene should also be evaluated. Improper housing and hygiene are important risk factors for poor kitten development and impaired health.

Physical Examination

The goals of the neonatal physical examination are to: 1) establish baseline data for future reference, 2) assess overall health and development of the kittens and 3) detect abnormalities that

Table 23-1. Normal physiologic values for neonatal kittens and data for neonatal care.

Litter size	-	Average: 3-5 (1-7)
Body weight	Birth weight	90-120 g
	Weeks 1-2	Double
	Weeks 3-4	Triple
Daily weight gain	Weeks 1-4	Average: 10-13 g/day
Body temperature	24 hr after birth	33.3-35.5°C (92-96°F)
	End of Week 1	36.6°C (98°F)
Heart rate	Weeks 0-4	>220 beats/min.
Respiratory rate	Weeks 1-2	15-35 breaths/min.
Shivering reflex develops	-	Week 1
Eyes	Eyelids open	8 days (5-14)
	Pupillary light response	24 hr after eyelids separate
Ears	Reaction to auditory stimuli	3 days
	External ear canals open	6-14 days (completely open by 17 days)
	Development functional hearing	21 days
Locomotion	Forelimbs start to support weight	3-4 days (1-10)
	Ability to stand	
	Sitting	10 days (5-25)
	Walking unsteadily	20 days
	Start climbing	21-22 days
Micturition and defecation	Voluntary control	3 weeks
Energy requirements	At birth	380 kcal/kg
	At 4 weeks	250 kcal/kg
Eating solid food	-	28-50 days
Deciduous teeth eruption	Incisors	2-3 weeks
	Canines	3-4 weeks
	Premolars	3-6 weeks
Permanent teeth eruption	Incisors	3-4 months
	Canines	4-5 months
	Premolars	4-6 months
	Molars	4-5 months

may impair normal development and health. During the physical examination, particular attention should be given to kitten behavior, body weight, body temperature and oral cavity health. Additionally, the umbilicus of each kitten should be closely evaluated. Normally, the queen will cut the umbilicus leaving approximately one and one-half inches. Occasionally, queens will remove excessive cord resulting in an umbilicus flush with the abdomen or an open hernia (**Figure 23-2**). Careful wound management and antibiotic therapy are often required to prevent omphalitis and/or septicemia. Umbilical cords left too long may wrap around the kitten's legs or paws cutting off circulation to the affected limb.

Kitten Behavior

Normal kittens are vigorous and have good muscle tone. They should nurse immediately or soon after parturition and have a strong sucking reflex. Well-fed kittens should have a distended abdomen and be quiet after feeding. Kittens that are hungry, cold, hot or in discomfort will cry continuously and should be closely monitored. Nursing behavior and milk intake should be carefully observed because some kittens develop rounded abdomens as a result of aerophagia. Kittens may have difficulty nursing queens of longhaired breeds due to hair accumulation or matting around nipples. In these cases, abdominal hair can be clipped to allow easier access to the queen's nipples. Care should be taken not to damage the queen's nipples during this process.

The behavioral response of kittens to the queen is also important. Poor maternal-kitten interaction may result in cannibalism or neglect. Kittens depend on the queen for food, antibodies, warmth and hygiene; therefore, serious metabolic alterations (e.g., hypoglycemia, hypothermia, dehydration and malnutrition), infectious disease and death are common sequelae to abnormal behavior and maternal neglect.

Body Weight

Monitoring initial and subsequent body weight is a good way to evaluate milk intake and health status of nursing and orphaned kittens. Healthy nursing kittens should be weighed at birth and weekly thereafter using a gram scale. Daily weighing is important to evaluate the queen's milk production and to help assess sick, weak and underweight kittens. Weight loss or slow weight gain in individuals or entire litters may indicate: 1) disease in kittens or the queen, 2) inability of kittens to suckle or 3) inadequate milk production.

Birth weights are normally between 85 to 120 g with mean weights of approximately 100 g. Kittens weighing less than 75 g have very high mortality rates and require extra care and monitoring if they are to survive. Low birth-weight kittens should be weighed every 24 to 48 hours for the first one to three weeks of life to ensure proper weight gain. Kittens gain an average of 100 g/week for the first six months of life. Minimally, they should gain 7 g/day (Lawler and Bebiak, 1986).

Body Temperature

Kittens regulate body temperature poorly during the first four

Table 23-2. Optimal environmental temperature for orphaned kittens.

Age	°C	°F
Immediate environment/incubator for orphans		
Week 1	32-34	89.5-93
Week 2	27-29	81-84
Week 3	24-27	75-81
Weeks 4-12	24	75
Environment around litter		
Week 1	24-27	75-81

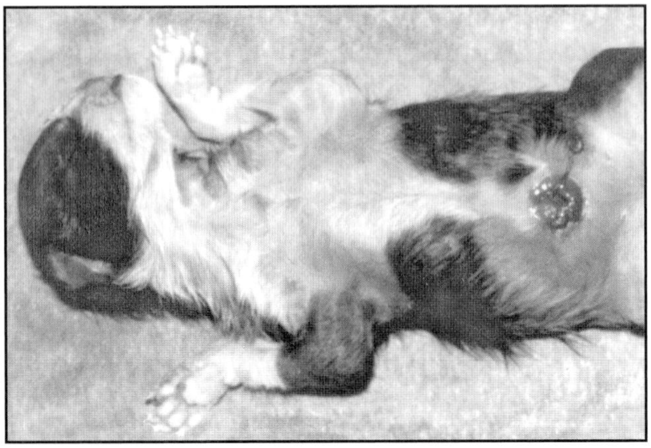

Figure 23-2. A neonatal kitten with an open umbilical hernia following excessive umbilical cord removal by the queen after parturition.

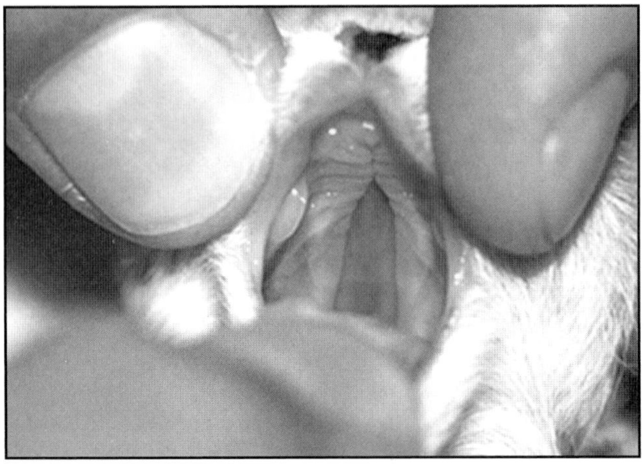

Figure 23-3. Cleft palate in a neonatal kitten. This is a common birth defect in kittens and may be associated with malnutrition of the queen during gestation. Nutrients commonly associated with a cleft palate include deficiencies of zinc and copper, as well as, vitamin A toxicosis during gestation.

weeks of life. Normal body temperature is approximately 36.0°C (96.8°F) at birth and increases to 37.5°C (100.0°F) by one week of age (Lawler and Bebiak, 1986). Extreme environmental conditions or abandonment by the queen may lead to hypothermia, which may quickly result in circulatory failure and death.

Normally the queen maintains the temperature and humidity in the nest box. Without the queen, kittens can quickly become hypothermic. Artificial heat should provide age-optimal environmental temperatures (**Table 23-2**). It is best to set heat sources to establish heat gradation in the nest box. This allows kittens to move away from the heat source as needed to avoid hyperthermia. Hyperthermia can be as detrimental as hypothermia; hyperthermic kittens can rapidly become dehydrated. Maintaining humidity near 50% helps reduce water loss in kittens and maintains the moisture and health of mucous membranes.

Oral Cavity

Examination of the oral cavity should include careful evaluation of the mucous membranes and hard palate. The mucous membranes should be light pink and moist. Cleft palates are relatively common defects in kittens (**Figure 23-3**). Vitamin A toxicity and trace mineral deficiencies (i.e., copper and zinc) during gestation have been associated with the development of cleft palates in kittens. However, in most cases, a cause is not identified. Most kittens with a cleft palate are unable to nurse effectively. Affected kittens must either be tube fed until the time of surgical correction or spontaneous closure, or they should be humanely euthanatized.

Laboratory Evaluation

Laboratory tests should be performed as needed to assess any abnormalities noted during the physical examination. Particular attention should be given to hydration status and serum glucose and electrolyte concentrations. When evaluating laboratory data in kittens, age-appropriate reference values should be used because concentrations of certain analytes (e.g., phosphorus, hematocrit, serum proteins) vary markedly from adult values (Hoskins, 1990).

Key Nutritional Factors

Colostrum and Milk

Colostrum is milk provided by the queen during the first 24 to 72 hours after parturition. Colostrum provides nutrients, water, growth factors, digestive enzymes and maternal immunoglobulins, all of which are critical to survival of neonatal kittens. Colostrum differs from mature milk in water and nutrient composition (**Table 23-3**). The dry matter (DM) content of colostrum is high, which accounts for its sticky, concentrated appearance compared with mature milk. The DM concentration declines as water content increases from Day 1 to 3 of lactation (Adkins et al, 1997). Lactose concentrations are low in colostrum (29.9 g/l or 23 mg/kcal) and increase as milk matures. Protein and lipid levels decline markedly from Day 1 to 3; however, this decline likely reflects the initial change in water content because nutrient levels rebound after Day 3 and increase slightly over the course of lactation. Like protein and lipid levels, the calculated gross energy of colostrum is high on Day 1 of lactation (1,300 kcal/l or 5.44 MJ/l) and falls significantly by Day 3. However, the energy content then increases throughout lactation. Changes in mineral content also vary with time. Calcium and phosphorus concentrations increase up to Day 14, whereas iron,

Table 23-3. Nutrient comparison among queen's colostrum, queen's milk and milk of selected species.

Nutrients	Queen's colostrum*	Queen's milk*	Bitch's milk**	Cow's milk***	Goat's milk***
Moisture (g/100 g)	–	79	77.3	87.7	87.0
Dry matter (g/100 g)	–	21	22.7	12.3	13
Crude protein (g/100 g)	8.3	7.5	7.5	3.3	3.6
Arginine (mg/100 g)	357	347	420	119	119
Taurine (mg/100 g)	26	27	–	0.13	–
Methionine (mg/100 g)	202	188	–	82	80
Crude fat (g/100 g)	9.3	8.5	9.5	3.6	4.1
Lactose (g/100 g)	3.0	4.0	3.3	4.7	4.0
Minerals					
Calcium (mg/100 g)	46	180	240	119	133
Phosphorus (mg/100 g)	114	162	180	93	111
Potassium (mg/100 g)	–	103	120	150	204
Magnesium (mg/100 g)	11	9	11	14	14
Copper (mg/100 g)	0.04	0.11	0.33	–	–
Iron (mg/100 g)	0.19	0.35	0.70	0.05	0.05
ME (kcal/100 g)	130	121	146	64	69
ME (kJ/100 g)	544	506	610	268	288

Key: ME = metabolizable energy.
*Adapted from Adkins Y, Zicker SC, Lepine A, et al. Changes in nutrient and protein composition of cat milk during lactation. American Journal of Veterinary Research 1997; 58: 370-375. Zottman B, Dobenecker B, Kienzle E, et al. Investigations on milk composition and milk yield in queens (abstract). In: Proceedings. The Waltham International Symposium, Orlando, FL, 1997.
**Adapted from Meyer H, Kienzle E, Dammers C. Milchmenge und Milchzusammensetzung bei und Hündin sowie Futteraufnahme und Gewichtsenwicklung ante und post partum.Fortschritte in der Tierphysiologie und tierernährung (Advances in Animal Physiology and Animal Nutrition) 1985; Suppl. No. 16: 51-72.
***Adapted from Pennington JA. Food Values of Portions Commonly Used. New York, NY: Harper Collins, 1989.

copper and magnesium concentrations decline. Early studies reported very low calcium concentrations and calcium-phosphorus ratios of 0.5:1 in queen's milk. These values likely represent colostral milk (calcium-phosphorus ratio = 0.4:1) (Baines, 1981). Recent studies of queen's milk report calcium-phosphorus ratios between 0.8:1 to 1:1 on Day 7; ratios reach 1.2:1 by late lactation (Dobenecker et al, 1998; Adkins et al, 1997). The variation in nutrient content with time probably explains the discrepancy in milk composition published by different investigators. Different values probably represent milk from different stages of lactation.

In addition to providing complete nutrition for nursing kittens, queen's milk also supplies non-nutritive factors that enhance food digestion, neonatal development and immune protection. The immunoglobulin concentration of cat colostrum and mature milk may not be significantly different as they are in most species (Casal et al, 1996). More studies are needed to further evaluate this difference; a decline in immunoglobulin concentrations and an increased casein-whey ratio with time contradict this finding (Adkins et al, 1997). Regardless, kittens acquire passive systemic and local immunity from ingesting either colostrum or mature milk (Casal et al, 1996). Kittens should receive colostrum within the first 12 hours of life to obtain adequate systemic immunity; after 16 hours, passive immunoglobulin transfer does not occur in kittens (Casal et al, 1996). During this time, kittens absorb intact immunoglobulins across the intestine. Failure to ingest colostrum or queen's milk during this absorptive window leaves kittens immunologically compromised and susceptible to infections and sepsis. Passive transfer of systemic immunity is particularly important to orphaned and hand-raised kittens that are fed only milk replacers. Consumption of queen's milk provides local concentrations of immunoglobulins within the gastrointestinal (GI) tract and helps prevent invasion of microorganisms into the bloodstream (passive local immunity). Local immunity persists as long as kittens receive queen's milk. Both systemic and local immunity are important in maintaining kitten health until maturation of the kittens' immune system.

Mature milk is a complete food for nursing kittens. Water, protein, fat, lactose, minerals and vitamins are provided in amounts sufficient for normal growth and development. As mentioned previously, mature milk may sustain high immunoglobulin levels similar to those provided by colostrum. Continued nursing provides high immunoglobulin levels for passive local immunity. Thus, the major feature differentiating mature queen's milk from colostrum is the nutrient content (**Table 23-3**). As lactation progresses, milk energy, protein, lactose, calcium and phosphorus levels increase whereas copper, iron and magnesium concentrations decrease (Adkins et al, 1997). The amino acid profiles of colostrum and mature milk also differ. Notable features include the relatively high concentrations of arginine and taurine in queen's milk, which likely reflect the unique metabolism of cats.

The nutrient requirements of nursing kittens have not been well studied. Although the nutrient profile of queen's milk is thought to provide optimal nutrition, faster growth rates are typically observed in kittens fed milk replacers (Remillard et al, 1993). Nevertheless, nutrient recommendations for neonates are based on the composition of queen's milk and growth studies in weaned kittens. Despite discrepancies in published nutrient values, queen's milk varies markedly from milk of other species (**Table 23-3**). Consequently, milk from other species is unsuitable for nursing kittens.

Table 23-4. Daily energy intake recommendations for orphaned kittens as a basis for determining food dose.*

Age (days)	kcal ME/100 g BW	kJ ME/100 g BW
1-3	15	60
4-6	20	85
>6	20-25	85-105

Key: ME = metabolizable energy, BW = body weight.
*Clients should not overfeed orphan formulas initially; the energy amounts listed for the first six days of the feeding period intentionally underfeed but then gradually increase so that the orphans' energy requirements are being met after about one week. Adapted from Mundt H-C, Thomée A, Meyer H. Zur Energie- und Eiweißversorgung von Saugwelpen über die Muttermilch. Kleintierpraxis 1981; 26: 353-360. Schaefers-Okkens AC. Pediatrie Post University Course, Ghent, Belgium, January 14, 1993. Sheffy BE. Nutrition and nutritional disorders. Veterinary Clinics of North America: Small Animal Practice 1978; 8: 7-29. Monson WJ. Orphan rearing of puppies and kittens. Veterinary Clinics of North America: Small Animal Practice 1987; 17: 567-576. Hoskins JD. Clinical evaluation of the kitten from birth to eight weeks of age. Compendium on Continuing Education for the Practicing Veterinarian 1990; 12: 1215-1225.

Replacement formulas with a nutrient profile similar to that of mature milk should be used for orphans and supplemental feedings. Thus, the nutrient content of queen's milk in **Table 23-3** provides a summary of the key nutritional factors for nursing kittens. For nutrients in which the concentration in mature milk is unknown, values recommended by the Association of American Feed Control Officials (AAFCO) for growth should suffice (2007). Also, the key nutritional factor discussion (Chapter 24) for postweaning kitten growth provides information that could be extrapolated to neonates, in lieu of other information.

Water

Kittens contain 78.8% body water at one week of age (Halle, 1992). Total body water decreases to 70.1% at weaning. By comparison, adult cats are composed of only 61.7% water (Halle, 1992). Water is one of the most important nutrients in orphan feeding. The normal water intake of kittens is relatively high. A normal kitten needs about 155 to 230 ml water/kg body weight/day (i.e., 4.4 to 6.5 ml water/oz. body weight). On average, orphaned kittens should receive about 180 ml of liquid/kg body weight to make orphan feeding successful. Water should be given until a total intake of 180 ml/kg body weight/day is reached if the milk replacer doesn't provide this much water at the recommended dilution.

Energy

Queen's milk typically meets the energy requirements of nursing kittens. Newborn kittens require about 24 kcal (100 kJ) metabolizable energy (ME)/100 g body weight for the first four weeks of life. **Table 23-4** provides recommended levels of energy intake for orphaned kittens from one to four weeks of age. By six weeks of age, male kittens are significantly heavier than female kittens and consume a proportionately larger quantity of food. As a rule, milk contains from 0.85 to 1.6 kcal/ml (3.6 to 6.7 kJ/ml) and milk replacers contain approximately 1 kcal/ml (4.2 kJ/ml) as fed. In general, kittens less than one week old will eat a volume equal to 10 to 15% of their body weight as milk or properly formulated milk replacer per day and a volume equal to 20 to 25% of their body weight per day between Weeks 1 to 4. This is also a reasonable target if the caloric content of the food is unknown. A very common mistake is to underestimate the energy requirements of neonates. In the beginning, however, it is better not to overfeed to avoid diarrhea. In most cases, it is best to follow label recommendations on commercial products or feed based on energy calculations.

Protein

The minimum protein requirement of nursing kittens has not been established. However, it is assumed to be comparable to that for weanling kittens, which is approximately 18 to 20% DM (Smalley et al, 1985). These requirements were established using purified diets and may not accurately reflect the needs of kittens fed commercial foods made from typical ingredients. The AAFCO recommendation of 30% DM appears adequate (2007); however, the protein content of queen's milk ranges from 33 to 44% DM (Adkins et al, 1997; Baines, 1981).

It is essential that commercial milk replacers and homemade replacer formulas have adequate protein and essential amino acid content. The arginine and histidine levels in the formula are particularly important. Deficiency of these amino acids can cause cataract development in neonates and contribute to anorexia and poor growth. The minimum recommended levels of these two amino acids for growth in kittens after weaning are 0.96 and 0.33% DM, respectively (NRC, 2006). These recommendations are based on a food with 22.5% DM crude protein. For foods with 30% crude protein, DM arginine should be increased to 0.975% (NRC, 2006).

Taurine

Taurine is important for normal growth and development of kittens. Fortunately, dietary taurine is more available to kittens than adult cats (Earle and Smith, 1994), presumably because of reduced bacterial degradation of taurine in the GI tract. Normal plasma taurine concentrations are maintained in 12- and 18-week-old kittens fed taurine at 150 to 197 mg/kg body weight/day (Earle and Smith, 1994). Queen's milk supplies about 300 mg taurine/liter (NRC, 1986; Adkins et al, 1997). Queens fed low-taurine foods have significantly lower milk taurine levels, which may impair normal growth and development.[a] Dietary taurine intake influences milk taurine concentrations, thus it is not surprising that cow's milk is a poor source of taurine (i.e., only 1.3 mg/l) (NRC, 1986). Therefore, homemade milk replacers based on cow's milk should be supplemented with taurine (30 mg taurine/100 ml milk replacer). Taurine is commercially available as crystalline taurine from veterinary pharmacies or health food stores.

Fat

Milk fat is an important source of energy and essential fatty acids for nursing kittens. The composition of the queen's diet can significantly influence milk fat quantity and quality, which translates into fat composition of the offspring (Pawlosky and Salem, 1996). The fat content of queen's milk increases throughout lactation. Average fat concentrations of 28% DM or 86 g/l appear typical (Dobenecker et al, 1998; Adkins et al, 1997; Baines, 1981). Queen's milk provides the essential fatty acids linoleic and arachidonic acid at 5.8 and 0.5% DM, respectively (Dobenecker et al, 1998). Docosahexaenoic acid (DHA) is also essential for normal retinal development and function in kittens (Pawlosky et al, 1997). Milk DHA concentrations reflect the dietary intake of the queen. The recommended DM level of DHA plus eicosapentaenoic acid (EPA) for kittens after weaning is 0.01%. EPA should not exceed 60% of the total DHA plus EPA (NRC, 2006). These levels are probably also suitable for orphan formulas.

Carbohydrate

No carbohydrate requirements have been established for nursing and growing kittens. However, the lactose concentration of queen's milk ranges from 14 to 26% DM. Intestinal lactase activity declines to adult levels very soon after weaning (Kienzle, 1987). Overfeeding cow's milk causes diarrhea, bloating and abdominal discomfort in kittens due to bacterial metabolism of undigested lactose in the large intestine. Owners who wish to offer cow's milk should be advised to limit the quantities given and to discontinue feeding cow's milk if intolerance occurs.

Calcium and Phosphorus

Calcium concentrations are low in colostrum (0.22% DM) and increase significantly to approximately 1% DM by mid to late lactation (Adkins et al, 1997). Thus, requirements appear limited early on and increase with bone mineralization and growth. Milk phosphorus concentrations do not vary to the same extent. Therefore, calcium-phosphorus ratios increase from a low of 0.4:1 to 0.8:1 on Day 1 of lactation to approximately 1:1, or higher, between one to three weeks of lactation and remain at that level throughout lactation (Adkins et al, 1997; Dobenecker et al, 1998).

Trace Minerals

Queen's milk contains iron, copper and zinc concentrations markedly higher than those in human and bovine milk but similar to those in canine milk. Copper and iron levels gradually decline throughout lactation, whereas zinc concentrations remain constant. Consequently, mineral deficiencies are rarely reported to occur in nursing kittens fed queen's milk. However, milk replacers made from cow's milk should be supplemented to levels typically found in queen's milk to avoid deficiency (**Table 23-3**).

Commercial milk replacers are often fortified with iron at concentrations higher than those found in queen's milk. Orphaned kittens, especially low birth-weight neonates born with low iron reserves, may benefit from iron intakes higher than those normally found in milk. The additional iron supports hematopoiesis and helps avoid anemia sometimes observed in three- to four-week-old neonates.

Digestibility

DM digestibility of queen's milk is very high (>95%). Digestibility of milk replacer formulas should also be high (>90%) to allow for smaller quantities to be fed and avoid diarrhea.

Osmolality

High osmolality should be avoided in milk replacers because it may cause hyperosmolar diarrhea and potentiate dehydration. High osmolarity may delay gastric emptying and predispose to regurgitation, vomiting and aspiration during the next meal, if the stomach is not completely empty. The osmolarity of queen's milk is approximately 329 mOsm/kg.

FEEDING PLAN

The feeding plan includes determining the best food and feeding method, under the prevailing circumstances. **Tables 23-5** and **23-6**, respectively, provide feeding plan summaries for nursing and orphaned kittens.

Assess and Select the Food

Foods should be liquid until kittens are three to five weeks old, then semi-solid to solid foods may be introduced, which marks the beginning of the weaning process (**Box 23-2**). Foods may consist of queen's milk, commercial milk replacers or homemade milk replacers (including supplemented human enteral formulas). **Table 23-7** provides a list of commercial milk replacers and compares their nutrient profiles (key nutritional factors) with queen's milk. **Table 23-8** provides two homemade milk replacer recipes and **Table 23-9** compares these recipes' nutrient profiles with that of queen's milk.

Kittens should receive colostrum within the first 12 to 24 hours after parturition. Subsequently, immunoglobulins are no longer absorbed from the GI tract and passive transfer will not occur (Casal et al, 1996). If colostrum is unavailable, milk collected from queens at any stage of lactation may be substituted. Antibody levels in non-colostral milk appear to adequately transfer passive immunity to kittens (Casal et al, 1996).

Alternatively, sterile serum may be given to kittens subcutaneously if milk is unavailable (Pedersen and Wastlhuber, 1991). To collect serum, using sterile technique, blood should be obtained from healthy, well-vaccinated donors free of communicable diseases. After the blood has clotted and been centrifuged, the serum is removed and administered in a sterile manner. Ideally, serum donors should be blood-typed to avoid neonatal isoerythrolysis. A dosage of 150 ml/kg/day is divided into three doses and given over a 24-hour period. This dose provides passive antibody concentrations that are similar to antibody concentrations of kittens that receive colostrum until at least six weeks of age (Levy et al, 2001). After the first 24 hours, kittens should be fed queen's milk or a complete and bal-

Table 23-5. Feeding plan summary for nursing kittens.

1. Ensure good husbandry practices are understood and in place (**Box 23-1**).
2. Ensure colostrum intake by the kittens within the first 12 hours.
3. Provide queen's milk only until three to four weeks of age, then initiate the gradual weaning process by introducing small amounts of semisolid to solid food to augment the queen's milk (**Box 23-2**).
4. The weaning food should be a good quality growth/reproduction type commercial food (Chapters 22 and 24).
5. Assess nursing kittens daily. Body weights should be obtained at birth then once weekly, if no complications are present. Normal birth weights range from 85 to 120 g and healthy kittens should gain approximately 100 g/week; minimally they should gain 7 g/day. Poor weight gain or failure to thrive should prompt the breeder/owner to seek an immediate evaluation by a veterinarian.
6. Kittens not thriving on queens' milk should be fed via partial or total orphan feeding techniques; check the queen, including its food, to ensure there are no health or nutrition issues to affect lactation.
7. Wean at six to nine weeks (**Box 23-2**) and feed according to recommendations in Chapter 24 (growing kittens).

Table 23-6. Feeding plan summary for orphaned kittens.

1. Ensure good husbandry practices are understood and in place (**Box 23-1**); have owner attempt to provide as much total care as would be expected from the queen.
2. Ideally, kittens should have had colostrum within the first 12 hours; if not, and if available, queen's milk is the second best choice provided if given in the same time frame; alternatively, sterile serum can be given subcutaneously (50 ml serum/kg body weight every eight hours for a total of three doses).
3. Use foster queen if possible; partial orphan feeding is next best and bottle feeding is the best of the hand-feeding techniques (**Figure 23-4** and Chapter 16).
4. **Table 23-7** lists commercial milk replacers and compares them to queen's milk; **Table 23-8** provides two homemade formulas and **Table 23-9** compares them to queen's milk. Commercial milk replacers are best.
5. Use **Table 23-4** to estimate kittens' daily energy requirement; divide the daily energy requirement by the energy density of the milk replacer to determine the daily amount to feed. Most milk replacers will provide about 1 kcal/ml when properly diluted. Besides energy and other nutrients, on average, orphaned kittens should receive about 180 ml/kg body weight/day; if necessary, add additional water to the milk replacer if the recommended dilution doesn't provide for this total fluid intake.
6. Milk replacers should be heated to 38°C (100°F) and the daily amount divided and fed four or more times/day at equal intervals.
7. Good hygiene is critical and includes: Washing/boiling feeding utensils before each feeding. Preparing no more than 24 hours worth of milk replacer and refrigerating unused portions. Carefully washing kittens with a moist, soft cloth twice weekly.
8. Gradually initiate the weaning process by introducing small amounts of semisolid to solid food to augment the milk replacer (**Box 23-2**).
9. Ensure the weaning food is a good quality growth/reproduction type commercial food (Chapters 22 and 24).
10. Assess orphaned kittens daily. Body weights should be obtained at birth then once weekly, if no complications are present. Normal birth weights range from 85 to 120 g. Healthy kittens should gain approximately 100 g/week; minimally they should gain 7 g/day. Poor weight gain or failure to thrive should prompt the breeder/owner to seek an immediate evaluation by a veterinarian. Weekly veterinary checks should be recommended for the first month.
11. For kittens failing to thrive when receiving the milk replacer, review the milk replacer quality (**Tables 23-7** and **23-9**), dilution calculations and feeding amounts; switch to a different milk replacer if necessary.
12. Wean at six to nine weeks (**Box 23-2**) and feed according to recommendations in Chapter 24 (growing kittens).

anced feline milk replacer.

Queen's milk is considered an ideal food for nursing kittens because it provides all essential nutrients, antibodies, enzymes and hormones. Commercial milk replacers and homemade replacer recipes may mimic the essential nutrient content of queen's milk but lack its other beneficial properties. However, queen's milk is rarely available in sufficient quantities to hand raise orphans. The next best option is to attempt to foster kittens to a surrogate queen. If milk replacers are used, generally commercial products are preferred although several homemade formulas have proved sufficient.

Commercial and homemade milk replacers should closely mimic the profile of queen's milk. Unsupplemented ruminant milk may be used as a base for homemade formulas but does not meet the nutritional needs of kittens. Goat's milk provides no nutritional benefit over cow's milk. **Tables 23-7** and **23-9** are useful for assessing and selecting milk replacers.

The quality of queen's milk and milk replacers is difficult to assess without analysis. Measurement of kitten growth is indirect, but probably the most practical method of assessment. Additionally, the queen's food should be assessed if the queen is losing excessive amounts of weight. A thin queen (body condition score 1/5 to 2/5) may not produce enough milk or may produce poor-quality milk. If milk analysis is required, a sample can be collected by manually expressing milk from the queen after preventing the kittens from nursing for a short time. Parenteral oxytocin (5 IU/queen) facilitates milk collection. Small samples (1 to 3 ml) are easily collected during normal lactation and should be frozen until analysis. Commercial laboratories do not routinely analyze such small milk samples; therefore, an appropriate research facility should be contacted ahead of time for specific information about sample size, preservation and shipping instructions.

Assess and Determine the Feeding Method

Nursing kittens should be allowed free access to the queen as the preferred feeding method. Kittens should be observed to ensure they have received colostrum by 12 hours after partu-

Box 23-2. Weaning.

Weaning is usually a gradual process that begins with the queen avoiding the kittens and kittens eating increasing amounts of solid food. Typically, weaning begins when kittens are three to four weeks old and is complete at six to nine weeks of age. At three to four weeks of age, kittens begin to eat solid foods, although approximately 95% of their caloric intake is still provided by the queen's milk. By five to six weeks of age, kittens eat nearly 30% of their caloric requirement as solid food and the remainder as milk. A progressive intake of solid food continues until the kittens are completely independent of the queen. Most domestic shorthair kittens are weaned by six weeks of age, whereas purebred kittens are usually weaned around eight to nine weeks of age. Later weaning allows more time for kitten growth and immune system maturation, which may help reduce kitten mortality in the postweaning period.

The weaning process may be initiated by the gradual refusal of the queen to allow the kittens to nurse or by the breeder who separates the kittens from the queen. During weaning, many queens will reduce food intake and milk production gradually. Regardless, the queen's energy requirement will decrease from lactation to maintenance levels after weaning is complete.

A commonly used schedule for the final phase of the weaning process follows. On the first day: 1) the kittens and food are withheld from the queen, 2) the kittens are allowed free access to their weaning food and 3) the kittens are returned to the queen at the end of the day and allowed to nurse. The following day: 1) the kittens are removed and allowed free access to their weaning food and not returned to the queen (they are weaned) and 2) the queen is given one-fourth of its ration. Over the next three days, food amounts for the queen are gradually increased to pre-breeding (maintenance) levels. The kittens should continue to be housed and fed separately. To minimize mammary gland engorgement in queens that are abruptly removed from their kittens and/or those that are heavy milk producers, have owners restrict food intake a day or two before the final weaning process is begun.

Weaning can be a stressful event in the kitten's life. Transition to independent feeding, greater environmental exposure and waning maternal antibodies result in reduced immune defense. These factors contribute to increased morbidity and mortality in the postweaning period. Proper nutrition and careful husbandry can reduce these events markedly.

Recommended nutrient allowances for weanling kittens are similar to those for lactating queens and for growing kittens, postweaning (Chapters 22 and 24). Energy requirements for weanling kittens are between 200 to 250 kcal/kg body weight (837 to 1,046 kJ/kg body weight). The stomach volume of kittens is small; therefore, feeding energy-dense foods helps meet the higher energy needs of weanling kittens without exceeding gastric capacity. Kittens from queens with lower body weights reportedly have limited growth. Milk production may be compromised in underweight queens. After weaning, however, smaller kittens compensate by increasing food intake and growth rate until they attain their expected size.

At the onset of weaning (three to four weeks of age), kittens should be offered moist foods or dry foods moistened with water or milk replacer. The food should be moistened until it forms a soft but not liquid gruel. Kittens at this stage lap at but do not prehend food. By six to eight weeks of age, most kittens have learned to eat solid, unmoistened foods; therefore, gruels are no longer necessary. The food should be highly digestible and complete and balanced for growth and reproduction. Semi-moist foods that promote a highly acidic urinary pH should not be fed as the sole food source for growing kittens. High levels of dietary acid may lead to metabolic acidosis and impaired bone mineralization.

The weaning process will be less stressful if kittens are initially offered the same food that will be fed after weaning. Using the same food facilitates the transition away from the queen and helps avoid gastrointestinal upsets associated with a food change. After three weeks of age, kittens should have water and food available at all times in addition to free access to the queen. Food and water should be easily accessible and offered in broad shallow pans. Food should be replenished three to four times daily. High-moisture foods begin to spoil and harbor high levels of bacteria when left at room temperature for prolonged periods (Chapter 11). Thus, washing pans between feedings is recommended. Ideally, food should be warmed to about 38ºC (100ºF) or at least brought to room temperature. Kittens first eat by accident, as they step into food and then ingest it during grooming. This process can be hastened by smearing small quantities of food around a kitten's mouth.

Daily monitoring of physical appearance, activity, stool quality and food intake is recommended. Kittens should be weighed and their body condition assessed weekly; they should continue to grow at approximately 100 g/week. Gender differences in growth rate are now evident; female kittens are normally smaller than males (Chapter 24). Kittens should demonstrate increasing activity and social and exploratory behavior. After a meal, the kittens' abdomen should be well rounded but not overly distended. Crying in neonates and older kittens usually indicates discomfort (e.g., cold, hunger, pain, disease or isolation).

The queen still consumes the kittens' feces to keep the nest box clean early during this phase. At about four weeks, the kittens begin to defecate outside the nest box and stools can be readily monitored. Kittens eating solid foods should have soft-formed stools, whereas those eating predominantly milk will have pasty yellow to light-brown stools. It is vital during this phase to practice good cattery husbandry and monitor kittens closely for disease. Weaning is a stressful event and outbreaks of diarrhea and disease are very common. Growth rate is universally impaired in sick and malnourished kittens.

The Bibliography for **Box 23-2** can be found at www.markmorris.org.

rition. Most neonatal kittens require feeding every two to four hours during the first week of life then every four to six hours until weaning. Weak kittens may need to be placed on the queen and held to facilitate nursing. Chilled kittens will not suckle and have reduced GI function. It is imperative to adequately warm weak kittens before they are fed. Hypoglycemia and hypothermia may occur simultaneously in neonates and have similar clinical signs. If kittens fail to respond to warm-

Table 23-7. Nutrient content of milk replacers compared with that of queen's milk/100 grams of milk, as fed.*

Nutrients**	Queen's milk	KMR Liquid	KMR Reconstituted Powder	Nurturall C Kitten Liquid†	Nurturall-C Reconstituted Powder†	Just Born Kitten Liquid†	Just Born Reconstituted Powder†
Manufacturer	-	**PetAg**	**PetAg**	**VPL**	**VPL**	**Farnam**	**Farnam**
Dilution***	na	na	1+2	na	1+1	na	1+1.33
Moisture (g)	79.0	81.7	na	80.1	74.0	80.1	79.1
Dry matter (g)	21.0	18.3	na	19.9	26.0	19.9	21.0
Crude protein (g)	7.5	7.7	7.7	7.7	9.8	7.7	7.9
Arginine (mg)	430	250	310	200	240	200	195
Taurine (mg)	10	10	10	na	na	na	na
Fat (g)	8.5	4.7	4.7	4.4	5.4	4.4	4.5
Linoleic acid (C18:2) (g)	na	na	0.31	na	na	na	na
Arachidonic acid (C20:4) (mg)	na	na	20	na	na	na	na
Carbohydrate							
NFE (g)	na	4.7	3.6	6.2	8.7	6.2	7.0
Lactose (g)	4.0	na	3.1	na	na	na	na
Crude fiber (g)	na	0	0	<0.1	<0.1	<0.1	<0.1
Minerals							
Total ash (g)	0.6	1.2	1.4	1.5	2.1	1.5	1.7
Calcium (mg)	180	190	200	252	373	252	300
Phosphorus (mg)	162	160	200	220	287	220	231
Sodium (mg)	90	80	70	na	na	na	na
Potassium (mg)	103	210	190	102	308	102	248
Magnesium (mg)	9.0	16.0	14.2	18.4	31.5	18.4	25.3
Copper (mg)	0.11	0.26	0.27	0.40	0.73	0.40	0.58
Iron (mg)	0.4	1.2	1.4	0.4	5.5	0.4	4.4
Energy							
ME (kcal)	121	83	79	86	111	86	91
ME (kJ)	505	347	332	360	464	360	379
Osmolarity (mOsm/kg, H_20±SD)	329±18.7	na	na	na	na	na	na
Nutrient content of milk replacers compared with that of queen's milk/100 kcal metabolizable energy††							
Crude protein (g)	6.3	9.3	9.7	9.0	8.9	9.0	8.7
Fat (g)	7.1	5.6	5.9	5.1	4.9	5.1	5.0
Linoleic acid (C18:2)	>1.1	na	390	na	na	na	na
Carbohydrate							
NFE (g)	na	5.71	4.54	7.21	7.85	7.21	7.71
Lactose (g)	3.3	na	3.9	na	na	na	na
Minerals							
Total ash (g)	0.5	1.4	1.8	1.7	1.9	1.7	1.8
Calcium (mg)	150.0	230	250	293	336	293	331
Phosphorus (mg)	135	190	250	256	259	256	255
Sodium (mg)	75	100	90	na	na	na	na
Potassium (mg)	86	250	240	119	278	119	273
Magnesium (mg)	7.5	19.3	17.9	21.4	28.4	21.4	27.9
Copper (mg)	0.10	0.31	0.34	0.50	0.66	0.47	0.64
Iron (mg)	0.3	1.4	1.7	0.5	5.0	0.5	4.9

Key: na = not applicable/available, NFE = nitrogen-free extract, ME = metabolizable energy, mOsm = milliosmoles.
*Manufacturers' data; nutrient content for reconstituted powdered products are manufacturers' calculations based on the recommended dilution. Nutrient data per 100 ml would be reduced slightly (between 1 to 2%), because the specific gravity of milk is greater than that of water.
**g/100 g = %.
***The first number is the milk powder, the second the water (e.g., 1+2 = one part of powder plus two parts of water).
†Nutrients in liquid and powder forms are averages from the yearly laboratory analyses of composite samples from 2004 to date.
††The nutrient levels per 100 kcal ME were calculated from the nutrient and energy levels in the top portion of the table.

ing, a dilute glucose solution (2.5% glucose) may be given orally. This should be repeated until kittens are able to initiate a strong sucking reflex. Because nursing kittens depend completely on queen's milk, the feeding plan for the queen should be evaluated and modified if necessary (Chapter 22).

It may be necessary to alter the feeding method when managing orphaned kittens, especially if they are hand reared. Evaluation of the current feeding method with foreknowledge of growth demands will facilitate this part of feeding plan development. Orphaned kittens and those too weak to nurse are candidates for fostering, partial orphan rearing or hand feeding. These feeding methods are discussed below.

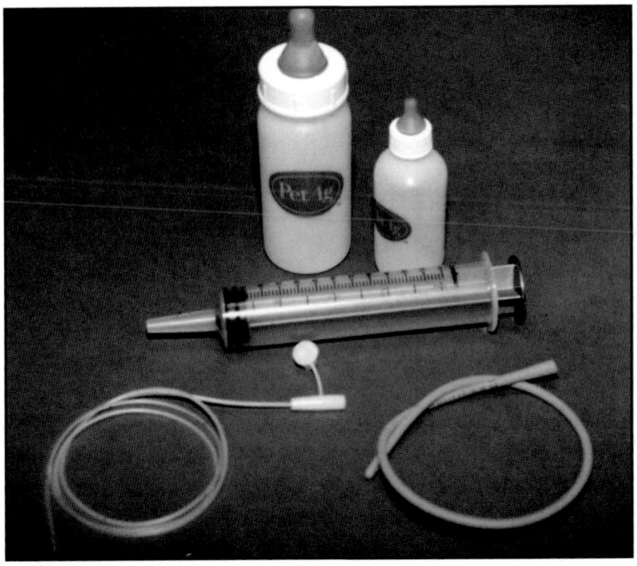

Figure 23-4. Various bottles and feeding tubes can be used for hand feeding orphaned kittens.

Fostering

The optimal means of feeding orphaned or rejected kittens is to foster them to another lactating queen. Fostering is the least labor intensive, provides optimal nutrition, reduces mortality, improves immune status, usually provides an optimal physical environment and promotes normal social development of kittens. Unlike large animals, queens readily accept additional kittens during lactation. If several foster mothers are available, it is best to place orphans in litters with fewer than 14 days age difference. Larger kittens often crowd out smaller individuals if the age discrepancy is too large. This situation can be managed by supervised feeding until the orphans can fend for themselves. Unfortunately, foster mothers are not normally available and alternative techniques must be used.

Partial Orphan Rearing

Kittens that cannot be successfully raised by the queen for reasons of health, poor lactation performance or too large of a litter, may be left with the mother but given supplemental feeding to support nutritional needs. Supplemental food may be given by hand feedings or timed feedings using a surrogate queen. Kittens may also be reared in a communal situation. Partial orphan rearing can be accomplished by dividing the litter into two groups of equal number and size. One group remains with the mother while the other is removed and fed milk replacer. The groups are exchanged three to four times daily. It is important to feed the separated group before it is returned to the mother. As a result, the group just placed with the dam will be less inclined to nurse immediately. It is better to supplement all the kittens in the litter rather than just a few. The advantages of partial orphan rearing are similar to those of fostering. In addition, continued access to the mother can help stimulate milk production and mothering behaviors. When using foster or surrogate mothers, it is important to monitor for signs of rejection and cannibalism. Partial orphan rearing may be necessary to assist the efforts of foster mothers. Unfortunately, foster and surrogate mothers are usually unavailable.

Table 23-8. Recipes for homemade kitten orphan formulas.

Recipe 1*		Recipe 2**	
Skim milk	70 g	One whole egg, fresh	15 g
Low-fat curd***	15 g	Protein supplement	25 g
Lean beef hash	8 g	Milk, sweetened, condensed	17 ml
Egg yolk (1/5)	3 g	Corn oil	7 ml
Vegetable oil	3 g	Water	250 ml
Lactose	0.8 g	-	-
Vitamin-mineral mix	0.2 g		
Total	100 g	Total	310 g

*Adapted from Kienzle E. Raising of motherless puppies and kittens. In: Proceedings. World Small Animal Veterinary Association Congress, Vienna, Austria, 1991: 240-242.
**Remillard RL, Pickett JP, Thatcher CD, et al. Comparison of kittens fed queen's milk with those fed milk replacers. American Journal of Veterinary Research 1993; 54: 901-907.
***Do not use cottage cheese because it may increase the risk of clotting in the neonate's stomach.

Table 23-9. Key nutritional factor content of homemade orphan formulas (**Table 23-8**) compared to key nutritional factor content of queen's milk.

Nutrients*	Queen's milk	Recipe 1**	Recipe 2**
Moisture (g)	79.3	83.1	86.4
Dry matter (g)	20.7	16.9	13.6
Crude protein (g)	7.5	7.1	6.4
Fat (g)	8.6	4.4	3.4
NFE (g)	4	4.7	2.9
Ash (g)	0.6	0.8	0.7
Calcium (mg)	180	96.2	109
Phosphorus (mg)	162	126	109
Sodium (mg)	90	33.5	90
Potassium (mg)	103	117	113
Copper (mg)	0.11	0.03	0.2
Iron (mg)	0.35	0.6	3.5
Zinc (mg)	na	0.7	1.9
Energy			
ME (kcal)***	121	80	62
ME (kJ)***	506	335	260

Key: NFE = nitrogen-free extract, ME = metabolizable energy.
*Calculated before addition of the vitamin-mineral mix.
**Calculated based on the addition of 2.5 g Pecutrin (Bayer).
***Calculated.

Hand Feeding

The most common method of raising orphaned kittens is hand feeding. Eyedroppers, syringes, bottles and stomach tubes are typically used to hand feed orphans. The method of choice largely depends on the age, vitality and adequacy of the sucking reflex of the kitten and the handler's expertise.

BOTTLE FEEDING

Bottle feeding is the preferred method for vigorous kittens with good nursing reflexes. Bottle feeding has the advantage that neonates will nurse until they are satiated and reject the milk or formula when full. However, bottle feeding can be time

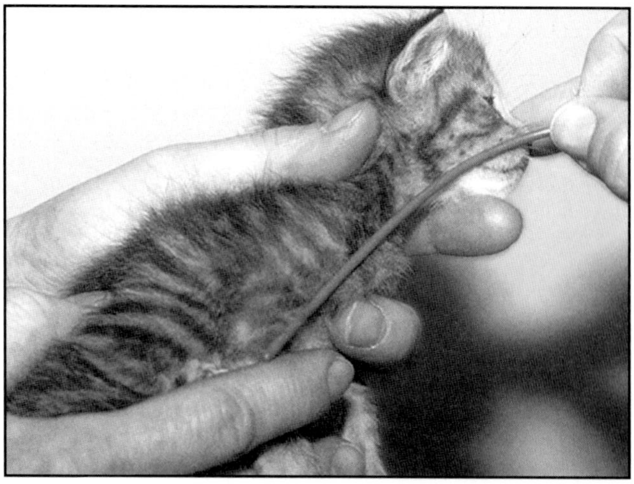

Figure 23-5. Feeding tubes should be premeasured and marked at a spot approximately 75% of the distance from the nose to the last rib. This placement will ensure the tube tip is in the distal esophagus.

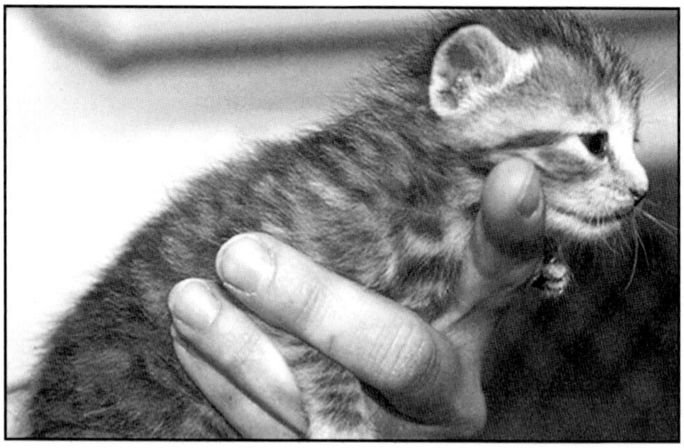

Figure 23-6. Kittens should be held horizontally in the palm of the hand for tube feeding.

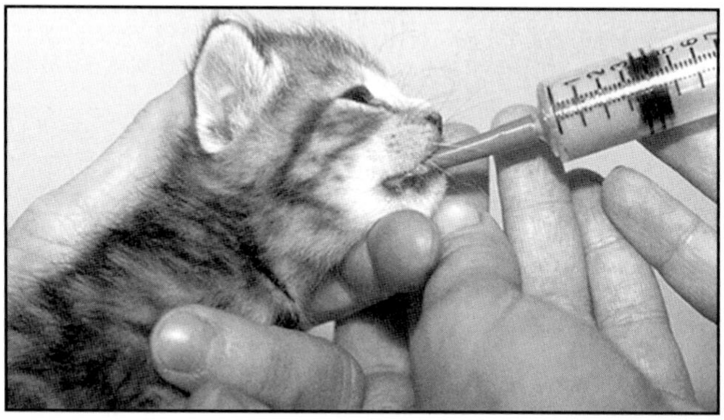

Figure 23-7. A lubricated tube is gently advanced to the premeasured mark and warm formula is administered over several minutes. The tube should be withdrawn and repositioned if resistance or struggling is encountered.

consuming, especially with large litters.

Most kittens will readily nurse small pet nursing bottles available in pet stores (**Figure 23-4**). Feeding bottles for dolls or bottles with nipples for premature human infants are alternatives. The opening should only allow one drop at a time to fall from the nipple when the bottle is inverted. A horizontal slit made with a razor blade instead of a round hole may make it easier for neonates to obtain milk or formula. Milk should be sucked-never squeezed-from the bottle. A rapid flow rate may lead to aspiration of milk resulting in pneumonia and/or death.

Kittens should normally be held horizontally with the head in a natural position. This position reduces the risk of aspiration (Figure 16-1).

TUBE FEEDING

Kittens that are weak or suckle poorly may need to be tube fed. Tube feeding is faster than bottle feeding and is often used when several orphans must be cared for by the same person. Bottle feeding allows kittens to control the amount of food intake, whereas tube feeding bypasses this control mechanism. Infant feeding tubes (5 to 8 Fr.) or soft urethral or intravenous catheters may be used (**Figure 23-4**).

The tube should be lubricated and placed in the lower esophagus, which is approximately 75% of the distance from the nose to the last rib (**Figure 23-5**). It is best to measure and mark the tube with an indelible marker or a piece of tape before insertion. Recheck measurements every few days to account for growth of the kitten. The orphan should normally be placed horizontally in the palm of the hand with its head in a natural position (**Figure 23-6**).

The mouth can be opened using the same hand that steadies the head. Gently advance the tube to the premeasured mark. If resistance is encountered or the kitten suddenly struggles, the tube may be in the trachea. It should be removed and repositioned into the esophagus. Do not feed until proper placement is ensured. After the tube is placed, attach the feeding syringe and slowly administer the warmed formula over one to two minutes (**Figure 23-7**). The stomach may be palpated to determine the degree of distention. Administration of formula should be stopped if the stomach becomes taut or there is resistance to formula flow. Continuation of feeding may result in gastric overdistention and regurgitation. If regurgitation occurs, withdraw the tube and discontinue feeding until the next meal.

Success of orphan rearing depends on how well the caregiver fulfills the daily routine of hygienic measures, strict feeding schedules and all aspects of care normally provided by the queen. These measures are vital for survival of kittens early in life.

Hygiene

Strict hygiene is especially important with hand feeding. Hygienic measures must be more stringent for orphaned kittens because they may have received less colostrum and be more susceptible to infections than other neonates.

- Feeding materials (e.g., bottles and nipples) should be cleaned thoroughly and boiled in water between uses.
- Ingredients for homemade milk replacers should be fresh and refrigerated until used.
- Clients should never prepare more milk replacer than can be used in 24 hours and refrigerate.
- Formulas should be discarded after one hour at room tem-

perature.
- At least twice a week, orphans should be washed gently with a soft moistened cloth to simulate cleaning by the dam's tongue.

Feeding Amount, Schedule and Rate and Formula Temperature

To determine the amount to feed, first use **Table 23-4** to estimate the kittens' daily energy requirement (DER). Then, divide the DER by the energy density of the milk replacer to determine the amount to feed. Most milk replacers provide about 1 kcal/ml when properly diluted. Orphaned kittens should receive about 180 ml/kg body weight/day (18 ml/100 g body weight). If necessary, add additional water to the milk replacer if the recommended dilution doesn't provide for this amount of total fluid intake. During the first week of life the capacity of milk intake is limited to about 10 to 15 ml per feeding.

The energy density of the milk replacer should be adequate at the recommended dilution. If the energy density is too low, the neonate's intake capacity may be exceeded. If this occurs, the neonates might not gain weight, and could actually lose weight, despite apparently adequate volume intake. Affected neonates may start vocalizing and become restless.

Orphans should be fed at least four times daily. Very young neonates and weak kittens should preferably be fed every two to four hours. Older kittens should be fed every four to six hours. Normally, one- to two-week-old kittens will obtain more than 90% of their normal daily intake in four to five meals.

Milk replacer should be warmed to 38°C (100°F) and delivered slowly. Cold foods, rapid feeding rates and overfeeding may result in regurgitation, aspiration, bloating and diarrhea.

Review and have clients correct the feeding methods if untoward signs develop. If diarrhea is observed, food volume should be reduced or diluted with water, then gradually returned to levels to meet caloric requirements over successive feedings. It is better to underfeed than overfeed neonatal kittens.

REASSESSMENT

Nursing kittens should be reassessed daily. Body weights should be obtained at birth then once weekly, if no complications are present. Poor weight gain or failure to thrive should prompt the breeder/owner to seek an immediate evaluation by a veterinarian.

Adequacy of the queen's milk production can be assessed by the growth rate of the kittens, kittens' contentment and, to some extent, the degree of mammary gland distention. Expressing milk from a queen's nipples demonstrates the functionality of individual mammary glands, but does not indicate adequate milk production.

Orphaned kittens should be evaluated daily for the first two weeks of life. They should remain normally hydrated, sleep quietly between feedings and gain weight at a rate similar to queen-raised neonates. Alertness, eagerness to suckle, general behavior, body temperature (i.e., temperature of skin and lower limbs), body weight and stool character should be recorded daily or more often if neonates appear weak or listless.

Orphan rearing permits precise measurement of food intake. Nursing kittens should grow about 100 g/week. If kittens do not thrive when fed a commercial milk replacer or homemade replacer, the nutrient content should be compared with mother's milk (**Tables 23-7** and **23-9**). The dilution recommended by the manufacturer should also be checked. In some cases, it may be necessary to switch to another formula.

Kittens with rectal temperatures less than 35°C (95°F) should not be fed. At this temperature, the sucking reflex is usually absent and normal gut motility has ceased. Neonates should first be warmed slowly after receiving a warm solution of 2.5% glucose by subcutaneous injection (1 ml/30 g body weight).

Weaning is an important event and is integral to successful feeding of nursing and orphaned kittens (**Box 23-2**).

ACKNOWLEDGMENTS

The authors and editors acknowledge the contributions of Drs. Claudia A. Kirk and P. Jane Armstrong in the previous edition of Small Animal Clinical Nutrition.

ENDNOTE

a. Kirk CA. Unpublished data. 1994.

REFERENCES

The references for **Chapter 23** can be found at www.markmorris.org.

Chapter 24

Feeding Growing Kittens: Postweaning to Adulthood

Kathy L. Gross
Iveta Becvarova
Jacques Debraekeleer

"Kittens are born with their eyes shut. They open them in about six days, take a look around, then close them again for the better part of their lives."
Stephen Baker

INTRODUCTION

The postweaning growth period includes kittens from weaning (about eight weeks of age) until adulthood (10 to 12 months). The nutritional needs of growing kittens include maintenance needs similar to those of adult cats and energy and substrates necessary for rapid tissue accretion (**Figure 24-1**). Growth rate slows if nutritional deficiencies exist. Thus, nutritional requirements are easiest to determine in growing animals using growth rates as a nutritional marker. The nutritional needs of postweaning, growing kittens are best understood by comparing their needs with those of other lifestages. Nevertheless, the optimal nutrient levels for growth may not represent the optimal levels for other physiologic functions. Further research may redefine nutrient requirements of growing kittens as physiologic parameters besides growth are studied. The ultimate goal of feeding kittens is to ensure they develop into healthy adults. The specific objectives, however, are to optimize growth, minimize risk factors for disease and achieve optimal health.

PATIENT ASSESSMENT

History and Physical Examination

The general health and risk factors should be determined for every kitten early in the growing phase. A thorough history and physical examination, including determination of body weight and body condition, are generally sufficient. Ideally, a veterinarian should assess the kitten at weaning and monthly thereafter until the kitten is four months old. This schedule coincides with typical vaccination protocols for young kittens. The veterinary health care team should educate the owner about nutrition, weight management, neutering and dental care during these examinations. The owner can then evaluate stool and appetite daily and body condition weekly or every two weeks.

Kittens should continue to grow at approximately 100 g/week until about 20 weeks of age. At 20 weeks, males typically gain 20 g/day whereas females gain 11 g/day (NRC, 1986). Growth rate slows as kittens approach 80% of adult size at 30 weeks and reach adult body weight at 40 weeks (10 months) (Figure 23-1). Most cats will achieve skeletal maturity at 10 months of age although some growth plates have yet to close. Additional weight gain may occur after 12 months of age and represents a phase of maturation and muscle development.

There is no evidence that the age at neutering alters growth rate. Investigators evaluating early neutering found kittens neutered at 12 weeks of age reached similar size as adults neutered at the more typical ages of six to nine months (Root, 1995). Unfortunately, energy requirements decline following

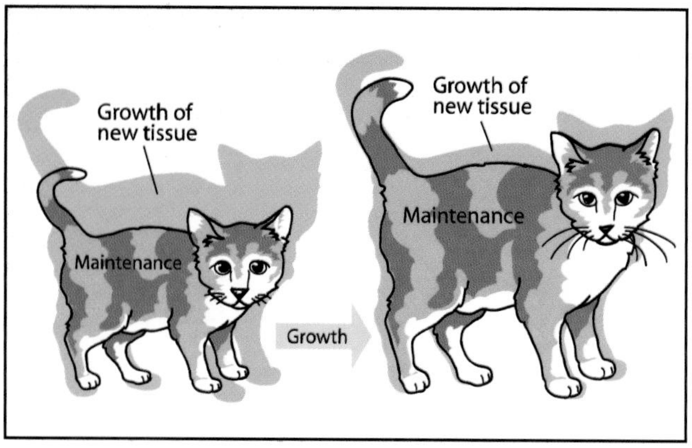

Figure 24-1. Representation of nutritional requirements of kittens. The nutritional needs of growing cats include maintenance requirements similar to those of adult cats (depicted here as the body of the cat) plus nutrients necessary for rapid tissue accretion (shaded area). The proportion of nutrient intake needed for maintenance vs. tissue accretion changes throughout growth as depicted here.

Table 24-1. Key nutritional factors for foods for growing kittens (postweaning to adult).*

Factors	Recommended food levels**
Energy density (kcal ME/g)	4.0-5.0
Energy density (kJ ME/g)	16.7-20.9
Protein (%)	35-50
Fat (%)	18-35
DHA (%)	≥0.004
Calcium (%)	0.8-1.6
Phosphorus (%)	0.6-1.4
Ca:P ratio	1:1-1.5:1
Potassium (%)	0.6-1.2
Average urinary pH***	6.2-6.5

Key: ME = metabolizable energy; DHA = docosahexaenoic acid.
*Concentrations presume an energy density of 4.0 kcal/g. Levels should be corrected for foods with higher energy densities. Adjustment is unnecessary for foods with lower energy densities.
**Dry matter basis.
***As determined in growing kittens.

neutering; therefore, the risk for obesity increases (Root, 1995; Flynn et al, 1996; Scarlett et al, 1994). Neutering, however, is not the only risk factor for obesity. Practitioners have noted an alarming increase in the number of young cats with marked abdominal fat accumulation before neutering. An indoor lifestyle, high-fat foods, overfeeding and certain feeding practices (e.g., free-choice feeding) are additional risk factors for obesity (Scarlett et al, 1994). Obesity should be prevented at an early age because it significantly affects the health, longevity and quality of life of cats (Scarlett and Donoghue, 1997). Therefore, the risks for obesity should be determined as part of each cat's health evaluation at each veterinary visit.

Key Nutritional Factors

Key nutritional factors for postweaning, growing kittens are reviewed below and in **Table 24-1**.

Energy Density

Growing kittens have high energy requirements to meet the needs of a rapid growth rate, thermoregulation and maintenance. Kittens may grow at rates from 14 to 30 g/day during the rapid growth phase. Although ensuring optimal growth is desired, excessive energy intake may lead to obesity. Ten-week-old kittens have a daily energy requirement (DER) of approximately 200 kcal/kg body weight (837 kJ/kg body weight), which declines to adult levels (80 kcal/kg body weight [335 kJ/kg body weight]) at 10 months of age. Age-related changes in energy requirement have not been observed after 10 months in young cats (Root, 1995). Neutering reduces energy requirements by 24 to 33% regardless of the age at neutering (Root, 1995; Flynn et al, 1996). After neutering, limiting food intake and/or feeding a food with a lower energy density may be required to prevent excessive weight gain. The energy density of the food fed to rapidly growing kittens should be between 4.0 to 5.0 kcal metabolizable energy (ME)/g (16.7 to 20.9 kJ ME/g). A higher energy density allows smaller volumes of food intake to satisfy caloric needs. However, foods with energy densities at the lower end of this range should be fed to neutered kittens and those with a body condition score (BCS) of 4/5 or greater. The prevalence of obesity increases dramatically after one year of age. Over-nutrition is of greater concern than undernutrition in growing kittens.

Foods with an energy density of at least 4 kcal ME/g (16.7 kJ ME/g) dry matter (DM) or greater are likely to have above average digestibility. The mean apparent digestibility of several nutrients was found to be lower in younger kittens but increased with age. Fat digestibility increased until kittens were 24 weeks of age (Harper and Turner, 2000). Bile salt-activated lipase is a component of queen's milk suggesting that it plays a role in facilitating fat digestion in nursing kittens (NRC, 2006). Besides the inherent issues of apparent digestibility in younger kittens, their small stomach capacity relative to their body size limits food intake in the face of relatively high-energy demands. Providing highly digestible foods maximizes use of the nutrients consumed.

Protein

The protein requirements of kittens reflect their essential amino acid requirements and minimal nitrogen needs. Protein also provides sulfur-containing amino acids, which are required in greater amounts in kittens than in other species (MacDonald et al, 1984). Carrying over from the nursing period, protein requirements are high at weaning then decrease gradually to adult levels as growth slows. Kittens fed purified foods meeting all essential amino acids at or above the requirement have minimum protein needs of 20% DM (MacDonald et al, 1984; Smalley et al, 1985). Protein biologic value and amino acid digestibility in practical cat foods are typically lower than in purified foods (NRC, 1986). The minimum recommended allowance for crude protein for commercial foods for growth of kittens after weaning is 22.5% (NRC, 2006). The Association of American Feed Control Officials (AAFCO) recommends a minimum crude protein level of 30% DM (2007). This same crude protein level resulted in growth rates of approximately 30 g body weight/day in kittens fed purified foods (Rogers et al, 1987). To provide sufficient sulfur-containing amino acids without additional supplementation, at least 19% of the food must come from animal protein (MacDonald et al, 1984). Thus, the recommended range of crude protein for practical foods for healthy kitten growth is 35 to 50% DM (**Table 24-1**). High-protein foods (56% DM) must contain the essential amino acid arginine at 1.5 times the requirement to maintain normal urea cycle function (Rogers et al, 1998).

In other species (swine and poultry), amino acid requirements as ratios to total energy intake are more important than protein content or protein calories. Eventually, protein and amino acid nutrition studies in cats and dogs will likely follow this approach.

Fat and Fatty Acids

Dietary fat serves three primary functions in growing kittens, it: 1) supplies essential fatty acids, 2) acts as a carrier for fat-soluble vitamins and 3) provides a concentrated source of energy in food. However, excessive fat and caloric intake may predispose young kittens to obesity. As kittens grow, body composition changes dramatically. In one study, fat comprised only 5.5% of body weight in eight-week-old kittens, increased to 14.6% of body weight by 18 weeks and was 24.3% by six months of age. This is the upper end of body fat for ideal body condition (Munday et al, 1994).

Kittens tolerate wide levels of dietary fat (NRC, 2006). When kittens are offered foods with differing levels of fat, they select foods with a fat content of 25% DM (Kane et al, 1981). True dietary fat requirements are much lower. The minimum recommended allowances for growth are 9% DM (AAFCO, 2007; NRC, 2006). However, optimal growth rates are achieved with higher fat intake. Unless excessive growth or weight gain is evident, feeding foods with 18 to 35% fat is preferred to enhance palatability, meet essential fatty acid needs and maintain the energy density of the food at or above 4.0 kcal ME/g (16.7 kJ ME/g). Overweight and neutered kittens may need foods with dietary fat levels well below this range to achieve ideal body condition (BCS 3/5) and/or they should be limit fed.

Kittens, like adult cats, require linoleic and arachidonic acid, and they also require fatty acids of the omega-3 (n-3) series (docosahexaenoic acid [DHA], 20:6n-3). Studies indicate DHA is essential for normal neural, retinal and auditory development in kittens (Pawlosky et al, 1997). Similar results have been found in other species (Pawlosky et al, 1997; Birch et al, 2002; Diau et al, 2003; Hoffman et al, 2003). The inclusion of fish oil as a source of DHA in foods for puppies improved trainability (Kelley et al, 2004). The need for DHA during growth in kittens may be even more important than in puppies considering the cat's reduced ability to convert shorter chain fatty acids to DHA. The minimum recommended allowance for DHA plus eicosapentaenoic acid (EPA) is 0.01% DM with EPA not exceeding 60% of the total (NRC, 2006). Thus, DHA needs to be at least 40% of the total DHA plus EPA, or 0.004% DM.

AAFCO recommendations for growth for linoleic acid and arachidonic acid are 0.5 and 0.02% DM, respectively (2007). The minimum recommended allowances are similar or the same: 0.55 and 0.02% DM, respectively (NRC, 2006). These levels will sustain adequate growth. The minimum recommended allowance for α-linolenic acid is 0.02% DM (NRC, 2006). Commercial cat foods that carry an "AAFCO approved" label statement should provide adequate amounts of these fatty acids.

Calcium and Phosphorus

Weaned kittens appear to be fairly insensitive to inverse calcium-phosphorus ratios (e.g., kittens have been fed foods with ratios as low as 0.38:1 with no deleterious effects) (Morris and Earle, 1996). The minimum requirement for dietary calcium in growing kittens is approximately 5 g/kg food (0.5% DM) (Morris and Earle, 1996). Thus, AAFCO minimum allowances for calcium (0.8% DM) and phosphorus (0.6% DM) (2007) and NRC minimum recommended allowances (0.8 and 0.72% [DM], respectively) are appropriate for postweaning kittens (2006). Unlike the situation with puppies, calcium excess in kittens is not associated with developmental orthopedic disease. However, very high concentrations of calcium significantly reduce magnesium availability (Howard et al, 1998). Dietary calcium concentrations of 2% resulted in a nearly twofold increase in the magnesium requirement of growing kittens. Providing calcium in amounts sufficient to meet the needs of growing kittens without impairing the availability of other nutrients is the basis for recommending ranges of 0.8 to 1.6% and 0.6 to 1.4% DM for calcium and phosphorus, respectively (**Table 24-1**). The calcium-phosphorus ratio should be between 1.1:1 to 1.5:1.

Calcium deficiency coupled with phosphorus excess occurs most commonly in kittens fed unsupplemented all-meat diets. Nutritional secondary hyperparathyroidism results in osteitis fibrosa and is manifested by limping, pain and reluctance to move. Kittens fed such foods should immediately be fed a commercial food that meets the recommended minimum requirements with a calcium-phosphorus ratio of 1.2:1 to 2:1. Additional supplementation of calcium is not recommended and may lead to hypercalcemia as a result of serum parathyroid hormone excess.

Potassium

The potassium requirement of kittens is highly dependent on the protein content of the food and the effect of the food on acid-base balance (Hills et al, 1982). Urinary potassium loss is markedly increased when kittens are fed high-protein, acidified foods. To avoid syndromes associated with hypokalemia, postweaning kittens should not be fed highly acidifying foods and potassium allowances should be between 0.6 to 1.2% of the DM intake. The minimum recommended allowance is 0.4% DM (NRC, 2006). Chloride levels of 0.1% DM also cause hypokalemia despite adequate potassium levels (Yu and Morris, 1998). Some foods intended for lifestage feeding target urinary pH levels more appropriate for adult cats. These foods

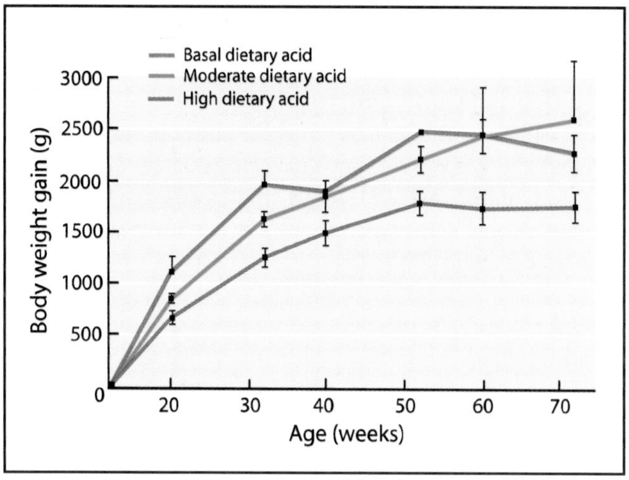

Figure 24-2. Effect of dietary acid load on body weight gain in kittens. Kittens fed highly acidifying foods grow more slowly and plateau at lower body weights than kittens fed more basic foods. (Adapted from Buffington CA, Rogers QR, Morris JG. Effects of age and food deprivation on urine pH of cats. Veterinary Clinical Nutrition 1994; 1: 12-17.)

Table 24-2. Feeding plan summary for growing kittens.

1. Using **Table 24-3** (or manufacturer's information), select a food with key nutritional factors closest to the target levels; remember urinary pH values are lower in kittens compared to those of adult cats; therefore, highly acidified foods should be avoided.
2. The selected food should also have been approved for kitten growth by a credible regulatory agency (e.g., AAFCO).
3. Determine the preferred feeding method. Generally, free-choice feeding is easiest but is best considered for kittens less than five months of age; free-choice feeding may predispose to overweight/obesity.
4. For food-restricted meal feeding, age, body condition and other assessment criteria will determine the DER. DER is calculated by multiplying resting energy requirement by a factor of 2.5 for kittens less than six months and by 2 for kittens between six months to adulthood. DER calculations should be used as guidelines, starting points and estimates for individual animals and not as absolute requirements. See **Table 24-4** for details about calculating DER for growing kittens.
5. If using food-restricted meal feeding, determine the quantity of food based on DER calculation (DER ÷ food energy density); divide between three to four feedings/day for younger kittens.
6. Regularly monitor body condition, weight gain and general health.

Key: DER = daily energy requirement, AAFCO = Association of American Feed Control Officials.

should be carefully assessed to ensure potassium is provided at appropriate levels.

Urinary pH
The urinary pH of growing kittens is lower than that of adult cats fed similar foods. Presumably, the lower pH is caused by hydrogen ions released during bone formation, which are excreted into urine. This increased response to dietary acidification continues until kittens are about 12 months old (**Figure 24-2**) (Buffington et al, 1994). Kittens fed highly acidifying foods (e.g., free-choice fed, urinary pH at or below 6.0) grow more slowly and plateau at lower body weights than kittens fed more basic foods. In addition to contributing to slow growth rates, feeding highly acidified foods results in poor bone mineralization in growing kittens (Buffington, 1988). To reduce the risk of acidification on bone mineralization and growth, kittens should not be fed foods that produce urinary pH values less than 6.2 when fed free choice. Because growing kittens have a reduced risk for developing struvite-mediated lower urinary tract disease (Bartges, 1996), an upper maximum for urinary pH is poorly defined. A urinary pH of 6.5 will reduce the risk of struvite precipitates in cats at risk for lower urinary tract disease and avoid over-acidification.

Other Nutritional Factor
Tyrosine is not an essential amino acid but is made from phenylalanine. Also, tyrosine spares about half of the needed phenylalanine. Therefore, it is appropriate to consider the amount of phenylalanine required as the sum of phenylalanine plus tyrosine. Although phenylalanine and tyrosine have not been shown to be the most limiting amino acids for growth in commercial foods, at least twice as much phenylalanine, or phenylalanine plus tyrosine, are required for maximal black hair color as for growth (Yu et al, 2001; Anderson et al, 2002). Phenylalanine and tyrosine are necessary for protein, thyroid hormone and catecholamine synthesis (NRC, 2006). The minimal recommended allowance for phenylalanine plus tyrosine in foods for kitten growth after weaning is 1.91% (DM) with 50% or more supplied by phenylalanine (NRC, 2006).

FEEDING PLAN

The feeding plan includes use of the best food and feeding method to ensure the goal of achieving a healthy adult. **Table 24-2** summarizes the feeding plan.

Assess and Select the Food
The two steps in assessing and selecting a food for healthy kitten growth include ensuring the nutrient profile is approved by a credible regulatory agency such as AAFCO and that the food's key nutritional factor profile closely fits the recommended levels for foods for healthy kitten growth (**Table 24-1**).

Proof that a food has AAFCO approval, or that of a similar regulatory agency, can be found on the label of commercial products. The label statement should note that the food is complete and balanced for kitten growth (Chapter 9). Such foods are often the same foods marketed for feeding reproducing queens and are sometimes referred to as growth/reproduction-type foods. Foods labeled for all lifestages should also have a nutrient profile to adequately support growth. But for optimal growth and long-term health, layering on the requirement of meeting the key nutritional factor profiles is an important part of the selection process.

The profile of key nutritional factors for the food being fed,

Table 24-3. Comparison of the key nutritional factors recommended for foods for healthy kitten growth to the key nutritional content of selected commercial foods.*

Dry foods	Energy density (kcal/cup)**	Energy density (kcal ME/g)	Protein (%)	Fat (%)	DHA (%)	Ca (%)	P (%)	Ca:P ratio	K (%)	Urinary pH
Recommended levels	**–**	**4.0-5.0**	**35-50**	**18-35**	**≥0.004**	**0.8-1.6**	**0.6-1.4**	**1:1-1.5:1**	**0.6-1.2**	**6.2-6.5**
Hill's Science Diet Kitten Healthy Development Original	510	4.5	42.3	26.1	0.24	1.28	1.13	1.1:1	0.9	6.4
Hill's Science Diet Kitten Indoor	510	4.5	42.2	26.1	0.24	1.28	1.14	1.1:1	0.9	6.4
Hill's Science Diet Nature's Best Chicken & Brown Rice Dinner Kitten	487	4.4	37.6	26.0	0.26	1.45	1.2	1.2:1	0.8	6.4
Iams Eukanuba Chicken Formula Kitten	469	4.5	40.0	25.7	na	1.29	1.07	1.2:1	0.97	na
Iams Kitten	470	5.0	37.8	24.6	na	1.15	0.94	1.2:1	0.86	na
Nutro Natural Choice Complete Care Kitten	463	4.4	40.7	24.2	0.077	1.32	1.21	1.1:1	0.71	na
Purina Kitten Chow	457	4.5	44.8	15.6	na	1.43	1.43	1:1	0.77	na
Purina ONE Healthy Kitten	512	4.8	45.5	21.1	na	1.33	1.20	1.1:1	0.98	na
Purina Pro Plan Kitten Chicken & Rice Formula	472	4.3	46.0	20.1	na	1.33	1.16	1.1:1	0.68	na
Royal Canin Babycat 34 Formula	531	4.8	37.4	27.5	na	1.29	1.12	1.1:1	0.67	na
Royal Canin Kitten 34 Formula	393	4.6	37.4	22.0	na	1.25	1.14	1.1:1	0.71	na
Moist foods	**Energy density (kcal/can)****	**Energy density (kcal ME/g)**	**Protein (%)**	**Fat (%)**	**DHA (%)**	**Ca (%)**	**P (%)**	**Ca:P ratio**	**K (%)**	**Urinary pH**
Recommended levels	**–**	**4.0-5.0**	**35-50**	**18-35**	**≥0.004**	**0.8-1.6**	**0.6-1.4**	**1:1-1.5:1**	**0.6-1.2**	**6.2-6.5**
Hill's Science Diet Kitten Healthy Development Liver & Chicken Entrée Minced	114/3 oz. 210/5.5 oz.	4.7	49.3	23.9	0.243	1.3	0.95	1.4:1	0.88	6.4
Hill's Science Diet Tender Chunks in Gravy Real Chicken Dinner Kitten	84/3 oz. (pouch)	4.3	47.8	22.6	0.087	1.17	1.09	1.1:1	1.04	6.3
Purina Pro Plan Kitten Chicken & Liver Entrée Classic	98/3 oz.	4.6	56.0	31.2	na	2.0	1.96	1:1	1.36	na

Key: ME = metabolizable energy, DHA = docosahexaenoic acid, Ca = calcium, P = phosphorus, K = potassium, na = not available from manufacturer.

*From manufacturers' published information or calculated from manufacturers' published as fed values; all values are on a dry matter basis unless otherwise stated.

**Energy density values are listed on an as fed basis and are useful for determining the amount to feed; cup = 8-oz. measuring cup. Energy density also reflects digestibility; foods with higher energy density are likely to have better digestibility than foods with lower energy density. To convert kcal to kJ, multiply kcal by 4.184.

or considered, should be compared to the recommended levels. **Table 24-3** provides this comparison for several commercial foods marketed for kitten growth. For foods not in this table, contact the manufacturer to obtain the food's key nutritional factor levels. This approach is usually necessary to obtain information about homemade foods. A more appropriate food should be selected if the current food does not adequately compare to the key nutritional factors listed in **Table 24-1**. It is better to change to a food formulated specifically for kittens than to try balancing an inappropriate food.

Both dry and moist foods are appropriate for weaned kittens. Dry foods are more energy dense per volume of food, which benefits small kittens with increased caloric needs. Moist foods tend to be more palatable and thus encourage food intake. Semi-moist foods that excessively acidify the urine (i.e., <6.0 pH units) should be avoided until skeletal growth is complete. Identification of health risks such as obesity and over-acidification necessitates a scrupulous review of foods provided for growth.

Treats are unnecessary but may be fed in small quantities (i.e., <10% of the daily caloric intake). Milk is commonly offered to kittens as a treat. Amounts offered should be limited because intestinal lactase levels decline shortly after weaning (**Box 24-1**) (Pawlosky et al, 1997). Fresh water should be provided daily and be available at all times.

Assess and Determine the Feeding Method

Feeding methods include the amount to feed and how the food is offered. Several feeding methods are appropriate for growing kittens. However, the overall feeding method should be tailored to the individual kitten's needs, the type of food being offered and the owner's preference.

Table 24-4. Daily energy requirements of growing kittens.

Age (months)	kcal/kg BW/day	kJ/kg BW/day
Birth	250	1,045
1	240	1,005
2	210	880
3	200	840
4*	175	730
5	145	610
6**	135	565
7	120	500
8	110	460
9***	100	420
10	95	400
11	90	375
12	85	355

Key: RER = resting energy requirement = $70(BW_{kg})^{0.75}$, BW = body weight.
*Up to 50% of adult BW (at about four months of age) or 3.0 x RER.
**Between 50 and 70% of adult BW (around six months of age) or 2.5 x RER.
***Between 70 and 100% of adult BW (around nine to 12 months of age) or 2 x RER.

Box 24-1. Feeding Cow's Milk to Growing Kittens.

Carbohydrates are not required in the food of growing kittens as long as an adequate supply of glucogenic amino acids is available. Nevertheless, cats can readily digest starch in cereal grains (i.e., >95% digestible). However, excessive feeding of poorly digestible carbohydrates may result in bloating, gas and diarrhea. These signs are often observed in kittens offered large quantities of cow's milk after weaning. The combination of high lactose levels with waning intestinal lactase levels results in carbohydrate overload.

To determine an amount to feed, the kitten's DER may be calculated based on the age-associated energy requirements listed in **Table 24-4**, divided by the caloric content of the food. The caloric content of many foods is not readily available; therefore, feeding guides on package labels and the manufacturers' literature are useful starting places. After an initial food amount is chosen, weight gain and body condition need to be regularly evaluated to provide a basis for tailoring the feeding amounts to individual cats. Young postweaning kittens should be evaluated weekly. Evaluations every two weeks are appropriate after kittens are about four months old. Owners can easily evaluate body weight and can be taught to determine body condition; however, a member of the veterinary health care team should confirm/reinforce the owner's findings during vaccination and wellness visits.

Free-choice feeding is often preferred because it reduces the risk of underfeeding and the marked gastric distention that sometimes accompanies rapid food consumption when food-restricted meal feeding regimens are used. The feeding frequency should be three to four times daily for meal-fed kittens less than six months of age. This frequency ensures sufficient food intake to meet the high nutritional demands of kittens without encouraging engorgement. By six months of age, most kittens will tolerate twice daily feeding. Free-choice feeding is preferred for kittens younger than five months.

If kittens are thriving on their current regimen, alterations in the feeding method are unnecessary. A more appropriate feeding method should be considered for kittens with poor growth rates and those with excess weight gain and obesity. Free-choice feeding methods should be used for underweight and slow-growing kittens. Providing unlimited food for free-choice intake is inappropriate for overweight and obese kittens. A defined food quantity should be measured then offered as meals or fed free choice until consumed. Neutering increases the risk for obesity; therefore, use caution when recommending free-choice feeding of high-fat foods to neutered kittens.

Young kittens should be fed in shallow pans to facilitate access to food. Food should be offered at room temperature; however, moist foods should not be left out for prolonged periods at room temperature because they may spoil (Chapter 11).

REASSESSMENT

After weaning, kittens should be weighed monthly until they are four to five months old. Weighing is usually performed at the time of vaccinations or veterinary examinations. The growth rate varies from ideal by gender, breed and nutritional status; however, it can be evaluated using Figure 23-1 as a guide. Owners should continue to monitor daily food and water consumption. Determination of total intake is necessary only if inappetence, illness or poor growth rate is evident. Body condition scoring every one to two weeks is a better means to assess growth and adequacy of food intake. Results of body condition assessment allow owners to monitor kitten growth and adjust food offerings as needed to maintain ideal body condition (BCS 2.5/5 to 3.5/5). Kittens provided proper nutrition are healthy and alert and have ideal body condition, steady weight gain and a clean, glossy coat. Normal stools are firm, well formed and medium to dark brown. The veterinarian should conduct a nutritional assessment at each visit, or approximately monthly from six to 16 weeks of age, and then annually. Instructions for nutritional modifications and dental care can be given at that time.

ACKNOWLEDGMENTS

The authors and editors acknowledge the contributions of Drs. Claudia A. Kirk and P. Jane Armstrong in the previous edition of Small Animal Clinical Nutrition.

REFERENCES

The references for **Chapter 24** can be found at www.markmorris.org.

CASE 24-1

Lumbar Pain in a Young Cat

M. Anne Hickman, DVM, PhD, Dipl. ACVN
Pfizer, Inc.
Groton, Connecticut, USA

Claudia A. Kirk, DVM, PhD, Dipl. ACVN and ACVIM (Internal Medicine)
College of Veterinary Medicine
University of Tennessee
Knoxville, Tennessee, USA

Patient Assessment

An eight-month-old castrated male domestic shorthair cat was examined for hind-limb stiffness, lethargy and a soft tissue mass in the lumbar region. The cat suffered a twisting fall one month earlier. It was subsequently stiff and lethargic and had some lumbar pain. An examination at that time revealed no significant findings. Treatment included exercise restriction, antibiotics (cefadroxil) and oral glucocorticoids (dexamethasone). No improvement occurred over the next month; therefore, the cat was presented for a second opinion.

Physical examination revealed a 3.2-kg cat with good body condition (body condition score [BCS] 3/5). The cat was stiff in the rear legs, had an arched back and a soft tissue swelling in the thoracolumbar region that was very sensitive to palpation. Neurologic evaluation was unremarkable. No other abnormalities were noted.

Results of a complete blood count were normal except for moderate Heinz body formation on red blood cells. Serum biochemistry analyses were within normal limits. Urinalysis results were normal. Radiographs of the spine revealed diffuse osteopenia, increased opacity over the caudal aspect of L_1 and a mild subluxation between L_1 and L_2. Ultrasonographic examination of the lumbar region and abdomen was unremarkable.

Assess the Food and Feeding Method

The cat was fed ground sirloin and beef and veal baby foods. These foods were offered in several meals throughout the day. No commercial foods were offered.

Questions

1. What is the approximate calcium-phosphorus ratio of this diet?
2. What is the tentative diagnosis for this patient?
3. What caused the Heinz body formation in this cat?
4. Outline a feeding plan, including an appropriate food and feeding method.

Answers and Discussion

1. This cat's diet consists of all-meat ingredients (beef and veal). In general, meat is relatively high in phosphorus and low in calcium, which gives an inverse calcium-phosphorus ratio, approximately 1:20.
2. A diagnosis of secondary nutritional hyperparathyroidism is likely based on the dietary history and generalized skeletal osteopenia. The clinical signs of thoracolumbar swelling and pain are probably related to a compression fracture of L_1 and L_1-L_2 subluxation that occurred during the fall. The osteopenia probably contributed to the injury.
3. Heinz body formation is caused by oxidative denaturation of hemoglobin in erythrocytes. In cats, the unusual metabolism and unique hemoglobin structure of erythrocytes increase their sensitivity to oxidant injury. Heinz bodies usually appear within 24 hours of exposure of erythrocytes to an intoxicant. Affected erythrocytes undergo hemolysis or are removed within several days. Mild to severe anemia may result. Causes of Heinz body formation include ingestion of onions, acetaminophen, phenacetin, phenazopyridine, methylene blue, D,L-methionine, propylene glycol, benzocaine, zinc toxicosis, excessive vitamin K_3, diabetes mellitus and other systemic diseases. Onion powder used in human baby foods has been implicated in excessive Heinz body formation in cats. This is the most likely cause in this patient because it was regularly fed two different baby foods.
4. The diet should be changed to a balanced commercial or homemade cat food. Homemade food recipes should have an obvious source of calcium such as dicalcium phosphate, bone meal or calcium carbonate. Changing the cat's food from an all-meat diet to a balanced food may be difficult. The new food should be introduced gradually over several weeks. If necessary, a nutritionist can be contacted to formulate a homemade food to include the cooked sirloin the cat is currently eating. If food refusal becomes a major problem, hand feeding or assisted feeding with a feeding tube may be necessary. Caloric requirements should be calculated to reflect a young cat that will probably be confined with limited opportunities for exercise.

Progress Notes

Cerebrospinal fluid was collected and analyzed to rule out central nervous system infection as a cause of back pain. Results were normal. Blood samples were collected to measure parathyroid hormone (PTH) concentrations. PTH concentrations were elevated, confirming a diagnosis of hyperparathyroidism.

A balanced commercial moist cat food formulated for growing cats was chosen (Science Diet Feline Growth[a]). The cat's daily energy requirement (DER) was estimated to be 1.4 x resting energy requirement because the cat was still maturing and would be strictly confined. DER for a 3.2-kg cat = 166 kcal (695 kJ) x 1.4 = 232 kcal (971 kJ) or one-half of a 5.5-oz. can twice daily. Increasing amounts of food were mixed with cooked ground sirloin for several weeks. Within three weeks, the cat was eating only the commercial moist food. The food was warmed to body temperature in a microwave oven and offered in several meals throughout the day to encourage acceptance.

Exercise was severely restricted. The owners were instructed to confine the cat to a small kennel or room to prevent jumping. The owners were also advised that the cat should be reassessed monthly. The reassessment should include a dietary history, physical examination and radiographs to monitor bone density. By 12 months of age, the cat's bone density should return to normal and the cat can then be fed a commercial or homemade food that meets adult maintenance requirements. At that time, the DER also could be increased to reflect normal activity levels.

Endnote

a. Hill's Pet Nutrition, Inc., Topeka, KS, USA. This food is currently available as Science Diet Kitten Original.

Bibliography

Cook JL, Gross MM. What is your diagnosis? Generalized loss of cortical bone density and a displaced compression fracture of 10th thoracic vertebra. Journal of the American Veterinary Medical Association 1996; 208: 1019-1020.

Johnson KA, Watson ADJ, Page RL. Skeletal diseases. In: Ettinger SJ, Feldman EC, eds. Textbook of Veterinary Internal Medicine, 4th ed. Philadelphia, PA: WB Saunders Co, 1995; 2077-2103.

Kaplan AJ. Onion powder in baby food may induce anemia in cats (Letter to the editor). Journal of the American Veterinary Medical Association 1995; 207: 1405.

Morris JG, Earle KE. Vitamin D and calcium requirements of kittens. Veterinary Clinical Nutrition 1996; 3: 93-96.

Robertson JE, Christopher MM, Rogers QR. Heinz body formation in cats fed baby food containing onion powder. Journal of the American Veterinary Medical Association 1998; 212: 1260-1266.

Section 6

Assisted Feeding

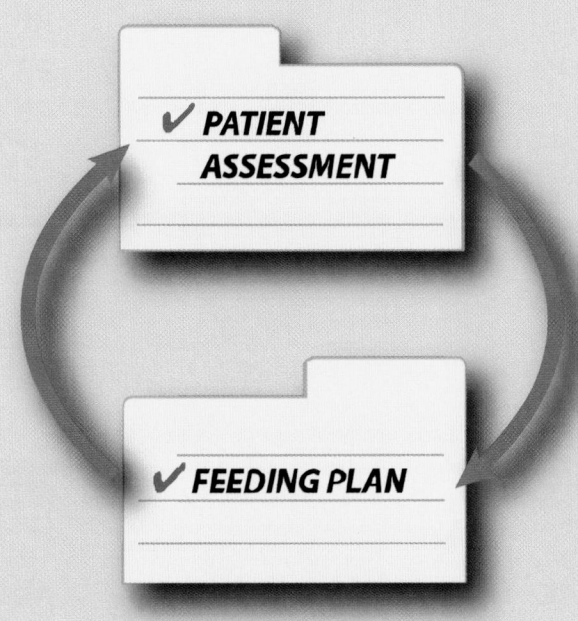

Chapter 25

Critical Care Nutrition and Enteral-Assisted Feeding

Korinn E. Saker

Rebecca L. Remillard

"Let food be your medicine and medicine be your food."
Hippocrates

CLINICAL IMPORTANCE

Patients of any age may become malnourished from inadequate nutrient intake. Malnutrition is any disorder with inadequate or unbalanced nutrition associated with either nutritional deficiencies or excesses. By most estimates, many hospitalized people and companion animals do not receive adequate nutrition. Hospitalized veterinary patients are more commonly malnourished due to decreased total food intake. The major consequences of malnutrition in all patients, but more prominently in sick or injured patients, are decreased immunocompetence, decreased tissue synthesis and repair and altered drug metabolism.

Immunocompetence

The reciprocal relationship between nutrition and immunity has been recognized for centuries. A malnourished patient is more susceptible to infections and a septic patient is more likely to be anorectic, which results in malnutrition. Nutrient imbalances suppress immune function, which increases the risk of disease; conversely, certain diseases alter some nutrient requirements (Semba et al, 1997; Burkholder and Swecker, 1990). Decreased protein-calorie intake is the most common cause of secondary immunodeficiency in people and can cause progressively poorer responses in several components of the immune system including significantly impaired cell-mediated responses, secretory IgA production, phagocytosis, complement function, antibody affinity and cytokine production (Shikora et al, 1994; Chandra, 1992; Redmond et al, 1991). Although fewer studies are available for review, similar alterations in the immune system are seen in pets with insufficient caloric intake (Freitag et al, 2000; Simon et al, 2000). Studies have shown that protein deficiencies that limit amino acid and nucleotide substrates for cell proliferation result in reduced numbers of circulating T-lymphocytes, helper cells and suppressor cells (Chandra and Kumari, 1994). Malnutrition also decreases immune function of existing cells through reduced complement secretions, less effective macrophage function and decreased killer cell activity (Saxena et al, 1984). Cytokine production and release are independently impaired in protein-calorie malnutrition and in several micronutrient (zinc, iron, pyridoxine, vitamin A, copper and selenium) deficiencies (Meydani, 1990; Chandra, 1992a).

Numbers of T_4 helper cells and T_8 cytotoxic suppressor cells in malnourished people return to normal quickly with refeeding (Chandra, 1983). Immunoglobulins and circulating antibodies are maintained at relatively low levels during malnutrition, but are highly responsive to appropriate refeeding stimuli. For example, investigators measured serum globulin concentrations in 12 healthy beagles before and 24 hours after small bowel resection. All dogs were fed via gastrostomy tube immediately after surgery. Six dogs received a monomeric food whereas the other six were fed an electrolyte solution. Twenty-four hours postoperatively, the dogs fed the monomeric food

Box 25-1. Regulation of Food Intake.

For many years it has been known that the hypothalamus is the center of appetite control. Although voluntary food intake can vary in amount and composition from day to day, over time, energy intake is matched to energy expenditure. Body weight is tightly conserved; therefore, food intake, meal frequency and size are highly regulated. The role of peripheral and central pathways involved in appetite control is being studied as obesity increases in human and pet populations.

Appetite is the desire for food and is often used synonymously with hunger. Satiety is the opposite of hunger and means that hunger has been satisfied. The body is normally in a state of hunger, which is intermittently relieved by eating. Hunger and satiety centers are found in the brain. The lateral hypothalamus contains the hunger center; stimulation of this area causes an animal to eat voraciously. The ventromedial hypothalamus contains the satiety center. Stimulation of this area causes complete satiety. Many neuroendocrine and metabolic factors affect these centers and therefore contribute to appetite control.

Short- and long-term input from the periphery including nutrients, gut vagal nerves, sensory spinal nerves, gut peptides and gut hormones act on the arcuate nucleus of the hypothalamus. The peptide, ghrelin, released from the stomach, is the "hormone of hunger." Ghrelin is released in response to gut nutrients rather than gastric distention. Peptide YY (PYY) is an appetite depressant. It affects gut motility centrally, acting as an "ileal brake." Neural control of PYY is demonstrated by its release shortly after food intake before nutrients reach the small intestine and colon, the site of highest PYY concentrations. Glucagon like peptide-1 (GLP-1) acts on the pancreas to cause release of insulin and inhibit food intake. Its rapid enzymatic breakdown has limited its potential use in Type II diabetics. Other gut peptides, pancreatic peptide (PP) and oxyntomodulin (oxm) play roles in decreasing food intake and homeostatic regulation of body weight. The peripheral appetite depressant, cholecystokinin (CCK) is secreted in the duodenum in response to fat and protein ingestion. CCK, gut vagal nerves and sensory spinal nerves travel to the nucleus tractus solitarius (NTS) satiety center in the brainstem.

Insulin, released peripherally in proportion to body fat mass and blood glucose levels, acts directly on hypothalamic appetite centers. Another gut hormone, leptin, is released from adipocytes in direct relationship to body fat. Leptin decreases appetite and increases thermogenesis. Obese patients appear to be leptin resistant, which may impede their ability to regulate body weight.

Gut peptides (ghrelin, PYY, GLP-1, PP, oxm) and hormones (insulin and leptin) act directly on the arcuate nucleus of the hypothalamus. The arcuate nucleus has two populations of neurons. The orexigenic neurons release two neuropeptides, neuropeptide Y (NPY) and agouti-related peptide (AgRP), which stimulate feeding and promote obesity. The anorexigenic neuron center acts as an appetite inhibitor with the neuropeptides alpha-MSH and cocaine and amphetamine-regulated transcript (CART).

These neuron centers of the arcuate nucleus project to the paraventricular nucleus of the hypothalamus. The paraventricular nucleus receives direct input from other peripheral signals. Peripheral CCK, nutrients, vagal and sensory spinal signals travel to the NTS, which then acts directly on the paraventricular nucleus.

Central signals to the paraventricular nucleus include the appetite stimulator, melanin-concentrating hormone (MCH) of the lateral hypothalamus. The cortex and limbic system integrate appetite signals with the paraventricular nucleus. The paraventricular nucleus then coordinates both central and peripheral signaling for feeding, energy metabolism, sympathetic nervous system activity and the endocrine axis.

In addition, the special senses of taste and smell are involved in the regulation of food intake. Taste is mediated through taste buds and free nerve endings. Taste bud cells are constantly renewed by dividing epithelial cells surrounding the taste buds. Taste buds are located on the tongue, soft palate, pharynx, larynx, epiglottis, cranial esophagus and even on the lips and cheeks of some species. Gustatory information received from taste buds is projected by cranial nerves to several areas of the brain including the lateral hypothalamus. Olfaction occurs via axons of bipolar neurons that course through the small holes of the cribriform plate of the ethmoid bone and form connections in the olfactory bulb. As with taste, there are olfactory projections to the hypothalamus.

Donna Raditic, DVM
Angell Animal Medical Center
Boston, MA, USA

The Bibliography for **Box 25-1** can be found at www.markmorris.org.

synthesized more than twice the amount of globulin (12 g) than those dogs fed the electrolyte solution (5.3 g) (Moss, 1978). Other cell populations and specific cell functions are likewise quickly responsive to daily nutrient intake. Cats fed 25% of their resting energy requirement (RER) for seven days had significantly decreased total white blood cell (WBC) count, lymphocytes and monocytes; major histocompatibility complex (MHC) class II expression; phagocytic activity; lymphocyte proliferative capacity and delayed-type hypersensitivity response by Day 4. These alterations were reversed by Day 4 of refeeding to meet RER (Freitag et al, 2000; Simon et al, 2000). The immune system depends on and is responsive to adequate nutrition.

Tissue Synthesis and Repair

Tissue synthesis and wound healing are a function of local and whole body nutritional status (Crane, 1989). On the cellular level, amino acids and carbohydrates are needed for collagen and ground substance synthesis. Fibroblasts require energy to synthesize the RNA, DNA and ATP necessary for protein anabolism. Migration of fibroblasts and epithelial and endothelial cells also requires energy. On the organ level, the liver has energy and protein needs specifically for synthesis of fibronectin, complement and glucose. The bone marrow requires nutrients for production of platelets, red blood cells (RBC) and leukocytes. Transportation of these necessary components and oxygen to wound sites requires the muscular activities of respiration and cardiac work. Tissue trauma and healing alter the normal cycle of protein turnover (synthesis and degradation) in the body. In rats, the rates of protein synthesis and degradation increased after trauma (Stein et al, 1976). Studies in perioperatively fed people indicate a 91% increase in protein synthesis with only a 10% increase in protein degradation (net synthesis) (Kien et al, 1978). Conversely, perioperatively fasted people had only a 50% increase in protein synthesis with a 79% increase in protein degradation (net loss) (Birkham et al, 1980). Therefore, proper nutrition on the cellular level depends on whole body nutrition for net tissue synthesis and wound healing.

Drug Metabolism

Cellular activities depend on and are regulated by the coordinated actions of peptides, lipids, vitamins and minerals as substrates, enzymes, coenzymes and cofactors of intermediary metabolism. Therefore, all nutrients are essential for the maintenance of normal cellular structure and function (Parke, 1991). Nutrient deprivation alters the normal metabolic synergy responsible for ion gradients, membrane potentials, production of high-energy phosphate compounds and antioxidant defenses. Enteral and parenteral nutritional support with products containing little or no lipid decreases hepatic cytochrome P-450 concentration and activity, which significantly decreases specific drug clearances (Knodell, 1990; Raftogianis et al, 1995). Protein-calorie deficiencies may result in decreased: 1) hepatic biotransformation of certain antibiotics, 2) concentrations of serum proteins that bind and transport drugs throughout the body and 3) renal blood flow, which decreases the rate of drug elimination and increases the possibility of drug overdose (Walter-Sack and Klotz, 1996). Therefore, protein-calorie malnutrition may alter the expected metabolism of certain drugs, which may increase or decrease their therapeutic effect even when given at recommended dosages (Pelissier et al, 1993; Krishnaswamy, 1989) (Chapter 69). Patients receiving sufficient calories and protein are expected to have better, or near normal, drug distribution, metabolism and elimination than patients with protein-calorie malnutrition.

Inadequate nutritional support can suppress the immune response, cause organ dysfunction, impair wound healing, result in muscle wasting and weakness, increase the incidence of acquired infections and increase mortality. As an example, a 50% decrease in jejunal mucosal mass and thickness normally occurs after burn injuries when no enteral feedings are given for 24 hours. Early feeding prevents this mucosal atrophy. Malnutrition in people, even imprecisely defined, is associated with prolonged ventilatory dependence and increased complication rates with longer hospital stays and higher costs (Remillard and Martin, 1990). Similarly in veterinary patients, malnutrition is thought to increase morbidity and mortality. Diseased and debilitated patients require nutrients daily to maintain optimal immune function, tissue synthesis and repair and proper drug metabolism.

ANOREXIA, CACHEXIA AND ACCOMMODATION

Normally, satiety occurs after a patient's caloric needs have been met. Conversely, anorexia is the loss of desire for food before caloric needs have been satisfied (**Box 25-1**). Anorexia may be partial or complete. The anorexia is complete if a patient consumes no food for a period beyond that considered normal. The anorexia is partial if the patient consumes some food but less than that considered a normal daily intake.

The flavor of food results from chemical stimulation of taste buds and free nerve endings in the nose, mouth and throat. "Taste" disorders often result from abnormalities in olfaction. Disorders of taste or smell can impair appetite and occur because of:

- Old age. The number of taste buds declines with age. Olfaction is usually the first sensory system to show an aging effect.
- Damage to neural connections due to surgery or traumatic head injury. Accidental blows to the head can shear the fine olfactory nerves that pass through the cribriform plate and are a common cause of anosmia (inability to smell) in people.
- Impaired renewal of taste buds and olfactory epithelium. Decreased chemosensory cell turnover is consistent with the decreased cell renewal reported to occur in the small intestinal epithelium as a result of food deprivation, radiation therapy, uremia, vitamin B_{12} deficiency and therapy with methotrexate. Many endocrine factors also depress cell proliferation. These factors and many conditions and drugs (**Table 25-1**) probably impair regeneration and function of taste buds and olfactory cells in the same manner that they impair regeneration of intestinal epithelium. The turnover time of taste buds and olfactory cells is about 10 days. Therefore, a return to normal taste function after mitosis is interrupted requires at least 10 days and usually longer.
- Modification of receptor cells as a result of a chronic change in local environment (e.g., an alteration in saliva or the fluids bathing the olfactory mucosa) due to drugs or metabolic agents such as urea.

Numerous medical problems including organic disease, inflammation, trauma and neoplasia can cause anorexia. In addition, pain, fear and other components of emotional stress inhibit the desire for food (Schiffman, 1983). If anorexia persists, depletion of body nutrient stores occurs. Nutritional depletion may also result from facial or oral injuries, or obstruction or dysfunction of the gastrointestinal (GI) tract, liver or pancreas so that the patient is incapable of ingesting, chewing, swallowing, digesting or absorbing food. In general, patients not eating for more than 48 hours or those consuming less than 50% of normal intake for more than three days should be of concern and noted as having a form of anorexia. Cats and dogs with a history of complete anorexia for three or more days or those with a history of partial anorexia for several weeks warrant further nutritional assessment.

Cachexia is a state of general illness, malnutrition and profound disability. For nearly 50 years, investigators and nutri-

Table 25-1. Disorders and drugs that affect taste and smell in people.*

Disorders		
Adrenocortical insufficiency	Cushing's syndrome	Nasal polyposis
Allergic rhinitis	Diabetes mellitus	Niacin deficiency
Bronchial asthma	Head trauma	Radiation therapy
Burns	Hepatic cirrhosis	Sinusitis
Cancer	Hypertension	Viral hepatitis (acute)
Chronic renal failure	Hypothyroidism	Zinc deficiency
Cobalamin deficiency	Influenza-like infections	

Drug classification	**Examples**
Amebicides	Metronidazole
Antiepileptic drugs	Phenytoin
Anesthetics (local)	Benzocaine, procaine hydrochloride, tetracaine hydrochloride
Antihistamines	Chlorpheniramine maleate
Antimicrobial agents	Amphotericin B, ampicillin, cephalosporins, chloramphenicol, gentamicin, griseofulvin, kanamycin, lincomycin, neomycin, nitrofurantoin, sulfonamides, streptomycin, tetracyclines
Antineoplastic agents	Doxorubicin, methotrexate, vincristine sulfate
Antirheumatic, analgesic, antipyretic, antiinflammatory, immunosuppressive agents	Allopurinol, azathioprine, colchicine, levamisole, D-penicillamine, phenylbutazone
Antithyroid agents	Propylthiouracil, thiouracil
Diuretics and antihypertensive agents	Captopril, furosemide, thiazides
Opiates	Codeine, morphine
Sympathomimetic drugs	Amphetamines, ephedrine
Others	Digitalis glycosides, estrogens, iron sorbitex, oral antidiabetic agents, vitamin D

*Adapted from Schiffman SS. Taste and smell in disease (first of two parts). New England Journal of Medicine 1983; 308: 1275-1279. Schiffman SS. Taste and smell in disease (second of two parts). New England Journal of Medicine 1983; 308: 1337-1343.

tionists have recognized that cachexia and a resultant low body condition score (BCS) are associated with increased risk of complications in people (Windsor, 1993). Loss of skeletal and visceral proteins can have adverse anatomic and functional consequences in food-deprived patients. These adverse effects include anemia, reduced heart muscle mass and function, decreased pulmonary mechanical function and diminished respiratory drive, altered intestinal morphology and mildly impaired absorptive abilities (Biden and Taylor, 1983). Cachexia may affect dogs and cats with long-standing cancer, cardiac disease or renal disease (Chapters 30, 36 and 37, respectively). A state of metabolic "accommodation" that prolongs survival has been recognized in people with chronic diseases. A similar state of metabolic accommodation probably occurs in chronically ill dogs and cats.

Accommodation occurs when the energy equilibrium is reestablished at a constant but lower food intake and lean-tissue wasting is arrested before protein deficiency becomes fatal. Accommodation in people is successful when: 1) total lean-tissue depletion is less than that considered critical, 2) weight is low but stable and 3) albumin levels and total peripheral WBC counts are normal with an intact delayed cutaneous hypersensitivity response (Hoffer, 1994).

Accommodation with the exception of an intact delayed cutaneous hypersensitivity response accurately describes the condition of some chronically ill patients (i.e., those with chronic renal, hepatic or cardiac insufficiency). Some chronically ill, cachectic cats and dogs may be maintained at a less than optimal body weight and condition for some time, even though important organ function deficits are apparent. In these cases, metabolic rate has been down regulated and protein turnover has been altered to establish a fragile homeostasis. This homeostasis can be maintained until a new stress supervenes. Affected patients very often do not survive additional stresses such as trauma, surgery, infection or tumors, as might a previously healthy dog or cat.

Metabolic Changes Through Days of Food Deprivation

Simple Starvation

Simple starvation includes metabolic changes that occur in mammals, in the absence of disease, as days of food deprivation continue. The time course of metabolic changes and associated alterations in nutrient usage should guide how these hospitalized patients are fed. An understanding of the metabolic changes that take place (particularly in the liver) during starvation is essential to understanding metabolic alterations present during anorexia and disease states.

In the postprandial period of well-fed patients, exogenous dietary nutrients are used to meet immediate metabolic needs, thus sparing endogenous fuels stored as glycogen, adipose and muscle protein. After these needs are met, replenishment of glycogen reserves (in the liver, fat and muscle) as well as proteins catabolized since the last meal, takes place. Any excess energy in the form of carbohydrate, fat or protein is then converted to triglycerides for storage as fat in adipose, muscle and liver tissue. In the fed state when serum glucose is high, the liver becomes a net importer of glucose, trapping it in hepatocytes by phosphorylation via glucokinase. Glucokinase is an inducible hepatic enzyme whose maximal enzymatic activity (Km = 180 mg/dl) for glucose is reached with the help of insulin, at high blood glucose concentrations (Engelking and Anwer, 1992).

Patients undergoing food deprivation display almost complete reversal of the metabolic processes described for the well-fed patient. Due to the lack of exogenous dietary sources, endogenous sources become the primary fuel for meeting immediate metabolic needs. Glycogen stores, instead of being replenished, become exhausted as the initial energy source. Then in order to preserve vital functions as long as possible, patients use different proportions of stored body fat and protein to maintain blood glucose concentrations. Which fuel or mixture of fuels the patient uses depends on the length of time the patient was food deprived and the quantity of each of the fuel stores available to the patient (**Figure 25-1**). The adaptation from fed to starved state is one in which fuel use by the patient shifts from primarily a mixture of fuels to one in which the primary fuel is fatty acids.

Carbohydrate metabolism is profoundly altered during the first week of starvation. During the first few days, omnivores (i.e., dogs) maintain blood glucose levels through glycogenolysis and gluconeogenesis. In simple, uncomplicated starvation of mammals, a decrease in blood glucose below 120 mg/dl decreases activity of hepatic glucokinase. This triggers hepatic glycogenolysis during which the liver becomes a net exporter of glucose to preserve serum glucose levels (**Figure 25-2**). This is observed after four to five hours of fasting and will only maintain blood glucose levels for another 12 to 28 hours (Cahill and Owen, 1968). Thereafter, gluconeogenesis must maintain blood glucose concentrations because hepatic glycogen stores will have been depleted. In contrast, carnivores (i.e., cats) must rely solely on gluconeogenesis, beginning intraprandially for maintenance of blood glucose levels because of their decreased hepatic glycogen reserves. This decreased reserve is due in part to lower glycogen synthase and glucokinase concentrations (**Table 25-2**).

Gluconeogenesis is initiated by glucagon and later glucocorticoids as serum glucose levels decrease (**Figure 25-3**). This process is carried out predominately in the liver and kidneys using substrates (glycerol, lactate and glucogenic amino acids) resulting from the catabolism of adipose and muscle tissue. Adipose tissue supplies glycerol for glucose production and fatty acids for oxidation to supply energy. Muscle catabolism releases glucogenic amino acids, lactic acid and pyruvate for glucose production by the liver (Welborn and Moldawar, 1997). Once available in the circulation, extrahepatic tissues are able to trap glucose intracellulary due to the presence of hexokinase, the enzyme present in all mammalian cells. Hexokinase has a low Km (1 mg/dl) for glucose compared to glucokinase and it does not require insulin to be effective. Therefore, intracellular trapping of glucose via hexokinase activity can happen at very low blood glucose levels (Engelking and Anwer, 1992).

In an effort to conserve circulating glucose for glucose-dependent tissues, the liver releases ketone bodies as an alternate fuel for non-glucose dependent tissues. Ketones are oxidation products of long-chain fatty acids, which originate from triglycerides in adipose stores. Unlike fatty acids, which are water insoluble and must be carried in the blood by albumin, ketones are water soluble and thus have a very wide distribution within the body and are able to diffuse across cell membranes. In this way they act to serve as a direct source of energy for vital organs such as the brain. Additionally the insoluble nature of fatty acids and their dependence on albumin limits their serum concentration. Thus the advantages of converting fatty acids to ketones are threefold: ketones are water soluble, not dependent on albumin for transport and can provide lipid fuel to cells at a much higher blood and interstitial fluid concentration. In

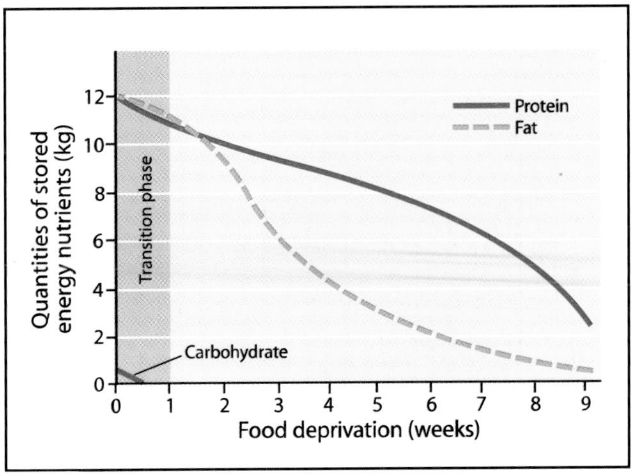

Figure 25-1. Disappearance of nutrient stores during starvation. (Adapted from Lewis LD, Morris ML Jr, Hand MS. Anorexia. In: Small Animal Clinical Nutrition III. Topeka, KS: Mark Morris Associates, 1987; 5-6.)

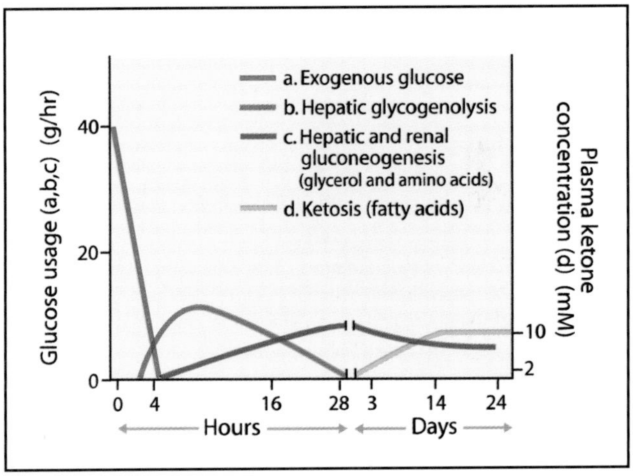

Figure 25-2. Graph of glucose use and source during starvation. (Adapted from Engelking LR, Anwer MS. Liver and biliary tract. In: Anderson NV, Sherding RG, Merritt AM, et al, eds. Veterinary Gastroenterology, 2nd ed. Philadelphia, PA: Lea & Febiger, 1992; 211-274.)

Table 25-2. Relative hepatic enzyme concentrations.

Enzymes	Dogs	Cats
Glycogen synthase	13*	1*
Glucokinase	55	5
Hexokinase	1.2	1

*Relative activity levels.

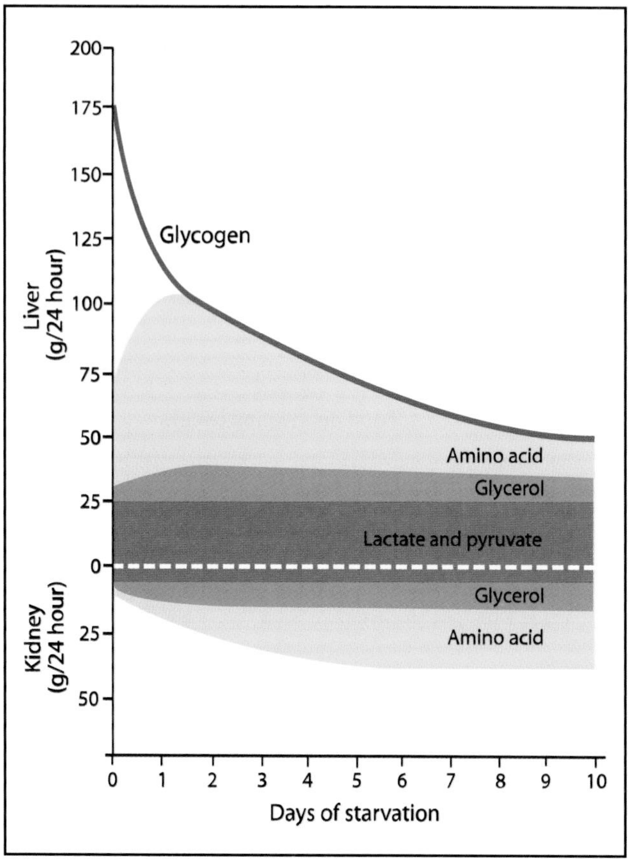

Figure 25-3. Graph of glucose production and source by the liver and kidneys. (Adapted from Owen OE, Felig P, Morgan AP, et al. Liver and kidney metabolism during starvation. Journal of Clinical Investigation 1969; 48: 574-583.)

mammals, serum ketones can reach 2 to 3 mM within a few days of starvation, with levels increasing to between 7 and 8 mM after one week. This is greater than the normal glucose concentration of 5 mM (Engelking and Anwer, 1992).

Increased serum ketones contribute to the adaptive response of the patient towards conservation of endogenous protein and glucose sparing for the non-adaptive, glucose-dependent tissues (erythrocytes and renal medullary cells). Enzymatic changes in peripheral tissues and brain caused by increased serum ketone concentrations promote ketone use and decrease the demand for glucose. Ketosis in food deprivation is an appropriate physiologic response and may not lead to severe ketoacidosis except in diabetic dogs and cats. Thus, ketone bodies serve as a readily diffusible lipid-source fuel for muscles, kidney cortex, peripheral nerves and the brain during periods of starvation. Ketone body production is usually maintained until adipose tissue is depleted.

In addition to adaptation from mixed fuels to fatty acids as a primary fuel source, as food deprivation continues metabolism begins to decrease. By the third day of food deprivation in all mammals, the basal metabolic rate decreases to promote conservation of resources for long-term survival. Decreases in blood glucose levels result in a decrease in serum insulin release. The conversion of thyroxine (T_4) to triiodothyronine (T_3) is insulin responsive and thus declines in the face of decreased insulin (Gavin and Moeller, 1983). T_3 levels begin to decrease within 24 hours of fasting and may be 40 to 50% lower as compared to values in fed animals by Day 3 of food deprivation (Vagenakis et al, 1975). Thus the net effect is a hypometabolic state, which becomes a beneficial adaptation allowing conservation of body functions until appropriate caloric intake resumes.

By Day 5 of food deprivation in all mammals, endocrine changes have mandated a metabolic shift from exogenous fuel usage in the fed state to endogenous fuel usage in the forms of fatty acids and ketone bodies. Decreased insulin levels trigger lipolysis in an effort to conserve protein stores and maintain blood glucose levels for glucose-dependent tissues. By undergoing fatty acid oxidation, amino acids are partially spared, which helps maintain muscle protein stores throughout starvation until the end stages. Body proteins are only partially spared because muscles will catabolize branched chain amino acids. Nitrogen is exported with pyruvate as alanine and to a lesser extent glutamine, which may be deaminated and transaminated for hepatic protein synthesis. Additionally, their ketoanalogs are used for hepatic and renal glucose synthesis (Felig et al, 1969).

The respiratory quotient (RQ) can provide an indication of which substrate(s) are undergoing catabolism. An RQ of 0.7 indicates fat catabolism, 0.8 indicates protein catabolism and 1.0 indicates that carbohydrates are being used as the primary fuel. Studies involving well-fed dogs measured an RQ of 0.94 at rest, indicating high carbohydrate use. The RQ of the same dogs after five to 15 days of starvation was 0.8 indicating a shift from primarily carbohydrate use to that of lipid and/or protein catabolism (Himwich and Rose, 1927). This is a testament to the importance of fat as a primary fuel source after three to five days of food deprivation.

Refeeding management of the food-deprived patient is aimed at matching the number of "no food" days with the pattern of fuel use (i.e., adaptation from using a mixture of fuels to primarily using fat). This is often in the patient's dietary history. As described, the different proportions of stored carbohydrate, fat and protein that is/are used to maintain blood glucose and provide an energy source mainly depends on the duration of food deprivation. To minimize the metabolic complications of refeeding, the refeeding formula should contain a complete balance of nutrients and should have a carbohydrate, fat and protein source similar to that which the liver has become adapted or is estimated to be using from body stores. Oftentimes this requires a feeding formula that is lower in carbohydrate and higher in fat and protein sources as compared to a maintenance-type food. As described, patients deprived of food are in a state of catabolism, which can often be reversed by refeeding if body protein losses have not exceeded 25 to 30%.

Disease State

In contrast to patients undergoing simple starvation, patients in disease states are often inappetent or anorectic due to their disease process. Although similar in their decreased dependence on glucose for fuel and increased propensity for lipolysis, patients in disease states have increased energy requirements and are more dependent on proteolysis than are patients that are simply food deprived. The hypermetabolic state that results from illness and anorexia is generated by general neuroendocrine responses and local mediators common to stressful stimuli. The specific hormonal and subsequent physiologic changes that occur in a stressed patient are unique to that disease condition, the time course of the disease process and other complicating diseases or conditions. The metabolic responses have best been characterized in conditions with a known acute onset such as trauma or infection (sepsis) (Cuthbertson, 1979). The response has been described as having an acute (ebb) phase followed by an adaptive (flow) phase (Popp and Brennan, 1983). These phases can vary in duration and intensity depending on the severity of the condition. Duration is usually shorter with trauma as compared to infection during which the acute phase remains until the infection has been eliminated.

The acute phase is characterized by catabolism and generally occurs within the first 24 to 72 hours. As mentioned, the hypermetabolic state that occurs results from a milieu of neuroendocrine and locally activated mediators stimulated by the sympathetic nervous system as part of the stress response. As in simple starvation, glucose use is somewhat reserved; however, part of this reservation is by consequence of increased cortisol levels perpetuating insulin resistance and hyperglycemia. Simultaneous sympathetic nervous system stimulation and release of catecholamines, cortisol, adrenocorticoids, glucagon, growth hormone and antidiuretic hormone induce metabolic and physiologic responses including:

- Insulin antagonism leading to insulin resistance.
- Hyperglycemia from glycogenolysis and gluconeogenesis, which provides an energy source for the "fight or flight" phenomenon.
- Increased lipolysis to provide fatty acids and glycerol for glucose and energy production.
- Increased proteolysis and net protein catabolism from albumin and skeletal muscle sources to supply gluconeogenic amino acids for glucose production and hepatic and immune cell proteins.
- Increased rate and depth of respiration and increased cardiac work to maintain perfusion to muscles and wound sites.

These responses are amplified in infection in which a toxic response results from invasive organisms and resorption of necrotic tissue. The amplification is caused by release of chemical mediators and lysosomal enzymes including histamine, kinins, prostaglandins, cytokines and serotonin. Interleukin-1 induces fever, which increases energy expenditure 10 to 13% per degree Celsius increase in body temperature. Endotoxins released from dying gram-negative bacteria trigger coagulation cascades that profoundly affect carbohydrate metabolism and cytokines stimulate production of hepatic acute-phase proteins. The net result is a hypermetabolic state with increased energy requirements that if not met, result in catabolism of endogenous fat and protein stores.

In the *acute phase*, glucose is the preferred fuel; however, muscles are insulin resistant and hyperglycemia is maintained for net immune and hepatic tissue anabolism. This is beneficial to the patient because it ensures an energy source in the face of hypoperfusion or poorly perfused organs (Daley and Bistrian, 1994). General feelings of malaise and anorexia signal the patient to reduce activity of skeletal muscle and signal the GI tract to conserve energy for essential tissue maintenance and repair. Although in the short-term, hyperglycemia appears to benefit the patient, maintaining this state is not conducive to recovery. Thus, the acute phase is characterized by decreased exogenous nutrients in the face of increased energy demands (hypermetabolic state) and a net negative energy balance. Breakdown or catabolism of protein and fat stores is necessary to address this imbalance between expenditure and intake.

This catabolic phase will continue until the neuroendocrine stimuli and cytokine mediators are removed. During severe head trauma, burns, multiple trauma and sepsis, lean tissue loss and overall body weight loss are rapid and unremitting in the absence of feeding. It is difficult to reverse the ongoing catabolism and achieve nitrogen balance in patients with these injuries and conditions. The goal in providing nutrition to these patients is to feed the catabolism with exogenous sources of protein and fat while sparing endogenous sources. The latter is critical because loss of 25 to 30% of body protein stores has been associated with reduced heart muscle mass and function, decreased pulmonary function, diminished respiratory drive, compromised immune function and therefore mortality (Matthews and Fong, 1993).

There is a definite turning point in which clinicians note a subjective improvement in their patients. This noted improvement is associated with the adaptive phase in which net anabolism occurs. The adaptive phase is characterized by increased metabolic rate, nitrogen gain and normal body temperature and may last for several days, weeks or years (Daley and Bistrian, 1994). The convalescent anabolic phase rebuilds damaged and catabolized lean tissue and therefore requires exogenous energy and protein sources. RQ values determined in resting postoperative and severely traumatized dogs were 0.76, indicating that fat was the preferred energy fuel, while dietary protein is used for anabolic processes (Walton et al, 1996).

In the catabolic and adaptive phases, fat and protein will more effectively address nutrient needs of the patient. Therefore, provision of dietary carbohydrates should be minimized, whereas fat and protein calories are maximized in refeeding formulas (provided there is no contraindication). Increased food carbohydrate fractions may lead to electrolyte disturbances and hyperglycemia, though the latter happens rarely in dogs. Cats, however, have very low glucokinase activity and cannot effectively transport glucose into hepatic cells given high intravenous and occasionally high enteral concentrations (**Table 25-2**). Subsequently, hyperglycemia is a commonly observed phenomenon during refeeding of cats. Additionally, specific disease states will affect the type and/or degree of metabolic and hormonal alterations in the patient, which subsequently influence substrate usage. In consideration of these factors, the recovery phase is patient dependent, which underscores the need for continual and consistent reassessment

Table 25-3. Examples of hospital feeding orders.

1. Offer 2 cans of product XX every 6 hr PO.
2. Give 100 ml of product YY gruel every 6 hr via PEG (percutaneous gastrostomy) tube.
3. Administer 300 ml of parenteral solution IV every 8 hr.

Sometimes the feeding orders should contain special conditions:

4. Begin feeding liquid product ZZ at 10 ml/hr via NG (nasogastric) tube. D/C (discontinue) all feeding if vomiting begins.
5. Administer 300 ml of parenteral solution IV every 8 hr. Check urine glucose and decrease rate to 150 ml every 8 hr if urine is positive. Recheck serum potassium daily and increase to 40 mEq/l if below normal.
6. Give 30 ml of product YY gruel every 6 hr by PEG. Increase meal volume fed by 10 ml every 24 hr. decrease volume by 50% if vomiting begins.

Table 25-4. Laboratory data of a dog after four months of starvation.

Tests	Results	Reference ranges
Complete blood cell count*		
RBC (x 10^6/mm^3)	2.73	4.62-8.3
HGB (g/dl)	6.5	11.6-20.6
HCT (%)	18.2	33.1-66.4
Reticulocyte (%)	0.0	0-3
WBC (x 10^3/mm^3)	3.4	4.8-16.2
Fibrinogen (mg/dl)	430	88-380
Serum biochemistry profile**		
Glucose (mg/dl)	172	65-110
AST (U/l)	79	9-43
ALT (U/l)	75	14-50
Alkaline phosphatase (U/l)	230	5-125
Total protein (g/dl)	4.0	4.6-7.0
Albumin (g/dl)	2.1	2.6-4.2
Calcium (mg/dl)	8.5	8.9-11.1
Phosphorus (mg/dl)	2.9	3.0-5.9
BUN (mg/dl)	28	7.0-25.0
Creatinine (mg/dl)	0.2	0.6-1.6
Urinalysis		
Specific gravity	1.052	1.015-1.045
pH	7.0	6.0-7.5
Ketones	Trace	-

Key: HGB = hemoglobin, HCT = hematocrit, AST = aspartate aminotransferase, ALT = alanine aminotransferase, BUN = blood urea nitrogen.
*MCV, MCH, MCHC, platelet numbers, WBC differential, blood lead and coagulation profile were normal.
**Serum K, Mg, Na, Cl and total bilirubin concentrations were normal.

of the patient to optimize the nutrition support plan.

PATIENT ASSESSMENT

Malnutrition can be recognized in patients through use of a nutritional assessment protocol. Nutritional assessment helps identify those patients that require assisted feeding to avoid or reduce nutrient deficiencies and the associated complications. Although inadequate nutrient intake may complicate many disorders, anorexia has been traditionally viewed as a secondary problem that will improve when the primary disease problem has resolved, i.e., "They'll eat when they feel better." However, it is better to be proactive and recognize the value of administering nutrients to veterinary patients and realize that, "They'll feel better sooner when they eat."

Diseased and debilitated patients (hospitalized or not) need to be assessed frequently, regardless of their age or lifestage. Assessment uses a number of parameters taken together to give an overall impression of whether a patient is experiencing malnutrition and requires specific nutritional intervention. Useful parameters to be assessed have been identified in large populations of people; however, no such parameters have been specifically formulated for dogs and cats. A veterinary nutritional assessment protocol should include history, physical examination (with special attention given to certain risk factors), body condition assessment (BCS) and laboratory tests (Buffington, 1994). Weight and dietary history, physical examination and body condition are relatively easy parameters to obtain. However, specific laboratory and immunologic tests that correlate well with nutritional status have not been identified. To date, very few clinical studies have been performed in veterinary patient populations to determine which parameters are applicable and their accuracy in determining nutritional status and predicting outcome (Michel, 1993).

History and Physical Examination

All patients should receive a physical examination including an accurate determination of body weight and an estimate of body condition. Weight changes must be viewed as a proportion or percentage of "normal, usual or optimal" weight within a certain time period as opposed to absolute changes in units (e.g., g or kg lost). Weight loss of more than 10% within a week is clinically significant and warrants further assessment. As a point of reference, a weight change of 10 to 15% within several days is most likely a hydration problem and should be corrected first with medical or fluid management. Pets on a designated weight-loss program can safely lose 1 to 4%, more typically 1 to 2%, of their body weight per week (Laflamme, 1993) (Chapter 27). A 10% (5 kg) weight loss within a week for a 50-kg dog is easily recognized as significant, but a similar percent weight loss over seven days for a 5-kg cat (i.e., 0.5 kg) is not easily recognized. This weight loss should be considered as serious as the same percentage weight loss in the dog. It is more difficult to accurately determine a 0.5-kg weight change than a 5-kg change; therefore, cats should be weighed on a scale that is accurate between 0 and 15 kg.

Body weight is an objective measurement, whereas body condition is a more subjective evaluation of the patient's tissue composition relative to its weight (i.e., fat, muscle and bone) (Chapter 1). Body condition scoring adds valuable information to body weight data. Decreasing fat stores indicate low energy intake and vice versa. Muscle wasting implies protein intake has been insufficient because skeletal muscle mass supports hepatic protein synthesis when dietary intake is inadequate. In one human study, using three independent clinicians' nutritional assessment of the same 64 patients, there was a 77% agreement among clinicians, and their clinical judgment of nutritional risk correlated well with objective data such as albumin, transferrin and cholesterol concentrations and weight loss history (Lupo et al, 1993).

Survival rates of people have been directly correlated with available muscle mass. Loss of more than 25 to 30% of body protein compromises the immune system and muscle strength, and death results from infection, pulmonary failure or both (Matthews and Fong, 1993). Decreased muscle mass may occur before serum protein levels drop below normal in chronic states because overall muscle wasting is less life threatening than decreased serum protein concentrations. Muscle atrophy due to protein malnutrition occurs bilaterally and should involve several muscle groups. Bedridden patients can develop muscle atrophy due to decreased use just as astronauts develop muscle atrophy of anti-gravity muscles because muscle size depends on exercise and gravity (Lane et al, 1993). Selected muscle groups may be atrophied in animals that have limited use of a limb. Therefore, lack of activity should be considered when evaluating the muscles of a patient, particularly one that is partially paralyzed or has a long-term illness.

Recording the food intake of hospitalized patients helps determine whether or not assisted feeding is necessary. In addition to having complete feeding orders, the medical record should also contain the time of day and amount of food actually consumed by the patient. Consumption can be simply recorded as some percentage of the food offered (e.g., 0%, 50%, 100%). If feeding orders are properly written and food consumption is recorded, it will be apparent after 24 hours of hospitalization whether or not the patient is consuming sufficient food to meet its RER, and whether assisted feeding is necessary. In a study of 276 hospitalized dogs, a positive-energy balance (>95% RER) was achieved in only 27% of 821 dog days recorded, whereas a negative-energy balance (<95% RER) was observed on the majority (73%) of the dog days. The primary reasons for the 601 negative-energy balance dog days were: 1) dogs refused to eat any or all of the food offered (43%) and 2) the attending veterinarian ordered nil per os (NPO) (34%) (Remillard et al, 1998). Currently, many hospitalized dogs do not consume their RER primarily because they refuse to eat the food offered to them. Also, feeding orders for hospitalized patients should be clear and complete. Properly written hospital feeding orders identify a specific food product with the amount, frequency and the route of intake specified, if not per os (**Table 25-3**). In the same study, fewer than 20% of approximately 1,000 written feeding orders were complete and accurate.

Assisted feeding should be considered for any patient with a suspected or documented food intake below the calculated daily RER for more than three days. Nutritional support should initially deliver sufficient amounts of a nutritionally balanced food to meet the RER of the patient at its current weight when the BCS is 3/5 or less. RER is primarily determined by total weight of metabolically active tissues such as skeletal and smooth muscle and visceral organs. BCS is primarily a measure of body fat stores. RER and BCS taken together are used to initially estimate the patient's daily caloric requirement. Animals with a BCS of 4/5 or 5/5 generally have the same muscle and organ mass as those with a BCS of 3/5; however, these animals have increased fat stores, which do not increase RER. It may be prudent, therefore, to calculate RER on an estimate of optimal weight in overweight patients to prevent overfeeding (Chapter 27). After several days, the food intake may be increased if warranted.

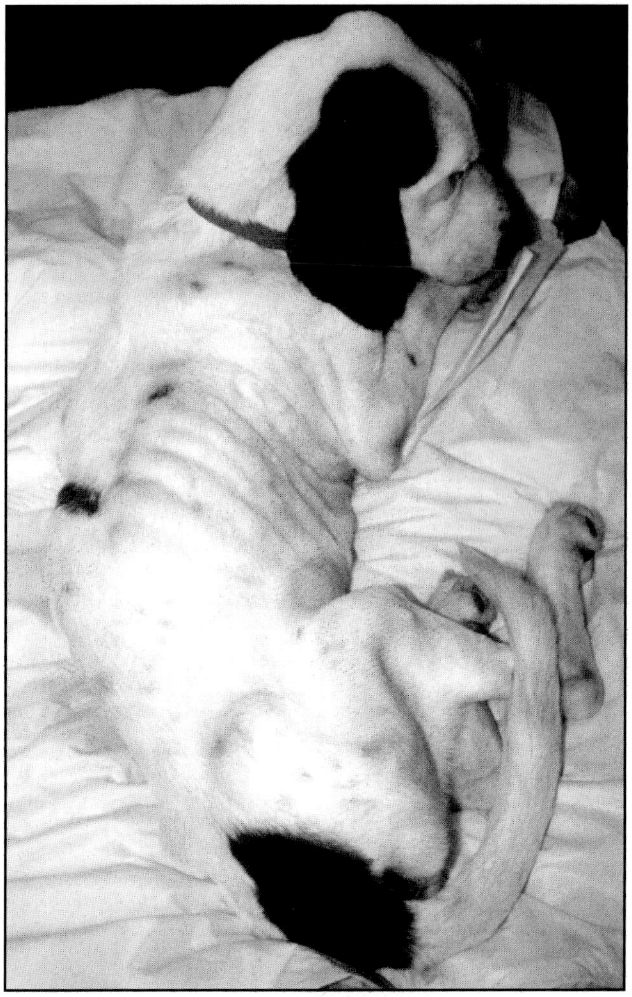

Figure 25-4. This dog experienced four months of starvation because its owner was unable to care for it due to a chronic terminal illness. **Table 25-4** presents laboratory data from this animal.

Laboratory Data and Other Clinical Information

The changes in most laboratory data due to malnutrition are indistinguishable from those occurring in some disease processes; however, malnutrition should be considered when examining the patient and reviewing the data (**Figure 25-4** and **Table 25-4**). RBC number, hemoglobin content, urea nitrogen, potassium, albumin and total protein concentrations, total WBC and lymphocyte count are useful in nutritional assessment of adequately hydrated patients. RBCs, hemoglobin, albumin and total protein have moderately long half-lives of one to eight weeks and are an indication of the energy and protein status of the patient over the preceding weeks to months. In one study, dogs fed a protein-deficient food (4% dry matter

Box 25-2. Future Laboratory Tests for Nutritional Assessment.

DELAYED-TYPE HYPERSENSITIVITY TESTING

The delayed-type hypersensitivity (DTH) skin test has been promoted as an inexpensive and simple bedside preoperative test for people with sepsis-related mortality risk, again relating the close tie between immunocompetence and patient outcome. Patients who did not have an appropriate skin reaction to a multi-antigen intradermal injection had a sepsis rate of 34% and a mortality rate of 38% vs. a 7% sepsis rate and 3% mortality rate for patients who reacted to the test injection. Several diseases and drugs, however, may alter the specificity of this test as an indicator of malnutrition.

Delayed-type intradermal hypersensitivity testing is not currently used in dogs and cats; however, some preliminary work in cats has shown promise. Cats infected with feline leukemia and feline immunodeficiency viruses had a DTH response less than that of normal cats. In another study, healthy cats receiving no food had a significantly reduced response to an intradermal injection of feline rhinotracheitis-calicivirus-panleukopenia antigens on Day 4 vs. when they received food daily.[a]

LYMPHOCYTE FUNCTION TESTING

Other promising indicators of nutritional status in the development stage for dogs and cats are specific immune function tests. A battery of immune function tests has been developed for use in cats, including: 1) immunophenotyping to identify relationships between immunosuppressor and helper cells, 2) measuring membrane calcium flux to evaluate membrane function, 3) immunophenotyping to identify cells expressing major histocompatibility class II surface antigen, 4) measuring phagocytic capabilities of monocytes and 5) assessing neutrophil activation. Preliminary data indicate differences in these lymphocyte function tests among normal-fed, normal-fasted and ill anorectic cats.[b]

ACUTE-PHASE PROTEIN TESTING

Laboratory tests available in other species, but not yet fully investigated as parameters of nutritional assessment in dogs and cats include serum prealbumin, transferrin, retinol-binding protein, fibronectin and cholesterol concentrations and total iron-binding capacity. A group of down-regulated proteins (prealbumin, transferrin, fibronectin and retinol-binding protein) and up-regulated proteins (ceruloplasmin, α-1-antitrypsin, α-1-acid glycoprotein and C-reactive protein) may prove useful in nutritional assessment. These proteins have relatively short half-lives (two hours to 10 days) in people, and have been suggested as indicators of the patient's energy and protein status. The half-lives of these proteins are unknown in cats and dogs but are assumed to be relatively short and related to the nutritional status of the patient.

GENE EXPRESSION TESTING

Gene expression of metabolic enzymes and hormones in the fed vs. fasted state can be differentiated. The means by which food affects genetic activity probably differs among responding organs but also depends on the duration of the fast and the composition of the refeeding food. Many nutritional studies using animals have demonstrated the expression of enzymatic genes using a three-day fast followed by refeeding specific dietary formulations. For example, this starvation-refeeding paradigm has demonstrated that fasting causes adaptive increases in the concentrations of many hepatic and renal enzymes that convert amino acids to precursors of glucose and fatty acids. Conversely, feeding a carbohydrate diet decreases the activity of those enzymes involved in gluconeogenesis and amino acid catabolism. Fasting and refeeding alter the structure of chromatin in regions near the structural genes involved in metabolic regulation. The alterations in chromatin also depend on the amount of carbohydrate, protein and fat in the refeeding food. The method of refeeding affects transcriptional regulation of certain genes. In the future, it should be possible to more accurately assess the metabolic state (i.e., nutritional status) of animal patients by measuring the activities of specific enzymes, cell receptors and gene signaling pathways and then to administer an appropriate refeeding formulation.

ENDNOTES

a. Saker KE, Virginia-Maryland Regional College of Veterinary Medicine, Blacksburg, VA, USA. Unpublished data. October 1997.
b. Saker KE, Remillard RL, Virginia-Maryland Regional College of Veterinary Medicine, Blacksburg, VA, USA, and Angell Memorial Animal Hospital, Boston, MA, USA. Unpublished data. January 1997.

The Bibliography for **Box 25-2** can be found at www.markmorris.org.

[DM] protein) with adequate caloric intake (19% DM fat) had below normal serum albumin and total protein levels but normal globulin concentrations after four weeks (Davenport et al, 1994). As an indicator of morbidity and mortality, serum albumin concentration is a reliable tool (Mendez et al, 2005). Numerous studies in people have demonstrated that a low serum albumin value correlates with complications during recovery. It is not recommended, however, to use serum albumin levels alone to determine nutritional status in critical care patients, because multiple factors can lead to hypoalbuminemia without malnutrition (Makhija and Baker, 2008). Establishment of an accurate and sensitive nutritional assessment protocol for veterinary patients, such as the Subjective Global Assessment used in people, would provide a valuable tool for veterinary practitioners.

Decreased serum protein levels may occur in more acute states of inadequate protein intake relative to a large protein loss (e.g., protein-losing enteropathies, open abdomen). In starving animals, loss of muscle mass decreases the body's protein reserves and, together with a slower rate of protein turnover in the remaining muscle, decreases the body's ability to synthesize proteins in response to metabolic needs (Tomkins et al, 1983). Such patients are poor surgical candidates because the body's protein reserves (muscle mass) have been catabolized to maintain the higher priority protein pools. If surgery can be safely postponed, several days of preoperative nutritional support in such patients is advisable. Only one to three days of adequate energy and protein intake may be required to up-regulate hepatic and muscle anabolic enzymes (Zeiderman et al, 1989).

Serum potassium and urea nitrogen concentrations may also be lower in anorectic patients because these variables are largely affected by food intake on a day-to-day basis. Urea nitrogen, however, tends to increase in endstage starvation because muscle is catabolized for energy when fat stores are depleted. Serum creatine kinase levels have also been evaluated as a possible marker in feline malnutrition and refeeding (Fascetti et al, 1997). Creatine kinase concentrations, however, will also increase and decrease in many disease states (Kitagawa et al, 1991). Several different types of tests that may lead to better nutritional assessment are currently under investigation (**Box 25-2**).

Risk Factors

Physiologic State

The physiologic status of the patient should be noted. This is relatively simple but rarely noted in the medical record. Knowing the gender, reproductive status, age and activity level of a patient aids in the nutritional evaluation. For example, a neutered bitch at less than optimal weight and body condition (BCS 2/5) is clearly very different from one currently lactating for eight puppies. Dietary recommendations should reflect the obvious difference in energy requirement. Neuter status can alter metabolic rate and energy needs (Root et al, 1996; Flynn et al, 1996). The metabolic processes of growth, gestation and lactation do not necessarily cease when a dog or cat becomes acutely ill. Several days of inadequate energy intake may be necessary before the hormonal milieu for growth, gestation or lactation is down regulated. Environmental temperature is usually a minor risk factor because most hospitalized dogs and cats are kept indoors.

History of Malnutrition

Patients fed homemade foods, table foods, vegetarian or single item foods are at greater risk for developing subclinical nutritional imbalances and warrant further nutritional assessment. Foods designed, formulated or prepared by owners may not be nutritionally complete, balanced or consistent (Chapter 10). These patients may not only have protein-calorie malnutrition, but are more likely to have several vitamin and mineral imbalances concurrently (e.g., calcium and certain micromineral deficiencies and/or subclinical vitamin A and D toxicoses).

Patients with a history of nausea, vomiting and diarrhea are at increased risk of malnutrition because nutritional intake probably has been less than optimal before admission. Nutrient intake may be voluntarily decreased with nausea, whereas vomiting and diarrhea can compromise nutrient digestion and absorption. Such clinical signs are also associated with additional losses of body protein.

Key Nutritional Factors

The primary focus of the key nutritional factor discussion is on enteral foods. However, some information regarding parenteral nutrition (Chapter 26) is included here and in the "Other Nutritional Factors" section that follows.

The Association of American Feed Control Officials (AAFCO) allowances (2008), and the "recommended allowances" listed in the National Research Council (NRC) Nutrient Requirements of Dogs and Cats (2006) are based on healthy animals, but are often referenced when estimating average nutrient requirements of critically ill dogs and cats to be fed enterally. This approach has been considered appropriate because most foods used in assisted feeding have nutrient digestibilities greater than those of typical pet foods (AAFCO, 2008) and, therefore, the actual available nutrient level provided by these foods would be greater than the referenced estimate. Assessment of the critical care patient may reveal nutritional factors that are not accounted for by AAFCO or the NRC; therefore, the practice of using these references for critically ill patients should be approached with caution. When estimating nutrient intakes for patients receiving parenteral nutrition, the NRC "minimal requirement" recommendations are probably better estimates than AAFCO allowances, because NRC minimum requirement recommendations were typically determined using synthetic foods, which better approximate 100% availability (2006). In addition to assuring that enteral foods intended for critically ill patients meet AAFCO (or some other credible regulatory agency) allowances, special emphasis is placed on the key nutritional factors and their recommended levels discussed below and summarized in **Table 25-5**.

Unlike the key nutritional factor recommendations for normal and clinical conditions described in the rest of this book, in critical care nutrition, nutrient requirements are conventionally expressed on an energy rather than on a DM basis (Chapter 1). This designation is primarily an extension of the units used in actual clinical metabolic trials. In addition, nutrient profiles of oral liquid products and parenteral solutions used in nutritional support/recovery are more commonly expressed on an energy rather than on a DM basis.

Fluid and Electrolyte Therapy

Initial support often involves management of fluid, electrolyte and acid-base disorders. The water requirements in ml for normal healthy animals approximate their daily energy requirement (DER) in kcal (i.e., 1 kcal [4.184 kJ] DER = 1 ml of water). Fresh, clean water should be available to patients at all times, unless the patient requires a period of nothing per os. Most patients in an intensive care unit (ICU) have venous catheters in place and receive crystalloid fluid therapy. These patients may have fluid restrictions or, conversely, may require diuresis. In these cases, the water or fluid administered will not be equal to the patient's DER. Daily maintenance fluid requirements are approximately 60 ml/kg body weight/day.

The patient's fluid and electrolyte (sodium, potassium, calcium, magnesium and phosphorus) balance should be near normal limits before assisted feeding is begun. Nutritional support

Table 25-5. Key nutritional factors for commercial liquid or blended foods for canine and feline patients requiring enteral nutrition (EN) support.

Factors	Recommended food levels
Water	Correct dehydration with parenteral fluid therapy before starting assisted feeding. Supply at 1 ml/kcal DER unless patient requires fluid restriction or diuresis. Typical daily maintenance fluid requirement is 60 ml/kg body weight.
Electrolytes	Major electrolyte disorders, acid-base abnormalities and blood glucose levels should be corrected before instituting EN support.
Osmolarity	250 (optimal) to 400 mOsm/liter.
Energy density	Supply 1 kcal/ml (as standard minimum). If the patient is not eating at least RER per os, provide nutritional support by assisted-feeding techniques to meet this requirement. By the fifth day of food deprivation or longer, patients should receive the majority (60 to 90%) of their calculated RER as lipid. If using a liquid or blended food, select a product that provides 1.0 to 2.0 kcal/ml (1.0 to 2.0 kcal/g), as fed.
Digestible carbohydrate	Dogs and cats: 2 to 4 g/100 kcal is a safe starting point for refeeding. Increase to 6 to 10 g/100 kcal 3 to 4 days into the refeeding process.
Protein	Dogs: Use a food that provides 5.0 to 12.0 g protein/100 kcal. Cats: Use a food that provides 7.5 to 12.0 g protein/100 kcal.
Arginine	≥146 mg arginine/100 kcal for dogs. ≥250 mg arginine/100 kcal for cats.
Glutamine	≥500 mg/100 kcal.
Fat	Provide a calorically dense food (5 to 7.5 g fat/100 kcal), except in cases in which high fat content is not tolerated. Provide a low-fat content food (2.0 to 3.5 g fat/100 kcal) if fat restriction required*

Key: DER = daily energy requirement, RER = resting energy requirement, to convert kcal to kJ, multiply kcal by 4.184.
*For example, patients with pancreatitis.

should not be initiated until the patient is hemodynamically stable because administering enteral or parenteral nutrition may further compromise the patient. Nutritional support should not be initiated as a "last ditch" effort in unstable patients. Major electrolyte disorders, acid-base abnormalities and blood glucose levels should be corrected before instituting enteral or parenteral nutritional support. It is also desirable to correct severe tachycardia, hypotension, colloid and volume deficits before starting assisted feeding (Minard and Kudsk, 1994). A practical goal is to begin nutritional assessment and support within 24 hours of hospitalization for the injury or illness (Burkholder, 1995).

Osmolarity

Osmolarity refers to or represents the number of solute particles per liter of solution. Serum concentrations greater than 310 mOsm/l in dogs and greater than 330 mOsm/l in cats are usually considered hyperosmolar (Tilley and Smith, 2004). During enteral nutritional support, the osmolarity of a food appears to have the most significant clinical impact on GI function and stool character (i.e., presence of diarrhea) (Pasulka and Crockett, 1994). In general, osmolarity of commercial pet foods is not reported. Instead digestibility of typical dry or moist foods is evaluated and, among other things, reflects the potential of a food to be tolerated by the GI tract. As digestibility increases, the osmolarity decreases, allowing for greater absorption of ingesta/digesta and minimizing the draw of excess water into the GI tract. Conversely, the osmolarity of liquid foods is reported for veterinary and human products. To optimize GI function, transit time and stool character, liquid foods of 250 to 400 mOsm/l are recommended.

Along with GI tolerance, another clinical concern affects critical care patients fed hyperosmolar foods. As described previously, these patients often exhibit insulin resistance associated with the stress response to illness and/or trauma. Liquid foods providing increased digestible (soluble) carbohydrate-derived calories are hyperosmolar (>400 mOsm/l). This promotes and perpetuates a hyperglycemic state, thus increasing the risk of the hyperglycemic hyperosmolar syndrome (Schaer, 2005). Specific concerns for delivery of hyperosmolar nutrient solutions intravenously are discussed in Chapter 26.

Energy and Energy Density

Knowing a patient's approximate caloric requirement is important because feeding more of any food than is necessary may cause metabolic complications. Overfeeding patients is possible through a feeding tube or with parenteral nutritional support. In people and several animal models, excessive carbohydrate intake was associated with hyperglycemia, hypercarbia, fatty liver, increased ventilatory drive and failure to wean from a ventilator (Deitel et al, 1983). Excessive fat administration has been associated with hyperlipidemia, hypoxia, increased rate of infection and higher postoperative mortality (Lowry and Brennan, 1979).

The proportion of fat and carbohydrate supplying calories to hospitalized patients should be similar to that which the liver is estimated to be using from body stores (**Figure 25-2**). Caloric density is important in both enteral and parenteral feedings when volume is limited. Enterally fed patients can be volume restricted by gastric or intestinal sensitivities. Parenterally fed patients can be fluid restricted due to cardiorespiratory diseases and functional disabilities. In general, most dogs and cats tolerate the volume of food or solutions that meet the patients' RER within easily tolerated volumes when the caloric density is approximately 1 kcal/ml.

In malnutrition, without disease or injury, decreased T_3 concentrations decrease the metabolic rate in an effort to conserve functional protein and energy stores. However, with an ongoing disease process or traumatic injury, the neuroendocrine responses to stress increase the metabolic rate above that found in simple starvation. Respiration calorimetry measurements of more than 3,000 people with a wide variety of diseases, specifically excluding hyperthyroidism, showed that 90% of the patients had energy requirements from 15% above to 15% below RER (Boothby and Sandiford, 1924). The energy expenditure in people with trauma peaks in three to four days and then subsides by Days 7 to 10 unless complicated by sepsis (Moore and Moore, 1994). Energy expenditure of people with other disease conditions probably follows a similar pattern with varying requirements above RER that may occur over time.

Hospitalized veterinary patients are assumed to be similar to ill people and their DER is very near their RER. Results of a few preliminary respiration calorimetry measurements in dogs with specific disease conditions suggested that most had requirements near RER (Walton et al, 1996; Ogilvie et al, 1996). Estimating the RER of hospitalized patients should be calculated by the equation RER = $70(BW_{kg})^{0.75}$ (Chapter 5). Most hospitalized veterinary patients should be fed at their calculated RER, realizing their actual energy requirement is likely to change over the course of the disease process and recovery. In human surgical patients, there was relatively little additional benefit to increasing intake after half of the caloric requirement of patients had been achieved (Elwyn et al, 1981). Therefore, initially feeding patients at RER, or at least 60% of RER, if 100% RER is not possible, is a rational and safe recommendation that decreases the probability of metabolic complications. Regular nutritional assessment of the patient is strongly recommended to adjust initial feeding rates.

There are exceptions when the caloric requirement will be greater than RER. Particular cases have energy requirements 1.3 to 2.1 x RER as determined by bedside respiration calorimetry in people (Moore and Moore, 1994). For example, according to indirect respiration calorimetry, people with severe closed-head and brain injury have energy requirements 40 to 60% above their calculated RER (Ott et al, 1990). Brain injury apparently increases oxygen consumption and acute-phase protein synthesis, which subsequently increase patients' caloric and protein requirements significantly above RER. Energy requirements of twice RER appear to be the upper limit in the most severe head injuries. Energy expenditure may be 30 to 50% above RER in patients with multisystem trauma. Severely burned patients also have energy and protein requirements 80 to 100% above RER, relative to the extent of skin damage and surface area exposed (Moore and Moore, 1994). The body loses heat, moisture and protein through wounds that have little or no epithelial covering. The patient's actual metabolic rate and resultant energy requirement are related to the degree of trauma, disease and/or complications and can only be approximated in a clinical setting.

The energy density of foods intended for patients requiring assisted feeding is often reported relative to the water or fluid content of the food. This is because an animal's energy requirement in kcal is approximately equal to its water requirement in ml and most critical care feeding is done in a liquid form. Thus, when patients are fed a sufficient amount of food to meet their energy requirements, they also meet their requirements for water. The recommended energy density of a food intended for assisted feeding (enteral or parenteral nutrition) is 1 to 2 kcal/ml.

Adjusting for Protein Calories

Calculating and adjusting for protein calories is of minor consequence when feeding at RER. If one assumes that part of the caloric intake is to be supplied by protein, then that fraction of protein intake that is used for energy vs. that which is used for protein synthesis must be estimated because the same amino acid cannot do both. Theoretically, if protein were supplied at 4 g/100 kcal to the patient but all of it was oxidized for energy with none going to synthesis, the protein could only account for 14% (4 g x 3.5 kcal/g) of the total caloric intake at best.

The most conservative and simplest method is to first provide the entire caloric need with fat and carbohydrate, and then meet the protein requirement entirely with amino acids, and not estimate the fraction of the protein that may be catabolized vs. anabolized. This method will not shortchange either the caloric or protein requirement because the fraction of amino acids actually used for energy will provide only a small amount (<15%) of additional calories. Essential amino acids provided by food are most efficiently used in protein synthesis and should not be used for energy, if at all possible. In summary, protein calories may be taken into account, however, the contribution is small and not significant.

Carbohydrate

Carbohydrate usage during the healthy fed state results in energy storage (glycogen) or energy production (ATP) in a very efficient manner. Conversely, use of this nutrient in refeeding scenarios during the unfed state is less efficient and can result in adverse metabolic and physiologic states, particularly in diseased or injured patients. Insulin resistance, presence of bacteria with infection, diminished production of digestive enzymes, altered GI absorptive capacity and alteration of gut microbiota complicate the recovery process and influence dietary carbohydrate tolerance. The two major clinical manifestations currently associated with carbohydrate intake include altered glucose control and diarrhea. Consequently, most foods formulated for recovery are low in carbohydrate content.

Tight glucose control in ICU patients has been regarded as beneficial because both hyperglycemia and hypoglycemia have detrimental effects on tissue function and clinical outcome, but recently this goal has been challenged (Elia and De Silva, 2008). Adverse effects of hyperglycemia that can predispose the patient to infection and delay recovery from illness include osmotic shifts, glucosuria, altered immune and endothelial cell function and promotion of free radicals. Conversely, hyperglycemia is a normal response to injury or stress. Glucose is needed for wound healing and inflammatory/immune cells that are involved in the metabolic response to injury, as well as other physiologic functions. A review of several human ICU-based studies indicated that narrowly controlled glucose did not significantly reduce hospital mortality (Elia and DeSilva, 2008). Circulating glucose is the major energy source for the brain. Although in most ICU patients, during the unfed state and during diabetic ketoacidosis, the brain can use ketones as an energy source. Once re-fed, the circulating insulin acts to suppress ketone body concentrations, which once again leaves glucose as the major energy source for the brain. Reducing the blood glucose concentration in some patients (lower than seen with stress/injury response) could have detrimental effects such as neuronal dysfunction, neuronal death or cerebral infarction (Gandhi et al, 2007). In contrast, partial or complete cessation of nutrition has been identified to be one of the major risk factors for developing hypoglycemia (Elia and De Silva, 2008). A low-carbohydrate food can amplify the onset of the hypoglycemic state, particularly in small-breed dogs.

Diarrhea appears to be a common problem in critically ill patients during refeeding. Malabsorption of dietary carbohydrate or fat, hyperosmolar formulas (generally high carbohydrate content), and feeding high volumes of enteral fluid have all been reported as causal factors (Mutlu et al, 2001). Complications of diarrhea include effects on hydration, acid/base status, mineral balance, contamination of wounds, decreased colonic fermentation and reduced butyric acid production (Thaklar et al, 2005; Kien et al, 1999). Traditional attempts to minimize the osmotic diarrhea, believed due to carbohydrate malabsorption, have focused on limiting the dietary carbohydrate intake (Kein et al, 2004). Small intestinal carbohydrate malabsorption (breath H_2) and colonic fermentation, stool volume and total enteral fluid volume were measured in burn patients receiving a high carbohydrate (Vivonex TEN) enteral food over a four-week period. Although all patients had diarrhea over several weeks, the lack of correlation of either carbohydrate intake or breath H_2 with stool volume suggested diarrhea was due to factors other than carbohydrate malabsorption (Thaklar et al, 2005). Notwithstanding, prevention and possibly treatment of osmotic diarrhea has been addressed by delivery of lower osmolarity nutrient solutions.

The value of dietary carbohydrate in maintaining an adequate and healthy population of gut microbiota cannot be overlooked. The intestinal microflora has been proposed as an environmental factor responsible for control of body weight and energy metabolism. Fermentation of non-digestible dietary fiber (insoluble carbohydrate) and resistant starches (oligosaccharides) along with numerous other mechanisms are linked to the health of gut microflora and energy metabolism. The major part of the microbiota is present in the colon where food products have escaped digestion, so the biologic functions controlled by this microflora seem to relate to effectiveness of bacteria to harvest energy that has been ingested, but not digested, by the patient. Human and rodent studies similarly conclude that microbiota can extract energy from non-digestible carbohydrate based on species (Turnbaugh et al, 2006; Ley et al, 2006), suggesting a benefit of providing adequate insoluble carbohydrate in the diet of critically ill patients. Additionally, fructooligosaccharides taken in the diet (5 to 20 g/day) improved mucosal barrier function, improved glucose tolerance and insulin homeostasis in human patients and rodents (Cani and Delzenne, 2007). Another study further highlights the value of resistant starches and dietary fiber as sources of short-chain fatty acids in critically ill/injured patients. Increased short-chain fatty acids, in particular butyrate, significantly enhanced colonic anastomosis healing and increased intestinal bursting pressure postoperatively in rats (Campos et al, 2008).

Perioperative carbohydrates minimize postoperative complications. Intracellular tight junctions maintain the intestinal epithelial barrier. Formation of dysfunctional tight junctions after stressful events such as surgery, contribute to postsurgical complications and delayed recovery (Bouritius et al, 2008). Adequate intestinal blood flow along with the mononuclear phagocytic system, located predominately in the liver, work in tandem to protect against bacterial translocation. Studies have indicated that glucose supplementation increases intestinal blood flow and that hepatic glycogen content contributes to increased survival rate by maintaining the liver system. Clinically these findings were substantiated when rats receiving a carbohydrate drink consisting of glucose, maltose and polysaccharides (12 g carbohydrate/100 ml) for six days before major abdominal surgery retained intestinal barrier function and were protected from translocation of bacteria to distant organs compared to cohorts not fed carbohydrates (Bouritius et al, 2008). Based on these studies, dietary carbohydrates maintain the mucosal barrier, hasten tissue healing, minimize complications and shorten hospital stays.

The dietary carbohydrate level in the initial refeeding of critically ill patients should be based on patient assessment and timing. Dampening the body's natural response of hyperglycemia to illness/stress may not be as beneficial as previously thought; carbohydrates in various forms have metabolic and physiologic value to patients. Conversely, promotion of a severe hyperglycemic state in these patients is contraindicated to recovery. On average, "recovery" type foods provide 2 to 4 g carbohydrate/100 kcal, with increased fat and/or protein content; this appears to be a safe starting point for refeeding. Then, consider transitioning to a higher carbohydrate food (6 to 10 g/100 kcal) and evaluating the insoluble carbohydrate (fiber) source three to four days into the refeeding process, based on patient reassessment.

Protein

Protein in the body is always in flux between synthesis and breakdown. Protein synthesis requires that amino acids be present within cells at the correct time and ratio so that a protein may be constructed successfully. Protein degradation involves the release of amino acids, and if the amino acid is deaminated, the ketoacid analog is converted to glucose or fat and the amino group enters the hepatic urea cycle and is ultimately excreted in the urine. Under most circumstances, about 15% of the RER comes from the oxidation of amino acids (Kinney, 1988). Providing a dietary protein source to patients in catabolic states spares endogenous skeletal muscle protein and supplies essential amino acids and amino groups for acute-phase proteins and the immune response. Excessive dietary protein should be avoided in patients with kidney or liver disease (Chapters 37 and 68). However, high dietary protein intakes are handled well by most canine and feline critical care patients to replace dietary carbohydrate when carbohydrates are not well tolerated.

Protein administration should complement nonprotein calories because amino acids will be oxidized for energy when a patient's total energy need has not been met first. Sufficient calories must be available from fat and/or glucose before ingested amino acids will be used for tissue synthesis and repair (Mallet, 1984). Excessive protein feeding requires energy expenditure to rid the body of excess nitrogen, which, in certain patients, may or may not be handled well by the liver (urea cycle) and kidneys and can result in hyperammonemia with accompanying clinical signs of encephalopathy. Conversely, insufficient protein has been linked to low albumin concentrations, poor immune response, impaired healing and increased risk of wound dehiscence and muscle wasting. The most efficient use of protein in people occurs when 2 to 6 g protein/100 kcal are administered (Stein, 1986).

Commercial products intended for enteral support of canine and feline critical care patients provide between 5.5 and 14.3 g protein/100 kcal. Due to a lack of evidence to the contrary and because these products appear to work well in critical care patients, a range of 5.0 to 12.0 g protein/100 kcal is recommended for canine patients and 7.5 to 12.0 g protein/100 kcal is recommended for feline patients. Because of the overlap of these recommendations, several commercial products intended for enteral support are designated for use in both canine and feline critical care patients.

When formulating parenteral nutritional support, it is prudent to first provide for total caloric needs with carbohydrate and fat, and then meet the protein requirement. If sufficient calories are supplied to patients as either fat or carbohydrate, then most of the essential amino acids will be used for protein synthesis and not burned for energy. A starting point of 2 to 3 g protein/100 kcal parenterally (Remillard and Thatcher, 1989) can be used for most dogs that can excrete protein waste products and do not have an extraordinary protein loss. A lower range (1 to 2 g/100 kcal parenterally) is a more reasonable estimate for patients with kidney or liver diseases. A higher range (3 to 4 g/100 kcal parenterally) is a more reasonable estimate for cats because of their constant state of gluconeogenesis from amino acids. Protein intake can then be adjusted based on the patient's needs and ability to handle the initial protein recommendation (e.g., decreasing serum albumin concentration or encephalopathic signs).

In addition, specific nutrients affect immunocompetence. Some nutrients act directly on the lymphoid system and immune cell function, thereby altering host immune response to pathogens. As an example, arginine, glutamine and dietary nucleotide-enriched foods are associated with significant reduction in wound infection and length of hospital stay in human burn patients.

Arginine

Arginine is essential to traumatized patients. It has a marked immunopreserving effect in the face of immunosuppression induced by protein malnutrition and cancer. In postsurgical patients, arginine supplementation enhances T-lymphocyte response and augments T-helper cell numbers, with a rapid return to normal T-cell function postoperatively, compared with findings in control patients (Bower et al, 1995). These data taken together suggest that arginine supplementation may increase or preserve function in high-risk surgical patients and theoretically enhance the host's capacity to resist infection. Arginine enrichment stimulates the immune system, improves wound healing and decreases morbidity and mortality in burn patients. A feeding regimen with arginine as 9% of the protein source has been suggested and tested in burn patients. Those receiving the arginine-enriched food had a significant reduction in the incidence of wound infection and shorter hospital stays. As a nutrient substrate, arginine appears nontoxic and may benefit surgical patients at increased risk of infection (Goffschlich et al, 1990). The optimal arginine intake for people is unknown, so selection of enteral foods based solely on arginine content is not recommended for human patients.

Numerous studies in a variety of animal models demonstrated the efficacy of arginine-supplemented foods in reducing the catabolic response to major trauma, sepsis and injury and in improving the immune response after a variety of adverse stimuli. For example, a food containing arginine as 2% of the total nonprotein calories significantly increased survival after 30% surface burns (Irenton-Jones and Baxter, 1990). Furthermore, in animal studies, exogenous arginine supplementation consistently improved nitrogen retention, protein turnover and wound healing. Arginine augments cellular immunity, as evidenced by enhanced skin allograft rejection in normal mice, and improves delayed hypersensitivity responses.

Arginine is an essential amino acid in dogs, cats and people. Therefore, most pet foods meeting AAFCO nutrient concentrations should contain at least 146 mg arginine/100 kcal for adult dogs and 250 mg arginine/100 kcal for adult cats (providing approximately 80 to 200 mg/kg body weight). Arginine content of human enteral products is variable but usually stated on the label. Human enteral products and parenteral nutrition solutions must contain at least adequate amounts of arginine if used for more than a few days in dogs or cats.

Glutamine

Glutamine is an amino acid that plays an important role in many cellular processes. Human studies suggest that glutamine concentrations in whole blood and skeletal muscle decrease markedly following injury and other catabolic states, thus making it "conditionally" essential during serious injury or illness (Lacey and Wilmore, 1990). Numerous clinical trials suggest that intervention with glutamine reduces rates of infectious complications in postsurgical patients and complications and mortality rates in critically ill patients (Novak et al, 2002). Replicating cells such as fibroblasts, lymphocytes and intestinal epithelial cells have high glutaminase activity and consume glutamine, but the intracellular level of glutamine remains low. The mechanism linking the beneficial effect of glutamine on attenuating cellular metabolic dysfunction and enhancing cell survival depends on glutamine-induced enhancement of specific heat shock proteins (Peng et al, 2006). These findings may be important for patients with large wounds or inflammation associated with infection.

The controversy persists as to which route of glutamine administration (enteral or parenteral) is most effective at improving clinical outcomes in critically ill patients. At least 80% of the published data in laboratory animals demonstrate a positive effect with glutamine-enriched feedings. Positive effects include enhanced protein metabolism, intestinal and pancreatic repair and regeneration, nutrient absorption, gut-barrier function, systemic and intestinal immune function and animal survival. The mechanism(s) for these effects are not well clarified, but studies suggest several possibilities. First is the inter-organ conversion of glutamine-derived citrulline to renal arginine synthesis (Ligthart-Melis et al, 2007). A second mechanism is through glutamine attenuation of the gut-derived inflammatory response (Wischmeyer, 2006).

Numerous animal studies have demonstrated the value of enteral glutamine during stress. For example, rats undergoing abdominal radiation and fed glutamine orally for eight days following the stress had significantly increased jejunal villous number and height and an increased number of mitoses per crypt, whereas non-irradiated control rats fed the same food without glutamine supplementation had no significant increase in mucosal cell activity (Klimberg et al, 1990). Similarly, dogs had an increased intestinal requirement for glutamine during the immediate postoperative phase (less than seven days), but uptake rates returned to normal later during the recovery phase (after 10 days) (Souba et al, 1987). Oral glutamine supplementation influences GI function, along with cell morphology. For example, rats undergoing ischemia-reperfusion injury maintained small intestinal barrier function when provided with enteral glutamine (Kozar et al, 2004).

Provision of exogenous glutamine to stressed patients might better support the metabolic requirements of the small intestine and possibly decrease the rate of systemic protein catabolism (Wischmeyer, 2006), therefore, supplementation is warranted. The optimal concentration of glutamine for different disease states is still under study. It is presently unclear whether glutamine must be in the free form to be beneficial or if the protein-bound form is also beneficial in maintaining gut integrity. Most enteral foods contain some protein-bound glutamine but the glutamine concentration of these products must be estimated. Some enteral products have added free glutamine. The glutamine content of these products is often stated on the label. Glutamine levels in commercial enteral foods intended for critical care canine and feline patients should be at least 500 mg/100 kcal.

Although based on human studies indicating the gut preferably takes up enterally administered glutamine compared with intravenously provided glutamine (Ligthart-Melis et al, 2007), evidence suggests intravenous glutamine can provide benefits as well. In protein-depleted rats, intravenous glutamine supplementation resulted in increased villous height, increased small-bowel mucosal weight, enhanced DNA activity (O'Dwyer et al, 1989) and improved DNA content and sucrase and lactase activities. Parenteral admixture supplemented with 2% glutamine and administered for 48 hours before and 72 hours postintestinal abdominal surgery in undernourished dogs improved ileal morphology, increased CD4:CD8 cells, select immunoglobulins and mononuclear cell function and resulted in fewer postsurgical diarrhea days compared to dogs administered non-glutamine supplemented parenteral admixture (Saker et al, 2001). In short-term studies in rats and pigs, adding glutamine to nutritional intravenous solutions reduced some aspects of disuse intestinal atrophy and enhanced intestinal immune function (Remillard et al, 1998). Intravenous glutamine supplementation immediately following hemorrhagic shock partially restored the depletion of hepatic ATP, reduced cellular apoptosis and oxidative stress-associated cell damage in rat and feline models (Yang et al, 2007; Krizova et al, 2004), suggesting additional benefit from intravenous-glutamine supplementation during critical illness. Intravenous glutamine should probably be limited to short-term use (one week or less) just before oral refeeding. Inclusion of 2% L-glutamine via the intravenous route has been safely used in human and veterinary patients. However, it should be noted that inclusion of glutamine in parenteral nutrition solutions can be difficult to achieve due to solubility constraints.

Fat

Supplying the majority of calories as fat to critically ill patients has several benefits. Fat contains 8.5 kcal metabolizable energy/g and is therefore calorically dense compared to carbohydrate and protein. Therefore, more calories may be provided in a smaller volume to patients. After three to five days of not eating, the liver has shifted from glucose to fat metabolism, therefore providing more fat and less dextrose at this time reduces metabolic complications of nutritional support. Additionally, providing calories as fat rather than dextrose reduces CO_2 production, which noticeably reduces respiratory work in patients requiring oxygen therapy. On average, "recovery" type foods provide 5 to 7.5 g fat/100 kcal; this appears to be a safe starting point for refeeding. The exceptions include patients with pancreatitis or other conditions in which enteral intake of a high-fat food is not tolerated.

Other Nutritional Factors

Other nutritional factors can be important considerations for enteral foods or parenteral fluids for critical care patients. Factors such as vitamins and minerals are typically included in adequate amounts in commercial veterinary therapeutic enteral foods formulated for dogs and cats. However, these nutrients are important to consider in parenteral nutrition support. Other factors (nucleotides, essential fatty acids and antioxidants) may benefit veterinary patients based on the human critical care literature and case reports. The optimal daily dose and duration of provision have yet to be standardized for dogs and cats. Typical ingredients used in many enteral foods contain nucleotides, essential fatty acids and antioxidants. Some critical care foods have been specifically enriched, whereas others have not been and would need exogenous supplementation if they were deemed valuable. Provision enterally is more efficient and practical than through parenteral fluids.

B Vitamins

Folic acid, thiamin, riboflavin, niacin, pantothenic acid, pyridoxine and B_{12} are essential for hepatic metabolism of glucose, fat and protein. These are coenzymes for the tricarboxylic acid (TCA) cycle, ATP production and RBC metabolism. B vitamins are required in small amounts relative to other nutrients, but they are required daily and are necessary for efficient energy metabolism. Most commercial pet foods contain adequate amounts of these nutrients, so deficiency should not be of concern if the patient is eating or being fed enough food to meet its RER. B vitamins should be added to the fluids (1 to 2 ml of vitamin-B complex/1,000 ml of crystalloid fluid) of all patients that are not eating but receiving fluid therapy or parenteral nutrition support.

Microminerals

Zinc, copper, manganese, chromium and selenium are vital cofactors for optimal hepatic and peripheral metabolism of energy substrates. Microminerals (i.e., trace minerals or trace elements) are important cofactors (metalloenzymes) and participate in tissue repair and albumin synthesis; therefore, zinc, copper and manganese should be included in all food forms used for assisted feeding. Most pet foods contain adequate amounts of these nutrients, thus deficiency should not be of concern if the patient is eating enough food to meet its RER. Specialized solutions containing essential trace (zinc, copper and manganese) minerals can easily be added to parenteral nutrition solutions at approximately 1 ml per 100 kcal of solution.

Fat-Soluble Vitamins and Macrominerals

Hospitalized patients rarely need fat-soluble vitamins and macrominerals. Most patients have fat and hepatic stores of the fat-soluble vitamins sufficient to meet metabolic needs for months to years. However, administering fat-soluble vitamins should be considered in cases of prolonged malnutrition in which the patient is severely underweight with little to no fat stores (i.e., BCS 1/5). Most pet foods contain adequate amounts of these nutrients, thus deficiency should not be of concern if the patient is eating enough food to meet its RER. Fat-soluble vitamins are not added to parenteral nutrition solutions due to insolubility problems. It is easiest to administer a single dose of vitamins A, D and E by deep intramuscular injection to patients needing these vitamins. Such an injection supplies approximately one to two months of daily requirements.

Macrominerals (i.e., calcium, phosphorus, magnesium, sodium and potassium) are rarely needed by patients above that required to maintain serum electrolyte levels. Whole body stores of these minerals can be depleted but are usually easily corrected by intravenous administration. The distribution between the intracellular and extracellular fluid space can be a problem and imbalances should be corrected before assisted feeding is begun (**Box 25-3**). Sodium, potassium and magnesium levels may

Box 25-3. Refeeding Syndrome.

Refeeding syndrome in people is characterized by generalized muscle weakness, tetany, myocardial dysfunction, dysrhythmias, seizures, excessive sodium and water retention, hemolytic anemia and death due to cardiac or respiratory failure. A similar syndrome occurs less commonly in veterinary patients. When it does occur, it is most often seen in patients receiving parenteral nutrition or during inappropriate assisted enteral feeding and most commonly presents as hypokalemia or hypophosphatemia. Significant electrolyte shifts occur from extracellular to intracellular compartments as energy and amino acids are reintroduced. This electrolyte shift will occur regardless of the route of administration (i.e., enteral or parenteral). Often serum ion levels are deceptively normal in anorectic patients before refeeding begins (**Table 25-4**). However, when calories are reintroduced, particularly from carbohydrate, potassium and phosphate shift intracellularly with glucose resulting in hypokalemia and hypophosphatemia.

Potassium moves into cells with refeeding because glucose stimulates insulin release, which in turn stimulates the Na-K ATPase pump and glycogen synthesis, which requires 0.33 mEq potassium/g of glycogen. Phosphate moves into cells with refeeding to support the increased production of phosphorylated intermediary compounds of energy metabolism. Severe hypophosphatemia, hemolytic anemia and death have occurred in cats within 12 to 72 hours of refeeding with either an apparently normal or phosphorus-deficient diet. The refeeding formula should contain at least the Association of American Feed Control Officials recommended minimum allowance of 0.5% dry matter phosphorus.

In people, hypomagnesemia is another common electrolyte complication that must be corrected. Hypomagnesemia increases urinary excretion of potassium, exacerbates hypokalemia and causes hypocalcemia, which is refractory to supplementation until the hypomagnesemia is corrected. Little information is available about magnesium status in hospitalized dogs and cats; however, serum magnesium levels should probably be monitored in veterinary patients with abnormal serum electrolytes.

RECOMMENDATIONS FOR AVOIDING COMPLICATIONS OF THE REFEEDING SYNDROME

1. Anticipate the potential for the problem and re-feed with formulations known to contain adequate potassium, phosphate and magnesium levels and lowered digestible (soluble) carbohydrate content.
2. Use initial nutritional refeeding rates that do not exceed the patient's resting energy requirement (RER) and 2 to 6 g protein/100 kcal (parenterally) or 5.5 to 7.5 g protein/100 kcal (enterally). These rates can be increased as needed over subsequent days. Consider refeeding a high-fat, low-carbohydrate formula to patients that have not eaten for four to five days or more.
3. Monitor serum potassium, phosphate and magnesium levels as needed. Once a day is sufficient for most cases.
4. Supply water-soluble vitamins free choice, particularly thiamin, to facilitate energy metabolism.
5. Monitor patients daily for signs of fluid overload and congestive heart failure.

The Bibliography for **Box 25-3** can be found at www.markmorris.org.

become a concern in patients experiencing excessive urinary loss of those minerals due to intensive diuretic therapy. Most pet foods contain adequate amounts of these nutrients, thus deficiency should not be of concern if the repleted patient continues eating enough food to meet its RER. Calcium and magnesium are not added to parenteral nutrition solutions due to insolubility problems; however, phosphorus, sodium and potassium can be added to parenteral nutrition solutions at maintenance concentrations or for repletion if needed.

Nucleotides

Nucleotides are precursors of DNA and RNA, but they also participate in a number of metabolic reactions fundamental to cellular activity. Dietary nucleotides appear to be important for maintenance of normal cellular immunity and are vital to maintain host defenses against bacterial and fungal pathogens. Dietary nucleotides appear essential to the normal maturation of lymphocytes (Hall et al, 1998). In vitro mixed lymphocyte culture response and mitogen stimulation are suppressed in patients supported on a casein-based laboratory food. Such foods are nucleotide free. Mice maintained on nucleotide-free foods are much more susceptible to lethal infections caused by *Candida albicans* and *Staphylococcus aureus* and exhibit depressed macrophage bactericidal activity compared to nucleotide-fed counterparts. Similarly, animals fed a nucleotide-free food for six weeks had significant immunosuppression as demonstrated by enhanced cardiac allografts and diminished ability to survive a fungal challenge. These findings are significant because all commercially available parenteral and nearly all enteral human products are devoid of nucleotides.

The clinical value of nucleotides was evaluated in two separate studies that investigated the effects of a human enteral product enriched with arginine, nucleotides and omega-3 fatty acids (Impact[a]). In one study, researchers investigated the effects of this enriched enteral product on immune parameters of patients undergoing major abdominal surgery. In general, patients receiving the enriched product had enhanced immunocompetence and fewer infectious complications than patients in other groups. In the other study, a subset of patients with sepsis who were fed the enriched enteral product (Impact) had shorter hospital stays and a major reduction in the frequency of acquired infections vs. other groups (Bower et al, 1995). Though clinical gain was evident from the nucleotide-enriched food, it is not clear if the benefit was from nucleotides alone or from the combination of special nutrients provided in the food. There are no reported studies evaluating the clinical value of nucleotide-enriched foods for critical care veterinary patients, likely because pet foods that use meats and cereal grains as ingredients should provide adequate levels of dietary nucleotides. Despite the limiting data substantiating their clinical value in veterinary patients, dietary nucleotides are a vital component of regimens to maintain or restore immune function and host defense and, therefore, should be considered when choosing a critical-care food.

Omega-3 Fatty Acids

The effect of dietary fatty acids on the immune system depends on which fatty acid is fed and what specific aspects of the immune system are evaluated. Dietary fatty acids are thought to affect the immune system by three mechanisms: 1) altered eicosanoid synthesis, 2) changes in cell membranes that affect membrane-associated protein and receptor function and 3) changes in intracellular nonesterified fatty acid pools that affect cytokine production. Generally, omega-3 (n-3) fatty acids produce fewer inflammatory cytokines, whereas omega-6 (n-6) fatty acids produce more proinflammatory cytokines (Lands, 1992).

The capacity of tissues and WBC to produce pro- or anti-inflammatory prostaglandins and lipoxygenase products is largely determined by the amount and type of fatty acids present, which is mostly determined by concentration of dietary fatty acids. Omega-3 fatty acids, once incorporated into the plasma membrane, affect immune cell function by altering membrane fluidity and second messenger function, and by increasing production of dienoic prostaglandins, the 3-series prostaglandins and 5-series leukotrienes. These changes may be responsible for alterations in such cell functions as phagocytosis, production of interleukins and production of superoxides. A significant reduction in dietary omega-6 polyunsaturated fatty acids will lower production of proinflammatory eicosanoids and appears to be a prudent approach in nutritional support of immunocompromised, traumatized, postoperative or infected patients. Conversely, the inclusion of omega-3 fatty acids in such foods would seem to be beneficial in increasing antiinflammatory eicosanoid production. Findings suggest that marked improvement can be made in foods by adjusting the omega-6 and omega-3 components to ensure optimal immune function.

Clinical evidence suggests that dietary omega-3 fatty acids may benefit the management of severe inflammatory and autoimmune disorders in rodents and people. These less inflammatory metabolites alter immune function and may improve survival in patients in which the inflammatory process threatens to cause irreversible damage, as in septic shock or endotoxemia. Omega-3 fatty acids shift the response away from intense inflammation. In other studies, fish oil protected guinea pigs from endotoxic shock and lactic acidosis, providing them with a survival advantage (Fritsche and McGuire, 1996).

Timing of dietary omega-6 and omega-3 fatty acid manipulation is critical to influencing patient inflammatory response. The literature varies when reporting dosing route, concentration and species. Nonesterified fatty acids in tissues have been effectively altered within hours of oral dosing with omega-3 fatty acids. In cats, concentrations of specific fatty acids were altered in immune cell membranes within 28 days of enteral feeding (Saker, 2002); whereas in pigs, plasma phospholipid profiles differed significantly within eight days (Murray et al, 1991). Intestinal mucosa and plasma had an altered fatty acid profile within four weeks, whereas an alteration in the fatty acid profile of skin generally occurred after six to 12 weeks of supplementation. In dogs, however, investigators found plasma fatty acid profile changes within two weeks after the onset of omega-3 dietary supplementation (Campbell and Dorn, 1992). Thus, there may not be enough time for dietary omega-3 fatty acid therapy to affect an acute inflammatory process, depending on the affected tissue unless the fatty acids were incorporated into the patient's dietary regimen before the onset of disease. The dietary dose that favors a less inflammatory cascade during a disease process is still not standardized across veterinary patients, but is suggested as an omega-6:omega-3 fatty acid ratio ranging between 5:1 to 1:1, depending on patient assessment.

On the other hand, chronic suppression of the inflammatory and/or immune response by feeding high levels of omega-3 fatty acids should be done cautiously and is not warranted in disease states in which a fully competent immune system is essential for survival and recovery. Studies in which mice were pre-fed (two to four weeks) extremely high levels of omega-3 fatty acids (40% of calories as fish oil) compromised their resistance in an infectious disease state (Chang et al, 1992). Platelet function was significantly diminished in healthy cats fed an enriched omega-3 fatty acid food (omega-6:omega-3 ratio of 1.3:1) for eight weeks (Saker et al, 1998). As with many other nutrients, excessive levels of omega-3 fatty acids can be detrimental.

FEEDING PLAN

The feeding plan discussion assumes that the health care team has determined that the patient is a candidate for nutritional support (see History and Physical Examination section, above).

Nutrients can be supplied enterally or parenterally (**Figure 25-5**). Enteral feeding provides adequate nutrition simply and cost effectively whether done orally or by feeding tube. Enteral feeding is usually preferred to parenteral feeding because it is less expensive, stimulates the systemic and GI immune systems, helps to maintain GI mucosal integrity and avoids most metabolic complications. However, nutrients must be administered parenterally when the GI tract is inaccessible or not functioning adequately enough to meet the patient's nutrient requirements enterally. Chapter 26 covers parenteral-assisted feeding.

Enteral-assisted feeding is providing nutrients to the patient using some portion of the GI tract. Patients that cannot or will not eat but who can digest and absorb nutrients from the small intestine should receive enteral-assisted feeding. Feeding via the GI tract is often the simplest, fastest, easiest, safest, least expensive and most physiologic method of feeding patients. Prior knowledge that a patient requires other medical and surgical procedures should also be considered when formulating an enteral assisted-feeding plan. For example, feeding tubes can easily be placed at the end of a procedure requiring anesthesia or tranquilization. Feeding tube placement must consider the treatment plan and owners' expectations. Some feeding tubes can only be used when the patient is in the hospital whereas other tubes may also be used for at-home feeding.

The two methods, enteral and parenteral, are not mutually exclusive; supplementing what the patient consumes voluntarily with parenteral calories and protein infusion is possible in many veterinary practices. Therefore, overall patient assessment, including evaluating a patient's ability to eat and assimilate food, is the first step in developing a feeding plan because it dictates the route, enteral, parenteral or both, for providing assisted feeding.

The food choice should be made based on a food's key nutritional factor profile and form of the food (i.e., liquid, moist) that best accommodates the specific nutritional support feeding method. For example, if a small nasogastric feeding tube were to be used, a liquid food of appropriate viscosity and key nutrient make-up would be selected. This is an added consideration compared to developing feeding plans for patients that do not require assistance.

Select the Feeding Method

Enteral Feeding Routes

ORAL FEEDING

Several routes exist for enteral feeding, but the first attempt usually should be oral feeding. Placing a bolus of food in the proximal portion of the mouth may stimulate the swallowing reflex and, if the patient offers no resistance, is a good method as long as the patient receives enough food to meet its RER. Simple syringe feeding of a liquid product is also a good method, if tolerated. For dogs, the syringe tip is placed between the molar teeth and cheek with the head held in a normal or lowered position; for cats, the syringe tip is placed between the four canine teeth (**Box 25-4**). The patient may choose to swallow the liquid or allow it to flow from the mouth down the esophagus by gravity. Some patients refuse to swallow boluses of food; therefore, forced feeding may increase the risk of food aspiration. Oral feeding should be discontinued if the patient does not swallow food voluntarily. Appetite stimulants may be used to induce food consumption in some patients; however, voluntary food intake rarely continues and their RER is often not met (**Table 25-6**).

Orogastric tubes require placement at each feeding but may provide a useful option for one or two days of feeding. They can be used as long as there is no nasal, pharyngeal or esophageal trauma or disease. Anesthesia is not required; therefore, this route can be used in patients that are an anesthetic risk. Neonates appear to tolerate multiple daily oral tube feedings better than adults. A red rubber or polyvinyl chloride tube (8 to 24 Fr.)[b] may be used with the tip placed in either the caudal esophagus or stomach. An indwelling feeding tube is the method of choice if enteral-assisted feeding is necessary for more than two days.

Feeding through an indwelling tube is easier and less stressful on the patient than forced feeding or repeated placement of an orogastric tube. Nasoesophageal, pharyngostomy, esophagostomy, gastrostomy and enterostomy are potential placement sites. Tubes should be placed in the most proximal functioning portion of the GI tract possible by the least invasive method. The stomach should be used whenever possible.

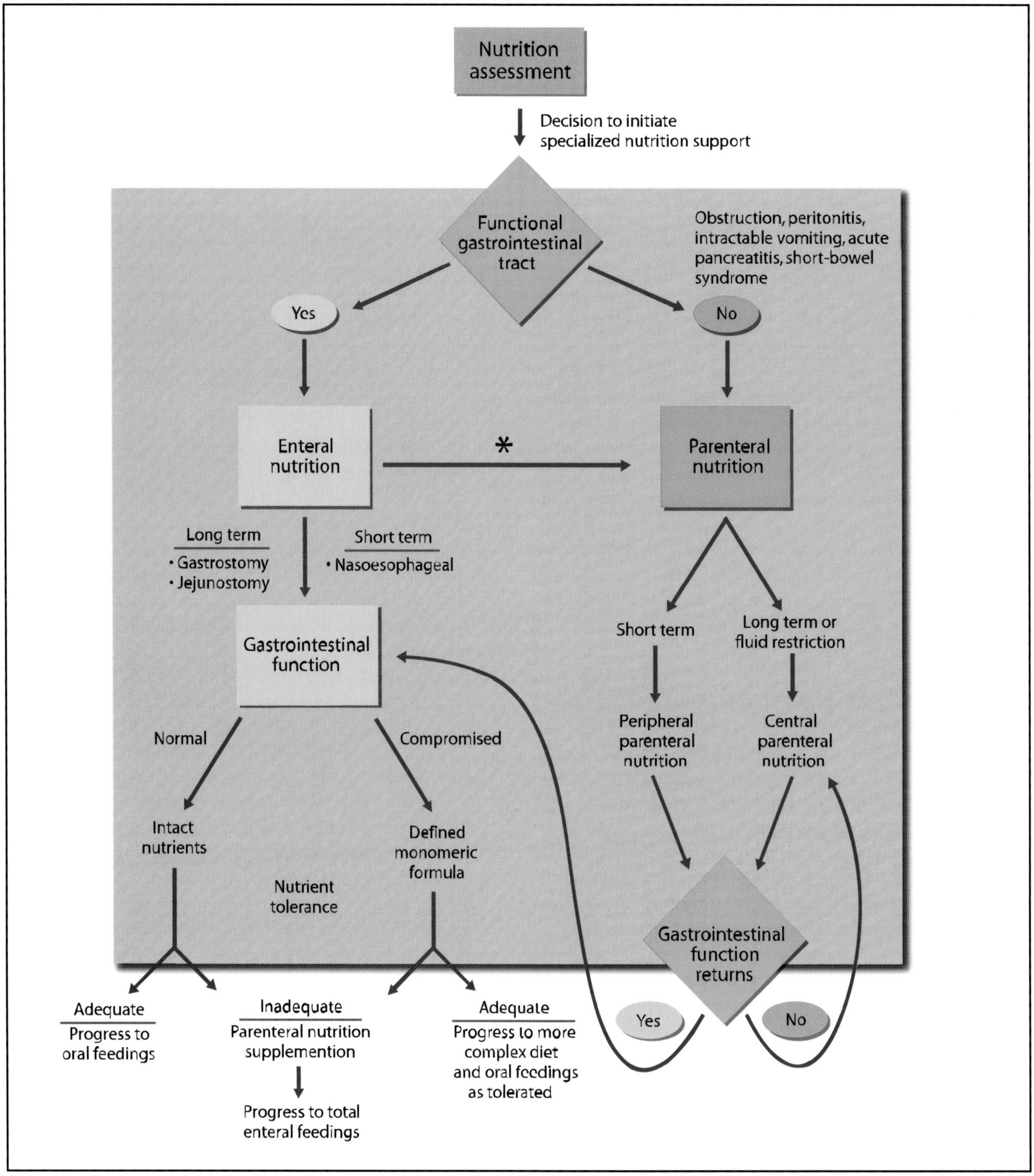

Figure 25-5. Clinical decision making algorithm for selecting the route of nutritional support. (Adapted from Hudak CM, Gallo BM, Gonce-Morton P, eds. Patient management: Gastrointestinal system. Critical Care Nursing, 7th ed. Philadelphia, PA: Lippincott, 1998; 771.)
*Nasoesophageal tube not tolerated or anesthesia not possible.

NASOESOPHAGEAL TUBES

Nasoesophageal tubes are generally used for three to seven days but are occasionally used longer (weeks, if moved to the opposite side every seven days). Polyurethane tubes (6 to 8 Fr., 90 to 100 cm) with or without a tungsten-weighted tip[c] and silicone[d] feeding tubes (3.5 to 10 Fr., 20 to 105 cm) may be placed in the caudal esophagus or stomach. The preferred placement of all tubes originating cranial to the stomach is in the caudal esophagus to minimize gastric reflux and subsequent esophagitis. An 8-Fr. tube will pass through the nasal cavity of most dogs. A 5-Fr. nasoesophageal tube is more comfortable for cats. Nasoesophageal feedings may be used in anorectic

Box 25-4. Syringe Feeding.

Patients are often fed a liquid or moist homogenized product by syringe on a short-term basis. For dogs, the syringe tip is placed between the molar teeth and cheek with the head held in a normal or lowered position (**Figure 1**). For cats, the syringe tip is placed between the four canine teeth (**Figure 2**). The patient may choose to swallow the liquid or allow it to flow down the mouth into the esophagus by gravity. Some patients refuse to swallow the liquid or food; therefore, force feeding may increase the risk of aspiration. Syringe feeding should be discontinued if the patient does not swallow food voluntarily.

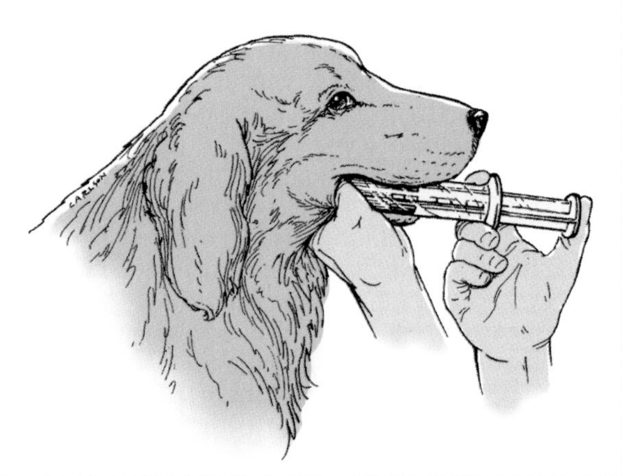

Figure 1. Syringe-feeding technique for administering liquid or moist homogenized foods to dogs.

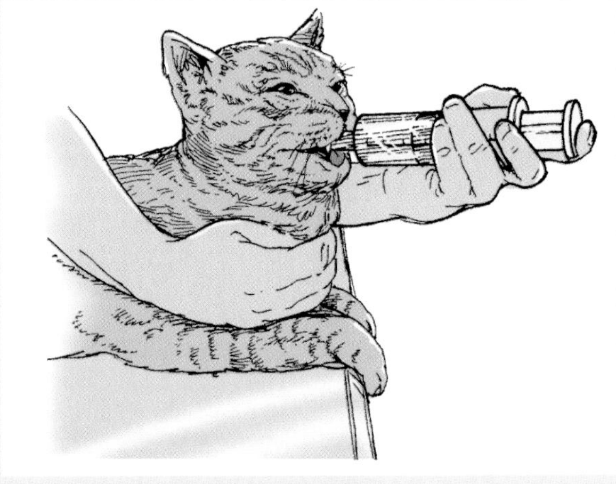

Figure 2. Syringe-feeding technique for administering liquid or moist homogenized foods to cats.

patients that do not have nasal, oral or pharyngeal disease or trauma. Anesthesia or tranquilization is not necessary to place a nasoesophageal tube, so this route provides enteral access to patients considered anesthetic risks. These tubes are most often used in the hospital, although conscientious owners can use nasoesophageal tubes at home (**Box 25-5**).

Table 25-6. Pharmacologic appetite stimulants.*

Cyproheptadine	Antihistamine and anti-serotonin effects. Dose cats at: a) 2 to 4 mg per cat per os once or twice daily, b) 2 mg per cat every 12 hours. May take up to 24 hours for a response. Give at this dosage for one week and then taper.
Diazepam	Short-lived appetite stimulant with sedative properties. Dose in cats varies: a) 0.05 to 0.15 mg/kg IV once daily to every other day or 1 mg per os once daily, b) 0.05 to 0.4 mg/kg IV, IM or per os. Eating may begin within a few seconds after IV administration. Food should be readily available.
Mirtazapine	Increases central nervous system serotonin while antagonizing serotonin activity in the GI tract. Dose cats at: 3.5 mg per cat per os every three days. May take up to 36 hours for a response.
Oxazepam	Short-lived appetite stimulant with sedative properties. Dose cats at 2 mg per cat (total dose) every 12 hours.
Prednisolone	Dose glucocorticoids at 0.25 to 0.5 mg/kg per os every day, every other day or intermittently as needed in dogs.

*Adapted from Plumb DC. Veterinary Drug Handbook, 3rd ed. White Bear, MN: Pharma Veterinary Publishing, 1999.

PHARYNGOSTOMY/ ESOPHAGOSTOMY/ GASTROSTOMY TUBES

Pharyngostomy and esophagostomy tubes (8 to 19 Fr.) may be placed in patients with disease or trauma to the nasal or oral cavity. The tip of the tube is placed in the caudal esophagus and the tube can be used for long-term (weeks to months) in-hospital or home feedings. **Boxes 25-6** and **25-7** describe pharyngostomy and esophagostomy tube placement, respectively.

For patients in which the pharynx and esophagus must be bypassed, gastrostomy tubes (mushroom-tipped, 16 to 28 Fr.)[e] can be placed either intraoperatively or percutaneously using an endoscope or a gastrostomy tube introduction device (Clary et al, 1996).[f] Gastrostomy tubes are also recommended for long-term feeding (weeks to months) if needed and have generally replaced pharyngostomy tubes, even when the esophagus is normal. Gastrostomy tubes are convenient and safe for in-hospital and at-home feedings.

There are two basic techniques for percutaneous placement of gastrostomy tubes. One technique uses an endoscope, whereas the other involves a "blind," nonendoscopic approach using a gastrostomy tube placement device or applicator. The advantages of percutaneous vs. surgical gastrostomy tube placement are ease and speed of placement, lower cost and less tissue trauma. **Boxes 25-8** through **25-10** describe these three methods of gastrostomy tube placement.

Any tube that has been placed into the esophagus or stomach allows for bolus or meal-type feeding schedules because the stomach acts as a food reservoir. Some patients, however, cannot tolerate bolus feeding into the stomach without vomiting. Such patients may benefit from a slow, continuous drip administration (by pump or gravity flow) of food into the stomach. Most veterinary patients tolerate bolus feedings of enteral nutritional support via nasoesophageal, esophagostomy or gastrostomy feeding tubes.

JEJUNOSTOMY TUBES

Jejunostomy tubes (J-tubes, 5 to 8 Fr.) are placed within the small intestine, ideally at the time of exploratory celiotomy, to bypass the proximal GI tract (Orton, 1986). J-tubes may also be placed by mini-laparotomy, or by threading a small feeding tube through a larger esophagostomy, pharyngostomy or gastrostomy feeding tube and placing the tip of the smaller tube in the jejunum (Crowe, 1986; Jergens et al, 2007). There is risk, however, that even a weighted-tip tube will be returned to the stomach by reverse peristalsis. Ideally, food should be administered through J-tubes at a slow, continuous drip delivered by a pump. Some patients, however, will tolerate frequent small-bolus feedings.

Amount to Feed and Feeding Schedule

Feeding plans require an understanding of the patient's metabolic state relative to changes in metabolism resulting from ongoing food deprivation. Estimating a patient's approximate caloric requirement is important because feeding more of any food than is necessary may cause metabolic complications. Overfeeding patients is possible through a feeding tube and should be avoided because it results in metabolic and mechanical complications. **Table 25-7** provides an example of using feeding guidelines to determine how much to feed and the feeding schedule.

The feeding schedule is often determined by the patient's ability to tolerate food and the logistics of feeding. Feeding an amount equal to the patient's RER during the first 24 hours of food reintroduction, if physically tolerated, is recommended. Feeding one-third of RER the first 24 hours and then increasing the amount by one-third every 24 hours until at RER is a more cautious approach to initial feeding, but is not always necessary. Foods should be warmed to room temperature, but not higher than body temperature, before feeding.

Food boluses must be infused slowly (over approximately one minute per 5 ml of food) to allow gastric expansion. Daily food dosage should be divided into several meals according to the expected stomach capacity. Gastric capacities for cats and dogs are typically 5 to 10 ml/kg body weight during initial food reintroduction. Maximum capacities as high as 45 to 90 ml/kg body weight have been measured in cats and dogs when fully re-alimented. Most often, the patient's RER can be met in volumes far less than these maximum gastric capacities. Salivating, gulping, retching and vomiting may occur when too much food has been infused or when the infusion rate is too fast.

Research in people has demonstrated that the stomach does not "shrink" during a prolonged fast, but rather the stretch receptors are more sensitive and stimulated by a smaller volume when refeeding occurs. Feeding should be stopped at the first sign of retching or salivating; then the meal size reduced by 50% for 24 hours and then increased by 25% gradually. Foods

Box 25-5. Nasoesophageal Tube Placement.

Nasoesophageal tubes are generally used for three to seven days, but are occasionally used longer (weeks if moved to the opposite side every seven days). Polyurethane tubes (6 to 8 Fr., 90 to 100 cm) with or without a weighted tip and silicone feeding tubes (3.5 to 10 Fr., 20 to 105 cm) may be placed in the caudal esophagus or stomach. The preferred placement of all tubes originating cranial to the stomach is in the caudal esophagus to minimize gastric reflux and subsequent esophagitis. An 8-Fr. tube will pass through the nasal cavity of most dogs; a 5- Fr. tube is more comfortable for cats.

The length of tube to be inserted is determined by measuring from the nasal planum along the side of the animal to the caudal margin of the last rib (**Figure 1**) and marking the tube at a point that is approximately three-fourths of the total measured length with a piece of adhesive tape or an indelible marker. This mark is how far the tube should be inserted. Tape will also provide a tab to secure the tube. The animal's nose is desensitized by placing a few drops of topical anesthetic (2% lidocaine or 0.5% proparacaine) into a nostril and tilting the head upward for a few seconds. The tip of the tube is lubricated with a water-soluble lubricant or 2 to 5% lidocaine ointment/jelly before passage.

To pass the tube, direct the tip in a caudoventral, medial direction into the ventrolateral aspect of the external nares. The head is generally held in a normal static position. As soon as the tip of the catheter reaches the medial septum at the floor of the nasal cavity in dogs, the external nares are pushed dorsally, which opens the ventral meatus, ensuring passage of the tube into the oropharynx (**Figure 2**). To aid passage, the proximal end of the tube is lifted as the nose is pushed upward (**Figure 2**). In cats, because of the lack of a well-developed alar fold, the tube can be inserted initially in a ventromedial direction and continued directly into the oropharynx. The tube is inserted until the adhesive tape tab or indelible mark is reached (**Figure 3**).

To evaluate proper tube placement, 3 to 15 ml of sterile water or saline solution may be injected through the tube and the animal evaluated for coughing (**Figure 4**). A lateral radiograph may be taken of the neck to confirm the tube is placed in the caudal esophagus (i.e., over the larynx). After confirmation of position, the tube is secured with either sutures or glue. The first tape tab is secured to the skin just lateral to the external nares. A second tape tab is secured to the skin on the dorsal nasal midline, just rostral to the level of the eyes. An Elizabethan collar is used in most animals to prevent inadvertent removal of the tube (**Figure 5**).

Complications of nasoesophageal intubation include epistaxis, lack of tolerance of the procedure and inadvertent removal of the tube by the animal. Incidence of tube removal by the animal has been reported to be as high as 50% even with use of collars. Nasoesophageal tubes should not be used in vomiting patients or those with respiratory disease.

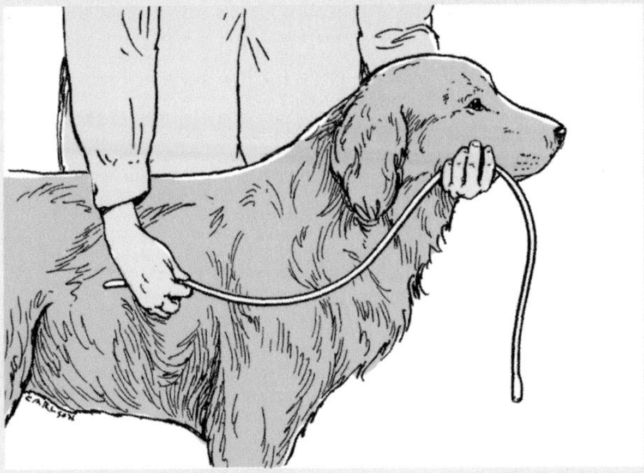

Figure 1. The length of tube to insert is determined by measuring from the nose to the last rib. Marking the tube at three-quarters of the distance between the last rib and the nose will place the end of the tube in the caudal esophagus. This location is marked with an indelible marker or a piece of adhesive tape. Tape can also serve as a suture tab to secure the tube.

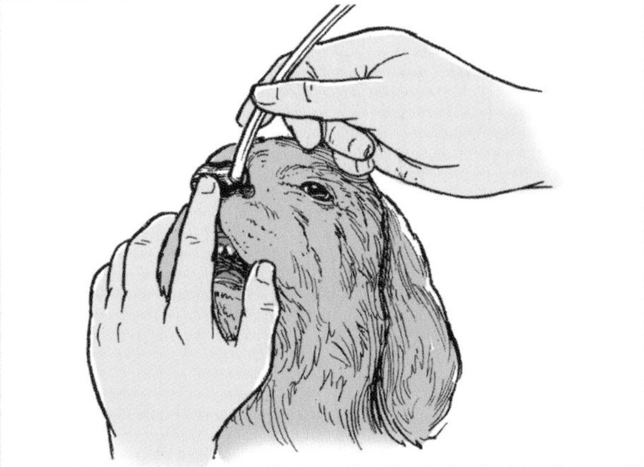

Figure 2. The external nares are pushed dorsally and the proximal end of the tube is lifted to facilitate passage of the tube into the ventral nasal meatus.

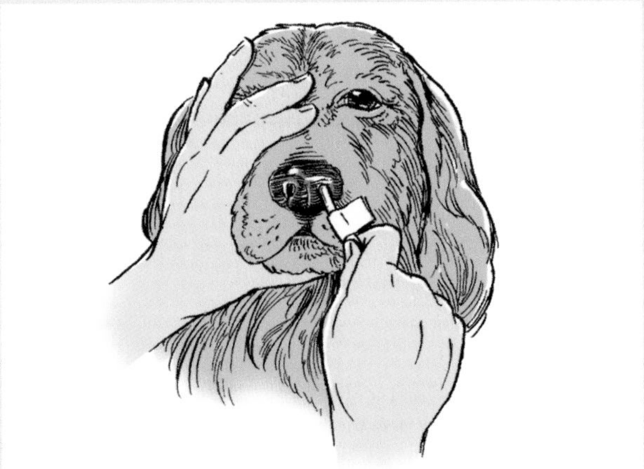

Figure 3. The tube is inserted until the indelible mark or adhesive tape tab is reached. Sutures or glue are used to secure the tape tab to the skin.

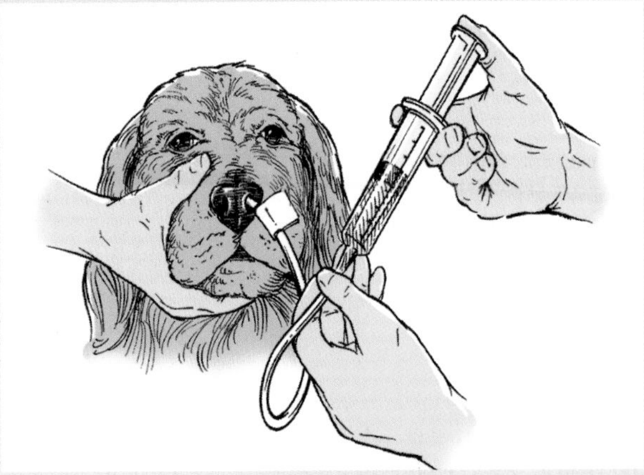

Figure 4. A test injection of sterile water or saline solution is made to ensure proper tube placement.

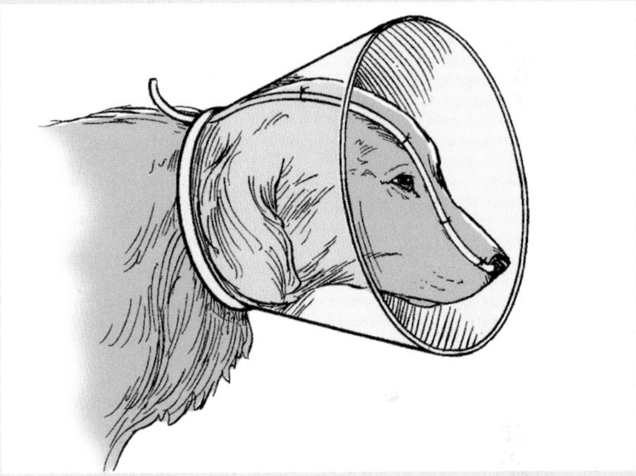

Figure 5. Securing the tube at several locations by suturing or gluing tape tabs to the skin and applying collars will help decrease inadvertent removal of the tube by the animal.

Box 25-6. Pharyngostomy Tube Placement.

In some instances, a pharyngostomy tube is used to bypass the nose and mouth of an animal requiring nutritional support (e.g., in cases of facial trauma) or when nasoesophageal tubes are not tolerated. Pharyngostomy tubes have been largely replaced by esophagostomy tubes or gastrostomy tubes placed percutaneously.

The patient is anesthetized, intubated and positioned in lateral recumbency. The area caudal to the mandible on either side is prepared for aseptic surgery. A 14- to 18-Fr. polyvinylchloride tube is premeasured as described in **Box 25-5, Figure 1**, except that the tube exit site will be caudal to the mandible.

With the mouth held open with a speculum, palpate the hyoid apparatus with one finger. The tube exit site must be carefully planned to avoid interfering with laryngeal opening and epiglottic movement. The tube should exit as far caudally and dorsally along the lateral pharyngeal wall as possible. The finger inside the mouth locates the hyoid apparatus and protrudes from the pharyngeal wall laterally at the selected exit site (**Figure 1**). Alternatively, forceps can be used to bulge the pharyngeal wall laterally. The finger locates the pulsating carotid artery, ensuring that it will be avoided, while providing a target for the tunneling forceps. A 1-cm skin incision is made over the bulging pharyngeal wall. Long, curved forceps are used to bluntly tunnel caudally through the tissues from outside to inside. Blunt dissection prevents injury to nearby nerves, carotid artery and jugular vein. Forceps are used to grasp one end of the feeding tube so it exits through the dissection site while the other end is advanced down the esophagus (**Figure 2**). The tube is then secured to the skin with tape and sutures.

Complications include airway obstruction, tube displacement, damage to cervical nerves and blood vessels and infection at the exit site. Placing the tube exit site caudal to the hyoid apparatus or use of very large diameter tubes is much more likely to result in airway obstruction or aspiration (**Figure 3**). The animal should be observed frequently for signs of respiratory embarrassment as it recovers from anesthesia. Frequent inspection and cleansing of the tube entrance/exit site help prevent skin infection. These tubes should not be used in vomiting patients or those with respiratory disease.

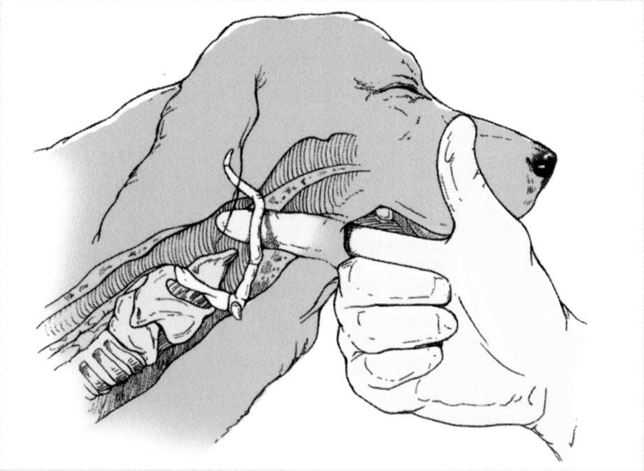

Figure 1. A finger is used to find the optimal exit site for the pharyngostomy tube. The tube should exit the pharyngeal wall as far caudally and dorsally as possible.

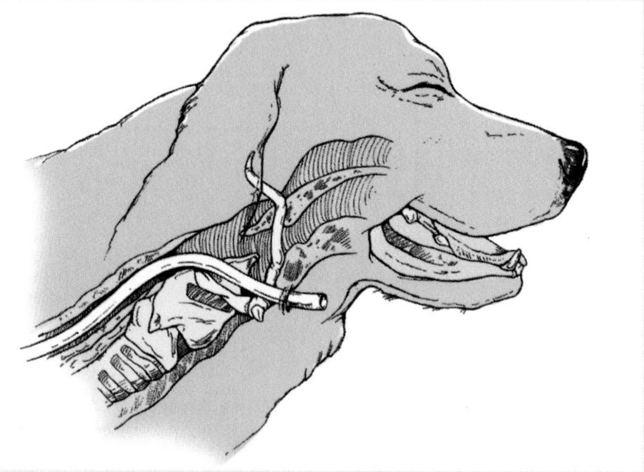

Figure 2. Proper placement of a pharyngostomy tube with the tube exiting dorsal and caudal to the larynx.

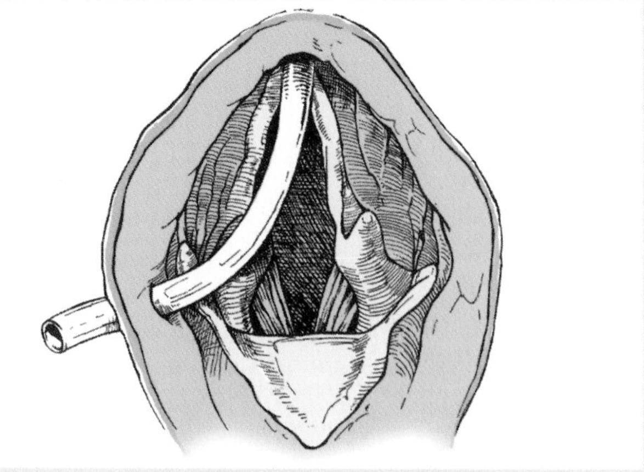

Figure 3. Inappropriate positioning of a pharyngostomy tube, as depicted here, causes the tube to course over the laryngeal opening and to interfere with movement of the epiglottis. This placement can lead to serious airway obstruction. The tube should exit the pharyngeal wall as far caudally and dorsally as possible.

Box 25-7. Esophagostomy Tube Placement.

Several techniques have been described for mid-cervical placement of esophagostomy tubes in dogs and cats. The animal receives light general anesthesia for esophagostomy tube placement. The entire lateral cervical region from the ventral midline to near the dorsal midline is clipped and aseptically prepared for surgery.

In one technique, appropriately sized, curved Kelly, Carmalt or similar forceps are inserted into the pharynx and then into the proximal cervical esophagus. The tip of the forceps is turned laterally and pressure is applied in an outward direction, thereby tenting up the cervical tissue so that the instrument tip can be seen and palpated externally. A small skin incision, just large enough to accommodate the feeding tube, is made over the tip of the forceps. In small dogs and cats, the tip of the forceps is forced bluntly through the esophagus. In larger dogs, a deeper incision is made to allow passage of the tip of the forceps through the esophagus. Tube sizes 12- to 19-Fr. are generally used. The tube is premeasured as described in **Box 25-5, Figure 1** so that the distal tip resides in the mid to caudal esophagus. The distal tip of the tube is grasped with forceps, pulled into the esophagus and out through the mouth, turned around and redirected into the esophagus. The tube is then secured with tape and sutures. A light circumferential bandage containing antibiotic-impregnated gauze is then placed at the exit site.

Another technique uses a percutaneous feeding tube applicator (ELD Gastrostomy Tube Applicator) (**Figure 1**).

Reported complications of tube esophagostomy for nutritional support include tube displacement due to vomiting or scratching by the animal and skin infection around the exit site.

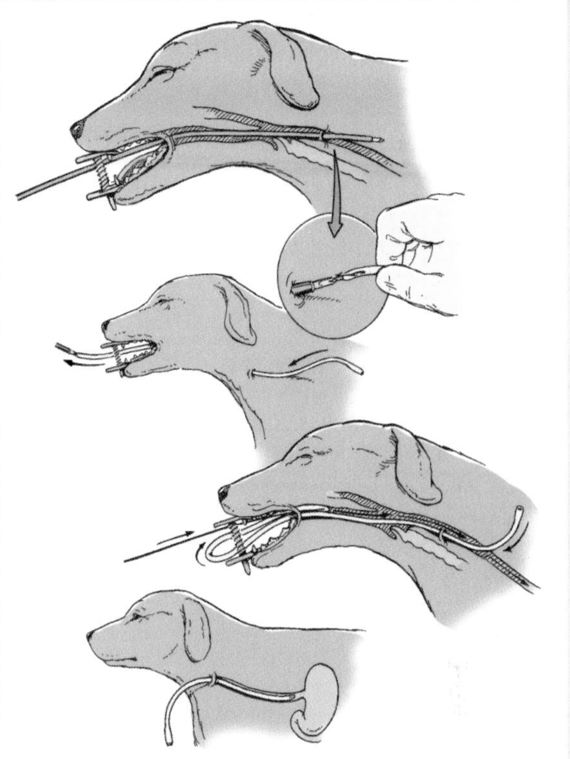

Figure 1. Insertion of a percutaneous feeding tube applicator into the mid-cervical esophagus. The distal tip is palpated and an incision is made through the skin and subcutaneous tissue over the tip of the applicator. The trocar is advanced through the esophageal wall and directed through the incision. The distal end of the feeding tube is secured to the eyelet of the trocar with suture material. The applicator and attached feeding tube are retracted into the esophagus and out the mouth. The feeding tube is redirected into the esophagus for final placement. A wire stylet can be inserted into the feeding tube if necessary to ease placement in the esophagus.

provided by J-tubes must be infused slowly and often in either very small quantities or preferably by a slow gravity drip or enteral pump with an hourly rate equal to RER/24 hours because the jejunum is volume sensitive.

Each bolus-fed meal must be followed by a water flush to clear the feeding tube of food residue. When the patient is volume sensitive, it is important to know the minimum volume required to effectively flush the tube. The patient's daily fluid requirement must also be met and additional water may be administered through the feeding tube to meet that requirement. Liquid oral medications may also be administered easily through feeding tubes. Plugged feeding tubes can be cleared by filling the tube with water or a nonalcoholic carbonated beverage and allowing time for the food plug to dissolve. End-port tubes are usually easier to maintain because food tends to become trapped in the blind end of side-port tubes. All tubes except orogastric and nasoesophageal tubes require standard every-other-day bandage care.

Assess and Select the Food

Selecting a food for hospitalized patients requires complete knowledge of the case, and often the food needs to be individually tailored because of each patient's unique circumstances. Refeeding patients in the early phase vs. refeeding in the later phases of food deprivation dictates the proportion of fat and carbohydrate in the refeeding formula. For example, the refeeding formula for a patient that has not eaten in seven days or more should contain predominantly fat as the energy fuel, as opposed to higher levels of carbohydrate (e.g., glucose). Pancreatitis patients, in which high-fat foods are contraindicated for dogs and presumably for cats, would be exceptions. In these cases, consider foods providing lower fat, low to moderate carbohydrate and increased protein calories. The food selection process should include a comparison of the key nutritional factor content of the food to the recommended levels. **Tables 25-8** and **25-9** list selected foods for assisted feeding and compares them to the recommended levels of key nutritional factors for dogs and cats, respectively.

Pre-existing conditions requiring specific nutritional modifications (e.g., renal insufficiency) or dietary modifications (e.g., adverse reactions to foods) must be understood and incorporated into selecting a food for the patient. For example, a cat diag-

Box 25-8. Surgical Gastrostomy Tube Placement.

A limited left flank celiotomy for gastrostomy tube placement provides an alternative when endoscopic or blind gastrostomy techniques are not performed. A gastrostomy tube may also be inserted when a celiotomy is performed for other reasons. General anesthesia is administered and the left flank is aseptically prepared for surgery. The prepared left paracostal area is draped and a 2- to 3-cm incision is made through the skin and subcutaneous tissue. The incision is made just caudal and parallel to the last rib, with its dorsal limit just below the ventral edge of the paravertebral epaxial musculature. The incision should be extended ventrally so that the intraperitoneal rather than the retroperitoneal space is accessed. The incision should be long enough to permit insertion of one or two fingers and a tissue forceps.

The greater curvature of the stomach is located and an Allis or Babcock tissue forceps is used to grasp and exteriorize the stomach through the incision. A stomach tube may be passed by an assistant and the stomach dilated with 10 to 15 ml of air/kg body weight if difficulty is encountered locating the stomach. Exteriorizing the stomach through a small flank incision can be difficult, especially in larger, deep-chested canine breeds. The left lateral aspect of the gastric body or the caudal aspect of the fundus is selected for the ostomy site. Two pursestring sutures are placed around the selected ostomy site (**Figure 1**). A stab incision is made through the ostomy site, the tube is inserted into the stomach and the pursestring sutures are tied snugly. Tube sizes 14 to 28 Fr. can be inserted.

The tube may exit the body wall through a separate stab wound or the original incision. The stomach is then fixed to the abdominal wall where the tube enters the peritoneum using a continuous suture pattern circling the gastrostomy tube placement (**Figure 2**). After the gastropexy sutures are placed, gentle traction is applied to the external end of the tube to ensure the stomach is adjacent to the abdominal wall (**Figure 3**). A rubber flange, which is slid down the tube to rest lightly against the skin, is sutured to the skin to secure the tube in place.

Potential risks with this procedure are the same as with any celiotomy and include wound infection, peritonitis and dehiscence. Pressure necrosis of the stomach may also occur if excessive tension is placed on the pursestring sutures. Wrapping the intraperitoneal tube with the omentum should contain leakage to a localized site. A layer of greater omentum can also be placed over the ostomy site before the stab incision is made into the stomach.

Percutaneous gastrostomy tube placement with gastropexy using a large-bore stiff plastic stomach tube has also been described. This technique is less invasive than the technique described here and may be more convenient for some veterinary practitioners.

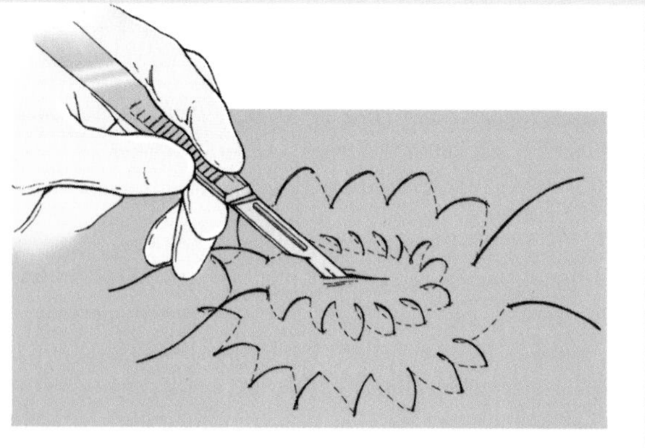

Figure 1. Two full-thickness pursestring sutures are placed concentrically around the selected gastrostomy site to help invert the stomach around the tube. A stab incision is made in the center of the suture pattern for tube placement.

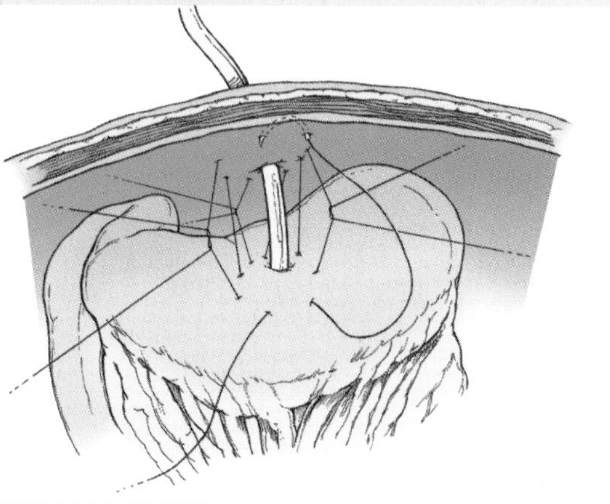

Figure 2. The stomach is sutured to the abdominal wall with four preplaced mattress sutures (or a simple continuous pattern). These sutures should include the strong abdominal fascia and the gastric submucosa. Tightening the loops brings the gastric serosa and omentum snugly in contact with the peritoneum.

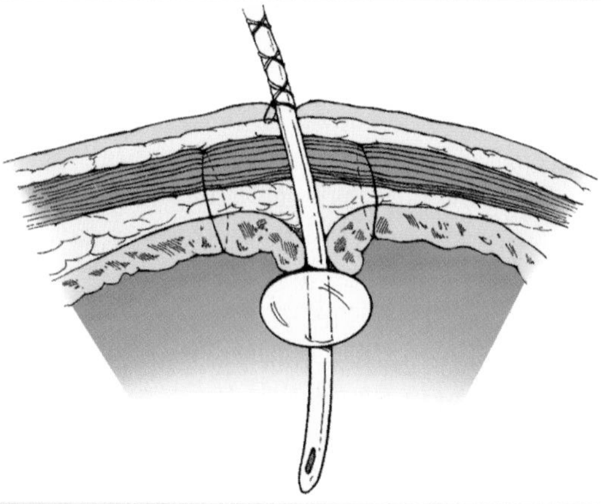

Figure 3. A mushroom-tip Pezzer catheter or one with an inflatable bulb is placed in the stomach. After the gastropexy sutures are placed, gentle traction is applied on the external end of the tube to ensure this area of the stomach is adjacent to the abdominal wall.

nosed with colitis that has a history of chronic renal insufficiency will require a feeding plan compatible with both diseases. Alternatively, the patient may be fed the food it was accustomed to eating before the injury or illness. The latter approach reduces the number of food changes that ultimately will need to be made.

Food selection will also depend on tube size and location within the GI tract, the availability and cost of products and the experience of the clinician. Commercial foods available for enteral use in veterinary patients can be divided into two major types: 1) liquid or modular products and 2) blended pet foods. Nasal and jejunostomy tubes usually have a small diameter (<8 Fr.), which requires use of liquid foods. Orogastric, pharyngostomy, esophagostomy and gastrostomy tubes have large diameters (>8 Fr.) and are suitable for blended pet foods.

Liquid Foods and Modules

Liquid foods consist of two basic types: 1) elemental or monomeric and 2) polymeric. Commercially available foods defined as "elemental" are not truly elemental, but contain nutrients in small hydrolyzed absorbable forms and are best described as monomeric. Protein requirements are usually met by free amino acids, dipeptides or tripeptides or larger hydrolyzed protein fractions. The fat source is often an oil of mixed (medium- and long-chain) fatty acids and the carbohydrate sources are mono-, di- and trisaccharides. Several liquid enteral feeding products on the human medical market are positioned as monomeric or hydrolyzed foods. They range between 270 to 550 mOsm/l and vary in protein and fat content based on the disease-specific formulation. These monomeric products are homogenized liquids that can be fed through any feeding tube including a J-tube. Monomeric foods are indicated in disease conditions such as inflammatory bowel disease, lymphangiectasia, refeeding parvoviral enteritis and pancreatitis cases and any other condition in which a patient's digestive capabilities are impaired. Most human liquid foods are adequate for adult dogs but are too low in protein for cats, puppies and adult dogs with increased protein losses (e.g., protein-losing enteropathies, drains). Most human liquid enteral products do not contain adequate concentrations of protein, taurine, arginine and arachidonic acid for long-term feeding of cats.

Polymeric products contain mixtures of more complex (less refined) nutrients. Protein is supplied in the form of large peptides (e.g., casein or whey). Carbohydrates are usually supplied as cornstarch or syrup, and fats are provided by medium-chain triglycerides (MCT) or vegetable oil. These foods require normal digestive function and are appropriate for most veterinary clinical situations, especially when a small tube (<8 Fr.) has been placed. In comparison to the rather vast selection of human polymeric diets, diets formulated for small animal veterinary patients are limited. Currently there are two liquid polymeric veterinary foods[g,h] that meet the current AAFCO nutrient allowances for adult dogs and cats. They are homogenized liquids providing between 1 to 1.25 kcal/ml, and one of these products[g] contains supplemental glutamine and carnitine.

Table 25-7. Example using enteral-assisted feeding guidelines.

Patient data needed	Canine patient example
1. Current body weight	12 kg
2. Calculate resting energy requirement (RER) as kcal/day	451 kcal/day
3. Expected daily fluid volume in ml/kg/day	60 ml/kg
4. Size (Fr.) and volume capacity of feeding tube	18-Fr., E-tube (10-ml volume)
Food information needed:	
Determine the caloric density of the food or food blend. Liquid foods have a set caloric density (kcal/ml) provided on the product information sheet. Moist foods need to be blended with a liquid (water or liquid food) to make a gruel (food blend) that can be delivered through a feeding tube or syringe.	
1. Determine gruel caloric density:	
Identify kcal per can of food	569 kcal/12.7 oz. can
Calculate ml/can (XX oz. in can x 30 ml/oz.); assumes 30 ml/weight/oz.	12.7 oz. x 30 = 383 ml
Determine ml of fluid needed to blend with canned food	100 ml warm water
Determine caloric density of fluid if not water*	–
Calculate caloric density of food blend. kcal/ml = (total kcal ÷ total ml)	569 ÷ (383 + 100) = 1.2 kcal/ml
2. Determine water provided in food or food blend:	
Calculate water in canned food (ml x % moisture); 75% moisture in canned food obtained from product information sheet	383 x 75% = 287 ml
Calculate water in liquid if not water**	–
Calculate % water in blend (ml total water ÷ total ml)	(287 + 100) ÷ 483 = 79%
3. Provide a feeding protocol:	
Method of food delivery (bolus feeding or constant rate infusion)	bolus
Beginning feeding rate (x % of RER)	25% RER
Daily caloric intake goal (kcal/day)***	113 kcal/day
Daily feeding rate	–
Calculate amount (kcal/day ÷ kcal/ml of food blend)	113 kcal ÷ 1.2 kcal/ml = 94 ml food blend/day
Determine meals/day (per 24 hr)	4
Determine feeding dosage (ml/meal/day)	94 ml ÷ 4 meals = 24 ml/meal; therefore, 24 ml q6hr
Water provided by food or food blend/day (ml)	94 ml x 79% = 74 ml water
Flush required after food delivery (ml)	4 x 10 ml flush = 40 ml water
Additional water needed to meet daily fluid volume (daily requirement = 60 ml/kg)	720 ml/day – (74 + 40) = 606 ml
Provide guidelines for residuals (see text)	–
Provide monitoring guidelines (see text)	–
Tube maintenance and removal guidelines (see text)	–

*If blending the canned food with a commercial liquid food, these foods provide a caloric density greater than 0. Determine the liquid food's caloric density and plug it into the top half of the equation. The caloric density can range between 0.8 to 1.9 kcal/ml depending on the commercial product.

**Every liquid food is part solids and part water, find this information about the product and calculate the absolute water contribution to the food blend, or assume the liquid food to be 100% water, if moisture content is 90% or greater.

***Increase this rate as tolerated by the patient or with a feeding goal to meet the patient's RER by Day 2 or 3.

Box 25-9. Percutaneous Endoscopic Gastrostomy Tubes.

Percutaneous endoscopic gastrostomy (PEG) tubes are inserted with the aid of general anesthesia. The patient is placed in right lateral recumbency and an area of the left flank extending 4 to 6 inches caudal to the last rib is surgically prepared. **Figures 1** to **7** describe tube placement technique in detail. Landmarks for feeding tube placement are usually 1 to 2 cm caudal to the last rib and one-third the distance from the ventral border of the epaxial musculature to the ventral midline. Commercial PEG catheter assembly kits, ranging in size from 16 to 28 Fr., are now available for small animal patients and provide cost-effective, convenient materials for PEG tube placement (**Figure 4**).

Following insertion, the tube is usually incorporated into a light bandage, with the free end brought to a convenient position for feeding. PEG tubes should be left in place for a minimum of five to seven days. Firm adhesions between the gastric serosa and the peritoneum have been reported to form within 36 to 48 hours of PEG tube placement in healthy dogs but do not reliably form in healthy cats. Adhesion formation may also be variable in undernourished animals.

The stomach should be empty when the tube is removed. Sedation or anesthesia is not generally required for tube extraction. Tubes are removed by exerting firm traction on the tube, while simultaneously applying counter-pressure around the exit site (**Figure 8**). An alternative method of removal, suitable for dogs weighing more than 10 kg, is to cut the catheter off flush with the skin, leaving the catheter tip to be passed in the feces. The resulting gastrocutaneous fistula usually heals rapidly.

Complications of PEG tube placement include vomiting, peristomal skin infection, cellulitis and pressure necrosis at the tube exit site.

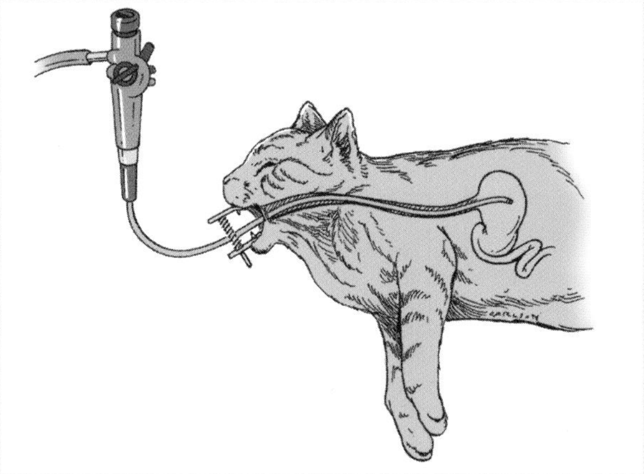

Figure 1. The animal is positioned in right lateral recumbency and an endoscope is introduced. The stomach is insufflated with air so that the gastric wall comes in contact with the body wall and the spleen is displaced caudally.

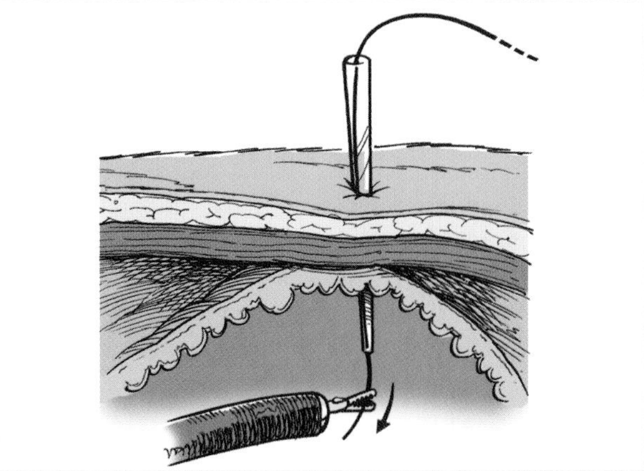

Figure 3. Nylon suture is advanced through the needle or catheter until it can be grasped with endoscopic retrieval forceps. The suture material is pulled out through the mouth as the endoscope is withdrawn.

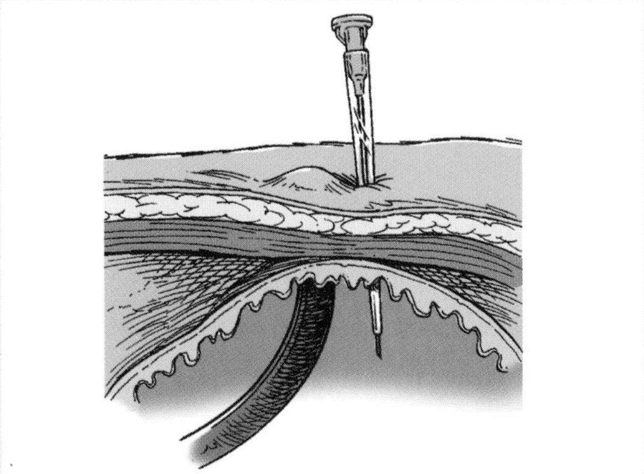

Figure 2. The lighted tip of the endoscope will be seen pressing outward against the abdominal wall. A large-bore needle or over-the-needle intravenous catheter is inserted into the stomach adjacent to the endoscope tip.

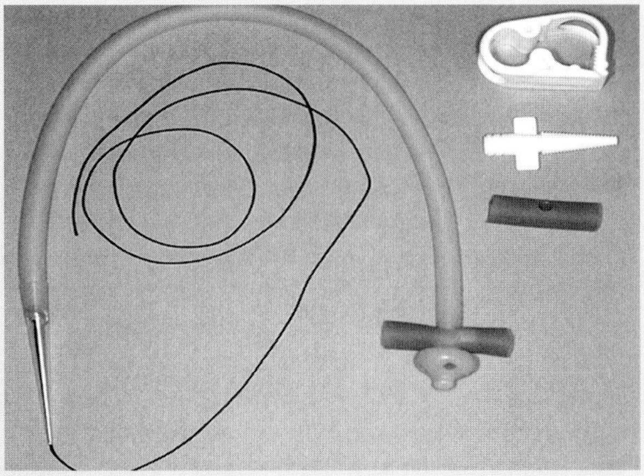

Figure 4. Commercial PEG catheter assembly kits provide the most convenient materials for PEG tube placement. The catheter guide is already secured to the free end of the feeding tube in commercial kits.

These products are usually accepted better than human liquid products containing MCT oil. In most critical care veterinary cases, these liquid foods are the best option currently available in North America when small-diameter nasogastric and jejunostomy feeding tubes have been placed, or when continuous drip feedings are necessary.

Liquid milk replacer products are generally inappropriate to feed to adult dogs and cats because they typically contain some lactose, have high (>300 mOsm/l) osmolarity and some are low in caloric density (<1.0 kcal/ml), which can result in RER constraints due to volume limitations.

Module products are concentrated powdered or liquid forms of nutrients and are primarily supplemental (**Table 25-10**). These products may be added to a liquid product to increase the concentration of a specific nutrient. Protein, fat and carbohydrate modules (e.g., casein powder, vegetable oil or corn syrup) are available. For example, a modular protein product may be added to a human liquid product for a patient with a high protein requirement. A vegetable oil or menhaden-fish oil can be added to increase omega-6 and/or omega-3 fatty acids. Soluble fiber (e.g., psyllium husk fiber or pectin) can be added to modular products, but requires greater than an 8-Fr. tube due to the increased viscosity of the food.

Blended Pet Foods

The term blended pet foods refers to commercial products that are nutritionally complete and balanced according to AAFCO allowances for dogs and cats. Moist veterinary therapeutic foods are available with nutrient profiles that assist in the management of various disease conditions in dogs and cats. Requirements for all other nutrients need not be calculated when the food contains non-energy nutrients properly balanced to the caloric density of the product. When the patient consumes the proper amount of a balanced food, all other

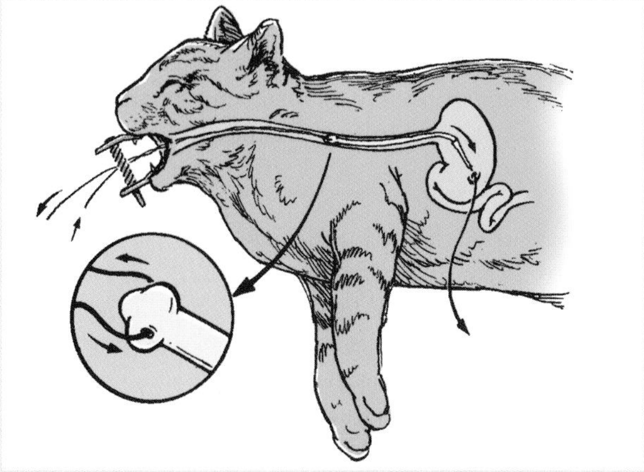

Figure 5. The lubricated catheter is drawn down the esophagus as the suture exiting the body wall is pulled. A second "safety" suture is placed through the openings in the mushroom-tip feeding tube (insert) and exits the mouth. This safety suture is used to retrieve the feeding tube from the stomach if problems occur during the placement procedure.

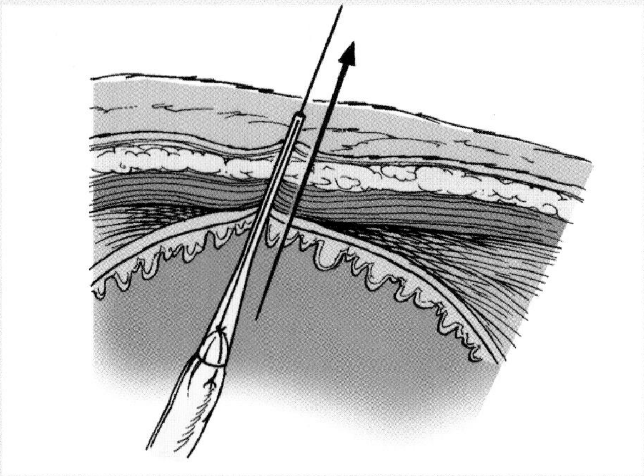

Figure 6. Resistance will be encountered when the catheter tip guide contacts the body wall. Steady traction and firm application of counter-pressure to the body wall will allow the guide tip to emerge through the skin (arrow). A small skin incision (2 to 3 mm) at the point of exit may help.

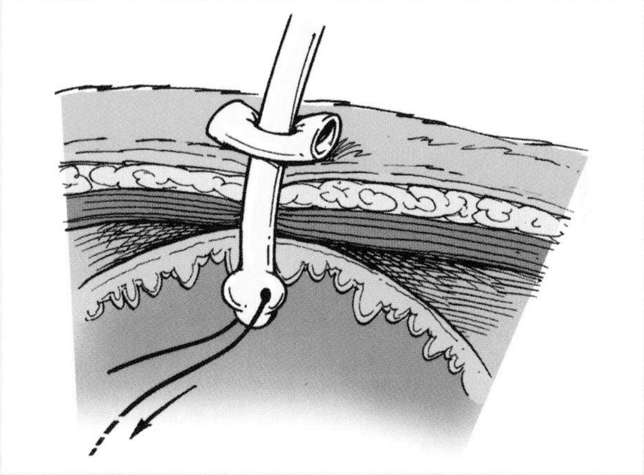

Figure 7. Gentle traction is used to bring the stomach and abdominal wall into loose contact. A rubber flange is fitted down the tube and a piece of tape attached to prevent tube slippage. The tube is not usually sutured or glued to the skin. The safety suture is removed via the mouth (arrow) after the feeding tube is secured.

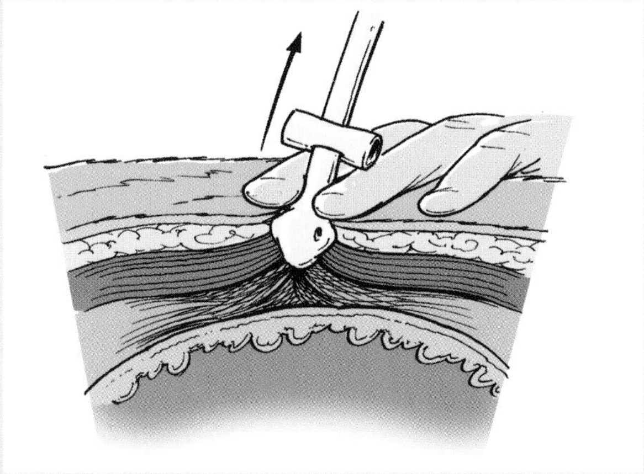

Figure 8. PEG tubes are usually removed by traction. The mushroom tip will usually collapse as it pulls through the abdominal wall. The resulting gastrocutaneous fistula usually heals rapidly.

Box 25-10. Percutaneous Nonendoscopic Gastrostomy Tubes.

Percutaneous gastrostomy techniques have been developed to allow convenient, cost-effective placement of feeding tubes without relying on availability of relatively expensive endoscopes. One nonendoscopic technique uses a commercial feeding tube applicator device (**Figure 1**) as described in **Box 25-7**. The other nonendoscopic technique uses a commercial gastrostomy tube placement device (**Figure 2**) pressed against the stomach wall. Use of either device allows suture material to be placed through the body wall into the stomach and retrieved through the mouth, and a gastrostomy tube to be inserted as described for PEG tube placement.

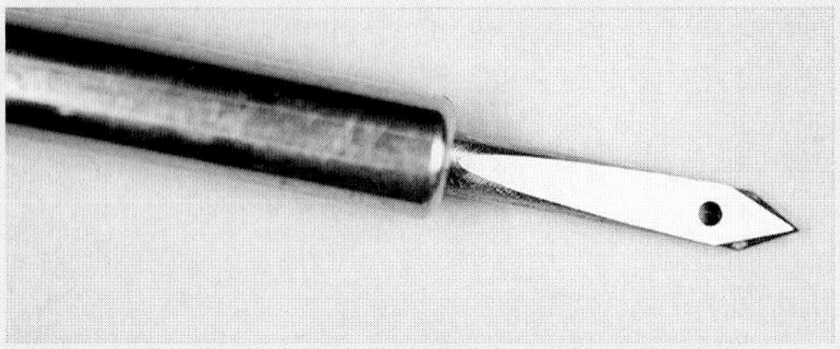

Figure 1. A commercial gastrostomy tube applicator can be used for percutaneous nonendoscopic gastrostomy tube placement in dogs and cats. The rigid outer tube encloses a trocar that can be pushed through the stomach and abdominal wall. A suture is placed through the small hole in the trocar tip, pulled into the stomach and then pulled antegrade out through the mouth. See **Box 25-7**, **Figure 1** for use of this device in esophagostomy tube placement.

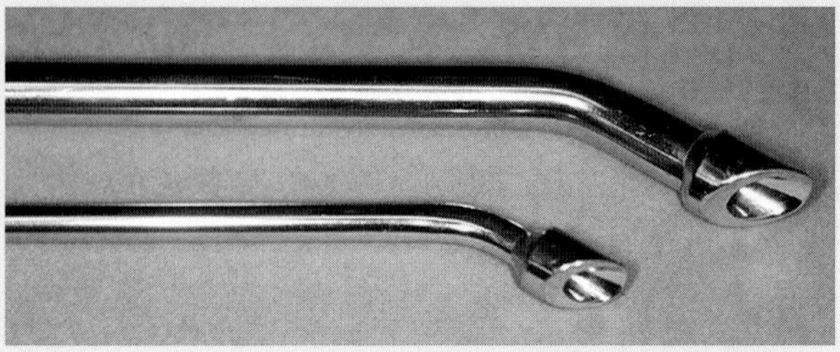

Figure 2. Commercial gastrostomy tube placement devices in various lengths and diameters can be used for percutaneous nonendoscopic gastrostomy tube placement in dogs and cats.

nutrient needs have been met, except when known losses of particular nutrients occur (e.g., protein and electrolytes).

Commercial products used as blended pet foods should provide complete and balanced nutrition for dogs or cats and should have passed AAFCO or equivalent feeding trials. These products are more readily available, better tolerated and less expensive than the human liquid foods. These pet food products contain essential amino acids and micronutrients properly balanced to the caloric density of the food. Fewer medical complications (e.g., diarrhea, hyperglycemia) are likely to result with blended pet foods. However, blended products are more likely to plug the feeding tube if the tube is not properly flushed after feeding and/or the blend is not of appropriate consistency to flow through the feeding tube. Patients may later consume the pet food orally, eliminating a food change when the patient's appetite returns and the tube has been removed. Blended pet foods, particularly the "recovery," "growth" or "performance" type foods, are appropriate for patients in catabolic states that are using fat and protein substrates from body stores.

These foods can be blended with a liquid to form a diet with a consistency that flows easily through a feeding tube. Some products have a blended texture, a high water content and very small particle size and may not need to be mixed with water or can easily be mixed with water depending on the size of the feeding tube. Most moist pet foods must be mechanically blenderized with water (or an appropriate liquid food) and strained to produce slurries or gruels that are administered through medium- and large-bore feeding tubes (i.e., 14 Fr. or larger). **Table 25-11** summarizes food blends commonly used for critical care tube feeding of feline and canine patients. Examples of patients that may benefit from these blended therapeutic formulas include those with renal or hepatic insufficiencies, diabetes mellitus, hyperlipidemia, pancreatitis, congestive heart disease and severe trauma. Appropriate moist foods are listed in the respective disease chapters.

Human Baby Foods

Some canine and feline patients voluntarily eat human baby foods packed in jars. In general, the meat and/or egg baby foods are high in protein (30 to 70% DM) and fat (20 to 60% DM), which, at the lower end of these ranges compares favorably with blended pet food products used for patients with increased protein and calorie needs. However, baby foods that provide upwards of 45% DM protein and 35% DM fat exceed the upper limits of veterinary critical care foods and would have little clinical value. Additionally, baby foods contain only one or two food types (protein, protein/grain) and do not contain a balanced mixture of other essential nutrients (amino acids, vitamins and minerals). For example, these products contain only 10% of the calcium required by dogs and cats and, therefore, have a large inverse calcium-phosphorus ratio. Some products contain onion powder, which can cause Heinz body formation in cats (Robertson et al, 1997). The human and veterinary liquid products have a better nutritional profile for feline and canine patients than do the human baby food products.

REASSESSMENT

Regular reassessment is a critical step in successful nutritional management of hospitalized patients, regardless of whether the enteral route, the parenteral route or both are used. Malnutrition in the form of insufficient nutrient intake to support tissue metabolism undermines medical and/or surgical management of a case. Malnutrition is far more common in veterinary patients than is currently recognized. Patients resting in a cage have been mistakenly assumed to require little or no nutrition when, in fact, the nutrient costs of tissue repair,

Table 25-8. Key nutritional factor content of selected commercial veterinary liquid foods, human liquid foods and moist veterinary foods used for enteral-assisted feeding of critically ill dogs compared to key nutritional factor recommended levels.*

Factors	Osmolarity (mOsm/l)	Energy density (kcal/ml)	CHO (g)	Protein (g)	Arginine (mg)	Glutamine (mg)	Fat (g)
Recommended levels	**250-400****	**1-2*****	**2-4**	**5-12**	**≥146**	**≥500**	**5-7.5**
Liquid veterinary products							
Abbott CliniCare Canine/Feline Liquid Diet	315	1.0	6.8	8.2	350	815	5.1
Abbott CliniCare RF Liquid Diet	235	1.0	5.9	6.3	350	615	6.8
PetAg Formula V Enteral Care HLP	312	1.2	4.2	8.5	413	na	4.8
PetAg Formula V Enteral Care MLP	256	1.1	5.8	7.5	392.6	na	5.7
Liquid human products							
Glucerna Shakes	355	1.0	9.6	4.2	na	na	5.4
Nestlé Impact Advanced Recovery	375	1.0	13.2	5.6	1,250	na	2.7
Nestlé Peptamen AF	390	1.2	8.9	6.3	na	na	4.6
Novartis Resource Diabetic	300	1.1	10.0	6.3	na	na	4.7
Moist veterinary foods†							
Hill's Prescription Diet a/d Canine/Feline	-	1.2	3.2	9.2	495	1,077	6.3
Hill's Prescription Diet n/d Canine	-	1.6	3.7	7.0	544	na	6.1
Iams Veterinary Formula Maximum-Calorie Canine & Feline	-	2.1	2.2	7.2	534	940	6.4
Purina Veterinary Diets Cardiovascular (CV) Feline Formula	-	1.4	4.7	8.8	469	1,169	5.5
Purina Veterinary Diets Dietetic Management (DM) Feline Formula	-	1.2	1.7	11.9	568	1,825	5.0
Royal Canin Veterinary Diet Feline and Canine Recovery RS	-	1.0	1.9	12.3	683	na	7.7

Key: CHO = digestible carbohydrate, na = information not available from the manufacturer.
*Liquid and moist veterinary foods in this table are formulated to meet minimum requirements of the Association of American Feed Control Officials; all nutrient values = units/100 kcal, unless otherwise stated; to convert kcal to kJ, multiply kcal by 4.184.
**250 is optimal.
***Energy density as fed basis.
†**Table 25-11** contains recipes for blending these foods for tube feeding.

immunocompetence and drug metabolism are significant. Therefore, reassessment of nutritional status is important whether the patient remains in the hospital or recovers at home.

Monitoring Parameters

Food intake or administration of nutritional support for hospitalized patients should be reviewed at least daily. Body weight should be recorded daily. Body condition should be noted; however, a patient's BCS is unlikely to change during the course of a hospital stay. Laboratory assessments specific for patients receiving nutritional support are generally not necessary beyond those tests already routinely performed for critically ill patients. The most common alterations that occur in laboratory parameters associated with nutrient administration are decreases in serum potassium, phosphate and magnesium levels, increases in serum glucose concentrations and hyperlipidemia. Even apparently stable patients might develop metabolic complications as a result of ongoing disease processes or from undiagnosed subclinical disease states. However, most patients show subjective improvement in attitude within 36 hours of refeeding.

Most parameters used to assess the nutritional status of patients will not change as a result of assisted feeding during the course of hospitalization. Laboratory parameters (e.g., albumin and total protein concentrations, RBC count and hemoglobin content) are unlikely to change in less than two weeks. Perhaps laboratory parameters that change during a hospital stay as a result of assisted feeding may be detected when acute-phase proteins with half-lives between two and 12 hours can be measured reliably in dogs and cats. The patient's body weight and condition and some laboratory parameters (albumin and total protein concentrations) should improve over the course of weeks (McAdams et al, 1996).

Residual Volume

Despite the numerous benefits of initiating enteral nutrition to hospitalized patients soon after admission, many critically ill patients are frequently intolerant of intragastric feeding due to GI motility dysfunction. The incidence of intolerance in human ICU settings is 43 to 63%, with the development of high gastric residual volumes accounting for 30 to 51% of cases (MacLaren et al, 2008). Although undocumented for veterinary patients, high gastric residual volume due to decreased GI motility is commonly encountered when refeeding. Adverse consequences for the patient include underfeeding needed calories, possible aspiration, increased mortality and prolonged hospital stay. Current therapeutic approaches for managing elevated gastric residual volumes involve administration of a prokinetic agent, alteration of the enteral feeding regimen (i.e., decreased volume, increased frequency, switch from intragastric to postpyloric site), or initiation of parenteral nutrition support. To maximize enteral support and limit complications associated with gastric residuals, measure the residual volume before each bolus tube feeding and intermittently during CRI feeding, then adjust the feeding schedule accordingly. Based on clinical experience, the authors suggest these

Table 25-9. Key nutritional factor content of selected commercial veterinary liquid foods, human liquid foods and moist veterinary foods used for enteral-assisted feeding of critically ill cats compared to key nutritional factor recommended levels.*

Factors	Osmolarity (mOsm/l)	Energy density (kcal/ml)***	CHO (g)	Protein (g)	Arginine (mg)	Glutamine (mg)	Fat (g)
Recommended levels	**250-400****	**1-2**	**2-4**	**7.5-12**	**≥250**	**≥500**	**5-7.5**
Liquid veterinary foods							
Abbott CliniCare Canine/Feline Liquid Diet	315	1.0	6.8	8.2	350	815	5.1
Abbott CliniCare RF Liquid Diet	235	1.0	5.9	6.3	350	615	6.8
PetAg Formula V Enteral Care HLP	312	1.2	4.2	8.5	413	na	4.8
PetAg Formula V Enteral Care MLP	256	1.1	5.8	7.5	392.6	na	5.7
Liquid human foods							
Glucerna Shakes	355	1.0	9.6	4.2	na	na	5.4
Nestlé Impact Advanced Recovery	375	1.0	13.2	5.6	1,250	na	2.7
Nestlé Peptamen AF	390	1.2	8.9	6.3	na	na	4.6
Novartis Resource Diabetic	300	1.1	10.0	6.3	na	na	4.7
Moist veterinary foods†							
Hill's Prescription Diet a/d Canine/Feline	-	1.2	3.2	9.2	495	1,077	6.3
Iams Veterinary Formula Maximum-Calorie Canine & Feline	-	2.1	2.2	7.2	534	940	6.4
Purina Veterinary Diets Cardiovascular (CV) Feline Formula	-	1.4	4.7	8.8	469	1,169	5.5
Purina Veterinary Diets Dietetic Management (DM) Feline Formula	-	1.2	1.7	11.9	568	1,825	5.0
Royal Canin Veterinary Diet Feline and Canine Recovery RS	-	1.0	1.9	12.3	683	na	7.7

Key: CHO = digestible carbohydrate, na = information not available from the manufacturer.
*Liquid and moist veterinary foods in this table are formulated to meet minimum requirements of the Association of American Feed Control Officials; all nutrient values = units/100 kcal, unless otherwise stated; to convert kcal to kJ, multiply kcal by 4.184.
**250 is optimal.
***Energy density as fed basis.
†**Table 25-11** contains recipes for blending these foods for tube feeding.

Table 25-10. Modules for augmenting foods.

Products	Key features
Arginine (various)	Available OTC as 500-mg capsules in most pharmacies and health food stores
Corn syrup (various)	Mostly maltose, 2.9 kcal/ml
Glutamine (various)	Available as powder from chemical catalogs and most pharmacies and health food stores; check label for concentration
Medium-chain triglyceride oil (Mead Johnson)	Fractionated coconut oil, 8.3 kcal/ml
Pectin (various)	Available OTC as a powder containing <1% crude protein and ~90% soluble fiber
ProMod (Ross Laboratories)	23.6 g protein/100 kcal, 18.2 g glutamine/100 g powder, 1.48 kcal/ml reconstituted
Psyllium fiber (FiberAll Regular, Rydelle Labs)	Available OTC as a powder containing 8% crude protein, 85% total dietary fiber, 72% soluble fiber
Psyllium fiber (Metamucil Regular, Searle)	Available OTC as a powder containing 17% crude protein, 53% total dietary fiber, 44% soluble fiber
Taurine (various)	Available OTC as 250-mg and 500-mg tablets in most pharmacies and health food stores

Key: OTC = over the counter; to convert kcal to kJ, multiply kcal by 4.184.

guidelines for monitoring residual fluid volumes:

1. Before a scheduled food delivery, attach an appropriate size syringe to the end of the feeding tube. Gently aspirate with the syringe. If more than 20 ml/kg body weight is aspirated, discard that fluid and/or place some portion of that fluid back into the tube and skip that scheduled tube feeding. If less than 20 ml/kg body weight is aspirated, proceed with the scheduled feeding.
2. If a feeding needs to be skipped due to high residual fluid volume, recheck residual volume just before the next scheduled feeding. If less than 20 ml/kg body weight is aspirated, proceed with food delivery at the predetermined volume or at a lesser volume. Slowly work back up to the daily RER feeding amount.
3. If a feeding needs to be skipped due to high residual fluid volume and the next recheck for residual volume yields more than 20 ml/kg body weight, consider diagnostics to evaluate and/or prokinetic agents to manage the GI dysmotility. Consider alternative approaches to nutritional support for the patient.
4. Check the residual fluid volume every 12 to 24 hours when using CRI.

Changing Foods

Sometimes, the patient only needs a specific therapeutic formula for a short time and then may be fed its regular food. Changing from a therapeutic formula to an over-the-counter brand may also be done according to the short schedule in Table 1-1. Should a problem such as vomiting, diarrhea or food refusal occur, the last successful food mixture should be

Table 25-11. Recipes for blending selected commercial moist veterinary therapeutic foods in **Tables 25-8** and **25-9** for use with feeding tubes.

Feeding tube size			20 Fr.		18 Fr.		16 Fr.		14 Fr.	
Moist veterinary foods	Can size (oz.)	No. of cans	Water added (ml)	Energy density (kcal/ml)*	Water added (ml)	Energy density (kcal/ml)*	Water added (ml)	Energy density (kcal/ml)*	Water added (ml)	Energy density (kcal/ml)*
Hill's Prescription Diet a/d Canine/Feline	5.5	2	30	1.00	40	0.97	45	0.96	50	0.95
Hill's Prescription Diet n/d Canine	12.7	1	95	1.20	100	1.18	110	1.16	120	1.14
Iams Veterinary Formula Maximum-Calorie Canine & Feline	6	2	30	1.74	35	1.72	40	1.70	45	1.68
Purina Veterinary Diets Feline CV	5.5	2	100	1.04	105	1.03	110	1.01	120	0.99
Purina Veterinary Diets Feline DM	5.5	2	55	1.01	60	1.00	70	0.97	75	0.96
Royal Canin Veterinary Diet Feline and Canine Recovery RS	6	2	30	0.88	32.5	0.88	35	0.87	37.5	0.87

*Predicted as fed energy density of blended mixture.

offered for several more days before proceeding with the food change. Most pets undergo food changes with few or no detectable GI disturbances.

SUMMARY

- The major consequences of malnutrition in all patients are decreased immunocompetence, decreased tissue synthesis and repair and altered drug metabolism.
- A nutritional assessment includes a patient history, a diet history, a physical examination with special attention given to certain risk factors, body condition scoring and laboratory tests.
- Patients with a history of nausea, vomiting and diarrhea are at increased risk for malnutrition because nutrient intake and/or usage has been suboptimal for some time before admission.
- Animals use body carbohydrate, fat and protein stores to maintain blood glucose concentrations throughout the course of food deprivation, trying to maintain vital functions for as long as possible. The proportion of each stored component used varies over the course of food deprivation.
- The adaptation from the fed to the fasting state is one in which fuel use by the patient shifts from primarily a mixture of fuels to one in which the primary fuels are glycerol and fatty acids (fat).
- An understanding of the metabolic changes that occur during simple starvation is essential to understanding the underlying metabolic alterations present during anorexia with concurrent illness.
- Major electrolyte and acid-base abnormalities and blood glucose levels should be corrected or near normal before instituting either enteral or parenteral nutritional support.
- A practical goal is to begin nutritional support within 24 hours of hospitalization for the injury or illness.
- Patients with a suspected or documented food intake less than their calculated daily RER for more than three days are candidates for assisted feeding.
- The optimal target feeding for hospitalized patients is their calculated RER, realizing their actual energy requirement is likely to change over the course of the disease process through the recovery period.
- Nutritional support by an enteral, parenteral or a combination method should initially deliver sufficient calories to meet the patient's RER at its current weight, adjusted for protein and body condition. To begin feeding patients at RER is a rational and safe estimate that decreases the probability of metabolic complications.

ACKNOWLEDGMENTS

The authors and editors acknowledge the contributions of Drs. P. Jane Armstrong and Deborah J. Davenport in the previous edition of Small Animal Clinical Nutrition.

ENDNOTES

a. Impact, Novartis, Minneapolis, MN, USA.
b. Sovereign Feeding Tube. Sherwood Medical, St. Louis, MO, USA.
c. Kangaroo Enteral Feeding Tube. Sherwood Medical, St. Louis, MO, USA. KeoFeed II Feeding Tube. IVAC Corp., San Diego, CA, USA.
d. Feeding Tube. Cook Veterinary Products, Bloomington, IN, USA.
e. Pezzar Model Catheter, C.R. Bard, Inc., Covington, GA, USA.
f. Gastrostomy Tube Introduction Set. Cook Veterinary Products, Bloomington, IN, USA.
g. CliniCare. Abbott Laboratories, North Chicago, IL, USA.
h. Formula V EnteralCare, PetAg, Hampshire,IL, USA.

REFERENCES

The references for **Chapter 25** can be found at www.markmorris.org.

CASE 25-1

Gastric Tube Feeding in a Cat

Stephen D. Gilson, DVM, Dipl. ACVS
Sonora Veterinary Surgery and Oncology
Scottsdale, Arizona, USA

Patient Assessment

A two-year-old castrated male Persian cat was examined for evaluation and treatment of suspected septic peritonitis secondary to dehiscence of an intestinal anastomosis. Eight days before, the cat had been diagnosed with an intestinal intussusception. A jejunal resection (6 cm) and anastomosis had been performed. After surgery, the cat remained depressed, weak and was intermittently febrile with rectal temperatures spiking at 41.6°C (107°F).

When examined, the cat was thin (body weight 3.5 kg, body condition score 2/5), febrile (41.2°C [106.2°F]), depressed and showed signs of circulatory shock. Ten ml of purulent fluid were recovered by abdominocentesis. Microscopically, the effusion contained 99% degenerative neutrophils. Bacteria were present in large numbers.

Assess the Food and Feeding Method

The owners reported that the cat was normally fed a commercial grocery brand dry food free choice and was a hearty eater before the intussusception occurred. Except for a small meal three days after surgery, the cat had not eaten for nine days.

Questions

1. What is an appropriate treatment plan for this patient?
2. What are the key nutritional factors to consider in this anorectic cat with sepsis?
3. What feeding techniques should be considered to support this patient?

Answers and Discussion

1. Septic shock should be managed very aggressively and management should precede surgical exploration of the abdomen. Intravenous fluid therapy helps maintain cardiac output and prevents further decline in cardiopulmonary function. Vasoactive drugs may also be needed to maintain cardiac output. Electrolyte imbalances and hypoglycemia are common in patients with peritonitis and should be corrected in addition to providing intravenous fluids. Standard shock therapy with corticosteroids and bicarbonate is usually indicated. To combat sepsis, antimicrobial therapy should be started while awaiting the results of specific culture and antimicrobial sensitivity testing from samples obtained by prior centesis of the peritoneal cavity. After the patient has been stabilized, exploratory surgery is indicated to drain and lavage the abdomen, find the cause of the sepsis (probably dehiscence of the previous anastomosis) and repair the defect. Aggressive nutritional support is also indicated in an underweight, septic patient recovering from major surgery. Nutritional support will help reverse the catabolic process associated with sepsis, improve the immune response and optimize healing.
2. Key nutritional factors in this patient include energy, carbohydrate, protein, arginine, glutamine and fat. Providing these nutrients in an energy-dense formula will aid in sparing lean body mass and maintain host defenses. Palatability is another key factor in anorectic patients; foods with high concentrations of protein, fat and water are usually palatable.
3. Intestinal function should be normal unless a large portion of the intestinal tract is removed during the second surgery. Therefore, assisted feeding using enteral techniques is recommended for this patient during the postoperative period. Nasoesophageal tube feeding is a short-term option (five to 10 days), does not require sedation or general anesthesia, takes less than 10 minutes to complete and is less expensive than placing other tubes. Nasoesophageal tubes could also be used if the patient is unable to tolerate anesthesia or if surgery had to be postponed. Enteral tube placement (i.e., esophagostomy, pharyngostomy or gastrostomy tubes) during surgery would be easy, convenient and allow enteral feeding to begin early in the recovery period. A gastrostomy tube would be large enough to handle a variety of commercial foods specifically formulated for cats. The daily energy requirement (DER) in the hospital should be equal to at least resting energy requirement (RER) at the patient's current weight. The amount of food provided daily should be divided into multiple small meals. Assisted feeding should be continued until the cat is eating at least 50% of DER voluntarily for two to three days.

Progress Notes

The cat was initially treated for septic shock. An exploratory celiotomy was performed after the cat's physiologic parameters stabilized. A small dehiscence at the anastomosis site and severe secondary generalized peritonitis were found. A partial omentectomy was performed, the affected portion of small intestine was resected and healthy bowel was anastomosed. A mushroom-tipped, 18-Fr. Pezzer gastrostomy tube was placed intraoperatively and the abdomen was copiously lavaged and closed routinely.

The cat's RER was calculated to be 180 kcal/day (753 kJ/day) at its current weight of 3.5 kg (RER = $70[3.5]^{0.75}$). Feeding was begun via the gastrostomy tube six hours postsurgery. A commercial moist homogenized recovery formula (Prescription Diet a/d Canine/Feline[a]) was chosen because it is complete and balanced for cats and can be administered through a gastrostomy tube. The food was made into a gruel by blending two 5.5-oz. cans with 50 ml water. The total volume was approximately 300 ml of liquid gruel that contained approximately 300 kcal (1.26 MJ) metabolizable energy. The feeding protocol for the first 24 hours of hospitalization included six 30-ml feedings of the gruel (i.e., every four hours). The gruel was given through the gastrostomy tube over three to five minutes while the cat was monitored for signs of intolerance (i.e., nausea, discomfort and vomiting). Although no signs of intolerance were noted, the appropriate strategy to follow should they occur is to discontinue feeding and attempt to feed the patient again 60 minutes later. Ten ml of water were flushed through the tube at the end of each bolus feeding. The cat's maintenance fluid requirement was approximately 210 ml/day (60 ml/kg body weight/day). The gruel provided approximately 180 ml of fluid plus six 10-ml water flushes through the gastrostomy tube per day for a total of 240 ml of fluid per day, which adequately maintained hydration.

The feeding protocol was modified to five 35-ml feedings of the same gruel during Day 2 of hospitalization. On Day 3, the feeding protocol was modified to four 45-ml feedings of the same gruel (i.e., every six hours). No problems with intolerance occurred. Fresh food (dry recovery formula cat food) and water were offered and the cat's voluntary food intake was monitored. Gastrostomy tube feedings were continued for eight days, but were gradually reduced as the cat voluntarily ate more dry food. The gastrostomy tube was removed 14 days after surgery, the patient's previous maintenance food was reintroduced gradually over several days and the cat made an uneventful recovery.

Endnote

a. Hill's Pet Nutrition, Inc., Topeka, KS, USA.

Bibliography

Abood SK, Mauterer JV, McLoughlin MA, et al. Nutritional support of hospitalized patients. In: Slatter DJ, ed. Textbook of Small Animal Surgery, 2nd ed. Philadelphia, PA: WB Saunders Co, 1993; 63-83.

Davenport DJ. Enteral and parenteral nutritional support. In: Ettinger SJ, Feldman EC, eds. Textbook of Veterinary Internal Medicine, 4th ed. Philadelphia, PA: WB Saunders Co, 1995; 244-252.

Gilson SD. Nutritional assessment and feeding of the anorectic acute care patient. In: Enteral Nutrition: Its Performance in Recovery (monograph). Topeka, KS: Hill's Pet Nutrition, Inc., 1992; 15-27.

CASE 25-2

Jejunostomy-Tube Feeding in a Dog

Korinn E. Saker, MS, DVM, PhD, Dipl. ACVN
College of Veterinary Medicine
North Carolina State University
Raleigh, North Carolina, USA

Patient Assessment

An 11-year-old neutered male cocker spaniel was presented with a six-month history of recurrent episodes of regurgitation upon eating solid food. The dog was able to drink and eat moist food blended with water, but ingestion of dry food or solid moist food consistently resulted in regurgitation. Three years earlier, the patient had been diagnosed with an esophageal stricture and secondary megaesophagus, which had been successfully managed with esophageal dilatation, medications (sucralfate[a], cimetidine[b], metoclopramide[c]), a sequence of dietary changes (see below) and elevated feeding for two and one-half years. At that time, a gastric mass 1 cm in diameter was detected. The owner elected to monitor the mass via endoscopy every three to four months rather than to have it resected.

On physical examination, the dog was alert with a normal temperature, pulse and respiratory rate. Results of serum biochemistry analysis, complete blood count and urinalysis were normal. Although mild right-heart enlargement was noted radiographically, the pulmonary parenchyma was normal and no esophageal abnormalities were detected. The dog weighed 8.6 kg and had a body condition score of 2/5 and had lost 3 kg over the last six months. An endoscopic examination revealed pyloric hypertrophy and a marked enlargement of the gastric mass. Two gastroesophageal masses were removed during an exploratory celiotomy. Biopsy specimens were also obtained from the pylorus. The histologic diagnosis of the gastric masses was leiomyoma; however, the pylorus was histologically normal. A 5-Fr. jejunostomy tube was placed intraoperatively.

Assess the Food and Feeding Method

After the initial esophageal dilatation procedure, chronic regurgitation in this patient was initially managed using a moist slurry made from 454 g of Prescription Diet i/d Canine[d] blenderized with 340-ml water and fed in an elevated position. The dog was transitioned from the slurry to moist food, then water-soaked kibbles and finally to small dry kibbles (Iams Mini-Chunks[e], 1 to 1.5 cups/day). Neither regurgitation nor vomiting was observed for 2.5 years after esophageal dilatation.

Jejunostomy-tube feeding was initiated 12 hours postoperatively using a polymeric canine liquid food (Canine CliniCare[f]), which supplied 1.0 kcal/ml (4.2 kJ/ml) with a nutrient profile of 27.2% protein, 30.8% fat, 33.4% carbohydrate and 4.8% ash on a dry matter basis. This food was delivered via an enteral pump system for a continuous rate infusion. In addition, fluid therapy was maintained through a peripheral venous catheter.

Questions

1. After the esophageal dilatation, chronic regurgitation was initially managed in this patient using a highly digestible moist slurry fed in an elevated position. How might the feeding schedule, form and nutrient composition of the dog's food have facilitated gastric emptying during this time?
2. A polymeric liquid food supplying 1 kcal/ml (4.2 kJ/ml) with an osmolality of 230 mOsm/kg was administered through the jejunostomy tube. Calculate the dog's resting energy requirement (RER) and maintenance fluid requirement. Write the feeding orders for the continuous rate infusion of a liquid enteral food and concurrent crystalloid intravenous fluid administration to meet the patient's fluid requirement and RER.
3. Potential complications of enteral feeding include vomiting, abdominal discomfort and diarrhea. How might the general characteristics, administration and infusion rate of polymeric foods have reduced these complications?

Answers and Discussion

1. In general, smaller meals have a faster rate of gastric emptying than larger meals. Increasing the moisture content of foods increases the rate of gastric emptying, suggesting that a moist food will leave the stomach faster than dry kibble. Increasing the fat content of the food slows gastric emptying. Therefore, feeding multiple small meals of a highly digestible, moderate-fat, low-fiber moist product facilitated gastric emptying when the dog was initially presented three years ago. An elevated feeding position is indicated in the dietary management of megaesophagus to allow gravitational forces to enhance passage of food into the stomach.
2. This patient's RER was 352 kcal/day (1,473 kJ/day) (RER = $70[BW_{kg}]^{0.75}$ or $[8.6]^{0.75} \times 70$). The caloric density of the liquid diet was 1 kcal/ml (4.184 kJ/ml). To meet the daily RER, the patient must be fed 352 ml of the food every 24 hours. On Day 1, 176 ml or 50% of RER were delivered at a continuous infusion rate of 7 ml/hour. This amount supplied approximately 170 ml of the patient's daily water requirement. The volume of liquid food was increased to supply 100% of the RER on Day 2 using an infusion rate of 14 ml/hour, which supplied 352 ml of the daily water requirement. Because the maintenance fluid requirement for this patient was 516 ml/day (516 ml = 8.6 kg x 60 ml/kg body weight/day), the infusion of crystalloid intravenous fluid was reduced to 340 ml/day and 180 ml/day on Days 1 and 2 of jejunostomy-tube feeding, respectively.
3. Food digestion begins in the oral cavity as the particle size of the meal is reduced through mastication and salivary enzyme secretions. Subsequently, gastric and pancreatic secretions further breakdown dietary protein and carbohydrate to dipeptides and tripeptides and monosaccharides and disaccharides, respectively. Bile salts, phospholipids and cholesterol from the gallbladder and liver solubilize dietary fat within the intestine. Water moves into the duodenum diluting the chyme and reducing the osmolarity from 1,200 to 1,500 mOsm/l to 300 to 350 mOsm/l. Peristalsis and segmentation in the duodenum deliver small volumes of an isosmolar, water-soluble chyme to the jejunum for further digestion and absorption. The isosmolar polymeric food administered to this patient was composed of small peptides, saccharides and emulsified long-chain triglycerides. Continuous infusion of small volumes of liquid food (14 ml/hour [0.23 ml/min.]) mimicked normal physiology of the jejunum, fostering nutrient absorption and lessening the likelihood of abdominal cramping and diarrhea.

Progress Notes

Jejunostomy-tube feeding was continued for four days postoperatively. On Day 2, the dog was offered, and drank, small amounts of water. On Day 3, one tablespoon of a moderate-fat, low-fiber moist food (Prescription Diet i/d Canine) was offered every four hours. No vomiting occurred. The jejunostomy-tube infusion rate was reduced by 50% on Day 4 as the dog ate increasing amounts of the moist food. Tube feeding was discontinued and the tube removed on Day 5 postoperatively. The dog was maintained on two-thirds of a 15-oz. can of Prescription Diet i/d Canine (supplying 362 kcal/day [1,515 kJ/day]; can size at the time the case was written), divided between four meals per day until it was discharged on Day 7. The owners were instructed to feed one can (544 kcal/day [2,276 kJ/day]) of food, divided equally between three daily meals to exceed the dog's daily energy requirement (DER) of 492 kcal/day (2,058 kJ/day) (DER = $1.4 \times 70[8.6]^{0.75}$). When the patient returned for suture removal 14 days later, the owners reported that regurgitation had not occurred and the patient had gained 0.8 kg. The owners were encouraged to continue feeding the moist food until the dog had returned to its ideal body condition.

Endnotes

a. Carafate. Marion Merrell Dow, Kansas City, MO, USA.
b. Tagamet. SmithKline Beecham, Philadelphia, PA, USA.
c. Reglan. A.H. Robins Co., Richmond, VA, USA.
d. Hill's Pet Nutrition, Inc., Topeka, KS, USA.
e. The Iams Co., Dayton, OH, USA.
f. Abbott Laboratories, North Chicago, IL, USA.

Bibliography

Abood SK, Mauterer JV, Melouglinin MA, et al. Nutritional support of hospitalized patients. In: Slatter DJ, ed. Textbook of Small Animal Surgery, 2nd ed. Philadelphia, PA: WB Saunders Co, 1993; 63-83.

Guilford WG, Strombeck DR. Chronic gastric diseases. In: Guilford WG, Center S, Strombeck DR, et al, eds. Strombeck's Small Animal Gastroenterology. Philadelphia, PA: WB Saunders Co, 1996; 275-302.

Khoury TL, Borlase BC, Forse RA, et al. Early enteral feeding: A safe technique in critically ill patients. In: Borlase BC, Bell SJ, Blackburn GL, et al, eds. Enteral Nutrition. New York, NY: Chapman & Hall, Inc, 1994; 142-151.

CASE 25-3

Gastric Tube and Parenteral Feeding in a Cat

Rebecca L. Remillard, PhD, DVM, Dipl. ACVN
Angell Animal Medical Center
Boston, Massachusetts, USA

Patient Assessment

A 13-year-old spayed female domestic longhaired cat was referred to the oncology service for radiation therapy of a nasal lymphoma. The owner traveled to the U.S. from Canada with the understanding that the cat would remain in the hospital for two weeks to receive daily radiation therapy. When admitted, the cat was thin (body weight 3.1 kg, body condition score 1/5) and depressed. The cat had a low albumin 2.6 g/dl (normal = 3.1 to 4.1), hemoglobin 9.4 g/dl (normal = 10.7 to 16.6) and hematocrit 27.2% (normal = 30.6 to 48.5).

Assess the Food and Feeding Method

The cat presented with a gastrostomy tube already in place. The owners reported that the cat had been receiving 30 ml of CliniCare[a] liquid food six times daily followed by 10-ml water flushes. The feeding protocol was changed to 30 ml of Prescription Diet a/d Canine/Feline[b] slurry six times daily and radiation therapy was initiated. The a/d slurry was made by mixing 30 ml of water with one can of a/d to make a 1 kcal/ml solution.

Questions

1. Was the G-tube feeding plan appropriate for this patient using the liquid food?
2. What are the key nutritional factors to consider in this anorectic cat with cancer?
3. What particular features of the a/d slurry were advantageous to the cat's progress?

Answers and Discussion

1. The cat's resting energy requirement (RER) was 163 kcal (682 kJ). The feeding protocol of 30 ml of CliniCare (1 kcal/ml) six times daily provided the cat with 180 kcal. The initial feeding protocol was appropriate.
2. Key nutritional factors in this patient include energy, carbohydrate, protein, arginine, glutamine and fat. The provision of food should help spare lean body mass while supporting repair of tissue damage due to the tumor and radiation therapy.
3. The Prescription Diet a/d product contained appropriate key nutritional factors and omega-3 fatty acids and antioxidants to facilitate tissue repair, inhibit tumor growth and reduce tissue damage due to the oxidizing effects of radiation therapy.

Progress Notes

A nutrition consult was requested on Day 10 of therapy because although the cat had been tolerating the G-tube feedings, it was losing weight. The cat now weighed 2.1 kg. A review of the medical record revealed that although six feedings a day had been ordered, on most days the patient only received four feedings due to daily anesthesia for radiation therapy. The cat was receiving

120 kcal per day through the G-tube. At 2.1 kg, the cat's RER = 122 kcal. Therefore, the patient was understandably losing weight due to insufficient daily caloric intake.

Further Question

How should this caloric deficiency be corrected while not interfering with the anesthetic and radiation procedures?

Answer and Discussion

The daily caloric deficiency of 50 kcal was corrected by administering 20% lipid solution intravenously over the 18 hours the cat was not undergoing therapy. The dose of lipids was initiated to ensure the cat received a total of 180 kcal per day from the combined enteral and parenteral feedings until discharge.

Endnotes

a. Abbott Laboratories, North Chicago, IL, USA.
b. Hill's Pet Nutrition, Inc., Topeka, KS, USA.

Chapter 26

Parenteral-Assisted Feeding

Rebecca L. Remillard
Korinn E. Saker

"When the facts change, I change my mind. What do you do?"
John Maynard Keynes

CLINICAL IMPORTANCE

Parenteral nutrition (PN) is valuable in meeting a patient's daily resting energy and amino acid requirements. In veterinary medicine, clinicians attempt to meet the patient's estimated resting energy requirement (RER) and most immediate requirements for essential amino and fatty acids, and selected water-soluble vitamins, electrolytes (macro) and trace minerals. PN does not consistently limit disease activity in patients and therefore is an adjunct (not a primary) therapy. PN support in veterinary patients may prevent nutrient deficiencies, preserve lean body mass and support the functional capacity of most body organs when nutrient intakes fall below requirements. The overriding rationale and criteria for using PN in veterinary patients is to treat subclinical undernutrition due to three or more days of decreased appetite and to avoid the development of clinical undernutrition resulting from insufficient energy intake in the face of increased energy needs (ASPEN, 2002). **Box 26-1** describes PN nomenclature.

Patient selection is very important to the successful use of PN support. Patients with impairment of the small intestine that is unlikely to resolve within three days are candidates for PN support. PN can be used initially to meet energy and amino acid requirements for cases in which enteral access cannot be safely acquired for several days. Depending on patient size, it may not be cost effective to use PN as a method of assisted feeding for less than a three-day course. There is a substantial startup cost to preparing the parenteral solution. The procedure becomes cost effective when the cost is spread over several days or more than one patient.

There is evidence that 48 to 72 hours are required to reverse a catabolic state and begin anabolism (Zeiderman et al, 1989; Wernerman et al, 1986). Thus, proper patient selection mandates that the patient be hospitalized for at least three days because instituting PN for only one or two days is of questionable cost benefit. However, when PN is done in conjunction with enteral feeding, a course shorter than three days may be cost effective and provide nutritional benefit. PN support should not begin until the patient is hemodynamically stable and electrolyte and acid-base abnormalities, severe tachycardia, hypotension and volume deficits have been corrected (**Table 26-1**).

There are many published lists of diseases, disorders and case examples in which PN could or should be instituted. The number and type of veterinary patients that would benefit from PN is greatly expanded; however, if the goal in assisted feeding is to deliver the patient's energy and amino acid needs daily by any means (Remillard and Thatcher, 1989). Parenteral administration of nutrients has value in patients with inflammatory (small and large) bowel disease, parvoviral enteritis and other causes of impaired gastrointestinal (GI) motility, peritonitis, pancreatitis, intestinal lymphosarcoma and short-bowel syndrome (small bowel resection). Neurologic patients and those that are comatose or receiving large doses of pain-control medications that

Box 26-1. Nomenclature.

The term "parenteral nutrition (PN)" indicates administration of nutrients in a manner other than through the gastrointestinal (GI) tract. PN could therefore be administration by intravenous, intramuscular, subcutaneous, intraosseous or intraperitoneal routes. PN has been further characterized in human medicine as total or partial (relative to meeting all nutrient requirements) and central or peripheral (relative to venous access). A common misnomer associated with PN, originally from the human literature, is the term "hyperalimentation." This term incorrectly implies the administration of nutrients via the GI tract in excess of need. The term "parenteral nutrition" is used throughout this text because it simply and accurately identifies a general method of administering nutrients to a patient.

Another common misnomer is total parenteral nutrition (TPN). In veterinary medicine, PN is not total because there is no immediate need to meet all the amino and fatty acid, fat- and water-soluble vitamin and macro, trace and ultra-trace element requirements as there is in people dependent on PN for years.

There are several valid reasons why partial PN, rather than TPN, is used in veterinary medicine. The foremost reason is the comparatively short period PN is administered to animals (three to 14 days for animals vs. weeks to years in people). In people, long-term feeding implies 10 days or longer. The shorter time frame of assisted feeding of pets allows omission of less immediately essential nutrients (e.g., fat-soluble vitamins). Until there is a demand by pet owners for a longer period of support (weeks to months), PN support in animals will remain cost effective by providing only the most immediately essential nutrients (i.e., electrolytes, energy and amino acids).

Only some of the nutrients needed by animals are readily available in water-soluble form for PN solutions. Some water-soluble nutrients are available as multiple single nutrients in specially prepared water-insoluble products. Such nutrients (vitamins A and E) are cost prohibitive and difficult to justify on a short-term basis. As more nutrient preparations are added to PN solutions, the risk for incompatibility and formation of insoluble precipitates increases. PN solutions currently used in veterinary medicine contain only the less expensive essential nutrients. PN solutions are therefore limited by necessity, pharmacokinetics, cost and current nutritional knowledge.

Table 26-1. Patient criteria for administration of parenteral nutrition.

1. The patient is hemodynamically stable and major electrolyte and acid-base abnormalities, severe tachycardia, hypotension and volume deficits have been corrected.
2. Actual or anticipated food intake is less than calculated resting energy requirement for more than three days.
3. Concurrent small intestinal disorder is known or suspected to be present, or a safe enteral nutritional access cannot be established.
4. The patient is expected to be hospitalized for at least the next three days.

cause lateral recumbency with questionable swallowing reflexes and/or risk of aspiration when oral or tube feedings are attempted also benefit from PN. PN has been used successfully in complicated cases of feline hepatic lipidosis, in patients with facial fractures, pneumonia, lung lobe torsion or contusion and diaphragmatic hernias, and in other patients that are poor anesthetic risks.

PN can be administered until patients are more stable and can tolerate placement of a feeding tube. Septic and anemic patients and those with severe upper respiratory infections that cause persistently poor appetites may benefit from PN. Sometimes PN support may be as simple as augmenting oral intake with intravenous lipids to meet RER. Patients with a poor appetite that also have large heat and/or protein losses (e.g., continuous-suction chest or abdominal drains, large areas of skin loss due to burns, degloving injuries) benefit from PN in addition to voluntary oral food intake.

The goal of assisted feeding is to provide adequate nutrition to meet the patient's RER. The logistics of that support should be determined on a case-by-case basis. The guidelines presented here are to help establish a foundation. But never underestimate the need for attentiveness, initiative and ingenuity in meeting the patient's nutritional needs; no two cases are alike.

Because enteral nutrition and PN are often used in conjunction, the reader may want to refer to Chapter 25 for information about:

- Consequences of malnutrition
- Patient assessment, including physiologic state and history of malnutrition
- Anorexia, cachexia and accommodation
- Metabolic changes through days of starvation (simple starvation and disease states)
- Key nutritional and other factors.

PARENTERAL PRODUCTS

Compounding a PN solution is beyond the scope of most veterinary practices; however, most veterinary practices can administer PN to patients. Individual dextrose, lipid and amino acid solutions can be combined as a "three-in-one" solution, also called a total nutrient admixture (TNA). TNA in veterinary medicine refers to one fluid bag containing a sufficient mixture of parenteral solutions to meet a particular patient's fluid, energy, amino acid, electrolyte and B-vitamin needs for a 24-hour period. This is a very convenient method requiring only one bag, one infusion pump and one administration set. Any opaque liquid infusion pump can be used. The formulation is designed specifically for the patient based on its current RER, daily fluid and electrolyte requirements, approximate protein need and ability to handle dextrose vs. lipid.

The TNA solution should be calculated to first meet the patient's RER and protein needs with essential water-soluble vitamins and trace mineral products (if available). The total fluid volume should then be adjusted with a standard crystal-

Table 26-2. Standard total nutrient admixture (TNA) formulations.

PART A. CALCULATION WORKSHEET	
Patient data needed	**Feline example**
1. Current body weight in kg	4.1 kg
2. Calculate resting energy requirement (RER) as kcal/day	200 kcal/day
3. Expected fluid volume in ml/kg/day	70 ml/kg
4. Calories from fat as a percent	80%
5. Protein-calorie ratio as g/100 kcal RER	4 g/100 kcal RER
6. Potassium concentration as mEq/l	30 mEq/l
Parenteral solution formula	
1. Determine volume of fat and dextrose needed daily	
Calculate RER calories from fat	200 x 0.80 = 160 kcal
Calculate volume of 20% lipid needed	160 kcal ÷ 2 kcal/ml = **80 ml/day**
Calculate RER calories from dextrose	200 - 160 = 40 kcal
Calculate volume of 50% dextrose needed	40 kcal ÷ 1.7 kcal/ml = **24 ml/day**
2. Determine volume of amino acid solution needed daily	
Calculate g of protein needed	RER x 4 g/100 kcal = 8 g protein/day
Calculate volume of 8.5% amino acid needed	8 g ÷ 0.085 g/ml = **94 ml/day**
3. Determine volume of B vitamins and trace minerals needed daily	
Calculate B vitamins needed	RER x 1 ml/100 kcal = **2 ml/day**
Calculate trace minerals needed	RER x 1 ml/100 kcal = **2 ml/day**
Daily parenteral nutrition formula	80 ml of 20% lipid emulsion 24 ml of 50% dextrose 94 ml of 8.5% amino acid with electrolytes 2 ml of vitamin-B complex 2 ml of trace elements **Total = 202 ml**
4. Determine volume of crystalloid solution needed to meet daily fluid requirement	
Daily fluid volume requested	4.1 kg x 70 ml/kg = 287 ml/day
Volume required is daily total – PN total	287 – 202 = 85 ml
5. Determine phosphorus supplementation	
Phosphorus from amino acids	94 x 30 mM/l = 2.8 mM
Desired final phosphorus concentration in the TNA	= 10 mM/l x 287 ml = 2.9 mM (no phosphorus is needed)
6. Determine potassium supplementation	
K^+ from lactated Ringer's solution	85 ml x 4 mEq/l = 0.3 mEq
K^+ from amino acid solution	94 ml x 60 mEq/l = 5.6 mEq
Total K^+ in TNA solution	0.3 mEq + 5.6 mEq = 5.9 mEq
Desired final K^+ concentration in TNA	30 mEq/l x 287 ml = 8.6 mEq
KCl (2.0 mEq/ml) required	8.6 mEq – 5.9 mEq = 2.7 mEq ÷ 2.0 = 1.4 ml
PART B. FELINE FORMULA EXAMPLE	
Animal data	
Body weight	4.1 kg
RER	200 kcal/day
Calories from fat	80%
Calories from glucose	20%
Protein-calorie ratio	4 g/100 kcal (adequate for most cats)
Fluid volume	70 ml/kg (maintenance fluid volume)
Potassium concentration	30 mEq/l
Parenteral solution	
50% dextrose	24 ml providing 41 kcal
20% lipid emulsion	80 ml providing 160 kcal
8.5% amino acids with electrolytes	94 ml providing 8 g of amino acids
Potassium chloride	1.4 ml
Vitamin-B complex	2 ml
Trace elements	2 ml
Lactated Ringer's solution	85 ml
Total fluid volume	288 ml
This final solution is a 500-ml bag containing 200 kcal (80% from fat), adequate nitrogen, major B vitamins with the following electrolyte profile	
Sodium	61.6 mEq/l
Potassium	29.5 mEq/l
Magnesium	3.3 mEq/l
Phosphorus	9.8 mM/l
Chloride	55.4 mEq/l
Calcium	0.8 mEq/l
Zinc	2 mg
Copper	1 mg
Manganese	0.2 mg

Table 26-2 continued

Chromium	8 mg
Final osmolarity	768
Approximate cost = $100 per day	
PART C. CANINE FORMULA EXAMPLE	
Animal data	
Body weight	14 kg
RER	507 kcal/day
Calories from fat	90%
Calories from glucose	10%
Protein-calorie ratio	3 g/100 kcal
Fluid volume	70 ml/kg
Potassium concentration	20 mEq/l
Parenteral solution	
50% dextrose	30 ml providing 51 kcal
20% lipid emulsion	227 ml providing 454 kcal
8.5% amino acids with electrolytes	176 ml providing 15 g of amino acids
Potassium phosphate	1.4 ml
Vitamin-B complex	5 ml
Trace elements	5 ml
NormaSol R	543 ml
Total fluid volume	987 ml
This final solution is a 1-liter bag containing 507 kcal (90% from fat), adequate nitrogen, major B vitamins with the following electrolyte profile	
Sodium	88.0 mEq/l
Potassium	20.3 mEq/l
Magnesium	3.5 mEq/l
Phosphorus	9.9 mM/l
Chloride	65.5 mEq/l
Calcium	0 mEq/l
Zinc	5 mg
Copper	2 mg
Chromium	20 mg
Manganese	0.5 mg
Final osmolarity	523 mOsm/l
Approximate cost = $100 per day	

loid solution (e.g., lactated Ringer's solution, Plasmalyte A) to meet the patient's daily fluid requirement. Then electrolytes are adjusted, if necessary (**Table 26-2**). Alternatively, crystalloid fluids with added potassium may be administered by a separate intravenous line piggybacked into the same catheter.

Energy Solutions

A TNA solution should supply sufficient energy to meet, but not exceed, the patient's daily RER. Negative consequences of PN administration (i.e., metabolic complications) are often due to administering energy in excess of the patient's expenditure (Deitel et al, 1983; Chang and Silvis, 1974; VA Study Group, 1991; Lippert et al, 1993). Early PN solutions for people contained dextrose and "liberal" amounts of protein. These solutions were administered at rates providing 3,000 to 5,000 kcal/day (12.55 to 20.92 MJ) to a 70-kg person (Solomon and Kirby, 1990). This "hyperalimentation" actually increased catabolism by exceeding the patients' endogenous usage of energy and produced multiple adverse metabolic effects. Human patients are given 1,000 to 2,400 kcal (4.2 to 10 MJ) with 75 to 100 g of protein per day with fewer metabolic complications (Woolfson, 1983). Currently, people are fed at RER instead of RER times a disease factor (McMahon, 1993; Forse, 1995; DeBiasse and Wilmore, 1994). Energy is routinely provided to veterinary patients receiving PN as a combination of dextrose and lipid. Several companies manufacture dextrose and lipid products of various strengths and attributes (**Table 26-3**). Most TNA solutions formulated for veterinary patients use 50% dextrose and 20% lipid. Dextrose solutions range from 2.5 to 70% glucose, which is usually derived from hydrolyzed cornstarch. Osmolarity ranges from 126 to 3,530 mOsm/l and is directly proportional to the glucose concentration (AHFS Drug Information, 1997). Dextrose solutions are maintained in the pH range of 3.5 to 5.5 and are sterilized by autoclave to prolong shelf life at room temperature.

Lipid (10, 20 or 30%) products (**Table 26-3**) contain emulsified fat particles (0.5 mm) of soybean oil and/or safflower oil, glycerin and linoleic and linolenic acids. Earlier formulations made with cottonseed oil were taken off the market in 1965 because they caused severe adverse reactions in people. Lipid emulsions are maintained in a pH range of 6.0 to 8.9 and have an osmolarity range of 260 to 310 mOsm/l, which effectively decreases the final osmolarity of the TNA (AHFS Drug Information, 1997). Dextrose and lipids are readily available and both are strongly recommended as sources of energy in a TNA solution.

Table 26-3. Nutritional comparison of parenteral products.

Products	Caloric density (kcal/ml)	Osmolarity (mOsm/l)	Amino acids (g/100 ml)	Fat (g/100 ml)	Carbohydrate (g/100 ml)	Electrolytes (kcal/ml)	Comments
Amino acids 8.5% without electrolytes	na	785-860	8.5	0	0	Few	Contains all essential amino acids except taurine, nitrogen 1.3 g/100 ml, pH 5.3-6.5, available in 500- and 1,000-ml sizes.
Amino acids 8.5% with electrolytes	na	1,160	8.5	0	0	Yes	Contains all essential amino acids except taurine, nitrogen 1.3 g/100 ml, pH 5.3-6.5, electrolytes Na, K, Mg, Cl, PO_4, available in 500- and 1,000-ml sizes.
ProcalAmine	0.25	735	3	0	3	Yes	Contains 3% glycerol and 3% amino acids, nitrogen 4.6 g/1,000 ml, pH 6.5-7.0, electrolytes Na, K, Mg, Cl, PO_4, available in 500- and 1,000-ml sizes. Contains 13 nonprotein kcal/ml and 22.5 g amino acids/100 nonprotein kcal as is. Mix 775 ml ProcalAmine with 300 ml 20% lipid to get 1,075 ml of a 3.2 g protein/100 nonprotein kcal solution.
Lipid 10%	1.1	268	0	10	0	No	Contains soybean and/or safflower oil, glycerin, linoleic and linolenic acids, egg yolk as phospholipid emulsifier, pH 6.0-8.9, available in 50-, 100-, 250- and 500-ml sizes.
Lipid 20%	2	268	0	20	0	No	Contains soybean and/or safflower oil, glycerin, linoleic and linolenic acids, egg yolk as phospholipid emulsifier, pH 6.0-8.9, available in 50-, 100-, 250- and 500-ml sizes.
Dextrose 2.5-70%	0.09-2.4	126-3,535	0	0	2.5-70	No	Contains hydrolyzed (various) cornstarch, pH 3.5-5.5, available in 50- and 500-ml sizes.

Key: na = not available.

Dextrose-Fat Ratio

When PN is begun, most patients have not consumed their daily RER for at least three days, and are more likely even further along in the course of food deprivation (Day 5 or more). The proportion of glucose to lipid in the PN solution should mirror the current metabolic condition of the liver. Fewer metabolic complications will arise if the liver tolerates the glucose-lipid ratio in the PN solution.

PN is rarely instituted during the early phases of food deprivation (fewer than three days of anorexia); however, if PN is indicated, canine patients should tolerate a moderate percentage of their calculated RER as dextrose. For example, dogs in

Box 26-2. Complications of Fat Administration.

LIVER PATHOLOGY

Administering parenteral total nutrient admixture (TNA) solutions to human adults and infants for long periods (weeks to months) has been reported to cause steatosis, intrahepatic cholestasis, periportal inflammation and even cirrhosis. Fatty infiltration of the liver is the earliest and most common change noted. This undesirable relationship between long-term parenteral feeding and hepatic changes is thought to be multifactorial, but is not yet well understood. These complications are not specific to parenteral nutrition (PN) or lipid emulsions. Lipid additions are now encouraged, even in patients with hepatic disease, because replacing a portion of the glucose with lipid ameliorates some hepatic pathology. Choline is not routinely included in TNA solutions but is a conditionally essential nutrient in people. Studies have correlated choline deficiency and hepatic steatosis in people receiving total parenteral nutrition (TPN). Investigators studying TPN-fed rats reported reversal of hepatic complications with both oral and intravenous choline administration. Today, it is extremely rare for a veterinary patient to receive a PN solution for more than two or three weeks; therefore, hepatic complications from prolonged PN administration are unlikely, although choline is an essential nutrient in dogs and cats.

COAGULOPATHIES AND THROMBOCYTOPENIA

Lipid infusions have been reported to cause fat overload syndrome in people and, in the past, were associated with hyperlipidemia, hemolytic anemia, coagulopathies, thrombocytopenia and respiratory impairment with liver and renal dysfunction. Most adverse reports were associated with the use of a cottonseed oil emulsion, which was withdrawn from the market in the 1960s. Only isolated cases have been reported to occur with the soybean or safflower oil emulsions used today, and no cases have been associated with the relatively limited use of medium-chain triglyceride (MCT) emulsions. Thrombocytopenia has been reported as a rare complication of soybean oil emulsions and is now considered an idiosyncratic reaction. In vitro, lipids have a limited effect on shortening prothrombin times, but this effect may be due to the phospholipids or vitamin K in emulsions. Reduced aggregation of platelets has also been produced in vitro and at high triglyceride concentrations. It is important to emphasize that slow continuous infusion of lipids has little or no effect on platelet numbers, aggregation or bleeding time. Fat infusion rates for people have been recommended at 0.10 to 0.15 g/kg body weight/hour. Infusing veterinary patients with PN solutions containing 80 to 90% of nonprotein calories as lipid over a 24-hour period is usually within these guidelines.

ALTERED IMMUNE FUNCTION

Lipid infusions have also been associated with altered and impaired immune function. Major controversies exist about the role lipid emulsions play in affecting reticuloendothelial cells and eicosanoid, cytokine and complement synthesis. Many of these effects have not been observed with slow infusion of pure soybean oil or during rapid infusion of MCT emulsions. One review of many studies concluded there was no evidence supporting the opinion that lipid infusions detrimentally alter immune function.

The Bibliography for **Box 26-2** can be found at www.markmorris.org.

the early phase of food deprivation maintain blood glucose levels by glycogenolysis and therefore should receive 60 to 90% of the RER as dextrose. However, feline patients in the early phases of food deprivation maintain blood glucose levels by lipolysis and gluconeogenesis, and should receive 60 to 90% of their RER from lipid.

By Day 5 of food deprivation or longer, patients should receive the majority (60 to 90%) of their calculated RER as lipid because the liver is using glycerol from endogenous fat for gluconeogenesis. Giving high doses of glucose at a time when the patient's natural metabolic response is to minimize glucose usage is unlikely to result in optimal glucose use. This is the most likely cause of hyperglycemia. There is evidence to suggest the proportion of calories needed from fat increases greatly (>60%) in starving and diseased states. For example, in an acute sepsis model, rats given a fat-free glucose solution parenterally had increased and extensive mobilization of endogenous fat. Control, nonseptic rats had no mobilization of endogenous fat when a high glucose solution was given (Stein, 1986). A measurable shift in the preferred fuel (from glucose to endogenous fat) occurred in these septic patients. In people, fat is well oxidized in the septic state, and as the sepsis worsens the amount of fat oxidized increases and the glucose oxidative capacity decreases (Stoner et al, 1983). Dogs with a septic abdomen receiving PN with both glucose and lipid maintained nitrogen balance better than dogs receiving glucose-only PN solutions (Iriyama et al, 1985).

The optimal caloric source is a mixture of glucose and fat; however, the precise ratio is unknown (Stein, 1986). A mixed fuel source should decrease the possibility of fat deposition in the liver when any metabolic pathway that handles either fat or glucose becomes overloaded. Studies have shown that serum glucose, lactate, pyruvate, free fatty acid, triglyceride and insulin concentrations were more stable and more closely approximated the normal postabsorptive state in people when all three substrates were administered (i.e., simultaneous lipid infusion with glucose and amino acids), as opposed to fat-free PN solutions (MacFie et al, 1991). The old recommendation that fat should not compose more than 4 g/kg body weight/day or 60% of the calories has been perpetuated many times.[a] Over the last decade or so, the recommended proportion of calories from fat supplied to burn victims has progressively increased from 5 to 15 to 50%. Furthermore, higher proportions of fat calories (75 to 80%) have been recommended in other disease states (Nordenstrom et al, 1983; Chiarelli et al, 1994; Deitel and Kaminsky, 1974).

The negative effects of high-fat infusions have included reports of liver pathology, coagulopathies, thrombocytopenia,

Table 26-4. Advantages to administering a high fat total nutrient admixture (TNA) solution.

1. The liver is metabolically geared for lipolysis and preferentially uses fat as a source of calories. Therefore, supplying a high-fat solution accommodates that profile, spares endogenous fat stores and does not raise insulin levels.*
2. The osmolarity of the fat solution is 260 mOsm/l and can be administered by peripheral catheter. Fat included in a TNA solution decreases the final osmolarity:

80% calories from 50% dextrose and 20% calories from 20% lipid	= 862 mOsm/l**
20% calories from 50% dextrose and 80% calories from 20% lipid	= 535 mOsm/l**
5% dextrose and lactated Ringer's solution	= 525 mOsm/l
Blood or plasma	= ~300 mOsm/l

3. The pH of the final TNA solution that includes fat is closer to 7.0 than solutions of dextrose and amino acids excluding fat, thus imposing less of an acid load.
4. Patients with compromised pulmonary function are prone to developing respiratory acidosis when given solutions containing a high dextrose concentration. High-fat solutions produce less carbon dioxide to be expelled than high dextrose solutions.***

*Stein TP. Protein metabolism and parenteral nutrition. In: Rombeau JL, Caldwell MD, eds. Clinical Nutrition; Parenteral Nutrition, 1st ed. Philadelphia, PA: WB Saunders Co, 1986; 100-134.
**These osmolarity examples are based on a total fluid volume of 70 ml/kg body weight, 3 g protein/100 kcal resting energy requirement and 30 mEq K^+/liter.
***Askanazi J, Nordenstrom J, Rosenbaum SH, et al. Nutrition for the patient with respiratory failure: Glucose vs. fat. Anesthesiology 1981; 54: 373-377.

altered immune function, atherosclerosis and the overall unknown effect of synthetic chylomicrons on blood vessels when administered to people for more than 10 days. These adverse effects occurred in people and other animals during high infusion rates in which lipids were provided in excess of energy need (Klein and Miles, 1994; Mashima, 1979; Meguid et al, 1984; Adamkin et al, 1984). In addition, some of the products used in these studies are no longer available (**Box 26-2**).

To date, there appears to be little in the veterinary literature documenting why lipids could not or should not provide more than 60% of a dog's or cat's RER. In fact, when central venous access is limited and the patient requires fluid therapy at or below maintenance rates, administering a lipid emulsion by peripheral access (providing 100% of the caloric intake as fat) is well tolerated. The use of solutions containing high-fat concentrations (60 to 90%) has gained a wider acceptance with fewer complications as compared to those containing high-glucose concentrations. PN may be successfully administered to ferrets and rabbits using the same overall guidelines. No unusual metabolic or hematologic complications have been associated with these infusions (**Table 26-4**).

Unlike patients in earlier reports, most patients receiving high-fat solutions today do not develop hyperglycemia, based on regular urine glucose checks (VA Study Group, 1991; Lippert et al, 1993). Glycemia is better controlled in patients with diabetes mellitus, pancreatitis and septicemia when a TNA solution is used that provides most of the calories as fat. A TNA solution with 80% fat calories contains 1 to 3% dextrose. Intravenous infusion of a lipid emulsion routinely increases plasma triglyceride levels transiently. However, this should not be considered a true hyperlipidemia because most patients can clear these chylomicron-size lipid particles within 30 minutes. The half-life of chylomicrons in the plasma of dogs from either diet or intravenous infusion of soybean oil and safflower oil emulsions ranges from seven to 16 minutes (Edgren and Meng, 1962; Kesterson, 1978). Therefore, it is sometimes necessary to turn off the TNA infusion pump 20 to 30 minutes before blood is drawn if hyperlipidemia is a problem. Lipid from the TNA solution does interfere with certain serum biochemistry tests (Chapter 28).

The PN guidelines for people state that the role of intravenous artificial lipid emulsions in influencing the course of pancreatitis is not defined. Lipid emulsions are safely used in hyperlipidemic people when serum triglyceride concentrations remain below 400 mg/dl (ASPEN, 2002). PN solutions containing a lipid portion do not stimulate the pancreas (Konturek et al, 1979; Kelly and Nahrwold, 1976; Edelman and Valenzuela, 1983) and should be implemented when enteral nutrition is not tolerated (ASPEN, 2002). Most people tolerate glucose- and lipid-based formulas well because hypertriglyceridemia-induced pancreatitis is rare unless serum concentrations exceed 1,000 mg/dl (Silberman et al, 1982). PN administration without lipid emulsions beyond two weeks is not advised because of the risk for developing essential fatty acid deficiency. There are no similar data available for dogs or cats; however, patients with hypertriglyceridemia and/or pancreatitis have routinely received a high-fat TNA at their RER with no additional problems.[b]

Protein Solutions

Patients must receive a source of essential and nonessential amino acids. Solutions are available containing 3.5 to 15% amino acids. These solutions are maintained in the pH range of 5.3 to 6.5, have an osmolarity between 300 and 1,400 mOsm/l and may contain various combinations of electrolytes and/or dextrose (AHFS Drug Information, 1997). Modified formulas are available with disproportionate concentrations of branched-chained vs. aromatic amino acids. These formulas are designed for patients with renal or liver failure or multiple trauma, but have not been widely used in veterinary medicine due to expense. The most commonly used product in veterinary medicine is the conventional 8.5% amino acid solution either with or without electrolytes (**Table 26-3**). Most amino acid solutions contain all the essential amino acids for dogs and cats, except

Table 26-5. Drug incompatibility with B-complex vitamins.*

Known incompatible	Suspected incompatible
2-PAM (pralidoxime chloride)	4-methylpyrazole
Aminophylline	Adriamycin
Asparaginase	Carboplatin
Bicarbonate	Cisplatin
Calcium versenate	Dobutamine
Cefazolin	Dopamine
Diazepam	Fentanyl
Digoxin (injectable)	Propranolol
Mannitol	
Nitroprusside	
Penicillin G	
Quinidine	

*Plumb DC. Veterinary Drug Handbook, 3rd ed. White Bear, MN: Pharma Veterinary Publishing, 1999.

taurine. However, some specialized pediatric amino acid products contain taurine.

Protein should be provided to the patient within a ratio of 1 to 6 g protein/100 kcal of nonprotein energy provided. Adult dogs and cats do well on 2 to 3 g/100 kcal and 3 to 4 g/100 kcal, respectively. Ferrets should receive protein intakes similar to those for cats (4 to 5 g protein/100 kcal), whereas rabbits should receive lower protein intakes (1 to 2 g protein/100 kcal). The lower protein-calorie ratios are recommended for patients with renal or hepatic insufficiency. The higher protein intakes are recommended for patients with increased protein needs (e.g., albumin losses, chest-tube drains). The exact protein intake for each patient cannot be determined prospectively but may have a significant effect on outcome. Postoperative patients receiving 1 g amino acids/kg body weight parenterally had less negative nitrogen balance and greater transferrin concentrations and lymphocyte counts compared with people receiving an isocaloric intake of calories as glucose without amino acids (Hwang et al, 1993). Therefore, the ratios recommended here should be used as guidelines only. A reasonable estimate of a patient's protein needs should be made, the patient's response to that particular protein intake should be monitored and the intake should be adjusted accordingly. Patients are rarely azotemic due to PN administration when amino acids are provided within these protein-energy ratios and a product is used that provides mostly essential amino acids.

There are some combination amino acid/glycerin products that provide amino acids and an energy source in a fixed ratio (**Table 26-3**). Some of these combinations are provided as a two-compartment bag with dextrose and amino acid solutions separated by a breakable divider. Most of these prepackaged dextrose/amino-acid mixes contain very high protein-calorie ratios and do not contain fat.

Electrolyte Solutions

The more common electrolyte abnormalities associated with PN occur with the major intracellular cation potassium and the anion phosphorus. Potassium and phosphorus rapidly move intracellularly with refeeding by either enteral or parenteral methods or with the administration of glucose or insulin (Forrester and Moreland, 1989). Potassium moves intracellularly when acidosis is corrected or when insulin is released. A TNA solution composed of 8.5% amino acids with electrolytes and lactated Ringer's solution contains approximately 12 mEq potassium/l, which is inadequate to maintain normal serum potassium levels. Potassium can be added to the PN solution using either a 2 mEq/ml potassium chloride solution or a 4.4 mEq/ml potassium phosphate solution.

If the patient is normokalemic when PN is initiated, 30 to 40 mEq potassium/l will usually maintain normokalemia. However, if the patient is hypokalemic when PN is started, 40 or more mEq potassium/l will be required. If the patient is hyperkalemic when PN is initiated, no additional potassium is recommended; however, serum potassium concentrations should be monitored daily. Administration of crystalloid solutions containing potassium by a second intravenous line is a convenient method of regulating serum potassium levels in difficult cases.

Phosphorus moves intracellularly with refeeding because of increased production of high-energy phosphate compounds (Hardy and Adams, 1989). Patients receiving PN rarely become hypophosphatemic. Sufficient quantities of phosphorus (10 mM/l) appear to be available in the TNA from lipid (15 mM/l) and amino acid/electrolyte (30 mM/l) solutions. However, adding a potassium phosphate solution containing 4.4 mEq potassium and 3 mM phosphorus/ml will increase the potassium and phosphorus content of the TNA. In cases of hyperphosphatemia, the quantity of amino acids, electrolytes and fat must be reduced to decrease phosphate concentrations in the TNA. Alternatively, an amino acid solution without electrolytes and potassium chloride can be used.

Vitamin Solutions

Very few veterinary patients receiving PN have a demonstrable need for fat-soluble vitamins unless there is a history of prolonged weight loss, inappetence and decreased fat absorption (diarrhea/steatorrhea). Dogs and cats usually have sufficient body stores of vitamins A, D, E, K and B_{12} to last several weeks to months if there is no increased demand or losses. Fat-soluble vitamin supplementation is warranted in cases with a history of long-term fat malabsorption (months). One-time administration of 1 ml of a vitamin A, D and E product,[c] divided into two intramuscular sites, is simple, cost effective and supplies fat-soluble vitamins for about three months. Vitamin K_1 injections (3 to 5 mg/cat, b.i.d., subcutaneously) reportedly improved abnormal coagulation times in cases of severe idiopathic hepatic lipidosis (Center, 1995, 1996). Most disease states are associated with increased oxidative stress and free radical-induced cell damage. Administering a PN solution with a high lipid concentration may provide nutritional support, but is also an oxide-rich nutrient source. Early work indicated patients administered highly oxidative nutrient solutions (lipids) may benefit from receiving the antioxidant d-α-tocopherol (24 to 48 IU/g lipid) (Becvarova et al, 2005).

Water-soluble vitamins, however, must be supplied daily by either the enteral or parenteral route. Most veterinary vitamin B-complex products do not contain all 11 B-complex vitamins, because some B vitamins are incompatible (e.g., folic acid and riboflavin in the same solution). Folic acid, therefore, must be administered separately if needed. Based on the National Research Council (NRC, 2006) daily vitamin recommendations for healthy dogs and cats and given the vitamin concentrations available in most solutions[d] the recommended dose of 1 ml of B vitamins/100 kcal exceeds daily B-vitamin requirements by several-fold, except for B_{12}. Most previously healthy patients, however, have sufficient hepatic stores of B_{12}.

Some B vitamins are light labile; therefore, most B-vitamin preparations should be kept in a light-resistant bottle and stored between 15 to 30°C (59 to 86°F). Riboflavin, perhaps the most light-labile B vitamin, still has 50% of its original activity after exposure to indoor fluorescent lighting for eight hours (Chen et al, 1983; Smith et al, 1988). Given the NRC (2006) recommended dose of riboflavin and the concentration of riboflavin in the TNA at 1 ml B vitamins/100 kcal, the patient would receive the daily recommended amount of riboflavin within the first two hours of TNA therapy. Thus, covering the intravenous fluid bag to protect B vitamins is unnecessary. Also, the addition of lipid increases the opacity of the final solution, reduces light penetration and precludes having to cover the PN solution from light (Smith et al, 1988). Adding B vitamins is a low-cost (pennies per day), effective means of improving energy metabolism. However, B vitamins are incompatible with some drugs commonly administered to veterinary patients by continuous intravenous infusion (**Table 26-5**).

Trace-Element Solutions

Trace-element requirements have not been determined for catabolic veterinary patients and dosing recommendations for zinc and copper in PN solutions are still evolving. In studies, dogs receiving a zinc-free PN solution had serum levels 50% of normal after one week; therefore, some zinc supplementation is recommended (Iriyama et al, 1982). Supplementing PN solutions with at least 0.1 to 0.2 mg zinc/100 kcal has been suggested (Buffington, 1991; Hill, 1994). Piglets receiving PN for four weeks with a solution containing 5 mg zinc and 0.3 mg copper/100 kcal had toxic zinc but normal copper hepatic concentrations and evidence of pancreatic necrosis associated with zinc toxicosis. Piglets receiving a similar PN protocol with 1.2 mg zinc and 0.3 mg copper/100 kcal had normal hepatic zinc and copper concentrations and no pancreatic pathology (Gabrielson et al, 1996). Based on the NRC (2006) daily zinc and copper recommendations for dogs and cats and one author's (RLR) experience, PN solutions containing 2 mg zinc and 0.2 mg copper/100 kcal RER approximate the patient's needs or approximately 1 ml of a trace-element solution may be added per 100 kcal RER daily. These elements can be added to the PN solution most economically (pennies per day) using a multiple trace-elemente combination available in multiple-dose or single-dose vials.[e]

Table 26-6. Drugs compatible with total nutrient admixtures.*

Aminophylline	Furosemide
Ampicillin	Gentamicin
Cefazolin	Heparin
Chloramphenicol	Insulin (regular)
Cimetidine	Lidocaine
Clindamycin	Metoclopramide
Digoxin	Penicillin G
Diphenhydramine	Phytonadione
Dopamine	Ranitidine
Erythromycin	Ticarcillin

*Dickerson RN, Brown RO, White KG. Parenteral nutrition solutions. In: Rombeau JL, Caldwell MD, eds. Clinical Nutrition; Parenteral Nutrition, 2nd ed. Philadelphia, PA: WB Saunders Co, 1993; 310-333.

DRUG ADDITIONS

Although it is very convenient to administer drugs intravenously with the PN solution, *extreme caution must be taken before any medications are added to the TNA.* Drug and TNA solution compatibility studies are ongoing, and there are published lists of drugs known to be compatible and safe (Trissel et al, 1999). **Table 26-6** lists drugs of most interest to veterinarians that can be incorporated into a three-in-one mixture. The *Handbook on Injectable Drugs* is updated and published every two years and is a good source for current information about drug compatibility with PN solutions (Trissel, 2007). After a medication has been added to the day's PN solution, a decision to discontinue that medication can be costly, because a new bag of PN solution must be compounded. Therefore, use of a second peripheral catheter or a multi-lumen central catheter may be preferable to adding drugs to PN solutions.

COMPOUNDING

PN solutions can be obtained from several sources. Some human hospitals and independent pharmaceutical companies will compound TNA solutions for veterinarians. A prescription must be written indicating the volume or final concentration of each nutrient (fat, dextrose, amino acids and each electrolyte), and the person preparing the TNA is likely to refer to the solution as "TPN." Some veterinary schools, large referral practices and private veterinary hospitals have parenteral solution compounders and supplies for their own use and will compound and sell TNA bags directly to practitioners. Several bags of PN solution (up to 10 days' worth) can be sent by overnight mail services directly to the practice. This is often the safest, most convenient and economical method of obtaining an all-in-one PN solution for the occasional patient in most practices.

TNA solutions can be compounded by one of three basic methods: 1) syringe, 2) gravity flow or 3) computerized flow (Remillard and Thatcher, 1989). All-in-one PN or TNA supplies can be purchased from the same sources that provide

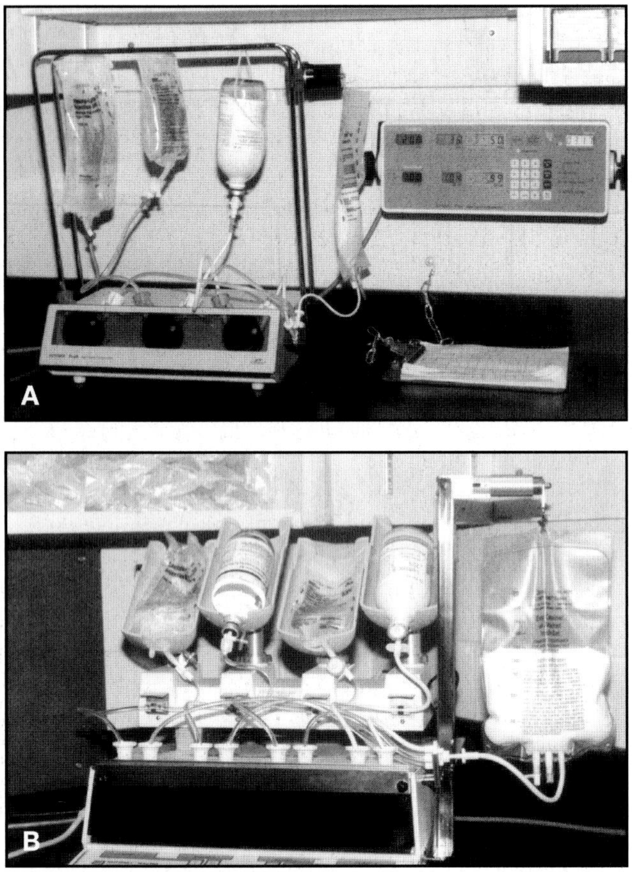

Figure 26-1. A three-station (A) and four-station (B) total nutrient admixture compounder.

nutrient solutions. The least desirable method uses a 35- or 60-ml syringe to transfer each nutrient solution (dextrose, amino acid and lipid) into a sterile, empty fluid bag. This method is the most time-consuming and carries the greatest risk of contamination because of the multiple transfers required. Transfers are ideally done under a laminar flow hood.

The second method uses a closed-circuit fluid system in which the all-in-one bag comes with a pre-attached three-lead transfer set. Each lead, with a vented filter spike, is inserted directly into the individual nutrient solutions (dextrose, amino acid and lipid), and the nutrients are transferred directly into the all-in-one bag by gravity flow. This method is faster and safer than the syringe method, but transfer of exact quantities is impossible. This method may be most economical when few patients require PN. Both syringe and gravity feed methods usually leave partially unused bottles of dextrose, lipid and amino acids.

The third and best method, used by most human hospitals and some large referral veterinary hospitals, employs a high-speed, closed-circuit fluid compounder that pumps three or four solutions (dextrose, amino acid, lipid and fluid) directly into one TNA bag within 60 seconds. Each solution is accurately transferred to within 1 ml. The method has a mean error of less than 3% (**Figure 26-1**). Multiple bags of TNA for several patients can be efficiently compounded at one time using partial bottles of dextrose, fat and amino acids. Making TNA bags with a compounder is safe, fast, accurate and efficient. Veterinary technicians can routinely accomplish this task (McClendon, 1981). A computerized compounder has been used to formulate in one author's (RLR) practice since 1993. To date, no confirmed or suspected cases of microbial contamination have occurred during formulation.[f] All-in-one or TNA solutions can be refrigerated for seven to 14 days (**Box 26-3**).

ADMINISTRATION

The first practical technique for PN administration was demonstrated in the late 1960s (Franga, 2002). At that time, the only form of concentrated non-protein calories for intravenous use was hypertonic dextrose; therefore, a large-diameter, high-flow central vein was needed to avoid phlebothrombosis. Thus, infusion of this high osmolarity PN solution was best delivered into the superior vena cava. The predominant clinical complication with this feeding system was hyperalimentation and subsequent hyperglycemia. It was quickly realized that intravenous delivery of excessive dextrose calories commonly resulted in metabolic and infectious complications. Development and availability of crystalline amino acid and fat solutions helped to address these adverse PN-associated sequelae, because admixtures of lower osmolarity could be formulated for peripheral vein delivery. Additionally, there have been infrequent reports of PN solution delivery through either an intraosseous or intraperitoneal catheter. These alternatives offer additional options for short-term nutritional support.

The route of PN delivery is chosen after consideration of several factors including the underlying disorder and its severity, therapeutic goals for the patient, admixture composition, patient characteristics (e.g., body composition, species, age, vein accessibility), clinician experience and complication risk level (Hansen, 2006; Gallivan and Benotti, 1997). If management of the disease or disorder is thought to require prolonged (more than seven days) parenteral feeding, then the admixture delivery system should be initiated through or changed over to a central venous route. The peripheral route of admixture delivery is best suited to a short-term (less than seven days) nutritional support scenario or when central venous access is unavailable.

Central Vein Infusion

Traditionally, the right external jugular vein is the preferred access route for central venous catheters (CVC). From this site, the external jugular vein joins the cranial vena cava in a straighter line through the brachycephalic trunk, which facilitates catheter passage (Hansen, 2006). Body composition (obese, cachexia) can complicate CVC placement. Imaging techniques help reduce multiple attempts at placing CVCs, thereby minimizing coagulative states (Hunter, 2007; Franga, 2002). The large diameter of a central vein allows for delivery of a high osmolarity solution without concerns about phlebitis caused by fluid shifts in the vein lumen. Practically speaking, the proportions of dextrose, lipid or amino acids in a PN admixture formulated for delivery through a central vein are not restricted. High- and low-dextrose admixtures are tolerated.

Central venous access can also be obtained by inserting a long catheter into the saphenous vein. This is commonly referred to as a peripherally inserted central catheter. Placing a 10- to 20-cm polyurethane[g] or silicone[h] catheter into the medial saphenous vein at the level of the tarsus and advancing the catheter up the vein places the tip of the catheter into the caudal vena cava of cats. A similar, but longer (20- to 30-cm) polyurethane or silicone catheter, placed in the lateral saphenous vein, is more useful in dogs weighing less than 20 kg. Parenteral admixtures can easily be administered to dogs and cats through a peripherally inserted central line. Cats, compared with most dogs, are smaller, have higher protein requirements and sometimes have restrictive fluid allowances. For cats (more so than for dogs), the final osmolarity of the PN solution will be greater than 600 mOsm/l; therefore, the solution should be administered into a large vein.

Catheters placed in a central vein can have a single lumen or multiple lumina. Although use of central catheters has not been adequately evaluated in veterinary patients, their use for PN administration in people is associated with an increase in septic complications (McCarthy et al, 1987). Many sources advocate that the central catheter must be "dedicated" to PN administration, and should not be used for blood sampling, medication or blood product administration or central venous pressure monitoring. However, when venous access is limited, the PN catheter may be used for blood sampling and administering medications if it is adequately flushed before and after PN administration is interrupted. It is imperative, as with any catheter, that proper aseptic handling technique be used during line interruptions. Likewise, the need for wiping PN lines after handling has not been substantiated; however, precautions are always warranted to reduce the risk of septic complications.

Peripheral Vein Infusion

The lateral saphenous (dog) and medial saphenous (cat) veins are most commonly used for peripheral catheter placement. These sites are preferred because the skin cover is thinner, thus providing better visualization and control over catheter insertion (Hansen, 2006). Less commonly used locations for catheter placement for delivery of PN include the cephalic and/or accessory cephalic veins, femoral veins in some dogs and cats and the ear veins in dogs with pendulous ears.

Based on peripheral vein diameter, there are limitations on the osmolarity of PN solutions that can be administered. In human patients, PN solutions with osmolarities ranging from 550 to 1,250 mOsm/l have been administered peripherally for short periods (three days) (Gazitua et al, 1979; Matsusue et al, 1995; Daly et al, 1985; Isaacs et al, 1977; Maden et al, 1992). Phlebitis, which occurred within the first 72 hours in 26 to 48% of human patients, was the principal complication (Bayer-Berger et al, 1989). Although peripheral vein administration of PN is not new in veterinary medicine, published studies are limited. One study of five dogs evaluated a 3-in-1 admixture delivered over various infusion time periods (Chandler and Payne-James, 2006). An 840 mOsm/l admixture was administered through a peripheral catheter for either 24 hours or 10 to 12 hours/day. Patency of the intravenous line was maintained for a median of 36 hours; no biochemical abnormalities were reported in study dogs. The incidence of line failure, due to thrombus or thrombophlebitis, was decreased by shorter infusion times. In another study, obese cats receiving a high-lipid, low-dextrose admixture through peripheral vein catheters for four days exhibited no mechanical, metabolic or septic complications (Becvarova et al, 2005).

Box 26-3. Complications of Total Nutrient Admixture Solutions.

The diverse composition of total nutrient admixture (TNA) solutions increases the risk of physiochemical incompatibilities. The most likely problem is deterioration of the lipid emulsion within the TNA in which individual fat particles collide forming larger particles creating a potentially dangerous intravenous mixture. TNA solutions containing 10 or 20% lipid have an osmolarity of about 300 mOsm/l, a pH of 7.0 and are stable when stored as directed at room temperature. An egg-yolk phospholipid emulsifier stabilizes the 4- to 5-mm lipid particles by giving the surface a negative charge to maintain a repulsive electrostatic force between particles. Fat breakdown in individual bottles of lipids rarely occurs.

In a TNA, however, fat particles can aggregate and larger particles will migrate to the surface of the solution, creating a whiter band at the top of the TNA solution. This process is called "creaming." It can be easily reversed by gently mixing the TNA solution, and is of no danger to the patient. However, when the negative surface charge is neutralized, the emulsion destabilizes irreversibly and, with repeated collisions between fat particles, the emulsion completely destabilizes. This irreversible coalescence process creates two immiscible oil and water phases. Coalescence is associated with a dark yellow color, either in a line across the top portion of the TNA or as large yellow globules throughout the TNA solution. Adding B-vitamins to a TNA solution gives the solution a light but uniform yellow color, and should not be confused with coalescence. Bags with evidence of coalescence should not be administered to patients because the larger particles can become fat emboli that will plug 5-mm pulmonary capillaries.

Adding divalent cations (e.g., calcium or magnesium) to the TNA solution is not advisable because the positive charge can destabilize the negatively charged surface of fat, break the emulsion and cause coalescence. Adding solutions that reduce the final pH of the TNA to 5 or less will also cause the emulsion to breakdown. Individual dextrose solutions are kept at a pH of 5 to minimize microbial growth, whereas amino acid solutions are buffered and have a pH of 6. When mixing a TNA solution, it is important to add the lipid last when there is a large volume of fluid with a higher pH already in the parenteral nutrition bag.

The Bibliography for **Box 26-3** can be found at www.markmorris.org.

Observed physiologic alterations in study cats were associated with obesity-induced oxidative damage. Calories can easily and safely be administered peripherally to dogs and cats using a TNA of 400 to 650 mOsm/l or an isomolar 20% lipid solution piggybacked with standard fluid therapy at volumes sufficient to meet RER.[1]

Other Routes of PN Infusion

Intravascular complications associated with repeated catheter placements, insufficient blood flow or coagulation abnormalities can limit vascular accessibility. Alternatives for PN support include the intraosseous and intraperitoneal (IP) routes, as reported in several laboratory species, people (adults and children) and dogs. In two separate studies, rats were infused with PN solutions through IP catheters for seven or more days. No adverse effects from the placement or use of IP catheters were found. Weight maintenance was dependent on the caloric profile of the admixture; a PN solution approximating 600 to 700 mOsm/l was preferred (Rubin et al, 1988; LeLeiko et al, 1983). PN solutions (850 mOsm/l) have been infused by IP routes for more than 20 days in 19 normal dogs and in 12 normal dogs that had undergone intestinal resection (Moran et al, 1989; Garcia-Gamito et al, 1991). IP infusion of a 10% lipid solution into three-month-old beagles demonstrated that fat was quantitatively absorbed from the peritoneal cavity over a four-hour period (Klein et al, 1983). Despite this apparent success, the IP route for PN support isn't widely used in veterinary medicine. Intraosseous infusion of drugs and fluids is used as an emergency, last resort access site for human and veterinary patients. Reports of short-term PN infusion (e.g., bolus) are limited, but encouraging. Tibial intraosseous infusion is the preferred site for critically ill children (Koenig, 2000), whereas the sternum is reported to be the most effective site for infusion of lipids in adults (Koenig, 2000). Likewise, a solution containing electrolytes, amino acids, dextrose and vitamins has been successfully infused intraosseously in dogs (Otto et al, 1989). Several precautions exist for intraosseous infusions including appropriate catheter placement, avoiding compromised skin areas and growth plates and extravasation of fluid around bone cortices or vessel foramina (Moss et al, 2005). Although fat embolization is a reasonable consideration, it has yet to be reported in the literature.

Risks and Complications

Catheter placement and management come with potential risks. The most clinically significant problem in administering PN solutions involves the catheter, including loss of access, thrombophlebitis and infection generally in that order of occurrence. Parenteral feeding can introduce additional risks not associated with non-caloric fluid delivery. An overview of the risks and complications associated with central and peripheral vein PN delivery follows.

Infection

Infectious complications with intravenous infusions have been recognized for more than 40 years and are now primarily associated with substandard catheter care. Most catheter-related septicemias are due to microbial invasion at the catheter wound either during or after insertion, but other risk factors include poor patient and personnel hygiene, operator inexperience, method and site of catheter insertion, duration of catheterization and number of catheter manipulations (Bozzetti, 1985; Yilmaz et al, 2007).

Catheters for PN administration must be placed using meticulous aseptic technique. Bandage contamination increases the risk of infection; peripheral vein catheters are more likely to be exposed to and soiled by feces, urine and vomitus compared to CVCs (Hansen, 2006). For either peripherally- or centrally-placed catheters, bandage and administration sets should be changed at least every other day, and preferably daily. When the bandage is changed, the venipuncture site should be cleaned with an iodine solution and examined for redness, edema or swelling. A topical antibiotic ointment (e.g., povidone iodine) that contains antifungal properties should be applied to the catheter-skin junction. If redness, edema or swelling is noticed, the catheter should be removed and cultured and the site should be kept clean and hot packed, if necessary, to reduce swelling. Appropriate antibiotics should be given if culture and antimicrobial sensitivity testing show the catheter or PN solution is contaminated.

Cut-down incisions may be necessary for catheter placement at any location and can increase the risk of infection. Infected or wounded skin at the catheter placement site increases the risk of infection (Hansen, 2006). If there is no other option for a catheter insertion site other than in close proximity to wounded or infected skin, aseptic placement is absolutely necessary. Extreme care should be exercised when assembling and disassembling the admixture flow system and frequent bandage changes are highly recommended. Tunneling or the "indirect catheterization" method forms a subcutaneous tunnel between the point of entry through the skin and the point of entry into the vein. Catheter tunneling helps prevent infection. This technique is more commonly performed when placing a CVC for long-term use. Tunnels serve as a barrier to bacterial migration (Hansen, 2006; Franga, 2002).

In human intensive care units, catheter-related infections are the third most common cause of nosocomial infections (CDC, 1997). Although these data are not reported for veterinary patients, the findings most likely would be similar. Catheter infections are either related to cellulitis from contamination at the catheter exit site (type I) or microorganism contamination within the catheter lumen (type II). Both are due to a failure in aseptic technique (Kaminski, 1997). Adding extra lumina to the same catheter appears to potentiate the risk for type II infections (Kaminski, 1997; Early, 1990; Kemp, 1994). Data are controversial regarding the practice of maintaining a dedicated catheter line for PN administration. In the event a line cannot be dedicated to PN administration, stopping PN delivery, flushing the line adequately before and after delivery of medications, then restarting the PN delivery, will help minimize complications associated with potential solution incompatibilities.

CVCs vary in size and composition (i.e., polyethylene, polyurethane, polyvinyl, silicone, Teflon). Selection of catheter material has implications for catheter-related infections. Silicone catheters reduce the sensitivity of *Staphylococcus aureus* to antibiotics (Williams, 1997). CVCs impregnated with antibiotics reduce the incidence of catheter-related infections (Hanley, 2000). Reports indicate that minocycline/rifampin-coated catheters are less likely to become colonized and have a significantly decreased number of catheter-related infections compared to chlorhexidine/silver sulfadiazine-impregnated catheters (Darouiche, 1999).

Other sources of catheter-related infection include urinary tract infections, abscesses, pneumonia, bacterial translocation from the GI tract or other infected sites (Ryan et al, 1974), resulting in thrombus formation at the catheter tip. Infusion of contaminated fluid is another potential source of infection. Using a closed-circuit fluid system minimizes this route of contamination. Whether individual nutrient solutions within the PN solution promote bacterial or fungal growth if stored inappropriately is still controversial. The crystalline amino acid products now used in PN formulations prohibit bacterial growth (Goldmann et al, 1971; Wilkinson et al, 1973). As a safety precaution, the Centers for Disease Control and Prevention has recommended that lipid-only emulsions be administered for no longer than 12 hours, except in PN systems, which can be administered over a 24-hour period (Simmons et al, 1982). Infection associated with PN administration is a rare complication, most often attributed to substandard catheter care.

Thrombosis

Thrombophlebitis is a response of the vein intima to the unique combination of the infusate, the catheter material and placement and the ratio of catheter to vessel size. Ideally, the smallest catheter necessary to deliver the desired therapy should be selected. Cannulating a vein always poses a risk for thrombosis formation. The longer the catheter remains in place, the greater the risk. Any indwelling catheter becomes covered by a fibrin sheath and platelets within several hours of placement (Hansen, 2006). The likelihood of thrombosis increases in a small vein (i.e., peripheral vein relative to catheter size) that has lower blood flow; when a catheter traverses a mobile joint, when a pre-existing disease exists such as glomerulonephritis, protein-losing enteropathy, autoimmune hemolytic anemia, phlebitis or any disorder causing systemic inflammation. The catheter material is thought to be the single most important factor in the severity of infusion thrombophlebitis (Gaukroger et al, 1988; McKee et al, 1989). Three major characteristics of catheter material have been identified that contribute to thrombus formation: roughness, stiffness and propensity for platelet adhesion (Linder et al, 1984). Numerous studies comparing catheter types are available for review. Catheter choice is multifactorial; minimizing thrombus formation during PN administration should an important consideration. The primary complication from thrombosis is loss of vessel patency, although other complications of deep venous thrombosis include septic thrombophlebitis, venous gangrene, extravasation of infusate, pulmonary embolism and death (Gallivan and Benotti, 1997). Although the risk of thrombosis in a catheterized jugular vein is much lower, the consequences are much more severe compared to those that might occur in a peripheral vein.

Extravasation

When a catheter is displaced, fluid leaks into or infiltrates surrounding tissues (extravasation) causing pain and swelling. Stiff plastic catheters are more likely to perforate vessels during and after placement compared to softer polyurethane or silicone catheters.

Complications with CVC extravasation may not become evident until large volumes of fluid are administered. Fluids (solution) tend to accumulate in the mediastinal and pleural spaces resulting in labored breathing. When catheters are advanced into the right atrium, blood and fluid will accumulate in the pericardial sac causing cardiac tamponade. Thoracic radiographs, physical signs and possibly fluid analysis can be used to document PN solution extravasation.

Swelling and tenderness at peripheral vein infusion sites may indicate extravasation of the PN admixture. The skin overlying the catheter tip may feel cool, and/or the catheter insertion site may be swollen, red and hot, and left unattended, may lead to tissue necrosis and sloughing.

Catheter Damage

Catheters placed in limbs are more accessible for patients to chew or tear. Placement of an Elizabethan collar may help prevent damage to the PN system after the catheter has been placed and the feeding system constructed. Catheters placed in an ear vein may be dislodged by scratching and head shaking. A well-fitted Elizabethan collar will minimize this concern. Catheters placed in the jugular vein are at least risk for damage because patients are less likely to disturb this site. Loss of venous access is caused by catheter kinking, catheter tip migration or blockage. In these instances, the catheter should be removed and a new catheter placed in another vein. Chewing and/or scratching at bandages that conceal a catheter may indicate that the catheter or bandage is irritating the patient. Check the bandage and catheter for tightness, wetness, inflammation or infection. Immediately remove the bandage if any of these problems arise. Assess catheter viability, vein patency, presence of inflammation or infection and immediately make changes to rectify the problem(s).

Guidelines for parenteral feeding of human patients clearly recommend central vein delivery for long-term (months) intravenous nutritional support. However, intravenous nutritional support for most companion animals lasts two to seven days; in some extreme cases, parenteral feeding may be used for several weeks. Catheter placement for PN delivery in small animals should be based on catheter complication risks, duration of feeding, catheter placement and monitoring experience and cost and solution composition (**Table 26-7**).

Table 26-7. Summary of catheter placement sites for parenteral nutrition administration in small animals.

Site/Technique	Pros	Cons	Indications
External jugular	Central vein (large) access Exchangeable High osmolar solution compatible Long-term use (>7 days) Less bandage damage	Placement technically difficult Infection rate higher Intensive patient monitoring required	Inability to use GI tract for nutritional support Electrolytes stable Interruption of oral alimentations for >7 days; catabolic <7 days Non-septic patients Hospitalization required
Tunneled catheters	Lower infection rate of CVC Long-term use (>7 days) Central venous access Hospitalization compatible	Operative placement recommended Placement technically difficult	Long-term CVC required for PN
PICC (femoral vein)	Central vein access Hospitalization compatible Exchangeable	Thrombophlebitis risk higher Infection rate higher Short-term use (<3 days) Blood draws not predictable	To accommodate hospitalization in cats and small dogs No jugular access
Peripheral (saphenous, cephalic)	Easy insertion Lower infection rate Amendable to 3-in-1 solutions Less intensive patient monitoring Exchangeable Lower cost	Requires low osmolar solution (<650 mOsm/l) Short-term use (<7 days) Increase risk of bandage damage Elizabethan collar recommended	High risk of catheter sepsis from CVC Patient can tolerate lipid emulsions Patient in mild metabolic stress/ malnutrition Central vein access not available/ contraindicated Short duration PN Adjunct to enteral or oral nutrition on short-term basis
IO, IP	Venous access not required	Ultra short-term use (IO) Placement technically difficulty (IO) Limited documentation	Emergency situations when venous access is unavailable

Key: GI = gastrointestinal, CVC = central venous catheter, PN = parenteral nutrition, PICC = peripherally inserted central catheter, IO = intraosseous, IP = intraperitoneal.

COMBINED ENTERAL AND PARENTERAL FEEDING

In human medicine, there has been increased acceptance and use of PN in combination with tube feeding (Adams et al, 1986; Moore and Jones, 1986). Feeding enterally minimizes the disadvantages of PN. Prolonged fasting (more than three days) results in enterocyte deterioration and decreased GI immunity (Alverdy et al, 1985). Translocation of enteric bacteria due to a compromised intestinal mucosal barrier represents a possible source of infection with PN administration. Enteral infusion of small quantities of a liquid diet helped prevent intestinal mucosal deterioration during PN administration in piglets (2 ml/kg body weight b.i.d.), human infants (4 to 5 ml/kg body weight/hour) and adults (0.7 ml/kg body weight/hour) (Remillard et al, 1998; Andrassy et al, 1979, 1985). Intestinal adaptations after disease and intestinal hypertrophy after surgery require intraluminal nutrients. Food intake promotes intestinal hyperplasia and brush border enzyme activity (Herman-Zaidius, 1986). Therefore, current recommendations encourage some enteral feeding for patients receiving PN support, if at all possible. Feeding both the small bowel and the patient is important (Daley and Bistrian, 1994).

Either central or peripheral vein delivery systems can be used together with enteral feeding (voluntary or assisted). If PN complements a tube feeding system, avoid the central vein-esophagostomy feeding tube combination. Close proximity of the jugular vein catheter and the feeding tube insertion site may increase the risk of infection and mechanical problems. Other PN and enteral feeding combinations work predictably to optimize nutritional support and GI health.

REASSESSMENT

Regular reassessment is a critical step in successful nutritional management of hospitalized patients, regardless of whether the enteral route, the parenteral route or both are used. Malnutrition in the form of insufficient nutrient intake to support tissue metabolism undermines medical and/or surgical management of a case. Malnutrition is far more common in veterinary patients than is currently recognized. Patients resting in a cage have been mistakenly assumed to require little or no caloric intake when, in fact, the nutrient costs of tissue repair, immunocompetence and drug metabolism are significant. Therefore, reassessment of nutritional status is important whether the patient remains in the hospital or recovers at home.

Monitoring Parameters

Food intake or administration of nutritional support for hospi-

Table 26-8. Metabolic complications of parenteral-nutrition administration, treatment and potential patient considerations.

Complications are listed in descending order of likely occurrence and treatments are listed from immediate to longer term solutions. To minimize complications, patients should be hemodynamically stable and any electrolyte and acid-base abnormalities, severe tachycardia, hypotension and volume deficits should be corrected before starting PN.

Complication	Treatment	Patient considerations
Hyperglycemia	Stop infusion, recheck in two to four hours, decrease PN infusion by 50% until normal, then increase infusion rate slowly Subcutaneous insulin therapy Change caloric sources: Increase lipid fraction of calories Decrease glucose fraction of calories	Glucose intolerance
Hypokalemia	Add KCl or KPO_4 to PN bag Correct serum magnesium as needed Change caloric sources: Increase lipid fraction of calories Decrease glucose fraction of calories	GI or renal losses Drug therapies that increase urinary excretion Insulin therapy
Hypophosphatemia	Add $NaPO_4$ or KPO_4 to PN bag	Diabetic ketoacidosis
Hyperlipidemia	Stop infusion, recheck in two to four hours, decrease infusion by 50% until normal, then increase infusion rate slowly Change caloric sources: Decrease lipid fraction of calories Increase glucose fraction of calories	Decreased lipid clearance
Phlebitis	Change catheter and infusion site Lower PN osmolality: Increase lipid fraction of calories Decrease glucose fraction of calories Add heparin to PN bag	Proper hydration Endogenous site of infection
Hyperkalemia	Change PN bag and decrease potassium	Acidosis, renal failure, sepsis Drug therapies that decrease urinary excretion
Hyperammonemia	Decrease PN infusion by 50% until normal Change PN bag, decrease amino acid concentration Use branched-chain amino acid sources	Liver dysfunction, GI bleeding
Hypomagnesemia	Add $MgSO_4$ to PN bag	GI or renal losses Drug therapies that increase urinary excretion
Hypoglycemia	Piggyback 50% dextrose drip until normal Change caloric sources: Decrease lipid fraction of calories Increase glucose fraction of calories	Sepsis Insulin therapy Insulinoma
Infected catheter site	Change catheter and infusion site Culture catheter and PN solution Give antibiotics based on culture and antimicrobial sensitivity tests Hot pack the site	Substandard catheter care Endogenous site of infection Properly hydrated

Key: PN = parenteral nutrition, GI = gastrointestinal.

talized patients should be reviewed at least daily. Body weight should be recorded daily. Body condition should be noted; however, an animal's body condition score is unlikely to change during the course of a hospital stay. Laboratory assessments specifically for patients receiving nutritional support are generally not necessary beyond those tests already routinely performed for critically ill patients. The most common alterations that occur in laboratory parameters associated with nutrient administration are decreases in serum potassium and phosphate levels, increases in serum glucose concentrations and hypertriglyceridemia (**Table 26-8**). Even apparently stable patients might develop metabolic complications as a result of ongoing disease processes or from undiagnosed subclinical disease states. However, most patients' attitude improves subjectively within 36 hours of refeeding.[j]

Most parameters used to assess the nutritional status of patients will not change as a result of assisted feeding during the course of hospitalization. Laboratory parameters (e.g., albumin and total protein concentrations, RBC count and hemoglobin content) are unlikely to change in less than two weeks. The patient's body weight and condition and some laboratory parameters (albumin and total protein concentrations) should improve over the course of weeks (McAdams et al, 1996). Laboratory parameters that change during a hospital stay as a result of assisted feeding may be detected when acute-phase proteins with half-lives between two and 12 hours can be measured reliably in dogs and cats.

Changing Foods

Parenterally fed patients should be fed enterally as soon as possible, but may continue to receive PN as enteral intake increases to meet RER. The food offered enterally may be a fixed-formula therapeutic food intended as the food to be fed to the patient at home because of an ongoing disease condition (Chapter 25). When the patient has a decreased appetite, a highly palatable, fixed-formula food may be offered initially to stimulate oral consumption. This food may then be mixed in gradually decreasing proportions with the food to be fed on a long-term basis (Chapter 1). Vomiting and diarrhea are the most common problems seen when refeeding patients orally. Foods should be introduced in amounts equal to RER in small frequent meals, and the amounts increased if well tolerated over several days.

ENDNOTES

a. Prescribing information for Intralipid Intravenous Fat Emulsion, 1981. Cutter Laboratories, Berkeley, CA, USA.
b. Remillard RL, Angell Animal Medical Center, Boston, MA, USA. Unpublished data.
c. Vital E-A+D containing 100 IU of D and 300 IU of alpha-tocopherol per ml. Schering-Plough Animal Health Corp., Kenilworth, NJ, USA.
d. B-Vitamin Complex containing 50 mg thiamin, 2 mg riboflavin, 100 mg niacin, 2 mg pyridoxine, 10 mg pantothenic acid, 0.4 µg B12 per ml. Butler Co., Columbus, OH, USA.
e. MTE-4 contains 1.7 mg zinc, 0.42 mg copper, 0.37 mg manganese and 6 µg chromium per ml containing the preservative benzyl alcohol. Abbott Laboratories, Chicago, IL, USA.
f. Remillard RL, Angell Animal Medical Center, Boston, MA, USA. Unpublished data.
g. L-Cath (16 and 18 ga.). Luther Medical Products, Inc., Santa Ana, CA, USA. Central venous (20 to 16 ga.) catheters. Cook Veterinary Products, Bloomington, IL, USA.
h. Silicone (20 to 16 ga.) catheters (50 to 60 cm) can be cut to appropriate lengths. Cook Critical Care, Bloomington, IL, USA.
i. Remillard RL, Angell Animal Medical Center, Boston, MA, USA; Saker K, North Carolina State University, Raleigh, NC, USA. Unpublished data.
j. Remillard RL, Armstrong PJ, Guilford WG. Personal clinical experience.

REFERENCES

The references for **Chapter 26** can be found at www.markmorris.org.

CASE 26-1

Peripheral Parenteral Nutrition in a Dog

Korinn E. Saker, MS, DVM, PhD, Dipl. ACVN
College of Veterinary Medicine
North Carolina State University
Raleigh, North Carolina, USA

Patient Assessment

A six-year-old, intact male, mixed-breed dog weighing 29.5 kg with a body condition score (BCS) of 3/5 was presented for evaluation of suspected sepsis following a severe neck wound. A large open wound on the right side of the dog's neck was first noticed five days earlier. The local veterinarian flushed and closed the wound and initiated antibiotic therapy (enrofloxacin[a], amoxicillin[b] and a single dose of cephalexin[c]). The dog's clinical condition continued to deteriorate; therefore, the dog was referred for further evaluation.

On physical examination, the dog was depressed and laterally recumbent. The wound on the right side of the dog's neck extended from the dorsal margin of the ear pinna to the ventral midline. There was a necrotic odor originating from the wound. A fluid-filled pocket ventral to the wound was incised, releasing a large volume of purulent material. Specimens were collected for bacteriologic studies. When skin sutures were removed, a large wound extending deep into the tissues on the left side of the neck was found. The trachea, jugular vein and several nerves were visible at the wound margins, along with large amounts of green necrotic tissue. Skin surrounding the wound was indurated and necrotic. The dog's right ear was swollen and edematous with a creamy exudate originating from wounds on the medial aspect. Crackles could be auscultated in the right caudal lung field and the patient was mildly dyspneic.

Laboratory abnormalities included neutrophilia with a left shift, thrombocytopenia, decreased total protein (5.2 g/dl [normal 5.5 to 7.4 g/dl]) and albumin (2.3 g/dl [normal 2.8 to 3.6 g/dl]) values, lymphopenia, elevated bilirubin (5.0 mg/dl [normal 0.1 to 0.5 mg/dl]) concentration and increased alanine aminotransferase (367 U/l [normal 13 to 100 U/l]) and alkaline phosphatase (2,954 [normal 20 to 167 U/l]) activities.

After initial presentation to the teaching hospital, the dog was sedated twice daily for aggressive wound management and bandage care with wet-to-dry bandages. Aerobic and anaerobic wound cultures grew *Pseudomonas aeruginosa, Eubacterium aureofaciens, Bacteroides bivius* and *Clostridium perfringens.* The patient regurgitated white foam numerous times during the first three days of hospitalization and was dysphagic.

Assess the Food and Feeding Method

The dog had not eaten during the five days before presentation and was not offered food for the first three days of hospitalization while undergoing wound exploration and débridement and diagnostic cultures, radiography, bronchoscopy and esophagoscopy. Although nutritional support was not offered, a physiologic replacement fluid (lactated Ringer's solution) containing 20 mEq of potassium chloride/l was administered in the first 12 hours to replace an estimated fluid deficit of 10%. Fluids were reduced to maintenance rates thereafter.

Questions

1. What techniques and parameters could be used to assess the nutritional status of this patient?
2. Which nutrients would be beneficial in enhancing tissue repair and immunocompetence?
3. When and by what method should nutritional support be initiated?

Answers and Discussion

1. Currently, nutritional assessment is limited to the veterinary equivalent of anthropometric measures (i.e., body weight and condition), routine laboratory tests (e.g., total protein and albumin levels, lymphocyte counts) and clinical examination. Weight loss of more than 10% in sick or injured patients is considered a guideline for implementing nutritional support. Albumin has a half-life of eight days in normal dogs, thus it may remain within the normal range during short-term (one week) nutritional deprivation. The albumin concentration will decrease as the period of anorexia and lack of nutritional support is prolonged. The lymphocyte count also is altered in a relatively short period (days) as a result of nutrient deprivation. However, both hypoalbuminemia and lymphopenia can result from non-nutritionally related causes.
2. The patient's immune system was not responding optimally because of the infection and sepsis related to the neck injury. As a result of eight days of nutritional deprivation, the patient's body was now metabolizing fat and protein stores for energy and tissue repair. The labile protein pool (free amino acids) was becoming depleted and visceral and muscle protein was mobilized, which will result in atrophy and wasting in prolonged states of food deprivation in the face of accelerated catabolism. Immune cells and damaged muscle tissue benefit from dietary protein and fat. Research has shown that protein-energy malnutrition (PEM) results in immune system dysfunction. PEM increases the risk of mortality from infection, because it compromises innate and adaptive barriers to disease challenges. Specific alterations include: 1) a decreased marrow pool of neutrophils, 2) depressed neutrophil and monocyte phagocytic activity, 3) depressed antigen-presenting capacity of macrophages, 4) atrophy of lymphoid organs, 5) alterations in critical CD4 and CD8 cell subsets, 6) increased adhesion of organisms to mucosal epithelia and 7) alterations in regulation of inflammatory mediators. Micronutrients such as zinc, copper, iron, selenium and vitamins A, E and C should also be supplied because they are integral components in enzyme systems that promote antioxidant activity, antibody formation, cell activation and proliferation and protein synthesis.
3. Nutritional support should be instituted immediately. The twice daily wound débridement and bandage changes with sedation limit the time this patient is alert enough to assimilate oral nutrients. Additionally, this patient has a history of regurgitation and dysphagia since being admitted to the teaching hospital. In light of these factors, as well as the physical inaccessibility to the neck region because of the wound and bandages, this patient is an excellent candidate for peripheral parenteral feeding. The peripheral route of intravenous feeding can supply 100% of resting energy requirement (RER), amino acids plus maintenance electrolytes, minerals, vitamins and trace elements.

   The intravenous admixture should be formulated as a high-fat, low-carbohydrate solution to mirror the patient's current metabolic profile. A total admixture containing 3 g protein/100 kcal with 80 to 90% fat calories and 10 to 20% dextrose calories plus maintenance fluid therapy will ensure an osmolarity less than 600 mOsm/l and that the admixture can be administered peripherally. This high-fat admixture will also reduce the incidence of hyperglycemia and hyperinsulinemia, and improve nitrogen balance, which is particularly important in this case because of the patient's extensive tissue necrosis. A high-fat diet has also been recommended in cases with pulmonary compromise as observed in this patient. Metabolism of fat calories produces less carbon dioxide for excretion than carbohydrate metabolism. Feeding fat decreases the pulmonary work to excrete carbon dioxide and thereby reduces ventilatory work.

   This nutrient admixture, administered through a peripheral access, should be done using a silicone or polyurethane catheter. Sodium heparin can be added to the admixture (0.5 to 1 U/ml of total admixture) to prevent formation of fibrin clots around the catheter tip when it is placed in a small vessel. To promote or maintain gastrointestinal health, the patient should also be fed small amounts of a high-protein, high-fat liquid or moist food per os as soon as clinically possible. The oral food should be enriched with glutamine, arginine and omega-3 fatty acids to enhance enterocyte proliferation and immune cell function.

Progress Notes

The patient received peripheral parenteral feeding (**Table 1**) for eight days during which time the frequency of wound débridement and bandage changes was decreased to once daily. The patient's food assimilation and swallowing reflex improved so that the patient was able to eat a food with high protein, fat and moisture content (Prescription Diet a/d Canine/Feline[d] gruel and then Prescription Diet p/d Canine[d] meatballs) to meet its RER. Just before the patient was discharged, its laboratory values were normal except for mild hypoalbuminemia (2.4 g/dl). The patient was discharged with antibiotic therapy and instructions to the owners for daily wound care. The dog returned for weekly evaluations. Tissue healing was marked but not complete four weeks after hospitalization. The owners were advised to feed 4.5 cups of a moderately high-protein, calorie-dense food (Science Diet Puppy Original[d] dry) to meet the dog's daily energy requirement (DER) of 1,595 kcal (DER = 1.8 x RER) (6.67 MJ) until tissue healing was complete.

Endnotes

a. Baytril. Bayer Animal Health, Shawnee, KS, USA.
b. Amoxi-Tabs. Pfizer Animal Health, Exton, PA, USA.
c. Cephalexin. Teva Pharm, Sellersville, PA, USA.
d. Hill's Pet Nutrition, Inc., Topeka, KS, USA.

Bibliography

Codina LM. Peripheral parenteral nutrition. In: Shikora SA, Blackburn GL, eds. Nutrition Support: Theory and Therapeutics. New York, NY: Chapman & Hall, 1997; 169-176.

Nelson KM, Long CL. Physiological basis for nutrition in sepsis. In: Schneider PD, Bell S, eds. Selected Reviews in Nutrition Support. Silver Spring, MD: Aspen Publications, 1993; 142-151.

Neuvonen PT, Salvo M. Effects of short-term starvation on the immune response. Nutrition Research 1984; 4: 771-776.

Zaloga G, Ackerman MH. A review of disease-specific formulas. American Association of Critical-Care Nurses: Clinical Issues 1994; 421-435.

Table 1. Peripheral parenteral TNA for one day.*

Nutrients/fluids	Quantities (ml)
50% dextrose	52
20% lipid emulsion	400
8.5% amino acids (with electrolytes)	312
Potassium phosphate (4.4 mEq K, 3 mM P/ml)	4.9
Potassium chloride (2 mEq/ml)	7.5
Vitamin-B complex**	9
Trace elements***	9
Lactated Ringer's solution	1,252

*RER ($[29.5]^{0.75}$ x 70) = 886 kcal ME/day (3.7 MJ). Calories from lipid = 90%. Calories from dextrose = 10%. Protein-calorie ratio = 3 g/100 kcal. [K] = 29.6 mEq/l. [P] = 11.8 mM/l. Osmolarity = 486 mOsm/l.
**B-vitamin complex contains 50 mg thiamin, 2 mg riboflavin, 100 mg niacin, 2 mg pyridoxine, 10 mg pantothenic acid and 0.4 µg B_{12} per ml. Butler Co., Columbus, OH, USA.
***MTE-4 contains 1.7 mg zinc, 0.42 mg copper, 0.37 mg manganese and 6 µg chromium per ml containing the preservative benzyl alcohol. Abbott Laboratories, Chicago, IL, USA.

CASE 26-2

Central Parenteral Nutrition in a Cat

Kathryn E. Michel, DVM, MS, Dipl. ACVN
School of Veterinary Medicine
University of Pennsylvania
Philadelphia, Pennsylvania, USA

Patient Assessment

A 10-year-old, spayed female, domestic shorthair cat presented to the emergency service with a three-week history of poor appetite and weight loss. The chief complaint was facial swelling (especially around the nose) and nasal discoloration. The cat's problems were originally associated with an episode of pollakiuria and inappropriate urination, which resolved with antimicrobial therapy (sulfadimethoxine[a]). About two weeks before presentation, the cat became lethargic and tachypneic and its appetite deteriorated further. At that time the owners noticed that the cat's normally pink nose had become discolored. They initially observed a small bloody spot on the bridge of the nose overlying bluish skin. Over the course of a week the nose became progressively swollen and the skin blackened. The cat developed mild epistaxis.

On physical examination, the patient was depressed, moderately dehydrated (8 to 10%) and hypothermic (36.7°C [98.2°F]). The cat weighed 3 kg and its body condition was considered cachectic (body condition score [BCS] of 1/5). Mucous membranes were pale and slightly tacky. Ecchymoses and petechiae were present on the sclera, pinnae and gingiva. Harsh lung sounds were auscultated bilaterally. Swelling and discoloration were noted on the nose, upper lip and tail.

Initial laboratory work included a serum biochemistry analysis, a complete blood count (CBC), a coagulation profile, activated clotting time (ACT) and blood typing. The cat had previously tested negative for feline leukemia virus and feline immunodeficiency virus. Results of the serum biochemistry profile were within normal limits. Abnormalities on the CBC included a hematocrit of 11% (normal 27 to 45%), hemoglobin of 3.5 g/dl (normal 8 to 15 g/dl) and an inflammatory leukogram with a left shift. The cat had a platelet count of 88,000/µl (normal 175,000 to 425,000/µl) and a corrected reticulocyte count of 8.28% (normal 1 to 10%). The coagulation profile was within normal limits, although the ACT was abnormal and the blood never completely clotted. Thoracic radiographs revealed an alveolar pattern in the cranioventral lung fields and overall increased density in the caudodorsal lung fields. Active inflammation and hemorrhage were noted on the tracheal wash. Biopsy specimens were submitted from the nose and upper lip. A cardiac consult revealed no evidence of primary heart disease and an occult heartworm test was negative.

The problem list included cachexia, anemia, neutrophilia, thrombocytopenia and alveolar disease. The differential diagnosis included thromboembolic disease, pneumonia and cold agglutinin disease. Microscopic thrombi consistent with cold agglutinin disease were found on biopsy specimens. Cold agglutinin disease was confirmed by a positive Coomb's test at 7°C (44.6°F).

Assess the Food and Feeding Method

The cat showed no interest in food even though a variety of foods were offered and efforts were made to coax it to eat. The cat had been fed a commercial grocery brand dry cat food (Purina Cat Chow[b]) free choice for several years. It would accept only a small amount of food when given by syringe. The necrotic condition of the cat's nose probably affected its ability to smell food and that in combination with dyspnea and anemia caused the lack of appetite. The cat's poor body condition, the severity of its illness and the likelihood of a prolonged clinical course prompted a more aggressive approach for providing nutrition to this patient.

Initial therapy included a maintenance infusion (65 ml/kg body weight/day) of 0.9% NaCl with 20 mEq K/l, antibiotic therapy (enrofloxacin[c] and ampicillin[d]) and a transfusion with whole blood and fresh frozen plasma. The cat was admitted to the intensive care unit where it was placed in an oxygen cage with orders to keep it warm. The cat was started on cyproheptadine[e] (2 mg per os, t.i.d.) with orders to offer a variety of warmed foods and to coax it to eat. A central venous polyurethane catheter was placed in the left femoral vein and a parenteral nutrition (PN) admixture containing 50% dextrose, 20% lipid emulsion, 8.5% amino acid solution without electrolytes, potassium phosphate, potassium chloride, trace elements and injectable B complex was begun (**Table 1**). The PN solution was delivered at a rate of 5 ml/hour for the first 24 hours to deliver two-thirds of the calculated resting energy requirement (RER). On subsequent days, it was delivered at a rate of 7 ml/hour (56 ml/kg body weight/day) to deliver 100% of the RER ($[3.0]^{0.75}$ x 70 = 160 kcal/day [670 kJ/day]). The peripheral catheter infusion rate of the NaCl solution was reduced to 9 ml/kg body weight/day to accommodate the central PN infusion and meet the cat's daily maintenance fluid requirement.

Table 1. Central parenteral TNA for one day.*

Nutrients/fluids	Quantities (ml)
50% dextrose	38
20% lipid emulsion	48
8.5% amino acids (without electrolytes)	113
Potassium phosphate (4.4 mEq K, 3 mM P/ml)	1.4
Potassium chloride (2 mEq/ml)	1.4
Vitamin-B complex**	1
Trace elements***	0.1

*RER ($[3.0]^{0.75}$ x 70) = 160 kcal ME/day (670 kJ/day). Calories from lipid = 60%. Calories from dextrose = 40%. Protein-calorie ratio = 6 g/100 kcal. [K] = 29.7 mEq/l. [P] = 11.8 mM/l. Osmolarity = 1,188 mOsm/l.
**B-vitamin complex contains 50 mg thiamin, 2 mg riboflavin, 100 mg niacin, 2 mg pyridoxine, 10 mg pantothenic acid and 0.4 µg B_{12} per ml. Butler Co., Columbus, OH, USA.
***MTE-4 contains 1.7 mg zinc, 0.42 mg copper, 0.37 mg manganese and 6 µg chromium per ml. Abbott Laboratories, Chicago, IL, USA.

Questions

1. Which other feeding routes might have been considered to support this patient and why were they rejected in favor of centrally administered PN?
2. Were any micronutrients absent from the PN formulation that might be important for erythropoiesis?
3. What types of metabolic complications should be anticipated in a critically ill patient receiving PN?

Answers and Discussion

1. A number of enteral feeding routes and PN infusion via peripheral venous access were considered for this patient. The nasoesophageal route was rejected for several reasons. The most obvious reason was the condition of the patient's nares, which were partially obstructed due to necrosis. Also, there was the concern of provoking epistaxis in a thrombocytopenic and severely anemic patient as the tube was advanced through the nose. Finally, there was the issue of blocking the nares in an animal already experiencing difficulty breathing through its nose. All other routes of enteral feeding (i.e., esophagostomy, pharyngostomy, gastrostomy and enterostomy) require heavy sedation or general anesthesia with varying degrees of surgical intervention. The cat's compromised pulmonary function and thrombocytopenia were considered contraindications for these procedures. (There was a missed opportunity later on in this case to place a less invasive type of enteral feeding tube [e.g., an esophagostomy tube]. On Day 10 of hospitalization the cat was anesthetized for a bronchioalveolar lavage and a bone marrow aspirate). Central infusion of PN was selected instead of peripheral infusion because there was a concern of fluid overload, given the extent of alveolar disease in this patient. Therefore, a more concentrated, smaller volume admixture was conservatively infused via a central vein rather than peripherally.

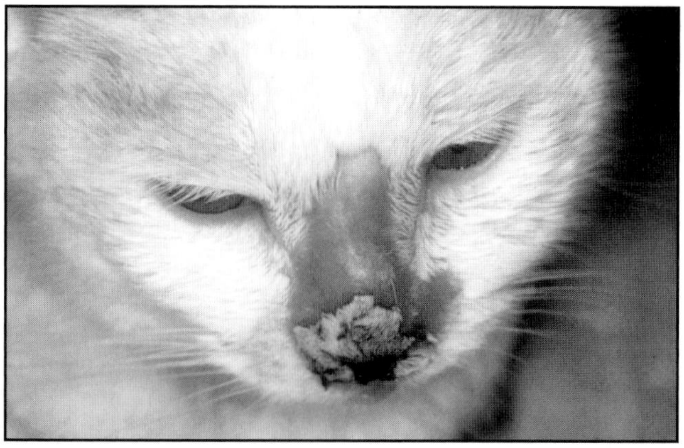

Figure 1. A 10-year-old, domestic shorthair cat with cold agglutinin disease on Day 19 of hospitalization.

2. Two micronutrients important for red blood cell production, and which are associated with anemia when deficient, were omitted from the PN admixture because of noncompatibility issues. The first was iron. Parenteral iron solutions are not approved for mixing with any vehicle including PN admixtures and are therefore commonly given separately by intramuscular or intravenous routes. However, the concern that this patient would become iron deficient was minor because the cat had received multiple red blood cell transfusions during the course of hospitalization.

   The other missing nutrient was folic acid. Folic acid is omitted from standard veterinary parenteral B-complex formulations because of noncompatibility and stability issues. Some human parenteral vitamin formulations contain folic acid; however, at the time this case presented, there was a severe shortage of these products and their use in a veterinary patient could not be justified. Although omission of folic acid from this cat's nutritional support was not optimal, the extent of folic acid deficiency may have been limited due to ongoing efforts to feed the cat per os throughout the time it received PN.
3. Common metabolic complications associated with PN include hyperglycemia, lipemia and electrolyte disturbances. Hyperglycemia and lipemia were not noted at any time during PN infusion in this patient, probably due in part to the conservative estimate of its caloric requirements and because the cat received only 40% of its nonprotein calories as dextrose. Serum potassium, sodium, chloride and ionized calcium levels were monitored daily. Serum phosphorus and magnesium levels were monitored two or three times per week.

Progress Notes

The patient continued to require oxygen therapy. The thrombocytopenia resolved, but the anemia persisted with a poor regenerative response. *Pasteurella multocida* was cultured from a tracheal wash but it was unknown whether this isolate was the cause of the alveolar disease or a contaminant. The patient's appetite was poor despite continued efforts to coax the cat to eat. The cyproheptadine was discontinued after four days. On Day 4 of PN, a low serum magnesium concentration was detected and corrected with an infusion of magnesium sulfate at a rate of 1 mg/kg body weight/day via the peripheral catheter. The serum magnesium level returned to normal within 24 hours and the magnesium sulfate infusion was discontinued. Mild hypokalemia also occurred and was corrected by increasing the admixture potassium concentration to 30 mEq/l. Low serum phosphorus levels were not detected in this patient.

On Day 7, the cat was still receiving most of its nutrition parenterally. Therefore, injections of fat-soluble vitamins were given (1,000 IU vitamin A, 100 IU vitamin D, 3 IU vitamin E intramuscularly and 7.5 mg vitamin K subcutaneously). On Day 10, the cat was anesthetized for bronchoscopy, an ultrasound-guided fine-needle lung aspirate and a bone marrow aspirate. There were no abnormalities found grossly at bronchoscopy and when the bone marrow aspirate was examined. Cultures of the bronchoalveolar lavage revealed different organisms from the tracheal wash; however, the pulmonary disease seemed to be improving. The decision was made to start immunosuppressive therapy (prednisolone acetate 1 mg/kg, subcutaneously, b.i.d.) because the cat's red blood cells were still agglutinating.

The patient started to improve, and by Day 13 no longer required oxygen therapy. The necrotic tissue on the cat's nose had begun to scab over. By Day 19 (**Figure 1**), the Coomb's test was negative at 4°C (39.2°F), the nares became clear of scabs and the cat's appetite returned. The patient started to eat a maintenance dry cat food (Science Diet Feline Maintenance[f]) voluntarily with an excellent appetite and consumed sufficient quantities of food to exceed its RER. On Day 20, central venous access was lost, but because the cat was eating well, there was no concern about continuing PN. On Day 22, the necrotic portion of the cat's tail was removed using local ring-block anesthesia. The patient continued to improve and was discharged from the hospital on Day 25. At the time of discharge, the cat weighed 3.2 kg and had a hematocrit of 19%. The cat continued to do well at home. At two weeks after discharge it weighed 3.4 kg, was still thin (BCS 2/5) but no longer cachectic and had a hematocrit of 22% with a corrected reticulocyte count of 6.2%. One year later on a routine annual examination, the cat weighed 4.1 kg (BCS 3/5), had a normal PCV with no reticulocytes and was reportedly doing very well.

Endnotes

a. Albon. Pfizer Animal Health, Exton, PA, USA.
b. Ralston Purina Co., St. Louis, MO, USA.
c. Baytril. Bayer Animal Health, Shawnee, KS, USA.
d. Amoxi-Tabs. Pfizer Animal Health, Exton, PA, USA.
e. Periactin. Merck and Company, Inc., Rahway, NJ, USA.
f. Hill's Pet Nutrition, Inc., Topeka, KS, USA.

Bibliography

Godfrey DR, Anderson RM. Cold agglutinin disease in a cat. Journal of Small Animal Practice 1994; 35: 267-270.
Lippert AC, Fulton RB, Parr AM. A retrospective study of the use of total parenteral nutrition in dogs and cats. Journal of Veterinary Internal Medicine 1993; 7: 52-64.

CASE 26-3

Combined Parenteral and Enteral Feeding in a Cat

Donna Raditic, DVM
MSPCA Angell Animal Medical Center
Boston, Massachusetts, USA

Patient Assessment

A five-year-old, neutered male, domestic shorthair cat was presented for anorexia and weight loss. The patient lived in a large multiple-cat household and had been missing for one week. The owners found the cat and thought it had lost weight, but couldn't coax the cat to eat. On physical examination, the cat was lethargic, dehydrated with a body weight of 4.5 kg and a body condition score of 2/5. The cat had excessive skin folds, which supported the owner's report of recent weight loss. The cat was icteric with palpable liver enlargement. All cats in the household were fed a dry grocery brand cat food fed free choice.

Results of a complete blood count included a regenerative anemia; *Bartonella* was detected on a blood smear. The patient also had elevated liver enzyme activities, increased blood urea nitrogen values and hypoalbuminemia. Serum electrolytes were within normal limits.

The patient was stabilized with an intravenous bolus of crystalloid solution followed by appropriate fluid management, antibiotics and antiemetics. Although therapy stabilized the cat's laboratory values, the patient continued to vomit bilious fluid throughout the day and evening. Plans included radiography, ultrasonography and liver biopsy.

Abdominal ultrasonography showed hepatic enlargement. An ultrasound-guided liver biopsy was performed. Histopathology revealed neutrophilic and lipid infiltrates. A diagnosis of hepatic lipidosis with *Bartonella* infection was made.

Because the patient's vomiting was unresponsive to antiemetics, a parenteral solution of Aminosyn II (a parenteral nutrition [PN] admixture containing 3.5% amino acids and 5% dextrose solution) was started. The PN was given at a rate of 20 ml per hour and supplied 144 kcal/day. The patient became more alert and seemed to be responding positively to PN feeding.

Two days later the cat was sedated for placement of an esophagotomy tube for possible home care. Feeding instructions were given early afternoon, to start a continuous rate infusion of a monomeric solution[a] that contained 1.3 kcal/ml. This solution was given at a rate of 5 ml/hour, providing the cat with 156 kcal/day (653 kJ/day). PN and supportive care were continued. The next day the cat was unresponsive, febrile, more anemic and had increased liver enzyme activities. An electrolyte panel was performed (**Table 1**).

Questions

1. What is this cat's resting energy requirement (RER)?
2. How many kcal did the combination of PN and enteral feedings provide?
3. How should the serum electrolyte abnormalities, seen after 24 hours of enteral feedings, be interpreted?
4. How should these electrolyte imbalances be addressed given the patient's deterioration?

Answers and Discussion

1. RER is calculated as 70(weight in kg)$^{0.75}$. This cat's RER was 216 kcal/day. PN and/or enteral feeding should begin at the patient's RER. No "illness factors" should be used to avoid possible complications.
2. The PN supplied 144 kcal/day and the enteral feedings added 156 kcal/day. Therefore, the patient was receiving 300 kcal/day or 1.4 times above its RER.
3. Potassium decreased to 2.7 mg/dl (normal = 3.5 to 5.2) and phosphorus decreased to 1.2 mg/dl (normal = 2.6 to 8.3), whereas sodium, chloride and magnesium remained normal.

   This cat's hypophosphatemia and hypokalemia are classic signs of refeeding syndrome. These electrolyte changes occur most commonly when a patient is force fed an amount that is greater than is needed (i.e., above RER). Initially the cat was fed below RER with PN alone, and then total caloric intake increased above RER with the addition of enteral feedings. All patients fed with PN, enteral nutrition or both should initially be fed at RER. Glycogen stores are first rapidly depleted in cats with anorexia. With ongoing anorexia, fat mobilization and skeletal muscle degradation provide energy and support blood glucose.

   When refeeding, potassium and phosphorus move into intracellular spaces as normal cellular function (gluconeogenesis and ATP production) returns. Providing calories in excess of whole body potassium and phosphorous stores drives these electrolytes into intracellular spaces creating a deficient in the vascular space. Hypophosphatemia is the most serious electrolyte imbalance because it can result in hemolytic anemia and even death.
4. The patient's PN was discontinued and an intravenous crystalloid solution supplemented with potassium and phosphorous was started to replete body stores and normal serum levels. Enteral nutrition was continued at 25% of RER for two days simultaneously to maintain intestinal integrity until serum electrolyte levels returned to normal. Intestinal absorption of potassium and phosphorus should not cause electrolyte imbalances at a flow rate below RER. **Table 2** depicts the electrolyte panel 24 hours after feeding adjustments were made.

Progress Notes

Phosphorus was delivered by intravenous administration for another 24 hours to correct deficits. The patient continued to eat well in the hospital and was discharged three days later.

Endnote

a. Perative. Abbott Laboratories, Abbott Park, IL, USA.

Table 1. Electrolyte values after presentation.

Electrolyte	Value	Reference range
Sodium (mEq/l)	147	146-158
Potassium (mEq/l)	2.7	3.5-5.2
Phosphorus (mg/dl)	1.2	2.6-8.3
Chloride (mEq/l)	125	114-126
Magnesium (mEq/l)	2.1	1.9-2.28

Table 2. Electrolyte values after feeding adjustments were made.

Electrolyte	Value	Reference range
Sodium (mEq/l)	148	146-158
Potassium (mEq/l)	3.1	3.5-5.2
Phosphorus (mg/dl)	2.4	2.6-8.3
Chloride (mEq/l)	122	114-126
Magnesium (mEq/l)	2.3	1.9-2.28

Section 7

Obesity

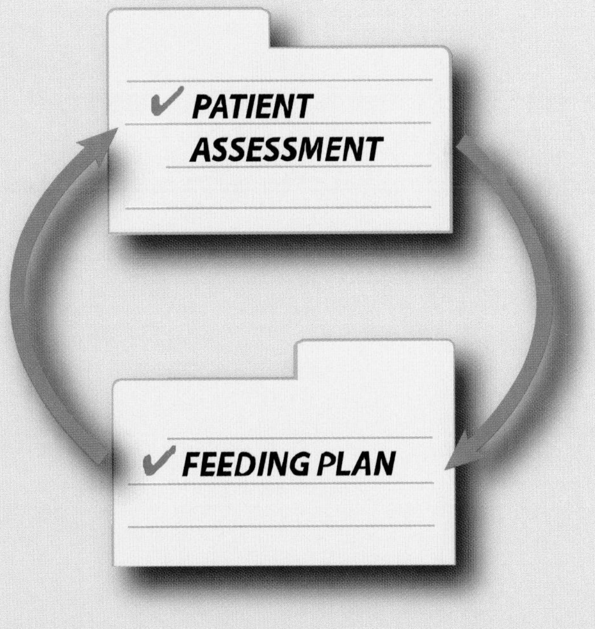

Chapter 27

Obesity

Philip W. Toll
Ryan M. Yamka
William D. Schoenherr
Michael S. Hand

"If we could give every individual the right amount of nourishment and exercise, not too little and not too much, we would have found the safest way to health."
Hippocrates

CLINICAL IMPORTANCE

Obesity is a real disease and is thought to be the most prevalent form of malnutrition in pets of westernized societies. Large studies in Great Britain and the United States indicate that the prevalence of overweight and obese dogs is between 24 to 30% (Lund et al, 2006; Armstrong and Lund, 1996; Mason, 1970; Meyer et al, 1978; Edney and Smith, 1986). Similar studies indicate the prevalence of overweight and obesity in cats is between 25 to 35% (Lund et al, 2005; Armstrong and Lund, 1996; Scarlett et al, 1994). Being overweight appears to be more problematic in middle-aged dogs and cats; 42% of dogs and 44% of cats between the ages of five and 11 years are overweight in the United States (Lund et al, 2005, 2006).

Deciding when a given animal is in ideal, overweight or obese body condition has clinical relevance because overweight and obesity may adversely affect an animal's health. By definition, obesity is the accumulation of excess body fat. Body weight increases as fat accumulates; thus, having excessive body fat and being overweight are related. Although body weight can increase for multiple reasons (Burkholder and Toll, 2000), the majority of overweight dogs and cats have excess body fat.

Body weight relative to an animal's optimal (ideal) weight has been used as a defining criterion for obesity because body weight is easier to measure than body fat. Relative body weight (RBW) is simply an animal's current weight divided by its estimated optimal weight. People are defined as mildly obese when actual body weight exceeds optimal body weight by 15 to 30% (NIH, 1985, 1998; Owen, 1988). Similar definitions have been proposed for dogs and cats (Joshua, 1970; Lewis et al, 1987). Arbitrary ranges for RBWs for overweight dogs and cats are between 10 and 20% above optimal weight. Obese dogs and cats are characterized by RBWs above 20%.

Fat mass, expressed as a percentage of body weight, can also be used to define obesity. People are considered obese when percent body fat (%BF) exceeds 20 to 30% of total weight (NIH, 1985; Owen, 1988). Body composition studies of dogs and cats indicate that animals judged to be in ideal body condition have 15 to 20% body fat (Stanton et al, 1992; Laflamme et al, 1994, 1995; Burkholder, 1994; Laflamme, 1997, 1997a).

Health Risks of Obesity

Excessive deposition of body fat has detrimental effects on health and longevity. In people, these detrimental effects begin, and thus obesity has been defined, when body fat exceeds 20 to 30% of body weight (NIH, 1985; Lew and Garfinkel, 1979).

Even being moderately overweight throughout life reduces lifespan. In a lifelong study of two groups of Labrador retriever dogs, the treatment group was fed 25% less than the control group (Kealy et al, 2002). Over the course of the study, the control group became moderately overweight. The median lifespan of the leaner group was 13.0 years compared to 11.2 years for the moderately overweight dogs. Many pet dogs and cats are

Table 27-1. Diseases associated with or exacerbated by obesity.

Metabolic alterations
Anesthetic complications
Dyslipidemia or hyperlipidemia
Glucose intolerance
Hepatic lipidosis (cats)
Insulin resistance
Endocrinopathies
Diabetes mellitus
Hyperadrenocorticism
Hypopituitarism
Hypothalamic lesions
Hypothyroidism
Insulinoma
Pituitary chromophobe adenoma
Functional alterations
Decreased immune function
Dystocia
Exercise intolerance
Heat intolerance
Hypertension
Osteoarthritis/joint stress/musculoskeletal pain
Respiratory distress or dyspnea
Other diseases
Altered kidney function
Cardiovascular disease
Dermatopathy
Neoplasia
Oral disease
Pancreatitis
Transitional cell carcinoma (bladder)
Urinary tract disease (cats)

Table 27-2. Selected adipocyte secretory products (fat-derived peptides).*

Adiponectin	Leptin
Angiotensinogen	Plasminogen activator inhibitor-1
Complement protein 3	Resistin
Insulin-like growth factor-1	Serum amyloid A
Interleukin β	Transforming growth factor β
Interleukin 6	Tumor necrosis factor

*Adapted from Coppack SW. Proinflammatory cytokines and adipose tissue. Proceedings of the Nutritional Society 2001; 60: 349-356. Gayet C, Bailhache E, Dumon H, et al. Insulin resistance and changes in plasma concentration of TNFα, IGF1, and NEFA in dogs during weight gain and obesity. Journal of Animal Physiology and Animal Nutrition (Berlin) 2004; 88: 157-165. Miller D, Bartges J, Cornelius L, et al. Tumor necrosis factor-α levels in adipose tissue of lean and obese cats. Journal of Nutrition 1998; 128 (Suppl.): 2751S-2752S. Trayhurn P. Inflammation in obesity: Down to the fat? Compendium on Continuing Education for the Practicing Veterinarian 2006; 28 (Suppl. 4): 33-36.

overweight to this degree (Lund et al, 2005, 2006).

Numerous diseases are associated with obesity (Laflamme, 2006). **Table 27-1** lists abnormalities associated with or exacerbated by obesity. Potential common threads exist between excess body fat and many of these diseases including cytokines, hormones and oxidative stress. A growing body of evidence suggests that body fat is no longer thought of as simply an energy storage depot. Adipocytes produce and secrete numerous cytokines and hormones, sometimes collectively referred to as fat-derived peptides (**Table 27-2**) (Trayhurn, 2006; Gayet et al, 2004; Coppack, 2001; Miller et al, 1998). Many of these fat-derived peptides are proinflammatory and probably are important in several of the diseases discussed below. Thus, obesity is likely a chronic, low-grade inflammation affecting many body systems.

Other studies show that obesity increases oxidative stress. The consequences of prolonged oxidative stress to cell membranes, proteins and DNA have been associated with cancer, diabetes mellitus, urinary tract disease, heart disease and liver disease (Tanner et al, 2006; Sonta et al, 2004; Urakawa et al, 2003; Ha and Le, 2000; Thamilselvan et al, 2000; Kesavulu et al, 2000; Freeman et al, 1999; Cheng et al, 1999; Center, 1999; Knight, 1999; Ames et al, 1993).

Obesity in people is closely associated with insulin resistance, type 2 diabetes mellitus, hypertension, hyperlipidemia and cardiovascular disease. In 1999, the World Health Organization (WHO) clustered these ailments and characterized the condition as metabolic syndrome. Metabolic syndrome was defined as impaired glucose tolerance/insulin resistance with two or more of the following: elevated blood pressure, obesity (body mass index [BMI] >30), reduced high-density lipoprotein cholesterol, high triglyceride concentrations and microalbuminuria. Although metabolic syndrome has not been identified in dogs and cats as defined by the WHO, they are prone to many diseases that have been linked to and are associated with obesity.

Similar to findings in people, obese dogs and cats have increased risk of dyslipidemia (high triglycerides and cholesterol). Obese dogs and cats have elevated levels of triglycerides, cholesterol and altered lipoprotein profiles (Yamka et al, 2006; Yamka and Friesen, 2006; Jeusette et al, 2004, 2005; Sunvold and Bouchard, 1998). As in people, cholesterol and triglyceride levels decrease in dogs undergoing weight loss (Diez et al, 2004). Note that in these studies, although triglyceride and cholesterol levels were elevated, both were still within normal published ranges.

Obese dogs have an increased prevalence of cardiovascular disease in the form of congestive heart failure (Edney and Smith, 1986). Increases in blood pressure have been documented to occur in dogs under experimental conditions immediately after increases in body weight (Rocchini et al, 1987, 1989; Buffington, 1994). Structural changes in the heart have been documented in as little as nine weeks in obesity-related hypertension in dogs. Pathology included marked changes in the right atrium and left ventricle (Philip-Couderc et al, 2003). The liver and adipose tissue produce the peptide angiotensinogen (**Table 27-2**). The strong correlation between obesity and hypertension implies that excess adipose tissue may play a direct role in blood pressure regulation (Frederich et al, 1992).

Grossly obese dogs have an increased prevalence of traumatic and degenerative orthopedic disorders (Edney and Smith, 1986). Furthermore, the severity of osteoarthritis is greater in dogs with body condition scores (BCS) above ideal. Also, the mean age at which 50% of dogs required long-term treatment for osteoarthritis was significantly younger (10.3 years) in moderately overweight dogs compared to dogs with normal BCS (13.3 years) (Kealy et al, 2002). In addition to increased mechanical stress on joints resulting from excess body weight, the associated body fat produces several inflammatory mediators (Eisele et al, 2005; Trayhurn and Wood, 2004) that could contribute to, or conceivably cause, osteoarthritis (Sowers et al, 2002). In a study that investigated multiple biomarkers for early indicators of disease, obese dogs had significantly higher levels of alkaline phosphatase and type 2 cartilage synthesis indicating increased risk for osteoarthritis (Yamka et al, 2006).

Obesity has also been reported to predispose dogs and cats to diabetes mellitus or exacerbate this illness (Mattheeuws et al, 1984, 1984a; Nelson et al, 1990; Nelson, 1990; Panciera et al, 1990). Certain of the hormones and inflammatory mediators produced by adipose tissue (**Table 27-2**) are thought to play a role (Plomgaard et al, 2005). For example, adiponectin is a non-cytokine, fat-derived peptide and is the only one protective against inflammation. Unlike most fat-derived peptides, circulating levels are inversely proportional to obesity; low levels of adiponectin cause insulin resistance (Pischon et al, 2004). Another fat derived peptide, resistin, is up-regulated in obesity. Increased resistin levels participate in the pathogenesis of insulin resistance (Muse et al, 2004; Steppan et al, 2001). Also, overweight dogs have increased levels of tumor necrosis factor-α, insulin-like growth factor-1 and glucagon-like protein-1; all of these peptides have been associated with insulin resistance (Gayet et al, 2004; Yamka et al, 2006).

Obesity is a predisposing factor to idiopathic hepatic lipidosis in anorectic cats (Armstrong, 1989; Biourge et al, 1994). A less well-documented effect of obesity in dogs and cats is an increased risk for anesthetic complications, a belief held by many veterinary practitioners (Clutton, 1988). Decreased heat tolerance and stamina are also purported consequences of obesity in dogs and cats (Anderson and Lewis, 1980; Edney, 1974). Other health problems thought to be associated with or exacerbated by obesity include dyspnea, dystocia, dermatologic problems and reduced immune function, although the association between obesity and these clinical effects is less than definitively documented (Buffington, 1994; Newberne, 1966; Williams and Newberne, 1971). Oral disease and urinary disease have also been linked to obesity (Lund et al, 2005). **Table 27-1** lists abnormalities associated with or exacerbated by obesity.

Overweight and obesity in people, dogs and cats are strongly associated with an increased risk for urinary stone formation. Overweight dogs have twice the risk for developing uroliths (Lekcharoensuk et al, 2000). Overweight cats have nearly three times the risk of calcium oxalate urolithiasis compared to lean cats (Lekcharoensuk et al, 2001). In people, this correlation is reported to be due to increased urinary excretion of promoters, but not inhibitors of calcium oxalate urolith formation. Also, a significant positive relationship was shown for BMI and urinary excretion of uric acid, sodium, ammonium and phosphate. An inverse correlation was shown between BMI and urinary pH (Siener et al, 2004).

An indirect relationship between obesity and cancer has been reported to occur in overweight dogs. A case control study was conducted to determine if exposure to secondhand cigarette smoke, household chemicals and topical insecticides was associated with transitional cell carcinoma of the urinary bladder. Bladder cancer risk was unrelated to cigarette smoke or household chemicals but was significantly increased by topical insecticide use, depending on the number of applications per year. This risk was enhanced in overweight and obese dogs (Glickman et al, 1989).

PATIENT ASSESSMENT

The assessment goals for overweight and obese patients should be to: 1) review the medical record for associated concurrent health issues, 2) conduct a thorough feeding assessment and 3) determine the degree to which the patient is overweight or obese. Attaining these goals is central to the development of an effective feeding plan for weight management.

History and Physical Examination

Medical Record Review

A review of the medical record provides objective historical information and documents the pet's previous health status and whether the pet is currently receiving any medications that might be associated with an overweight or obese condition.

Obesity can be a clinical sign accompanying the endocrinopathies listed in **Table 27-1**. Hyperadrenocorticism, hypothyroidism and diabetes mellitus are the endocrinopathies most amenable to treatment. In these cases, obesity is caused by the physiologic alterations resulting from hyperadrenocorticism and hypothyroidism. Although hypothyroidism is commonly associated with obesity in dogs, hypothyroidism is not a common cause of obesity. The prevalence of hypothyroidism in dogs is only 1% (Chastain and Panciera, 1995). No more than one-fourth of hypothyroid dogs are obese, whereas the prevalence of obesity in dogs is 25% (Chastain and Panciera, 1995). Obesity may either cause or occasionally result from diabetes mellitus. In either case, weight loss in an obese diabetic will improve the chances for better regulation of blood glucose concentrations and perhaps decrease or eliminate the need for insulin administration to achieve glycemic control (Chapter 29).

Treatment of the remaining endocrinopathies in **Table 27-1** is often unrewarding. They are listed for completeness and reference, and should be considered after the more common diagnoses are excluded and when patients do not lose weight with even the most severe caloric restriction. A veterinarian presented with an obese patient should use historical information and physical and clinical pathologic findings to include or exclude the possibility of a systemic problem causing or contributing to the obesity.

Current Feeding Plan Assessment

A thorough feeding assessment should be conducted, particularly in regards to food intake, physical activity and changes in body weight. The food history should include the name of the

Box 27-1. Feeding History and Food Records.

A quantitative food record can provide important information for use in a weight-loss program. Knowledge of total calories being consumed can be used to determine the amount to feed for weight loss. The process of a pet owner providing a feeding history to a veterinary health care team can help with compliance to a weight-loss program by making pet owners aware of all the sources of calories that could conceivably contribute to the pet's overweight condition.

The food record should include amounts of all foods and account for all calories the patient consumes. Caloric content of commercial pet foods and treats can be obtained from the manufacturer or calculated (Chapter 1). Tables 13-4 (dogs) and 20-4 (cats) list caloric content for several commercial foods. Most packaged human foods include caloric content on the label. The clinical cases at the end of this chapter demonstrate the utility of a quantitative food record for determining appropriate amounts of food for achieving weight loss.

The owner's quantitative descriptions of how much pet food, how many treats and access to table food and consumable chew toys must be evaluated. Terms such as "bowls," "cups" and "handfuls" reported by owners come in all sizes; thus, the amount of food and calories these objects can hold varies as well. The veterinary nutritionist's "cup" is a standard 8-oz. volume measure. The amount of dry dog or cat food reportedly fed by owners needs to be converted to this standard or to weight (as fed) for accurate determination of caloric intake. Treats, consumable chew toys and table food can supply significant calories, especially if the owner is unaware of their caloric content or how many the animal eats daily.

Whether the pet has access to any other sources of food also needs to be determined. Other sources include other pets' food in multi-pet households. Having multiple people feed the pet can result in multiple sources of food, particularly if different people have different opinions about the body condition of the pet. The previous two situations can condemn a weight-reduction program to failure before it ever begins if the owner cannot, or will not, feed the overweight pet separately and keep the overweight pet from eating other pets' food. Dogs and cats that roam unsupervised also have the opportunity to obtain other sources of food.

If an owner insists on feeding treats to a pet entering a weight-loss program, the number can be controlled by placing a specific quantity of treats containing the number of calories reserved for treats in a "treat container" each day. No additional treats are allowed for that day after the treat container is empty.

food, its form and how much is fed. Also, it should be determined whether commercial treats and/or table foods are fed and if so, how much. Accurate accounting of the total amount of food (calories) fed can be very important in the development of a feeding plan for weight loss (**Box 27-1**). It is also important to know what feeding methods are used for the pet and who feeds and/or provides treats. Most owners supplement their pets' food regimen with treats and/or table foods (Buffington et al, 2004).

Determining the Degree of Overweight and Ideal Body Weight

Determining whether a cat or dog is overweight is usually not difficult. However, accurately determining the degree of overweight and the patient's ideal weight can be challenging. In the clinical setting, the subjectivity inherent in determining the degree of body fat makes irrefutable, objective measurement difficult. This subjectivity results from variation in body conformation across breeds, variation of frame size within breeds, especially for dogs and the veterinarian's and owner's bias for what constitutes a patient's ideal body weight and conformation. For example, most dog and cat owners underestimate their pet's body condition (Singh et al, 2002; Allan et al, 2000). Even veterinarians overlook obesity (Lund et al, 1999). There is no ideal, definitive method for deciding whether a dog or cat is in a thin, ideal, overweight or obese body condition. In reality, a continuum exists from emaciation to morbid obesity, making absolute definitions and divisions arbitrary.

Clinically, it is important to assess body condition of cats and dogs objectively. The ability to assess body condition is necessary to determine when a dog or cat is likely to benefit from weight loss, and to substantiate a diagnosis of obesity for the patient's owners and convince them that their pet needs to lose weight. Radiographic and ultrasound images can be used to help convince an owner his or her pet is overweight (**Box 27-2**); however, these aids do not quantify the degree to which a pet is overweight. Quantifying excess body weight and determining ideal body weight are essential to the effectiveness of a weight-loss program. The most practical method for making these determinations is body condition scoring.

BODY CONDITION SCORING

The BCS is a subjective assessment of an animal's body fat, and to lesser extent its protein stores, that takes into account the animal's frame size independent of its weight. Scoring systems using defined criteria help objectify the process, but cannot remove all subjectivity involved in assigning a score to a given patient. Body condition scoring like other physical examination techniques is a learned skill. Within the range of defined criteria, the scorer still must learn by experience what visual and palpable characteristics correspond with a given BCS. Standardization of scores between observers scoring a given animal can be problematic. What one scorer feels to be an excessive amount of fat covering the ribs, another scorer may assess as appropriate. However, once learned, body condition scoring is a reliable indicator for determining the proportion of body fat or body composition (Mawby et al, 2004; Laflamme, 1993, 1997, 1997a; Laflamme et al, 1994; Graham et al, 1982; Croxton and Stollard, 1976).

Different body condition scoring systems for dogs and cats

Box 27-2. Other Diagnostic Procedures.

Radiographic or sonographic images can often help an owner appreciate the degree of excess fat deposited subcutaneously or intra-abdominally, particularly when viewed next to radiographs or sonograms of similar size animals that are in optimal body condition (**Figures 1A** and **B** and **2A** and **B**). However, radiographs should not be taken solely for diagnosing obesity. Many veterinary schools now have dual energy x-ray absorptiometry, which can be effectively used for weight-reduction/maintenance programs.

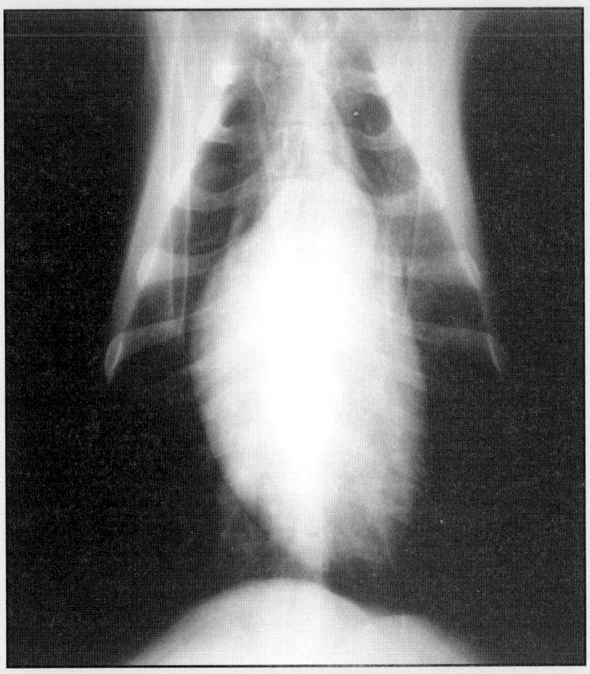

Figures 1A and 1B. Ventrodorsal radiographs of a normal dog (BCS 3/5, above) and an obese dog (BCS 5/5, below). Compare the body wall thickness of the two dogs.

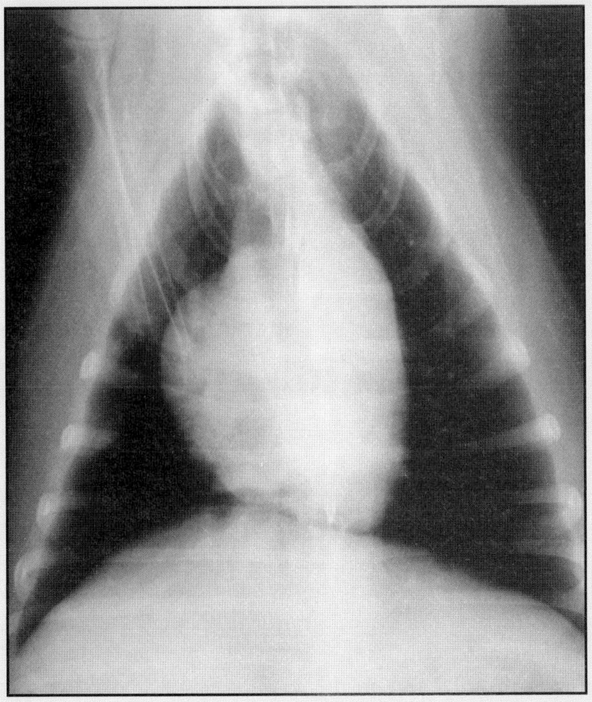

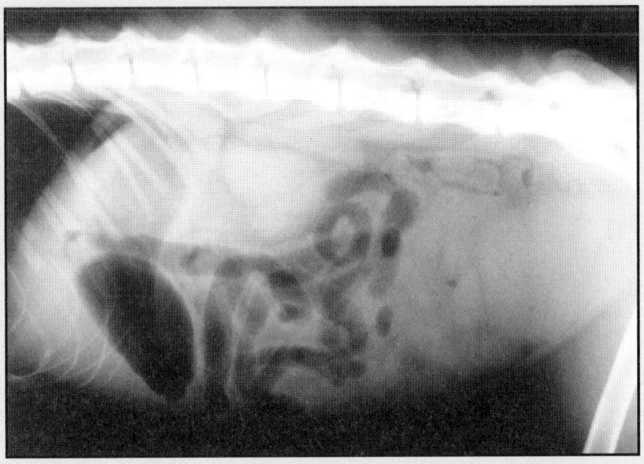

Figures 2A and 2B. Lateral abdominal radiographs of a normal cat (BCS 3/5, above) and an obese cat (BCS 5/5, below). Note the enlarged abdomen and ventral fat deposition in the obese cat.

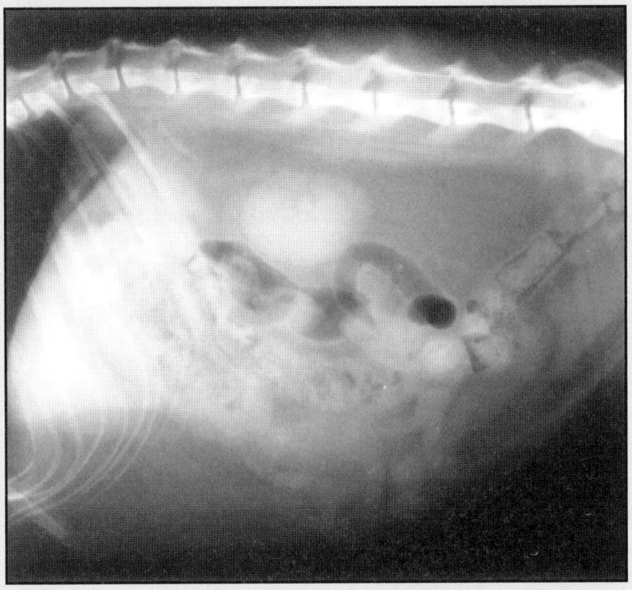

Table 27-3. Relationships between body condition score (BCS; 5-point system) and actual body weight, ideal body weight, resting energy requirement (RER; kcal metabolizable energy [ME]/day) and estimated percent body fat (%BF). Actual body weight and BCS can be used to estimate a patient's ideal weight* and associated RER, which can be further used for determining the amount of food to feed for weight loss.

BCS	Body weight (kg)											
5	2	2.5	3	3.5	4	4.5	5	5.5	6	6.5	7	7.5
4	1.7	2.1	2.6	3	3.4	3.9	4.3	4.7	5.1	5.6	6	6.4
3	1.5	1.9	2.3	2.6	3	3.4	3.8	4.1	4.5	4.9	5.3	5.6
RER	95	112	129	144	160	174	189	203	216	230	243	256
BCS	**Body weight (kg)**											
5	8	8.5	9	9.5	10	10.5	11	11.5	12	12.5	13	13.5
4	6.9	7.3	7.7	8.1	8.6	9	9.4	9.9	10.3	10.7	11.1	11.6
3	6	6.4	6.8	7.1	7.5	7.9	8.3	8.6	9	9.4	9.8	10.1
RER	268	281	293	305	317	329	341	352	364	375	386	397
BCS	**Body weight (kg)**											
5	14	14.5	15	15.5	16	16.5	17	17.5	18	18.5	19	19.5
4	12	12.4	12.9	13.3	13.7	14.1	14.6	15	15.4	15.9	16.3	16.7
3	10.5	10.9	11.3	11.6	12	12.4	12.8	13.1	13.5	13.9	14.3	14.6
RER	408	419	430	441	451	462	472	483	493	503	513	524
BCS	**Body weight (kg)**											
5	20	21	22	23	24	25	26	27	28	29	30	31
4	17.1	18	18.9	19.7	20.6	21.4	22.3	23.1	24	24.9	25.7	26.6
3	15	15.8	16.5	17.3	18	18.8	19.5	20.3	21	21.8	22.5	23.3
RER	534	553	573	593	612	631	650	668	687	705	723	741
BCS	**Body weight (kg)**											
5	32	33	34	35	36	37	38	39	40	41	42	43
4	27.4	28.3	29.1	30	30.9	31.7	32.6	33.4	34.3	35.1	36	36.9
3	24	24.8	25.5	26.3	27	27.8	28.5	29.3	30	30.8	31.5	32.3
RER	759	777	794	812	829	846	863	880	897	914	931	947
BCS	**Body weight (kg)**											
5	45	47	49	51	53	55	58	61	64	67	70	73
4	38.6	40.3	42	43.7	45.4	47.1	49.7	52.3	54.9	57.4	60	62.6
3	33.8	35.3	36.8	38.3	39.8	41.3	43.5	45.8	48	50.3	52.5	54.8
RER	980	1,013	1,045	1,077	1,108	1,139	1,186	1,231	1,277	1,321	1,365	1,409

BCS	%BF	BCS	%BF	BCS	%BF
5	**≥40**	**4**	**30**	**3**	**20**

*The formula used to derive the relationship between body weight and BCS is described in **Box 27-3**.

Example: A 32-kg dog has a BCS of 4/5. What is its ideal weight and associated RER and approximate %BF?

1. Find the closest value for its current body weight (31.7 kg) in the row for BCS 4/5.
2. Locate the corresponding body weight for BCS 3/5 (ideal weight) in the same number column. In this case it is 27.8 kg.
3. Below the ideal body weight of 27.8 kg, find the RER value for that weight; in this case it is 846 kcal/day (to convert to kJ, multiply kcal by 4.184).
4. At its current BCS (4/5), the dog's approximate %BF is 30.

contain from three to nine categories for body condition and have been assessed to different extents for precision, accuracy and repeatability (Armstrong and Lund, 1996; Mason, 1970; Edney and Smith, 1986; Scarlett et al, 1994; Joshua, 1970; Laflamme et al, 1994, 1995; Burkholder, 1994; Laflamme, 1993). Chapter 1 presents a 5-point body condition scoring system in detail. Systems with either five or nine categories are used most commonly. A 5-point system scored to the nearest half score and a 9-point system scored to the nearest whole score each have nine total scores for body condition. A 5-point system scored to the nearest half score subdivides into three categories each for insufficient, ideal and excess body conditions, with a score of 3.0 falling in the middle of the optimal range.

In general, dogs and cats in ideal body condition have: 1) normal body contours and silhouettes, 2) bony prominences that can be readily palpated but not seen or felt above skin surfaces and 3) intraabdominal fat insufficient to obscure or interfere with abdominal palpation. The most critical division points in a 5-point system are between the scores of 2.0 vs. 2.5 and 3.5 vs. 4.0, because assignment of a BCS less than 2.5 or greater than 3.5 suggests action should be taken to return the patient's BCS to the optimal range. These same criteria (i.e., what contours are absent that otherwise should be present and what bony prominences should be easily felt but are not readily palpable) can be demonstrated to the patient's owner as part of the educational process to obtain agreement that the patient needs to lose weight.

BCS and body weights should always be recorded in the hospital record whenever a veterinarian or another health-care team member examines a patient. An accurate estimate of the patient's ideal weight is important for a successful weight-loss program. Deciding on an optimal weight can be problematic for the veterinarian and the pet owner, especially if the two disagree. However, after a patient's BCS has been determined, its ideal body weight can be estimated using **Table 27-3**. This is done by locating the patient's body weight for the BCS determined during the physical examination and finding the patient's corresponding body weight for its ideal BCS (3/5) on the table.

BCS can also be used to estimate %BF because body condition can be defined as the ratio of fat to nonfat tissues (Murray, 1919). If 15 to 20% body fat is accepted as optimal for dogs and cats, then a patient with a BCS of 3 out of 5 (3/5) should have between 15 to 20% body fat. Research to critically assess the capability of BCS to predict body composition suggests that %BF changes by roughly 10% for each change in BCS on a 5-point scale (or 5% on a 9-point scale) (Laflamme et al, 1994; Laflamme, 1997, 1997a). Using the upper end of the range of %BF (20% body fat) for dogs and cats with a BCS of 3/5, a BCS of 4/5 correlates with approximately 30% body fat and a BCS of 5/5 correlates with 40% (or more) body fat (**Table 27-3**). Thirty percent body fat (BCS 4/5) is similar to the critical %BF for assessing when people are at risk for ill effects from being overweight. Most studies critically assessing the precision of BCS against some criterion measure of body fat indicate that %BF is estimated with a standard deviation of ± 4 to 5% (Laflamme et al, 1994; Burkholder, 1994; Laflamme, 1993; Graham et al, 1982; Croxton and Stollard, 1976).

One misconception that could arise about body condition scoring is the implication that some maximum amount of body fat corresponds to the maximum BCS. BCS have a maximum upper number assigned to the fattest animals used to define the scoring criteria, which consequently is associated with the mean %BF of those animals. However, the maximum amount of body fat compatible with life is unknown and is very likely more than the approximate value of 40% body fat of all dogs or cats with a BCS of 5/5. The correct interpretation for %BF based on assigning a maximum BCS should be that the animal has at least 40% body fat, but the %BF could be considerably higher. **Box 27-3** reviews obesity classification in people and proposes a similar method be considered for obese dogs and cats.

OTHER METHODS

Although not as practical as BCS, other means exist to determine whether a dog or cat is at optimal weight, overweight or obese. These include ultrasound, morphometric analysis and methods that are currently too expensive or otherwise impractical for use in private practice.

Ultrasound has been used to estimate back fat thickness in livestock including swine, cattle, sheep, horses and ponies. Ultrasound has also been used in people to determine %BF (Stouffer, 2004). Because ultrasound is routinely used as a diagnostic tool in small animal medicine, it has potential for determining %BF in dogs and cats. In combination with specific morphometry, it predicts %BF in beagles (Yamka et al, 2007).

%BF can also be estimated with morphometry (i.e., measurement of form). Morphometric analyses are routinely used in people to estimate body composition and %BF from measurements of various anatomic circumferences and lengths (Houmard et al, 1991; Weltman et al, 1987, 1988; Davis et al, 1985). The success for measurements made in specific locations to estimate overall body composition depends on correlation of measurements to total body composition. In people, BMI is practical because of the small range of body types. Even in people, the accuracy of BMI is influenced by differences in bone size. However, because of the immense diversity of body types within the canine species (e.g., English bulldog vs. greyhound), the use of morphometric analysis to estimate body fat requires more measurements and complex math to provide reasonable estimates of body fat than it does in people. Furthermore, fat is deposited in slightly different body sites in cats compared to dogs. Cats store most of their fat subcutaneously along their ventral abdomen, in their faces and intra-abdominally. Dogs deposit significant amounts of fat intra-abdominally and subcutaneously in thoracic, lumbar and coccygeal areas.

Methods for morphometric analysis of dogs and cats have been determined (Laflamme et al, 2001; Burkholder, 1994; Stanton et al, 1992). Besides the shortcomings mentioned above of using this technology in dogs and cats, repeatability is a concern. Differences in measurements occur due to: 1) variations in coat thickness, 2) operator variability (i.e., tension on the tape measure), 3) operator variability in determining the precise location of anatomic landmarks for measurement and 4) patient restraint, particularly in cats. Cats usually require anesthesia to obtain accurate measurements (Burkholder and Toll, 2000).

Weight at the time the dog or cat reaches adult age is often a good indicator of optimal weight if body condition assessments are unavailable. However, weight at maturity may not automatically be optimal if the animal was underfed or overfed during growth. For most dogs and cats, maturity occurs around 12 months of age. Giant-breed dogs, however, may require up to 18 months to reach mature adult weight.

For purebred dogs, determining optimal weight from published optimal weights by breed is often not accurate enough for an individual within a breed. A similar approach has been considered for cats based on body type and the fact that cats have less variability of body weights than dogs (Burkholder and Toll, 2000). Neither method is accurate enough to be used routinely as the basis for an effective weight-reduction feeding plan. Appendices 14 and 15 list proposed optimal weights for dog breeds by gender based on data from the American Kennel Club and other sources.

There are multiple methods that vary widely in cost, sophistication and precision for estimating %BF in people (Brodie, 1988, 1988a; Lukaski, 1987). Some are used for determining %BF in dogs and cats in research settings. Several methods are available for determining body composition, and thus, %BF: 1) magnetic resonance imaging, 2) computed tomography, 3) neutron activation, 4) hydrodensitometry, 5) total body water by isotope dilution, 6) total body potassium, 7) ultrasound, 8) bioelectrical impedance and 9) dual energy x-ray absorptiometry (Brodie, 1988, 1988a; Lukaski, 1987). Unfortunately, at this time, most of these methods are impractical for use in private veterinary hospitals.

Box 27-3. Proposed Refinement of Body Condition Score (BCS) Classification of Obese Dogs and Cats (BCS 5/5).

In people, body mass index (BMI) is a very useful tool for classifying the degree of overweight and obesity. Furthermore, BMI is related to the risk for the development of diseases associated with obesity, because BMI, which describes relative weight for height, is significantly correlated with body fat content. BMI is calculated by dividing body weight (kg) by height squared (m^2). The resultant BMI value is not the same as percent body fat. In people, **Table 1** is used for classification of overweight and obesity, by BMI.

The rationale behind these definitions is based on epidemiologic data that show increased mortality with BMIs greater than 25. The increase in mortality, however, tends to be modest until a BMI of 30 is reached. For persons with a BMI greater than 30, mortality rates from all causes, but especially from cardiovascular disease, are generally increased by 50 to 100% above that of people with BMIs in the range of 20 to 25. For people with BMIs greater than 35 (obesity II) and 40 (extreme obesity), mortality rates are further increased.

BMI has not been determined for dogs and cats. Morphometric measures established for companion animals are similar but much more complicated to obtain and therefore, less reliable.

Assessing BCS combined with data from **Table 27-3** (See text.) is a simple and reliable method for determining the degree of overweight and obesity in dogs and cats. However, after a patient reaches a BCS of 5, there is potential for considerable variability regarding how obese the patient could be. Thus, as for obesity classifications in people using BMI, the BCS 5/5 (>40% body fat) could be further categorized to indicate degrees of obesity in cats and dogs. **Table 2** presents such a proposed classification.

The added dimension of BCS 5/5 subcategories 5 (a,b,c) would better define the degree of obesity and could be used to improve the estimation of ideal weight in very obese and extremely obese patients, which could lead to a more appropriate amount of food to feed these patients for weight loss.

The discrepancy in food dosage that can result from whether a patient with a BCS of 5/5 has 40% body fat or 60% body fat is significant. For example, if a patient has 40% body fat and a current (obese) weight of 30 kg, its estimated ideal (target) weight would be 22.5 kg and its estimated resting energy requirement (RER) would be 745 kcal/day. However, a 30-kg patient with 60% body fat would have an ideal weight of 15 kg and its RER would be 520 kcal/day; a considerable difference of 225 kcal/day (**Table 27-3** and **Table 3**).

However, currently there are no descriptive and/or visual standards for subdividing the obese category of either the 5-point or 9-point systems. Until such tools are developed, the initial phases of weight-loss programs should be closely monitored and further restrictions of caloric intake should be instituted if weight loss does not occur within two weeks (**Figure 27-1**). Underestimation of percent body fat and resultant overestimation of ideal weight can be problematic when designing weight-loss programs for extremely obese patients.

Philip W. Toll, DVM, MS
William D. Schoenherr, PhD
Hill's Science and Technology Center
Topeka, KS, USA

Table 1. Human overweight and obesity classifications.

Class	Obese class	BMI (kg/m²)
Underweight	-	<18.5
Normal	-	18.5 to 24.9
Overweight	-	25.0 to 29.9
Obesity	I	30.0 to 34.9
	II	35.0 to 39.9
Extreme obesity	III	≥40

Table 2. Proposed classification scheme for BCS and degrees of obesity in companion animals.

Class	BCS	Body fat (%)
Very thin	1	<5
Underweight	2	10
Normal	3	20
Overweight	4	30
Obese	5(a)	40
Very obese	5(b)	50
Extremely obese	5(c)	≥60

Table 3. The ideal weight formula used to develop the body weights in **Table 27-3** and in the examples above.

Ideal weight = current weight x (100 - percent body fat [%BF]) ÷ 0.80

The assumptions and definitions used to derive this formula include:

a) Current weight (overweight due to excess adipose tissue); obtain by weighing patient
b) Body weight = fat mass + lean body mass (LBM)
c) LBM is constant between ideal and current weights
d) %BF can be estimated from BCS
e) Ideal %BF = 20%; thus, ideal LBM = 80%
f) %LBM = 100 - %BF
g) Ideal weight = LBM ÷ 0.80
h) LBM = current weight x %LBM

The steps for deriving the formula include:
Ideal weight = current weight (100 - %BF) ÷ 0.80

a) If ideal weight = LBM (g)* ÷ 0.80
b) And if LBM = current weight x %LBM (h)*
c) Then, ideal weight also = current weight x %LBM ÷ 0.80
d) And if %LBM also = 100 - %BF (f)*
e) Then ideal weight also = current weight (100 - %BF) ÷ 0.80

*Letters refer to the assumptions and definitions immediately above.

The Bibliography for **Box 27-3** can be found at www.markmorris.org.

Etiopathogenesis and Risk Factors

Energy Balance and Body Composition Control

Positive energy balance results when consumption of calories exceeds daily energy expenditure. This may result from energy intake increases and/or energy expenditure decreases. When positive imbalance is sustained, excess energy is stored in adipose tissue and overweight or obese body conditions develop due to excess body fat. An understanding of the components that contribute to the energy input side of the equation (i.e., the daily energy requirement [DER]), explains why animals of similar body weight and frame size can have different caloric requirements independent of genetics or neuter status. Understanding DER components simplifies the rationale behind recommendations and alterations made to correct obesity. Multiple components contribute to DER. The DER to maintain body weight of an animal can be subdivided into: 1) resting energy requirement (RER), 2) exercise energy requirement (EER), 3) thermic effect of food (TEF) and 4) adaptive thermogenesis (AT). In people, RER correlates closely with lean body mass and accounts for 60 to 80% of the total DER for adult maintenance (Danforth, 1985; Horton, 1983; Wilson, 1990). RER represents energy used to maintain normal physiologic functions at rest in a thermoneutral environment several hours after eating (Horton, 1983). Very little energy is required to maintain adipose tissue.

EER is the energy expended for muscular activity. The contribution of EER to DER is determined by the animal's body weight plus the duration and intensity of muscular activity. Animals that are less active or have little opportunity to exercise expend less energy compared with active animals of similar size. EER can account for 10 to 20% of total daily energy expended by nonathletic people (Danforth, 1985).

TEF represents the obligatory cost of digesting and absorbing food. TEF constitutes approximately 10% of total expenditure and is affected by food composition and the number of meals eaten per day (Danforth, 1985; Horton, 1983). The obligatory cost associated with digesting and absorbing each meal is the reason weight-reduction programs recommend multiple small meals per day rather than one or two large meals. RER, EER and TEF make up the majority of DER; thus, these are the components that can be manipulated to affect the amount and rate of weight loss.

AT makes up the smallest proportion of the DER for most pets. AT is the energy expended to regulate body temperature during exposure to ambient temperatures below or above the thermoneutral zone or during transient periods of excess caloric consumption.

Most dogs and cats maintain an ideal, constant body weight due to a complex system of neural, hormonal and biochemical mechanisms that keep the balance between energy intake and expenditure within fairly precise limits (**Boxes 27-4** and 25-2) (Druce and Bloom, 2003). Thus, under normal circumstances, homeostatic mechanisms control energy intake and maintain body composition at or near some "set point." Set point can be defined as the physiologic regulation of energy balance that maintains stable body condition. When certain abnormal conditions are imposed on these set point mechanisms, positive energy balance occurs and excess body fat accumulates. Several of these risk factors are discussed below.

Box 27-4. Central Regulators of Food Intake and Energy Balance.

Numerous feedback mechanisms exist to control eating and energy stores (Box 25-2). These mechanisms are designed to store energy as fat when energy sources are plentiful so animals can survive when food is not readily available (famine or hibernation). Three regulators of food intake and energy balance that have received attention recently include neuropeptide Y (NPY), leptin and ghrelin.

NPY is a hypothalamic hormone; its synthesis increases when an animal is deprived of food. Repeated injections of NPY into the brain results in consumption of larger meals, weight gain and obesity.

Leptin is a polypeptide hormone synthesized by white adipose tissue and secreted into the bloodstream. Leptin regulates energy intake, energy expenditure and acts at the hypothalamus to reduce synthesis of NPY, thereby down regulating food intake. Leptin secretion is proportional to the amount of lipid stored in adipocytes. As a result, serum leptin concentrations are highly correlated with obesity in rodents, dogs, cats and people.

The obese gene ("ob gene") codes for leptin and is absent in one strain of genetically obese mice ("ob mice"), thus this mouse strain readily becomes obese. Long-term treatment of ob mice with exogenous leptin causes a decline in eating and is associated with loss of body weight. In dogs, leptin injections resulted in decreased food intake and body weight. The reduction in body weight and food intake in both species is believed to be an attempt by the animal to limit weight gain.

Ghrelin is a gastric peptide and a secretagogue of growth hormone. Ghrelin controls feeding behavior, energy homeostasis, gastric acid secretion and gastric motor activity and is essential for growth hormone release. Ghrelin levels increase during fasting and decline shortly after eating. In obese dogs and cats, ghrelin and leptin levels are inversely related. The lower ghrelin levels observed in obese animals likely result from down regulation of this peptide due to excess energy storage.

The Bibliography for **Box 27-4** can be found at www.markmorris.org.

Risk Factors

Several risk factors contribute to positive energy balance and affect the body's compositional set point. They can be grouped under the headings of genetic and environmental. Although genetic risk factors make it easier for positive energy balance and obesity to develop, environmental risk factors dictate the expression of that potential and, thus, the overweight/obesity condition. Although the greater opportunity for intervention is in managing environmental risk factors, the opportunity for prevention includes management of both. Prevention of obesity is critical (Chapters 13 through 17 and

Box 27-5. Lipoprotein Lipase and Obesity Recurrence.

Following weight loss of an obese patient, weight regain is likely if there is not strict adherence to appropriate diet and exercise programs. This may be due in part to the change in lipoprotein lipase (LPL) activity.

After digestion and absorption, dietary fat is transported to adipose tissue via chylomicrons. LPL is an enzyme located in the capillaries of body fat and facilitates removal of dietary fat (triglycerides) from the chylomicrons in the bloodstream and its entry through capillary walls into adipocytes. LPL hydrolyzes triglycerides into free fatty acids and glycerol. Fatty acids enter adipocytes, where they are re-esterified into triglycerides and stored. When needed by other body cells for energy, stored triglycerides are hydrolyzed once again to fatty acids and glycerol by hormone sensitive lipase (HSL) and reenter the circulation.

LPL increases during periods of weight gain in both obese and non-obese people. After weight is lost, LPL returns to normal levels in non-obese people; however, in obese patients that have lost weight, LPL increases. This increase is probably one of the factors contributing to the rapid weight regain that is common in obese human patients and could also be a culprit in weight regain in previously overweight dogs and cats.

The Bibliography for **Box 27-5** can be found at www.markmorris.org.

20 through 24); weight loss is more difficult after body fat is gained and maintained (Laquatra, 2000) (**Box 27-5**). Under these conditions, the body essentially has a new set point. All risk factors should be understood if obesity is to be prevented and treated effectively.

Genetics

Obesity in people has a large propensity for being heritable, accounting for 37 to 40% of BMI (Coady et al, 2002). Genetics likely determine the concentration and activity of various metabolic regulators, their receptors and, thus, metabolic efficiency (Bogardus et al, 1986; Campfield et al, 1995; Halaas et al, 1995; Pelleymounter et al, 1995). Various genetic factors also influence the risk of obesity in dogs; breed accounts for 30 to 70% of the risk (Buffington et al, 2004). Some breeds are more likely to be overweight. Breed prevalence within a geographic area influences the prevalence of obesity in specific breeds. Labrador retrievers, golden retrievers, Cairn terriers, cocker spaniels, long-haired dachshunds, Shetland sheepdogs, basset hounds, cavalier King Charles spaniels, pugs, Dalmatian dogs and beagles have a greater prevalence of obesity than other breeds (Mason, 1970; Edney and Smith, 1986; Lund, 2007). In contrast to dogs, cats of mixed breeding are more likely to be obese than purebred cats (Scarlett et al, 1994). These findings suggest that genetics influence body condition set points and the tendency for weight gain or loss in dogs and cats.

Certain genes appear to be related to obesity. Compared to lean beagles (BCS 2.2/5), overweight beagles (BCS 4.3/5) had higher expression of genes associated with fatty acid metabolism, purine metabolism and platelet-derived growth factor signaling. In addition, the overweight beagles had lower expression of genes associated with nucleotide metabolism, carbohydrate metabolism, peroxisome proliferator-activated receptor signaling, insulin-like growth factor-1 signaling, insulin receptor signaling, amino acid metabolism, branched-chain amino acid degradation and lipid metabolism (Yamka et al, 2007a).

Food and Feeding

Specific attributes of foods and how foods are fed can overwhelm normal body condition set point systems and result in positive energy balance. Such food attributes include palatability and energy density. Feeding methods that further aggravate food attributes include how much is fed and how it is offered (e.g., free-choice feeding of highly palatable, energy-dense foods).

Food palatability is a highly competitive attribute in the pet food industry. Feeding pets and watching them eagerly eat is part of the pleasure people derive from having pets and apparently contributes to the human-animal bond. Palatability is also an attribute that owners perceive reflects a food's quality. Thus, pet food companies continuously strive to improve the palatability of their food, because having a highly palatable food is a competitive advantage. If the amount of a highly palatable food isn't limited, it stands to reason that a pet is more likely to overeat. Normal body condition set point systems may not have been designed to deal with some of the highly palatable foods that exist today.

Caloric density of a food is primarily a function of its dietary fat content. On a weight basis, in typical commercial pet foods, dietary fat provides 8.5 kcal (35.6 kJ) metabolizable energy (ME)/g compared to 3.5 kcal (14.6 kJ) ME/g for carbohydrate and protein. Most of the lipid in fat cells comes directly from dietary fat. In general, the fatty acid composition of body fat mirrors the fatty acid composition of the food (Laquatra, 2000). Conversely, inclusion of dietary fiber, water or air can decrease caloric density by taking up space in the food while providing few to no calories.

One study found no difference in types of food given to overweight pets compared with foods given to those in optimal body condition (Edney and Smith, 1986). Other studies demonstrated an increased risk for being overweight when certain food categories were fed (Mason, 1970; Scarlett et al, 1994). In these studies, all of the associated foods, whether commercial or home prepared, were considered calorically dense, although caloric density per se was not the variable tested for increased risk of being overweight.

Free-choice feeding can also contribute to excessive caloric intake. Feeding unlimited amounts of highly palatable, energy-dense foods to dogs and cats may encourage energy consumption that exceeds requirements, particularly if a genetic predisposition exists. Likewise, excessive use of treats or substitution of food (and treats) for other types of interaction between the owner and pet may also encourage excess energy intake.

Determining amounts to feed based on manufacturer recommendations may also lead to excessive caloric intake. This results not because manufacturers make inappropriate or self-serving recommendations, but rather because manufacturers base recommendations on ranges and average caloric requirements for a given body weight. Recommendations often list a minimum and maximum amount of food to feed within a given range of body weights (e.g., two to four cups for a 5.9- to 11.4-kg dog). The maximum amount can be one and one-half to four times the minimum amount listed for a given range of body weights. Excess caloric intake can occur if pet owners interpret that a smaller dog should be fed the larger amount. Furthermore, excess caloric intake can occur because pet owners overestimate the activity of their pet. Many pets today are relatively inactive due to the lifestyle of their owners. (See Activity below.) Also, cat and dog owners underestimate the body condition of their pets (Singh et al, 2002; Allan et al, 2000), increasing the likelihood that pets will be overfed.

Activity

Many pets, particularly cats, live indoors, which is often associated with reduced physical activity. Physical activity is the most variable component of energy expenditure. Adequate exercise can contribute markedly to daily energy expenditure. Furthermore, the risk of obesity decreases with each hour of weekly exercise in dogs (Robertson, 2003). Thus, it is not surprising that animals with decreased activity or restricted opportunities for exercise are at greater risk for becoming overweight (Scarlett et al, 1994). Unfortunately, most owners consider their dogs to be moderately or very active (Slater et al, 1995).

Caloric intake can also become excessive if changes occur in a pet's lifestyle or daily routine that markedly reduce activity without reducing calories. Such changes include moving to smaller dwellings, musculoskeletal injuries and diseases that require persistent long-term use of central nervous system depressants or corticosteroids.

Age

Caloric requirements decrease as some animals age. Requirements for a given weight are less for maintenance of adults than for growing individuals of similar weight. Age has been correlated with the prevalence of excess body weight in dogs and cats (Armstrong and Lund, 1996; Mason, 1970; Scarlett et al, 1994; Sloth, 1992; Kronfeld et al, 1991). Dogs and cats have the highest prevalence of obesity from five to 11 years of age (Lund et al, 2005, 2006). After about 12 years of age, the prevalence tends to decrease markedly in most cross-sectional studies (Armstrong and Lund, 1996; Scarlett et al, 1994; Sloth, 1992; Kronfeld et al, 1991). These observations have bearing on two theories concerning obesity and aging. First, one theory suggests that aging causes a decrease in energy requirement as a result of concomitant loss of lean body tissue and that obesity will result if energy intake fails to decrease. Except for one study (Mason, 1970), the data from other cross-sectional studies appear not to support this theory on initial examination (Armstrong and Lund, 1996; Scarlett et al, 1994; Sloth, 1992; Kronfeld et al, 1991). Instead, dogs and cats 12 years of age or older become thinner and tend to be in less than optimal body condition (Armstrong and Lund, 1996; Scarlett et al, 1994; Kronfeld et al, 1991).

However, an alternate hypothesis suggests that overweight dogs and cats die sooner and do not reach ages attained by thinner animals because excess weight is detrimental to overall health (Armstrong and Lund, 1996). Caloric consumption has been inversely related to lifespan of dogs (Kealy et al, 2002), rodents (Masoro, 1984, 1988, 1992) and rhesus monkeys (Lane et al, 1997). Cats may be similarly affected.

Gender and Neuter Status

Small differences in body composition and energy intake between intact male and intact female cats have been reported (NRC, 1986; Jewell et al, 1996). The differences in energy intake appear to be due to gender-related differences in lean body mass (Jewell et al, 1996; Klausen et al, 1997).

No controlled studies have been done in dogs to measure differences between energy requirements of intact males compared to intact females. As in other mammals (e.g., cats) intact females probably require less caloric intake than intact males. This assumption is probably due to gender-related differences in lean body mass. The lean body mass of an animal accounts for nearly all of its RER (Blaxter, 1989).

One study showed that female dogs had an average of 16% more body fat than male dogs (Meyer and Stadtfeld, 1980). These findings suggest that intact female dogs need fewer calories than intact male dogs. Surveys found a much higher prevalence of overweight and obese female than male dogs (Edney and Smith, 1986; Mason, 1970).

Neutering increases the risk of obesity in dogs and cats (Jeusette et al, 2006; Lund et al, 2005; McGreevy et al, 2005; Kanchuk et al, 2003; Scott et al, 2002; Martin et al, 2001; Harper et al, 2001; Robertson, 1999; Fettman et al, 1997; Root et al, 1996). Neutered cats are more likely to be overweight than are intact cats of either gender (Scarlett et al, 1994; Root and Johnston, 1995; Flynn et al, 1996). Neutered female dogs are about twice as likely to be overweight than are intact female dogs (Edney and Smith, 1986). A similar trend occurs in castrated male dogs (Edney and Smith, 1986). Neutering predisposes dogs and cats to weight gain and eventual obesity for several reasons. Neutered cats had resting metabolic rates 20 to 25% below those of intact cats of similar age, as measured by indirect calorimetry (Root et al, 1996). In practical terms, this finding indicates that neutered cats require only 75 to 80% of the food needed by intact cats to maintain optimal body weight. These studies confirm the previously suspected decrease in metabolic rate caused by loss of estrogens and androgens from neutering. This reduction in resting metabolic rate appears to be in addition to any decrease in physical activity that might occur from decreased roaming and sexual behavior (Hart and Barrett, 1973; Hopkins et al, 1976).

Furthermore, estrogens suppress appetite in several animal species (Czaja and Goy, 1975). Neutered female beagles and cats will eat more food and gain more weight than sham-operated females fed an identical food (Flynn et al, 1996; Houpt et

Table 27-4. Key nutritional factors for calorie-restricted dog foods for weight loss and prevention of weight regain.

Factors	Dietary recommendations (dry matter basis)
Energy density	Foods for weight loss and prevention of weight regain should contain ≤3.4 kcal (≤14.2 kJ) metabolizable energy (ME)/g
Fat	Foods for weight loss should contain ≤9% Foods for prevention of weight regain should contain ≤14%
Fiber	Foods for weight loss should contain 12 to 25% Foods for prevention of weight regain should contain 10 to 20%
Protein	Foods for weight loss should contain ≥25% Foods for prevention of weight regain should contain ≥18%
Lysine	Foods for weight loss should contain ≥1.7%
Carbohydrate	Foods for weight loss should contain ≤40% Foods for prevention of weight regain should contain ≤55%
L-carnitine	Foods for weight loss and prevention of weight regain should contain ≥300 ppm
Antioxidants	Foods for weight loss and prevention of weight regain should contain:
Vitamin E	≥400 IU vitamin E/kg
Vitamin C	≥100 mg vitamin C/kg
Selenium	0.5 to 1.3 mg selenium/kg
Sodium	Foods for weight loss and prevention of weight regain should contain between 0.2 to 0.4%
Phosphorus	Foods for weight loss and prevention of weight regain should contain between 0.4 to 0.8%

Table 27-5. Key nutritional factors for calorie-restricted cat foods for weight loss and prevention of weight regain.

Factors	Dietary recommendations (dry matter basis)
Energy density	Foods for weight loss should contain ≤3.4 kcal (≤14.2 kJ) metabolizable energy (ME)/g Foods for prevention of weight regain should contain ≤3.8 kcal (≤15.9 kJ) ME/g
Fat	Foods for weight loss should contain ≤10% Foods for prevention of weight regain should contain ≤18%
Fiber	Foods for weight loss should contain 15 to 20% Foods for prevention of weight regain should contain between 6 to 15%
Protein	Foods for weight loss and prevention of weight regain should contain ≥35%
Carbohydrate	Foods for weight loss should contain ≤35% Foods for prevention of weight regain should contain ≤40%
L-carnitine	Foods for weight loss and prevention of weight regain should contain ≥500 ppm
Antioxidants	Foods for weight loss and prevention of weight regain should contain:
Vitamin E	≥500 IU vitamin E/kg
Vitamin C	100 to 200 mg vitamin C/kg
Selenium	0.5 to 1.3 mg selenium/kg
Sodium	Foods for weight loss and prevention of weight regain should contain between 0.2 to 0.6%
Phosphorus	Foods for weight loss and prevention of weight regain should contain between 0.5 to 0.8%

al, 1979). Thus, removal of the metabolic effects of estrogens and androgens by gonadectomy may lead to increased food consumption, when at the same time the animal's energy requirement is lower because of its decreased metabolic rate and physical activity.

Thus, prudent postneutering feeding recommendations for young adult dogs and cats include: 1) feeding low-calorie foods or restricted feeding of regular foods (three-fourths of previous amount) and 2) obtaining body weight and BCS every two weeks for four or five months after neutering to ensure maintenance of normal body weight and condition.

Viral Infections

To date, eight viruses have been shown to cause obesity in animals (Atkinson, 2008). Several viruses cause obesity in laboratory animals (Dhurandhar, 2001). Canine distemper virus can disrupt hypothalamic function and down regulation of genes for melanin production, causing obesity (Verlaeten et al, 2001). Adenoviruses have been associated with viral-induced obesity in people, monkeys, chickens, mice and rats (Atkinson, 2007).

Key Nutritional Factors: Calorie-Controlled Foods for Weight Loss and Prevention of Weight Regain in Dogs and Cats

The traditional method to achieve weight loss in overweight pets and to prevent regain of lost weight is to feed calorie-restricted foods. Such foods should provide amounts of the key nutritional factors listed in **Tables 27-4** (dogs) and **27-5** (cats). Key nutritional factors are described in more detail below.

Energy Density

Decreasing the daily caloric intake of overweight dogs and cats is the primary strategy for producing weight loss and subsequently maintaining reduced body weight. Most typical maintenance-type pet foods are nutritionally balanced according to their energy density and the expected intake required to support a given body weight. If energy restriction is attempted by simply reducing the amount of the maintenance food currently being fed, the intake of all nutrients is restricted, not just energy. A deficiency in energy and other nutrients can occur if the amount of a maintenance food being fed is markedly decreased to produce weight loss.

A better approach is to use an energy-restricted food. A properly formulated restricted-calorie food will be replete in all nutrients except energy so that protein, essential fatty acids, vitamins and minerals are present in amounts sufficient to support normal physiologic processes and retention of lean body tissue, even when calorie intake is insufficient to maintain body weight. The goal of a weight-management food should be to restrict only energy, not other nutrients.

Thus, foods sufficiently restricted in energy content are more suitable for weight management. Pet foods marketed as restricted in calories can vary widely in caloric content, including the proportion of nutrients contributing calories, fiber and digestibility. Regulatory definitions for the terms "light," "lean," "reduced calorie" and "reduced fat" have been implemented in the United States (**Box 27-6**).

For optimal performance, the energy content of dog foods for weight loss and prevention of weight regain should be no

Box 27-6. Regulatory Definitions for Descriptive Terms Indicating Restricted Calories or Fat.

Model Pet Food Regulation PF10 of the Association of American Feed Control Officials (AAFCO) defines limits and labeling requirements for claims related to restricted calorie and fat content. The regulation was implemented in the United States in January 1998.

Maximum calories or fat allowed for "light" or "lean" claims depending on moisture content and intended species*

	Dry foods (<20% moisture)	Semi-moist foods (20 to <65% moisture)	Moist foods (≥65% moisture)
		Dogs	
Light (also "lite," "low calorie")	3,100 kcal ME/kg as fed	2,500 kcal ME/kg as fed	900 kcal ME/kg as fed
Lean (also "low fat")	9% fat as fed	7% fat as fed	4% fat as fed
		Cats	
Light (also "lite," "low calorie")	3,250 kcal ME/kg as fed	2,650 kcal ME/kg as fed	950 kcal ME/kg as fed
Lean (also "low fat")	10% fat as fed	8% fat as fed	5% fat as fed

Key: ME = metabolizable energy.
*"Light" (or similar terms) on pet food labels must bear a calorie content statement as described in AAFCO PF9. "Lean" and "low fat" pet food labels must bear a maximum percentage crude fat guarantee.

"Less" or "Reduced Calories"
For dog or cat food labels bearing a claim of "less calories," "reduced calories" or similar words, a maximum level of calories is not stipulated in the regulations. However, the percentage of reduction and the product of comparison must be explicitly stated on the label. The product label must also bear a calorie content statement and feeding directions should reflect a reduction in calories compared with feeding directions for the product of comparison. Comparisons between products in different categories of moisture content are considered misleading.

"Less" or "Reduced Fat"
For dog or cat food labels bearing the claims of "less fat," "reduced fat" or similar words, a maximum percentage of fat is not stipulated in the regulations. However, the percentage of reduction and the product of comparison must be explicitly stated on the label. The product label must also bear a maximum crude fat guarantee immediately after the minimum crude fat guarantee in the mandatory guaranteed analysis information. Comparisons between products in different categories of moisture content are considered misleading.

The Bibliography for **Box 27-6** can be found at www.markmorris.org.

David A. Dzanis, DVM, PhD, Dipl. ACVN
Dzanis Consulting & Collaborations
Santa Clarita, CA, USA

more than 3.4 kcal (14.2 kJ) metabolizable energy (ME)/g on a dry matter (DM) basis.

For energy-restricted foods for weight loss in cats, the energy density should be no more than 3.4 kcal (14.2 kJ) ME/g DM. For prevention of weight regain in cats following weight reduction, the energy density of the food should be no more than 3.8 kcal (15.9 kJ) ME/g DM. Pet food manufacturers decrease the energy density of foods by reducing fat and simultaneously increasing the fiber, air or moisture content of the food.

Fat

Most typical maintenance-type pet foods contain more fat than do energy-restricted foods. Fat has about 2.25 times the calories of an equivalent weight of carbohydrate or protein. In addition, fat is a very efficiently digested and metabolized source of energy. In one study, overweight dogs fed restricted calories from a food containing more fat lost less body weight and body fat than did overweight dogs fed equivalent calories from a food containing less fat (Borne et al, 1996). The thermal effect of dietary fat is less than the TEF of dietary carbohydrate or protein in obese people (Swaminathan et al, 1985). Studies in people have also determined that the lipid in body fat stores comes primarily from dietary fat, whereas an increased TEF is more closely correlated with carbohydrate intake (Danforth, 1985). Thus, a food with more calories supplied from fat will tend to support retention of body weight and body fat even when total calories consumed are reduced.

The recommended upper limit for dietary fat for weight loss in dogs is 9%, DM; for preventing regain of weight, the upper limit is 14% DM fat. The recommended upper limit for dietary fat for weight loss in cats is 10%, DM; foods for preventing weight regain should contain no more than 18% DM fat.

Fiber, Water and Air

There is some debate regarding the use of calorie-diluting agents in foods intended for weight management. Typical calorie-diluting agents are dietary fiber, water and air. Air is sometimes used to reduce caloric density in dry foods only. Water is a factor in moist foods. Water and air are removed from the gastrointestinal (GI) tract and contribute only transiently to GI fill. However, dietary fiber, besides diluting calories (Laflamme and Jackson, 1995; Jackson et al, 1997; Fekete et al, 2001), offers several physiologic and nutritional effects.

Dietary fiber helps produce weight loss by diluting calories, increasing satiety and limiting food consumption as a result of more bulk being present during its transit through the GI tract (Levine and Billington, 1994). Fiber may also help produce weight loss by decreasing the availability of calories by interfering with the digestion and absorption of fat, protein and digestible carbohydrate (Levine and Billington, 1994). Many of the effects of dietary fiber depend on the specific type, form and amount of fiber used.

Increased levels of dietary fiber contribute to satiety via prolonged distention of the GI tract. Fiber types affect the duration of gastric and intestinal distention differently. Insoluble fibers have little effect on gastric emptying, whereas soluble fibers slow gastric emptying (Levine and Billington, 1994; Vahouny, 1987; de Haan et al, 1990). Although both soluble and insoluble fibers slow intestinal transit, insoluble fiber (e.g., purified cellulose) produces the greater effect (Bueno et al, 1981). Thus, even though the type of fiber affects the two segments of the GI tract differently, total transit time through the entire GI tract is increased and is approximately the same for soluble and insoluble fibers.

Besides affecting transit time, mixed fibers are thought to promote weight loss through delayed gastric emptying, increased ileal transit time and increased gastric distention. Gastric distention stimulates cholecystokinin secretion, thus affecting appetite. However, the ratio of slowly to rapidly fermentable fibers is important (Kritchevsky, 2001). Dog foods with mixed fiber sources provide good weight loss performance (Yamka et al, 2007b).

Actual documentation of increased satiety from dietary fiber is difficult to prove in people and more so in other animals, because satiety is a subjective feeling of fullness and a lack of desire to eat. Indirect evidence for satiety can be obtained from animals by measuring decreases in food consumption and food-seeking activities. In people, increased intake of dietary fiber decreases food intake for variable periods lasting up to eight hours (Burley et al, 1987; Delargy et al, 1993; Stevens et al, 1987). Studies in dogs have produced variable results. Some studies in dogs showed no effect on caloric intake when foods containing 12 to 14% of DM as soluble or insoluble fibers were fed (Fahey et al, 1990, 1990a). In one study, foods containing either 2.2 or 15.6% fiber did not produce any measurable difference in satiety (Butterwick et al, 1994). However, the dogs in this study were fed quantities of food supplying only 40% of calories for adult maintenance, and this degree of caloric restriction may have overshadowed any effect of fiber between the two groups. In another study, dogs offered maintenance calories from food containing 21% insoluble fiber consumed significantly less food and calories than when offered equivalent calories from foods containing less fiber (Jewell and Toll, 1996). These dogs also ate less food when subsequent meals were offered 30 to 45 minutes after consuming the high-fiber food, indicating a satiety effect (Jewell and Toll, 1996). Other reports support a satiety effect of dietary fiber in dogs and cats (Jackson et al, 1997; LaFlamme and Jackson, 1995; Fekete et al, 2001).

Fiber decreases the apparent digestibility of energy-providing nutrients in the food by 2 to 8% (Levine and Billington, 1994; de Haan et al, 1990; Fahey et al, 1990a; Kelsay et al, 1978; Farrell et al, 1978). Fiber decreases pancreatic enzyme activity in vitro and pancreatic lipase secretion in vivo (Isaksson et al, 1982; Stock-Damge et al, 1983). Fiber also increases the fecal excretion of bile acids and fat (Vahouny, 1987). It is well documented that some dietary fibers slow the absorption rate of carbohydrate and fat, but the total quantity absorbed during the entire period of digestion is not significantly less than the quantity absorbed from fiber-free foods (de Haan et al, 1990; Edwards, 1992; Nelson et al, 1991). Increased dietary fiber decreases the apparent digestibility of dietary protein when fecal nitrogen is measured (de Haan et al, 1990; Fahey et al, 1990a; Kelsay et al, 1978; Farrell et al, 1978). However, it is unclear whether the increased fecal nitrogen is from dietary protein that would normally be digested and absorbed, or whether the nitrogen is from increased numbers of fecal bacteria, endogenous loss of mucosal cells or a component of the fiber itself. The effect of dietary fiber on mineral availability depends on the specific fiber(s) and mineral(s). In general, insoluble fibers such as cellulose are less likely to reduce mineral availability than are soluble fibers (Chapter 5).

Pet owners need to be advised that increased levels of dietary fiber will have noticeable effects on normal defecation habits. Dietary fiber increases the amount of fecal material and frequency of defecation (Vahouny, 1987; Fahey et al, 1990a). Dogs fed soluble fiber produced more feces than dogs fed similar amounts of predominantly insoluble fiber (Fahey et al, 1990). Dogs may not tolerate beet pulp and pectin when fed in amounts greater than 10% (Fahey et al, 1990a) or 13% DM (Nelson et al, 1991). Pet owners should be informed that the quantity of feces the animal produces will probably increase when their cats and dogs are fed foods containing more than 10% DM fiber. Excessive flatus can also be an unwelcomed side effect of feeding high-fiber foods. Fiber solubility roughly equates with fiber fermentability (Chapter 5). Increased amounts of highly fermentable fiber in a food are more likely to result in excessive flatulence than if insoluble fibers are used.

Depending on the combination, mixed fibers would be likely to result in less flatulence than using only soluble fibers and less fecal volume than using only insoluble fibers.

Taken together, study results support the use of dietary fiber in foods intended for weight loss and weight maintenance. For the reasons noted above, most commercial calorie-restricted foods with increased fiber contain primarily insoluble fiber.

The recommended range for fiber content of dog foods intended for weight loss is between 12 and 25% DM; for prevention of weight regain, the range is between 10 to 20% DM. The range for dietary fiber content of cat foods used for weight loss is between 15 and 20% DM; for prevention of weight regain following weight loss, the range is between 6 and 15% DM.

Protein and Amino Acids

Dietary protein has several effects that benefit weight loss. Increased dietary protein and amino acids are necessary for animals undergoing a weight-loss regimen to prevent loss of lean body mass (Hannah and Laflamme, 1998; Bierer and Bui, 2004; Laflamme and Hannah, 2005). Dog foods for weight loss should contain at least 25% DM crude protein (higher is better) to help prevent loss of lean body mass (Jewell and Toll, 2007). Dog foods intended for prevention of weight regain should contain at least 18% crude protein (higher is better). Cat foods for weight loss should contain at least 35% DM crude protein (higher is better) for the same reason. These same values are recommended for prevention of weight regain in cats.

Not only is the amount of protein important in protecting against loss of lean body mass during weight loss, so is the protein quality (Yamka et al, 2007b). The quality of a protein depends on the makeup of its constituent amino acids. When amino acids are used for protein synthesis, each necessary amino acid must be available in adequate amounts. The amino acid that is in the shortest supply is referred to as the first limiting amino acid. The idea of an ideal or perfect protein was first established in swine. The purpose of optimizing the amino acid profile of feeds for swine was to maximize lean tissue and minimize fat in finished swine carcasses. This required determining the first limiting amino acid, usually lysine, then balancing the content of the other essential amino acids in the feed to the lysine content. This resulted in swine feeds with ideal or perfect protein content; protein for which the potential for amino acid antagonism and imbalances were minimized (Chapter 5). The result was a leaner, more readily marketable carcass and more efficient growth. Later, researchers used the same idea for determining the ideal or perfect amino acid profile for dogs and cats (Baker and Czarnecki-Mauldin, 1991).

The use of this technology in foods for overweight dogs has shown promising results in weight loss and maintenance of lean body mass during weight loss. Overweight dogs (>30% body fat) were fed either a commercial veterinary therapeutic weight-loss food (control food) or two experimental weight-loss foods for two months. The control food provided 28% DM protein and 21% DM crude fiber. The two experimental foods were only slightly different and contained about 33.5% DM protein and about 10.5% DM crude fiber; the soluble fiber fraction was increased vs. the control food. The experimental foods also had optimized amino acid ratios based in part on higher lysine content. Compared to dogs fed the control food, dogs fed the experimental foods lost significantly more body weight (-2.1 kg vs. -1.3 kg, respectively) and had better lean body mass responses (approximately +0.3 kg vs. -1.1 kg, respectively) (Yamka et al, 2007b).

The lysine content of a food for weight management is not reflected by crude protein content. Individual ratios of essential amino acids to lysine are useful but are cumbersome to use for key nutritional factor targets. Although not an ideal representation of how "perfect" a food's protein content is, the total amount of lysine in dog foods for weight management is somewhat indicative. The recommended amount of DM lysine in dog foods for weight loss is at least 1.7% (Yamka et al, 2007). Dietary protein stimulates increased postprandial thermogenesis and protein turnover. The heat generated during the postprandial period is approximately 68% greater than that generated from carbohydrate sources. Therefore, when an animal consumes protein, it burns more energy (more heat), which appears to be associated with increased protein turnover (increased protein synthesis). Also, the efficiency of the body to convert protein to ATP via oxidation is decreased substantially when compared to fat or carbohydrate. Thus, less net energy is available when animals consume high-protein compared to high-carbohydrate foods (Laflamme and Hannah, 2005).

Carbohydrates

Carbohydrates are an excellent source of energy in canine and feline foods. There are three main categories of carbohydrates: simple sugars, complex carbohydrates and dietary fiber (Flickinger and Sunvold, 2005) (Chapter 5). The importance of dietary fiber has been discussed above.

Simple sugars and complex carbohydrates (grain sources) have received much attention in human nutrition and weight loss because of their effects on the glycemic index. The glycemic index is a ranking system for carbohydrates based on their immediate effect on blood glucose levels. Similar to effects in people, consumption of different sugars and carbohydrate sources alters postprandial glucose levels and insulin secretory patterns in dogs and cats (Flickinger and Sunvold, 2005; Bouchard and Sunvold, 2000; Nguyen et al, 1998; Sunvold and Bouchard, 1998). As a result, it has been suggested that foods producing low glycemic responses be fed to animals that are diabetic, obese and for the prevention of both conditions. Consumption of foods with a low glycemic index improves blood glucose and lipid control (Nguyen et al, 1998).

In a study that evaluated the effects of feeding five different carbohydrate sources (corn, wheat, barley, rice and sorghum) on glucose and insulin responses in dogs, rice had the highest postprandial glycemic response (i.e., increased postprandial glucose and insulin response). Barley, corn and sorghum were the best carbohydrate sources for dogs with impaired glucose control (i.e., diabetes and obesity) because of their low-insulinogenic responses (Sunvold and Bouchard, 1998).

Another study evaluated the effects of feeding the same five carbohydrate sources on glucose and insulin responses in cats. Rice had the highest postprandial insulin response and higher glucose levels early in the postprandial period. This study found that barley, corn and sorghum were the best carbohydrate sources for cats with impaired glucose control (Bouchard and Sunvold, 2000). When considering which weight-management food to use in a canine or feline weight-loss program, it is important to evaluate the carbohydrate sources. Based on these data, it is best to avoid foods based primarily on rice when selecting weight-loss foods. Note that the earlier listing of rice on a specific product's ingredient label, the more rice the product contains. Arbitrarily, rice should not be one of the first three or four non-water ingredients on a weight-loss or weight-control food's label (Chapter 9).

The recommended upper limit for DM carbohydrates in foods for weight loss in dogs is 40%; for prevention of weight regain, the upper recommended limit should not exceed 55% DM. For cat foods intended for caloric-restriction weight loss, the DM carbohydrate content should not exceed 35%; for prevention of weight regain, the recommended upper limit should not exceed 40% (DM).

L-Carnitine

L-carnitine is a vitamin-like, amino acid compound present in all animal cells. Biochemically, it is involved in a variety of functions including fat metabolism and energy production (Chapter 6). In food animals during active growth, among other things, L-carnitine improves nitrogen balance, increases protein accretion and reduces fat deposition (Odle et al, 2000).

The food animal industry has long been interested in nutrients that influence partitioning away from body fat and toward muscle deposition. L-carnitine supplementation results include improved nitrogen balance, increased protein accretion and reduced body fat (Gross et al, 1998). In a 12-week study involving obese dogs (>1.3 RBW) fed a dry, low-fat, high-fiber food with or without added L-carnitine, dogs were fed to achieve weight loss equal to 2.5% of their initial obese weight per week. Food, energy and protein intakes were similar in both groups. Although dogs in control and study groups lost similar amounts of weight, the L-carnitine-supplemented dogs maintained lean body mass and had a trend towards greater body weight loss (Gross et al, 1998).

Results were similar in another controlled study of obese dogs (42 to 43% body fat) in a 19-week weight-loss program. Dogs were fed dry, low-fat, high-fiber foods with or without added L-carnitine. In the first seven-week phase of the study, both groups were fed free choice. The L-carnitine-supplemented dogs lost more body weight. During the last 12 weeks of the study, the dogs' food intake was adjusted to provide just less than 1% loss of their initial body weight per week. The L-carnitine-supplemented dogs tended to have a higher lean body mass percentage, lower percent fat mass and lost more weight than the other group (Sunvold et al, 1998, 1999). Another study in healthy obese-prone dogs fed a low-fat, high-fiber, L-carnitine-supplemented food for six months showed similar results (Allen et al, 1998).

Several studies demonstrated the effectiveness of L-carnitine supplementation for overweight cats. One 18-week study of obese (>1.2 RBW) pet cats either supplemented with an aqueous source of L-carnitine or a placebo, were fed a moist, high-protein, low-carbohydrate commercial cat food intended for weight loss. Weight loss was safely achieved in study and control groups; however, the L-carnitine-supplemented cats had significantly more weight loss than the placebo group (Center et al, 2000). In a study involving obese colony-housed cats, cats receiving L-carnitine supplements lost significantly more weight than cats without supplements (both groups were fed a low-fat food) (Ibrahim et al, 2003). Thus, weight-loss foods with supplemental L-carnitine have improved weight-loss performance in overweight dogs and cats.

L-carnitine supplementation during fasting and experimental induction of hepatic lipidosis may be protective (Armstrong et al, 1992; Blanchard et al, 2002).

The recommended level of L-carnitine in foods intended for weight loss in dogs is at least 300 ppm (DM). For cat food intended for weight loss, the recommended level is at least 500 ppm (DM). The recommended levels for prevention of weight regain in dogs and cats are the same as for weight loss.

Antioxidants

Obesity increases oxidative stress, which may also contribute to diseases associated with obesity (Tanner et al, 2006; Sonta et al, 2004; Urakawa et al, 2003). Studies also show supplemental antioxidants help blunt oxidative stress. For example, serum levels of vitamin E and β-carotene were significantly lower in obese children than for normal weight cohorts consuming similar amounts of these nutrients (Strauss, 1999). Obese rats receiving dietary vitamin E supplementation had lowered oxidative stress biomarkers compared to those in similarly supplemented lean rat cohorts (Laight et al, 1999; Blakely et al, 2003). Furthermore, as in other species, antioxidant combinations seem to work best because they participate in networks to regenerate and/or spare each other to extend/improve their positive effects on oxidative stress in dogs and cats (Jewell et al, 2000; Milgram et al, 2002; Devlin et al, 2001). Effective inclusion levels have been studied for vitamins E and C and selenium for their antioxidant benefits in dog and cat foods. Although other sources of antioxidants are available (e.g., carotenoids, thiols and various fruits and vegetables), the following discussion focuses on vitamins E and C and selenium as antioxidant key nutritional factors because: 1) they are biologically important, 2) they act synergistically (e.g., vitamin C regenerates vitamin E after reacting with free radicals), 3) they are safe and 4) information about inclusion levels in pet foods is usually readily available.

VITAMIN E

Vitamin E is the main lipid-soluble antioxidant in plasma, erythrocytes and tissues (NRC, 2006). It functions as a chain-breaking antioxidant that prevents propagation of free radical damage of biologic membranes. Vitamin E inhibits lipid peroxidation by scavenging lipid peroxyl radicals much faster than these radicals can react with adjacent fatty acids or membrane proteins. Levels of vitamin E higher than recommended requirements confer specific biologic benefits. Based on antioxidant biomarker studies in dogs and cats, for improved antioxidant performance, weight-management foods for dogs and cats should contain at least 400 and 500 IU/kg (DM), respectively (Jewell et al, 2000).

VITAMIN C

Besides regenerating vitamin E, vitamin C (ascorbic acid) also: 1) regenerates glutathione and flavonoids, 2) quenches free radicals intra- and extracellularly, 3) protects against free radical-mediated protein inactivation associated with oxidative bursts of neutrophils, 4) maintains transition metals in reduced form and 5) may quench free radical intermediates of carcinogen metabolism.

Dogs and cats can synthesize required amounts of vitamin C. However, their ability to synthesize vitamin C may be much less than for other mammalian species (Chatterjee et al, 1975). Dogs can rapidly absorb supplemental vitamin C (Wang et al, 2001). In people, high levels of oral vitamin C increased urine oxalate excretion and risk of urolithiasis (Massey et al, 2005). Cats given vitamin C supplements (0, 200, 400 and 1,000 mg/day) had a small progressive reduction of urinary pH from 6.9 to 6.5 (Kienzle and Maiwald, 1998). Moderate supplementation (193 mg vitamin C/kg of food, DM; approximately 10 mg/day) of foods for healthy adult cats with vitamin C did not seem to increase the risk of oxalate production (Yu and Gross, 2005). Supplemental vitamin C (224 mg/kg DM), in combination with supplemental vitamin E and β-carotene improved antioxidant status in dogs (Wedekind et al, 2002). Until more studies are available, for improved antioxidant performance, and in conjunction with recommended levels of vitamin E, weight-management foods for adult dogs and cats should contain at least 100 mg vitamin C/kg DM and 100 to 200 mg vitamin C/kg DM, respectively.

SELENIUM

Glutathione-peroxidase is a selenium-containing antioxidant enzyme that defends tissues against oxidative stress by catalyzing the reduction of H_2O_2 and organic hydroperoxides and by sparing vitamin E. In addition to the antioxidant function of selenium-dependent glutathione-peroxidase, it affects regulation of proinflammatory cytokines including leukotrienes, thromboxanes and prostaglandins, which might benefit the adipokine component of the pathology associated with obesity (**Table 27-2**) (Surai, 2002, 2003). The minimum requirements for selenium in foods for dogs and cats are 0.10 and 0.13 mg/kg (DM), respectively (Wedekind et al, 2002a, 2003, 2003a). Animal studies and clinical intervention trials in people have shown selenium to be anticarcinogenic at much higher levels (five to 10 times) than recommended human allowances or minimal requirements (Combs, 2001; Neve, 2002). Several mechanisms have been proposed for this effect, including enhanced antioxidant activity via glutathione peroxidase (Neve, 2002). Therefore, for increased antioxidant benefits, the recommended range of selenium for weight-management dog and cat foods is 0.5 to 1.3 mg/kg (DM). There are no data to base a safe upper limit of selenium for dogs or cats, but for regulatory purposes, a maximum standard of 2.0 mg/kg (DM) has been set for dog foods in the United States (AAFCO, 2007).

SODIUM AND PHOSPHORUS

Dogs and cats that are overweight may be experiencing some degree of hypertension (See Health Risks of Obesity discussion, above and **Table 27-1**). Also, because they may be fed weight-management foods for extended periods of time, and subclinical renal disease is relatively common, sodium and phosphorus levels in weight-management foods are important. Therefore, the recommendations for sodium in foods for weight management in dogs and cats are 0.2 to 0.4% and 0.2 to 0.6% (DM), respectively. The recommended phosphorus levels for weight-management foods for dogs and cats are 0.4 to 0.8% and 0.5 to 0.8% (DM), respectively.

Key Nutritional Factors: Metabolic-Control Foods for Weight Loss in Cats

The use of metabolic-control foods is an alternative to calorie-control foods for weight loss in overweight cats. This approach is similar to the "low carb" human weight-loss programs that have resurged in popularity. The first low-carbohydrate diet that enjoyed popular success in people was used in the 1860s (Bravata et al, 2003). Contemporary variations on the low-carbohydrate theme for people include programs such as the Atkins and South Beach diets. The metabolic approach to weight loss in cats is probably more like the South Beach diet in that it is less restrictive in carbohydrate and lower in fat than the Atkins diet approach. Although the popular emphasis is on lowering carbohydrate intake, both the Atkins and South Beach diets rely on a multifaceted approach. Dietary protein is also important, as with traditional calorie-restricted foods discussed above. The South Beach diet recommends less fat, lower glycemic index carbohydrate sources and, to a lesser extent, increased dietary fiber. The basic premise of the metabolic approach is to shift energy metabolism from energy storage to energy use.

Clinical trials have shown the efficacy of metabolic-control foods to be equivalent to traditional low-calorie foods for safe weight loss in cats.[a] The key nutritional factors for metabolic-control cat foods for weight loss are discussed below and summarized in **Table 27-6**.

Carbohydrate

Limiting dietary carbohydrate is an important component of metabolic control for weight loss. There are three key advantages to limiting dietary carbohydrate to 20% (DM) or less: 1) lower glycemic index, 2) metabolic shift from energy storage to energy usage and 3) increased satiety.

As discussed for the key nutritional factors for calorie-

Table 27-6. Key nutritional factors for metabolic-control cat foods for weight loss.

Factors	Dietary recommendations (dry matter basis)
Carbohydrate	≤20%
Protein	At least 47% but not exceed 55%
Fat	≤25%
Fiber	≥5%
L-carnitine	≥500 ppm
Antioxidants	Foods for weight loss and prevention of weight regain should contain:
Vitamin E	≥500 IU vitamin E/kg
Vitamin C	100 to 200 mg vitamin C/kg
Selenium	0.5 to 1.3 mg selenium/kg
Sodium	Foods for weight loss should contain between 0.2 to 0.6%
Phosphorus	Foods for weight loss should contain between 0.5 to 0.8%

restricted foods, simple sugars and complex carbohydrates (i.e., grain sources) have received much attention in human weight-loss programs because of the known effects of various carbohydrates on the glycemic index. As in people, consumption of different sugars and carbohydrate sources alters postprandial glucose levels and insulin secretory patterns in cats and dogs (Flickinger and Sunvold, 2005; Bouchard and Sunvold, 2000; Nguyen et al, 1998; Sunvold and Bouchard, 1998). Therefore, foods producing low glycemic responses should be recommended for obese or diabetic patients.

The stimulatory effect of increased carbohydrate intake on insulin secretion provides for a metabolic shift to support fat deposition, given the potent lipogenic effects of insulin. In contrast, low-carbohydrate foods, particularly in combination with fat, protein and fiber, result in a more blunted insulin response that helps set the stage for fat use. Also, as discussed above, by using less available carbohydrate sources, the glycemic index can be modified to further shift energy use to be more dependent on amino acids (protein), fat and ketones. Furthermore, in the calorie-restriction approach to weight loss, different sugar and starch sources variably affect postprandial glucose levels and insulin secretory patterns in cats (Bouchard and Sunvold, 2000). Carbohydrate sources that result in a lower glycemic index are more desirable for metabolic weight control. Compared to barley, corn and sorghum, rice as a starch source produces the highest glycemic index in cats. Therefore, as with energy-restricted foods, it is probably best if rice is not one of the first three or four non-water ingredients on the product's label (Chapter 9).

A reduced ratio of dietary carbohydrate to protein in people has a satiety effect (Layman et al, 2003). Lowering the glycemic index could have an effect on satiety because a rapid increase in blood glucose typically evokes an equally intense insulin response that can lead to a period of hypoglycemia followed by hunger. In people, this occurs approximately two hours after a meal (Roberts, 2000). However, increasing protein can also have a satiety effect (see below). The satiety effect of a reduced dietary carbohydrate to protein ratio may be due to both components.

For metabolic weight-loss foods for cats, dietary digestible carbohydrates should not exceed 20% (DM); lower is probably better. When foods containing this level of dietary carbohydrate in combination with increased protein and moderate fat are fed in appropriate amounts, they result in controlled weight loss in cats (Butterwick and Markwell, 1994, 1996).[a]

Protein

Cats have an innate metabolic capacity to readily use protein (amino acids) for energy (Chapter 19). The natural diet of cats is primarily animal tissue and contains only small amounts of digestible carbohydrate. Cats, therefore, typically have lower levels of hepatic glucokinase than do omnivorous species and have higher levels of transaminases and deaminases that do not down regulate, even when protein intake is reduced. Thus, cats have a higher protein requirement and are metabolically geared to use protein for energy. Cats rely heavily on glucogenic amino acids to generate glucose for glucose-dependent tissues (Macdonald et al, 1984) (Chapter 19).

Increasing its protein content can reduce the carbohydrate content of a food. As discussed for the key nutritional factors for the energy-restriction approach to weight loss, relying on dietary protein as a major energy source has beneficial metabolic effects for weight loss. These effects include reduced energy efficiency, satiety effects and preservation of lean body mass.

In people, increasing a food's protein content increases its thermic and satiety effects (Crovetti et al, 1998). The TEF is the obligatory cost of digesting and absorbing food. TEF constitutes approximately 10% of total expenditure. Thus, increasing a food's thermic effect reduces its energy efficiency (Danforth, 1985; Horton, 1983). In a human study, 10 people received, in randomized order, high-protein, high-fat and high-carbohydrate meals. The high-protein meal was the most thermogenic ($p < 0.001$) and it determined the highest sensation of fullness ($p = 0.002$). There were no differences in the sensation and thermic effects between the high-fat and high-carbohydrate meals. A significant relationship linked TEF to fullness sensation ($r = 0.41$, $p = 0.025$) (Crovetti et al, 1998).

Increasing the dietary protein level during weight loss spares lean body mass. In one study in cats, 47% DM dietary crude protein preserved lean body mass during controlled weight loss (1% per week). In this study, weight loss did not differ significantly between cats fed a high-protein food and those fed a control food with less protein. However, the high-protein group had significantly greater loss of body fat and significantly less loss of lean body mass (Laflamme and Hannah, 2005).

Theoretically, prolonged, excessive protein intake poses some risks. Consumption of high-protein diets in people (i.e., two to three times the U.S. Recommended Daily Allowance) increases urinary calcium loss and may, over time, predispose to bone loss (Eisenstein et al, 2002). However, cats have a relatively high protein requirement because of their obligatory use of amino acids in gluconeogenesis (Chapter 19) and are well adapted to using dietary protein. The protein requirement for an adult cat is twice as much as that for an adult dog (NRC, 2006).

The recommended dietary protein level for cat foods for metabolic-control weight loss is at least 47%, but should probably not exceed 55% (DM).

Fat
When dietary digestible carbohydrate is limited, cats rely more on fat as an energy source. This approach, to a degree, mimics fasting metabolism. During fasting, carbohydrate intake is interrupted and plasma insulin levels decrease while glucagon levels increase. Body fat is then stimulated to release long-chain fatty acids that are transported to the liver where some are converted to ketones, which can be used as energy to fuel hepatic gluconeogenesis. Those ketones not used by the liver are released into the bloodstream for use by peripheral tissues, some of which cannot use long-chain fatty acids for fuel. Fasting ketosis is physiologic and is not harmful because ketones do not reach the level they do during diabetic ketoacidosis (Bruss, 1997). Typically, fasting ketosis results in ketone levels of only 7 to 20% of the levels associated with diabetic ketoacidosis. Thus, low dietary carbohydrate intake sets the stage for a greater reliance on fat and protein for energy usage. Ketones reduce protein catabolism, which may in part explain the preservation of lean body mass observed when low-carbohydrate/high-protein foods are used for weight loss (Volek and Westman, 2002).

In cats, high dietary fat, low-carbohydrate intake (29.5 and 11.8%, DM, respectively) results in a lower glycemic index than low dietary fat, high-carbohydrate intake (15.1 and 38.4%, DM, respectively). Higher dietary fat also reduces the digestibility of the carbohydrate portion of the food (Thiess et al, 2004). However, as has been discussed, dietary fat provides considerably more energy per unit weight than does protein or carbohydrate. Therefore, as in energy-restricted foods, dietary fat levels in metabolic weight-loss foods should be kept as low as possible. However, metabolic-control foods containing 20% fat (DM) have achieved weight-loss performance equivalent to that of low-fat, energy-restricted foods.[a]

Thus, dietary fat should not exceed 25% (DM).

Fiber
Dietary fiber promotes weight loss by diluting calories, increasing satiety and limiting food consumption due to more bulk in the GI tract (Levine and Billington, 1994). Fiber may also help produce weight loss by decreasing the availability of calories by interfering with the digestion and absorption of fat, protein and digestible carbohydrate (Levine and Billington, 1994). Refer to the fiber discussion above in the Key Nutritional Factors: Calorie-Controlled Foods for Weight Loss and Prevention of Weight Regain in Dogs and Cats section, for detailed information about the advantages of dietary fiber in weight-loss foods. Inclusion of fiber in metabolic-control foods for weight loss in cats allows for further reduction of digestible carbohydrate and/or fat content.

Dietary fiber levels in metabolic-control foods for weight loss in cats should be at least 5% (DM).

L-Carnitine
L-carnitine nutriture is important for safe weight loss in overweight cats (see expanded discussion of L-carnitine in the Key Nutritional Factors: Calorie-Controlled Foods for Weight Loss and Prevention of Weight Regain in Dogs and Cats section, above). Adequate intake of L-carnitine protects against the development of hepatic lipidosis and improves weight-loss performance in cats fed high-protein, low-carbohydrate, low-fat foods (Center et al, 2000). The recommended level of dietary L-carnitine should be at least 500 ppm.

Antioxidants
Because oxidative stress is increased in overweight patients and oxidative stress contributes to diseases associated with obesity, supplemental antioxidants are recommended for weight-loss foods. Also, combinations of antioxidants are more effective in relieving oxidative stress than are individual antioxidants. Thus, for improved antioxidant performance, weight-loss foods for cats should contain at least 500 IU vitamin E/kg DM (Jewell et al, 2000); 100 to 200 mg vitamin C/kg DM and 0.5 to 1.3 mg selenium/kg DM. (See the Antioxidant section in the Key Nutritional Factors: Calorie-Controlled Foods for Weight Loss and Prevention of Weight Regain in Dogs and Cats section, above.)

Sodium and Phosphorus
Overweight cats may also be experiencing some degree of hypertension. (See Health Risks of Obesity discussion, above and **Table 27-1**.) Also, because these patients may be fed weight-management foods for extended periods of time, and subclinical renal disease is relatively common (Chapters 20, 21 and 37), sodium and phosphorus levels in metabolic weight-control foods are important. Therefore, the recommendations for sodium and phosphorus in foods for metabolic weight loss for cats are 0.2 to 0.6% (DM) and 0.5 to 0.8% (DM), respectively.

FEEDING PLANS FOR OVERWEIGHT AND OBESE DOGS AND CATS

Weight Reduction
A successful weight-reduction program is a multi-step process that requires: 1) pet owner commitment (**Box 27-7**), 2) proper food, 3) an appropriate feeding method, 4) an exercise plan (**Box 27-8**), 5) pet owner communication (**Box 27-9**) and 6) patient monitoring (reassessment). This six-step program is listed in **Figure 1, Box 27-9**.

In people, the combination of reduced-calorie foods, regular exercise and behavior modification has the greatest chance of achieving and maintaining weight loss (Wilson, 1990; Vasselli et al, 1983; Leaf, 1990; Caterson, 1990; Council on Scientific Affairs, 1988). For overweight dogs and cats, formulation of a program for achieving weight reduction consists first of select-

Box 27-7. Obtaining Pet Owner Commitment.

An important step in a successful weight-loss program is for everyone who feeds the pet to recognize, accept and understand the reason why the pet should lose weight, and to make a commitment to accomplish that goal. Satisfactory weight loss is unlikely to occur unless the pet owners recognize the problem and are committed to take corrective steps. Such commitment will greatly improve compliance (Chapter 3) with a feeding plan and increase the likelihood of a successful outcome. The good news is that owners care whether or not their pets are overweight as evidenced by the results of a survey of cat owners: more than 90% said that maintaining their pets' proper weight was important or extremely important.[a]

Several techniques can be used to help owners recognize and accept that their pet is overweight and not just "stocky." Some of these techniques have already been discussed in the accompanying chapter. Past body weights and body condition scores (BCS) in the patient's medical record can be used along with relative body weights to show an owner how excessive present body weight relates to the animal's frame size and optimal body weight (Appendices 14 and 15). BCS illustrations may help (Chapter 1). Because they typically underestimate their pets' body condition, owners should be taught to feel where bony structures should be readily palpable but are not, and where body contours differ from optimal. The BCS can be used to estimate percent body fat; for additional body composition information, see **Table 27-3**.

If thoracic or abdominal radiographs have been taken, a side-by-side comparison with similar radiographic views from an animal of similar size at optimal body weight can quite effectively demonstrate to the owner the pet's excess subcutaneous or intra-abdominal fat (**Figures 1** and **2** in **Box 27-2**). Practitioners should consider keeping a reference set of radiographs for cats and dogs in optimal body condition for this specific purpose. Also, a side-by-side comparison of the overweight animal and one of the same breed and frame size in optimal body condition can serve the same purpose if an animal of optimal weight is available. Sequential dual energy x-ray absorptiometry scans can also be used for this purpose.

A free web-based program is available in which the patient's silhouette is matched to a dog/cat visual and an ideal weight is automatically calculated; this program could also be a persuasive aid (**Box 27-10**).

After the owners recognize and accept that the pet is overweight, the next step is for them to commit to a weight-loss program. There are several strategies to help owners make this commitment. Owners can be informed about documented problems associated with obesity and how returning the animal to optimal weight will reduce the risk of one or more of these problems. The risks can be quantified economically for animals likely to suffer orthopedic or metabolic problems because of their degree of obesity. Often, a strong motivating factor for commitment is to improve or even resolve a problem caused or exacerbated by obesity. Weight loss in these cases becomes part of the overall therapeutic plan and can be crucial for realizing clinical improvement and benefit from other treatments.

ENDNOTE

a. Weight Management Study, Pet Owner Summary #D02-284. Hill's Pet Nutrition, Inc. September 2002.

The Bibliography for **Box 27-7** can be found at www.markmorris.org.

ing a specific food and determining the feeding method. The feeding method includes setting a goal for the amount of weight to lose and determining how much of the new food to feed to achieve the weight loss. Although not a nutritional consideration, obtaining owner agreement about a realistic exercise plan should be part of the process. Reassessment of the weight-loss part of weight management should include monitoring the progress of weight loss and, as necessary, adjusting food intake and exercise to achieve the agreed upon weight-loss goal. Finally, it is very important to stabilize caloric intake of the animal at its reduced weight to ensure that weight is not regained.

Assess and Select the Food for Weight Reduction

The calorie-restriction strategy should be used for overweight dogs and, initially, for overweight cats. **Tables 27-7** for dogs and **27-8** for cats compare the key nutritional factor targets to the key nutritional factor content of selected commercial veterinary therapeutic foods marketed for weight loss. Select the food that is most similar to the key nutritional factor targets and/or has the best efficacy evidence for managing weight loss in dogs or cats (Roudebush et al, 2008).

If an energy-restriction strategy has been tried in cats, but has not achieved the desired weight loss, a metabolic weight-loss program should be considered. **Table 27-9** compares the key nutritional factor targets to the key nutritional factor content of available veterinary therapeutic cat foods marketed for a metabolic approach to weight loss. Again, select the food that is most similar to the key nutritional factor targets and/or has the best efficacy data (Roudebush et al, 2008).

Another criterion for selecting a food that may become increasingly important in the future is evidence-based clinical nutrition. Practitioners should know how to determine risks and benefits of nutritional regimens and counsel pet owners accordingly. Currently, veterinary medical education and continuing education are not always based on rigorous assessment of evidence for or against particular management options. Still, studies have been published to establish the nutritional benefits of certain pet foods. Chapter 2 describes evidence-based clinical nutrition in detail and applies its concepts to various veterinary therapeutic foods.

Ideally treats, snacks and human foods should be eliminated from the feeding plan to maximize the chances for successful

Box 27-8. Exercise and Environmental Enrichment Programs as Part of a Weight-Loss Plan.

Moderate, regular exercise is advocated in all pet weight-management programs because increased physical activity can enhance weight loss. Exercise is the only practical means of increasing energy expenditure to create or widen a deficit between energy consumed and energy expended for overweight patients. The metabolic rate of people undergoing weight reduction decreases more than expected after corrections have been made for decreased thermogenic effects of food due to decreased intakes and decreased resting energy requirement (RER) due to loss of lean body mass. The only way to successfully sustain or increase overall energy expenditure during weight reduction is to increase the amount of physical activity. Exercise may also benefit obese patients by supporting retention of lean body mass and maintaining or increasing RER. In some cases, pets fail to lose weight unless exercise is part of the weight-reduction plan, regardless of the severity of caloric restriction. Thus, modifying physical activity has been a key target of behavioral intervention to change body weight in people and pets.

Besides increasing energy expenditure, moderate, regular physical activity can help regulate food intake and improve lean body mass. This seems to hold true for weight-loss and weight-maintenance programs. Exercise improves insulin sensitivity, partially reverses leptin resistance and suppresses the enhanced proinflammatory burden induced by obesity. In obese people, physical activity appears to have an independent effect on health-related outcomes compared to body weight. It is unknown if exercise creates beneficial health effects in obese or overweight pets independent of weight loss.

In people, exercise appears to be critical for prevention of significant weight gain and maintenance of weight loss. In dogs, the risk of obesity appears to decrease with each hour of weekly exercise. Owners of overweight cats play less with their cats than do owners of normal weight cats. In people, concomitant changes in food and exercise are more important in women than men.

Specific recommendations for increasing exercise should consider the patient's previous level of activity, presence of any physical problems for which exercise is contraindicated and time constraints of the owner.

For dogs, 15- to 30-minute walks at least five to seven times per week are recommended. Up to an hour of walking has been reported to be practical and enjoyable for some owners and pets. The daily energy requirements of dogs covering 5 km per day are estimated to increase between 7 to 15%. Exercise should be implemented gradually, starting with amounts the patient can comfortably tolerate, especially if orthopedic, cardiovascular or pulmonary disease is also present. It is more important that the animal increase its activity by some amount each day even if it initially is able to walk only out the door to the sidewalk and back inside. The goal should be to work up to 15 to 30 minutes of uninterrupted walking if the animal cannot do this initially. Exercise may need to be omitted initially for patients recovering from orthopedic surgery because walking may exacerbate joint pain. Swimming is an alternative to walking that sometimes works for orthopedic patients if facilities are available to the owner. Because swimming uses more calories per minute than walking, the same number of calories can be expended in less time (5- to 15-minute swim vs. 15- to 30-minute walk).

Some creativity is often required to increase the activity of an overweight cat. Although cats do not readily walk on a leash, they can be trained to do so if the owner is patient and persistent. Sometimes a cat will walk back home on a leash if an exceptionally dedicated owner is willing to carry the cat on the out-bound half of the walk. The type of harness used for cats to be walked on a leash should be secure so the cat cannot escape the leash. This can be a challenge. Less extraordinary ways of increasing a cat's daily activity are to engage the cat in supervised play with string, balls, laser "mice," other toys or other pets. Such methods can make a difference. In a study of overweight cats, encouragement to play and environmental enrichment increased activity enough to cause a 1% loss in body weight over a four-week period.

Options exist for indoor cats to safely be outdoors. Being outdoors provides cats with more opportunity for spontaneous exercise, compared to that which occurs with their typical indoor lifestyle. Such experiences have the additional benefit of environmental enrichment. The outdoor options for indoor cats include a wide variety of pet doors and safe cat-proof fencing. **Table 1** provides a partial listing of websites for doors and fencing; internet searches and pet supply stores are additional sources.

Environmental enrichment can be important to a weight-loss program. A recent study evaluated the effects of environmental enrichment on weight loss in cats. Cat owners were given feeding guidelines to reduce their obese cats' body weight and were randomly assigned to either include environmental enrichment or not. Enrichments included additional food dishes, water bowels and litter boxes, plus climbing towers, window perches, scratching posts, cat spas, grooming supplies and toys. Cats were weighed weekly and some were monitored for activity levels. Environmentally enriched cats had increased activity levels and a trend towards increased weight loss. Owners of the environmentally enriched cats had a more positive image of their cat and felt they were playing a more active role in their cat's weight loss.

There may also be benefits when people and pets exercise together during weight loss. In one study, people exercising with their dogs reported a significantly improved quality of life for themselves and a combined dog/owner weight-loss program was more effective at maintaining participation in a canine weight-loss program.

Table 1. Cat doors and cat-proof fencing.

Websites for cat doors
Catdoors.com
Petdoors.com
Solopetdoors.com
Websites for cat fences
Catfence.com
Catfencein.com
Feralcat.com/fence.html
Purrfectfence.com
Websites for electronic cat fences
Hitecpet.com
Radiofence.com

The Bibliography for **Box 27-8** can be found at www.markmorris.org.

weight loss. A portion of the total daily calories for weight loss (10% or less) can be reserved if the owner insists on feeding treats or snacks (Yaissle et al, 2004). Some treats are specifically formulated for use in veterinary patients and are appropriate for overweight pets (**Table 27-10**). Treats can also be low-calorie foods such as the dry form of the reducing food, popcorn (air popped), low-fat, low-starch vegetables or low-fat commercial treats. The calories supplied by the treats must be accounted for within the total calories allowed in the feeding plan. (See below.) Cats in a metabolic weight-loss program should not receive treats, unless the treats conform nutritionally to the key nutritional factor content of the food.

Assess and Determine the Feeding Method for the Weight-Reduction Program

Feeding method considerations include determining the amount of food to feed for weight loss and selecting the way the food is fed. Determining the amount of food to feed is essential to the success of the plan and is based on the estimate of caloric restriction necessary to safely achieve weight loss. If body fat were the only tissue component lost during weight reduction, then simply starving dogs, *but not cats*, would be an acceptable option for weight loss from a strictly physiologic perspective. There are several disadvantages; however, to using starvation for weight reduction in dogs including loss of lean body mass; therefore, it is not recommended (Burkholder and Toll, 2000).

Even when body weight is lost using more conventional weight-loss programs, 10 to 25% of the loss comes from lean tissues (Burgess, 1991; Butterwick and Markwell, 1996). This loss of lean body mass ultimately decreases an animal's RER and the number of calories required for DER, unless the level of activity is increased to that associated with athletic training. Therefore, one underlying objective in setting the number of daily calories for weight loss is to restrict calories enough to produce weight loss, but still provide enough calories, protein, vitamins and minerals to prevent or minimize nutrient deficiencies and subsequent loss of lean body tissue. As mentioned above, foods properly formulated for weight loss minimize loss of lean body mass (See Assess and Select the Food section above).

Studies in people indicate that loss of more than 2% of body weight per week is unhealthy (Weinsier et al, 1984, 1995). A greater proportion of lean body mass is lost when more than 2% of body weight is lost per week. This ultimately reduces the RER and works against the goal of maintaining the greatest metabolic rate possible in a patient undergoing weight reduction. A 2% loss of initial body weight per week is a reasonable estimate of the maximum acceptable rate of weight loss. However, the impact of losing more than 2% of the initial body weight per week on the proportion of fat vs. lean tissue loss and on the metabolic rate has not been reported from weight-loss studies using dogs or cats. Very few animals fed reduced-calorie foods by the methods discussed above will lose more than 2% of their initial body weight per week. At the other extreme, a rate of loss of at least 0.5% of the initial body weight per week is needed to maintain owner interest and complete the weight-reduction program within a reasonable period. When weight is lost at the rate of 0.5% per week, it may take a year or more to achieve the target body weight, especially in cats. Owners should be apprised of this to manage their expectations and maintain their involvement.

How to Estimate the Amount of Food to Feed for Controlled Weight Loss

Several methods exist for determining the caloric need, and therefore, the quantity of food necessary for weight loss. Four of the more common methods are reviewed below. They are recommended for energy-restricted foods for dogs and energy-restricted and metabolic weight-loss foods for cats. They include: 1) using product information, 2) calculations based on estimated ideal weight, 3) calculations based on current food intake and 4) calculations based on current (obese) weight. All generate estimates, and thus, should be considered starting points, which will likely need adjustment with time. For dogs, the goal is an average weight loss of 1 to 2% of the obese body

Box 27-9. Pet Owner Communication.

Educating pet owners about obesity is important to the successful outcome of weight-control programs. Clients usually enroll their pets in weight-loss programs because of veterinary recommendation, access to support and supervision by the hospital's health care team and the perception that weight loss will improve their pet's health. Retention in a weight-loss program improves when the program includes daily recording of food intake in a diary by the client and scheduling regular trips to the hospital for progress checks. However, there is a point of diminishing returns. Owner education programs that provide monthly classes for nutrition-related topics failed to improve average weight loss or body condition scores compared to weight-control programs without the monthly classes. An obesity-treatment program that included an appropriate feeding plan and monthly hospital rechecks during weight-loss and subsequent weight-maintenance periods was sufficient to achieve good results.

Recommendations for feeding, exercising and rechecking the patient need to be provided in clear, concise terms. These directions should be verbal and written, and the owner should be able to demonstrate understanding by verbal recall. Pet food companies have brochures that explain obesity and its associated health risks. Some brochures provide space to write individual instructions for feeding, exercise and recheck appointments and provide ways of visually documenting progress (**Table 1**). A veterinary practice may also elect to design and distribute its own printed or computer-generated material for this purpose.

The Bibliography for **Box 27-9** can be found at www.markmorris.org.

Box 27-9 continued

Table 1. Canine and feline fact and monitoring sheet.

Customized Pet Weight-Loss Plan

A weight-reduction program has been designed to improve your pet's quality of life. An optimal body weight, specific food(s) and amount(s) have been determined for your pet, along with a recommended exercise regimen.

To successfully manage a weight-reduction program for your pet, you should:

1. Feed only the prescribed food(s).
2. Feed your pet alone; away from other pets.
3. Do not feed table scraps, treats, snacks or other food unless your veterinary health-care team approves them and the amount(s) to be fed.
4. Exercise your pet as prescribed.
5. Do not handle, prepare or eat food in the presence of your pet.
6. Have your pet rechecked on a regular basis by a member of your veterinary health-care team to monitor progress of the weight-loss program.

To be filled out by your veterinary health-care team:

Patient's name________________________________ Dog___ Cat___

Beginning date: _____/_____/_____

Beginning body weight: _________lb/kg Target (optimal) body weight _________ lb/kg

Prescribed food(s)____

Amount of food per meal __________________ Number of meals per day__________________

Amount and type of exercise per day ____

Estimated time to reach optimal weight *if all instructions are followed* __________months

Weigh your pet every _________weeks, and record the weight in the chart below.

Weight Loss Chart

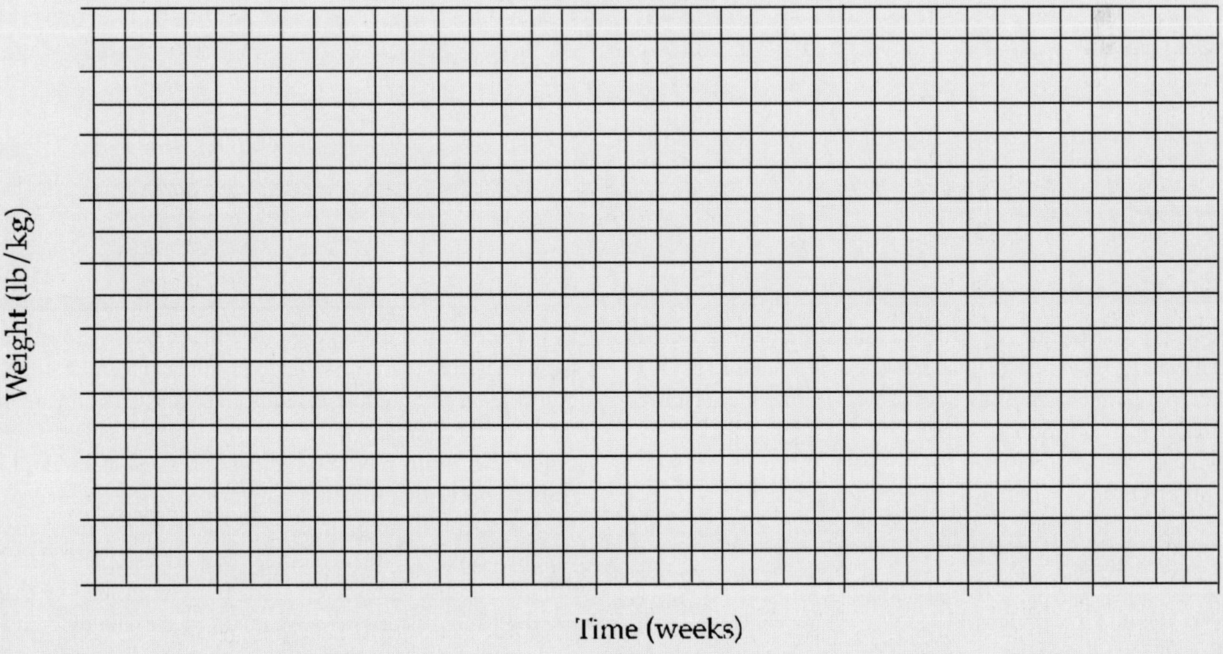

Table 27-7. Levels of key nutritional factors in selected commercial foods marketed for calorie-restricted weight loss in dogs compared to recommended levels.*

Dry foods	Energy density (kcal/cup)**	Energy density (kcal ME/g)	Fat (%)	Fiber (%)	Prot (%)	Lys (%)	Carb (%)	Carn (ppm)	Vit E (IU/kg)	Vit C (mg/kg)	Se (mg/kg)	Na (%)	P (%)
Recommended levels	-	≤3.4	≤9	12-25	≥25	≥1.7	≤40	≥300	≥400	≥100	0.5-1.3	0.2-0.4	0.4-0.8
Hill's Prescription Diet r/d Canine	242	3.3	8.2	13.5	34.3	1.91	38.7	301.1	618	262	1.37	0.24	0.66
Hill's Prescription Diet r/d with Chicken Canine	241	3.3	8.8	13.6	35.2	1.86	36.0	300.0	620	266	1.49	0.40	0.75
Iams Veterinary Formula Weight Control D/ Optimum Weight Control	209	3.5	9.5	3.0	28.7	na	51.2	na	na	na	na	0.51	1.0
Iams Veterinary Formula Weight Loss/Restricted-Calorie	217	3.7	9.1	2.4	25.0	na	58.0	na	na	na	na	0.24	0.83
Medi-Cal Calorie Control	238	na	10.4	4.1	30.2	na	na	na	na	na	na	0.4	1.4
Medi-Cal Fibre Formula	266	na	10.6	14.3	26.2	na	na	na	na	na	na	0.3	0.9
Purina Veterinary Diets OM Overweight Management	266	3.0	7.2	10.3	31.1	na	44.2	na	na	na	na	0.31	0.89
Royal Canin Veterinary Diet Calorie Control CC 26 High Fiber	232	3.1	10.4	17.6	30.9	1.37	33.7	na	962	na	0.33	0.33	0.77
Royal Canin Veterinary Diet Calorie Control CC 32 High Protein	234	3.9	10.4	3.3	37.4	1.42	38.6	na	962	na	0.38	0.38	1.42
Moist foods	**Energy density (kcal/can)****	**Energy density (kcal ME/g)**	**Fat (%)**	**Fiber (%)**	**Prot (%)**	**Lys (%)**	**Carb (%)**	**Carn (ppm)**	**Vit E (IU/kg)**	**Vit C (mg/kg)**	**Se (mg/kg)**	**Na (%)**	**P (%)**
Recommended levels	-	≤3.4	≤9	12-25	≥25	≥1.7	≤40	≥300	≥400	≥100	0.5-1.3	0.2-0.4	0.4-0.8
Hill's Prescription Diet r/d Canine	257/12.3 oz.	3.0	8.6	21.2	25.3	1.39	39.2	370.9	731	131	0.86	0.24	0.53
Iams Veterinary Formula Weight Loss/Restricted-Calorie	397/14 oz.	3.9	14.9	3.2	34.4	na	40.8	na	na	na	na	0.46	0.93
Medi-Cal Calorie Control	212/360 g	na	23.2	1.6	59.2	na	na	na	na	na	na	1.2	1.7
Medi-Cal Fibre Formula	350/396 g	na	9.1	15.0	24.8	na	na	na	na	na	na	0.5	0.8
Purina Veterinary Diets OM Overweight Management	189/12.5 oz.	2.5	8.4	19.2	44.1	na	21.7	na	na	na	na	0.28	1.06
Royal Canin Veterinary Diet Calorie Control CC High Fiber	346/14 oz.	3.6	12.5	8.8	25.9	1.48	46.3	na	271	na	0.41	0.53	0.62
Royal Canin Veterinary Diet Calorie Control CC High Protein in Gel	263/12.7 oz.	4.8	28.5	3.0	51.5	3.1	5.1	na	396	na	na	0.99	1.58

Key: ME = metabolizable energy, na = information not available from manufacturer, Fiber = crude fiber, Prot = protein, Lys = lysine, Carb = digestible carbohydrate, Carn = L-carnitine, Se = selenium, Na = sodium, P = phosphorus, g = grams.

*From manufacturers' published information or calculated from manufacturers' published as-fed values; all values are on a dry matter basis unless otherwise stated.

**Energy density values are listed on an as fed basis and are useful for determining the amount to feed; cup = 8-oz. measuring cup.

To convert to kJ, multiply kcal by 4.184.

weight per week until the patient reaches the desired weight. Also, in dogs, as in people, gradual weight loss is more likely to result in maintenance of the target body weight, once achieved (Laflamme and Kuhlman, 1995).

For cats, a safer and more realistic goal is 0.5 to 1% per week. Again, a weight loss of 0.5% per week for either dogs or cats is acceptable as long as the owner knows that it will take much longer to achieve the desired results.

PRODUCT INFORMATION

For dogs and cats, the simplest and probably the most common method for determining the amount to feed for weight loss is to obtain the food dose recommendation from the company that manufactures the food. This information may be available on the product label, from published company literature, on the company website or by using "calculators" or proprietary software programs. However, the last method often requires an estimate of the patient's ideal or optimal weight. Free web-based programs are available for estimating ideal weight (**Box 27-10**). A simple way to estimate ideal body weight is to use **Table 27-3**. This is accomplished by correlating the patient's current weight with its current BCS and then finding the weight in the same line that corresponds to the ideal BCS (3/5). This and other methods are listed in **Table 27-11**.

Table 27-8. Levels of key nutritional factors in selected commercial foods marketed for calorie-restricted weight loss in cats compared to recommended levels.*

Dry foods	Energy density (kcal/cup)**	Energy density (kcal ME/g)	Fat (%)	Fiber (%)	Prot (%)	Carb (%)	Carn (ppm)	Vit E (IU/kg)	Vit C (mg/kg)	Se (mg/kg)	Na (%)	P (%)
Recommended levels	-	**≤3.4**	**≤10**	**15-20**	**≥35**	**≤35**	**≥500**	**≥500**	**100-200**	**0.5-1.3**	**0.2-0.6**	**0.5-0.8**
Hill's Prescription Diet r/d Feline	263	3.3	9.3	13.6	36.9	33.5	538.6	614	80	0.66	0.35	0.81
Hill's Prescription Diet r/d with Chicken Feline	266	3.4	9.8	13.8	37.7	32.2	556.3	716	120	0.70	0.35	0.84
Iams Veterinary Formula Weight Control D/ Optimum Weight Control	326	3.8	12.2	1.5	38.6	41.2	na	na	na	na	0.39	1.01
Iams Veterinary Formula Weight Loss/Restricted-Calorie	268	3.7	11.0	2.5	35.2	44.5	na	na	na	na	0.37	0.92
Medi-Cal Calorie Control	230	na	9.7	5.1	43.5	na	na	na	na	na	0.8	1.3
Medi-Cal Fibre Formula	280	na	12.2	14.9	34.2	na	na	na	na	na	0.5	0.8
Medi-Cal Reducing Formula	250	na	9.6	5.2	41.8	na	na	na	na	na	0.3	1.2
Purina Veterinary Diets OM Overweight Management Feline Formula	321	3.6	8.5	5.6	56.2	22.4	na	693	116	na	0.57	1.19
Royal Canin Veterinary Diet Calorie Control CC 29 High Fiber	251	3.3	10.2	14.0	33.5	34.5	na	1,065	na	0.32	0.51	0.81
Royal Canin Veterinary Diet Calorie Control CC 38 High Protein	235	3.7	10.2	4.2	43.5	31.5	na	1,124	na	0.38	0.70	1.40
Moist foods	**Energy density (kcal/can)****	**Energy density (kcal ME/g)**	**Fat (%)**	**Fiber (%)**	**Prot (%)**	**Carb (%)**	**Carn (ppm)**	**Vit E (IU/kg)**	**Vit C (mg/kg)**	**Se (mg/kg)**	**Na (%)**	**P (%)**
Recommended levels	-	**≤3.4**	**≤10**	**15-20**	**≥35**	**≤35**	**≥500**	**≥500**	**100-200**	**0.5-1.3**	**0.2-0.6**	**0.5-0.8**
Hill's Prescription Diet r/d with Liver & Chicken Feline	114/5.5 oz.	3.1	9.2	15.4	37.5	31.3	512.5	746	108	1.67	0.29	0.62
Iams Veterinary Formula Weight Loss/Restricted-Calorie	172/6 oz.	4.3	15.5	1.7	44.2	32.3	na	na	na	na	0.43	0.86
Medi-Cal Calorie Control	99/165 g	na	26.0	1.3	49.6	na	na	na	na	na	1.9	1.6
Medi-Cal Fibre Formula	130/170 g	na	17.1	16.7	40.0	na	na	na	na	na	0.4	0.9
Medi-Cal Reducing Formula	111/170 g	na	27.2	1.3	54.3	na	na	na	na	na	1.0	1.6
Purina Veterinary Diets OM Overweight Management Feline Formula	150/5.5 oz.	3.9	14.6	10.2	44.6	23.2	na	na	na	na	0.31	0.99
Royal Canin Veterinary Diet Calorie Control CC High Fiber	164/6 oz.	4.1	21.3	7.7	33.5	32.5	na	276	na	0.43	0.38	0.81
Royal Canin Veterinary Diet Calorie Control CC High Protein	130/5.8 oz.	4.7	24.4	2.4	53.5	7.0	na	562	na	na	1.50	1.68

Key: ME = metabolizable energy, na = information not available from manufacturer, Fiber = crude fiber, Prot = protein, Carb = digestible carbohydrate, Carn = L-carnitine, Se = selenium, Na = sodium, P = phosphorus, g = grams.

*From manufacturers' published information or calculated from manufacturers' published as-fed values.

**Energy density values are listed on an as fed basis and are useful for determining the amount to feed; cup = 8-oz. measuring cup. To convert to kJ, multiply kcal by 4.184.

CALCULATION BASED ON ESTIMATED IDEAL WEIGHT

A second method also depends on an estimate of the patient's ideal weight (**Table 27-12**) but requires a few simple calculations. Pets at ideal body weight in a thermoneutral environment will typically expend about 70% of their DER for maintenance of lean body tissue (RER). Maintaining adipose tissue in obese pets requires relatively little energy; therefore, most calories consumed by an overweight patient, regardless of the degree of obesity, are used to support lean body tissues. Although the lean body mass of an overweight patient is greater than the lean body mass of the same patient at its optimal weight, the relationship is not linear. This method, then, assumes the RER for the optimal weight and RER for obese

Table 27-9. Levels of key nutritional factors in selected commercial foods marketed for the metabolic approach to weight loss in cats compared to recommended levels.*

Dry foods	Energy density (kcal/cup)**	Carb (%)	Prot (%)	Fat (%)	Fiber (%)	Carn (ppm)	Vit E (IU/kg)	Vit C (mg/kg)	Se (mg/kg)	Na (%)	P (%)
Recommended levels	-	**≤20**	**≥47-≤55**	**≤25**	**≥5**	**≥500**	**≥500**	**100-200**	**0.5-1.3**	**0.2-0.6**	**0.5-0.8**
Hill's Prescription Diet m/d Feline	480	14.7	51.5	22.0	5.9	551.1	946	234	0.79	0.40	0.74
Purina Veterinary Diets DM Dietetic Management Formula	592	15.0	57.8	17.9	1.3	18.0	109	na	1.26	0.60	1.52

Moist foods	Energy density (kcal/can)**	Carb (%)	Prot (%)	Fat (%)	Fiber (%)	Carn (ppm)	Vit E (IU/kg)	Vit C (mg/kg)	Se (mg/kg)	Na (%)	P (%)
Recommended levels	-	**≤20**	**≥47-≤55**	**≤25**	**≥5**	**≥500**	**≥500**	**100-200**	**0.5-1.3**	**0.2-0.6**	**0.5-0.8**
Hill's Prescription Diet m/d Feline	156/5.5 oz.	15.7	52.8	19.4	6.0	524.2	810	125	1.77	0.36	0.69
Purina Veterinary Diets DM Dietetic Management Formula	194/5.5 oz.	8.1	56.9	23.8	3.7	na	214	na	na	0.39	1.10

Key: na = information not available from manufacturer, Carb = digestible carbohydrate, Prot = protein, Fiber = crude fiber, Carn = L-carnitine, Se = selenium, Na = sodium; P = phosphorus.

*From manufacturers' published information or calculated from manufacturers' published as-fed values; all values are on a dry matter basis unless otherwise stated.

**Energy density values are listed on an as fed basis and are useful for determining the amount to feed; cup = 8-oz. measuring cup. To convert to kJ, multiply kcal by 4.184.

Table 27-10. Selected commercial treats marketed for weight management in dogs and their respective levels of key nutritional factors (levels for maintenance of target weight (**Table 27-4**).*

	Energy per treat (kcal)	Energy density (kcal ME/g)	Fat (%)	Protein (%)	Fiber (%)	Phosphorus (%)	Sodium (%)
Recommended levels	**na****	**≤3.4**	**≤14**	**≥18**	**10-20**	**0.4-0.8**	**0.2-0.4**
Hill's Prescription Diet Canine Treats	13	2.9	7.3	14.6	17	0.45	0.11
Royal Canin Veterinary Diet Canine Treats	14	3.4	6.3	10.9	6.8	0.47	0.19

Key: na = not applicable, ME = metabolizable energy.

*All values are on a dry matter basis except for energy (kcal)/treat, which is on an as fed basis.

**This information is for feeding purposes only. Treats should not make up more than 10% of the total caloric intake and these calories should be accounted for by reducing the amount of kcal fed as food, accordingly.

weight are similar enough to be representative of one another. If lean body mass is similar at ideal and obese body conditions, the energy required to maintain each body condition should also be similar; this assumption is the basis for this approach to calculating the initial food dosage for controlled weight loss. Because the lean body mass for a patient at its optimal weight will be less than when it is overweight, this method provides a more aggressive initial food dosage for weight loss than calculations based on the patient's obese weight. Also, as mentioned above, web-based programs exist for determining ideal or target weight of obese patients (**Box 27-10**).

For dogs and cats, use RER for optimal weight as an initial estimate of calories required for appropriate weight loss. RER can be obtained directly from **Table 27-3** or calculated as shown in **Table 27-13**. RER should provide approximately 70 to 80% of DER for optimal weight or 60 to 70% of DER for obese weight, assuming the animal is only 20% over optimal weight. This level of restriction should provide about 1 to 2% loss of obese body weight per week. Because this level of restriction will make caloric intake nearly equal to the calories required to support lean body mass at optimal weight, energy for physical activity must subsequently be supplied by further catabolizing fat stores. See **Box 27-8** for a discussion of exercise for weight loss.

After the caloric intake for weight loss is calculated, it is divided by the calorie content of the selected food to determine the actual daily amount to feed. **Table 27-12** provides an example of this method for calculating initial food dosage.

CALCULATION BASED ON CURRENT FOOD INTAKE

A third method requires knowledge of the number of calories the patient is currently eating based on information obtained from the patient history (**Box 27-1**) and feeding a reduced number of calories in the food form selected for weight loss. (See Assess and Select the Food section, above.) **Table 27-**

Box 27-10. Web-Based Programs for Obesity Management.

www.PetFit.com
This is a commercial pet food company sponsored free program for determining ideal (target) body weight for overweight/obese dogs and cats. The visuals in this program include a profile and dorsal view of a dog and cat with a slide bar beneath. The body condition score of the initial view is 3/5. The patient's current weight is entered and the slide bar is moved to the right (or left) to match the dimensions of the patient. After the operator is satisfied with the match, an ideal body weight is automatically calculated.

Balance IT (info@dvmconsulting.com)
Balance IT is a fee-based program designed to help veterinary health care teams with calculation-based weight-loss feeding plans. The user can select/enter all the foods a patient is currently fed (based on the diet history) and the program will then determine the caloric needs of the patient for weight loss. Users can set the desired weight-loss rates and select the commercial weight-loss food they wish to feed (along with any treats up to 10% of daily calories). The program calculates the amount to feed and enters this information into a report to be printed for clients. Based on weight rechecks, the software adjusts the amount to feed the patient.

14 provides more details and an example of this method. **Box 27-10** includes a web-based program that will perform calculations based on the current food information obtained from the diet history. This can be an excellent way to calculate the initial food dose if the recorded amount fed in the feeding history is complete and accurate. If the food history is incomplete, the owner can be instructed to return home and record actual amounts fed for a three-day period and either phone in the information or schedule a followup visit. Potential shortcomings of this approach include losing the attention and commitment of the owners due to busy schedules, inaccurate owner reports due to concerns of having been "feeding too much" and having to convert volume measures to calories if energy density on a volume basis is not readily available.

Table 27-11. Methods for determining ideal/optimal body weight.

1. Consult the patient's medical record to determine if a body condition score (BCS) of 3/5 was recorded with a simultaneous ideal body weight.
2. Consult the patient's medical record to see if the patient's body weight was recorded at about the time the patient reached one year of age. Such a body weight would likely be near ideal (but not always). Thus, this method might not be as reliable as Method 1 above.
3. Consult **Table 27-3** in this text.
   a. Determine patient's current BCS and obtain current body weight.
   b. Locate the current BCS and body weight in **Table 27-3.**
   c. Note the weight in **Table 27-3** that coincides with a BCS of 3/5 in the same column.
4. Consult web-based programs (**Box-27-10**).

Table 27-12. Using ideal body weight to determine initial food dosage for controlled weight loss.

The following steps represent the process for estimating the initial amount to feed for weight loss using ideal body weight:
1. Determine the patient's current weight and BCS.
2. Consult **Table 27-3**; for current BCS, find current weight and read associated ideal weight (BCS 3/5) from same column.
3. Determine RER for ideal weight (also from **Table 27-3**, immediately below ideal weight) = initial estimated daily energy intake.
4. Divide RER by the as fed energy density of selected food = initial daily food dose.

An example case follows:
An obese dog weighs 30 kg and has a BCS of 5/5. Consulting **Table 27-3**, we determine that the dog's ideal body weight (BCS 3/5) is 22.5 kg. In **Table 27-3**, the RER for a 22.5-kg dog is located immediately below the weight. In this case it is 723 kcal/day.*
The food selected for weight loss provides 220 kcal/cup; 723 kcal/day ÷ 220 kcal/cup = 3.3 cups/day. This amount is a starting point and may need to be modified to achieve the desired weight loss.
Recheck body weight after two to three weeks. The weight-loss target should be between 0.5 and 2% per week of initial obese body weight.
Key: BCS = body condition score (Figures 1-2 and 1-3), RER = resting energy requirement.
*To convert to kJ, multiply kcal by 4.184.

CALCULATION BASED ON OBESE WEIGHT

A fourth method for determining the amount to feed for controlled weight loss is based on obese weight, which is more straightforward to obtain than optimal weight. This method also includes a calculation for the amount of desired weekly weight loss.

With this method, the DER for obese weight is calculated. Then the caloric equivalent of adipose tissue to be lost per week is determined using a target of 1 to 2% of weight loss per week. This weekly amount of desired calorie deficit is converted to a daily amount and is subtracted from the previously calculated DER to provide the daily number of calories to feed for controlled weight loss. After the caloric intake for weight loss is calculated, it is divided by the calorie content of the selected food to determine the actual daily amount to feed. **Table 27-15** provides an example calculation using this method. Because the amount of lean body mass does not increase linearly with the degree of obesity, this method could overestimate the initial food dose for weight loss of very obese patients.

A reminder: all four methods generate what should be considered as starting points. Individual animals of the same weight have a wide variation of energy requirements (Figure 1-5). Thus, in actual practice, individual animals are encountered that need the same, markedly fewer and, occasionally, markedly more calories than product literature or calculations suggest. Caloric restriction may be insufficient to produce weight loss or may even produce weight gain in some patients (Laflamme et

Table 27-13. Two alternative methods for estimating resting energy requirement (RER).*

1) RER (kcal/day) = $70(BW_{kg})^{0.75}$. This calculation can be performed with a calculator that has a fractional exponent key or by cubing the body weight and taking its square root twice.
2) RER (kcal/day) = $30(BW_{kg}) + 70$. Results using this formula correlate well with results derived from Formula 1 above for body weights greater than 2 kg. Alternatively Table 5-2 provides this information for dogs weighing up to 70 kg.
*__Table 27-3__ provides RER estimates without requiring calculations.

Table 27-14. Using the food history to determine the initial food dosage for controlled weight loss.

The following steps represent the process for estimating the initial amount to feed for weight loss based on the amount of calories currently being fed to maintain the patient's obese weight.

1. Determine the food/treats currently being fed and, as close as possible, the exact amounts (volume and/or weight) being fed (**Box 27-1**).
2. Calculate the total calories currently being fed by obtaining calorie content information for the pet foods, treats and snacks from Chapters 13 (dogs) and 20 (cats) or product information; use Appendices 16 through 19 for the energy content of human food sources or consult product label information. This is done by multiplying the volume or weight of the food, treats and snacks by their caloric content and summing them. The sum is the calorie intake used to maintain the pet's current body weight.
3. Multiply the calorie sum obtained in Step 2 by 70% to obtain the initial number of calories to feed dogs and cats for controlled weight loss.
4. Convert the calorie target to a food dosage by dividing the calorie target by the energy density of the food selected for weight loss (kcal/cup for dry or kcal/can for moist). The answer will be the amount of food to feed per day.

An example case follows:
An obese dog weighs 30 kg and has a body condition score of 5/5.* According to the pet owner, the dog is fed only commercial food. The food history indicates the following daily intake: two cups of dry food (Brand A), one can (14.75 oz.) of moist food (Brand B) and four to five Brand C treats. Manufacturer's information regarding these foods indicates the following calorie content: 350 kcal/cup of dry food, 400 kcal/14.75-oz. can moist food, 50 kcal per treat. The total daily calorie intake is:
350 kcal/cup x two cups = 700 kcal**
+ 400 kcal/can x one can = 400 kcal
+ 5 treats x 50 kcal/treat = 250 kcal
Sum = 1,350 kcal/day

To determine the target number of calories to feed per day:
70% x 1,350 kcal = 945 kcal/day
To convert this to an amount of a selected weight-loss food to feed daily (in this case, the owner chose to feed a combination of moist (300 kcal/can) and dry (220 kcal/cup) weight-loss foods plus low-calorie treats (16 kcal/treat):
1 can x 300 kcal/can = 300 kcal
945 kcal weight-loss target – 300 kcal = 645 kcal left for dry food and treats
Feed 10 treats/day x 16 kcal/treat = 160 kcal
645 kcal – 160 kcal for treats = 485 kcal remaining for dry food
485 kcal ÷ 220 kcal/cup dry food = 2.2 cups dry food
Recheck body weight after two to three weeks to determine if adjustments need to be made.
Weight-loss target should be between 0.5 and 2% per week of initial obese body weight.
*(Figures 1-2 and 1-3)
**To convert to kJ, multiply kcal by 4.184.

Table 27-15. Using obese body weight and desired rate of weight loss to determine initial amount to feed for controlled weight loss.

The following steps represent the process for estimating the initial amount to feed for weight loss using obese body weight and a desired rate of weight loss:

1. Obtain current (obese) body weight.
2. Calculate DER for current body weight = estimated current daily energy intake.
3. Calculate the energy content of body fat (7,920 kcal/kg adipose tissue) to be lost weekly, assuming a target weight loss of between 0.5 to 2% initial body weight per week.
4. Divide the weekly amount of adipose calories by 7 to obtain desired daily calorie deficit.
5. Subtract the daily calorie deficit from the DER to obtain the number of calories to feed per day.
6. Divide the number of calories to feed per day by the energy density of the selected food to determine the amount of food to feed per day.

An example case follows:
An obese dog has a body weight of 30 kg and a BCS of 5/5. The DER for the dog's obese weight is calculated using the formula DER = RER x 1.4. RER (kcal/day) = $30(BW_{kg}) + 70$. RER = 30(30 kg) + 70 = 970 kcal/day. DER = 1.4 x RER = 1.4 x 970 = 1,358 kcal/day. RER can also be obtained directly from **Table 27-3**.
A targeted weight loss of 1.5% of the dog's obese weight per week would be 0.45 kg/week.
The energy density of adipose tissue is 7,920 kcal/kg; 7,920 kcal/kg x 0.45 kg = 3,564 kcal/week or 509 kcal/day (3,564 kcal/week ÷ 7 days/week).
The calculated daily energy intake for this rate of weight loss = 1,358 kcal/day – 509 kcal = 849 kcal/day.
The food selected for weight loss provides 220 kcal/cup; 849 kcal/day ÷ 220 kcal/cup = 3 and 7/8 cups/day. This amount is a starting point and may need to be modified to achieve the desired weight loss. Recheck body weight after two to three weeks.
Key: DER = daily energy requirement, BCS = body condition score (Figures 1-2 and 1-3), RER = resting energy requirement, BW = body weight.

al, 1997). Patients will need to be rechecked regularly, initially every two to three weeks, so that modifications, if necessary, can be made to their food intake (Saker and Remillard, 2005). **Figure 27-1** is an algorithm for monitoring progression of weight loss and making decisions to keep weight loss progressing toward the target (ideal) weight. The pet owner's clear understanding that the initial amount to feed might need revision is more important than whether the veterinarian's initial recommendation is correct. Continually managing the client's expectations is very important.

Finally, a cautionary reminder about food restriction in cats: restricting calories for DER at optimal weight of a cat by more than 70% effectively makes caloric intake less than RER because DER for neutered adult cats is only 1.2 to 1.4 x RER. RER represents a theoretical minimum for daily energy consumption for cats because of the risk for hepatic lipidosis (Biourge et al, 1994). However, experimental and clinical trials using caloric restrictions between 59 and 80% of RER produced acceptable rates of weight loss in overweight cats with no biochemical evidence of hepatic lipido-

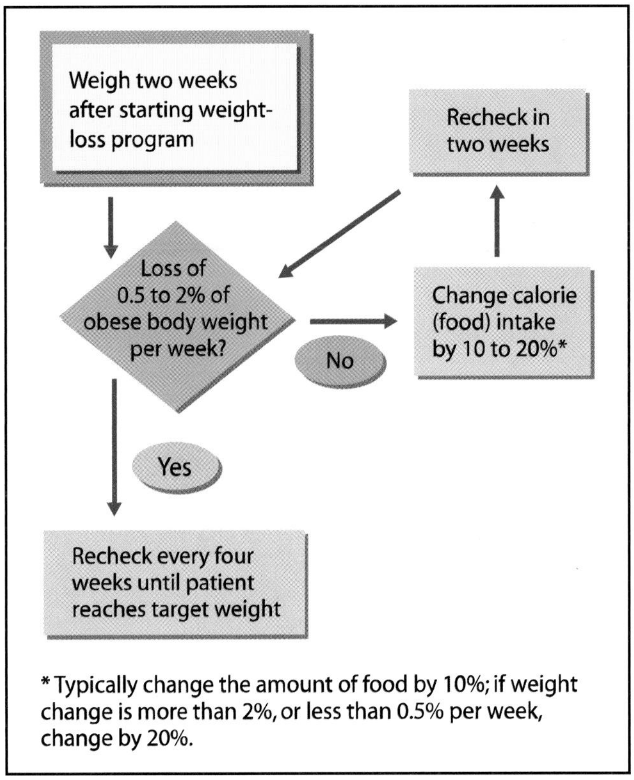

Figure 27-1. Algorithm for decision making and patient monitoring during weight loss.

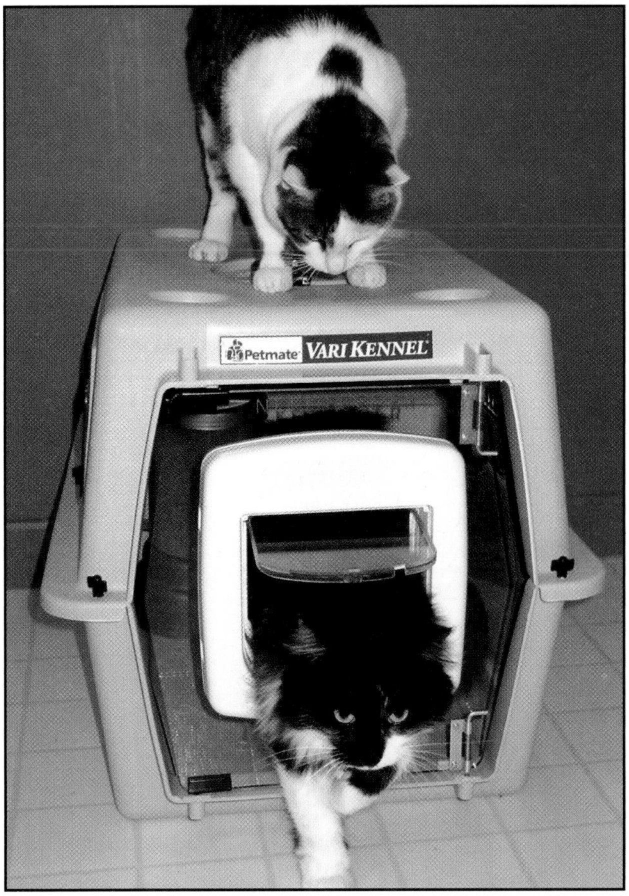

Figure 27-2. A commercial feeding system for cats and small dogs. Close proximity of a special collar unlocks the feeder door and the pet wearing the collar simply pushes the door open and enters the feeder. More than one pet can have access to one feeder. (Courtesy of NekoFeeder, LLC. www.nekofeeder.com [802-264-6055] 6D Laurette Drive, Essex Junction, VT.)

sis (Markwell et al, 1996). Thus, when feeding obese cats for weight loss, be sure they are eating at least 50% of their estimated food dose to prevent development of hepatic lipidosis. A weight loss goal of 0.5 to 1% per week is safer.

Feeding Methods for Weight Reduction

Consideration should be given to how the owner feeds the pet. Feeding foods free choice may work for individual cats and dogs that can self-regulate their daily intake of food to match their DER. However, free-choice feeding rarely works for weight loss or for maintenance of reduced body weight even with the most calorie-restricted foods.

Dogs and cats on weight-reduction programs should be fed multiple small meals during the day rather than a single large meal to take advantage of the obligatory energy cost for digesting and absorbing food. The optimal number of meals for maximizing caloric expenditure from TEF has not been determined. However, the total daily food should be divided into at least two portions fed eight to 12 hours apart. Most pet owners can feed two meals per day without disrupting their schedules. Clients who can conveniently feed three or more meals per day should do so.

Meal sizes should be in portions that are practical to measure (i.e., to the nearest one-fourth cup or can). If the daily amount of food does not divide evenly into portions that are readily measurable, some meals will contain less and others more food. The meals containing more food should be fed when the owner will be with the pet for the longest time between meals. The pet should be kept out of the kitchen and dining areas during preparation and consumption of family meals. These practices can help reduce the pet's begging and the owner's urge to give the pet additional food or treats.

As with any food change, it is best to transition the patient to the new weight-loss food gradually over a period of several days (Table 1-1).

In multi-pet households, care must be taken to ensure that obese patients being treated for weight loss do not have access to other pets' food. This can be challenging. Commercial feeders are available for pets that limit access to food. Internet searches can be conducted to locate sources of commercial automatic feeders that might make it easier to feed an individual dog or cat for weight loss in a multi-pet household. **Figure 27-2** shows an example of a commercial feeder for cats and small dogs that selectively restricts access to food. Also, feeders for cats in multi-cat households can be constructed from a cardboard box. The box should be of sufficient size for one cat and its bowl of food. An opening small enough to allow a thin cat, but not the overweight cat, to enter and exit is cut into the closed box. The food intended for the thinner

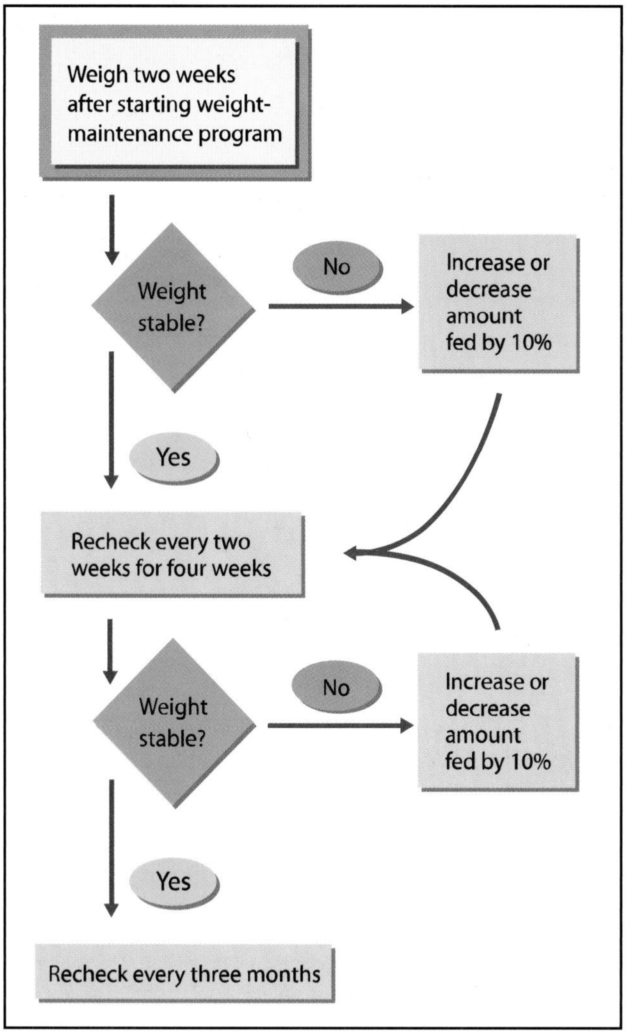

Figure 27-3. Algorithm for stabilizing body weight after weight loss.

cat is placed in the box, limiting access by the overweight cat. However, industrious overweight cats sometimes defeat such a system.

REASSESSMENT

Assess the Performance of the Weight-Loss Program

Regular monitoring of patient weight loss is important to ensure the prescribed program is effective and to motivate the owner. Simply telling a patient's owner to feed a certain quantity of a calorie-restricted food and increase the patient's activity is unlikely to produce weight loss for several reasons. Office rechecks or "weigh-ins" to monitor patient progress throughout weight loss are an integral component of a weight-reduction program, equal in importance to diet and exercise (**Box 27-11**). There are three critical times during a weight-reduction program when rechecks can prevent the program from failing. These are at the very beginning, the very end and anytime in between when weight loss slows or stops (**Figure 27-1**).

The focus should be on acceptable rates of weight loss instead of calculating a specific number of days that pet owners view as the time it will take to complete the weight-loss program. It can be disheartening to pet owners and harmful to the veterinarian's credibility, and thus the weight-loss program, if a single specific time is projected for returning the animal to optimal weight and then, as in most cases, it actually takes more time. The minimum and maximum acceptable times for a cat or dog to complete a weight-loss program can be calculated (**Box 27-12**). Realistically, eight to 12 months will be required to complete the weight reduction of most dogs and cats that are truly obese and that have metabolic rates lower than predicted by standard equations; some will take even take longer.

If weight loss is not proceeding at a rate between 0.5 to 2% per week, decrease the amount being fed by 10 to 20% and recheck body weight in two weeks. Continue this cycle until the desired rate of weight loss is obtained. After the desired rate is obtained, continue feeding that amount of food until the target weight is obtained, rechecking progress every four to six weeks.

Adjunctive Therapy

Box 27-13 reviews a new drug that may help manage overweight and obese conditions in dogs and cats.

FEEDING PLANS FOR WEIGHT MAINTENANCE

After the patient reaches the target weight, a weight-maintenance program should be initiated to ensure that the target weight is maintained and weight regain does not occur. The success of the weight-maintenance program, like that of the weight-loss program, depends on continued pet owner commitment (**Box 27-7**), proper food and feeding plan, exercise (**Box 27-8**), pet owner communication (**Box 27-9**) and patient monitoring (reassessment). These patients, like human patients, are at considerable risk for weight regain and resumption of their previous overweight condition.

Assess and Select the Food for Weight Maintenance

Simply feeding the animal its previous food, even at reduced amounts, may lead to weight regain, negating the effort required to produce weight loss and the resulting benefits. Thus, the strategy of energy restriction is also used to avoid weight regain. The same nutritional principles discussed for weight loss are employed, but energy is less restricted. **Tables 27-16** for dogs and **27-17** for cats compare the key nutritional factor targets to the key nutritional factor content of selected commercial veterinary therapeutic foods marketed for maintenance of target weight after weight loss or prevention of weight gain in patients not previously overweight. Select the food that

Box 27-11. Rechecks and the Overall Success of a Weight-Loss Program.

Rechecks accomplish several things necessary to ensure success of a weight-loss program. When done timely and properly, rechecks improve compliance and ensure the program is conducted efficiently and effectively. Rechecks reinforce the commitment of owners and the veterinary health care team in helping patients lose weight. Also, rechecks give pet owners an opportunity to see the results of their efforts or, on the contrary, to see the impact of inadvertently or purposefully feeding extra calories or not ensuring that the pet performed the specified amount of exercise since the last recheck.

During rechecks, the veterinary health care team can adjust the caloric intake, feeding plan and exercise recommendations to get or keep weight loss proceeding at a desirable rate. The opportunity to make these adjustments is a key iterative step in a weight-loss program. The initial considerations and calculations for caloric restriction and the feeding plan, no matter how carefully or scientifically made, are only an educated guess at what the caloric restriction should be for a safe and reasonable rate of weight loss for an individual patient. The appropriateness of this educated guess is ultimately determined by changes in the body weight and body condition score. Pelvic and abdominal girth measurements, determined with a tape measure, can also be used to track progress.

Pet owners need reinforcement in the form of compliments and encouragement even when their overweight pets lose weight. Such pet owners are likely to be experiencing one or more negative consequences as a result of changing what and how they feed their pet. The dog or cat can manifest hunger. As a result, some pet owners will feel they are depriving their pet of needed food or affection. The pet owner's resistance to acquiescing to the pet's behavior and the urge to feed the pet more food should be acknowledged and reinforced.

Reinforcement and encouragement are certainly required when weight remains the same, or worse, increases from one recheck to the next. The reason for lack of progress needs to be determined and explained. Sometimes the animal is actually losing weight and it is simply not detected, either because the scale is not sensitive enough or the gastrointestinal or urinary tract has above average contents at the time of the weighing. If this is the case, the weight is likely to be decreased at the next recheck. A true lack of progress can be due to consumption of additional food, either because the patient had unlimited access to food while unsupervised, or the owners fed more treats or snacks than recommended. Insufficient exercise will also slow, or stop, weight loss. In any of these cases, owners need to understand what caused the observed results and efforts should be redoubled to assist the patient and the owner in adhering to the feeding and exercise plan.

However, insufficient weight loss could occur despite what any calculation would suggest and despite 100% compliance by the owner. Problems with caloric restriction can occur initially or after some period of weight loss, perhaps because of a decreasing metabolic rate from the weight loss. If monitoring and counseling in the form of rechecks are not being done, these problems will not be detected until the patient is seen some time in the future weighing the same or more than when the weight-loss program was started. The opportunity to promote weight loss in such patients will probably be lost because the pet owner will conclude that switching the food and tolerating undesirable behaviors did not produce results and was not worth the trouble and/or expense involved.

The best reinforcement and encouragement come initially from seeing the pet's body weight decrease, and later from seeing the return of normal body contours and resolution of clinical signs (e.g., better exercise tolerance, reduced lameness or decreased insulin doses). However, if the period of time between rechecks is short, or the rate of weight loss is particularly slow, progress based on body weight alone may not be readily apparent.

When dogs and cats lose or gain weight, the body dimension that changes most is the abdominal (pelvic) circumference. The thoracic circumference will also change somewhat, but the magnitude will not be as great or the change as readily measurable as in the pelvic region. If progress is slow, sometimes the pelvic circumference will decrease between rechecks even when body weight remains constant or vice versa. The decrease in circumference indicates progress and does not need to be converted into a decrease in body fat to be interpreted. In fact, simply measuring pelvic and thoracic circumferences at each recheck and periodically reevaluating the patient's body condition score could track progression of weight loss. These methods of assessing weight loss should be considered in settings such as house-call practices where veterinarians may not have scales capable of measuring the change in a pet's body weight.

Rechecks should be scheduled to allow enough time for detectable progress, but not so much time that the pet owner becomes dismayed at the lack of progress when problems are finally detected. Shorter intervals between rechecks are needed at the beginning and end of a weight-reduction program when the caloric content and amounts of food are changed. Initially two weeks is a reasonable recheck interval for most patients. Cats and some small dogs may take three weeks to lose enough weight for scales to measure the loss. At the most, no more than four weeks should pass before the patient is rechecked. However, four weeks may be too long for some patients if changes need to be made to the feeding or exercise plans.

Ideally, three body weights would be used to establish a true trend for, and an accurate rate of, weight loss. Thus, a determination that initial caloric restriction is insufficient to produce weight loss can be made sooner with a two-week recheck interval than with a four-week interval, saving at least two and perhaps six weeks, during which the animal is not losing weight. Intervals between rechecks can be increased to every four weeks after weight loss is documented to occur at a steady rate acceptable to the pet owner and veterinary health care team. If the animal fails to lose weight during a four-week interval with no apparent explanation (i.e., more calories or less exercise) then the rechecks need to be more frequent to determine if weight loss has stopped and to assess the degree of caloric restriction needed for weight loss to recur (**Figure 27-3**).

Box 27-12. Calculating Time for Weight Loss and its Use in Monitoring Patients.

The loss of 2% of initial body weight per week can be used as the maximum desired rate of weight loss in typical obese patients and a loss of 0.5% of initial body weight per week can be used as the minimum desired rate of weight loss. These two weight-loss rates can be used to calculate the minimum and maximum time expected for a dog or cat to reach its ideal or target body weight. The following case will demonstrate a simple method for determining this time interval and show its use in monitoring response to therapy in an obese cat.

METHOD
Obese weight – desired weight = A (kg)
Obese weight x 2% = B (kg/week)
A ÷ B = C (number of weeks necessary for weight loss at 2% rate)
C x 4 = D (number of weeks necessary for weight loss at 0.5% rate)
Desired weight loss should occur within these two time frames.

CASE
Patient Assessment
A three-year-old, neutered female domestic shorthair cat weighing 5.9 kg is presented for annual vaccinations. The owner had recently acquired the cat from her parents and was concerned that the cat was overweight compared with a cat owned by her roommate. All physical examination findings were normal except for obesity. Results of a complete blood count, serum biochemistry profile and urinalysis were normal.

The cat's body condition was assessed as 4.5/5. Ideal body weight was estimated to be 4.5 kg (**Table 27-3**).

Assess the Food and Feeding Method
The cat was fed one-half cup of a dry specialty brand cat food and 3 oz. of various brands and flavors of moist cat foods once daily. The cat consumed at least 400 kcal (1,674 kJ) of metabolizable energy (ME) daily.

Feeding Plan
The resting energy requirement (RER) at the estimated optimal body weight was calculated as follows: RER optimal weight = $70(4.5)^{0.75}$ = 218 kcal ME (912 kJ). Daily energy requirement (DER) would be approximately 1.4 x RER or 305 kcal ME (1,276 kJ). The daily caloric intake was much higher than the estimated DER.

The initial caloric restriction was set at RER calculated for optimal body weight. The owner was also instructed to increase the cat's activity as much as possible. The food was changed to commercial products containing less fat and more fiber. The owner was asked to return every two weeks for the first two months to monitor progress.

Calculations for Weight Loss
Obese weight = 5.9 kg
Desired weight = 4.5 kg
Desired weight loss = 1.4 kg

5.9 x 2% = 0.12 kg/week
1.4 kg ÷ 0.12 = 12 weeks at 2% rate
12 weeks x 4 = 48 weeks at 0.5% rate

Reassess
The accompanying figure shows the weight loss that occurred with this feeding plan and exercise. The actual body weight loss for this cat falls nicely within the calculated minimum and maximum rates. The feeding plan was changed at 22 weeks to stabilize the body weight at 4.5 kg.

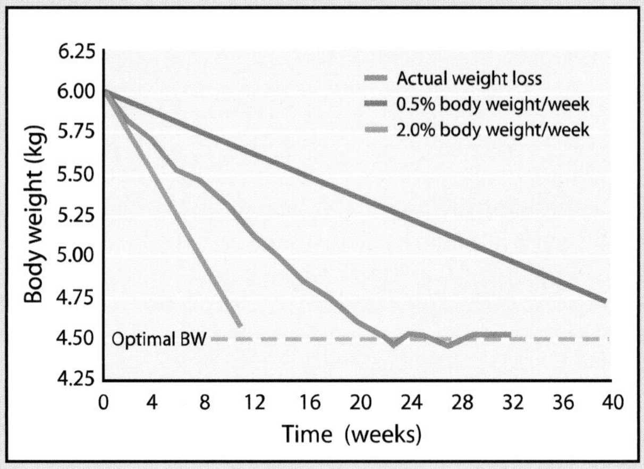

is most similar to the key nutritional factor targets for managing weight maintenance in dogs or cats.

If a metabolic weight-control food was used for an overweight feline patient, it is also appropriate to switch to a calorie-restricted food for maintenance of the target weight, after the target weight has been achieved.

If the owner intends to feed treats or snacks, the same treats (**Table 27-10**) and snacks (the dry form of the weight-maintenance food, popcorn (air popped), low-fat, low-starch vegetables) recommended for weight loss can be considered for use in the weight-maintenance program. As with the weight-loss program, the calories supplied by the treats must be accounted for within the total calories allowed in the feeding plan.

Assess and Determine the Feeding Method for Weight Maintenance

Feeding method considerations include determining the amount of food to feed for weight maintenance and selecting the way the food is to be fed.

How to Estimate the Amount of Food to Feed for Weight Maintenance

The following methods for determining the amount to feed for maintenance of target weight after weight loss provide best estimates. Patients should initially receive frequent rechecks (every one to two weeks for four to six weeks) (**Figure 27-3**) to guard against weight regain.

Box 27-13. Pharmacologic Approach to Obesity in Dogs: Dirlotapide.

Given the growing health problem of obesity in people, dogs and cats, pharmacologic investigations to manage obesity have been underway for many years. There are numerous receptors in the hypothalamus that have been identified as possible targets of a pharmacologic remedy to obesity. Hypothalamic receptors appear to be reasonable targets given the role of the hypothalamus in controlling appetite, food intake and energy expenditure.

During dietary fat digestion and absorption, lipids enter an enterocyte and are repackaged as chylomicrons by a microsomal triacylglycerol transfer protein (MTP). From there they are transferred to the lymphatics and blood. Dirlotapide[a] is a MTP inhibitor that is highly selective for enterocytes when taken orally. Dirlotapide partially inhibits MTP resulting in an accumulation of lipid within the mucosal cell lining. Triglyceride accumulation within enterocytes triggers secretion of hypothalamic satiety hormones (PYY and GLP-1), which ultimately leads to a voluntary decrease of food and calorie intake. The dirlotapide label insert states that the "...mechanism for producing weight loss is not completely understood, but seems to result from reduced fat absorption and a satiety signal from lipid-filled cells lining the intestine." It has been estimated that 90% of the weight lost is due to decreased food intake and 10% is due to reduced lipid absorption. Fecal fat increases in dogs given dirlotapide because enterocytes containing fat are normally shed as part of fecal material.

Weight-loss programs that incorporate MTP inhibitors will almost certainly be successful initially and may help dogs with immediate medical concerns related to excessive weight. But it is imperative that weight-loss programs incorporating MTP inhibitors take advantage of this initial short-term success and capitalize on the opportunity to change owner behaviors, which will then foster long-term success. If this opportunity is not captured, weight gain (rebound) will be inevitable when the MTP inhibitors are withdrawn because appetite returns within days of discontinuing the drug. If used incorrectly, and not integrated into an overall plan of proper food, food dosage and exercise, weight loss with MTP inhibitors will be cyclic and results will be just as frustrating as current programs.

ENDNOTE

a. Slentrol. Pfizer Animal Health, New York, NY, USA.

The Bibliography for **Box 27-13** can be found at www.markmorris.org.

Rebecca L. Remillard, PhD, DVM, Dipl. ACVN
MSPCA Angell Animal Medical Center
Boston, MA, USA

Table 27-16. Levels of key nutritional factors in selected commercial foods marketed for weight maintenance in dogs after a weight-loss program compared to recommended levels.*

Dry foods	Energy density (kcal/cup)**	Energy density (kcal ME/g)	Fat (%)	Fiber (%)	Prot (%)	Carb (%)	Carn (ppm)	Vit E (IU/kg)	Vit C (mg/kg)	Se (mg/kg)	Na (%)	P (%)
Recommended levels	**-**	**≤3.4**	**≤14**	**10-20**	**≥18**	**≤55**	**≥300**	**≥400**	**≥100**	**0.5-1.3**	**0.2-0.4**	**0.4-0.8**
Hill's Prescription Diet w/d Canine	243	3.3	8.8	16.4	18.9	51.2	349.5	574	274	1.34	0.22	0.56
Hill's Prescription Diet w/d with Chicken Canine	239	3.2	8.7	17.1	19.1	50.1	328.0	611	298	1.52	0.27	0.56
Iams Veterinary Formula Weight Control D/ Optimum Weight Control	209	3.5	9.5	3.0	28.7	51.2	na	na	na	na	0.51	1.00
Medi-Cal Weight Control/ Mature	320	na	8.5	4.0	19.5	na	na	na	na	na	0.2	0.8
Purina Veterinary Diets OM Overweight Management	266	3.0	7.2	10.3	31.1	44.2	na	na	na	na	0.31	0.89
Moist foods	**Energy density (kcal/can)****	**Energy density (kcal ME/g)**	**Fat (%)**	**Fiber (%)**	**Prot (%)**	**Carb (%)**	**Carn (ppm)**	**Vit E (IU/kg)**	**Vit C (mg/kg)**	**Se (mg/kg)**	**Na (%)**	**P (%)**
Recommended levels	**-**	**≤3.4**	**≤14**	**10-20**	**≥18**	**≤55**	**≥300**	**≥400**	**≥100**	**0.5-1.3**	**0.2-0.4**	**0.4-0.8**
Hill's Prescription Diet w/d Canine	329/13 oz.	3.5	12.7	12.4	17.9	52.6	364.1	614	116	0.72	0.24	0.52
Medi-Cal Weight Control/ Mature	370/396 g	na	10.0	5.5	21.5	na	na	na	na	na	0.3	0.6
Purina Veterinary Diets OM Overweight Management	189/12.5 oz.	2.5	8.4	19.2	44.1	21.7	na	na	na	na	0.28	1.06

Key: ME = metabolizable energy, na = information not available from manufacturer, Fiber = crude fiber, Prot = protein, Carb = digestible carbohydrate, Carn = L-carnitine, Se = selenium, Na = sodium, P = phosphorus, g = grams.

*From manufacturers' published information or calculated from manufacturers' published as-fed values. All values are on a dry matter basis unless otherwise stated.

**Energy density values are listed on an as fed basis and are useful for determining the amount to feed; cup = 8-oz. measuring cup.

To convert to kJ, multiply kcal by 4.184.

Table 27-17. Levels of key nutrients in selected commercial foods marketed for weight maintenance in cats after a weight-loss program compared to recommended levels.*

Dry foods	Energy density (kcal/cup)**	Energy density (kcal ME/g)	Fat (%)	Fiber (%)	Prot (%)	Carb (%)	Carn (ppm)	Vit E (IU/kg)	Vit C (mg/kg)	Se (mg/kg)	Na (%)	P (%)
Recommended levels	-	**≤3.8**	**≤18**	**6-15**	**≥35**	**≤40**	**≥500**	**≥500**	**100-200**	**0.5-1.3**	**0.2-0.6**	**0.5-0.8**
Hill's Prescription Diet w/d Feline	281	3.5	9.8	7.6	39.0	37.4	498.9	692	117	0.85	0.30	0.77
Hill's Prescription Diet w/d with Chicken Feline	278	3.5	9.9	7.6	39.9	35.4	500	721	122	0.70	0.35	0.86
Iams Veterinary Formula Weight Control D/ Optimum Weight Control	326	3.8	12.2	1.5	38.6	41.2	na	na	na	na	0.39	1.01
Medi-Cal Weight Control	325	na	11.8	3.4	34.4	na	na	na	na	na	0.3	1.0
Purina Veterinary Diets OM Overweight Management Feline Formula	321	3.6	8.5	5.6	56.2	22.4	na	693	116	na	0.57	1.19
Moist foods	**Energy density (kcal/can)****	**Energy density (kcal ME/g)**	**Fat (%)**	**Fiber (%)**	**Prot (%)**	**Carb (%)**	**Carn (ppm)**	**Vit E (IU/kg)**	**Vit C (mg/kg)**	**Se (mg/kg)**	**Na (%)**	**P (%)**
Recommended levels	-	**≤3.8**	**≤18**	**6-15**	**≥35**	**≤40**	**≥500**	**≥500**	**100-200**	**0.5-1.3**	**0.2-0.6**	**0.5-0.8**
Hill's Prescription Diet w/d with Chicken Feline	127/5.5 oz.	3.5	16.6	10.6	39.6	26.4	514.9	745	115	1.70	0.38	0.68
Medi-Cal Weight Control	144/170 g	na	22.6	4.2	40.0	na	na	na	na	na	0.5	1.1
Purina Veterinary Diets OM Overweight Management Feline Formula	150/5.5 oz.	3.9	14.6	10.2	44.6	23.2	na	na	na	na	0.31	0.99

Key: ME = metabolizable energy, na = information not available from manufacturer, Fiber = crude fiber, Prot = protein, Carb = digestible carbohydrate, Carn = L-carnitine, Se = selenium, Na = sodium, P = phosphorus, g = grams.
*From manufacturers' published information or calculated from manufacturers' published as-fed values. All values are on a dry matter basis unless otherwise stated.
**Energy density values are listed on an as fed basis and are useful for determining the amount to feed; cup = 8-oz. measuring cup. To convert to kJ, multiply kcal by 4.184.

For both dogs and cats, the simplest method for determining the amount to feed for weight maintenance is to obtain the food dose recommendation from the company providing the food. As with foods intended for weight loss, this information may be available on the product label, from product literature, from the company website or by using specially designed "calculators" or proprietary software programs (**Box 27-10**). The last method should only be considered if the amount fed for weight loss was determined this way and was appropriate (i.e., successful) for weight loss.

A more reliable, safer method is to feed 10% more calories than were required for weight loss. After the initial caloric intake for weight maintenance is calculated, divide it by the calorie content of the selected food to determine the actual daily amount to feed. **Table 27-18** provides an example of this method for calculating initial food dosage. Rechecks and adjustments will likely need to be made. (See Reassessment.)

How the Food is Fed

Free-choice feeding is a risk factor for becoming overweight. As with weight-loss programs, free-choice feeding rarely works for maintenance of reduced body weight even with the most calorie-restricted foods. Thus, as with the weight-loss program, patients being fed to maintain their target weight should be fed multiple small meals during the day to take advantage of the obligatory energy cost for digesting and absorbing food. The total daily food should be divided into at least two portions fed eight to 12 hours apart. Most pet owners can feed two meals per day without disrupting their schedules. Clients who can conveniently feed three or more meals per day should do so.

Meal sizes should be in portions that are practical to measure (i.e., to the nearest one-fourth cup or can). If the daily amount of food does not divide evenly into portions that are readily measurable, some meals will contain less and others more food. The meals containing more food should be fed when the owner will be with the pet for the longest time between meals. As with the weight-loss program, the patient should be kept out of the kitchen and dining areas during preparation and consumption of family meals. These practices can help reduce the pet's begging and the owner's urge to give the pet additional food or treats.

As with any food change, it is best to transition the patient to the new weight-maintenance food gradually over a period of a few days (Table 1-1).

REASSESSMENT

Assess the Performance of the Weight-Maintenance Program

Figure 27-3 is a simple algorithm that outlines the reassessment process for weight maintenance after successful weight

Table 27-18. Using number of calories fed for weight loss to determine the initial amount of food to feed for target weight maintenance.

The amount of food fed for weight loss at the time the target weight was achieved is the basis for a method of determining the amount of food to feed initially to avoid weight regain. The following steps are involved in this process:

1. First, the daily number of calories fed for weight loss is calculated by multiplying the amount of the weight-loss food fed (usually a volume measure) by its caloric density. Caloric density can be obtained from **Tables 27-16** (dogs) or **27-17** (cats) or from product information.
2. Next, increase the number of calories by 10% to determine the estimated daily number of calories to feed (initially at least) to maintain the target weight.
3. Finally, divide the daily number of calories by the energy density of the food selected for weight maintenance to determine the amount of this food to feed per day.

An example case follows:

Through a well-executed weight-loss program, a previously obese dog achieved the target weight of 25 kg. It was being fed 3.5 cups of an appropriate energy-restricted food formulated for weight loss.

The energy density of the weight-loss food is 220 kcal/cup. The amount of food fed is multiplied by the energy density of the food (3.5 cups x 220 kcal/cup) to yield approximately 770 kcal/day.*

The daily number of calories fed for weight loss is increased by 10% (10% x 770 kcal = 77 kcal; 770 kcal + 77 kcal = 847 kcal) to yield the number of calories to feed as a starting point for weight maintenance.

The selected weight-maintenance food provides 243 kcal/cup (obtained from product information). The daily calories for weight maintenance are divided by the energy density of the weight-maintenance food to yield the daily amount to feed (847 kcal/day ÷ 243 kcal/cup = 3.5 cups/day).

Note that this is the same volume of food that was being fed for weight loss. This is because the weight-maintenance food contains 10% more calories/cup than the weight-loss food.

This calculation assumes that if treats were fed during the weight-loss program that the same amount or fewer are fed during the weight-maintenance program. The same is true for the amount of exercise.

At least three days should be spent transitioning to the new food. Body weight should be rechecked every week or two for four to six weeks. Adjustments in increments of 10% should be made until body weight stabilizes at the target weight.

*To convert to kJ, multiply kcal by 4.184.

loss. Rechecks are essential after the pet attains its target weight. More frequent rechecks are needed when the animal reaches its target weight and calories are increased to maintain that weight. Rechecks should occur every two weeks to assess the appropriateness of caloric intake in conjunction with continued exercise. During this stage of the weight-maintenance program, no more than two weeks should elapse between weigh-ins because weight regain can rapidly occur. If changes in food intake are necessary to maintain the target weight, increase or decrease the amount in 10% increments; be careful not to allow weight regain.

Maintain the every two-week recheck schedule until the patient's body weight has stabilized at the desired weight for at least three consecutive weighins. Then, rechecks can occur every three months for a year and finally to six months thereafter. The precise timing of the rechecks isn't as important as the general notion of the timely tracking of the patient's body weight and adjusting the amount of food to feed, as necessary. Such rechecks also help reinforce compliance as with the weight-loss program (**Box 27-11**).

ACKNOWLEDGMENT

The authors and editors thank Dr. William J. Burkholder for his contribution to this chapter in the previous edition.

ENDNOTE

a. Schoenherr WD. Hill's Science and Technology Center, Topeka, KS, USA. Unpublished data. 2003.

REFERENCES

The references for **Chapter 27** can be found at www.markmorris.org.

CASE 27-1

Respiratory Distress in an Obese Miniature Poodle

William J. Burkholder, DVM, PhD, Dipl. ACVN*
College of Veterinary Medicine
Texas A & M University
College Station, Texas, USA

Patient Assessment

A four-year-old intact male miniature poodle weighing 17.3 kg was admitted for coughing, dyspnea, cyanosis and exercise intolerance. Physical examination findings were normal except for obesity. Results of a complete blood count, serum biochemistry profile, urinalysis, thoracic radiography and fluoroscopic examination of the trachea were normal. Bronchoscopy revealed no abnormalities. Cultures of tracheal and bronchial washings were negative for growth of pathogenic organisms. Lung scintigraphy showed no pulmonary vascular deficits.

Body condition score was 5/5. Morphometric measures estimated 47% of the dog's weight was fat. Optimal body weight was estimated to be 9.1 kg, making the patient's initial body weight 90% above optimal.

Assess the Food and Feeding Method

Table 1 lists the dietary history.

Questions

1. Estimate the amount of energy consumed by this patient each day.
2. Calculate the daily energy requirement (DER) for this patient at its estimated optimal body weight and compare this number with the energy estimate in Question 1.
3. Outline a feeding, exercise and monitoring plan for weight reduction for this dog.

Answers and Discussion

1. The energy consumed by the dog each day is at least 1,247 kcal (5.22 MJ). This is estimated from the moist food (one can, 556 kcal/can [2.33 MJ/can]), dry food (one cup, 327 kcal/cup [1.37 MJ/cup]), commercial treats (five treats, 20 kcal/treat [84 kJ/treat]) and ice cream (one cup, 264 kcal/cup [1.11 MJ/cup]). The daily caloric consumption was probably higher because the dog also ate various meats from the owner's meals.
2. The resting energy requirement (RER) at the estimated optimal body weight is calculated as follows: RER optimal weight = $70(9.1)^{0.75}$ = 367 kcal (1.54 MJ). DER would be approximately 1.4 to 1.6 x RER or 514 to 587 kcal (2.15 to 2.46 MJ). The daily caloric intake estimated in Question 1 is much higher than the estimated DER (about double).
3. The initial caloric restriction was set at an amount slightly above RER calculated for optimal body weight. The owners were instructed to feed no ice cream, meat or other table foods. The commercial treats were continued but fewer were given per day. The food was changed to a commercial product containing less fat and more crude fiber. Caloric restriction was accomplished using the specific foods and feeding methods listed in **Table 2**.

   The owners were also instructed to walk the dog on a leash daily. Initially they were to walk only as far as the dog could tolerate without becoming dyspneic. The walks were gradually increased to 20 to 30 minutes per walk, once or twice a day. The owners were asked to return every two weeks for the first couple of months to weigh the dog and monitor progress.

Progress Notes

Figure 1 shows the weight loss that occurred with this feeding plan and exercise. The coughing and dyspnea gradually resolved after the dog lost approximately 2 kg. The owners noticed a dramatic increase in the dog's activity after three months. The food was changed on Week 34 of the weight-reduction program to the foods and feeding methods listed in **Table 3**. Body weight stabilized (**Figure 1**) and the dog remained free of respiratory signs and distress.

Animals that are obese because of gross overfeeding are the

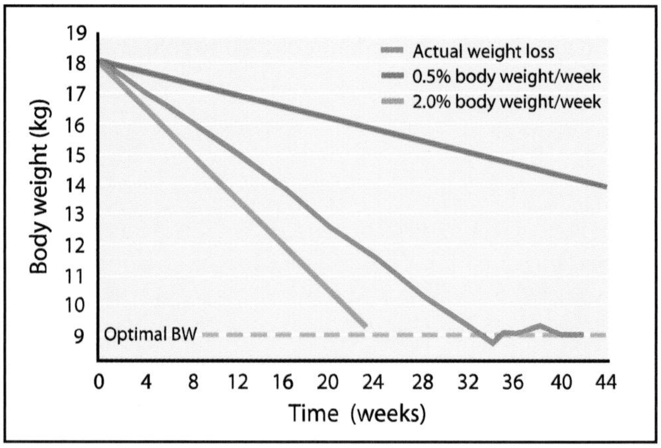

Figure 1. Progression of body weight loss compared with the minimum (loss of 0.5% of initial body weight/week) and maximum (loss of 2% of initial body weight/week) rates of weight loss.

patients most likely to achieve expected rates of weight loss when owners comply with caloric restriction.

*Dr. Burkholder's current affiliation is:
Division of Animal Feeds, HFV-228
Center for Veterinary Medicine
7519 Standish Place
Rockville, MD, USA 20855

Endnotes

a. Hill's Pet Nutrition, Inc., Topeka, KS, USA. Science Diet Canine Maintenance, moist and Science Diet Canine Maintenance, dry are currently marketed as Science Diet Beef & Chicken Entrée Adult Canine and Science Diet Adult Original Formula. Science Diet Canine Maintenance Light, dry is currently marketed as Science Diet Light Adult Canine.

b. Nabisco, East Hanover, NJ, USA.

Table 1. Foods and feeding method assessment of an obese miniature poodle with respiratory distress.

Foods	Feeding method
Science Diet Canine Maintenance, moist[a]	One can, once daily
Science Diet Canine Maintenance, dry[a]	One cup, once daily
Milk-Bone treats (small)[b]	Five, daily
Ice cream	One cup, once daily
Various meats from owner's meals	Once or twice daily

Table 2. Feeding plan for weight reduction.

Foods	Feeding method	kcal (kJ)
Prescription Diet r/d Canine, moist[a]	Three-fourths can, once daily	150 (628)
Science Diet Canine Maintenance Light, dry[a]	One cup, once daily	221 (925)
Milk-Bone treats (small)	Two treats, daily	40 (167)
Total = 411 kcal/day (1.72 MJ)		

Table 3. Feeding plan to stabilize reduced body weight.

Foods	Feeding method	kcal (kJ)
Science Diet Canine Maintenance, moist	One-half can, once daily	278 (1,163)
Science Diet Canine Maintenance, dry	One cup, once daily	327 (1,368)
Milk-Bone treats (small)	Four treats, daily	80 (335)
Total = 685 kcal/day (2.87 MJ)		

CASE 27-2

An Overweight Cat

William J. Burkholder, DVM, PhD, Dipl. ACVN*
College of Veterinary Medicine
Texas A & M University
College Station, Texas, USA

Patient Assessment

An eight-year-old neutered male domestic longhair cat weighing 6.6 kg was diagnosed with asymmetric hypertrophy of the interventricular septum via echocardiography. No abnormalities were noted on physical examination except for excessive body weight. Complete blood count, serum biochemistry profile and urinalysis results were normal.

The cat's body condition was assessed as 4.5/5. Optimal body weight was estimated to be 5.5 kg, making the initial body weight 20% above ideal.

Assess the Food and Feeding Method

The cat was fed a commercial food that was lower in fat and higher in crude fiber than regular commercial cat foods (Science Diet Feline Maintenance Light;[a] one-third cup, twice daily).

Questions

1. Estimate the amount of energy consumed by this patient each day.
2. Calculate the daily energy requirement (DER) for this patient at its estimated optimal body weight and compare this number with the assessment in Question 1.
3. Outline a feeding and monitoring plan for weight reduction for this cat.

Answers and Discussion

1. The energy consumed by the cat each day was approximately 168 kcal (703 kJ). This is estimated from the dry food (two-thirds cup, 248 kcal/cup [1,038 kJ]).
2. The resting energy requirement (RER) at the estimated optimal body weight is calculated as follows: RER optimal weight = $70(5.5)^{0.75}$ = 250 kcal (1,046 kJ). DER at optimal body weight would be approximately 1.2 x RER or 300 kcal (1,255 kJ). The daily caloric intake estimated in Question 1 is actually lower than the RER for optimal body weight.
3. The cat was switched to a commercial dry feline food that had a slightly higher fiber content but approximately the same fat content and caloric density as the current food (Prescription Diet w/d Feline;[a] one-third cup twice daily, 165 kcal/day [690 kJ]). This food supplied only 66% of the calories estimated for RER at the optimal body weight. The owner was instructed to increase the cat's activity as much as possible and asked to return every two weeks for the first couple of months to weigh the cat and monitor the progress.

Progress Notes

Figure 1 shows the weight loss that occurred with this feeding and exercise plan. Note that the initial weight loss stopped by Week 13. At that time, the amount of food was reduced to one-fourth cup, twice daily, which supplied 123 kcal (515 kJ) or 49% of RER at optimal body weight. The two times when body weight increased were associated with the cat being fed by other people because the owner was out of town for several weeks. These lapses emphasize the need to have everyone understand the need for adhering to and measuring the prescribed amounts of food. The cat's owner understood the need for strict adherence to the feeding schedule, but those who fed the cat in the owner's absence did not. Some decrease in exercise level may also have occurred in the owner's absence.

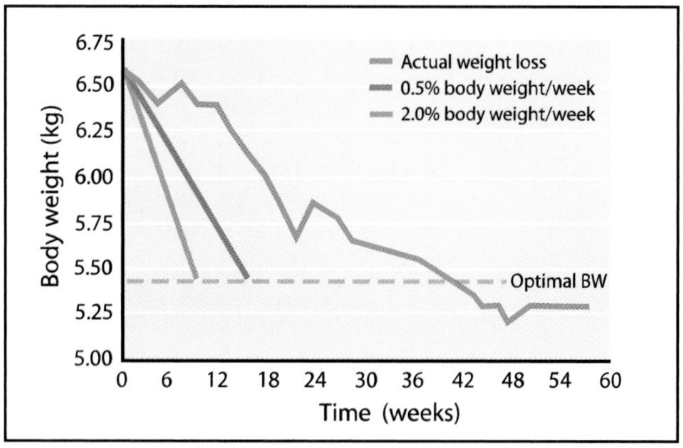

Figure 1. Progression of body weight loss compared with minimum and maximum rates of weight loss.

Figure 2 compares weight loss with measurements of the cat's pelvic circumference. This shows how the pelvic circumference can be used along with body weight to track relative progression of weight loss.

Weight was stabilized at 5.3 kg by returning the cat to the original food and increasing daily caloric intake to 165 kcal (690 kJ). This was done in two steps. On Week 43, the food was changed to Science Diet Feline Maintenance Light;[a] one-fourth cup was fed in the morning and one-third cup in the evening. This feeding plan provided 144 kcal (602 kJ) per day. Weight loss slowed but body weight still tended to decrease. On Week 47, the food was increased to one-third cup twice daily and body weight stabilized.

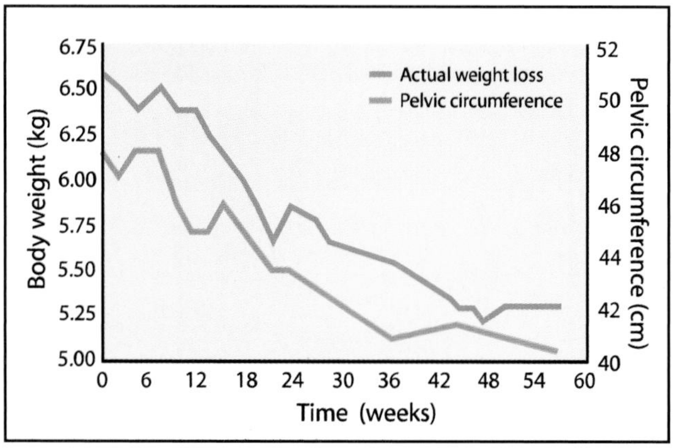

Figure 2. Comparison of body weight loss and decrease in pelvic circumference during the weight-reduction program.

*Dr. Burkholder's current affiliation is:
Division of Animal Feeds, HFV-228
Center for Veterinary Medicine
7519 Standish Place
Rockville, MD, USA 20855

Endnote

a. Hill's Pet Nutrition, Inc., Topeka, KS, USA. Science Diet Feline Maintenance Light is currently marketed as Science Diet Light Adult Feline.

CASE 27-3

Lameness in an Obese Labrador Retriever

William J. Burkholder, DVM, PhD, Dipl. ACVN*
College of Veterinary Medicine
Texas A & M University
College Station, Texas, USA

Patient Assessment

A nine-year-old neutered female Labrador retriever weighing 41.8 kg was admitted six months after repair of a ruptured left anterior cruciate ligament. The dog was still limping on its left rear leg. Radiographs of the stifle showed evidence of mild osteoarthrosis. Orthopedic examination of the stifle for stability and range of motion was normal. No other abnormalities were found on physical examination. Results of a complete blood count, serum biochemistry profile, urinalysis and serum T_3 and T_4 concentrations were normal.

The dog's body condition was assessed as 4.5/5. Ideal body weight was estimated to be 34 kg (**Table 27-3**). Morphometric measures estimated 35% of the dog's body weight was fat.

Assess the Food and Feeding Method

Caloric restriction had been initiated after surgery in an attempt to promote weight loss. **Table 1** lists the assessment of the foods and feeding management. No weight loss had occurred in the last three to four months.

Questions

Table 1. Foods and feeding method assessment of an obese Labrador retriever with lameness.

Foods	Feeding method
Prescription Diet r/d Canine, moist[a]	One can, twice daily
Prescription Diet r/d Canine, dry[a]	One cup, twice daily
Milk-Bone treats (small)[b]	One treat, once daily

1. What are some risk factors for obesity that can be identified from the animal assessment?
2. Estimate the amount of energy consumed by this patient each day.
3. Calculate the daily energy requirement (DER) for this patient at its estimated optimal body weight and compare this number with the assessment in Question 2.
4. Outline a feeding, exercise and monitoring plan for weight reduction for this dog.

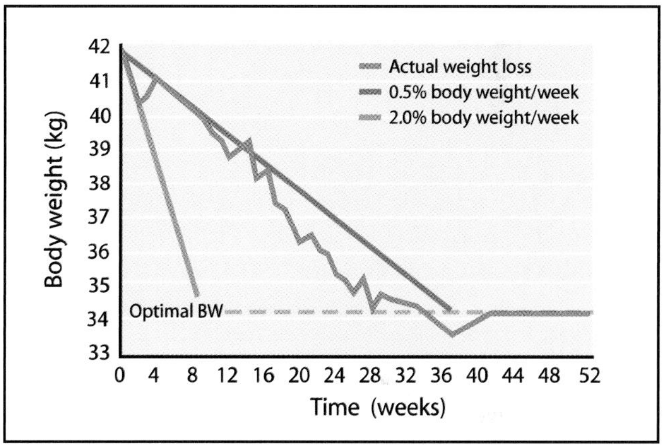

Figure 1. Progression of body weight loss compared with minimum and maximum rates of weight loss.

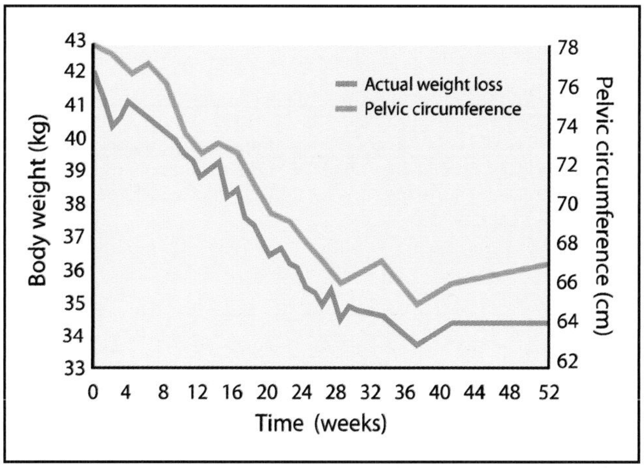

Figure 2. Comparison of body weight loss and pelvic circumference during the weight-reduction program.

Answers and Discussion

1. Risk factors for obesity in this patient include age (middle-aged dogs are more prone to obesity than younger animals), gender (female dogs are at higher risk than male dogs), reproductive status (neutered dogs are at more risk than intact animals), breed (Labrador retrievers are considered an obesity-prone breed) and exercise level (the dog had been sedentary since the knee surgery). Obesity may have contributed to the anterior cruciate rupture and restricted exercise since surgery may have contributed to persistent obesity despite recent caloric restriction.
2. The energy consumed by the dog each day was approximately 920 kcal (3.85 MJ). This is estimated from the moist food (two cans, 250 kcal/can [1.05 MJ/can]), dry food (two cups, 200 kcal/cup [837 kJ/cup]) and commercial treats (one treat, 20

kcal/treat [84 kJ/treat]).

3. The resting energy requirement (RER) at the estimated optimal body weight is calculated as follows: RER optimal weight = $70(34)^{0.75}$ = 988 kcal (4.13 MJ). DER at optimal body weight would be approximately 1.4 to 1.6 x RER or 1,383 to 1,581 kcal (5.79 to 6.62 MJ). The daily caloric intake estimated in Question 2 is actually lower than RER for optimal body weight.
4. Because the current intake of 920 kcal (3.85 MJ) was slightly less than RER for an optimal weight of 34 kg, this level of caloric restriction was not initially changed. Because the dog had been minimally active since the knee surgery, 20 to 60 minutes of persistent leash walking per day was initiated. The owners were instructed to work up gradually to whatever amount of walking the dog could do comfortably without soreness. The owners were asked to return every two weeks for the first couple of months to weigh the dog and monitor progress.

Progress Notes

Figure 1 shows the weight loss that occurred with this feeding and exercise plan. Loss of almost 2% of starting weight (the maximum acceptable rate of weight loss) was achieved during the first two weeks by the addition of exercise. Unfortunately, weight was actually gained during Weeks 3 and 4, which greatly discouraged the owners. The owners were counseled to persist with the leash walking and the daily caloric intake was decreased to 725 kcal/day (3.03 MJ) (approximately 80% of calories indicated by the dietary assessment) using the foods and feeding methods listed in **Table 2**.

After the dog had lost approximately 3 kg by Week 10, it ceased to limp and had a normal gait thereafter. The owners were unable to walk the dog during Weeks 12 to 14 and some weight gain occurred. Weight loss continued when leash walks were resumed. This finding demonstrates the importance of exercise as a component of daily energy expenditure, especially during weight reduction of calorically efficient animals.

Figure 2 compares weight loss with measurements of the dog's pelvic circumference. This shows how the pelvic circumference can be used with body weight to track relative progression of weight loss.

Calories were increased on Week 28 to maintain a body weight of 34 kg (**Table 3**). This dog maintained the reduced weight on the same number of kcal as it used to maintain the obese weight. This indirectly supports the assertion that adipose tissue requires very few calories to maintain its mass.

*Dr. Burkholder's current affiliation is:
Division of Animal Feeds, HFV-228
Center for Veterinary Medicine
7519 Standish Place
Rockville, MD, USA 20855

Endnotes

a. Hill's Pet Nutrition, Inc., Topeka, KS, USA.
b. Nabisco, East Hanover, NJ, USA.

Table 2. Feeding plan for further weight reduction.

Foods	Feeding method	kcal (MJ)
Prescription Diet r/d Canine, moist	One-half can, morning	125 (0.52)
Prescription Diet r/d Canine, dry	One and one-half cups, twice daily	600 (2.51)
Total = 725 kcal/day (3.03 MJ)		

Table 3. Feeding plan to stabilize reduced body weight.

Foods	Feeding method	kcal (MJ)
Prescription Diet r/d Canine, moist	One-half can, twice daily	250 (1.05)
Prescription Diet r/d Canine, dry	One and two-thirds cups, twice daily	668 (2.80)
Total = 918 kcal/day (3.85 MJ)		

CASE 27-4

Weight Loss in a Domestic Shorthair Cat

Philip Roudebush, DVM, Dipl. ACVIM (Small Animal Internal Medicine)
Hill's Scientific Affairs
Topeka, Kansas, USA

William D. Schoenherr, PhD
Hill's Pet Nutrition Center
Topeka, Kansas, USA

Patient Assessment

A 10-year-old, neutered female domestic shorthair cat was examined for routine geriatric health maintenance. The patient weighed 4.8 kg and its ribs were very difficult to feel under a thick fat cover. A moderate-to-thick fat layer covered bony prominences. The cat's abdomen was pendulous with no obvious waist. A marked abdominal fat pad was present and the cat's back was broadened when viewed from above. The cat's limbs also had fat deposits. Results of a complete blood count, serum biochemistry profile and urinalysis were normal.

Assess the Food and Feeding Method

The cat was fed a dry, specialty brand adult cat food free choice and was given one can of moist, grocery store brand cat food twice weekly as a treat.

Questions

1. What is the body condition score (BCS) for this patient?
2. What are risk factors for obesity in cats?
3. What types of therapeutic foods are available to help manage overweight or obese cats?
4. Are there clinical studies supporting the use of therapeutic foods for effective weight loss in cats?

Answers and Discussion

1. The physical examination findings support a diagnosis of obesity (BCS 5/5).
2. This cat has several risk factors for obesity. Middle-aged and older cats are more prone to obesity than younger animals. Female cats are at higher risk than male cats. Neutered cats are at greater risk than intact animals. Studies have shown that neutered cats require up to 30% fewer calories per day than before they were neutered. Strictly indoor cats usually are less active.
3. Traditional methods of weight management include use of low-calorie, high-fiber foods. Added fiber increases bulk and reduces hunger, while diluting calories. Weight-management foods often contain added L-carnitine, which helps cats lose fat safely, while maintaining lean body mass. An alternative weight-management concept for cats includes using a low-carbohydrate, high-protein food to alter a cat's metabolism for effective weight loss. When carbohydrates are unavailable, the body burns body fat and dietary protein as energy sources. When fed this type of food, cats lose weight and have improved glucose and lipid control. Food choice is based on veterinarian discretion and response to previous weight-management programs. Regardless of the food chosen, caloric restriction should be instituted and the amount of food fed should be closely monitored.
4. A study was conducted in which middle-aged or senior domestic shorthair cats with more than 30% body fat were fed either a low-calorie, high-fiber formula (Prescription Diet r/d Feline[a]) or a low-carbohydrate, high-protein formula (Prescription Diet m/d Feline[a]) for 24 weeks. Cats were fed to achieve ideal body weight and condition, which typically means 20% body fat. Each cat was fed its assigned food until it achieved 20% body fat or completed the 24-week study. More than 70% of each group reached ideal body weight within 20 weeks. Weight loss was well within the 0.5 to 2% of initial body weight per week recommended for safe weight loss by veterinary nutritionists. Importantly, both groups maintained lean body mass.

   After two months of feeding, cats fed the moist, low-carbohydrate, high-protein formula had twice the levels of beta-hydroxybutyrate (a ketone) as cats fed the moist, low-calorie, high-fiber formula. This finding signals a metabolic shift from using dietary carbohydrates to body fat as a primary energy source. These metabolic changes contributed to the weight loss in cats fed the low-carbohydrate, high-protein formula. Biochemistry profile data indicated no abnormal changes in organ function in either study group. Both the traditional, low-calorie, high-fiber food, and the low-carbohydrate, high-protein, metabolic control food, were safe and effective for weight loss in cats.

Progress Notes

The cat was fed a dry, low-carbohydrate, high-protein food (Prescription Diet m/d Feline) to help achieve weight loss. The amount of food was calculated based on an ideal body weight of 3.41 kg (daily energy requirement for weight loss = 0.8 x resting energy requirement). The amount of food was carefully measured and divided into at least two or more daily meals (typically, 1/8th cup of food, twice daily). The owners were told that successful weight loss depends greatly on avoiding common pitfalls such as feeding their cat treats.

After three months, the cat weighed 3.95 kg, which represented a loss of 0.86 kg or 18% of its original body weight. After four months, the cat weighed 3.82 kg, and was losing 1.3% of initial body weight per week. Serum biochemistry, urinalysis and physical examination findings remained normal during the weight-loss period, proving the safety and efficacy of the program. This feeding plan was continued until the cat reached an ideal weight of 3.41 kg. The cat was transitioned to a dry, low-calorie, moderate-fiber food (Prescription Diet w/d Feline[a]) over seven days to help maintain ideal weight. A moist, low-calorie, moderate-fiber food (Prescription Diet w/d Feline) was recommended as snack offerings in place of the previous moist, grocery brand products.

Endnote

a. Hill's Pet Nutrition, Inc., Topeka, KS, USA

Bibliography

Fettman MJ, Stanton CA, Banks LL, et al. Effects of neutering on bodyweight, metabolic rate and glucose tolerance of domestic cats. Research in Veterinary Science 1997; 62: 131-136.

Schoenherr WH. Feline weight-loss studies. Clinical Evidence Report TD-1002. Hill's Pet Nutrition, Inc., Topeka, Kansas, 2003.

Section 8

Lipid and Endocrine Disorders

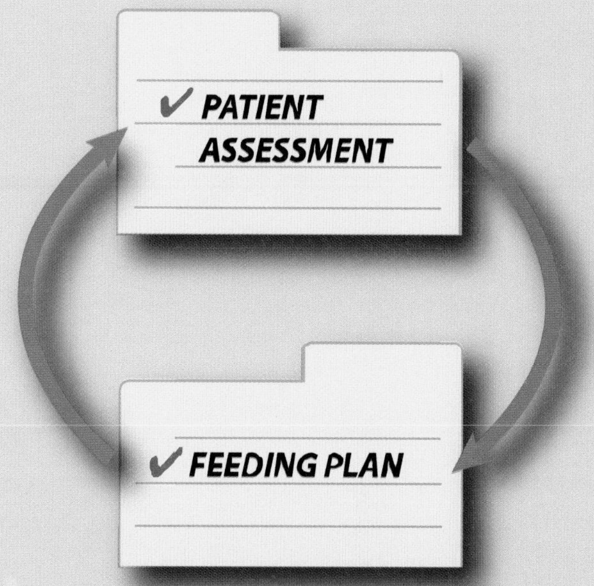

Chapter 28

Disorders of Lipid Metabolism

Richard B. Ford
Chris L. Ludlow

"It is a scientific fact that your body will not absorb cholesterol if you take it from another person's plate."
Dave Barry

CLINICAL IMPORTANCE

Hyperlipidemia (also called hyperlipoproteinemia) refers to a disturbance of lipid metabolism that results in an elevated concentration of blood lipids, particularly triglycerides, cholesterol or both. In the fasted state, hyperlipidemia is an abnormal laboratory finding that represents either accelerated synthesis or retarded degradation of lipoproteins (Brown and Goldstein, 1987). Among dogs and cats, the most common, clinically important type of hyperlipidemia is characterized by an excess concentration of triglycerides in blood, a condition referred to as hypertriglyceridemia (Ford, 1993, 1996). The serum and plasma of affected animals typically appear milky white and turbid, or lipemic. In cases of extreme hypertriglyceridemia, the patient's serum can be so lipemic that it is opaque, or lactescent (**Figure 28-1**).

Hypercholesterolemia is an excess concentration of cholesterol in blood. Most of the circulating cholesterol in dogs and cats is carried on high-density lipoprotein (HDL), the smallest lipoprotein (Ford, 1996; Mahley and Weisgraber, 1974; Mahley et al, 1974). Because HDL particles are small and do not refract light, patients with extreme cholesterol elevations will not have lipemic serum unless the triglyceride concentration is also elevated.

The clinical importance of hyperlipidemia in companion animal medicine centers around four facts: 1) lipemic serum may positively or negatively interfere with quantitative analyses of other serum analytes, 2) hyperlipidemia in fasted (>12 hours) dogs or cats is abnormal and should be addressed as a significant clinical finding, 3) hyperlipidemic patients are at risk for developing significant clinical illness, including acute pancreatitis and 4) specific dietary and/or drug intervention can eliminate or at least diminish the morbidity associated with hyperlipidemia.

PATIENT ASSESSMENT

History and Physical Examination

The major clinical manifestations of hyperlipidemia include intermittent vomiting, diarrhea and abdominal discomfort and seizures in dogs; cutaneous xanthomata (**Figure 28-2**) and peripheral neuropathy in cats and lipid keratopathies (**Figure 28-3**) and lipemia retinalis in both species (**Figure 28-4**). Some hyperlipidemic dogs and cats do not manifest clinical signs but are considered to be at risk for developing overt signs in the future. Atherosclerosis is a rare manifestation of hyperlipidemia in dogs and cats as opposed to people.

Dogs with Hyperlipidemia

Table 28-1 lists the clinical signs associated with hypertriglyceridemia in dogs. The most common presenting complaints are vague and intermittent but usually center around vomiting and diarrhea. Accompanying signs include non-localizing abdominal discomfort and occasional pain, accompanied by a transient

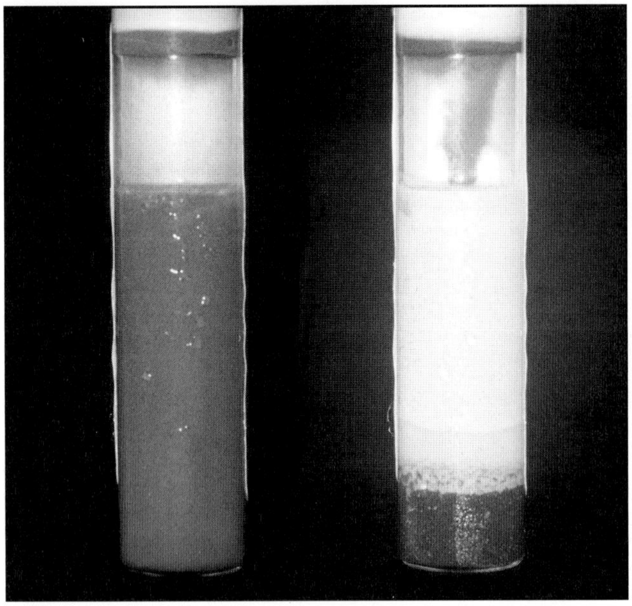

Figure 28-1. Blood samples from a Doberman pinscher with hypothyroidism and severe lipemia. The picture on the left was taken immediately after the sample was drawn. Note that the lipid content is so high that even in black and white photography the blood has a "tomato soup" appearance. The blood sample on the right was allowed to separate forming a "cream layer" of triglyceride-rich chylomicrons on top.

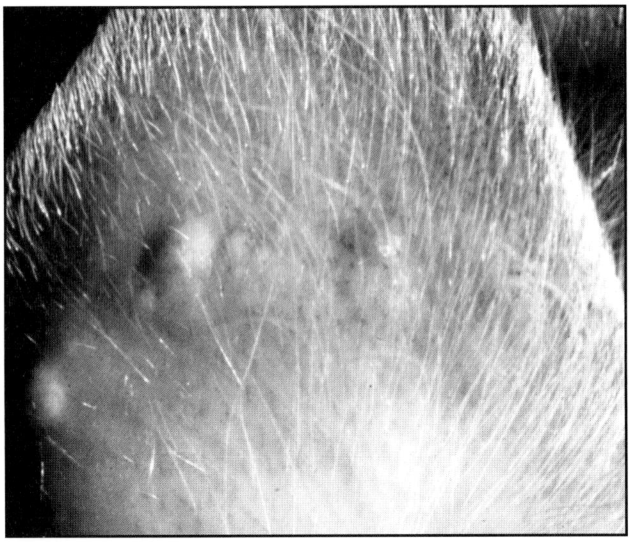

Figure 28-2. Xanthomas on the pinna of a cat with hyperlipidemia. Xanthomas are tumors composed of lipid-laden foam cells, which are histiocytes containing cytoplasmic lipid material. These lesions resolved with use of a low-fat, high-fiber food.

decrease in appetite. The owner may report episodic signs, lasting a few hours to a few days that may resolve spontaneously with fasting. Abdominal distention is occasionally reported. There appears to be no gender predilection. Affected dogs are usually four years of age and older although younger dogs may be affected.

On physical examination, dogs may appear lethargic and may or may not manifest abdominal pain. Clinical signs and history are compatible with acute pancreatitis; however, abdominal radiographs, ultrasound and laboratory evidence supporting a diagnosis of pancreatitis are typically lacking. The term pseudopancreatitis has been used to describe the clinical manifestations associated with hypertriglyceridemia (Ford, 1993, 1996).

Lipemia retinalis, a condition characterized by pale pink retinal arterioles and venules, is an incidental finding seen on funduscopic examination of lipemic dogs and cats (**Figure 28-4**). This condition does not affect vision. Laboratory analysis of affected animals will verify extreme hypertriglyceridemia, typically greater than 1,000 mg/dl.

Sustained hypertriglyceridemia is a principal risk factor among people and dogs for developing acute pancreatitis (Brown and Goldstein, 1987; Ford, 1993; Armstrong and Ford, 1989; DeBowes, 1987; Sanfey and Cameron, 1985; Whitney et al, 1987; Williams, 1995). Dogs with acute abdominal pain and vomiting should be evaluated for hyperchylomicronemia at the time of presentation and during the recovery phase when food intake is restored.

Hypertriglyceridemia should be considered in patients presenting with a history of seizures. A small number of patients, many of them miniature schnauzers, diagnosed with idiopathic epilepsy have elevated fasting triglyceride concentrations and lipemic serum (Rogers et al, 1975, 1975a). In some dogs, dietary therapy has successfully reduced blood triglyceride levels and eliminated seizures without concomitant use of anticonvulsant drugs. Interestingly, seizures associated with hyperlipidemia are not necessarily associated with other signs typically attributed to hyperlipidemia (e.g., vomiting and diarrhea).

Although owners of hypertriglyceridemic dogs rarely express concern about their pet's inactivity or lethargy at the time of initial presentation, owners often remark that the pet's activity level increased as a result of lowering circulating triglyceride levels.[a]

Cats with Hyperlipidemia

Clinical signs in hyperlipidemic cats are different than those reported to occur in dogs (**Table 28-1**). The most common clinical finding in affected cats is cutaneous xanthoma, a painless, raised lesion caused by accumulation of lipid-laden macrophages or foam cells in the skin (**Figure 28-2**) (Jones and Watson, 1995; Jones et al, 1983; Jones, 1995). Xanthomas are most likely to occur over bony prominences and areas of skin subject to chronic pressure or direct injury.

Xanthomata may also occur in other tissues such as liver, spleen, kidney, heart, skeletal muscle and intestines. Uniquely, xanthomata can form at the point where spinal nerves emerge through the vertebral foramina (Jones, 1993), the point at which nerves and vascular tissue are subject to mild injury associated with the movement of adjacent vertebrae. Peripheral neuropathy caused by neuronal xanthoma is characterized by motor paralysis. Signs vary depending on the specific nerves involved. Horner's syndrome, tibial nerve paralysis and radial nerve paralysis have been reported most often (Jones, 1993, 1995). In cases in which mixed motor and sensory nerves have been affected, sensation to painful stimuli was retained.

Lipemia retinalis is more common in cats than dogs (**Figure 28-4**). Other ocular manifestations of hyperchylomicronemia in cats are uncommon but include iridocyclitis, arcus lipoides corneae and lipemic aqueous and lipid keratopathy (**Figure 28-3**). These lesions are thought to occur subsequent to existing ocular disease in lipemic cats (Jones, 1995; Crispin, 1993).

Laboratory Evaluation

Veterinarians assessing a dog or cat for hyperlipidemia should submit serum or plasma rather than whole blood (**Box 28-1**). Plasma or serum samples for cholesterol and triglyceride determinations can be refrigerated or frozen for several days without significant effect.

The presence of excess triglycerides, particularly if associated with retention of chylomicrons, is an important source of either positive (falsely increased) or negative (falsely decreased) interference for analytes determined by colorimetric methods (Whitney et al, 1987). The effect of lipemia on individual analytes is variable and depends on the degree of lipemia, the analyte being measured and the analytic method used. Lipemia also causes in vitro hemolysis, a phenomenon induced by the effect of lipid on erythrocyte membrane fragility, which may also induce interference when performing laboratory profiles (Allerman, 1990). The extent to which in vitro hemolysis affects determination of hemoglobin and hematocrit values has not been established. The amount of red-cell hemolysis appears to be proportional to the length of time red cells are in contact with the lipemic serum and the degree of lipemia. The type and extent of interference induced by lipemia varies from one laboratory to another, depending on the analytical instrumentation and methodologies used. Visual inspection of the patient's serum provides valuable physical evidence about the presence or absence of an excessive concentration of triglycerides. In fasting patients (i.e., 24-hour fast or longer), lipemia or lactescent serum denotes hypertriglyceridemia and is usually associated with triglyceride concentrations in excess of 2,000 mg/dl (canine normal = 50 to 150 mg/dl, feline normal = 50 to 100 mg/dl). A diagnosis of hypertriglyceridemia should be based on laboratory determination of serum triglycerides in uncleared serum. By laboratory methods used in North America, serum triglyceride concentrations greater than 500 mg/dl are abnormal for fasted dogs and cats. Although a correlation has not been observed between triglyceride concentrations and the severity of clinical signs, dogs with a triglyceride concentration of 1,000 mg/dl or higher are at risk for developing clinical signs and, as such, are candidates for dietary intervention (Armstrong and Ford, 1989; Rogers et al, 1975a; Chapman, 1980). Maintaining triglyceride levels less than 500 mg/dl in lipemic (familial) patients may be difficult with nutritional management alone. A more reasonable target range for dietary control is 500 to 1,000 mg/dl postprandially. Furthermore, clinical signs of hypertriglyceridemia appear to be uncommon in patients with postprandial triglyceride levels less than 1,000 mg/dl.

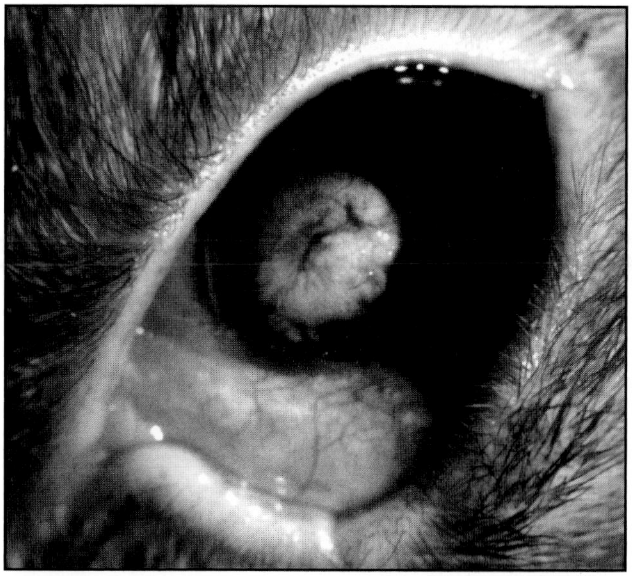

Figure 28-3. Lipid keratopathy in a rabbit. Note the white lipid accumulation in the corneal stroma. Corneal vascularization may precede or follow lipid deposition. Lipid keratopathy has been described in several species including human beings, rabbits, cats and dogs.

Table 28-1. Clinical signs and diseases associated with hypertriglyceridemia in dogs and cats.

Dogs
Abdominal discomfort*
Acute pancreatitis
Behavior (lethargy, inactivity)
Crystalline stromal dystrophy (especially cavalier King Charles spaniels)
Cushing's syndrome
Fasting lipemia (six to 12 hours)
Intermittent diarrhea*
Intermittent vomiting*
Lipemia retinalis
Lipemic aqueous
Lipid corneal dystrophy/arcus lipoides corneae
Seizures
Cats
Cutaneous xanthomata
Lipemia retinalis
Lipid keratopathy
Peripheral nerve paralysis
Horner's syndrome
Tibial nerve paralysis
Radial nerve paralysis
Splenomegaly

*These clinical signs may occur concomitantly in the same patient. The collective term used to describe these signs is "pseudopancreatitis."

Significant hyperlipidemia characterized by lipemic serum and hypertriglyceridemia has been observed as an incidental finding in fasted adult dogs and cats. The absence of clinical signs at the time of presentation does not justify ignoring the significance of the lipemia. Because of the risks associated with hypertriglyceridemia, patients that behave normally but have persistent lipemia should be managed in the same manner as

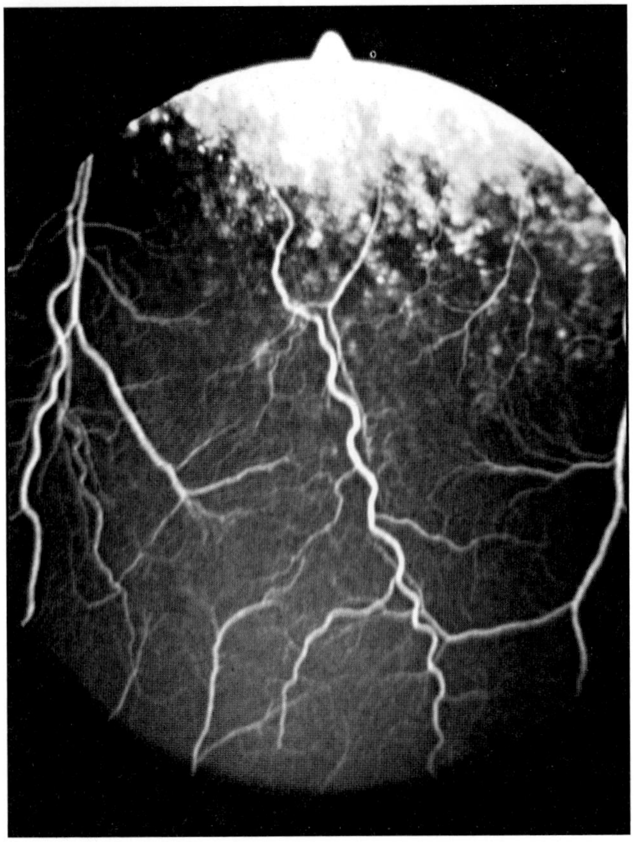

Figure 28-4. Lipemia retinalis in a cat with hyperlipidemia. Note the white, milky appearance of the retinal blood vessels.

Box 28-1. Handling Lipemic Samples.

Submission of lipemic blood to a commercial laboratory necessitates knowing how the sample will be processed. Because of the interference induced by lipemia, some laboratories will simply reject lipemic samples. Many laboratories, however, will attempt to clear lipemic serum (by removing chylomicrons) before performing any biochemical assays. Unfortunately, there is neither a standardized method for clearing lipemic serum nor do commercial laboratories consistently report whether or not an attempt was made to clear the sample. For veterinarians, however, knowledge of the fact that a lipemic sample was cleared before determining the triglyceride concentration is critical in making reasonable interpretations. Although clearing a lipemic sample eliminates interference associated with chylomicrons, it effectively eliminates a critical element of clinical information (i.e., that the patient is hypertriglyceridemic).

Ideally, two aliquots of a serum sample from a lipemic patient should be submitted simultaneously. One sample, if effectively cleared, can be used to perform routine biochemical testing, including triglyceride levels. Determining triglyceride concentrations in the second, lipemic (uncleared) sample documents the true extent of triglyceride excess, serves as an important baseline value for assessing response to therapy and can, when compared to the triglyceride value in the cleared sample, characterize the nature of the hyperlipidemia.

those presenting with clinical signs.

Hyperchylomicronemia is confirmed in fasted dogs with lipemic serum, hypertriglyceridemia (in uncleared serum) greater than 500 mg/dl and a positive chylomicron test. Clinical signs are not prerequisite for diagnosis nor for recommending therapeutic intervention. However, therapy in dogs that do not have associated signs is generally reserved for those having fasting hypertriglyceridemia on two consecutive samples two to four weeks apart.

Chylomicrons will normally appear in the serum of dogs and cats within 30 minutes to one hour after ingestion of a meal containing fat. This finding is associated with a transient (i.e., six to 12 hours) increase in serum triglycerides after which triglyceride levels rapidly return to baseline values. Physiologic hyperlipidemia is easily excluded from consideration if the patient is known to have fasted throughout the 12-hour period before blood collection. In normal, postprandial animals, serum turbidity is associated with a modest elevation of serum triglycerides (from 150 to 400 mg/dl) that typically returns to normal within 10 hours.

Lipoprotein Electrophoresis

Lipoprotein electrophoresis (LPE) has been used as a means of characterizing abnormalities in lipid metabolism (Ford, 1993; Armstrong and Ford, 1989; Whitney, 1992). The value of LPE has been in question in human medicine for several years and is justifiably questioned in veterinary medicine. Compared to the quantitative assays currently available, LPE appears to have limited value in the clinical evaluation of lipid disorders in dogs and cats.

The Chylomicron Test

Knowing that the patient has fasting lipemia provides immediate evidence of hypertriglyceridemia. The lipid disorder may be further characterized by performing a simple, in-hospital test for the presence of chylomicrons. The lipemic serum, separated from red cells, is refrigerated and allowed to stand undisturbed for six to 12 hours. Chylomicrons, if present, will float to the surface of the sample forming an opaque "cream layer" over a clear infranatant (**Figure 28-5**). This finding suggests a disorder of chylomicron metabolism, the most common form of hyperlipidemia in dogs. If the sample remains turbid, but doesn't form a cream layer, retention of very low-density lipoproteins (VLDL), rather than chylomicrons, is suggested. This finding also suggests that the hyperlipidemia is secondary to an underlying disorder. In some dogs, particularly poorly regulated diabetics, a cream layer may form over turbid, lipemic serum suggesting retention of chylomicrons and VLDL (Armstrong and Ford, 1989; Chapman, 1980).

Risk Factors

Familial (primary) hyperchylomicronemia in cats has been reported as an autosomal recessive trait limited to certain lines of cats. The trait is thought to be present in mixed-breed cats throughout much of the world; therefore, clinically affected cats appear sporadically. Certain dog breeds, most notably miniature schnauzers, are also at increased risk of clinical illness associated with hypertriglyceridemia characterized by the inability to degrade chylomicrons. Though not definitively proven, familial traits are thought to cause these disorders. Results of a limited survey of healthy adult dogs suggested that primary hypercholesterolemia might occur within some families of Doberman pinschers, rottweilers,[a] Shetland sheepdogs (Sato et al, 2000), rough collies (Jeusette et al, 2004) and briards (Watson et al, 1993).

Secondary risk factors (i.e., particularly endocrine disorders, certain drugs and possibly certain diets leading to hyperlipidemia) are known to occur but have not been well studied. For example, profound fasting hypertriglyceridemia occurs inconsistently in dogs with unregulated diabetes mellitus. Clinical signs associated with excess triglyceride concentrations typically include vomiting, diarrhea and abdominal discomfort. Approximately 30% of untreated hypothyroid dogs and from 25 to 30% of untreated dogs with pituitary-dependent hyperadrenocorticism have excess serum cholesterol concentrations. However, the relationship between clinical signs, if any, and the hyperlipidemia has not been established.

Obesity is known to cause abnormalities of lipid metabolism in people. Experimentally induced chronic obesity in otherwise normal dogs fed a complete and balanced maintenance food resulted in significantly higher concentrations of cholesterol in total plasma (+41%) and in VLDL (+125%), HDL (+45%) and low-density lipoprotein (LDL) (+58%) fractions and significantly higher concentrations of triglycerides in total plasma (+75%) and in the VLDL (+118%). When switched to a low-energy, high-fiber diet that resulted in overall decreased energy intake, plasma lipid values decreased (Jeusette et al, 2005).

In some animals, drugs are known to either decrease lipoprotein degradation or increase lipoprotein production, thereby causing hyperlipidemia. For example, dogs receiving long-term phenobarbital therapy for regulation of idiopathic epilepsy may develop hypercholesterolemia. The clinical significance is unknown and may, in fact, be related to thyroid-hormone production or activity. Cats receiving megestrol acetate may secondarily develop diabetes mellitus, which may culminate in altered lipoprotein lipase activity and hyperchylomicronemia.

Etiopathogenesis

Normal Lipid Metabolism

LIPOPROTEINS

Cholesterol and triglycerides are hydrophobic molecules; therefore, they cannot circulate in the aqueous milieu of blood without being incorporated into complex, spherical macromolecules called lipoproteins (Brown and Goldstein, 1987; Chapman, 1980; Schaefer and Levy, 1985; Weinberg, 1987; Watson and Barrie, 1993). The water-soluble outer coat of the lipoprotein is comprised of phospholipids, nonesterified (free) cholesterol and several unique proteins called apolipoproteins (**Figure 28-6**). Cholesterol, in the form of cholesterol esters, and triglycerides are carried within the nonpolar core of spherical lipoprotein macromolecules. Abnormally high concentra-

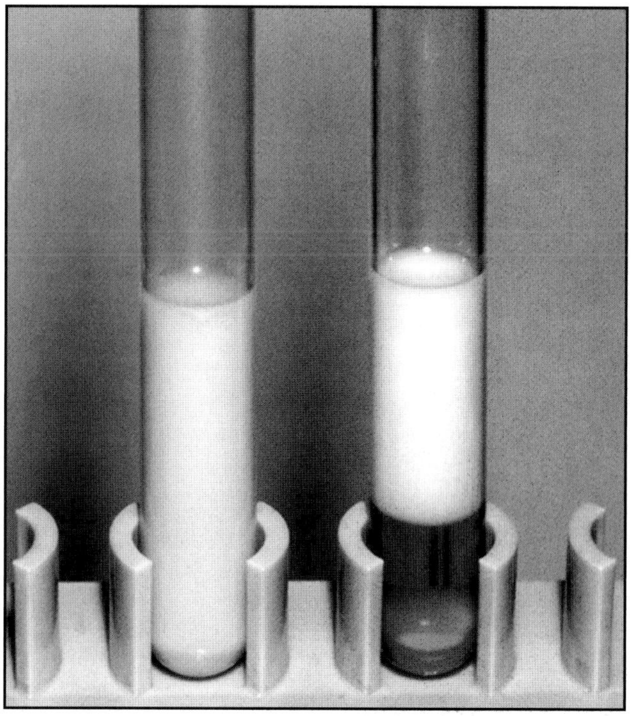

Figure 28-5. The positive chylomicron test. The lactescent serum in both tubes was obtained from a dog with hypertriglyceridemia. The sample on the left is the serum immediately after separation from the red blood cells whereas the sample on the right was allowed to stand undisturbed for 10 hours. The so-called "cream layer" is comprised of triglyceride-rich chylomicrons. (Reprinted with permission from Ford RB. Canine hyperlipidemia. In: Ettinger SJ, Feldman EC, eds. Textbook of Veterinary Internal Medicine, 4th ed. Philadelphia, PA: WB Saunders Co, 1995; 1417.)

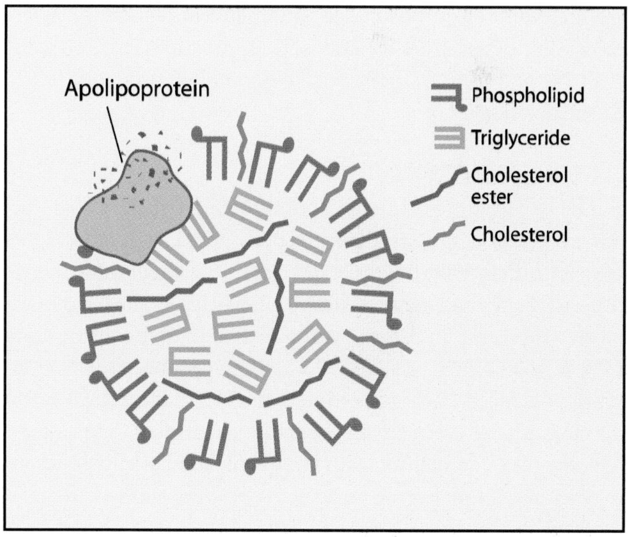

Figure 28-6. Diagram illustrating the composition and structure of lipoproteins. Cholesterol and triglycerides comprise much of the lipoprotein core and are present in varying proportions. (Adapted from Brody T, ed. Nutritional Biochemistry. New York, NY: Academic Press Inc, 1994; 276.)

tions of cholesterol or triglycerides, as measured in routine biochemical assays, actually reflect increased synthesis or decreased degradation of lipoproteins.

APOLIPOPROTEINS

It is well recognized that the apolipoproteins (commonly referred to as apoproteins), contained within the outer coat of lipoproteins, bind to specific enzymes or transport proteins on cell membranes (Brown and Goldstein, 1987; Chapman, 1980; Naito, 1986). Thus, they are responsible for directing the lipoprotein to various sites of metabolism. Several apoproteins have been recognized in dogs and cats. Abnormalities or deficiencies in specific apoproteins are likely to be responsible for altered lipoprotein metabolism that culminates in hyperlipidemia.

Apoprotein C-II (also called apo C-II) (**Figure 28-6**) activates lipoprotein lipase and is very much involved in triglyceride metabolism during the postprandial period. An inherited deficiency in apo C-II is one of the proposed mechanisms responsible for hyperchylomicronemia in dogs.

Classes of Lipoproteins

Four major lipoprotein classes in dogs and cats can be separated by preparative nonionic precipitation and ultracentrifugation: 1) chylomicrons, 2) VLDL, 3) LDL and 4) HDL (Mahley et al, 1974; Armstrong and Ford, 1989; Barrie et al, 1993). A comprehensive lipoprotein profile consists of determining the concentration (mg/dl) of triglycerides and cholesterol in each lipoprotein class. Through lipoprotein profiling, it is possible to categorize hyperlipidemic patients according to lipoprotein phenotype, facilitate diagnosis of primary and secondary lipid disorders and even prescribe therapy. Unfortunately, uniform standards for performing lipoprotein profiles are not commercially available. Alternatively, laboratory determinations of total cholesterol and triglycerides are routinely available and can be used to make good diagnostic and therapeutic decisions.

CHYLOMICRONS

The largest and least dense lipoprotein particles are chylomicrons. These large, triglyceride-rich lipoprotein complexes transport dietary fat (triglycerides) from the small intestine via the lymphatics and general circulation to various sites of metabolism. Appearing in plasma within one hour after consumption of a fat-containing meal, chylomicrons can be visually confirmed as turbid or cloudy serum, a finding that corresponds to a transient (i.e., six to 12 hours postprandial), physiologic hypertriglyceridemia. A cream layer comprised of chylomicrons may form over a clear infranatant if serum is allowed to stand undisturbed for six to 10 hours.

In dogs, and probably cats, only about 10% of the lipid contained in chylomicrons is cholesterol (cholesterol ester). After a meal, hypertriglyceridemia is associated with transient increases in serum cholesterol that may exceed the normal reference range.

Chylomicrons transport fat to the capillaries of adipose tissue and skeletal muscle where they are exposed to the enzyme lipoprotein lipase. The enzyme, once activated by apo C-II, hydrolyzes triglycerides into glycerol and free fatty acids. What remains of the chylomicron is a remnant particle, rich in cholesteryl esters, that subsequently delivers cholesterol to the liver (Schaefer and Levy, 1985; Weinberg, 1987; Gotto, 1988; Eckel, 1989). Chylomicron hydrolysis is normally complete within six to 12 hours following a meal, after which the plasma will again become clear. Fasting hyperchylomicronemia is an abnormal condition resulting from decreased clearance of chylomicrons in the circulation. It is recognized in dogs, cats and people. Although clinical manifestations recognized in dogs are quite different from those in cats, hyperchylomicronemia is the most common lipid disorder recognized in companion animals.

VERY LOW-DENSITY LIPOPROTEINS

Produced in the liver and containing a predominance of triglycerides, VLDL are transported to tissue capillaries where they are catabolized by lipoprotein lipase in the same manner as chylomicrons (Brown and Goldstein, 1987; Eckel, 1989). Retention of VLDL, and the resulting hypertriglyceridemia, occurs frequently in dogs with insulin-dependent diabetes mellitus. Although serum turbidity is manifest in the fasted patient, a cream layer will not separate when the sample is left undisturbed, even when refrigerated.

LOW-DENSITY LIPOPROTEINS

Like VLDL, LDL is responsible for transporting endogenously synthesized lipids (especially cholesterol) from the liver to target tissues. Subsequent to the hydrolysis of VLDL and the removal of triglycerides from its core, a short-lived intermediate-density lipoprotein is ultimately processed by hepatic lipase to form LDL. Delivery of LDL to peripheral tissues is facilitated by the interaction of the structural protein of LDL with a specific receptor, called the LDL receptor. In people, approximately 70% of total cholesterol is carried within LDL, which is sometimes referred to as the atherogenic lipoprotein (Mahley et al, 1974). However, most cholesterol in dogs and cats is carried on HDL.

HIGH-DENSITY LIPOPROTEINS

Newly formed HDL, secreted by the liver and the intestine, binds with unesterified cholesterol released from peripheral tissues during normal cellular turnover (Brown and Goldstein, 1987; Barrie et al, 1993; Gotto, 1988; Eckel, 1989). The conversion process from nascent HDL to mature, spherical HDL particles is mediated by the enzyme lecithin-cholesterol acyltransferase (LCAT) (Brown and Goldstein, 1987; Gotto, 1988). As members of the antiatherogenic lipoprotein family, HDL is recognized for its ability to remove excess cholesterol from tissues and transport it to the liver.

A number of subgroups of HDL have been recognized in people (HDL_2 and HDL_3) (Brown and Goldstein, 1987) and dogs (HDL_1 and HDL_2) (Mahley et al, 1974; Rogers et al, 1975, 1975a). In both dogs and cats, a large HDL molecule (HDL_1) is formed as HDL acquires free cholesterol and expands under the influence of LCAT. However, the actual role of HDL subgroups in predicting or diagnosing disease in animals has not been defined. Because commercial laboratories do not routinely isolate HDL subgroups, subgroup analyses in veterinary medicine have not been found to have immediate application in clinical practice.

Classification of Hyperlipidemic States

Hyperlipidemic states can be classified as postprandial, familial or acquired. Familial hyperlipidemia, also called primary hyperlipidemia, refers to those defects in lipoprotein metabolism that are known or suspected to be inherited. Fasting lipemia is frequently recognized in miniature schnauzers and is possibly linked to a familial defect in chylomicron metabolism. Feline hyperchylomicronemia is the only hyperlipidemic state proven to be familial (Jones and Watson, 1995; Jones et al, 1983; Jones, 1993, 1995).

Acquired hyperlipidemia, also called secondary hyperlipidemia, refers to an excess concentration of lipid in blood resulting from an underlying disease in which normal lipoprotein metabolism is markedly altered. Several endocrine diseases alter lipid metabolism leading to secondary hyperlipidemia. For example, insulin-deficient states alter carbohydrate and lipid metabolism. Animals with insulin-dependent diabetes mellitus may have either hypertriglyceridemia or hypercholesterolemia. Hyperadrenocorticism, renal disease and hypothyroidism are variably associated with secondary hyperlipidemia (Ford, 1996; DeBowes, 1987; Whitney, 1992; Barrie et al, 1993; Rogers, 1977; Zerbe, 1986).

In clinical practice, it is not unusual to encounter a patient with both primary and secondary hyperlipidemia. A miniature schnauzer presented with diabetes mellitus is likely to have extreme elevations in serum triglycerides and lactescent serum. From the clinician's perspective, hyperlipidemia, whether primary or secondary, can be associated with undesirable clinical effects. The ability to recognize the signs associated with hyperlipidemia and to make appropriate dietary or therapeutic recommendations becomes fundamental to the management of these cases.

Postprandial Hyperlipidemia

Triglycerides are the predominant dietary fat in pet food. Subsequent to consuming a meal, dogs and cats will experience transient, physiologic hyperlipidemia characterized by increased triglyceride concentration (circulating chylomicrons) and, depending on the amount of fat consumed, serum turbidity (lipemia). However, postprandial hyperlipidemia does not necessarily imply that a disorder of lipid or lipoprotein metabolism exists. In normal dogs and cats, postprandial hyperlipidemia normally persists from six to 12 hours after a meal. Even when a high-fat food is consumed, serum triglyceride levels are not expected to exceed 500 mg/dl in normal animals. In dogs and cats, hyperlipidemia associated with serum triglyceride levels greater than 1,000 mg/dl, whether fasted or not, is likely to result from an underlying disorder of lipid metabolism (Ford, 1996). Because chylomicrons carry only a fraction of circulating cholesterol, consumption of a meal has little impact on cholesterol during the six- to 12-hour postprandial period.

Postprandial hyperlipidemia, although physiologic, must be distinguished from intrinsic causes (primary or secondary). Confirming that a hyperlipidemic patient has fasted for 10 to 12 hours before collection of blood effectively excludes a recent meal as the cause for increased blood lipids and, therefore, justifies further evaluation in an attempt to determine the source of the hyperlipidemic state.

Canine Familial Hyperchylomicronemia

Hypertriglyceridemia, particularly that associated with retention of chylomicrons, is the most prevalent lipid disorder recognized in dogs and cats and is associated with the greatest health risk (Ford, 1993, 1995). In dogs, the precise mechanism has not been elucidated; however, this disorder of lipoprotein metabolism is believed to be caused by either the lack of lipoprotein lipase activity or the absence of apo C-II (Brown and Goldstein, 1987; Schaefer and Levy, 1985; Gotto, 1988; Zerbe, 1986). Several reports have been published suggesting that miniature schnauzers are predisposed to primary or familial hyperlipidemia (Ford, 1993, 1995, 1996; Rogers et al, 1975; Rogers, 1975a). Although it is not definitively known that hyperlipidemia is an inherited disorder of miniature schnauzers, there appears to be a higher than expected prevalence of hypertriglyceridemia in the breed (Ford, 1993).[a] Several other purebred and mixed-breed dogs have been identified as having fasting hyperchylomicronemia with significant clinical illness, but have no detectable underlying disease.

Canine Idiopathic Hypercholesterolemia

Results of a limited survey of healthy, adult dogs suggested that primary hypercholesterolemia might occur within some families of Doberman pinschers and rottweilers (Armstrong and Ford, 1989). A relationship between the presence of peripheral corneal dystrophy, regarded by some ophthalmologists as containing cholesterol, and excess serum cholesterol concentration (>300 mg/dl) is of noteworthy interest. Lipoprotein profiles of affected dogs demonstrate elevations of LDL-cholesterol.[a] To date, no studies have demonstrated whether or not administration of cholesterol lowering drugs (e.g., fibrates, statins) would either decrease the cholesterol concentration of hypercholesterolemic dogs or cause regression of the corneal dystrophy. Dietary management with a low-fat veterinary therapeutic food was successful in treatment of bilateral lipid keratopathy in one dog (Linton et al, 1994). In a family of rough collies, treatment with a low-fat, energy-restricted food had no effect on serum total cholesterol or corneal lipidosis. The addition of short-chain fructooligosaccharides resulted in regression of corneal lipidosis, but had a variable and transient effect on total serum cholesterol (Jeusette et al, 2004).

Occasionally, extreme elevations of cholesterol will be discovered incidentally in healthy, adult dogs with normal triglyceride values. The clinician is justified in evaluating the patient for evidence of an underlying disorder, such as diabetes mellitus or hyperadrenocorticism. However, in some dogs, hypercholesterolemia cannot be explained. Unless clear evidence of underlying disease exists, treatment specifically intended to lower serum cholesterol does not appear warranted.

Table 28-2. Key nutritional factors for hyperlipidemia.

Disorder	Factor	Dietary recommendations
Hyperlipidemia	Triglycerides	Feed a food that reduces serum triglycerides Restrict dietary fat (<12% dry matter [DM]) Feed a food that reduces serum triglycerides and binds cholesterol and bile acids Increase dietary fiber: Dogs: ≥10% DM Cats: ≥7% DM Add lipid-reducing drugs (fibrates) if dietary management alone is unsuccessful in controlling hyperlipidemia

Feline Inherited Hyperchylomicronemia

A primary, genetic disorder of young cats was found to alter chylomicron metabolism (Jones et al, 1983). Cats that had inherited this disorder developed a form of hyperlipidemia similar to that reported to occur in miniature schnauzers.

Secondary Disorders of Lipid Metabolism

Considering the prevalence of metabolic diseases that affect lipid metabolism, it is possible that secondary hyperlipidemia affects more animals than primary hyperlipidemia. Several endocrine diseases, as well as renal and hepatic diseases, variably alter lipoprotein metabolism resulting in either hypertriglyceridemia or hypercholesterolemia.

DIABETES MELLITUS

Hyperlipidemia secondary to diabetes mellitus in dogs and cats may be characterized by hypertriglyceridemia and moderate hypercholesterolemia (Ford, 1996; Armstrong and Ford, 1989; Barrie et al, 1993). In insulin-deficient states, clearance of chylomicrons is impaired due to insufficient activation of lipoprotein lipase in vascular endothelial cells by insulin (Brown and Goldstein, 1987). Examination of lipid profiles of diabetic dogs reveals lipemia, an increase in chylomicrons and VLDL and a corresponding increase in triglyceride concentration. In some diabetic dogs, excess serum cholesterol concentrations will be present independent of hypertriglyceridemia. In one study, diabetic dogs did not have cholesterol levels significantly different from those of a control population (Barrie et al, 1993). LDL-cholesterol, on the other hand, was increased presumably as a result of increased LDL synthesis. The clinical significance of this finding is unknown.

Although a relationship between the quality of glucose regulation and serum triglyceride levels has been recognized in people, it is unknown whether a similar relationship exists in dogs and cats. Lipemia retinalis in dogs and cutaneous xanthomatosis in cats are associated clinical findings that may be apparent among insulin-dependent diabetics, particularly those with severe hypertriglyceridemia. The hyperlipidemia associated with diabetes mellitus usually improves or resolves as glycemic control is achieved.

Diabetic dogs with excess serum triglyceride concentrations appear to be at risk for developing acute pancreatitis or pseudopancreatitis. Dietary fat restriction can be expected to lower the serum triglyceride concentration and may facilitate glycemic regulation in dogs receiving insulin.

PROTEIN-LOSING NEPHROPATHY

Hyperlipidemia, characterized by increased serum cholesterol or triglyceride levels, may be detected in patients with proteinuria due to glomerulonephritis or amyloidosis. An inverse relationship between elevated blood lipids/lipoproteins and decreased plasma albumin concentration has been reported to occur in patients with nephrotic syndrome. The actual pathogenesis whereby the hyperlipidemia develops is complex and appears to be due to a combination of factors involving altered metabolism of lipoproteins (Bernard, 1982). Hypercholesterolemia occurs inconsistently in dogs with heavy proteinuria. The lipoprotein profile of dogs and cats with nephrotic syndrome has not yet been characterized. The influence of hyperlipidemia on morbidity and mortality in nephrotic syndrome is unknown.

HYPERADRENOCORTICISM

Hypercholesterolemia has been recognized in dogs with hyperadrenocorticism (Cushing's syndrome) without concomitant diabetes mellitus (Armstrong and Ford, 1989; DeBowes, 1987; Barrie et al, 1993). Affected dogs have clear serum, increased plasma cholesterol and LDL-cholesterol levels, but no discrete clinical signs specifically attributable to excess cholesterol. In a limited study of adult dogs confirmed to have hyperadrenocorticism, only 30% were hypercholesterolemic.[a] There appears to be little diagnostic value to performing lipid determinations in dogs suspected of having endogenous cortisol excess. However, monitoring changes in a given patient's cholesterol profile may have prognostic value in dogs undergoing treatment.

HYPOTHYROIDISM

Hypercholesterolemia is present in up to two-thirds of hypothyroid dogs and is believed to result from impaired LDL clearance from the general circulation. It has been suggested that an absolute triiodothyronine deficiency may lead to an increased hepatic cholesterol pool. In turn, LDL-receptor activity is down regulated preventing excess sterol accumulation in the liver (Barrie et al, 1993). Atherosclerotic-type arterial lesions have occasionally been reported (DeBowes, 1987). This finding has led to the suggestion that cholesterol be included in an initial diagnostic screening for hypothyroidism. However, superior laboratory tests are available for evaluating thyroid disease in cats and dogs and should be considered before serum cholesterol evaluation. Therapy should be directed towards correcting the thyroid-hormone deficiency. Although hypothyroid people may experience decreased cholesterol levels after thyroid-replacement therapy is started, there is no apparent value in monitoring cholesterol in affected dogs.

Table 28-3. Selected commercial foods used in dogs with hyperlipidemia compared to recommended levels of key nutritional factors.*

Dry foods	Energy density (kcal/cup)**	Fat (%)	Crude fiber (%)
Recommended levels	-	**<12**	**≥10**
Hill's Prescription Diet r/d Canine	242	8.2	13.5
Hill's Prescription Diet r/d with Chicken Canine	241	8.8	13.6
Iams Veterinary Formula Weight Loss/Restricted Calorie	217	9.1	2.4
Purina Veterinary Diets EN GastroENteric Formula	397	12.6	1.5
Purina Veterinary Diets HA HypoAllergenic Formula	311	10.5	1.6
Purina Veterinary Diets OM Overweight Management Formula	266	7.2	10.3
Royal Canin Veterinary Diets Digestive Low Fat LF	226	6.6	2.3
Moist foods	**Energy density (kcal/can)****	**Fat (%)**	**Crude fiber (%)**
Recommended levels	-	**<12**	**≥10**
Hill's Prescription Diet r/d Canine	257 (12.3-oz. can)	8.6	21.2
Iams Veterinary Formula Weight Loss/Restricted Calorie	397 (14-oz. can)	14.9	3.2
Purina Veterinary Diets EN GastroENteric Formula	423 (12.5-oz. can)	13.8	0.9
Purina Veterinary Diets OM Overweight Management Formula	189 (12.5-oz. can)	8.4	19.2
Royal Canin Veterinary Diets Digestive Low Fat LF	442 (13.6-oz. can)	6.9	3.0

*From manufacturers' published information; all values expressed on a dry matter basis unless otherwise stated.
**Energy density values are listed on an as fed basis and are useful for determining the amount to feed (the amount to feed = the daily energy requirement ÷ the energy density [kcal/cup or can]); cup = 8-oz. measuring cup. To convert to kJ, multiply kcal by 4.184.

Key Nutritional Factors

Fat

Chylomicrons are exclusively of dietary origin; therefore, the amount and type of dietary fat is of primary importance. Foods containing less than 12% dry matter (DM) fat are most commonly recommended (**Table 28-2**).

Marine fish oils are rich in omega-3 (n-3) fatty acids, which effectively decrease production of triglyceride-rich VLDL. Marine fish oils have been recommended as the first line of medical treatment for idiopathic hypertriglyceridemia in dogs. Suggested doses range from 10 to 30 mg/kg to 200 mg/kg body weight. Experience with marine fish oils is limited and most reported successes are based on anecdotal reports.

Fiber

Many low-fat foods also have increased levels of dietary fiber. The contribution of fiber in low-fat foods and fiber's ability to reduce serum lipids is unclear. At this time, no studies have been done in animals to evaluate the effects of dietary fiber type or amount on reducing serum triglyceride levels. Multiple studies in people have shown that dietary fiber, regardless of type or amount, has no significant effect on serum triglyceride levels. Increasing dietary fiber, however, can lower serum cholesterol levels. Furthermore, primarily soluble fibers of differing types have been evaluated. Psyllium, oat bran, guar gum and pectin are a few that effectively reduce cholesterol in people. Reports have shown cholesterol reductions with fiber range from 3 to 10%, depending on fiber type and amount (Hunninghake et al, 1994; Anderson et al, 2000). In some studies, the amount of dietary fiber was high and patient compliance may have been reduced due to increased gastrointestinal side effects (i.e., diarrhea, flatulence, abdominal distention).

Several mechanisms have been suggested for the cholesterol-reducing effects of soluble fiber. Fiber binds dietary cholesterol in the intestine thereby reducing absorption and binds bile acids in the intestine resulting in increased gastrointestinal excretion and increased cholesterol usage to synthesize more bile acids (Marlett, 1997). Some investigators suggest that the cholesterol-lowering effect is due to the substitution of dietary fiber for higher fat content foods (Swain et al, 1990). Studies with prebiotic fibers have shown similar cholesterol-reducing effects (Maki et al, 2003; Behall et al, 2004). Similar effects may occur in animals. Short-chain fructooligosaccharides are reportedly effective in reducing serum cholesterol concentrations and treating corneal lipidosis (Diez et al, 2000); however, when used to treat long-term corneal lipidosis in a rough collie dog the serum cholesterol-lowering effects were transient although the corneal lipidosis resolved (Jeusette, 2004).

Several low-fat veterinary therapeutic foods that have been used successfully to treat hyperlipemic dogs and cats also include increased levels of dietary fiber. The effect of fiber in low-fat foods on further reduction of serum lipids is unclear. However, responses of hyperlipemic patients to dietary intervention with low-fat, high-fiber foods have been positive, including significant decreases in serum triglycerides (**Case 28-1**) (Jeusette et al, 2005; Linton et al, 1994; Rogers et al, 1975). Therefore, based on the lipid-lowering effects observed clinically when commercial low-fat, high-fiber foods have been used, including knowledge of the fiber content of these foods, fiber levels of at least 10% DM are recommended for dogs and at least 7% are recommended for cats.

FEEDING PLAN

Assess and Select the Food

Long-term dietary management of dogs and cats with lipemia caused by primary hypertriglyceridemia is indicated only after secondary causes of hypertriglyceridemia have been ruled out. Food is the single most important element in managing primary hyperlipidemia, particularly in hypertriglyceridemic patients. **Tables 28-3** and **28-4** list commercially available foods marketed for the management of primary hyperlipidemia for dogs and cats, respectively, and compare their key nutritional

Table 28-4. Selected commercial foods used in cats with hyperlipidemia compared to recommended levels of key nutritional factors.*

Dry foods	Energy density (kcal/cup)**	Fat (%)	Crude fiber (%)
Recommended levels	-	<12	≥7
Hill's Prescription Diet r/d Feline	263	9.3	13.6
Hill's Prescription Diet r/d with Chicken Feline	266	9.8	13.8
Purina Veterinary Diets OM Overweight Management Formula	321	8.5	5.6
Moist foods	**Energy density (kcal/can)****	**Fat (%)**	**Crude fiber (%)**
Recommended levels	-	<12	≥7
Hill's Prescription Diet r/d with Liver & Chicken Feline	114 (5.5-oz. can)	9.2	15.4
Purina Veterinary Diets OM Overweight Management Formula	150 (5.5-oz. can)	14.6	10.2

*From manufacturers' published information; all values expressed on a dry matter basis unless otherwise stated.
**Energy density values are listed on an as fed basis and are useful for determining the amount to feed (the amount to feed = the daily energy requirement ÷ the energy density [kcal/cup or can]); cup = 8-oz. measuring cup. To convert to kJ, multiply kcal by 4.184.

factor content with the recommended levels of key nutritional factors (**Table 28-2**). The patient's current food should be compared to the foods in **Tables 28-3** and **28-4** and a new food selected if the key nutritional factors in the patient's current food do not closely match the levels recommended in the tables. Selection of a new food should be made on the basis of the closest match to the recommended key nutritional factors.

The approach to treating any patient with secondary hypertriglyceridemia includes managing the underlying disease; an appropriate response to the medication should include resolution of the lipemia. Concurrent disorders may also influence the key nutritional factors and lead to other food and feeding method choices. Depending on their underlying disease, dogs and cats with secondary hyperlipidemia may benefit from foods listed in **Tables 28-3** and **28-4**. However, there may be other nutritional factors to consider in some diseases, for example, key nutritional factors important for patients with protein-losing nephropathy should also be considered when making food selections (Chapter 37).

Assess and Determine the Feeding Method

The method of feeding is often not altered in the nutritional management of lipid disorders. If a new food is fed, the amount to feed can be determined from the product label or other supporting materials. The food dosage may need to be changed if the fat level in the food is reduced, because the caloric density of the new food will probably differ from that of the previous food (i.e., the caloric density will usually be lower). The patient's body condition score (BCS) and body weight should be recorded before initiating dietary management because these become important parameters to monitor during reassessment. If body weight and BCS are optimal initially, the dosage of the new food should reflect the amount of energy (kcal or kJ) consumed by the animal previously.

Dogs and cats with hyperlipidemia due to diabetes mellitus may benefit from a feeding protocol that matches their insulin therapy (Chapter 29). Good compliance is necessary for effective clinical nutrition. Enabling compliance includes limiting access to other foods and knowing who feeds the animal. If the dog or cat comes from a household with multiple pets, access to other pets' food should be denied.

MEDICAL MANAGEMENT OF SECONDARY HYPERLIPIDEMIC STATES

Hyperlipidemic states associated with a primary underlying disorder (e.g., diabetes mellitus or hyperadrenocorticism) can cause clinical signs in dogs and cats indistinguishable from those caused by primary hyperlipidemic states. Accurate diagnosis and treatment of the underlying disorder should resolve the hyperlipidemia and any associated signs. However, dietary therapy as outlined above should still be implemented. Dogs and cats with clinical signs associated with persistent hyperlipidemia, whether primary or secondary, should benefit from appropriate dietary therapy (**Tables 28-3** and **28-4**) as long as optimal weight is maintained.

REASSESSMENT

The effect of dietary therapy on hyperlipidemic patients is best determined three to four weeks after the feeding plan is initiated. Reassessment includes reviewing the client's assessment of the patient's response, documenting body weight and condition and evaluating the extent outward manifestations (i.e., ocular or cutaneous lesions) have resolved. Laboratory assessment involves: 1) collecting a blood sample from a fasted animal (10 to 12 hours), 2) evaluating the appearance of the serum for lipemia, 3) determining the triglyceride level in uncleared serum and 4) performing a chylomicron test. The veterinary health care team should assess the client's compliance with the outlined feeding plan. Feeding high-fat snacks and treats and access to other pet foods, even infrequently, can markedly increase circulating triglyceride levels in affected patients.

The goals of dietary therapy are to achieve: 1) a clear serum sample, 2) a total triglyceride concentration less than 500 mg/dl, 3) a negative chylomicron test, and, most importantly 4) amelioration or elimination of clinical signs. Amelioration or elimination of clinical signs can be expected within two weeks (dogs with pseudopancreatitis) to as long as three months (cats with cutaneous xanthomata) after initiation of appropriate dietary therapy.

Most dogs and cats with primary hyperlipidemia will experience a marked reduction in serum triglyceride and cholesterol concentrations if appropriate dietary management is employed

Box 28-2. Medical Management of Primary Hyperlipidemia.

Although dietary therapy is recommended as the initial means of managing primary hypertriglyceridemia, up to 10% of dogs with idiopathic hyperlipidemia are unresponsive to dietary fat restriction and may require pharmacologic supplementation. A variety of medical treatments for reducing lipid levels in dogs and cats have been recommended. However, the efficacy and pharmacokinetics of these treatments in animals have not been well researched. Furthermore, cost, dosage and toxicity are factors that must be considered when recommending long-term drug therapy to manage primary hyperlipidemic states.

FIBRATES

Gemfibrozil is the most commonly recommended drug to lower serum triglyceride levels in dogs and cats when dietary management fails. The drug is administered to dogs at doses ranging from 200 mg/day, orally, to 150 to 300 mg every 12 hours. The dosage of gemfibrozil for cats is 7.5 to 10 mg/kg body weight every 12 hours. Side effects in cats and dogs appear to be minimal; however, reports have suggested a long-term cancer risk associated with its use in people.

DIETARY SUPPLEMENTS

Massive doses of nicotinic acid (niacin) have also been recommended for reducing serum cholesterol concentrations in people and thereby reducing the risk of coronary artery disease. There is no known value in using nicotinic acid to manage primary hyperlipidemic states in dogs and cats.

Dietary supplementation with aged garlic extract has beneficial effects on the lipid profile and blood pressure of moderately hypercholesterolemic human patients. The effect of garlic extracts on hyperlipidemic animals has not been investigated.

STATINS

The 3-hydroxy-3-methylglutaryl coenzyme A (HMG CoA) reductase inhibitors, commonly referred to as "statins," effectively reduce hepatic cholesterol synthesis and enhance excretion of LDL-cholesterol from the circulation. Because of their ability to reduce the risk of coronary artery disease, the HMG CoA reductase inhibitors are the preferred class of drug prescribed to manage hypercholesterolemia in people. Although these drugs are generally well tolerated by dogs, the actual therapeutic advantage associated with lowering circulating levels of LDL-cholesterol is unknown. Dogs and cats normally have very low levels of LDL-cholesterol. Specific dosages for dogs and cats have not been reported.

CHOLESTEROL ABSORPTION INHIBITORS

Drugs such as ezetimibe inhibit dietary cholesterol and bile acid cholesterol uptake in the intestine and have been an effective tool for reducing serum cholesterol levels. In people, the use of statin drugs markedly reduces cholesterol production; however, there is a resultant increase in cholesterol uptake from the gastrointestinal tract. Similar compensatory mechanisms have been demonstrated in dogs. Combining statins with drugs that selectively inhibit cholesterol uptake from the digestive tract is more effective than statins alone at lowering serum cholesterol concentrations. Safety and similar synergistic effects have been shown in normal dogs. The application and dosages of these combination drugs in clinical patients have not been evaluated. Because these drugs (especially statins) can have serious side effects, their use is currently not recommended.

BILE ACID SEQUESTRANTS

The bile acid sequestrants, categorized as ion exchange resins, effectively reduce serum cholesterol concentrations through their ability to reduce enterohepatic circulation of bile salts and enhance cholesterol excretion. Cholestyramine has been recommended for dogs with persistent idiopathic hypercholesterolemia at dosages of 1 to 2 g every 12 hours. However, the associated side effects, principally gastrointestinal discomfort and diarrhea, combined with the fact that actually reducing serum cholesterol levels may not resolve clinical signs, limits the clinical value of these drugs.

The Bibliography for **Box 28-2** can be found at www.markmorris.org.

and rigorously followed. A reasonably acceptable goal is slight serum turbidity, a triglyceride concentration less than 1,000 mg/dl and an incomplete cream layer at the top of the sample.

Unless weight loss is desired, the patient's body weight and BCS should be the same as it was before the feeding plan was initiated.

For reasons currently unknown, some patients remain profoundly hyperlipidemic despite excellent owner compliance in feeding an appropriate food. However, these animals should continue to receive the appropriate low-fat food; human table food should not be fed. The patient should be reassessed in one to two months. If a demonstrable reduction in fasting serum triglyceride concentrations still hasn't occurred, drug therapy should be added to the dietary therapy. Drug therapy for patients with primary hypertriglyceridemia has included clofibrate, niacin, gemfibrozil and dietary supplementation with omega-3 fatty acids from fish oils (**Box 28-2**) (Logas et al, 1991; Levy, 1988; Schaefer, 1988; Watson, 1996).

Patients that lose a significant amount of weight (more than 1% of body weight per week) should receive gradually increasing amounts of the recommended food until desired weight can be maintained. In these cases, caloric intake may be inadequate.

ENDNOTE

a. Ford RB. Unpublished observation. April 1994.

REFERENCES

The references for **Chapter 28** can be found at www.markmorris.org.

CASE 28-1

Episodic Diarrhea in a Mixed-Breed Dog

Richard B. Ford, DVM, Dipl. ACVIM (Internal Medicine)
School of Veterinary Medicine
North Carolina State University
Raleigh, North Carolina, USA

Patient Assessment

A seven-year-old, female, mixed-breed dog was initially examined for a four-month history of episodic diarrhea accompanied by lethargy and a decreased appetite. The owner reported that the frequency of the episodes had gradually increased to once weekly over the last two months. Clinical signs would spontaneously resolve within 24 to 48 hours.

The initial physical examination revealed an active, alert dog. Abdominal palpation was unremarkable and well tolerated. The dog weighed 11.8 kg and appeared thin (body condition score 2/5) although the owner had not reported weight loss.

A presumptive diagnosis of dietary intolerance was made and empiric treatment with a veterinary therapeutic food for management of gastrointestinal (GI) disease was initiated. Ten days later the dog was examined for significant lethargy and abdominal discomfort. The owner indicated that the dog had eaten nothing during the past 24 hours but did drink water. Soft feces were noted occasionally. Abdominal palpation was associated with discomfort; however, the source of the abdominal pain could not be localized.

Results of an abdominal radiograph, urinalysis and fecal flotation for intestinal parasites were normal. Blood collected for analysis was profoundly lipemic and moderately hemolyzed. Test results were obtained from a commercial laboratory on the following day. Results of a complete blood count were normal. Abnormal serum biochemistry profile results included hypocalcemia (8.5 mg/dl, normal 9.2 to 11.2). Serum cholesterol (278 mg/dl) and triglyceride (96 mg/dl) concentrations were normal.

Assess the Food and Feeding Method

The dog was normally fed a combination of dry and moist commercial grocery store brand foods with occasional snacks. The food was offered once daily. The dog's diet had been consistent for several years until the change 10 days ago to a moist veterinary therapeutic food (Prescription Diet i/d Canine[a]) designed for the management of GI disorders.

Questions

1. Why is the serum triglyceride concentration normal in a patient with lipemia?
2. What is the tentative diagnosis in this patient?
3. What is an appropriate feeding plan (food and feeding method) for this dog?

Answers and Discussion

1. In an attempt to avoid lipid interference with other biochemical assays, many commercial laboratories will use ultracentrifugation to clear chylomicrons before performing any tests on a lipemic serum sample. This process removes excess triglycerides before testing. Thus, the triglyceride concentration reported by the laboratory may be normal. Simply observing a lipemic sample in a fasted (six to 12 hours) animal is sufficient clinical evidence to document hypertriglyceridemia. The low serum calcium concentration was probably an artifact due to interference from the lipemia.
2. The predominant cause of hyperlipidemia in dogs is excess concentrations of triglyceride-rich chylomicrons. Thus, canine hyperchylomicronemia (hypertriglyceridemia) is the most likely diagnosis, after the clinician has observed the serum sample and confirmed the presence of lipemia (i.e., a cream layer denoting hyperchylomicronemia) or measured triglyceride levels (i.e., levels exceeding 500 mg/dl). Fasting lipemia can be a significant clinical problem associated with episodic diarrhea, inappetence, abdominal discomfort and occasional vomiting. The collective term to describe this syndrome is "pseudopancreatitis." The rapid worsening of clinical signs justifies expanding the differential diagnosis to include pancreatitis, hypoadrenocorticism, neoplasia and primary intestinal disease (e.g., inflammatory bowel disease, etc.). Additional endocrine testing may be indicated to rule out secondary causes of hyperlipidemia.
3. For any patient with fasting hyperlipidemia, regardless of the cause, food with a fat content less than 12% dry matter is recommended. Foods designed for empiric management of GI disorders often have a fat content that exceeds this recommendation. Multiple small meals rather than one large meal per day may be helpful in patients with GI signs.

Progress Notes

After fasting hypertriglyceridemia (hyperchylomicronemia) was confirmed, the initial treatment prescribed was limited to dietary intervention with low-fat, high-fiber food. Prescription Diet w/d Canine[a] dry was recommended because of its palatability, low-fat content (approximately 9.0% dry matter [DM]) and high-fiber level (17.6% DM). The owner was advised that: 1) dietary management is the most reasonable, economical means of controlling this potentially serious condition, 2) dietary fat restriction would be a life-long requirement, if treatment were successful and 3) even a single high-fat meal (e.g., eating from the trash) could acutely exacerbate clinical signs and cause pancreatitis.

The patient was reexamined after consuming the veterinary therapeutic food for three weeks to assess dietary compliance and serum triglyceride levels. A fasting (overnight) blood sample was collected. The serum triglyceride (uncleared) concentration was determined and compared to that obtained during the initial examination (**Table 1**).

Results suggested excellent dietary control of the hyperlipidemic state and good dietary compliance. Specific drug intervention was deemed unnecessary at the time the patient was rechecked. However, the owner was advised that although the risk of serious illness (pancreatitis) had been markedly reduced, follow-up examinations twice yearly, including fasting triglyceride measurements, would be a prudent course to follow.

Endnote

a. Hill's Pet Nutrition, Inc., Topeka, KS, USA.

Bibliography

Ford RB. Canine hyperlipidemia. In: Ettinger SJ, Feldman EC, eds. Textbook of Veterinary Internal Medicine, 4th ed. Philadelphia, PA: WB Saunders Co, 1995; 1414-1419.

Table 1. Serum triglyceride levels before and after three weeks of treatment with a low-fat, high-fiber veterinary therapeutic food.*

Initial level	2,350 mg/dl**
Three-week level	477 mg/dl**

*Prescription Diet w/d Canine. Hill's Pet Nutrition, Inc., Topeka, KS, USA.
**Uncleared specimen.

Chapter 29

Endocrine Disorders

Steven C. Zicker
Richard W. Nelson
Claudia A. Kirk
Karen J. Wedekind

"Truth is what stands the test of experience."
Albert Einstein

INTRODUCTION

The interactions of carbohydrate and lipid metabolism and their control by hormones comprise the basis for metabolic homeostasis in health and disease. Diagnosing and treating these disorders requires a working knowledge of cellular changes and the role of hormones in controlling nutrient flux. This chapter covers the nutritional aspects of diabetes mellitus, hyperthyroidism and hypothyroidism.

DIABETES MELLITUS

Diabetes mellitus describes an alteration in cellular transport and metabolism of glucose, lipids and amino acids wherein insulin-dependent tissues (e.g., skeletal and cardiac muscle, adipose tissue) either never receive the signal or fail to properly interpret the signal. Altered metabolism results in either an absolute or relative deficit in insulin secretion by pancreatic beta cells as perceived by insulin-dependent cells in the periphery of the body. Causative pathophysiologic mechanisms include: 1) insufficient insulin release from the pancreas (e.g., glucose toxicity, beta-cell degeneration or islet amyloid deposition), 2) decreased number of functional insulin receptors (down regulation) and 3) problems with transduction of the insulin signal following binding of insulin to insulin receptors (**Table 29-1**) (Feldman and Nelson, 2004, 2004a).

Classification

In people, diabetes mellitus is usually classified as: 1) type I, 2) type II, 3) secondary (type S), 4) impaired glucose tolerance (e.g., gestational diabetes) (type IGT) and 5) previous abnormality of glucose tolerance (type PrevAGT) based on the pathophysiologic mechanisms and pathogenic alterations affecting beta cells (Stogdale, 1986). Type I diabetes is characterized by a combination of genetic susceptibility and immunologic destruction of beta cells, with progressive and eventually complete insulin insufficiency. The presence of circulating autoantibodies against insulin, beta cells and/or glutamic acid decarboxylase usually precedes the development of hyperglycemia or clinical signs.

Type II diabetes mellitus is characterized by insulin resistance and "dysfunctional" beta cells; defects thought to be genetic in origin and which are evident for a decade or longer before hyperglycemia and clinical signs of diabetes develop. Deleterious effects of type II diabetes mellitus can be accentuated by environmental factors such as obesity (Warram et al, 1990; Martin et al, 1992). Type II diabetes mellitus has been referred to as a relative insulin deficiency because the amount of insulin actually secreted by the beta cells may be increased, decreased or normal. The concentration of glucose in serum is thus determined by the relative response of peripheral tissues to the secreted insulin, which is usually blunted.

People with type I diabetes depend on insulin to control the disease (i.e., insulin-dependent diabetes mellitus [IDDM]),

Table 29-1. Possible causes of diabetes mellitus in dogs and cats.*

Concurrent illness (hyperadrenocorticism, acromegaly)
Drugs (glucocorticoids, progestins)
Genetics
Immune-mediated insulitis
Infection
Islet amyloidosis
Obesity
Pancreatitis

*Adapted from Feldman EC, Nelson RW, eds. Diabetes mellitus. Canine and Feline Endocrinology and Reproduction, 3rd ed. Philadelphia, PA: WB Saunders Co, 2004; 489.

Table 29-2. Differential diagnosis for hyperglycemia in dogs and cats.*

Acromegaly
Diabetes mellitus
Diestrus (bitch)
Drug therapy (glucocorticoids, progestogens, megestrol acetate)
Exocrine pancreatic insufficiency
Glucose-containing fluids
Hyperadrenocorticism
Hyperthyroidism (cats)
Laboratory error
Pancreatitis
Pheochromocytoma
Renal insufficiency
Stress

*Adapted from Feldman EC, Nelson RW, eds. Diabetes mellitus. Canine and Feline Endocrinology and Reproduction, 3rd ed. Philadelphia, PA: WB Saunders Co, 2004; 493.

whereas control of the diabetic state in people with type II diabetes is usually possible through diet, exercise and oral hypoglycemic drugs. Insulin treatment may be necessary in some type II diabetics if insulin resistance and beta-cell dysfunction are severe. As such, people with type II diabetes mellitus can have IDDM or non-insulin-dependent diabetes mellitus (NIDDM).

Classifying diabetic dogs and cats as type I or type II based on criteria established for people is difficult, in part, because: 1) familial history is rarely available for diabetic dogs and cats, 2) the clinical presentation is usually unhelpful in differentiating type I from type II diabetes, 3) insulin secretagogue tests are not routinely performed and their results may be misleading and 4) autoantibody tests for type I diabetes are not readily available (Nelson et al, 1993; Kirk et al, 1993). It is probably more clinically relevant to classify dogs and cats as insulin-dependent and non-insulin dependent based on their need for insulin.

The overwhelming majority of dogs have IDDM at the time diabetes is diagnosed. Cats are more confusing because islet pathology may be mild to severe and progressive or static; reversible suppression of beta-cell function occurs with chronic hyperglycemia (glucose toxicity), and responsiveness of tissues to insulin varies, often in conjunction with the presence or absence of concurrent inflammatory, infectious, neoplastic or hormonal disorders. These variables affect a cat's need for insulin, insulin dosage and ease of diabetic regulation. Furthermore, these variables may change with time. Cats may have IDDM or NIDDM at the time diabetes is diagnosed. Cats with NIDDM may progress to IDDM with time, cats with apparent IDDM may revert to a non-insulin requiring state after initiation of treatment and cats may have IDDM or NIDDM as severity of insulin resistance and impairment of beta-cell function waxes and wanes.

Patient Assessment

History

Dogs and cats with diabetes mellitus are usually examined because of polydipsia, polyphagia, weight loss and diminished activity. Care should be taken to differentiate between polyphagia from underfeeding compared to polyphagia associated with disease (true polyphagia). Less commonly, complaints of blindness (dogs), rear-limb weakness (cats) and lethargy (dogs and cats) may be identified. If diabetic ketoacidosis (DKA) develops, affected animals are often examined for anorexia, vomiting, diarrhea, weakness and a moribund state. DKA may be precipitated by infection, severe stress, hypokalemia, hypomagnesemia, renal failure, drugs that decrease insulin secretion, drugs that cause insulin resistance or inadequate fluid intake (Nichols and Crenshaw, 1995). Concurrent disease such as pancreatitis and bacterial infection is common in dogs and cats developing DKA and often accentuates the clinical signs of DKA, prompting owners to seek veterinary care. A thorough assessment of the patient is critically important for developing an appropriate management protocol for dogs and cats diagnosed with DKA (Feldman and Nelson, 2004, 2004a; Plotnick and Greco, 1995).

Physical Examination

Body condition scores (BCS) for diabetic dogs and cats range from emaciated (BCS 1/5) to obese (BCS 5/5) depending on the severity and duration of disease. Weight loss, which becomes obvious with time, is a hallmark sign of diabetes mellitus. Other physical findings may include lethargy, unkempt coat (cats), hepatomegaly, cataracts (dogs), rear-limb weakness (cats) and dehydration (Plotnick and Greco, 1995; Feldman and Nelson, 2004, 2004a).

Diagnostic Testing

HEMOGRAMS

Results of complete blood counts are usually within normal ranges in uncomplicated cases of diabetes mellitus. An increase in packed cell volume may be present in dogs and cats with DKA due to decreased extracellular water attributable to osmotic diuresis. Occasionally, increased numbers of Heinz bodies may be noticed in cats with diabetes mellitus. Leukocytosis or shifts of white cell morphology to more immature types may indicate an underlying infectious process that confounds the diagnosis of uncomplicated diabetes mellitus.

SERUM BIOCHEMISTRY PROFILES

The most consistent and requisite feature of diabetes mellitus is persistent fasting hyperglycemia and glucosuria in the absence of other disease processes. Hyperglycemia, however, may be caused by other disease or physiologic states and drugs (**Table 29-2**). A thorough assessment may help identify the underlying cause of hyperglycemia. Repetitive determination of serum glucose concentrations may be required in cats to differentiate diabetes mellitus from stress hyperglycemia. A diagnosis of DKA is established if ketonuria is present with systemic metabolic acidosis.

Other commonly identified abnormalities include increased serum concentrations of cholesterol and triglycerides. Increased serum concentrations of urea nitrogen and creatinine may be present when dehydration becomes severe enough to impair renal diffusion (prerenal azotemia). Electrolyte and acid-base alterations are more common in animals with DKA and include: 1) hyponatremia, 2) hypokalemia, 3) hypocalcemia, 4) hypomagnesemia, 5) hypophosphatemia and 6) hypochloremia. A shift in acid-base balance towards metabolic acidosis with a compensatory respiratory alkalosis may occur.

Increased activity of alanine aminotransferase in serum may be present in cases in which hepatic lipidosis has resulted in hepatocellular damage. Activity of serum alkaline phosphatase may also be increased. Increased serum alkaline phosphatase activity is primarily associated with hepatomegaly and biliary stasis; however, pancreatic inflammation resulting in extrahepatic biliary obstruction may also be present. Less commonly, serum concentrations of bile acids and total bilirubin may be elevated.

Dogs and cats with diabetes mellitus may present with concurrent exocrine pancreatic insufficiency or pancreatitis (Williams and Minnich, 1990). Increased activity of amylase and lipase in serum may indicate pancreatitis; however, the correlation of these two enzyme activities with pancreatitis is poor, especially in cats. Other disease processes may also result in increased activity of these enzymes in serum.

OTHER BIOCHEMICAL TESTS

Determination of insulin concentration in serum is not routinely performed in suspected cases of diabetes mellitus. A reliable radioimmunoassay must be used when measuring serum insulin, especially in cats. Insulin exhibits variance in the primary amino acid sequence between species; therefore, the test methodology must be validated for each species. Serum insulin concentrations, when they are determined, may be high, normal or low. Concentrations of insulin greater than 15 μU/ml in animals not receiving exogenous insulin indicate the presence of functional beta cells. Conversely, concentrations of insulin less than 10 μU/ml do not preclude the possibility of functional beta cells. Serum pancreatic lipase immunoreactivity (increased activity) and trypsin-like immunoreactivity (decreased activity) can help identify pancreatitis and exocrine pancreatic insufficiency, respectively (Chapters 66 and 67).

Serum thyroid-hormone concentrations are usually normal in diabetic dogs and cats. However, both hypothyroidism and hyperthyroidism may be associated with insulin resistance and can occur in conjunction with diabetes mellitus. As such, evaluation of thyroid function may be useful in patients with diabetes mellitus that are difficult to control with insulin and dietary intervention (**Case 29-2**). Care must be exercised in the interpretation of serum thyroxine (T_4) concentrations in sick dogs and cats because concentrations of T_4 may be falsely low in poorly regulated cases of diabetes mellitus. This alteration is presumed to be attributable to the euthyroid sick syndrome (Feldman and Nelson, 2004c).

URINALYSES

Urine specific gravity is typically greater than 1.025 in diabetic dogs and cats. Urine specific gravity less than 1.015 should increase suspicion for concurrent disorders, such as renal insufficiency or hyperadrenocorticism. Glucosuria is a hallmark finding in untreated diabetic dogs and cats. Lack of glucosuria rules out diabetes mellitus as the cause of polydipsia and polyuria. Other common urinalysis findings include ketonuria, proteinuria and changes consistent with urinary tract infection (i.e., bacteriuria and pyuria). Proteinuria may result from either bacterial infection or glomerulopathy secondary to basement membrane damage from the primary disease process.

Risk Factors

Risk factors for development of diabetes mellitus in dogs and cats include genetics, age, sex, obesity and concurrent problems causing insulin resistance. Although diabetes can occur in dogs and cats of any age, gender and breed, the disease is more common in older dogs and cats with a peak prevalence of seven to nine years of age in dogs and nine to 11 years in cats (Panciera et al, 1990; Goossens et al, 1998). Juvenile-onset diabetes occurs in dogs and cats less than one year of age, but is uncommon. In dogs, females are affected about twice as frequently as males, whereas in cats, diabetes occurs predominately in neutered males (Panciera et al, 1990; Goossens et al, 1998). Breeds of dogs at risk for diabetes mellitus include Australian terriers, standard and miniature schnauzers, bichons frisés, spitz, fox terriers, miniature and toy poodles, Samoyeds, Cairn terriers, keeshonds, Maltese, Lhasa apsos and Yorkshire terriers (Guptill, 1999; Hess et al, 2000). There is no apparent breed predisposition in cats; however, Burmese cats may be overrepresented in Australia (Rand et al, 1997).

The presence and severity of insulin resistance is an important variable in the development and successful treatment of diabetes mellitus in dogs and cats. Insulin resistance increases the demand for insulin secretion. A sustained demand for insulin secretion in response to insulin resistance can lead to islet pathology and loss of beta cells. The more severe and chronic the insulin resistance and the more severe the loss of islets, the more likely hyperglycemia will develop. Persistent hyperglycemia can, in turn, suppress function of remaining beta cells, causing hypoinsulinemia, worsening hyperglycemia and further reducing the population of beta cells. Any chronic insulin-resistant disorder can have a deleterious effect on the population and function of beta cells and play a role in the development of NIDDM or IDDM (**Figure 29-1**). Examples include obesity, chronic pancreatitis, acromegaly, hyperadreno-

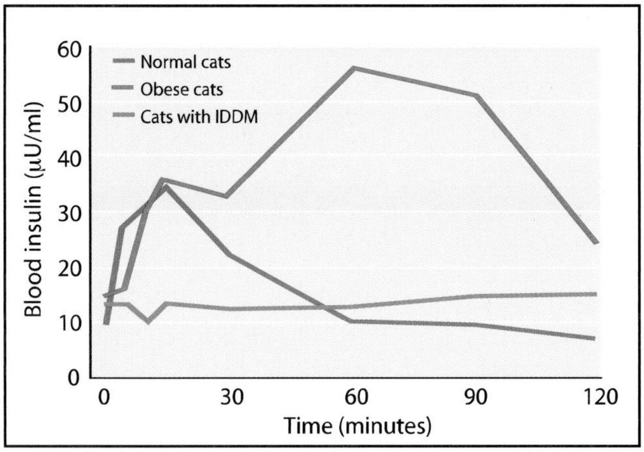

Figure 29-1. Mean blood insulin concentrations following the intravenous injection of 0.5 g glucose/kg body weight in normal cats, extremely obese cats and cats with type I diabetes mellitus. The insulin secretory pattern in obese cats is similar to that of people with NIDDM. (Adapted from Nelson RW. Disorders of the endocrine pancreas. In: Ettinger SJ, ed. Textbook of Veterinary Internal Medicine, 3rd ed. Philadelphia, PA: WB Saunders Co, 1989; 1676.)

corticism and long-term administration of glucocorticoids or progestagens. Obesity-induced carbohydrate intolerance is the classic insulin-resistant disorder affiliated with development of NIDDM in people and increases the risk for diabetes in cats by fourfold (Scarlett, 1997).

Etiopathogenesis

INSULIN PHYSIOLOGY

Insulin is produced in the beta cells of the endocrine pancreas and is released in response to increased concentrations of glucose in plasma. Active insulin is a dipeptide that is linked by disulfide bonds between cysteine amino acid side chains. Insulin is first synthesized as proinsulin in beta cells and is subsequently processed by a cleavage step that produces C-peptide and active insulin (Muench, 1986).

Active insulin released into the bloodstream normally interacts at target tissues via cell surface receptors specific for insulin. Most tissues have insulin receptors but some (e.g., skeletal and cardiac muscle and adipose tissue) depend more on insulin for the acquisition of glucose and amino acids than others, and are classified as insulin-dependent tissues (Harris, 1986; Granner, 1988). For example, brain tissue has insulin receptors, but is quite capable of transporting glucose intracellularly without the help of hormonal stimuli; therefore, it is considered an insulin-independent tissue.

Insulin receptors are membrane glycoproteins composed of two subunits; a larger alpha subunit that extends extracellularly, which is involved in binding the insulin molecule, and a smaller beta subunit that is predominately cytoplasmic, which is responsible for activating the signaling cascade that ultimately leads to increased glucose transport, increased glycogen and lipid synthesis and stimulation of other metabolic pathways (Masharani and Karam, 2001). Because cell membranes are impermeable to glucose, all cells require carrier proteins to transport glucose across the lipid bilayers into the cytosol. At least five glucose transporters have been described, to date, in people, each having a different affinity for glucose. GLUT 1 and GLUT 3 are present in all tissues and mediate basal glucose uptake and neuronal uptake of glucose, respectively. GLUT 2 is the major glucose transporter in beta and hepatic cells. It has a low affinity for glucose, and acts as a transporter during periods of hyperglycemia. GLUT 5 is found on the brush border of human small intestinal cells and is mainly a fructose transporter. GLUT 4 is found intracellularly in insulin-dependent tissues, most notably skeletal muscle and adipose tissue. Activation of the insulin signaling cascade results in movement of GLUT 4 transporters to the cell surface where the transporter facilitates glucose entry into cells (James et al, 1988; Thorens et al, 1990).

DIABETES MELLITUS IN DOGS

The most common clinically recognized form of diabetes mellitus in dogs is IDDM. In our hospital (School of Veterinary Medicine, University of California, Davis), virtually all dogs have IDDM when diabetes mellitus is diagnosed. IDDM is characterized by permanent hypoinsulinemia and an absolute necessity for exogenous insulin to maintain glycemic control. The etiology of IDDM has been poorly characterized in dogs, but is undoubtedly multifactorial and may be similar to human type I diabetes. Genetic predispositions have been suggested by familial associations (Guptill, 1999; Hess et al, 2000). Common histologic abnormalities in dogs include a reduction in the number and size of pancreatic islets, a decrease in the number of beta cells within islets and beta-cell vacuolation and degeneration. In some dogs, an extreme form of the disease may occur, represented by a congenital absolute deficiency of beta cells and pancreatic islet hypoplasia or aplasia. Less severe pancreatic islets and beta-cell changes may predispose adult dogs to diabetes mellitus after exposure to environmental factors, such as insulin-antagonistic diseases and drugs, obesity or pancreatitis. Environmental factors may induce beta-cell degeneration secondary to chronic insulin resistance or may cause release of beta-cell proteins that induce immune-mediated destruction of the islets (Nerup et al, 1994). Studies designed to detect anti-beta-cell autoantibodies in diabetic dogs have been conflicting; they were identified in newly-diagnosed diabetic dogs with IDDM in one study (Hoenig and Dawe, 1992) but not in another (Haines, 1986). Immune-mediated insulitis has also been described in diabetic dogs (Alejandro et al, 1988). Seemingly, autoimmune mechanisms, in conjunction with genetic and environmental factors, may play a role in the initiation and progression of diabetes in dogs.

DIABETES MELLITUS IN CATS

Common histologic abnormalities in cats with diabetes mellitus include islet-specific amyloidosis, beta-cell vacuolation and degeneration and chronic pancreatitis (Goossens et al, 1998). The cause of beta-cell degeneration is unknown. Still, other diabetic cats have reduced numbers of pancreatic islets and/or insulin-containing beta cells based on immunohisto-

Table 29-3. Key nutritional factors for diabetic dogs and cats.*

Factors	Dogs (increased-fiber/ high-carbohydrate food)	Cats (increased-fiber/ high-carbohydrate food)	Cats (low-carbohydrate/ high-protein food)
Water	Fresh, clean water should be available at all times	Fresh, clean water should be available at all times	Fresh, clean water should be available at all times
Digestible carbohydrate	Avoid simple sugars Provide foods with no more than 55% digestible carbohydrate	Avoid simple sugars and starch Provide foods with less than 40% digestible carbohydrate	Avoid simple sugars and starch Provide foods with less than 20% digestible carbohydrate
Fiber	7 to 18%	7 to 18%	–
Fat	<25%	<25%	<25%
Protein	15 to 35% Dogs with renal failure should be fed protein at the low end of the range	28 to 55% Cats with renal failure should be fed protein at the low end of the range	28 to 55% Cats with renal failure should be fed protein at the low end of the range
Food form	Avoid semi-moist foods	Avoid semi-moist foods	Avoid semi-moist foods

*Nutrients expressed on a dry matter basis.

chemical evaluation, suggesting additional mechanisms may be involved in the physiopathology of diabetes mellitus in cats. Although lymphocytic infiltration of islets, in conjunction with islet amyloidosis and vacuolation, has been described in two diabetic cats (Nakayama et al, 1990), this histologic finding is very uncommon. Beta-cell and insulin autoantibodies have not been identified in newly diagnosed diabetic cats (Hoenig et al, 2002). The role of genetics remains to be determined.

Non-insulin-dependent type II diabetes may be identified in as many as 50 to 70% of newly-diagnosed diabetic cats. In contrast, clinical recognition of NIDDM is very uncommon in dogs and is usually associated with a concurrent insulin antagonistic disease or drug. Islet amyloidosis is an important factor in the development of non-insulin-dependent type II diabetes in people and presumably cats. Islet-amyloid polypeptide (IAPP), or amylin, is the principal constituent of amyloid in people with NIDDM and in adult cats with diabetes (Johnson et al, 1989). IAPP is stored in beta-cell secretory granules (Westermark et al, 1987, 1987a; Johnson et al, 1988), and is co-secreted with insulin by beta cells (Lutz and Rand, 1996). Stimulants of insulin secretion also stimulate amylin secretion. Increased long-term secretion of insulin and amylin, as occurs with obesity and other insulin resistant states, results in aggregation and deposition of amylin in the islets as amyloid. IAPP-derived amyloid fibrils are cytotoxic and associated with apoptotic cell death of islet cells (Hiddinga and Eberhardt, 1999). If amyloid deposition is progressive, islet cell destruction progresses and eventually leads to diabetes mellitus. The severity of islet amyloidosis determines, in part, whether diabetic cats have IDDM or NIDDM. Total destruction of the islets results in IDDM and the need for insulin treatment for the rest of the cat's life. Partial destruction of the islets may or may not result in clinically-evident diabetes; insulin treatment may or may not be required to control glycemia, and transient diabetes may or may not develop after treatment is initiated. If amyloid deposition progresses, cats will progress from a subclinical diabetic state to NIDDM and ultimately to IDDM. The presence and severity of insulin resistance are important variables that influence the clinical picture in cats. A sustained demand for insulin secretion in response to insulin resistance can lead to worsening islet pathology and further reduce the population of beta cells. Our current understanding of the etiopathogenesis of diabetes in cats suggests that the difference between IDDM and NIDDM is primarily a difference in the severity of beta-cell loss and severity and reversibility of concurrent insulin resistance.

Key Nutritional Factors

Key nutritional factors consist of nutrients of concern and other factors such as food type. This section emphasizes key nutritional factors that vary significantly in commercial foods and markedly affect management of diabetes mellitus (**Table 29-3**). The degree to which any of these factors affects management of diabetes mellitus greatly depends on the efficacy of primary disease control through insulin or other pharmacologic treatment. However, it has been shown that appropriate nutritional support may allow for less medical intervention, and in some cases, precludes the need for medical intervention (Bennett et al, 2006; Farrow et al, 2002; Frank et al, 2001; Nelson et al, 1998, 2000; Rand et al, 2004; Thiess et al, 2004).

WATER

Increased water loss due to osmotic diuresis from glucose, and ketone bodies if DKA is present, must be compensated. Generally, a source of potable water is recommended in amounts sufficient to meet the increased water requirement. This is usually accomplished via free-choice access to water. Dehydrated patients and those with DKA may require parenteral fluid administration. Caution should be observed with type and rate of fluid replacement because of electrolyte perturbations. Rapid replacement of fluid loss with hypotonic solutions may lead to water intoxication and cerebral edema (Schaer, 1975).

DIGESTIBLE CARBOHYDRATE

Concerns have been raised about the composition of carbohydrate in cat foods because cats have a different capacity to metabolize carbohydrates than dogs (Maskell and Graham,

Table 29-4. Effect of feeding insoluble dietary fiber to dogs and cats with diabetes mellitus.*

	Mean daily insulin dose (U/kg/day)	Mean fasting blood glucose (mg/dl)	Mean blood glucose/24 hrs (mg/dl)	Mean urine glucose excretion (g/24 hrs)	Mean glycosylated hemoglobin (%)
Dog food**					
Low-fiber food (1% DM)	1.9 ± 0.6	247 ± 99	246 ± 100	9.3 ± 14.0	6.9 ± 1.8
High-fiber food (13% DM)	1.7 ± 0.5	164 ± 69	184 ± 71	2.8 ± 3.3	5.9 ± 1.4
Cat food**					
Low-fiber food (1% DM)	1.2 ± 0.7	328 ± 153	285 ± 131	Not done	2.7 ± 0.8
High-fiber food (12% DM)	1.0 ± 0.6	191 ± 118	182 ± 99	Not done	2.1 ± 0.4

Key: DM = dry matter.
*Adapted from Nelson R, Duesberg C, Ford S, et al. Dietary insoluble fiber and glycemic control of diabetic dogs (abstract). In: Proceedings. Twelfth Annual Veterinary Medical Forum, American College of Veterinary Internal Medicine, San Francisco, CA, 1994: 993. Nelson R, Scott-Moncrief C, DeVries S, et al. Dietary insoluble fiber and glycemic control of diabetic cats (abstract). In: Proceedings. Twelfth Annual Veterinary Medical Forum, American College of Veterinary Internal Medicine, San Francisco, CA, 1994: 996.
**By the parameters shown here, dogs and cats eating the higher fiber food had better glycemic control than comparable animals eating the low-fiber food.

1994). The composition and quantity of carbohydrates in foods for management of diabetes mellitus differ between dogs and cats, in part, because dogs are omnivores and tolerate digestible (soluble) complex carbohydrates better than diabetic cats. In general, foods containing 55% or less digestible carbohydrate on a dry matter (DM) basis are acceptable for dogs with diabetes mellitus, especially when the food also contains an increased amount of dietary fiber (Nelson et al, 1991, 1998). In contrast, cats are carnivores and have higher dietary protein requirements than omnivores such as people and dogs. The activity of hepatic enzymes responsible for the phosphorylation of glucose for subsequent storage or oxidation (glucokinase, hexokinase) and the conversion of glucose to glycogen for storage in the liver (glycogen synthetase) are lower in cats, compared with that for carnivores with omnivorous dietary habits (Zoran, 2002). The low activity of these hepatic enzymes suggests that cats primarily use gluconeogenic amino acids and fat rather than starch in their diet for energy, and suggests that diabetic cats may be predisposed to developing higher postprandial blood glucose concentrations following consumption of foods containing a high carbohydrate load and vice versa.

The optimal level of digestible carbohydrates for foods for diabetic cats has not been determined. Currently there are two acceptable approaches: low-carbohydrate/high-protein foods and increased-fiber/high-carbohydrate foods. Limiting carbohydrate intake results in blood glucose being maintained primarily via hepatic gluconeogenesis. The advantage is that glucose resulting from gluconeogenesis is released into the circulation at a slow and steady rate. Wider fluctuations in postprandial blood glucose levels, such as would be expected from feeding higher-carbohydrate foods, are avoided (Kirk, 2006). The end result of feeding increased-fiber/high-carbohydrate foods is similar. Increased dietary fiber also reduces fluctuations in postprandial blood glucose levels (Chandalia et al, 2000; Nelson et al, 2000), even though such foods provide more carbohydrate. Both approaches (low-carbohydrate/high-protein and increased-fiber/high-carbohydrate improve glycemic control in diabetic cats (Mazzaferro et al, 2001; Frank et al, 2001; Bennett et al, 2006; Nelson et al, 2000). In one of the studies comparing the two types of foods, diabetic cats from both groups were able to discontinue insulin and revert to a non-diabetic state; 41% of the cats fed an increased-fiber/high-carbohydrate food vs. 68% of the cats fed a low-carbohydrate/high-protein food (Bennett et al, 2006). Other studies have shown improved glycemic control in both healthy and diabetic cats fed low-carbohydrate/high-protein foods (Massaferro et al, 2003; Frank et al, 2001).

In general, digestible carbohydrates should be less than 20% DM in low-carbohydrate/high-protein foods for diabetic cats, and increased-fiber/high-carbohydrate foods for diabetic cats should contain less than 40% digestible carbohydrates DM (Nelson et al, 2000; Bennett et al, 2006). Digestible carbohydrate content of increased-fiber/high-carbohydrate foods for dogs should probably not exceed 55% DM.

Foods and snacks containing simple sugars rapidly increase blood glucose concentration and should be avoided for diabetic dogs and cats. Fructose should also be avoided in cats. Cats do not appear to metabolize fructose, which leads to fructose intolerance, polyuria and potential renal damage (Kienzle, 1994). Fructose may be found in commercial semi-moist foods, as a humectant in the form of sucrose, or high-fructose corn syrup. The potential effects of fructose in foods for dogs with diabetes mellitus have not been evaluated.

FIBER

As mentioned above, studies in diabetic cats have documented glycemic improvement in response to consumption of foods containing increased amounts of fiber (Nelson et al, 2000; Bennett et al, 2006). Foods containing increased fiber content also benefit glycemic control of diabetes in dogs (**Table 29-4**) (Nelson et al, 1991, 1998). The ability of fiber to form a viscous gel and thus impair convective transfer of glucose and water to the absorptive surface of the intestine appears to be the most important mechanism for slowing intestinal glucose absorption. The more viscous soluble fibers (e.g., gums, pectins) slow glucose diffusion to a greater degree than do the less viscous insoluble fibers (e.g., lignin, cellulose). Studies in diabetic dogs have documented glycemic improvement in response to the consumption of foods containing increased amounts of soluble and insoluble fiber (Nelson et al, 1991, 1998, 2000a; Graham et al, 1994, 2002).

Although an ideal fiber content has not been established, it is evident that including moderate amounts (approximately 7 to 18% DM) of insoluble or mixed insoluble and soluble dietary fiber in high-carbohydrate foods aids nutritional management of type I and type II diabetes mellitus in dogs and cats. Low-carbohydrate/high-protein foods intended for diabetic cats typically contain lower levels of fiber; between 2 to 7% DM. Whether such levels are important in the efficacy of these type foods for the management of diabetes is unknown. Thus, at this time, dietary fiber is not considered to be a key nutritional factor in low-carbohydrate/high-protein foods for management of diabetes in cats.

Some soluble fibers and mixtures of soluble/insoluble fibers may decrease small intestinal digestion of certain nutrients without affecting total tract digestibility (Muir et al, 1996). Caution should be exercised with use of either fiber type in the management of diabetes mellitus because hyperglycemia inhibits the gastrocolic response, which may predispose to constipation (Sims et al, 1995). In addition, increased fiber levels may trap water in the gastrointestinal tract; therefore, water balance may need to be more closely monitored in patients with poorly controlled diabetes mellitus fed foods with moderate fiber levels.

FAT

Derangements in fat metabolism are common in diabetic dogs and cats and include increased serum concentrations of cholesterol, triglycerides, lipoproteins, chylomicrons and free fatty acids; hepatic lipidosis, atherosclerosis and a predisposition for development of pancreatitis may also occur (DeBowes, 1987; Hess et al, 2003). Feeding high-fat food may also cause insulin resistance and promote hepatic glucose production (Massillon et al, 1997). Feeding a low-carbohydrate, high-protein, high-fat food also increases concentrations of fat metabolites in healthy male cats (Thiess et al, 2004). These findings strongly support feeding foods that are relatively low in fat content, i.e., less than 25% DM. Feeding lower fat foods will help minimize the risk of pancreatitis, control some aspects of hyperlipidemia and reduce overall caloric intake to favor weight loss or maintenance. Foods with a higher fat content may be needed for weight gain in thin or emaciated diabetic dogs and cats.

PROTEIN

Diabetic dogs and cats may have increased loss of amino acids in urine attributable to inappropriate or inadequate hormonal signals and renal glomerulopathy. It is important to provide protein quantity and quality that will meet the requirements of diabetic animals in the face of increased amino aciduria while avoiding excess protein content that may enhance renal damage or contribute to excessive insulin secretion.

As mentioned above, in cats, two basic nutritional approaches are used for diabetes management (and weight loss, see Chapter 27). These include increased-fiber/high-carbohydrate foods and low-carbohydrate/high-protein foods. In one study, obese cats fed isocaloric amounts of a low-carbohydrate/high-protein food vs. obese cats fed a low-protein/high-carbohydrate food, researchers concluded that the low-carbohydrate/high-protein food was beneficial through maintenance of normal insulin sensitivity of fat metabolism, facilitating the loss of body fat during weight loss. Whether or not the beneficial effects were due to high protein, low carbohydrate, or both, was not determined (Hoenig et al, 2006).

Also, as mentioned above, as true carnivores, cats primarily use gluconeogenic amino acids rather than dietary carbohydrates for energy, which suggests that diabetic cats may be predisposed to developing higher postprandial blood glucose concentrations following consumption of high-carbohydrate/lower-protein foods, and vice versa.

The protein content of foods for diabetic patients should be approximately 15 to 35% of the food DM for dogs and 28 to 55% of the food DM for cats.

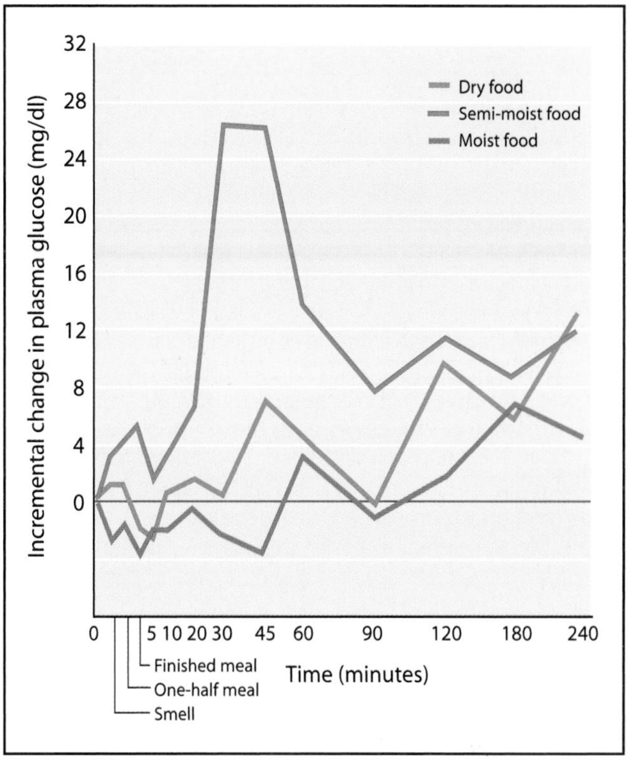

Figure 29-2. Changes in postprandial plasma glucose concentrations in healthy dogs fed commercial dry, semi-moist or moist dog food. Each dog consumed 50 kcal/kg body weight. Results are expressed as means compared with respective time-0 values. Note the profound increase in plasma glucose concentrations that follow consumption of semi-moist foods, which makes them an inappropriate food form for diabetic animals. (Adapted from Holste LC, Nelson RW, Feldman EC, et al. Effect of dry, soft moist, and canned dog foods on postprandial blood glucose and insulin concentrations in healthy dogs. American Journal of Veterinary Research 1989; 50: 987.)

Box 29-1. Trace Minerals and Vitamins in Diabetes Mellitus.

Changes in trace mineral nutrition status associated with diabetes mellitus have been evaluated in multiple species. The role of zinc in diabetes mellitus is controversial; however, it may affect insulin release from the pancreas, glucose tolerance and insulin resistance through changes in insulin binding and activity. Zinc appears to have biphasic activity; low concentrations enhance insulin secretion and activity whereas higher levels reverse this effect. Whole body zinc stores are often low in patients with diabetes mellitus.

Chromium has been proven to be an essential trace element and is thought to have a role in glucose homeostasis. Chromium has no known enzymatic cofactor function, but it may exist as a complex with nicotinic acid and amino acids to form a "glucose tolerance factor" that may aid insulin action. Chromium supplementation may improve glucose tolerance in malnourished subjects and subjects with poor glucose tolerance. Chromium supplements given to diabetic people have mostly proven ineffective in improving glycemic control; however, efficacy may vary on a case-by-case basis and chromium may prove beneficial in some individuals. At present, there is no reliable method to detect marginal chromium deficiency. Cats may display some gastrointestinal side effects when supplemental chromium is administered.

Manganese deficiency has been associated with perturbations in insulin secretion and carbohydrate and lipid metabolism, including impaired glucose usage in laboratory animals; however, its importance in the etiopathogenesis of diabetes is controversial. Repletion of manganese in deficient animals restores normal glucose tolerance and improves insulin secretion. However, treatment of diabetic subjects with manganese supplements had no impact on glycemic control; therefore, it is inferred that manganese deficiency is not a major factor in the pathophysiology of diabetes mellitus.

Iron overload can cause glucose intolerance due to pancreatic damage secondary to hemochromatosis. Overall, iron status does not seem to play a role in diabetes mellitus. Other trace element deficiencies such as vanadium and selenium have been associated with changes in glucose tolerance or insulin-like activity. Vanadium administered to healthy cats caused vomiting and diarrhea but also lowered blood glucose levels in one diabetic cat. Selenium appears to play no role in the development or manifestation of diabetes mellitus.

Substantiation of trace mineral benefits in diabetic dogs and cats has been confounding. Improvement with supplementation appears to occur on a case-by-case basis. In general, until otherwise proven, providing a food with microminerals supplied according to Association of American Feed Control Officials (AAFCO) recommendations for the appropriate lifestage should suffice for most animals with diabetes mellitus.

Diabetes mellitus may increase or decrease vitamin balance (**Table 1**). Conversely, vitamin status may affect the development and manifestations of diabetes mellitus. Much of the investigative work in this area is controversial and needs to be clarified. In general, foods that contain AAFCO recommended levels of vitamins for adult maintenance should meet most of the altered requirements induced by diabetes. In some cases of diabetes mellitus, it may be necessary to supplement the food with exogenous B vitamins.

Diabetic osteopenia is fairly well-documented in people and has a rational paradigm. Diabetes mellitus may lead to hypomagnesemia, which leads to decreased parathyroid hormone secretion and action, which then results in decreased formation of 1,25-dihydroxyvitamin D_3. Insulin deficiency further impairs formation of 1,25-dihydroxyvitamin D_3. The resultant impaired ability to enhance calcium absorption and retention in the face of hypercalciuria leads to calcium depletion.

Vitamin A homeostasis and status may influence development and control of diabetes mellitus. However, studies have yielded conflicting results; therefore, the effect of vitamin A on diabetes mellitus remains clouded. Most commercial pet foods provide abundant vitamin A.

Table 1. Micronutrient status in people with diabetes mellitus.*

Minerals	**IDDM**	**NIDDM**
Chromium	Normal to increased	Normal
Copper	Normal	Normal to increased
Iron	Normal	Normal
Manganese	Normal to decreased	Increased
Selenium	Increased	?
Zinc	Decreased	Decreased
Vitamins		
Thiamin	Normal	Normal
Vitamin A	Decreased?	Normal
Vitamin B_{12}	Normal to decreased	Normal
Vitamin B_6	Normal to decreased	Normal to decreased
Vitamin C	Normal to decreased	Normal to decreased
Vitamin E	Increased	Increased

Key: IDDM = insulin-dependent diabetes mellitus, NIDDM = non-insulin-dependent diabetes mellitus.
*Adapted from Mooradian AD, Morley JE. Micronutrient status in diabetes mellitus. American Journal of Clinical Nutrition 1987; 45: 877.

The Bibliography for **Box 29-1** can be found at www.markmorris.org.

FOOD FORM

Semi-moist foods tend to have a hyperglycemic effect compared to dry foods because they contain increased levels of simple carbohydrates and other ingredients used as humectants (**Figure 29-2**). Semi-moist foods should be avoided in dogs and cats with diabetes mellitus (**Table 29-3**).

Other Nutritional Factors

ELECTROLYTES

The osmotic diuresis induced by glycosuria and ketonuria results in urinary loss of electrolytes such as sodium, potassium, chloride, calcium, phosphorus and magnesium. Total body deficits in electrolytes often exist in poorly-regulated and ketotic diabetic dogs and cats, even when serum concentrations are within the normal range (Feldman and Nelson, 2004b). In addition, treatment of DKA may result in shifts of serum electrolytes between the intracellular and extracellular compartments. Perhaps the most clinically relevant is the shift of potassium, phosphorus and magnesium into intracellular compartments following initiation of insulin treatment for DKA, which can lead to severe reductions in serum concentrations of these cations. Frequent monitoring of serum electrolytes and adjustments in the electrolyte composition of the intravenous fluids helps prevent life-threatening deficiencies of these electrolytes from developing during treatment of DKA.

Feeding foods containing appropriate amounts of electrolytes is important to achieve and maintain normal homeostasis in diabetic dogs and cats. However, no studies have been performed to establish recommended levels of minerals in foods for animals with diabetes mellitus. Dogs and cats without renal impairment should be fed foods with adequate amounts of phosphorus to avoid and replace whole body phosphorus deficits. However, excess dietary phosphorus should be avoided in animals with renal impairment. Diabetic cats fed foods with low magnesium content should be monitored carefully to avoid magnesium depletion. In general, foods that meet Association of American Feed Control Officials (AAFCO) recommendations for adult maintenance should supply adequate amounts of cations and anions to compensate for the increased losses described above. Most, if not all, commercial veterinary therapeutic foods will provide adequate amounts of these minerals. Diabetes mellitus may also affect micromineral and vitamin status (**Box 29-1**).

OMEGA-3 FATTY ACIDS

Omega-3 (n-3) fatty acids have been used in people with diabetes mellitus to decrease the incidence of atherosclerotic disease (Nettleton, 1995). At present, the recommendation of fish oil (enhanced with omega-3 fatty acids) for management of type I diabetes mellitus is more accepted than for type II diabetes mellitus in people. The dose of fish oil, diet composition and type of diabetes have resulted in confounding results. Administration of supplemental omega-3 fatty acids to diabetic people generally increased high-density lipoprotein concentrations, improved blood viscosity, reduced triglyceride levels and reduced blood pressure. However, reports of reduced glycemic control, increased apolipoprotein B levels and increased low-density lipoprotein levels with concomitant increases in cholesterol concentrations have dampened enthusiasm for the use of omega-3 fatty acids in diabetic people (Nettleton, 1995). Administration of omega-3 fatty acids to diabetic dogs and cats has not been evaluated, but may prove to have benefits similar to those shown in other species.

Feeding Plans

Treatment for diabetes mellitus usually involves a combination of commonly available options. Treatment with injectable insulin or oral sulfonylurea agents has been the mainstay of pharmacologic intervention for uncomplicated diabetes mellitus (Feldman and Nelson, 2004, 2004a). Nutritional intervention is the major non-pharmacologic treatment modality for diabetes mellitus and plays an important role in the successful management of diabetic dogs and cats. Adjustments in food and feeding methods (amount fed and timing of feedings) should be considered when insulin therapy is initiated and should be directed at correcting or preventing obesity, maintaining consistency in the timing and caloric content of the meals and furnishing a food that helps minimize postprandial hyperglycemia.

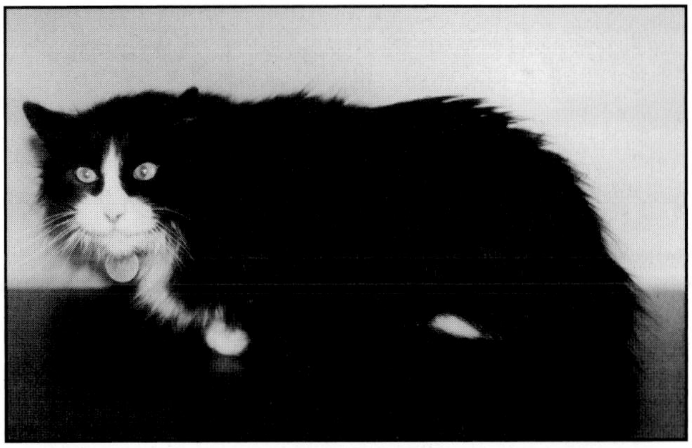

Figure 29-3. This nine-year-old, neutered male domestic longhair cat presented for polydipsia, polyuria, polyphagia and weight loss. The initial diagnoses were diabetes mellitus and concurrent hyperthyroidism. The cat was treated with methimazole for the hyperthyroidism; however, the diabetes mellitus persisted. The diabetes mellitus was controlled with a combination of oral glipizide and a veterinary therapeutic food containing low-fat and moderate fiber levels. Methimazole therapy was continued.

The nutritional plan for cats with non-insulin-dependent type II diabetes is similar to that for type I diabetes mellitus. In many diabetic cats, clinical signs and hyperglycemia resolve with appropriate dietary treatment and proper case management (**Figure 29-3**) (Bennett et al, 2006; Reusch et al, 2006).

Exercise also plays an important role in improving and maintaining control of glycemia by helping promote weight loss, eliminating insulin resistance induced by obesity and promoting glucose usage by muscle (Nishida et al, 2001). The amount and timing of exercise should be consistent from day to day to avoid unpredictable fluctuations in blood glucose that may result in potentially severe hypoglycemia. Finally, changes in diet, body weight and exercise may alter insulin requirements and should be accompanied by concurrent monitoring to assess if glycemic control has been affected. For example, an increase in dietary fiber may decrease blood glucose concentrations and lead to hypoglycemia or the Somogyi response. Similarly, loss of body weight will improve insulin sensitivity and may lead to hypoglycemia unless the insulin treatment regimen is modified.

Assess and Select the Food

Levels of the key nutritional factors should be evaluated in foods currently being fed to diabetic patients. Semi-moist foods should be avoided. Amounts and levels of key nutritional factors should be compared to those established for diabetic dogs and cats (**Table 29-3**). Information from this aspect of assessment is essential for making any changes to foods currently provided. If key nutritional factors in the current food do not match the recommended levels, then changing to a more appropriate food is indicated. **Tables 29-5** through **29-7** list the recommended key nutritional factors for diabetic dogs and cats

Table 29-5. Selected commercial veterinary therapeutic foods marketed for dogs with diabetes mellitus compared to recommended levels of key nutritional factors.*

Dry foods	Energy density (kcal/cup)**	Carbohydrate (%)	Fiber (%)	Fat (%)	Protein (%)***
Recommended levels	**-**	**≤55**	**7-18**	**<25**	**15-35**
Hill's Prescription Diet r/d Canine	242	38.7	13.5	8.2	34.3
Hill's Prescription Diet r/d with Chicken Canine	241	36	13.6	8.8	35.2
Hill's Prescription Diet w/d Canine	243	51.2	16.4	8.8	18.9
Hill's Prescription Diet w/d with Chicken Canine	239	50.1	17.1	8.7	19.1
Iams Veterinary Formula Weight Control D/Optimum Weight Control	209	51.2	3.0	9.5	28.7
Iams Veterinary Formula Weight Loss/ Restricted-Calorie	217	58.0	2.4	9.1	25.0
Purina Veterinary Diets DCO Dual Fiber Control	320	47.8	7.6	12.4	25.3
Royal Canin Veterinary Diet Diabetic HF 18	186	48.6	12.1	9.9	22.0
Moist foods	**Energy density (kcal/can)****	**Carbohydrate (%)**	**Fiber (%)**	**Fat (%)**	**Protein (%)*****
Recommended levels	**-**	**≤55**	**7-18**	**<25**	**15-35**
Hill's Prescription Diet r/d Canine	257/12.3 oz.	39.2	21.2	8.6	25.3
Hill's Prescription Diet w/d Canine	329/13 oz.	52.6	12.4	12.7	17.9
Iams Veterinary Formula Weight Loss/Restricted-Calorie	397/14 oz.	40.8	3.2	14.9	34.4

Note: Fresh water should be available at all times; semi-moist foods should be avoided.
*From manufacturers' published information or calculated from manufacturers' published as fed values; all values are on a dry matter basis unless otherwise stated.
**Energy density values are listed on an as fed basis and are useful for determining the amount to feed; cup = 8-oz. measuring cup. To convert to kJ, multiply kcal by 4.184.
***Dogs with renal failure should be fed protein at the low end of the range.

and selected commercial veterinary therapeutic foods often fed to patients with either insulin-dependent type I, or non-insulin-dependent type II, diabetes mellitus.

There are two types of foods for diabetic cats: increased-fiber/high-carbohydrate foods and low-carbohydrate/high-protein foods (**Tables 29-6** and **29-7**, respectively). Both have been shown to improve glycemic control in diabetic cats (Mazzaferro et al, 2001; Frank et al, 2001; Bennett et al 2006; Nelson et al, 2000). In one of the studies comparing the two types of foods, diabetic cats from both groups were able to discontinue insulin and revert to a nondiabetic state. Forty-one percent of the cats fed an increased-fiber/high-carbohydrate food and 68% of the cats fed a low-carbohydrate food became nondiabetic (Bennett et al, 2006). On the basis of calculated odds ratios, cats fed a low-carbohydrate food are three times more likely to discontinue insulin therapy and revert to a nondiabetic state (Kirk, 2006). Other studies have shown improved glycemic control in both healthy and diabetic cats fed low-carbohydrate foods (Massaferro et al, 2003; Frank et al, 2001). When choosing a type of food to feed diabetic cats, besides considering the aforementioned study results, the clinician's personal experience with a given approach is also important.

Another criterion for selecting a food that may become increasingly important in the future is evidence-based clinical nutrition. Practitioners should know how to determine risks and benefits of nutritional regimens and counsel pet owners accordingly. Currently, veterinary medical education and continuing education are not always based on rigorous assessment of evidence for or against particular management options. Still, studies have been published to establish the nutritional benefits of certain pet foods. Chapter 2 describes evidence-based clinical nutrition in detail and applies its concepts to various veterinary therapeutic foods.

Assess and Determine the Feeding Method

Determining the amount to feed diabetic dogs and cats requires special consideration. Patients with diabetes mellitus display a classic clinical picture of polyphagia with weight loss. Before making recommendations for daily energy requirement (DER), it is important to emphasize that the clinical response of patients with diabetes mellitus to dietary manipulation depends on the level of control of the primary disease process and the presence or absence of concurrent disease. For example, if weight loss or weight gain is a continuing problem, it may be due to poorly controlled diabetes mellitus or concurrent disease such as thyroid disorders (dogs and cats), lymphoplasmacytic enteritis (cats) or hyperadrenocorticism (dogs), rather than inappropriate calculation of DER. Consistent reevaluation and owner education are important tools in adjusting food dose and managing diabetes mellitus. After a patient's DER is estimated, the amount of food to feed (cups and/or cans) can be determined by dividing the DER by the as fed energy density of the food which can be found in **Tables 29-5** through **29-7**.

The basal metabolic rate may actually be decreased in patients with poorly controlled diabetes mellitus because of the euthyroid sick syndrome. Caution should therefore be taken to

Table 29-6. Selected commercial fiber-enhanced veterinary therapeutic foods marketed for cats with diabetes mellitus compared to recommended levels of key nutritional factors.*

Dry foods	Energy density (kcal/cup)**	Carbohydrate (%)	Fiber (%)	Fat (%)	Protein (%)***
Recommended levels	**–**	**<40**	**7-18**	**<25**	**28-55**
Hill's Prescription Diet r/d Feline	263	33.5	13.6	9.3	36.9
Hill's Prescription Diet r/d with Chicken Feline	266	32.2	13.8	9.8	37.7
Hill's Prescription Diet w/d Feline	281	37.4	7.6	9.8	39.0
Hill's Prescription Diet w/d with Chicken Feline	278	35.4	7.6	9.9	39.9
Iams Veterinary Formula Weight Control D/Optimum Weight Control	326	41.2	1.5	12.2	38.6
Iams Veterinary Formula Weight Loss/ Restricted-Calorie	268	44.5	2.5	11.0	35.2
Purina Veterinary Diets OM Overweight Management	321	22.4	5.6	8.5	56.2
Moist foods	**Energy density (kcal/can)****	**Carbohydrate (%)**	**Fiber (%)**	**Fat (%)**	**Protein (%)*****
Recommended levels	**–**	**<40**	**7-18**	**<25**	**28-55**
Hill's Prescription Diet r/d with Liver & Chicken Feline	114/5.5 oz.	31.3	15.4	9.2	37.5
Hill's Prescription Diet w/d with Chicken Feline	127/5.5 oz.	26.4	10.6	16.6	39.6
Iams Veterinary Formula Weight Loss/ Restricted-Calorie	172/6 oz.	32.3	1.7	15.5	44.2
Purina Veterinary Diets OM Overweight Management	150/5.5 oz.	23.2	10.2	14.6	44.6

Note: Fresh water should be available at all times; semi-moist foods should be avoided.
*From manufacturers' published information or calculated from manufacturers' published as fed values; all values are on a dry matter basis unless otherwise stated.
**Energy density values are listed on an as fed basis and are useful for determining the amount to feed; cup = 8-oz. measuring cup. To convert to kJ, multiply kcal by 4.184.
***Cats with renal failure should be fed protein at the low end of the range.

avoid over diagnosis of true hypothyroidism in light of the prevalence of euthyroid sick syndrome. Hyperthyroidism is rare in dogs but may occur in some cats with diabetes mellitus.

The energy intake of diabetic patients must be assessed in relation to body condition. For most patients (BCS 2/5 to 4/5), feeding at the daily energy requirement (DER) for ideal body weight in conjunction with adequate control of diabetes mellitus will achieve desired body weights. It is best to calculate a DER as a multiple of resting energy requirement (RER) based on the standard formulas for normal dogs and cats (Chapter 1). For neutered dogs, a factor of 1.6 x RER, and for intact dogs, a factor of 1.8 x RER are good initial estimates of DER. For inactive/obese-prone dogs (most dogs), a range of 1.2 to 1.4 x RER is suggested. Factors of 1.2 x RER and 1.4 x RER for neutered and intact cats, respectively, are appropriate starting points. For inactive/obese-prone cats (most cats), using 1.0 x RER is appropriate. All patients should be reevaluated regularly with food doses adjusted based on body condition.

Diabetic dogs and cats often present with an obese body condition. For overweight and obese diabetic patients, a conservative weight-loss protocol may need to be instituted after medical problems are stabilized. For controlled weight loss in overweight/obese dogs, a starting point for DER is 1.0 x RER and for overweight/obese cats 0.8 x RER. These calculations assume RER for ideal body weight and are a good initial estimate for calculation of food doses. Frequent monitoring and readjustment should be the norm rather than the exception in weight-loss programs for patients with concurrent disease such as diabetes mellitus. Note that in these patients, improvement in insulin resistance is often accomplished with weight loss. Because many cats with type II diabetes mellitus are obese, caloric restriction may be a requisite part of their dietary management. In cats, care must be taken to avoid rapid weight loss that may predispose to hepatic lipidosis. Loss of 0.5 to 1% of initial body weight per week is considered safe (Chapter 27). Hepatic lipidosis does not seem to be a weight-loss concern for dogs. See **Box 29-2** for a feeding plan for DKA.

Feeding a food with moderate to high levels of fiber may pose problems for weight gain or even maintenance of current weight in diabetic patients that are too lean. These patients may need to be fed a food with less than 10% DM crude fiber and/or with slightly increased fat content to increase food energy density to a level where body weight is increased or maintained. Also, in these cases, feeding an increased quantity of food may prove useful. However, increasing the amount of food may not result in desired effects on body weight and condition if diabetes is poorly controlled.

Regarding when to feed, the feeding schedule should be designed to enhance the actions of insulin, maximize food usage and minimize postprandial hyperglycemia (**Figure 29-4**). The development of postprandial hyperglycemia depends, in part, on the amount of food consumed per meal, the rate at which glu-

Table 29-7. Selected commercial low-carbohydrate/high-protein veterinary therapeutic foods marketed for cats with diabetes mellitus compared to recommended levels of key nutritional factors.*

Dry foods	Energy density (kcal/cup)**	Carbohydrate (%)	Fat (%)	Protein (%)***
Recommended levels	**-**	**<20**	**<25**	**28-55**
Hill's Prescription Diet m/d Feline	480	14.7	22.0	51.5
Medi-Cal Diabetic DS 44	247	25.6	12.9	49.5
Purina Veterinary Diets DM Dietetic Management	592	15.0	17.9	57.8
Royal Canin Veterinary Diet Diabetic DS 44	239	25.6	12.9	49.5
Moist foods	**Energy density (kcal/can)****	**Carbohydrate (%)**	**Fat (%)**	**Protein (%)*****
Recommended levels	**-**	**<20**	**<25**	**28-55**
Hill's Prescription Diet m/d Feline	156/5.5 oz.	15.7	19.4	52.8
Iams Veterinary Formula Stress/Weight Gain Formula	333/6 oz.	12.2	37.2	41.8
Purina Veterinary Diets DM Dietetic Management	194/5.5 oz.	8.1	23.8	56.9

Note: Fresh water should be available at all times; semi-moist foods should be avoided.
*From manufacturers' published information or calculated from manufacturers' published as fed values; all values are on a dry matter basis unless otherwise stated.
**Energy density values are listed on an as fed basis and are useful for determining the amount to feed; cup = 8-oz. measuring cup. To convert to kJ, multiply kcal by 4.184.
***Cats with renal failure should be fed protein at the low end of the range.

cose and other nutrients are absorbed from the intestine and the effectiveness of exogenous insulin during this time. The daily caloric intake should be ingested when insulin is still present in the circulation and is capable of disposing of glucose absorbed from the meal. If meals are consumed while exogenous insulin is still metabolically active, the postprandial increase in blood glucose concentration will be minimal or absent. In contrast, feeding diabetic dogs and cats after insulin action has waned results in increasing blood glucose concentration shortly after consumption of the food. Ideally, several small meals given at regular intervals throughout the day with and following insulin administration result in minimal hyperglycemia (Ihle, 1995; Nelson, 1988). Diabetic dogs and cats that nibble throughout the day should be allowed to continue their pattern of eating (Martin and Rand, 2000). For these dogs and cats, the food should be available at the time of each insulin injection and the dog or cat allowed to choose when and how much to eat. The process is repeated at the time of the next insulin injection. In contrast, diabetic dogs and cats that eat all of the food when offered should be fed a set amount of food (calories) at defined times during the day. Generally, for patients receiving once-a-day insulin, half of the caloric requirement should be fed at the time of exogenous insulin administration and the other half eight to 10 hours later. If insulin is given twice daily, half of the caloric requirement should be fed with each injection. For finicky eaters, food is usually offered before insulin administration to avoid insulin-induced hypoglycemia if the animal does not eat.

Reassessment

Clinical Signs and Physical Examination

The most important initial parameters to assess when evaluating control of glycemia are the owners' subjective opinion of presence and severity of the pet's clinical signs and the overall health of their pet, findings on physical examination and stability of body weight. If the owner is satisfied with the results of treatment, the physical examination is supportive of good glycemic control and the body weight is stable, the diabetic dog or cat is usually adequately controlled. Poor control of glycemia should be suspected and additional diagnostics or a change in therapy considered if: 1) the owner reports persistent clinical signs suggestive of hyper- or hypoglycemia such as polydipsia, polyuria, lethargy, lack of grooming behavior (cats), weakness, ataxia or changes in jumping ability (cats), 2) the physical examination identifies problems consistent with poor control of glycemia such as an unthrifty or thin appearance, poor coat or plantigrade stance caused by peripheral neuropathy in diabetic cats or 3) the dog or cat is losing weight when it should not. Veterinary reassessment should take place every three to four months if the patient is stable and doing well. If the patient is persistently symptomatic, veterinary reassessment should take place every one to two weeks until control of the diabetic state is attained.

Body Weight and Condition

Achievement of weight goals can be measured through assessing body condition and weight. These measurements may also provide insight about the degree of glycemic control and the presence of other disease processes, especially in cases in which adjustments in food dose do not produce expected changes in body condition. Patients should be weighed every two weeks and have body condition assessed at least monthly. The owner should be encouraged to keep a chart of body weights and BCS. It may take several months to achieve weight-loss goals in obese patients. A loss of 10% body weight in already thin animals indicates a need for reassessment of the dietary and pharmacologic regimens.

Food Intake

Food intake, with maintenance of body weight, should decrease in patients with a favorable response to exogenous insulin administration. This response is caused by increased nutrient usage associated with hormonal treatment. If patients are anorectic or have depressed food intake, the relative palatability of the food may be poor and another food should be tried after ruling out medical causes. It is especially important to monitor food intake in cats because prolonged anorexia is a risk factor for hepatic lipidosis (Barsanti et al, 1977).

Urine Glucose and Ketones

Although most owners can monitor urine for glucose and ketones, urine testing for glucose is a crude indicator of glycemic control status. In the newly-diagnosed or ketotic diabetic dog or cat, a decrease in urinary ketone bodies and glucose signals a favorable response to treatment. Well-controlled diabetic dogs and cats should not have ketone bodies in their urine. Occasional monitoring of urine for glycosuria and ketonuria in the home environment is helpful in those diabetic dogs and cats that have problems with recurring ketosis or hypoglycemia to determine if ketonuria or persistent negative glycosuria is present, respectively. In cats that have reverted to a non-insulin-requiring diabetic state, monitoring helps determine if glycosuria has recurred; in cats treated with oral hypoglycemic drugs, it helps determine if glycosuria has improved or worsened; and in cats with suspected stress-induced hyperglycemia, monitoring helps differentiate transient from persistent hyperglycemia. Owners should not adjust daily insulin dosages based on results of urine glucose testing, except to decrease the insulin dose in dogs or stop insulin treatment in cats with recurring hypoglycemia and persistent negative glycosuria.

Biochemistry Profiles

The biochemistry profile should return to normal with well-controlled diabetes and adequate nutritional intake. The primary exception is hyperglycemia that may or may not be present depending on when the blood sample is obtained in relation to insulin administration. Abnormalities of biochemical constituents in the face of controlled diabetes mellitus should be evaluated as separate disease entities.

Serum Fructosamine

Measurement of glycated proteins (e.g., glycosylated hemoglobin and serum proteins [fructosamine]) is a common method of monitoring glycemic control in diabetic people and animals. Glycosylated hemoglobin is the most common glycated protein measured in diabetic people, but assays are time-consuming, often of questionable accuracy and not routinely evaluated in diabetic dogs and cats. Serum fructosamine is the most common glycated protein measured in diabetic dogs and cats (Reusch et al, 1993; Crenshaw et al, 1996; Elliott et al, 1999). Fructosamines result from an irreversible, nonenzymatic, insulin-independent binding of glucose to serum proteins. Serum fructosamine concentrations are a marker of mean blood glucose concentration during the circulating lifespan of the protein, which varies from one to three weeks, depending on the protein. The extent of glycosylation of serum proteins is directly related to the blood glucose concentration; the higher the average blood glucose concentration during the preceding two to three weeks, the higher the serum fructosamine concentration, and vice versa. Serum fructosamine concentrations increase when glycemic control of diabetic dogs and cats worsens and decrease when glycemic control improves. Serum fructosamine concentration is unaffected by acute increases in blood glucose concentration, as occurs with stress or excitement-induced hyperglycemia, but can be affected by hypoalbuminemia (<2.5 g/dl), hyperlipidemia (triglycerides >150 mg/dl) and hyperthyroidism (Lutz et al, 1995; Crenshaw and Peterson, 1996; Reusch and Haberer, 2001). Interpretation of serum fructosamine in diabetic dogs and cats should consider the fact that hyper-

Box 29-2. Feeding Plan for Diabetic Ketoacidosis.

Intensive care and intravenous fluid administration are not required if the patient is bright, alert and well-hydrated. Administration of short- or intermediate-acting insulin can be initiated in conjunction with feeding recommendations similar to those for type I and type II diabetes mellitus. Some patients with diabetic ketoacidosis may require in-hospital intensive care. Goals are to correct dehydration, electrolyte disorders (hypokalemia, hypophosphatemia, hyponatremia, hypochloremia, hypomagnesemia), ketonuria and acidosis while initiating a feeding plan. Nutritional recommendations are similar to those for type I and type II diabetes mellitus after the patient is stabilized (**Table 29-3**).

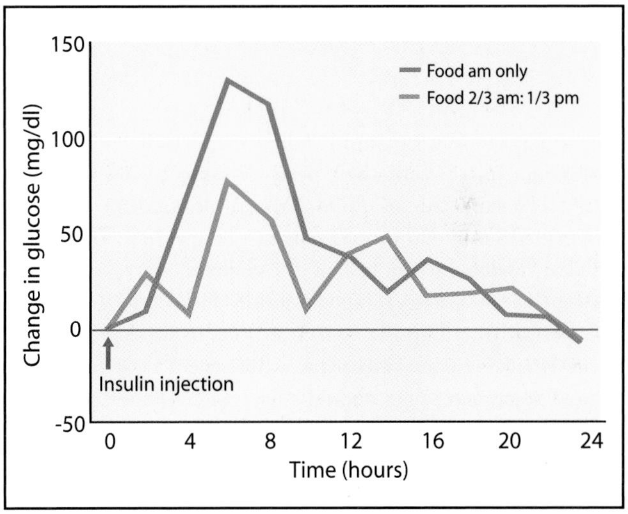

Figure 29-4. Mean change in blood glucose concentrations in eight dogs with insulin-dependent diabetes mellitus (type I) fed 66 kcal/kg body weight of a commercial moist dog food. A fixed amount of NPH insulin was administered to each dog at 8:00 a.m. Food was given either in one meal at 8:00 a.m. or in two meals at 8:00 a.m. (two-thirds of the food) and 6:00 p.m. (one-third of the food). Note the reduction in the mean blood glucose excursion merely by feeding multiple rather than one meal daily. (Adapted from Nelson RW. Disorders of the endocrine pancreas. In: Ettinger SJ, ed. Textbook of Veterinary Internal Medicine, 3rd ed. Philadelphia, PA: WB Saunders Co, 1989; 1694.)

Table 29-8. Clinical signs associated with hypothyroidism and hyperthyroidism.

Clinical signs	Hyperthyroidism	Hypothyroidism
Appetite	Increased to decreased	Normal to decreased
Behavior	Nervous, hyperactive to lethargic, excess vocalization, aggressive, heat intolerance	Lethargy, mental dullness, inactivity, cold intolerance
Coat	Dry/greasy/patchy alopecia/unkempt	Dry/sparse (endocrine alopecia), seborrhea
Eyes	Normal	Normal or corneal lipid deposits, corneal ulceration/uveitis
Heart rate/rhythm	Increased with possible dysrhythmias	Normal to decreased with possible dysrhythmias
Neck	Normal/mass	Normal/mass
Neuromuscular	Weakness, tremors, ventriflexion of head, muscle wasting	Seizures, ataxia, circling, vestibular signs, weakness, knuckling, facial nerve paralysis
Respiratory	Panting, respiratory distress, dysphonia (dogs)	Normal
Skin	Normal	Hyperpigmentation
Stools	Bulky to diarrhea	Constipation to diarrhea
Thirst	Increased	Normal to decreased
Urine	Excess urination	Normal
Vomiting	Possible	No
Weight	Normal to decreased	Normal to increased
Other	Reproductive dysfunction	Reproductive dysfunction, poor growth

glycemia is common, even in well-controlled diabetics. Most owners are happy with their pet's response to insulin treatment if serum fructosamine concentrations can be kept between 350 and 450 µmol/l. Values greater than 500 µmol/l indicate inadequate control of the diabetic state and values greater than 600 µmol/l indicate serious lack of glycemic control. Serum fructosamine concentrations in the lower half of the normal reference range (i.e., <300 µmol/l) or below the normal reference range should raise concern for significant periods of hypoglycemia in diabetic dogs and cats. Increased serum fructosamine concentrations (i.e., >500 µmol/l) suggest poor control of glycemia and the need for insulin adjustments, but do not identify the underlying problem.

Serial Blood Glucose Curves

Serial blood glucose curves are indicated during the initial regulation of newly-diagnosed diabetic dogs and cats and whenever an adjustment in insulin therapy is deemed necessary after reviewing the history, physical examination, changes in body weight and serum fructosamine concentration. Results of the serial blood glucose curve provide guidance when adjusting the insulin treatment regimen, unless blood glucose measurements are unreliable because of stress, aggression or excitement. Reliance on history, physical examination, body weight and serum fructosamine concentration to determine when a blood glucose curve is needed helps reduce the frequency of performing blood glucose curves, reduces the number of venipunctures and shortens the time the dog or cat spends in the hospital, thereby minimizing the patient's aversion to these evaluations and improving the chances of obtaining meaningful results when a blood glucose curve is needed.

When assessing glycemic control, the insulin and feeding schedule used by the owner should be maintained. The dog or cat should be dropped off at the hospital early in the morning, and blood obtained every one to two hours throughout the day for glucose determination. The marginal ear vein prick technique for blood sampling can be used in diabetic cats to minimize problems with stress-induced hyperglycemia. Home monitoring of blood glucose concentrations using the marginal ear vein prick technique is also a viable option. Details on adjustment and in-depth analysis of serial glucose curves are provided elsewhere (Feldman and Nelson, 2004, 2004a).

FELINE HYPERTHYROIDISM

Hyperthyroidism is a clinical condition that results from excessive production and secretion of thyroxine (T_4) and triiodothyronine (T_3) by the thyroid gland. Hyperthyroidism is the most common endocrine disease affecting cats. The first clinical reports appeared in the late 1970s and early 1980s (Peterson et al, 1979; Holzworth et al, 1980). Disease prevalence has been estimated at one in 300 from necropsy findings (Ferguson, 1993). In a 1993 survey conducted at the Animal Medical Center in New York City, approximately 22 cats with hyperthyroidism were identified monthly (Broussard et al, 1995). It is unclear whether the prevalence of hyperthyroidism continues to escalate; however, there is no doubt that feline hyperthyroidism is now commonly recognized throughout the world and is one of the most frequently diagnosed diseases in small animal practice.

In contrast, hyperthyroidism is uncommon in dogs and is caused by functional thyroid adenomas and carcinomas, not adenomatous hyperplasia as typically occurs in cats (See below.) (Feldman and Nelson, 2004d). Thyroid carcinomas are highly malignant tumors that spread quickly in dogs. Thyroid carcinoma should always be assumed in any dog diagnosed with hyperthyroidism until histopathologic evaluation of the thyroid mass proves otherwise. Diagnosis is based on presence of clinical signs similar to those seen in hyperthyroid cats (See below.), identification of a thyroid mass with digital palpation and cervical ultrasound and documentation of increased serum T_4 and free T_4 and non-detectable serum thyroid-stimulating hormone (TSH) concentration. Surgical removal of the thyroid mass is the treatment of choice whenever possible. Radiation therapy, chemotherapy, radioactive iodine-131, methimazole or a combination of these treatment modalities is usually indicated following removal of a thyroid carcinoma, especially if surgical debulking is incomplete or metastasis is suspected.

The remainder of this chapter will focus on feline hyperthyroidism.

Patient Assessment

History and Physical Examination

Hyperthyroidism is a disease of older cats. The average age at the time of diagnosis is 13 years with a range of four to 20 years. Fewer than 5% of cats with this disorder are younger than eight years (Feldman and Nelson, 2004e). There is no sex-related predisposition and domestic shorthair and longhair cats are the most frequently affected breeds. Clinical signs result from excessive secretion of thyroid hormone by the thyroid mass and typically include weight loss (which may progress to cachexia), polyphagia and restlessness or hyperactivity (**Table 29-8**). Polyphagia is due to increased cellular metabolism. In some hyperthyroid cats, appetite may be decreased following a prolonged period of polyphagia. Decreased appetite is usually associated with weakness, muscle wasting and severe weight loss. The most common finding on physical examination is digital palpation of one or more discrete thyroid masses in the ventral neck. Because of the multisystemic effects of hyperthyroidism, the variable clinical signs and its resemblance to many other feline diseases (**Table 29-9**), hyperthyroidism should be suspected in any aged cat with medical problems.

Table 29-9. Differential diagnoses for hyperthyroidism.*

Non-thyroid endocrine disease
Acromegaly (rare)
Diabetes insipidus (rare)
Diabetes mellitus
Hyperadrenocorticism (rare)
Renal disease
Heart disease
Congestive cardiomyopathy
Hypertrophic cardiomyopathy
Idiopathic dysrhythmia
Gastrointestinal disease
Cancer
Diffuse gastrointestinal disorders
Inflammatory
Pancreatic exocrine insufficiency
Hepatopathy
Cancer
Inflammatory
Pulmonary disease

*Adapted from Feldman EC, Nelson RW, eds. Feline hyperthyroidism (thyrotoxicosis). Canine and Feline Endocrinology and Reproduction, 2nd ed. Philadelphia, PA: WB Saunders Co, 1996; 135.

Laboratory and Other Diagnostic Testing

The primary purpose of laboratory testing is to confirm the diagnosis of hyperthyroidism and screen the cat for concurrent disease, most notably renal insufficiency, which is common in geriatric cats and often present in conjunction with hyperthyroidism. Any number of abnormalities may be present in individual cats; however, clinical studies have elucidated common changes (**Table 29-10**). Specific diagnostics for thyroid dysfunction should be performed if thyroid disease is still consistent with and suspected from results of the initial screening of blood and urine tests.

SERUM THYROID HORMONE TESTING

The diagnosis of hyperthyroidism is based on identification of appropriate clinical signs, palpation of a thyroid nodule and documentation of an increased serum T_4 concentration. Measurement of random baseline serum T_4 concentrations has been extremely reliable in differentiating hyperthyroid cats from those without thyroid disease. Cats with early disease may have serum T_4 concentrations within the upper portion of the reference range (i.e., 2.5 to 5.0 µg/dl). Serum T_4 concentrations that fall within the upper portion of the reference range can create a diagnostic dilemma, especially when clinical signs suggest hyperthyroidism and a nodule is palpated in the ventral region of the neck. Cats with mild or occult hyperthyroidism and hyperthyroid cats with significant non-thyroidal illness can have normal serum T_4 concentrations. The diagnosis of hyperthyroidism should not be excluded on the basis of one normal test result, especially in a cat with appropriate clinical signs and a palpable neck mass. Additional diagnostics to consider include measurement of the non-protein-bound fraction of T_4 (i.e., free T_4) in the circulation, the T_3 suppression test, sodium pertechnetate thyroid scan or repeating the serum T_4 test three to six months later. Measurement of serum free T_4 using an equilibrium dialysis technique is the current recommendation of choice to confirm hyperthyroidism in cats with non-diagnostic serum T_4 test results (Peterson et al, 2001). Measurement of serum free T_4 is a more reliable means of assessing thyroid gland function than serum T_4 concentration, in part, because non-thyroidal illness has less of a suppressive effect on serum free T_4 than T_4 and serum free T_4 is increased in many cats with occult hyperthyroidism and normal T_4 test results (Peterson et al, 2001). Occasionally, concurrent illness will cause an increase in serum free T_4 concentration in cats; an increase that can exceed the reference range. For this reason, serum free T_4 should always be interpreted in conjunction with T_4 measured from the same blood sample.

TRIIODOTHYRONINE (T_3) SUPPRESSION TEST

The T_3 suppression test is used to distinguish euthyroid from mildly hyperthyroid cats in cases in which T_4 and free T_4 test results are nebulous. The T_3 suppression test is based on the theory that oral administration of T_3 will suppress pituitary TSH secretion in euthyroid cats, resulting in a

Table 29-10. Laboratory findings in animals with hypothyroidism and hyperthyroidism.

Laboratory tests	Feline hyperthyroidism	Canine and feline hypothyroidism
Biochemical analysis	Increased ALT, ALP, creatinine, urea nitrogen, glucose, bilirubin and phosphate values	Increased cholesterol, triglyceride, ALT (mild), ALP (mild) and CK (mild, variable) values
Cardiac diagnostics	Tachycardia, PVCs, hypertrophic cardiomyopathy	Bradycardia, inverted T waves
Complete blood count	Erythrocytosis, leukocytosis, lymphopenia, eosinopenia, increased MCV	Normocytic, normochromic, nonregenerative anemia with leptocytes possible
Imaging	Normal or cardiac/respiratory abnormalities	Normal/thyroid mass, metastatic lesions, thoracic or abdominal effusion
Urinalysis	Increased or decreased specific gravity, glucosuria, signs of inflammation	Normal to nonspecific increase in white blood cells

Key: MCV = mean corpuscular volume, ALT = alanine aminotransferase, ALP = alkaline phosphatase, PVC = premature ventricular contraction, CK = creatine kinase.

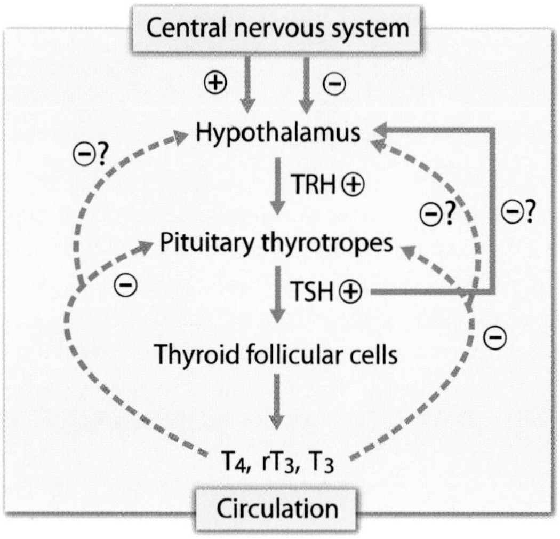

Figure 29-5. Schematic of the hypothalamic-pituitary-thyroid axis. Key: TRH = thyrotropin-releasing hormone, TSH = thyroid-stimulating hormone (thyrotropin), T_4 = thyroxine, T_3 = 3,5,3'-triiodothyronine, rT_3 = reverse T_3, + = stimulation, – = inhibition.

decrease in circulating T_4. In contrast, pituitary TSH secretion is already suppressed in cats with hyperthyroidism, oral administration of T_3 will not cause further suppression and serum T_4 will not decrease following T_3 administration. In this test, T_3 is administered orally three times daily for seven treatments and serum T_4 concentration is determined before and eight hours after the last T_3 administration (Feldman and Nelson, 2004e).

SODIUM PERTECHNETATE THYROID SCAN

The sodium pertechnetate thyroid scan is used to identify functional thyroid tissue. Radioactive sodium pertechnetate is administered intravenously and uptake by thyroid tissue is assessed by scintillation scan. Uptake of sodium pertechnetate will be greater and the distribution and size of functioning thyroid tissue will be abnormal in hyperthyroid cats, compared with scans obtained in euthyroid cats. Sodium pertechnetate uptake is useful for diagnosing unilateral vs. bilateral thyroid lobe involvement, identifying ectopic thyroid tissue and identifying sites of metastasis in cats with thyroid carcinoma.

Etiopathogenesis

NORMAL THYROID FUNCTION

The thyroid gland is the site of thyroid hormone synthesis and is regulated by integration of cortical and substrate feedback signals (**Figure 29-5**) (Feldman and Nelson, 2004c; Kaptein et al, 1994). The thyroid gland concentrates iodide under the influence of TSH for thyroid hormone synthesis. Iodide anions undergo peroxidation and linkage to tyrosine residues, which are components of larger acceptor proteins (i.e., primarily thyroglobulin). Excess absorbed iodine is eliminated primarily in urine; however, unabsorbed amounts may be found in feces (Kaptein et al, 1994).

Tyrosine residues attached to thyroglobulin may be either monoiodinated (monoiodotyrosine [MIT]) or diiodinated (diiodotyrosine [DIT]) and subsequent dimerization results in formation of the iodothyronines T_3 and T_4. Thyroglobulin is subsequently processed so that T_4, and to a much lesser degree T_3, are eventually released into the bloodstream. The thyroid gland directly produces all T_4 and approximately 20% of T_3 found in serum; 99% of these hormones are bound to serum proteins (Kaptein et al, 1994). The portion of T_4 and T_3 partitioned into serum, and not associated with protein, is often called free or fT_4 and fT_3. Some biologically inactive MIT and DIT and intact thyroglobulin may be released into the circulation. Reverse T_3 (rT_3) is another inactive thyroid metabolite found in serum and is formed from the deiodination of T_4.

T_3, the more active form of thyroid hormone, is primarily produced from thyroxine via deiodinase enzymes in target tissues. Deiodinase I, a selenoprotein, is located primarily in the kidneys and liver (Larsen and Berry, 1995). Deiodinase I prefers rT_3 as a substrate, releasing DIT; therefore, it may be important in the deactivation process of thyroid hormone. Deiodinase I also has activity for T_4, producing active T_3; however, this is an order of magnitude less than the rT_3 affinity. The T_3 produced by the liver may be released into the general circulation to exert its biologic activity. The exact physiologic importance of deiodinase I in the liver has yet to be elucidated (Larsen and Berry, 1995).

The enzyme deiodinase II is specific for production of T_3 from T_4 and is found in low concentrations in most cells including those of the brain, skin, muscle and placenta (Larsen and Berry, 1995; Freake and Oppenheimer, 1995). Deiodinase II is responsible for the intracellular production of T_3, which may subsequently be moved to the nucleus of these cells (**Figure 29-6**). Production of T_3 and subsequent nuclear binding is probably the major physiologic route of thyroid action. Preliminary evidence suggests deiodinase II is a selenoprotein (Davey et al, 1995).

The major route of thyroid hormone action is thought to be via nuclear interaction at peripheral tissues. As a result, cells increase consumption and production of energy and exert hormonal effects for normal growth and development of skeletal muscle and neural tissues. The exact mode of this action has yet to be elucidated; however, it is thought to involve the key enzymatic controls of carbohydrate, fat and protein metabolism. In addition, investigators have proposed a possible uncoupling of oxidative phosphorylation and modulation of Na/K-ATPase activity at the cellular membrane (Kaptein et al, 1994).

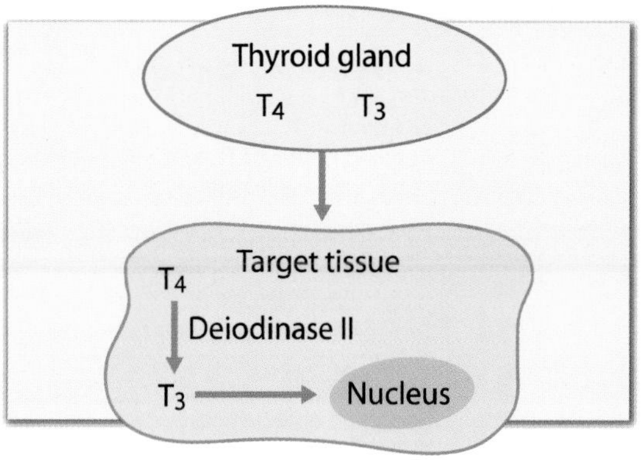

Figure 29-6. Deiodinase II enzyme is found in low concentrations in most cells and is responsible for the intracellular production of T_3 from T_4. The production of T_3 and subsequent nuclear binding is probably the major physiologic route of thyroid action.

Table 29-11. Goitrogenic factors in foods and the environment.*

Nutrients or food types
Cabbage (goitrin)
Canned foods
Cassava (linamarin)
Cyanides
Excess iodine
Iodine deficiency
Millet
Rutabagas
Sweet potatoes
Turnips
Seaweed
Various beans (including soybeans)
Environmental
Polychlorinated biphenyls (fish-containing foods)
Pesticides
Phthalates
Polyphenols (fish-containing foods)
Propylthiouracil (drug)
Resorcinols (fish-containing foods)

*Epidemiologic associations and risk factors.

Risk Factors

Although the clinical aspects of feline hyperthyroidism have been well characterized, the etiology of hyperthyroidism remains unknown. The presence of adenomatous hyperplasia rather than neoplasia in most affected cats, bilateral thyroid lobe involvement with differences in severity of involvement between the lobes and the initial involvement of one thyroid lobe progressing to involvement of both lobes suggests the presence of a goitrogenic factor that may influence development of thyrotoxicosis in a species that may be predisposed to the disease. It has been postulated that immunologic, infectious, nutritional, environmental or genetic factors may interact to cause pathologic changes (Scarlett, 1994; Gerber et al, 1994). Epidemiologic studies have identified consumption of commercial canned cat foods as a risk factor for development of hyperthyroidism, suggesting that a goitrogenic compound may be present in the diet (**Table 29-11**) (Scarlett et al, 1988; Kass et al, 1999; Martin et al, 2000; Edinboro et al, 2004). Environmental factors such as use of kitty litter may also be involved. The increase in the number of cats housed indoors and the corresponding change in quality of care and the types of cat food in the late 1960s and early 1970s followed by the sudden recognition of the disorder in the late 1970s supports a role for diet or the environment in the pathogenesis of hyperthyroidism. Iodine is one potential dietary goitrogen. Most commercially prepared cat foods contain adequate amounts of iodine, with measured levels ranging from three to 100 times recommended amounts (Mumma et al, 1986; Johnson et al, 1992). Variability in iodine intake has resulted in iodine-induced hyperthyroidism in people (Jodbasedow syndrome) (Skare and Frey, 1980; Fradkin and Wolff, 1983). In addition, deficient or excessive iodine intake in homemade or poorly formulated foods may also be goitrogenic (Scarlett, 1994). Soybean is another potential dietary goitrogen that is commonly used as a high quality vegetable protein in commercial cat foods (Court and Freeman, 2002; White et al, 2004). The goitrogenic effect of soybeans has been attributed to an inhibitory effect of the soy isoflavones genistein and daidzein on thyroid peroxidase, an enzyme essential to thyroid hormone synthesis (Divi et al, 1997). In a recent study, short-term administration of dietary soy to healthy cats resulted in a modest increase in serum T_4 and free T_4 concentrations relative to serum T_3 concentrations (White et al, 2004). One epidemiologic study found consumption of pop-top canned (compared to dry) food was associated with a greater risk of developing hyperthyroidism and speculated that the chemicals lining the cans, specifically bisphenol A, may have migrated into the food and served as a goitrogen (Edinboro et al, 2004). Bisphenol A reduces binding of T_3 to

Table 29-12. Key nutritional factors for hyperthyroid cats.*

Factors	Recommended food levels
Water	Fresh, clean water should be available at all times
Energy	Feeding at the DER for ideal weight in conjunction with adequate control of hyperthyroidism will result in desired body weight: Neutered cats: 1.2 x RER Intact cats: 1.4 x RER
Fat	Provide increased dietary fat for underweight cats Fat levels for normal cats are usually adequate until normal body condition is achieved (Tables 20-3 and 21-2)
Protein	Provide increased dietary protein for underweight cats The following levels are adequate unless renal function is compromised: 28 to 45%
Fiber	Avoid fiber levels >8 in cats with poor body condition
Macrominerals	Ensure food meets AAFCO recommendations for adult maintenance to compensate for increased losses of magnesium, potassium, chloride, calcium and phosphorus
Trace minerals	Generally, foods that meet AAFCO minimum allowances for trace minerals are adequate; however, commercial products vary greatly in trace mineral content It may be necessary to contact product manufacturers to determine iodine and selenium levels

Key: DER = daily energy requirement, RER = resting energy requirement, AAFCO = Association of American Feed Control Officials.
*Nutrients expressed on a % dry matter basis.

thyroid receptors and interferes with signal transduction in rats (Moriyama et al, 2002) and has been detected in canned cat foods (Kang and Kondo, 2002).

Recent studies have also identified overexpression of the *c-ras* oncogene in areas of nodular follicular hyperplasia in feline thyroid glands, suggesting that mutations in this oncogene may play a role in the etiopathogenesis of hyperthyroidism in cats (Merryman et al, 1999). In normal cells, activation of the *ras* protein leads to mitosis. Mutations of the *ras* oncogene produce mutated *ras* proteins, which are not subject to the normal cellular feedback mechanisms that prevent uncontrolled mitosis. Altered expression of G proteins involved in the signal transduction pathway that stimulates growth and differentiation of thyroid cells has also been identified in adenomatous thyroid glands obtained from hyperthyroid cats (Hammer et al, 2000; Ward et al, 2005). Decreased inhibitory G protein expression has been identified; a decrease that creates a relative increase in stimulatory G protein expression, which may stimulate unregulated mitogenesis and thyroid hormone production in hyperthyroid cells. Future studies will hopefully clarify the significance of these findings and the relationship between abnormalities identified in thyroid cells from hyperthyroid cats, potential dietary or chemical goitrogens identified in canned cat foods and the development of hyperthyroidism in cats.

Key Nutritional Factors

The key nutritional factors for foods for cats with hyperthyroidism are summarized in **Table 29-12** and discussed in more detail below. Some references are made to the key nutritional factor tables for young adult and mature adult cats that are of normal body weight (Tables 20-3 and 21-2).

WATER

Cats with hyperthyroidism often exhibit polydipsia and polyuria. Therefore, a readily available source of potable water is recommended for free-choice access.

ENERGY/FAT

Uncompensated hyperthyroid patients are usually in an increased metabolic, energy-deficit state. Treatment of the primary disease usually results in equilibration of energy requirements to what is expected for age and physiologic status. Therefore, primary emphasis should be directed at regulation of the disease process rather than nutritional intervention. Provision of DER at the calculated ideal body weight of the patient should result in rapid return to normal body weight if primary disease processes are controlled. DER: neutered cats = 1.2 x RER, intact cats = 1.4 x RER.

Hyperthyroid patients may have decreased fat stores because they are in an increased metabolic state. Treatment of the primary disease and use of a food that meets AAFCO nutrient allowances for the desired physiologic state should result in rapid normalization of body weight. If severe wasting of body mass has occurred, the fat content of foods may be increased to achieve higher energy density and enhance weight gain. See Tables 20-3 and 21-2 for recommended levels of dietary fat for foods for normal weight young adult cats and mature adult cats, respectively.

PROTEIN

Hyperthyroid cats are in a hypercatabolic state and may exhibit signs of protein wasting and deficiency. Increased protein intake may be needed during the recovery period to replenish body protein. However, hyperthyroidism is frequently associated with renal failure, which should prompt a complete evaluation of renal function before feeding higher protein foods (Chapter 37).

Provide increased dietary protein for underweight animals. The following DM levels are adequate unless renal function is compromised: 28 to 45%. True protein digestibility should be greater than 85%.

FIBER

Avoid food with DM fiber levels greater than 8% in patients with poor body condition (**Table 29-12**).

Other Nutritional Factors

MACROMINERALS

Because hyperthyroidism may result in macromineral abnormalities (i.e., phosphorus, potassium, sodium, calcium), it is best to avoid foods with excess (all-purpose foods) or deficient levels. Decreased sodium chloride intake may benefit some cases in which hypertension and cardiac disease are primary problems (Chapter 36). Foods that exceed AAFCO minimum nutrient allowances should suffice in most cases. Most commercial cat foods will provide adequate levels of these nutrients. A more refined recommendation would be the mineral key nutritional factor recommendations for normal weight young adult and mature adult cats (Tables 20-3 and 21-2).

TRACE MINERALS

Iodine may be excessive or deficient in different states of thyroid disease. Iodine intake should be thoroughly evaluated to determine adequacy. Generally, foods that meet AAFCO minimum allowances for trace minerals are adequate; however, some commercial products vary greatly in trace mineral content (**Box 29-3**).

Feeding and Treatment Plan for Hyperthyroid Cats

The success of nutritional management of hyperthyroidism depends to a great degree on the effectiveness of medical/surgical treatment for the primary disease. Three modes of treatment are generally accepted for hyperthyroidism in cats: 1) long-term antithyroid medication, 2) surgical thyroidectomy and 3) radioactive iodine (Kintzer, 1994).

Assess and Select the Food

Information obtained from assessing the food is essential for making changes to foods currently fed. Compare the current food's key nutritional factor content with the recommendations in **Table 29-12** and those in Tables 20-3 and 21-2 for healthy young adult and mature adult cats in the sections for normal body weight and condition. Identify any discrepancies between the recommended levels of key nutritional factors and current intake. If discrepancies exist, consider selecting a food that more closely matches the key nutritional factor targets from Tables 20-3 and 21-2. During the convalescent period, in those cases that require additional protein and energy to regain body weight, commercially prepared maintenance-type foods may be mixed with growth/reproduction-type formulas to achieve higher protein and fat intakes (Feldman and Nelson, 2004e). However, growth/reproduction-type foods may add excessive sodium and phosphorus possibly complicating concurrent renal disease or primary cardiac disease, if present.

Assess and Determine the Feeding Method

It may not always be necessary to change the feeding method when managing animals with hyperthyroidism. However, a thorough evaluation includes verification that an appropriate feeding method is being used. Any deviations from ideal feeding methods should be identified and changes made as required.

Patients will usually return to normal body weight if provided energy at the calculated DER for ideal body weight. Small amounts in several feedings may need to be fed during recovery. Two daily feedings are adequate after a patient resumes normal eating behavior.

Reassessment

Patient response to treatment is assessed by owner observation of clinical signs, bimonthly body weight charting and monitoring food intake, findings on physical examination and measurement of serum T_4 concentrations. Return to normal activity, body condition and appearance, and normal serum T_4 concentration indicate a successful response to treatment. Treatment is inadequate if clinical signs persist, body weight and body condition remain poor and serum T_4 concentration remains increased. Adjustments in the treatment regimen and problems with owner compliance should be considered if the cat is being treated with oral methimazole. Remnants of hyperfunctioning thyroid tissue should be considered if thyroidectomy was performed or radioactive iodine-131 was administered.

HYPOTHYROIDISM

Adult-onset hypothyroidism may be the most common endocrine disease affecting dogs and results from destruction of the thyroid gland. Two histologic forms of primary hypothyroidism predominate in dogs: lymphocytic thyroiditis and idiopathic atrophy. Lymphocytic thyroiditis is an immune-mediated disorder that appears to have a genetic component based on breed predisposition for the disease (Nachreiner et al, 2002). Idiopathic atrophy of the thyroid gland may be a primary degenerative disorder or an endstage of lymphocytic thyroiditis (Gosselin et al, 1981; Conaway et al, 1985). In contrast, naturally-acquired adult-onset hypothyroidism occurs rarely in cats, but iatrogenic hypothyroidism may occur following treatment of hyperthyroidism. Congenital hypothyroidism is very uncommon in dogs and cats and usually results from thyroid dysgenesis or dyshormonogenesis (Feldman and Nelson, 2004c).

The diagnosis of hypothyroidism is based on the presence of appropriate clinical signs (**Table 29-8**), findings on physical examination, results of routine blood and urine tests and tests of thyroid gland function, including serum T_4, free T_4 and TSH (**Table 29-10**). Treatment involves oral administration of sodium levothyroxine once or twice daily. In adult dogs, all abnormalities caused by hypothyroidism will resolve with appropriate thyroid hormone replacement therapy. A tendency to gain weight and development of hyperlipidemia are two problems associated with untreated hypothyroidism that may require dietary intervention. Weight gain often occurs without a corresponding increase in appetite or food intake. In one study, energy expenditure, as measured by indirect calorimetry, was approximately 15% lower in hypothyroid dogs, compared with healthy dogs (Greco et al, 1998). Energy expenditure returned to normal after initiating levothyroxine sodium treatment. Initiating a weight-loss program in conjunction with thyroid hormone replacement therapy is warranted in obese

Box 29-3. Role of Selenium and Iodine Excess in Hyperthyroid Disease.

Since the first clinical reports in 1979 and 1980, pathologic and epidemiologic studies of hyperthyroidism have indicated that the incidence of the disease has increased. A recent study showed that the prevalence of this disease increased 20% over a 20-year period and the estimated overall prevalence is 2%. The cause of this epizootic is important, particularly because this disease has become a leading cause of morbidity in middle-aged and older cats.

A number of epidemiologic studies indicate a greater incidence of hyperthyroidism in cats consuming canned foods (i.e., two- to fourfold higher incidence in cat populations consuming canned foods relative to cats consuming dry foods only). **Figures 1** and **2** show that selenium concentrations are markedly higher in canned cat foods vs. dry cat foods, suggesting that selenium could be a factor in this disease. Selenium concentrations in cat foods are also higher than in dog foods. This selenium difference may explain why hyperthyroidism is prevalent in cats, but not dogs. There is also a known metabolic basis for selenium's involvement in thyroid hormone metabolism. Iodothyronine deiodinase, the enzyme that converts thyroxine (T_4) to the metabolically active 3,3'-5 triiodothyronine (T_3), is a selenium-containing enzyme.

Iodine is another nutrient that can profoundly affect thyroid gland function. Iodine concentrations in pet foods can vary widely from deficient to excess (100x the minimum recommended dietary allowance). This variation may be of importance; people living in iodine-deficient areas who later become exposed to normal or excessive amounts of iodine can present with signs of hyperthyroidism.

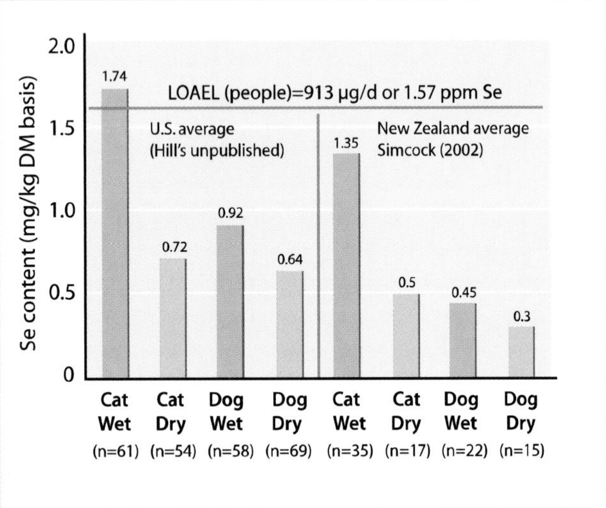

Figure 1. Selenium (Se) concentrations in U.S. vs. New Zealand pet food. Bars represent average Se concentration (dry matter basis) for four categories: Wet (canned) cat food, dry cat food, wet dog food and dry dog food and compare U.S. products (left) vs. New Zealand products (right) (n = number of samples). Se concentrations in U.S. wet and dry cat food ranged from 0.81 to 5.0 and 0.43 to 1.9 mg/kg Se, respectively. Se ranges were not given for New Zealand products. Regardless of country, Se concentrations in wet cat food are generally two- fourfold higher than those of dry cat food. Furthermore, Se concentrations in most wet cat foods exceed safe upper limits established for people, but vary widely among products of pet food companies. Key: LOAEL = lowest observable adverse effect level.

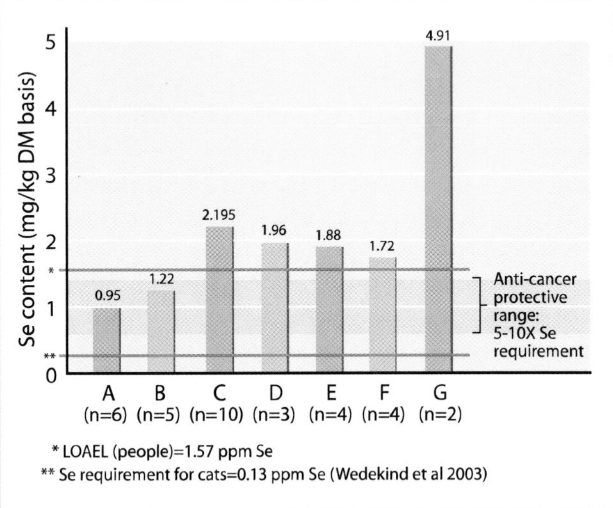

Figure 2. Selenium (Se) concentrations in U.S. feline canned foods. Companies are not identified, but noted as A to G; (n = number of samples). Bars represent average Se concentrations (dry matter [DM] basis). Se concentrations ranged from 0.81 to 5.0 mg/kg. The minimum Se requirement of adult cats is 0.13 mg/kg DM Se (Wedekind et al, 2003). According to sources, beneficial anti-cancer effects are observed when Se is fed at 5 to 10x the requirement (Combs, 2000; Neve, 2002). For cats, this optimal range is 0.65 to 1.3 mg/kg. However, the safe upper limit for Se for cats should probably be set at 1.3 mg/kg Se. There is probably little benefit of additional Se above this range and possibly harm. In people, the lowest observable adverse effect level (LOAEL) occurs at 913 μg/d and the no observable adverse effect level (NOAEL) occurs at 800 μg/d (DRI, 2001), which equates to 1.57 mg/kg Se (metabolic equivalent for cats) and 1.38 mg/kg Se, respectively. Overt signs of selenosis in people include hair loss and nail sloughing.

Figures 3 and **4** confirm the variability and excessive levels of iodine concentrations that exist in some commercial pet foods. There have been several theories regarding the role of diet and environment in hyperthyroid disease: 1) iodine excess, 2) immunoglobulins, 3) goitrogenic compounds and 4) environmental exposure to chemicals and infectious agents. However, none of these theories have conclusively identified the factor or factors involved in this disease.

The evidence presented below suggests selenium as a factor in the disease. One other study evaluated the role of selenium in hyperthyroid cats, but these researchers were unable to document a link between selenium status and hyperthyroid incidence.

Evidence of selenium's role in feline hyperthyroidism:

1. Serum T_3 increases with increasing selenium intake. There is a metabolic basis for selenium's role in thyroid hormone metabolism.
2. Serum T_3 is highly correlated with serum selenium concentration.
3. Serum selenium concentrations are higher in cats (approximately fivefold greater) than levels in other species. Cats fed foods containing similar selenium levels as dogs have significantly higher serum selenium concentrations (**Table 1**).
4. A dose-titration study in dogs showed excess selenium produces changes in thyroid hormone profiles directionally similar to those cited for hyperthyroid cats (**Table 2**).
5. Higher selenium concentrations are present in canned cat foods relative to dry cat foods and dry or canned dog foods (**Figure 1**).

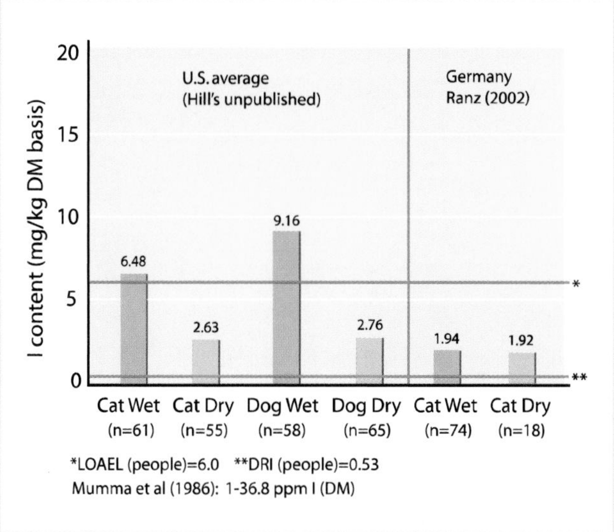

Figure 3. Iodine (I) concentrations in U.S. pet foods vs. cat foods in Germany. Bars represent average I concentration (dry matter basis) for four categories: Wet (canned) cat food, dry cat food, wet dog food and dry dog food and compare U.S. products (left) vs. Germany products (cat foods only) (right) (n = number of samples). I concentrations in U.S. cat foods ranged from 1.1 to 52.3 mg/kg; I concentrations in U.S. dog foods ranged from 0.8 to 196.8 mg/kg. Cat foods from Germany ranged from 0.22 to 6.4 mg/kg I. Likewise, other investigators found highly variable and high I concentrations in U.S. pet foods (e.g., 1 to 36.8 mg/kg I) (Mumma et al, 1986). In the U.S., wet pet foods are typically higher in I than dry pet foods. Also, U.S. dog foods were generally higher in I than cat foods, but were highly variable. In people, the no observable adverse effect level (NOAEL) and lowest observable adverse effect level (LOAEL) for I are 1,000 and 1,700 μg/day, respectively (DRI, 2001). According to research, there is good agreement between people and cats with regards to measures of I status; thus, the human guidelines should be applicable to cats, and would equate to 3.5 and 6.0 mg/kg I, respectively (Wedekind et al, In press). Note that a number of pet foods exceed the safe upper limit established for people. High I intakes in people have been associated with thyroiditis, goiter, hypothyroidism, hyperthyroidism, thyroid papillary cancer and iodermia, a dermatologic reaction to iodine (DRI, 2001).

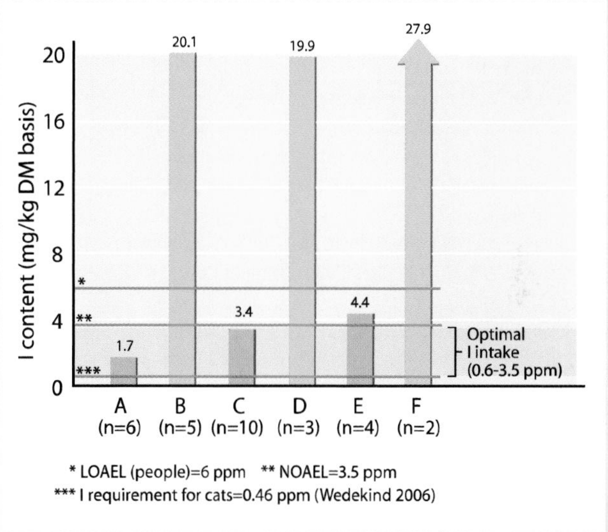

Figure 4. Iodine (I) concentrations in U.S. feline canned foods. Companies are denoted as A to F and not identified by name (n = number of samples). Bars represent average I concentrations (dry matter basis). I concentrations ranged from 1.1 to 52.3 mg/kg. The minimum I requirement of adult cats is 0.46 mg/kg (Wedekind et al, In press). For cats, the recommended optimal I range is between 0.60 to 3.5 mg/kg. The lower end is based on the experimentally derived requirement, plus 30% overage to allow for lower availability in certain foods, whereas the upper limit is extrapolated from people and is based on the no observable adverse effect level (NOAEL). In people, 10x the daily I requirement may lead to goiter and hypothyroidism (Pennington, 1990). Therefore, the upper limit should probably be less than 10x the cat requirement (i.e., 1,000 μg/day or 3.5 mg/kg I). Note that I concentrations vary widely by products from different companies and may greatly exceed safe upper limits established for people.

Box 29-3 continued

Selenium concentrations in canned cat foods are two times greater than those in dry cat foods. A two- to fourfold greater incidence of hyperthyroidism occurs in cats consuming canned foods.

6. Selenium concentrations in a number of feline canned foods (**Figure 2**) average 1.74 mg/kg selenium. This equates to 517 µg/day (i.e., the metabolic equivalent for people). This level is 19-fold higher than the human dietary reference intake (DRI) (55 µg selenium/day) and 13 to 15x higher than canine and feline selenium requirements. Similarly, other researchers have suggested that selenium concentrations in feline canned foods are excessive. Safe upper limits for selenium have not yet been defined for foods for cats.

Despite the high-selenium concentrations in commercial cat foods, no reported cases of clinical selenium toxicity in cats could be found. One possible explanation is that high-protein foods may be protective against selenium toxicity. For example, 10 mg/kg selenium was toxic in rats fed foods containing 10% crude protein, but not when fed foods that contained 20% crude protein. Because cats are strict carnivores, protein requirements are higher than for dogs or people. Although clinical signs of selenium toxicity have not been reported in cats, consuming high dietary selenium may result in changes in thyroid hormone metabolism that predispose cats to hyperthyroidism.

The cause of hyperthyroidism in cats is unknown. Previous research suggested iodine as a factor, but findings were inconclusive. The studies reported here point to excess selenium as a factor in this disease. Optimal ranges and consistent levels of selenium and iodine in commercial pet foods may prevent or decrease the prevalence of hyperthyroidism in cats.

Table 1. Serum selenium (Se) concentrations in cats and dogs fed foods with similar Se content.

Dietary Se* (mg Se/kg food)	Serum Se (cats) (µmol/l)	Serum Se (cats) (µg/ml)	Serum Se (dogs) (µmol/l)	Serum Se (dogs) (µg/ml)
0.1	5.18	0.41	3.42	0.272
1.0	7.12	0.56	4.18	0.332
5.0	11.2	0.88	6.97	0.554

*Se provided as selenomethionine and fed to dogs and cats for six months.

Table 2. Similarities between thyroid hormone profiles of hyperthyroid cats vs. those of adult dogs fed excessive selenium.

Thyroid hormone profile	Hyperthyroid cats	Hormone profile difference (%)*
Total T_4	High	↑ 21
Free T_4	May be elevated	↑ 12
Total T_3	May be elevated	↑ 44 (significant)
Free T_3	May be elevated	↑ 33 (outside normal range)
cTSH	Depressed	↑ 16 (significant)
Reverse T_3	?	↑ 29 (significant)

*Dogs fed 5 mg/kg selenium compared to dogs fed a control food (0.12 mg/kg selenium).

The Bibliography for **Box 29-3** can be found at www.markmorris.org.

dogs diagnosed with hypothyroidism (Table 27-7).

Fasting hypercholesterolemia, hypertriglyceridemia and lipemia are classic clinical chemistry findings in dogs with hypothyroidism. Hyperlipidemia can become severe with serum cholesterol and triglyceride concentrations exceeding 1,000 mg/dl. Thyroid hormones stimulate virtually all aspects of lipid metabolism, including synthesis, mobilization and degradation (Mahley et al, 2003). Both synthesis and degradation of lipids are depressed in hypothyroidism, with degradation affected more than synthesis. The net effect is an accumulation of plasma lipids and the potential for development of atherosclerosis (Hess et al, 2003). Fortunately, hyperlipidemia resolves fairly quickly after initiation of thyroid hormone replacement therapy. Regardless, feeding lower fat-containing foods to hyperlipidemic dogs diagnosed with hypothyroidism is warranted to help correct the hyperlipidemia, minimize problems associated with hyperlipidemia (e.g., atherosclerosis, abdominal discomfort, neurologic signs, pancreatitis) and reduce caloric intake to favor weight loss.

REFERENCES

The references for **Chapter 29** can be found at www.markmorris.org.

CASE 29-1

Polydipsia/Polyuria in a Cat

Richard W. Nelson, DVM, Dipl. ACVIM (Internal Medicine)
School of Veterinary Medicine
University of California, Davis
Davis, California, USA

Patient Assessment

A six-year-old, neutered female domestic shorthair cat was examined for polydipsia and polyuria of two weeks' duration, lethargy and anorexia. The cat remained indoors at all times and had been overweight for several years.

Physical examination revealed an alert, hydrated cat. Body weight was 4.8 kg with a body condition score (BCS) of 5/5. The optimal body weight was estimated to be 3.5 kg. The abdomen was tense when palpated but nonpainful. The borders of the liver were palpable beyond the margins of the rib cage and the bladder was distended. The coat had a greasy appearance with slight dander.

Results of a complete blood count were normal. Abnormal serum biochemistry profile results included increased glucose (398 mg/dl, reference interval = 70 to 110 mg/dl) and cholesterol (416 mg/dl, reference interval = 90 to 250 mg/dl) concentrations. Urinalysis revealed glucosuria and a urine specific gravity of 1.019. The tentative diagnoses were diabetes mellitus and obesity.

Assess the Food and Feeding Method

The cat was normally fed a commercial specialty brand dry cat food (Science Diet Feline Maintenance[a]) free choice and one can of a commercial grocery brand "gourmet" cat food (Fancy Feast Chunk Chicken Feast[b]) twice daily. **Table 1** lists nutrient levels in these foods. The gourmet food contained approximately 85 kcal (356 kJ) per can. Water was available free choice. The cat's appetite had always been very good until yesterday.

Questions

1. What factors may have predisposed this cat to developing diabetes mellitus?
2. What key nutritional factors should be considered for this patient?
3. Outline an appropriate feeding plan (foods and feeding method) for this cat.
4. How should this patient be monitored?

Answers and Discussion

1. Obesity is a known risk factor for development of non-insulin-dependent diabetes mellitus (type II), especially in cats. Type II diabetes mellitus may occur in obese animals subsequent to down regulation of peripheral insulin receptors, as occurs in people.
2. The key nutritional factors for patients with uncomplicated diabetes mellitus are water, digestible (soluble) carbohydrate, fiber, fat, protein and food form (avoid semi-moist foods). Dietary minerals and vitamins may also be important in patients with some forms of diabetes mellitus (ketoacidosis) and those with prolonged polydipsia and polyuria. Water should always be available free choice and in abundant amounts. The amount of energy and source of energy substrates (e.g., avoid simple sugars and fat) are also important. Complex carbohydrates and protein best supply energy for this patient. Excess dietary fat should also be avoided as part of a weight-reduction program. Increased dietary fiber helps reduce the caloric density of the food and helps maintain glycemic control in conjunction with medical management.
3. The goals of dietary management for this cat include: 1) reducing weight to improve or eliminate peripheral insulin resistance and other metabolic abnormalities, 2) providing consistent daily energy intake and 3) minimizing postprandial fluctuations in serum glucose concentrations. The cat should be fed a food that contains lower energy density, lower fat and higher crude fiber levels than the foods currently being offered. The amount of food should be divided and offered at least twice daily immediately after treatment with insulin or oral hypoglycemic agents. Daily food dosage should be calculated for optimal body weight. Many well-regulated overweight diabetic cats lose weight when fed at optimal body weight. An energy calculation of 1.2 x resting energy requirement (RER) for the estimated optimal body weight is a reasonable starting point.
4. Response to treatment can be assessed through careful owner observation. Favorable response to treatment is indicated by decreased water intake, decreased urination, decreased food intake (in animals that exhibit polyphagia), achievement of weight goals and a generalized increased thriftiness. Unfavorable responses include continuation of polydipsia, polyuria, polyphagia and inability to achieve weight goals. If the animal is stable and doing well then veterinary reassessment should take place every three to four months. If the animal is symptomatic then veterinary reassessment should take place every one to two weeks until stable.

   Achievement of weight goals can be measured through BCS and body weight. Cats should be weighed and have body condition assessed at least once a month. The owner may keep a chart of body weight and BCS. Weight loss will usually take six to 12 months to occur. A loss of 10% body weight in already thin animals indicates a need for reassessment of the dietary regimen and diabetic regulation.

Maintenance of body weight with a reduction in food intake should occur in polyphagic animals responding favorably to exogenous insulin administration. This response occurs due to increased nutrient usage associated with hormonal treatment. If animals exhibit anorexia or depressed food intake then the relative palatability of the food may be poor and another food should be tried after ruling out medical causes. It is especially important to monitor food intake in cats because prolonged anorexia can lead to hepatic lipidosis.

Abnormalities in the serum biochemistry profile should return to normal with well-controlled diabetes and adequate nutritional intake. The major exception to this is hyperglycemia, which may or may not be present depending on when the blood sample is obtained in relation to when insulin is administered. Abnormalities of biochemical constituents in the face of controlled diabetes mellitus should be evaluated as separate disease entities.

Progress Notes

An oral hypoglycemic sulfonylurea drug (glipizide[c]) was chosen (5 mg per os, twice daily) because the owners did not want to give insulin injections. The food was changed to a commercial moist veterinary therapeutic food (Prescription Diet w/d Feline[a]) that was lower in fat (16.6% dry matter [DM]) and higher in crude fiber (approximately 10% DM) than the previous foods. The digestible carbohydrate content of the new food was approximately 27% DM. The daily food amount was divided into two meals and offered 30 minutes after the drug treatment each morning and evening. Total daily energy intake was initially calculated at 1.2 x RER for a body weight of 3.5 kg (210 kcal/day, 880 kJ/day).

The cat lost weight over the next six months. It reached a body weight of 3.8 kg (BCS 3/5) and glipizide was eventually discontinued because normal glucose tolerance was maintained with dietary management alone. The lower fat, higher fiber food was continued but the amount fed was increased to maintain optimum body weight and condition.

Endnotes

a. Hill's Pet Nutrition, Inc., Topeka, KS, USA. This product is currently available as Science Diet Adult Original.
b. Friskies Petcare Co, Glendale, CA, USA.
c. Glucotrol. Roerig Division, Pfizer Inc., New York, NY, USA.

Bibliography

Kirk CA, Feldman EC, Nelson RW. Diagnosis of naturally acquired type-I and type-II diabetes mellitus in cats. American Journal of Veterinary Research 1993; 54: 463-467.

Nelson RW, Feldman EC, Ford SL, et al. Effect of an orally administered sulfonylurea, glipizide, for treatment of diabetes mellitus in cats. Journal of the American Veterinary Medical Association 1993; 203: 821-827.

Table 1. Nutrient levels in foods fed to a diabetic cat.

Nutrients (DM)	Dry specialty brand food*	Moist grocery brand food**
Crude fat (%)	23.0	34.0
Crude fiber (%)	1.0	0.4
Energy (kcal/g)	4.5	4.9
NFE (%)	37.0	5.3
Protein (%)	33.8	50.8

Key: DM = dry matter, NFE = nitrogen-free extract.
*Science Diet Feline Maintenance, Hill's Pet Nutrition, Inc., Topeka, KS, USA.
**Fancy Feast Chunk Chicken Feast, Friskies Petcare Co, Glendale, CA, USA.

CASE 29-2

Insulin Resistance in a Labrador Retriever

Richard W. Nelson, DVM, Dipl. ACVIM (Internal Medicine)
School of Veterinary Medicine
University of California, Davis
Davis, California, USA

Patient Assessment

A five-year-old, 39-kg, castrated male Labrador retriever was admitted to a referral institution because of difficulty in controlling diabetes mellitus. Insulin-dependent diabetes mellitus (type I) had been diagnosed one year before referral. The dog had initially responded well to 25 IU of beef/pork NPH insulin administered once daily. During the two months before referral, the dog developed progressively worsening polydipsia and polyuria despite receiving 50 IU of insulin once daily. The owner and referring veterinarian reported no other abnormalities.

The dog was alert and responsive with normal temperature, pulse and respiratory rate. Abnormalities identified included obesity (body condition score 5/5), hepatomegaly and a dry lusterless coat. The estimated optimal body weight was approximately 32 kg.

Abnormalities of the serum biochemistry profile included hyperglycemia, preprandial lipemia, hypercholesterolemia and increased alanine aminotransferase activity. Urinalysis revealed glucosuria and bacteriuria and a urine culture isolated *Escherichia coli.* Abdominal ultrasonography and thoracic radiographs were unremarkable. An initial blood glucose curve revealed persistent hyperglycemia at all time points (greater than 300 mg/dl).

Assess the Food and Feeding Method

The dog was fed a mixture of commercial moist and dry food twice daily. One can of a grocery brand dog food (Cycle Adult[a]) mixed with one to two cups of a dry grocery brand dog food (Alpo Beef Flavored Dinner[a]) was offered at the time of the insulin injection in the morning. A second portion of the same dry and moist food mixture was offered eight hours later. **Table 1** lists nutrient levels in these foods. The dog was eating approximately 1,600 to 1,800 kcal/day (6.69 to 7.53 MJ).

Questions

1. What factors may be contributing to the apparent insulin resistance in this dog?
2. What are the key nutritional factors that should be considered in this patient?
3. Outline an appropriate feeding plan (food and feeding method) for this dog.
4. What concurrent therapy should be used in this patient?

Answers and Discussion

1. Insulin resistance exists whenever normal concentrations of insulin produce a less than normal biologic response. Proposed mechanisms for insulin resistance include: 1) an abnormal insulin molecule, 2) increased insulin degradation, 3) insulin antibodies, 4) insulin-receptor antibodies, 5) high circulating levels of counter-regulatory hormones, 6) insulin-receptor defects (altered numbers or affinity) and 7) postreceptor defects. In diabetic dogs and cats, insulin resistance has been arbitrarily defined to exist when therapeutic doses of insulin exceed 2.0 to 2.5 units/kg body weight per day. Conditions that can contribute to insulin resistance include obesity, hyperadrenocorticism, acromegaly (excess growth hormone), hyperthyroidism (cats), hypothyroidism, renal failure, liver disease, bacterial infections, pregnancy and anti-insulin antibodies.
2. The key nutritional factors for patients with uncomplicated diabetes mellitus are water, digestible (soluble) carbohydrate, fiber, fat, protein and food form (avoid semi-moist foods). Water should always be available free choice and in abundant amounts. The source of energy substrates (e.g., avoid simple sugars) are also important. Excess dietary fat should be avoided as part of a weight-reduction program. Increased dietary fiber helps reduce the caloric density of the food and helps maintain glycemic control in conjunction with medical management.
3. The goals of dietary management in this dog include: 1) decrease obesity, which may improve or eliminate peripheral insulin resistance and other metabolic abnormalities, 2) provide consistent daily energy intake and 3) minimize postprandial fluctuations in serum glucose concentrations. The dog should be fed a food that contains lower energy density, lower fat and higher crude fiber levels than the foods currently being offered. The amount of food should be divided and offered at least twice daily immediately after treatment with insulin. Daily food dosage should be calculated; a starting energy calculation of 1.0 x resting energy requirement (RER) for the estimated optimal body weight is a reasonable starting point.
4. The bacterial urinary tract infection may be contributing to insulin resistance and should be eliminated with appropriate antimicrobial therapy. The beef/pork insulin should also be changed to another insulin type in case anti-insulin antibodies are contributing to the problem.

Progress Notes

The urinary tract infection was treated with oral cefadroxil[b] for 10 days and the insulin was changed to 55 IU recombinant human Lente insulin[c] every 12 hours, subcutaneously. The food was changed to a commercial dry veterinary therapeutic food that was lower in fat, higher in digestible carbohydrates and higher in dietary fiber (Prescription Diet w/d Canine[d]) than the current foods (**Table 1**). The estimated daily energy requirement for weight loss was 1,000 kcal/day (4.18 MJ); this was met by feeding 2.25 cups twice daily shortly after insulin administration.

Reassessment one month later showed that insulin continued to be ineffective despite increasing the dose to 60 IU every 12 hours, subcutaneously. The owner reported recent lethargy, weakness and excessive shedding in addition to continuing polydipsia and polyuria. Results of serum biochemistry analysis, urinalysis, blood glucose curves and a complete blood count had not changed from those values at the initial presentation. Baseline serum thyroxine concentration was low (0.6 µg/dl, reference = 1.5 to 3.5 µg/dl) and decreased to 0.5 µg/dl four hours following administration of 200 µg of thyrotropin-releasing hormone (TRH). Hypothyroidism with insulin resistance, diabetes mellitus and obesity became the working diagnoses. Levothyroxine sodium[e] (0.8 mg, per os, every 12 hours) was initiated and the insulin dosage was reduced (30 IU, subcutaneously, every 12 hours). The feeding plan was unchanged.

Over the next three months the insulin dosage was stabilized at 28 IU, subcutaneously, every 12 hours. The dog's activity level and coat improved. A weight loss of 5 kg was attained as well. Abnormalities in the serum biochemistry profile were alleviated except for the hyperglycemia. Serum thyroxine concentration six hours after levothyroxine administration was 4.8 µg/dl (normal = 1.5 to 3.5 µg/dl).

Additional Comments

Diabetes mellitus in dogs is most often insulin-dependent. When conventional therapy fails to work, other disease processes should be considered as well as other modalities of treatment for diabetes control. The use of a low-fat, high-fiber food in this case was beneficial for weight reduction and maintaining glycemic control.

Endnotes

a. Friskies Petcare Co, Glendale, CA, USA.
b. Cefa-Tabs. Fort Dodge Laboratories, Fort Dodge, IA, USA.
c. Humulin L. Eli Lilly & Co, Indianapolis, IN, USA.
d. Hill's Pet Nutrition, Inc., Topeka, KS, USA.
e. Soloxine. Daniels Pharmaceuticals, St. Petersburg, FL, USA.

Bibliography

Nelson RW. Insulin resistance in diabetic dogs and cats. In: Bonagura JD, ed. Current Veterinary Therapy XII. Philadelphia, PA: WB Saunders Co, 1995; 390-393.

Peterson ME, Sampson GR. Insulin and insulin syringes. In: Bonagura JD, ed. Current Veterinary Therapy XII. Philadelphia, PA: WB Saunders Co, 1995; 387-390.

Table 1. Nutrient levels in foods fed to a diabetic dog.

Nutrients (DM)	Dry grocery brand food*	Moist grocery brand food**	Dry veterinary therapeutic food***
Crude fat (%)	13.3	21.8	9.0
Crude fiber (%)	4.3	1.1	17.6
Energy (kcal/g)	3.7	4.4	3.3
Protein (%)	24.8	39.7	18.9
Digestible carbohydrate (%)	52.2	28.3	50.1

Key: DM = dry matter.
*Alpo Beef Flavored Dinner. Friskies Petcare Co, Glendale, CA, USA.
**Cycle Adult. Friskies Petcare Co, Glendale, CA, USA.
***Prescription Diet w/d Canine. Hill's Pet Nutrition, Inc., Topeka, KS, USA.

Section 9

Neoplastic Disorders

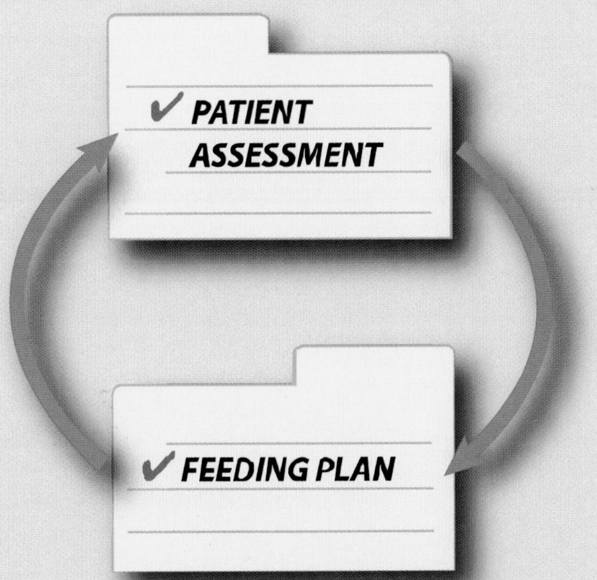

Chapter 30

Cancer

Korinn E. Saker
Kimberly A. Selting

"Life well spent is long."
Leonardo da Vinci

CLINICAL IMPORTANCE

Cancer is among the most common causes of nonaccidental death of dogs and cats, often ranking first or second (Bonnett et al, 2005; Egenvall et al, 2005; Proschowsky et al, 2003; Moore et al, 2001). One study documented that 23% of 2,000 pets examined at necropsy died of cancer (Bronson, 1982). Additionally, in a more recent study of more than 350,000 insured dogs, cancer was the most common cause of death, accounting for 18% of deaths; cancer occurred more commonly in females than in males for most breeds (Egenvall et al, 2005).

In cats, cancer also commonly threatens life and quality of life. Cats have the largest number of different retroviruses of any companion animal and these are closely linked to feline leukemia virus infection (FeLV). The overall prevalence (number of diagnosed cases/year) of FeLV infection in the United States is between 1 and 3%; however, the prevalence may be as high as 30% in multi-cat households and 11.5% in sick cats (Macy, 1996). In addition, known carcinogens can affect animals as well as people. Recent studies have investigated the link between environmental tobacco smoke and the development of cancers such as lymphoma and squamous cell carcinoma (SCC) in cats, and respiratory tumors in dogs (Snyder et al, 2004; Bertone et al, 2002, 2003; Reif et al, 1998). Additional environmental risk factors for SCC in cats include consumption of canned food and tuna fish, and the use of flea collars. For dogs, the indoor use of kerosene or coal also increased the risk of sinonasal cancer. Furthermore, obesity and insecticide use have been linked to bladder cancer (Bukowksi et al, 1998; Glickman et al, 1989).

Often, cancer results in either rapid weight loss or an inability or unwillingness to eat that is difficult to circumvent. Nutritional options for cats with cancer are less well studied though equally important. Because of their size, cats may necessitate increased frequency of nutritional support. The overall prevalence of cancer in pets appears to be increasing (Macy, 1996) for a variety of reasons, including greater longevity, improved veterinary care and an increased awareness of veterinarians through specialty services and advanced diagnostics.

Cancer incidence continues to increase in the human population as well. Statistics show that approximately 38% of women and 45% of men will develop cancer in their lifetime (Jemal et al, 2007). An estimated 1.3 million people were projected to be newly diagnosed with cancer in 2006, and more than a half million people were projected to die (Jemal et al, 2007). Therefore, it is not unusual to realize that many pet owners have had a personal experience with cancer affecting themselves, family members, friends or acquaintances. Veterinarians and health care teams should approach pets with cancer, and their owners, in a positive, compassionate and knowledgeable manner. Many owners understand or are willing to be educated about the importance of nutrition and how proper feeding can enhance the quality and length of life for

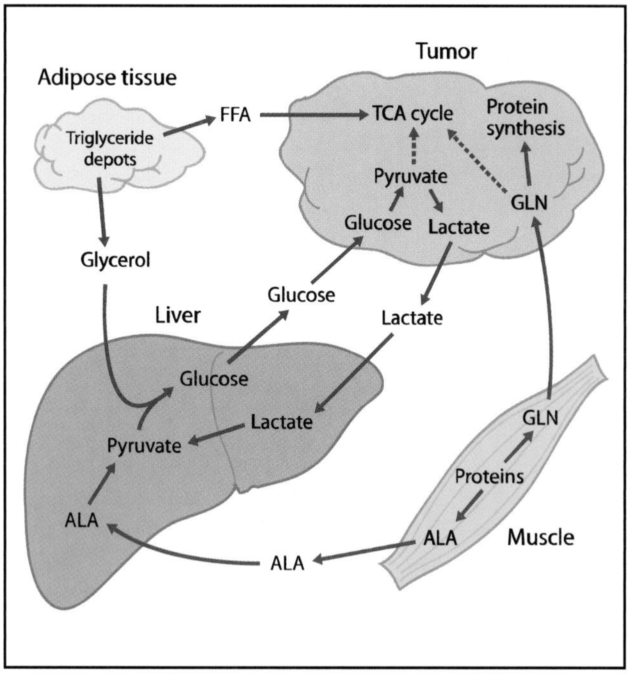

Figure 30-1. Metabolic relationships in cancer lead to increased proteolysis in the host's tissues, especially skeletal muscle. The Cori and glucose-alanine cycles undergo increased activity. High circulating concentrations of alanine (ALA) and glutamine (GLN) result, helping to feed the high glucose demand of the tumor.

pets with cancer.

Nutritional support can reduce or prevent toxicoses associated with cancer therapy and ameliorate the metabolic alterations induced by cancer in dogs and cats. Additionally, there is growing evidence that specific nutrients can be used to treat cancer directly or indirectly. This chapter focuses on the nutritional management of patients with cancer rather than on cancer prevention.

PATIENT ASSESSMENT

History and Physical Examination

The metabolic and clinical alterations in cancer patients have been described in four phases (**Table 30-1**) (Ogilvie and Vail, 1996, 1992, 1990; Ogilvie and Moore, 1995, 1995a; Shein et al, 1976; Theologides, 1979; Buzby and Steinberg, 1981; Landel et al, 1985; Bray and Campfield, 1975; Vail et al, 1990). The first phase is a preclinical "silent" phase in which patients do not exhibit overt clinical signs of disease, but subtle changes in behavior can often be observed. As the underlying malignancy progresses, owners often state that their pet seems to be "slowing down" or aging more rapidly, or is less active and less willing to engage in normal activities. Despite normal clinical appearances, patients in Phase 1 have quantifiable metabolic changes such as hyperlactatemia, hyperinsulinemia and alterations in blood amino acid profiles (**Figure 30-1**).

The second phase is a clinical phase in which patients begin to exhibit anorexia, lethargy and early evidence of weight loss. These patients are likely to exhibit side effects associated with chemotherapy, radiation therapy, immunotherapy and surgery that may alter nutrient intake and use, and thus the nutrition support plan.

The third phase (cancer cachexia) is characterized by marked debilitation, weakness and biochemical evidence of negative nitrogen balance such as hypoalbuminemia. In this phase, cancer patients begin to lose body protein and fat stores. Chronic vomiting, diarrhea, weakness, lethargy and weight loss are reported by owners of dogs and cats with endstage cancer.

A fourth phase (recovery or remission) occurs in those patients undergoing treatment with apparent elimination of their disease. Metabolic alterations persist in some patients despite elimination or control of the cancer via chemotherapy, radiation or surgery. Here again, the therapy itself may cause changes that affect the feeding plan. Animals may develop food aversions at any time because of treatment-induced alterations in taste and smell.

Clinical staging of cancer is performed by assessing tumor size, depth of tumor invasion, presence of tumor in regional lymph nodes and by identifying tumors in distant sites. This information is used to stage tumors by the TNM system: T (tumor size and/or invasion), N (nodal involvement) and M (distant metastasis). Tumor staging may correlate with clinical behavior in certain types of cancer and, in the future, may help determine whether a tumor will respond to nutritional management. To date, body condition scoring and body weight changes are the most practical tools for monitoring the overall nutritional effects of cancer and cancer treatment in dogs and cats (Chapter 1).

Laboratory and Other Clinical Information

Laboratory evaluation of total lymphocyte count, hematocrit, serum glucose, albumin, urea nitrogen concentrations and thyroid hormone levels can be helpful to further evaluate nutritional status. Toxic changes in neutrophils have been seen in cats with cachexia, and were significantly associated with longer hospitalization and higher treatment cost (Segev et al, 2006). Use of these parameters is somewhat limited because they may have causes unrelated to cancer. Albumin also has a relatively long half-life (eight days in normal dogs; the half-life of albumin in cats is unknown, but suspected to be between 5.7 and 8.2 days) and is slow to respond to changes in nutritional status. Plasma levels of triiodothyronine (T_3), reverse T_3, free thyroxine (T_4) and thyroid stimulating hormone (TSH) were severely altered in malnourished patients undergoing surgery for T_1 to T_4 carcinomas of the head and neck, as compared to well-fed cohorts. This study suggests, as starvation and overfeeding modulate thyroid hormone metabolism, thyroid hormone status can potentially be used to evaluate nutritional status of cancer patients (Siroen et al, 2006).

Body weight becomes an insensitive index in patients with severe intestinal malassimilation including marked hypoalbuminemia and ascites due to changes in total body water rather than lean body mass. Apart from this, body weight is a very sensitive long-term (weeks to months) indicator of decline or recovery of animals. Dogs and cats in the pre-clinical or "silent" phase may appear clinically normal but may gradually lose weight despite a good appetite.

Plasma amino acid profiles and serum lactate concentrations, parameters associated with tumor cell progression in the canine cancer model, have not been used clinically to assess the nutritional status of veterinary cancer patients. Likewise, biomarkers associated with tumor growth and subsequent nutritional support such as serum creatine kinase (Fascetti et al, 1997); mitogen-activated protein kinase (MAPK) (Saker et al, 2002); serum mineral content including zinc, chromium, iron and total iron-binding capacity (Kazmierski et al, 2001) and the vascular endothelial growth factor (VEGF) system, including VEGF and the VEGF receptors, Flt-1and KDR (Millanta et al, 2006) have yet to be instituted clinically. Acute-phase reactant proteins, although not specific for cancer, can be measured in serum and can predict prognosis and response to therapy. The combination of certain acute-phase proteins can be more powerful than one assay (others include C-reactive protein and alpha-fetoprotein). Alpha 1-acid glycoprotein is an acute-phase protein that is increased in cats with cancer, and has been used to predict loss of remission for dogs (but not cats) with lymphoma (Selting et al, 2000; Correa et al, 2001; Hahn et al, 1999).

In certain tumors, grading the degree of malignancy histologically predicts biologic behavior. Although a direct relationship between tumor grade and nutritional status including cancer cachexia has not been established, it is thought that more aggressive cancers tend to cause more pronounced systemic effects on body condition. Conversely, even a benign tumor can significantly affect the nutritional status of a dog or cat if it interferes with intake or assimilation. Oral tumors such as SSC in cats may inhibit food intake, and intestinal tumors such as lymphomas can cause poor nutrient absorption, decreased appetite and diarrhea. Tumor grade may correlate with survival, metastatic rate, disease-free interval or with frequency or speed of local recurrence. Not only can a prognosis be determined based on tumor grade, but more aggressive nutritional therapies may be applied to higher grade tumors. Clearly, no single "gold standard" test exists for determining a cancer patient's nutritional status.

Risk Factors

Numerous studies have outlined risk factors of certain nutrients and their relationship to development of cancer. For example, decreased fiber and increased fat have been most commonly incriminated as causal factors for the development of a wide variety of malignant conditions of the gastrointestinal (GI) tract, breast and urinary bladder in people.

Existing data are controversial regarding the cause and effect relationship between diet and cancer in pets. One group of investigators conducted a case-controlled study of nutritional factors and canine breast cancer (Sonnenschein et al, 1991). Neither a high-fat diet nor obesity one year before diagnosis increased the risk of breast cancer. However, the risk of breast cancer was significantly reduced among neutered dogs that had been thin at nine to 12 months of age. Among intact dogs, a thin body condition at nine to 12 months of age reduced the risk of breast cancer. Results of this study suggest that nutritional factors resulting in altered body composition early in life may be important in canine breast cancer. A case-control study evaluated the possible relationship between diet and dietary management in 86 healthy control dogs and 102 dogs with mammary gland tumors or mammary gland dysplasia (Perez-Alenza et al, 1998). Body composition, diet and reproductive history were reviewed. Nutritional status was evaluated from serum selenium and retinol values and adipose fatty acid profiles. Obesity at one year of age and an obese body condition score (BCS) one year before diagnosis are significantly related to a higher prevalence of mammary tumors and cell dysplasias in dogs. Additionally, intake of homemade meals vs. commercial foods is significantly related to a higher incidence of tumors and dysplasias; increased intake of red meat (beef, pork) strongly influences disease incidence. Results from this study indicated that obesity at one year of age was independently and significantly associated with risk of developing mammary tumors and dysplasia. A five-year retrospective study evaluated the distribution of BCS values for dogs with and without histologically and behaviorally malignant neoplasms (Weeth et al, 2007). A total of 14,760 dogs (1,777 with cancer; 12,893 controls) met the inclusion criteria. Dogs with cancer were further allocated into the general categories of sarcoma (n = 582), carcinoma (n = 428) or round cell tumor (n = 767) based on histologic classification of tumor cells. Using a 9-point BCS system, 21.6 and 14.8% of dogs were classified as overweight or obese, respectively. Overall, the mean BCS of all dogs with cancer was 5.4 ± 1.2 vs. 5.3 ± 1.2 for noncancer controls. Investigators reported a significantly lower prevalence of overweight and obese dogs with cancer compared to control dogs without cancer. The

Table 30-1. Phases of clinical and metabolic alterations in cancer patients.

Phase	Clinical changes	Metabolic changes
1	Preclinical, silent phase No obvious clinical signs	Hyperlactatemia Hyperinsulinemia Altered blood amino acid profiles
2	Early clinical signs Anorexia Lethargy Mild weight loss More susceptible to side effects from chemotherapy, etc.	Similar metabolic changes
3	Cachexia Anorexia Lethargy More susceptible to side effects from chemotherapy, etc.	Similar changes but more profound
4	Recovery Remission	Metabolic changes may persist Changes secondary to surgery, chemotherapy or radiation therapy

study revealed a lower prevalence of overweight and obese dogs with sarcomas and carcinomas, but no difference in distribution of BCS in dogs with round cell tumors compared to controls.

Overweight or obese body condition in dogs may also influence the risk of bladder cancer. Investigators have evaluated the role of diet in preventing bladder cancer in Scottish terriers, a breed predisposed to the development of transitional cell carcinoma of the urinary bladder. This survey-based study evaluated each dog's diet for one year before diagnosis and compared data to that from non-neoplastic counterparts. Results were adjusted for age, sex and weight. There was a statistically significant decreased risk of developing transitional cell carcinoma in dogs fed green leafy and yellow-orange vegetables and for dogs fed vegetables at least three times per week. Although the risk of transitional cell carcinoma was lower in dogs fed cruciferous vegetables, the finding was insignificant. These results suggest diet may play a role in the prevention or management of bladder cancer (Raghavan et al, 2005).

Currently, there is no common thread or single measurable parameter that defines the population at risk for or experiencing cancer. Risk assessment for cachexia and nutritional support for cancer must be tailored to each patient with consideration for breed, age, tumor type and other factors.

Etiopathogenesis

There are three basic steps that ultimately lead to generation of a cancer cell from a normal cell: 1) initiation, 2) promotion and 3) progression (London and Vail, 1996). Initiating agents induce permanent and irreversible changes in the DNA of affected cells. Promoting agents cause reversible tissue and cellular changes up to development of the first autonomous tumor cell. Promoting action generally occurs over a long latency period and requires nearly continuous exposure to the promoting agent. Progressing agents convert initiated cells, or cells undergoing promotion, into cells that exhibit the malignant phenotype capable of developing into a mature neoplasm.

Multi-step carcinogenesis occurs through five basic pathways; more than one pathway may be involved in the generation of a particular tumor (London and Vail, 1996). The five carcinogenic pathways are: 1) heritable, 2) passive, 3) biologic, 4) chemical and 5) physical.

Although little is known about breed-specific genetic alterations that may predispose domestic pets to develop neoplastic disease, certain breeds of dogs have a higher incidence of cancer than others. Recent studies have examined breed-specific predispositions to certain types and subtypes of cancer, such as lymphoma (Modiano et al, 2005). Breeds commonly overrepresented in tumor-bearing cohorts include boxers, rottweilers, German shepherd dogs, Scottish terriers and golden retrievers. Siamese cats appear to be at more risk than other feline breeds. Perhaps the best characterized genetic mutation suspected to cause a specific cancer is found in German shepherd dogs with renal cystadenocarcinoma and nodular dermatofibrosis. The chromosomal region that overlaps the human Birt-Hogg-Dubé (BHD) locus responsible for a phenotypically similar syndrome in people, showed mutation of exon 7 of the canine BHD gene. Genetic analysis and pedigree evaluation support this mutation as causative for this cancer (Lingaas et al, 2003).

Point mutations, chromosomal translocations and gene amplification occur as spontaneous events in any dividing cell population. These changes accumulate over a lifetime, possibly explaining why many cancers arise in mature or aged individuals.

Carcinogens can be found in many different aspects of the environment. The most common biologic agents capable of inducing cancer are retroviruses, DNA tumor viruses and some parasites. Various chemical compounds, some naturally occurring and some synthetic, are capable of inducing malignant neoplasia. In most cases, chemical carcinogens require repeated administration or exposure to demonstrate an effect. Physical carcinogens include ultraviolet radiation, ionizing radiation and foreign materials (London and Vail, 1996).

Cancer Cachexia

Cancer cachexia is a complex paraneoplastic syndrome that adversely alters the functional status of the patient (**Figure 30-2**). It manifests as weight loss, reduced food intake and systemic inflammation as a consequence of the cancer disease process (Fearon et al, 2006). This syndrome differs from simple starvation in that both protein and fat stores are lost almost simultaneously in cachectic patients. Initially in simple starvation, fat stores are lost preferentially followed later by loss of protein stores. The time frame for onset of noticeable cachexia-induced weight loss in dogs and cats with cancer can vary. One survey-based study examined dogs as they were presented to the oncology service (Michel et al, 2004). Body weight before cancer diagnosis was available for 64 of 100 dogs. Twenty-three percent had lost more than 10% of their body weight before diagnosis. Body condition scoring, however, found only 4% of dogs with cachexia and 15% with clinically evident muscle wasting; 29% were markedly overweight (Michel et al, 2004). Although body condition scoring and changes in weight are good clinical measures of body condition, they do not consider the complexity of factors influencing the cachectic state such as the metabolic alterations that can occur even before any overt clinical signs associated with cancer cachexia are identified (Ogilvie and Vail, 1996, 1992; Ogilvie and Moore, 1995).

Cancer cachexia may be partly due to negative energy balance secondary to decreased energy intake or altered energy expenditure (Lawson et al, 1982; Dempsey et al, 1984). Investigators have found alterations in basal metabolic rate and resting energy requirement (RER) that were associated with altered carbohydrate, protein and lipid metabolism in human patients with cancer cachexia (Lawson et al, 1982; Dempsey et al, 1984). Additionally, resting energy expenditure and caloric requirements are increased in some tumor-bearing people and animals when compared to healthy individuals (Dempsey et al, 1986; Hansell et al, 1986; Fredrix et al, 1991; Zyliez et al, 1990; Delarue et al, 1990).

Several studies have evaluated energy expenditure in dogs with lymphoma and non-hematopoietic malignancies. Dogs with osteosarcoma have been compared to normal beagles to evaluate metabolic alterations using indirect calorimetry (resting energy expenditure and respiratory quotient), stable isotope tracers (protein synthesis and glucose flux) and dual x-ray absorptiometry scans (body composition). Dogs with osteosarcoma were described as being "weight-stable." These dogs had higher resting energy expenditure before and after surgery, decreased rates of protein synthesis, increased urinary nitrogen loss and increased glucose flux postoperatively (Mazzaferro et al, 2001).

Earlier studies evaluated energy expenditure in dogs with carcinomas and sarcomas (Ogilvie et al, 1997; Walters et al, 1993). These studies found no significant differences in energy expenditure (and presumably caloric requirements) in dogs with a wide range of malignancies compared to healthy, client-owned dogs. This finding suggested that, in general, dogs with cancer and no evidence of weight loss do not have energy requirements higher than those of apparently healthy dogs without cancer. Furthermore, these parameters did not change significantly in dogs with cancer when the tumor was removed surgically (Ogilvie et al, 1996).

Because the thyroid gland and its hormones are intimately involved in the control of energy homeostasis (Premachandra et al, 1981; Sestoft, 1980), investigators have speculated that perturbations in thyroid function or thyroid hormone concentrations play a role in altering energy states in tumor-bearing individuals. In one study, researchers compared thyroid hormone concentrations in dogs with cancer (with and without chronic weight loss) with those in nontumor-bearing dogs (with and without chronic weight loss) (Vail et al, 1994). Diminished serum concentrations of T_4, T_3 and free T_3 occurred in proportion to the degree of weight loss, regardless of tumor-bearing status. Apparently, these reductions in hormone concentrations are related to the abnormal nutritional state or severity of illness rather than to a tumor-related phenomenon. This has been termed "euthyroid sick syndrome." Taken together, these studies illustrate that daily energy requirement (DER) in animals with uncomplicated cancer are similar to those of normal animals, and there is a complexity of metabolic alterations that can occur in cancer patients even in the absence of clinically evident cachexia.

The endstage of cancer cachexia is weight loss that is due not only to primary effects of the tumor, such as compression or infiltration of the alimentary tract, but also to: 1) therapy (e.g., chemotherapy-induced anorexia, nausea or vomiting) or 2) alteration of metabolic pathways composing this paraneoplastic syndrome (**Figure 30-2**) (Ogilvie and Vail, 1996, 1992; Ogilvie and Moore, 1995). Many tumor-bearing animals have altered metabolism, which necessitates special methods for delivering nutrients and specific types of fluid and nutrient support (Ogilvie and Vail, 1996, 1992, 1990; Ogilvie and Moore, 1995, 1995a; Shein et al, 1976; Theologides, 1979; Buzby and Steinberg, 1981; Landel et al, 1985; Bray and Campfield, 1975; Vail et al, 1990, 1990a, 1990b; Ogilvie et al, 1992).

Nutritional Effects from Cancer Treatment

Besides the effects of cancer itself, various modalities used to treat cancer (radiation, chemotherapy and surgery) may

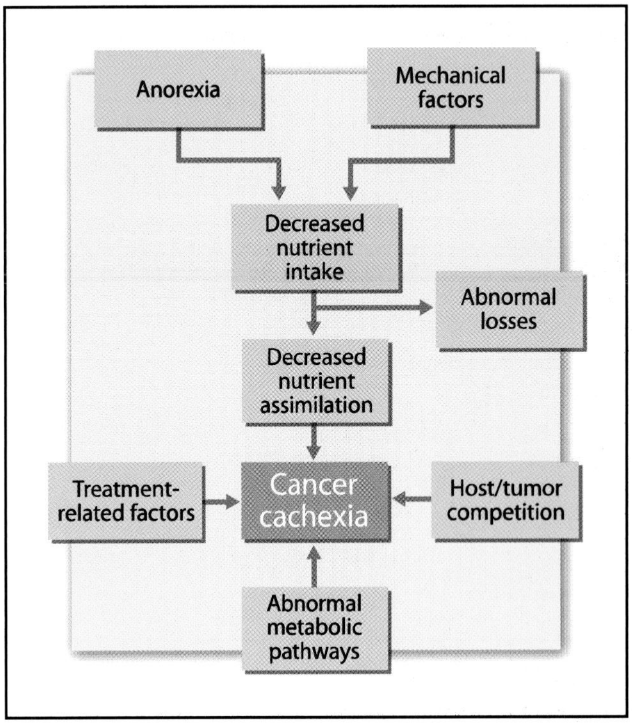

Figure 30-2. Mechanisms of cancer cachexia.

adversely affect a patient's nutritional status. The malnutrition that results from treatment assumes even more importance given that many cancer patients are already debilitated from their disease. Anticancer therapy may produce only mild, transient disturbances, such as mucositis, or it may lead to severe, permanent problems, as in small bowel resection or disabilities of mastication and swallowing after head and neck surgery or radiation. Generally, nutritional problems should be anticipated, feeding tubes placed and patients fed earlier to lessen the adverse effects of treatment.

Surgery

Surgery is used in the treatment of cancer in an attempt to remove tumors or alleviate clinical signs (e.g., intestinal or urinary tract obstruction). Nutritional problems that may develop depend on the surgical location and type of procedure performed (**Table 30-2**). Preliminary studies in dogs suggest that metabolic alterations associated with cancer persist even after tumors are removed surgically (Ogilvie et al, 1997). In general, feeding tubes (esophagostomy, gastrostomy, jejunostomy) should be placed at the time of surgery to avoid additional anesthesia and to allow early feeding.

Radical head or neck surgery may lead to significant malnutrition by altering a patient's ability to eat. Although some of these changes are temporary, many patients have permanent difficulty with chewing and/or swallowing with subsequent risk of aspiration. Proactive placement of gastrostomy tubes (Chapter 25) during head and neck surgery will facilitate enteral feeding during the immediate postoperative period. These tubes may be used for long-term enteral feeding of some cancer patients (Chapter 25). In one retrospective study of cats

Table 30-2. Effects of surgery that may have nutritional implications for cancer patients.

Cancer sites	Surgical procedures	Possible nutritional problems
Head, neck, tongue	Mandibulectomy Maxillectomy Glossectomy	Difficulty prehending, chewing and swallowing food
Esophagus	Esophagectomy, with or without reconstruction	Dysphagia Regurgitation
Stomach	Gastrectomy, partial or complete	Altered gastric emptying Diarrhea
Small intestine	Resection	Malabsorption Diarrhea Intestinal obstruction
Large intestine	Colectomy, partial or complete	Fluid and electrolyte imbalances
Pancreas, liver	Pancreatectomy Cholecystectomy Cholecystoduodenostomy	Diabetes mellitus Maldigestion

Table 30-3. Effects of chemotherapy that may have nutritional implications for cancer patients.

Alterations in smell or taste
Constipation
Decreased appetite
Diarrhea
Food aversions
Nausea
Stomatitis, glossitis, pharyngitis
Vomiting

undergoing mandibulectomy for oral neoplasia, nearly half had an enteral feeding tube placed at the time of surgery, and tubes were used for a median of 74 days postoperatively. Tube placement was deemed an appropriate aspect of management for oral neoplasia as 72% of the cats experienced dysphagia postoperatively, and 12% never regained the ability to eat. Additionally, 83% of owners were satisfied with the outcome of treatment (Northrup et al, 2006).

The nutritional sequelae of gastric and intestinal resection are directly related to the site and extent of resection and to the individual functions of the various segments. The ability of various segments of the small intestine to increase absorptive capabilities over a period of several months prevents major clinical problems after small bowel resection unless the resection is massive. With massive resection, malabsorption (short bowel syndrome) becomes the primary nutritional problem (Chapter 59). In people, colon surgery is usually well tolerated. The large water and electrolyte losses in the early postoperative period decrease rapidly after surgery. Feeding frequency and nutrient composition of the diet should be closely managed to optimize nutritional support for patients with surgical treatment of GI cancers.

Chemotherapy

Chemotherapeutic agents may contribute to malnutrition through a variety of direct and indirect mechanisms (**Table 30-3**). These problems should be anticipated and feeding tubes placed before therapy because early feeding lessens the adverse effects of therapy. Chemotherapeutic agents affect normal and malignant cells but have the greatest effect on rapidly proliferating cells such as epithelial cells of the GI tract. The degree to which GI function is affected depends on the chemotherapeutic agent, drug dosage, duration of treatment, rate of metabolism and the individual animal's susceptibility.

Small bowel villous damage is a major side effect of some chemotherapeutic agents and may be greatly intensified when radiation therapy is given concurrently. The rapid renewal rate of the alimentary tract epithelium usually means that clinical problems from drug-induced mucositis are short-lived.

Nausea and vomiting commonly accompany the administration of many anticancer drugs. Alterations in smell and taste are reported to occur in people and may occur in animals. Side effects experienced during chemotherapy make it difficult for some patients to consume adequate amounts of food.

Corticosteroids such as prednisone are used in chemotherapeutic protocols for some cancers, most notably lymphoma. High doses or prolonged therapy with corticosteroids causes profound polydipsia and polyuria and increased loss of water-soluble vitamins.

It is important to consider the effects of nutritional manipulation and supplemental therapies on the pharmacokinetics and pharmacodynamics of standard cytotoxic chemotherapy. Clients often regard supplements as harmless and may not report their use to the treating clinician in both human and veterinary medicine. However, growing evidence suggests that certain supplements may have toxicity of their own, and may interact with other drugs, including chemotherapeutic agents. Herbal supplements may affect metabolizing enzymes, interfering with pharmacokinetics of some drugs. Antioxidants may squelch free radicals responsible for the anticancer effect.

Because omega-3 (n-3) fatty acids have been associated with improved survival and decreased side effects in dogs with lymphoma, and have many possible anticancer properties, the effect of these fatty acids on the handling of doxorubicin was recently examined. Dogs with lymphoma were enrolled prospectively and randomized to receive a food either high or low in omega-3 fatty acids. There was no significant difference between food groups in this study (Selting et al, 2006).

Fatty acids, vitamins and herbal remedies are readily available over the counter and it is important to understand the possible effects of these and other supplements, such as singular amino acids, antioxidants and flavonoids on cancer therapy.

Radiation

Veterinary patients receiving radiation therapy may have complications that affect food intake. The complications of radiation vary according to the region of the body radiated, dose, fractionation and associated antitumor therapy such as surgery or chemotherapy. Complications may develop acutely during radiation or become chronic and progress even after radiation therapy has been completed (**Table 30-4**).

Radiation to the head and neck affects the oral mucosa and salivary secretions. Saliva production decreases in conjunction with an increase in saliva viscosity, when the salivary glands are in the field of radiation. In addition to causing mouth dryness (xerostomia) and impairing swallowing, the decrease in saliva-tion alters the oral bacterial flora, which in turn may promote dental disease and stomatitis. In people, the thick, scant secre-tions may also create a feeling of nausea (Ross, 1990).

The mucosa of the mouth and oropharynx is sensitive to radiation, which can produce a sore mouth or throat, painful ulcerations, bleeding or even chronic radiation ulcers. Radionecrosis of oral tissue may result from the combination of trauma and infection superimposed on highly radiated tissues. Radiation damage alters or suppresses taste and smell sensa-tions and affects sensitivity to food texture and temperature. In people, taste returns gradually within two to four months after radiation therapy is completed, but may take up to one year (Sandow et al, 2006). Alterations in smell and taste undoubt-edly occur in animals but have not been well documented. These changes create a potentially serious situation because patients are often already anorectic and undernourished.

Radiation to the thoracic area induces esophagitis and dys-phagia. These lesions and signs usually disappear after cessation of therapy. Tumor necrosis, however, may produce delayed complications such as ulceration, fistula formation and obstruc-tion from fibrosis and stricture.

Abdominal or pelvic radiation may alter intestinal function. Patients receiving upper abdominal radiation may experience nausea and vomiting whereas those receiving radiation to the lower abdomen often experience diarrhea due to intestinal mucosal damage, loss of villi and accompanying malabsorption. Acute radiation enteritis usually disappears after therapy is dis-continued. However, late effects of abdominal radiation may occur months to years after completion of radiation therapy and are manifested as intestinal obstruction, fistula formation and chronic enteritis (Kokal, 1985).

Radiation therapy in animals is usually performed on five successive days per week with patients restrained by general anesthesia, which presents an opportunity to place a feeding tube (Chapter 25). This treatment schedule requires careful planning of the feeding method to ensure that patients con-sume their required amount of food each day.

Unless nutritional intervention is provided, many patients lose weight during radiation therapy. Assisted feeding is indi-cated if food intake is inadequate (Chapters 25 and 26).

Table 30-4. Effects of radiation therapy that may have nutritional implications for cancer patients.

Treatment areas	Acute effects	Chronic effects
Head and neck	Mucositis of mouth, tongue, esophagus	Dry mouth Dental disease Alterations in smell Alterations in taste
Thorax	Esophagitis	Esophageal fistula Esophageal stricture
Abdomen	Nausea, vomiting Enteritis, diarrhea Malabsorption	Intestinal obstruction Fistula formation Chronic enteritis

Table 30-5. Key nutritional factors for foods for canine and feline cancer patients.

Factors	Dietary recommendations
Digestible carbohydrate (NFE)*	Avoid excess digestible carbohydrate NFE = ≤25% DM or <20% of the food's ME
Fat	Provide a large proportion of energy from fat Fat = 25 to 40% of DM or 50 to 65% of the food's ME
Omega-3 fatty acids	Provide foods with increased levels of omega-3 fatty acids (>5% DM)
Omega-6: omega-3 fatty acid ratio	Provide foods with an omega-6:omega-3 ratio as close to 1:1 as possible
Protein	Avoid protein deficiency Provide protein in excess of adult requirements Dogs: protein = 30 to 45% of DM or 25 to 40% of the food's ME Cats: protein = 40 to 50% of DM or 35 to 45% of the food's ME (Taurine is always a necessary inclusion in feline diets)
Arginine	Provide foods with arginine DM levels >2%

*Key: NFE = nitrogen-free extract, DM = dry matter, ME = metabolizable energy.

Key Nutritional Factors

Alterations in carbohydrate, lipid and protein metabolism pre-cede obvious clinical disease and cachexia in cancer patients. These metabolic alterations may persist in patients with clini-cal remission or apparent recovery from their cancer. Key nutri-tional factors in cancer patients include digestible (soluble) car-bohydrate, fat, fatty acids and protein, including a few specific amino acids, notably arginine. Several other amino acids have been identified as potentially imparting benefits to cancer patients; however, evidence-based studies in companion ani-mals are not yet available. The key nutritional factors for the dietary management of cancer and their recommended amounts are discussed below and listed in **Table 30-5**. Additional nutrients and nutritional factors that have been identified in human cancer nutrition research include polyphe-nols, flavonoids and specific vitamin and mineral antioxidants. Veterinary patient data are not currently available to recom-mend specific dietary levels of these other nutrients, but research is ongoing to clarify their benefit or potential harm in the dietary management of veterinary cancer patients.

Digestible Carbohydrate

The complex role of carbohydrates in mammalian tumor cell metabolism was identified more than 50 years ago by bio-chemist Otto Warburg (Ristow, 2006). Warburg noted that tumor cells have high rates of anaerobic glycolysis and impaired respiration. Others have since confirmed these metabolic alter-ations and numerous mechanisms have been proposed to explain oxidative metabolism in cancer cell growth. Recent studies indicate that neoplastic cells require not only ATP derived from glycolysis, but also biosynthetic precursors from

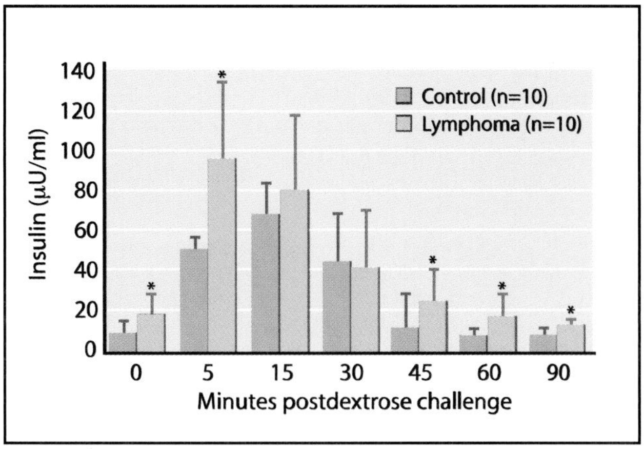

Figure 30-3. Serum insulin concentrations from dogs with and without lymphoma before and after intravenous administration of 500 mg glucose/kg body weight. Asterisks indicate values from dogs with lymphoma that differ significantly (p <0.001) from control dog values obtained at the same time. (Adapted from Vail DM, Ogilvie GK, Wheeler SL, et al. Alterations in carbohydrate metabolism in canine lymphoma. Journal of Veterinary Internal Medicine 1990; 4: 307.)

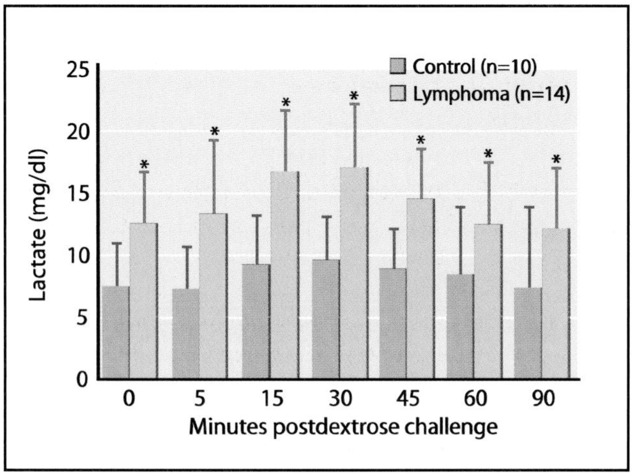

Figure 30-4. Serum lactate concentrations from dogs with and without lymphoma before and after intravenous administration of 500 mg glucose/kg body weight. Asterisks indicate values from dogs with lymphoma that differ significantly (p <0.001) from control dog values taken at the same time. (Adapted from Vail DM, Ogilvie GK, Wheeler SL, et al. Alterations in carbohydrate metabolism in canine lymphoma. Journal of Veterinary Internal Medicine 1990; 4: 307.)

glycolytic intermediates in order to proliferate and invade (Chesney, 2006). One such intermediate, fructose-2,6-biphosphate, controls the overall rate of glycolysis in tumor cells. A second intermediate, 6-phosphofructo-2-kinase/fructose-2,6-bisphosphatase, controls the intracellular concentration of glucose in tumor cells and is constitutively expressed by several leukemias and solid tumor cells (Chesney, 2006). The high glycolytic flux to pyruvate/lactate observed in tumors also alters intracellular pH, causing apoptosis in normal surrounding cells. Increased glucose transport (Birnbaum et al, 1987) and overexpression of oncogenes associated with glucose transport (Flier et al, 1987) have also been associated with tumors cells. Increased glycolysis in tumors may also be a consequence of hexokinase redistribution in subcellular and mitochondrial compartments, or the altered ability of mitochondria to metabolize substrates other than carbohydrates or their derivatives for energy (Ristow, 2006). Numerous mechanisms have been proposed and studied to clarify the altered mitochondrial metabolism in tumor cells.

Regardless of the exact mechanism(s) involved, increasing the rate of glycolysis in tumor cells promotes tumor cell growth in several species including dogs (Ogilvie and Vail, 1992; Heber et al, 1986), forming lactate as an end product. The host must then expend energy to convert lactate to glucose via the Cori cycle, resulting in a net energy gain by the tumor and a net energy loss by the host (Vail et al, 1990b; Heber et al, 1986; Bozzetti et al, 1980; Dempsey and Mullen, 1985). Abnormalities in dogs have been documented in peripheral glucose disposal, hepatic gluconeogenesis, insulin effects and whole body glucose oxidation and turnover (Vail et al, 1990a, 1990b; Ogilvie et al, 1992).

Following a 90-minute intravenous glucose tolerance test, serum lactate and insulin concentrations were significantly higher in dogs with lymphoma when compared with control values (**Figures 30-3** and **30-4**) (Vail et al, 1990). The noted hyperlactatemia and hyperinsulinemia did not improve when these dogs achieved remission with doxorubicin chemotherapy (Ogilvie et al, 1992). Additionally, a subset of dogs with nonhematopoietic malignancies (e.g., osteosarcoma, mammary adenocarcinoma and pulmonary bronchogenic adenocarcinoma) demonstrated hyperlactatemia and hyperinsulinemia, which did not improve when their tumors were completely excised (Ogilvie et al, 1997). The same metabolic alterations are suspected to occur in cats, but there are no published reports to date to verify this assumption.

The clinical significance of altered mitochondrial respiration and increased glycolysis resulting in altered carbohydrate metabolism is highlighted by hyperlactatemia and its sequelae. Foods high in carbohydrate also appear to increase the total amount of lactate produced when fed to dogs with lymphoma. Mean blood glucose, lactate and insulin concentrations obtained during food tolerance testing were often higher in dogs fed a high-carbohydrate, low-fat food (9% dry matter [DM] fat, 58% DM carbohydrate) compared to those fed a low-carbohydrate, high-fat food (37% DM fat, 14% DM carbohydrate) (Ogilvie et al, 1992). However, although there was a positive initial response to chemotherapy, there was no difference in the duration of remission between the two groups.

Blood lactate concentrations in dogs with lymphoma were significantly elevated compared to values in controls before, during and after lactated Ringer's solution was infused (4.125 ml/kg body weight/hr) (**Figure 30-5**). This lactated Ringer's-induced increase in lactate concentration may create an additional metabolic burden, requiring the host to convert lactate back to glucose, further exacerbating energy demands. This finding may be even more important for septic, critically ill cancer patients that require more intensive fluid therapy. It is also important to consider that glucose-containing fluids delivered to septic, critically ill patients can exacerbate the septic state.

Because alterations in insulin and glucose metabolism occur in cancer patients, concerns about dietary carbohydrate (glucose) are further warranted from the perspective of oxidative metabolism of tumor cell growth and metabolic mechanisms of stress hyperglycemia (Mechanick, 2006). In acute and chronic cancer patients, as with all critically ill patients, the stress response leads to a plurality of organ-system derangements including glucose allostasis, immune-neuroendocrine axis activation and insulin receptor signal transduction (Mechanick and Brett, 2005). The concurrent inflammation, tissue catabolism and hyperglycemia should be evaluated when designing a feeding protocol. Manipulating the dietary fat, protein (amino acids) and digestible carbohydrate concentrations can potentially minimize physiologic sequelae resulting from the stress response and slow tumor progression. Digestible carbohydrates may be poorly used because of peripheral insulin resistance. Feeding high levels of digestible carbohydrate may lead to hyperglycemia, glucosuria, hyperosmolarity, hepatic dysfunction, respiratory insufficiency and hyperlactatemia. More specifically, until further information is known about the effects of hyperlactatemia on critically ill animals with cancer, glucose- and lactate-containing fluids should generally be avoided. Carbohydrate levels in foods for canine cancer patients should contain no more than 25% DM digestible carbohydrate.

The specific role of dietary carbohydrates has not been reported in feline cancer patients. Although carbohydrate metabolism in healthy cats differs from that of healthy dogs, it is suspected that tumors in cats use carbohydrates as an energy source. Redistribution of hexokinase and its influence on the rate of glycolysis in tumor cells may be of particular interest for managing the nutritional aspect of feline cancer patients. Based on guidelines discussed below for dietary fat of 25 to 40% DM and protein of 40 to 50% DM, the caloric contribution from digestible carbohydrate is limited to 25% DM or less.

Fat and Fatty Acids

In contrast to the ready use of carbohydrates and proteins by tumor cells, some tumor cells have difficulty using lipids as a fuel source. Theoretically, this preferential use of digestible carbohydrates and proteins leaves lipids available as an energy source for the host (Shein et al, 1986). This finding led to the hypothesis that foods relatively high in fat may benefit patients with cancer compared to foods relatively high in carbohydrates. Recent studies have identified alterations of lipid metabolism in canine cancer patients; this knowledge is paramount for developing feeding protocols. An overview of the current literature may help determine if the focus should be on total amount of fat, specific sources of fat or both for cancer patients.

Highly malignant tumors, in rodent models and in vitro cell cultures, can exhibit up to an 85% decrease in the rate of fatty acid usage. This decrease is linked to decreased activity of the key activating enzyme of β-oxidation, acyl thiokinase (Ristow, 2006). Conversely, well-differentiated tumors can retain the ability to metabolize fatty acids, especially under hypoxic conditions (Ristow, 2006; Swinnen et al, 2006; Menendez and Lupu, 2006). Although tumor type may influence fat usage, a high proportion of weight loss in cachectic cancer patients is attributed to loss of body fat. Not surprisingly, people and animals with cancer have marked abnormalities in lipid metabolism (Chlebowski and Heber, 1986; Dewys, 1982; McAndrew, 1986; Ogilvie et al, 1994; Shein et al, 1986; Tisdale et al, 1987; Daly et al, 1991).

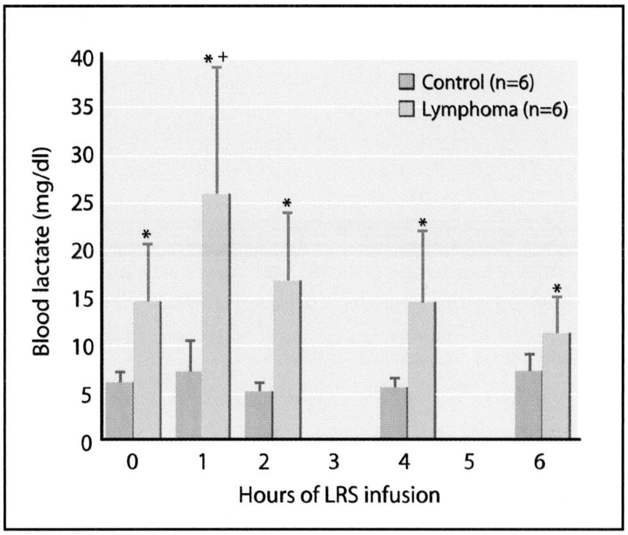

Figure 30-5. Blood lactate concentrations from dogs with and without lymphoma before and during intravenous infusion of lactated Ringer's solution (LRS). Asterisks indicate values from dogs with lymphoma that differ significantly ($p < 0.05$) from control dog values obtained at the same time. Plus signs indicate values that differ significantly ($p < 0.05$) from pre-infusion baseline values within the same test group. (Adapted from Vail DM, Ogilvie GK, Fettman MJ, et al. Exacerbation of hyperlactatemia by infusion of lactated Ringer's solution in dogs with lymphoma. Journal of Veterinary Internal Medicine 1990; 4: 228-232.)

The decreased lipogenesis and increased lipolysis observed in people and rodents with cancer cachexia alter the lipid profile dramatically. Changes include increased blood concentrations of free fatty acids, very low-density lipoproteins (VLDL), triglycerides (TG), plasma lipoproteins and hormone-dependent lipoprotein lipase activity and decreased concentrations of endothelial-derived lipoprotein lipase (McAndrew, 1986). Lipid profiles have been evaluated in dogs with lymphoma to determine if alterations similar to those reported in other species are present (Ogilvie et al, 1994). In contrast to healthy controls, dogs with lymphoma had significantly altered concentrations of cholesterol-associated VLDL, TG, VLDL-TG, low-density lipoprotein (LDL-TG) and high-density lipoprotein (HDL-TG). In dogs with lymphoma, HDL-TG and VLDL-TG concentrations were significantly increased above pretreatment values after remission was lost. Additionally, dogs developed overt signs of cancer cachexia. These abnormalities did not normalize when clinical remission was obtained. The clinical significance of the previously mentioned lipid parameters in dogs with lymphoma is unknown.

Epidemiologic studies and meta-analyses examining the

effects of dietary fat and cancer in people have produced conflicting results. Despite this lack of consensus regarding human data, murine and experimental studies have shown suppression of tumor growth by specific fatty acids, particularly in breast, colon and prostate cancers. Omega-3 fatty acids (eicosapentaenoic acid [EPA], docosahexaenoic acid [DHA]) generally have an inhibitory effect on tumor growth, whereas omega-6 (n-6) fatty acids (linoleic acid, γ-linolenic acid) enhance metastases. In vivo studies have shown that EPA has selective tumoricidal action without harming normal cells (Lowell et al, 1990; Ramesh et al, 1992; Dippenaar and Booyenes, 1982; Begin et al, 1986, 1985; Plumb et al, 1993; Mengeaud et al, 1992; Pascale et al, 1993; Jenski et al, 1993; Roush et al, 1991; Holian and Nelson, 1992).

Similar findings have been reported to occur in canine patients with lymphoma and non-hematopoietic malignancies (Ogilvie et al, 2000). Dogs receiving chemotherapy for lymphoma and fed a food supplemented with arginine and omega-3 fatty acids had elevated plasma arginine, EPA and DHA levels. Plasma levels of arginine and omega-3 fatty acids were positively correlated with survival time. Similarly, in dogs undergoing radiation therapy for nasal carcinomas, plasma levels of arginine, EPA and DHA were positively correlated with quality of life and negatively correlated with inflammatory mediators and mucositis in irradiated areas (Anderson et al, 1997).

Focus on nutritional support of feline cancer patients involves fatty acid influence on the mechanisms of tumor cell signaling. Human estrogen receptor insensitive breast tumor cells have nearly identical histology to feline malignant mammary tumor cells (Perez-Alenza et al, 2004). This provides a two-way model for mammary tumor research. Estrogen receptor insensitive breast tumor cell lines maintained in omega-3 enriched media exhibited significantly reduced activation of MAPK pathway intermediates (Ras, Raf, MEK and MAPK), increased apoptosis, decreased cell proliferation and decreased cyclooxygenase-2 (COX-2) pathway inflammatory eicosanoid expression compared to cells in omega-6 enriched media (Phipps et al, 2004; Saker et al, 2002, 2002a, 2004). Feline feeding studies associated with MAPK expression and dietary fatty acids are equally as compelling.

Healthy adult cats fed diets providing varying omega-6:omega-3 fatty acid ratios (5:1 to 0.4:1) exhibited a ratio dependent decrease in MAPK activation. In addition, omega-6 concentrations decreased and omega-3 concentrations increased in mammary adipose tissue and leukocytes (Saker et al, 2002). Furthermore, a threefold decrease in MAPK activity was detected along with stasis of tumor cell growth as measured by ultrasound and caliper readings in cats with either pancreatic masses or inflammatory mammary carcinomas when the fatty acid content of their food was changed from enriched omega-6 (16:1) to enriched omega-3 (<1:1). MAPK activity increased by 3.5-fold when the original food enriched with omega-6 fatty acids (16:1) was reintroduced. Taken together, these data support the value of enhanced omega-3 fatty acid diets as antitumorigenic and antiinflammatory (**Box 30-1**).

Fish oil may also affect colon cancer development, depending on dietary fiber source. The effect of either omega-3 or omega-6 fatty acids in combination with different fiber types in a rat model of carcinogen-induced colon cancer was reported. Dietary fish oil in combination with pectin was more protective against colon cancer than omega-3 fatty acids with cellulose or omega-6 fatty acids with any fiber type (Chang et al, 1998). The mechanism of enhanced protection appeared to be due to increased colonocyte apoptosis through simultaneously increased reactive oxygen species production and decreased antioxidant enzyme activity (Sanders et al, 2004).

Other potential benefits of omega-3 fatty acids focus on their reported anticachectic effect and association with decreased blood lactate levels. EPA decreases protein degradation without altering protein synthesis; the net effect is anticachectic (Beck et al, 1991; Jho et al, 2002). **Box 30-1** explores suggested mechanism(s) by which fatty acids influence tumor growth and cachexia.

Foods with high omega-3 fatty acid concentrations ameliorate endotoxin-induced lactic acidosis in guinea pigs (Pomposelli et al, 1989). This finding may be of clinical importance because hyperlactatemia occurs commonly in dogs with lymphoma.

Although studies have identified some of the mechanisms involved in lipid use by cancer patients, much more research is needed to match dietary fat levels and omega-6:omega-3 fatty acid ratios to specific tumor types and cancer stages in cats and dogs. Currently, recommendations for canine and feline cancer patients continue to be focused on foods with increased fat calories (25 to 40% DM fat); increased levels of dietary omega-3 fatty acids (>5.0% DM) and an omega-6:omega-3 fatty acid ratio approximating 1:1.

Protein and Arginine

Altered nitrogen balance is observed in human cancer patients, which appears to be a consequence of decreased body muscle mass and skeletal protein synthesis. Increased skeletal protein breakdown, liver protein synthesis and whole body protein synthesis apparently promote tumor growth because tumors often use amino acids for energy (Heber et al, 1986; Bozetti et al, 1980; Dempsey and Mullen, 1985; Chory and Mullen, 1986; Langstein and Norton, 1991; Kurzer and Meguid, 1986; Teyek et al, 1986; Oram-Smith and Stein, 1977). Tumor use of amino acids for energy becomes clinically significant when protein degradation exceeds protein intake. This imbalance can alter immune response, GI function and surgical wound healing (Langstein and Norton, 1991; Kurzer and Meguid, 1986).

In one study, cancer-bearing dogs had significantly lower plasma concentrations of threonine, glutamine, glycine, valine, cystine and arginine and significantly higher concentrations of isoleucine and phenylalanine than did normal control dogs (Ogilvie and Vail, 1990). The results were the same for different types of tumors, and observed alterations in plasma amino acid profiles did not normalize after tumors were surgically removed. This finding suggests that cancer induces

Box 30-1. Omega-3 Fatty Acids, Tumor Growth, Cachexia and Inflammation.

Polyunsaturated omega-6 (n-6) and omega-3 (n-3) fatty acids alter protein-lipid interactions and lipid-based signal transduction pathways in cells. The simultaneous generation of inositol phosphates and diacylglycerol, yielding the secondary release of intracellular calcium and activation of protein-kinase C (PKC) depend on phospholipase C, a lipid-comprised phosphatidylinositol. In addition, the specific lipid composition of the diacylglycerol (i.e., omega-6 vs. omega-3) results in a differing affect on the mitogen activated protein kinase (MAPK) signal transduction pathway. MAPK, one of several cell signal transduction pathways, is paramount in regulating tumor (mammary, uterine, prostate, lung) cell proliferation. Numerous human and murine studies have reported the value of omega-3 fatty acids (eicosapentaenoic acid [EPA], docosahexaenoic acid [DHA]) in inhibiting tumor growth and metastasis through alterations in expression of the pro-angiogenic vascular endothelial growth factor (VEGF) and down-regulation of the proinflammatory regulator cyclooxygenase 2 (COX-2). COX-2 enzyme activity promotes proinflammatory eicosanoid production, which stimulates VEGF and vascularization of tumor tissue. Fatty acids attenuate transcriptional activity of COX-2 and VEGF through anti-MAPK and -AP-1 mechanisms in breast cancer cell lines.

The anticachectic effect of EPA has been reported to influence cytokine release from tumor cells. Administration of omega-3 fatty acids reduced secretion of tumor necrosis factor-alpha (TNF-α), interleukin-1β (IL-1β), interleukin-1α (IL-1α) and interleukin-2. This may be especially important because IL-1 and TNF are important mediators of cachexia and may act as tumor growth factors.

The onset and perpetuation of the anorectic state in cancer and critically ill patients can be influenced through omega-3 fatty acid supplementation. Studies have demonstrated that omega-3 fatty acids modulate changes in the concentrations and actions of several orexigenic and anorexigenic neuropeptides in the brain. These peptides include neuropeptide Y, α-melanocyte stimulating hormone, serotonin and dopamine. In patients with acute or chronic inflammatory conditions, as is thought to occur in many cancer patients, omega-3 fatty acid supplementation suppresses proinflammatory cytokine production and improves food intake by normalizing hypothalamic orexigenic peptides and neurotransmitters.

The Bibliography for **Box 30-1** can be found at www.markmorris.org.

long-lasting changes in protein metabolism.

The anorexia-cachexia syndrome prevalent in cancer patients is associated with profound metabolic perturbations including increased muscle proteolysis. Thus, decreased lean body mass and increased protein requirements in cancer patients are driven by amino acid redistribution for: 1) synthesis of hepatic acute-phase-reactant proteins, 2) support of the cellular immune response, 3) provision of gluconeogenic substrates and 4) direct oxidation for fuel.

To date, there appears to be less of a focus on protein metabolism in cancer patients compared to the focus on fat metabolism. Despite the unique protein requirements of cats, protein use studies in companion animals have been limited to canine cancer patients. Current recommendations for dietary protein are based on a limited number of companion animal cancer studies, well-founded knowledge of protein metabolism in critically ill patients and extrapolation from non-veterinary species.

Dietary protein levels in foods for cancer patients should exceed levels normally used for maintenance of adult animals, assuming renal and liver function is adequate to tolerate enhanced protein. If signs of intolerance are observed, titrate down to tolerable protein levels. Currently, recommended protein levels in foods for dogs with cancer are 30 to 45% DM. Based on dietary protein requirements for critically ill cats, suggested protein levels in foods for cats with cancer are 40 to 50% DM.

Arginine is an essential amino acid for cats and is considered to be a conditionally essential amino acid for dogs. Arginine is synthesized endogenously in the kidney from gut-derived citrulline and is converted by the enzyme arginase into ornithine and urea. Arginine has potent secretagogue effects on several endocrine and neuroendocrine glands. Intravenous administration of arginine induces secretion of growth hormone, prolactin, insulin, glucagon, insulin-like growth factor-1, pancreatic polypeptide, somatostatin and catecholamines (Barbul, 1986). Arginine, given in large doses, exerts numerous beneficial effects on the immune system, particularly on thymus-dependent and T-cell-dependent immune reactions. The exact mechanism whereby arginine stimulates T-cell function is unknown. In addition to its positive effects on immune function, arginine may also influence tumor growth, metastatic rate and survival time in patients with cancer.

Adding arginine to parenteral solutions decreases tumor growth and metastatic rate in rodent cancer models (Tachibana et al, 1985). Increased dietary arginine, in conjunction with increased dietary omega-3 fatty acid intake, influenced clinical signs, quality of life and survival time in dogs with lymphoma (Ogilvie et al, 2000) and enhanced quality of life for dogs undergoing radiation therapy for nasal carcinomas (Anderson et al, 1997). The minimum effective level of dietary arginine for cancer patients is unknown; however, based on work in other species, it is thought appropriate to provide more than 2% DM arginine in foods for dogs with cancer. There are no reports demonstrating efficacy of additional arginine in feline cancer patients. The minimum recommended allowance for queens in late gestation and peak lactation is 1.5% (DM) (NRC, 2006). Therefore, this same recommendation (>2%, DM) is probably minimally satisfactory for dietary arginine in feline cancer patients.

Other Nutritional Factors

Several amino acids, vitamins, minerals and novel foods and ingredients have received considerable attention in cancer prevention and therapy (**Boxes 30-2** through **30-5**).

Box 30-2. Amino Acids and Cancer.

GLUTAMINE

Glutamine may have specific therapeutic value. Glutamine is an essential precursor for nucleotide biosynthesis and is an important oxidative fuel for enterocytes. Supplementation of enteral preparations with glutamine has benefited several animal models of intestinal injury by improving intestinal morphometry, reducing bacterial translocation, enhancing local immunity and improving survival. Glutamine has only recently been recognized as a conditionally essential amino acid in certain pathophysiologic states including stress. Glutamine is added to most human enteral formulas, and has been evaluated in parenteral formulations for its potential to protect intestinal integrity in critically ill, anorectic patients. The parenteral studies have most consistently delivered a 2% solution of L-glutamine.

One study using a feline model of methotrexate-induced intestinal injury failed to demonstrate a beneficial role for glutamine supplementation to an amino acid-based purified food. A recent review indicated glutamine and glutamate metabolism appears to be intact in tumor mitochondria, suggesting that the mitochondrial activity of tumor cells can be restored by using supplemental glutamine as a fuel source. Contrary to these findings, dietary glutamine was reported to suppress mammary carcinogenesis in a 7,12-dimethylbenz[a]anthracene (DMBA)-induced breast cancer animal model. Glutamine supplemented at 1 g/kg/day to tumor-induced rats for 11 weeks significantly decreased tumor glutathione (GSH) levels, altered tumor GSH/GSSG status and enhanced tumor apoptotic activity by Bax, caspase-3 and Bcl-2. Additional studies are needed to determine the potential mechanism(s) by which glutamine alters tumor cell growth, and if commercially available foods supplemented with glutamine improve intestinal integrity during cancer treatments.

BRANCHED-CHAIN AMINO ACIDS

Branched-chain amino acids (BCAA), notably leucine, isoleucine and valine, are neutral amino acids with clinically relevant metabolic effects. Their potential role as anti-anorexia and anticachectic agents has been reported. Numerous human clinical trials indicate anorexia is associated with deranged brain tryptophan/serotonin metabolism. Tryptophan crosses the blood-brain barrier via a specific transport mechanism shared with other neutral amino acids. Therefore, supplementation with competing neutral amino acids (BCAA) reduces tryptophan entry into the brain, thereby inhibiting hypothalamic serotonin synthesis and release with subsequent amelioration of anorexia. Supplemental oral BCAA given to cancer patients at a dose of 14.4 g/day for seven days significantly improved energy intake by Day 3.

The anticachectic value of BCAA, particularly leucine, was evaluated in experimental studies and human clinical trials. Tumor-bearing rats fed a leucine-enriched diet had a 1.4-fold higher rate of protein synthesis and decreased expression of the ubiquitin-proteosome system and chymotrypsin-like activity. Bed-rested, catabolic patients receiving 18 g BCAA/day for a month exhibited improved lean leg mass, strength and protein synthetic rate. The long-term benefit of BCAA administration was evaluated in patients with hepatocellular carcinoma. Those who received 11 g BCAA supplementation/day for one year had lower morbidity, higher serum albumin concentrations and a better quality of life compared to values in control group patients. These findings indicate BCAAs appear to have specific anticachectic effects.

BCAA appear to influence cell growth in canine tumor cell lines. Canine osteosarcoma, bronchoalveolar carcinoma and Madine-Darby kidney cells were cultured under the influence of 0 to 100 mM concentrations of leucine, isoleucine or valine to evaluate the anti-proliferative effects of these BCAAs. Study results were tumor-type dependent; leucine appeared to have the most significant effect in diminishing neoplastic cell growth at supraphysiologic concentrations. Additional studies are needed to establish relevancy in the management of veterinary cancer patients. Available human trial data suggest supplementation with 10 to 15 g/day of BCAA as leucine, isoleucine and valine may provide anti-anorexic and anticachectic benefits.

METHIONINE AND ASPARAGINE

Certain tumor cell lines require methionine for growth. Replacing methionine with its precursor, homocysteine locks these tumor cells into late S and G2 phases of the cell cycle. Because certain cancer chemotherapeutic agents are cell-cycle specific, the percentage of tumor cells sensitive to chemotherapy increases, improving the therapeutic index. Asparagine is essential for tumor cell growth in lymphoma. Treatment of dogs and cats with L-asparaginase has induced complete remissions in up to 80% of dogs and cats with lymphoma.

TYROSINE AND PHENYLALANINE

Tyrosine and phenylalanine restriction has been reported to suppress melanoma cell growth in tissue cultures and in rodent tumor models. Administration of tyrosine and phenylalanine increased the survival of melanoma tumor-bearing mice and increased the effectiveness of levodopa against melanoma.

GLYCINE

Some amino acids may decrease the toxicity associated with chemotherapy. For example, glycine reduces cisplatin-induced nephrotoxicity.

The Bibliography for **Box 30-2** can be found at www.markmorris.org.

FEEDING PLAN

Although cancer and traditional cancer treatments in dogs and cats result in a spectrum of metabolic/nutritional derangements, a number of these derangements are common to most types of cancer and provide the basis for development of a general feeding plan.

The previous sections discussed the clinical fundamentals of cancer from clinical importance to patient assessment and determination of key nutritional factors. This section describes how to feed patients with cancer. It continues the iterative process by developing these feeding plan topics: 1) assess and select the food, 2) assess and determine the feeding method and

Box 30-3. Vitamins and Cancer.

Retinoids, β-carotene, vitamin C and vitamin E all appear to influence the growth and metastasis of cancer cells by a variety of mechanisms. Some of these mechanisms include selected receptor-mediated anti-proliferative activities. These vitamins have been reported to bind their cytosolic receptors followed by translocation of the bound complex to the nucleus where the receptors mediate gene regulation. Other effects result from antioxidant, hormone-like and immunomodulator capabilities.

RETINOIDS

"Retinoids" refer to the entire group of naturally occurring and synthetic vitamin A derivatives, including retinol, retinal and retinoic acid. Retinoids appear to have the potential for regulating cancer cells either alone or in combination with other agents. Specific studies in human and veterinary medicine suggest that retinoids alone or with other agents can be effective for the treatment of certain types of malignancies. The synthetic retinoids, isotretinoin and etretinate, have been used successfully in some dogs with intracutaneous cornifying epitheliomas, other benign skin tumors, cutaneous lymphoma, solar-induced squamous cell carcinoma and associated preneoplastic lesions. The retinoids promote cellular differentiation and may enhance the susceptibility of neoplastic cells to chemotherapy and radiation therapy.

VITAMIN C

Vitamin C (ascorbic acid) has been reported to inhibit nitrosation reactions and prevent chemical induction of cancers of the esophagus and stomach. Processed foods high in nitrates and nitrites, such as bacon and sausage, are often supplemented with vitamin C to reduce the carcinogenic capability of the resultant nitrosamines.

Ascorbic acid may be one therapeutic alternative for overcoming drug resistance in some cancer cells. Studies suggest that an ascorbic acid-sensitive mechanism may be involved in drug resistance to vincristine in certain cancer cell lines. Despite the extensive amount of vitamin C research, few direct data exist proving its efficacy in dogs and cats.

VITAMIN E

Vitamin E (α-tocopherol) can also inhibit nitrosation reactions. Vitamin E also has a broad capacity to inhibit mammary tumor and colon carcinogenesis in rodents. Research indicates that vitamin E influences a variety of cell functions including free-radical scavenging, which can prevent oxidative damage that leads to cell death.

In addition to its anticancer properties, vitamin E may potentially convey therapeutic efficacy against certain malignancies. Vitamin E has been reported to have anti-proliferative activity, which involves the binding of the vitamin to salicylic receptors, followed by translocation to the nucleus where DNA binds on the domains of receptors that mediate gene regulatory events. Recent evidence suggests that the two prominent vitamin E isoforms, vitamin E succinate (VES) and α-tocopherol acetate (α-TEA) have specific anticancer activity. Both isoforms increased apoptosis in human breast cancer cell lines, ovarian and cervical cancer cell lines, mesothelioma cells, lung cancer cells and gastric cells without affecting surrounding normal cells.

Retrovirus-induced tumorigenesis involves transformation of normal cells into tumor cells. Evidence suggests that vitamin E may normalize the immune system by interacting with macrophages and T lymphocytes to inhibit retroviral-induced infections.

The Bibliography for **Box 30-3** can be found at www.markmorris.org.

Box 30-4. Minerals and Cancer.

Minerals that have been suggested as being important in patients with cancer include selenium, iron and zinc. Optimal levels of specific minerals for cancer prevention and treatment have not been established for pet animals.

SELENIUM

Selenium has been one of the most heavily studied minerals associated with the development of cancer. Low serum selenium levels have been observed in human patients with gastrointestinal cancer. In rodents, dietary supplementation with selenium inhibits colon, mammary gland and stomach carcinogenesis.

IRON

Iron transferrin and ferritin have been linked to cancer risk and cancer cell growth. Lung, colon, bladder and esophageal cancer in people have been highly correlated with increased serum iron concentrations and increased transferrin saturation. Because many tumor cells require iron for growth, it has been suggested that the increased use of iron by the tumor depresses serum iron levels in human cancer patients. Mice with low levels of iron have slow tumor growth compared to those with normal iron levels.

ZINC

In people, low levels of zinc in blood and diseased tissue have been observed in esophageal, pancreatic and bronchial cancer. Zinc deficiency appears to enhance carcinogenesis in laboratory animals.

The Bibliography for **Box 30-4** can be found at www.markmorris.org.

3) reassess and modify the feeding plan, as necessary. The key nutritional factors identified in the previous section are used here as benchmarks for comparing selected foods marketed for the dietary management of cancer.

Nutritional support of cancer patients must be individualized. Nutritional therapy should be undertaken with the overall prognosis of the patient clearly in mind so that the aggressiveness of dietary intervention (e.g., supportive, adjunctive, defin-

Table 30-6. Selected commercial foods for canine cancer patients compared to recommended levels of key nutritional factors.*

Dry food	Energy density (kcal/cup)**	Carbohydrate (%)	Fat (%)	Omega-3 fatty acids (%)	Omega-6: omega-3 ratio	Protein (%)	Arginine (%)
Recommended levels	**-**	**≤25**	**25-40**	**>5**	**~1:1**	**30-45**	**>2**
Medi-Cal Development Formula	425	na	17.5	na	na	28.4	na
Moist foods	**Energy density (kcal/can)****	**Carbohydrate (%)**	**Fat (%)**	**Omega-3 fatty acids (%)**	**Omega-6: omega-3 ratio**	**Protein (%)**	**Arginine (%)**
Recommended levels	**-**	**≤25**	**25-40**	**>5**	**~1:1**	**30-45**	**>2**
Hill's Prescription Diet a/d Canine/Feline	180/5.5 oz.	15.4	30.4	2.62	2.3:1	44.2	2.37
Hill's Prescription Diet n/d Canine	569/12.7 oz.	19.9	33.2	7.29	0.3:1	38.0	2.95
Iams Veterinary Formula Maximum Calorie/Canine & Feline	333/6 oz.	12.2	37.2	na	na	41.8	na
Medi-Cal Development Formula	445/396 g	na	14.1	na	na	32.2	na
Medi-Cal Recovery Formula/ Canine & Feline	185/170 g	na	32.1	na	na	53.4	na
Purina Veterinary Diets DM Dietetic Management Feline Formula	194/5.5 oz.	8.1	23.8	0.88	3.8:1	56.9	na

Key: na = Information not available from manufacturer; values were obtained from manufacturers' published information, g = grams.
*Nutrients expressed on % dry matter basis, unless otherwise stated.
**As fed energy density is useful for determining amount to feed; cup = 8-oz. measuring cup; to convert to kJ, multiply by 4.184.

Table 30-7. Selected commercial foods for feline cancer patients compared to recommended levels of key nutritional factors.*

Dry foods	Energy density (kcal/cup)**	Carbohydrate (%)	Fat (%)	Omega-3 fatty acids (%)	Omega-6: omega-3 ratio	Protein (%)	Arginine (%)
Recommended levels	**-**	**≤25**	**25-40**	**>5**	**~1:1**	**40-50**	**>2**
Medi-Cal Development Formula	425	na	23.9	na	na	34.7	na
Purina Veterinary Diets DM Dietetic Management Feline Formula	592	15.0	17.9	0.39	5.6:1	57.8	3.57
Moist foods	**Energy density (kcal/can)****	**Carbohydrate (%)**	**Fat (%)**	**Omega-3 fatty acids (%)**	**Omega-6: omega-3 ratio**	**Protein (%)**	**Arginine (%)**
Recommended levels	**-**	**≤25**	**25-40**	**>5**	**~1:1**	**40-50**	**>2**
Hill's Prescription Diet a/d Canine/Feline	180/5.5 oz.	15.4	30.4	2.62	2.3:1	44.2	2.37
Iams Veterinary Formula Maximum Calorie/ Canine & Feline	333/6 oz.	12.2	37.2	na	na	41.8	na
Medi-Cal Development Formula	216/170 g	na	27.5	na	na	45.0	na
Medi-Cal Recovery Formula/Canine & Feline	185/170 g	na	32.1	na	na	53.4	na
Purina Veterinary Diets CV Cardiovascular Feline Formula	223/5.5 oz.	23.1	26.8	na	na	42.5	na
Purina Veterinary Diets DM Dietetic Management Feline Formula	194/5.5 oz.	8.1	23.8	0.88	3.8:1	56.9	na

Key: na = Information not available from manufacturer; values were obtained from manufacturers' published information, g = grams.
*Nutrients expressed on % dry matter basis, unless otherwise stated.
**As fed energy density is useful for determining amount to feed; cup = 8-oz. measuring cup; to convert to kJ, multiply by 4.184.

itive) can be adjusted appropriately. Owners of cancer patients should be educated about the integral role nutrition plays in the total management of their pet's disease, but at the same time should understand the limitations of the dietary management component of the overall treatment plan. The feeding plan depends on the extent of disease, anorexia, nausea, weight loss and consequences of treatment.

Assess and Select the Food

There is only one veterinary therapeutic commercial food[a] that has been specifically developed for canine cancer patients. This food has been shown to improve the longevity and quality of life of selected canine patients with cancer. However, other veterinary therapeutic foods provide certain key nutritional factors at near recommended levels. **Tables 30-6** (dogs) and **30-7** (cats) include the key nutritional factors from **Table 30-5** and compares them to the levels in selected commercial foods. The food selected should most closely fit the recommended levels for patients with cancer.

Another criterion for selecting a food that may become increasingly important in the future is evidence-based clinical nutrition. Practitioners should know how to determine risks and benefits of nutritional regimens and counsel pet owners accordingly. Currently, veterinary medical education and continuing education are not always based on rigorous assessment of evidence for or against particular management options. Still, studies have been published to establish the nutritional benefits of certain pet foods. Chapter 2 describes evidence-based clinical nutrition in detail and applies its concepts to various veterinary therapeutic foods. Evidence Grade 1 (the highest level) exists for at least one food used for canine cancer patients.[a] See Case 2-1.

Some owners feed debilitated or cachectic pets home-cooked foods to enhance palatability and food intake and as a means of bonding with their pet. Interest in homemade diets has peaked in recent years as a feeding alternative for healthy and ill pets. Numerous references are available that contain published recipes or provide computer-based recipes. Homemade diets must be nutritionally balanced. Adequate provision of protein and energy to maintain the cancer patient and consideration of key nutrient concerns should be the focus of home-cooked diet formulations. (See Chapter 10 for basic guidelines for formulating and evaluating homemade diets.) Research efforts to identify optimal foodstuffs and levels of nutrients for veterinary cancer patients are ongoing. As more experimental and clinical trial data become available, diet selection for cancer patients will expand and likely become tumor-type and disease-stage specific. **Tables 30-6** and **30-7** list commercially available diet choices; however, when selecting a diet, the overall goal of supplying daily water, protein and energy requirements to sustain an acceptable quality of life should not be overlooked. Patient assessment and owner constraints may affect diet selection.

Assess and Determine the Feeding Method

The feeding method includes the amount to feed as well as how often and by what route. Careful assessment of the feeding method is important to determine whether the patient is currently receiving its caloric requirement and if it is able to prehend, masticate, swallow and assimilate its food.

How Much to Feed

Calculation of the patient's energy requirement, determination of the energy density of the food, careful measurement of the amount of food eaten by the animal and body condition scoring will help establish whether cancer patients with weight loss are actually receiving sufficient calories and nutrients. Limitations to the accurate calculation of RER or DER in veterinary patients can offer a challenge to maintaining or improving the patient's body weight and condition. Again, routine assessment is paramount to fine-tuning the feeding protocol for each patient. The general "rule of thumb" is to feed ill, hospitalized patients at RER for their current body weight, and increase to DER for a more optimal body weight during "at home" feeding. As feeding for cancer patients is individualized, these guidelines do not hold true for all cases, but rather should be considered as starting points.

Hospitalized patients should eat enough food to at least meet their estimated RER. Calculations for determination of energy requirements can be reviewed in Chapters 1 and 5. Initiate an assisted-feeding protocol for hospitalized patients that fail to consume enough food to meet RER for three or more days. (See How to Feed below.)

Patients managed at home should eat enough food to meet their estimated DER, which takes into account increased activity and a less controlled environment. Determination of DER should start at current body weight using a species-specific factor that accounts for low activity. As the patient tolerates this intake, a gradual increase in daily calories can be attempted with a goal of feeding DER at a more optimal body weight. Based on individual assessment (including activity, attitude, age, prognosis, etc.) the DER factor typically ranges from low activity (1.1 to 1.3 x RER) to adult maintenance (1.4 x RER for cats and 1.6 x RER for dogs). Frequent recording of body weight and condition helps ascertain the appropriateness of the feeding plan.

Some underweight animals with cancer will stabilize at a less than optimal BCS (2/5 rather than 3/5). It may be difficult to achieve weight gain in these patients; therefore, the goal should change to maintaining this leaner body condition (Chapter 25, Accommodation).

How to Feed

Enteral feeding is the preferred route for providing nutritional support because it is less complicated and safer for patients fed at home. Additionally, enteral feeding is more physiologic because it improves intestinal mucosal thickness, stimulates gut trophic hormones and stimulates IgA production. Enhancing food palatability is the simplest means of increasing voluntary intake. A food can sometimes be made more palatable by heating to improve its aroma and mouth feel. Hand feeding critically ill, weak or depressed pets may enhance intake. Human companionship appears to increase the pet's interest in food. It

Box 30-5. Novel Foods, Ingredients and Cancer.

PROTEASE INHIBITORS

Much information suggests that soybean-derived Bowman-Birk inhibitor can inhibit or suppress carcinogenesis in vivo and in vitro. Extracts of the Bowman-Birk inhibitor suppress carcinogenesis in several animal model systems, including colon- and liver-induced carcinogenesis in mice, anthracene-induced cheek pouch carcinogenesis in hamsters, lung tumorigenesis in mice and esophageal carcinogenesis in rats. Bowman-Birk inhibitor concentration inhibits metastases and weight loss associated with radiation-induced thymic lymphoma in mice. Irradiated rodents treated with dietary Bowman-Birk inhibitor have fewer deaths, lower average grade of lymphoma and larger fat stores than controls. Various soy products produce dramatic protection against methotrexate (MTX)-induced enterotoxicity in rodent models.

One study was performed using a feline model of MTX-induced enteritis to determine the impact of purified foods containing intact protein sources (soybean protein or casein) or crystalline amino acids on intestinal structure and function. Cats receiving a commercially available (complex) food served as the control group. MTX administration was associated with severe enterotoxicity manifested by vomiting and diarrhea, especially in cats receiving crystalline amino acid and casein-based purified foods. Cats receiving the casein-based purified food had the largest decrease in total white blood cell (WBC) and platelet counts, the greatest villous atrophy (**Figure 1**) and the highest incidence of positive mesenteric lymph node and hepatic bacterial cultures (50 and 33%, respectively). Cats fed the soybean protein-based purified food had the least villous atrophy (**Figure 2**) and a significantly smaller magnitude of reduction in WBC counts compared with cats receiving the crystalline amino acid (**Figure 3**) and casein-based purified foods. Feeding complex (**Figure 4**) and soybean protein-based foods was also associated with the greatest secretagogue activity on plasma cholecystokinin (CCK) concentrations after ingestion of the respective meals, compared with concentrations in cats receiving the amino acid and casein-based purified foods. This study showed an association between feeding a soybean protein-based purified food and improved intestinal integrity. These findings might be associated with a greater secretogogue effect in stimulating trophic gut hormones such as CCK. In contrast, the casein-based purified food was associated with increased morbidity, villous atrophy, increased bacterial translocation and decreased secretogogue activity on CCK. Additional studies may determine the underlying mechanism of protection and the exact compound(s) responsible for soybean protein's protective effects.

POLYPHENOLIC COMPOUNDS AND FLAVONOIDS

Numerous health benefits result from consumption of diets rich in phytochemicals such as polyphenolic compounds. Polyphenolic compounds are potent dietary antioxidants and it is thought that

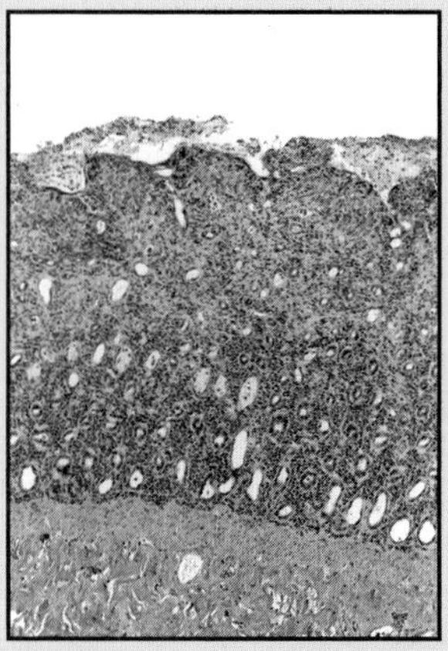

Figure 1.

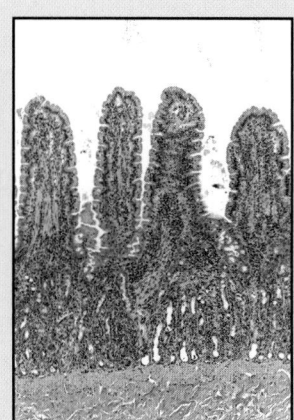

Figure 2.

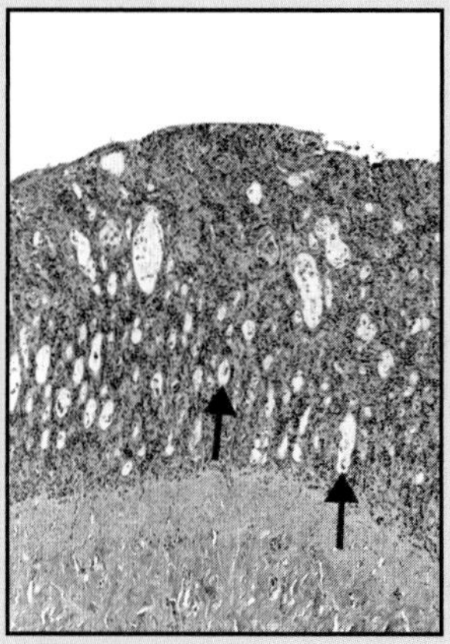

Figure 3.

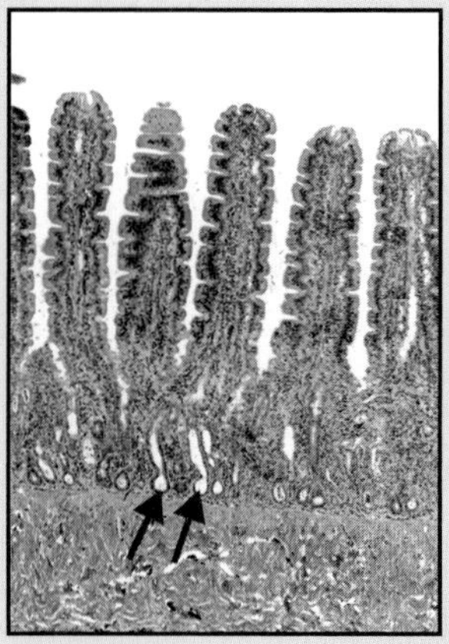

Figure 4.

Figure 1. Distal duodenal section obtained 72 hours postmethotrexate administration from a cat fed a casein-based purified diet. The villi are severely blunted and fused with multifocal ulceration. Crypt loss is marked and the remaining crypts are severely dilated.

Figure 2. Proximal duodenal section obtained 72 hours postmethotrexate administration from a cat fed a soybean protein-based purified diet. Villi have normal architecture and crypts are moderately dilated.

Figure 3. Proximal duodenal section obtained 72 hours postmethotrexate administration from a cat fed a purified diet containing free amino acids. Villi are completely effaced. The surface is covered with an intermittent layer of attenuated enterocytes. Crypts are severely dilated and distorted (arrows).

Figure 4. Distal duodenal section obtained 72 hours postmethotrexate administration from a cat fed a commercial food containing intact protein sources. Villi have normal architecture. Crypts in the lamina propria are moderately dilated (arrows).

(**Figures 1** to **4** adapted from: Marks SL. Dietary modulation of methotrexate-induced enteritis in cats. PhD Dissertation, University of California, Davis, 1996.)

Box 30-5 continued

the antioxidant properties of these compounds confer protection against certain chronic diseases such as cancer. Antioxidants may act directly by limiting oxidative stress and indirectly through preserving protective enzymatic pathways and modulation of signaling pathways. Flavonoids added to neoplastic cell lines have shown promising results. An interesting example is the phytochemical activity of pomegranate fruit. Pomegranate polyphenolic extracts inhibit growth in human leukemia cells, prostate cancer cell lines and suppress formation of chemically induced skin tumors and colon carcinogenesis in rodent models.

Supplementation of estrogen receptor sensitive and insensitive cells with a 1 or 5% commercial juice extract or fresh fruit extract inhibited in vitro cell proliferation by up to 90%. Although investigations to identify the mechanism(s) of action are ongoing, the potential for using natural food products to manage cancer patients is encouraging.

GARLIC

Epidemiologic studies have suggested a correlation between high garlic consumption and reduced risk of cancer. Garlic, garlic extracts and several thioalkyl compounds inhibit the activation of carcinogens and carcinogen-induced aberrations in the cell nucleus. Garlic extracts have an anti-promotion effect in animals exposed to carcinogens. Furthermore, garlic exerts direct cytolytic effects against cultured human breast cancer and melanoma cells. The concentrations of garlic used in these studies to arrest cancer cell growth had no effect on normal cells.

Pretreatment with garlic protects rodents against subsequent induction of tumors by a variety of carcinogens. There are no studies demonstrating the safety and efficacy of garlic for the prevention or treatment of cancer in people, dogs and cats.

The Bibliography for **Box 30-5** can be found at www.markmorris.org

has been suggested that critically ill patients often have a diminished will to live; their bodily energy and normal GI function including motility, digestion and absorption are likewise diminished. Building a patient's Zheng Qi, or bodily energy, has been addressed using herbs and herbal formulas. This approach to managing critically ill patients by enhancing use of enteral nutrition requires a substantial knowledge of herbs and drug interactions. References and individuals experienced in the area of veterinary botanical medicine are available for consultation by interested pet guardians. Acupuncture appears to have a cumulative "feel good" affect on pets following chemotherapy (Wurth, 2003). The better patients feel, the more likely they are to have interest in eating.

If necessary, drug therapy can be attempted before offering food. Administration of a benzodiazepine derivative (diazepam or oxazepam) or cyproheptadine increases appetite transiently; however, these drugs are unreliable for ensuring adequate caloric intake. Benzodiazepine derivatives are contraindicated in patients with severely reduced hepatic function, especially when signs of hepatic encephalopathy are present. In addition, the appetite-stimulating properties of these agents appear to wane with time when used in sick animals. Megestrol acetate causes weight gain and increases appetite in people with cancer. The clinical benefit of this drug in veterinary patients remains to be determined. Controlled studies with human cancer patients have revealed that cyproheptadine, corticosteroids and nandrolone decanoate have little to no impact on improving food intake, body weight and clinical outcome (Kardinal et al, 1990; Chlebowski et al, 1986; Willcox et al, 1984). A deficiency of B vitamins is associated with anorexia and may occur in some cancer patients fed unbalanced homemade foods or patients that have decreased food intake.

Assisted-feeding techniques should be considered if these appetite-stimulating efforts fail and/or the patient has not voluntarily eaten for three or more days. Enteral and/or parenteral techniques can be used for nutritional support while patients are hospitalized (Chapters 25 and 26). As noted in previous sections, before starting a treatment regimen (i.e., chemotherapy, radiation, surgery), an assisted-feeding device can be proactively placed to ensure adequate nutrition regardless of treatment side effects. Examples include placing a gastrostomy tube in patients with oral tumor resections or before radiation treatment to the nose, oral cavity or neck.

If feeding assistance is required at home, syringe or tube feeding (i.e., nasoesophageal, esophagostomy, gastrostomy tube) protocols can be established to allow the owner to successfully deliver nutritional support to the pet.

Parenteral nutrition (PN) is a more complex system in terms of formulation and delivery of the admixture, as well as patient monitoring (Chapter 26). PN is less physiologic with respect to gut health; however, evaluation of admixture supplementation with specific nutrients to promote gut integrity is ongoing (Burke et al, 1989; Sheng-Long et al, 1992), which may help promote the efficacy of PN for critically ill patients. Nevertheless, PN is generally reserved for patients that are unable to assimilate nutrients or those with intractable vomiting. An example is a patient with GI lymphoma that is stabilized with PN until remission is obtained with chemotherapy. Optimally, the next step would entail DER being met with a combination of PN and enteral nutrition. Eventually, as appetite and tolerance improve, the enteral route can be used exclusively. PN in human cancer patients is still controversial; some clinical trials have failed to demonstrate benefit, whereas others demonstrate a positive effect with respect to nutritional parameters, survival or tumor response (McGeer et al, 1990; Chlebowski, 1991). Large clinical trials have not been performed with veterinary cancer patients; however, one author (KES) has reported PN to be beneficial for managing individual canine and feline cancer patients. Benefits have been assessed by weight maintenance, enhanced immunocompetence and wound healing, improved attitude, maintenance of normoglycemia and hydration status and successful transition from the ICU to at home feeding.

REASSESSMENT

Reassessment of cancer patients should include monitoring the effects of: 1) cancer on the animal, 2) treatment and nutritional management on the tumor and 3) treatment and nutritional support on the patient. The frequency of reassessment depends on each patient's treatment protocol, response to treatment, the complexity of the feeding plan and prognosis. Initially, reassessment may be required daily or multiple times per day. After the patient is discharged and managed at home, reassessment may be conducted weekly, monthly or quarterly until the patient's condition stabilizes.

Comparing the current body weight and BCS with previous assessments best assesses the overall effects of cancer, cancer treatment and nutritional management on the animal. The patient's appetite should be assessed and the daily caloric intake monitored closely. These parameters are most accurately assessed by frequent (daily) record keeping by the pet owner. The veterinarian can review these records and correlate them with recheck physical examination and diagnostic findings to ascertain the adequacy of the overall treatment and feeding plan. Additionally, nutrient status influences stabilization of organ function, protein status, leukocyte number, hydration, blood glucose and electrolyte status; these parameters are easily monitored through routine blood work and urinalysis. Additional markers of tumor growth and disease staging, which are currently more amendable to monitoring in a research setting, have been reviewed in previous sections. Appropriate modifications to the feeding plan should be made as the patient's status changes.

Food and feeding method changes may be part of the management plan. An important goal of assisted feeding is to transition the patient to voluntary intake. This can be facilitated by: 1) decreasing the amount of food administered and/or the feeding frequency and 2) offering an appropriate palatable form of food for voluntary consumption before, or in place of, the scheduled tube feeding. As the patient increases voluntary caloric intake, calories delivered via the assisted route should be decreased proportionately. After the patient is consuming 75% of DER calories voluntarily, assisted-feeding devices can be removed.

Patient management may require diet alternatives due to physiologic changes that result in food aversion or inability of the patient to consume a certain form of diet. In the case of suspected food aversion, first choose an alternate diet with novel protein sources. A second attempt might include increasing the fat and/or sodium content. If aversions persist with commercial diet options, consider a home-cooked diet.

Assess the patient's ability to adequately prehend and swallow the form of diet offered. Moist diets may be easier to consume in adequate amounts compared to dry kibble. Moistening dry food with warm water or a flavored broth may enhance intake.

ACKNOWLEDGMENTS

The authors and editors acknowledge the contributions of Drs. Gregory K. Ogilvie and Stanley L. Marks in the previous edition of Small Animal Clinical Nutrition.

ENDNOTE

a. Prescription Diet n/d Canine. Hill's Pet Nutrition, Inc., Topeka, KS, USA.

REFERENCES

The references for **Chapter 30** can be found at www.markmorris.org.

CASE 30-1

Diarrhea and Weight Loss in a Gordon Setter

Stanley L. Marks, BVSc, PhD, Dipl. ACVIM (Internal Medicine, Oncology) and ACVN
School of Veterinary Medicine
University of California, Davis
Davis, California, USA

Patient Assessment

A seven-year-old, 23-kg, intact male Gordon setter was examined for anorexia, lethargy, diarrhea and weight loss of six weeks' duration. Physical examination revealed a depressed, cachectic dog (body condition score 1/5). The remainder of the physical examination was unremarkable except for mild dehydration (5%). Abnormal results of a complete blood count, serum biochemistry profile and urinalysis included hypoalbuminemia (2.1 g/dl, normal 2.8 to 3.5) and hypoglobulinemia (2.3 g/dl, normal 3.0 to 3.5). Thoracic and abdominal radiographs were normal. Intestinal lymphoma was confirmed based on histopathologic evaluation of biopsy specimens taken from the small intestine during flexible endoscopy of the upper gastrointestinal (GI) tract.

The cachexia was likely due to a combination of diminished caloric intake, malassimilation and altered metabolism secondary to malignancy (**Table 1**). The anorexia was probably associated with the intestinal lymphoma, secondary abdominal pain and hyperlactatemia. The dehydration and lethargy were probably secondary to the underlying problems causing cachexia.

Assess the Food and Feeding Method

The dog was normally fed one cup of a dry specialty brand food twice daily (810 kcal [3.39 MJ]) with occasional table foods. The food had the following nutrient profile (% dry matter basis):

Protein	29	Sodium	0.4
Crude fat	19	Phosphorus	1.3
Crude fiber	3.5	Potassium	0.6
Calcium	1.6	Magnesium	0.1
Chloride	0.5	NFE (carbohydrate)	44

Questions

1. What indices can be used to assess this dog's nutritional status in the face of severe cachexia?
2. What are the types and amounts of macronutrients that should be fed to this dog?
3. What is this patient's caloric requirement?
4. What food and feeding method should be used for this dog?

Answers and Discussion

1. Because anthropometric measurements are usually not performed in dogs and cats, nutritional status is determined by a thorough history and physical examination. Laboratory evaluation of total lymphocyte count, hematocrit and serum albumin and urea nitrogen concentrations can be helpful to further evaluate nutritional status. These parameters have limited usefulness because hypoalbuminemia and lymphopenia have many causes unrelated to nutritional status. Albumin also has a relatively long half-life (eight days in normal dogs) and is slow to respond to changes in nutritional status. In the face of severe intestinal malassimilation with marked hypoalbuminemia and ascites, body weight becomes an insensitive index. Body condition assessment is the best means of assessing nutritional status of patients with cancer.
2. Some tumor cells preferentially use carbohydrates and protein, but have difficulty using lipids. Host tissues can continue to oxidize lipids for energy. This phenomenon has led to the hypothesis that foods relatively high in fat benefit animals with cancer compared with foods high in easily digested carbohydrates. Dietary carbohydrates should be reduced to limit the tumor from metabolizing glucose for energy by anaerobic glycolysis with the formation of lactate as an end product. Fluid therapy to correct dehydration should avoid fluids containing lactate. High concentrations of carbohydrate may result in peripheral lactate production and energy loss by futile cycling through the Cori cycle. Other complications of excess dietary carbohydrate include hyperglycemia, hyperosmolar states, excess CO_2 production and hepatic steatosis. An appropriate formulation for supporting canine cancer patients contains 30 to 45% protein calories, 50 to 65% fat calories and fewer than 20% carbohydrate calories.
3. The estimated resting energy requirement (RER) for this dog at its current weight is RER = $70(BW_{kg})^{0.75}$ or 735 kcal (3.08 MJ). Daily energy requirement (DER) would be approximately 1,000 kcal (4.15 MJ) (1.35 x RER). This amount could be increased if activity level were higher or if weight gain was being promoted.
4. Although the cure for intestinal lymphoma remains elusive, it is clear that adequate, aggressive nutritional support is a key adjuvant to the treatment plan for cancer patients with chronic diarrhea. The enteral route is the preferred route of nutritional support because it is easier, less expensive and more physiologic than parenteral administration. However, some animals are temporarily unable to assimilate nutrients administered into the GI tract because of functional (severe malassimilation secondary to intestinal lymphoma), anatomic (short bowel syndrome) or mechanical (ileus or obstruction) reasons.

   Patients with intractable vomiting or diarrhea, severe malabsorption and severe pancreatitis may also benefit from parenteral nutrition (PN). PN is indicated in this dog because of the absence of available functional bowel to digest and absorb sufficient nutrients to promote recovery. It is well documented; however, that patients receiving long-term PN develop intestinal mucosal atrophy, bacterial translocation and reduced concentrations of secretory IgA.

   Beause enteral feeding improves mucosal thickness, stimulates gut trophic hormones and stimulates IgA production, partial enteral feeding via nasoesophageal intubation is recommended. PN can be used to supply the majority of the dog's energy and protein requirements, whereas enteral feeding can be used to help maintain intestinal mucosal integrity and limit bacterial translocation. Nasoesophageal tubes are an excellent first choice for the short-term (i.e., less than 10 days) enteral feeding of most critically ill dogs and cats. One disadvantage of nasoesophageal tubes is their small diameter (3- to 8-Fr. tubes), necessitating the use of a liquid enteral formula.

Treatment and Feeding Plan

PN was initiated on Day 2 of hospitalization at a rate of 20 ml/hr (50% of the estimated DER). The rate was increased to 40 ml/hr on Day 3 of hospitalization. The parenteral solution consisted of 8.5% crystalline amino acids, 20% lipid, 50% dextrose and B-complex vitamins. Body weight, attitude, rectal temperature and concentrations of serum total protein, glucose and electrolytes were monitored to allow for early recognition and management of complications. A multi-drug approach to treat lymphoma was started on Day 2 of hospitalization.

Nasoesophageal feeding was instituted on Day 3 using an energy-dense (1.3 kcal/ml, 5.44 kJ/ml) commercial enteral formula

(Prescription Diet a/d Canine/Feline[a]) that contains high levels of protein (44.2% dry matter [DM]), fat (30.4% DM), glutamine (5.2% DM), arginine (2.4% DM) and omega-3 fatty acids (2.6% DM). The enteral formula was tube-fed four times daily (50 ml per feeding) to supply 20% of the dog's estimated caloric requirement. Although low fat foods are better tolerated in a variety of GI disorders, the multiple small feedings and slow rate of administration were felt to abrogate this concern. The dog was receiving its DER on Day 4 of hospitalization through the combined use of enteral and parenteral routes. No complications were observed with the feeding regimen. The dog appeared brighter and had gained 1.1 kg of body weight.

The dog gained an additional 1.5 kg of body weight over the next four days of hospitalization and its attitude and diarrhea continued to improve. On Day 8 of hospitalization, the PN administration rate was decreased to 20 ml/hr (50% of estimated caloric requirement). In place of the nasoesophageal feedings, small frequent feedings of a moist commercial veterinary therapeutic food (Prescription Diet n/d Canine[a]) were given to meet 50% of the dog's caloric requirement. The dog was discharged 10 days after initial hospitalization following discontinuation of parenteral feeding. The moist veterinary therapeutic food was continued at home. DER was increased to 1,300 kcal (5.44 MJ).

The dog continued to do well throughout the rest of the induction period (six weeks), and was seen weekly for physical examinations, complete blood counts and chemotherapy administration. Apart from continued mild nonregenerative anemia, and mild neutropenia on Day 31, the dog maintained in complete remission and showed no adverse effects to chemotherapy. The dog had gained 6 kg of body weight at the end of the induction period (Day 45) and its body condition score had improved to 2/5. Reassessment on Day 180 revealed a bright, alert and responsive dog that appeared to be in complete remission.

Further Discussion

It is imperative that a cancer patient's response to dietary therapy be evaluated and modified if needed. The DER can vary by as much as 20% between different dogs with the same body weight and catabolic insult. Thus, the patient's caloric intake may need to be increased or decreased depending on body weight and condition. Long-term administration of chemotherapeutic agents such as prednisone or other immunosuppressive therapy could further worsen malnutrition and predispose patients to significant infective complications.

Endnote

a. Hill's Pet Nutrition, Inc., Topeka, KS, USA.

Bibliography

Matus RE. Chemotherapy of lymphoma and leukemia. In: Kirk RW, ed. Current Veterinary Therapy X. Philadelphia, PA: WB Saunders Co, 1989; 482-488.

Table 1. Nutritional problems associated with gastrointestinal neoplasia.

Anorexia with progressive weight loss and dehydration
Taste changes causing reduced food intake
Alterations in fat, carbohydrate and protein metabolism
Intestinal malabsorption associated with:
Protein-losing enteropathy
Electrolyte and fluid loss

CASE 30-2

Chronic Vomiting in a Cat

Gregory K. Ogilvie, DVM, Dipl. ACVIM (Internal Medicine, Oncology)
California Veterinary Specialist's Angel Care Cancer Center
San Diego Valley, California, USA

Patient Assessment

A 10-year-old, neutered female domestic shorthair cat was examined for persistent vomiting of 10 days' duration. The vomiting occurred most commonly after meals, was projectile at times and was becoming more frequent. Two months earlier, another veterinarian removed an "abscessed lymph node" found during an exploratory celiotomy that was performed to determine the cause of intermittent vomiting. Histopathology was not performed on the excised lymph node.

The cat appeared very depressed, slightly dehydrated and was breathing slowly (10 breaths/min.). Dried vomitus was adhered to its lower jaw and chest. Rectal temperature was 38.8°C (102°F). The pulse rate was 180/min. Mucous membranes were tacky and pale pink. Body weight was 3 kg and the body condition score was 2/5.

A complete blood count, serum biochemistry profile, urinalysis, chest and abdominal radiographs and feline leukemia virus and feline immunodeficiency virus tests were performed. Results of these tests were negative or within normal limits except for the following values: hypoalbuminemia (2.1 g/dl, normal 2.8 to 3.5), hypochloremia (109 mEq/l, normal 118 to 125), hyponatremia (120 mEq/l, normal 147 to 156), hypokalemia (3.0 mEq/l, normal 4.0 to 4.5) and metabolic alkalosis (bicarbonate 39 mEq/l, normal 17 to 24). A dilated stomach and proximal duodenum were noted on radiographs. Very little abdominal fat was present. A tentative diagnosis of proximal gastrointestinal obstruction was made.

The metabolic problems were treated with intravenous fluids (0.9% NaCl with 40 mEq KCl/l) in anticipation of an exploratory celiotomy. A "napkin ring" stricture of the proximal duodenum was surgically resected. Intraoperative cytology and subsequent histopathology confirmed a diagnosis of intestinal lymphoma.

Assess the Food and Feeding Method

The cat was normally fed a commercial dry specialty brand cat food formulated for adult cats. The food was offered free choice.

Questions

1. Why is nutritional management important for recovery of this patient?
2. What short- and long-term feeding methods should be used for this patient?
3. Chemotherapy is indicated in this cat to control systemic disease. Can the adverse effects of chemotherapy be managed nutritionally?

Answers and Discussion

1. Hypoalbuminemia, reduced fat mass and less than ideal body condition indicate significant malnutrition in this patient. Cancer cachexia is associated with slow wound healing, decreased immune response, increased toxicity from chemotherapy and decreased survival. Nutritional support of cancer patients maximizes healing, decreases side effects of chemotherapy and prolongs the disease-free interval and survival.
2. Feeding tubes and enteral nutritional support should always be considered in cancer patients undergoing surgery. Placement of feeding tubes at the time of surgery is convenient and allows both short- and long-term nutritional management of patients. It is far easier to prevent development of cancer cachexia than to return a patient with cancer cachexia to a more normal state. Feeding tubes are also convenient to ensure that medications (e.g., antiemetics, antibiotics) are administered without the need for central venous access. Chemotherapy, radiation therapy and cachexia are associated with poor wound healing in cancer patients. Because of these factors, gastrostomy tubes may be associated with higher complication rates such as leakage and development of peritonitis. Esophagostomy tubes may be preferred in these types of patients for enteral nutritional support.
3. Well-controlled studies in human cancer patients show that adequate nutritional support is associated with decreased toxicity from chemotherapy. Although similar studies have not been performed using dogs and cats, it is likely that side effects of chemotherapy would also be minimized in animals receiving appropriate food in adequate amounts.

Progress Notes

Jejunostomy and esophagostomy tubes were placed during surgery. Within 24 hours after surgery, feeding was started with a commercial human liquid food (Osmolite HN[a]) supplemented with protein (Promod[a]). Chemotherapy was started for lymphoma even though no obvious disease was found outside the intestinal tract. The cat was treated initially with cyclophosphamide, vincristine, prednisone and doxorubicin at the time of suture removal.

As soon as vomiting subsided (one week after surgery), jejunostomy tube feeding was discontinued and feeding through the esophagostomy tube was initiated. Metoclopramide was given via the tubes as needed to control further vomiting. After four weeks, the cat had gained weight and was able to maintain improved body condition with voluntary oral feeding of a veterinary enteral product (Prescription Diet a/d Canine/Feline[b]). This food was fed for three months during chemotherapy. The original dry specialty food was fed when chemotherapy was discontinued. The cat has remained in clinical remission for three years.

Endnotes

a. Ross Laboratories, Columbus, OH, USA.
b. Hill's Pet Nutrition, Inc., Topeka, KS, USA.

Section 10

Adverse Food Reactions and Skin and Hair Disorders

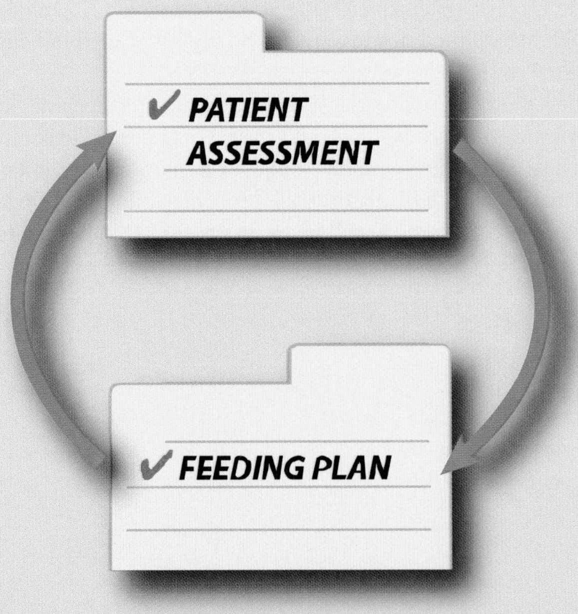

Chapter 31

Adverse Reactions to Food

Philip Roudebush
W. Grant Guilford
Hilary A. Jackson

"For this changed concept of reactivity, I propose the term allergy. 'Allos' implies deviation from the original state, from the behavior of the normal individual..."
Von Pirquet, 1906

CLINICAL IMPORTANCE

An adverse reaction to food is an abnormal response to an ingested food or food additive. Adverse reactions to food are composed of a variety of subclassifications based on pathomechanisms (**Figure 31-1**) (Anderson, 1986; Strombeck and Guilford, 1991). The terms food allergy and food hypersensitivity should be reserved for those adverse reactions to food that have an immunologic basis. Food intolerance refers to a large category of adverse food reactions due to nonimmunologic mechanisms. Traditionally, the terms food hypersensitivity and food allergy have been used to describe all adverse reactions to food in dogs and cats, including reactions that were truly food intolerances.

In view of the number of diverse foods that are routinely ingested by dogs and cats, it is not surprising that adverse reactions develop. That food-related reactions appear relatively infrequently is testimony to the effectiveness of the gastrointestinal (GI) mucosal barrier and oral tolerance. Adverse reactions to food were reported in dogs and cats as early as 1920 and have been blamed for a variety of clinical syndromes usually involving the skin and GI tract.

Carefully controlled prevalence studies of adverse food reactions in dogs and cats have not been performed. The major problem with establishing prevalence is that adverse food reactions mimic other diseases, especially other pruritic dermatoses, and they often coexist with other allergic conditions. Veterinary dermatologists suggest that adverse food reactions account for 1 to 6% of all dermatoses in general practice and that food allergy constitutes 10 to 49% of allergic responses in dogs and cats (MacDonald, 1993; Scott et al, 2001; Chesney, 2002; Loeffler et al, 2004; Jackson et al, 2005). Several investigators have suggested that adverse food reactions are relatively more common in cats than in dogs (MacDonald, 1993; Scott et al, 2001). Food allergy is one of the most common causes of hypersensitive skin disease in dogs and cats along with arthropod (flea) hypersensitivity and atopic dermatitis triggered by environmental allergens (MacDonald, 1993; Scott et al, 2001; Jackson et al, 2005). Adverse food reactions can cause a wide variety of cutaneous lesions and should be considered as a cause of any pruritic disease in dogs or cats. Most of the reported adverse food reactions causing dermatoses have been termed food allergy or food hypersensitivity, although no specific tests were performed to confirm an immunologic basis for the clinical signs.

Adverse reactions to foods also appear to be an important cause of GI signs in cats and dogs. In one study of chronic idiopathic GI problems in cats, 16 of 55 cats (29%) were diagnosed as food sensitive by elimination-challenge tests (Guilford et al, 2001). Furthermore, the clinical signs of 11 cats (20%) in this

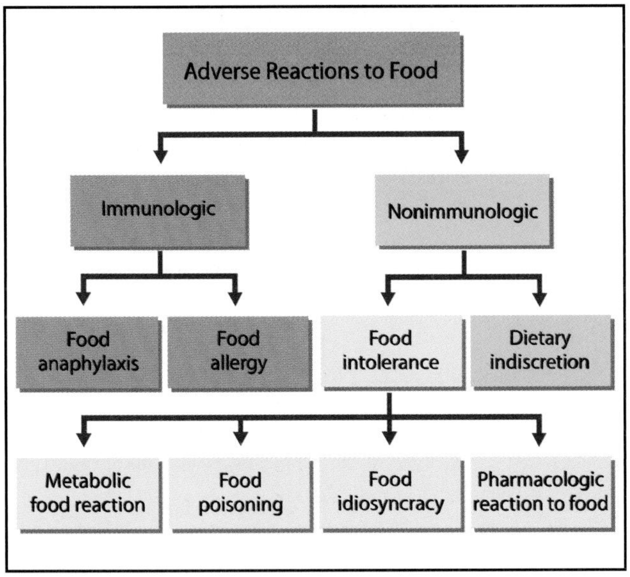

Figure 31-1. Classification of adverse reactions to food.

study resolved when they were fed the elimination food but signs did not recrudesce when the previous food was fed. Food sensitivity may also be involved in some cases of inflammatory bowel disease (IBD) in dogs and cats, particularly lymphocytic-plasmacytic enteritis and eosinophilic gastroenteritis (Elwood et al, 1994; Rutgers et al, 1995; Guilford, 1996). Clinical response to a modification in the feeding plan suggests that hypersensitivity to food antigens plays a role in dogs with chronic idiopathic or lymphocytic-plasmacytic colitis (Simpson et al, 1994; Leib et al, 1989; Nelson et al, 1988). It is unknown if chronic colitis or other forms of inflammatory disease of the small bowel are a direct manifestation of an adverse food reaction or if modifying the feeding plan is merely palliative in some patients.

PATIENT ASSESSMENT

Nutritional History

The authors of two series of dermatologic cases due to adverse food reactions could not relate the onset of clinical signs with recent food changes (Walton, 1967; Baker, 1974). This finding suggests that dogs and cats may develop food allergies after prolonged exposure to one brand, type or form of food. In contrast, adverse reactions due to food intolerance may occur after a single exposure to a food ingredient because immune amplification is unnecessary.

The nutritional history of the patient should be reviewed carefully for ingredients thought to be commonly associated with adverse food reactions. The nutritional history should include a complete list of the foods used in the pet's regular feeding plan or as treats including: 1) specific commercial foods, 2) commercial snacks and treats, 3) supplements, 4) chewable medications, 5) chew toys, 6) human foods and 7) access to other food sources. As an example, a dog might be given a dry commercial food as its main source of nutrition, but may also be given rawhide chews, commercial dog biscuits, flavored monthly oral heartworm prophylactic medication and leftover foods from human meals, and it may have access to commercial food fed to cats in the household. All of these ingested items could be sources of adverse food reactions. It is often helpful to have the pet owner keep a diary for several weeks documenting the types of food and other items the pet ingests daily. Nutritional assessment is described in more detail later in this chapter.

History and Physical Examination

Dermatologic Responses to Adverse Food Reactions in Dogs

Reports of adverse food reactions in dogs with cutaneous disease did not document a gender predisposition and ages ranged from four months to 14 years (MacDonald, 1993; Scott et al, 2001; Walton, 1967; Baker, 1974; August, 1985; White, 1986; Carlotti et al, 1990; Jeffers et al, 1991; Kunkle and Horner, 1992; Rosser, 1993; Harvey, 1993; Paterson, 1995; Roudebush and Schick, 1995). Up to one-third of cases, however, may occur in dogs less than one year of age (Rosser, 1993; Harvey, 1993). Most investigators have not found a breed predilection, although when compared to the local hospital case population, West Highland white terriers were found to be at increased risk (Rosser, 1993; Chesney, 2002; Jackson et al, 2005).

Adverse food reactions in dogs typically occur as nonseasonal pruritic dermatitis, occasionally accompanied by GI signs (MacDonald, 1993; Scott et al, 2001; Walton, 1967; Baker, 1974; August, 1985; White, 1986; Carlotti et al, 1990; Jeffers et al, 1991; Kunkle and Horner, 1992; Rosser, 1993; Harvey, 1993; Paterson, 1995; Roudebush and Schick, 1995). The pruritus varies in severity. Lesion distribution is often indistinguishable from that seen with atopic dermatitis triggered by environmental allergens; feet, face, axillae, perineal region, inguinal region and ears are often affected (MacDonald, 1993; Scott et al, 2001; Walton, 1967; Baker, 1974; August, 1985; White, 1986; Carlotti et al, 1990; Jeffers et al, 1991; Kunkle and Horner, 1992; Rosser, 1993; Harvey, 1993; Jackson, 2005). The similarity of clinical presentation has prompted the International Task Force on Canine Atopic Dermatitis to publish a position statement to the effect that canine atopic dermatitis should be considered a disease condition that can be triggered by environmental and or food allergens and both should be considered in dogs with nonseasonal disease (Olivry et al, 2007).

In one report, one-fourth of dogs with adverse food reactions had lesions only in the region of the ears (Rosser, 1993). This finding suggests that adverse food reactions should always be suspected in dogs with pruritic, unilateral or bilateral otitis externa, if accompanied by secondary bacterial or *Malassezia* infections (MacDonald, 1993; Scott et al, 2001). Unusual or atypical dermatologic responses to adverse food reactions in dogs include: erythema multiforme (Scott and Miller, 1999), claw disease (Mueller et al, 2000) and generalized erythematous wheals (urticarial vasculitis) (Nichols et al, 2000).

Adverse food reactions in dogs produce no set of pathognomonic cutaneous signs. A variety of primary and secondary skin lesions occur and include: 1) papules, 2) erythroderma, 3) excoriations, 4) hyperpigmentation and 5) seborrhea sicca. Adverse food reactions often mimic other common canine skin disorders including pyoderma, pruritic seborrheic dermatoses, folliculitis and ectoparasitism (MacDonald, 1993; Scott et al, 2001). Twenty to 30% or more of dogs with suspected adverse food reactions may have concurrent allergic disease, such as flea-allergic or atopic dermatitis (Baker, 1974; Jeffers et al, 1991; Rosser, 1993; Hillier and Griffin, 2001; Jackson et al, 2005). Some dogs present with only recurrent bacterial pyoderma, with or without pruritus, wherein all clinical signs resolve temporarily with antibiotic therapy (Scott et al, 2001; White, 1986; Harvey, 1993).

Food anaphylaxis is an acute reaction to food or food additives with systemic consequences. The most common clinical manifestation in dogs occurs in localized form referred to as angioedema or facioconjunctival edema (Scott et al, 2001; Thompson, 1995). Angioedema is typically manifested by large edematous swellings of the lips, face, eyelids, ears, conjunctiva and/or tongue, with or without pruritus (Scott et al, 2001; Thompson, 1995). The same types of substances that induce systemic anaphylaxis evoke angioedema (Thompson, 1995). Most veterinary practitioners attribute angioedema solely to insect envenomation (biting or stinging insects) but a number of other common causes include food, drugs, vaccines, infections and blood transfusions (Scott et al, 2001; Thompson, 1995; Nichols et al, 2001). These reactions usually occur within minutes of allergen exposure and generally subside after one to two hours.

One of the authors (PR) has seen angioedema of the tongue, palate and throat repeatedly in the same dogs after ingestion of mushrooms, domestic flowers or other plants. This presentation resembles the oral allergy syndrome in people, which is a form of contact urticaria confined almost exclusively to the oropharynx (Sampson, 1993). Clinical signs in people include rapid onset of pruritus and angioedema of the lips, tongue, palate and throat. Signs usually resolve rapidly. This syndrome is most commonly associated with ingestion of various fresh fruits and vegetables. Affected people are often primarily sensitized to certain airborne pollens (especially birch or ragweed pollen); the immunologic basis for this syndrome is IgE cross reactivity. One report details the clinical and immunologic findings in a dog that developed oral allergy syndrome to tomato after prior sensitization with Japanese cedar (Fujimora et al, 2002).

Dermatologic Responses to Adverse Food Reactions in Cats

The age of cats affected with food sensitivity has ranged from six months to 12 years; a gender predisposition has not been documented (Carlotti et al, 1990; White and Sequoia, 1989; Rosser, 1993a; Guaguere, 1995; Roudebush and McKeever, 1993; Medleau et al, 1986). In one study, almost half the cats developed the disease by two years of age (Rosser, 1993a). Siamese or Siamese cross cats accounted for nearly one-third of cases in two studies, suggesting a potential increased risk (Carlotti et al, 1990; Rosser, 1993a).

Dermatologic signs include several different clinical reaction patterns such as: 1) severe, generalized pruritus without lesions, 2) miliary dermatitis, 3) pruritus with self trauma centered around the head, neck and ears, 4) self-induced alopecia, 5) pyotraumatic dermatitis and/or 6) scaling dermatoses (MacDonald, 1993; Scott et al, 2001; Carlotti et al, 1990; White and Sequoia, 1989; Rosser, 1993a; Guaguere, 1995; Roudebush and McKeever, 1993; Medleau et al, 1986). In one study, angioedema, urticaria or conjunctivitis occurred in one-third of cats with adverse food reactions (Rosser, 1993a). Adverse reactions to food may also be implicated in cats with the so-called eosinophilic skin diseases such as eosinophilic plaques, eosinophilic granulomas and indolent ulcers of the lips (MacDonald, 1993; Scott et al, 2001; Roudebush and McKeever, 1993; Waisglass et al, 2006). Concurrent flea-allergy or atopic dermatitis triggered by environmental allergens may occur in up to 30% of cats with suspected adverse food reactions (Carlotti et al, 1990; Rosser, 1993a).

It has been suggested that moderate to marked peripheral lymphadomegaly is found in up to one-third of cats with dermatologic manifestations of food allergy (Scott et al, 2001). Absolute peripheral eosinophilia occurs in 20 to 50% of feline cases (Scott et al, 2001; White and Sequoia, 1989; Medleau et al, 1986).

GI Responses to Adverse Food Reactions in Dogs and Cats

Gender predilections have not been established for GI disease resulting from adverse reactions to foods (Walton, 1967; Baker, 1974). Similarly, there are no well-documented breed predispositions to GI food allergy, but Chinese Shar-Pei and German shepherd dogs are commonly affected. Furthermore, gluten-sensitive enteropathy has been well documented in Irish setter dogs (Batt et al, 1984). A wide age range of patients can be affected, including dogs and cats as young as weaning age.

Every level of the GI tract can be damaged by food allergies. In dogs, cats and people, clinical signs usually relate to gastric and small bowel dysfunction, but colitis can also occur (Heyman, 1989; Guilford and Badcoe, 1992; Sampson et al, 2001). Vomiting and diarrhea are prominent features. The diarrhea can be profuse and watery, mucoid or hemorrhagic (Guilford and Badcoe, 1992; Baker, 1990). Intermittent abdominal pain, intermittent diarrhea, weight loss, flatulence, irritable demeanor, soft feces and increased frequency of defecation are also seen (Guilford et al, 2001; Loeffler et al, 2004). Concurrent cutaneous signs may be seen. GI disturbances occur in up to half of dogs and cats with cutaneous manifestations of food hypersensitivity (MacDonald, 1993; Scott et al, 2001; Loeffler et al, 2004, 2006). In experimentally induced food hypersensitivity, the most common clinical signs are diarrhea, an increase in the number of bowel movements and occasional vomiting (Roudebush and McKeever, 1993; Frick, 1991). Pruritic dogs with more than three bowel movements per day are more likely to have an adverse reaction to food as part of the reason for

Box 31-1. Gastroscopic Food Sensitivity Testing.

Gastroscopic food sensitivity testing (GFST) is a diagnostic technique in which food extracts (5,000 to 15,000 protein nitrogen units/ml) are dripped onto the gastric mucosa by means of the operating channel of an endoscope. The site is then observed for two to three minutes. Mucosal swelling suggests an immediate sensitivity to the food extract tested. Erythema, blanching, edema and petechiation at the mucosal site also suggest the test subject is hypersensitive to the food, and the food, therefore, should not be used as part of the sensitive patient's diet. Sampling of the mucosal site with subsequent measuring of histamine levels, other mediator levels or mast cell degranulation can be used to determine whether the response was immune mediated. The diagnostic accuracy of GFST isn't known.

The Bibliography for **Box 31-1** can be found at www.markmorris.org.

their dermatoses (Scott et al, 2001; Paterson, 1995; Loeffler et al, 2004, 2006). The increased frequency of defecation will normalize with use of an appropriate elimination food (Loeffler et al, 2004).

There are at least five subacute to chronic GI conditions thought to involve food allergy in people: 1) food protein-induced enterocolitis, 2) food-induced colitis syndrome, 3) food-induced malabsorption syndrome, 4) gluten-sensitive enteropathy and 5) allergic eosinophilic gastroenteritis (Sampson, 1991; Sampson et al, 2001; Motala, 2008). All of these conditions can occur in dogs and cats. The role of food allergy in canine and feline IBD is unknown. Hypersensitivity to food is probably involved in the pathogenesis of this syndrome; at least some affected animals could be more appropriately diagnosed as suffering from food protein-induced enterocolitis. Dogs with GI diseases, including IBD, have more food allergen-specific serum IgG than normal dogs, a finding that may reflect increased antigen exposure due to increased mucosal permeability (Foster, 2003). Currently, 10% of dogs with IBD diagnosed by one of the authors (WGG) have positive gastroscopic food sensitivity tests (GFST) to food antigens (**Box 31-1**). Positive GFST results to foods used in the treatment of the disease are often detected during followup endoscopic studies. This finding strongly implies that food allergy is involved in the perpetuation of IBD but that it may not be the primary cause. That is, inflammation of the mucosa predisposes animals to the development of acquired food allergies. Therefore, a change in food antigens may temporarily reduce the immune-mediated mucosal inflammatory response. The longevity of this amelioration is questionable; however, because most of the so-called "hypoallergenic" foods commonly used in veterinary medicine contain intact proteins that are hypoallergenic primarily by virtue of their novelty to the host's immune system. The duration of protein novelty to the gut-associated lymphoid tissue (GALT) is likely to be very limited if the antigen is fed to a patient with a highly porous mucosal barrier. Irritable bowel syndrome is a disease of dogs characterized by chronic recurrent abdominal pain and large bowel diarrhea (Guilford, 1996a). Feeding changes will often alleviate the signs of irritable bowel disease, implying that food sensitivity plays a role in this syndrome. In the experience of one of the authors (WGG), avoiding gas-producing foods (e.g., homemade vegetable-based foods) or foods with a high fat content is particularly advantageous in the management of dogs with irritable bowel syndrome. In affected dogs, the adverse reactions to these nutrients are most likely due to food intolerance rather than food allergy.

Diagnostic Methods

The diagnosis of an adverse reaction to a food is confirmed by elimination-challenge trials (Jackson, 2009). In food-sensitive patients, resolution of clinical signs occurs after elimination of the responsible food from the diet followed by a return of the signs when the patient is challenged with the original food. Subsequently, feeding the elimination food should again alleviate clinical signs. Correct design of elimination-challenge trials is imperative for reliable diagnosis and is described below in the Feeding Plan section.

Failure to challenge a suspected food-sensitive patient will lead to marked over diagnosis of food sensitivity (Guilford et al, 2001). However, whether to challenge the patient or not is a decision that needs to be made collectively with the owner. Many owners are happy with a presumptive diagnosis of food sensitivity and do not wish to undertake a challenge test. After a diagnosis of food sensitivity is made, further cycles of elimination-challenge trials may then be undertaken in an attempt to identify the responsible food ingredients. It is noteworthy that dietary trials confirm or rule out adverse reactions to food but do not indicate the underlying mechanism (allergy or intolerance).

The place of skin tests, laboratory assays and endoscopic provocation tests remains uncertain in the diagnosis of food sensitivity. None of these are suitable as screening tests for adverse reactions to food because they do not screen for the entire spectrum of adverse reactions to foods (both allergy and intolerance). Some tests (e.g., measurement of food-specific serum IgE) suggest that an adverse reaction to a particular food (identified in an elimination-challenge trial) may be due to a type-1 hypersensitivity response rather than another type of allergic reaction or a food intolerance. However, at the present time, intradermal testing, radioallergosorbent tests (RASTs) and enzyme-linked immunosorbent assays (ELISAs) for food hypersensitivity are considered unreliable in patients with dermatologic (Jeffers et al, 1991; Kunkle and Horner, 1992) and GI disease (Foster, 2003). Although it is sensible to avoid feeding proteins that have caused positive gastroscopic or colonoscopic food sensitivity tests (especially more severe reactions such as edema and petechiation), the diagnostic accuracy of these endoscopic provocation tests requires further evaluation (Guilford et al, 1994; Vaden et al, 2000; Allenspach et al, 2006) as does the diagnostic accuracy of ultrasonography for food sensitivity, which has recently shown some promise (Arslan et al, 2006; Gaschen et al, 2008).

Risk Factors

Risk factors for adverse food reactions in animals are currently unknown but may include: 1) certain foods or food ingredients (see below), 2) poorly digestible proteins, 3) any disease that increases intestinal mucosal permeability (e.g., viral enteritis), 4) selective IgA deficiency, 5) genetic predisposition, 6) age (six months to four years) and 7) concurrent allergic disease.

Etiopathogenesis

Normal Mucosal Barrier and Oral Tolerance

Ingested food represents the greatest foreign antigenic load confronting the immune system. The defense against hypersensitivity to food antigens includes an effective mucosal barrier and oral tolerance generated by the cellular immune system of GALT (Strombeck and Guilford, 1991; Sampson, 1993; Walker, 1987; Murphy and Walker, 1991).

An important adaptation of the GI tract is the development of a mucosal barrier that prevents the overwhelming uptake of food antigens (Sampson, 1993; Walker, 1987; Murphy and Walker, 1991). Efficient functioning of the mucosal barrier excludes the majority of ingested antigens, thus minimizing antigen exposure to GALT. The concept of a mucosal barrier includes effective digestion, the mucous layer, intact and functioning epithelial cells and IgA (**Table 31-1** and **Figure 31-2**).

Complete digestion of food protein results in free amino acids and small peptides that are poor antigens. An incompletely digested food protein has the potential to incite an allergic response because of residual antigenic proteins and large polypeptides. The composition of the mucous coat overlying the intestinal surface contributes to the defense against antigen attachment and penetration. Mucus contains carbohydrate moieties that may act as receptor inhibitors, thereby interfering with attachment of antigens to the intestinal microvillous surface (Sampson, 1993; Walker, 1987; Murphy and Walker, 1991). A direct association between intestinal cell membrane protein/phospholipid ratios and antigen uptake has been demonstrated in some species. Changes in cell membrane composition and function occur early in life, but how these changes affect food antigen uptake is unknown. IgA is the major immunologic component of the mucosal barrier because it is present in high concentrations in intestinal secretions. IgA may complex with food antigens in the intestinal lumen or within the mucous coat, thereby preventing their transport.

Despite these defense mechanisms, the mucosal barrier is not completely impervious to macromolecules; food proteins cross the intact intestinal mucosa in small but significant amounts. Antigens that enter and pass through the lamina propria are removed by the mononuclear-macrophage (reticuloendothelial) system of the liver and mesenteric lymph nodes.

The intestine, traditionally viewed as an organ of digestion and absorption of nutrients, maintains an indispensable immunologic function (Walker, 1987; Murphy and Walker, 1991). The gut is probably one of the largest immune organs in the body. GALT is composed of four distinct lymphoid compartments: 1) aggregates of lymphoid follicles throughout the intestinal mucosa, 2) lymphocytes and plasma cells scattered throughout the lamina propria, 3) intraepithelial lymphocytes interdigitated between enterocytes and 4) mesenteric lymph nodes (**Figure 31-3**) (Sampson, 1993).

Although GALT must mount a rapid and potent response against potentially harmful foreign substances and pathogenic organisms, it also must remain unresponsive to enormous quantities of food antigens. Absorbed food antigens (Van Wijk and Knippels, 2007) are presented to GALT in such a manner that a potent gut-associated, cell-mediated suppressive response develops (**Figure 31-4**).

Table 31-1. Gastrointestinal barriers to ingested food antigens.

Physiologic barriers
Breakdown ingested antigens
Gastric acid and pepsin
Pancreatic enzymes
Intestinal enzymes
Intestinal epithelial cell lysozyme activity
Block penetration of ingested antigens
Unstirred water layer
Intestinal mucous coat (glycocalyx)
Intestinal microvillous membrane composition
Intestinal peristalsis
Immunologic barriers
Block penetration of ingested antigens
Antigen-specific secretory IgA in gut lumen
Clear antigens penetrating GI barrier
Monocyte-macrophage system
Serum antigen-specific IgA and IgG

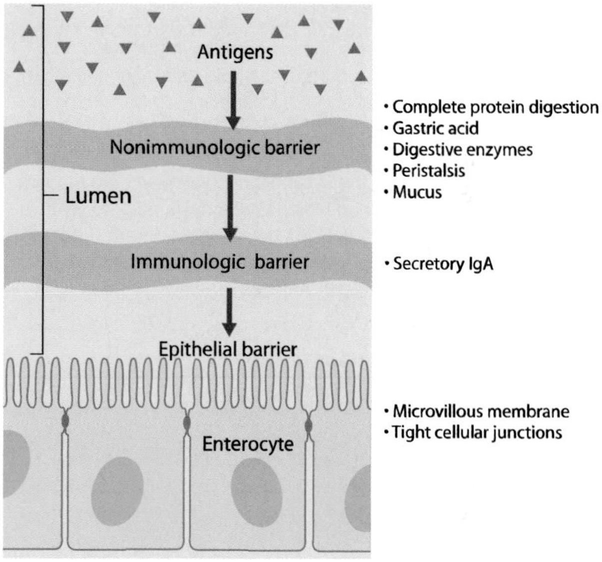

Figure 31-2. Diagrammatic representation of barriers to antigen penetration of the intestinal mucosa. Antigens are prevented from entering the mucosa by nonimmunologic and immunologic mechanisms and the physical structure of the epithelium. (Adapted from Iyngkaren N, Abidin Z. Intolerance to food proteins. In: Lifshitz F, ed. Pediatric Nutrition. New York, NY: Dekker, 1981; 453.)

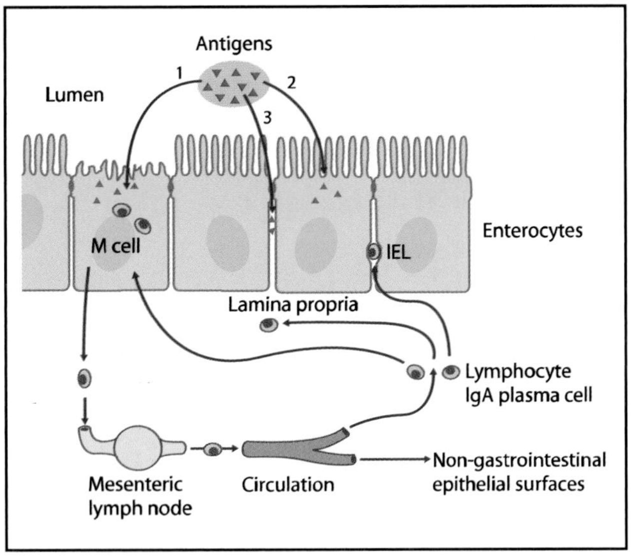

Figure 31-3. Diagrammatic representation of the gut-associated lymphoid tissue (GALT) and the mucosal immune cycle. GALT is composed of Peyer's patches, lamina propria lymphocytes and plasma cells, intraepithelial lymphocytes (IEL) and mesenteric lymph nodes. Food antigens are absorbed via specialized M cells (1) or enterocytes (2,3). These antigens stimulate lymphocytes, which migrate by way of the intestinal lymphatics to mesenteric lymph nodes, ultimately reaching the systemic circulation via the thoracic duct. Specific immune-primed lymphocytes cycle back to GALT or are deposited at other mucosal surfaces. (Adapted from Patrick MK, Gall DG. Protein intolerance and immunocyte and enterocyte interaction. Pediatric Clinics of North America 1988; 35: 17-34.)

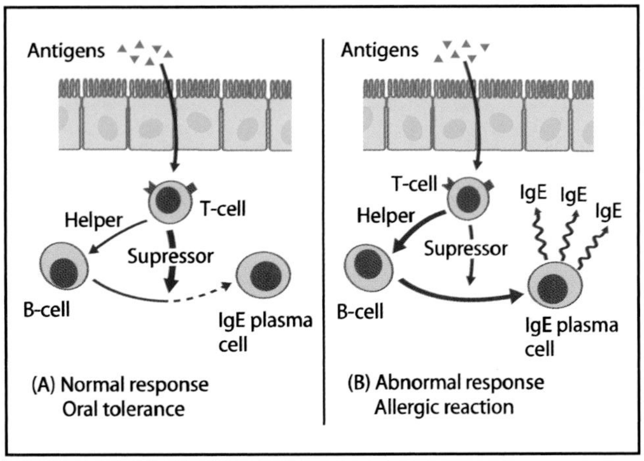

Figure 31-4. Diagrammatic representation of food antigen absorption under different conditions. With a normal response (A), T-cell suppressor activity occurs and contributes to oral tolerance. In (B), an abnormal immune response contributes to production of excess IgE and may result in allergic disease. (Adapted from Walker WA. Pathophysiology of intestinal uptake and absorption of antigens in food allergy. Annals of Allergy 1987; 59: 7-16.)

This immune suppressor response, along with anergy and cell deletion is the basis of oral tolerance. Conversely, an allergic response may result if the antigen encounters a defective suppressor arm of GALT or escapes into the systemic circulation. The concept of "immune exclusion" of food antigens is important because systemic lymphoid tissue responds by active immunoreactivity, which could lead to allergic clinical signs rather than immune suppression (tolerance).

Immunologic Reactions to Food

FOOD ALLERGENS

The specific food allergens or ingredients that cause problems in animals have been poorly documented (**Table 31-2**). In general, the major food allergens that have been identified in people are water-soluble glycoproteins that have molecular weights ranging from 10,000 to 70,000 daltons and are stable to treatment with heat, acid and proteases (Sampson, 1993). Other physiochemical properties that account for their unique allergenicity are poorly understood (Aalberse, 2000; Breiteneder and Ebner, 2000).

The most common food allergens in children are found in chicken egg, peanut, cow's milk, fish, soy and wheat (Sampson, 1993, 1991a, 1988; Yunginger, 1991). In human adults, various fruits, tree nuts, peanut, fish, seafood (mollusks, crustaceans) and cow's milk are confirmed most often as causing food allergy (Sampson, 1993, 1991a, 1988; Yunginger, 1991). Discussion of the specific protein fractions and allergens in these foods that are thought to cause problems are reviewed elsewhere (Sampson, 1993; Yunginger, 1991; Breiteneder and Ebner, 2000; Sicherer, 2001; www.allergen.org).

Fifteen different studies, representing 278 dogs, described primarily cutaneous lesions associated with adverse reactions to specific foods or ingredients (Elwood et al, 1994; Walton, 1967; Carlotti et al, 1990; Jeffers et al, 1991, 1996; Kunkle and Horner, 1992; Harvey, 1993; Paterson, 1995; Mueller and Tsohalis, 1998; Mueller et al, 2000; Chesney, 2002; Tapp et al, 2002; Ishida et al, 2003, 2004) (**Table 31-2**). Beef, dairy products and wheat are most commonly reported as ingredients causing adverse food reactions in dogs. After analysis, specific food allergens identified in dogs include chicken serum albumin, bovine IgG (cow's milk, beef), ovine IgG (lamb), muscle phosphoglucomutase (beef, lamb) and Gly proteins 50 and 75 kD (soy) (Cave et al, 2000; Cave, 2001; Cave and Guilford, 2004; Martin et al, 2004; Serra et al, 2006).

Ten different studies or case reports, representing 56 cats, described cutaneous lesions and/or GI disorders associated with adverse reactions to specific foods or ingredients (Walton, 1967; Carlotti et al, 1990; White and Sequoia, 1989; Guaguere, 1995; Walton et al, 1968; Stogdale et al, 1982; Reedy, 1994; Guilford et al, 1996b, 2001)[a] (**Table 31-2**). Beef, dairy products and fish are most commonly reported as ingredients causing adverse food reactions in cats. Specific food allergens have not been identified in cats.

Human allergy reference books often contain phylogenetic tables of animal and vegetable foods, so food-allergic persons can avoid other closely related foods. In clinical practice, human patients often report cross reactivity among various fish and crustaceans, but less cross reactivity within vegetable food groups (Sicherer, 2001). Results of oral food challenges in children demonstrate that clinically important cross reactivity to legumes (peanuts, soybeans, green beans, lima beans, peas, lentils) is very rare (Bernhisel-Broadbent and Sampson, 1989). Wheat, rye and barley cross react in allergic people, but oat allergens appear to cross react only weakly (Varjonen et al, 1994). Cross reactivity between milk proteins from cows, goats and sheep is common. In children, chicken egg cross reacts with egg proteins of other birds (Sampson, 1993). Cross reactivity among food allergens has only been investigated to a minor degree in pet animals (Jeffers et al, 1996; Martin et al, 2004).

PATHOPHYSIOLOGIC MECHANISMS

Abnormalities in GI defense mechanisms may predispose patients to food allergies (Strombeck and Guilford, 1991). Predisposing factors for food allergy include: 1) mucosal barrier failure (poorly digestible proteins, incomplete protein digestion, increased intestinal mucosal permeability, age-related changes in microvillous cell membrane composition, inflammatory-induced changes in mucus composition) and 2) defective immunoregulation (decreased IgA secretion, deranged cell-mediated responses of GALT, monocyte-macrophage system dysfunction) (**Figure 31-4**). Which of these pathomechanisms are important predisposing factors in dogs and cats awaits further investigation. The most extensively studied and best-defined food allergic reactions in people and laboratory animals involve IgE-mediated responses that result in clinical signs of immediate hypersensitivity (within minutes to hours) (Sampson, 1993). IgE-activated mast cells also may release a variety of cytokines that mediate a late-phase response (within several hours to days). With repeated ingestion of a food allergen, mononuclear cells are stimulated to secrete histamine-releasing factors that interact with IgE bound to the surface of basophils and mast cells and increase their releasability (Sampson et al, 1989). This in vitro phenomenon has been associated with increased cutaneous reactivity in children with atopic dermatitis (Sampson et al, 1989).

Unlike food allergy in people, the pathogenesis of adverse food reactions in dogs and cats has not been fully elucidated. Canine models of IgE-mediated food hypersensitivity have been developed by repeated exposure to food allergens and adjuvant (Guilford and Badcoe, 1992; Schiessl et al, 2003; Buchanan and Frick, 2002; Kennis, 2001; Cave and Guilford, 2004). More recent reports describe spontaneous food allergy in dogs in which food-allergen specific IgE responses can be demonstrated in association with clinical disease (Ishida, 2003; Jackson and Hammerberg, 2002; Jackson et al, 2003). However, other studies have been unable to detect clinically relevant food antigen-specific IgE in client-owned dogs with known adverse food reactions (Mueller and Tsohalis, 1998; Hillier and Kunkle, 1994). Although IgE may be involved in the pathogenesis of food allergy in some dogs, it is unlikely to be the sole immunologic mechanism of disease, particularly in chronic situations (Foster et al, 2003).

Type II (cytotoxic), Type III (immune complex) and Type IV (cell-mediated) hypersensitivity reactions have been implicated less commonly in food-allergic disorders in people (Sampson, 2004).

Table 31-2. Ingredients commonly associated with adverse food reactions.*

Dogs	
Ingredients	***% of reported cases***
Beef, dairy products, wheat	69
Lamb, chicken egg, chicken, soy	25
Cats	
Ingredients	***% of reported cases***
Beef, dairy products, fish	80

*Data from cases reported in North America, Europe, Australia, Japan and New Zealand. Common food allergens may differ in other geographic locations.

GLUTEN (GLIADIN) ENTEROPATHY

Gluten-induced enteropathy (celiac disease) is an important chronic inflammatory disease of the small intestine of people. The prevalence of gluten intolerance in dogs and cats is unknown. Research has conclusively demonstrated that an analogous disorder affects Irish setter dogs (Batt et al, 1984), and clinical experience suggests that other breeds may also be affected.

Flour from cereal grains contains various proteins including: 1) water-soluble albumins, 2) saline-soluble globulins, 3) ethanol-soluble prolamins and 4) acid- or alkali-soluble glutelin (Yunginger, 1991). Prolamins of wheat, rye and barley have marked sequence homology, but not the prolamins of rice and corn, which do not exacerbate the disorder (Kasadra et al, 1976). The prolamin and the glutelin proteins of wheat are gliadin and glutenin. Gliadin is a glutamine- and proline-rich polypeptide with a molecular weight of 15,000 daltons. Gliadin is composed of four major electrophoretic fractions, the most toxic of which in people appears to be α-gliadin (Kasadra et al, 1976). "Gluten" is a crude mixture of gliadin and glutenin. Pancreatic enzymes in the intestinal lumen and intracellular enzymes of the mucosal brush border normally digest these peptides. Completely hydrolyzed gliadin is nontoxic.

The cause of gluten sensitivity is unknown. Studies involving gluten-intolerant Irish setters have demonstrated that increased mucosal permeability predates development of the disease (Hall and Batt, 1990). The pathogenesis of gluten-sensitive enteropathy has been debated for many years, but researchers now think gluten sensitivity in people is probably mediated by the immune system. Knowledge of the complete sequence of immunologic events is incomplete, but it appears IgE mediates acute responses to gluten whereas the delayed hypersensitivity (and mucosal atrophy) is mediated by IgA and IgG (Vojdani et al, 2008). Gliadin-activated macrophages may possibly recruit lamina propria lymphocytes resulting in a delayed hypersensitivity response and various inflammatory changes such as infiltration of inflammatory cells, mast cell degranulation, production of eicosanoids, increased microvascular permeability and complement activation (Marsh, 1992; Loft et al, 1989). The lymphocyte density of the mucosal intraepithelium is increased and serum total IgA levels are elevated in gluten-sensitive dogs (Hall et al, 1992).

In contrast to findings in people, antigliadin antibody (IgG) levels are lower in affected dogs than in age-matched control dogs. In addition, serum immune complex levels are not elevated in dogs whereas they are frequently elevated in people (Hall et al, 1992). These findings do not support a role for a systemic immune response in the pathogenesis of canine gluten-sensitive enteropathy but do not rule out a mucosal delayed hypersensitivity response.

Nonimmunologic Reactions to Food

Nonimmunologic, abnormal reactions to food include food intolerance and dietary indiscretion (**Figure 31-1**). Like the terms food allergy and food hypersensitivity, the term food intolerance has been applied inappropriately to any and all adverse reactions to food. Food intolerance mimics food allergy except that it can occur on the first exposure to a food or food additive, because nonimmunologic mechanisms are involved. The incidence of food intolerance vs. food hypersensitivity or food allergy is unknown.

FOOD POISONING

Food poisoning or food toxicosis is an adverse effect caused by the direct action of a food or food additive on the host. Examples of food poisoning include ingestion of: 1) nutrient excesses (vitamin A or vitamin D toxicosis), 2) food contaminated with microorganisms or their toxic metabolites (scavenging putrefied material, vomitoxin), 3) specific foods (onions, chocolate) or 4) toxic food preservatives (benzoic acid or propylene glycol in cats) (Chapter 11).

Food poisoning is a frequent cause of GI disease in dogs and cats. In addition to ingestion of pathogenic microorganisms or their toxins, food poisoning can result from the ingestion of plant-derived toxins or irritants. For example, high levels of oxalates and anthraquinone glycosides contained in rhubarb, spinach and beets can lead to a corrosive gastroenteritis, and large quantities of spices such as peppers can cause abdominal discomfort in people.

REACTIONS TO FOOD ADDITIVES

Idiosyncratic adverse reactions to food additives often occur in people (Hannuksela and Haahtela, 1987; Simon and Stevenson, 1993; Metcalfe et al, 1991; Fuglsang et al, 1994). Food additives frequently incriminated in human adverse reactions include sulfites, monosodium glutamate, tartrazine and other azo or non-azo dyes, benzoates, parabens and spices (Hannuksela and Haahtela, 1987; Simon and Stevenson, 1993; Metcalfe et al, 1991; Fuglsang et al, 1994). Few of the adverse reactions to food additives appear to involve an immunologic mechanism, although IgE-mediated reactions may occur (Hannuksela and Haahtela, 1987; Simon and Stevenson, 1993; Metcalfe et al, 1991; Fuglsang et al, 1994). Confirmed reactions to food additives are best described as food intolerances or food idiosyncrasies because clinical signs resulting from their ingestion are not thought to be immunologically mediated. Examples are reactions to azo dyes, non-azo dyes and antioxidants that can directly cause histamine release from leukocytes of clinically normal people (Murdoch et al, 1987).

Although food additives are frequently incriminated as causing problems in dogs and cats, few data confirm this perception (Roudebush and Cowell, 1992; Roudebush, 1993). Propylene glycol has been documented to cause hematologic abnormalities in cats and subsequently has been eliminated from cat foods sold in the United States and some other countries (Hickman et al, 1990; Weiss et al, 1990). Disulfides found in onions (onion powder, onion-based broth and baby foods containing onion) promote oxidative damage to hemoglobin in canine and feline red blood cells (Robertson et al, 1998). The result is Heinz body production and red cell destruction.

REACTIONS TO VASOACTIVE AMINES IN FOOD

Another cause of food intolerance is pharmacologic reactions to substances found in food. Vasoactive or biogenic amines such as histamine cause clinical signs in people when present in excessive levels in food (Taylor, 1986; Morrow et al, 1991). Scombroid fish such as tuna, mackerel, skipjack and bonito that spoil before consumption are a frequent cause of histamine toxicosis in people (Taylor, 1986; Morrow et al, 1991). Clinical signs usually include diarrhea, flushing, sweating, nausea, vomiting, urticaria, facial swelling and erythroderma.

The role of histamine and other vasoactive amines in food intolerance in dogs and cats is unknown. Adverse reactions to ingested scombroid fish have been observed in cats and dogs (Guilford et al, 1994a). Surveys to detect histamine in pet foods found the highest levels of histamine in moist fish-based cat foods and those cat foods containing fish solubles (Guilford et al, 1994a; Guraya and Koehler, 1991). Vasoactive amines such as cadaverine may also exacerbate adverse reactions to spoiled fish by inhibiting histamine metabolism (Taylor, 1986; Bjeldanes et al, 1978). Tyramine, spermine, spermidine, phenethylamine, putrescine and cadaverine are other vasoactive amines found in low levels in pet foods (Paulsen, 2000).[b] Vasoactive or biogenic amines may not be present in levels high enough to cause clinical signs, but could lower the threshold levels for allergens in individual dogs and cats. Idiosyncratic intolerances to small quantities of histamine have been reported to occur in people and animals (Guilford et al, 1994a).

CARBOHYDRATE INTOLERANCE

Adult hypolactasia, infantile lactase deficiency, congenital lactose intolerance and congenital glucose-galactose malabsorption are disorders of carbohydrate intolerance in people (Halliwell, 1992). Fewer conditions are associated with recognized carbohydrate intolerance in dogs and cats. However, neonatal death following episodes of diarrhea is common and the same spectrum of metabolic disorders resulting in carbohydrate intolerance in people may occur in dogs and cats (Strombeck and Guilford, 1991; Halliwell, 1992).

The diarrhea, bloating and abdominal discomfort that occur when animals with lactose intolerance ingest milk are relatively common metabolic adverse reactions in dogs and cats (Hill and Kelley, 1974; Mundt and Meyer, 1989). Puppies and kittens normally have adequate levels of intestinal lactase to permit digestion of lactose in the dam's milk. In many subjects, brush border disaccharidase activity decreases after weaning to a fraction of the activity found in young animals. Osmotic diarrhea will often occur when excessive levels of lactose are consumed. Puppies, kittens or adult animals may develop diarrhea when given cow's or goat's milk because these milk sources contain more lactose than either bitch's or queen's milk. One study showed that adult dogs were able to use up to 1 g of lactose/kg body weight/day (Meyer et al, 1984), an amount equivalent to 20 to 22 ml/kg of cow's or goat's milk. Greater amounts increased intestinal lactose and lactic acid concentrations, fecal water content and frequency of defecation.

Intolerance to disaccharides commonly occurs secondary to enteritis or rapid food changes. Loss of intestinal brush border disaccharidase activity contributes to the diarrhea associated with enteritis. Inadequate intestinal disaccharidase activity is also one of the factors responsible for diarrhea following rapid food changes. Several days are required for intestinal disaccharidase activity to adapt to changes in food carbohydrate sources.

DIETARY INDISCRETION

Dietary indiscretions such as gluttony, pica and garbage ingestion usually cause GI signs and can be suspected based on the environmental and nutritional history. The clinical signs may be caused by ingestion of excessive fat, bacterial or fungal toxins, vasoactive amines or indigestible materials such as bone, plastic, wood and aluminum foil. Note that underlying disease such as hyperadrenocorticism can also induce polyphagia and resultant dietary indiscretion.

Key Nutritional Factors

Because most food allergens are thought to be glycoproteins, dietary protein in food is the nutrient of most concern in patients with suspected food allergy. The number of different proteins in the food, protein sources and amount of protein comprise the key nutritional factors for foods for diagnosis and management of adverse food reactions. Whether the patient has been exposed previously to the protein is also important.

Because elimination foods replace regular maintenance foods and are fed long term, several key nutritional factors are included because of their relationship to other common health issues rather than specific benefits for patients suffering from adverse food reactions. **Table 31-3** summarizes the key nutritional factors, which are discussed in more detail below.

Table 31-3. Key nutritional factors for foods for the diagnosis and management of adverse food reactions in dogs and cats.

Factors	Dietary recommendations
Dogs	
Protein	Limit dietary protein to one or two sources Use protein hydrolysate or protein sources to which the dog has not been exposed previously Avoid excess levels of dietary protein (dermatologic cases only): protein should be 16 to 22% DM Use a food that is nutritionally balanced for dogs Avoid foods that contain wheat, barley or rye (dogs with diarrhea)
Vasoactive amines	Avoid foods that contain certain fish ingredients (e.g., tuna, mackerel, skipjack, bonito)
Total omega-3 fatty acids	0.35 to 1.8% DM
Phosphorus*	0.4 to 0.8% DM
Sodium*	0.2 to 0.4% DM
Cats	
Protein	Limit dietary protein to one or two sources Use protein hydrolysate or protein sources to which the cat has not been exposed previously Avoid excess levels of dietary protein (dermatologic cases only): protein should be 30 to 45% DM Use a food that is nutritionally balanced for cats
Vasoactive amines	Avoid foods that contain certain fish ingredients (e.g., tuna, mackerel, skipjack, bonito)
Total omega-3 fatty acids	0.35 to 1.8% DM
Phosphorus*	0.5 to 0.8% DM
Sodium*	0.2 to 0.6% DM
Magnesium*	0.04 to 0.1% DM
Urinary pH*	6.2 to 6.4

Key: DM = dry matter.
*Not related to adverse reactions to food but important when elimination foods are used for long-term feeding: phosphorus and sodium are considered key nutritional factors for apparently healthy adult dogs and cats for purposes of ameliorating or slowing the progression of subclinical kidney disease and/or hypertension; magnesium and urinary pH are important for reducing the risk of feline lower urinary tract disease.

Protein

Commercial veterinary therapeutic foods containing unique or novel protein ingredients have been available for more than 40 years. Novel protein sources are usually defined as animal or vegetable ingredients containing protein that are not commonly used in pet foods and/or are not commonly associated with adverse food reactions. Examples of such protein sources include lamb, venison, rabbit, various fish, rice, potato and green peas. Beef, dairy products and wheat in dogs, and beef, dairy products and fish in cats are the most commonly reported ingredients causing adverse reactions and should be avoided in patients with adverse reactions to foods. A careful dietary history should disclose these protein sources. Several published clinical studies support the use of commercial foods containing novel protein sources in the management of adverse food reactions in cats and dogs (Roudebush et al, 2002).

Using the product label to determine whether a potentially offensive protein source(s) is/are present in a patient's current food can be challenging. A large number of protein ingredients are used to manufacture typical commercial pet foods. Many protein ingredients differ from those commonly used for human consumption and may be unfamiliar to veterinarians, veterinary health care team members and animal owners. For example, chicken for human consumption, chicken used in moist pet foods and poultry by-product meal used in dry pet foods may each contain unique allergens. Chapter 8 discusses pet food ingredients and reviews several of the more commonly used protein sources. In the U.S., most commercial foods must adhere to the Association of American Feed Control Official (AAFCO) guidelines for label ingredient listings and definitions (AAFCO, 2008). The definitions can help determine what specific protein sources are in a given ingredient. This information might not be obvious from reading a product's label (Chapter 9).

Another approach to providing novel protein ingredients is the use of hydrolyzed protein(s). Protein hydrolysates offer several hypothetical advantages over intact protein sources. Protein hydrolysates of appropriate molecular weight (<10,000 daltons) are less likely to elicit an immune-mediated response. For example, complete digestion of an initially intact food protein results in free amino acids and small peptides that are poor antigens (Yunginger, 1991). In contrast, poorly digested protein has the potential to incite an allergic response because of residual antigenic proteins and large polypeptides.

Several published clinical studies document the efficacy of foods containing protein hydrolysates in veterinary patients. Clinical improvement was seen in 50 to 80% of dogs allergic to the intact protein (Beale et al, 2001; Jackson et al, 2003; Puigdemont et al, 2006; Serra et al, 2006). Additionally, several clinical trials with protein hydrolysate-type foods have been conducted in canine and feline patients seen in private and specialty practices with dermatologic or GI disease. The results of these studies show similar efficacy of hydrolysates as compared with the more traditional novel protein sources (Loeffler et al, 2004, 2006; Ishida et al, 2004; Biourge et al, 2003; Rosser, 2001). Protein hydrolysates have also been used successfully in cats with self-inflicted alopecia (psychogenic alopecia) and chronic GI disorders (Waly et al, 2006; Waisglass et al, 2006).

Foods containing protein hydrolysates may also benefit patients with increased GI permeability, in which enhanced protein absorption contributes to the pathogenesis of the disease. One study showed positive responses in a small number of dogs with IBD (Marks et al, 2002). Protein hydrolysates have been used for many years in human infant formulas and for human patients with various GI diseases. Novel or unique protein sources are less important with protein hydrolysates. Total protein content, average molecular weight of the hydrolyzed protein and digestibility of nutrients vary among these products.

The value of high protein digestibility in foods with intact protein ingredients has been documented for some commercial pet foods marketed as hypoallergenic or elimination foods (Roudebush et al, 1995). As noted above, more complete digestion of an initially intact food protein results in more free amino acids and small peptides that are poor antigens (Yunginger, 1991). Protein digestibility of at least 87% is recommended for such foods. This degree of protein digestibility is typically met by most veterinary therapeutic pet foods.

Elimination foods that use intact novel proteins should contain preferably only one but no more than two protein sources to which the patient has not been previously exposed. This recommendation includes commercial or homemade foods and either animal or vegetable protein sources.

Excess protein levels should be avoided to reduce the amount of potential allergens to which the patient is exposed. Foods for dogs should provide between 16 to 22% dry matter (DM) protein and foods for cats should provide between 30 to 45% DM protein. A higher protein level may be necessary to counteract losses from the GI tract or impaired absorption in patients with hypoproteinemia and weight loss associated with severe GI disease. Certain protein ingredients are more likely sources of excessive levels of vasoactive or biogenic amines such as histamine. The highest levels of histamine occur in moist fish-based cat foods and cat foods containing fish solubles (Guilford et al, 1994a; Guraya and Koehler, 1991). Pet foods containing these fish may be a source of such amines and probably should be avoided. Human foods that may contain excessive levels of vasoactive or biogenic amines include tomato, avocado, cheese, liver, processed meats such as sausage and certain fish. As mentioned above, vasoactive or biogenic amines may not be present in levels high enough to cause clinical signs, but could lower the threshold levels for allergens in individual dogs and cats.

Omega-3 Fatty Acids

Omega-3 (n-3) fatty acids exhibit multiple antiinflammatory and immunomodulating effects. They have the potential to affect allergic and other inflammatory diseases through modulating cytokine production, inhibiting cellular activation and cytokine secretion, altering the composition and, in the case of dermatologic disease, function of the epidermal lipid barrier (Olivry et al, 2001). Their mechanisms of action, therefore, are likely to be explained by a combination of effects. Generally, however, omega-3 fatty acids are thought to produce less inflammatory cytokines (Sigal, 1991; Lands, 1989; Lokesh et al, 1988; Lokesh and Kinsella, 1987; Broughton et al, 1991; Croft et al, 1987).

Based on levels of omega-3 fatty acid supplementation recommended for use in the management of inflammatory skin diseases (Chapter 32), veterinary therapeutic foods for dogs and cats with inflammatory disease related to adverse food reactions should provide 0.35 to 1.8% DM of total omega-3 fatty acids. However, because of their potential benefit in inflammatory diseases, inclusion of omega-3 fatty acids could confuse the diagnostic phase of managing food sensitivity. The ratio of omega-6 to omega-3 fatty acids that should be included in foods for patients with adverse food reactions is currently unknown.

Phosphorus, Sodium, Magnesium and Urinary pH

Elimination foods used to diagnose patients with possible food sensitivity are fed for short time periods. However, if there is a positive diagnosis of food sensitivity, appropriate veterinary therapeutic foods are fed for prolonged periods of time, in the place of regular maintenance foods. Phosphorus and sodium are recommended as key nutritional factors for maintenance foods for apparently healthy adult dogs and cats for purposes of ameliorating, or slowing the progression of possible concurrent subclinical kidney disease and/or hypertension. Thus, even though phosphorus and sodium are not associated with food sensitivity, they are included as key nutritional factors for overall health. The recommended allowances for phosphorus and sodium in foods for adult dogs are 0.4 to 0.8% DM and 0.2 to 0.4% DM, respectively. For foods for adult cats, the recommended allowances for phosphorus and sodium are 0.5 to 0.8% DM and 0.2 to 0.6% DM, respectively. In addition, for adult cats, magnesium and urinary pH are also key nutritional factors for foods intended for long-term feeding, based on their role in feline lower urinary tract disease. The recommended allowance for magnesium in foods for adult cats is 0.04 to 0.1% DM. Foods for adult cats should produce a urinary pH in the range of 6.2 to 6.4. Chapters 13 and 20 discuss the rationale for including these key nutritional factors for dogs and cats, respectively.

Other Nutritional Factors

Carbohydrate and Fat

Modification of the total dietary fat and carbohydrate content of foods is usually not required in the management of food-sensitive dermatologic patients. However, choosing foods with highly digestible fat and carbohydrate can be important in the management of food-sensitive GI patients because of the enteropathy and malassimilation that may result from allergic inflammation of the GI tract. Furthermore, a reduction in the content of one or both of these macronutrients may be required in patients with nonimmunologic food intolerances to fat and carbohydrate.

Food Additives

Pet food additives such as antimicrobial preservatives, colorants, antioxidant preservatives and emulsifying agents rarely cause food intolerance or allergy. Additives are found least often in moist pet foods and most commonly in semi-moist foods, treats, snacks and dry foods. Many moist commercial pet foods are free of additives. Two of the most frequently incriminated additives in human foods, benzoates and tartrazine, are rarely found in commercial pet foods. However, other additives that have been documented to cause problems in people are found in pet foods (**Table 31-4**). These include azo dyes, non-azo dyes, sodium bisulfite, sodium glutamate, sodium nitrate, butylated hydroxyanisole (BHA), spices, sodium alginate, guar gum and propylene glycol (Fuglsang et al, 1994).

Table 31-4. Food additives that have been reported as occasional causes of food intolerance in people and that are sometimes present in pet foods or treats.*

Antioxidant preservatives
Butylated hydroxyanisole (BHA)
Butylated hydroxytoluene (BHT)
Antimicrobial preservatives
Sodium nitrite
Humectants
Propylene glycol
Coloring agents/preservatives
Azo dyes
Tartrazine (FD&C No. 5)
Sunset yellow (FD&C No. 6)
Allura red (FD&C No. 40)
Non-azo dyes
Brilliant blue (FD&C No. 1)
Indigotin (FD&C No. 2)
Flavors/flavor enhancers
Monosodium glutamate
Spices
Emulsifying agents, stabilizers, thickeners
Seaweed extracts (carrageenan, alginates)
Seed gums (guar gum)

*These additives are frequently incriminated as causing adverse food reactions in dogs and cats, but there are no well-documented case reports to substantiate this perception.

FEEDING PLAN

Unlike most other clinical conditions, the feeding plan for possible food sensitivity patients includes a diagnostic phase. At the present time, intradermal testing, RASTs and ELISAs for food hypersensitivity are considered unreliable for patients with dermatologic disease (Jeffers et al, 1991; Kunkle and Horner, 1992). Dietary elimination trials are the primary diagnostic method used in dogs and cats with suspected adverse food reactions (Jackson, 2009) and are discussed below in the Assess and Determine the Feeding Method section.

Assess and Select the Food

Commercial Elimination Foods

Ingredient statements on commercial pet food labels in the U.S. are sources of information for identifying all the food ingredients that might cause adverse reactions. An individual dog or cat may develop an adverse reaction to virtually any pet food ingredient. However, particular attention should be directed at those ingredients that contain protein. Unfortunately, pet food labeling requirements in other countries are not necessarily as stringent and ingredient statement information is often incomplete (Chapter 9). Contact the manufacturer or distributor for more detailed ingredient information when the ingredient statement is incomplete.

Several companies manufacture a variety of foods with limited and different protein sources (**Tables 31-5** and **31-6**). These commercial veterinary therapeutic products are convenient, contain protein hydrolysates and/or novel protein sources and are nutritionally complete and balanced for either dogs or cats (approved for long-term feeding of healthy adults by a credible regulatory agency such as AAFCO). Unfortunately, few of these commercial foods have been adequately tested in dogs and cats with known adverse food reactions; only a limited number of foods (approximately 15 of more than 50 veterinary therapeutic foods marketed for adverse food reactions) have undergone the scrutiny of clinical trials using patients with dermatologic or GI disease (Rutgers et al, 1995; Simpson et al, 1994; Nelson et al, 1988; Jeffers et al, 1991; Rosser, 1993; Paterson, 1995; Roudebush and Schick, 1995; Guilford et al, 2001; Loeffler et al, 2004, 2006). In published clinical trials,

Table 31-5. Selected commercial veterinary therapeutic foods marketed as elimination foods for dogs with adverse food reactions compared to key nutritional factor recommendations.*

Dry foods	Protein ingredients	Protein (%)**	Omega 3 (%)***	P (%)†	Na (%)†
Recommendations	**Maximum of 1-2 protein sources Avoid scombroid fish†† Avoid wheat, barley and rye†††**	**16-22**	**0.35-1.8**	**0.4-0.8**	**0.2-0.4**
Hill's Prescription Diet d/d Potato & Duck Formula Canine	Potato, duck	18	0.35	0.58	0.36
Hill's Prescription Diet d/d Potato & Salmon Formula Canine	Potato, salmon	18.4	0.995	0.58	0.37
Hill's Prescription Diet d/d Potato & Venison Formula Canine	Potato, venison	18	0.337	0.57	0.36
Hill's Prescription Diet d/d Rice & Egg Formula Canine	Rice, egg	18.8	0.366	0.5	0.28
Hill's Prescription Diet z/d Low Allergen Canine	Potato, hydrolyzed chicken/chicken liver	19.6	na	0.57	0.36
Hill's Prescription Diet z/d ULTRA Allergen-Free Canine	Hydrolyzed chicken/chicken liver	19	na	0.51	0.29
Iams Veterinary Formula Skin & Coat/ Response FP Canine	Potato, herring meal, beet pulp	25.0	na	0.99	0.35
Iams Veterinary Formula Skin & Coat/ Response KO Canine	Oat flour, kangaroo, canola meal, beet pulp	22.7	na	1.01	0.44
Medi-Cal Hypoallergenic Formula	Oat flour/hulls, rice, duck meal	21.3	0.7	0.8	0.4
Medi-Cal Hypoallergenic HP	Rice, soy protein isolate hydrolysate, beet pulp	23.1	0.4	0.9	0.4
Medi-Cal Sensitivity RC 21	Rice/rice gluten, catfish meal	25.8	na	1.3	0.5
Medi-Cal Vegetarian Formula	Oat flour, rice, potato protein, flax meal, beet pulp, tomato pomace	20.9	na	0.9	0.4
Natural Balance Limited Ingredient Diet Potato & Duck Formula	Potato, duck/duck meal, flaxseed	na	na	na	na
Natural Balance Limited Ingredient Diet Sweet Potato & Fish Formula	Sweet potato, salmon/salmon meal, flaxseed	na	na	na	na
Natural Balance Limited Ingredient Diet Sweet Potato & Venison Formula	Sweet potato, venison/venison meal, potato protein, flaxseed	na	na	na	na
Purina Veterinary Diets DRM Dermatologic Management Canine Formula	Rice, salmon meal, trout, canola meal, brewers yeast	30.2	na	1.16	0.24
Purina Veterinary Diets HA Hypoallergenic Canine Formula	Soy protein isolate	21.3	na	0.87	0.24
Royal Canin Veterinary Diet Canine Hypoallergenic HP 19	Rice, soy protein hydrolysate, beet pulp	23.1	0.901	0.88	0.44
Royal Canin Veterinary Diet Canine Potato & Duck Formula	Potato/potato protein, duck/duck by-product meal	22.2	na	0.68	0.33
Royal Canin Veterinary Diet Canine Potato & Duck Formula Light	Potato/potato protein, duck/duck by-product meal	26.9	na	0.81	0.38
Royal Canin Veterinary Diet Canine Potato & Rabbit Formula	Potato/potato protein, rabbit/rabbit meal	23.1	na	0.67	0.33
Royal Canin Veterinary Diet Canine Potato & Venison Formula	Potato/potato protein, venison/venison meal	22.3	na	1.01	0.24
Royal Canin Veterinary Diet Canine Potato & Venison Formula Large Breed	Potato/potato protein, venison/venison meal	23.6	na	1.08	0.45
Royal Canin Veterinary Diet Canine Potato & Whitefish Formula	Potato, herring meal, whitefish	22.5	na	0.66	0.44

usually two-thirds to three-fourths of patients with suspected adverse food reactions had significantly improved clinical signs when fed commercial veterinary therapeutic elimination-type foods. **Tables 31-5** and **31-6** compare the recommended key nutritional factors to those in selected commercial veterinary therapeutic foods intended for patients with adverse food reactions.

Novel or unique protein sources are less important when the patient's nitrogen and amino acid requirements are met by protein hydrolysates. Clinical trials with protein hydrolysates show similar efficacy to more traditional novel protein-source foods (Loeffler et al, 2004, 2006; Ishida et al, 2004; Biourge et al, 2003; Rosser, 2001). Protein hydrolysate foods have also been used successfully in cats with self-inflicted alopecia and chronic GI disorders (Waly et al, 2006; Waisglass et al, 2006).

In general, snacks, chews and treats should be avoided.

Royal Canin Veterinary Diet Canine Skin Support SS 21	Menhaden fish meal, rice/brown rice, beet pulp	25.3	0.714	1.21	0.44
Royal Canin Veterinary Diet Canine Vegetarian Formula	Oat flour, rice, yeast culture, tomato pomace, beet pulp, flaxseed, carrot pomace	19.1	na	0.56	0.15
Wellness Simple Food Solutions Rice + Duck Formula	Rice/rice protein concentrate, duck, flaxseed	na	na	na	na
Wellness Simple Food Solutions Rice + Venison Formula	Rice/rice protein concentrate, venison, flaxseed	na	na	na	na
Moist foods	**Protein ingredients**	**Protein (%)****	**Omega 3 (%)*****	**P (%)†**	**Na (%)†**
Recommendations	**Maximum of 1-2 protein sources** **Avoid scombroid fish††** **Avoid wheat, barley and rye†††**	**16-22**	**0.35-1.8**	**0.4-0.8**	**0.2-0.4**
Hill's Prescription Diet d/d Duck Formula Canine	Duck/duck liver, potato	17.4	0.384	0.69	0.36
Hill's Prescription Diet d/d Lamb Formula Canine	Rice, lamb/lamb liver	15.8	0.395	0.31	0.34
Hill's Prescription Diet d/d Salmon Formula Canine	Salmon, potato	18.9	1.787	0.7	0.33
Hill's Prescription Diet d/d Venison Formula Canine	Venison, potato	18.9	0.328	0.53	0.37
Hill's Prescription Diet z/d ULTRA Allergen-Free Canine	Hydrolyzed chicken liver	19.6	na	0.57	0.2
Iams Veterinary Formula Skin & Coat/Response FP Canine	Catfish, herring meal, potato starch, beet pulp	35.5	na	0.92	0.60
Medi-Cal Hypoallergenic Formula	Pheasant, rice flour, duck meal, oat hulls	20.1	0.006	1.0	0.5
Medi-Cal Sensitivity VR	Venison/venison by-products, rice	35.8	na	2.4	1.2
Medi-Cal Vegetarian Formula	Rice/brown rice, soy protein isolate	26.4	na	0.7	0.5
Natural Balance Duck & Potato Formula	Duck/duck liver, potato	na	na	na	na
Natural Balance Fish & Sweet Potato Formula	Ocean white fish, sweet potato, salmon, potato, fish meal	na	na	na	na
Natural Balance Venison & Sweet Potato Formula	Venison/venison liver, sweet potato, potato	na	na	na	na
Royal Canin Veterinary Diet Canine Duck Formula	Potato, duck/duck by-products	18.5	na	0.86	1.45
Royal Canin Veterinary Diet Canine Venison Formula	Potato, venison/venison by-products	18.5	na	0.86	1.45
Royal Canin Veterinary Diet Canine Whitefish Formula	Potato, whitefish	18.5	na	0.86	1.45
Wysong Duck Au Jus	Duck, animal plasma	na	na	na	na
Wysong Rabbit Au Jus	Rabbit	na	na	na	na
Wysong Turkey Au Jus	Turkey/turkey liver, animal plasma	na	na	na	na
Wysong Venison Au Jus	Venison/venison liver, animal plasma	na	na	na	na

Key: Omega 3 = total omega-3 fatty acids, P = phosphorus, Na = sodium, na = not available from manufacturer.
*Values are on a dry matter basis unless otherwise stated.
**A higher protein level may be necessary to counteract protein losses from the GI tract or impaired absorption in patients with hypoproteinemia and weight loss associated with severe GI disease.
***Omega-3 fatty acids are important for dermatologic cases.
†Phosphorus and sodium are not important for adverse food reactions but are important for overall health when feeding these foods long-term.
††Fish source ingredients that can be a source of vasoactive amines.
†††For dogs with diarrhea.

Another criterion for selecting a food that may become increasingly important in the future is evidence-based clinical nutrition. Practitioners should know how to determine risks and benefits of nutritional regimens and counsel pet owners accordingly. Currently, veterinary medical education and continuing education are not always based on rigorous assessment of evidence for or against particular management options. Still, studies have been published to establish the nutritional benefits of certain pet foods. Chapter 2 describes evidence-based clinical nutrition in detail and applies its concepts to various veterinary therapeutic foods.

Homemade Elimination Foods

Results of a survey of veterinarians in the American Academy of Veterinary Dermatology (AAVD) showed that homemade foods were often recommended as the initial test

Table 31-6. Selected commercial veterinary therapeutic foods marketed as elimination foods for cats with adverse food reactions compared to key nutritional factor recommendations.*

Dry foods	Protein ingredients	Protein (%)**	Omega 3 (%)***	P (%)†	Na (%)†	Mg (%)†	Urinary pH†
Recommendations	**Maximum of 1-2 protein sources Avoid scombroid fish††**	**30-45**	**0.35-1.8**	**0.5-0.8**	**0.2-0.6**	**0.04-0.1**	**6.2-6.4**
Hill's Prescription Diet d/d Duck & Green Pea Formula Feline	Peas, duck/duck meal	32	0.353	0.72	0.4	0.111	6.30
Hill's Prescription Diet d/d Rabbit & Green Pea Formula Feline	Peas, rabbit/rabbit meal	32	0.336	0.73	0.34	0.118	6.38
Hill's Prescription Diet d/d Venison & Green Pea Formula Feline	Peas, venison/venison meal	32	0.34	0.74	0.3	0.116	6.32
Hill's Prescription Diet z/d Low Allergen Feline	Rice, hydrolyzed chicken liver/hydrolyzed chicken	33	0.102	0.67	0.34	0.068	6.30
Medi-Cal Hypoallergenic HP 23	Rice/rice gluten, soy protein isolate hydrolysate	27.4	0.3	0.8	0.5	na	na
Medi-Cal Hypoallergenic/Gastro	Potato meal/potato protein, duck meal, rice	29.8	0.24	0.9	0.4	na	6.2
Medi-Cal Sensitivity RD 30	Rice/rice gluten, duck by-product meal	34.4	na	1.3	0.6	na	na
Natural Balance Limited Ingredient Diets Duck & Green Pea Formula	Peas, duck meal, flaxseed	na	na	na	na	na	na
Royal Canin Veterinary Diet Feline Green Peas & Duck Formula	Peas, duck meal/duck	34.9	na	1.45	0.77	0.118	na
Royal Canin Veterinary Diet Feline Green Peas & Lamb Formula	Peas/pea protein, lamb meal/lamb	34.9	na	1.43	0.76	0.129	na
Royal Canin Veterinary Diet Feline Green Peas & Rabbit Formula	Peas/pea protein, rabbit meal/rabbit	34.9	na	1.13	0.77	0.172	na
Royal Canin Veterinary Diet Feline Green Peas & Venison Formula	Peas/pea protein, venison meal/venison	34.9	na	1.81	0.87	0.129	na
Moist foods	**Protein ingredients**	**Protein (%)****	**Omega 3 (%)*****	**P (%)†**	**Na (%)†**	**Mg (%)†**	**Urinary pH†**
Recommendations	**Maximum of 1-2 protein sources Avoid scombroid fish††**	**30-45**	**0.35-1.8**	**0.5-0.8**	**0.2-0.6**	**0.04-0.1**	**6.2-6.4**
Hill's Prescription Diet d/d Duck Formula Feline	Duck/duck liver, peas	38.1	0.479	0.75	0.3	0.083	6.38
Hill's Prescription Diet d/d Rabbit Formula Feline	Rabbit, peas	36	0.594	0.73	0.27	0.08	6.24

food for dogs and cats with suspected food allergy (Roudebush and Cowell, 1992). Homemade test foods usually include a single protein source or a combination of a single protein source and a single carbohydrate source. Ingredients typically recommended for homemade feline foods include lamb baby food, lamb, rice and rabbit. Lamb, rice, potato, fish, rabbit, venison, various beans and tofu are often recommended for homemade canine foods.

Most of the homemade foods recommended in the AAVD survey for initial management of dogs and cats with suspected food allergy were nutritionally inadequate for growth or adult maintenance (Roudebush and Cowell, 1992). Most homemade foods fail to meet nutritional requirements because they are made from a minimum of ingredients. In general, homemade foods lack a source of calcium, essential fatty acids, certain vitamins and other micronutrients and contain excessive levels of protein, which are contraindicated in food allergy cases.

Feeding nutritionally inadequate homemade foods to dogs less than 12 months of age and cats for more than three weeks may result in clinical problems. Anorexia and poor growth occur in puppies within 10 to 20 days of feeding a thiamin-deficient food (NRC, 2006). Anorexia and emesis occur within one to two weeks after a thiamin-deficient food is fed to cats (NRC, 2006). Many previously recommended homemade elimination foods have a severe inverse calcium-to-phosphorus ratio of 1:10. Skeletal disease in young dogs can occur within four weeks of feeding a food with severe mineral imbalances (Goddard et al, 1970; Morris et al, 1971). Such foods should not be fed for longer than three weeks (Codner and Thatcher, 1990).

This book and other references contain complete and balanced homemade food recipes (Lewis et al, 1987; Remillard and Thatcher, 1989; Meyer, 1990; Roudebush, 1994; Brown et al, 1995; Strombeck, 1999). Non-flavored vitamin and mineral supplements are not perceived as causes of adverse food reactions. Additive-free supplements that do not contain animal or vegetable proteins are unlikely to be sources of ingested allergens. Intolerance to calcium supplements has been reported to occur in atopic children, but is rare (Devlin and David, 1990). Homemade rations should also contain a source of essential fatty acids, such as vegetable oil. Vegetable oils are not a routine source of ingested allergens; studies show that people allergic to

Hill's Prescription Diet d/d Venison Formula Feline	Venison/venison liver, peas	37.3	0.654	0.73	0.35	0.088	6.45
Hill's Prescription Diet z/d ULTRA Allergen-Free Feline	Hydrolyzed chicken liver	33.7	na	0.64	0.3	0.064	6.28
Iams Veterinary Formula Skin & Coat/Response LB Feline	Lamb/lamb liver/lamb by-products/lamb meal, barley, beet pulp	43.4	na	1.02	0.34	0.085	na
Medi-Cal Hypoallergenic/Gastro	Duck/duck meal, rice	35.5	0.16	1.7	0.7	na	6.4
Medi-Cal Sensitivity CR	Chicken, rice	34.5	na	1.6	1.1	na	na
Medi-Cal Sensitivity VR	Venison by-products/ venison, rice	43.0	na	1.6	1.0	na	na
Natural Balance Limited Ingredient Diets Duck & Green Pea Formula	Duck/duck liver/duck meal, peas/pea protein	na	na	na	na	na	na
Natural Balance Limited Ingredient Diets Venison & Green Pea Formula	Venison/venison liver, venison meal, peas, flax-seed	na	na	na	na	na	na
Royal Canin Veterinary Diet Feline Duck Formula	Duck/duck by-products, peas	44.1	na	0.74	0.47	0.078	na
Royal Canin Veterinary Diet Feline Lamb Formula	Lamb by-products/lamb, peas	44.1	na	0.74	0.47	0.078	na
Royal Canin Veterinary Diet Feline Venison Formula	Venison by-products/ venison, peas	44.1	na	0.74	0.47	0.078	na
Wysong Duck Au Jus	Duck, animal plasma	na	na	na	na	na	na
Wysong Rabbit Au Jus	Rabbit	na	na	na	na	na	na
Wysong Turkey Au Jus	Turkey/turkey liver, animal plasma	na	na	na	na	na	na
Wysong Venison Au Jus	Venison/venison liver, animal plasma	na	na	na	na	na	na

Key: Omega 3 = total omega-3 fatty acids, P = phosphorus, Na = sodium, Mg = magnesium, na = not available from manufacturer.
*Values are on a dry matter basis unless otherwise stated.
**A higher protein level may be necessary to counteract protein losses from the GI tract or impaired absorption in patients with hypoproteinemia and weight loss associated with severe GI disease.
***Omega-3 fatty acids are important for dermatologic cases.
†Phosphorus, sodium, magnesium and urinary pH are not important for adverse food reactions but are important for overall health when feeding these foods long-term.
††Fish ingredients that can be a source of vasoactive amines.

peanuts and soybeans can safely ingest peanut oil or soybean oil (Taylor et al, 1981; Nordlee et al, 1981; Bush et al, 1985; Bock, 1991). Homemade food recipes should provide an optimal amount of protein and foods for cats should be supplemented with taurine.

Assess and Determine the Feeding Method

Feeding method factors to consider include how the food is offered, amount fed, access to other food and who feeds the pet. All of this information should have been gathered when the history of the patient was obtained. If the patient has a normal body condition score (2.5/5 to 3.5/5), the amount of food it was fed previously (energy basis) was probably appropriate. There are two basic phases to the feeding method for patients suspected of having adverse food reactions: the diagnostic phase and the treatment phase.

Diagnostic Phase

PERFORMING AN ELIMINATION TRIAL IN PATIENTS WITH DERMATOLOGIC DISEASE

Before an elimination trial is initiated, the clinician should discuss potential sources of food allergens with the client (**Figure 31-5**). The patient is then fed a controlled elimination food for six to 12 weeks. In addition to the feeding change, no other substances should be ingested including treats, flavored vitamin supplements, chewable medications, fatty acid supplements and chew toys. Flavored chewable medications (e.g., oral heartworm preventive medications) have been proven to cause adverse reactions in dogs and should be changed or discontinued in patients with suspected food allergy or intolerance (Jackson and Hammerberg, 2002a). During the elimination trial, the client should document daily the type and amount of food ingested and the occurrence and character of adverse reactions (**Figure 31-6**). A daily food diary helps document progression of clinical signs during the elimination trial and whether a strict elimination trial was performed in the home environment. The diary will often reveal different findings than those offered to the clinician by the client during the recheck examination.

A tentative diagnosis of an adverse food reaction in dermatologic patients is made if the level of pruritus markedly decreases. This improvement may be gradual and may take four to 12 weeks to become evident. In many cases, concurrent

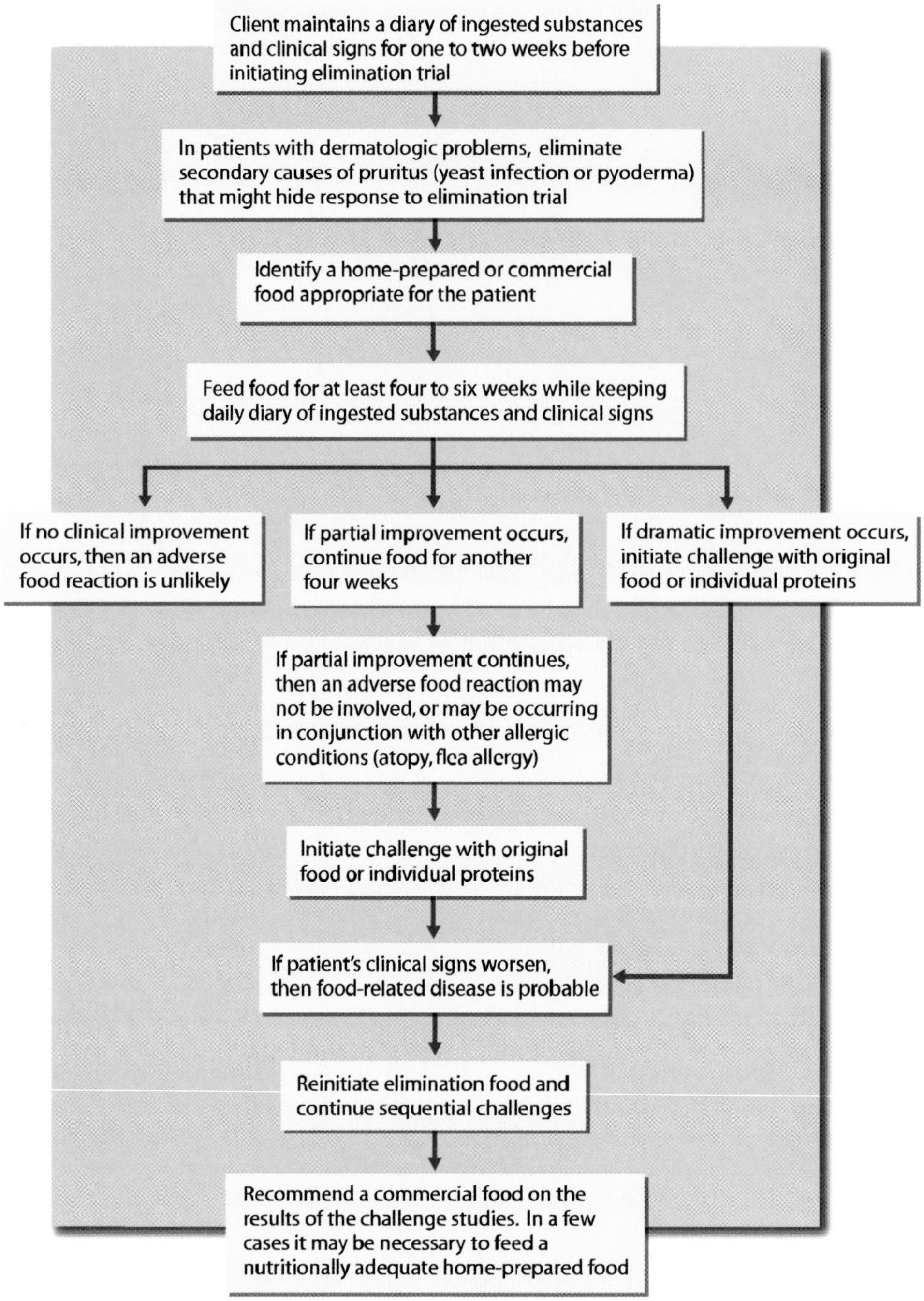

Figure 31-5. Protocol for elimination-challenge trials for the diagnosis of adverse reactions to food.

Malassezia dermatitis, pyoderma and/or otitis externa are present at the time of initial presentation. Treatment for these conditions may be prescribed concurrent with the elimination trial, but after therapy is completed the patient should be fed the elimination food only for two to three weeks before challenge (see below) to ensure that any improvement is maintained. It is also prudent to check that the client is not administering prescribed medications in elicit foods. Patients with chronic otitis externa due to adverse food reactions may require four to six month for obvious improvement to be noted, especially if proliferative lesions are present.

A diagnosis of an adverse food reaction is confirmed if clinical signs reappear after the patient's former food and other ingested substances are offered as a challenge. Clinical signs may be evident within hours of challenge or take up to 14 days. Reinstituting the elimination food should resolve the clinical signs induced by the food challenge. Food challenges can be performed in an "open," "single-blind" or "double-blind" manner. In an open food challenge, both the client and veterinarian are aware that a specific food or previous food is being fed. In a single-blind food challenge, only the veterinarian is aware of what food is being given. In a double-blind food challenge, neither the client nor veterinarian is aware of whether a specific food is being given. Double-blind, placebo-controlled food challenges are considered to be the "gold standard" for the diagnosis of adverse food reactions in people (Sampson, 1993; Bock, 1991). Only half of human patients thought to be allergic to a food react to the food when challenged in controlled, blinded conditions (Bock, 1991). Unfortunately, all reports and most food challenge recommendations in the veterinary literature have been open challenges. Open challenges will continue as the most practical method of establishing tentative diagnoses of adverse food reaction in dogs and cats, but are subject to false interpretation by clients and veterinarians.

Provocation involves introducing single ingredients until as many positive reactions as possible can be documented. Clients and veterinarians are often reluctant to pursue challenge and provocation after clinical signs have improved or have been eliminated. Provocation may also be difficult to perform in many dogs and cats because commercial pet foods contain large numbers of ingredients and feeding the same ingredients often cannot be duplicated in challenge studies. As an example, use of chicken meat in a provocative food challenge may not duplicate the types or levels of antigens found in poultry by-product meal.

Elimination trials are often difficult to interpret because of concurrent allergic skin disease. In several studies, up to 30% of dogs and cats with adverse food reactions had concurrent hypersensitivities (White, 1986; Carlotti et al, 1990; Rosser, 1993, 1993a; Paterson, 1995; Roudebush and Schick, 1995). These patients may only partially respond to an elimination trial. Flea-allergy and atopic dermatitis triggered by environmental allergens are the most common concurrent diseases and should be eliminated through other diagnostic testing.

PERFORMING AN ELIMINATION TRIAL IN PATIENTS WITH GI DISEASE

Elimination-challenge trial designs for patients with GI disease are similar to those for patients with dermatologic problems. However, shorter elimination periods are usually satisfactory (two to four weeks). One study in cats with GI sensitivity showed that vomiting stopped almost immediately in all affected cats and diarrhea resolved within two or three days (Guilford et al, 2001). In chronic relapsing conditions, the elimination period chosen must be longer than the usual symptom-free period of the patient to allow reliable assessment of how food sensitivity contributes to the patient's signs.

As with skin disease, the degree of clinical improvement during the elimination trial will be 100% only if food sensitivity is the sole cause of the patient's problems. For instance, resolution of allergies acquired as a *result* of GI disease will not eliminate the clinical signs due to the primary GI disease process. A return of GI signs after challenge with the responsible allergen will usually occur within the first three days, but may take as long as seven days, particularly if the responsible allergen was removed from the food for longer than one month (Guilford et al, 2001; Walton, 1967).

Treatment Phase

For most adverse food reactions, avoiding the offending foods or food additives is the most effective treatment. Thus, after a diagnosis of adverse food reaction has been made through the proper use of elimination-challenge trials, the elimination food, if nutritionally complete and balanced, should be fed for maintenance. Ideally, when used for long-term feeding, the food choice should also have appropriate levels of phosphorus and sodium for dogs and cats, and magnesium and the recommended urinary pH range for cats (**Tables 31-5** and **31-6**). An attempt should always be made to find an acceptable commercial food that will increase owner compliance with the feeding change.

REASSESSMENT

How selective or meticulous an avoidance food must be depends on the individual patient's sensitivity. Some dogs and cats may suffer adverse reactions to even trace quantities of an offending food or food additive, whereas others may have a higher tolerance level. Concurrent allergies may influence the threshold level of clinical signs in some patients. Symptomatic therapy for pruritic patients may also include corticosteroids and antihistamines. Corticosteroids along with feeding changes are often used in cats with IBD. One-third of people fed a strict avoidance food for one to two years have tolerated the reintroduction of food allergens (Pastorello et al, 1989). Whether this is the case in dogs and cats is not known.

ACKNOWLEDGMENT

The authors and editors acknowledge the contribution of Dr. Kevin J. Shanley in the previous edition of Small Animal Clinical Nutrition.

ENDNOTES

a. Ishida R, Masuda K, Kurata K, et al. Lymphocyte blastogenic responses to inciting food antigens in cats with food sensitivity. Unpublished data. University of Tokyo, Japan, 2002.

b. Roudebush P. Unpublished data. May 1992.

REFERENCES

The references for **Chapter 31** can be found at www.markmorris.org.

Diary for Dietary Elimination Trial							
Day	Date	Food Offered	Food Consumed	Other Items Ingested*	Clinical Signs (Scale 0-5 and Comments)**	Feces (Scale 1-5 and Comments)***	Other Observations
1							
2							
3							
4							
5							
6							
7							
8							
9							
10							
11							
12							
13							
14							
15							
16							
17							
18							
19							
20							
21							
22							
23							
24							
25							
26							
27							
28							
29							
30							

Figure 31-6. Example of a diary that can be maintained at home by clients during a food elimination trial.

31							
32							
33							
34							
35							
36							
37							
38							
39							
40							
41							
42							
43							
44							
45							
46							
47							
48							
49							
50							
51							
52							
53							
54							
55							
56							
57							
58							
59							
60							

***Other Items Ingested**
List rawhide chews, vitamin supplements, chewable medications, treats or snacks, fatty acid supplements, table foods, fresh food or access to other food sources (e.g., dog eating cat food or cat eating an animal it has captured outdoors).

****Clinical Signs**
0 = no clinical signs
5 = severe clinical signs
Itching (scratching, rubbing face, chewing, licking, head shaking); hair loss; skin lesions (scabs, scales, bleeding, red skin, pimples)

*****Feces**
1 = liquid feces that have lost all form
2 = soft-liquid feces with no form
3 = soft feces that form a pile
4 = mixture of soft and firm feces with a cylindrical shape
5 = firm feces with cylindrical shape
Presence of mucus or fresh blood; number of daily bowel movements

CASE 31-1

Pruritic Dermatitis in a Domestic Shorthair Cat

Philip Roudebush, DVM, Dipl. ACVIM (Small Animal Internal Medicine)
Hill's Scientific Affairs
Topeka, Kansas, USA

Patient Assessment

A five-year-old neutered female domestic shorthair cat was referred for severe pruritus with self-trauma around the head, neck, forelimbs and ventral abdomen. The owner reported that intense pruritus had been evident for several weeks and that antihistamines given by another veterinarian had been only partially effective in decreasing the itching. The owner took systemic corticosteroids herself several years ago and developed severe side effects. Because of her experience, she was very reluctant to give corticosteroids to her cat. The owner was very upset about the intense pruritus and apologized for her cat's appearance.

The medical history was unremarkable except for intermittent bouts of lower urinary tract disease that had been treated with antibiotics and a veterinary therapeutic food. The cat spent almost all of its time indoors; no other animals were in the home.

Physical examination revealed excoriations and evidence of self-trauma around the face, neck, ventral abdomen and posterior aspects of the forelimbs (**Figures 1** to **3**). No other abnormalities were noted. There was no evidence of flea infestation. The cat weighed 3.2 kg and had a body condition score of 3/5.

Assess the Food and Feeding Method

The cat was currently fed a dry veterinary therapeutic food (Prescription Diet c/d Feline[b]) and various commercial moist cat foods from the grocery store. The dry food was available free choice and small amounts of the moist foods were offered each day.

Questions

1. What are the major rule outs (differential diagnoses) for this cat's generalized pruritus?
2. If an adverse reaction to food is suspected as a cause of this cat's problem, then an elimination trial would be appropriate. What criteria should be used to select a food for the elimination trial?
3. Describe the feeding method and reassessment plan for this patient.
4. How will the history of lower urinary tract disease influence the feeding plan for this patient?

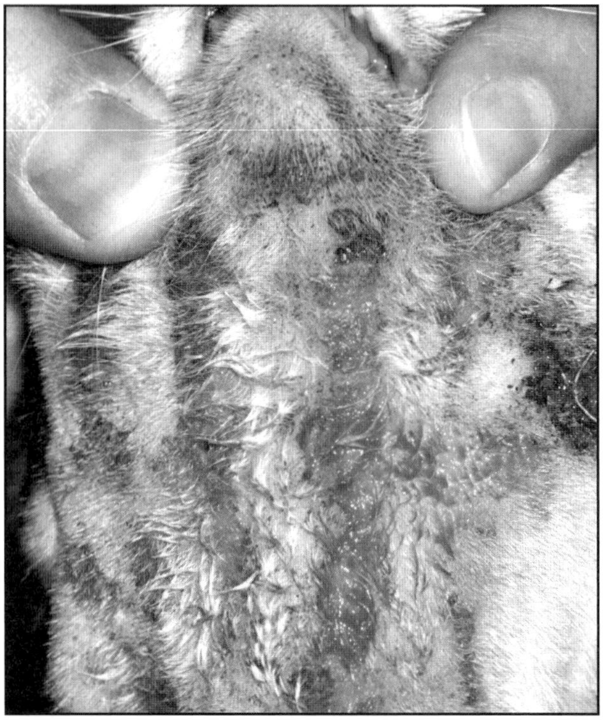

Figure 1. The ventral neck of a five-year-old female domestic shorthair cat showing evidence of severe pruritus with self-trauma.[a]

Answers and Discussion

1. The major rule outs for pruritic dermatitis in this cat include 1) otodectic mange, 2) flea-allergy dermatitis, 3) adverse food reaction, 4) atopic dermatitis triggered by environmental allergens, 5) secondary infections with *Malassezia* spp., and staphylococci spp. and 6) dermatophytosis.

Otodectic mange. Otodectes cynotis (ear mite) is a nonburrowing, psoroptid mite that lives on the surface of the skin. Lesions are usually restricted to the ear canal (otitis externa) but mites are commonly found on other areas of the body, especially on the neck, rump and tail. These ectopic mites often cause no disease but some animals have a pruritic dermatitis that may resemble flea-bite hypersensitivity, atopy or food allergy.

Arthropod hypersensitivity. Flea-bite hypersensitivity (flea-allergy dermatitis) is the most common feline hypersensitivity disease in areas where fleas are present, causing a variety of clinical syndromes all characterized by pruritus. No age, breed or gender predilections have been reported in cats. Papulocrustous eruptions are the most typical lesions, although alopecia, excoriations, crusts and scales may also be found. The presence of fleas, flea dirt, flea eggs or infection with the tapeworm *Dipylidium caninum* provide circumstantial evidence of flea allergy. Recent bathing or grooming may, however, remove all evidence of fleas. In this case, there was no history of flea exposure and no evidence of fleas on the cat.

Adverse reaction to food (food allergy or food intolerance). The intense pruritus in this patient with traumatic alopecia centered around the head, neck and ears is one of the more common clinical manifestations of adverse food reactions in cats. Other dermatologic signs of adverse food reactions in cats include severe, generalized pruritus without significant lesions, miliary dermatitis, moist dermatitis and scaling dermatoses. Angioedema, urticaria and conjunctivitis may occur in up to one-third of cats with adverse food reactions. Concurrent flea-allergy dermatitis and atopy also commonly occur in these patients.

Atopic dermatitis. Feline atopic dermatitis is caused by an exaggerated or inappropriate response of the affected cat to environmental allergens. It is considered the second most common hypersensitivity in cats after flea-allergy dermatitis. The most common clinical signs are noninflammatory alopecia, eosinophilic granuloma complex lesions, miliary dermatitis and pruritus of the face or pinnae. The clinical signs in this patient are compatible with those of feline atopic dermatitis although concurrent flea-bite hypersensitivity and adverse food reactions may also occur.

Secondary infections. Malassezia spp. or staphylococci infections are common and may contribute to the pruritus. Skin surface cytology should be performed to detect these organisms and treatment instituted if necessary.

Dermatophytosis. Feline dermatophytosis most often appears as one or more irregular or annular areas of alopecia on the head, pinnae or paws. The alopecia may be severe and widespread, accompanied by little evidence of inflammation. Pruritus is usually absent to minimal although some cats have a more inflammatory reaction with pruritus and widespread papulocrustous dermatitis. Dermatophytosis is more common in young cats.

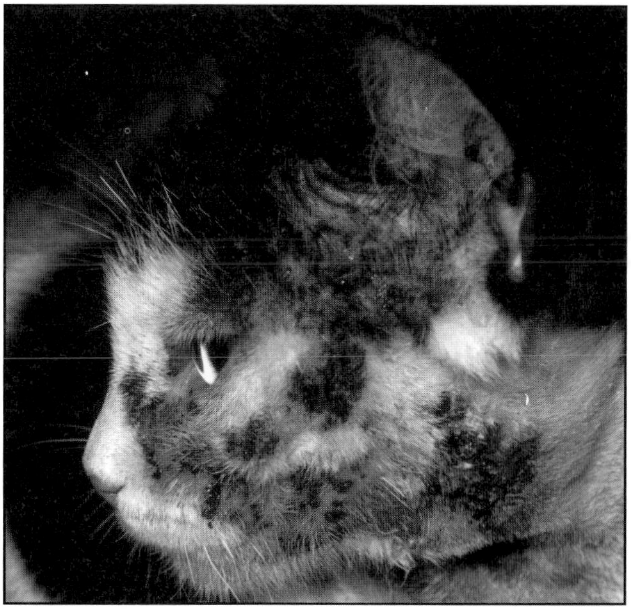

Figure 2. The head and face of the cat in Figure 1 with evidence of intense pruritus and self trauma.[a]

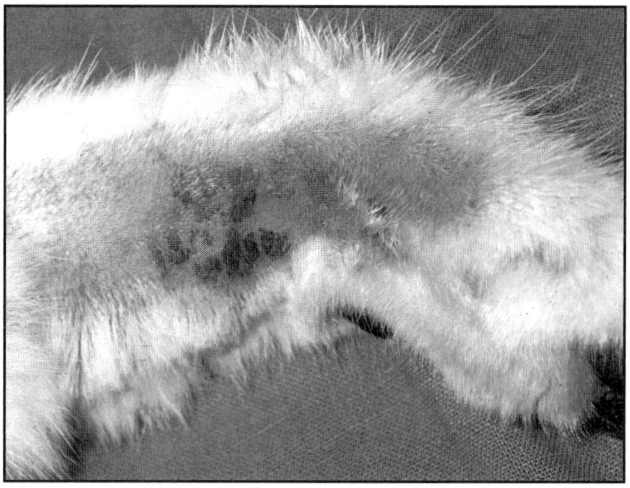

Figure 3. The antebrachium of the cat in Figure 1 showing erythroderma and hair loss due to excessive licking.[a]

2. The key nutritional factors for elimination foods for feline patients with dermatologic disease should: 1) have a limited number of protein sources, 2) have protein hydrolysates or novel protein sources to which the patient has not been previously exposed, 3) avoid excess levels of protein (30 to 45% dry matter), 4) avoid excessive levels of biogenic amines such as histamine, putrescine, cadaverine, etc., 5) have increased levels of omega-3 fatty acids and be nutritionally appropriate for long-term feeding of adult cats (including these key nutritional factors: phosphorus, sodium, magnesium and urinary pH). **Table 31-6** lists selected commercial veterinary therapeutic foods that meet many of these criteria.
3. Before an elimination trial is initiated, the client should be instructed to feed the cat its usual food for several days. During this time the client should record the type and amount of food ingested, any other ingested food items such as table scraps, treats or snacks and the occurrence and character of adverse reactions. The patient should then be fed a controlled elimination food for four to 12 weeks. No other substances such as treats, flavored vitamin supplements or heartworm prophylaxis, fatty acid supplements or toys should be offered. During the elimination trial, the client should document daily the type and amount of food ingested, and the occurrence and character of adverse reactions (**Figure 31-6**). This daily diary is important for documenting the progression of clinical signs during the elimination trial and determining whether a strict elimination trial was performed in the home environment. The diary will often document different findings than those described by the client during the recheck examination.

   A tentative diagnosis of an adverse food reaction is made if the level of pruritus markedly decreases. Improvement may take four to 12 weeks to become evident.
4. Further questioning revealed that this cat had previous problems with struvite urinary precipitates. The struvite precipitates had been well controlled by the veterinary therapeutic food. Offering a food that avoids excess magnesium and produces normal acidic urine helps prevent struvite precipitates (Chapter 46). Therefore, commercial elimination foods used in this patient should also

avoid excess magnesium (<0.1% dry matter magnesium) and produce normal acidic urine (urinary pH 6.2 to 6.4). The urinary pH can be checked periodically as part of the reassessment.

Progress Notes
Diagnostic evaluation included multiple skin scrapings (negative), cytologic evaluation of ear swabs and skin cytology (negative). Intradermal skin testing revealed a few positive reactions to house dust mite antigen and several mold antigens. The cat was treated with an anthelmintic twice at three-week intervals.

Food and Feeding Method
The cat was fed a homemade lamb-based food for four weeks. The food dosage was calculated to maintain current body weight and optimum body condition.

Reassessment
The cat improved slightly after being fed the homemade food for four weeks. Severe pruritus with self-trauma occurred when the previous dry veterinary therapeutic food and one of the moist grocery store foods were fed. The owner refused further testing to establish exactly which ingredients in these foods were causing the problem. Nutritional therapy with a commercial canned lamb and rice food was begun and the cat again responded partially.

A tentative diagnosis of atopic dermatitis, initiated by environmental and food allergens, was made based on the positive skin test results and partial response to a dietary elimination trial. Concurrent allergies occur in up to 20% of cats with adverse reactions to food. The commercial lamb and rice food was continued at the same dosage and an antihistamine (chlorpheniramine) was used to manage periods of intermittent pruritus.

Endnotes
a. Adapted with permission from Roudebush P. Nutritional management of the allergic patient. In: August JR, ed. Consultations in Feline Internal Medicine, 2nd ed. Philadelphia, PA: WB Saunders Co, 1994; 201-208.
b. Hill's Pet Nutrition Inc., Topeka, KS, USA.

Bibliography
Guaguere E. Food intolerance in cats with cutaneous manifestations: A review of 17 cases. European Journal of Companion Animal Practice 1995; 5: 27-35.
Rosser EJ. Food allergy in the cat: A prospective study of 13 cats. In: Ihrke PJ, Mason IS, White SD, eds. Advances in Veterinary Dermatology, vol. 2. New York, NY: Pergamon Press, 1993; 33-39.
Roudebush P, McKeever PJ. Evaluation of a commercial canned lamb and rice diet for the management of cutaneous adverse reactions to foods in cats. Veterinary Dermatology 1993; 4: 1-4.
White SD, Sequoia D. Food hypersensitivity in cats: 14 cases (1982-1987). Journal of the American Veterinary Medical Association 1989; 194: 692-695.

CASE 31-2

Allergic Dermatitis in a German Shepherd Dog
Kevin J. Shanley, DVM, Dipl. ACVD
West Chester, Pennsylvania, USA

Patient Assessment
A seven-year-old neutered male German shepherd dog weighing 37 kg (body condition score of 3/5) was admitted with the primary complaint of moderate to severe pruritus during the previous two years. The pruritus began on the face and feet, and progressed to involve the axillae, ears and abdomen. The pruritus was nonseasonal, but worsened slightly in the summer when it also involved the dorsal lumbosacral area.

The dog spent most of its time indoors but also had access to a fenced yard for several hours a day. The other household pet, a cat, had no dermatologic disease or pruritus. None of the people associated with the dog had pruritus or dermatologic disease. The dog had three episodes of bilateral ear infections the previous year that were treated with unknown topical medications that resolved the problem. Prior treatment with injectable and oral glucocorticoids provided marked relief but not complete remission of the pruritus. The pruritus returned within a few days after discontinuing corticosteroid therapy. Oral antihistamines (diphenhydramine and hydroxyzine) and various medicated shampoos and topical sprays provided little benefit.

Dermatologic examination revealed marked traumatic and complete alopecia with hyperpigmentation and erythema involving the periocular areas, inner pinnae, axillae, feet and ventral abdomen (**Figures 1** to **3**). Small numbers of papules were found on the ventral abdomen. Excoriations were present in the axillae and periocular areas.

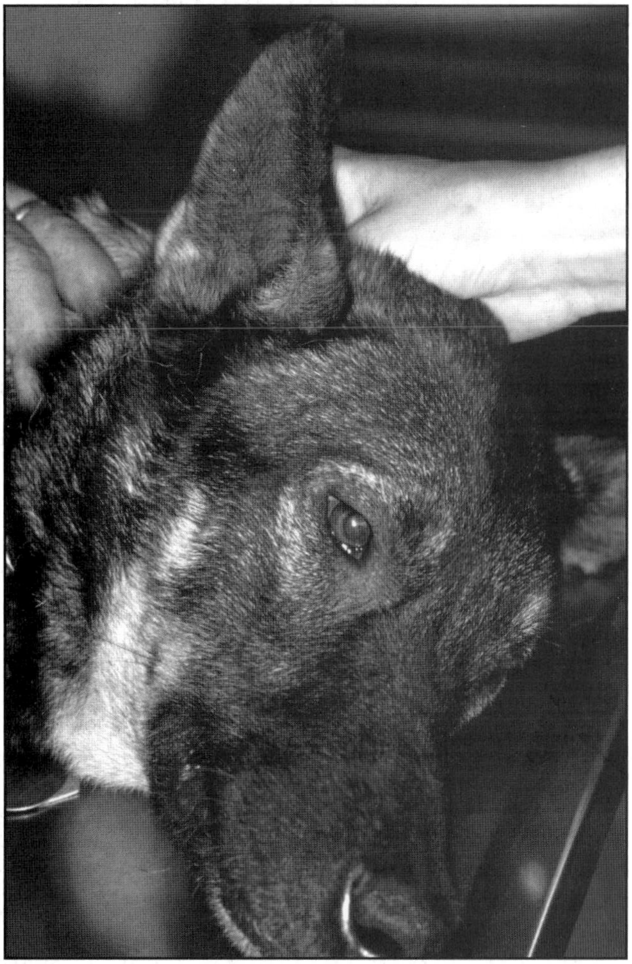

Figure 1. View of the lateral face and right pinna of a seven-year-old male German shepherd dog with periocular alopecia, hyperpigmentation, erythema and mild excoriations. The inner pinnal surface was hyperpigmented, erythematous and alopecic.

Assess the Food and Feeding Method

The dog was fed a variety of commercial dry foods; the client changed brands frequently. The dry food was fed free choice. Other food sources included occasional table food, commercial canine biscuit treats, rawhide chews and flavored heartworm preventive medication, which was given monthly for nine months of the year.

Questions

1. What are the primary diseases in the differential diagnosis of this patient? What secondary diseases may be present?
2. What food and feeding method is appropriate for this patient?
3. How might the dog's otitis externa correlate with the other evidence of dermatologic disease?

Answers and Discussion

1. The primary diseases in the differential diagnosis include:

Atopic dermatitis. Most patients with atopic dermatitis have pruritus and clinical disease at six months to three years of age. A seasonal history also suggests atopic dermatitis. This dog's dermatologic problems began at five years of age and the pruritus is nonseasonal, which is still compatible with atopic dermatitis. Atopic dermatitis is more common than food allergy but less common than flea allergy.

Adverse reaction to food (food allergy or food intolerance). The typical age at onset of food allergy is unclear. A recent report described an age predilection of several months to three years of age whereas previous reports did not find an age predilection. The pruritus associated with food allergy is nonseasonal and a variety of clinical presentations and distribution of lesions may be seen. The response to corticosteroid therapy is variable. Food allergy is not as common as flea allergy or atopy.

Flea-allergy dermatitis. Flea allergy usually begins at three to seven years of age and has a marked predilection for the dorsal lumbosacral area, the ventral abdomen and legs. This dog is the correct age for development of flea-allergy dermatitis, but the distribution of lesions on the face, feet and ears is not likely without more prominent disease on the dorsal lumbosacrum. The increased pruritus and involvement of the dorsal lumbosacrum in the summer suggests that flea allergy may be adding to the pruritus seasonally.

Scabies. Infestation with *Sarcoptes scabiei* is often difficult to prove. Pruritus is usually severe and nonseasonal. No age, breed or gender predilection is present. The pinnal margins, periocular areas, elbows, hocks and ventrum are usually involved. Contagion or zoonosis is present in approximately 30% of the cases. Skin scrapings are positive in 25% of affected dogs. Response to therapy may be the only way to diagnose many cases.

Dermatophytosis. The dermatologic lesions typically seen with dermatophyte infections include many of those seen in this patient. Although no strong breed or gender predilection exists, young animals are affected most often. Pruritus is variable. The distribution of lesions is quite variable but usually is not bilaterally symmetric as seen in this patient.

The secondary diseases in the differential diagnosis include:

Superficial pyoderma (bacterial folliculitis). Superficial pyoderma is a secondary infection seen with many pruritic skin diseases, including food allergy and food intolerance. *Staphylococcus intermedius* is the most common causal bacteria in dogs. Typical lesions include follicular papules, pustules, complete alopecia, epidermal collarettes, erythema and focal circular postinflammatory hyperpigmentation. Oral antibiotic therapy should clear the lesions and pruritus associated with the pyoderma.

Malassezia dermatitis. Pruritus associated with *Malassezia* infection is common. *Malassezia* species proliferate in moist, hyperplastic apposed skin surfaces, particularly lip folds, nasal folds, interdigital areas, axillae, ventral abdominal skin, ear canals and the

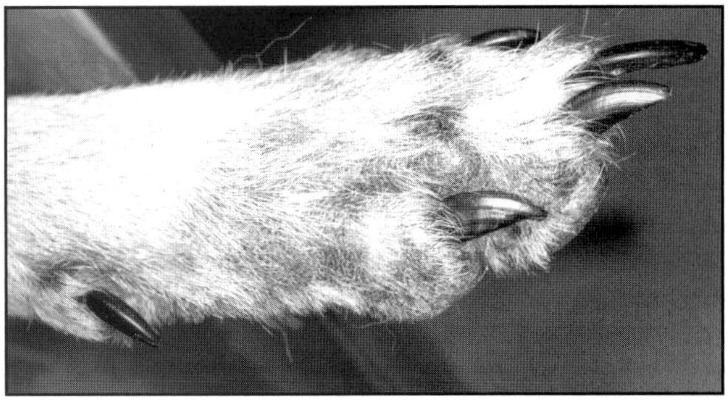

Figure 2. View of the left front foot showing traumatic alopecia with hyperpigmentation and focal excoriations.

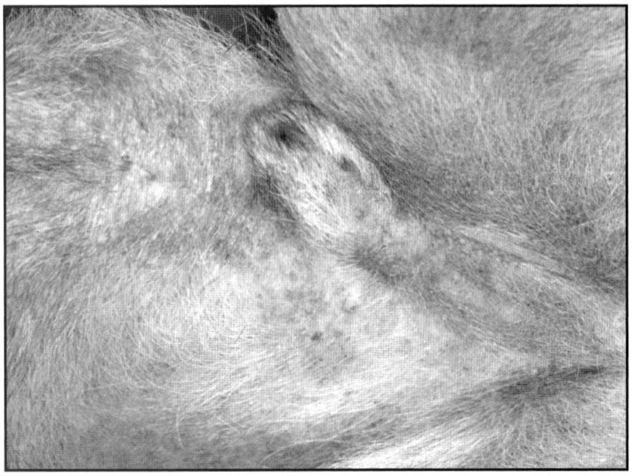

Figure 3. The ventral abdomen and medial thighs showing mild alopecia, hyperpigmentation, erythema and papules.

ventral neck. Underlying allergies, including adverse reactions to food, are common diseases that predispose animals to yeast infection. Topical and oral therapy may be necessary to correct the yeast infection and will also control any pruritus associated with the *Malassezia* infection.

2. An appropriate food for an elimination trial should include limited numbers of ingredients, particularly protein sources. The protein sources should be novel (not ingredients that the patient has been exposed to previously). The food should avoid excessive levels of protein, should be free of excessive levels of biogenic amines, have increased levels of omega-3 fatty acids and be nutritionally appropriate for long-term feeding of adult dogs (including phosphorus and sodium). **Table 31-5** lists selected commercial veterinary therapeutic foods that meet many of these criteria.

   The elimination food should be gradually introduced over several days as the current food is discontinued. The pet owner should feed only the elimination food for up to three months. For this patient, the table food, biscuit snacks, rawhide chews and flavored heartworm medication should also be discontinued. A nonchewable heartworm medication can be used. The client should keep a daily diary to record the clinical progress and degree of pruritus, as well as any other foods, table scraps, treats or snacks given in addition to the elimination food (**Figure 31-6**).

   The client should be instructed to watch for a marked (at least 50%) decrease in the pruritus. Periodic reexamination by the veterinarian will help monitor the patient's progress and help reinforce the feeding restrictions.

3. Otitis externa is a frequent clinical presentation with atopic dermatitis and adverse food reactions. One study found that many dogs with adverse food reactions presented with only ear problems and no other dermatologic disease. Food allergy and food intolerance should always be suspected in dogs with chronic or recurrent otitis externa. Although otitis externa is usually bilateral, some patients may present with unilateral otitis.

   Diagnosis of otitis externa is best accomplished with otoscopic examination and impression smears of aural exudate. Underlying allergies often predispose the animal to chronic or recurrent otic bacterial and yeast infections.

Progress Notes

Flea combing revealed no fleas or flea dirt; skin scrapings were also negative. Impression smears of the affected areas revealed few cocci or neutrophils. No *Malassezia* spp. were present. Intradermal allergy testing revealed no reactions to any of the inhaled allergens that were tested.

Food and Feeding Method

A commercial dry food composed of lamb meal and rice was initiated and fed exclusively for six weeks. The food dosage was calculated to maintain the dog's current body weight and optimal body condition.

Reassessment

The pruritus decreased dramatically over several days. After minimal pruritus was noted for one week, one of the previously fed dog foods was given for seven days. By the third day, there was a significant return of the pruritus at all of the previously affected sites. The elimination food was reinitiated and the pruritus resolved in 10 days.

After the pruritus decreased, individual food ingredients were added to the elimination food for up to seven days each. These challenge ingredients were derived from the list of foods and ingredients that had been fed previously. The ingredients included beef, chicken, corn, wheat, eggs and milk. Marked pruritus occurred when beef was fed and moderate pruritus when corn was fed. The final diagnosis was an adverse reaction (food allergy or food intolerance) to beef, corn and possibly other ingredients that were not tested. The commercial food used in the elimination trial was continued because it was complete and balanced for maintenance of adult dogs.

Bibliography

Carlotti DN, Remy I, Prost C. Food allergy in dogs and cats. A review and report of 43 cases. Veterinary Dermatology 1990; 1: 55-62.
Harvey RG. Food allergy and dietary intolerance in dogs: A report of 25 cases. Journal of Small Animal Practice 1993; 34: 175-179.
Jeffers JG, Shanley KJ, Meyer EK. Diagnostic testing of dogs for food hypersensitivity. Journal of the American Veterinary Medical Association 1991; 189: 245-250.
Rosser EJ. Diagnosis of food allergy in dogs. Journal of the American Veterinary Medical Association 1993; 203: 259-262.
White SD. Food hypersensitivity in 30 dogs. Journal of the American Veterinary Medical Association 1986; 188: 695-698.

CASE 31-3

Protein-Losing Enteropathy in a Dog

W. Grant Guilford, BVSc, BPhil, PhD, FACVSc, Dipl. ACVIM (Small Animal Internal Medicine)
School of Veterinary Medicine
Massey University, New Zealand

Patient Assessment

An eight-year-old, male English setter was referred with the primary complaints of diarrhea and weight loss of six months' duration. The diarrhea had been continuous over this period but varied in severity. The feces were very liquid, increased in volume and pale yellow. No fecal blood or mucus had been seen. The dog defecated four to five times per day. The owner classified the weight loss as moderately severe. There had been no vomiting. The dog's appetite and demeanor remained normal. Past treatments included a variety of antibiotics and gut protectants to which there had been no response. Physical examination revealed a thin (body condition score [BCS] of 2/5), bright, alert dog that weighed 27 kg. The remainder of the physical examination was normal.

The problems identified were chronic small bowel diarrhea with associated weight loss. Diagnostic procedures included fecal flotations, fecal culture, serum trypsin-like immunoreactivity, complete blood count, serum biochemistry profile, gastroduodenoscopy, endoscopic pinch biopsy of the stomach and duodenum, quantitative bacterial culture of the small intestine and rectal mucosal biopsy.

The most significant laboratory abnormality was panhypoproteinemia (albumin 1.51 g/dl [reference range = 2.2 to 3.5 g/dl]; globulin 2.39 g/dl [reference range = 2.2 to 4.5 g/dl]). Endoscopic findings included mildly increased duodenal mucosal granularity and friability. Results of histopathologic examination of gastric biopsy specimens showed a very mild lymphocytic gastritis; duodenal and rectal histopathologic results included mild to moderate lymphocytic-plasmacytic enteritis and colitis. Results of quantitative bacterial culture of the small intestine were normal. The tentative diagnosis was mild inflammatory bowel disease (IBD) and protein-losing enteropathy.

Assess the Food and Feeding Method

The dog ate a variety of moist and dry commercial foods fed free choice before and during the diarrheic episode. The dog's water intake was increased but there had been no polyuria.

Questions

1. What are the key nutritional factors to consider for this patient?
2. Calculate the energy requirements for this patient.

Answers and Discussion

1. The ideal food for dogs with chronic small bowel-type diarrhea should: 1) be highly digestible, 2) be free of gluten (gliadin), 3) have a limited number of protein sources to which the dog has not been recently exposed (novel proteins), 4) be isoosmolar and 5) avoid excess fat and lactose.

   Protein requirements increase in patients with protein-losing enteropathy because of excessive protein loss. Excess fat should be avoided during gastrointestinal (GI) dysfunction because malabsorbed fatty acids and bile acids cause secretory diarrhea.
2. The patient's resting energy requirement (RER) calculated at the current weight (27 kg) would be approximately 880 kcal/day (3,682 kJ/day), but that would increase to 1,000 kcal/day (4,184 kJ/day) for the patient's ideal body weight of 30 kg. To calculate this dog's daily energy requirement (DER) to achieve optimal body condition, the factor used to multiply times the RER must be greater than that used in calculations for normal mature dogs. The DER would be 1,600 to 2,000 kcal (6,694 to 8,368 kJ).

Therapy Including Feeding Plan

The dog was initially treated with prednisone for five weeks (60 mg twice daily for 14 days; then 40 mg once daily for 14 days; then 20 mg once daily for one week) but the feeding plan was not modified. At five weeks, the dog was reexamined. Its body weight remained constant despite an improved appetite. The diarrhea had improved to a "cow pat" consistency. Albumin (2.58 g/dl) and globulin (2.91 g/dl) concentrations had improved markedly. When the dog was reexamined endoscopically, scattered shallow erosions were visible in the gastric antrum; these were attributed to the prednisone therapy. Histopathologic examination of biopsy specimens taken from the small intestine during endoscopy showed that the prednisone therapy had had little effect. The histologic diagnosis remained mild to moderate lymphocytic-plasmacytic enterocolitis.

When the dog was discharged after the five-week recheck, the owner was instructed to prepare a homemade food of chicken and rice with added vitamins and minerals. Food dosage was calculated to achieve optimal body condition. Within three days of this food change, the dog's stools became firm and remained normal thereafter. Nine months later, the dog's body weight had improved to 31 kg and the BCS was 3/5. Serum albumin and globulin levels were 2.71 g/dl and 4.21 g/dl.

Further Discussion

This case suggests that protein-losing enteropathy can accompany food sensitivity. Protein exudation into the bowel has been demonstrated during GI type I hypersensitivity responses in laboratory animals and may occur in clinical patients.

The lack of complete response to prednisone emphasizes that corticosteroids often will not control the clinical signs of food-sensitive patients without concurrent feeding of a suitable hypoallergenic food. This case also illustrates how closely food sensitivity can mimic the clinical and histologic findings of idiopathic IBD.

Bibliography

Guilford WG. Adverse reactions to food: A gastrointestinal perspective. Compendium on Continuing Education for the Practicing Veterinarian 1994; 16: 957-969.

Patrick MK, Gall DG. Protein intolerance and immunocyte and enterocyte interaction. Pediatric Clinics of North America 1988; 35: 17-34.

CASE 31-4

Pruritus and Dermatitis in a Labrador Retriever

Philip Roudebush, DVM, Dipl. ACVIM (Small Animal Internal Medicine)
Hill's Scientific Affairs
Topeka, Kansas, USA

Patient Assessment

A nine-year-old neutered male Labrador retriever was examined for chronic recurrent episodes of pruritus and dermatitis. The dog had been treated for acute pyotraumatic dermatitis ("hot spots") around the face four months previously and had a chronic lesion of acral lick dermatitis ("lick granuloma") on the left metatarsus. The owner was concerned about face rubbing, excessive licking and scratching, skin redness and an overall dull coat. The only other significant medical problem was bilateral hip osteoarthritis.

The dog weighed 39 kg and had a body condition score of 4/5. Physical examination revealed multiple subcutaneous lipomas and evidence of moderately severe acute inflammation in the bilateral axillary and inguinal regions. Moderate inflammation was noted in the interdigital region of the right forefoot and in the perianal area. The initial evaluation of these problems included skin scrapings (negative) and interdigital skin cytology (no abnormal findings).

Assess the Food and Feeding Method

The dog had been fed a commercial dry food with lower fat and calorie content for the past year to help manage its overweight condition (Exclusive Reduced Fat Chicken & Rice Adult Formula[a]). Dry food was offered twice daily and a commercial canine treat was offered occasionally. The dog would also sometimes eat food available for other pets in the household. The dog had lost approximately 4.5 kg with this feeding regimen.

Questions
1. What additional diagnostic tests would be helpful for this patient?
2. What dietary changes may help manage the pruritus and dermatitis in this patient?

Answers and Discussion
1. Underlying allergic disease such as atopic dermatitis, flea allergy or food allergy could cause the pruritus and dermatitis seen in this patient. Labrador retriever dogs are at increased risk for atopic dermatitis and adverse food reactions. These allergic conditions often occur concurrently in the same patient and the clinical signs often mimic one other. Atopic dermatitis is primarily a clinical diagnosis; intradermal and in vitro allergy testing is used to confirm reactions to individual allergens and determine specific therapy (e.g., hyposensitization injections [allergy shots] or allergen avoidance [environmental control of house dust mites]). There was no evidence of past or current flea infestation on the patient. An adverse reaction to food is best confirmed with an elimination food trial using novel- or hydrolyzed-protein ingredients.
2. Allergic skin disease such as atopic dermatitis and/or adverse food reaction was strongly suspected in this dog. Enhanced dietary levels of omega-3 fatty acids may help control inflammation, clinical signs and improve skin barrier function. In general, it is more convenient and cost effective to deliver these nutrient enhancements as part of a food rather than using supplements. Use of foods containing novel or hydrolyzed protein sources is important in patients with suspected or confirmed food allergy.

Progress Notes
The food was changed to one with novel protein ingredients and enhanced levels of omega-3 fatty acids. The owner chose to offer both dry (Prescription Diet d/d Potato & Venison Formula Canine[b]) and canned (Prescription Diet d/d Venison Formula Canine[b]) formulas divided into two equal meals (two cups plus one-half can per meal). No treats were offered during an eight-week feeding trial and the owners were asked to eliminate access to food for other household pets.

An examination four weeks after changing the food revealed no inflammation in the axillary regions and less inflammation in the inguinal and interdigital areas. The owner thought there was noticeable improvement in the dog's overall coat condition. An examination eight weeks after changing the food revealed no inflammatory skin lesions and the acral lick dermatitis lesion was healed. The owner thought there was moderate overall improvement in the dog's condition and that it was more active and felt better. A recommendation was made to continue the venison-based foods with higher levels of omega-3 fatty acids. Food dosage calculations were based on an obese-prone dog in an effort to also manage the overweight condition. The owner was also given a recipe for making homemade treats from the canned venison food.

Endnotes
a. PMI Nutrition, Henderson, CO, USA.
b. Hill's Pet Nutrition, Inc., Topeka, KS, USA.

Chapter 32

Skin and Hair Disorders

Philip Roudebush
William D. Schoenherr

"Dermatoses affecting various species of animals are more commonly associated with malnutrition than they are with . . . a good state of nutrition."
F. Kral and B.J. Novak, Veterinary Dermatology, 1953

CLINICAL IMPORTANCE

Very little information is available concerning the demographics of canine and feline skin and hair disorders. Surveys and textbooks suggest that skin disorders are the most common reason for patient visits to the veterinarian's office (Scott et al, 2001). Surveys also indicate that 15 to 25% of all small animal practice activity is involved with the diagnosis and treatment of problems with the skin and coat (Scott et al, 1995).

The most commonly diagnosed canine skin disorders are: 1) allergy (flea-bite hypersensitivity, atopic dermatitis), 2) cutaneous neoplasms, 3) bacterial pyoderma, 4) seborrhea, 5) parasitic dermatoses, 6) adverse reactions to food (food hypersensitivity or food intolerance), 7) immune-mediated dermatoses and 8) endocrine dermatoses (Sischo et al, 1989; Scott and Paradis, 1990). The most common feline skin disorders are: 1) abscesses, 2) parasitic dermatoses, 3) allergy (flea-bite hypersensitivity, atopic dermatitis), 4) miliary dermatitis, 5) eosinophilic granuloma complex, 6) fungal infections, 7) adverse reactions to food, 8) psychogenic dermatoses, 9) seborrheic conditions, 10) neoplastic tumors and 11) immune-mediated dermatoses (Scott and Paradis, 1990; Nesbitt, 1982).

Clearly, skin and hair disorders are an important part of small animal practice; bacterial infections, ectoparasitism, allergies, fungal infections and neoplasia are common problems. Aside from adverse reactions to food, nutritional skin diseases in pets fed nutritionally adequate commercial pet food appear to be very uncommon. However, the skin and coat can be affected by many nutritional factors (**Table 32-1**), and many pet owners want to improve the quality and appearance of their pet's coat. The tactile and visual interactions between people and pets are among the greatest pleasures of the companion animal-human bond (Credille et al, 2000). This emphasizes the importance of understanding the nutritional factors that affect normal skin and hair and the nutritional factors that should be investigated in patients with skin disorders. This chapter discusses the nutritional factors that affect skin and hair, except for adverse reactions to food, which are specifically addressed in Chapter 31.

This chapter is divided into two sections: 1) nutrient-deficient dermatoses and 2) fatty acids for inflammatory skin disease. The first section covers dermatoses related to nutrient deficiencies. These deficiencies usually occur when pets in a nutritionally demanding lifestage are fed homemade foods, poor quality commercial foods, commercial foods that contain nutrient excesses or even high quality commercial foods that are inappropriately supplemented. Breed predilection can also be a factor. The second section focuses on the use of antiinflammatory fatty acids in the management of skin diseases that have an inflammatory or pruritic component. These dermatoses are responsive or partially responsive to antiinflammatory intervention. Many commonly diagnosed skin disorders have an inflammatory component.

Table 32-1. Key nutritional factors for foods and supplements for dogs and cats with nutrient-responsive dermatoses.

Factors	Associated conditions	Nutritional recommendations
Protein and fat	Keratinization abnormalities Loss of normal hair color Secondary bacterial or yeast infection Impaired wound healing Decubital ulcers Telogen defluxion Anagen defluxion	Avoid protein and energy deficiency Adult maintenance Dogs: Protein = 25 to 30% dry matter (DM) Fat = 10 to 15% DM Cats: Protein = 30 to 45% DM Fat = 10 to 15% DM Growth/lactation Dogs: Protein = 30 to 35% DM Fat = 15 to 30% DM Cats: Protein = 35 to 50% DM Fat = 20 to 35% DM Phenylalanine + tyrosine >1.3% DM Use a food with DM digestibility >80%
Essential fatty acids (EFA)	Excessive scales (seborrhea sicca) Alopecia Dry, dull coat Lack of normal hair growth Erythroderma Interdigital exudation	Avoid fatty acid deficiency Dogs: Linoleic acid >1.0% DM Cats: Linoleic acid >0.5% DM Some dogs and cats respond to levels in excess of those listed above Provide adequate levels and availability of zinc, B-complex vitamins and vitamin E to ensure adequate use of EFA
Zinc	Alopecia Skin ulceration Dermatitis Paronychia Footpad disease Slow hair growth Buccal margin ulceration Hyperkeratotic plaques Secondary bacterial or yeast infection	Avoid zinc deficiency Dogs: 100 to 200 mg/kg food DM Cats: 50 to 150 mg/kg food DM Avoid excess calcium Higher levels of zinc are required in foods with calcium >1.5% DM Avoid excess copper (copper <200 mg/kg food DM) Avoid EFA deficiency (see above) Zinc supplementation (Do not give with food) Zinc sulfate: 10 mg/kg body weight/day per os 10 to 15 mg/kg body weight/week IV Zinc methionine: 2 mg/kg body weight/day
Copper	Loss of normal color Dull or rough coat Reduced density of hair Alopecia	Avoid copper deficiency Dogs: >5 to 10 mg/kg food DM Cats: >15 mg/kg food DM Avoid excess zinc (zinc <1,000 mg/kg food DM) Avoid ingredients that have low copper availability Copper oxide Liver from simple-stomached mammals Avoid excess calcium Higher levels of copper are required in foods with calcium >1.5% DM
Vitamin A	Seborrheic skin disease (mainly cocker spaniel breed) Keratinization disorders Chin acne Nasodigital hyperkeratosis Ear margin seborrhea/dermatosis Callus Actinic keratosis Cutaneous neoplasms Schnauzer comedo syndrome Sebaceous adenitis Lamellar ichthyosis	Treatment with retinoids (**Table 32-5**): Vitamin A alcohol 625 to 1,000 U/kg body weight, q24h, per os 10,000 U q24h, per os (cocker spaniel, miniature schnauzer) 50,000 U q24h, per os (Labrador retriever) Tretinoin Apply topically q12 to 24h Isotretinoin 1 to 3 mg/kg body weight, q24h, per os Acitretin 0.75 to 1.0 mg/kg body weight, q24h, per os
Vitamin E	Discoid lupus erythematosus Systemic lupus erythematosus Pemphigus erythematosus Sterile panniculitis Acanthosis nigricans Dermatomyositis Ear margin vasculitis	Treatment with vitamin E: Dogs: 200 to 800 IU twice daily, per os

NUTRIENT-DEFICIENT DERMATOSES

Patient Assessment

History

The signalment (species, breed, age, gender, reproductive status, hair color) is an important part of the historical information that should be obtained for patients with dermatologic problems, especially those with possible nutritional disorders (**Table 32-2**). Both dogs and cats develop nutritionally related skin and hair disorders, although certain conditions such as zinc-responsive dermatoses are best characterized in dogs.

The age of the patient is important; most skin and coat changes due to nutritional deficiencies occur in young growing animals or adult females during gestation and lactation. The requirement for most nutrients is highest during growth and reproduction, which accounts for the increase in nutritionally related skin and hair problems seen during these lifestages. As an example, a biotin-deficient food will cause dermatitis, alopecia, dull fur and achromotrichia when fed to young growing kittens but will not cause similar clinical signs when fed to non-lactating adult cats (Pastoor et al, 1991). Many other examples of nutritional skin diseases exist that occur during periods of increased nutritional demand but do not occur during normal adult lifestages. This age-related phenomenon is complicated by the fact that congenital defects of the integument and certain parasitic, fungal and bacterial infections of the skin are also more common in dogs and cats younger than six months. Gender and reproductive status affect the prevalence of certain skin problems, but they are not usual risk factors in nutritional skin disorders, unless the increased nutritional demands of pregnancy or lactation are present.

The clinician should obtain a complete medical history in all cases. Specific details of the dermatologic history are found elsewhere (Scott et al, 2001). The nutritional history should focus on the adequacy of the specific food for the patient's lifestage, and types and dosages of nutritional supplements. The veterinarian or a veterinary nutritionist should evaluate homemade foods for nutritional adequacy (Chapter 10) because nutrient deficiencies or imbalances are more likely to occur in dogs or cats eating homemade vs. commercial foods. Excessive nutrient levels in food can cause skin disease due to direct toxicosis or interaction/interference with the use of other nutrients in the food.

Table 32-2. Breed predilection for non-neoplastic skin diseases often managed by food changes or supplementation.*

Breed	Disease
Airedale terrier	Atopic dermatitis
Akita	Sebaceous adenitis
Basenji	Atopic dermatitis
Basset hound	Atopic dermatitis
Beagle	Atopic dermatitis
Boston terrier	Atopic dermatitis
Boxer	Adverse reactions to food Atopic dermatitis
Bull terrier	Acrodermatitis Atopic dermatitis Zinc-responsive dermatosis
Chesapeake Bay retriever	Atopic dermatitis
Dalmatian	Atopic dermatitis
English bulldog	Atopic dermatitis
German shepherd dog	Adverse reactions to food Atopic dermatitis Seborrhea, primary
Golden retriever	Atopic dermatitis
Gordon setter	Atopic dermatitis
Irish setter	Atopic dermatitis Seborrhea, primary
Labrador retriever	Adverse reactions to food Atopic dermatitis Seborrhea, primary
Lhasa apso	Atopic dermatitis
Malamute	Zinc-responsive dermatosis
Old English sheepdog	Atopic dermatitis
Poodle, standard	Sebaceous adenitis
Pug	Atopic dermatitis
Schnauzer, miniature	Atopic dermatitis
Shar Pei	Adverse reactions to food Atopic dermatitis
Shih Tzu	Atopic dermatitis
Siberian husky	Zinc-responsive dermatosis
Spaniels	Adverse reactions to food Atopic dermatitis (American cocker) Seborrhea, primary
Terriers	Atopic dermatitis
Vizsla	Sebaceous adenitis

*Atopic dermatitis is often managed with fatty acid supplementation, sebaceous adenitis and primary seborrhea with retinoid supplementation, zinc-responsive dermatosis with zinc supplementation and adverse reactions to food with dietary changes. Specific nutrient deficiencies are usually not breed-specific.

Physical Examination

A comprehensive physical examination that evaluates all body systems should be performed on patients with skin or hair disease. Internal disease is often manifested as skin and coat disease, and this diagnostic possibility should not be overlooked by concentrating on the integumentary changes alone.

The skin can be affected by many nutritional factors, but usually responds in a limited number of ways. The cutaneous changes associated with nutritional abnormalities are often indistinguishable from those caused by other more common skin diseases. Changes that raise the suspicion for nutritional abnormalities include: 1) a sparse, dry, dull and brittle coat with hairs that epilate easily, 2) slow hair growth or regrowth from areas that have been clipped, 3) abnormal scale accumulation (seborrhea sicca), 4) loss of hair, erythema or crusting in areas of friction or stretch such as the distal extremities, 5) decubital ulcers and poor wound healing and 6) loss of normal hair color. Primary lesions such as papules and pustules rarely occur with nutritional abnormalities, but can occur with bacterial pyoderma secondary to nutritional, allergic or other underlying problems.

Laboratory and Other Clinical Information

Common laboratory evaluations including a complete blood count, serum biochemistry profile, urinalysis and thyroid panel are rarely helpful in evaluating nutritional skin disease. However, these tests can be used to rule out internal or metabolic diseases as causes of cutaneous problems.

Routine laboratory procedures for patients with dermatologic problems include skin scrapings for parasites, hair examination, cytologic examination of tissue or fluids, fungal culture, bacterial culture and biopsy for dermatohistopathologic examination. Of these procedures, hair examination and dermatohistopathology are most helpful for evaluation of potential nutritional problems.

HAIR EXAMINATION

Plucking hairs from the skin and examining them microscopically is termed trichography. This procedure helps diagnose a number of conditions including nutritional diseases. Trichography is performed by grasping a small number of

Box 32-1. The Hair Cycle.

HAIR FOLLICLE STRUCTURE

Most omnivores and herbivores have "simple" hair follicles, which means that each infundibulum contains a single hair shaft. In contrast, dogs, cats and carnivores have "compound" hair follicles, where multiple follicles grow closely together and share a common infundibulum; multiple hairs exit through a common opening. By convention, the largest hairs in a compound follicle are called primary or guard hairs and the smaller hairs that make up the majority of the hair shafts in a compound follicle are called secondary or undercoat hairs. There is a distinct orientation of primary and secondary hairs. Primary hairs are always the most cranial (toward the head) with secondary hairs caudal (toward the rear) of the primary hairs. The secondary hairs that are closest to the primary hairs are the largest and become progressively smaller the more caudally they are positioned. In this way, hair follicles are designed so that hairs will lie down smoothly, with guard hairs on top of the fine undercoat. The ratio of secondary to primary hairs can be greater than 10 to 1.

THE HAIR CYCLE

The growth of hair is cyclical and each cycle consists of an active growth phase (anagen), a transitional involutionary phase between active and no growth (catagen) and a stage of senescence (telogen), during which hair is retained in the follicle. The length of time required to complete the hair cycle varies between different species and is different among dog breeds. In human scalp hair, anagen is the longest phase of the cycle; thus, hair grows almost constantly. In most mammals, the hair cycle is telogen based; hairs grow to a predetermined length and then enter a long period of inactivity during which the telogen hair follicle firmly retains the hair shaft. Most dogs and cats appear to have telogen-dominant hair cycles in which the hair shafts are retained in telogen follicles for long periods of time. How long the follicle remains in telogen appears to be a breed-specific phenomenon. Some breeds of dogs, such as poodles and schnauzers, have anagen-dominant hair cycles with hair that grows almost constantly. Hair follicles have an intrinsic rhythm that can be altered by intrinsic (local growth factors, cytokines) and extrinsic (photoperiod, hormones, nutrition) factors.

One theory for why many canine breeds have such a long telogen phase is conservation of energy and protein required for active hair growth. For example, Nordic breeds appear to have a longer telogen phase than other canine breeds. They need a thick coat to provide insulation during cold weather and conserve the energy and protein needed to grow hair during the winter months when food may be more difficult to obtain. These breeds may benefit from maintaining hair in a state of "suspended animation." Preliminary studies have been conducted on the nutritional effects on canine hair follicles of various breeds. Further studies are needed to document how nutrition might influence hair follicle function, the hair cycle of various breeds and shedding.

The Bibliography for **Box 32-1** can be found at www.markmorris.org.

hairs with the fingertips or hemostats, pulling them out completely, placing them on a microscope slide, adding mineral oil and examining them with the low-power objective of the microscope. One study evaluated the impact of anatomic location on trichogram analysis. Results of this study indicated that the shoulder was the site of choice for plucking hair (Diaz et al, 2004).

The hair bulbs are examined first. Hairs do not grow continuously but rather in cycles. Each cycle consists of a growing period (anagen), during which the follicle is actively growing hair, a transitional period (catagen) and a resting period (telogen), during which the hair is retained in the follicle as a dead or club hair that is subsequently lost (Scott et al, 2001). More details about hair follicles and normal hair-growth cycles can be found in **Box 32-1**. Anagen hair bulbs are rounded, smooth, shiny, glistening, often pigmented and soft, so the root may bend. In some cases, the end of the anagen bulb is tightly attached to the dermal papilla and when plucked the hair appears squared at the tip with a slight flair (i.e., like a "pant's leg"). Telogen bulbs are club- or spear-shaped, rough-surfaced, nonpigmented and generally straight. Normal adult dogs and cats have a mixture of anagen and telogen hairs, the ratio of which varies with the season and other factors. Estimation of the ratio of anagen to telogen hair bulbs can be useful. All the hair of normal patients should not be in telogen; this finding suggests a diagnosis of telogen defluxion or follicular arrest. Inappropriate numbers of telogen hairs (e.g., mostly telogen hairs during the summer when the ratio should be about 50:50) suggest a diagnosis of nutritional, endocrine or metabolic disease (Scott et al, 2001). In people, the ratio of telogen to anagen hair increases with prolonged protein deficiency (Bradfield et al, 1967). Unfortunately, well-established normal trichogram values are not available in veterinary medicine, limiting their usefulness. The use of site, age, breed and climate matched controls, if possible, may increase the usefulness of this diagnostic procedure.

Examination of the hair shaft follows bulbar examination. A normal hair shaft is uniform in diameter and tapers gently to the tip. The hairs may be straight or twisted depending on the coat type of the patient. All hairs should have a clearly discernible cuticle, and a sharply demarcated cortex and medulla. Hair pigmentation depends on coat color and breed. Hairs that are inappropriately curled, misshapen and malformed suggest an underlying nutritional or metabolic disease (Scott et al, 2001). When unusual pigmentation is observed, external sources (salivary staining, chemicals, topical medications), nutritional disorders, color dilution/color mutant disorders and endocrine disorders should be considered (Scott et al, 2001).

Hairs with a normal shaft that are suddenly and cleanly broken indicate external trauma from licking, scratching or grooming. Breakage of hairs with abnormal shafts suggests nutritional disorders, dermatophytosis or congenitohereditary disorders such as color dilution alopecia. Morphologic changes in the hair bulb and hair diameter are sensitive indicators of overall protein status. Hair bulb atrophy, constriction and hair depigmentation may be seen in people after as little as two weeks of protein deprivation (Bradfield et al, 1967). Protein deprivation may not produce changes as rapidly in dog and cat hair because the hair in these species spends more time in telogen and less time in anagen.

BIOPSY AND DERMATOHISTOPATHOLOGY

The following are general guidelines for when a skin biopsy should be performed: 1) all obviously neoplastic or suspected neoplastic lesions, 2) all persistent ulcerations, 3) any case involving a major disease that is most readily diagnosed by biopsy (e.g., immune-mediated skin disease), 4) a dermatosis that is unresponsive to conventional therapy, 5) any unusual or serious dermatosis and 6) vesicular dermatitis. Some nutritional skin diseases, such as zinc-responsive dermatosis, have clearly delineated histopathologic lesions that are easily recognized during microscopic examination of a skin biopsy specimen. In general, the skin should be biopsied within three weeks for any dermatosis that does not respond to appropriate therapy. This includes those dermatoses that do not respond to initial management with a food change or supplementation.

CHEMICAL COMPOSITION OF HAIR

Some investigators and clinicians have advocated the use of chemical analysis of hair as a useful diagnostic technique. Hair is a complex tissue consisting of several morphologic components (epicuticle, exocuticle, endocuticle, medulla); each component has a different chemical composition. Genetic factors, nutrition, environmental effects and cosmetic treatment affect the chemical composition of hair (Robbins, 1988; Stafforst, 1982; Mundt and Stafforst, 1987). These complex factors and the expense of analysis make it unlikely that chemical composition of hair will be routinely useful as a diagnostic technique.

Hair, depending on its moisture content, consists of 65 to 95% protein. The remaining constituents are water, lipids, pigment and trace elements. The amount of moisture in hair plays a critical role in its physical and cosmetic properties. Moisture of hair often depends on relative humidity; as relative humidity increases from 29 to 70%, the approximate moisture content of hair increases from 6 to 14% (Robbins, 1988).

Hair consists of surface (external) lipid and internal lipid. In addition, part of the internal lipid is free lipid and part is structural lipid of the cell membrane complex. Skin surface lipids of cats and dogs contain more sterol esters, free cholesterol esters and diester waxes, but fewer triglycerides, monoglycerides, free fatty acids, monoester waxes and squalene than do skin surface lipids of people (Scott et al, 2001; Dunstan et al, 2000; Watson, 2003). It has been suggested that the skin surface lipids of cats and dogs are mainly of epidermal origin, whereas those of people are mainly of sebaceous gland origin (Scott et al, 2001).

Hair generally has very low mineral content (less than 1%), and it is difficult to determine whether this inorganic matter is derived from extraneous sources or whether it arises during fiber synthesis. Hair length and pigmentation intensity have been reported to affect concentrations of zinc and other trace elements, as well as certain macro elements, in canine hair (Stafforst, 1982; Mundt and Stafforst, 1987). Zinc and copper concentrations in hair from normal cats have also been documented (van den Broek et al, 1992).

SKIN AND HAIR BIOPHYSICAL PARAMETERS

Several studies have evaluated typical skin and hair biophysical parameters in cats and dogs such as skin pH, thickness, hydration, elasticity, transepidermal water loss, coat thickness, hair regrowth and hair length. These parameters are used most often in research studies and are not yet available for routine clinical practice. The skin and hair biophysical parameters measured to date differ widely according to breed, gender, gonadal status and age of the animal, as well as, the season of the year, limiting their routine use (Young et al, 2003; Schroeder et al, 2003; Watson et al, 2001, 2002; Cline et al, 2003; Matousek and Campbell, 2002; Hester et al, 2003; Bourdeau et al, 2004, 2004a; Diaz et al, 2003). Various nutritional studies using these parameters have been published or reported and are described below.

Risk Factors for Nutritionally Related Skin Disease

Genotype, lifestage, food type and food supplementation are risk factors for nutritionally related skin disease. Breed predilection determines the prevalence of some skin disorders. Tables of common skin diseases categorized by breed are readily available (**Table 32-2**). In general, more than 30 canine breeds are at increased risk for skin diseases (Ihrke and Franti, 1985). The nutrient-sensitive skin diseases such as zinc-responsive dermatoses and retinoid-responsive dermatoses often occur in specific breeds. As an example, one form of zinc-responsive dermatosis is frequently seen in arctic-type breeds such as malamutes and Siberian husky dogs.

As mentioned before, nutrient deficiencies that cause skin disease are more likely to occur during growth, gestation, lactation and illness when nutritional requirements are highest.

Some dry, commercial, generic, private label brand and grocery pet foods have lower fat content, lower nutrient digestibility and higher mineral content than other grocery and specialty brands. Low amounts of fat and poor-quality fat are risk factors for essential fatty acid (EFA) deficiency; poor nutrient digestibility contributes to protein-energy malnutrition, especially during growth and lactation; and high levels of minerals such as calcium inhibit the absorption of nutrients such as zinc, which are essential for normal, healthy skin.

A pet that obtains most of its nutrients from homemade foods is at increased risk for several nutritional problems (Chapter 10). In general, homemade foods are more likely to lack adequate calcium, EFA, certain vitamins and other micronutrients (Roudebush and Cowell, 1992). Homemade foods should include: 1) a calcium source such as bone meal,

Box 32-2. Red Coat Syndrome.

The quantity and type of melanin pigments synthesized by follicular melanocytes and deposited in keratinocytes are the prime determinant of mammalian hair color. Hair or fur color is genetically controlled but can be affected by various extrinsic factors, including nutrition. The two melanin pigments, eumelanin and phaeomelanin, are synthesized from a common precursor, dopaquinone, which is a product of tyrosine oxidation.

Reports from breeders and pet owners have identified some cats and dogs that have had their coat change from black to a reddish-brown color or have had hair stripes become less noticeable. Controlled studies in cats and dogs suggest that dietary deficiency of the amino acid tyrosine or its precursor phenylalanine is a significant factor causing black hair to change to a reddish-brown color. When tyrosine is limiting, there is insufficient dopaquinone for full expression of eumelanin formation and the yellow to reddish-brown phaeomelanin is the predominant pigment observed.

Tyrosine has not been regarded as an essential amino acid because phenylalanine is metabolized to tyrosine in all mammals and can supply the total tyrosine needs. Tyrosine contributes to the total aromatic amino acid (phenylalanine plus tyrosine) requirement and can spare about half the phenylalanine requirement. This appears to be a unique situation in which the need for a dispensable amino acid to support maximal melanin synthesis in cats and dogs is much greater than that required for nitrogen balance or maximal growth. Dietary phenylalanine plus tyrosine levels greater than 2% dry matter or addition of L-tyrosine to the food should provide optimal amino acid levels for maximal melanin synthesis in cats and dogs.

The Bibliography for **Box 32-2** can be found at www.markmorris.org.

oyster shell or dicalcium phosphate, 2) a source of EFA such as corn oil, safflower oil or some other vegetable oil and 3) a multivitamin-trace mineral supplement. Also, homemade cat foods should be supplemented with taurine. The final risk factor for nutritionally related skin disease is oversupplementation using naturally occurring foods or commercial supplements. Vitamin A toxicosis is associated with excessive use of liver as a supplement. High levels of minerals such as calcium in commercial supplements can interfere with absorption of essential trace elements such as zinc.

The Skin as a Metabolic Organ

The skin is the largest organ of the body and the anatomic and physiologic barrier between the animal and its environment. The skin protects against water loss and physical, chemical and microbiologic injuries while its sensory components perceive heat, cold, pain, touch, pruritus and pressure (Scott et al, 2001). In addition, the skin is contiguous with several internal organs and may reflect internal pathologic processes. The subcutis, skin and hair of a newborn puppy represent 24% of its body weight, which decreases in some breeds to only 12 to 14% of mature body weight (Miller et al, 1964).

The skin and coat significantly influence nutrient requirements. The ability of an animal's coat to regulate body temperature and energy requirements in cold environments correlates closely with hair length, thickness and density and with the medullation of individual hair fibers. In general, coats composed of long, fine, poorly medullated fibers are the most efficient for thermal insulation at low environmental temperatures and thus help modulate energy requirements. The skin also influences water requirements by minimizing transepidermal moisture loss. Loss of this normal barrier function as a result of fatty acid deficiency can increase a patient's water requirement, which is clinically manifested as polydipsia (Burr and Burr, 1929, 1930; Basnayake and Sinclair, 1956).

The hair cycle, and thus the coat, is influenced by the general state of health, genetics, photoperiod, ambient temperature, hormones, nutrition and poorly understood intrinsic factors (Scott et al, 2001; Scott, 1990). **Box 32-1** provides more details.

Dog breeds can be classified as having high, moderate and low weights of hair. Longhaired breeds with relatively large body surface areas per body weight, such as Pomeranians, have the largest relative amount of hair. Estimates indicate that as much as 30% of protein in food is needed to maintain daily hair growth in small breeds with long coats (Stafforst, 1982; Mundt and Stafforst, 1987). On the other hand, larger dogs with short coats may use less than 10% of food protein to maintain daily hair growth (Stafforst, 1982; Mundt and Stafforst, 1987). Whether dogs of similar body surface areas have different requirements for protein and other nutrients based solely on their type of coat is unknown, but of possible clinical significance. For example, there may be differences in nutrient requirements during peak hair growth for a Pomeranian vs. a Chihuahua or an Old English sheepdog vs. a German shorthaired pointer based on coat type alone.

The epidermis has a renewable cell population. Keratinocytes migrate from the mitotically active pool in the basal layer of the epidermis, through the spinous layer and granular layer, and finally into the superficial stratum corneum, followed by normal exfoliation. The normal canine epidermis has a very slowly renewing cell population. Only 1.5% of epidermal basal cells undergo DNA replication at any point in time (Kwochka and Rademakers, 1989; Kwochka, 1990, 1991). In dogs, it takes approximately 22 days for cells to migrate from the basal layer to, but not through, the stratum corneum.

The upper external root sheath of the hair follicle and sebaceous gland have essentially the same cell kinetic growth characteristics as the surface epidermis (Kwochka and Rademakers, 1989; Kwochka, 1990, 1991). Conversely, the root matrix of anagen hairs is one of the most rapidly renewing cell populations of the body (Kwochka, 1990). In actively growing hair, up to 24% of cells are undergoing DNA replication.

Key Nutritional Factors

The key nutritional factors for foods and nutritional supplements and the recommended amounts and doses for dogs and cats with nutrient deficiency dermatologic problems are summarized in **Table 32-1** and discussed in more detail below.

PROTEIN AND FAT

As mentioned previously, the integument is a metabolically active organ that is affected by the nutritional status of the animal. Protein and energy are required for the development of new hair and skin; fat is the most concentrated source of dietary energy. Developing hair requires sulfur-containing and other amino acids. Therefore, for normal skin and hair, it is important for the pet's food to provide optimal protein quantity, quality (appropriate levels of essential amino acids) and digestibility. Dogs and cats have increased protein and energy requirements during growth, gestation, lactation and some illnesses. Abnormal skin and hair will often be noted if nutritionally inadequate foods are fed during these stages (Ralston Purina Company, 1987; Huber et al, 1991). Key nutritional factor profiles for various lifestages of dogs and cats are listed in Chapters 13 through 24. Optimal levels of protein and fat, and minimum dry matter (DM) digestibility of foods for dogs and cats with skin and hair disorders are listed in **Table 32-1**.

Foods inadequate in protein and energy can cause keratinization abnormalities, depigmentation of hair and changes in epidermal and sebaceous lipids (**Box 32-2**). The skin loses its protective barrier function in patients with protein-energy malnutrition and becomes more susceptible to secondary bacterial or yeast infection. Impaired wound healing and decubital ulcers are also sequelae to protein-energy malnutrition. Protein-deficient dogs and cats have patchy alopecia and coats that are dry, dull and brittle.

Telogen defluxion is usually recognized as hair loss associated with a stressful event (e.g., pregnancy, severe illness, surgery) that causes the abrupt, premature cessation of growth of many anagen hair follicles and the synchronization of these hair follicles in catagen, then in telogen (Scott et al, 2001; Harvey, 1994). Short-term increased requirements of energy, protein and other nutrients during growth, gestation, lactation and illness may cause telogen defluxion if appropriate nutritional changes are not instituted. Bitches and queens in late gestation and lactation, and growing puppies and kittens are at risk unless they are fed nutritionally balanced, highly digestible foods that meet their increased nutritional requirements.

Anagen defluxion is a sudden loss of hair due to an unusual event (e.g., antimitotic drugs, infectious disease, metabolic disease) that interferes with anagen, resulting in abnormalities of hair follicles and shafts. Patients suffering from the stress of illness, injury and surgery often require increased amounts of energy, protein, specific amino acids and other nutrients. Patients with severe illness that do not receive adequate nutritional support are at risk for telogen defluxion, anagen defluxion or other coat abnormalities.

Dogs with severe primary seborrhea may have increased protein and other nutrient requirements. The calculated epidermal cell renewal time is approximately seven to eight days for dogs with primary seborrhea (Kwochka and Rademakers, 1990; Baker and Maibach, 1987). The hyperproliferative nature of the skin of dogs with primary seborrhea, with at least a threefold increase in epidermal cell renewal, may change the nutrient requirements of these dogs. However, no studies to date have evaluated the specific nutrient requirements of dogs with severe primary seborrhea vs. age- and breed-matched controls. Some authors suggest that primary seborrhea worsens greatly in dogs with nutritional inadequacies (Scott et al, 1995). Dogs with severe deep pyoderma secondary to generalized demodicosis or other underlying diseases may have increased nutrient requirements above those found in the normal adult animal.

Metabolic Epidermal Necrosis

Metabolic epidermal necrosis is a rare cutaneous disease that in most cases is a marker for a serious underlying metabolic disorder. In dogs, this syndrome has findings similar to those of necrolytic migratory erythema of people and has also been termed hepatocutaneous syndrome or superficial necrolytic dermatitis. Clinical features include crusting acral dermatopathy with erosions around the mouth, eyes, legs, feet and genitalia (Scott et al, 2001; Angarano, 1993). Hyperkeratosis, ulceration of footpads or both conditions is also prominent. The cutaneous syndrome is typically diagnosed in older dogs and is often associated with hepatic cirrhosis, other hepatopathies, diabetes mellitus, hyperadrenocorticism, and rarely, glucagon-secreting pancreatic tumors. Metabolic changes often include carbohydrate intolerance and marked hypoaminoacidemia (Outerbridge et al, 2002).

Specific treatment is aimed at correcting the underlying metabolic disease. Unfortunately, most cases are associated with irreversible chronic liver disease and hepatic cirrhosis (Chapter 68). Symptomatic treatment includes antimicrobials for secondary infections, insulin therapy as needed for diabetes mellitus, hydrotherapy to help remove crusts and lessen pruritus and glucocorticoids. Treatment of hypoaminoacidemia may reverse the skin lesions. Anecdotal reports suggest that foods for repletion/recovery containing moderate protein levels (Prescription Diet a/d Canine/Feline[a]), zinc, egg yolks or intravenous administration of crystalline amino acid solutions will reverse the skin lesions in some patients.[b,c] A review of 36 canine cases showed that dogs responded better to therapy with intravenous amino acid infusions rather than oral protein hyperalimentation (Outerbridge et al, 2002).

ESSENTIAL FATTY ACIDS

Functions in the Skin

EFA are polyunsaturated fatty acids (PUFA) derived from and including the parent EFA, cis-linoleic acid (LA) and α-linolenic acid (ALA). **Figure 32-1** summarizes the metabolic pathway of EFA. The skin of adult mice, guinea pigs and presumably other animals lacks Δ-6-desaturase and Δ-5-desaturase activity (Chapkin et al, 1987). Thus, the epidermis depends on food to supply EFA or the continuous formation of γ-linolenic acid (GLA), arachidonic acid (AA) and eicosapentaenoic acid (EPA) by the liver, with subsequent transportation to the skin by the blood (Chapkin et al, 1987; Horrobin, 1989; Campbell, 1990).

In the skin, EFA are principally found in phospholipids, and

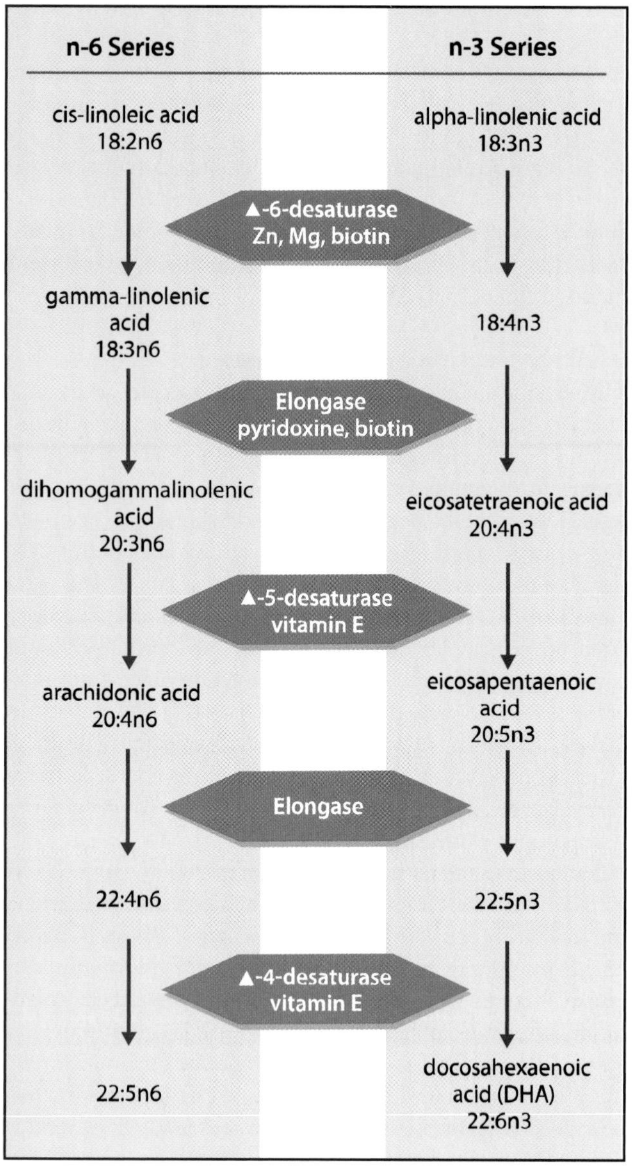

Figure 32-1. Diagram of metabolic pathways for essential fatty acids.

so have an accepted structural function in the lipoproteins of cell membranes. The high degree of unsaturation of EFA bestows fluidity to these structures at physiologic temperatures, allowing conformational changes to occur (Prottey, 1976). One of the most important skin-related functions of EFA is the incorporation of LA into the ceramides of the lipid portion of the epidermal cornified envelope. This envelope serves an essential barrier function to prevent loss of water and other nutrients. EFA are a source of energy for the skin and serve as precursors to a variety of potent, short-lived molecules including prostaglandins (PG), leukotrienes (LT) and their metabolites.

Essential Fatty Acid Deficiency

When mammals are deprived of fats, among other things, they develop characteristic signs of EFA deficiency. The existence of EFA was first recognized when rats deprived of fat had poor weight gain, increased water intake, necrosis of the tail and scaly skin (Burr and Burr, 1929, 1930). The skin scaliness was exacerbated by low ambient humidity or restricted access to water. The increased water intake was later linked to increased transepidermal water loss (Basnayake and Sinclair, 1956). When newly weaned rats were fed foods devoid of EFA, LA and AA levels in the skin rapidly declined (Basnayake and Sinclair, 1956). After five weeks, these acids were virtually absent from the skin, weight loss and increased water intake ensued and scaly skin developed. After 10 weeks, the rate of transepidermal water loss began to increase rapidly to values about 10 times those of normal rats. Growth stunting caused by EFA deficiency is predominantly due to the increase in thermogenesis required to counter heat loss from accelerated transepidermal water evaporation (Phinney et al, 1993).

Cutaneous changes have been described in fatty acid deficiency in dogs (Hansen and Weise, 1951) and cats (Frankel and Rivers, 1978). These cutaneous abnormalities include scaliness (seborrhea sicca), matting of hair, loss of skin elasticity, alopecia, a dry and dull coat, erythroderma, hyperkeratosis, epidermal peeling, interdigital exudation, otitis externa and lack of hair regrowth following plucking. These changes are associated with epidermal and dermal metabolic effects leading to: 1) increased transepidermal water loss, 2) increased epidermal cell turnover, 3) sebaceous gland hypertrophy, 4) increased sebum viscosity, 5) poor wound healing, 6) increased susceptibility to infection and 7) weakening of cutaneous capillaries.

Dogs with cutaneous abnormalities due to low-fat foods have lower levels of fatty acids in serum, skin, liver, kidneys and heart muscle than do animals with healthy skin (Hansen and Weise, 1951). Cats fed an EFA-deficient food developed moderate seborrhea sicca and mild hair loss after six months (MacDonald et al, 1984). Severe seborrhea sicca with large scales developed in EFA-deficient cats when the environmental relative humidity decreased from approximately 75 to 55% (MacDonald et al, 1984). Hair loss is extensive and stroking causes clumps of hair to epilate.

Deficiency of other nutrients, particularly zinc (Ohlen and Scott, 1986), vitamin E (Scott and Sheffy, 1987) and pyridoxine (Cunnane et al, 1984) can cause clinical signs similar to those caused by experimental EFA deficiency. EFA intake influences the requirement of these nutrients. In rodents, clinical signs of zinc deficiency can be largely prevented by EFA supplementation (Cunnane and Horrobin, 1980).

Fatty acid deficiency is rapidly reversible if EFA are introduced orally, parenterally or topically. Various abnormal cutaneous parameters of dogs (Hansen and Weise, 1951) and cats (Frankel and Rivers, 1978; MacDonald et al, 1984) are restored within a few days by LA supplementation.

Supplementation with EFA will increase fatty acid levels in serum of dogs (Campbell et al, 1992; Campbell and Roudebush, 1995) and cats (MacDonald et al, 1984), and in the skin of normal and seborrheic dogs (Campbell et al, 1992; Campbell and Roudebush, 1995; Rees et al, 2001; Marsh et al, 2000). Optimal food levels of EFA for normal dogs and cats and those with skin and hair disorders are listed in **Table 32-1**.

Use of Fatty Acids for Seborrhea

Fats and fatty acids have been recommended for many years as supplements to improve the sheen and luster of hair. In the past, animal and vegetable sources of fat were recommended to improve coat quality.

Dogs with seborrhea have abnormally low cutaneous levels of LA and increased cutaneous levels of oleic acid (Campbell et al, 1992). These low cutaneous levels are found despite normal food and serum fatty acid concentrations. Following supplementation for 30 days with a vegetable oil high in LA (sunflower oil), the cutaneous fatty acid concentrations return to near normal and clinical signs of seborrhea improve. The clinical signs of seborrhea in dogs may be partly attributable to a localized deficiency of LA, elevated levels of AA in the skin or both (Campbell et al, 1992). However, one study noted no significant differences in the serum and skin fatty acid profiles of normal and a small number of seborrheic dogs (White, 1990).

Seborrhea sicca is also associated with increased transepidermal water loss, which can be reversed with cutaneous administration of vegetable oils rich in LA (Campbell and Kirkwood, 1993). Supplementing food with ALA can also decrease transepidermal water loss (Campbell and Roudebush, 1995). Dietary supplementation with EFA also appears to improve skin and coat condition in normal animals consuming otherwise complete and balanced commercial pet foods (Rees et al, 2001; Marsh et al, 2000).

Antiinflammatory Fatty Acids

See the Fatty Acids for Inflammatory Skin Disease section below.

MINERALS

Minerals in food interact with one another (**Figure 32-2**) and this interaction must be kept in mind when assessing integumentary problems that might be associated with certain homemade foods, commercial foods or nutritional supplements. Skin manifestations of mineral imbalances are seen most commonly with primary (nutritional inadequacy) or secondary (nutrient interaction) deficiencies of copper and zinc.

Copper

Copper is an essential trace element of all plant and animal cells (Brewer, 1987). Copper is involved in various biologic functions, primarily as a component of storage and transport proteins and cuproenzymes. One of the enzymes is lysyl oxidase, which is required for maturation of connective tissue and the cross-linking of aldehydes in collagen and elastin (Brewer, 1987). Copper-containing enzymes also catalyze the conversion of carotene to retinal, the formation of keratin from prekeratin and the biosynthesis of melanin from L-tyrosine.

Cutaneous manifestations of copper deficiency include achromotrichia or loss of normal hair coloration, reduced density or lack of hair and a dull or rough coat. Pigmented hair on the head and face loses its normal color, develops a "washed

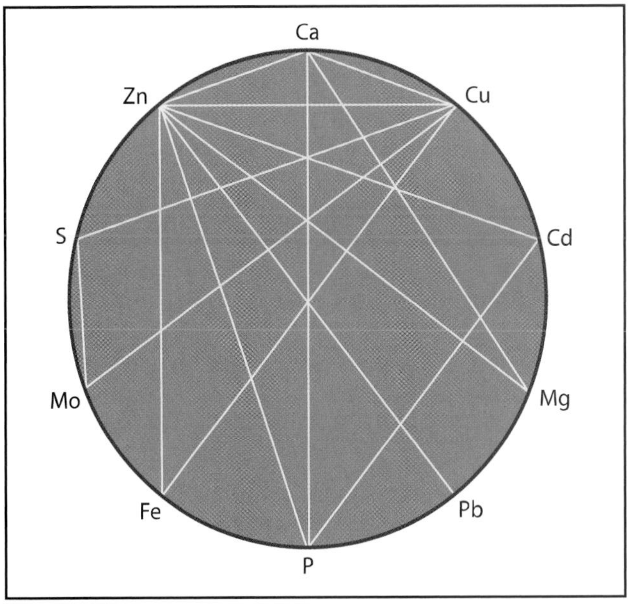

Figure 32-2. Diagram of clinically important mineral interactions in patients with cutaneous disease.

out" appearance and becomes gray (Zentek and Meyer, 1991; Morris and Rogers, 1995; van den Broek and Thoday, 1986). This change may extend over the entire body (Ralston Purina Company, 1987; Morris and Rogers, 1995). In dogs and cats with cutaneous manifestations of copper deficiency, copper concentrations are significantly reduced in plasma, hair, liver, kidney and heart muscle (Zentek and Meyer, 1991; Morris and Rogers, 1995; van den Broek and Thoday, 1986). Copper deficiency is seen most commonly in young puppies and kittens.

Dogs and cats can develop copper deficiency due to: 1) inadequate copper in food, 2) poor availability of copper in food or 3) an excess of competing minerals. Zinc, in particular, can adversely affect copper homeostasis. Zinc is thought to inhibit copper absorption by its action on intestinal metallothioneins, which sequester copper in the intestinal epithelial cells and make copper unavailable for use elsewhere in the body (Fosmire, 1990). The greater the intake of zinc and the lower the intake of copper (absolute or relative), the greater the potential for copper sequestration and ultimately, copper deficiency. Studies involving people and foals have shown increased nutritional copper requirements as the amount of zinc in the food increases (Fosmire, 1990; Bridges and Moffitt, 1990). Optimal levels of copper in foods for dogs and cats with skin and hair disorders are listed in **Table 32-1**.

Copper availability varies widely among feed ingredients (Aoyagi et al, 1993). Copper availability is relatively high in poultry by-product meal, avian liver (chicken and turkey) and ruminant liver (beef and sheep); copper from soybean meal and corn gluten meal is moderately available; copper from monogastric mammalian liver (pork and rat) and copper oxide is poorly available (Morris and Rogers, 1995; Aoyagi et al, 1993; Aoyagi and Baker, 1993; Czarnecki-Mauldin et al, 1993). Risk factors for copper deficiency in dogs and cats include: 1) rapid

Table 32-3. Classification scheme for zinc-related cutaneous disorders in dogs.

Previous classification schemes
Acrodermatitis of bull terriers
Dry juvenile pyoderma
Generic dog food syndrome
Syndrome I (Siberian husky, malamute, other breeds)
Syndrome II (growing dogs)
Proposed classification
Animal abnormalities
Acrodermatitis of bull terriers
Zinc malabsorption (Siberian husky, malamute)
Nutritional abnormalities
Primary zinc deficiency
Secondary zinc deficiency
Essential fatty acid deficiency

Table 32-4. Risk factors for zinc-related skin disease in dogs.

Certain breeds
Siberian husky
Malamute
Bull terrier
Great Dane
Labrador retriever
Other rapidly growing large and giant breeds
Food
High mineral levels (calcium, phosphorus, magnesium)
High phytate levels (high levels of cereal ingredients)
Low essential fatty acid levels
Dietary supplements
Calcium and/or other mineral supplements
Cottage cheese or other dairy products
Small intestinal disease
Viral enteritis
Malassimilation (malabsorption, maldigestion)

growth, 2) unsupplemented homemade foods, 3) commercial or homemade foods supplemented with copper oxide and 4) homemade or commercial foods supplemented with excessive levels of zinc, calcium or iron.

Zinc

Zinc Deficiency

Zinc is an important cofactor of numerous metalloenzymes and modulator of many critical biologic functions. Numerous reports have linked zinc deficiency to many dermatoses in dogs and cats.

Zinc deficiency in animals has been well documented through experiments in numerous species including dogs and cats. Investigators reported decreases in plasma zinc concentrations, a dull and rough coat and skin lesions on the abdomen and hind limbs after feeding a calcium-supplemented, zinc-deficient, corn-soy food to dogs (Robertson and Burns, 1963). Another study documented the progressive development of cutaneous lesions when young puppies were fed a corn-soy, zinc-deficient food (Sanecki et al, 1982). Puppies developed alopecia, skin ulceration, dermatitis, parakeratotic hyperkeratosis, follicular hyperkeratosis and generalized acanthosis similar to lesions described in other animals with zinc deficiency (Sanecki et al, 1982). These changes were prominent in areas of contact and trauma (footpads), areas of stretch (skin over joints), areas of friction (axillae, groin), distal extremities and tail, mucocutaneous junctions and ear canals. The feet were severely affected with paronychia and fissured, cracked and focally eroded footpads. The cutaneous lesions were completely reversible within six weeks of adding zinc to the food.

Dogs fed a zinc-deficient food developed skin lesions, which improved dramatically within 72 hours of adding zinc to the food (Banta, 1989). A study in kittens fed a zinc-deficient food described poor coats characterized by hair thinning, slow hair growth, scaliness and buccal margin ulcerations (Kane et al, 1981).

Studies in rodents demonstrated the close linkage of zinc and EFA metabolism (Cunnane and Horrobin, 1980; Cunnane, 1982; Huang et al, 1982). Zinc deficiency accelerates development of clinical signs of EFA deficiency; conversely, supplementing with EFA can largely reverse clinical signs of zinc deficiency. Several of the manifestations of zinc deficiency are mediated by a relative state of EFA deficiency attributed, in part, to reduced Δ-6-desaturase enzyme activity (Cunnane and Horrobin, 1980; Cunnane, 1982; Huang et al, 1982). Zinc deficiency may impair the absorption of EFA and vice versa (Huang et al, 1982). Low zinc intake during pregnancy prevents the normal accumulation of long-chain fatty acids and differentially depletes maternal whole-body stores of LA and ALA (Cunnane et al, 1993). This finding suggests that low zinc intake during pregnancy and lactation may be a risk factor for fatty acid deficiency. It is unknown whether similar interactions of zinc and EFA also occur in dogs and cats.

Zinc-Related Dermatoses

A variety of cutaneous diseases in dogs have been described that are thought to be primary or secondary zinc deficiency, or that respond to zinc supplementation. The classification of these skin diseases is confusing and often overlaps (**Table 32-3**). A crusted dermatosis has been reported to occur in young shorthaired dog breeds termed dry juvenile pyoderma or juvenile hyperkeratosis (Baker, 1974; Anderson, 1977). Many cases were not caused by primary bacterial infection and often resolved spontaneously at sexual maturity. In retrospect, these case reports most likely represent the first clinical descriptions of cutaneous disease caused by zinc deficiency in young dogs. A classification scheme was proposed in 1980 for zinc-responsive dermatoses that included two syndromes (Kunkle, 1980). Syndrome I included Siberian husky and malamute dogs, which usually developed lesions in early adulthood and responded to zinc supplementation. Syndrome II included rapidly growing puppies that developed lesions due to zinc deficiency and responded to food change, zinc supplementation or both. Later, a generic dog food syndrome was described in adult dogs and rapidly growing puppies consuming a poor quality food (Sousa et al, 1988). These animals had lesions consistent with zinc deficiency and responded to a food change. Simultaneously, acrodermatitis was described in bull terriers and linked to abnormal zinc absorption and metabolism (Jezyk et al, 1986; Mundell, 1988).

In all of these syndromes, the dermatoses were clearly associated with zinc deficiency and possibly a deficiency or abnormal metabolism of other nutrients. A more practical classification scheme for zinc-related cutaneous changes in dogs includes clinical syndromes due to nutritional abnormalities (primary or secondary zinc deficiency) or abnormalities of zinc metabolism (**Table 32-3**).

Zinc-Related Dermatoses Associated with Nutritional Abnormalities. Zinc-responsive cutaneous lesions have been frequently described in rapidly growing puppies and less frequently in adult dogs. Many breeds may be affected, but Great Danes, Doberman pinschers, German shepherd dogs, German shorthaired pointers, beagles, standard poodles, Rhodesian ridgebacks and Labrador retrievers are reportedly affected more often (Scott et al, 1995; Ohlen and Scott, 1986; van den Broek and Thoday, 1986; Kunkle, 1980; Sousa et al, 1988; Fadok, 1982; Wright, 1985; Wolf, 1987; Gross et al, 1992; Degryse et al, 1987). Lesions somewhat resemble those of experimental zinc deficiency in puppies and include erythroderma, alopecia and hyperkeratotic plaques (exudative crusts) on the face, head, distal extremities and mucocutaneous junctions (Scott et al, 1995; Gross et al, 1992). Thickened, fissured footpads are also frequently seen. Severely affected animals have systemic signs of lymphadomegaly, poor growth, fever, depression and anorexia. Microscopic examination of skin biopsy specimens shows hyperplastic superficial perivascular dermatitis with diffuse parakeratotic hyperkeratosis.

Risk factors for development of zinc-responsive cutaneous disease are listed in **Table 32-4**. Foods with high mineral levels (calcium, phosphorus, magnesium), poor digestibility, high levels of phytate and/or low levels of total fat and EFA are significant risk factors, especially when fed to puppies during the rapid growth phase. As shown in **Figure 32-2**, other minerals in the food influence zinc absorption. Foods high in calcium, phosphorus and magnesium adversely affect absorption of zinc. Excessive use of mineral supplements containing calcium in large- and giant-breed puppies is common and can inhibit zinc absorption.

Phytin, phytate and phytic acid are different forms of organic phosphorus, presumably inositol hexaphosphate, found in plant proteins. Foods high in cereal ingredients often have excessive levels of phytate that complex with and prevent normal absorption of zinc. Phytate and calcium also interact to affect zinc absorption (Forbes et al, 1984). The relative effect of phytate on zinc absorption increases with the calcium level in the food. Thus, foods high in phytate and calcium have an even greater negative impact on zinc absorption.

Low-cost commercial generic or private label brand dry pet foods are often low in total fat and EFA because fat is an expensive ingredient. Zinc and EFA metabolism interact and foods with marginal concentrations of zinc and EFA may be more likely to cause clinical disease.

Viral enteritis and prolonged diarrhea adversely affect zinc absorption in swine and similar changes may occur in other animals (Whiteneck et al, 1978).

Zinc Deficiency Associated with Metabolic Abnormalities. Lesions attributed to zinc deficiency develop early in adulthood in Siberian huskies, malamutes and bull terriers and progress at a variable rate (Scott et al, 2001). Skin lesions develop in these breeds despite consumption of well-balanced commercial foods containing adequate levels of zinc. Lesions include erythroderma, alopecia, crusting, scaling and suppuration involving the head, extremities and mucocutaneous junctions. The footpads may become hyperkeratotic. Secondary Malassezia and bacterial infections are common. Some malamute and Siberian husky dogs appear to have a decreased capability for zinc absorption (Brown et al, 1978; Willemse, 1992). Bull terriers that are siblings of those with acrodermatitis may also be affected and probably have abnormal zinc absorption and metabolism (Scott et al, 1995). These patients will probably require zinc supplementation for life to maintain normal tissue zinc concentrations and to avert clinical disease.

Acrodermatitis is an inherited, autosomal recessive metabolic disease reported to occur in bull terriers in the United States, Canada and the United Kingdom (Jezyk et al, 1986; Mundell, 1988; Smits et al, 1991; McEwan, 1993). The syndrome develops shortly after birth and is associated with defects in zinc absorption and metabolism. The condition has been termed lethal acrodermatitis because homozygously affected dogs rarely live beyond 18 months of age.

Cutaneous and systemic clinical signs resemble those of severe zinc deficiency, including growth retardation, gastrointestinal disease, chronic bacterial infections and progressive, erythematous, exfoliative, papular to pustular dermatitis of the distal extremities and skin surrounding the mucocutaneous junctions (Jezyk et al, 1986; Mundell, 1988; Smits et al, 1991; McEwan, 1993). Surface crusts usually contain numerous bacteria and yeast organisms (Smits et al, 1991). Owners complain that their dogs have difficulty eating and are affected by skin disease, poor growth and large, splayed, painful feet (McEwan, 1993). Ulcerated and thick, crusted lesions are prominent on the muzzle and ears. Abnormal keratinization of the footpads, severe nail dystrophy and paronychia are also common. Histopathologic examination of skin reveals massive parakeratotic hyperkeratosis.

A study showed that two affected dogs had significantly lower plasma zinc concentrations, lower zinc and copper concentrations in the kidneys and liver and lower zinc absorption when compared with age-matched control dogs (Mundell, 1988). Serum zinc concentrations may also be normal (Smits et al, 1991; McEwan, 1993). Supplementation with oral or intravenous zinc fails to ameliorate clinical signs. Treatment with systemic antimicrobials, especially for secondary superficial yeast infections, may result in marked improvement, although systemic and cutaneous infections recur. Some apparently normal littermates may develop a zinc-responsive dermatitis (Scott et al, 2001).

Diagnosis and Management of Zinc-Responsive Skin Disease

Diagnosis of zinc-responsive cutaneous disease is based on the history, physical examination and results of skin biopsy evaluation. Hyperplastic superficial perivascular dermatitis with marked diffuse and follicular parakeratotic hyperkeratosis is suggestive of zinc deficiency (Gross et al, 1992a). In general, zinc concentrations in serum, leukocytes and hair are not good indicators of zinc status in dogs (van den Broek and Thoday, 1986; Wolf, 1987; van den Broek et al, 1988; Logas et al, 1993). Age, seasonal variation and many diseases affect serum zinc concentrations (Fisher, 1977; Keene et al, 1981). One study found no significant difference in serum zinc concentrations between normal dogs, dogs that were ill without skin disease, dogs with allergic skin disease and dogs with other dermatoses (Logas et al, 1993).

Treatment generally includes changing to a food that avoids excess minerals and contains adequate amounts of zinc and EFA. Optimal levels of zinc and EFA in foods for dogs and cats with skin and hair disorders are listed in **Table 32-1**. This type of change will usually result in rapid improvement in puppies and some adult dogs. Zinc supplementation will be necessary in those breeds in which decreased ability to absorb zinc is suspected. Oral supplementation with zinc sulfate (10 mg/kg body weight/day) or zinc methionine (2 mg/kg body weight/day) is adequate in most cases. Zinc absorption is maximal if supplements are given between, rather than with, meals. Supplemental zinc from zinc amino acid chelates may be more available to dogs than are inorganic zinc sources (Lowe et al, 1994). Some dogs, especially Siberian huskies, do not respond to oral zinc supplementation. Intravenous injection of sterile zinc sulfate solutions at dosages of 10 to 15 mg/kg body weight has been effective in these dogs (Willemse, 1992). Weekly injections for at least four weeks are necessary to resolve the lesions, and maintenance injections every one to six months may be necessary to prevent relapses.

Existing skin lesions can be improved by hydrating the crusts with wet dressings, applying petrolatum or petrolatum-based topical agents or whole-body warm water soakings. Dogs with evidence of superficial pyoderma or *Malassezia* infections should be treated with appropriate antimicrobials. Some authors also recommend low doses of oral, short-acting glucocorticoids (Kwochka, 1993).

VITAMINS

Vitamin A

Retinol, retinal and retinoic acid are three natural compounds that have vitamin A activity in mammals. Food sources include retinyl esters (vitamin A palmitate) in animal tissues and carotenoids (β-carotene) in vegetables. These sources are assimilated and ultimately stored as retinyl palmitate in the liver. Cats require preformed vitamin A because they lack the ability to effectively convert β-carotene to vitamin A (NRC, 2006).

The general functions of vitamin A include growth promotion, differentiation and maintenance of epithelial tissue and maintenance of normal reproductive and visual functions. Retinoic acid affects differentiation and proliferation of epithelial cells by binding to and activating a specific set of cell nuclear receptors (Wolf, 1990; Blumenberg et al, 1992). In particular, epithelial cells have a specific nuclear receptor for retinoic acid (Blumenberg et al, 1992). The mechanism of action of retinoic acid is similar to that of steroid hormones and thyroxine, and involves activation of specific genes. Retinoic acid and thyroid hormone control overlapping gene networks, regulating growth and differentiation through nuclear receptors that can modify rates of gene transcription.

Retinoic acid influences epidermal differentiation and directly affects keratinization by action of retinoic acid receptors on regulatory sites in keratin genes. Retinoic acid may also influence hair growth through activity at the hair bulb.

Vitamin A deficiency in dogs was among the first of the vitamin deficiencies to be studied experimentally (NRC, 2006). Skin lesions and focal atrophy of the skin have been reported with experimental vitamin A deficiency in dogs and cats, although it is seldom encountered clinically (NRC, 1986, 1985). Some of the earliest work with vitamin A showed that puppies had heavier, more lustrous coats when foods were supplemented with vitamin A (Bradfield and Smith, 1938). It is unlikely that vitamin A deficiency would occur in dogs and cats eating typical commercial pet foods because these foods contain several times the minimum daily requirement of vitamin A (Kallfelz and Dzanis, 1989). The minimum recommended allowance for vitamin A in foods for dogs is 5,050 IU/kg of food (DM) (growth/reproduction and maintenance requirements are the same) and 3,333 and 6,666 IU/kg of food (DM) for growth/maintenance and gestation/lactation for cats, respectively (NRC, 2006).

Retinoid-Responsive Dermatoses

The term "retinoids" refers to the entire group of naturally occurring and synthetic vitamin A derivatives. These therapeutic agents should be reserved for cases in which there are clinical and histopathologic abnormalities most consistent with primary keratinization disorders of the surface and/or follicular epithelium or abnormalities of the sebaceous glands (Power and Ihrke, 1990; Kwochka, 1993a). Other causes of clinical scaling (ectoparasitism, allergies, infections, endocrinopathies) should first be eliminated through other diagnostic testing.

A vitamin A-responsive dermatosis has been described primarily in cocker spaniels but it has also been recognized in a Labrador retriever and a miniature schnauzer (Scott et al, 2001; Kwochka, 1993a). The condition is characterized by adult-onset, medically refractory seborrheic skin disease with marked follicular plugging and hyperkeratotic plaques, primarily on the ventral and lateral thorax and abdomen (Scott et al, 2001; Kwochka, 1993a). A ceruminous otitis externa and unthrifty appearing coat are often present. The clinical lesions are characterized histologically by marked follicular orthokeratotic hyperkeratosis. Improvement is noted within three to four weeks of starting oral vitamin A alcohol (retinol) with complete remission by eight to 10 weeks (Scott et al, 2001; Kwochka,

1993a). It is important to remember that this syndrome represents only a small subset of seborrheic disease in cocker spaniels. However, it is logical to try a four- to eight-week course of vitamin A in dogs with ventral hyperkeratotic plaques that do not respond well to other therapy (Kwochka, 1993a).

Many synthetic retinoids have been developed to offer better therapeutic response and less toxicity than naturally occurring vitamin A compounds. The most commonly used synthetic retinoids include tretinoin, isotretinoin and etretinate.

Tretinoin is effective topically as therapy for localized follicular and epidermal keratinization disorders such as chin acne, nasodigital hyperkeratosis, calluses and ear margin seborrhea/dermatosis (Scott et al, 2001; Power et al, 1990; Kwochka, 1993a). Isotretinoin and etretinate are given orally, in combination with food, and may be useful to manage primary idiopathic seborrhea in cocker spaniels, keratinization disorders in other breeds, schnauzer comedo syndrome, sebaceous adenitis, lamellar ichthyosis, actinic keratosis (solar-induced precancerous lesions) and various cutaneous neoplastic disorders (squamous cell carcinoma, cutaneous T-cell lymphoma, multiple keratocanthomas). Etretinate is no longer available but has been replaced by acitretin, a metabolite of etretinate (Scott et al, 2001).

Retinoid dosages commonly recommended by veterinary dermatologists are outlined in **Table 32-5**. Side effects that occur commonly with retinoids include conjunctivitis, decreased tear production, vomiting, diarrhea, arthralgia/myalgia, moderate to marked elevations in serum triglyceride levels, elevations in liver enzyme activity and teratogenic effects.

Table 32-5. Indications and dosages for retinoids in primary keratinization disorders.

Vitamin A alcohol (retinol)
Subset of seborrheic skin disease, primarily in cocker spaniels
Dosage: 625 to 1,000 IU/kg q24h per os
10,000 IU q24h per os in cocker spaniels and miniature schnauzers
50,000 IU q24h per os in Labrador retrievers
Tretinoin (all-trans retinoic acid)
Chin acne of dogs and cats
Nasodigital hyperkeratosis
Ear margin seborrhea/dermatosis
Dosage: Apply topically q12 to 24h to control; then decrease frequency for maintenance
Isotretinoin (13-cis retinoic acid)
Lamellar ichthyosis
Schnauzer comedo syndrome
Sebaceous adenitis
Dosage: 1 to 3 mg/kg q24h per os with food for control; then try to decrease to alternate-day therapy
Acitretin (analogue of retinoic acid ethyl ester)
Actinic keratosis
Idiopathic seborrhea, especially of cocker spaniels
Lamellar ichthyosis
Sebaceous adenitis
Dosage: 0.75 to 1.0 mg/kg q24h per os for control; then try to decrease to alternate-day therapy

Vitamin E

Eight isomeric forms of tocopherol represent vitamin E activity, with α-tocopherol being most important biologically. Vitamin E quenches free radicals in PUFA of membrane phospholipids. The nutritional requirement of vitamin E is closely related to the dietary intake of PUFA.

Naturally occurring vitamin E deficiency has only been reported to occur in cats. Steatitis occurs when sources of highly unsaturated fatty acids, such as red meat tuna, are fed to cats without adequate vitamin E. Clinical signs and laboratory findings include anorexia, fever, hyperesthesia, hemolytic anemia, leukocytosis and firm subcutaneous nodules. Diagnosis is confirmed by microscopic examination of biopsy specimens from adipose tissue. Typical lesions are firm, yellow to orange-brown fat with lobular panniculitis and ceroid within lipocytes, macrophages and giant cells. Treatment includes a change of food to a complete and balanced ration, supplemental vitamin E (25 to 75 mg/kg body weight/day), corticosteroids and supportive care.

Naturally occurring vitamin E deficiency has not been reported to occur in dogs, but experimentally induced vitamin E deficiency does produce skin lesions (Scott and Sheffy, 1987). Initial lesions consist of a keratinization defect (seborrhea sicca), followed by a greasy and inflammatory stage (erythroderma and seborrhea oleosa) and secondary bacterial pyoderma. The dermatosis rapidly responds to vitamin E supplementation. All lesions respond within eight to 10 weeks. It is unlikely that vitamin E deficiency would occur in dogs and cats that eat typical commercial pet foods because such foods contain three to five times the minimum daily requirement of vitamin E (Kallfelz and Dzanis, 1989).

Because of its role as a barrier, the skin is uniquely challenged by oxidants (i.e., free radicals). The skin is continuously exposed to an oxidative environment, including high oxygen tensions, air pollutants, ultraviolet (UV) radiation, parasites, aerobic microorganisms and oxidants released as a result of normal metabolism. UV radiation causes tissues to produce reactive oxygen species, eicosanoids and cytokines, which can result in acute adverse effects (e.g., sunburn, photosensitivity) as well as long-term sequelae (e.g., actinic keratosis, solar dermatitis, malignant skin tumors) (Scott et al, 2001; Nikula et al, 1992; Kimura and Doi, 1994). Because of the high lipid content of skin, lipophilic antioxidants such as α-tocopherol are expected to play a major role in scavenging reactive oxygen species during oxidative stress (Thiele et al, 2001). Vitamin E protects against UV-induced skin damage through a combination of antioxidant and UV-absorptive properties (Thiele et al, 2001). One study revealed that increasing vitamin E amounts in food significantly increased vitamin E concentrations in serum and skin of cats and dogs (Jewell et al, 2002). Previous studies have shown that increased vitamin E levels decrease serum levels of some biomarkers associated with oxidative stress (Jewell et al, 2000). This suggests that increases in dietary vitamin E concentrations are likely to be beneficial. However, the relationship between increases in serum and skin vitamin E concentrations and the prevention, development and treatment of specific skin diseases remains to be elucidated by intervention studies. The recommendation for vitamin E in foods is at least 400 IU/kg of food (DM) for dogs and at least 500 IU/kg of food (DM) for cats (Chapters 13 and 20). The minimum recommended allowances for foods for adult dogs and cats for maintenance is 30 IU/kg (DM) and 38 IU/kg (DM), respectively (NRC, 2006).

Vitamin E-Responsive Dermatoses

A number of inflammatory dermatoses in animals have been treated with oral vitamin E, including discoid lupus erythematosus, systemic lupus erythematosus, pemphigus erythematosus, sterile panniculitis, acanthosis nigricans, dermatomyositis and ear margin vasculitis. Vitamin E is often used in conjunction with systemic glucocorticoids, topical steroids and other immunosuppressive agents. Large doses of vitamin E may stabilize cell and lysomal membranes against damage induced by free radicals and peroxides, modulate AA and PG metabolism, inhibit proteolytic enzymes, enhance phagocytic activity and enhance humoral and cellular immunity.

Vitamin E appears to have limited value as an antipruritic agent. One uncontrolled study in allergic dogs that received vitamin E failed to document a reduction in pruritus (Miller, 1989). A well-controlled study in adult people with atopic dermatitis also failed to demonstrate improvement with vitamin E or selenium supplementation (Farris et al, 1989).

The oral dosage of vitamin E for inflammatory dermatoses is 200 to 800 IU twice daily (Scott et al, 2001; Rosenkrantz, 1993). This dose is seven to 27 times higher than the lower end of the recommended daily amount (≥400 IU/kg food [DM]) for a 10-kg dog (Chapters 13 and 14). Anecdotal reports suggest that topical vitamin E may help resolve discoid lupus erythematosus lesions (Rosenkrantz, 1993). Vitamin E is one of the least toxic vitamins.

B-Complex Vitamins

Experimental deficiencies of biotin and riboflavin can cause cutaneous lesions in dogs and cats (NRC, 2006). The most common clinical signs include anorexia, weight loss, diarrhea, alopecia and dry, flaky seborrhea. Clinical lesions are more likely to occur in young, growing animals than in adults (Pastoor, et al, 1991).

Several B-complex vitamins act as cofactors in EFA metabolism. LA desaturation and GLA elongation may be impaired in pyridoxine deficiency (Cunnane et al, 1984). EFA may have a sparing effect on the cutaneous lesions caused by B-complex vitamin deficiency and vice versa (Cunnane et al, 1984).

It is unlikely that B-complex vitamin deficiency would occur in dogs and cats that eat commercial pet foods, because most foods contain several times the minimum daily requirement of these vitamins. However, supplementation of complete and balanced pet foods with biotin, pantothenic acid, inositol, choline, other B vitamins, zinc and fatty acids has been shown to alter skin function (reduce transepidermal water loss) and improve coat softness and appearance (Markwell et al, 2004; Watson and Marsh, 2001). Thus, for some patients with skin/coat problems, feeding foods with additional amounts of these nutrients may be beneficial. B-complex deficiency could occur in animals eating homemade foods inadequately supplemented with vitamins.

Feeding Plan

Assess and Select the Food

In general, a patient's food should be changed if one of the following skin or coat conditions develops:

- Loss of normal hair color, especially lightening, graying or reddish-brown discoloration of normally pigmented hair,
- Brittle and easily broken hair,
- Generalized scaling, crusting, alopecia or loss of normal hair sheen for which no underlying skin disorder can be identified through routine diagnostic evaluation,
- Poor wound healing or decubital ulcers,
- Severe, generalized inflammatory skin disease such as deep pyoderma or immune-mediated skin disease,
- Hyperproliferative skin disorder such as primary seborrhea,
- Abnormal hair growth or failure of hair to regrow where clipped or lost.

Table 32-1 summarizes the key nutritional factors for foods for patients with nutrient responsive-dermatoses. A food for patients with skin and hair problems should include the recommended levels of these nutrients, and the nutrients should be available to the patient. Digestibility and assimilation of nutrients are especially important during periods of increased nutrient demand such as growth, gestation and lactation. Use of maintenance-type foods (which are usually lower in protein, fat, minerals, vitamins and digestibility than growth/lactation or foods for repletion/recovery) may be a risk factor for nutritional skin disease during these lifestages. Levels of these nutrients can be found in food tables for normal dogs and cats (Chapters 13 and 20). Otherwise, they can be obtained by contacting the manufacturer or distributor of the food.

A detailed assessment of nutritional supplements is also important. Vitamin supplements are rarely indicated except in those nutrient-sensitive disorders that respond to high levels of vitamins A or E. Excessive use of mineral supplements can interfere with assimilation of zinc and copper. Besides recommended key nutritional factors for foods for patients with nutrient-deficiency dermatologic conditions, **Table 32-1** also provides information about nutritional supplements for patients with skin and hair disorders. When appropriate, nutritional supplements can be used in conjunction with the food change or can be added to the original food. Changing to a food appropriate for the patient's lifestage will usually reverse cutaneous signs associated with a relative nutrient deficiency. Select a food whose nutritional adequacy was determined by animal tests (Chapter 9). This helps ensure that the nutrients in the food are available to the animal. Foods formulated to meet the nutrient profiles set forth by the Association of American Feed Control Officials might be nutritionally adequate but this form of establishing nutritional adequacy cannot ensure nutrient availability. Supplementation alone will not usually improve a poor-quality food. Supplementation with fatty acids, zinc, retinoids and vitamin E usually exceeds levels used to meet nutrient requirements. In these cases, nutrient supplements are being used as therapeutic agents.

Another criterion for selecting a food that may become increasingly important in the future is evidence-based clinical nutrition. Practitioners should know how to determine risks and benefits of nutritional regimens and counsel pet owners accordingly. Currently, veterinary medical education and continuing education are not always based on rigorous assessment of evidence for or against particular management options. Still, studies have been published to establish the nutritional benefits of certain pet foods. Chapter 2 describes evidence-based clinical nutrition in detail and applies its concepts to various veterinary therapeutic foods.

Assess and Determine the Feeding Method

The method of feeding is often not altered in the nutritional management of skin and hair disease. If a new food is fed, the amount to feed can be determined from the product label or other supporting materials. The food dosage may need to be changed if the caloric density of the new food differs from that of the previous food. The food dosage is usually divided into two or more meals per day. The food dosage and feeding method should be altered if the patient's body weight and condition are not optimal.

For clinical nutrition to be effective, there needs to be good compliance. Enabling compliance includes limiting access to other foods and knowing who feeds the animal. If the patient comes from a household with multiple pets, it should be determined whether the pet with skin disease has access to the other pets' food.

Reassessment

Cutaneous disease due to a nutrient deficiency will usually respond rapidly and dramatically to appropriate nutritional change or supplementation. Patients will usually improve within a few days to weeks. Nutrient-sensitive disorders usually respond to supplements more slowly, over several weeks to several months. After a nutritional change or supplementation has been started, the patient should be examined monthly for significant changes in skin lesions and hair quality. Trichograms can be repeated in those patients that have abnormal hair quality or hair growth.

FATTY ACIDS FOR INFLAMMATORY SKIN DISEASE

Clinical Importance

EFA exhibit multiple antiinflammatory and immunomodulating properties. They have the potential to affect allergic and other forms of skin inflammation through modulating cytokine production, inhibiting cellular activation and cytokine secretion and altering the composition and function of the epidermal lipid barrier (Olivry et al, 2001). Their mechanisms of action, therefore, are likely to be explained by a combination of effects.

The most commonly proposed mechanism of action of EFA in the treatment of inflammatory skin diseases is the modulation of cutaneous production of PG and LT (Olivry et al, 2001). AA is the major PUFA in cell membrane phospholipids (Stossel et al, 1974). The normal response of injured tissue is inflammation, a tissue protective mechanism. Under these circumstances, phospholipases are activated and act on phospholipids of cell membranes to release constituent fatty acids. AA, the fatty acid in greatest concentration, is released and converted into eicosanoids, which mediate inflammation.

Eicosanoids are also derived from GLA and EPA. They also include PG, thromboxanes, LT, hydroperoxyeicosatetraenoic acids (HPETE) and hydroxyeicosatetraenoic acids (HETE). Macrophages are the most significant sources of eicosanoids (Lokesh et al, 1988; Meydani et al, 1991; Hwang, 1989; Magrum and Johnston, 1983).

Four AA-derived LT and one PG play a central role in the inflammatory process. LTB_4 stimulates neutrophil and eosinophil chemotaxis and increases vascular permeability. LTC_4, LTD_4 and LTE_4 encourage smooth muscle contraction and increase vascular permeability. PGE_2 inhibits T and B lymphocyte proliferation, reduces cytokine production and limits natural killer cell activity. However, these proinflammatory eicosanoids can result in pathologic conditions when produced in excessive amounts and/or prolonged periods of time (Sigal, 1991; Lands, 1989). Increased production of LT and PGE_2 has been reported in many chronic inflammatory diseases (Goodwin and Ceuppens, 1983).

Modulating the PUFA content of cell membrane phospholipids by dietary means can alter eicosanoid production. Such modulation can affect the intensity and duration of inflammatory and immune responses (Lokesh et al, 1988; Meydani et al, 1991; Hwang, 1989; Magrum and Johnston, 1983). Generally, omega-3 fatty acids are thought to produce less inflammatory cytokines (Sigal, 1991; Lands, 1989; Lokesh et al, 1988; Lokesh and Kinsella, 1987; Broughton et al, 1991; Croft et al, 1987).

Consumption of flax or fish oils with omega-3 PUFA results in replacement of AA in the macrophage membrane with ALA, docosahexaenoic acid (DHA) or EPA. The result is production of fewer AA- (omega-6) derived eicosanoids and more ALA- (omega-3) derived eicosanoids, thereby reducing the inflammatory response (Meydani et al, 1991; Calder et al, 1990; Endres et al, 1989, 1993; Baldie et al, 1993; Lee et al, 1985). Studies using neutrophils from normal dogs have shown that enhanced levels of dietary omega-3 fatty acids inhibit leukotriene generation (Byrne et al, 2000; Vaughn et al, 1994). Studies have also shown alterations in inflammatory response and immune function in normal cats fed foods with enhanced levels of omega-3 fatty acids (Chew et al, 2000). Consequently, changing the type of eicosanoid production and the subsequent alteration in cytokine production can reduce inflammation by eicosanoid-mediated effects (Horrobin and Manku, 1990; Calder et al, 1990; Endres et al, 1989, 1993; Baldie et al, 1993; Lee et al, 1985; Watson et al, 1990). This premise is the basis for using omega-3 fatty acids for treatment of chronic inflammatory conditions.

A similar effect is proposed for the use of GLA, an omega-6 derivative of LA. GLA and DHA reduce histamine release and alter cell mediator production in canine mast cells (Gueck et al, 2004). If similar changes occur in dermal mast cells from patients with atopic dermatitis, these results suggest that GLA and omega-3 fatty acid supplements or similarly enriched foods might be beneficial. Black currant oil, borage oil and evening primrose oil are sources of GLA (Meydani et al, 1991; Calder et al, 1990; Endres et al, 1989, 1993; Baldie et al, 1993; Lee et al, 1985).

Besides affecting LT and PG production, EFA exhibit numerous additional immunomodulating properties. They have been reported to decrease the synthesis of proinflammatory cytokines, decrease T-cell lymphocyte proliferation and activation, affect expression of cell adhesion molecules, influence signaling within cells of the immune system and regulate cytotoxic activity of phagocytes by modulating the production of reactive oxygen species (Olivry et al, 2001a). Preliminary investigations suggest that dogs with atopic dermatitis also may exhibit abnormal epidermal lipid levels and metabolism (Olivry and Hill, 2001a). EFA have the potential to modulate this abnormal skin lipid barrier function in animals with inflammatory skin disease.

For more information about fatty acid metabolism and fatty acid modulation of the inflammatory response see the Lipids section in Chapter 5.

Patient Assessment

History and Physical Examination

Numerous skin diseases have an inflammatory component. However, dietary fatty acid therapy has been used primarily in patients with allergic skin disease or patients with pruritus or papulocrustous dermatitis for which a specific cause has not been identified.

Pruritus is the most common historical feature of allergic skin disease in dogs and cats. Clinical signs reportedly first occur in most dogs and cats with atopic dermatitis between six months and three years of age (Scott et al, 2001; Griffin et al, 1993; Griffin and DeBoer, 2001). Lesions of canine atopic dermatitis usually involve the muzzle, periocular region, pinnae and external ear canals, paws, axillae, groin and abdomen. Although the face and paws are most commonly involved, many animals will have generalized pruritus by the time they are examined. Chronic licking, rubbing, chewing or scratching can result in alopecia, lichenification, hyperpigmentation, scaling and excoriation. Other common lesions in atopic dogs include papules and erythematous macules, secondary superficial pyoderma, secondary *Malassezia* dermatitis, chronic otitis externa and seborrhea.

Cats with atopic dermatitis most commonly exhibit symmetric alopecia, miliary dermatitis, eosinophilic plaques, indolent ulcer of the lip, pruritus of the head and neck with excoriations or generalized pruritus (Scott et al, 2001; Sousa, 1995). Atopic cats are pruritic, but many are secretive and groom or traumatize themselves without the owner's knowledge.

Cats with miliary dermatitis have numerous small erythematous papules with adherent brownish crusts and various degrees of alopecia and pruritus (Scott et al, 2001; Sousa, 1995). These lesions can usually be palpated over the dorsal lumbar and cervical regions long before they are visualized. Feline miliary dermatitis is most commonly a manifestation of flea allergy, but may occur with other ectoparasite infestations, dermatophytosis, bacterial folliculitis, adverse food reactions, atopic dermatitis, drug eruptions and immune-mediated skin disease.

Canine flea-bite hypersensitivity is characterized by a pruritic, papular dermatitis (Scott et al, 2001). Flea bites induce an initial papule that may then form a crust. Chronic pruritus may lead to alopecia, lichenification, severe crusting and hyperpigmentation. Lesions are typically confined to the dorsal lumbosacral area, caudomedial thighs, ventral abdomen and flanks. Pyotraumatic dermatitis ("hot spots"), secondary bacterial pyoderma and secondary seborrhea are common in chronic cases. The presence of otitis externa, severe pedal pruritus or facial pruritus strongly suggests concurrent atopic dermatitis or adverse food reaction.

Numerous insects besides fleas and arachnids in the normal dog and cat environment can stimulate hypersensitivity reactions. Blackfly, deerfly, horsefly, mosquito, red ant, black ant and tick bites may all contribute to allergic skin disease in dogs and cats (Griffin et al, 1993). The primary clinical sign is pruritus, although an erythematous maculopapular dermatitis may be present (Scott et al, 2001). Nodules and papules induced by mosquito bites are usually found on the bridge of the nose and pinnae of cats. Stable flies occasionally induce a granulomatous reaction, producing nodules or plaques and varying degrees of alopecia on the pinnae. Ticks may induce nodules due to granuloma formation at the site of attachment. Acute-onset nasal dermatitis has also been observed in dogs; pruritic papules and nodules are found on the bridge of the nose.

Adverse reactions to food mimic other allergic diseases. The clinical features and management of adverse food reactions are described in detail in Chapter 31.

Laboratory and Other Clinical Information

Skin biopsy and histopathology can be used to confirm the presence of inflammatory skin disease. Chronic hyperplastic dermatitis is a common histopathologic reaction pattern seen in dogs with chronic allergy (Gross et al, 1992; Olivry and Hill, 2001b). The predominant types of inflammatory cells may suggest the specific allergic disease. However, many chronic dermatoses have similar histopathologic features, making specific diagnosis difficult. The nature of epidermal and dermal inflammatory cell infiltrates in canine atopic dermatitis has recently been characterized using modern immunologic techniques and is described in other sources (Olivry and Hill, 2001b).

Two methods of allergy testing are available to practitioners. Intradermal testing has been performed for many years. More recently, in vitro tests for detection of allergen-specific IgE have become commercially available.

Intradermal testing is widely used by veterinary dermatologists for making a definitive diagnosis of canine atopic disease and for selecting allergens for hyposensitization (Scott et al, 2001; Hillier and DeBoer, 2001). Intradermal allergy tests detect the allergen-specific IgE fixed to the surface of mast cells in the dermis, and assess the ability of IgE to fix allergen and cause mast cell degranulation and subsequent vasodilatation. In a well-controlled study using allergen mixes, 59% of dogs responded to hyposensitization that was formulated on the basis of intradermal testing results (Willemse et al, 1984).

Intradermal allergy testing has several disadvantages (Hillier and DeBoer, 2001). Negative intradermal results occur in some dogs strongly suspected to have atopic dermatitis. Anti-inflammatory and antihistamine drugs must be withdrawn before testing to prevent false-negative results. The test cannot be performed on dogs with generalized dermatitis. Shaving of the coat and sedation are usually required. Intradermal allergy testing is time-consuming and not cost-effective when performed infrequently. The usefulness of intradermal allergy testing is also limited by lack of standardized allergy extracts and no homogeneous criteria for the interpretation of results. Most intradermal testing is performed at dermatologic referral centers because of these disadvantages. Intradermal testing for food hypersensitivity is unreliable in animals with dermatologic disease (Chapter 31).

In vitro "allergy" tests measure serum concentrations of allergen-specific IgE and avoid many of the disadvantages of intradermal allergy tests (Codner and Griffin, 1996). In vitro tests require only a serum sample; so they are readily available to private practitioners and can be used on patients with generalized dermatitis. Laboratories use several different techniques to detect circulating IgE levels, including a radioallergosorbent test (RAST), enzyme-linked immunosorbent assay (ELISA) or liquid-phase enzyme immunoassay (EIA). Problems with in vitro testing include poor reproducibility and a high false-positive rate (Codner and Lessard, 1993). Results to date suggest that more than 60% of atopic dogs respond to hyposensitization formulated on the basis of in vitro results (Anderson, 1993; Sousa and Norton, 1990). In vitro testing is also available for confirming flea-allergic dermatitis (Cook et al, 1996) but is unreliable for diagnosing food hypersensitivity (Chapter 31).

Controversy continues over whether intradermal or in vitro testing is the better method for confirming a diagnosis of atopic dermatitis and for selecting allergens for hyposensitization (DeBoer and Hillier, 2001). Furthermore, long-term studies are needed to evaluate responses of allergic animals to hyposensitization based on both types of testing.

Risk Factors

Atopy (atopic state) is a genetically-predisposed tendency to develop IgE-mediated allergy to environmental allergens (Olivry et al, 2001c). Atopic disease is any clinical manifestation of atopy including most commonly atopic dermatitis, atopic conjunctivitis and/or atopic rhinitis (Olivry et al, 2001c). Atopic dermatitis is a genetically predisposed inflammatory and pruritic allergic skin disease with characteristic clinical features (Olivry et al, 2001c). It is associated most commonly with IgE antibodies to environmental allergens. Although the exact mode of inheritance is unknown, strong breed predilection and familial involvement in dogs indicate a genetically determined cause. Canine breeds reported to be predisposed to atopy include Cairn terriers, West Highland white terriers, Scottish terriers, wire-haired fox terriers, Boston terriers, Sealyham terriers, Lhasa apsos, Dalmatians, pugs, Irish setters, English setters,

Table 32-6. Key nutritional factors for foods and supplements for dogs and cats with inflammatory dermatoses.

Factors	Nutritional recommendations
Omega-3 fatty acids (ALA, EPA and/or DHA)	Supplements or foods should initially provide 50 to 300 mg total omega-3 fatty acids/kg body weight/day Foods should contain between 0.35 to 1.8% dry matter

Key: ALA = α-linolenic acid, EPA = eicosapentaenoic acid, DHA = docosahexaenoic acid.

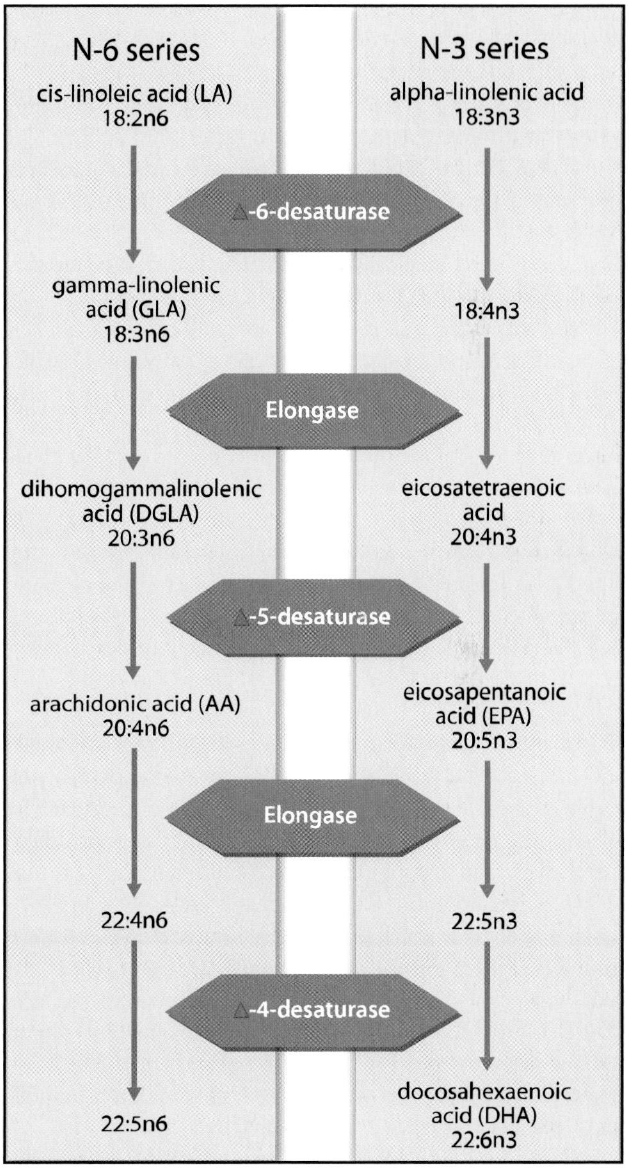

Figure 32-3. Metabolic transformation of two major unsaturated fatty acid families by desaturation and elongation.

Table 32-7. Fatty acids found in pet food ingredients and supplements.

Fatty acids	Ingredients/supplements
Linoleic acid (omega-6)	Vegetable oils (soy oil, corn oil, safflower oil, canola oil, etc.)
	Grains (corn, soybeans)
γ-linolenic acid (GLA, omega-6)	Black currant oil
	Borage oil
	Evening primrose oil
α-linolenic acid (ALA, omega-3)	Flax
	Flax (linseed) oil
Eicosapentaenoic acid (EPA, omega-3)	Fish meal
	Cold water marine oils
Docosahexaenoic acid (DHA, omega-3)	Fish meal
	Cold water marine oils

golden retrievers, Labrador retrievers, boxers, miniature schnauzers, English bulldogs, Bichon Frise, Chinese Shar-Pei, Shih Tzu, German shepherd dogs, Belgian Tervuren, beauceron and cocker spaniels (Scott et al, 2001; Griffin et al, 1993; Anderson, 1993). However, canine atopic dermatitis may be seen in any breed, including mixed breeds. Breed predisposition has not been reported for atopic cats (Scott et al, 2001).

Hypersensitivity requires environmental exposure to flea, other biting insect or arachnid allergens. Depending on the offending allergen, these cases may be seasonal in temperate climates; worse clinical signs occur during warm weather. The onset of clinical signs may be historically correlated with an increase in insect or arachnid numbers in the environment.

Key Nutritional Factors

The key nutritional factors for foods and dietary supplements for omega-3 fatty acid-responsive skin diseases are summarized in **Table 32-6** and are discussed in more detail below.

OMEGA-3 FATTY ACIDS

The use of omega-3 fatty acids as antipruritic agents in dogs and cats has been the subject of numerous studies and considerable debate. The inflammation and dermatitis associated with allergic skin disease may be partially caused by abnormal EFA metabolism and inappropriate eicosanoid synthesis (White, 1993). A unique feature of skin is that it lacks Δ-6- and Δ-5-desaturase enzyme activity, and thus is incapable of making AA from LA or EPA from ALA (**Figure 32-3**) (Campbell, 1990). Skin can elongate GLA to dihomogammalinolenic acid (DGLA) and EPA to DHA. Normal dogs metabolize dietary sources of ALA to EPA and DHA elsewhere in the body. These fatty acids are then incorporated into the skin (Campbell and Roudebush, 1995).

DGLA, EPA and DHA in cutaneous cellular membranes may decrease inflammation through competition with AA for metabolic enzymes or because of the antiinflammatory nature of the eicosanoids produced (White, 1993). The rationale for specifically administering products high in GLA (an omega-6 [n-6] fatty acid) is that GLA can be incorporated into the skin, where it is rapidly elongated to DGLA. Because skin lacks desaturase enzymes, DGLA is not further metabolized to AA. As a result, DGLA competes with AA for metabolic enzymes. Thus there is a decrease in AA-derived eicosanoids and an increase in the antiinflammatory eicosanoids PGE_1 via the cyclooxygenase cascade and 15-HETE via the lipoxygenase pathway. Specific recommendations for food amounts for GLA have not yet been determined. Thus, GLA is not listed as a key nutritional factor at this time. However, evening primrose, borage or black currant oils are used to increase dietary GLA intake.

ALA is an omega-3 (n-3) PUFA that is metabolized to EPA and DHA, and incorporated into the skin of normal dogs (Manku et al, 1982). Findings suggest that atopic dermatitis in human beings is associated with a deficiency of Δ-6-desaturase activity, which prevents the rapid conversion of ALA to EPA and DHA in atopic individuals (Manku et al, 1982, 1984). Comparable studies using atopic dogs and cats have not been published. However, one study suggested that subsets of atopic dogs exist with different fatty acid metabolic capabilities (Scott et al, 1997). Other studies suggest that ALA can modulate inflammatory and immune responses in normal cats (Chew et al, 2000). Flax, flax oil or linseed oil is typically used to provide ALA for supplements or foods.

The use of fatty acids for treating atopic dermatitis and chronic pruritus has been extensively studied in dogs (Scott et al, 1992, 1997; Scott and Buerger, 1988; Miller et al, 1989, 1992; Lloyd and Thomsett, 1989; Lloyd, 1989; Scott and Miller, 1990; Scarff et al, 1990; Paradis et al, 1991; Scarff and Lloyd, 1992; Bond and Lloyd, 1992, 1992a, 1993; White, 1992; Logas and Kunkle, 1994; Schick et al, 1995). Unfortunately, most of these studies have been uncontrolled, masked clinical trials using low doses of fatty acids for short periods. In these studies, 0 to more than 75% of pruritic patients had degrees of clinical improvement. Clinical studies using randomization, placebos and high doses of fatty acids for six weeks or more showed decreased pruritus in 0 to more than 50% of patients (Scarff and Lloyd, 1992; White, 1992; Logas and Kunkle, 1994). Dogs that did not have decreased pruritus still showed improvement in other clinical signs, including less erythroderma and skin edema. The benefit of fatty acid supplementation is maximized in dogs if other contributing diseases such as adverse reactions to food, flea hypersensitivity, bacterial pyoderma and *Malassezia* dermatitis are controlled. Overall, it is probably safe to inform clients that up to 50% of dogs with allergic pruritus will improve with modification in fatty acid intake, if secondary bacterial and yeast infections are controlled. Synergistic effects have been documented between fatty acids and other antipruritic agents such as antihistamines and glucocorticoids (Scott et al, 2001; Scott and Miller, 1990; Paradis et al, 1991). Fatty acid supplementation may also allow lower doses of antihistamines and glucocorticoids to be used to control clinical signs (Sævik et al, 2004; Bond and Lloyd, 1994; Paterson, 1995; Scott et al, 2001).

The use of fatty acids for management of allergic skin disease and papulocrustous (miliary) dermatitis in cats has been reported (Harvey, 1991, 1993, 1993a; Miller et al, 1993). More than

Table 32-8. The total essential fatty acid intake for a 10-kg adult dog eating 600 kcal (2,510 kJ) per day of selected commercial foods or being given one of the selected supplements.*

Dry foods	**Food consumed (g)**	**Total omega-6 consumed (mg)**	**Total omega-3 consumed (mg)****
Hill's Prescription Diet b/d Canine	165	4,884	1,548
Hill's Prescription Diet d/d Potato & Duck Formula Canine	161	4,854	1,164
Hill's Prescription Diet d/d Potato & Salmon Formula Canine	162	4,206	2,100
Hill's Prescription Diet d/d Potato & Venison Formula Canine	161	4,932	1,146
Hill's Prescription Diet d/d Rice & Egg Formula Canine	154	4,692	990
Hill's Prescription Diet j/d Canine	176	4,032	5,688
Hill's Prescription Diet z/d Canine Low Allergen	163	4,812	618
Hill's Prescription Diet z/d ULTRA Allergen Free Canine	161	6,222	804
Hill's Science Diet Canine Active Adult	130	5,976	678
Hill's Science Diet Canine Adult Original	162	5,310	726
Hill's Science Diet Canine Lamb Meal & Rice Recipe Adult	162	4,815	1,002
Hill's Science Diet Canine Light Adult	200	5,988	618
Hill's Science Diet Canine Senior 7+ Original	163	4,590	1,710
Hill's Science Diet Sensitive Skin Dog	158	7,392	2,166
Iams Eukanuba Adult Maintenance Formula	139	4,800	600
Iams Eukanuba Reduced Fat Adult Formula	155	3,600	600
Iams Eukanuba Senior Maintenance Formula	142	3,600	600
Iams Veterinary Formulas Joint/Articulation	142	4,200	600
Iams Veterinary Formulas Response FP	147	1,600	400
Nutro Ultra Adult	166	7,998	1,290
Nutro Ultra Senior	168	7,392	1,380
Purina Veterinary Diets DRM Dermatologic Management Canine Formula	151	1,680	1,680
Royal Canin IVD Limited Ingredient Diets Potato & Duck Canine Formula	175	2,940	1,020
Royal Canin IVD Limited Ingredient Diets Potato & Rabbit Canine Formula	177	3,120	1,380
Royal Canin Veterinary Diet Hypoallergenic HP19	143	7,158	1,158
Royal Canin Veterinary Diet Sensitivity RC21	168	3,354	1,512
Royal Canin Veterinary Diet Skin Support SS21	153	4,884	1,758
Moist foods	**Food consumed (g)**	**Total omega-6 consumed (mg)**	**Total omega-3 consumed (mg)****
Hill's Prescription Diet a/d Canine/Feline	521	6,882	3,126
Hill's Prescription Diet d/d Duck Formula Canine	624	4,932	1,248
Hill's Prescription Diet d/d Lamb Formula Canine	451	3,972	1,488
Hill's Prescription Diet d/d Salmon Formula Canine	613	5,148	4,350
Hill's Prescription Diet d/d Venison Formula Canine	550	4,950	1,098
Hill's Prescription Diet j/d Canine	446	4,104	6,066
Hill's Prescription Diet n/d Canine	380	2,772	8,088
Hill's Prescription Diet z/d ULTRA Allergen Free Canine	617	6,102	738
Iams Veterinary Formulas Response FP	475	9,600	1,200
Royal Canin IVD Limited Ingredient Diets Duck Canine Formula	536	5,340	720
Royal Canin IVD Limited Ingredient Diets Whitefish Canine Formula	522	6,600	3,300
Supplements			
3V Caps for Large & Giant Breeds	1 capsule	0	417
3V Caps for Medium & Large Breeds	1 capsule	0	300
3V Caps for Small & Medium Breeds	1 capsule	0	171
3V Caps Liquid	0.75 ml	0	187
3V Caps Liquid HR	1 ml	0	450
DermCaps 100 lb	1 capsule	402	252
DermCaps ES	1 capsule	368	123
DermCaps ES Liquid	1 ml	375	130
DermCaps Liquid	1 ml	621	65
DermCaps Regular	1 capsule	402	108
Nutrived O.F.A. Granules	1 scoop	539	129
EicosaDerm	1 pump	0	600
Welactin	1 pump	0	330-364
Omegaderm – Small Dogs & Cats	1 packet (4 ml)	1,488	300
Nordic Naturals Omega-3	1 capsule	0	350
Nordic Naturals Arctic Cod Liver Oil	1 capsule	0	280
Nordic Naturals Ultimate Omega	1 capsule	0	700

*Adapted from Roudebush P. Consumption of essential fatty acids in selected commercial dog foods compared to dietary supplementation: An update. In: Proceedings. Annual Members Meeting AAVD & ACVD, Norfolk, VA, 2001: 53-54.

**Laboratory and clinical studies in a number of species have established a daily dosage for total omega-3 fatty acids that seems to be a reasonable starting point in patients with inflammatory disease. An initial dose of 50 to 300 mg of total omega-3 fatty acids/kg body weight/day seems to be effective in a large number of studies.

Table 32-9. The total essential fatty acid intake for a 4.5-kg cat eating 260 kcal (1,088 kJ) per day of selected commercial foods or being given one of the selected supplements.

Dry foods	Food consumed (g)	Total omega-6 consumed (mg)	Total omega-3 consumed (mg)*
Hill's Prescription Diet d/d Duck & Green Pea Formula Feline	68	2,254	473
Hill's Prescription Diet d/d Rabbit & Green Pea Formula Feline	69	2,304	460
Hill's Prescription Diet d/d Venison & Green Pea Formula Feline	67	2,142	458
Hill's Prescription Diet z/d Low Allergen Feline	69	3,630	419
Hill's Science Diet Adult Original Cat Food	64	2,301	140
Hill's Science Diet Mature Adult 7+ Original Cat Food	66	2,114	146
Hill's Science Diet Sensitive Skin Adult Cat Food	67	3,123	294
Iams Eukanuba Chicken & Rice Formula Cat Food	55	2,158	302
Iams Eukanuba Mature Care Formula for Cats	61	2,049	411
Royal Canin Adult Fit 32 Cat Food	68	2,462	322
Royal Canin Indoor 27 Cat Food	70	2,395	408
Royal Canin IVD Limited Ingredient Diets Green Pea & Venison Feline Formula	73	1,794	624
Royal Canin Persian 30 Cat Food	60	2,889	481
Royal Canin Skin Care 30 Cat Food	63	2,951	499
Royal Canin Veterinary Diet Feline Hypoallergenic HP 23	63	3,003	486
Royal Canin Veterinary Diet Feline Sensitivity RD 30	67	2,140	213
Moist foods	**Food consumed (g)**	**Total omega-6 consumed (mg)**	**Total omega-3 consumed (mg)***
Hill's Prescription Diet a/d Canine/Feline	226	3,344	1,422
Hill's Prescription Diet d/d Duck Formula Feline	215	3,354	666
Hill's Prescription Diet d/d Rabbit Formula Feline	233	3,403	699
Hill's Prescription Diet d/d Venison Formula Feline	206	4,178	988
Hill's Prescription Diet z/d ULTRA Allergen Free Feline	241	2,574	289
Hill's Science Diet Savory Salmon Entrée Adult Cat Food	250	2,072	1,147
Iams Veterinary Formulas Response LB/Feline	199	2,600	520
Supplements			
3V Caps for Small & Medium Breeds	1 capsule	0	171
3V Caps Liquid HR	1 ml	0	450
DermCaps ES Liquid	1 ml	375	130
DermCaps Liquid	1 ml	621	65
DermCaps Regular	1 capsule	402	108
Nutrived O.F.A. Granules	1 scoop	539	129
EicosaDerm	1/2 pump	0	300
Welactin	1 pump	0	330-364
Nordic Naturals Omega-3	1 capsule	0	350

*Laboratory and clinical studies in a number of species have established a daily dosage for total omega-3 fatty acids that seems to be a reasonable starting point in patients with inflammatory disease. An initial dose of 50 to 300 mg of total omega-3 fatty acids/kg body weight/day seems to be effective in a large number of studies.

50% of allergic cats may improve, based on the results of uncontrolled, masked clinical trials published to date. Better clinical studies using randomization, placebos and masked protocols are needed in cats with allergic and other forms of dermatitis.

Laboratory and clinical studies in a number of species have established a daily dosage for total omega-3 fatty acids that seems to be a reasonable starting point in patients with inflammatory disease. An initial dose of 50 to 300 mg of total omega-3 fatty acids (ALA, EPA and/or DHA)/kg body weight/day seemed to be effective in a large number of studies (Endres et al, 1989; Lee et al, 1985; Logas and Kunkle, 1994; Kremer et al, 1987, 1995; Geusens et al, 1994; Hawthorne et al, 1992; Vaughn and Reinhart, 1994; Lorenz et al, 1989; Stenson et al, 1992).[d,e] As a food amount, this dose range translates to approximately 0.35 to 1.8% total omega-3 fatty acids (DM). Also, this total dose can be supplied through a combination of appropriate foods and supplements.

Dietary omega-3 fatty acid supplements are usually derived from cold-water marine fish oils. Food ingredient sources of EPA and DHA are usually fish meal or fish oil. Most commercial pet foods already exceed the omega-6 EFA requirement for LA by using vegetable oil and/or vegetable ingredients in their formulas.

Feeding Plan

Assess and Select the Food and/or Supplement

Patients with dermatitis having an inflammatory component may benefit from changes in dietary fatty acid intake. The most common modification is to increase omega-3 fatty acid intake and/or increase intake of GLA, an omega-6 fatty acid. **Table 32-7** lists typical pet food ingredients and supplements with their associated fatty acids.

Changing the food, adding a supplement or both can modify fatty acid levels in the overall diet. Initially, the EFA levels in the current food should be assessed. Unfortunately, information about fatty acid concentrations in commercial pet foods is sometimes difficult to obtain. This information is not typically found in guaranteed or typical analysis statements on pet food

Table 32-10. Summary of randomized, masked clinical studies using fatty acid supplements or fatty acid-enhanced foods in dogs with dermatologic disease.

Reference*	Dogs (no.)	Type of trial	Duration of therapy (weeks)	Control of pruritus (%)**	Control of clinical signs***
Scott et al, 1992	20	R,DB	2	25	–
Scarff and Lloyd, 1992	35	R,DB,PC	9	0	+
Bond and Lloyd, 1992a	21	R,DB,PC	8	76	+
Bond and Lloyd, 1992b	37	R,SB	16	64	+
Bond and Lloyd, 1993	28	R,DB	16	67	+
White, 1992	10	R,DB,PC	8	0	+
Logas and Kunkle, 1994	16	R,DB,X	6	56	+
Harvey, 1999	18	R,DB,PC	8	50	+
Paterson, 1995	32	R,SB,PC	12	50-75	+
Sævik et al, 2004	60	R,DB,PC	12	57	–
Taugbøl et al, 2004	24	R,DB,PC	10	53	–
Noli and Banni, 2004	24	R,DB,PC	8	50	–
Mueller et al, 2003	29	R,DB,PC	NR	9-15	–
Mueller et al, 2005	30	R,DB,PC	10	40-50	+
Nesbitt et al, 2003	58	R,DB	8	50	+
Sture and Lloyd, 1995	25	R,DB,PC,X	9	40	+

Key: NR = not reported, DB = double blind, PC = placebo controlled, SB = single blind, R = randomized, X = cross-over.
*The references for **Table 32-10** are available at www.markmorris.org.
**Percentage of dogs in which good to excellent pruritus control was reported.
***A + symbol indicates that improvement in clinical signs other than pruritus was noted (e.g., less erythroderma, less edema, less scale).

Table 32-11. Summary of clinical studies using fatty acid supplements in cats with dermatologic disease.

Reference*	Cats (no.)	Type of trial	Duration of therapy (weeks)	Control of pruritus (%)**	Control of clinical signs***
Harvey, 1991	8	Open	6	75	+
Harvey, 1993	11	Open	12	100	+
Harvey, 1993a	14	Open	12	78	+
Miller et al, 1993	28	Open	6	57	–

Key: Open = nonblinded.
*The references for **Table 32-11** are available at www.markmorris.org.
**Percentage of cats in which good to excellent pruritus control was reported.
***A + symbol indicates that improvement in clinical signs other than pruritus was noted (e.g., less erythroderma, less edema, less scale).

labels and is often not published by the manufacturer. In those cases, the manufacturer should be contacted directly to obtain information about fatty acid concentrations in specific products. **Tables 32-8** and **32-9** contain information about fatty acid concentrations in selected commercial dog and cat foods, respectively. These tables compare the fatty acid intake of dogs and cats eating specific foods and supplements. If the patient is given a supplement, the fatty acid concentrations in the supplement should also be determined. Most supplements marketed to improve skin and coat list the fatty acid concentrations on the product label or in published technical information. **Tables 32-8** and **32-9** also contain information about fatty acid concentrations in selected commercial fatty acid supplements.

In many cases, fatty acid supplements contain much lower concentrations of fatty acids than concentrations already found in the food being consumed by the patient (**Tables 32-8** and **32-9**). Thus, it may be more appropriate and convenient to change the patient's food to one with higher concentrations of appropriate fatty acids rather than adding a fatty acid supplement to the current food. In some clinical cases, changing the food and simultaneously adding a fatty acid supplement may be appropriate.

The optimal concentrations and ratios of fatty acids have not been established for normal dogs and cats or patients with clinical disease. Trial and error with various food and supplement combinations may be needed in an individual patient to achieve the best clinical response.

The risks and side effects of high levels of dietary fatty acids are few. Soft feces, overt diarrhea, flatulence and oral malodor ("fishy breath") are most commonly noted at levels of fatty acid supplementation used in most patients. These risks and side effects are outweighed by the possibility that fatty acid supplements will allow practitioners to reduce or discontinue corticosteroid therapy for pruritic dogs and cats. Other nutrients such as zinc, magnesium, biotin, pyridoxine, vitamin E and vitamin C are important cofactors in fatty acid metabolic pathways. Most commercial pet foods have adequate levels of these nutrients; routine supplementation would not be expected to improve clinical response. Many fatty acid supplements contain additional amounts of these cofactor nutrients.

Another criterion for selecting a food that may become increasingly important in the future is evidence-based clinical nutrition. Practitioners should know how to determine risks and benefits of nutritional regimens and counsel pet owners accordingly. Currently, veterinary medical education and continuing education are not always based on rigorous assessment of evidence for or against particular management options. Still, studies have been published to establish the nutritional benefits of certain pet foods. Chapter 2 describes evidence-based clinical nutrition in detail and applies its concepts to various veterinary therapeutic foods.

Assess and Determine the Feeding Method

Other than supplementation, the method of feeding is often not altered in the nutritional management of allergic dermatitis. If a new food and/or a supplement is fed, the amount to feed can be determined from the product label or other supporting materials. The food dosage may need to be changed if the caloric density of the new food differs from that of the previous food. The food dosage is usually divided into two or more meals per day. The food dosage and feeding method should be altered if the animal's body weight and body condition are not optimal.

For clinical nutrition to be effective, there needs to be good client compliance. Enabling compliance includes limiting the patient's access to other foods and knowing who is responsible for feeding the food. If the patient comes from a multiple-pet household, it should be determined whether the pet with dermatitis has access to the other pets' food.

Reassessment

Allergic dermatitis patients receiving appropriate omega-3 fatty acid dietary intervention will usually respond over several weeks to several months (**Tables 32-10** and **32-11**). After a dietary change or supplement has been started, the patient should be examined every four weeks for significant improvement in pruritus or skin erythema. Some patients may not respond for several months or may need concurrent therapy with antihistamines, topical agents (medicated shampoo) or corticosteroids.

ACKNOWLEDGMENTS

The authors and editors thank Drs. Candace A. Sousa, Dawn E. Logas and William S. Swecker for their contribution to this chapter in the previous edition.

ENDNOTES

a. Hill's Pet Nutrition, Inc., Topeka, KS, USA.
b. Byrne K. University of Illinois, Urbana, IL, USA. Personal communication. 1995.
c. Power HT. What's up about the hepatocutaneous syndrome? Derm Dialogue, Winter 1999: 13-14.
d. Logas DB. Veterinary Dermatology Center, Winter Park, FL, USA. Personal communication. September 1997.
e. Schoenherr WD. Unpublished data. September 1997.

REFERENCES

The references for **Chapter 32** can be found at www.markmorris.org.

CASE 32-1

Seborrheic Dermatitis in a Cocker Spaniel

Dawn E. Logas, DVM, Dipl. ACVD
College of Veterinary Medicine
University of Florida
Gainesville, Florida, USA

Patient Assessment

A four-year-old spayed female cocker spaniel had a two-year history of seborrhea. The dog had previously been treated with antibiotics, steroids and topical antiseborrheic shampoos with minimal improvement. The dog weighed 10 kg and had a body condition score of 3/5.

The only abnormalities noted on physical examination were an odoriferous generalized dermatosis and bilateral otitis externa. The dermatosis was characterized by erythematous and hyperpigmented hyperkeratotic plaques in which the hairs were coated with keratinaceous casts that formed "fronds" (**Figure 1**). Multiple papules and pustules were noted on the ventrum and dorsum. Both ear canals were mildly erythematous and swollen with a thick, yellow waxy discharge.

Skin scrapings for parasites and fungal culture for dermatophytes were negative. Tape preparations of the skin revealed many cocci. Ear cytology revealed numerous yeast organisms. A culture specimen from a pustule grew moderate numbers of *Staphylococcus intermedius* colonies that were sensitive to all antibiotics except penicillin, amoxicillin and tetracycline. Histopathologically, the hyperkeratotic plaques were characterized by marked follicular hyperkeratosis with distended follicular ostia, orthokeratotic hyperkeratosis of the epidermis and irregular epidermal hyperplasia (**Figure 2**).

Assess the Food and Feeding Method

For the three years before presentation, the dog had eaten a commercial specialty brand dry dog food supplemented with table foods.

Therapy Including Feeding Plan

The tentative diagnosis was vitamin A-responsive dermatosis with superficial pyoderma and yeast otitis. Treatment was initiated with 10,000 IU of vitamin A orally along with the dog's original food. The patient was also given an appropriate antibiotic for the pyoderma and a topical antifungal for the yeast otitis.

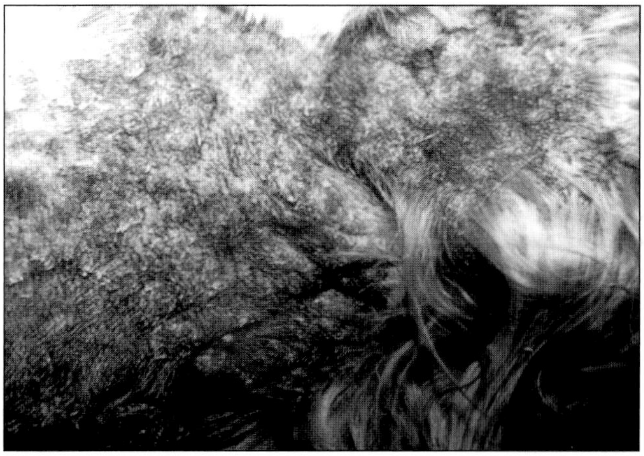

Figure 1. Hyperpigmented, hyperkeratotic plaques with fronding on the ventrum of a four-year-old cocker spaniel.

Questions

1. Why is vitamin A essential for normal epidermal function?
2. Why is this condition referred to as vitamin A-responsive dermatosis?
3. What are possible mechanisms by which vitamin A might correct the keratinization defect of this dermatosis?
4. How long must vitamin A be given to this dog and what potential side effects of vitamin A therapy might be expected?

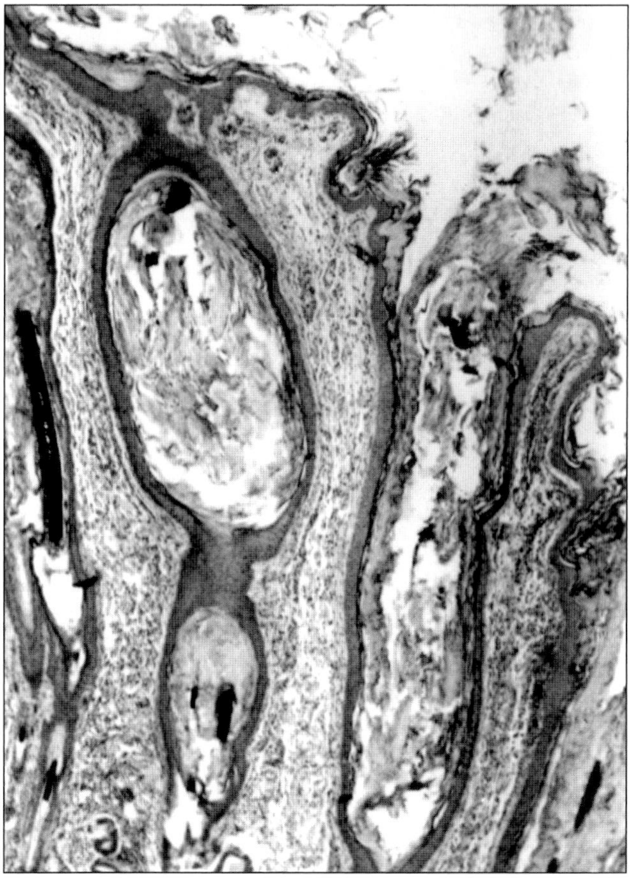

Figure 2. Skin biopsy specimen from a seborrheic cocker spaniel. The epidermis is mildly hyperplastic and hyperkeratotic. There is severe follicular hyperkeratosis and dilatation. (Magnification 10X.)

Answers and Discussion

1. Vitamin A appears essential in the control of epidermal differentiation from basal cells to corneocytes. This is best illustrated by comparing the dermatologic signs of vitamin A deficiency with the signs associated with vitamin A excess. Mucous membrane epithelium is normally composed of nonkeratinizing cells. In vitamin A deficiency, nonkeratinizing mucous membrane cells are replaced by keratinizing cells and cells that normally keratinize in the skin become hyperkeratotic. The opposite response occurs when vitamin A is given in excess; mucous or ciliated squamous cells replace cells that normally keratinize.
2. Serum vitamin A levels have been normal in all of the reported cases of vitamin A-responsive dermatosis. This finding suggests that systemic vitamin A deficiency is an unlikely cause of the dermatosis. These cases also fail to show other clinical signs associated with vitamin A deficiency such as retinal degeneration, hind leg weakness and keratinization of mucous membranes. Improvement is noted within three to four weeks of starting oral vitamin A alcohol (retinol) supplementation, with complete remission by eight to 10 weeks. The specific cause of the dermatosis is unknown but may represent a local or functional deficiency of vitamin A.
3. Vitamin A may be able to correct this dermatosis via anti-keratinization effects. Vitamin A normalizes the proliferation of keratinocytes and decreases the epidermal hyperproliferation. Vitamin A also alters the expression of certain structural genes that are important in epidermal differentiation and cornification. Examples include the suppression of transglutaminase, which is important in cell envelope formation, and the alteration of keratins to K19 and K13, which are normally not found in adult skin but are in fetal skin. Finally, vitamin A induces growth factors and the expression of growth factor receptors that also suppress epidermal differentiation.
4. These dogs usually must be given vitamin A for life. Discontinuing vitamin A supplementation usually results in recrudescence of dermatologic signs. Dogs generally tolerate vitamin A therapy quite well with minor side effects. Vitamin A should be used with caution in breeding animals because it may be teratogenic.

Progress Notes
The dog has done very well as long as vitamin A supplementation has been maintained. Cutaneous lesions reappeared when vitamin A supplementation was discontinued.

Bibliography
Ihrke PJ, Goldschmidt MH. Vitamin A-responsive dermatosis in the dog. Journal of the American Veterinary Medical Association 1983; 182: 687-690.
Kwochka KW. Retinoids and vitamin A therapy. In: Griffin CE, Kwochka KW, MacDonald JM, eds. Current Veterinary Dermatology. St Louis, MO: Mosby-Year Book Inc, 1993; 203-210.
Parker W, Yager-Johnson JA, Hardy MH. Vitamin A-responsive seborrheic dermatosis in the dog: A case report. Journal of the American Animal Hospital Association 1983; 19: 548-554.
Scott DW. Vitamin A-responsive dermatosis in the cocker spaniel. Journal of the American Animal Hospital Association 1986; 22: 125-129.

CASE 32-2

Recurrent Pyoderma in a Chesapeake Bay Retriever
Dawn E. Logas, DVM, Dipl. ACVD
College of Veterinary Medicine
University of Florida
Gainesville, Florida, USA

Patient Assessment
A two-year-old intact male Chesapeake Bay retriever was presented with a 12-month history of recurrent bacterial pyoderma and seborrhea sicca. The dog had previously been treated with two- to three-week courses of various antibiotics at appropriate doses. Response to therapy was partial; papules and pustules would resolve but epidermal flakes and dry brittle hair persisted. All dermatologic signs including papules and pustules would return within weeks after antibiotic therapy was discontinued. Historically, the dog had no other problems.

The dog was slightly underweight (body condition score 2/5), normothermic, alert and well hydrated. Mucous membranes were pink and capillary refill time was 1.5 seconds. Lymph node size, chest auscultation and abdominal palpation were all within normal limits. No abnormalities were noted on ocular or musculoskeletal examination. Both ears had a slight accumulation of yellow waxy exudate but were not inflamed. The coat was thin, dry and lacked sheen. The dermatosis was generalized, sparing only the head and feet. It consisted of large white flakes, papules, pustules, epidermal collarettes and crusts. The dog was only mildly to moderately pruritic; the pruritus historically abated with antibiotic therapy.

Skin scrapings for parasites and fungal culture for dermatophytes were negative. Tape preparation of the skin revealed moderate numbers of cocci bacteria. *Staphylococcus intermedius* was cultured from a pustule. Thyroid profile results were within normal limits.

Assess the Food and Feeding Method
The dog was fed a grocery store brand dry puppy food until 10 months of age at which time the client switched to a generic dry adult dog food. The owner would often purchase whatever generic dog food was on sale.

Therapy Including Feeding Plan
The dog was diagnosed as having a recurrent pyoderma possibly secondary to malnutrition associated with consumption of generic dog food. The pyoderma was treated for six consecutive weeks with an appropriate antibiotic. The food was changed to a grocery brand dry adult dog food supplemented with one tablespoon of corn oil for 12 weeks.

Questions
1. Which major nutrients are essential for normal epidermal function and how might dermatoses due to malnutrition occur in patients eating generic pet foods?
2. How might consumption of generic food have contributed to the dog's recurrent pyoderma?
3. Could nutritional deficiencies account for the dermatologic signs (other than the pyoderma) observed in this dog?

Answers and Discussion

1. Nutrients of special concern for maintaining normal skin and hair include protein, essential fatty acids (EFA), copper, zinc and certain vitamins. A previous report summarized the dermatologic signs that occurred in 13 dogs fed generic pet foods. Generic pet foods are marketed based on low daily cost of feeding. The low cost of the food is usually achieved by using ingredients that often have low total digestibility, low nutrient availability, high mineral content and low quantities of fat and EFA. Foods with high mineral levels (calcium, phosphorus, magnesium), poor digestibility, high levels of phytate and/or low levels of total fat and EFA are a significant risk factor for zinc-responsive cutaneous disease. See the section of this chapter that discusses the dermatologic signs associated with fatty acid and zinc deficiency.
2. Malnutrition resulting from consumption of generic dog food may have contributed to the recurrent pyoderma in this dog. Decreases in zinc and EFA can lead to changes in the microenvironment of the stratum corneum, which allow pathogenic bacteria to colonize the surface of skin. Once colonized, the skin may also be less able to control the infection because decreases in zinc, protein and EFA may diminish normal humoral and cellular immunity. Zinc deficiency impairs macrophage phagocytosis, diminishes chemotaxis and leads to lymphopenia. Decreased levels of EFA, which are normally converted to potent inflammatory mediators called eicosanoids, lead to decreases in chemotaxis, margination and killing ability of leukocytes, particularly neutrophils. Inadequate protein intake, particularly of essential amino acids, can alter the immune response.
3. EFA and zinc deficiency could account for the dry dull coat, fine scale and hyperkeratotic crusts. EFA are necessary for the formation of lamellar granules, which contain much of the epidermal lipids in dogs. These lipids are essential for the formation of the transepidermal water barrier. Without these lipids, the stratum corneum water loss increases and fine scales are formed. EFA are also necessary for the formation of normal sebaceous gland lipids. The sebaceous lipids are important for coating hairs and giving them their sheen.

   Zinc is necessary for normal keratinization. Although the exact mechanisms of zinc's effect on keratinization are unknown, they may be related to the many zinc metalloenzymes, which are found in the epidermis and are essential for epidermal cell differentiation. Therefore, zinc deficiency could lead to the hyperkeratotic crusts noted in this case.

Progress Notes

After six weeks of therapy there was no evidence of bacterial pyoderma or dry flakes. The patient's coat was much softer, shinier and fuller. Eight months after discontinuing antibiotic therapy, the dog's coat and skin remained normal with no recurrence of the pyoderma.

Bibliography

Sousa CA, Stannard AA, Ihrke PJ, et al. Dermatosis associated with feeding generic dog food: 13 cases (1981-1983). Journal of the American Veterinary Medical Association 1988; 192: 676-680.

CASE 32-3

Crusting Dermatitis in a Bull Terrier

Candace A. Sousa, DVM, Dipl. ABVP and ACVD
Pfizer Animal Health
Sacramento, California, USA

Patient Assessment

A four-year-old spayed female bull terrier was examined for severe skin crusting. The crusting had been present since the dog was five months old and had progressively worsened. Previous diagnostic tests included multiple skin scrapings for parasites (negative), a fungal culture (negative) and failure of a clinical response to several empirical therapies (antibiotics, shampoos).

Physical examination demonstrated a mature bitch that was well fleshed but smaller than breed standards (11.7 kg, body condition score 3/5). There were no abnormal physical findings other than those related to the integument. The coat was dull and brittle. Cream-colored patches of thick, tightly-adherent crusts were present above each eye, within the inner pinnae (**Figure 1**) and overlying the elbows and hocks. All of the footpads were thickened and cracked with "feathers" of adherent keratin extruding from the edges (**Figure 2**).

Results of a complete blood count, serum biochemistry profile and urinalysis were normal. Histopathology of skin biopsy specimens revealed marked parakeratotic hyperkeratosis. Neutrophils infiltrated the superficial dermis with some exocytosis, spongiosus and scattered individual dyskeratotic keratinocytes in the epidermis.

Assess the Food and Feeding Method

The dog had been fed a dry commercial food formulated for puppies for the first 10 months of life and several different dry dog foods formulated for adult maintenance for the next three years.

Therapy Including Feeding Plan

Based on the age at onset, breed, diagnostic results and a lack of response to various therapies, a tentative diagnosis of acrodermatitis of bull terriers was made.

Questions

1. What nutritional therapy should be recommended for this dog?
2. What other information should the owner be given regarding this disease and the prognosis for the dog?

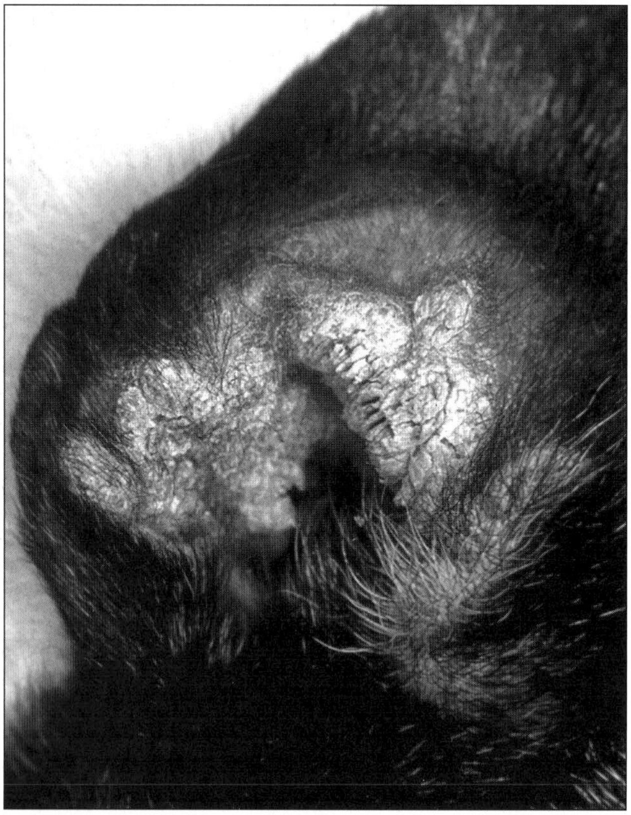

Figure 1. A four-year-old bull terrier with thick crusts in the inner pinna at the ear canal entrance.

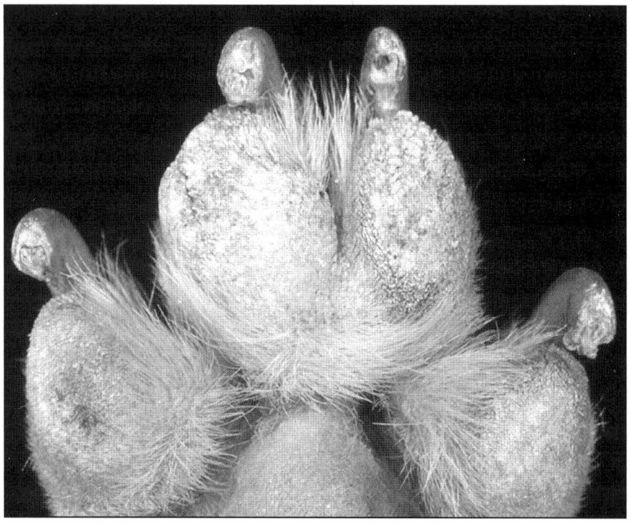

Figure 2. The same dog with hyperkeratosis of the footpads.

Answers and Discussion

1. Acrodermatitis develops in bull terriers shortly after birth and is associated with defects in zinc absorption and metabolism. Cutaneous and systemic clinical signs resemble severe zinc deficiency with growth retardation, gastrointestinal disease, chronic bacterial infections and progressive, erythematous, exfoliative, papular to pustular dermatitis of the distal extremities and skin surrounding the mucocutaneous junctions. Surface crusts usually contain numerous bacteria and yeast organisms.

   Supplementation of the food with oral or intravenous zinc usually fails to ameliorate clinical signs. Treatment with systemic antimicrobials, especially for secondary superficial yeast infections, may result in marked improvement, although systemic and cutaneous infections recur. This dog was treated with a zinc methionine supplement (50 mg once daily) and oral cephalexin (250 mg b.i.d.) for secondary pyoderma.
2. Acrodermatitis is an inherited, autosomal recessive metabolic disease reported to occur in bull terriers in the United States, Canada and the United Kingdom. This bitch had already been spayed but further breeding of this dog's parents should be discouraged. The condition has been termed lethal acrodermatitis because homozygously affected dogs rarely live beyond 18 months of age. Some of the apparently normal littermates may develop zinc-responsive dermatitis. Owners of affected dogs usually complain that their pets have skin disease, stunting, difficulty with eating and large, splayed, painful feet. Ulcerated and thick, crusted lesions are prominent on the muzzle and ears. Abnormal keratinization of the footpads, severe nail dystrophy and paronychia are also common. Prognosis is guarded to poor for severely affected dogs.

Progress Notes

After eight weeks of therapy, the crusting shown in the pictures had decreased about 30%. At that point, the dog was lost to further evaluation.

Bibliography

Jezyk PF, Haskins ME, Mackay-Smith MA, et al. Lethal acrodermatitis in bull terriers. Journal of the American Veterinary Medical Association 1986; 188: 833-839.

McEwan NA. Confirmation and investigation of lethal acrodermatitis of bull terriers in Britain. In: Ihrke PJ, Mason IS, White SD, eds. Advances in Veterinary Dermatology, vol. 2. New York, NY: Pergamon Press, 1993; 151-156.

Mundell AC. Mineral analysis in bull terriers with lethal acrodermatitis (abstract). In: Proceedings. Annual Members Meeting AAVD & ACVD, Washington, DC, 1988: 22.
Smits B, Croft DL, Abrams-Ogg ACG. Lethal acrodermatitis in bull terriers: A problem of defective zinc metabolism. Veterinary Dermatology 1991; 2: 91-95.

CASE 32-4

Crusting Dermatosis in a Siberian Husky Crossbred Dog

Candace A. Sousa, DVM, Dipl. ABVP and ACVD
Pfizer Animal Health
Sacramento, California, USA

Patient Assessment

A four-month-old male Siberian husky crossbred dog weighing 18 kg was presented for evaluation of an eight-week history of variable but persistent crusting. The lesions were first noticed above the eyes and around the mouth, but now extended to the chin and neck. A fungal culture was negative for dermatophytes. Therapy with topical agents, cephalexin and griseofulvin resulted in no clinical improvement. No history was available for either the parents or related dogs.

Physical examination revealed a bright, active and alert puppy with a body condition score of 3/5 (ideal). The only abnormalities noted were limited to the skin. Thick, tightly adherent white crusts were noted above both eyes. The outer ear pinnae were alopecic and crusty. Scattered, white, tightly adherent crusts 1 to 3 cm in diameter were found around the lip margins (**Figure 1**) and ventral neck.

Histopathology of multiple skin biopsy specimens demonstrated severe irregular acanthosis accompanied by prominent parakeratosis and marked serocellular crusting. The parakeratosis extended into the superficial hair follicles. A mixed inflammatory infiltrate, which included lymphocytes, macrophages, neutrophils, plasma cells and scattered eosinophils, was found beneath the acanthotic and multifocally spongiotic epidermis.

Assess the Food and Feeding Method

The owners fed the dog a combination of commercial moist and dry foods formulated for puppies after they obtained it from a private home at nine weeks of age.

Questions

1. Given the signalment and clinical signs, what diseases should be considered?
2. What are the risk factors for development of zinc-responsive cutaneous disease in dogs?
3. What are the best methods to diagnose zinc-related cutaneous disease in animals?
4. Outline an appropriate feeding plan for this puppy.

Answers and Discussion

1. The list of differential diagnoses for this dog should include demodicosis, dermatophytosis, bacterial pyoderma, primary keratinization defect (e.g., ichthyosis), nutritional dermatosis (vitamin A-responsive or zinc-responsive dermatosis) and autoimmune skin disease (e.g., pemphigus foliaceus, pemphigus erythematosus and lupus erythematosus). The histopathologic changes were most compatible with a zinc-responsive dermatosis and secondary pyoderma.
2. Risk factors for zinc-responsive skin disease in dogs include breed, high mineral or phytate levels in the food, low essential fatty acid levels, supplementation with calcium or other minerals and small intestinal disease resulting in malabsorption or maldigestion. Breeds in which zinc-responsive disease has been reported to occur include Siberian huskies, malamutes, bull terriers, Great Danes, Labrador retrievers and other rapidly growing large- and giant-breed dogs.
3. Diagnosis of zinc-responsive cutaneous disease is based on the history, physical examination and skin biopsy results.

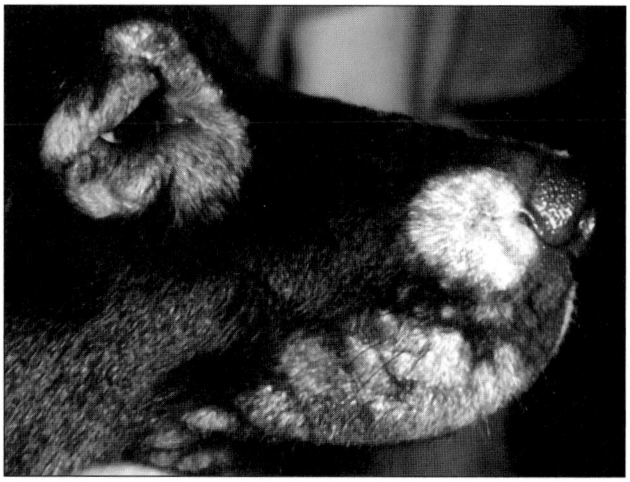

Figure 1. A four-month-old male Siberian husky cross with marked alopecia, lichenification and crusting of the periocular and perioral skin.

Hyperplastic superficial perivascular dermatitis with marked diffuse and follicular parakeratotic hyperkeratosis is suggestive of zinc deficiency. In general, concentrations of zinc in serum, leukocytes and hair are not good indicators of zinc status in dogs.

4. The tentative diagnosis was zinc-responsive dermatosis, which is often seen in Siberian husky dogs. Treatment generally includes changing to a food that avoids excess minerals and contains adequate amounts of zinc and essential fatty acids. Zinc supplementation will be necessary in those breeds in which decreased ability to absorb zinc is suspected. Siberian huskies are one such breed.

Progress Notes

Initial therapy consisted of feeding the moist food supplemented with 50 mg of zinc given orally once daily. Within two months, the lesions disappeared and the dog's coat had returned to normal. When the dog was 10 months old, the owner discontinued the zinc supplement and lesions began to return. Based on this finding, the dog will probably need zinc supplementation for the remainder of its life. Some Siberian huskies do not respond to oral zinc supplementation; however, intravenous injections of zinc sulfate solutions may be effective in these animals.

Bibliography

Brown RG, Hoag GN, Smart ME, et al. Alaskan malamute chondrodysplasia. V. Decreased gut zinc absorption. Growth 1978; 42: 1-6.

Degryse AD, Fransen J, van Cutsem J, et al. Recurrent zinc-responsive dermatosis in a Siberian husky. Journal of Small Animal Practice 1987; 28: 721-726.

Gross TL, Ihrke PJ, Walder EJ. Veterinary Dermatopathology. St Louis, MO: Mosby-Year Book Inc, 1992; 102-108.

Scott DW, Miller WH, Griffin CE. Small Animal Dermatology, 5th ed. Philadelphia, PA: WB Saunders Co, 1995; 897-899.

Willemse T. Zinc-related cutaneous disorders of dogs. In: Kirk RW, Bonagura JD, eds. Current Veterinary Therapy XI. Philadelphia, PA: WB Saunders Co, 1992; 532-534.

CASE 32-5

Pruritus and Seborrhea in a Wire-Haired Fox Terrier

Kevin P. Byrne, DVM, Dipl. ACVD
Bensalem, Pennsylvania, USA

Patient Assessment

A four-and-one-half-year-old, castrated male wirehaired fox terrier was examined for a two-year history of pruritus, oily coat and red skin bumps. Initially, the problems had been seasonal (occurring in the summer), but this year they did not clear up during the winter months. The pruritus had been responsive to oral prednisone. Physical examination revealed diffuse mild seborrhea oleosa with moderate erythema and scaling. These lesions were worse on the dorsum. Hypotrichosis with pustules and crusts were also found on the dorsum and in the axillae. Interdigital erythema was also present. The dog weighed 14 kg and had a body condition score of 4/5.

The initial evaluation of these problems included skin scrapings (negative) and interdigital skin cytology (no abnormal findings). Diagnosis was superficial bacterial pyoderma with seborrheic dermatitis and possible underlying allergic disease. Treatment was initiated with an oral antibiotic (cephalexin, 250 mg, t.i.d.), an antiseborrheic/antibacterial shampoo (twice weekly baths), and a six-week dietary elimination trial using a combination of commercial moist and dry therapeutic foods containing venison and potato.[a]

Six weeks later the dog weighed 13.5 kg and the owner reported a 50% improvement in the pruritus. Examination revealed no visible signs of bacterial pyoderma but erythema persisted in the axillary and interdigital areas.

Assess the Food and Feeding Method

The dog was normally fed a mixture of various dry and moist commercial grocery brand foods supplemented with occasional table foods (rice, potatoes, pasta) and various commercial biscuit snacks. The commercial venison and potato veterinary therapeutic foods were used for six weeks as part of a dietary elimination trial. The owners were instructed not to feed any other commercial foods, table foods or snacks during this trial.

Questions

1. What additional diagnostic tests would be helpful in this patient?
2. What dietary changes may help manage the pruritus and dermatitis in this patient?

Answers and Discussion

1. Underlying allergic disease due to atopy, flea allergy or food allergy could cause the pruritus, dermatitis and seborrhea seen in this patient and predispose the dog to secondary pyoderma. Atopy can be ruled out with intradermal and in vitro allergy testing. There was no evidence of flea infestation. The clinical improvement was probably due to elimination of the superficial bacterial pyoderma.
2. Supplementing the current food with fatty acids or changing to another food with higher fatty acid levels may benefit this patient. Fatty acid therapy alone is rarely successful in controlling moderate to severe pruritus in most patients with skin disease, but may be effective when used concurrently with other therapies. A synergistic effect between fatty acid and antihistamine administration has been documented in some clinical trials involving allergic dogs.

Progress Notes

Intradermal skin testing was positive for a few weed antigens. Blood was drawn for in vitro (ELISA) allergy testing. Positive reactions were found to house dust mites, several trees, several grasses and several weeds, including ragweed. The probable diagnosis was atopy with secondary superficial pyoderma and seborrhea. Treatment was initiated with an antihistamine (hydroxyzine, 25 mg, t.i.d.) and a fatty acid supplement[b] (1 capsule twice daily with food) that delivered 500 mg of eicosapentaenoic acid (EPA) daily in addition to the fatty acids in the food. Bathing with the shampoo was continued.

Eight weeks later the owners reported some improvement in the level of pruritus, but evidence of self-induced alopecia persisted (barbered hairs on the dorsal lumbar region). The skin was also erythematous; salivary staining was evident in these areas. The bathing, fatty acid supplementation and hydroxyzine administration were continued. Hyposensitization injections were started using allergens identified by the ELISA performed two months earlier. The veterinary therapeutic foods were fed until they were gone (about two weeks). At that time, the owner began feeding the dry and moist grocery store brand foods fed previously.

The owner reported significant improvement eight weeks later. There were no areas of visible erythema on the skin, but salivary staining persisted on all four feet. There was mild oiliness and scale accumulation on the dorsum. Bathing, hydroxyzine administration, hyposensitization injections and fatty acid supplementation were continued.

Further Discussion

The optimal dose of omega-3 fatty acids and γ-linolenic acid for control of inflammation and pruritus has not been established. The levels of these fatty acids in the grocery brand foods the patient was eating were unknown. The venison and potato veterinary therapeutic foods provided approximately 50 mg of omega-3 fatty acids per day to the patient. The supplement provided an additional 500 mg of EPA, which markedly increased total omega-3 intake. This dosing level may have been enough additional omega-3 fatty acids (36 to 40 mg EPA/kg body weight) to benefit this patient. The clinical improvement was probably attributable to the combination of all therapies used in this dog.

Endnotes

a. IVD Limited Ingredient Diets. Nature's Recipe Pet Foods, Corona, CA, USA.
b. 3V Caps Skin Formula. DVM Pharmaceuticals, Miami, FL, USA.

Bibliography

Paradis M, Scott DW. Nonsteroidal therapy for canine and feline pruritus. In: Kirk RW, Bonagura JD, eds. Current Veterinary Therapy XI. Philadelphia, PA: WB Saunders Co, 1992; 563-566.

Roudebush P. Consumption of essential fatty acids in selected commercial dog foods compared to dietary supplementation: An update. In: Proceedings. Annual Members Meeting AAVD & ACVD. Norfolk, VA, 2001: 53-54.

Scott DW, Miller WH, Griffin CE. Small Animal Dermatology, 5th ed. Philadelphia, PA: WB Saunders Co, 1995; 211-218.

Section 11

Musculoskeletal Disorders

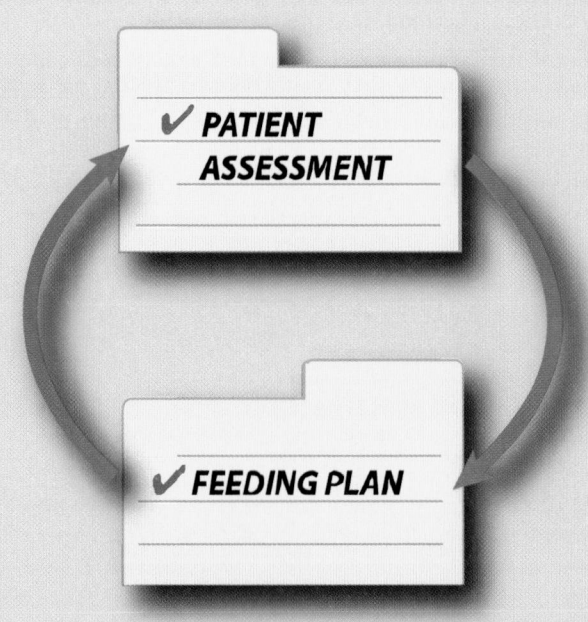

Chapter 33

Developmental Orthopedic Disease of Dogs

Daniel C. Richardson
Jürgen Zentek
Herman A. W. Hazewinkel
Richard C. Nap
Philip W. Toll
Steven C. Zicker

"The beginning is the most important part of the work."
Plato

The Dance of the Solids
The Polymers, those giant Molecules
Like Starch and Polyoxymethylene,
Flesh out, as protein serfs and plastic fools,
This Kingdom with Life's Stuff. Our time has seen
The synthesis of Polyisoprene
And many cross-linked Helixes unknown
To Robert Hooke; but each primordial Bean
Knew Cellulose by heart. Nature alone
Of Collagen and Apatite compounded Bone.
John Updike

CLINICAL IMPORTANCE

The prevalence of musculoskeletal disorders for all dogs at multicenter referral practices has been reported to be approximately one in four, with 70% of these disorders involving the appendicular skeleton (Johnson et al, 1994; LaFond et al, 2002). Furthermore, the prevalence of musculoskeletal problems in dogs less than one year old in all breeds is about 22%, with 20% possibly having a nutrition-related etiology.[a] Developmental orthopedic disease (DOD) includes a diverse group of musculoskeletal disorders that occur in growing animals (most commonly fast-growing, large- and giant-breed dogs whose adult weight will exceed 25 kg) and that are sometimes related to nutrition. Canine hip dysplasia and osteochondrosis make up the overwhelming majority of the musculoskeletal problems with a possible nutrition-related etiology.[a]

Canine Hip Dysplasia

Canine hip dysplasia is the most frequently encountered orthopedic disease in veterinary medicine with heritability and a potential nutrition-related etiology (Johnson et al, 1994). Canine hip dysplasia is an abnormal development, or growth, of the hip joint (**Figure 33-1**) manifested by varying degrees of laxity of surrounding soft tissues, instability of the joint and malformation of the femoral head and acetabulum with osteoarthrosis (Brinker et al, 1990). The number of cases of canine hip dysplasia is estimated to be in the millions worldwide (Corley and Hogan, 1985).

Osteochondrosis

Osteochondrosis is widespread among people and young, rapidly growing, domesticated species. Generally, osteochondrosis is a disruption in endochondral ossification that results in a focal lesion (Brinker et al, 1990a). Osteochondrosis occurs in the physis and/or epiphysis of growth cartilage, and may be considered a generalized or systemic disease. Clinical signs of osteochondrosis are related to the severity and location of disease.

When osteochondrosis affects physeal cartilage, it may cause growth abnormalities in long bones such as angular limb deformities. Osteochondrosis of articular epiphyseal cartilage

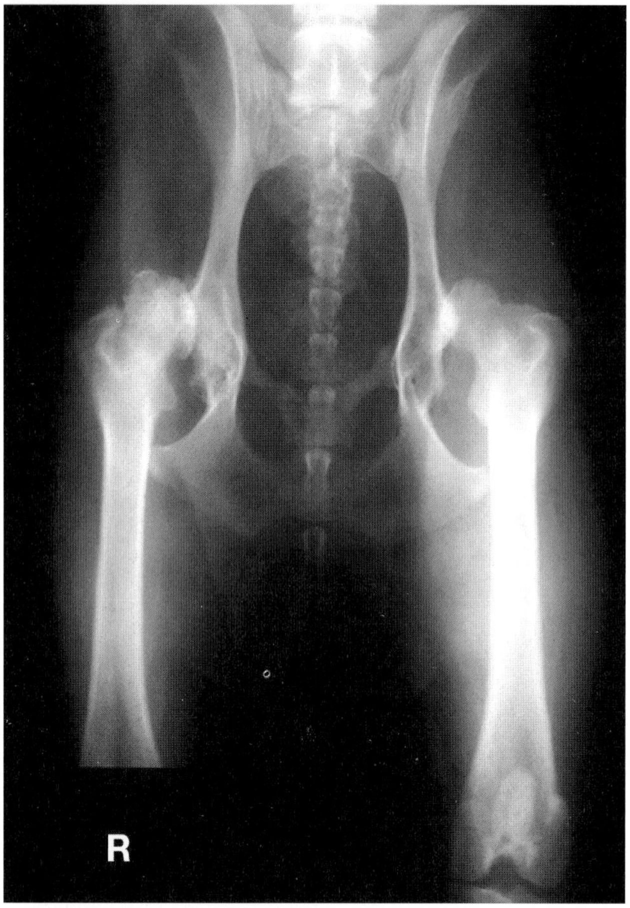

Figure 33-1. Progression of joint disease in a dog with rear-limb lameness due to severe bilateral hip dysplasia. This ventrodorsal radiograph shows degenerative joint disease in both coxofemoral joints. The right hip has advanced osteophyte formation on the femoral neck. The right acetabular cup and femoral head have remodeled to form a pseudoarthrosis. The left femoral neck also has osteophyte formation and the hip is luxated craniodorsally.

commonly occurs in the shoulder (proximal humerus, **Figure 33-2**), stifle (distal femur), hock (talus) and elbow (distal humerus). Acute inflammatory joint disease (or degenerative joint disease) may ensue subsequent to development of osteochondrosis when the cartilage surface is disrupted and subchondral bone is exposed to synovial fluid. Inflammatory mediators and cartilage fragments are released into the joint (osteochondritis dissecans), which perpetuates the cycle of degenerative joint disease (Hill et al, 1984) (Chapter 34). Other disease processes such as spondylolisthesis, intra-articular fracture, complete or partial epiphysiolysis and deformed joint surfaces have been associated with osteochondrosis but their etiology is still undetermined.

Elbow Dysplasia

Elbow dysplasia describes the four main developmental dysplastic conditions that are frequently diagnosed in the elbow joint: 1) osteochondrosis of the medial condyle, 2) fragmented medial coronoid process, 3) ununited anconeal process and 4) elbow incongruency, due to a relatively short ulna. These conditions result in severe lameness although the clinical manifestation varies with the breed, the underlying diagnosis, the typical exercise pattern and the amount of osteoarthritis.

Breed specific distribution of the elbow dysplasia types has been recognized and elbow dysplasia has a complex hereditary background. Each of the conditions included may occur independently in the canine population, although they can occur in the same elbow in different combinations.

The frequency and severity of elbow dysplasia are also subject to environmental factors such as nutrition, body weight and exercise. The etiology is similar to what has been described for osteochondrosis-related conditions. It seems that fragmented medial coronoid process is not influenced by nutrition as much as the other three conditions.

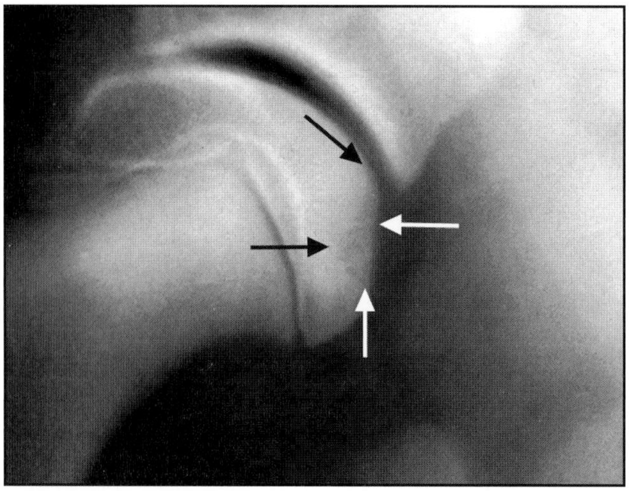

Figure 33-2A. Radiograph of the proximal humerus of a nine-month-old male Labrador retriever examined for forelimb lameness. The radiolucent area (arrows) indicates disrupted endochondral ossification and subchondral bone necrosis associated with osteochondrosis.

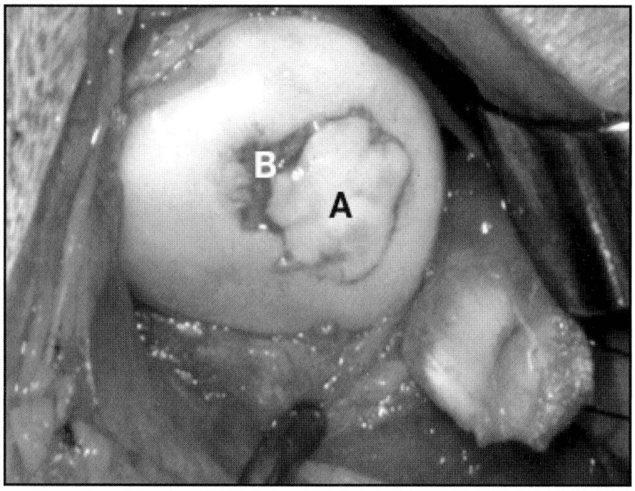

Figure 33-2B. Intraoperative view of an osteochondritis dissecans lesion in the articular epiphyseal cartilage of the proximal cartilage of the same dog. Note the cartilage flap (A) and exposed subchondral bone (B) where a portion of the cartilage flap is missing.

Growth Velocity
Puppy growth can be measured in height/length and body weight. Typically, when discussing growth in people, we assume an increase in height. Rapid growth in children means they reach an above average height at a certain age. Growth curves have been established per population and gender. However, in dogs, growth is usually measured in terms of body weight. When considering rapid growth, the risk is that real growth (increased height/length) becomes confused with the development of relative overweight during growth, resulting from excess food intake. This can become an issue when discussing risk factors for developmental disease conditions of the skeleton. The statement in the literature that overnutrition results in rapid growth is typically supported by body weight data and not by height/length measures. Because osteochondrosis conditions may be related to disturbed height/length growth and not just excessive weight, this discrepancy between human and canine growth references needs to be taken into account when interpreting growth. Some breed standards for popular dogs (including Labrador retrievers) tend to reflect overweight. This has to be taken into account when calculating energy requirements during growth relative to adult body weight.

Box 33-1. Use of DEXA to Assess the Skeleton.

The ability to make repeated, accurate assessments of body composition is crucial to the investigation of many key nutritional issues of cats and dogs. In a research setting, dual energy x-ray absorptiometry (DEXA) allows the body to be viewed as three compartments: bone mineral, fat tissue and lean tissue. The ability to evaluate changes in these three compartments independently greatly benefits the study of growth, obesity and geriatrics.

DEXA uses x-rays of two different energy levels (70 and 140 kVp) to distinguish the nature and amount of each tissue in the part of the body being scanned. The x-ray source below the table and the detector above the table move in concert to measure the amount of radiation passing through the subject. Because x-rays of different energy levels are impeded differently by bone mineral, fat and lean tissue, it is possible to calculate the quantity of each tissue in each area scanned.

The accuracy of DEXA in companion animals is supported by the good correlation between values obtained from DEXA and chemical analysis.

The Bibliography for **Box 33-1** can be found at www.markmorris.org.

PATIENT ASSESSMENT

History and Physical Examination
Breed and familial history are important predisposing factors for DOD. For mixed-breed dogs, it is useful to know the breed of the stud and bitch as well as historical wellness of offspring. If possible, it may be helpful to gather information pertaining to skeletal abnormalities of previous litters from the same bitch and stud. If it is anticipated that the puppy will have an adult weight of more than 25 kg, it should probably be considered at risk.

Food intake and history should be evaluated as described in Chapter 1. Any treats and supplements fed to the patient should be scrutinized closely, paying special attention to the calcium and energy intake. It is critical to calculate, or closely estimate, metabolizable energy (ME) and calcium and phosphorus intake to provide good advice for feeding growing large- and giant-breed dogs.

Puppies should be weighed during the initial visit and all subsequent visits to help monitor their growth rate. A body condition score (BCS) should be determined and recorded at each visit (Chapter 1). Attention to abnormal changes in weight or BCS will help in assessing and managing growing dogs. In some cases, graphs of body weight and BCS may prove useful in recognizing variances from desired goals. BCS does not always reliably indicate overfeeding, because many young dogs react to higher energy intake with an accelerated growth rate.

Before a physical examination is conducted, historical information should be gathered about the degree, if any, of perceived lameness, the affected limb(s), duration of lameness and any peculiarities regarding the lameness. Following historical evaluation, the patient should be observed at rest for any gross conformational abnormalities. Next, the patient should be observed in motion to ascertain the degree of lameness and location of involvement (Brinker et al, 1990b).

If a locomotor defect is confirmed, the etiology should be determined. To determine the cause, the examination should include: 1) palpation of limbs for asymmetry, swelling, heat and sensitivity, 2) deep palpation of long bones, 3) flexion/extension of joints to determine range of motion, crepitation, instability and sensitivity and 4) neurologic evaluation. Even after a thorough physical examination, the exact cause of the lameness may remain undetermined.

Radiography
Radiographs should be taken to further define the clinical diagnosis. Radiographic identification of lesions aids in confirming the disease. However, inability to identify lesions by survey radiography does not always negate the presence of disease (Henry, 1992) (**Box 33-1**).

Laboratory Information
Diagnostic tests to detect other diseases that may result in skeletal abnormalities should be considered when appropriate. Confounding diseases such as osteomyelitis, septic emboli and mycotic infection should be considered. DOD is usually typified by a lack of abnormal laboratory findings (Hazewinkel, 1994; Nap and Hazewinkel, 1994).

Uncomplicated cases of DOD rarely have altered complete blood counts. Severe elevations or decreases in white blood cell counts usually indicate other disease processes. If anemia is present, classifying the type may give insight to other causes for select skeletal disorders (e.g., copper deficiency) (Zentek et al,

Table 33-1. Parathyroid hormone (PTH), ionized calcium and 1,25-dihydroxyvitamin D_3 concentrations in different physiologic/disease states.*

States	PTH	Ionized calcium	1,25-dihydroxyvitamin D_3
Apocrine gland tumors of the anal sacs	Low	High	Low
Chronic renal failure	High	Low/normal	Normal/low
High calcium intake	Low	High	Normal/low
Hypervitaminosis D	Low	High	Normal/high
Hypoparathyroidism	Low	Low	Low
Lymphosarcoma	Low	High	Low
Primary hyperparathyroidism	High	High	Normal/high

*Adapted from Feldman EC, Nelson RW, eds. Canine and Feline Endocrinology and Reproduction, 2nd ed. Philadelphia, PA: WB Saunders Co, 1996; 455-493. Hazewinkel HAW. In: Bojrab MJ, ed. Disease Mechanisms in Small Animal Surgery, 2nd ed. Philadelphia, PA: Lea & Febiger, 1993; 1119-1128. Chastain CB, Ganjam VK, eds. Clinical Endocrinology of Companion Animals. Philadelphia, PA: Lea & Febiger, 1986; 192-217.

1991; NRC, 2006).

Occasionally, serum concentrations of calcium and phosphorus may be elevated or decreased during the genesis of DOD. However, absence of calcium or phosphorus perturbations does not rule out a diagnosis of DOD. Conversely, many other disease processes may result in altered calcium or phosphorus homeostasis, which indicates abnormal values are not pathognomonic for a diagnosis of DOD (Nap and Hazewinkel, 1994).

Increased bone remodeling may result in increased serum alkaline phosphatase activity. This parameter is already high in young, growing animals and may not be a very sensitive indicator of ongoing metabolic bone disease. Other enzyme activities in serum are not very useful for diagnosis of DOD. Biochemical markers of human bone metabolism such as type I collagen propeptides, tartrate-resistant acid phosphatase and osteocalcin are useful in research studies; however, the significance for veterinary diagnostics remains to be proven (Robey and Termine, 1990).

Serum and urinary assays of bone markers are of interest as noninvasive alternatives to bone biopsy. Assays that were developed for people have been shown to cross-react in dogs. Serum bone-specific alkaline phosphatase, urinary deoxypyridinoline and N-terminal telopeptide of collagen were measured in dogs with commercial enzyme immunoassays designed for people. Serum osteocalcin and carboxy-terminal cross-linked telopeptide of type I collagen were measured with commercial radioimmunoassays. Significant diurnal rhythms were identified for osteocalcin, bone-specific alkaline phosphatase, carboxy-terminal cross-linked telopeptide of type I collagen and urinary deoxypyridinoline. No clear rhythm was evident for N-terminal telopeptide of collagen. Due to the variability in marker excretion in individual animals, the most appropriate use for these assays is as a screening tool for cohort studies, rather than as a diagnostic or prognostic tool in individual animals (Ladlow et al, 2002). Breed effects cannot be excluded; however, for serum alkaline phosphatase and carboxyl-terminal cross-linked telopeptide of type I collagen, the concentrations were comparable in giant and toy breeds and in beagles (Breur et al, 2004).

Urinalysis results are usually within normal limits for animals with DOD. Advanced techniques, including measurement of calcium and phosphorus partial clearance ratios, may add insight about calcium and phosphorus nutrition, but repeated measurements may be needed for accurate interpretation. Evaluation of other mineral partial clearances may give some insight into dietary excesses or deficiencies. Analysis of urine for markers of bone turnover such as hydroxylysine glycosides, free pyridinolines or pyridinoline cross-links of collagen may prove useful in the future (Eyre, 1996).

Measuring and Interpreting Specific Laboratory Tests

PARATHYROID HORMONE

Interpretation of serum parathyroid hormone (PTH) concentrations from other species has proven that evaluation must be made in conjunction with presenting signs and other biochemical tests such as concentrations of ionized calcium and 1,25-dihydroxyvitamin D_3 (**Table 33-1**). PTH values may be increased, decreased or normal in DOD depending on the etiology. Increased PTH concentrations may be observed in association with renal disease, vitamin D deficiency and states in which insufficient calcium is present in foods. Decreased PTH concentrations may be observed when excess calcium or vitamin D is present in foods, and in other metabolic diseases.

PTH concentration is most accurately measured by a "two-site" immunoassay. This assay eliminates interference by mid-region or terminal fragments that are abundant in animal serum. Single time-point evaluations of PTH may not prove useful in determining the etiology of DOD. Repeated evaluations may yield more useable information, but are probably not cost effective.

CALCITONIN

Calcitonin, a peptide hormone, is released primarily from C-cells of the thyroid gland in response to sudden increased concentrations of ionized calcium in serum. Calcitonin may also be released in response to other stimuli such as gastrin secretion stimulated by food intake (Azria, 1989). Calcitonin is measured by radioimmunoassay (Hazewinkel et al, 1985, 1999). The test is not commercially available and rational interpretation requires multiple sample evaluations. If calcitonin levels are evaluated to investigate the etiology of DOD, results should be compared to normal values for the laboratory and interpreted in conjunction with results of other tests (e.g., PTH, ionized calcium and vitamin D_3 analyses).

VITAMIN D

Vitamin D_3 may be required in foods for dogs because endogenous synthesis may be limited (Hazewinkel et al, 1987; How et al, 1994). Because commercial foods contain added vitamin D_3, and in light of potentially limited endogenous synthesis, measurement of vitamin D_3 in serum may reflect dietary changes rather than specific disease states. 25-hydroxyvitamin D_3 is produced in the liver from vitamin D_3 and is a good indicator of general vitamin D_3 deficiency (Hazewinkel and Tryfonidou, 2002) or excess (Tryfonidou et al, 2003a). Another useful indicator of vitamin D_3 status is measurement of the most biologically active metabolite of vitamin D_3, 1,25-dihydroxyvitamin D_3, which is produced in the kidneys via the 1-α-hydroxylase enzyme. The concentration of 1,25-dihydroxyvitamin D_3 in serum is not a good indicator of vitamin D_3 toxicity (Tryfonidou et al, 2003a); however, it is a more sensitive indicator of deficiency than serum concentrations of 25-hydroxyvitamin D_3.

All metabolites of vitamin D_3 in serum may be measured by high-pressure liquid chromatography. Concentrations should be compared with reference values from laboratories performing the analysis, preferably derived from healthy dogs fed similar foods (Tenenhouse, 1990). A multitude of factors affect production of 1,25-dihydroxyvitamin D_3 including breed differences (Hazewinkel and Tryfonidou, 2002; Tryfonidou et al, 2003a) and laboratory results should be interpreted in conjunction with other physical and biochemical findings (**Table 33-2**). Generally, high concentrations of 1,25-dihydroxyvitamin D_3 indicate low availability of calcium to animals, normal concentrations indicate adequate calcium availability and low concentrations may indicate vitamin D_3 deficiency.

The amount of growth hormone and IGF-1 (insulin-like growth factor-1) may also directly influence vitamin D metabolism. In puppies, these hormones are inherently associated with growth rate and breed, with large-breed puppies having higher levels of these hormones than small breeds. Therefore, both dietary content and breed may influence metabolism of vitamin D and resultant bone development (Tryfonidou et al, 2003b).

Table 33-2. Factors affecting activity of 25-hydroxyvitamin D_3 renal 1-α-hydroxylase.*

Factors	Changes
Acidosis	Decrease
Alkalosis	Increase
Decreased ionized calcium	Increase
Decreased parathyroid hormone	Decrease
Increased 1,25-dihydroxyvitamin D_3	Decrease
Increased calcitonin	Increase/decrease/ no effect
Increased growth hormone	Increased vitamin D intake
Increased ionized calcium	Decrease
Increased parathyroid hormone	Increase
Increased phosphate (serum)	Decrease
Increasing age	Decrease
Insulin	Increase
Insulin-like growth factor-1	Increase
Pregnancy	Increase
Prolactin	Increase/no effect
Sex steroids	Increase

*Adapted from Tenenhouse HS. In: Simmons DJ, ed. Nutrition and Bone Development. New York, NY: Oxford University Press, 1990; 164-201. Hazewinkel HAW, Tryfonidou MA. Vitamin D3 metabolism in dogs. Molecular and Cellular Endocrinology 002; 197: 23-33.

Table 33-3. Composition of bone.

Bone is composed of a mineral phase, a non-mineral (organic) phase and a cellular phase

Mineral phase
99% of body calcium
85% of body phosphorus
40-60% of body sodium and magnesium
Ca-P ratio 1.67:1 on a molar basis. Ratio is 2.15:1 on a weight basis (hydroxyapatite crystals = $[Ca_{10}(PO_4)_6(OH)_2]$)

Organic phase
Type I collagen (90% of bone protein)
Noncollagenous protein (cell attachment proteins, proteoglycans, gamma carboxylated gla proteins, growth-related proteins)

Cellular phase
Osteoclasts
Osteoblasts
Osteocytes

CALCIUM

Bone contains 99% of the calcium in the body with the majority in the form of hydroxyapatite crystals (**Table 33-3** and **Box 33-2**). Bone functions physiologically as a structural material and an ion reservoir. When bone acts as an ion reservoir, it is in equilibrium with ionized calcium in serum and under tight homeostatic control.

Calcium homeostasis is maintained by the sum of physiochemical and calciotropic hormonal processes. Calcium in blood is in equilibrium between the ionized state (45 to 50%), a protein-bound state (40 to 45%) and a complexed or chelated state (5 to 10%). Generally, the concentration of ionized calcium is approximately 45 to 50% of the total concentration of calcium in serum over a wide range of total calcium concentrations. The concentration of ionized calcium is the most important determinant of calciotropic homeostatic regulation initiated by the parathyroid gland and the C-cells of the thyroid gland. Sudden increases in ionized calcium concentrations stimulate release of calcitonin from the thyroid gland, whereas decreases in concentrations of ionized calcium stimulate release of PTH from the parathyroid gland. The total concentration of calcium in serum is affected by the interplay of the homeostatic mechanisms involving influx (gastrointestinal [GI] absorption and bone resorption), efflux (GI and renal loss) and skeletal mineralization of the less labile bone pool as outlined below.

When concentrations of ionized calcium are below the normal range:

1. PTH secretion is stimulated, which in turn stimulates conversion of 25-hydroxyvitamin D_3 to the biologically more potent 1,25-dihydroxyvitamin D_3 in the kidneys.

Table 33-4. Summary of reports delineating risk factors for developmental orthopedic disease in dogs.

Diseases	Key points	Interpretation	Risk factors	References*
Hip dysplasia	Rapid weight gain German shepherd dogs First 60 days of age	Rapid weight gain increased risk of hip dysplasia. Dysplastic parents increased risk	Breed Rapid weight gain	Riser et al, 1964
Hip dysplasia	Pups born by cesarean section-hand reared Vaginally born pups, pair-fed bitch milk at 70% free choice	Free-choice feeding resulted in increased weight gain and increased occurrence of hip dysplasia	Free-choice feeding Rapid weight gain	Lust et al, 1973
Hip dysplasia	Labrador retrievers Rapid growth rate	Early fusion of triradiate growth plate in acetabulum	Breed Rapid weight gain	Lust et al, 1985
Hip dysplasia	Weight gain >breed standards	Increased occurrence of hip dysplasia	Rapid weight gain	Kässtrom, 1975
Hip dysplasia	Restricted feeding Labrador retrievers	Restricted feeding decreased occurrence of hip dysplasia	Breed Rapid weight gain	Kealy et al, 1992
Osteochondrosis	Epidemiologic study	Labrador retrievers, Great Danes, Newfoundlands, rottweilers at greatest risk All large breeds at increased risk	Breed Gender Anatomic location	Slater et al, 1991; Slater et al, 1992
Osteochondrosis	Epidemiologic study	Males at higher risk of OCD in shoulder	Gender Calcium content Well water	Dobenencker et al, 1997; Slater et al, 1991; Slater et al, 1992
Osteochondrosis	Great Danes Rapid growth Overnutrition	Rapid growth increased occurrence of developmental orthopedic disease	Breed Rapid growth	Daemmrich, 1991; Hedhammar et al, 1974; Meyer and Zentek, 1992
Osteochondrosis	Great Danes Excess calcium	Excessive calcium intake increased occurrence of developmental orthopedic disease	Breed Excessive calcium	Hazewinkel et al, 1985
Osteochondrosis	Great Danes Excess calcium and phosphorus intake	Excessive mineral intake at young age leads to hypercalcitoninism	Breed Excess minerals	Schoenmakers et al, 2000
Osteochondrosis	Great Danes Excess vitamin D intake	Imbalance of vitamin D metabolites at chondrocytes	Breed Excess vitamin D	Tryfonidou et al, 2003
Developmental orthopedic disease	Large breeds Rapid growth	Excessive energy intake increased occurrence of developmental orthopedic disease	Breed Rapid growth High energy density food	Richardson and Toll, 1997

*Adapted from Hedhammar A, Wu F, Krook L, et al. Overnutrition and skeletal disease. An experimental study in growing Great Dane dogs. Cornell Veterinarian 1974; 64 (Suppl. 5): 1-160. Meyer H, Zentek J. Über den Einfluß einer unterschiedlichen Energieversorgung wachsender Doggen auf Körpermasse und Skelettentwicklung. Journal of Veterinary Medicine A 1992; 39: 130-141. Lust G, Geary JC, Sheffy BE. Development of hip dysplasia in dogs. American Journal of Veterinary Research 1973; 34: 87-91. Lust G, Rendano VT, Summers BA. Canine hip dysplasia: Concepts and diagnosis. Journal of the American Veterinary Medical Association 1985; 187: 638-640. Kasström J. Nutrition, weight gain and development of hip dysplasia. Acta Radiologica Suppl. (Stockholm) 1975; 344: 135-179. Kealy RD, Olsson SE, Monti KL, et al. Effects of limited food consumption on the incidence of hip dysplasia in growing dogs. Journal of the American Veterinary Medical Association 1992; 210: 857-863. Daemmrich K. Relationship between nutrition and bone growth in large and giant dogs. Journal of Nutrition 1991; 121: S114-S121. Dobenencker B, Kienzle E, Matis U. Mal- and overnutrition in puppies with and without clinical disorders of skeletal development (abstract). In: Proceedings. European Society of Veterinary and Comparative Nutrition, Munich, Germany, 1997: 25. Riser WH, Cohen D, Linquist S, et al. Influence of early rapid growth and weight gain on hip dysplasia in the German Shepherd dog. Journal of the American Veterinary Medical Association 1964; 145: 661-668. Richardson DC, Toll PW. Relationship of nutrition to developmental skeletal disease in young dogs. Veterinary Clinical Nutrition 1997; 4: 6-13. Hazewinkel HAW, Goedgebuure SA, Poulos PW, et al. Influences of chronic calcium excess on the skeletal development of growing Great Danes. Journal of the American Animal Hospital Association 1985; 21: 377-391. Schoenmakers I, Hazewinkel HAWH, Voorhout G, et al. Effects of diets with different calcium and phosphorus contents on skeletal development and blood chemistry of growing Great Danes. Veterinary Record 2000; 147: 652-660. Slater MR, Scarlett JM, Donoghue S, et al. Diet and exercise as potential risk factors for osteochondritis dissecans in dogs. American Journal of Veterinary Research 1992; 53: 2119-2124. Slater MR, Scarlett JM, Kaderly RE, et al. Breed, gender, and age risk factors for canine osteochondritis dissecans. Journal of Veterinary Comparative Orthopedics and Traumatology 1991; 4: 100-106. Tryfonidou MA, Stevenhagen JJ, Buurman CJ, et al. Dietary 135-fold cholecalciferol supplementation severely disturbs the endochondral ossification in growing dogs. Domestic Animal Endocrinology 2003; 24(4): 265-285.

2. 1,25-dihydroxyvitamin D_3 stimulates calcium uptake in the gut via receptor-mediated mechanisms.
3. 1,25-dihydroxyvitamin D_3, in conjunction with PTH, stimulates bone resorption and calcium reabsorption in the kidneys.
4. PTH induces phosphaturia.

When concentrations of ionized calcium are above the normal range:

1. Calcitonin secretion is stimulated, PTH secretion is suppressed and 1,25-dihydroxyvitamin D_3 production is not stimulated. Instead, the kidneys produce 24,25-dihydroxyvitamin D_3, which is generally considered biologically inactive.
2. Gut absorption and bone resorption of calcium are not stimulated.
3. Calcitonin decreases osteoclastic activity.
4. Renal calcium excretion is increased.

The equilibrium between the protein-bound and ionized fraction of calcium is affected by a variety of physiologic conditions. Alterations of serum proteins usually do not affect the equilibrium of bound to ionized calcium, but the total calcium may be increased or decreased. Alterations in albumin or total serum protein concentrations should be corrected before calcium values are evaluated (Feldman and Nelson, 1996).

Albumin correction:

Corrected total calcium (mg/dl) = Total calcium (mg/dl) – albumin (g/dl) + 3.5

Total serum protein correction:

Corrected total calcium (mg/dl) – (0.4 x total protein [g/dl]) + 3.3

The percent of total calcium bound to protein may be roughly estimated using differential binding affinities of albumin and globulin (Arnaud and Kolb, 1991).

% protein-bound calcium = 8 x albumin (g/dl) + 2 x globulin (g/dl) + 3

Acidosis shifts the equilibrium toward ionized calcium and is not accounted for by the above equation. Other physiologic perturbations, such as alkalosis, chloride ion concentration and phosphate ion concentration may also affect the equilibrium and are not accounted for by the above equation. Accurate determination of ionized calcium is best performed using ion selective electrodes.

Risk Factors

The genesis of DOD is presumed to be a multifactorial process. The most critical period for development of DOD is during the growth phase, before physeal closure (**Figure 33-3**). Specific factors that are currently thought to increase the risk of DOD in young dogs include: 1) belonging to a large or giant breed (genetics) (>25 kg adult weight), 2) free-choice feeding (management), particularly of high-energy foods (nutrition) and 3) excessive intake of calcium and vitamin D from food, treats and supplements (nutrition) (**Table 33-4**) (Hazewinkel et al, 1985; Daemmrich, 1991; Dobenencker et al, 1997; Hedhammar et al, 1974; Kasström, 1975; Kealy et al, 1992; Lust et al, 1973, 1985; Meyer and Zentek, 1992; Riser et al, 1964; Slater et al, 1991, 1992; Richardson and Toll, 1997; Tryfonidou et al, 2003a).

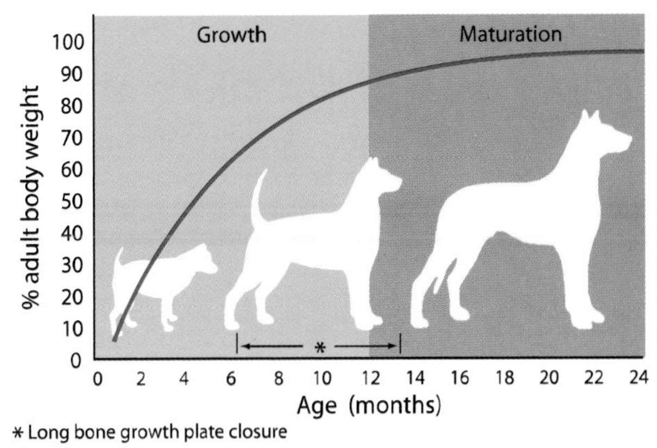

Figure 33-3. Growth phase vs. long bone physeal closure in dogs. Note that weight gain still occurs under the maturation phase although growth plate closure is complete. This is attributable to bone remodeling and especially to the acquisition of adult body mass, with the possible consequence of overweight/obesity.

Box 33-2. Calcium Deposition in Bone.

The actual physical mechanism of calcium deposition in bone is controversial. Evidence suggests the following:

- Calcium and phosphorus exist in metastable equilibrium in solution.
- A nucleation molecule initiates precipitation of solid calcium in collagen.
- Calcium is deposited initially as poorly crystalline type B (carbonate) apatite.
- Initial crystals have brushite properties but as they mature they become more hydroxyapatite in nature.
- Initial nucleation sites are within collagen fibrils.
- Nucleation sites are independent of each other (multicentric).
- Nucleation initiating molecules may include phosphoproteins, proteolipids and complex acidic phospholipids.
- Proteoglycans may inhibit or promote calcification centers.

The Bibliography for **Box 33-2** can be found at www.markmorris.org.

Etiopathogenesis

A variety of mechanisms are plausible in considering the pathogenesis of DOD. No one specific etiology is considered ultimately responsible for all observed clinical manifestations of DOD. Historically, feeding dogs imbalanced foods, especially those deficient in calcium, phosphorus or vitamin D_3, was the main risk factor predisposing them to skeletal diseases such as secondary hyperparathyroidism with subsequent development of osteodystrophia fibrosa (Daemmrich, 1991). Dietary deficiencies are rare in young, growing dogs fed commercial growth foods because most foods are formulated to meet or exceed allowances for specific nutrients (Kallfelz and

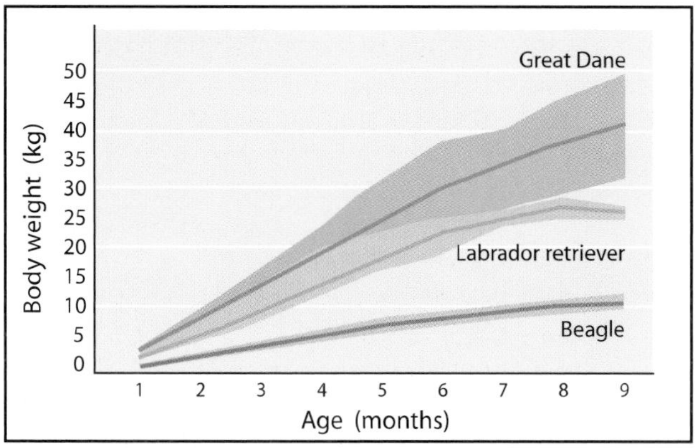

Figure 33-4. Growth curves (weight vs. age) for Great Dane, Labrador retriever and beagle dogs. Note that rapid growth occurs during the first few months in all breeds, but is prolonged in giant-breed dogs such as Great Danes.

Dzanis, 1989). Two popular theories for the pathogenesis of some types of DOD are discussed in the following sections. Specific nutrients are addressed in the Key Nutritional Factors section.

Theory 1: Energy/Growth/Biomechanical Stress

The musculoskeletal system changes constantly throughout life with the most rapid changes occurring during the first few months (**Figure 33-4**) (Hedhammar et al, 1974; Lust et al, 1973; Alexander et al, 1988; Allard et al, 1988; Booles et al, 1991; Booles et al, 1994; Meyer and Zentek, 1989; Romsos et al, 1976; Sheng and Huggins, 1971; Chakraborty et al, 1983; Lavelle, 1989; Rainbird and Kienzle, 1990). The skeletal system apparently is most susceptible to physical, nutritional and metabolic insults during the first 12 months of life because of heightened metabolic activity. Large- and giant-breed dogs are most susceptible to DOD, presumably because of their genetic propensity for rapid growth (Daemmrich, 1991; Meyer and Zentek, 1991).

Present knowledge about energy intake effects on bone growth gives rise to an hypothesis for the etiopathogenesis of growth disorders associated with overfeeding of energy to young, large- and giant-breed dogs. High energy intake directly affects growth velocity via nutrient supply and indirectly through changes in concentrations of growth hormone, IGF-1, triiodothyronine (T_3), thyroxine (T_4) and insulin (Blum et al, 1992; Danforth and Burger, 1989; Eigenmann et al, 1985; Nap, 1993). Dysregulation of these endocrine factors, whether attributable to nutrition, feeding management or genetics, during this critical period of skeletal growth may be responsible for producing an environment in which DOD develops.

Growth hormone and IGF-1 stimulate chondrocyte proliferation and differentiation (Daughaday et al, 1972; Froesch et al, 1985; Glade, 1984; Harris and Heaney, 1969; Hochberg et al, 1989; Isaksson et al, 1987; Eigenmann, 1986). Growth hormone release in non-canids is influenced primarily by energy intake but may also be affected by food protein content, specific amino acids or peptides, exercise and environmental factors (Nap and Hazewinkel, 1994; Blum et al, 1992; Glade, 1984; Eigenmann, 1986). IGF-1 is released systemically primarily from the liver but also locally from chondrocytes in response to growth hormone stimulus. Little is known about dietary influences on growth hormone secretion in dogs; however, young Labrador retrievers had a temporal decrease in concentrations of growth hormone from weaning to 14 weeks of age, followed by an increase in the prepubertal period (Chakraborty et al, 1983). IGF-1 was found in significantly higher concentrations in growing dogs fed free choice compared with animals on restricted feed allowance (Blum et al, 1992), whereas dietary protein intake only weakly influenced IGF-1 levels (Nap et al, 1993).

Free-choice feeding of dogs that results in excess energy intake is also accompanied by higher circulating concentrations of T_3 and T_4 compared with levels in food-restricted controls, reflecting a general stimulation of metabolic processes (Blum et al, 1992). Thyroid hormones are not only general stimuli for metabolic processes, including increasing the rate of bone formation and resorption, but are also important for capillary penetration of degenerating cartilage cells and the final stage of endochondral bone formation (Glade, 1984). In conjunction with the food-hormone relationships summarized here, additional endocrine or autocrine factors are involved in cartilage and bone metabolism (Glade, 1984); unfortunately, relevant data for growing dogs are unavailable. The result of these hormon-

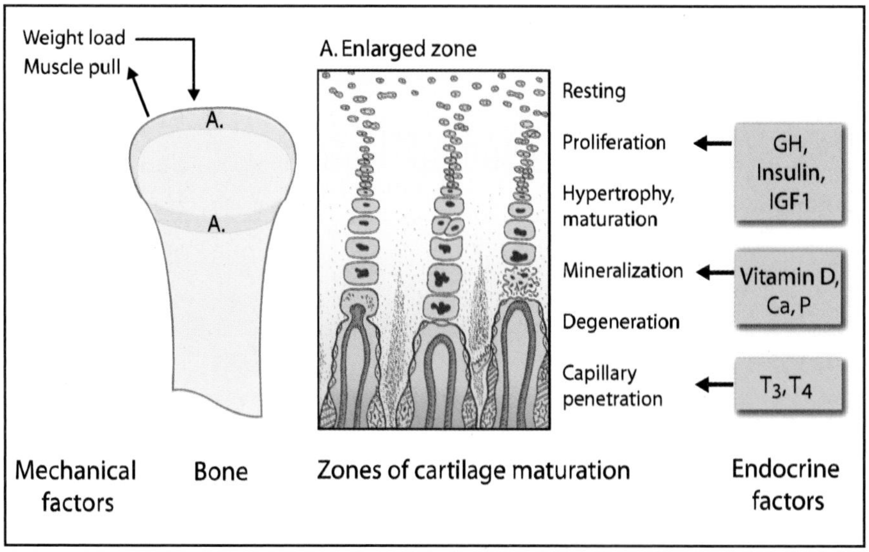

Figure 33-5. Biomechanical and endocrinologic influences on the growing skeleton are depicted. Biomechanically, excessive static (weight load) and dynamic (muscle pull) forces can damage immature skeletons. Note the various zones of cartilage maturation (resting zone, proliferation, hypertrophy and maturation, mineralization, degeneration and capillary penetration) where hormonal influences are thought to occur.

al influences is enhanced mitotic activity of proliferative cartilage cells, which may enlarge the width of the inherently mechanically unstable zone of chondrocyte growth.

Histologic examinations have revealed articular cartilage is less well supported by solid bone plates in rapidly growing dogs, compared with smaller breeds or to littermates fed restricted amounts after weaning (Daemmrich, 1991). The epiphyseal spongiosa of giant-breed dogs is inherently less dense and therefore assumed to be weaker than the spongiosa in small breeds, a tendency that may be exaggerated by overnutrition. Free-choice feeding may lead to a mismatch between bone growth and body growth, resulting in a lower ratio of long bone diaphyseal shaft cross-sectional area to body weight and also a less dense epiphyseal spongiosa.

The biomechanical stress induced by rapid weight gain during growth as discussed above has been cited as an etiology for DOD. It is unknown whether small focal cartilaginous lesions occur first and are then exacerbated by biomechanical stress (Daemmrich, 1991; Carlson et al, 1991), or if biomechanical stress first induces cartilaginous lesions (Hazewinkel et al, 1985; Hedhammar et al, 1974). In either case, increased static forces (weight load) and dynamic forces (muscle pull) may damage immature skeletons, especially in large- and giant-breed dogs. These dysregulations of nutrient supply, bone formation and endocrine regulation may interfere with skeletal maturation, thus increasing the risk for DOD in young animals (**Figure 33-5**).

Theory 2: Excess Calcium and Hypercalcitoninism

A contrasting theory to the preceding theory about high energy intake and rapid growth rate stems from the observation that the rate of DOD is increased in dogs with high calcium intakes (Dobenencker et al, 1997; Slater et al, 1992; Schoenmakers et al, 1997; Voorhout and Hazewinkel, 1987). Young Great Dane puppies fed a food high in energy and minerals free choice (Hedhammar et al, 1974), or high in calcium alone (Hazewinkel et al, 1985), developed osteochondrosis lesions with overt clinical signs of disease (**Figure 33-6**). These lesions appeared at both weight-bearing sites and sites where weight bearing was of no influence, such as the growth plates of ribs.

Feeding high-calcium foods to growing small-breed dogs results in histologic lesions but no clinical manifestations of DOD (Nap et al, 1993a). Large-breed dogs raised on food with a high calcium content or high calcium and phosphorus content had disturbed endochondral ossification (Nunez et al, 1974; Goedegebuure and Hazewinkel, 1986), retained cartilaginous cores in the distal radius and ulna (Schoenmakers et al, 1997; Voorhout and Hazewinkel, 1987) and delayed skeletal

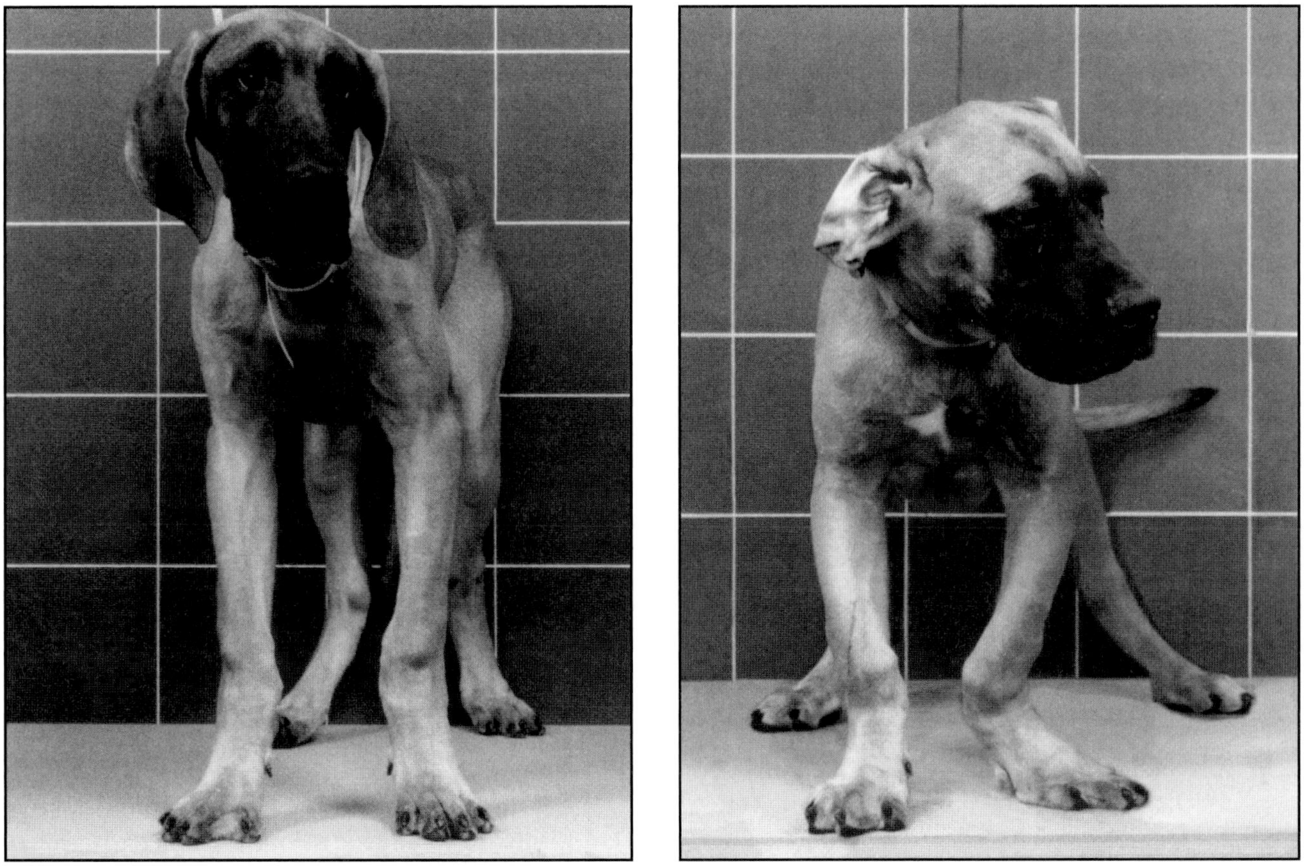

Figure 33-6. Littermate Great Dane puppies fed two different levels of dietary calcium. The puppy on the left was fed a growth food containing 1.1% dry matter calcium. The puppy on the right was fed a similar growth food containing 3.3% dry matter calcium. Note the poor growth and angular limb deformities in the puppy consuming excess calcium.

Table 33-5. Key nutritional factors for foods for growth (postweaning) of large- and giant-breed puppies.*

Factors	Dietary recommendations
Energy density	Energy density = 3.2 to 4.1 kcal/g; recommend the lower end of range if clients use free-choice feeding**
Fat	8.5 to 17%
Docosahexaneoic acid***	≥0.02%
Calcium	0.8 to 1.2% calcium
Phosphorus	Phosphorus amount is based on calcium amount to maintain recommended Ca-P ratio (below)
Ca-P ratio	1.1:1 to 2:1 (the lower end of range is preferred)
Supplements	None recommended if a commercial food is fed

Key: Ca = calcium, P = phosphorus.
*Dry matter basis.
**To convert kcal to kJ, multiply kcal by 4.184. Free-choice feeding is not recommended. Energy intake can be better controlled through food-limited feeding.
***For improved learning.

maturation and growth of bone length (Voorhout and Hazewinkel, 1987). Calcium intake, therefore, seems to be a significant determining factor in DOD. This may occur either directly by calcium competing with other minerals or indirectly by stimulating hormonal effects (PTH or calcitonin) or acid-base balance (**Box 33-3**). Accordingly, hypercalcitoninism may be a contributing factor to DOD in dogs (Hazewinkel et al, 1985; Hedhammar et al, 1974). Dogs ingesting excessive amounts of calcium for a prolonged period exhibited hyperplastic C-cells in their thyroid glands (Goedegebuure and Hazewinkel, 1986; Martin and Moseley, 1990). Great Dane puppies, with access to food with increased calcium content from three to six weeks (i.e., partial weaning), had significantly higher calcitonin release after challenge with calcium infusion, compared with the response of littermates that had access to food containing 1% calcium (Schoenmakers et al, 2000). These same dogs had clinical and radiographic evidence of DOD when compared with controls (Hazewinkel et al, 1985; Goedegebuure and Hazewinkel, 1986; Martin and Moseley, 1990).

Calcitonin is released into blood, where it has a half-life of a few minutes, and reduces concentrations of calcium and phosphorus (Hazewinkel, 1994; Martin and Moseley, 1990). Extrapolation of calcitonin action in other species indicates that increased osteoblastic activity and decreased osteoclastic activity are responsible for shifts in plasma concentrations of calcium and phosphorus, which in turn may affect production of 1,25-dihydroxyvitamin D_3 (**Table 33-2**) (Weisbrode and Capen, 1990). It has been proposed that the physiologic action of calcitonin on bone turnover (decreased skeletal remodeling) and endochondral ossification are inciting causes of DOD in dogs. Commercial foods with increased levels of calcium, calcium and phosphorus or vitamin D are associated with severe disturbances in endochondral ossification, with subsequent osteochondrosis and radius curvus syndrome (Schoenmakers et al, 2000; Tryfonidou et al, 2003).

Key Nutritional Factors

Nutrients must be provided in appropriate amounts and balances for optimal bone development. Excesses of calcium and energy, together with rapid growth, appear to predispose dogs to certain musculoskeletal disorders such as osteochondrosis and hip dysplasia (Hedhammar et al, 1974; Meyer and Zentek, 1991). However, severe excesses, deficits and imbalances of any nutrient may affect bone development. The recommended levels of key nutritional factors are summarized in **Table 33-5**.

Energy and Fat

Energy intake is a major determinant of growth rate. The detrimental influence of excess energy intake on skeletal development during growth has been demonstrated in dogs (Hedhammar et al, 1974; Kealy et al, 1992; Daemmrich et al, 1992; Zentek et al, 1995) and other animals (e.g., chickens, turkeys, pigs) (Carlson et al, 1988; Hester et al, 1990; Nakano and Aherne, 1994; Oviedo-Rondon et al, 2006). Associated lesions appear in physeal and/or articular epiphyseal cartilages as disturbances of endochondral ossification (Daemmrich, 1991). The best method for avoiding excess energy intake is to limit it quantitatively by means of food-limited (food-restricted) feeding.

The risk of DOD appears to be increased in large- and giant-breed puppies fed highly palatable, energy-dense foods, free choice. This is sometimes true even if foods are well balanced (Lavelle, 1989; Daemmrich, 1991; Kealey et al, 1992; Meyer and Zentek, 1992; Hoefling, 1989; Meyer, 1990; Richardson, 1992). However, when large-breed puppies were fed a very low energy density food (3.16 kcal [13.22 kJ]/g ME, 8.0% fat dry matter [DM] basis free choice vs. a food of higher energy density and increased fat (3.98 kcal [16.65 kJ]/g ME, 23.9% DM fat), the puppies eating the low energy density food had less body fat but not slower growth (no difference between groups in radius/ulnar lengths) (Richardson et al, 2000). It should be noted that none of the puppies in either group developed signs of DOD. The results of this report suggest that if free-choice feeding is used, it should only be done in combination with a low energy density food to decrease the risk for DOD and obesity. However, generally, free-choice feeding is risky and is not recommended for large- and giant-breed puppies until they have attained adulthood. Furthermore, commercial foods for large- and giant-breed puppies typically have energy densities of approximately 4 kcal (16.7 kJ) ME/g (DM) and should be food-limited fed.

Dietary fat is an important contributor to the energy density of a food. Dietary fat yields 8.5 kcal ME/g, whereas dietary digestible carbohydrate and protein each yield 3.5 kcal ME/g. Thus, as the fat content of a food is increased, the energy density is also increased (unless sufficient fiber is substituted for either carbohydrate or protein). Furthermore, when the energy density of a food is increased, concentrations of other essential nutrients need to be increased accordingly so that requirements for these nutrients are met at a lower food intake. The minimum recommended allowance for dietary fat in foods for growing puppies is 8.5% (DM) (NRC, 2006). Upper limits for dietary fat in foods intended for large- and giant-breed puppies have not been established but a dietary fat level of 17% is acceptable as long as the puppies are fed properly (food-limited feeding). The associated energy density range would be between 3.2 and 4.1 kcal ME/g (DM). Besides being an important energy source, dietary fat is necessary for the absorption of fat-soluble vitamins. Dietary fat is also important from the standpoint of its constituent fatty acids and their effects on bone metabolism.

Some dietary fatty acids may play a role in preventing DOD. Metabolism of lipid in bone is thought to be under the same regulatory controls as in other tissues (Gilder and Boskey, 1990). Lipid content of mineralized tissues ranges from 1.7% of dry weight for cartilage to 0.2% for bone and dentin. Although specific studies on long bone growth have not been performed, interesting results have been obtained in studies of dentin formation. Essential fatty acid deficiency leads to abnormal calculus deposition, loosened teeth and poor gingival color in rats (Prout and Tring, 1971). Other lipids may play equally important roles in several metabolic aspects of tissue calcification:

1. Phospholipids form matrix vesicles that may be important in new calcification sites.
2. Calcium-acidic phospholipid phosphate complexes may signal nucleation and apatite formation under appropriate conditions.
3. Proteolipids may help initiate apatite formation and calcification.
4. Prostaglandins may influence calcium resorption similar to PTH, and affect collagen synthesis.
5. Inositol phospholipids may mediate calcium transport in and out of cell organelles via second messenger systems.
6. Glycolipids are important constituents of most cell membranes and are found in high concentrations in epiphyseal cartilage. Their specific function is not understood.
7. Phosphatidylserine may act as an ionophore to mediate calcium translocation.

Although no specific studies have been performed in growing dogs to assess the effect of omega-3 (n-3) or omega-6 (n-6) fatty acids on musculoskeletal growth, studies in other species may prove important. Rats fed foods high in lard (animal fat) compared with those fed foods high in linolenic acid (vegetable fat) had increased weight gain and depressed T_3 concentrations (Takeuchi et al, 1995). Chicks fed four different lipid sources had the highest bone formation rate when fed butter and corn oil as the dietary fat (Watkins et al, 1997). Dietary lipids modulate bone prostaglandin E and IGF-1 production, and bone formation rate in chicks. Changing dietary omega-6 and omega-3 fatty acid concentrations alter eicosanoid production in dogs and help manage osteoarthritis. Omega-3 fatty acids are used to help manage osteoarthritis (Hansen et al, 1990). In a double-blind efficacy study with 36 osteoarthritic dogs, increased omega-3 fatty acid intake increased plasma concentrations of LTB_5 (a less inflammatory leukotriene), although these findings did not coincide with improved ground reaction forces (locomotion) (Hazewinkel et al, 1998) (Chapter 34).

It is difficult to determine the appropriate daily energy requirement (DER) for growing dogs because few well-controlled studies have been conducted. Energy intake reaches a maximum, as related to body weight, in the second to fourth month of life (<45% adult body weight) (**Figure 33-7**). The data used to develop **Figure 33-7** were free-choice energy intakes from several breeds. These average intakes may be used as a crude guideline for determining energy requirements in growing puppies of different breeds.

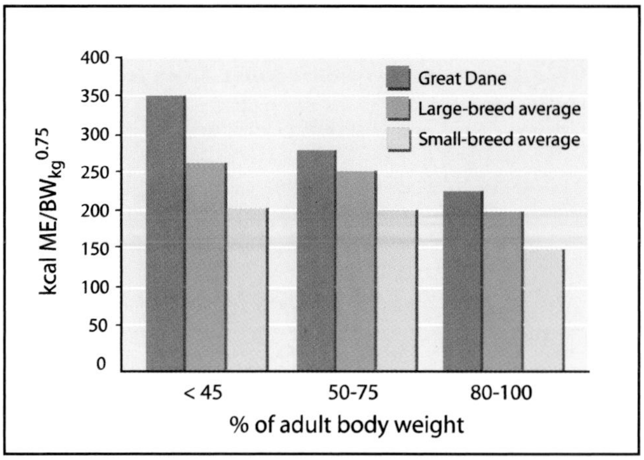

Figure 33-7. Average free-choice energy intake of Great Dane, large-breed and small-breed dogs in kcal metabolizable energy (ME)/$BW_{kg}^{0.75}$ as a percent of adult body weight. Note that energy intake is highest at <45% of adult body weight, which, on an age basis, is between the second and fourth month of life. Great Dane puppies appear to have higher energy requirements for growth than other large-breed dogs. (Adapted from Hedhammar A, Wu F, Krook L, et al. Overnutrition and skeletal disease. An experimental study in growing Great Dane dogs. Cornell Veterinarian 1974; 64 (Suppl. 5): 1-160. Meyer H, Zentek J. Über den Einfluß einer unterschiedlichen Energieversorgung wachsender Doggen auf Körpermasse und Skelettentwicklung. Journal of Veterinary Medicine A 1992; 39: 130-141. Meyer H. In: Ernährung des Hundes, 2nd ed. Stuttgart, Germany: Auflage. Eugen Ulmer, 1990. Rainbird A, Kienzle E. Untersuchungen zum Energiebedarf des Hundes in Abhängigkeit von Rassezugehörigkeit und Alter. Kleintierpraxis 1990; 35: 149-158. Zentek J, Meyer H, Daemmrich K. Untersuchungen einer Unterschiedlichen Energieversorgung auf die Wachstumsintensität und Skelettentwicklung bei Wachsenden Doggen. 3. Mitteilung: Klinisches Bild und chemische Skelettuntersuchungen. Journal of Veterinary Medicine A 1995; 42: 69-80.)

Breed differences in DER during growth may occur, but it is difficult to give specific recommendations because of the lack of quality data. Based on a small number of observations in dogs over eight months of age, the average ME intake for Great Dane puppies ranged from 311 kcal (1,300 kJ)/$(BW_{kg})^{0.75}$ at weaning to 263 kcal (1,100 kJ)/$(BW_{kg})^{0.75}$ at six months of age. These values are higher than for other large breeds and are consistent with reports of higher energy requirements for Great Dane puppies (Rainbird and Kienzle, 1990; Meyer, 1990; Zentek and Meyer, 1992; Zentek et al, 1995). Marked restriction of ME intake (191 kcal/$(BW_{kg})^{0.75}$ [800 kJ/$(BW_{kg})^{0.75}$]) for Great Dane puppies may lead to unacceptable body composition (Zentek and Meyer, 1992).

Unrelated to DOD, but considered important for all grow-

Box 33-3. Dietary Cation-Anion Balance.

Alteration of dietary cation-anion balance (DCAB) has been reported to influence skeletal development in several species. The DCAB of a food can be described, most simply, by the equation ([Na] + [K] – [Cl] mEq)/100 g dry matter (DM). As the DCAB increases, the net physiologic effect is alkalinization. Conversely, as it decreases an acidification effect is observed and calcium excretion in urine is increased. Acidification will be buffered by carbonate liberated from bone by increased osteoclasia, thus increasing osteoporosis in adult and bone remodeling in young animals. The mechanism for these effects on skeletal development is unclear. In addition, regulation of body acid-base balance, calcium homeostasis and osmolality of the synovial fluid compartment may be influenced.

The role of electrolyte balance in canine nutrition appears to be most relevant to preventing canine hip dysplasia. Investigators have associated the DCAB with the radiographic changes of subluxation in the coxofemoral joints in several canine breeds. A food with a DCAB ([Na] + [K] – [Cl]) <23 mEq/100 g DM fed to large-breed puppies was associated with less severe femoral head subluxation, on average, when the puppies reached six months of age. The slowed progression of subluxation was also observed in dogs fed a food with a reduced DCAB from 33 to 45 weeks of age. Hip joint laxity was determined using Norberg hip scores computed from radiographs. Significant correlation between radiographic findings (e.g., Norberg hip scores) and progression of canine hip dysplasia, either radiographic or clinical, was not proved. The authors proposed the balance of anions and cations in the food (specifically Na, K, Cl) influenced the electrolytes and osmolality in joint fluid. The joint fluid of dysplastic dogs has higher osmolality and is increased in volume when compared with that of disease-free hips from dogs of the same breed. The changes in osmolality and fluid volume could be a result rather than a cause of canine hip dysplasia. These studies suggest an association between DCAB and joint laxity without proving a mechanism of action. Most commercial growth foods encompass a very small range of DCAB and probably do not vary greatly in risk.

In commercial dog foods, the relation between cations and anions is 22 to 46 mEq/100 g DM. The balance of only the electrolytes Na, K, Cl, calculated as equivalents, will be between 15 to 42 mEq/100 g DM. Feeding foods with a dietary anion gap of 8 mEq/100 g DM lowered the severity of subluxation of the femoral head in growing dogs of different breeds. Increasing this relation to 41 mEq/100 g food was accompanied by a higher degree of subluxation as determined by the Norberg angle on radiography. Because the knowledge and experimental databases are very small in dogs, mineral salts should not be added in large amounts to nutritionally balanced foods. Problems may arise not only from the addition of anions, but also from increasing the amounts of cations. Further research is needed in this field but it seems prudent to avoid excessive acidifying foods or acidifying agents in growing puppies.

The Bibliography for **Box 33-3** can be found at www.markmorris.org.

ing puppies, are the effects of specific fatty acids on trainability and the development of special senses. Studies indicate that docosahexaneoic acid (DHA) is essential for normal neural, retinal and auditory development in puppies (Pawlosky et al, 1997). Similar results have been found in other species (Pawlosky et al, 1997; Birch et al, 2002; Diau et al, 2003; Hoffman et al, 2003). The inclusion of fish oil as a source of DHA in puppy foods improved trainability (Kelley et al, 2004). The conversion of short-chain polyunsaturated fatty acids to DHA is an inefficient process in puppies (Bauer et al, 2005). Thus, the essentiality of adding a source of DHA should be considered for this growth phase. The minimum recommended allowance for DHA plus eicosapentaenoic acid (EPA) is 0.05% (DM) with EPA not exceeding 60% of the total (NRC, 2006). Thus, DHA needs to be at least 40% of the total DHA plus EPA, or 0.02% (DM).

Calcium, Phosphorus and the Ca-P Ratio

The amount of true calcium absorption in dogs ranges from 25 to 90% depending on the amount of intake and the age of the animal (Nap and Hazewinkel, 1994; Hazewinkel et al, 1991). Calcium is absorbed via three mechanisms: 1) active absorption, 2) facilitated absorption and 3) passive diffusion. Passive diffusion is especially important in young animals. Active absorption is most important in the proximal GI tract. Passive diffusion and facilitated absorption, however, are important in the distal GI tract, primarily because of prolonged transit time and increased calcium concentration through that section. Vitamin D_3 metabolites, especially 1,25-dihydroxyvitamin D_3, are the most important hormonal regulators of GI calcium absorption (Birge and Avioli, 1990). Analysis of 90 dogs revealed that active calcium absorption decreases with increasing age, whereas passive absorption remains constant during the period of rapid growth. When calcium intake is high, active absorption becomes negligible and passive absorption accounts for up to 53% of total absorption of the amount eaten. There is no difference between breeds (Tryfonidou et al, 2002). Previous studies showed serious consequences for skeletal development in large-breed dogs (Hazewinkel et al, 1985) but not for small breeds (Nap et al, 1991). PTH, vitamin D_3 and dietary cation-anion balance modulate renal handling of calcium (**Box 33-3**), whereas calcitonin does not play a significant role in this aspect in dogs.

In the face of adequate levels of calcium in the food, the absolute level of calcium, rather than an imbalance in the calcium-phosphorus ratio, influences skeletal development (Hazewinkel et al, 1985; Hazewinkel et al, 1991) (**Boxes 33-4** and **33-5**). In one study, the prevalence of DOD was significantly increased in young, giant-breed dogs fed a food containing excess DM calcium (3.3%) with either normal DM phosphorus (0.9%) or high DM phosphorus (3%, to maintain a normal calcium-phosphorus ratio) (Hazewinkel et al, 1991). These puppies apparently were unable to protect themselves against the negative effects of long-term calcium excess (Hazewinkel et al, 1985; Tryfonidou et al, 2002). Furthermore, long-term calcium intake increases the frequency and severity of osteochondrosis (Nap and Hazewinkel, 1994). The minimum calcium requirement for growth in puppies of both large and small breeds is 0.8% DM and the recommended allowance for calcium in foods for puppies is 1.2% DM. These recommendations are for foods with an energy density of 4 kcal ME/g (DM) (NRC, 2006). There should be no supplementation of such foods with additional calcium.

Excessive as well as inadequate phosphorus intake may affect calcium homeostasis and thus bone development. Chronic, inadequate phosphorus intake, to a lesser degree than calcium depletion, may stimulate 1,25-dihydroxyvitamin D_3 synthesis (**Table 33-2**), which stimulates calcium and phosphorus resorption from bone and absorption in the gut (Tanaka and DeLuca, 1977). Mobilization of calcium and phosphorus decreases PTH secretion, increases the renal threshold for phosphorus and eliminates excess calcium in the urine. The result is an increase in serum phosphorus concentration while maintaining serum calcium levels (Broadus, 1996).

Conversely, excessive phosphorus intake with inadequate calcium intake may result in nutritional secondary hyperparathyroidism. The excess phosphorus in food reduces the ionized calcium concentration in serum via mass action equilibrium, thus resulting in hypersecretion of PTH. The end result is a decreased renal threshold for phosphorus and excessive osteoclasia and pathologic fractures of growing bone.

The phosphorus level recommended must be considered in conjunction with calcium recommendations. The calcium-phosphorus ratio should be maintained at 1.1:1 to 2:1; however, the lower end of the range is preferred (NRC, 2006). The absolute amount of calcium in the food is more important than the calcium-phosphorus ratio in young growing dogs (Schoenmakers et al, 1997; Hazewinkel et al, 1991). Great Dane puppies raised on food with a calcium to phosphorus ratio of 1.1:1 but with an excessive absolute amount of calcium (3.3% DM calcium:3.0% DM phosphorus) developed more severe signs of DOD than did control dogs (1.1% DM calcium:1.0% DM phosphorus) or dogs raised on low-calcium food (0.55% DM calcium:0.9% DM phosphorus). The last group (e.g., those fed the lowest calcium level) developed pathologic fractures due to hyperparathyroidism as described above. When calcium intake is set at 0.8 to 1.2% DM of the food, as recommended previously for large breeds at risk for DOD, the calcium-phosphorus ratio should be kept within physiologic limits (1.1:1 to 2:1).

Box 33-4. Dangers of Feeding Puppies Adult Maintenance Foods to Decrease Energy Intake.

Often puppies are switched from growth to adult maintenance-type foods under the pretense it will help avoid calcium excess and skeletal disease. However, because some maintenance foods have much lower energy density than most growth foods, the puppy must consume more dry matter (DM) volume to meet its energy requirement. If the DM calcium levels are similar between the two foods, the puppy may actually consume more calcium when fed the maintenance food.

This point is exemplified in the case of switching a 15-week-old, 15-kg, male rottweiler puppy from a growth food containing, on an as fed basis, 4.0 kcal (16.74 kJ)/g metabolizable energy and 1.35% calcium (1.5% DM) to a maintenance food containing the same amount of calcium but at a lower energy density (3.2 kcal [13.4 kJ]/g). The puppy would require approximately 1,600 kcal/day (6.69 MJ). To meet this energy need, the puppy would consume approximately 400 g of the growth food (containing 5.4 g of calcium) vs. 500 g of the maintenance food (containing approximately 6.7 g of calcium).

Box 33-5. Dangers of Feeding Calcium Supplements to Dogs.

Feeding dogs treats that contain calcium or providing calcium supplements further increases daily calcium intake. Two level teaspoons of a typical calcium supplement (calcium carbonate) added to the growth food of a 15-week-old, 15-kg rottweiler puppy more than doubles its daily calcium intake. This calcium intake is well beyond levels shown to increase the risk for developmental orthopedic disease. A review article best summed up the need for calcium supplements: "Because virtually all dog foods contain more calcium than is needed to meet the requirement, the use of a calcium supplement certainly is unnecessary. Now that the deleterious effects of excess dietary calcium have been delineated, we can say that the feeding of calcium supplements not is unnecessary, but, in fact, contraindicated!"

The Bibliography for **Box 33-5** can be found at www.markmorris.org.

Other Nutritional Factors

Other nutritional factors may be conditionally important in some animals. For example, animals fed improperly formulated homemade foods may receive insufficient calcium and excessive phosphorus. Animals fed such foods may develop nutritional secondary hyperparathyroidism as described above. Other nutritional factors are described below.

Digestibility

Digestibility is a nutritional factor that becomes important in certain physiologic states such as growth. Apparent digestibility is the difference between the amount of food ingested and that excreted in feces. During the growth period, the ability to ingest and absorb adequate amounts of various nutrients depends on food intake capacity and the quality of ingredients. It is especially important to consider quality of ingredients when trying to limit energy intake for at-risk dogs. The goal of energy restriction is not to provide low-quality foods that are poorly digestible, but to provide high-quality foods in a low energy density package that will promote appropriate growth. It is important to assess digestibility and recommend foods with at least average or above average digestibility for growth. Typically, foods that are highly digestible are also higher in energy density.

Copper

Copper plays an important role in the metabolism of collagen and elastin. The copper-dependent lysyl oxidase is specific for connective tissue and functions biologically to catalyze the oxidative deamination of the ε-amino groups of lysine and hydroxylysine to form allysyl or hydroxyallysyl residues (Harris et al, 1980; Siegel, 1979). This step forms intermolecular cross links between collagen fibrils, and is therefore essential for stabilization of connective tissues (Eyre et al, 1984).

In several animal species and in people, copper deficiency induces severe skeletal disease (Danks, 1980). Dietary copper levels less than 1 mg/kg DM were related to severe growth deformities, fractures, wide "knotty" epiphyses and especially severe hyperextension of the limb axis in growing dogs (Baxter and Van Wyk, 1953). In young beagles, clinical signs of copper deficiency were less severe than those previously reported; however, hyperextension of the forelegs was a characteristic feature (Zentek et al, 1991). Feeding a low-copper food (1.2 mg/kg DM) vs. a normal copper food (14.1 mg/kg DM) resulted in depletion of plasma (1.4 vs. 9.7 µmol/l) and liver copper stores (19 vs. 246 mg copper/kg DM). Secondary copper deficiency resulted in osteoporotic lesions in growing Great Dane puppies, which could be attributed to impaired osteoblastic function (Read et al, 1989). These dogs were fed an experimental food containing high concentrations of molybdate, which strongly impaired copper absorption and induced secondary copper deficiency.

The overall prevalence of primary copper deficiency (i.e., a dietary deficiency) should not be overestimated. Most common ingredients are rich in copper; however, some homemade, unsupplemented foods (made of rice, dairy products, fat, starch) may contain low or suboptimal copper concentrations. Under certain circumstances, these foods may contribute to the development of skeletal disease, even if copper levels are higher than in deficient experimental foods. A suboptimal copper supply could evoke negative effects especially if combined with high growth intensity or other dietary imbalances (e.g., calcium, zinc or carbohydrates). The possibility that large dogs are more susceptible to a low dietary copper intake cannot be excluded. Impaired copper absorption may also occur with high dietary calcium or zinc levels; the latter induces copper binding metallothionein in the gut mucosa (Brewer et al, 1992). High amounts of poorly digestible carbohydrates or foods that are rich in certain types of dietary fiber may also reduce copper absorption (Zentek, 1995).

The recommendation for copper in canine growth foods is 11 mg/kg (DM) (NRC, 2006). Most commercial canine growth foods deliver copper in the range from 11 mg/kg to 20 mg/kg (DM) and, therefore, meet this recommendation.

Zinc

Zinc is an essential trace element that is widely distributed in the body. It serves as an important coenzyme in numerous biochemical processes. The zinc concentration in newborn puppies is about 22 mg/kg body weight and concentrations increase to 120 mg/kg in tissues formed during the growth phase (GfE, 1989). Inadequate zinc supply, especially in growing animals, causes severe clinical signs within days, including growth depression, skin defects, impaired immune function and growth disorders of the skeleton. These disorders may be linked to the role of zinc as a cofactor in enzymes that are important for connective tissue metabolism. A low activity of alkaline phosphatase (<300 IU/l) is a good indicator of a low zinc status (i.e., deficient zinc intake) in growing animals and young dogs (Kirchgessner, 1987).[b] There are no reports that excessive zinc intake is detrimental to skeletal development in dogs; however, excess zinc is presumed to be toxic at higher levels, as observed in other species.

The essentiality of zinc for skeletal development is unequivocal; reports are available for many species describing severe growth disorders induced by zinc deficiency (Hambidge et al, 1986). Zinc deficiency in dogs is of practical importance mainly with regard to skin diseases (NRC, 2006) (Chapter 32). Skeletal abnormalities have been described in Alaskan malamutes with an inborn error in zinc metabolism (Smart and Fletch, 1971; Brown et al, 1978) and skeletal malformation in bull terriers with lethal acrodermatitis enteropathica, a genetically determined defect of zinc metabolism (Jezyk et al, 1986). Experimental zinc deficiency in beagles leads to a significant decrease of zinc concentrations in the skeleton especially in metaphyseal bone, which represents newly formed tissue. It is unknown to what extent marginal zinc intake, due to either subnormal dietary zinc concentrations or high concentrations of interacting substances (e.g., phytic acid, calcium, copper, low digestible carbohydrates) (Zentek, 1995), contributes to DOD. Foods for growing dogs should contain enough zinc to compensate for negative interactions with other dietary ingredients, especially if the originally balanced food is "improved" by dog owners who add large amounts of calcium carbonate or other calcium salts.

Canine growth foods should contain 100 mg/kg DM zinc (NRC, 2006). Most commercial canine growth foods contain higher levels of zinc to ensure this recommendation is met.

Iodine

Iodine is essential for function of the thyroid glands (Belshaw et al, 1975). The amino acid tyrosine is iodinated and, in subsequent metabolic steps, T_4 and the biologically more active form T_3 are formed. Both hormones, but particularly T_3, influence normal maturation of growing cartilage, penetration of capillaries and mineralization of newly formed bone. Thyroid hormones stimulate formation and resorption of bone, which results in remodeling of the skeleton (High et al, 1981). Boxers with congenital hypothyroidism were found to have shortened limb bones and severe disturbances of the ossification and mineralization process, problems that were alleviated by L-thyroxine supplementation (Saunders and Jezyk, 1991).

Low dietary iodine induces dysfunction of the thyroid glands. Goiter (enlarged thyroid glands) develops with extreme deficiency. In some regions of the world, goiter still occurs in dogs because they are fed unbalanced, homemade rations (Kienzle and Hall, 1994). Stunted limb development, hyperplasia of the thyroid glands and myxedema with no loss of hair typically occur in young puppies born to bitches that were iodine deficient during pregnancy. Most commercial foods meet the recommended iodine level of 0.88 mg/kg (DM) (NRC, 2006).

Manganese

Manganese acts as a coenzyme in glycosyl transferases in the metabolism of the ground substance in cartilage. In different species, experimental dietary deficiency leads to disproportionate shortened and thickened long bones, defective skull development and otoliths in the inner ear (Hurley and Keen, 1986). Currently, no reports describing manganese deficiency in dogs exist. Less than 5% of dietary manganese is absorbed in the canine intestinal tract and the process seems to be strictly regulated (Zentek, 1995). The dietary requirement of manganese for dogs appears to be lower than that of most other species (1.4 mg/1,000 kcal [0.33 mg/MJ] ME) (Meyer, 1990). Most commercial foods meet or exceed the recommended allowance of 5.6 mg/kg (DM) (NRC, 2006).

Protein

Protein is required for a variety of structural and functional molecules to achieve proper growth. The minimum adequate level of dietary protein depends on digestibility, amino acid composition, proper ratios among the essential amino acids, energy density of the food and amino acid availability from protein sources. The dietary protein requirements of healthy growing dogs decrease as they approach adulthood (Richardson and Toll, 1997).

Protein excess has not been shown to negatively affect health or skeletal development during growth of Great Dane puppies when compared with isoenergetically fed controls (Nap et al, 1993b). Protein deficiency may affect the general health of developing puppies, decrease plasma growth hormone levels and reduce skeletal growth (NRC, 2006; Gessert and Phillips, 1956). In Great Dane puppies, a DM protein level of 14.6% with 13% of the dietary energy derived from protein resulted in significant decreases in body weight and plasma albumin and urea concentrations with no increased frequency of osteochondrosis (Nap et al, 1993b, 1991). A growth food with average energy density should contain 22 to 32% DM protein of high biologic value (Dzanis, 1995). The recommended allowance for dietary protein (of high biologic value) for growth of puppies after weaning is at least 17.5% (DM) (NRC, 2006).

Vitamins

VITAMIN D

Metabolites of vitamin D_3 act in concert with other hormones to regulate calcium metabolism and therefore skeletal development in dogs. Vitamin D_3 metabolites aid in calcium and phosphorus absorption from the gut and influence bone cell activity (Hazewinkel, 1993). The vitamin D requirement of dogs may be met from food sources from plants (vitamin D_2) or animals (vitamin D_3) (How et al, 1994).

Clinical cases of vitamin D_3 deficiency (rickets) are extremely rare in dogs fed commercial foods (Kallfelz and Dzanis, 1989). Measuring circulating levels of vitamin D_3 metabolites can help make a diagnosis of vitamin D_3 deficiency. Increased growth plate width and thin bone cortices are not associated with low-calcium, high-phosphorus foods, but are strong indicators of rickets (Hazewinkel, 1993).

Vitamin D excess (i.e., 135x the recommended amount of 550 IU/kg food [DM]), in growing Great Dane puppies, caused no increase in calcium or phosphorus plasma concentrations and no increase in intestinal calcium absorption; however, severe disturbances occurred in endochondral ossification, resulting in osteochondrosis and radius curvus syndrome (Tryfonidou et al, 2003). Vitamin D intoxication can cause hypercalcemia, hyperphosphatemia, anorexia, polydipsia, polyuria, vomiting, muscle weakness, generalized soft tissue mineralization and lameness. In growing dogs, excessive supplementation with vitamin D can markedly disturb normal skeletal development because of increased calcium and phosphorus absorption (Richardson and Toll, 1997; Hazewinkel, 1993). The minimum recommended allowance is 13.8 µg/kg food (DM) or 550 IU/kg of food (DM) (NRC, 2006). The safe upper limit is 3,200 IU/kg (DM) (NRC, 2006). In a study published in 1989, commercial pet foods were shown to contain from two to 10 times the recommended amount (Kallfelz and Dzanis). Therefore, it is best to recommend against providing supplements that contain vitamin D to growing dogs fed commercial foods.

VITAMIN A

Vitamin A is an essential factor in bone metabolism, especially osteoclastic activity (Hayes, 1971). Deficiency or excess may lead to severe metabolic bone disease in growing dogs (NRC, 2006). Concentrations of vitamin A in canine serum range from 1,800 to 18,000 IU/l (Keane et al, 1947); however, with higher intakes, most of the retinol is bound to esters, making dogs relatively insensitive to higher intakes.

Hypervitaminosis A may result in anorexia, decreased weight gain, hyperesthesia, narrowing of long bone epiphyseal cartilage, ankylosis, new bone formation without osteolysis and thin bone cortices (Hazewinkel, 1994). High doses of vitamin A given to pregnant bitches may result in cleft palates in puppies (Wiersig and Swenson, 1967). Adult beagles fed at maintenance levels for 26 weeks demonstrated a very high tolerance to 200,000 IU of vitamin A/kg body weight with no detrimental effects on selected parameters (Goldy et al, 1996).

Hypovitaminosis A results in a variety of clinical signs including anorexia, weight loss, ataxia, xerophthalmia, metaplasia of bronchiolar epithelium, conjunctivitis and increased susceptibility to infection. In addition, faulty bone remodeling may constrict nerves passing through bone foramina resulting in neural degeneration.

The recommended concentration of vitamin A (all *trans*-retinol) in dog foods is 1,515 µg/kg DM or 5,050 IU/kg DM (NRC, 2006). Most commercial dog foods are supplemented well above the minimum requirement for vitamin A. The safe upper limit of vitamin A is 15,000 µg/kg DM (NRC, 2006). In

Table 33-6. Recommended levels of key nutrients for dogs at risk for developmental orthopedic disease compared to levels in selected dry commercial foods marketed for large- and giant-breed puppies.*

	Energy density (kcal/cup)**	Energy density (kcal/g) DM	Fat (%)	DHA (%)	Ca (%)	Ca-P ratio
Recommended levels	-	3.2-4.1	8.5-17	≥0.02	0.8-1.2	1.1:1–2:1***
Hill's Science Diet Puppy Lamb Meal & Rice Recipe Large Breed	357	3.9	18.0	0.220	1.17	1.1:1
Hill's Science Diet Puppy Large Breed	357	3.9	16.8	0.223	1.20	1.4:1
Iams Eukanuba Large Breed Puppy Formula	362	4.4	17.2	na	0.88	1.2:1
Iams Smart Puppy Large Breed	368	4.5	16.1	na	1.0	1.3:1
Nutro Natural Choice Large Breed Puppy	346	3.9	15.4	0.011	1.32	1.1:1
Purina ONE Large Breed Puppy Formula	404	4.1	16.7	na	1.44	1.1:1
Purina Pro Plan Large Breed Puppy Formula	377	4.0	16.4	na	1.37	1.1:1
Royal Canin Maxi Large Breed Puppy 32	365	4.3	15.6	na	1.12	1.2:1

Key: DM = dry matter, DHA = docosahexaneoic acid, na = not available from manufacturer.
*Nutrients are expressed on dry matter basis except for energy density, which is expressed on an as fed basis.
**Energy density values are as fed and are useful for determining the amount to feed; cup = 8-oz. measuring cup. To convert to kJ, multiply kcal by 4.184.
***The lower end of the range is preferred.

Box 33-6. Treatment of Dogs Affected with Developmental Orthopedic Disease.

1. If possible, determine if a nutritional imbalance is causing the skeletal disease observed. The feeding history, clinical signs, radiographic changes and laboratory values may be helpful.
2. To correct either deficiencies or excesses, recommend the pet owner feed a nutritionally adequate growth food designed for large- and giant-breed puppies (**Table 33-6**).
3. If a well-balanced growth food is being fed and skeletal diseases occur, reduce food intake up to 25%.
4. Do not give vitamin or mineral supplements to dogs eating commercial foods, particularly calcium, phosphorus, vitamin D and vitamin A. If a nutritionally adequate commercial growth food is being fed, supplementation is contraindicated.
5. Provide appropriate treatment for specific problems, such as pathologic fractures. Remember, dietary recommendations are inferred from limited group/breed observations and applied to individual animals. All feeding programs need to be tailored to individual animal and client situations. Initial dietary recommendations are a generalized starting point for veterinary/client interactions. Monitoring the body condition score, which necessitates veterinarian-client interaction at regular intervals, assesses dietary adequacy.

the rare case of suspected vitamin A toxicosis, foods low in vitamin A should be fed until signs diminish (Donoghue et al, 1987).

VITAMIN C

L-ascorbic acid (vitamin C) is integral to hydroxylation of proline and lysine during biosynthesis of collagen, of which type I collagen is the most widely distributed in connective tissue (primarily in bone and ligaments). Foods devoid of vitamin C and fed to puppies for 147 to 154 days neither affected growth nor caused skeletal lesions (Dzanis, 1995). Dogs supplemented with vitamin C had transiently elevated plasma vitamin C concentrations; however, long-term supplementation did not increase concentrations much above normal. Excess vitamin C supplementation is generally considered to have little or no effect on the skeleton but may enhance calcium absorption in some cases, thus increasing the risk for DOD (Teare et al, 1979). The relationship between vitamin C and DOD in dogs is unproved; therefore, supplementation is not recommended (Richardson, 1995).

FEEDING PLAN

Assess and Select the Food

To help prevent DOD in large- and giant-breed puppies (>25 kg adult weight), it is best to feed a commercial food specific for their unique nutrient requirements. The recommended intake of most nutrients in fast-growing, large- and giant-breed puppies is similar to that of other breeds (Chapter 17). However, recommendations are more stringent for dietary fat, energy, calcium and the calcium-phosphorus ratio (**Table 33-5**) in dogs at risk for DOD. Several commercial foods are available that have been formulated for fast-growing, large- and giant-breed puppies and their key nutritional factor profiles are compared to the key nutritional factor targets developed above (**Table 33-6**). A food should be selected that is most similar to the key nutritional factor benchmarks.

Foods for growth should have passed an Association of American Feed Control Officials or similar feeding trial specific for that lifestage, or at the very least have a formula that is approved by such an agency (AAFCO, 2007). For feeding trials to be meaningful, they should be conducted in large-breed puppies. However, even feeding trials do not ensure adequacy or safety for every breed. Generally, dry foods are more economical than moist foods. Considering most DOD occurs in large- and giant-breed puppies, the usual type of food selected is a dry formulation. However, moist foods may be fed as long as special attention is paid to key nutritional factors and successful feeding tests.

Owners should not add vitamin or mineral supplements to balanced foods, particularly calcium, phosphorus, vitamin D and vitamin A. If a nutritionally adequate growth food is being fed, supplementation is contraindicated.

Box 33-6 describes treatment plans often prescribed for dogs with DOD.

Assess and Select the Feeding Method

Both the key nutritional factor profile of a food and how it is fed (feeding method) are risk factors for DOD. Assessment of the feeding method requires owner knowledge of current feeding practices, which includes the amount being fed. If owners do not know how much food their puppies are consuming, they should measure how much is being ingested for several days under the current feeding regimen. This information will help when making recommendations for future feeding plans.

Ideally, the food selected for feeding large- and giant-breed puppies should also be fed during the weaning process (Chapters 16 and 17), either throughout weaning or for the last week or so. The advantage of the former is that a food change is unnecessary during or at weaning. The advantage of the latter is that a food change is unnecessary at the stressful time of weaning. Both ensure that appropriate food is being fed during a period of rapid growth.

There are three basic feeding methods: 1) free choice (ad libitum), 2) time limited or 3) food limited. In any feeding regimen an initial estimate of the amount to be fed is required.

Food-Restricted Meal Feeding

The method of choice for feeding puppies at risk for DOD is limiting food intake to maintain optimal growth rate and body condition. Food-limited feeding requires feeding a measured amount of food based on the puppy's DER divided into two or three meals per day.

There are several ways to determine a puppy's initial DER. However, all methods are estimates and even if a puppy's DER is determined accurately, it must be revised continually as the puppy grows.

One way to determine a DER starting point is based on a puppy's age. From weaning to four months of age, consider a puppy's DER to be three times its resting energy requirement (RER), followed by two times the RER until about one year of age (**Table 33-7**). RER can be calculated using either of the following equations: RER (kcal/day) = $70(BW_{kg})^{0.75}$ or RER (kcal/day) = $30(BW_{kg}) + 70$ or it can be obtained from Table 5-2.

Another method for determining a starting point for a puppy's DER is based on its relative body weight. At 15% of adult body weight, energy intake should be 2.5 x the maintenance energy requirement (MER) (MER = 130 x RER), at 30% it should be 2.1 x MER, at 60% 1.6 x MER and at 80% 1.3 x MER (**Table 33-8**) (NRC, 2006).

Table 33-7. Worksheet for determining the daily amount to feed for large- and giant-breed puppies.

I. **Weigh** (determine body weight in kg)
II. Estimate the initial amount to **feed** (starting point)
  A. Determine RER (use tabulated values or energy formulas) Table 5-2 or RER formulas:
    Linear formula: RER (kcal/day*) = $30(BW_{kg}) + 70$
    Exponential formula: RER (kcal/day) = $70(BW_{kg})^{0.75}$
  B. Determine DER
    DER = RER x 3.0 (2 to 4 months of age)
    = RER x 2.0 (4 to 12 months of age)
    = RER x 1.2 to 1.4 (inactive/obese prone adult)
    = RER x 1.6 (neutered adult)
    = RER x 1.8 (intact adult)
  C. Convert DER to 8-oz. measuring cups, cans or grams (divide DER by energy density of food as fed)
III. Reassess (**evaluate**) every two weeks
  A. Weigh
  B. BCS
  C. Clinical judgment
IV. **Adjust** amount to feed (as needed)
  A. If BCS >3/5, decrease amount fed by 10%
  B. If BCS <2/5, increase amount fed by 10%

Key: DER = daily energy requirement, RER = resting energy requirement, BCS = body condition score, BW = body weight.
*To convert kcal to kJ, multiply kcal by 4.184.

Table 33-8. A method for estimating daily energy requirement (DER) for growth of puppies after weaning.*

Puppy weight as a percent of anticipated adult body weight	MER factor**
15	2.5
30	2.1
43	1.9
60	1.6
71	1.4
80	1.3
100	1.0

Example calculation:
A puppy that has a current weight of 5.25 kg with an expected adult body weight of 35 kg would be at 15% of its anticipated adult weight. The corresponding MER factor from above would be 2.5.
The puppy's MER = $130(5.25_{kg})^{0.75} = 130(3.47) = 450$ kcal/day. Multiply MER by the MER factor to obtain the puppy's estimated DER for this stage of growth = 450 kcal/day x 2.5 = 1,127 kcal/day. Extrapolate MER factors for % anticipated adult weights not shown in table.
To convert kcal to kJ, multiply kcal by 4.184.
*Adapted from NRC, 2006.
**MER = maintenance energy requirement; MER (kcal/day) = $130(BW_{kg})^{0.75}$

After the DER is determined, it is converted to a daily amount of food to feed by dividing the DER by the energy density of the food on an as-fed basis (i.e., kcal/cup, kcal/can or kcal/g). The as-fed energy density of the food under consideration can be obtained from **Table 33-6**, the product label or the manufacturer (toll-free customer service telephone number on label, other published information or website content). **Table 33-9** provides an example calculation.

Great Dane puppies are the exception to the previous recom-

Table 33-9. Example calculation for converting estimated daily energy requirement (DER) to a daily amount of food to feed.

To determine the daily amount to feed, divide the estimated DER by the as-fed energy density of the food. For example, if a puppy's estimated DER is 1,127 kcal/day and the food selected provides 375 kcal/8-oz. measuring cup, feed three cups/day (1,127 kcal ÷ 375 kcal/cup = three cups). This amount would be divided into two or three meals per day. Regardless of how the DER is estimated, or if the manufacturer's recommendations are used as a starting point, adjust the amount to feed (as needed) every two weeks based on the puppy's body condition score (BCS). If the BCS is >3/5, decrease the amount fed by 10%; if the BCS is <2/5, increase the amount fed by 10%.
To convert kcal to kJ, multiply kcal by 4.184.

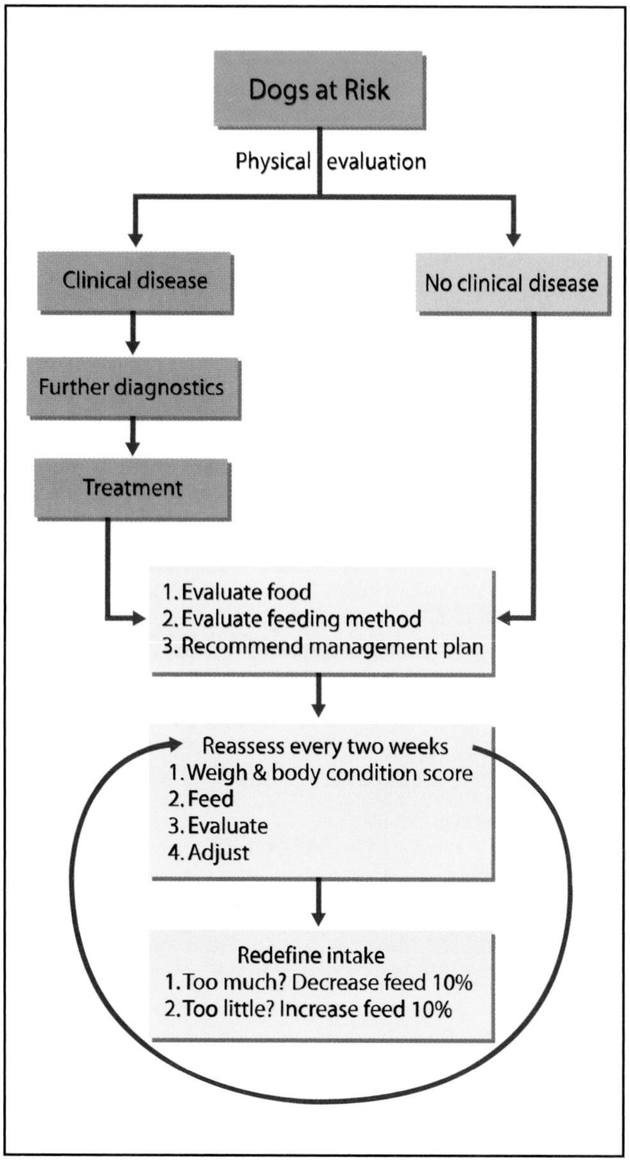

Figure 33-8. Flowchart for assessing dogs at risk for developmental orthopedic disease.

mendations because they may require 20% more energy than other large/giant breeds. Marked restriction (191 kcal [800 kJ]/$BW_{kg}^{0.75}$) of ME intake for Great Dane puppies may lead to unacceptable body condition (Zentek and Meyer, 1992).

Regardless of which method is used to determine an initial amount to feed, it is critical that subsequent regular (every two weeks) body condition assessment is done to ensure the amount being fed is appropriate (**Table 33-7** and **Figure 33-8**). Large- and giant-breed puppies should maintain a body condition score of 2/5 to 3/5.

Most large- and giant-breed puppies will increase body weight and muscle mass after 12 months of age, but the growth rate is reduced and most, if not all, growth plates are closed. At 12 months, these puppies can be fed as adults (1.6 x RER for neutered dogs and 1.8 x RER for intact dogs). Slower growth during the first year does not deleteriously affect final adult body size (**Figure 33-9**).

Free-Choice Feeding

Free-choice feeding is relatively effortless and may reduce abnormal behavior such as barking at feeding time. Additionally, frequent trips to the food bowl may help reduce boredom and timid or unthrifty puppies experience less competition when eating. Coprophagy may be decreased and frequent small meals may result in a more constant blood level of nutrients and hormones.

Disadvantages of free-choice feeding include food wastage, only dry or semi-moist forms of pet food can be fed and competition or boredom may stimulate overeating. The most serious disadvantage is increased risk of DOD because of potential overconsumption by large- and giant-breed puppies (Hedhammar et al, 1974; Kealy et al, 1992; Lavelle, 1989; Meyer and Zentek, 1991). If free-choice feeding is used, it is especially important to recommend a food with an energy density less than 3.8 kcal/g (15.9 kJ) (<12% DM fat) to decrease the risk of excess energy intake.

However, free-choice feeding is not recommended for large- and giant-breed puppies until they have reached skeletal maturity (about 12 months of age or at least 80 to 90% of adult weight).

Time-Restricted Meal Feeding

Time-limited feeding is a method in which dogs are allowed access to food for a defined period, usually 10 to 15 minutes, once or twice daily (three times per day for the first month after weaning, then twice per day). In some cases, the feeding periods may need to be even shorter.

Some investigators have proposed that puppies fed in this way consume less food because they have a smaller stomach volume than that of adults. The energy requirement of young animals may be two to three times that of adult dogs of the same weight, but the stomach volume may be smaller on a per body weight basis.

Investigators who advocate this feeding method suggest that puppies have slightly reduced growth rates, but achieve similar adult size and lean body mass when compared with puppies fed free choice (Alexander and Wood, 1987). Other studies have shown that feeding 15 minutes twice daily does not reduce food intake between free-choice and time-restricted groups (Toll et al, 1993). Again, it is important in this type of feeding program to recommend foods with a lower energy density (<12% DM fat) to decrease the risk of overconsumption.

Time-limited feeding may also help in disciplining and housetraining young puppies. The owner interacts with the puppy during this time and is able to observe its general condition and behavior, which may lead to earlier detection of health problems. A routine of feeding a puppy and then taking it outdoors can assist housetraining by taking advantage of the gastrocolic reflex. Advocates of this feeding method suggest that when some puppies fed in this manner reach adulthood they may voluntarily limit their feeding to once or twice a day and thus avoid overeating.

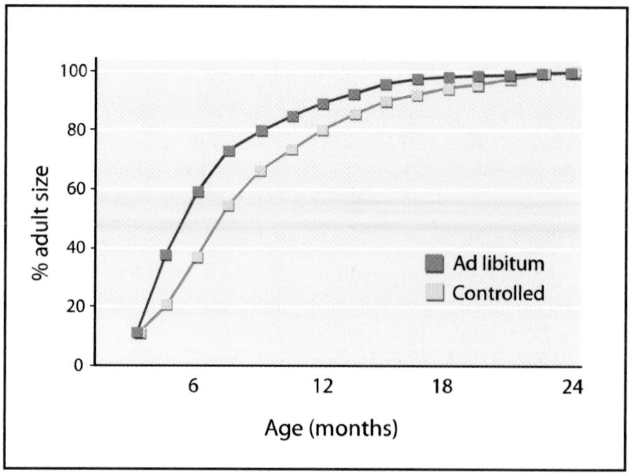

Figure 33-9. Comparison of growth curves of large-breed dogs fed free choice vs. those in a food-restricted feeding regimen.

REASSESSMENT

Regular clinical evaluation of growing puppies and adjustments in the food offered are crucial. Rapidly growing, large- and giant-breed dogs have a very steep growth curve and their intake requirements can change dramatically over short periods. These puppies should be weighed, their body condition evaluated and their daily feeding amount adjusted at least once every two weeks (**Figure 33-8** and **Table 33-7**). Large- and giant-breed puppies should be fed to maintain a BCS between 2/5 to 3/5.The veterinary health care team can perform this evaluation in the hospital and owners can be taught to perform this evaluation at home.

Skeletal disease can be influenced during growth by feeding technique and nutrient profile. However, nutritional management alone will not completely prevent DOD because there is a hereditary component (i.e., canine hip dysplasia and osteochondrosis can develop in genetically affected animals fed balanced foods). Additionally, the occurrence and clinical signs of DOD can be aggravated when forced exercise or environment are not adapted to the vulnerability of the young skeleton. Dietary deficiencies are of minimal concern in this age of commercial foods specifically prepared for young, growing dogs; the major potential for harm results from excess consumption of energy and calcium.

A balanced food fed in appropriate quantities will help optimize skeletal development and decrease the risk of DOD. After DOD has manifested, nutritional management becomes a minor component of treatment unless obesity is a contributing factor.

ENDNOTES

a. Breuer GJ. Purdue University, West Lafayette, IN, USA. Unpublished data. 1997.

b. Zentek J. Unpublished data, 1996.

REFERENCES

The references for **Chapter 33** can be found at www.markmorris.org.

CASE 33-1

Lameness in a Labrador Retriever

H.A.W. Hazewinkel, DVM, PhD, Dipl. ECVS, Dipl. ECVCN
Faculty of Veterinary Medicine
University of Utrecht
Utrecht, The Netherlands

Patient Assessment

A four-year-old female Labrador retriever was examined for difficulty in rising (standing up) and walking, especially the first few minutes of a walk. These problems were worse after the patient had been out for a long walk or played with other dogs, as often happened on weekends. The current exercise program included three 15- to 30-minute walks per day, free exercise in the yard between walks and two 60-minute walks in the woods on weekends.

Physical examination was unremarkable except for moderate obesity (body weight 45 kg, body condition score [BCS] 4/5) and abnormalities identified in the musculoskeletal system. The range of motion of both hip joints was diminished, crepitation was palpated and the dog reacted painfully when its hips were extended. Neither hind limb could be abducted normally in the sagittal plane when the dog was in dorsal recumbency. A thorough examination of limbs and lumbosacral area revealed no other abnormalities.

Radiographs of the coxofemoral joints confirmed a diagnosis of severe osteoarthritis due to hip dysplasia (**Figure 1**).

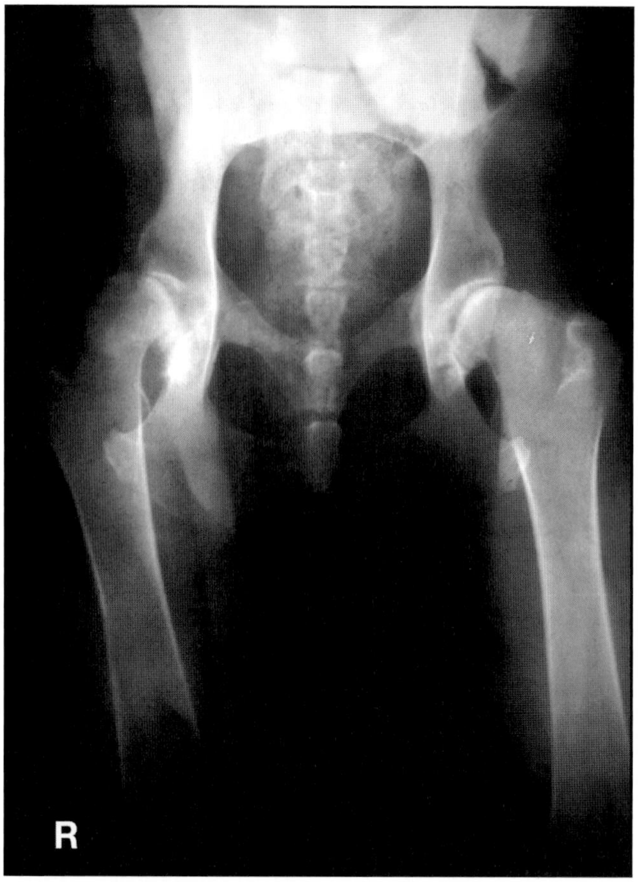

Figure 1. Ventrodorsal radiograph of a four-year-old Labrador retriever with bilateral hip dysplasia. Degenerative joint disease is evident in both coxofemoral joints. Note that the femoral heads have remodeling changes, the acetabuli are shallow and subchondral sclerosis and osteophyte formation are present in the femoral and acetabular components of the joint.

Assess the Food and Feeding Method

The dog was fed four cups (1,500 kcal [6.28 MJ]) of a commercial dry dog food and table foods. The dry food was fed once daily. The table foods were leftovers from the childrens' food; the amount varied daily. The owners indicated the dog gained most of its weight after an ovariohysterectomy two years earlier and during the summer holidays when the dog spent a month with the owners' parents who lived in an apartment for retired people. The food intake during that month was unknown.

Questions

1. What feeding plan should be implemented to improve the condition of this patient?
2. What non-nutritional management practices can be used to reduce the biomechanical stress on the hip joints of this patient?

Answers and Discussion

1. The biomechanical stress induced by rapid weight gain during growth has been cited as a popular etiology for canine developmental orthopedic disease (DOD). It is unknown, and somewhat contested, whether skeletal lesions occur first and are then exacerbated by biomechanical stress, or if biomechanical stress first induces cartilaginous lesions. In either case, increased static forces (excessive weight load) or dynamic forces (excessive muscle pull) may damage immature skeletons.

   In older overweight dogs with established osteoarthritis, biomechanical stress can be diminished with weight reduction. Weight reduction should be continued until very little subcutaneous fat is evident (BCS 2/5).

   Dietary fatty acid changes may provide antiinflammatory benefits that result in clinical improvement in some dogs with osteoarthritis. Changing the food or adding a supplement can manipulate fatty acid levels in the diet.
2. Biomechanical stress on the hip joints can also be reduced through alterations in the exercise protocol for the dog. Exercise is an important component of weight-loss and weight-control programs but must be carefully managed in patients with arthritis. Swimming is an excellent form of exercise that builds cardiovascular endurance and hastens weight loss without overloading the joints. Short, frequent walks on a leash should also be encouraged to prevent overloading of the joints, rather than long walks or unsupervised exercise. Nonsteroidal antiinflammatory drugs can be prescribed as needed for joint pain and lameness.

Progress Notes

A weight-reduction program was outlined for the owners. All table scraps were eliminated and the owners chose to feed a reduced quantity of the dog's current food (two cups [750 kcal, 3.14 MJ] per day divided into two equal feedings). The owners were advised to take the dog for daily swims or as often as possible. In addition, the owners walked the dog on a leash several times daily for approximately 20 minutes or for shorter periods when they recognized the dog was having difficulty rising. The target weight loss was 1% of body weight per week. The owners were instructed to return to the clinic every two weeks for body weight recordings and reinforcement of the program.

The target weight of 35 kg was reached in four months with this controlled exercise and feeding plan. The owners reported the dog could more easily accompany them on long walks. Few signs of lameness were present after the dog reached target weight.

CASE 33-2

Feeding a Golden Retriever Puppy

Daniel C. Richardson, DVM, Dipl. ACVS*
Hill's Science and Technology Center
Topeka, Kansas, USA

Patient Assessment

A 10-week-old male golden retriever puppy was presented for examination and routine health maintenance procedures. The owner had purchased the puppy from a breeder in a neighboring state. The dog was to be used as a family pet and for occasional hunting. The puppy was housed indoors and in an outdoor fenced enclosure.

Physical examination revealed a normal 6.7-kg puppy with a body condition score (BCS) of 3/5. Results of a fecal flotation test were negative. The puppy was vaccinated with an appropriate product and heartworm preventive medication was dispensed. Routine grooming procedures and socialization were discussed with the owner.

Assess the Food and Feeding Method

The breeder had given the owner a bag of a commercial dry specialty brand food (NutroMax Puppy[a]) specifically formulated for growing dogs. The owner brought the bag of food with him to the veterinary clinic. The guaranteed analysis was: crude protein, 28% minimum; crude fat, 17% minimum; crude fiber, 4% maximum; moisture, 10% maximum and ash, 8% maximum (8.9% on a dry matter [DM] basis). The breeder had instructed the owner to offer as much of this food as the dog would eat each day.

The owner was also given a dietary supplement, which was to be added to the food each day. The supplement powder was to be sprinkled over the food (1.5 scoops/day) or moistened to make a broth. The supplement's guaranteed analysis was: crude protein, not less than 42%; crude fat, not less than 19%; crude fiber, not more than 1% and moisture, not more than 4%.

Questions

1. What key nutritional factors are important to consider for this puppy?
2. What additional information is important to obtain about the food and supplement that have been recommended for this puppy?
3. Outline an appropriate feeding (food and feeding method) and monitoring plan for this patient.

Answers and Discussion

1. The key nutritional factors for growing, large- and giant-breed puppies at risk for developmental orthopedic disease (DOD) include energy, fat and calcium. Excessive intake of energy (fat is the primary contributor to energy intake) during growth directly affects growth velocity, contributes to rapid weight gain and may contribute to endocrine dysregulation. Abnormalities of nutrient supply, bone formation and endocrine regulation may interfere with skeletal maturation, thus increasing the risk for DOD in young animals.

   Dogs that ingest excessive amounts of calcium for prolonged periods may develop hypercalcitoninism. The physiologic action of calcitonin on bone turnover (decreased skeletal remodeling) has been proposed as an inciting cause of DOD in dogs.

   Adequate dietary protein is necessary for growth; however, excessive protein intake is not considered a risk factor for canine DOD.
2. The food should be assessed for energy density and specific levels of fat, calcium, phosphorus and protein. These nutrient levels should then be compared with those levels known to be optimal for growth and development of large- and giant-breed puppies. Most of this information is not found on the guaranteed analysis of the package label. The information should be obtained by contacting the manufacturer, reading manufacturers' technical information or consulting other published information or website content. A food for growing dogs should also have passed an Association of American Feed Control Officials (AAFCO) or similar feeding trial. Similar information should be obtained for the supplement.
3. The feeding and monitoring plan should include these steps:
   - Weigh the patient.
   - Estimate the caloric requirement (daily energy requirement [DER] = 3 x resting energy requirement [RER]).
   - Choose a food with metabolizable energy of 3.2 to 4.1 kcal/g (13.4 to 17.15 kJ/g), not more than 17% DM fat, 0.8 to 1.2% DM calcium and 22 to 32% DM protein.
   - Advise the owner to feed the calculated amount of food (energy basis) divided into two to three feedings per day.
   - Reassess the patient every two weeks by weighing it and evaluating its body condition (dogs should have a BCS of 2/5 to 3/5).
   - Adjust the amount of food offered if the BCS is greater than 3/5 or less than 2/5.

Progress Notes

The manufacturers of the food and supplement were contacted. The food had the following nutrient profile (DM): fat = 20.3%, calcium = 1.67%, energy density = 4.4 kcal/g (18.4 kJ). All other nutrient levels exceeded minimum recommendations established by AAFCO for growing dogs. The supplement had the following nutrient profile (DM): fat = 19%, calcium = 3.3%. The supplement also contained essential amino acids, essential fatty acids, vitamins and other minerals.

The combination of the food, supplement and free-choice feeding method probably provided excessive amounts of energy and calcium for optimal growth. The food was changed to another commercial dry specialty brand food (Science Diet Puppy Large Breed[b]), which is specifically formulated to reduce nutritional risk factors for DOD in dogs. This food contains 1% DM calcium, 14.8% DM fat and has an energy density of 3.6 kcal/g (15.0 kJ/g). The DER was estimated (3 x RER = 800 kcal/day [3.35 MJ]) and the owner was asked to discontinue free-choice feeding and begin meal feeding (DER divided into two or three meals per day). The owner was shown how to assign a BCS, asked to record the weight and BCS of his puppy every two weeks and to adjust the amount of food to maintain a BCS of 2/5 to 3/5. The weight and BCS were also recorded in the medical record at 10, 20 and 30 weeks of age when the puppy returned for further vaccinations and other health maintenance procedures. The supplement was discontinued. The owner was also encouraged to maintain a regular exercise and obedience program with the puppy.

Table 1 shows growth data for the puppy during the next 12 months. When the dog was 12 months old, its food was changed to a commercial dry specialty brand food for adult dogs (Science Diet Adult Large Breed[b]). At two years of age, there was no radiographic evidence of hip dysplasia and no clinical problems associated with the musculoskeletal system.

*Dr. Richardson's current address is:
K-State Olathe Innovation Campus, Inc.
18001 W. 106th St, Suite 160
Olathe, KS, USA 66061

Endnotes

a. Nutro Products Inc., City of Industry, CA, USA.
b. Hill's Pet Nutrition, Inc., Topeka, KS, USA.

Bibliography

Richardson DC. Developmental orthopedics: Nutritional influences in the dog. In: Ettinger SJ, Feldman EC, eds. Textbook of Veterinary Internal Medicine, 4th ed. Philadelphia, PA: WB Saunders Co, 1995; 252-258.

Table 1. Body weights and body condition scores (BCS) for a golden retriever puppy at 10-week intervals.

Age (weeks)	Weight (kg)	BCS (1-5)
10	6.7	3
20	16.3	3
30	24.0	3
40	28.2	3
50	28.8	3

CASE 33-3

Forelimb Lameness in a Great Dane Puppy

Jürgen Zentek, Dr med vet
Department of Animal Nutrition
Tierarztliche Hochschule
Hanover, Germany

Patient Assessment

An eight-month-old, male Great Dane puppy was examined for a stiff gait at the outset of walking and right forelimb lameness after taking a long walk. The dog was otherwise healthy but slightly overweight (body weight 48 kg, body condition score [BCS] 4/5). The owner reported that the dog was one of the largest of the litter and that it grew very fast from four to six months of age.

Physical examination was normal except for the musculoskeletal system. Palpation of the scapular region revealed bilateral muscle atrophy that was more pronounced on the right side. Passive movement of all the digits, carpi and elbow joints allowed full range of motion with no pain. Deep palpation of the radius, ulna and humerus did not elicit pain. Movement of both shoulder joints caused slight crepitation and elicited a painful response, especially with hyperflexion of the joint. Radiographs of the shoulder joints were obtained (**Figure 1**).

Assess the Food and Feeding Method

The puppy was initially fed a commercial dry food formulated for growth (protein = 29%, fat = 18%, calcium = 1.6%, phosphorus = 1.2%, all values listed on a dry matter basis) free choice. Because the puppy was "such a good eater," the owner supplemented the food occasionally with meat and table foods. When the puppy was 14 weeks old, the owner switched foods because the puppy developed abnormal locomotion, which members of the owner's dog club attributed to excessive protein intake. The new food was a commercial dry product formulated for adult maintenance (protein = 20%, fat = 13.3%, calcium = 1.7%, all values listed on a dry matter basis). The new food was offered free choice because of the puppy's "good appetite."

Questions

1. What is the tentative diagnosis and how does this condition cause the clinical signs in this dog?
2. How should this patient be managed?
3. Outline an appropriate feeding plan for this dog.

Answers and Discussion

1. Great Danes and other large- and giant-breed dogs are prone to osteochondrosis in the shoulder joints, especially when excessive energy and calcium are consumed during the period of rapid growth (two to six months of age). Osteochondrosis is a disturbance in endochondral ossification that can result in localized separation of articular cartilage and subchondral bone, and may lead to splitting of cartilage fragments into the joint, i.e., osteochondritis dissecans. Osteochondrosis is not painful; osteochondritis dissecans causes osteoarthritis and inflammation of subchondral bone, which is painful. A diagnosis of osteochondritis dissecans is very likely in this case based on the clinical (painful shoulder joints) and radiologic findings (indentation in the caudal humeral head).

   Because flexion and extension of both shoulder joints is painful with osteochondritis dissecans, dogs will shift their body weight to the rear limbs, resulting in abnormal locomotion. Dogs with osteochondritis dissecans of the shoulder joints also appear stiff because of the limited range of joint motion and have variable degrees of lameness.
2. Surgical treatment is indicated for most cases of shoulder joint osteochondritis dissecans when lameness is present and persisting, and when manipulation of the joint is painful. The loose cartilage flap is removed and the flap bed curetted until the subchondral bone bleeds. Granulation tissue and, ultimately, fibrocartilage fill the curetted defect in the articular surface. The joint is thoroughly irrigated and any floating "joint mice" or bony ossicles attached to the joint capsule are removed. Recovery is predictable with appropriate surgical treatment. Osteochondrosis and osteochondritis dissecans of the shoulder joint will cause secondary osteoarthritis, possibly causing clinical problems in later years, although osteoarthritis of the shoulder joint is usually well tolerated by dogs.
3. Altering the feeding plan may have no beneficial effects on osteochondrosis or osteochondritis dissecans at this stage of the disease process. Excess energy and calcium intake should be avoided during the rapid growth phase between two and six months of age. This puppy is slightly overweight; therefore, feeding to maintain a BCS of 2/5 can reduce biomechanical stress on the shoul-

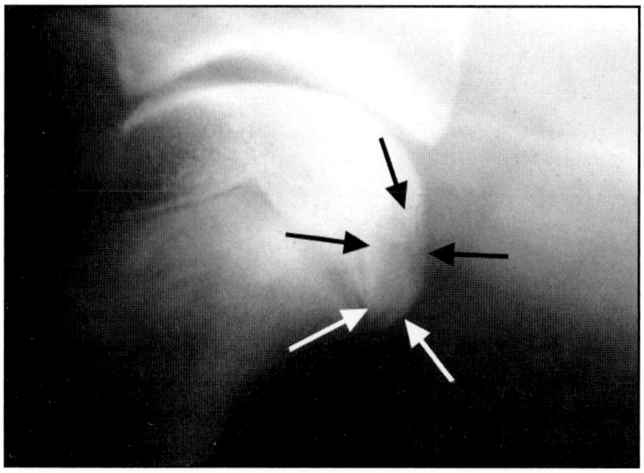

Figure 1. Radiograph of the proximal humerus of an eight-month-old male Great Dane puppy examined for forelimb lameness. The radiolucent area (arrows) is associated with disrupted endochondral ossification (osteochondrosis).

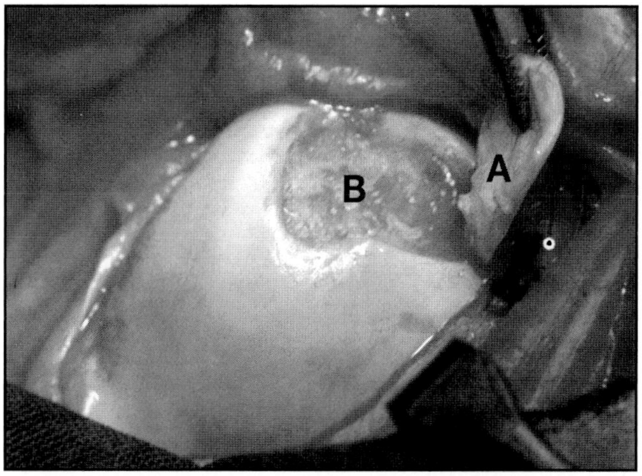

Figure 2. Intraoperative view of an osteochondritis dissecans lesion in the articular epiphyseal cartilage of the proximal cartilage of the same dog. Note the cartilage flap (A) and exposed subchondral bone (B) where a portion of the cartilage flap is missing.

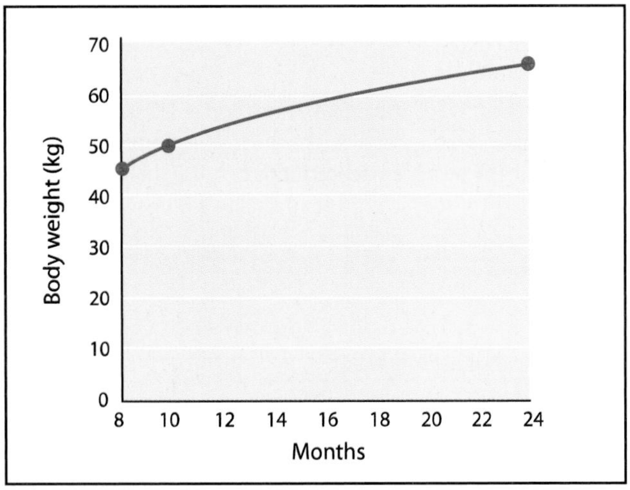

Figure 3. Growth curve recommended for an overweight eight-month-old Great Dane puppy with osteochondrosis.

der joints. Appropriate body condition is especially important considering 60 to 65% of the body weight is normally carried by the forelimbs of walking dogs. Daily energy requirement (DER) should be estimated for the ideal weight at the current age. The owner should discontinue free-choice feeding the puppy and begin meal feeding (DER divided into two or three meals per day). The owner should be shown how to assess body condition, and should record the weight and BCS of his puppy every two weeks. He should adjust the amount of food as necessary to obtain a BCS of 2/5.

Decreasing energy intake by decreasing food intake (meal feeding) and switching to a food with a lower fat level should effectively slow this puppy's growth rate. Adequate dietary protein is necessary for growth; however, excessive protein intake is not considered a risk factor for canine DOD.

Progress Notes

An arthrotomy was performed on the right shoulder and confirmed a diagnosis of osteochondritis dissecans (**Figure 2**). The cartilage flap was removed and the lesion curetted. Examination six weeks later revealed normal locomotion. A decision was made not to perform surgery on the left shoulder.

Because the puppy weighed more than the upper limit for its age, a feeding plan was implemented to slow growth for the next few months. The dog's mature body weight was estimated to be 65 kg, based on knowledge of adult body weights of its parents. The puppy should attain this target body weight at 18 to 24 months of age and have a BCS of not more than 3/5. The owner was given a recommended growth curve (**Figure 3**), taught body condition scoring techniques and given a new feeding plan.

The food was changed to a commercial dry food with 4.14 kcal (17.29 kJ)/g, 25% protein, 12% fat and 1.1% calcium, all values reported on a dry matter basis. No other foods or supplements were fed. The initial DER was estimated to be 1.6 x resting energy requirement at the current body weight or 2,484 kcal (10.37 MJ). It was emphasized to the owner that this was only a starting point and that he would need to monitor body weight and condition carefully, and compare body weights with values on the recommended growth curve. Food intake should be increased 10 to 15% if poor body condition occurred.

Bibliography

Zentek J, Daemmrich K, Meyer H. Zur pathogenese futterungsbedingter skeletterkrankungen bei junghunden grobwuchsiger rassen. Kleintierpraxis 1995; 40: 469-482.

CASE 33-4

Front-Leg Lameness in an Eight-Month-Old Rottweiler

H.A.W. Hazewinkel, DVM, PhD, Dipl. ECVS, Dipl. ECVCN
Faculty of Veterinary Medicine
University of Utrecht
Utrecht, The Netherlands

Patient Assessment

An eight-month-old rottweiler was presented for repetitive front-leg lameness. Signs first appeared when the dog was six months old. According to the owner, although the lameness had no effect on the patient's temperament and playfulness, the puppy had lameness especially after vigorous exercise with other dogs. There were no complaints about the patient's general health; however, the lameness episodes had become more frequent, and no differences in locomotion were noticed when the dog was exercised on different surfaces. The dog had no history of trauma.

When examined, the dog had no signs of impaired health. However, the patient bore more weight on its left than its right front leg. The dog's right elbow joint bulged slightly more at the site of the anconeal muscle than could be palpated on the ipsilateral side. No temperature differences or pain were detected on palpation. More distally, no differences were noticed between the right and left front legs. No abnormalities were found in either hind leg. When examined in lateral recumbency, the dog did not exhibit pain upon passive movement of the shoulder joint, but did on hyperextension of the right elbow joint especially when the antebrachium was concomitantly supinated; no crepitation was evident during the whole range of motion of the elbow joint. Thorough inspection, palpation and passive movement of all joints of the left front leg and both hind legs did not elicit abnormalities.

Mediolateral flexed (ML_{flexed}) and anterior-posterior (AP) radiographic views of the elbow joint were taken. The ML_{flexed} view revealed subtle sclerosis of the ulna in the region of the caudal end of the semilunar notch, but neither elbow radiograph showed signs of osteoarthrosis (OA) (**Figure 1**). An ununited anconeal process or indentation of the contours of the medial humeral condyle was excluded radiographically. Additional radiographs were taken of the elbow joint, including a mediolateral view with the elbow joint naturally extended, and a mediolateral oblique view. The normal contour of the coronoid process was visible and an incongruity of the joint was excluded as a diagnostic possibility; also the $ML_{extended}$ view did not reveal any irregularity at the medial humeral condyle or the margin of the medial condyle or ulna.

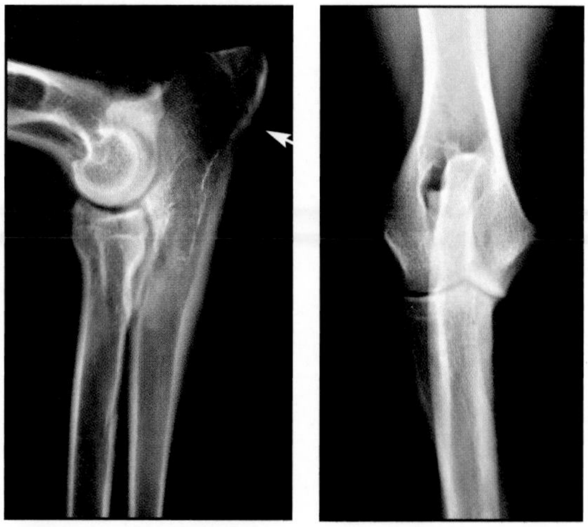

Figure 1. Mediolateral extended view, with sclerosis (arrow) at the ulnar trochlea. No other signs of osteoarthritis are present. The anterioposterior view reveals no abnormalities.[b]

In conclusion, the dog was lame on the right front leg, showed slight bulging over the right anconeal muscle and was painful when the elbow was hyperextended. Radiographs revealed subtle sclerosis of the ulna in the area of the coronoid process. A large percentage of rottweilers have OA of the elbow joint due to a fragmented coronoid process. Epidemiologic studies showed an incidence of more than 50% of elbow OA due to fragmented coronoid process in rottweilers in Scandinavia. The fragmentation occurs at four to six months of age and may cause irritation of the joint with signs of OA (pain, joint effusion, osteophyte formation), although not all dogs are affected to the same degree. Early diagnosis and removal of the fragmented coronoid process will relieve pain and possibly slow, but not prevent, the OA process. Late removal may cause severe cartilage damage, especially at the opposite (humeral) side. It is not advocated to perform invasive diagnostic procedures (i.e., arthrotomy or arthroscopy) when other options exist to further investigate the elbow joint for fragmented coronoid process. Noninvasive approaches include: 1) conservative therapy for an additional period (i.e., four to six weeks) with repeated clinical and radiologic investigation to reveal other abnormalities (e.g., panosteitis, osteochondritis of the shoulder joint), 2) computed tomography scanning to visualize fragmented coronoid process, which is located between the radius and the medial aspect of the ulna and 3) bone scintigraphy to visualize remodeling processes, which are increased in growth, infection, fracture and tumor formation. Bone scintigraphy makes visible different locations that could be overlooked clinically or radiographically.

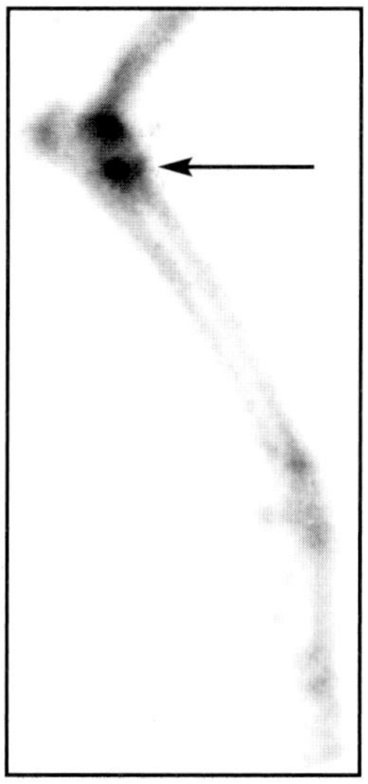

Figure 2. A botscintigram reveals increased calcium turnover irrespectible of its cause. A hot spot (black arrow) appears just distal to the overlapping humeral condyles.[b]

The owner agreed to a bone scan and a computed tomography scan if the bone scan was positive. Scintigraphy revealed hot spots at the coronoid process (**Figure 2**). Computed tomography scanning of the elbow joint revealed fragmentation of the medial coronoid process (**Figure 3**). The fragmented coronoid process was surgically removed and the dog was put on a diet for young, large-breed puppies to optimize skeletal development during the remaining part of its growth phase (**Case 33-2**).

Assess the Food and Feeding Method

The patient was meal fed a food with reduced amounts of calcium and energy (Science Diet Puppy Large Breed[a]).

Questions

1. How is fragmented coronoid process diagnosed?
2. What is the heritability of fragmented coronoid process, and which environmental factors play a role?
3. Outline an appropriate feeding plan for this dog.

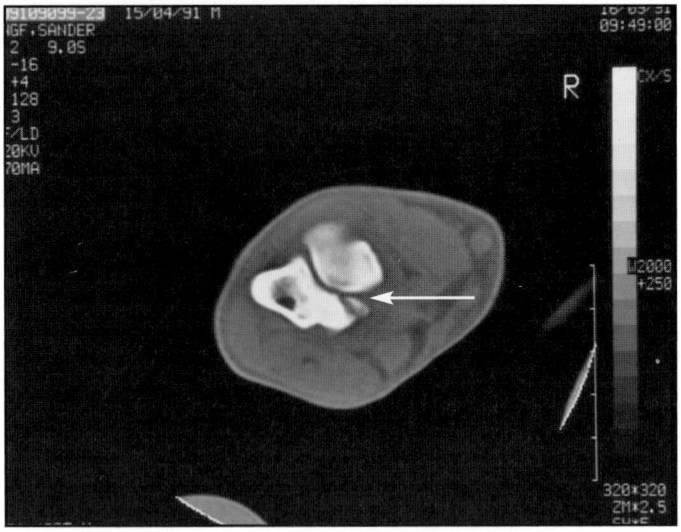

Figure 3. A fragmented coronoid process is evident (white arrow) on a computed tomography scan as cause of the lameness.[b]

Answers and Discussion

1. A good clinical examination will disclose abnormalities in the elbow joint including: more or less joint effusion due to over- or under-production of synovial fluid. In more advanced cases, osteophytes at the joint margins cause slight crepitation during extension, flexion with and without pronation and supination and pain upon hyperflexion and hyperextension, often more prevalent with concomitant pronation. Because 70% of fragmented coronoid process cases can be bilateral it is important to investigate the ipsilateral elbow for a prognosis and therapeutic plan. Hyperextension can be painful in dogs with panosteitis, which occurs in the same breeds and age category as those with fragmented coronoid process; therefore, it is important to rule out deep bone pain here and in other extremities. Also, hip dysplasia and osteochondritis dissecans in the shoulder, stifle and hock joints are seen in rottweilers of this age and warrant extra consideration.

   When no diagnosis can be made, despite serious complaints, clinical and further diagnostic procedures can be postponed for a reasonable period allowing bony changes to develop without much irreversible damage. It is at the discretion of the veterinarian to decide if, during this period, analgesics with provocative activity or rest with confinement should be advised.

   Noninvasive procedures include radiology, computed tomography scanning, bone scanning, sonography and magnetic resonance imaging. The last two are especially informative for soft tissue disorders, whereas the two scanning methods are available in some specialty practices. Radiology, in many cases, helps differentiate the different entities grouped together as elbow dysplasia (i.e., incongruity [visible at $ML_{extended}$ views], ununited anconeal process [visible at the ML_{flexed} view] and osteochondritis dissecans [visible at the AP and/or APMO view]). Damage to growing cartilage, due to a fragmented coronoid process, may cause an indentation at the medial humeral condyle near the location of the osteochondritis dissecans lesion and can, in some instances, be the only indication of a fragmented coronoid process.
2. Because it is difficult to evaluate entire litters and parent animals (i.e., complete clinical and radiologic investigations) information about elbow dysplasia is often incomplete; information about littermates is incomplete, the entities are grouped together or both parents aren't thoroughly investigated. From what is known, the h^2 is between 0.28 and 0.40, indicating that between 28 and 40% of the phenotype is influenced by the genotype and that the remaining depends on environmental influences. In addition to the thought that environment may play a major role in the occurrence of the disease, it has been demonstrated that not all animals with a positive genotype may express the entity. Excessive food intake, excessive mineral intake and excessive body weight have all been mentioned as factors that can play a role in the expression of disturbances in skeletal development. Altered growth in length and thus elbow incongruity and local disturbed endochondral ossification (due to genetic diseases, natural influence, under loading during early development or overloading when vulnerable) are possible causes.

   For screening the population and understanding the etiology, further molecular and population genetic investigations are necessary.
3. Although it is questionable whether dietary changes at this stage of life will prevent other expressions of disturbed endochondral ossification (including osteochondritis dissecans in the shoulder, stifle and hock joints), it is very important to avoid elbow joint stress after surgery. It is clear that an overweight condition coincides with the development of osteoarthritis, possibly in joints without a primary cause. A caloric intake adapted to the changing activity of the patient (decreased activity before surgery and during the recovering period) to prevent excess weight gain is of extreme importance. A balanced, high quality food especially designed for fast growing, large- and giant-breed dogs, characterized by a relatively low calcium content, should be fed until 18 months of age. After 12 to 14 months, dogs will not grow in height, but body conformation will change due to muscle development; a high quality food will support this conformational growth. Frequent palpation of the ribcage and inspection of abdominal lines should help the owner raise a healthy dog. Eventually this patient can be fed a balanced, high-quality diet containing chondroprotective agents (chondroitin sulfate and glucosamine glycans) with increased levels of omega-3 fatty acids to provide constituents that may support cartilage repair and thus help prevent osteoarthritis development.

Progress Notes

After surgery, the patient's leg was bandaged for three days. Exercise was restricted for three weeks after which the dog was exercised on a leash for three more weeks. The owner started a swimming program to help the dog gain musculature without overloading the leg. No lameness was present when sutures were removed 10 days after surgery; the dog was completely recovered after six weeks. Two years later, the dog was castrated and developed a tendency to become overweight. When the dog was 10% overweight, it developed clinical signs of osteoarthritis (i.e., lameness after intense exercise). A weight-reduction program was implemented and nonsteroidal antiinflammatory drugs were prescribed. The owner was advised to feed the dog a "joint-care" diet characterized by omega-3 fatty acids, chondroprotective nutraceuticals (chondroitin sulfate and glucosamine) and L-carnitine to assist in maintaining a healthy weight.

Endnotes

a. Hill's Pet Nutrition, Inc., Topeka, KS, USA.

b. ©Radiographs, bone scintigraphy and computed tomography are kindly provided by the section of diagnostic imaging of the Department of Clinical Sciences of Companion Animals, Utrecht University, The Netherlands.

Bibliography

Kealy RD, Lawler DF, Ballam JM, et al. Evaluation of the effect of limited food consumption on radiographic evidence of osteoarthritis in dogs. Journal of the American Veterinary Medical Association 2000; 217: 1678-1680.

Chapter 34

Nutritional Management of Osteoarthritis

Todd L. Towell
Daniel C. Richardson

"I don't deserve this award,
but I have arthritis and I don't deserve that either."
Jack Benny

CLINICAL IMPORTANCE

Osteoarthritis, also referred to as degenerative joint disease, is a chronic, progressive disease characterized by pathologic changes of movable joints and clinical signs of pain and dysfunction. Osteoarthritis is associated with degeneration of articular cartilage and loss of proteoglycan and collagen, proliferation of new bone and a variable inflammatory response. In the United Kingdom, osteoarthritis is the most commonly observed nontraumatic orthopedic condition of dogs (Clements et al, 2006). Osteoarthritis has been estimated to affect up to 20% of dogs over one year of age in the United States.[a] This finding is supported by the fact that osteoarthritis was in the top 10 most common medical conditions reported in a 2006 survey of insurance claims in the United States.[b] The most common risk factors for osteoarthritis in dogs are developmental orthopedic diseases, trauma including cruciate ligament rupture and obesity.

The extent to which the general population of cats is affected by osteoarthritis is unknown but the disease is thought to be common. Radiographic surveys suggest that approximately 20% of cats older than one year may be affected (Godfrey, 2005). In a study of 100 well cared for cats over 12 years of age, 90% had radiographic evidence of osteoarthritis (Hardie et al, 2002). The most common sites of radiographic osteoarthritis in cats are the elbow, vertebral column and hips. In addition to age, obesity appears to be a risk factor.

Because osteoarthritis is a heterogeneous disease with diverse origins, it can present with a range of clinical manifestations. As a result, therapeutic recommendations should be customized for each patient. When appropriate, surgical correction of underlying conditions should be considered. After osteoarthritis is diagnosed, clients should be educated to foster realistic expectations. Osteoarthritis is usually irreversible but good management can minimize pain and slow progression of the disease. The goals of management include: 1) mitigation of risk factors, 2) controlling clinical signs and 3) slowing progression of the disease. Thus, effective treatment requires a multifaceted approach, of which therapeutic nutrition is an important component (**Figure 34-1**). Foods designed for patients with osteoarthritis should supply age-appropriate nutrition and specific nutrients that may help reduce inflammation and pain, slow the degradative process, complement prescribed medications and provide tangible improvement in clinical signs.

PATIENT ASSESSMENT

History and Physical Examination

Osteoarthritis in dogs and cats tends to be slowly progressive and clinical signs are often subtle early in the course of the disease. As a result, many owners are unaware that a problem exists or may attribute changes in their pet's behavior to normal

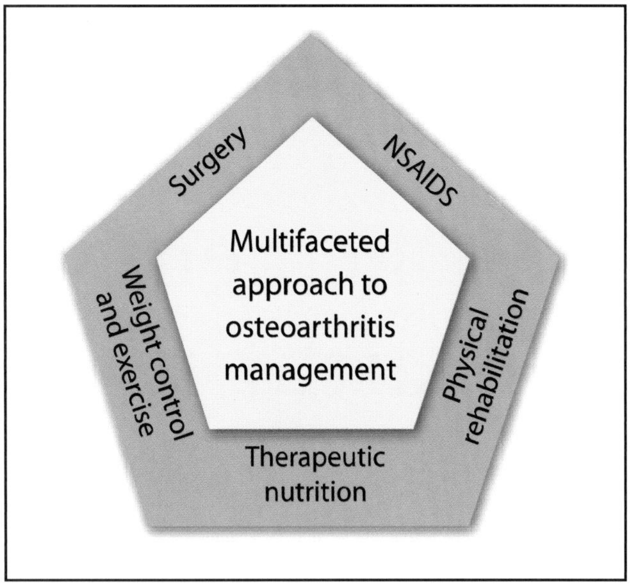

Figure 34-1. Treatment for osteoarthritis includes surgical correction, nonsteroidal antiinflammatory drugs (NSAIDs), physical rehabilitation, therapeutic nutrition and weight control and exercise. Most patients will benefit from a combination of these treatment options.

aging. Careful evaluation of pets whose owners report changes typically attributed to aging is warranted. Obtaining a complete history is important. The use of an owner questionnaire may facilitate recognition of these subtle changes (**Figure 34-2**) (Hielm-Bjorkman et al, 2003).

In dogs, clinical signs of osteoarthritis include reluctance to walk, run, use stairs, jump or play. Owners may also notice other signs including difficulty rising from rest, stiffness or lameness. They may describe their dog as lagging behind on walks or having decreased mobility that is attributed to age. Generally, signs of lameness are described as intermittent and progressive. Typically lameness or stiffness is worse after rest and improves with activity. The time it takes for activity to improve lameness or stiffness in affected dogs will frequently increase as the disease progresses. Pain is often difficult to assess and owners may be unaware of it unless a dog vocalizes (e.g., yelping or whimpering). Personality changes such as withdrawal or aggressive behavior may also be symptomatic of pain.

Clinical signs of osteoarthritis in cats are even more elusive. Most cats with osteoarthritis do not exhibit localizing lameness (Clarke and Bennett, 2006). The most common clinical signs are reduced activity and reluctance and/or inability to jump on or off elevated surfaces or travel up and down stairs. The inability to perform these activities may be related to the most common sites of osteoarthritis, which include elbows, vertebral column and hips. Many owners do not recognize decreased activity as problematic. Furthermore, if jumping or using stairs is not a normal part of a cat's daily routine its owners may not appreciate any abnormalities (Roe, 2006). Other behavioral changes that may be related to osteoarthritis include incomplete grooming, inappropriate elimination and aggression (Hardie, 1997). If mobility and flexibility are reduced, cats may be unable to groom completely and be either unable or unwilling to navigate stairs to reach the litter box or to enter litter boxes with tall sides. Stroking or combing over arthritic joints may be painful. Some cats may resent this type of attention and even demonstrate aggression as a result of pain (Overall et al, 2005). **Table 34-1** summarizes common clinical signs for dogs and cats (Beale, 2004).

Physical examination should include neurologic assessment and a thorough orthopedic examination. Joints, muscles, tendons, ligaments and long bones should be palpated for evidence of swelling, heat or pain. Joints should be assessed for crepitus, range of motion, collateral stress, abduction and adduction (instability). Muscle atrophy, hypertrophy or asymmetry should be noted because these findings may indicate the most clinically affected joint.

Circle the index score that best represents your dog's behavior or locomotion.

1. Rate your dog's mood.

Very alert	Alert	Neither alert nor indifferent	Indifferent	Very indifferent
0	1	2	3	4

2. Rate your dog's willingness to participate in play.

Very willingly	Willingly	Reluctantly	Very reluctantly	Does not participate at all
0	1	2	3	4

3. Rate your dog's vocalization (audible complaining, such as whining or crying out).

Never	Hardly ever	Sometimes	Often	Very often
0	1	2	3	4

4. Rate your dog's willingness to walk.

Very willingly	Willingly	Reluctantly	Very reluctantly	Does not participate in action at all
0	1	2	3	4

5. Rate your dog's willingness to trot.

Very willingly	Willingly	Reluctantly	Very reluctantly	Does not participate at all
0	1	2	3	4

6. Rate your dog's willingness to run.

Very willingly	Willingly	Reluctantly	Very reluctantly	Does not participate at all
0	1	2	3	4

7. Rate your dog's willingness to jump.

Very willingly	Willingly	Reluctantly	Very reluctantly	Does not participate at all
0	1	2	3	4

8. Rate your dog's ease in lying down.

With great ease	Easily	Neither easily nor with difficulty	With difficulty	With great difficulty
0	1	2	3	4

9. Rate your dog's ease in rising from lying down.

With great ease	Easily	Neither easily nor with difficulty	With difficulty	With great difficulty
0	1	2	3	4

10. Rate your dog's ease of movement after a long rest.

Never difficult	Hardly ever difficult	Sometimes difficult	Often difficult	Very often difficult
0	1	2	3	4

11. Rate your dog's ease of movement after major activity or heavy exercise.

Never difficult	Hardly ever difficult	Sometimes difficult	Often difficult	Very often difficult
0	1	2	3	4

Figure 34-2. Osteoarthritis pain assessment questionnaire. Dogs with total index scores greater than six are presumed to have chronic pain. (Adapted from Hielm-Björkman AK, Kuusela E, Liman KE, et al. Evaluation of methods for assessment of pain associated with chronic osteoarthritis in dogs. Journal of the American Veterinary Medical Association 2003; 222(11): 1552-1558.)

Radiography

Diagnosis of osteoarthritis generally requires a combination of history, physical examination findings and radiographic evidence. Clinical and radiographic signs of osteoarthritis are not always congruent. In one study, as few as 33% of cats with radiographic evidence of osteoarthritis also had clinical signs (Godfrey, 2005). In dogs, a study designed to evaluate the relationship between limb function and radiography of stifle osteoarthritis found that radiographic evidence of osteoarthritis did not correlate with clinical function (Gordon et al, 2003). Because the earliest changes in osteoarthritis occur at the level of the articular cartilage, and radiographs do not accurately assess this structure, changes may not be detected early in the course of the disease. As osteoarthritis progresses, typical radiographic changes include evidence of effusion, osteophytosis and subchondral sclerosis. Intraarticular ossific bodies are seen more commonly in cats. Synovial effusion and thickened periarticular soft tissue occur less commonly in cats than in dogs (Allan, 2000). Collapse of the radiolucent joint space and subchondral osseous cystic lesions may be observed in advanced cases of osteoarthritis.

Bony changes occur relatively late in the disease process and are largely irreversible. Early diagnosis of osteoarthritis by clinical signs and/or radiographic changes is hampered by the insidious onset and relatively silent progression of this disease. As a result, treatment that might prevent further cartilage destruction is often delayed. Recent efforts have concentrated on techniques to allow earlier diagnosis of osteoarthritis. Two methods of early recognition that have received considerable attention are radiographic predictors and biomarkers.

Because canine hip dysplasia (CHD) is one of the most common causes of osteoarthritis in dogs, it has been the focus of multiple studies designed to evaluate early predictors of osteoarthritis. Traditional subjective radiographic evaluations used to predict the presence of CHD include hip-extended radiographs evaluated by criteria established by either the Orthopedic Foundation for Animals (OFA) at two years of age or the British Veterinary Association Kennel Club (BVA/KC) scores at one year of age. Both underestimate the susceptibility to CHD and their use, therefore, has underestimated the development of osteoarthritis in affected populations (Kapatkin et al, 2004). As a result, these screening techniques have not reduced the incidence of CHD in affected populations when used as criteria for breeding selection. Hip joint laxity is a prominent feature of the pathogenesis of CHD; a variety of techniques to measure laxity have been described (Farese et al, 1999; Farese et al, 1998; Fluckiger et al, 1999; Smith et al, 1990; Todhunter et al, 2003). Several of these studies have documented that objective measurements of hip joint laxity such as the distraction index and dorsolateral subluxation score are better predictors of the presence of CHD and subsequent development of osteoarthritis than subjective evaluations. These techniques allow dogs to be evaluated as early as four months of age, which makes them more appropriate as screening tools for breeding populations (Adams et al, 1998; Lust et al, 2001; Smith, 1997; Smith et al, 1993; Smith et al, 2004; Todhunter et al, 2003a). One study evaluated the relationship between the presence of degenerative joint disease and radiographic measures of joint laxity in cats. Cats with increased laxity in the coxofemoral joint detected by objective measurements had an increased risk of osteoarthritis (Langenbach et al, 1998).

Table 34-1. Common clinical signs of osteoarthritis (OA).*

Stage	Dogs	Cats
Mild OA	Stiffness, decreased activity, limping	Decreased activity
Moderate OA	Pain, muscle atrophy, difficulty rising	Reluctance to jump, climb stairs, groom
Severe OA	Loss of range of motion, vocalization, crepitus, lethargy, inappetence	Limping, muscle atrophy, inappropriate elimination

*Adapted from Beale B. Orthopedic problems in geriatric dogs and cats. Veterinary Clinics of North America: Small Animal Practice 2005; 35: 655-674.

Laboratory Information

Routine complete blood counts, serum biochemistry profiles and urinalyses serve as a baseline for evaluation of overall health. Synovial fluid analysis can help confirm the presence or absence of septic, immune-mediated, acutely traumatic or neoplastic processes (Harari, 1997).

Biomarkers

Osteoarthritis biomarkers are molecules whose concentrations in a body fluid (synovial fluid, blood or urine) reflect a specific biologic or pathologic process, consequence of a process or a response to therapeutic intervention. Theoretically, biomarkers should be able to detect osteoarthritis at a very early stage. For biomarkers to successfully detect osteoarthritis, they must differentiate between arthritic and non-arthritic joints, be sensitive to change, have low variability and be reproducible. Although several candidates for osteoarthritis biomarkers exist for people, none have been found to be specific. Evaluation of a profile of biomarkers in combination with genetic analysis may prove to be more useful for risk assessment and evaluation of treatment effects (Haq et al, 2003). Most canine studies have examined the association of biomarkers with some aspect of the progression of either experimental or naturally occurring osteoarthritis (Arican et al, 1996; Budsberg and Bartges, 2006; de Rooster et al, 2000; Fujita et al, 2006; Fujita et al, 2005; Innes et al, 2005; Johnson et al, 2002; Matyas et al, 2004; Misumi et al, 2002; Trumble et al, 2004). Two articles have demonstrated changes in biomarkers as an indication of therapeutic intervention success in cats and dogs (Yamka et al, 2006; Yamka et al, 2006a). One obstacle to identifying reliable biomarkers is that most of the cartilage in the body is found in intervertebral disks and costochondral junctions. Joints typically affected by osteoarthritis represent a fraction of the total body cartilage and may develop only subtle biochemical changes in early disease. However, the expanding base of information about osteoarthritis-related biomarkers should positive-

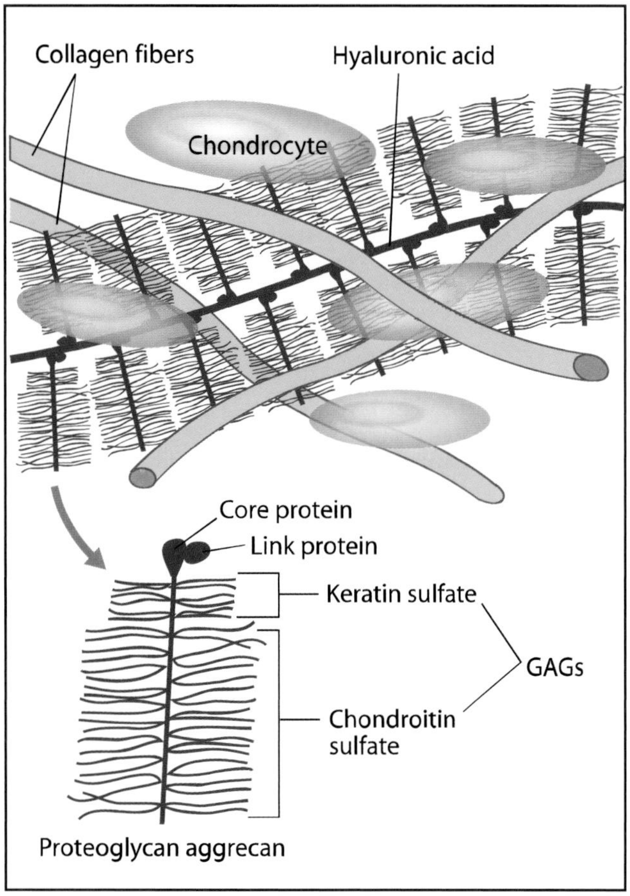

Figure 34-3. Microstructure of cartilage. Key: GAGs = glycosaminoglycans. (Adapted from White GW. DVM Best Practices. Nov. 2003.)

ly affect early diagnosis, development of therapeutics and ultimately clinical care.

Risk Factors

Dogs

Risk factors for developing osteoarthritis include age, breed (large or giant breeds), genetics, developmental orthopedic disease, trauma and obesity. Breeds with the greatest risk tend to be large and fast growing with genetic predispositions for developmental orthopedic diseases. These breeds include German shepherd dogs, rottweilers, Labrador retrievers and golden retrievers (Smith et al, 2001). Developmental orthopedic diseases are a heterogenous group of musculoskeletal disorders of growing dogs that can be affected by nutrition (Chapter 33). CHD, osteochondrosis, elbow dysplasia, fragmented medial coronoid process and ununited anconeal process are common developmental orthopedic diseases that can lead to osteoarthritis. The radiographic prevalence of CHD has been reported to be as high as 70% in golden retrievers and rottweilers (Paster et al, 2005). However, because CHD is a polygenic disease with complex inheritance, environmental factors such as nutrition and lifestyle can have a meaningful influence on its incidence and severity (Smith et al, 2006). Rupture of the cranial cruciate ligament is the most common cause of lameness in dogs and even with surgical correction, the most common traumatic cause of osteoarthritis in dogs (Hayashi et al, 2004; Wilke et al, 2005).

One long-term study documented that the prevalence and severity of osteoarthritis is greater in dogs with body condition scores above normal (Kealy et al, 2000). The mean age at which 50% of the dogs in this study required long-term treatment for clinical signs attributable to osteoarthritis was significantly younger (10.3 years, $p < 0.01$) for the overweight dogs compared to dogs with normal body condition scores (13.3 years) (Kealy et al, 2000). Traditionally, the mechanical stress of excess weight has been thought to be the primary perpetrator of the pathophysiology and progression of osteoarthritis. However, recent studies have documented metabolic activity in adipose tissue that may be of equal or greater importance. Adipocytes secrete several hormones including leptin and adiponectin and produce a diverse range of proteins termed adipokines. Among the currently recognized adipokines are a growing list of mediators of inflammation: tumor necrosis factor-α, interleukin-6, interleukin-8 and interleukin-10. These adipokines are found in human and canine adipocytes (Eisele et al, 2005; Trayhurn and Wood, 2004). Production of these proteins is increased in obesity, suggesting that obesity is a state of chronic low-grade inflammation. Low-grade inflammation may contribute to the pathophysiology of a number of diseases commonly associated with obesity including osteoarthritis. This might explain why relatively small reductions in body weight can result in significant improvement in clinical signs (Burkholder et al, 2000; Impellizeri et al, 2000).

Cats

Overweight cats are reported to be 2.9 times more likely to present for lameness not associated with cat bite abscesses (Scarlett and Donoghue, 1998). In one study, cats older than 12 years were examined for reasons other than lameness. Ninety percent of the radiographs taken documented at least one area of degenerative joint disease (Hardie et al, 2002). Radiographic evidence of osteoarthritis was found in 22% of the general population of cats, greater than one year of age, evaluated at primary care cat clinics in the United Kingdom over a four-year period. The highest incidence of osteoarthritis was found in cats older than 10 years (Godfrey, 2005). In both of these studies, the highest frequency of disease occurred in the elbow, with the vertebral column and stifle being the next most common sites, respectively. One prospective study of osteoarthritis in cats documented the elbow and hip as most commonly affected joints (Clarke and Bennett, 2006). Additional risk factors for osteoarthritis in cats include age-related cartilage degeneration, developmental and traumatic causes of joint instability, chondro-osseous dysplasia of Scottish fold cats, the storage disease mucopolysaccharidosis, nutritional imbalances (hypervitaminosis A), neuropathic diseases (diabetes mellitus) and immune-mediated polyarthritides (Allan, 2000).

Etiopathogenesis

The normal joint is composed of articular cartilage, subchondral bone, joint capsule and supporting ligaments and tendons. The normal joint provides low friction motion and transfer of body weight across the articular surface during movement. Articular cartilage is made up of chondrocytes and extracellular matrix. Chondrocytes are terminally differentiated cells that are highly metabolically active throughout life (Roush et al, 2002). Normal cartilage is dynamic and is replaced over a one- to two-year period by the balance of the catabolic action of degradative enzymes on the extracellular matrix with the anabolic synthesis of matrix components by chondrocytes.

The extracellular matrix is composed of collagen, proteoglycans and water (**Figure 34-3**). Chondrocytes produce and maintain the extracellular matrix. Collagen fibrils (primarily collagen type II) provide structural support for the cartilage matrix. Proteoglycans are composed of glycosaminoglycan (GAG) chains attached to a central core protein. Chondroitin sulfate, keratin sulfate and dermatan sulfate are the most common GAGs in articular cartilage. Aggrecan is the shortened name for the large aggregating chondroitin sulfate proteoglycan. Aggrecan is the most common and well-defined proteoglycan in articular cartilage and is comprised of a core protein to which as many as 100 GAG chains are attached (Lepine and Hayek, 2001). Because GAGs are anionic and hydrophilic, they attract and hold water in a gel-like consistency. Aggrecans, with their hydrophilic GAGs, are normally contained within the framework of collagen fibrils, which limit their expansion when hydrated.

In the normal joint, cartilage must withstand both compressive and shearing forces. The unique relationship between collagen and proteoglycans provides the biomechanical properties necessary to withstand these forces. Collagen fibrils alone cannot resist compressive forces without collapse but tolerate tensile forces well, whereas hydrated aggrecan complexes weakly resist shear forces but withstand compressive forces (Johnston, 2005). When the normal distribution of collagen, proteoglycans and water is disturbed, the function of articular cartilage is altered, leading to changes typically associated with osteoarthritis.

Normal cartilage metabolism is a highly regulated balance between synthesis and degradation of the various matrix components. Osteoarthritis can be initiated by a variety of physical stresses that damage chondrocytes such as trauma, obesity or developmental orthopedic diseases. Despite the variety of initiating events, there seems to be common pathways that lead to the destruction of articular cartilage (Johnston, 1997). Once initiated, these molecular and cellular pathways interact to form a self-perpetuating cycle.

The instigating event of this cycle is thought to be loss of proteoglycans (aggrecans) (Caterson et al, 2000; Hegemann et al, 2002). Damage to chondrocytes causes up-regulation of catabolic enzymes, particularly aggrecanases (enzymes that cleave aggrecans at specific peptide bonds). This shift from anabolic to catabolic pathways is responsible for the loss of proteoglycans. Damaged chondrocytes also produce inflammatory mediators. Inflammatory cytokines contribute to the perpetuation and progression of arthritis by sustaining catabolic processes (Curtis et al, 2002). Initially, damaged chondrocytes attempt to compensate for this imbalance by producing increased quantities of proteoglycans and collagen. This may lead to an initial thickening of the articular cartilage; however, the quantity and quality of the proteoglycans and collagen produced are abnormal (Renberg, 2005). Eventually aggrecanases destroy proteoglycans faster than new ones can be formed. This imbalance escalates the deterioration of the extracellular matrix and cartilage's normal physiologic properties.

Without a healthy extracellular matrix, cartilage is unable to withstand the compressive forces of weight bearing. The net result is cartilage with decreased load bearing capacity and localized areas of softening (Vaughan-Scott and Taylor, 1997). Fibrillations and microfractures are early histopathologic changes. With progression of osteoarthritis, gross evidence of damage to articular cartilage becomes obvious. The normally smooth glistening surface becomes dull and rough. Fissures become evident and ultimately areas of cartilage erosion develop (**Figure 34-4**) (Renberg, 2005). Osteoarthritis affects not only the articular cartilage, but also the underlying bone and adjacent joint structures. Stiffening of the subchondral bone occurs concurrently with changes in the articular cartilage matrix. Osteoblasts in the trabecular portion of underlying bone begin to form new bone and the subchondral region is often thickened and sclerotic. Although changes in subchondral bone may not be necessary for the development of osteoarthritis, these changes may play an important role in the progression of the disease (Johnston, 1997).

Osteophytes are commonly associated with osteoarthritis. Generally, they develop at the periphery of the joint and are thought to form as a result of joint instability. Although they normally form over weeks to months, experimental models have demonstrated formation as early as three days after creation of instability (Johnston, 1997). However, osteophytes have been documented to develop in the presence of inflammation without instability, suggesting that synovial membrane inflammation may play a role (Johnston, 1997). Osteoarthritis and the accompanying inflammation also cause changes in the joint capsule. These changes may include thickening of the synovium and increased vascularity. Conversely, synoviocytes contribute to the progression of osteoarthritis by producing cytokines and leukotrienes, which attract inflammatory cells and the release of prostaglandins and other inflammatory mediators. This inflammation of the synovium contributes to decreased elasticity and viscosity of synovial fluid. Synovitis can either precede or follow observable cartilage changes and is likely secondary to exposure of neoantigens on the cartilage or release of inflammatory mediators by damaged synovium or chondrocytes (Renberg, 2005).

Key Nutritional Factors

Besides supplying age-appropriate nutrition, foods designed for companion animals with osteoarthritis need to provide specific nutrients that may help reduce inflammation and pain, enhance cartilage repair, slow the degradative process, complement prescribed medications and provide tangible improvement in clinical signs. Because foods for osteoarthritis are fed in place of

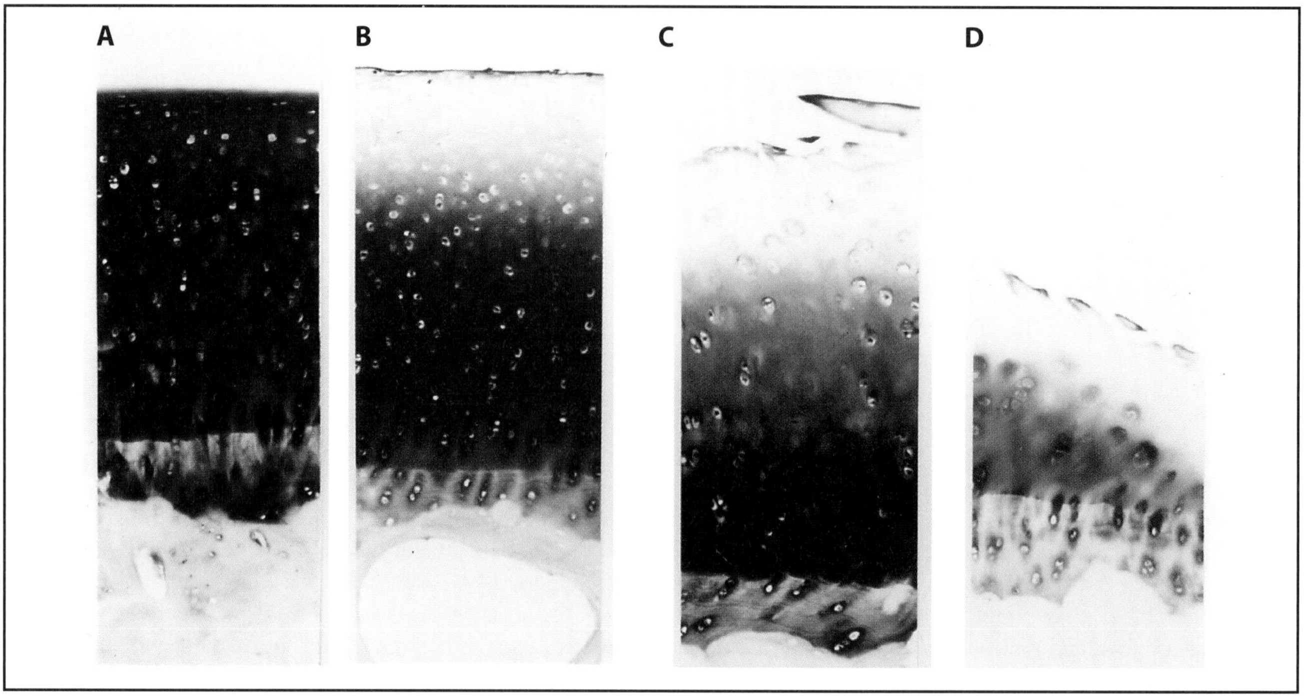

Figure 34-4. Toluidine blue-stained sections of canine articular cartilage from normal joints (A) and joints with early- (B), mid- (C) or late- (D) stage osteoarthritis (OA); the articular surface is at the top of each picture and subchondral bone is at the bottom. In the normal cartilage (A), the articular surface is smooth, the matrix (proteoglycans, collagen and water) is darkly stained and chondrocytes are visible in their lacunae. In early OA (B), proteoglycans and water are lost from the superficial layers (indicated by reduced stain uptake). As OA progresses (C, D), there is further loss of matrix accompanied by articular cartilage surface fibrillation and erosion due to collagen degradation and mechanical disruption of the tissue. (Used with permission from Caterson B, Flannery CR, Hughes CE, et al. Mechanisms involved in cartilage proteoglycan catabolism. Matrix Biology 2000; 19(4): 333-344.)

regular maintenance foods, several key nutritional factors are included due to their relationship to general health rather than specific benefits for osteoarthritis. Nutraceutical, or functional food additives, may also contribute to the management of osteoarthritis. **Table 34-2** summarizes key nutritional factors.

Omega-3 Fatty Acids

All mammals synthesize fatty acids de novo up to palmitic acid, which may be elongated to stearic acid and converted into oleic acid. Plants, unlike mammals, can insert additional double bonds into oleic acid and produce the polyunsaturated fatty acids linoleic acid (LA, 18:2n-6) and α-linolenic acid (ALA, 18:3n-3). Linoleic acid and α-linolenic acid are considered essential fatty acids because animals cannot synthesize them from other fatty acids; therefore, they must be supplied by food.

In most animals, linoleic acid can be converted into arachidonic acid (AA, 20:4n-6) via desaturation and elongation. However, in cats, these conversions are greatly limited because of low Δ-6 desaturase activity (Bauer, 2006). As a result, cats are unable to synthesize other physiologically important long-chain polyunsaturated fatty acids, such as arachidonic acid and docosahexaenoic acid (DHA, 22:6n-3), in amounts sufficient for certain lifestages or processes. For cats, marine fish oils, rather than plant oils, are a more appropriate source of these fatty acids. Many marine plants, especially algae in phytoplankton, carry out chain elongation and desaturation of α-linolenic acid to yield omega-3 (n-3) fatty acids with 20 and 22 carbon atoms and five or six double bonds. Formation of these long-chain omega-3 fatty acids by marine algae and their transfer through the food chain to fish accounts for the abundance of eicosapentaenoic acid (EPA, 20:5n-3) and DHA in certain marine fish oils.

Arachidonic acid and EPA act as precursors for the synthesis of eicosanoids, a significant group of immunoregulatory molecules that functions as local hormones and mediators of inflammation. The amounts and types of eicosanoids synthesized are determined by the availability of the fatty acid precursor and by the activities of the enzyme systems that synthesize them. In most conditions, the principal precursor for these compounds is arachidonic acid, although EPA competes with arachidonic acid for the same enzyme systems. The eicosanoids produced from arachidonic acid are proinflammatory and when produced in excess amounts may result in pathologic conditions. In contrast, eicosanoids derived from EPA promote minimal to no inflammatory activity. Ingestion of oils containing omega-3 fatty acids results in a decrease in membrane arachidonic acid levels because omega-3 fatty acids replace arachidonic acid in the substrate pool. This produces an accompanying decrease in the capacity to synthesize eicosanoids from arachidonic acid (**Figure 34-5**). Studies have documented that inflammatory eicosanoids produced from arachidonic acid are depressed when dogs consume foods with high levels of omega-3 fatty acids (Wander et al, 1997).

The effect of dietary fish oil on the expression and activity of matrix metalloproteinases (MMP), tissue inhibitors of MMP-2 and urokinase plasminogen activator in synovial fluid from

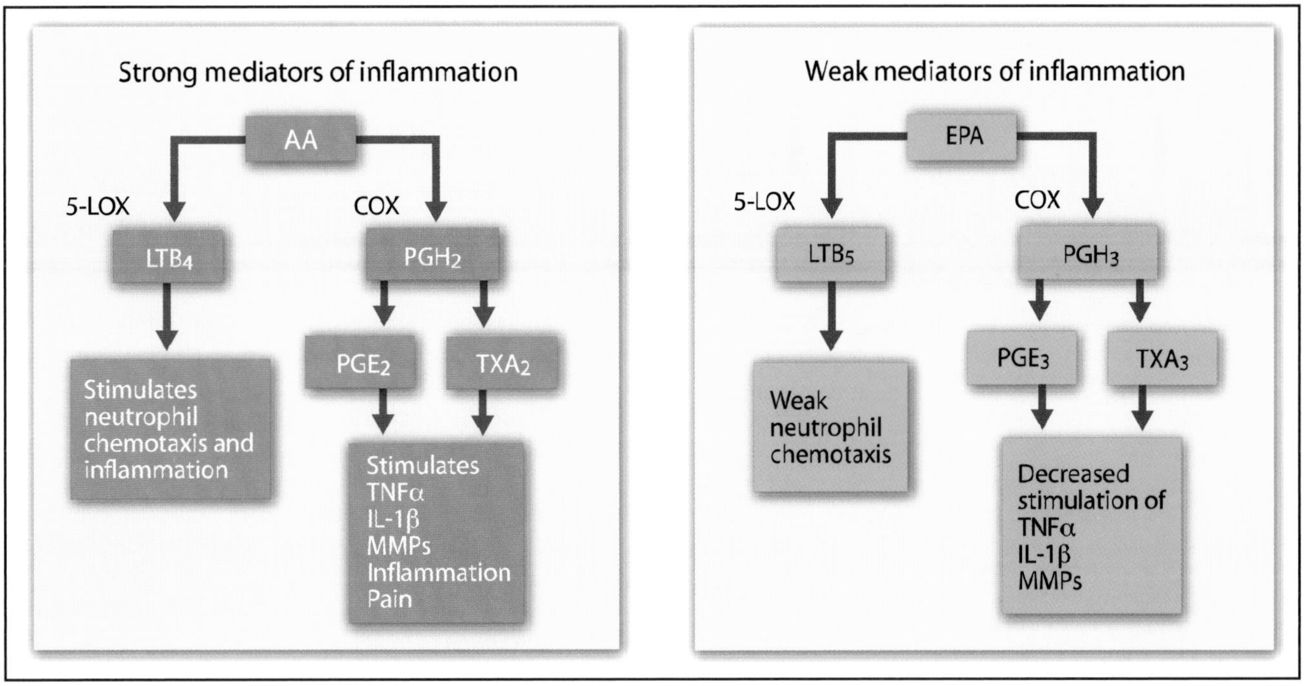

Figure 34-5. Eicosapentaenoic acid (EPA) competes with arachidonic acid (AA) for cyclooxygenase (COX) and lipoxygenase (5-LOX) pathways. Eicosanoids produced from AA are strong mediators of inflammation whereas those derived from EPA promote minimal to no inflammatory activity (sometimes referred to as antiinflammatory). Key: AA = arachidonic acid, LOX = lipoxygenase, COX = cyclooxygenase, LTB = leukotrienes, PGH/PGE = prostaglandins, TXA = thromboxanes, TNF = tumor necrosis factor, MMP = matrix metalloproteinase.

dogs with acute cranial cruciate ligament injury has been evaluated (Hansen et al, 2008). Two groups of 12 dogs with spontaneous cranial cruciate ligament injury were randomized to receive either a fish oil-supplemented food or control food from one week before surgery on the affected knee to 56 days postsurgery. The fish oil and control foods provided 90 and 4.5 mg of combined EPA and DHA/kg body weight per day, respectively. There were no changes in these biomarkers in the synovial fluid from the surgical joint at any time during the study. The authors suggested that the severe inflammation from cranial cruciate ligament injury and subsequent surgery was too great to be affected by the combined levels of EPA/DHA provided in the test food. However, dogs randomized to the fish oil food group had episodic but significantly ($p < 0.05$) decreased pro-matrix metalloproteinases and urokinase plasminogen activator and increased tissue inhibitors of MMP-2 in the synovial fluid from the nonsurgical knee. The fish oil food may have moderated the mild to moderate inflammation in the nonsurgical knee through suppression of inflammatory cytokines by EPA and DHA.

Reducing the production of proinflammatory mediators is only one mechanism by which omega-3 fatty acids promote the termination of inflammation and the return to homeostasis. Although it is true that the inflammatory response is essential to health and disease, sustained inflammatory responses are generally detrimental to the host. In people, in modern western civilization, unresolved inflammation has emerged as a central component of many diseases (e.g., arthritis, periodontal disease, cardiovascular disease, cancer and Alzheimer's disease) (Schwab and Serhan, 2006). Research has demonstrated that resolution of inflammation is an active, endogenous process aimed at protecting the individual from an excessive inflammatory response. The first endogenous local counter-regulatory mediators recognized were the lipoxins, which are derived from arachidonic acid (Serhan, 2005). Subsequently, two new families of lipid mediators derived from omega-3 fatty acids, resolvins and protectins, have been identified. Resolvins derived from EPA are denoted as resolvins of the E series (RvEs) and those derived from DHA acid are resolvins of the D series (RvDs) and protectins. These bioactive mediators have potent antiinflammatory, neuroprotective and pro-resolving properties (Schwab and Serhan, 2006). Further elucidation of the molec-

Table 34-2. Key nutritional factors for foods for canine osteoarthritis patients.*

Factors	Dietary recommendations
Total omega-3 fatty acids	3.5 to 4.0%
Eicosapentaenoic acid	0.4 to1.1%
Omega-6:omega-3 fatty acid ratio	<1:1
L-carnitine	≥300 mg/kg
Glucosamine HCl	≤0.10%
Chondroitin sulfate	≤0.08%
Antioxidants	
Vitamin E	≥400 IU/kg
Vitamin C	≥100 mg/kg
Selenium	0.5 to 1.3 mg/kg
Phosphorus**	0.3 to 0.7%
Sodium**	0.2 to 0.4%

*All values are expressed on a dry matter basis unless otherwise stated.
**Dogs with osteoarthritis are often in age groups at risk for kidney and/or heart disease.

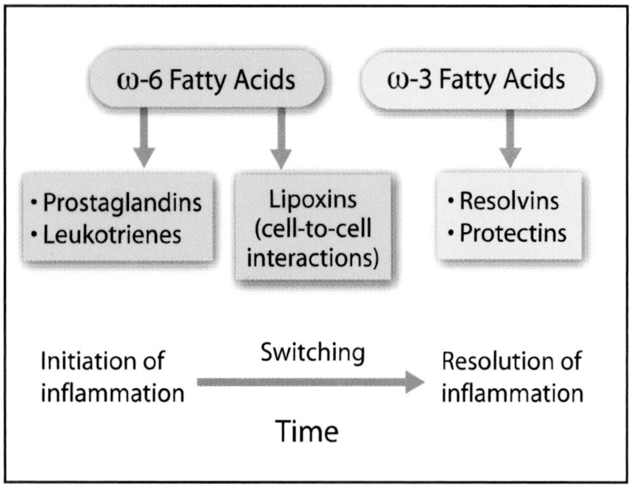

Figure 34-6. The role of omega-6 and omega-3 fatty acids in the initiation and resolution of inflammation over time. Resolution of inflammation is a progressive process involving a switch in the production of lipid-derived mediators over time. Pro-inflammatory products of omega-6 fatty acid metabolism (PGE2, PGE12, LTB4) are thought to initiate this sequence. Arachidonic acid-derived mediators foster the extravasation and homing of inflammatory cells at the site of the lesion. Cell-to-cell interactions exemplified by platelet-leukocytes within the vasculature and/or PMN-mucosal interactions enhance generation of lipoxins. With time, a class shift occurs towards domination by pro-resolving omega-3 derived mediators (resolvins, protectins). These mediators serve as endogenous stop signals by preventing inflammatory cell recruitment and stopping "cell entry" and promoting resolution by removing inflammatory cells from the lesion site through phagocytosis of PMNs and promotion of "cell exit." Key: PGE = prostaglandin, LTB = leukotriene. (Adapted from Schwab JM, Serhan CN. Lipoxins and new lipid mediators in the resolution of inflammation. Current Opinion in Pharmacology 2006; 6: 414-420.)

ular actions of these previously unappreciated families of lipid-derived mediators may shed light on the clinically recognized beneficial effects of omega-3 fatty acids (**Figure 34-6**).

The interaction between nutrients found in certain foods and the expression of genes responsible for certain disease conditions is known as nutrigenomics (Chapter 4). Progression from a healthy to a disease state occurs through changes in gene expression, which can be influenced through ingestion of specific nutrients. The capacity of specific omega-3 fatty acids (EPA in dogs) to alter the expression of genes responsible for progression of cartilage degradation is an example of one application of nutrigenomics to pet foods.

Mechanisms of cartilage metabolism in canine osteoarthritis and the potential role of omega-3 fatty acids to ameliorate the early events in the disease have been investigated using in vitro models. These studies identified some similarities and distinct differences between cartilage from dogs and other species in the response to catabolic agents and omega-3 fatty acids. Numerous catabolic agents significantly decreased canine cartilage proteoglycan synthesis. However, proteolysis and loss of aggrecan could only be stimulated by oncostatin M, leukemia inhibitory factor and retinoic acid. Stimulated aggrecan loss was associated with increased cleavage by aggrecanases and not matrix metalloproteinases. EPA was the only omega-3 fatty acid able to significantly decrease the oncostatin M-stimulated loss of aggrecan in the canine cartilage in vitro model (Caterson, 2005; Caterson et al, 2000; Curtis et al, 2002). In canine cartilage, EPA inhibits the up regulation of aggrecanases by blocking the signal at the level of messenger RNA (Curtis et al, 2000). Altering the expression of this messenger RNA signal by EPA is an example of how nutrigenomics can aid in the management of disease.

The application of nutrigenomic concepts can be applied to foods designed to aid in the nutritional management of osteoarthritis. Ideally, these foods should control clinical signs and moderate the progression of the disease and their efficacy should be demonstrated in well-controlled clinical studies. One veterinary therapeutic food[c] designed to aid in the management of osteoarthritis in dogs has been evaluated in multiple clinical studies. Specifically, four randomized, double-masked, controlled studies were completed in arthritic dogs fed either a control or test food. The foods had similar nutrient content with the exception of total levels of omega-3 fatty acids: 0.09% (dry matter [DM]) control vs. 3.48% DM test food and levels of EPA less than 0.01% DM vs. 0.38% DM, respectively. The ratio of omega-6 to omega-3 fatty acids was also markedly different in the two foods: 22.8:1 in the control vs. 0.7:1 in the test food (**Table 34-3**). Pet owners were given the option of feeding dry or a combination of moist and dry foods. One six-month and two three-month prospective studies were conducted in veterinary hospitals across the United States.[d-f] A fourth study was conducted as a three-month prospective study in two academic specialty practices in the United States.[g]

In all studies, osteoarthritis was diagnosed based on compatible history, clinical signs and radiographic evidence of arthritis in one or more joints of the clinically affected limb. To be eligible for inclusion, dogs had to be at least one year of age, weigh 12.5 kg or more, consume at least some dry dog food and be free of systemic disease as determined by history, physical examination, complete blood count, serum biochemistry analysis and urinalysis. Exclusion criteria included acute traumatic injuries, complicating disease conditions, preexisting conditions for which corrective surgery was anticipated during the feeding period and recent intraarticular injection or arthrocentesis.

Change in arthritic condition over time was evaluated in these studies and was based on owner observations of clinical signs and veterinary clinical evaluations. Variables were assessed at the beginning of the study and at set time intervals after onset of feeding the control or therapeutic food. Additionally, veterinary clinical evaluations were conducted at each time interval. These consisted of an orthopedic examination with a specific emphasis on lameness and pain, limitation in weight-bearing ability, range of motion of the affected joint(s) and willingness to bear weight on the most affected limb when the contralateral limb was elevated.

Investigators in the three studies conducted in veterinary hospitals[d-f] reported that the animals fed the EPA-supplemented food improved in several parameters throughout the studies. Veterinarians reported improvement in range of motion and ability to bear weight, along with a decrease in pain (upon palpation of the affected joint) and lameness as compared to evaluations of these dogs before they participated in the studies. Dogs fed the EPA-supplemented food had significantly ($p < 0.05$) improved ability to rise from a resting position, in running and playing at six weeks and improvements in walking at 12 and 24 weeks compared to dogs fed the control food.

In the academic specialty practice clinical study,[g] variables were assessed at the beginning of the study and at 45 and 90 days after onset of feeding the control or test food. Additionally, gait analyses using a computerized biomechanical force plate were conducted at the same time intervals. For each dog, five valid force-plate trials were obtained during each test period for the most severely affected and ipsilateral limbs. Orthogonal ground reaction forces of peak vertical force, vertical impulse, braking and propulsion peak force and braking and propulsive force were measured and recorded. All forces were normalized with respect to body weight in kg. Data from valid trials for each limb were averaged to obtain a mean value at each time period.

On clinical orthopedic examination, a significantly ($p < 0.05$) greater percent of dogs consuming the test food were evaluated as "improved" vs. those consuming the control food. In addition, more dogs in the test group had a reduction in pain at the end of the 90-day trial when the affected joint was palpated. Vertical peak force was the key parameter measured to determine weight bearing of affected limbs. There was no significant change in mean peak force over the duration of the 90-day feeding trial for the control group. The mean vertical peak force increased significantly ($p = 0.01$) for the test group over the same time interval. The percent mean change in vertical peak force was also significantly ($p = 0.04$) different between groups, indicating that the test group increased weight bearing on the affected limb over the course of the study. Additionally, only 31% of dogs in the control group had improved weight bearing after the 90-day feeding trial, whereas 82% of dogs in the test group increased weight bearing; this difference was also statistically significant ($p = 0.003$).

These clinical studies indicate that nutritional management using a veterinary therapeutic food supplemented with omega-3 fatty acids helped improve the clinical signs of osteoarthritis in dogs as noted by pet owners, clinical orthopedic examination and gait analysis of ground reaction forces. Based on these studies, a food designed to aid in the management of osteoarthritis in dogs should provide levels of total omega-3 fatty acids between 3.5 to 4.0% DM and specifically 0.4 to 1.1% DM EPA. The omega-6 to omega-3 fatty acid ratio should be less than 1:1. Dogs consuming the therapeutic food should receive an average of 50 to 100 mg EPA/kg body weight/day.

Supplements have traditionally been used to provide a source of omega-3 fatty acids to pets. However, using supplements to provide levels of EPA documented to have a clinical effect may prove cumbersome. Many supplements designed to provide omega-3 and omega-6 fatty acids are available in both human and veterinary formulations. Concentrations in these supplements range from 50 to 375 mg of EPA per dose. To achieve EPA concentrations of 50 mg/kg body weight/day, a 27-kg dog would require four to 27 doses of a supplement (**Table 34-4**). Long-term compliance with this dosing regimen is likely to be poor. Providing a food with the recommended levels of EPA and total omega-3 fatty acids is preferable and likely improves compliance.

One study in osteoarthritic geriatric cats evaluated the effects of feeding an omega-3 fatty acid-supplemented food on cartilage protection (Yamka et al, 2006). Increased levels of EPA (3.2% DM), DHA (0.23% DM), methionine (1.32% DM) and manganese (104 mg/kg DM) and no synthetic glucosamine or chondroitin sulfate were associated with decreased values for arthritic biomarkers in these cats. Changes in clinical signs were not noted during the 60-day study.

Anecdotally, radiographic signs of osteoarthritis in cats have been managed with a combination of calorie restriction plus supplementation of the food with omega-3 fatty acids (75 to 110 mg/kg body weight/day). Over eight weeks of evaluation, there were no changes in radiographic appearance, but therapy resulted in a more natural gait and increased voluntary activity

Table 34-3. Nutrient comparison of control and test foods.*

Nutrients	Control food	Test food**
Protein (%)	23.2	20.0
Fat (%)	13.9	13.6
NFE (%)	54.7	53.3
Total omega-3 fatty acids (%)	0.09	3.48
EPA (%)	<0.01	0.38
Omega-6:omega-3 fatty acid ratio	22.8	0.7

Key: NFE = nitrogen-free extract (digestible carbohydrate), EPA = eicosapentaenoic acid.
*All values are expressed on a dry matter basis unless otherwise stated.
**Prescription Diet j/d Canine dry. Hill's Pet Nutrition, Inc., Topeka, KS, USA.

Table 34-4. Fatty acid concentration of a therapeutic food vs. supplements for a 27-kg dog.

	Therapeutic food* (4 cups)	GNC Preventative Nutrition Multi Oil Formula (300 mg/capsule)	3V Caps for Large & Giant Breeds (DVM Pharmaceuticals) (1,488 mg capsule)	Welactin (Nutramax) Liquid (1.5 ml/pump)
EPA content	1,578 mg	180 mg/capsule	250 mg/capsule	97-120 mg/pump
Amount/day to equal intake from j/d Canine	-	9 capsules	6 capsules	13 pumps

Key: EPA = eicosapentaenoic acid.
*Prescription Diet j/d Canine dry. Hill's Pet Nutrition, Inc., Topeka, KS, USA.

(Saker, 2006). This treatment is similar to protocols recommended for management of dogs with osteoarthritis. Adverse effects on platelet function have been reported in cats fed a food with a 1.3:1 omega-6 to omega-3 ratio (1.03 g omega-3 fatty acids/kg food), but not in cats fed a food with 12:1 omega-6 to omega-3 ratio (0.07 g omega-3 fatty acids/kg food) (Saker et al, 1998). More studies are needed to confirm these findings; however, based on results in other species, providing enhanced levels of omega-3 fatty acids to cats with osteoarthritis seems promising.

L-Carnitine

Maintaining a healthy weight throughout life will delay the onset and minimize clinical signs of osteoarthritis. Achieving an ideal body weight in dogs diagnosed with osteoarthritis will improve clinical signs and long-term management. Paradoxically, many dogs diagnosed with osteoarthritis are either overweight or obese prone as a result of breed, age and/or decreased activity. One key nutrient in weight loss and weight maintenance foods is L-carnitine. It plays a vital role in a variety of physiologic processes related to fat metabolism and energy production; specifically L-carnitine mediates the transfer of long-chain fatty acids into mitochondria. This action promotes oxidation of fatty acids as an energy source. Perhaps more importantly, weight-loss foods with appropriate levels of L-carnitine (≥300 mg/kg DM) aid in the retention of lean body mass during weight loss in dogs (Allen, 1998). Additionally, L-carnitine supplementation of obese-prone dogs led to a reduction in fat mass and increase in lean body mass through an extended feeding period (Gross, 1998). Obese cats supplemented with L-carnitine have been reported to lose weight faster and have less ketogenesis (Center et al, 2000), suggesting that increasing the L-carnitine level of foods for cats at risk for becoming overweight, such as after neutering, could be beneficial. Because lean tissue uses more calories than fat, increased lean body mass is desirable for long-term maintenance of an ideal body weight in dogs and cats. Achieving and maintaining a healthy weight is critical to the successful management of osteoarthritis.

Because many patients with osteoarthritis need support to achieve or maintain a healthy body weight and L-carnitine supports both weight loss and maintenance of weight after weight loss, foods intended for the dietary management of osteoarthritis should contain at least 300 mg of L-carnitine/kg DM.

Chondroitin Sulfate and Glucosamine Hydrochloride

Chondroitin sulfate is a GAG consisting of repeating disaccharide subunits of glucuronic acid and N-acetylgalactosamine sulfate (Schoenherr, 2005). Commercially available chondroitin sulfate is generally derived from bovine cartilage. However, porcine and chicken cartilage and chondroitin from perna mussels and algae have also been used. Chondroitin sulfate decreases interleukin-1 production, blocks complement activation, inhibits metalloproteinases, inhibits histamine-mediated inflammation and stimulates GAG production and collagen synthesis (Beale, 2004). Both the molecular weight and species of derivation affect the bioavailability of chondroitin sulfate products. The low molecular weight form appears to be absorbed more readily. Some sources such as perna mussels contain only trace amounts of high molecular weight chondroitin sulfate and avian sources have not proven any more effective than placebo (Millis, 2006). **Box 34-1** contains additional information about commercially available glucosamine and chondroitin sulfate products.

Glucosamine hydrochloride is one of the basic sugar component precursors of the disaccharide units that make up all of the glycosaminoglycans in cartilage. Proposed mechanisms of action of glucosamine include a reduction of proteoglycan degradation and inhibition of the synthesis and activity of degradative enzymes (aggrecanases/matrix metalloproteinases) and inflammatory mediators (nitric oxide and prostaglandin E_2). Anabolic effects include stimulation of GAG and proteoglycan production (Neil et al, 2005). Glucosamine hydrochloride and glucosamine sulfate appear to be more efficacious than N-acetylglucosamine.

Glucosamine hydrochloride and chondroitin sulfate, taken in appropriate doses, are considered safe for dogs and cats. Safety studies of one proprietary formulation using oral administration in excess of the recommended daily dose for 30 days documented no clinically important alterations in hematologic indices or biochemistry and clotting profiles in dogs and cats (McNamara et al, 1996; McNamara et al, 2000). Although no coagulation abnormalities were recognized, because of the structural similarities of glycosaminoglycans and heparin, the concurrent use of other platelet inhibitors, such as phenylbutazone or aspirin, may be contraindicated. Some dogs and cats may experience mild gastrointestinal upset, which can be managed by offering the product with a meal.

Meta-analysis of randomized, double-blind, placebo-controlled studies evaluating the effectiveness of glucosamine and chondroitin sulfate supplements in people demonstrated moderate to large reductions of pain and disability in osteoarthritis compared with placebo; however, these effects may have been exaggerated as a result of publication bias. Greater effects have been detected for chondroitin sulfate than glucosamine (McAlindon et al, 2000). The Glucosamine/Chondroitin Arthritis Intervention Trial (GAIT) evaluated over 1,500 human participants with osteoarthritis of the knee who were randomly assigned to one of five treatment groups: 1) glucosamine alone, 2) chondroitin sulfate alone, 3) glucosamine and chondroitin sulfate in combination, 4) celecoxib or 5) a placebo. Patients were assessed at intervals over six months. Patients taking the positive control (i.e., celecoxib) experienced statistically significant pain relief vs. placebo. Overall, there were no significant differences between the other treatments tested and placebo. For a subset of participants with moderate-to-severe pain, glucosamine combined with chondroitin sulfate provided statistically significant ($p = 0.002$) pain relief compared to placebo. According to the researchers, because of the small size of this subgroup, these findings should be considered preliminary and need to be confirmed in further studies. For participants in the mild pain subset, glucosamine and chondroitin sulfate together or alone did not provide statistically sig-

Box 34-1. All Nutraceutical "Chondroprotective Agents" Are Not Created Equal.

Veterinary nutraceuticals have been defined as "a non-drug substance that is produced in a purified or extracted form and administered orally to a patient to provide agents required for normal body structure and function and administered with the intent of improving the health and well-being of animals." Because the term nutraceutical has no regulatory definition and is not recognized by the FDA, these products are not subject to a pre-market approval process. As a result the safety, efficacy and manufacturing quality of these products cannot be ensured and there is evidence that this lack of regulatory oversight should be of concern to consumers.

In the United States, although there is no mandatory regulatory oversight, manufacturers of nutraceuticals can voluntarily submit their products for quality assurance. A variety of independent groups such as Consumer Laboratory (www.consumerlab.com) and the Institute for Nutraceutical Advancement (www.nsf.org) or trade associations such as the National Animal Supplement Council (www.nasc.cc) provide independent quality assurance testing and certification programs. The two substances most commonly used for treatment of osteoarthritis in veterinary medicine are glucosamine HCl and chondroitin sulfate either alone or in combination. Chondroitin sulfate is an expensive ingredient of many "joint" targeted products and serves as an example of the need for careful evaluation of these unregulated products.

A 1999 study partially funded by Nutramax Laboratories found that 26 of 32 (81%) commercially available human products contained less than 90% of the chondroitin sulfate stated on the label and 17 (53%) of those products contained less than 40% of label claim. This study documented that products costing ≤$1/1,200 mg chondroitin sulfate were critically deficient; on average less than 10% of the label claim. Interestingly, expense did not guarantee content because several of the most expensive products also contained less than 10% of label claim (**Figure 1**). ConsumerLab.com (accessed 11/16/06) found similar problems with glucosamine HCl/chondroitin sulfate combination products. Initially, on November 2, 2003, two of three veterinary combination products evaluated were found to have no chondroitin sulfate despite each displaying a "guaranteed analysis." One of these companies has since produced a re-formulated product that did pass Consumer Lab testing. Glucosamine hydrochloride, unlike chondroitin sulfate, is much more likely to be present in the amounts indicated on product labels. Information about specific products and testing procedures can be accessed at the Consumer Lab website for a fee. Because of these inconsistencies, consumers are cautioned against extrapolating results from clinical and experimental studies comparing one product to other similar products. Based on this information, when prescribing nutraceuticals, preference should be given to those products whose quality assurance and efficacy can be verified.

The Bibliography for **Box 34-1** can be found at www.markmorris.org.

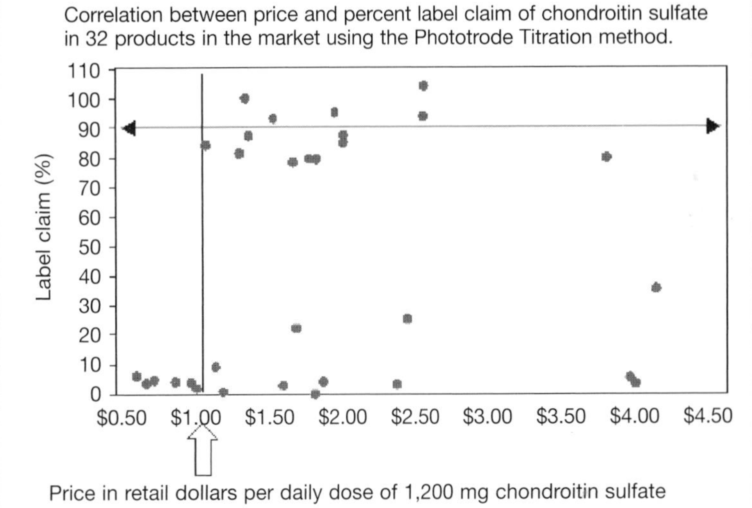

Figure 1. Relationship between products' label claims and standard retail prices. (Adapted from Adebowale AO, Cox DS, Liang Z, et al. Analysis of glucosamine and chondroitin sulfate content in marketed products and the Caco-2 permeability of chondroitin sulfate raw materials. Journal of the American Nutraceutical Association 2000; 3(1): 37-44.)

nificant pain relief (Clegg et al, 2006). The authors also noted that the elevated placebo response seen in this study may have dampened the ability to differentiate among the treatments (60% of patients receiving placebos had at least a 20% decrease in pain scores after 24 weeks) (Clegg et al, 2006). These studies suggest that glucosamine and chondroitin sulfate may offer clinically relevant reductions in pain for some patients with osteoarthritis. However, despite a large number of clinical trails in human medicine, there is still no consensus about the effectiveness of these compounds. In veterinary medicine, there is a lack of consensus and a lack of clinical trials to evaluate.

In veterinary medicine, claims of efficacy for glucosamine/chondroitin sulfate supplements are often based on subjective methods of assessment, in vitro testing or testimonials. Two studies evaluated the efficacy of supplements containing the combination of glucosamine/chondroitin sulfate in client-owned dogs with naturally occurring osteoarthritis compared to positive controls. These two trials evaluated 106 dogs with confirmed osteoarthritis. Nonsteroidal antiinflammatory drugs (carprofen and meloxicam) were used for positive controls. One study evaluated ground reaction forces and subjective owner and veterinary evaluations in 71 dogs randomized to receive meloxicam, carprofen, a combination glucosamine/chondroitin sulfate product or placebo (Moreau et al, 2003). After 60 days, dogs in the meloxicam and carprofen groups had improved ground reaction forces and clinical improvement. Owners noted subjective improvement only in the meloxicam group; dogs in the glucosamine/chondroitin sulfate and placebo groups were not different on any evaluation at the conclusion of the study. In the second study, subjective veterinary and owner evaluations were used to assess 35 dogs randomized to receive either a combination of glucosamine/chondroitin sulfate supplement or carprofen for 70 days (McCarthy et al, 2007). Dogs in the carprofen group improved in all five parameters with the onset for some parameters occurring as early as 14 days. Dogs in the glucosamine/chondroitin sulfate group showed significant ($p < 0.001$) improvements at the conclusion of the study in pain, weight bearing and overall condition compared to pre-treatment evaluations, but no improvement in lameness or joint mobility. One explanation for the lack of improvement in lameness and joint mobility may be the insensitivity of the subjective scoring system in dogs with mild disease (low scores). The strong positive correlation ($rs > 0.55$) between the pre-treatment disease score and the Day 70 change score ($p < 0.02$) for all parameters independent of treatment group suggests that dogs with higher pre-treatment scores tended to have higher positive changes in their scores. The authors suggested that future clinical studies evaluating glucosamine and chondroitin sulfate should monitor dogs for a minimum of 70 days and include an objective measurement of lameness such as force-plate gait analysis. In addition to these two studies, numerous uncontrolled studies, anecdotal evidence and case reports support the use of glucosamine and chondroitin sulfate (Anderson et al, 1999; Hoffman, 2001; Lippiello and Prudhomme, 2005; Moore, 1996).

Beneficial effects of glucosamine and chondroitin sulfate alone and in combination have been documented in in vitro studies in several species, but to date, well-designed clinical studies in dogs and cats with naturally occurring disease are sparse. The current evidence suggesting beneficial effects warrants further investigation into the mechanism of actions, pharmacokinetics and possible disease-modifying activities of these compounds. Addition of glucosamine and chondroitin sulfate to a therapeutic food for dogs with osteoarthritis seems safe and potentially beneficial.

Dosages can be based on studies documenting positive effects with supplements. Currently the best evidence in dogs suggests that providing glucosamine HCl at approximately 25 to 50 mg/kg body weight/day and chondroitin sulfate at approximately 15 to 40 mg/kg body weight/day may benefit some patients with osteoarthritis (McCarthy et al, 2007; Moreau et al, 2003). Glucosamine HCl and chondroitin sulfate are not currently included in the federal GRAS (Generally Recognized as Safe) listing. Furthermore, the Association of American Feed Control Officials (AAFCO) does not provide limits for inclusion levels in commercial foods sold in the United States. However, at least one regulatory agency has provided upper limits for intake of these substances in foods sold in its state. On that basis, glucosamine HCl and chondroitin sulfate should not exceed 15 mg and 12 mg/kg body weight/day, respectively.[h] Based on anticipated food intake for dogs whose daily energy requirement (DER) is 1.8 times their resting energy requirement, and in a food with an energy density of 4 kcal/g DM, glucosamine HCl and chondroitin sulfate should not exceed 0.10 and 0.08% DM, respectively.

Antioxidants

Free radicals are chemically unstable molecules that contain an unpaired free electron. Byproducts of mitochondrial respiration are the primary source of free radicals in mammals. In health, the potential destructive effects of free radials are mitigated by endogenous antioxidant systems. Imbalances between the concentrations of free radicals and availability of antioxidant defenses may be related to a variety of processes such as aging, cancer, diabetes mellitus, lupus and arthritis (Budsberg and Bartges, 2006). Chapter 7 discusses antioxidants in detail.

The generation of free radicals in synoviocytes and chondrocytes is an important factor in the development and maintenance of rheumatoid arthritis in people and animal models (Darlington and Stone, 2001). Free radicals are also implicated in aging of cartilage and in the pathogenesis of osteoarthritis. Increased oxidative activity in chondrocytes has a damaging effect on matrix, which may play an important role in matrix degradation, which is characteristic of osteoarthritis. Studies in animal models indicate that antioxidants can prevent matrix degradation and therefore may have a preventive or therapeutic value in osteoarthritis (Tiku et al, 1999). Clinical response to antioxidant supplements has been demonstrated in people with rheumatoid arthritis and osteoarthritis (Budsberg and Bartges, 2006). Methyl-sulfonyl-methane (MSM), a sulfur donor, and a normal oxidation product of dimethyl sulfoxide (DMSO), has not been studied in dogs and cats, but has been reported to be of benefit in the treatment of many human disorders including osteoarthritis (Parcell, 2002). The rationale for its use lies in the possibility of a dietary sulfur deficiency, with a resultant deficiency of sulfur-containing compounds in the body, such as antioxidants and chondroitin sulfate (Parcell, 2002). Additionally, organic sulfur as sulfur-containing amino acids can theoretically be used for the formation of connective tissue and repair of damaged protein. Damaged cartilage from osteoarthritic human patients has been shown to have approximately one-third the concentration of sulfur as normal cartilage (Rizzo et al, 1995). In a human study of 16 patients with osteoarthritis, 10 patients were randomly selected to receive 2,250 mg of MSM per day for a six-week trial; eight of the 10 patients experienced some relief of ostearthritis symptoms compared to placebo controls (Lawrence and Lignisul, 2002). A study in rats, administered MSM at 5 to 7 times the maximum recommended human dose as a single gavage of 2 g/kg or as a daily dose of 1.5 g/kg for 90 days, resulted in no adverse effects and was well-tolerated (Horvath et al, 2002).

Although there are no controlled studies in dogs or cats specifically assessing the efficacy of dietary antioxidants, there is a growing scientific rationale for their use as adjuncts in the treatment of inflammatory disorders including osteoarthritis. Thus, antioxidants are also recommended for inclusion in foods for general health.

The body synthesizes many antioxidants but relies on food

for others. The following discussion will focus on vitamins E and C and selenium as antioxidant key nutritional factors for foods for osteoarthritis because: 1) they are biologically important, 2) they act synergistically (e.g., vitamin C and selenium-containing glutathione peroxidase regenerate vitamin E after it has reacted with a free radical), 3) much is known about their safety and 4) information regarding inclusion levels in pet foods is usually available.

VITAMIN E

Vitamin E is the main lipid-soluble antioxidant present in plasma, erythrocytes and tissues (NRC, 2006). It is one of the most effective antioxidants for protecting cell membrane constituent polyunsaturated fatty acids from oxidation. Vitamin E inhibits lipid oxidation by scavenging lipid peroxyl radicals much faster than these radicals can react with adjacent fatty acids or with membrane proteins (Gutteridge and Halliwell, 1994).

Research indicates that a level of vitamin E higher than the requirement confers specific biologic benefits (Hayes et al, 1969; Hall et al, 2003; Meydani et al, 1998; Jewell et al, 2002). Based on antioxidant biomarker studies in dogs and cats, for improved antioxidant performance, veterinary therapeutic foods for osteoarthritis should contain at least 400 IU/kg DM (dog foods) and at least 500 IU/kg DM (cat foods) (Jewell et al, 2000).

VITAMIN C

Vitamin C is the most powerful reducing agent available to cells. Ascorbic acid: 1) regenerates oxidized vitamin E, glutathione and flavonoids, 2) quenches free radicals both intra- and extracellularly, 3) protects against free radical-mediated protein inactivation associated with oxidative bursts of neutrophils, 4) maintains transition metals in reduced form and 5) may quench free radical intermediates of carcinogen metabolism.

Although dogs and cats can synthesize enough vitamin C to fulfill minimum requirements (Innes, 1931; Naismith, 1958), in vitro studies indicated that both species have from one-quarter to one-tenth the ability to synthesize vitamin C as other mammals (Chatterjee et al, 1975). Whether or not this translates to a reduced ability in vivo is unknown. For improved antioxidant performance, and in conjunction with levels of vitamin E recommended above, foods for adult dogs and cats should contain at least 100 mg vitamin C/kg DM.

SELENIUM

Glutathione peroxidase is a selenium-containing antioxidant enzyme that defends tissues against oxidative stress by catalyzing the reduction of H_2O_2 and organic hydroperoxides and by regenerating vitamin E. The minimum requirement for selenium in foods for dogs and cats is 0.13 mg/kg DM (Wedekind et al, 2002; Wedekind et al, 2003). Animal studies and clinical intervention trials in people have shown selenium to be anticarcinogenic at levels much higher (five to 10 times) than the recommended allowances for people or the minimal requirements for animals (Combs, 2001; Neve, 2002). Therefore, for increased antioxidant benefits, the recommended range of selenium for dog and cat foods is 0.5 to 1.3 mg/kg DM.

Phosphorus, Sodium and Urinary pH

Because foods for osteoarthritis patients are fed in the place of regular maintenance foods and general health is the overall goal, key nutritional factors unrelated to osteoarthritis should also be considered. Besides being a risk factor for osteoarthritis, age is a risk factor for kidney and heart disease in dogs and cats. Phosphorus and sodium are considered key nutritional factors for apparently healthy adult dogs and cats for purposes of ameliorating or slowing the progression of subclinical kidney and heart disease. Phosphorus levels in foods for older dogs and cats should be within the range of 0.3 to 0.7% DM and 0.5 to 0.7% DM, respectively. Sodium levels should be between 0.2 to 0.4% DM for dog and cat foods. Urinary pH in older cats should be somewhat higher than for young cats (i.e., in the range of 6.4 to 6.6). For detailed discussions of the rationale for the inclusion of these key nutritional factors in foods for middle-aged to older dogs and cats, see Chapters 13 and 14 (dogs) and Chapters 20 and 21 (cats). These key nutritional factors are listed in **Table 34-2** along with the key nutritional factors for managing osteoarthritis.

FEEDING PLAN

Providing appropriate nutrition during growth and maintaining a healthy weight throughout life will minimize the expression of underlying genetic tendencies for the development of osteoarthritis. Current evidence suggests that the manifestation of developmental orthopedic diseases is affected by rate of growth, specific nutrients, food consumption and feeding methods (Chapter 33). Nutrition during growth of large- and giant-breed dogs requires providing nutrients in appropriate amounts and balances for optimal bone development. Excesses of calcium and energy, together with rapid growth, appear to predispose dogs to certain musculoskeletal disorders such as osteochondrosis and CHD (Hedhammar et al, 1974; Meyer and Zentek, 1991). Refer to Chapter 33 for additional information about nutritional management to prevent developmental orthopedic diseases of dogs.

Developmental orthopedic diseases have also been recognized in cats. Because cats seldom present with clinical signs referable to hip lameness, hip dysplasia in cats has received little attention. However, hip dysplasia has been documented in cats. Over a 21-year period (1974 to 1995) 21% of 284 radiographs of Maine Coon cats submitted for evaluation to the OFA were judged dysplastic. A 6.6% incidence of hip dysplasia was documented in 684 cats of various breeds. Much like in dogs, the frequency appears to be breed dependent with increased risks in Siamese, Persian and Himalayan breeds (Keller et al, 1999). A cross-sectional prevalence study designed to evaluate simultaneous patellar luxation and hip dysplasia in 78 cats of various breeds reported a 32% incidence of hip dysplasia, 58% incidence of patellar luxation and 24% incidence of concurrent hip dysplasia and patellar luxation (Smith et al,

Box 34-2. Physical Rehabilitation for Osteoarthritis.

The chronic pain associated with osteoarthritis often results in diminished use of the affected joints. With disuse, muscle mass, tone and function are typically reduced. As a result, added stress is placed on arthritic joints during locomotion. This creates additional pain and dysfunction, which may lead to immobility of the joint. Mobility is one of the most important aspects of a patient's quality of life and severe limitations may be a cause for elective euthanasia. Lack of mobility may also contribute to obesity or complicate weight-reduction protocols. Physical rehabilitation has been successfully used to manage pain and improve mobility in human osteoarthritis patients. In canine patients, physical rehabilitation has been evaluated and shown to be beneficial in laboratory and clinical settings.

The goals of physical rehabilitation programs include protecting and promoting mobility, assisting weight-reduction protocols and reducing joint pain. A variety of treatments are available including passive therapeutic options (cold therapy, heat therapy, stretching, massage and electrical stimulation), therapeutic exercises (land or water based) and the use of ambulation assistance devices.

Weight reduction in arthritic patients can be challenging. Successful weight-management programs typically include recommendations to increase exercise. This may be difficult for some arthritic patients. One study evaluated the effects of combining an intense physical rehabilitation program with a weight-reduction program in overweight dogs with osteoarthritis. The duration of the study was six months. Twenty-nine client-owned overweight dogs with clinical and radiographic evidence of osteoarthritis were randomized to participate in a weight-control program with a home-based physiotherapy protocol alone (Group 1) or a weight-control program with a home-based physiotherapy protocol with an additional intensive clinic-based physiotherapy program including transcutaneous electrical nerve stimulation (TENS) (Group 2). The combination of caloric restriction and intensive physiotherapy improved mobility as assessed by ground reaction forces and facilitated more effective weight loss. The authors attributed the more pronounced weight loss in Group 2 to enhanced owner compliance resulting from increased owner-patient-veterinary interactions and decreased pain sensations from TENS therapy, which promoted increased physical activity. Interestingly, even when dogs in both groups reached a goal of approximately 9% reduction in initial body weight, weight loss alone did not result in the same significant improvement of lameness as measured by ground reaction forces, in Group 1 compared to Group 2.

Physical rehabilitation should be considered as part of a multifaceted approach to the management of patients with osteoarthritis. Before initiating a rehabilitation program, patients should be thoroughly evaluated by a veterinarian and client education should include a clear understanding of the pathogenesis of the disease, typical disease progression and the anticipated benefits and potential complications of all treatment options.

The Bibliography for **Box 34-2** can be found at www.markmorris.org.

1999). Osteochondrosis dissecans was reported to occur in multiple joints of one cat (Ralphs, 2005). These sporadic reports suggest that developmental orthopedic disease may be more common in cats than previously thought. Increased awareness will undoubtedly lead to better characterizations of these diseases in cats. Appropriate nutrition in kittens should be focused on maintaining a healthy body weight and providing age-appropriate nutrition.

Although prevention of osteoarthritis is ideal, it is not always possible. After osteoarthritis is diagnosed, therapeutic recommendations should be customized for individual patients. The goals of management include: 1) mitigating risk factors, 2) controlling clinical signs and 3) moderating progression of the disease. These goals are best achieved by employing a multifaceted approach, which includes therapeutic nutrition, obesity management, analgesic medications, disease-modifying supplements and physical rehabilitation. The goals of nutritional management include reducing inflammation and pain, enhancing cartilage repair, slowing cartilage degradation and providing tangible improvement in clinical signs of osteoarthritis. After a patient has been diagnosed with osteoarthritis, or a condition that predisposes it to the development of osteoarthritis, initiating therapeutic nutrition is warranted.

Maintaining a healthy weight throughout life will delay the onset and minimize clinical signs of osteoarthritis. Achieving an ideal body weight in dogs diagnosed with osteoarthritis will improve clinical signs and long-term management. Although similar studies have not been conducted in cats, given that obesity is a risk factor in cats, similar effects can be expected. Obese patients diagnosed with either a concurrent risk factor or osteoarthritis should be managed with a weight-control program aimed at increasing mobility and restoring normal body condition. Weight control is best achieved by initiating an individualized weight-management program including the use of foods specifically designed for weight loss. Severely restricting the amount of a maintenance food to reduce energy intake will alter the intake and balance of other essential nutrients. It is important to remember that weight reduction alone may result in marked clinical improvement in patients suffering from osteoarthritis and should be a fundamental part of disease management. Refer to Chapter 27 for additional information about overweight/obesity and weight control.

Although calorie restriction is important, success in dogs and cats generally requires participation in an appropriate exercise program. Therapeutic exercise has been shown to help patients reduce body weight, increase joint mobility, reduce joint pain and strengthen supporting muscles. However, initiating an exercise program in overweight dogs suffering from osteoarthritis may be problematic (**Box 34-2**). If clinical signs are mild and reductions in body weight of 10% or less are necessary, patients can be managed with an appropriate therapeutic ostearthritis food fed at approximately 80% of DER for the ideal weight (Table 27-3). If reductions greater than 10% of body weight are necessary or if clinical signs are severe, dogs

Table 34-5. Key nutritional factor content of selected veterinary therapeutic foods marketed for osteoarthritis in dogs compared to reommended levels.*

Dry foods	Energy density (kcal/cup)**	Energy density (kcal ME/g)	Total omega-3 FAs (%)	EPA (%)	Omega-6: omega-3 ratio	Carn (mg/kg)	Gluc (%)	Chon (%)	Vit E (IU/kg)	Vit C (mg/kg)	Se (mg/kg)	P (%)	Na (%)
Recommended levels	**-**	**-**	**3.5-4.0**	**0.4-1.1**	**<1:1**	**≥300**	**≤0.1**	**≤0.08**	**≥400**	**≥100**	**0.5-1.3**	**0.3-0.7**	**0.2-0.4**
Hill's Prescription Diet j/d Canine	356	3.9	3.8	0.5	0.7:1	351	0.1	0.07	585	225	0.43	0.54	0.2
Iams Veterinary Formulas Joint	294	3.75	na	na	na	na	0.5	na	na	na	na	1.04	0.47
Medi-Cal Mobility Support	271	na	na	na	na	na	na	na	na	na	na	0.60	0.30
Purina Veterinary Diets JM Joint Mobility	351	4.2	1.07	na	1.8:1	na	0.14	na	1,073	133	na	1.07	0.39
Royal Canin Veterinary Diet Mobility Support JS 21	322	4.2	na	na	na	na	0.1	na	725	na	0.44	0.60	0.29
Royal Canin Veterinary Diet Mobility Support JS 21 Large Breed	332	4.3	na	na	na	na	0.22	na	725	na	0.43	0.60	0.40

Moist food	Energy density (kcal/can)**	Energy density (kcal ME/g)	Total omega-3 FAs (%)	EPA (%)	Omega-6: omega-3 ratio	Carn (mg/kg)	Gluc (%)	Chon (%)	Vit E (IU/kg)	Vit C (mg/kg)	Se (mg/kg)	P (%)	Na (%)
Recommended levels	**-**	**-**	**3.5-4.0**	**0.4-1.1**	**<1:1**	**≥300**	**≤0.1**	**≤0.08**	**≥400**	**≥100**	**0.5-1.3**	**0.3-0.7**	**0.2-0.4**
Hill's Prescription Diet j/d Canine	498/13 oz.	4.2	4.24	0.85	0.7:1	316.8	0.07	0.04	698	128	0.81	0.56	0.19

Key: ME = metabolizable energy, FAs = fatty acids, EPA = eicosapentaenoic acid, Gluc = glucosamine hydrochloride, Chon = chondroitin sulfate, Se = selenium, Carn = L-carnitine, P = phosphorus, Na = sodium, na = not available from manufacturer.

*Dry matter basis unless otherwise indicated.

**Energy density values are listed on an as fed basis and are useful for determining the amount to feed; cup = 8-oz. measuring cup.

To convert to kJ, multiply kcal by 4.184.

may be unwilling or unable to engage in even mild exercise. For these dogs, it may be prudent to initially provide a combination of appropriate analgesia and therapeutic ostearthritis food. The daily intake of the therapeutic ostearthritis food should be based on 80% of the DER for an ideal body weight and fed for approximately one month. During this time chondrocytes will selectively concentrate EPA in their membranes, aiding in modulating the inflammatory process and minimizing the destruction of cartilage matrix by degradative enzymes. Based on clinical studies[d-g] with a commercial veterinary therapeutic food,[c] dogs can be expected to have increased mobility in approximately one month, facilitating initiation of an exercise program. At the end of the month, body weight, body condition and mobility should be reevaluated. If additional weight reduction is necessary, the dog should be transitioned to a food specifically designed for weight loss and an exercise program initiated. Rechecks should be performed at monthly intervals to assess body weight, body condition and mobility. The veterinary therapeutic food for osteoarthritis and the food designed for weight

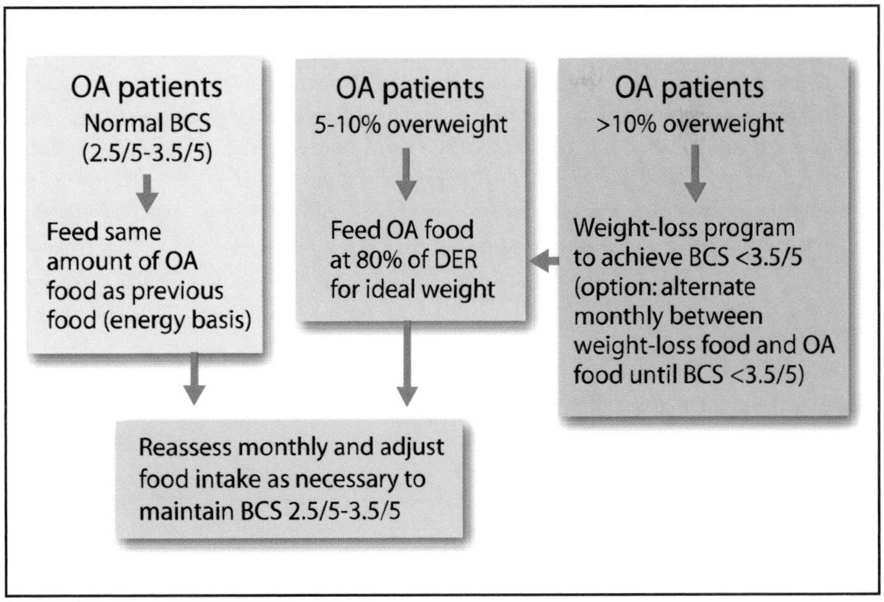

Figure 34-7. Overview of feeding regimen recommendations for osteoarthritis (OA) patients based on body weight/body condition scores (BCS). See Chapter 1 for methods for determining BCS. DER = daily energy requirement (Chapter 5).

Box 34-3. NSAIDs and NSAID Dosage When Feeding a Veterinary Therapeutic Food Designed for Patients with Osteoarthritis.

Nonsteroidal antiinflammatory drugs (NSAIDs) are the most common class of analgesics used to control pain in canine patients with osteoarthritis. In dogs, the efficacy of NSAIDs for relief of clinical signs of osteoarthritis is well documented. However, in some patients, glucocorticoids, narcotic and non-narcotic medications may be indicated for control of pain and clinical signs. Pain control in cats is more challenging because of their limited ability to metabolize drugs requiring glucuronide conjugation. Currently in the United States, there are no NSAIDs labeled for long-term use in cats. However, with careful dosing regimens both aspirin and meloxicam have been used for management of chronic pain and osteoarthritis in cats. Although they are an effective part of multifaceted therapy, NSAIDs have not been shown to alter the progression of osteoarthritis. As a class, NSAIDs may cause side effects related to gastrointestinal, hepatic, renal and hematopoietic systems. Because of their unique metabolism, cats are more sensitive to these side effects than dogs. When NSAIDs are prescribed, owners should be made aware of clinical signs indicative of adverse side effects of these products. Careful titration of the dosage of NSAIDs is recommended for each individual patient. The addition of other therapeutic modalities may affect the appropriate NSAID dose. Dogs in the initial phases of physical rehabilitation will benefit from effective analgesia. Conversely, the initiation of appropriate therapeutic nutrition may allow for a reduction in the daily NSAID dose.

In a 90-day prospective, randomized (dietary treatments), double-masked, controlled study designed to evaluate the effect of a veterinary therapeutic food[a] on the dose of an NSAID (carprofen) required to manage clinical signs in dogs with osteoarthritis,[b] significant effects were noted in the dogs consuming the therapeutic food. Pet owners observed significantly greater pain reduction in dogs consuming the veterinary therapeutic food compared to the control food. Carprofen dose reductions were possible in 43% of dogs consuming the therapeutic food vs. 32% of dogs eating the control food. Carprofen dose increases were necessary in 11% of the dogs consuming the control food and in only 2% of dogs consuming the therapeutic food. For the group receiving the therapeutic food, the mean carprofen dose reduction was 25%. Significantly greater reductions in carprofen dose (mg/lb body weight) were possible in the dogs consuming the therapeutic food compared with the control group. This study indicates that nutritional management using a food with high levels of total omega-3 fatty acids and eicosapentaenoic acid may allow for reduction in the dose of NSAIDs necessary to control clinical signs in dogs with osteoarthritis.

ENDNOTES

a. Prescription Diet j/d Canine. Hill's Pet Nutrition, Inc., Topeka, KS, USA.

b. Allen TA. A multi-center practice-based study of a therapeutic food and a non-steroidal anti-inflammatory drug in dogs with osteoarthritis. Hill's Pet Nutrition, Inc., Topeka, KS, USA. 2004.

The Bibliography for **Box 34-3** can be found at www.markmorris.org.

loss can be alternated at monthly intervals until ideal body weight is achieved. This approach will maximize the benefits of the weight-reduction food and the therapeutic food for osteoarthritis. Combining the foods (i.e., providing half the calories from each food each day) is not recommended and would be expected to compromise the benefits of both foods. **Figure 34-7** provides an overview of these feeding options.

Assess and Select the Food

After the patient has been assessed and, if necessary, body condition returned to normal, an appropriate veterinary therapeutic food should be selected to aid in the long-term management of osteoarthritis. The steps to assessing foods include: 1) ensuring the nutritional adequacy of the food has been determined by a credible regulatory agency such as AAFCO (See product label.) and 2) comparing the food's key nutritional factors with the recommended levels. Because foods for the management of osteoarthritis are used in place of regular maintenance foods, the key nutritional factors include those for promoting long-term general health by managing nutrition-related risk factors for kidney and heart disease.

Table 34-5 provides key nutritional factor profiles for selected commercial canine veterinary therapeutic foods marketed to provide an arthritis benefit and compares them to the key nutritional factors for osteoarthritis. Currently there are no veterinary therapeutic foods marketed in North America for cats with osteoarthritis. If the food in question cannot be found in this table, the manufacturer should be contacted. Manufacturers' addresses, websites and toll-free customer service numbers are listed on pet food labels. If the manufacturer cannot provide the necessary information, food selection should be limited to foods for which this information is available. Comparing a food's key nutritional factor content with the recommended levels is fundamental to food selection.

Another criterion for selecting a food that may become increasingly important in the future is evidence-based clinical nutrition. Practitioners should know how to determine risks and benefits of nutritional regimens and counsel pet owners accordingly. Currently, veterinary medical education and continuing education are not always based on rigorous assessment of evidence for or against particular management options. Still, studies have been published to establish the nutritional benefits of certain pet foods. Chapter 2 describes evidence-based clinical nutrition in detail and applies its concepts to various veterinary therapeutic foods.

Treats should not be fed in excessive amounts, if at all. It is best to limit treats to less than 10% of the total food fed on a volume, weight or calorie basis. Consider having owners switch to smaller treats or break larger treats in half and feed pieces instead of full treats. Too many treats will dilute the beneficial effects of a properly formulated veterinary therapeutic food. The key nutritional factors important for osteoarthritis are not included in most commercial treats, particularly at the necessary levels.

Assess and Determine the Feeding Method

It may not always be necessary to change the feeding method when managing a patient with osteoarthritis. However, a thorough assessment should be made to verify that an appropriate feeding method is being used. Items to consider include amount fed, how the food is offered, access to other food and who feeds the patient. If a new food is introduced, the amount to feed can be determined from the product label or other supporting materials. The food dosage may need to be changed if the caloric density of the new food differs from that of the previous food. The food dosage is usually divided into two or more meals per day. The food dosage should be altered if the patient's body weight and condition are not optimal.

For clinical nutrition to be effective there needs to be good client compliance. Ensuring compliance requires good client communication, both oral and written, regarding the benefits of, and instructions on, transitioning to the new food. Incorporating followup calls to clients within three days of initiating a new food and again in three weeks has been shown to dramatically improve client and patient acceptance of new foods (AAHA, 2003). Limiting the patient's access to other foods and providing both dry and wet products to satisfy owner and patient preferences may also promote compliance.

REASSESSMENT

Clinical studies suggest that dogs with signs of osteoarthritis will respond to appropriate therapeutic foods within four to six weeks. Normal weight dogs should be evaluated for changes in lameness. Orthopedic examinations and owner quality of life assessments at this time can help determine the efficacy of the therapeutic food for osteoarthritis. After a response is noted, patients can be evaluated semiannually for overall health and disease progression.

Overweight dogs with osteoarthritis should be evaluated monthly to assess body weight, body condition and mobility until ideal body condition (~3/5) is achieved. After patients reach an ideal body condition they should be maintained on a veterinary therapeutic food properly formulated for osteoarthritis. These obese-prone patients should be evaluated every three to six months to assess body weight, body condition and mobility. Careful monitoring will encourage compliance and prevent weight regain.

Because management of osteoarthritis often involves a multifaceted approach, dosages of concurrent analgesics or supplements should be reevaluated within the first four to six weeks of initiating an appropriate therapeutic food (**Box 34-3**), weight loss or physical rehabilitation program. Adjustments to the dose of concurrent analgesics or supplements should be based on response to therapy.

Maintaining cats at a healthy body weight should be of paramount concern until additional options such as therapeutic foods are available. Cats participating in weight-loss programs should be evaluated monthly until ideal body condition is achieved then semiannually for overall health and disease progression.

ENDNOTES

a. Proprietary market research. Veterinary sample size: 200. Data on file. Pfizer Animal Health, Exton, PA, USA. 1996.
b. www.press.petinsurance.com. Accessed September 2007.
c. Prescription Diet j/d Canine. Hill's Pet Nutrition, Inc., Topeka, KS, USA.
d. Allen TA. Dose titration effects of omega-3 fatty acids fed to dogs with osteoarthritis. Hill's Pet Nutrition, Inc., Topeka, KS, USA. 2004.
e. Allen TA. A multi-center practice-based study of a therapeutic food and a non-steroidal anti-inflammatory drug in dogs with osteoarthritis. Hill's Pet Nutrition, Inc., Topeka, KS, USA. 2004.
f. Dodd CE, Fritsch DA, Allen TA. Omega-3 fatty acids in canine osteoarthritis: A randomized, double-masked, practice-based, 6-month feeding study. Hill's Pet Nutrition, Inc., Topeka, KS, USA. 2004.
g. Allen TA. Effects of feeding omega-3 fatty acids on force plate gait analysis in dogs with osteoarthritis, 3-month feeding study. Hill's Pet Nutrition Inc., Topeka, KS, USA. 2003.
h. Eugster AK. Memorandum: Distributing Products Containing Glucosamine Hydrochloride and/or Chondroitin Sulfate. Texas Agricultural Experiment Station. The Texas A&M University, College Station, TX, USA. Office of the State Chemist. May 11, 1999.

REFERENCES

The references for **Chapter 34** can be found at www.markmorris.org.

CASE 34-1

Lameness in a Labrador Retriever Mixed-Breed Dog

Todd L. Towell, DVM, MS, Dipl. ACVIM (Small Animal Internal Medicine)
Hill's Pet Nutrition
Topeka, Kansas, USA

Patient Assessment

A six-year-old neutered female Labrador retriever mix, was examined for rear limb lameness of two years' duration. Clinical signs were mild to moderate in severity and included difficulty in rising from rest, limping, stiffness and reluctance to run, jump or play. The owner was giving no medications or supplements. The patient weighed 34 kg, but was considered overweight with a body condition score of 4 on a 5-point scale. The rest of the physical examination revealed no other abnormal findings. A thorough orthopedic examination disclosed the following abnormalities: slight left rear limb lameness at a walk, normal weight-bearing at rest, mild limitation in range of motion of the left hip joint and mild resistance to elevation of the right rear limb with full weight bearing on the left hind limb. Mild pain was elicited upon palpation of the left hip joint.

Results of a complete blood count, serum biochemistry profile and urinalysis were within normal limits. Radiographic changes were consistent with bilateral hip dysplasia and degenerative joint disease with the left coxofemoral joint more severely affected.

Assess the Food and Feeding Method

The patient was fed a low-calorie dry dog food but had access to food sources for other dogs and cats in the household.

Questions

1. What are the therapeutic goals for managing patients with osteoarthritis or degenerative joint disease of coxofemoral joints?
2. How might the overweight body condition contribute to the clinical problems in this dog?
3. Could this condition have been prevented with proper nutritional management?
4. Outline a comprehensive nonsurgical management plan for this patient.

Answers

1. Therapeutic goals for managing chronic osteoarthritis or degenerative joint disease in the coxofemoral joints include: 1) eliminating underlying causes (e.g., femoral head and neck excision for aseptic necrosis of the femoral head), 2) setting realistic treatment outcome expectations with the patient's owner, 3) enhancing the dog's quality of life by reducing pain, maintaining or improving activity level and joint function and 4) slowing disease progression by modifying cartilage structure and function. Most patients with chronic osteoarthritis or degenerative joint disease have irreversible changes with no opportunity to eliminate or cure the condition. This makes client education very important. The patient's owner should be made aware that degenerative joint disease is controllable but not curable and that a comprehensive management plan needs to include long-term pain management. The goals are to alter disease progression and improve the patient's quality of life.
2. Osteoarthritis is often associated with abnormal forces acting on normal joints or normal forces acting on abnormal joints. Obesity may contribute to progression of degenerative joint disease and clinical signs by causing excess physical stress on either normal or abnormal joints. In addition, excess body fat is a source of inflammatory cytokines. Multiple studies have shown that weight loss helps decrease lameness and pain in overweight dogs with existing hip osteoarthritis. In these studies, even mild weight loss was associated with clinical improvement.

   Large- and giant-breed dogs are at risk for developmental orthopedic disease including hip and elbow dysplasia, osteochondrosis and other conditions associated with joint instability or incongruity. Nutritional risk factors for developmental orthopedic disease include excess energy, fat and calcium intake during growth. Use of foods specifically formulated for large-breed puppies and avoiding free-choice feeding helps manage these nutritional risk factors and ensure a normal, healthy growth rate. An overweight body condition is recognized as a risk factor for development of degenerative joint disease in dogs; maintaining a normal body condition can help reduce the incidence and severity of osteoarthritis. A study found that when at-risk puppies were fed free choice during growth, they exhibited an increased incidence and severity of hip joint laxity and hip dysplasia compared to puppies fed in a restricted fashion. Over time, those dogs fed to maintain a lean body condition throughout life exhibited reduced severity of osteoarthritis and a delayed need for medication compared to their heavier siblings.
3. Nonsurgical management of osteoarthritis should focus on three main aspects: 1) activity modification, 2) medications and supplements to modify joint pain and function and 3) nutritional management that emphasizes weight control and modifying joint inflammation and cartilage degradation. Previously, limiting activity levels in patients with osteoarthritis and degenerative joint disease was considered important. However, studies in human patients with osteoarthritis have shown the benefits of exercise including decreased pain scores and improved joint function scores. Furthermore, exercise reduced the need for analgesic med-

ications. Today, veterinary specialists recommend therapeutic exercise as a way to improve quality of life for dogs with chronic osteoarthritis. A variety of medications and supplements are available to manage pain and joint function. Responses to medications and supplements vary markedly in patients with osteoarthritis and specific products and doses need to be individually tailored for each dog.

4. New information has been generated about canine osteoarthritis from in vitro studies with cartilage models and clinical studies in dogs with various forms of arthritis. In vitro cartilage studies have shown that canine chondrocyte membranes selectively store the omega-3 fatty acid eicosapentaenoic acid (EPA), but not other omega-3 fatty acids. EPA is the most important fatty acid for helping manage inflammation in cartilage of dogs. EPA is also the only omega-3 fatty acid shown to inhibit activity of enzymes that degrade cartilage and helps turn off the signal to make degradative enzymes. Based on these in vitro studies, clinical trials were performed in dogs with arthritis using a veterinary therapeutic food enhanced with levels of EPA. The food also contained high levels of total omega-3 fatty acids, an omega-6 to omega-3 fatty acid ratio less than 1.0, high L-carnitine levels, added glucosamine hydrochloride and chondroitin sulfate, added antioxidant nutrients and added lysolecithin. Feeding this food to dogs with arthritis resulted in higher serum EPA concentrations, significant improvements in clinical signs observed by pet owners, improved clinical assessments of arthritis by veterinarians and improved weight bearing on affected limbs as measured by force-plate gait analysis. Many of the dogs in the studies were not receiving medications or supplements in conjunction with the food.

Feeding Plan and Progress Notes

Prescription Diet j/d Canine dry food[a] was dispensed for the owners to feed. The amount of food was calculated for an obese-prone dog. The owners were encouraged to deny access to other sources of dog and cat food in the household. Controlled exercise was also encouraged using walks on a leash. Six weeks later the owners reported improvements in all clinical signs associated with arthritis and improvements in the patient's overall personality. The improvements observed by the owner continued at the three-month recheck and no pain was elicited on palpation of the left hip joint by the attending veterinarian. These improvements were noted without concurrent use of medications or supplements. Body weight and body condition score remained the same so client education focused on the importance of continued weight management with appropriate reductions in food, limiting access to other pet food and increased levels of exercise.

Acknowledgements

Thanks to Drs. James Roush of Kansas State University, Manhattan, and Tara Enwiller of Gilbert, Arizona, for providing information about this patient.

Endnote

a. Hill's Pet Nutrition, Inc., Topeka, KS, USA.

Bibliography

Budsberg S, Bartges J, Schoenherr B, et al. Effects of different n6:n3 fatty acid diets on canine stifle osteoarthritis (abstract). In: Proceedings. Veterinary Orthopedic Society Annual Conference 2001; 28: 40.

Burkholder WJ, Taylor L, Hulse DA. Weight loss to optimal body condition increases ground reactive forces in dogs with osteoarthritis (abstract). In: Proceedings. Purina Nutrition Forum; 2000: 74.

Caterson B, Flannery CR, Hughes CE, et al. Mechanisms involved in cartilage proteoglycan catabolism. Matrix Biology 2000; 19: 333-344.

Curtis CL, Hughes CE, Flannery CR, et al. N-3 fatty acids specifically modulate catabolic factors involved in articular cartilage degradation. Journal of Biological Chemistry 2000; 275: 721-724.

Curtis CL, Rees SG, Cramp J, et al. Effects of n-3 fatty acids on cartilage metabolism. Proceedings of the Nutrition Society 2002; 61: 381-389.

Dodd CE. Multicenter clinical study on the effect of an investigational food containing elevated omega-3 fatty acids on canine osteoarthritis clinical signs. Final report. Hill's Pet Nutrition Center, 2004.

Hansen RA, Allen KGD, Pluhar EG, et al. N-3 fatty acids decrease inflammatory mediators in arthritic dogs (abstract). FASEB Proceedings; 2003.

Impellizeri JA, Tetrick MA, Muir P. Effect of weight reduction on clinical signs of lameness in dogs with hip osteoarthritis. Journal of the American Veterinary Medical Association 2000; 216: 1089-1091.

Kealy RD, Olsson SE, Monti JL, et al. Effects of limited food consumption on the incidence of hip dysplasia in growing dogs. Journal of the American Veterinary Medical Association 1992; 201: 857-863.

Kealy RD, Lawler DF, Ballam JM, et al. Five-year longitudinal study on limited food consumption and development of osteoarthritis in coxofemoral joints of dogs. Journal of the American Veterinary Medical Association 1997; 210: 222-225.

Section 12

Neurologic Disorders

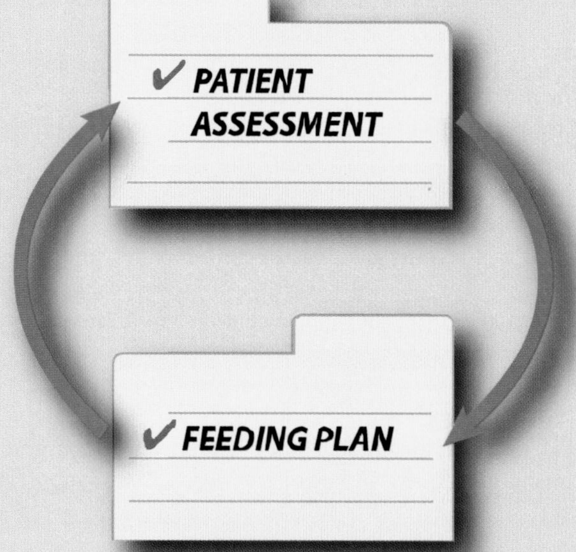

Chapter 35

Cognitive Dysfunction in Dogs

Lori-Ann Christie
Gary M. Landsberg
Viorela Pop
Steven C. Zicker
Elizabeth Head

"Dogs' lives are too short. Their only fault, really."
Agnes Sligh Turnbull

CLINICAL IMPORTANCE

Current estimates suggest that approximately 20 to 30 million dogs over the age of seven years live in the United States, representing 30 to 40% of the total canine population (AVMA, 2002). Behavioral changes, the development of new behavioral problems and the exacerbation of previous behavioral problems occur commonly with increasing age. At one animal behavior referral clinic, the most common complaints cited by pet owners included increased incidence of separation anxiety, house soiling, phobias, waking at night and excessive vocalization (Chapman and Voith, 1990). In addition, memory impairments, symbolic recognition and object permanence were associated with aging in dogs (Dehasse, 2005).

Canine cognitive dysfunction syndrome (CDS) is the name proposed to describe behavioral changes noted in client-owned aged dogs (Ruehl et al, 1995). Numerous owner-based observational studies have assessed the prevalence of CDS. For example, 180 dogs that had been determined to be healthy at their annual visit were reevaluated by client telephone followup; 28% of owners of 11- to 12-year-old dogs and 68% of owners of 15- to 16-year-old dogs reported at least one sign of CDS (Neilson et al, 2001). (See disorientation, alterations in interactions with people and other pets, alterations in sleep-wake cycles and house soiling [DISH] below.) In another study of 102 dogs eight years old and older, in which underlying medical problems had been ruled out, 41% had alterations in one category, whereas 32% had alterations in two or more categories of DISHA (See definition below) (Osella et al, 2007).

PATIENT ASSESSMENT

History, Screening Questionnaires and Other Clinical Information

Behavioral signs reported by pet owners are the primary criterion upon which to base a diagnosis of cognitive dysfunction (**Table 35-1**). However, the diagnosis can only be made after exclusion of all other medical problems that may cause similar clinical signs. For example, any change in personality or mood, inability to recognize or respond appropriately to stimuli or loss of previously learned behavior may indicate diseases of the forebrain or may arise from sensory system deficits. Diseases of virtually any other organ system can also affect behavior and these are discussed in more detail elsewhere (Landsberg and Araujo, 2005; Landsberg et al, 2003). Chronic or recurrent stress and anxiety can also affect health and behavior, in part by affecting the hypothalamic-pituitary axis and possibly by overstimulation of the noradrenergic system. Therefore, reporting any change in behavior is essential for the health and well-being of all pets, and, in particular, for senior pets, in which degenerative diseases, tumors, pain and discomfort are increasingly common.

In 2005, the American Animal Hospital Association senior care task force published guidelines that recommend yearly

Table 35-1. Behaviors evaluated in dogs to assess age-related cognitive decline.*

1. Confusion, awareness, spatial orientation
Gets lost in familiar locations
Goes to wrong side of doors (e.g., hinge side)
Gets stuck and cannot navigate around or over obstacles
Less responsive to stimuli
Decreased recognition of familiar people, pets or places
2. Relationships and social behavior
Decreased interest in petting or contact
Decreased greeting behavior
Alterations or problems with social hierarchy
In need of constant contact (e.g., over dependent or "clingy")
3. Activity: Increased, decreased or repetitive
Decreased daytime sleep/increased wandering or pacing
Decreased exploration (apathy)
Staring, fixation or snapping at objects
Licking owners or household objects
4. Agitation or anxiety
Inappropriate vocalization
Restless sleep
Increased irritability/aggression
Aimless pacing and wandering
Increased/new fears or phobias
Separation anxiety
5. Appetite
Increased interest (volume eaten or speed of eating)
Decreased interest
Anxiety–conflict behaviors at food bowl
6. Decreased responsiveness to stimuli
May seem to have a decline in vision, hearing or odor perception
7. Decreased self-care
8. Sleep-wake cycle
Restless sleep or awake at night
Increased daytime sleep
9. Learning and memory
a) House soiling: Indoor elimination at random sites or in view of owners
Decreased or no signaling
Goes outdoors, eliminates indoors upon return
Elimination in crate or sleeping area
Incontinence
b) Works, tasks, commands
Impaired working ability
Impaired responsiveness to known commands or tricks
Decreased ability to perform tasks
Inability or slow to learn new tasks (must retrain)

*Adapted with permission from Landsberg G, Hunthausen W, Ackerman L. The effects of aging on behavior in senior pets. Handbook of Behavior Problems of the Dog and Cat. Edinburgh, Scotland: Elsevier Health Sciences, 2003.

wellness screening for healthy middle-aged pets and twice yearly screening for senior pets (i.e., last 25% of predicted lifespan). At each visit, the pet should receive a physical examination and laboratory tests and the owner should be extensively questioned about changes in behavior and health (Epstein et al, 2005). Most of these changes would not be detected during a veterinary visit because they can be intermittent, subtle in onset and only noticeable in other environments. Therefore a senior care program should include use of a screening questionnaire (**Table 35-1**). (Landsberg and Araujo, 2005; Landsberg et al, 2003; Pfizer Animal Health) and/or allow sufficient time for interactive history taking. If problems are identified, early intervention may improve quality of life and longevity.

The reliability and usefulness of brain imaging for detection of CDS has not been systematically examined. However, in some cases, a magnetic resonance imaging (MRI) scan might be useful for differential diagnosis. Imaging might allow practitioners to rule out alternative explanations for changes in behavior, such as the presence of gliomas, tumors or damage due to stroke. Note that a normal MRI scan cannot be used to rule out CDS. However, with increased age, there is a tendency toward ventricular dilatation and neuronal loss. (See macroscopic changes below.) Although these changes might be expected to correlate with increasing cognitive dysfunction, this has not been validated. Traditionally, the signs of canine CDS, hypothesized to be caused by brain aging, were described by the acronym DISH. (See above.) Alterations in activity levels including increased restlessness and pacing have also been identified; therefore, an "A" for activity has more recently been added to the acronym (Landsberg and Araujo, 2005; Landsberg et al, 2003; Neilson et al, 2001; Osella et al, 2007). These signs, however, do not necessarily reflect all of those associated with CDS and brain aging.

In a review of 50 recent Veterinary Information Network (VIN) postings of behavioral signs in senior dogs (aged nine to 17), many of the reported problems were related to agitation and anxiety including fear, excessive vocalization, salivation, destructiveness, hypervigilance, over-attachment, separation anxiety, night-time waking and anxiety, restlessness, wandering, pacing, confusion, noise phobias, increased sensitivity to sound, compulsive licking and aggression (sometimes concurrent with and sometimes independent of other signs of DISH). Each case received the guidance of one or more of the VIN specialists in neurology, internal medicine or behavior. Seizures, hypertension, sensory decline, arthritis, pituitary-dependent hyperadrenocorticism and cerebral disease were the most commonly suggested rule outs. There was no identifiable medical cause in 24 of the 50 cases, and medical problems were deemed unlikely to have contributed to the behavioral signs in another nine cases. Of the remaining cases, arthritis, hearing loss, renal insufficiency, lymphadenopathy, mild anemia and pharmaceutical therapy such as phenylpropanolamine and prednisone were considered as possible contributing factors. This underscores the importance of ruling out medical problems that might cause clinical signs, and the fact that anxiety and agitation are commonly reported signs in senior pets.

A number of cognitive disorders have been described in the French literature including confusional syndrome, dysthymic disorder and involutive depression (which may be associated with compulsive and stereotypical behavior, hyper-attachment, vocalization and anxiety) (Landsberg and Araujo, 2005). In addition, laboratory studies indicate that there is a measurable decline in learning and memory associated with brain aging. Laboratory-based systematic studies of changes in behavior and cognition also provide evidence that behavioral changes in senior dogs observed clinically have a neurobiological basis. Thus the acronym DISHA may not sufficiently and accurately reflect all of the clinical signs associated with brain aging and cognitive dysfunction in older pets. Because these signs are generally noticed by pet owners and seldom in the veterinary clinic, pet owners should be counseled to immediately report any changes in behavior or health in older pets. In turn, veterinarians should use these signs, along with results of physical and neurologic examinations and results of other diagnostic testing to diagnose or rule out possible systemic causes, and to determine if the signs may be associated with brain aging. The use of a cognitive assessment questionnaire may help facilitate the process (**Table 35-1**).

Although feline data are much more preliminary, **Box 35-1** describes clinical observations of CDS, age-related neuropathology and treatment of CDS in cats.

Table 35-2. Laboratory deficits and tentative clinical correlates in age-related cognitive dysfunction syndrome in dogs.

Laboratory deficit	Clinical signs
Impaired spatial learning	Disorientation in space, time
Impaired spatial memory	Disorientation in familiar surroundings
Impaired oddity and discrimination learning	Impaired symbolic recognition, object permanence
Executive dysfunction	Deterioration of social skills, increased house soiling
Disrupted sleep-wake cycle	Wandering at night
Altered locomotion in open field	Altered activity levels

Relationship Between Age, Cognitive Dysfunction and Pathology: Laboratory Studies

Changes in Cognitive and Non-Cognitive Behaviors with Age

Although owner-based survey studies are informative for assessing global brain function, using laboratory-based neuropsychological tests represents a more systematic approach to detect subtle and early changes in learning and memory with age that might go unreported in the clinic. By contrast, owner assessment is generally unable to detect changes in learning or memory, because house soiling and the level and extent of commands that the pet has learned are the only values that can be assessed, except perhaps in performance, working or assistance dogs in which a higher degree of training and learning has been attained. A modified Wisconsin General Testing Apparatus (**Box 35-2**) is one laboratory-based method used to detect early changes and systematically characterize changes in cognition in aging beagles (Milgram et al, 1994). An array of tasks has been developed to measure specific cognitive abilities in dogs. These tests include assessment of associative learning in which a dog must learn that only one of two objects hides a food reward based on shape (Head et al, 1998), size (Head et al, 1998; Tapp et al, 2003) or spatial location (Christie et al, 2005; Milgram et al, 1999) of the object. There are also tasks that assess how long a dog can remember if it has seen a particular object (Callahan et al, 2000) or spatial location (Adams et al, 2000; Chan et al, 2002) and tests of executive function that assess how readily it can learn a particular rule or strategy for solving a task (Tapp et al, 2003a, 2004a).

Cross-sectional and longitudinal studies using these tests indicate that cognition declines with age in dogs, but that the decline is selective to certain cognitive abilities and tasks. Procedural learning, or the ability to remember particular skills or habits necessary for success in the Toronto General Testing Apparatus, remains relatively intact in old dogs (Milgram et al, 1994), whereas tests of executive function and working memory are highly sensitive to aging (Christie et al, 2005; Tapp et al, 2003, 2004). For example, young and old dogs are easily trained to associate one object in a pair of stimuli with a food reward when the object pair is presented repeatedly over several test trials (Adams et al, 2000; Christie et al, 2005; Milgram et al, 1994). At this stage, no age differences in learning are found, suggesting that simple visual processing remains intact in aged animals. If, however, the reward contingency is reversed such that the opposite stimulus becomes associated with food reward, some senior dogs are unable to change their response pattern (Christie et al, 2005; Head et al, 1998; Tapp et al, 2003, 2004). This indicates that age affects cognitive flexibility, or the ability to modify previously formed associations, which suggests changes in frontal lobe function in aged dogs (Tapp et al, 2004).

Aged dogs also have impaired ability to acquire and remember an oddity discrimination task (Milgram et al, 2002). In this paradigm, the animal is presented with three objects; two are identical but one differs in size, shape and color. The dog must learn that the odd object hides a food reward and remember to choose the odd object when tested at a later occasion on other oddity discrimination levels. There are four levels to the oddity task and each successive level becomes more difficult by increasing the similarity of the odd object to the identical pair of objects. Old dogs learn all oddity levels more slowly than young dogs. Furthermore, this age effect is particularly pronounced as the task increases in difficulty (Milgram et al, 2002).

The precise link between clinical measures of CDS and systematic laboratory cognitive tests is unknown. Currently, we can only speculate as to which laboratory-based deficits might correspond to clinical signs reported to occur in dogs with CDS (**Table 35-2**). For example, the owner-observed disorientation in space and time might correspond most closely with neuropsychological tests of spatial learning and memory. More research is needed to determine if results from the laboratory translate directly to the clinic and if tests of cognitive function in laboratory-based tasks involve the same brain circuits that are compromised in CDS. This would be accomplished, in part, by conducting both neuropsychological tests and in-home behavioral questionnaires on the same group of dogs. Currently, this is not a practical option because home tests would need to be developed and standardized.

Laboratory studies provide evidence that aged dogs develop changes in overall activity and in cognition. Studies identify differences in young and aged beagles in exploration (as measured by response to novel toys) and social responsiveness to a passive human subject. Although aged dogs with minimal evidence of cognitive impairment may have decreased activity, cognitively impaired aged dogs show increased sporadic activity levels, but decreased social responsiveness and exploratory behavior (Siwak et al, 2001, 2003). This may correlate with the initial decline in activity and increased sleep reported clinically in

Box 35-1. Clinical Observation of Cognitive Dysfunction Syndrome in Cats.

The presenting complaints of 83 senior cats referred to veterinary behaviorists were house soiling (73%), intraspecies aggression (10%), aggression toward people (6%), excessive vocalization (6%), restlessness (6%) and excessive grooming (4%). However, there is a much wider range of subtler and more frequent behavioral changes seen by owners that may not be reported and are unlikely to require referral.

A second study was intended to evaluate the prevalence of clinical signs in a population of otherwise healthy cats that were presented for annual examination or other routine care. Owners of 154 cats aged 11 and older were asked, using a questionnaire (similar to the canine questionnaire in **Table 35-1**), about whether their cats showed any behavioral signs such as altered activity levels, increased anxiety, night waking, increased vocalization, house soiling, altered responsiveness to stimuli, alterations in interactions with people or other cats and evidence of confusion or disorientation. After removing cats with medical problems, 50% of those aged 15 years or older were diagnosed with cognitive dysfunction syndrome (CDS); altered activity levels, aimless activity and excessive vocalization were reported most commonly. Additionally, 28% of cats aged 11 to 15 years had signs of CDS; altered social interactions were reported most commonly.

In an attempt to further determine some of the more common behavioral problems for which owners seek veterinary advice, 100 recent Veterinary Information Network (VIN) postings about senior cat (aged 12 to 22 years) behavioral problems were reviewed. The most common complaints were vocalization, altered sleep-wake cycles, night-time anxiety, nighttime restlessness, inappropriate elimination including spraying, confusion, disorientation, wandering, pacing, anxiousness, restlessness, irritability, aggression, fear/hiding, increased attachment/"clingy" behavior and decreased interaction with owners. A few problems were reported in only single cats. These included departure anxiety, pica (cardboard) and scratching. Pain (e.g., arthritis, dental), decreased mobility, metabolic problems including hyperthyroidism, renal and hepatic disease, hypertension, concurrent drug therapy, vision or hearing loss and forebrain lesions (particularly meningiomas) were the primary rule outs suggested by VIN specialists. Although many of these cases had sufficient workups to rule out all possible medical causes including physical and neurologic examinations, urinalyses, blood tests (including thyroxine measurement), radiographs and blood pressure evaluation, few cats had magnetic resonance imaging. Furthermore, the effects of arthritis and hearing and vision loss were difficult to assess. In 11 cases, a recent change in the household including the death of another pet may also have contributed to anxiety. In comparison to the canine data (See text.), there were far more feline cases in which concurrent medical conditions could not be entirely ruled out. Thus, although signs of anxiety are common in aging cats, age-related brain pathology (CDS), environmental changes and medical problems might be factors. Conversely, the diagnosis of a medical problem does not exclude CDS because both could exist concurrently.

To date, few systematic laboratory studies have looked at changes in cognition across the lifespan of cats. As described above, however, owners of senior cats report age-related behavioral problems. It is also known that cats develop age-related neuropathology that theoretically underlies cognitive decline (described in detail below). For example, one study found that development of diffuse senile plaques in the brains of three aged cats was correlated with behavioral changes including wandering, confusion and inappropriate vocalization. In a more recent study, a range of cognitive deficits from mild to severe, including wandering, inappropriate vocalization, confusion/getting lost, decreased grooming, lethargy, loss of housetraining and decreased affection and recognition of owners, was reported in four out of five cats aged 16 years and older. Development of laboratory-based tests for cats will allow the correlation of age-related behavioral problems with neuropathological changes and may allow detection of cognitive decline in younger cats, as has been found in dogs.

AGE-RELATED NEUROPATHOLOGY IN CATS

Beta-amyloid (Aβ) has also been studied in the brains of cats although not as extensively as in dogs. The first study to look at Aβ pathology in cats consisted of immunohistochemical staining of the brain of three family cats aged 15, 16 and 20 years old. According to their owners, all cats exhibited abnormal behavior within the final years of life including wandering, confusion and night-time howling. The 20-year-old cat was specifically described as having behavior "suggestive of Alzheimer's Disease." Pathologic analyses revealed that all three cats displayed age-dependent increases in Aβ pathology very similar to that found in aged dogs, with diffuse deposits (sometimes spanning the entire cortical depth) and smaller, denser deposits in various cortical layers. Senile plaques were also assessed in seven aged cats of various breeds (12 to 20 years old) that had no abnormal behavioral reports when they were alive. In this study, only three aged cats, two 18 year olds and one 20 year old, had senile plaques that were immunoreactive for Aβ in the temporal and occipital cortex. In another study in which the brains of seven Siamese and seven domestic shorthair cats (aged 7.5 to 21 years old) were examined, Aβ deposition was detected by various antibodies in different brain structures of all 14

aging dogs, which then progresses to repetitive behaviors, restless pacing and compulsive disorders.

Risk Factors

Age is a risk factor for CDS. Behavioral disturbances are reported with increasing frequency in dogs around 11 years of age (Bain et al, 2001; Landsberg et al, 2003; Neilson et al, 2001). Initially, these changes might be subtle and seem innocuous to the client; however, in many cases they progress to include more clinical signs and/or signs of increasing severity that affect the pet's quality of life and the owner's ability to care for the pet. For example, in one study, 22% of senior dogs that had no impairments at an initial interview developed at least one sign of CDS at a followup interview 12 to 18 months later. In the same study, 48% of dogs that initially displayed one behavioral disturbance had impairments in two or more categories at followup (Bain et al, 2001).

To date, age is the only risk factor for CDS that has been systematically studied in the clinic and laboratory, although other risk factors are possible, such as breed (larger breeds might have an earlier age of onset), previous head trauma or occurrence of microvascular accidents. Consistent breed differences in susceptibility to CDS have not been reported; however, a potential genetic predisposition for development of CDS can be inferred cats. One 12-year-old Siamese cat had a notable amount of Aβ plaques in the hippocampus, but diffuse Aβ plaque pathology was most likely to occur after 17 years of age. A study looking at very young and very old cats found that Aβ abnormalities were not observed in very young cats (<4 years old), but diffuse plaques were common in the brains of aged cats (16 to 21 years old). A more comprehensive study involving 19 cats (aged 16 weeks to 14 years old) found that 17 cats had clinical signs of neurologic dysfunction. Diffuse Aβ plaque deposition was observed beginning at 10 years of age and increased with age. Collectively, the Aβ neuropathological findings in cats show that, in comparison to dogs, which have Aβ deposition beginning at middle age, feline Aβ plaques appeared towards the end of the lifespan.

TREATMENT OF CDS IN CATS

Although no food is commercially available for cats with cognitive dysfunction, it is not unreasonable to believe that many of the same therapeutic options may be effective because cats have many of the same brain changes and behavioral signs associated with age as dogs and people. However, care must be taken when recommending off-label inclusion of some supplements such as α-lipoic acid because it is not metabolized as quickly in cats as in dogs. Therefore, although there is only anecdotal evidence of efficacy, some dietary supplements such as Senilife[a] are marketed for use in cats. There are no drugs licensed for treatment of cognitive dysfunction in cats, but selegiline, propentofylline and nicergoline have been used in cats with varying degrees of success.

As in dogs, treatment of clinical signs associated with brain aging such as vocalization, night waking or an increase in anxiety may also necessitate the use of anxiolytics drugs such as buspirone, benzodiazepines that have the least potential for hepatotoxicity such as oxazepam and antidepressants with no anticholinergic effects such as fluoxetine or pheromones such as Feliway.[b] It would be prudent to evaluate the effects of possible feline therapies either in the laboratory or clinic because aged cats may have compromised function and dose response data are limited.

ENDNOTES

a. Ceva Sante Animale, Libourne Cedex, France.
b. Veterinary Products Laboratories, Phoenix, AZ, USA.

The Bibliography for **Box 35-1** can be found at www.markmorris.org.

from reports of increased concordance rates of beta-amyloid plaque pathology (discussed in detail below) in littermates. In one study of aged dogs, the authors reported significant familial influence on plaque development by observing congruence in 15 of the 16 litters examined (Russell et al, 1992). Previous head trauma or occurrence of microvascular accidents may predispose animals to CDS by affecting the integrity of the blood-brain barrier (BBB), although no clinical data are available for definitive conclusions. In laboratory beagles, increases in BBB permeability with age in conjunction with the presence of vascular amyloid pathology suggest that disruptions to vascular integrity may be a risk factor for development of CDS (Su et al, 1998).

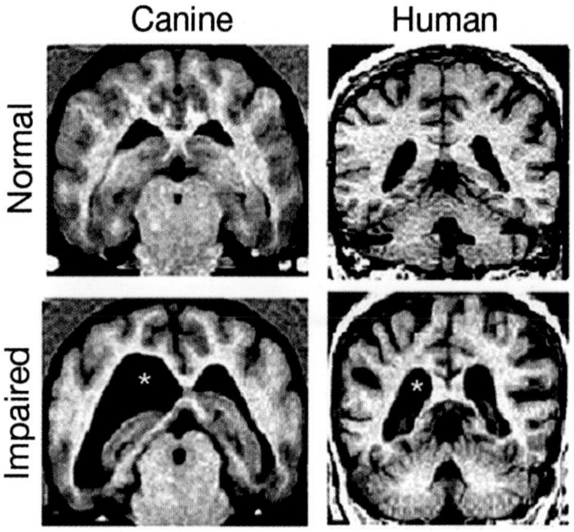

Figure 35-1. Magnetic resonance imaging of canine and human brain. Coronal sections of a cognitively normal beagle and person reveal structural similarities and a well-developed cortex. However, cognitive impairments are associated with enlarged ventricles (*) and general cortical atrophy of the gray and white matter, resulting in deep gyri and widened sulci. (Courtesy Dr. Min-Ying Su, University of California-Irvine.)

Etiopathogenesis

Cognitive changes in learning and memory often coincide with neuropathological changes in the brain. Despite the concomitant and statistically significant occurrence of various pathologic changes with deficits in cognition, to date, these studies remain largely correlative rather than directly causative. The following sections describe macroscopic and microscopic changes in the brains of dogs with cognitive dysfunction. See **Box 35-1** for information about age-related development of neuropathology in cats.

Macroscopic Changes in the Aging Brain

Changes in overall brain structure and volume can be seen using noninvasive techniques such as MRI. MRI studies in dogs reveal decreased brain volume, increased ventricular volume, increased perivascular space, lesions and cortical atrophy of the gray and white matter that often correlate with increasing age and cognitive decline (Su et al, 1998, 2005) (**Figure 35-1**). In 18 beagles (four to 15 years old), ventricular size increased slowly until 10 years of age and progressed very rapidly thereafter. In a longitudinal study using 47 beagles (eight to 11 years old at the first MRI), serial MRIs over four years revealed yearly increases in ventricular volume. Furthermore, different regions of the canine brain may have differing vulnerabilities to the aging process. An MRI study of 66 beagles (three months to 15 years) revealed decreases in total brain volume in dogs 12 years and older, whereas frontal lobe atrophy began much earlier, at eight years of age and correlated with impaired cognitive functions thought to be mediated by the frontal cortex (Tapp et al, 2004).

Lesions in aged beagles can be detected visually by MRI or by postmortem analysis of the brain. The cause and effect of these apparently spontaneous lesions is unclear; however, they have the morphologic appearance of lacunar infarcts or cysts

Box 35-2. The Toronto General Testing Apparatus.

The Toronto General Testing Apparatus (TGTA) is a canine-modified version of the Wisconsin General Testing Apparatus used for nonhuman primates. During testing, this wooden apparatus (**Figure 1**) houses the dog in a space (A) that contains no distinguishing features that a dog can use as cues for solving tasks. The experimenter is separated from the dog by a screen with a one-way mirror and a hinged door (B) that is opened for presentation of a sliding stimulus tray (C). The front of the TGTA is equipped with height- and width-adjustable bars (D) through which the dog accesses the stimulus tray, which contains one medial and two lateral food wells. The dog uses its nose to displace a stimulus and retrieves a highly-palatable cube of wet dog food when it makes a correct response. No food reward is given for an incorrect response. All stimuli used in tasks are baited with the same food in such a way that the dog can smell it but not see or eat it. This has the effect of masking any odor from the reward food cube so that it cannot be used as a cue to locate the correct stimulus.

Dogs first undergo a pretraining period during which they are exposed to the testing room and TGTA. They are encouraged to climb the stairs, enter the apparatus and eat food from the wells of the stimulus tray. After the pretraining phase is complete, a battery of cognitive tasks ranging from simple two-choice discrimination tasks to complex tests of executive function can be employed to provide objective and quantifiable measures of learning, memory and cognition. In addition, the TGTA can be used to assess attention, sensory and motor function, and recently, a paradigm was developed for evaluating dog food palatability. Cross-sectional studies using dogs of various ages are used to determine how learning is affected by age, and longitudinal studies are used to assess task retention across the lifespan.

The Bibliography for **Box 35-2** can be found at www.markmorris.org.

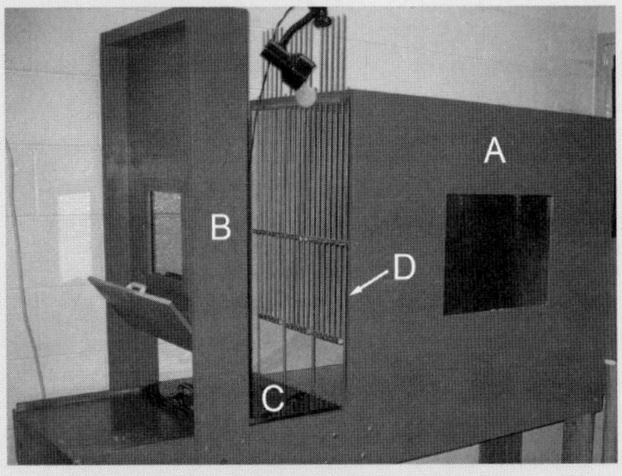

Figure 1. The Toronto General Testing Apparatus used to conduct cognitive testing in dogs. Test apparatus (A) where the dog is housed during testing, screen (B) to separate dog from experimenter with one-way mirror, sliding stimulus tray (C) with three food wells, height- and width-adjustable gates (D) allowing access to stimulus tray. (Courtesy Dr. Lori-Ann Christie, University of California-Irvine.)

and may be related to cerebrovascular changes in the aging brain. MRI lesions in beagles appear as hypointense cavities distributed throughout the brain, but are found most commonly in the frontal cortex and caudate nucleus (Su et al, 2005). In a group of 47 beagles imaged longitudinally over four years, lesions were observed starting at 11 years of age and became increasingly common by the time dogs were 14 years old (Su et al, 2005). Currently, the exact implications of these lesions are unknown and they may be clinically "silent."

Microscopic Changes in the Aging Brain

Microscopic signs of brain pathology can be observed in aged beagles with cognitive dysfunction. One type of pathology of significant interest is the accumulation of a protein fragment called beta-amyloid (Aβ). Aβ contains 39 to 43 amino acids and is the primary constituent of amyloid plaques in the brains of people with Alzheimer's disease (**Box 35-3**). Aβ is toxic to neurons in the brain and accumulates in diffuse proteinaceous plaques that are thought to play a causative role in the development of Alzheimer's disease in people (Selkoe, 2000).

Aged dogs naturally accumulate Aβ protein, with the exact same amino acid sequence, and with a similar extracellular pattern of deposition as occurs in people (Head et al, 2000; Johnstone et al, 1991). The brains of 40 beagles (two to 18 years old) were assayed for Aβ deposition; it was found that cortical Aβ is deposited in a specific spatial and temporal pattern. The earliest and most consistent area of Aβ, deposition was in the frontal cortex beginning at eight years of age, spreading caudally into the parietal and temporal/entorhinal regions by age 10 to 12 years, with the occipital cortex being the last to develop deposition at 13 years of age (Head et al, 2000). Other studies involving larger cohorts (more than 100 dogs) confirm that Aβ deposition is an accumulative and age-dependent process (Russell et al, 1996; Czasch et al, 2006). The Czasch et al 2006 study involving 130 dogs (one month to 18 years) revealed only one dog with pathology in the one month to seven years of age category, whereas 47% had Aβ deposition between the ages of eight to 10 years, 79% between 11 to 13 years and 91% between 14 to 18 years. Other studies involving dogs of different breeds (i.e., German shepherd dog, sheepdog, schnauzer, Doberman pinscher, poodle, Pekingese, fox terrier, beagle, caniche, boxer, Labrador retriever, collie, cocker spaniel, Irish setter, husky, mixed breed, etc.) also confirmed that Aβ deposition increases with age and severity of cognitive deficits (Anderson et al, 2000; Borras et al, 1999; Colle et al, 2000; Cummings et al, 1996; Hou et al, 1997; Pugliese et al, 2006, 2006a).

Aβ deposition has been studied more thoroughly in beagles than in other dogs. In this breed there are significant correlations with increased age and cognitive dysfunction (Cummings et al, 1996; Head et al, 1998; Tapp et al, 2004) and with decreased brain volume as determined by MRI (Tapp et al, 2004). Investigators selected 20 dogs (11 beagles) in one study and all dogs received a battery of six cognitive tasks (i.e., reward and object approach learning, discrimination and reversal learning, object recognition and spatial learning and memory). In this study, increased Aβ deposition was strongly associated with

Box 35-3. Similarities Between Neurologic Diseases in People and Those Found in Dogs.

The original rationale for conducting laboratory-based studies on canine cognition was to develop a model of human age-related cognitive dysfunction. The population of aged dogs tested to date display many similar characteristics to those observed in the aged human population. Like people, dogs show age-related individual variability in their learning, memory and cognitive abilities, and these impairments vary as a function of task. Some old dogs perform neuropsychological tests quite well for their age (successful agers), others are mildly impaired (similar to age-associated memory impairments in people) and still others are severely impaired (similar to dementia in people). Furthermore, neuropsychological tests developed for use in dogs have been adapted to test people. Preliminary evidence suggests that these adapted canine tasks are successful in discriminating healthy and cognitively impaired subpopulations of people.

Aged dogs develop similar neuropathological features to those in both successfully aging people and patients with Alzheimer's disease. As in people, beta-amyloid (Aβ) protein is deposited in the aging dog brain, and shows a selective distribution that changes as a function of age. Immunostaining of the frontal cortex with an anti-Aβ marker reveals morphologic similarities between Aβ plaques in the brains of normal and cognitively impaired people and beagles, making it very difficult to distinguish one species from another based on plaque deposition (**Figure 1**). Furthermore, the extent to which they possess these biologic markers is correlated with their cognitive abilities across the lifespan. For instance, results from a recent study show that decreased brain volume and increased Aβ load accumulation in the frontal cortex of aged dogs are correlated with deficits in complex discrimination and reversal learning.

Taken together, these findings suggest that the canine model can be used effectively for studying the etiology of age-related cognitive decline and dementia and their prevention and treatment in people. There are many research endeavors currently underway to determine if similar positive effects on cognition with antioxidant dietary intervention will be evident in people. This research represents a unique and exciting approach in translating what we know in dogs to aged and diseased human populations.

The Bibliography for **Box 35-3** can be found at www.markmorris.org.

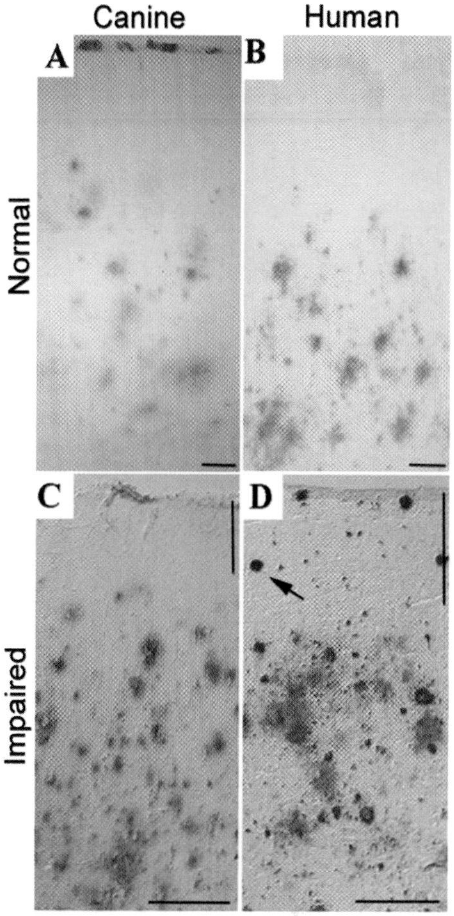

Figure 1. Comparable beta-amyloid (Aβ) immunostaining in the canine and human brain. The frontal cortex of a cognitively normal 13-year-old beagle (A) and 90-year-old female (B) illustrates a similar pattern of senile Aβ plaque deposition in the deeper cortical layers. Frontal cortex sections of a severely impaired 12-year-old beagle (C) and 86-year-old individual (D) with Alzheimer's disease show extensive Aβ pathology throughout all layers of cortex, whereas the molecular layer is largely spared (vertical line = molecular layer, arrow = compact plaque, all bars = 200 mm). (Reproduced with permission from Head E, Milgram NW, Cotman CW. Neurobiological models of aging in the dog and other vertebrate species. In: Hof P, Mobbs C, eds. Functional Neurobiology of Aging. New York, NY: Academic Press, 2001; 457-468.)

increased error scores across all tasks (Cummings et al, 1996) (**Figure 35-2**).

Functional Changes in the Aging Brain

In addition to macroscopic and microscopic morphologic changes in the aging canine brain, there is also evidence of functional change.

CHANGES IN THE BLOOD-BRAIN BARRIER WITH AGE

The BBB is a collective term for the complex vascular system of endothelial cells, astrocytes, pericytes and basement membranes surrounding the brain. The BBB allows for selective transport of nutrients from the blood to neuronal cells (Khan, 2005). An MRI study involving 18 beagles (four to 15 years old) showed a non-significant increase in BBB permeability with age; surprisingly, one six-year-old beagle, in which no pathology was expected, had severe BBB leakage and dysfunction, enlarged ventricles, Aβ deposition and cognitive dysfunction (Su et al, 1998). Another study reported a direct link between vascular Aβ deposition and vessel wall integrity; leptomeninges obtained from old dogs affected by cerebral amy-

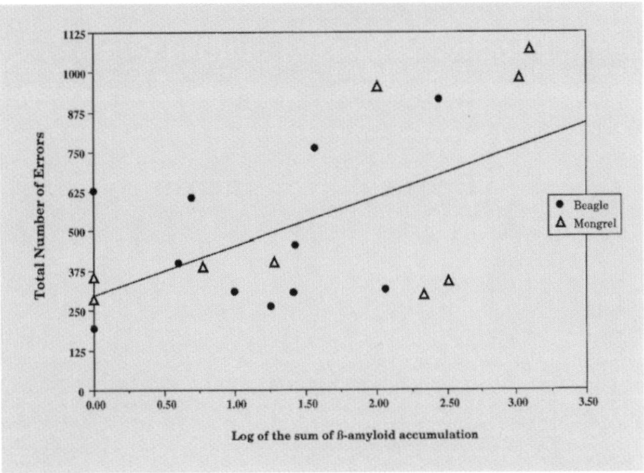

Figure 35-2. Correlations between cognitive task errors and beta-amyloid (Aβ) accumulation in beagles and mixed-breed dogs. The y-axis represents the summed error scores for a series of cognitive tasks and the x-axis represents the overall log scores of the Aβ load measurements from the frontal cortex, entorhinal cortex and cerebellum for each individual animal. Increased cognitive error scores were significantly correlated with increased Aβ measurements ($r = 0.66$, $p \leq 0.01$). (Reproduced with permission from: Cummings BJ, Head E, Afagh AJ, et al. Beta-amyloid accumulation correlates with cognitive dysfunction in the aged canine. Neurobiology of Learning and Memory 1996; 66: 11-23.)

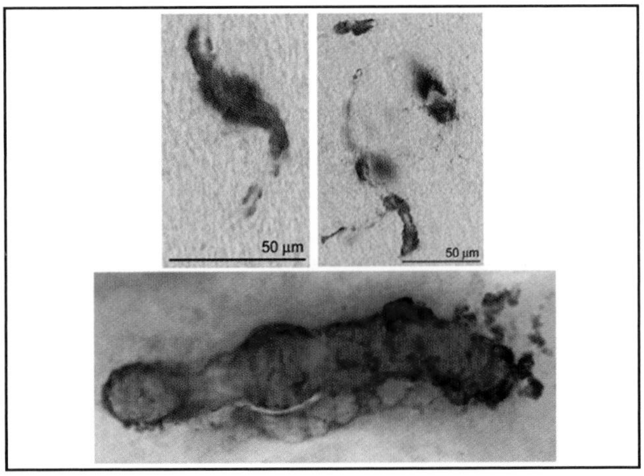

Figure 35-3. Amyloid angiopathy in the canine brain. All three panels illustrate immunostaining with beta-amyloid (Aβ) antibodies in the aged (~10 years old) canine cortex with vessels that are severely affected by Aβ deposition. Angiopathy can impair vascular function and damage the blood-brain barrier, leading to increased permeability of substances in and out of brain cells. (Courtesy Viorela Pop, University of California-Irvine.)

loid angiopathy showed segmental loss of vessel integrity at sites of Aβ deposition, suggesting that the presence of Aβ in old dogs disrupts the BBB (Prior et al, 1996). A study investigating the white matter of 31 dogs of various breeds (six months to 18 years old) found that age-related morphologic changes in the capillaries were associated with BBB permeability dysfunction. Specifically, aging dogs had degeneration of axons, perivascular infiltration of macrophages and iron and sometimes small foci of hemorrhages and infarction (Morita et al, 2005).

Recently, BBB permeability studies involving aged beagles treated with a food containing enhanced levels of antioxidants and/or behavioral enrichment found that, overall, there was a higher permeability index in the occipital lobe compared to the frontal and parietal regions (Su et al, 2006). In this same analysis, the occipital cortex had the highest amount of vascular Aβ pathology (**Figure 35-3**), which may have contributed to the increased BBB index in this region. Furthermore, yearly increases and worsening of BBB permeability were slowed in groups given antioxidant and/or enrichment treatment. Another study involving 25 dogs of various breeds (three to 19 years of age) found that scores on cognitive status questionnaires (Age-Related Cognitive and Affective Disorders) correlated with increased vascular Aβ deposition (Colle et al, 2000). More studies are underway to better understand BBB changes with increased age; interventions may prevent or delay BBB dysfunction and reduce the secretion of serum containing harmful substances that may further induce tissue damage and oxidative stress.

INCREASED OXIDATIVE DAMAGE WITH AGE

Oxidative damage is one possible mechanism that contributes to neuronal dysfunction and the progression of neuropathology with age. Normal metabolic processes in the brain lead to the production of oxidants, or reactive oxygen species (ROS). The free radical theory of aging (Harman, 1956) was the first to propose that excessive production of ROS leads to cell damage and that this damage accumulates over time and inevitably leads to age-dependent pathology in multiple tissues. ROS are the byproducts of mitochondrial aerobic respiration (Beckman and Ames, 1998), and include any atoms or molecules that contain one or more unpaired electrons. ROS are unstable because their unpaired electrons thermodynamically seek to pair with other electrons. This increases unregulated/nonspecific reactions that have enhanced potential for interaction, damage and dysfunction inside cells. Overproduction of ROS results in oxidative damage to proteins, lipids and nucleotides, which, in the brain, lead to neuronal dysfunction and untimely neuronal death. Therefore, the aging process might be mitigated by appropriate reduction of excessive ROS (Chapter 7).

Normal aerobic metabolism in mitochondria generates the superoxide ion, the ROS molecule of central interest. An appropriate balance between superoxide production and detoxification systems is essential to cellular health and intracellular metabolic signaling. Under normal circumstances, cells have a variety of mechanisms to detoxify superoxide (Head and Zicker, 2004). As mitochondria age or become dysfunctional from disease, defense mechanisms are compromised and/or overwhelmed and superoxide is produced in excess leading to uncontrolled reactions in cells (Ames et al, 1993; Cottrell and Turnbull, 2000).

In dogs, at least one defense system declines with age. Superoxide dismutase is present normally in the brain and acts to convert reactive superoxide ions to hydrogen peroxide, thereby decreasing oxidative damage to surrounding tissues. In fact, one approved treatment for cognitive dysfunction, selegiline, has been shown to increase levels of superoxide dismutase in the brain (Carillo et al, 1994). This compensatory mechanism appears to be compromised in older dogs (Kiatipattanasakul et al, 1997). It has also been shown that oxidative damage to proteins (Head et al, 2002) and lipids (Rofina et al, 2004) accumulates in older dogs. These findings, in combination with age-related cognitive dysfunction and pathologic changes, suggest that decreasing oxidative damage in the brain might improve cognitive function in older dogs. Thus, dietary interventions that decrease specific types of oxidative damage may slow the progression of age-related cognitive decline in dogs.

Key Nutritional Factors

A longitudinal laboratory-based study and a randomized, controlled clinical field trial of the effects of a food enriched in a broad spectrum of antioxidants were conducted as described below. Subjects were assigned to receive either an enriched food (test food) or an extruded senior food (control food). The enriched food was supplemented with vitamins C and E, selenium, L-carnitine, α-lipoic acid, omega-3 fatty acids and a mixture of fruits and vegetables. Key nutritional factors for cognitive dysfunction are listed in **Table 35-3** and discussed in more detail below.

Table 35-3. Key nutritional factors for foods for dogs with brain aging and associated behavioral changes (cognitive dysfunction).*

Factors	Dietary recommendation
Vitamin E	Increase dietary antioxidants Provide foods with ≥750 mg/kg
Vitamin C	Increase dietary antioxidants Provide foods with ≥150 mg/kg
Selenium	Increase dietary antioxidants Provide foods with 0.5 to 1.3 mg/kg
L-carnitine	Increase mitochondrial cofactors Provide foods with 250 to 750 IU/kg
α-lipoic acid	Increase mitochondrial cofactors Provide foods with ≥100 mg/kg
Omega-3 fatty acids (docosahexaenoic and eicosapentaenoic acids)	Total omegas-3 >1%
Fruits and vegetables	1% of each of five vegetable and fruit ingredients

*Dry matter basis.

Antioxidants and Mitochondrial Cofactors

Antioxidants are substances that scavenge ROS and decrease the overall number of oxidants in a system (Ames et al, 1993; De Ruvo et al, 2000). Many antioxidant compounds such as vitamin E, vitamin C and trace minerals (e.g., selenium) are derived from food sources. Vitamin C is a water-soluble vitamin that helps replenish vitamin E. Mitochondrial cofactors (α-lipoic acid and L-carnitine) act to enhance the function of aged mitochondria so that fewer ROS are produced during aerobic respiration (i.e., they work to increase mitochondrial efficiency). L-carnitine is involved in lipid metabolism within mitochondria; α-lipoic acid participates in redox reactions and increases intracellular concentrations of glutathione, a primary water-soluble antioxidant within cells. Fruits and vegetables contain flavonoids and carotenoids, which have antioxidant activities as well.

One hypothesis is that adding increased amounts of these components to a food would reduce the amount of oxidative damage in two ways, by: 1) decreasing the production of ROS and 2) increasing the capacity to clear ROS, and that this would slow the progression of age-related pathologic changes and cognitive decline by reducing overall oxidative damage.

A longitudinal laboratory-based study and a blinded veterinary clinical field trial were conducted to assess the effectiveness of a food supplemented with antioxidants and mitochondrial cofactors in ameliorating cognitive decline in older dogs (Dodd et al, 2003). Results were used as grade 1 evidence-based nutritional research for the development of a commercial, antioxidant-enriched food.[a]

Investigators conducting the clinical field trial recruited dogs over seven years of age that had clinical signs in two or more DISH categories. The dogs were randomly assigned to two groups: one that was fed a commercial control food (n = 64) and one that was fed an antioxidant fortified test dog food[a] (n = 61). Owners rated their pet's behaviors before and on Days 30 and 60 of the dietary intervention. After 30 days of dietary intervention, owners reported significant improvements in the following categories: disorientation, interactive changes, sleep patterns and house soiling. By Day 60, owners reported that dogs receiving the test food improved in all four DISH categories (plus activity) whereas those fed the control food improved in only two categories. Dogs receiving the fortified food had improvements in awareness of their surroundings, family and animal recognition and interaction, enthusiasm in greeting and agility, and were reported to circle and house soil less frequently. Overall, the test food was better than the control food; dogs receiving it improved in 13 of 15 behaviors (87%) compared to four of 15 behaviors (27%) for dogs in the control group (Dodd et al, 2003; Zicker, 2005).

The laboratory-based study included 48 aged beagles (10 to 13 years old) and 17 young dogs (three to five years). Each age group was divided into an enriched food group (antioxidant) and a control food group; both groups were balanced for age and initial cognitive performance. The enriched food consisted of a variety of antioxidants, mitochondrial cofactors and dried fruits and vegetables. The control food was an identical base food adequate for senior dogs; however, it was not fortified with additional antioxidants and mitochondrial cofactors. Dogs were tested at several time points over two years after initiation of dietary intervention. Old dogs receiving the antioxidant food had improved learning and memory as measured by several cognitive tasks. The oddity discrimination task was administered, as described above, six months after the dietary intervention began (Milgram et al, 2002). Both age and food effects were observed (**Figure 35-4**); old dogs made more errors at learning all levels of the task compared to young dogs. However, old dogs fed the antioxidant food made significantly

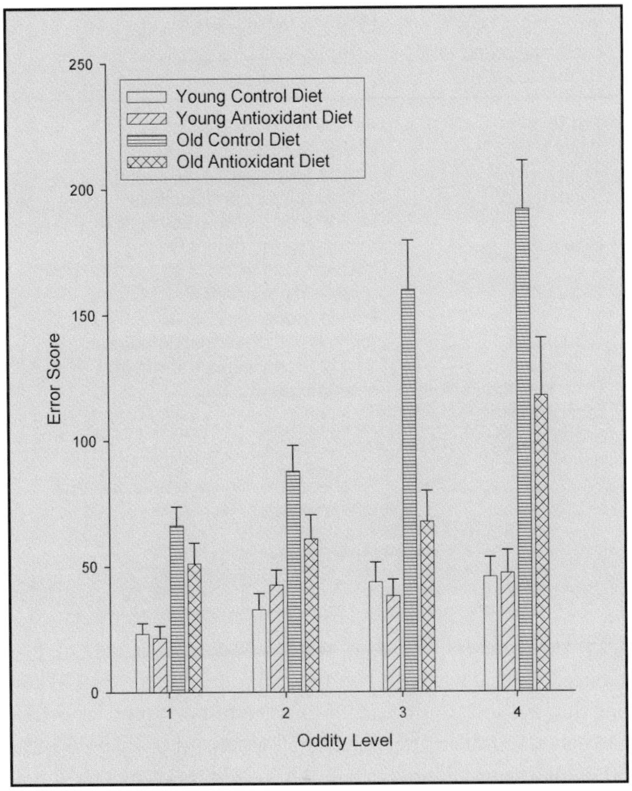

Figure 35-4. Effect of age, food and task difficulty on acquisition of an oddity discrimination learning task. Overall, the number of errors made to achieve the criterion increased with increasing oddity level; old dogs made more errors compared to young dogs on all levels. A food with enhanced levels of antioxidants and mitochondrial cofactors significantly reduced the number of errors made by old dogs to acquire the task. (Courtesy Dr. Elizabeth Head, University of California-Irvine.)

fewer errors than old dogs fed the control food. This effect was particularly pronounced at the most difficult oddity levels. Furthermore, the beneficial effect of the antioxidant food on oddity discrimination learning was not observed in young dogs, presumably because they did not have significant oxidative damage that could be reduced by dietary intervention like the older dogs (Head and Zicker, 2004; Milgram et al, 2002).

Positive antioxidant food effects were also observed selectively in old dog's reversal learning performance (Milgram et al, 2004, 2005). Dogs were first taught to respond to one of two stimuli to receive a food reward, as described above. There was no significant effect of diet at this stage of learning, which was anticipated given that simple discrimination learning, in general, remains intact in old animals (Milgram et al, 2005). However, when the reward contingencies for the task were reversed so that dogs had to suppress their tendency to respond to the previously rewarded stimulus and learn to choose the opposite stimulus, old dogs receiving the antioxidant food had improved learning compared to old dogs fed the control food. This effect of the antioxidant food on reversal learning was found when stimuli differed in size after one year of treatment and when they differed in intensity (e.g., black/white discrimination) after two years of treatment, indicating that the improvement in cognitive function was maintained over time (Milgram et al, 2005). Similar beneficial effects of the antioxidant food in old dogs have been observed with other cognitive tests, including a landmark spatial discrimination task as early as two months after the start of the trial (Ikeda-Douglas et al, 2004; Milgram et al, 2002), a complex size concept task (Siwak et al, 2005) and in contrast sensitivity discrimination (de Rivera et al, 2005).

Overall, the results demonstrate that the rate of cognitive decline observed in old dogs can be slowed by dietary intervention, and that the positive effects on cognition occur relatively rapidly. The findings also suggest that feeding a food containing a mixture of specific antioxidants and mitochondrial cofactors may act synergistically to reduce oxidative damage and increase mitochondrial efficiency, and that oxidative damage and mitochondrial function are fundamental mechanisms contributing to age-associated cognitive dysfunction in older dogs. More studies are currently underway to determine the specific combinations of ingredients that are most effective at ameliorating cognitive dysfunction in older dogs.

In the same laboratory-based intervention study in beagles described above, analyses of Aβ plaque deposition revealed that only dogs given the antioxidant food had less Aβ in the parietal and entorhinal cortex, but not in the prefrontal cortex (Pop et al, 2003). The food may prevent production of Aβ from its larger parent protein, Aβ precursor protein (APP), by increasing the activity of the alpha-secretase enzyme responsible for non-amyloidogenic APP cleavage (Pop et al, 2005). The results of the antioxidant study suggest that food can slow or prevent Aβ, deposition in regions actively accumulating Aβ (e.g., parietal and entorhinal), but cannot reverse existing deposits (e.g., those in the prefrontal cortex).

Appropriate levels of antioxidants and mitochondrial cofactors should be: vitamin E = ≥750 mg/kg; vitamin C = ≥150 mg/kg; selenium = 0.5 to 1.3 mg/kg; L-carnitine = 250 to 750 IU/kg; α-lipoic acid = ≥100 mg/kg; total omega-3 fatty acids = 1% added for docosahexaenoic and eicosapentaenoic acids; fruits and vegetables = 5% added for flavonoids and polyphenols, all on a dry matter basis. No minimum or maximum effective levels for fruits and vegetables have been established. The test food contained 1% of each of five vegetable and fruit ingredients as a substitute for corn.

A careful and detailed analysis of the concentrations of carotenoids, flavonoids and oxygen radical absorbance capacity of individual ingredients was necessary to develop the test food (Zicker, 2005). Studies of commodities with naturally occurring and synthetic antioxidants were conducted to ensure stability through processing, absorption from the gastrointestinal tract, safety and potential antioxidant biologic benefit. The results of these analyses highlighted that the mere presence of a fruit or vegetable on a label was not always indicative of high antioxidant content, an observation that practitioners and pet owners should take into account when choosing food for their senior pets.

Besides their apparent value in the dietary management of

Table 35-4. Recommended levels of key nutritional factors compared to the nutrient profile of a dry commercial food for canine cognitive dysfunction patients.*

	Energy density (kcal/cup)**	Energy density (kcal ME/g)	Vitamin E (mg/kg)	Vitamin C (mg/kg)	Selenium (mg/kg)	L-carnitine (mg/kg)	α-lipoic acid (mg/kg)	Total omega-3 fatty acids (%)	Fruits/ vegetables
Recommended levels	**-**	**-**	**≥750**	**≥150**	**0.5-1.3**	**250-750**	**≥100**	**>1%**	**Added**
Hill's Prescription Diet b/d Canine	358	4.0	1,075	109	na	299	na	1.02	Added

Key: na = not available from manufacturer
*Values obtained from manufacturer's published information. Nutrients expressed on a dry matter basis, unless otherwise stated.
**Energy density as fed is useful for determining the amount to feed; cup = 8-oz. measuring cup; to convert to kJ, multiply by 4.184.

CDS, antioxidants have been shown to play a role in the prevention of certain cancers through various mechanisms (Chapter 30). As in people, increasing age is a general risk factor for cancer in dogs.

Other Nutritional Factors

Older dogs are at increased risk for other diseases, including chronic periodontitis and osteoarthritis. Therefore, the clinician must choose the food based on which medical condition is of greatest priority for the pet. For example, cardiovascular and chronic renal failure may become more of a priority than cognitive dysfunction, necessitating reduced levels of sodium and phosphorus in the food. When the pet's health necessitates the use of a food other than one designed to promote optimal cognitive function, then specific supplements may need to be considered. However, the clinician should evaluate the evidence supporting the efficacy of any supplements that might be added to the feeding plan regimen and ensure there is no contraindication to their use.

FEEDING PLAN

The dietary goals are to provide a food that meets the patient's nutrient requirements and blunts the vulnerability of nervous tissue to ROS as the brain ages. Free radical damage can be manifested by behavioral changes or CDS. The food selected should contain levels of nutrients that protect against free radical damage and improve learning ability and alertness of older pets. Antioxidants and mitochondrial cofactors have demonstrated efficacy when fed in amounts as described in the Key Nutritional Factors section and shown in **Table 35-3.** Behavioral enrichment and medical therapy as described below may augment treatment.

Assess and Select the Food

Levels of key nutritional factors in foods currently fed to patients with cognitive dysfunction should be evaluated and compared with recommended levels. Information from this aspect of assessment is essential for making any changes to foods currently provided. Changing to a more appropriate food is indicated if key nutritional factors in the current food do not match recommended levels. **Table 35-4** provides the key nutritional factors recommended for foods for dogs with CDS and compares them to the key nutritional factor content of a commercial food developed specifically for dogs with CDS.[a]

Another criterion for selecting a food that may become increasingly important in the future is evidence-based clinical nutrition. Practitioners should know how to determine risks and benefits of nutritional regimens and counsel pet owners accordingly. Currently, veterinary medical education and continuing education are not always based on rigorous assessment of evidence for or against particular management options. Still, studies have been published to establish the nutritional benefits of certain pet foods. Chapter 2 describes evidence-based clinical nutrition in detail and applies its concepts to various veterinary therapeutic foods. Evidence Grade 1 (the highest level) exists for at least one food used for dogs with CDS.[a]

Assess and Determine the Feeding Method

A thorough assessment should include verification of the feeding method currently being used. Items to consider include feeding frequency, amount fed, how the food is offered, access to other food and who feeds the animal. All of this information should have been gathered when the history of the animal was obtained. If the animal has a normal body condition score (2.5/5 to 3.5/5), the amount of food previously fed (energy basis) was probably appropriate.

Adjunct Therapy

Behavioral Enrichment

Environmental enrichment (EE) also appears to play an important role in preserving cognitive abilities in old age. In dogs, there is laboratory-based evidence suggesting that an enriched environment acts synergistically with an antioxidant food to slow cognitive decline in older animals (Milgram et al, 2004, 2005). In the same study in which the fortified food was administered (described above), dogs in each of the food groups were further divided to include one group that received EE and one that did not. The EE program consisted of increased activity (i.e., exercise twice weekly), enriched kennel environments (i.e., toys and housing with kennelmates) and regular cognitive testing (i.e., neuropsychological testing five or six times weekly). In combination with the antioxidant food, positive effects of EE were observed after one year in the old dogs; size discrimination and reversal learning were improved. After two years of EE, the enrichment alone was sufficient to detect improved performance on the intensity discrimination and reversal tasks. On both of these tasks, the investigators found that combined antioxidant dietary and EE intervention were more effective than either treatment alone. The authors concluded that a prolonged period of EE has substantial effects on cognitive performance in older beagles, and like the antioxidant food, appears to slow development of age-related cognitive decline in old dogs (Milgram et al, 2004, 2005).

Supplements

A number of complementary therapies are marketed as treatments for cognitive dysfunction. These products may contain mixtures of herbal extracts, vitamins, phospholipids, fatty acids, antioxidants and mitochondrial cofactors believed to act in a synergistic or potentiating manner to slow the progression of or improve clinical signs associated with brain aging. Although there is little evidence to support the efficacy of most of these products, three clinical trials have recently reported improvements in clinical signs of CDS in pets given dietary supplements containing phosphatidylserine (Osella et al, 2007; Cena et al, 2005; Heath et al, 2007). Phosphatidylserine, *Gingko biloba*, pyridoxine and vitamin E are distributed in Italy as a neuroprotective dietary supplement for senior dogs and cats.[b] In a preliminary laboratory evaluation, dogs were tested after administration of a placebo or the product for 60 days, in a crossover design using spatial memory assessments (Araujo et al, 2006). Performance accuracy was significantly improved in the treated group compared to the baseline group. In addition, dogs receiving the supplement in the first portion of the study maintained their improved performance (Araujo et al, 2006). This product was recently reformulated and now contains resveratrol.

Other commercially available supplements contain docosahexaenoic acid, eicosapentaenoic acid and acetylcysteine, which is a primary precursor to glutathione and coenzyme Q10. Fatty acids and glutathione may be beneficial in slowing brain aging in people (Horrocks and Yeo, 1999; Pocernich et al, 2000). Preliminary work also showed an improvement in memory and health status in dogs receiving a docosahexaenoic acid supplement (Araujo et al, 2005). S-adenosyl-methionine (SAMe) may be useful in elderly pets because it has been shown to be helpful for treating cognitive dysfunction in people. Furthermore, in a preliminary open label clinical trial, SAMe improved activity levels, sleep-wake cycles, playfulness and fecal elimination disorders in elderly depressed or confused pets[c] (Arnold, 2005).

Drug Therapy

Selegiline is licensed for treatment of cognitive dysfunction in dogs in North America.[d] Selegiline is a selective and irreversible inhibitor of MOA-B in dogs (Milgram et al, 1993). It increases 2-phenylethylamine in the canine brain. This drug is a neuromodulator; therefore, the primary mode of action may be to enhance dopamine and catecholamine function in the cortex and hippocampus to improve cognitive function (Milgram et al, 1993; Knoll, 1998). Selegiline may also contribute to a decrease in ROS in the brain by decreasing production of free radicals, scavenging oxygen free radicals and enhancing the scavenging action of enzymes such as catalase and superoxide dismutase (Carillo et al, 1994; Heinonen and Lammintausta, 1991). Selegiline is given at a dose of 0.5 to 1 mg/kg per os each morning. Although selegiline can be used concurrently with most veterinary therapeutic foods and supplements, it should not be combined with narcotics, antidepressants or monoamine oxidase inhibitors. Therefore, it should probably not be used with supplements containing tryptophan, St. John's wort or *Ginkgo biloba.*

Propentofylline and nicergoline, which may enhance cerebrovascular transmission, are licensed in some European countries and Australia for signs of brain aging in senior pets (Penaliggon, 1991; Kapl and Rudolphi, 1998). The efficacy of nicergoline has been demonstrated in at least one clinical trial (Penaliggon, 1991). It was recently determined that senior dogs display a greater sensitivity to the memory impairment effects of scopolamine (an anticholinergic drug) than younger dogs and show a positive response to experimental cholinomimetics (Araujo et al, 2005a). A major focus of drug therapy for Alzheimer's disease in people is to enhance cholinergic transmission. Therefore, drugs that act to augment cholinergic transmission might have application for clinical use in dogs with cognitive decline; however, no available drugs have been sufficiently investigated (Araujo et al, 2005a). This may, however, explain why some of the natural supplements (e.g., those containing phosphatidylserine) are effective by enhancing cholinergic transmission or helping protect cholinergic neurons (Vannucchi et al, 1990; Gelbann and Mullet, 1992).

In addition to preventive therapy, it may be necessary to consider medications to treat specific signs such as anxiety, restlessness, night waking and agitation. Selection of the appropriate medication should consider the pet's health and any concurrent medications. In general, anxiolytics that are less likely to cause hepatic complications (e.g., clonazepam, oxazepam, lorazepam or buspirone), natural products such as DAP, and antidepressants that have little or no anticholinergic effects, such as fluoxetine might be the most appropriate options.

REASSESSMENT

Improvements in abnormal behavior associated with brain aging may be noted within six to 12 weeks after making a dietary change. If improvements are not noted with 12 weeks, then it is unlikely that nutritional management alone will result in significant improvement. Therapy with supplements and drugs appears to be safe to use in conjunction with nutritional management. Reassessment of behavioral changes can also occur during routine health maintenance protocols established for mature or geriatric pets in each hospital.

As mentioned above, in 2005, the American Animal Hospital Association senior care task force published guidelines that recommended yearly wellness screening for healthy middle-aged pets and twice yearly screening for senior pets (i.e., last 25% of predicted lifespan). At each visit, the pet should receive a physical examination and laboratory tests and the owner should be extensively questioned about changes in behavior and health (Epstein et al, 2005). However, patients with health problems and those receiving drugs or medications may need to be assessed more frequently or have more extensive testing (e.g., blood pressure measurement, radiographs). For example, semiannual visits may be adequate for dogs with CDS; however, if signs worsen or new signs arise, the owners should schedule a more immediate reassessment to ensure that new diseases are not emerging and to assess whether additional therapeutics might be needed. When drugs are dispensed, followup visits should be scheduled based on the specific drug and disease. For example, dogs receiving selegiline should be reassessed after the first month, whereas dogs receiving most nonsteroidal antiinflammatory drugs should be reassessed within a few weeks to establish therapeutic effect and reassess liver enzyme activity.

ENDNOTES

a. Prescription Diet b/d Canine. Hill's Pet Nutrition Inc., Topeka, KS, USA.
b. Senilife. Innovet Italia S.r.l., Milano, Italy.
c. Novofit Product Profile. Virbac Corporation, Fort Worth, TX, USA.
d. Anipyrl. Pfizer Animal Health, Exton, PA, USA.

REFERENCES

The references for **Chapter 35** can be found at www.markmorris.org.

CASE 35-1

Behavioral Changes in an Older Beagle

Philip Roudebush, DVM, Dipl. ACVIM (Small Animal Internal Medicine)
Hill's Scientific Affairs
Topeka, Kansas, USA

Patient Assessment

A 13-year-old intact female beagle was admitted for routine health maintenance procedures. The owners reported no obvious health problems with the dog other than halitosis and masses under the skin of the ventral abdomen. As part of the geriatric health maintenance program administered at this hospital, the owners were asked to complete a behavioral questionnaire and checklist (**Table 35-1**). On this questionnaire, the owners noted that the dog had shown decreased greeting behavior when they returned home, had less interest in being petted by the owners or their children, paced aimlessly in the fenced backyard at times, often refused to play with the younger dog at home and occasionally woke up at night and paced in their bedroom. The owners attributed these changes to aging and did not consider them major problems.

Physical examination revealed a geriatric dog with a body weight of 12.0 kg and an ideal body condition score of 3 on a 5-point scale. Abnormalities include moderate periodontal disease with extensive bilateral calculus formation on the premolars and molars and reddening and mild swelling of the gingival margins, a small, soft 2 x 2 cm subcutaneous mass at the left sternal border and a small, firm mammary tumor in the third right gland.

Routine preventive health testing included a complete blood count, serum biochemistry profile, heartworm check, urinalysis, fecal examination and fine-needle aspiration of the two masses for cytologic evaluation. Results of blood work, parasite exams and urinalysis were normal. Fine-needle aspiration cytology was consistent with a lipoma and benign mixed mammary tumor.

Assess the Food and Feeding Method

The dog was fed a combination of dry and moist commercial grocery brand dog foods supplemented with occasional table scraps.

Questions

1. What are potential causes and ways to evaluate the behavioral problems noted in this dog?
2. Outline a comprehensive medical and nutritional management plan for this patient.

Answers

1. Aged dogs are susceptible to a number of neurologic disorders with a wide variety of clinical presentations. Behavioral changes, alterations in mental status, seizures, loss of vision or hearing, pain, tremors, stiffness, weakness, gait abnormalities and motor dysfunction are associated with a variety of neurologic diseases. A screening neurologic examination that evaluates mental status, cranial nerve function and gait often can detect neurologic deficits. When deficits are present, a complete neurologic examination

is indicated to further characterize the abnormalities and localize the lesion.

Older dogs are also at risk for developing a variety of age-related behavioral disorders. Aged dogs exhibit deficits in learning and memory similar to those in people, and the underlying mechanisms that produce the cognitive deficits may affect behavior. Common behavioral problems in older dogs include decrements of attention and activity, inability to navigate stairs, wandering and disorientation and disturbances of the sleep-wake cycle. Older dogs lose housetraining habits and are less interactive with people, toys and other animals. Some dogs also exhibit decreased exploratory behavior. This spectrum of behavioral problems parallels many changes that occur in human dementia.

Many owners of older dogs are aware of behavioral changes but do not report them to veterinarians because they think it is part of the normal aging process. This emphasizes the importance of using behavioral or cognitive dysfunction checklists routinely as part of the screening process during geriatric health exams. In this case, the dog's owners noted mild behavioral alterations that should be discussed further.

2. As noted earlier, a neurologic examination should be performed to rule out significant neurologic disease. Normal results of routine blood, urine and fecal tests make serious underlying metabolic disorders unlikely at this time. Dental prophylaxis and excision of the masses can be accomplished during one anesthetic event. Medical and/or nutritional management can be used if brain aging and cognitive dysfunction are considered likely causes of the behavioral changes. Medical treatment includes use of drugs such as selegiline hydrochloride (Anipryl[a]) to alter brain neuropeptide levels.

Nutritional strategies are based on studies showing that oxidative damage to the canine brain increases with age and precedes morphologic brain changes associated with cognitive dysfunction and age-associated behavioral changes. Brain tissue is especially vulnerable to free radical damage because of its high metabolic activity, high fat content, naturally low levels of protective antioxidants and limited regenerative capabilities. Foods rich in antioxidants such as vitamin E, vitamin C, and flavonoids and carotenoids from fruits and vegetables, and rich in mitochondrial cofactors such as L-carnitine and α-lipoic acid will decrease signs of brain aging, improve cognitive ability and provide noticeable change in behaviors. Laboratory studies have shown that foods rich in antioxidants and mitochondrial cofactors improve learning in older dogs with cognitive dysfunction. In clinical studies, dogs with aged-related behavioral changes consuming an enriched food showed improvements in disorientation, family and animal recognition and interaction, sleep patterns, housetraining and activity level.

Epilogue

A neurologic examination was normal and the dog was hospitalized for a dental prophylaxis and tumor excision. The patient recovered uneventfully from these procedures and was discharged with Prescription Diet b/d Canine.[b] The dog's owners were instructed to feed the food enriched with antioxidants and mitochondrial cofactors for at least three months and then return for further evaluation. They were also instructed on how to brush the dog's teeth and appropriate oral care products were dispensed for home use. Phone calls to the owners over the next couple of months confirmed that they were brushing the dog's teeth, feeding the enriched food exclusively and that some behaviors were improving. At the three-month recheck examination, the patient's owners reported that the dog was wagging its tail for the first time in many years, was interacting with family members and the other dog more often and sleeping through the night without waking or pacing excessively.

Acknowledgement

Thanks to Joe Hosey of Topeka, KS, for providing case information.

Endnotes

a. Pfizer Animal Health, Exton, PA, USA.
b. Hill's Pet Nutrition Inc., Topeka, KS, USA.

CASE 35-2

Extending the Length and Quality of Life of an Aging Female Bichon Frise

Gary Landsberg, BSc, DVM, Dipl. ACVB (Behavior)
Doncaster Animal Clinic
Thornhill, Ontario, Canada

Patient Assessment

A 15.5-year-old, spayed female Bichon Frise was presented for euthanasia due to its age, multiple behavioral signs, its owner's age, financial considerations and household factors, which included the inability of a single elderly women in a small detached home to live with the dog's poor health and behavior. Previously, the dog received regular, quality care throughout its life.

At age 10, the dog developed calcium oxalate uroliths, which were removed surgically. Following surgery the dog was fed Prescription Diet u/d Canine[a] as an aid in preventing recurrence of uroliths. At age 12, the dog required surgery to repair a ruptured cruciate ligament. At age 14, the owner began to report a decrease in activity and responsiveness to stimuli. On examination, the dog had moderately decreased vision and some arthritis in the leg that had been surgically repaired. Results of all laboratory tests (complete blood count, serum biochemistry profile, urinalysis, endocrine screening) were within normal limits; no other physical abnormalities or neurologic deficits were identified. Because no other cognitive signs were evident, a nonsteroidal antiinflammatory drug (meloxicam) was prescribed for the stifle arthritis, which improved the dog's activity and mobility and the dog appeared to adapt well to its decreasing vision.

One year later, at age 15, the dog was presented because of newly emerging multiple behavioral signs. With the aid of the cognitive assessment table (**Table 35-1**), the owner reported an increase in anxiety, agitation, restless pacing, house soiling, a decreased responsiveness to stimuli and alterations in sleep with shorter, more frequent sleep periods during the daytime and waking throughout the night. All laboratory tests were within normal limits. Physical and neurologic examinations were also unremarkable except for the previously diagnosed vision loss and stifle arthritis. A neurologic referral and magnetic resonance imaging were declined; however, the owner consented to a selegiline[b] trial. Over the next two months, the owner noticed an increase in the pacing and house soiling, a further decrease in awareness, decreased responsiveness to the owner, a decline in hearing, a decreased tolerance to being left alone and a loss of learned commands. The dog also developed signs of colitis and intermittent vomiting. The owner discontinued the selegiline, which did not appear effective at controlling any of the behavioral signs, and then discontinued the meloxicam. Although the vomiting resolved, the colitis persisted.

Assess the Food and Feeding Method

The dog was fed one-half cup and one-half can of Prescription Diet u/d Canine daily.

Question

At this point, considering the uroliths were no longer a priority, could a trial of Prescription Diet b/d Canine[a] ameliorate some of this patient's behavioral problems before any final decisions were made regarding euthanasia?

Answer

A urinalysis and a fecal examination (to rule out parasites) were the only tests approved by the owner; results were within normal limits. The dog began to show some improvement within the first week of changing to Prescription Diet b/d Canine. At the end of two months, the owner reported that the dog was more aware, active and interactive with its owner and that wandering had decreased. The dog slept through most nights and was able to be retrained to paper to eliminate the house soiling. The owner also reported that the dog was barking at squirrels and other stimuli that passed the property, which it had ignored for more than two years. Therefore, an improved awareness and responsiveness to stimuli seemed to be emerging despite the apparent decline in vision and hearing. The owner also commented that the dog's stools were regular; however, the dog was experiencing increasing hind-leg discomfort as mobility increased. A glucosamine hydrochloride/chondroitin sulfate combination (Cosequin[c]) was dispensed because the owner was unwilling to try other pharmaceutical options.

Epilogue

The dog was maintained on Prescription Diet b/d Canine and Cosequin for almost a year before problems again began to emerge. At approximately 16.5 years of age, the dog was presented for evaluation of hematuria, decreased activity and further deterioration of vision and hearing. The owner reported that the dog was again more anxious, pacing when awake, seeking out the owner more, increasingly disoriented and sleeping much more. House soiling and waking at night had not recurred. The hematuria was caused by bacterial cystitis (with no evidence of calculus recurrence), and the arthritis and sensory decline were likely responsible for some of the decrease in activity levels. Euthanasia was discussed; however, the owner consented to concurrent trials with antibiotics and

Senilife.[d]

After one month, the owner reported that the dog was far less confused. It had been going to the opposite side of exit doors but was now entering and exiting properly. It was also more active and alert, sleeping less during the day, less dependent on the owner and appeared to be more aware of visual stimuli and odors. The dog maintained this improvement for several months but was euthanized at the age of 17, primarily due to extensive loss of vision and hearing, hind-leg weakness, inability to interact with its owner and find its paper for elimination.

In this case, the ongoing assessments (i.e., the cognitive assessment table [**Table 35-1**]), and interaction between the dog's owner and the veterinarian allowed for therapeutic adjustments. It might have been justified to intervene with a food such as Prescription Diet b/d Canine at an earlier age; however, preventing recurrence of uroliths had initially been a greater priority. When multiple problems exist, dietary decisions must be made according to the condition with the highest priority. Therefore, in this case, the patient was maintained on Prescription Diet u/d Canine and a drug approach (selegiline) was used for the behavioral problems. When selegiline was ineffective and the cognitive signs advanced, changing to Prescription Diet b/d Canine became the higher priority. Additionally, the pharmaceutical regimen may have contributed to the increase in wandering and gastrointestinal side effects. Selegiline is metabolized to amphetamine, which is expected to increase activity, and meloxicam is known to aggravate gastrointestinal problems. Additionally, some nonsteroidal antiinflammatory drugs may increase brain deposition of beta-amyloid. In addition, S-adenosyl-methionine may be useful to treat cognitive dysfunction in elderly pets.[e] It is also interesting to note that this was the first case in which the veterinarian saw improvement in cognitive signs with Prescription Diet b/d Canine but not selegiline.

By regularly and immediately attending to emerging health problems, monitoring each new therapeutic agent for effects and side effects and changing or adding new therapeutic options, the owner and veterinarian helped to maintain the patient's longevity and quality of life for almost seven years from the first onset of clinical problems.

Endnotes

a. Hill's Pet Nutrition, Inc., Topeka, KS, USA.
b. Pfizer Animal Health, Exton, PA, USA.
c. Nutramax Laboratories, Inc., Edgewood, MD, USA.
d. Innovet Italia S.r.l., Milano, Italy.
e. Novofit Product Profile. Virbac Corporation, Fort Worth, TX, USA.

Section 13

Cardiovascular Disorders

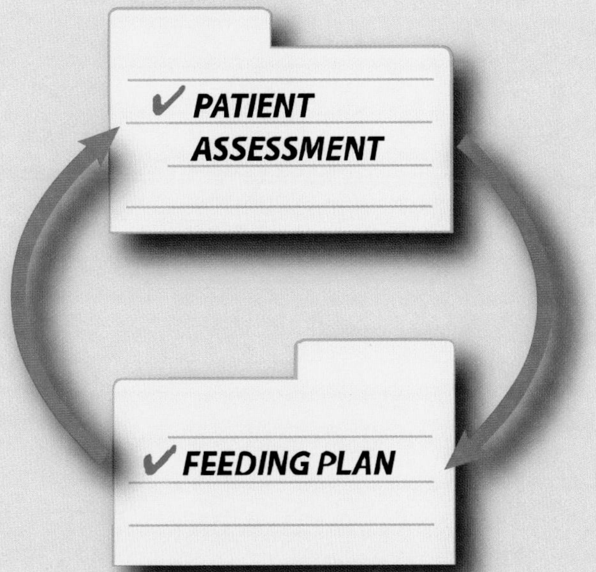

Chapter 36

Cardiovascular Disease

Philip Roudebush
Bruce W. Keene

"Give neither advice nor salt, until you are asked for it."
English Proverb

CLINICAL IMPORTANCE

Cardiovascular disease and congestive heart failure (CHF) are common conditions in dogs and cats. The types and prevalence of heart disease in dogs in the United States were characterized more than 40 years ago in a survey of 5,000 dogs at the University of Pennsylvania (Detweiler and Patterson, 1965). Eleven percent of dogs had reliable signs of heart disease and another 9% had possible heart disease. Congenital heart disease has been recognized in 0.56 to 0.85% of dogs and 0.2% of cats (Detweiler and Patterson, 1965; Harpster and Zook, 1987; Buchanan, 1992). These results predominantly reflect the prevalence of congenital disease in the necropsy populations of referral institutions, and may significantly underestimate the prevalence of heart diseases in the general pet population.

The overall prevalence of heart disease appears to be similar today, but comparable epidemiologic data for acquired heart disease in the U.S. are not available (Buchanan, 1992). A clinical review in Italy found heart disease in 11% of 7,148 dogs (Fioretti et al, 1988). One informal survey identified heart problems as the third leading cause of nonaccidental death of dogs (MAF, 1991). The results of a more recent informal survey of veterinary clinics performed by a pharmaceutical company also suggest that the prevalence of cardiovascular disease among dogs has probably not changed dramatically from these earlier estimates.[a]

Chronic mitral valvular disease (endocardiosis) is by far the most common acquired cardiac abnormality in dogs, affecting more than one-third of patients over 10 years of age (Buchanan, 1992, 1977). The tricuspid valve is also frequently involved (in approximately 30% of cases), but disease of the tricuspid valve is usually less severe. Chronic valvular disease occurs with relatively greater frequency in small dogs, especially poodles, miniature schnauzers, Chihuahuas, cocker spaniels, fox terriers, Boston terriers, dachshunds, Pekingese, miniature pinschers and whippets (Buchanan, 1977; Thrusfield et al, 1985). Mitral valvular disease has been identified in more than 50% of cavalier King Charles spaniels in the United Kingdom, Sweden and the U.S. (Darke, 1995; Beardrow and Buchanan, 1993). Acquired valvular disease in cats is rare.

Since 1987, the prevalence of dilated (congestive) cardiomyopathy in cats has decreased markedly following the discovery that taurine deficiency was the principal cause (Pion et al, 1987, 1989), and the subsequent supplementation of most commercial feline foods with taurine. One study documented that the prevalence of dilated cardiomyopathy as a cause of myocardial failure in cats decreased from 28% in 1986 to only 6% in 1989, whereas the occurrence of hypertrophic cardiomyopathy did not change (Skiles et al, 1990). Referral institutions continue to observe several individual cases of dilated cardiomyopathy in cats each year, only a few of which are now associated with taurine deficiency. Hypertrophic and restrictive cardiomyopathies are now the most common causes of myocardial failure in cats.

Various types of myocardial disease that were not recognized 40 years ago are now seen relatively commonly in dogs (Buchanan, 1992). Large-breed dogs, especially males, are predisposed to dilated cardiomyopathy. Doberman pinscher dogs are particularly susceptible. Hypertrophic cardiomyopathy occurs rarely in dogs. Arrhythmogenic right ventricular cardiomyopathy is common among boxer dogs (Meurs and Spier, 2009).

Pulmonary vascular disease with secondary cor pulmonale is most commonly associated with *Dirofilaria immitis* infection (heartworm disease). The prevalence of this disease is high in endemic areas in those dogs that do not receive appropriate preventive medication. Pulmonary hypertension unrelated to heartworm disease appears to be more common than previously believed and the frequency of diagnosis has increased because of heightened awareness about the condition (Henik, 2009) and the more widespread application of Doppler echocardiography. Pulmonary thromboembolism is most commonly associated with renal disease, hyperadrenocorticism, corticosteroid therapy, neoplasia, nephrotic syndrome, pancreatitis and immune-mediated hemolytic anemia. Primary systemic vascular disease is uncommon, but atherosclerosis and aortic or coronary thrombosis are occasionally recognized, particularly in dogs with hypothyroidism and elevated serum cholesterol concentrations. Secondary aortic thromboembolism in cats may occur with any of the forms of cardiomyopathy and is the most frequently acquired feline vascular abnormality.

Systemic hypertension in dogs and cats appears to be more common than studies indicated 40 years ago (Brown et al, 2007). Because blood pressure measurement in dogs and cats is technically challenging compared to measurement in people, and because of the prominent "white coat effect" in animals (elevations in measured blood pressure associated with the stress of the clinical visit) the actual prevalence of systemic hypertension in dogs and cats is still unknown. Spontaneous essential hypertension occurs in dogs, but hypertension most commonly develops secondary to chronic kidney disease in dogs and cats, hyperadrenocorticism in dogs and hyperthyroidism in cats (Littman and Drobatz, 1995). The demographic characteristics of dogs and cats at risk for the diseases that predispose to systemic hypertension overlap with those of dogs and cats with acquired heart disease. Although hypertensive dogs and cats may present at any age, most often they are middle-aged to geriatric (mean age: dogs nine years; cats 15 years, Littman and Drobatz, 1995). The strength of the peripheral pulses does not help detect systemic hypertension; absolute blood pressure numbers need to be determined. Retinal hemorrhages and detachments are common end-organ changes in patients with moderate to severe hypertension. These ocular signs are often the first evidence of hypertensive disease, which suggests that a fundic examination should be included in the routine evaluation of all dogs and cats. Other clinical signs of hypertension are most often related to the underlying disease that causes systemic hypertension.

The effects of long-term or severe systemic hypertension may cause significant heart disease (e.g. left ventricular concentric hypertrophy), and hypertension may complicate the treatment of chronic mitral valvular disease in dogs by worsening valvular regurgitation. It makes good clinical sense to screen dogs and cats with significant heart disease for the presence of systemic hypertension (by repeated blood pressure measurements), and also makes sense to search for underlying heart disease in patients with known hypertension, especially those exhibiting clinical signs that may be referable to heart disease.

The most frequently encountered problems associated with cardiovascular disease that require nutritional modification are fluid retention states associated with chronic CHF, primary or secondary hypertension, obesity, cachexia and myocardial diseases related to a specific nutrient deficiency (taurine- and carnitine-associated cardiomyopathy and electrolyte disorders that may predispose to cardiac dysrhythmias.

PATIENT ASSESSMENT

History and Physical Examination

Heart failure is a condition characterized by inadequate cardiac output and insufficient delivery of nutrients relative to tissue metabolic needs. Heart failure is not a specific disease, but a clinical syndrome caused by a variety of structural and functional disorders of the heart or great vessels. Clinical manifestations of heart failure are due to reduced cardiac output (weakness, exercise intolerance, syncope), pulmonary congestion (dyspnea, orthopnea, cough, abnormal breath sounds with crackles and wheezes), systemic fluid retention (jugular venous distention, hepatomegaly, ascites, pleural effusion) or a combination of these conditions.

In general, the clinical manifestations of heart failure are similar irrespective of the underlying cause, although the onset may vary. Occasionally, for example, heart failure may occur abruptly and lead to acute pulmonary edema (e.g., ruptured mitral valve chorda tendineae). Diagnosis of this fulminant form of heart failure is based on the history and overt, acute clinical signs. In many instances, however, heart failure becomes evident gradually; a long asymptomatic period (years) following the diagnosis of chronic valvular heart disease based on the presence of the typical murmur of mitral valve insufficiency is typical–this period may be followed by the onset of mild clinical signs that worsen gradually, or by the sudden onset of severe pulmonary edema. Most of the clinical signs used as the basis for diagnosing chronic heart failure may also occur as a result of other conditions.

Validity of a clinical diagnosis of heart failure in human patients was studied in a primary health care setting (Remes et al, 1991). One-third of human patients who were initially diagnosed with heart failure were subsequently found to have other conditions that caused their clinical problems. Obesity and pulmonary diseases were the most important conditions leading to false-positive diagnoses of heart failure in this population of human patients. Obesity and chronic bronchitis often occur in dogs and cats with heart disease and cause clinical manifestations similar to those of heart failure, thereby complicating the diagnosis. As an example, a small-breed dog may be admitted with moderate obesity, cough, tachypnea, exercise intolerance, abnormal breath sounds with crackles and a holosystolic murmur loudest over the mitral valve. It is important that this patient be evaluated thoroughly to determine whether the cause of the clinical signs is: 1) chronic bronchitis, 2) early heart failure, 3) obesity or 4) a combination of these conditions.

Human patients with heart disease and failure are categorized according to functional and structural schemes. The functional scheme is based on the clinical signs and symptoms evident at rest and during exercise (New York Heart Association functional classes). Members of the International Small Animal Cardiac Health Council popularized a functional classification scheme that is applicable to veterinary patients (**Table 36-1**) (ISACHC, 1994). Although patients with heart disease may follow an orderly progression though a functional classification, animals may change classifications in both directions–e.g., from Class III or IV to Class II or III following therapy, or from Class I to Class III or IV following a salty meal.

In 2001, the American College of Cardiology (ACC) and the American Heart Association (AHA) developed a staging scheme for heart failure patients emphasizing the progressive nature of the diseases that cause heart failure. This scheme has been adapted as follows for veterinary use (Keene and Bonagura, 2009):

- Stage A–patients at high risk for the development of heart failure, but without currently apparent structural heart abnormalities (e.g., cavalier King Charles spaniels, boxers, Doberman pinschers and other animals belonging to breeds, families or demographic groups known to be predisposed to heart disease).
- Stage B–patients with a structural heart abnormality, but without past or current symptoms of heart failure (e.g., patients with an asymptomatic murmur of mitral regurgitation).
- Stage C–patients with a structural abnormality and current or previous clinical signs of heart failure (this stage includes all patients that have experienced clinical signs of heart failure, and they stay in this stage despite resolution of their clinical signs with standard therapy).
- Stage D–patients with clinical signs of heart failure that have become refractory to standard treatment (defined practically as standard doses of furosemide, angiotensin-converting enzyme [ACE] inhibitor and pimobendan).

The ACC/AHA staging system emphasizes that progressive structural abnormalities of the heart underlie the pathogenesis of heart failure. This scheme is meant to encourage a program of client education and heart failure management that supports early screening for heart disease and provides a loosely defined plan for therapeutic intensification, including nutritional intervention, as heart disease progresses. This staging system further departs from functional classifications in that while a patient can still progress suddenly from Stage B to Stage C (or D, for example, if a previously asymptomatic dog with chronic valvular heart disease experiences a ruptured mitral valvular chorda tendineae), that path cannot be traveled in reverse.

Table 36-1. Functional classes of heart failure.*

Class I. The asymptomatic patient
Heart disease is detectable (cardiac murmur, dysrhythmia), but the patient is not overtly affected and does not demonstrate clinical signs of heart failure.

a. Heart disease is detectable but no signs of compensation are evident, such as volume or pressure overload ventricular hypertrophy.
b. Heart disease is detectable in conjunction with radiographic or echocardiographic evidence of compensation, such as volume or pressure overload ventricular hypertrophy.

Class II. Mild to moderate heart failure
Clinical signs of heart failure are evident at rest or with mild exercise and adversely affect the quality of life. Typical clinical signs include exercise intolerance, cough, tachypnea, mild respiratory distress and mild to moderate ascites. Hypoperfusion at rest is generally not present.

Class III. Advanced heart failure
Clinical signs of CHF are immediately evident. These clinical signs include respiratory distress (dyspnea), marked ascites, profound exercise intolerance and hypoperfusion at rest. In the most severe cases, the patient is moribund and suffers from cardiogenic shock.

*Adapted from International Small Animal Cardiac Health Council. In: Recommendations for the Diagnosis of Heart Disease and the Treatment of Heart Failure in Small Animals. Academy of Veterinary Cardiology, 1994.

The ACC/AHA scheme provides a framework for thinking about heart disease that is more analogous to the clinical approach to cancer, i.e., the identification of patients who are known to be at risk for cancer and who might benefit from more intensive screening to identify disease at an early stage (Stage A); the identification and treatment of patients with in-situ disease (Stage B); and the identification and treatment of patients with established (Stage C) or widespread (Stage D) disease. As our knowledge of the pathophysiology of heart disease and the progression of heart disease to heart failure expands, there is hope that early pharmacologic and/or nutritional intervention (often possible before the onset of clinical signs in heart disease) might significantly affect the eventual course of disease and survival in an individual patient. Currently, however, there are essentially no well-defined, effective therapies that prevent or delay the onset of heart disease or failure in either dogs or cats.

In assessing the nutritional status of patients with cardiovascular disease, overall body condition is the most important indicator of nutritional status and it appears to be an important, independent prognostic indicator. As will be discussed later, obesity causes cardiovascular changes that can complicate the management of cardiovascular disease, but in dogs and cats, significant weight loss is a far more common problem after the onset of heart failure. Although treatment of obesity is occasionally necessary in the management of patients with significant cardiovascular disease, it is relatively uncommon that clinically significant obesity coexists with life-threatening cardiovascular disease in dogs and cats. Cachexia is a syndrome of severe wasting seen clinically in a variety of diseases, especially chronic heart failure, cancer and acquired immunodeficiency syndrome. Cachexia is an additional risk factor in people with heart failure; loss of lean body mass is a negative predictor of survival (Freeman and Roubenoff, 1994). Systems for accurately assessing and scoring body condition are available for dogs and cats (Chapter 1). The body condition of dogs and cats with cardiovascular disease should be followed closely as part of reassessment.

Laboratory and Other Clinical Information

Measurement of Systemic Blood Pressure

Hypertension is often defined as that blood pressure two standard deviations above the mean for the population (Littman and Drobatz, 1995). Most investigators agree that the systemic systolic/diastolic blood pressure in awake, untrained dogs and cats normally should not exceed 180/100 millimeters of mercury (mm Hg), with values up to 200/110 mm Hg considered borderline or mild hypertension (Littman and Drobatz, 1995), especially in cats.

Direct blood pressure measurement is obtained by inserting a needle or catheter into an artery. The needle or catheter is connected to a pressure transducer and the result displayed on an oscilloscope/recording device. Anxiety and pain may falsely elevate the blood pressure of awake, restrained or uncooperative patients when measured by direct techniques.

Indirect blood pressure measurement is noninvasive and obtained with a cuff constricting a peripheral artery (leg or tail). An ultrasonic, oscillometric or photoplethysmographic transducer distal to the cuff is used to detect blood flow or arterial wall motion (Hansen, 1995). Blood pressure values obtained by direct and indirect methods generally correlate well, but indirect methods may produce values less than those obtained simultaneously by direct methods. In general, blood pressure measurements obtained routinely during hospital visits are reasonable estimates of a dog's true blood pressure (Remillard et al, 1991). Uncooperative, anxious patients may have elevated blood pressure measurements in the hospital setting that do not reflect normal values. A review of blood pressure measurements describes these techniques (Hansen, 1995). Comprehensive, current guidelines for the diagnosis and management of hypertension have recently been published (Brown et al, 2007).

Screening for Concomitant Disease

Cardiovascular disease is frequently associated with or exacerbated by underlying chronic renal disease in dogs and cats. All patients with cardiovascular disease should be screened for concomitant renal disease. This is best accomplished with a urinalysis and a serum biochemistry profile, which includes urea nitrogen, creatinine, electrolyte, calcium and phosphorus concentrations.

Hyperthyroidism in cats is a risk factor for secondary thyrotoxic cardiomyopathy and systemic hypertension. Cats over the age of seven years with evidence of cardiovascular disease should be screened for hyperthyroidism (Chapter 29).

Measuring and Interpreting Tissue Nutrients and Hormones

ELECTROLYTES AND MAGNESIUM

Serum electrolyte and magnesium concentrations are important factors to assess in patients with cardiovascular disease. Abnormalities in electrolyte and magnesium homeostasis can cause or contribute to the progression or severity of cardiac dysrhythmias, and decreased myocardial contractility associated with severe electrolyte abnormalities may cause profound heart muscle weakness. Electrolyte and magnesium abnormalities can also potentiate adverse effects from cardiac glycosides and other cardiac drugs. Unfortunately, the precise diagnosis of potassium and magnesium depletion can be difficult to make because these are primarily intracellular constituents. Normal serum potassium and magnesium concentrations can occur in the presence of total body depletion of these elements; therefore, serum potassium and magnesium concentrations do not always reflect total body stores.

TAURINE

Plasma and whole blood taurine concentrations are routinely measured to evaluate the taurine status of cats and dogs. Most early experimental and clinical studies used plasma taurine concentration to define taurine status. Values for plasma taurine of less than 20 to 30 nmol/ml (µmol/l) have been associated with deficiency in clinical studies involving client-owned cats (Pion et al, 1987; Sisson et al, 1991) and dogs (Kramer et al, 1995).

Studies involving laboratory cats have shown that plasma, but not whole blood taurine concentrations are affected by meals and food deprivation (Trautwein and Hayes, 1991; Pion et al, 1991). Therefore, whole blood taurine concentration is a more reliable index of taurine status in cats. In general, the whole blood taurine pool is remarkably stable and declines only during prolonged depletion, whereas plasma taurine concentrations fluctuate acutely depending on availability in food. Cats with whole blood taurine concentrations consistently less than 150 nmol/ml should be considered taurine deficient (Pion et al, 1989, 1991). Whole blood taurine concentrations have also been adopted by the Association of American Feed Control Officials (AAFCO) as part of its feeding protocols for cats. To successfully complete an AAFCO feeding protocol, no individual cat, kitten or queen can have a whole blood taurine concentration less than 200 nmol/ml (AAFCO, 2008).

Assessment of urinary taurine excretion has also been advocated as an alternative to measuring plasma or whole blood taurine concentrations (Glass et al, 1992). Urinary taurine excretion may provide vital information in the experimental setting for proper formulation of feline foods, but this assessment is probably not a practical technique for use with client-owned cats.

In North America, several laboratories routinely perform plasma and whole blood taurine assays. These laboratories are most easily accessed through regional veterinary reference laboratories that perform routine diagnostic services.

CARNITINE

Many investigators have reported blood and tissue carnitine concentrations in animals. The lowest levels are usually found in serum; in contrast, heart and skeletal muscle contain very high levels of carnitine, which underscores its importance in these tissues. Normal canine and feline values are similar for total, free and esterified carnitine concentrations in plasma based on measurements from a small number of healthy dogs and cats fed a standard dry commercial food (Jacobs et al, 1990, 1990a; Keene, 1992; Shelton, 1995). Total carnitine concentrations in plasma are influenced by intake of carnitine in food. Plasma concentrations will be elevated in animals that eat foods high in carnitine (e.g., raw meat or moist foods high in skeletal muscle content). To measure carnitine concentration, approximately 1 ml of heparinized plasma should be immediately separated, frozen and submitted to an appropriate laboratory.[b]

Carnitine concentrations can also be measured in cardiac muscle, skeletal muscle and liver (Jacobs et al, 1990, 1990a; Keene, 1992; Shelton, 1995). Cardiac tissue is obtained by using a modified transvenous endomyocardial biopsy technique (Keene et al, 1990). Skeletal muscle and liver tissue are obtained using standard biopsy techniques. Tissue specimens are blotted dry, immediately frozen in liquid nitrogen and stored at –70°C (–94°F) until the carnitine concentration is measured at an appropriate laboratory.[b] Tissues for carnitine assay should not be placed in formalin. Dogs with confirmed lipid storage myopathy should have plasma and tissue carnitine assays performed in the hope of identifying a potentially treatable cause of an otherwise difficult to manage disease (Shelton, 1995).[c]

BLOOD CONSTITUENTS ASSOCIATED WITH NEUROHUMORAL ACTIVATION

It is well established that activity of several neurohumoral systems is increased in many patients with chronic CHF. Elevated levels of renin, angiotensin, aldosterone and arginine vasopressin (AVP; antidiuretic hormone [ADH]) occur in both spontaneous and experimental canine models of CHF (Watkins et al, 1976; Riegger and Liebau, 1982; Riegger et al, 1988; Maher et al, 1989; Villarreal et al, 1990; Himura et al, 1994). Increased concentrations of renin, aldosterone, norepinephrine and brain or atrial natriuretic peptide or atrial natriuretic factor (BNP, ANP or ANF) occur in dogs with spontaneous heart disease and failure (Knowlen et al, 1983; Ware et al, 1990; Takemura et al, 1991; Vollmar et al, 1991; Buoro et al, 1992; Haggstrom et al, 1994; Pederson et al, 1995). Aldosterone, norepinephrine and ANP concentrations also increase with the severity of heart failure (Knowlen et al, 1983; Ware et al, 1990; Haggstrom et al, 1994). Aldosterone concentrations may offer some prognostic information about the severity of heart failure (Knowlen et al, 1983). Measurement of n-terminal BNP or troponin-I (a calcium regulatory protein that leaks from myocytes in many heart diseases) in the serum of dogs or cats shows significant promise as a means of identifying patients with either clinical or subclinical heart disease; however, the optimal application of these techniques awaits the availability of a reliable point-of-care test with proven positive predictive value in a variety of clinical settings (Prosek et al, 2007; Oyama et al, 2007). Norepinephrine, angiotensin, ANP and AVP analyses are only available through research laboratories. Plasma renin activity and aldosterone measurements are available through several reference laboratories.

Risk Factors

Risk factors for causing or complicating cardiovascular disease include breed, gender, obesity, renal disease, drug therapy, endocrinopathies and heartworm infection. Breed and gender appear to be the most important risk factors for cardiovascular disease in dogs. A number of breeds are at increased risk for several different congenital cardiovascular malformations, including patent ductus arteriosus, portacaval shunts, aortic stenosis, pulmonic stenosis, ventricular septal defects, tricuspid dysplasia and persistent aortic arch and related vascular abnormalities. Estimated relative risks (odds ratios) are listed elsewhere by breed for many of these congenital abnormalities (Buchanan, 1992). Chronic valvular heart disease occurs with relatively greater frequency in small dogs, whereas large dogs, especially males, are predisposed to dilated cardiomyopathy. Certain canine breeds also have characteristic cardiac dysrhythmias that may occur with or without significant cardiomegaly or signs of CHF. Finally, an increased risk of pericardial effusion is noted in golden retrievers, Labrador retrievers, German shepherd dogs, German shorthaired pointers and Akitas (Buchanan, 1992).

Obesity occurs frequently in dogs and cats with cardiovascular disease. Obesity not only produces clinical signs that mimic those of early heart failure (i.e., exercise intolerance, tachypnea, weakness), but also causes cardiovascular changes that can exacerbate underlying cardiovascular disease.

Chronic progressive kidney disease and failure often occur in dogs and cats with cardiovascular disease, especially in older patients. Cardiac disease often exacerbates underlying renal disease because a large proportion of the cardiac output is normally destined for the kidneys. Renal disease influences the types and dosages of medications that are used to treat patients with cardiovascular disease. Chronic kidney disease is also a risk factor for secondary hypertension in dogs and cats.

Therapy for CHF often includes: 1) diuretics and salt restriction to reduce preload and venous congestion, 2) pimobendan to increase contractility and dilate veins and arteries to increase contractility and decrease preload and afterload and 3) ACE inhibitors, which also act as arterial and venous dilators to reduce venous congestion, preload and afterload, but more importantly appear to have long-term survival benefits from inhibiting the activity of the renin-angiotensin-aldosterone (RAA) system. Dehydration, systemic hypotension, renal insufficiency, electrolyte abnormalities, acid-base disturbances, arrhythmias and loss of appetite are all potential complications of combined pharmacologic and nutritional therapy for patients with CHF.

Hyperthyroidism is a risk factor for hypertrophic cardiomyopathy and secondary hypertension in older cats. Hyperadrenocorticism is a risk factor for pulmonary thromboembolism. Heartworm infection is a risk factor for pulmonary vascular disease, cor pulmonale, right-sided CHF and pulmonary thromboembolism.

Table 36-2. Compensatory mechanisms in heart failure.

Autonomic nervous system
Heart
Increased heart rate
Increased myocardial contractile stimulation
Peripheral circulation
Arterial vasoconstriction (increased afterload)
Venous vasoconstriction (increased preload)
Kidney (renin-angiotensin-aldosterone)
Arterial vasoconstriction (increased afterload)
Venous vasoconstriction (increased preload)
Sodium, chloride and water retention (increased preload and afterload)
Increased myocardial contractile stimulation
Endothelin 1 (increased preload and afterload)
Arginine vasopressin (increased preload and afterload)
Atrial natriuretic peptide (decreased afterload)
Prostaglandins
Frank-Starling law of the heart
Increased end-diastolic fiber length, volume and pressure (increased preload)
Hypertrophy
Peripheral oxygen delivery
Redistribution of cardiac output
Altered oxygen-hemoglobin dissociation
Increased oxygen extraction by tissues
Anaerobic metabolism

Etiopathogenesis

Compensatory Mechanisms in Heart Failure

The first priority of the cardiovascular system is to provide oxygen and nutrients to critical organs such as the brain, kidneys and heart. The next priority is to supply nutrients to all other tissues; a final priority is to maintain normal venous pressure. In heart failure, these cardiovascular priorities are often lost in reverse order. The body will sacrifice normal venous pressure to provide nutrients to tissues. Increased venous pressure values above normal often result in clinical signs of CHF. The first and second cardiovascular priorities are maintained through compensatory responses from several neurohumoral mechanisms (**Table 36-2**), including the sympathetic nervous system, AVP secretion and the RAA system (Schlant and Sonnenblick, 1994; Kubo, 1990; Knight, 1995). In some animals, these compensatory changes ultimately result in: 1) sodium and water retention, 2) expanded extracellular fluid volume, 3) increased venous filling pressure and 4) clinical signs of cough, dyspnea, orthopnea, tachypnea, hepatomegaly and ascites.

SYMPATHETIC NERVOUS SYSTEM

The entire myocardium and peripheral vascular system are supplied with sympathetic nerve terminals. When cardiac output falls, the sympathetic nervous system coordinates increases in heart rate, strength of cardiac contraction and selective peripheral vascular vasoconstriction to restore hemodynamic equilibrium. Increased sympathetic discharge causes: 1) vasoconstriction of arterial resistance vessels with increased cardiac afterload, 2) increased renal neural traffic, which stimulates renin release and thus activation of the RAA system, 3) direct stimulation of renal sodium and water reabsorption and 4) splanchnic venoconstriction with central translocation of blood volume and increased cardiac preload (**Figure 36-1**). Sympathetic stimulation also causes the nonosmotic release of AVP. Diminished circulatory perfusion of arterial baroreceptors appears to activate simultaneously the three major vasoconstrictor systems: 1) the sympathetic nervous system, 2) the RAA system and 3) the nonosmotic release of AVP.

Generalized neurohumoral excitation occurs with impaired parasympathetic control of heart rate (Floras, 1993). The pathophysiologic implications of parasympathetic withdrawal in patients with heart failure have not been fully investigated.

Excessive sympathetic drive to the periphery can exacerbate the hemodynamic derangements of heart failure by increasing preload and afterload. Sympathetic activation occurs in dogs with spontaneous heart failure (Ware et al, 1990). Compared with clinically normal dogs, dogs with heart failure due to chronic mitral valvular disease or dilated cardiomyopathy have increased plasma norepinephrine concentrations that correlate positively with the clinical severity of disease (Ware et al, 1990). Dogs with the most severe degree of heart failure have mean norepinephrine concentrations significantly greater than those of dogs with all other functional classes of heart failure.

RENAL-ADRENAL-PITUITARY INTERACTIONS

In normal hearts and in those patients affected with mild disease, sympathoadrenal stimulation is the primary mechanism for adjusting to transient increases in workload (Schlant and Sonnenblick, 1994). However, as cardiovascular disease progresses, it imposes chronic, sustained changes in hemodynamics that require more stable, long-term adaptations. In this regard, the kidney plays a pivotal role in expanding blood volume and facilitating ventricular filling (increased preload).

Blood volume expansion results from renal conservation of sodium, chloride and water brought about by a combination of intrarenal hemodynamic alterations and neurohumoral stimulation. A decrease in cardiac output and blood pressure decreases renal perfusion pressure, which triggers renin release from the adjacent juxtaglomerular cells. Renin release is also stimulated by a decrease in the amount of sodium and chloride delivered to the distal renal tubules and by direct adrenergic stimulation of the juxtaglomerular cells. (See Sympathetic Nervous System above.) Renin acts on the circulating substrate angiotensinogen to produce angiotensin I. This relatively inactive decapeptide is converted by a peptidase enzyme, ACE, to the octapeptide angiotensin II.

Figure 36-1. (Opposite) Mechanisms for generalized sympathetic activation and parasympathetic withdrawal in heart failure. Normally (top figure), inhibitory input from arterial and cardiopulmonary receptors is high and heart rate is controlled by parasympathetic input (heavy lines). With progressing heart failure (bottom figure), sympathetic activity increases with resulting increases in vascular resistance, heart rate and adverse cardiac effects (heavy lines). Key: Ach = acetylcholine, E = epinephrine, NE = norepinephrine, CNS = central nervous system. (Adapted from Floras JS. Journal of the American College of Cardiology 1993; 22 [Suppl. A]: 72A-84A.)

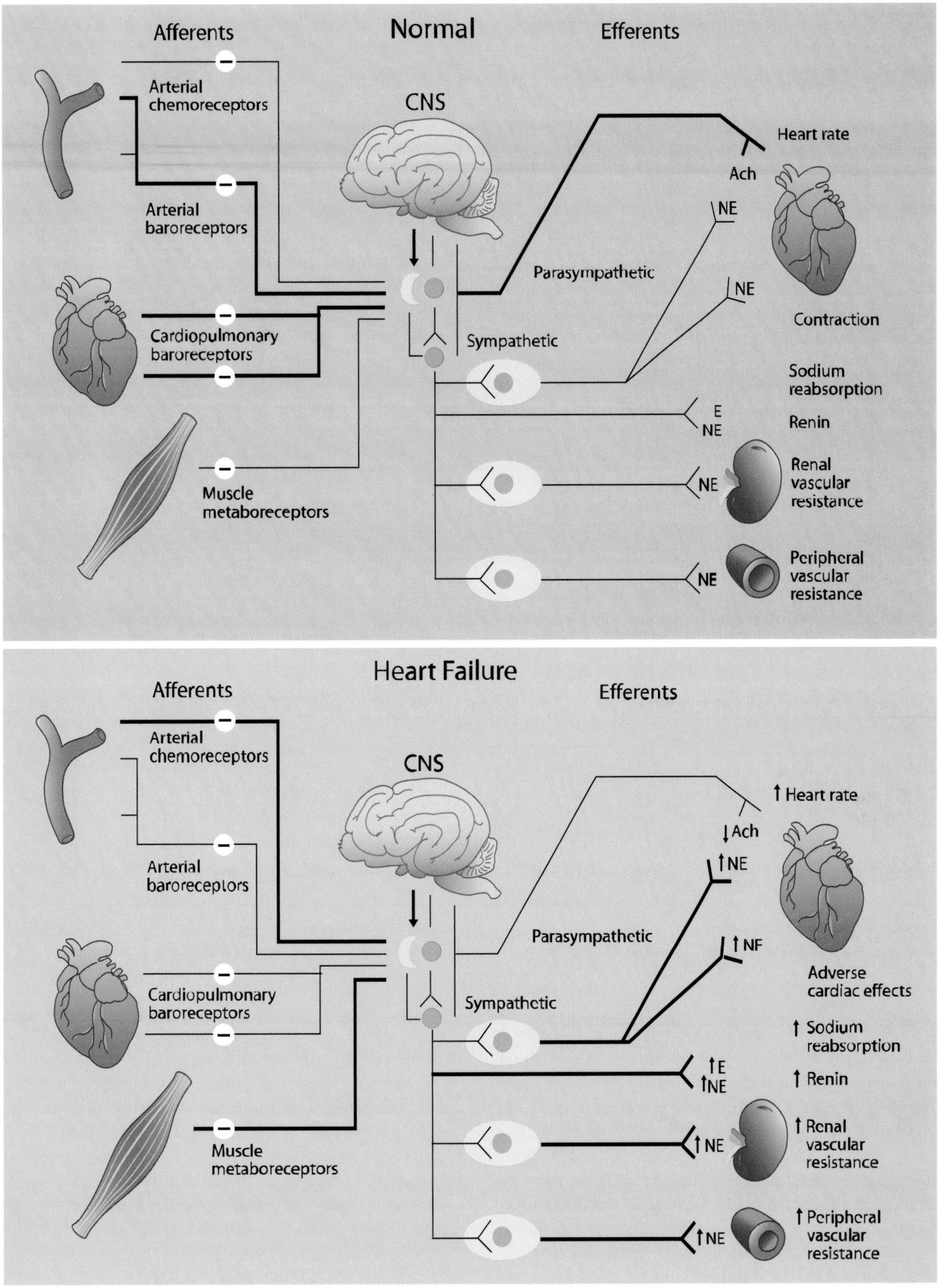
Normal
Afferents
Efferents
Arterial chemoreceptors
Arterial baroreceptors
Cardiopulmonary baroreceptors
Muscle metaboreceptors
CNS
Parasympathetic
Sympathetic
Heart rate
Ach
NE
NE
Contraction
Sodium reabsorption
E
NE
Renin
NE
Renal vascular resistance
NE
Peripheral vascular resistance
Heart Failure
Afferents
Efferents
Arterial chemoreceptors
Arterial baroreceptors
Cardiopulmonary baroreceptors
Muscle metaboreceptors
CNS
Parasympathetic
Sympathetic
↑ Heart rate
↓ Ach
↑ NE
↑ NE
Adverse cardiac effects
↑ Sodium reabsorption
↑ E
↑ NE
↑ Renin
↑ NE
↑ Renal vascular resistance
↑ NE
↑ Peripheral vascular resistance

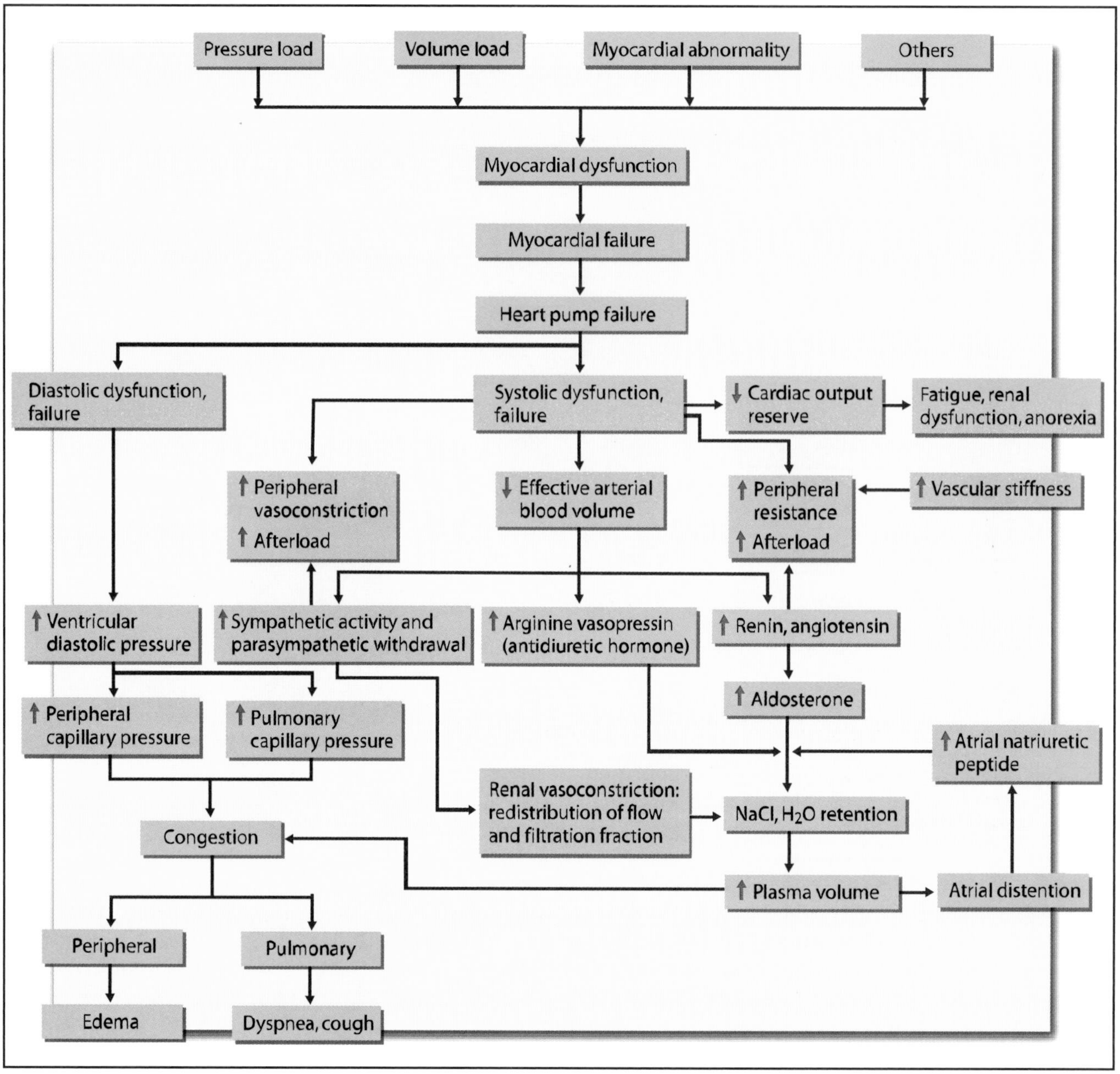

Figure 36-2. Schema of the sequence of events in heart failure. An increased load or myocardial abnormality leads to myocardial failure and eventually to heart failure. This results in increased sympathetic activity, increased levels of renin-angiotensin-aldosterone, pulmonary and peripheral congestion and edema and decreased cardiac output reserve. (Adapted from Schlant RC, Sonnenblick EH. Pathophysiology of heart failure. In: Schlant RC, Alexander RW, eds. The Heart, 8th ed. New York, NY: McGraw-Hill, 1994; 525.)

Angiotensin II counters a decline in effective arterial blood volume by serving as a potent constrictor of veins and arteries, and as a regulator of sodium-potassium homeostasis. Venoconstriction facilitates the return of blood to the heart and increases cardiac preload. Arteriolar vasoconstriction helps maintain systemic blood pressure. Angiotensin II also plays an important role in maintaining blood pressure and volume by stimulating secretion of aldosterone from the adrenal cortex. Aldosterone promotes reabsorption of sodium and chloride, and thus water, from the distal renal tubules and collecting ducts. The effects of aldosterone on sodium excretion may be less important than the direct intrarenal actions of angiotensin II. Studies in dogs support the theory that the intrarenal action of angiotensin II increases sodium and water retention (Hall and Brands, 1992). Angiotensin II also stimulates thirst, which facilitates expansion of blood and interstitial fluid volume. Blood levels of aldosterone tend to parallel those of renin and angiotensin II (Riegger and Liebau, 1982). If effective blood volume is restored, the stimulus for RAA secretion is withdrawn. However, if cardiovascular disease is severe, these hormones continue to stimulate the kidneys and tissue edema ensues or worsens (**Figures 36-2** and **36-3**).

In addition to the RAA system, a locally active paracrine renin-angiotensin system may exist in a number of tissues, par-

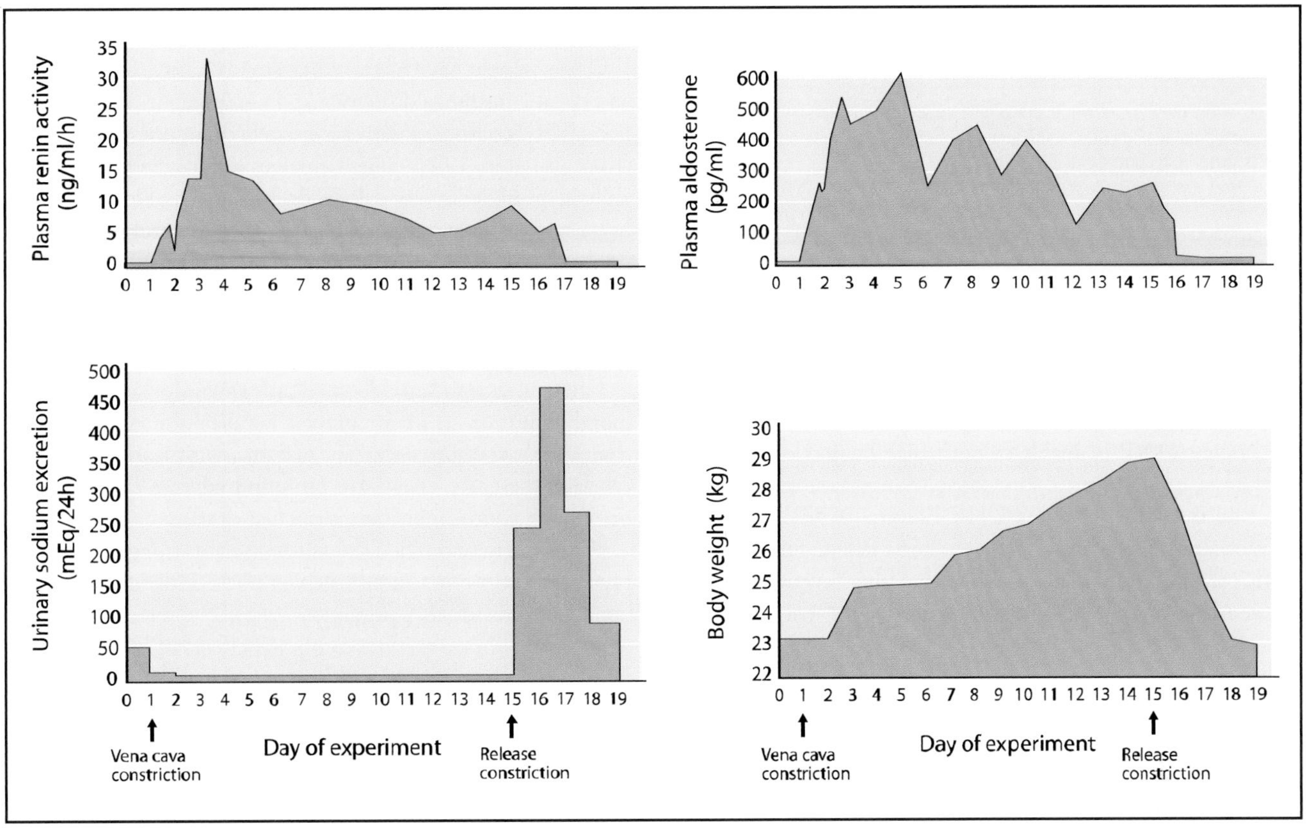

Figure 36-3. The response of a dog to thoracic vena cava constriction and the development of moderate to severe CHF. The first arrow indicates when vena cava constriction was applied. Note the persistent elevation in plasma renin activity (PRA) and plasma aldosterone (PA) concentration with a subsequent decrease in urinary sodium excretion and increase in body weight. The second arrow denotes when vena cava constriction was released. Note the rapid decrease in PRA and PA concentration with marked excretion of excess sodium in the urine and decrease in body weight. (Adapted from Watkins L, et al. Journal of Clinical Investigation 1976; 57: 1606-1617.)

ticularly those associated with cardiovascular homeostasis (MacFadyen, 1993; Straeter-Knowlen et al, 1995). ACE activity, renin substrate and renin-like enzymatic activity have been found in a number of sites including vascular, cardiac, renal, brain and adrenal tissues. Tissue renin-angiotensin activity may contribute to the pathophysiology of heart failure, but this is a topic of considerable debate (Hall and Brands, 1992). Further studies are needed to elucidate the role of extrarenal renin in the development and progression of heart failure.

AVP is secreted by the posterior lobe of the pituitary gland in response to nonosmotic stimuli. (See Sympathetic Nervous System above.) AVP is a potent vasoconstrictor and increases thirst and permeability of cortical and medullary collecting tubules, which allows reabsorption of free water. AVP secretion does not play a major role in the pathogenesis of edema. However, inappropriate AVP secretion probably plays a role in the pathogenesis of the hyponatremia associated with CHF.

Elevated levels of renin, angiotensin, aldosterone and AVP occur in experimental models of CHF in dogs (Watkins et al, 1976; Riegger and Liebau, 1982; Riegger et al, 1988; Maher et al, 1989; Villarreal et al, 1990; Himura et al, 1994). Plasma renin activity and aldosterone concentrations are also increased in dogs with spontaneous heart disease and failure (Knowlen et al, 1983; Buoro et al, 1992; Pederson et al, 1995). As disease in human patients progresses from early asymptomatic (heart disease but no heart failure) or mildly symptomatic left ventricular dysfunction to symptomatic heart failure, neuroendocrine mechanisms are progressively activated (Francis et al, 1990). The point at which significant neuroendocrine activation occurs in dogs and cats with spontaneous heart disease and failure has not been well documented.

CARDIORENAL INTERACTIONS

The volume expansion induced by activation of the RAA system is helpful to a point, after which deleterious clinical signs of pulmonary and peripheral edema begin to develop. ANP, primarily of atrial origin, counteracts these effects. An increase in transmural pressure (atrial distention or stretch) causes release of ANP, which triggers natriuresis and vasodilatation. ANP acts directly on the kidneys to: 1) cause diuresis through increased sodium and chloride excretion, 2) promote vasodilatation and 3) suppress aldosterone secretion and plasma renin activity. The last effect is presumably a result of the increase in sodium and chloride delivery to the distal tubules and macula densa. Studies have demonstrated a significant natriuretic and diuretic response using physiologic levels of ANP in normal dogs and dogs with experimental heart failure (Riegger and Liebau, 1982; Scriven and Burnett, 1985; Zimmerman et al, 1987). The renin-inhibiting effects of ANP may be dependent on the degree of activation of the RAA sys-

Table 36-3. Cardiovascular and neurohumoral adaptations that occur during the transition from lean to obese body condition.

Increased perfusion requirements of expanding adipose tissue
Elevated cardiac output
Abnormal left ventricular function
Variable blood pressure response (normotensive to hypertensive)
Increased retention of sodium and water by the kidney with subsequent increase in plasma volume
Increased plasma aldosterone and norepinephrine concentrations
Increased left atrial pressure
Increased heart rate
Exercise intolerance

tem (Kivlighn et al, 1990).

Although ANP is unable to normalize hemodynamics and natriuresis, it appears to provide an important modulating effect on the pathogenesis of CHF. Elevated ANP concentrations occur in dogs with spontaneous heart failure; furthermore, ANP concentration increases with increasing severity of heart failure (Takemura et al, 1991; Vollmar et al, 1991; Haggstrom et al, 1994).

CHF-ASSOCIATED HYPONATREMIA

Although the precise pathogenesis of CHF-associated hyponatremia remains controversial, the important factors can be divided into two categories (Oster et al, 1994). First, the increase in plasma angiotensin II concentration promotes thirst resulting in greater water intake. Second, renal diluting ability is impaired because the delivery of glomerular filtrate to the distal renal tubules is decreased (resulting from a reduced glomerular filtration rate and enhanced reabsorption proximally) and the plasma levels of AVP are increased. Both of these abnormalities might be mediated in part by angiotensin II. The osmotically inappropriate increase in plasma AVP concentration may be caused by a downward resetting of the osmostat because of a reduction in the effective blood volume (Oster et al, 1994). Aggressive use of diuretics may also contribute to the pathogenesis of hyponatremia in some patients.

CHF-associated hyponatremia is an important marker of poor prognosis in people with heart failure; it is seen almost exclusively in decompensated patients (Lee and Packer, 1986). People with heart failure and hyponatremia seem to have decreased renal blood flow, higher serum urea nitrogen concentrations, lower blood pressure and higher plasma renin activity (Oster et al, 1994; Lee and Packer, 1986). Anecdotal reports also suggest that hyponatremic patients in CHF have a poorer prognosis.

Obesity

Obesity has potentially profound cardiovascular consequences. From a cardiovascular perspective, obesity is a disease of blood volume expansion with: 1) elevated cardiac output, 2) increased plasma and extracellular fluid volume, 3) increased neurohumoral activation, 4) reduced urinary sodium and water excretion, 5) increased heart rate, 6) abnormal systolic and diastolic ventricular function, 7) exercise intolerance and 8) variable blood pressure response (**Table 36-3**) (Alexander, 1986; Crandall and DiGirolamo, 1990).

Obese people have increased plasma volume, cardiac output and plasma insulin, aldosterone and norepinephrine concentrations when compared with age-matched nonobese individuals (Rocchini et al, 1989). These changes occur whether the individuals eat high- or low-salt foods. Increases in blood pressure, heart rate, cardiac output, left atrial pressure and extracellular fluid volume also occur in dogs with experimentally induced obesity (Hall et al, 1993; Mizelle et al, 1994). Blood pressure always increases with increasing weight in dogs, regardless of the initial blood pressure.

The tendency toward blood volume expansion and neurohumoral activation in obese animals parallels the compensatory changes that often occur in patients with cardiac disease. Obesity, therefore, may have profound adverse effects in patients with concomitant cardiovascular disease.

Body weight and blood pressure correlate strongly in people. Hypertension occurs more often in obese individuals than in nonobese individuals (Alexander, 1986). The increase in blood pressure may be due to the combined effects of hyperinsulinemia, hyperaldosteronemia and increased sympathetic nervous system activity that characteristically occur in obesity (Rocchini et al, 1989). Hyperinsulinemia and blood pressure elevation also occur in dogs that have become rapidly obese (Rocchini et al, 1987). Hyperinsulinemia markedly reduces urinary sodium excretion (antinatriuresis) with resultant sodium and water retention (Hall et al, 1990, 1990a; Brands et al, 1991), possibly contributing to blood pressure changes. However, hyperinsulinemia for up to 28 days at levels comparable to those found in obese hypertensive people does not elevate mean arterial pressure in dogs with reduced renal mass even when sodium intake is high (Hall et al, 1990). This finding suggests that chronic hyperinsulinemia per se cannot account for obesity-associated hypertension. Further studies are needed to elucidate the pathophysiology of blood pressure responses and hypertension in obese patients.

Cachexia

Cachexia is a syndrome of weight loss (defined generally as unintentional loss of more than 10% body weight), lean tissue wasting and anorexia seen clinically in a variety of diseases, including chronic heart failure. The loss of lean body mass seen in cachexia is caused by a mismatch between food intake and nutritional requirements, resulting in negative nitrogen and energy balances (Freeman and Roubenoff, 1994). These imbalances may be due to inadequate intake, excessive losses or altered metabolism (**Figure 36-4**).

In patients with heart failure, anorexia may be due to the clinical signs of heart failure itself (dyspnea, fatigue), the presence of concomitant disease (nausea associated with renal failure), use of drugs that cause nausea (e.g., toxic doses of cardiac glycosides), the presence of elevated levels of inflammatory cytokines or sudden nutritional changes. The rate of loss of lean body mass with cardiac cachexia exceeds that attributable to anorexia alone, and reflects in part the excessive caloric expenditures of the increased work of respiration and elevated heart

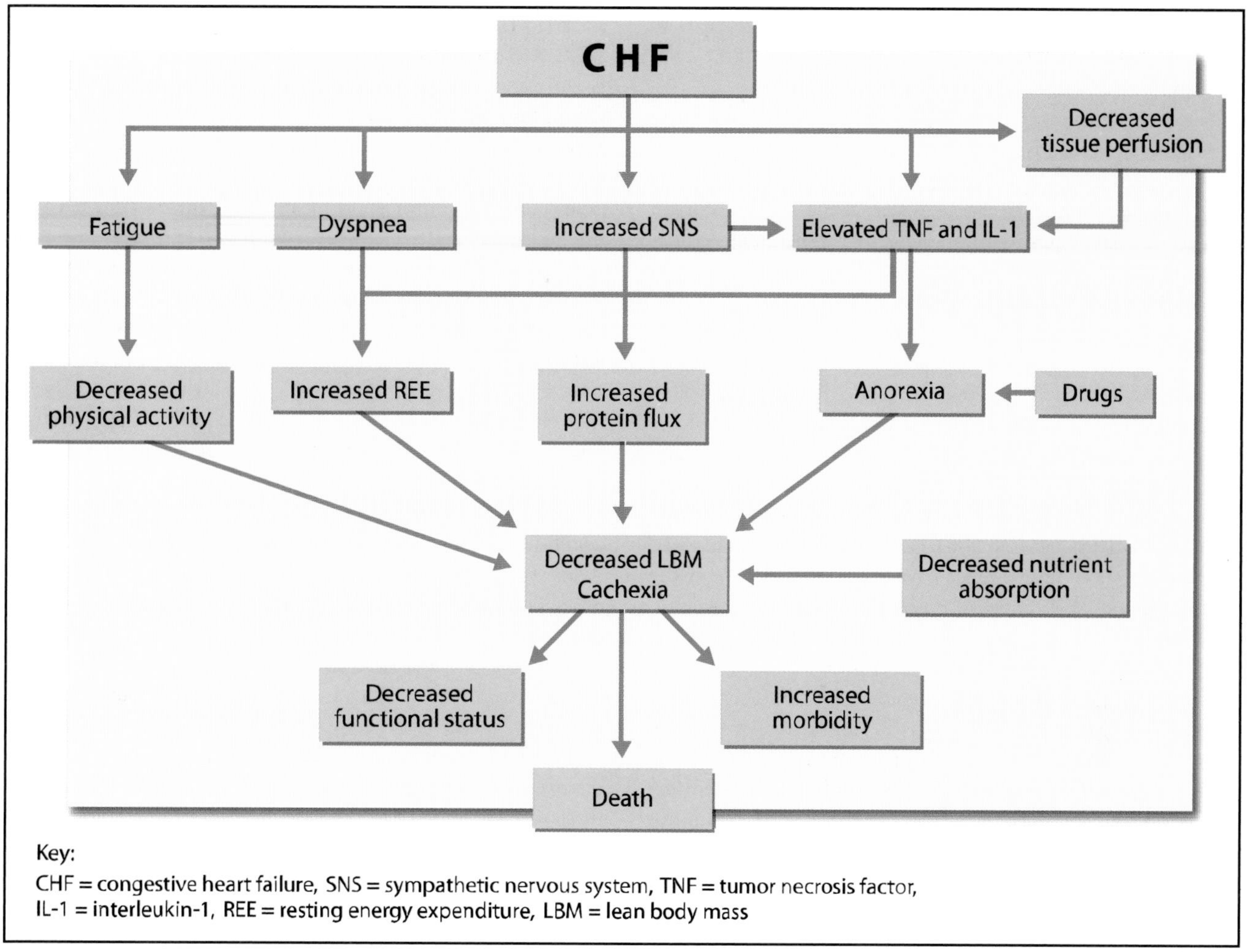

Figure 36-4. The cascade of factors in CHF that contributes to loss of lean body mass and cardiac cachexia. (Adapted from Freeman LM, Roubenoff R. Nutrition Reviews 1994; 52: 340-347.)

rate and in part, more complex metabolic issues. With simple starvation, most weight loss is loss of fat mass, whereas lean tissue is relatively spared, at least early on. Cachexia involves depletion of lean body mass. Physical inactivity may also contribute to loss of lean body mass because exercise is routinely restricted in patients with moderate to severe heart failure.

Altered metabolism appears to play a role in the pathogenesis of cachexia (**Figure 36-4**). Resting energy expenditure is elevated in some people with heart failure (Riley et al, 1991), and may be caused by increased ventilatory effort, sympathetic nervous system activity and concentrations of certain cytokines, specifically tumor necrosis factor (TNF, cachectin) and interleukin-1 (IL-1). Elevated serum TNF concentrations occur in people, dogs and cats with CHF (Levine et al, 1990; Freeman et al, 1994; Meurs et al, 1995). Both TNF and IL-1 cause cachexia by suppressing food intake and altering metabolism (Le and Vilcek, 1987; Oliff, 1988; Tracey et al, 1988, 1988a; Schollmeier, 1990). TNF suppresses the expression of several genes that encode for essential lipogenic enzymes, including lipoprotein lipase, and promotes the breakdown of adipose tissue and skeletal muscle (Le and Vilcek, 1987; Oliff, 1988; Tracey et al, 1988, 1988a; Schollmeier, 1990). TNF may also change the normal metabolic adaptation that accompanies caloric restriction and thus contribute to the nutritional imbalances observed in cachectic patients (Oliff, 1988).

As heart failure worsens, tissue perfusion and renal blood flow decline progressively. The kidneys release renin and prostaglandins, particularly prostaglandin E2, into the circulation in response to decreased renal blood flow. Prostaglandin E2 stimulates production of TNF from monocytes in vitro (Levine et al, 1990). Further studies are needed to confirm whether this pathogenic mechanism occurs in animals with cardiac cachexia and to explore the interaction of TNF with IL-1 and other cytokines.

Relationship of Taurine Deficiency to Myocardial Disease

Taurine is an essential amino acid in cats. Cats have a limited ability to synthesize taurine from cysteine and methionine because their tissues contain low concentrations of cysteine dioxygenase and cysteine sulfinate acid decarboxylase, key enzymes in the synthesis of taurine. Cats must also use taurine exclusively for conjugation of bile acids, which contributes to an obligatory loss of taurine. The decreased ability to synthesize taurine and the continuous obligatory losses predispose cats to taurine deficiency when they eat foods with low taurine concentrations.

The association of feline dilated cardiomyopathy with low plasma concentrations of taurine was first reported in 1987 (Pion et al, 1987). This observation was subsequently confirmed by large studies in North America and Europe (Sisson et al, 1991). Treatment with oral taurine supplements significantly improved clinical signs, restored myocardial function and improved survival of cats with dilated cardiomyopathy. Since 1987, supplementation of most commercial cat foods with taurine has resulted in a marked decline in the number of feline dilated cardiomyopathy cases. Several controlled experiments support the clinical studies. Myocardial taurine concentrations are reduced and left ventricular dilatation and myocardial dysfunction occur in cats fed foods low in taurine (Pion et al, 1992, 1992a; Fox and Sturman, 1992). However, idiopathic dilated cardiomyopathy is occasionally diagnosed in cats that show no evidence of taurine deficiency, and the condition does not improve with taurine supplementation (Sisson et al, 1991).

Dilated cardiomyopathy has also been associated with plasma taurine deficiency and low myocardial taurine concentrations in captive foxes (Moise et al, 1991) and a small number of dogs (Kramer et al, 1995; Kittleson et al, 1997; Pion et al, 1998). A retrospective study was conducted to determine dietary taurine concentrations in dogs with dilated cardiomyopathy and compare clinical outcomes (Freeman et al, 2001). Taurine concentrations were low in blood samples from 20 of 37 dogs with dilated cardiomyopathy but there was no correlation between dietary and circulating taurine concentrations. Other studies have confirmed that there is no clear and constant association between diet and taurine status in dogs with dilated cardiomyopathy (Vollmar and Biourge, 2004).

The mechanism of heart failure in taurine-deficient cats and dogs is poorly understood. Taurine may function in osmoregulation, calcium modulation and inactivation of free radicals (Pion et al, 1998). Other unidentified factors may be involved in the development of myocardial failure in patients with taurine deficiency. Many cats fed taurine-deficient foods for prolonged periods fail to develop clinical myocardial dysfunction. Dilated cardiomyopathy and heart failure may result from an inciting or contributing factor or factors in combination with taurine deficiency (Fox and Sturman, 1992).

Several studies have demonstrated an association between taurine and potassium balance in cats (Dow et al, 1992). Inadequate potassium intake may be sufficient to induce significant taurine depletion and cardiovascular disease in healthy cats (Dow et al, 1992). Female cats with dilated cardiomyopathy have significantly lower plasma taurine concentrations than do similarly affected male cats (Fox et al, 1994). This finding suggests that male cats are more prone to developing taurine-dependent dilated cardiomyopathy than are female cats, or they are more prone to developing clinical signs associated with cardiac decompensation at higher plasma taurine concentrations (Fox et al, 1994).

Relationship of L-Carnitine Deficiency to Myocardial Disease

L-carnitine is a small, water-soluble, vitamin-like quaternary amine found in high concentrations in mammalian heart and skeletal muscle. In dogs, L-carnitine is synthesized from the amino acids lysine and methionine, primarily in the liver. A poorly understood transport mechanism concentrates L-carnitine in cardiac and skeletal myocytes.

Although the heart uses various metabolic substrates to maintain the constant energy supply needed to sustain effective contraction and relaxation, it is well established that long-chain fatty acids are quantitatively the most important. Carnitine is a critical component of the mitochondrial membrane enzymes that transport activated fatty acids in the form of acyl-carnitine esters across the mitochondrial membranes to the matrix, where β-oxidation and subsequent high-energy phosphate generation occur (**Figure 36-5**). In addition to its role in fatty acid transport, free L-carnitine serves as a mitochondrial detoxifying agent by accepting (or "scavenging") acyl groups and other potentially toxic metabolites and transporting them out of the mitochondria as carnitine esters (Pion et al, 1998).

A subset of dogs with dilated cardiomyopathy apparently suffers from myopathic L-carnitine deficiency and may respond to L-carnitine supplementation (Keene, 1992; Pion et al, 1998). Plasma L-carnitine deficiency appears to be a specific but insensitive marker for myocardial L-carnitine deficiency in dogs with dilated cardiomyopathy (Keene, 1992; Pion et al, 1998); unfortunately, dogs with myocardial L-carnitine deficiency do not always have low plasma L-carnitine concentrations. Most dogs in which myocardial L-carnitine deficiency has been associated with dilated cardiomyopathy fall into the classification of myopathic L-carnitine deficiency (i.e., decreased myocardial L-carnitine concentrations in the presence of normal or elevated plasma L-carnitine concentrations). Many of these dogs may suffer from a membrane transport defect that prevents adequate amounts of L-carnitine from moving into the myocardium from the plasma at plasma L-carnitine concentrations found in dogs fed most commercial foods. Systemic L-carnitine deficiency (decreased plasma and myocardial L-carnitine concentrations) accounts for approximately 20% of the cases.

Hypertension

Regulation of systemic blood pressure involves complex relationships between central and peripheral nervous, renal, endocrine and vascular systems (Littman and Drobatz, 1995). Most people with hypertension have essential hypertension, which means their hypertension occurs without a discernible organic cause (primary or idiopathic hypertension). Hypertension secondary to an identifiable underlying cause is more common in dogs and cats.

The kidneys ultimately provide long-term control of blood pressure because they are able to excrete sodium and water (Guyton, 1981). This control is accomplished by manipulating the determinants of systemic blood pressure: cardiac output and total peripheral resistance (BP = CO x TPR). Cardiac output is

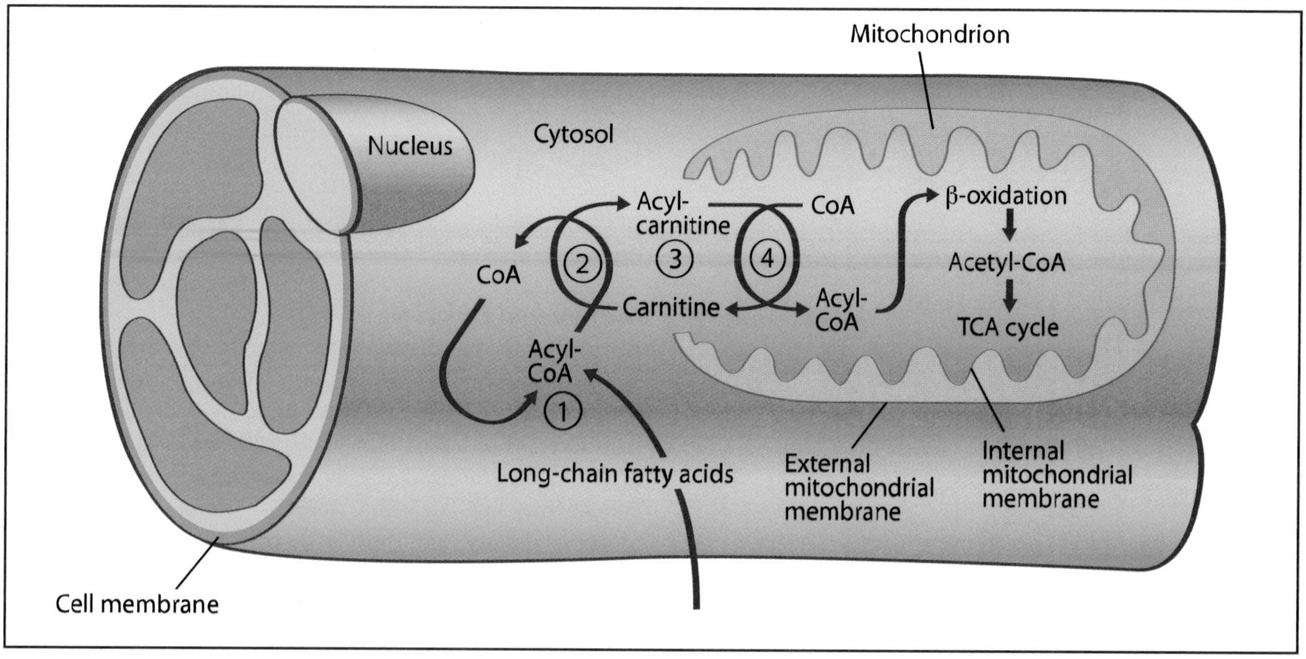

Figure 36-5. L-carnitine is essential for aerobic mitochondrial energy production and assists in the transit of energy (ATP) into the cytoplasm, where it provides the fuel for cellular functions. After entry into the cell, fatty acids are activated to form acyl-CoA (1). The acyl-CoA can then be transported into the mitochondrion as acyl-carnitine (2) via a carnitine-dependent shuttle (3). Acyl-carnitine then undergoes beta-oxidation to acetyl-CoA on the inner mitochondrial membrane (4) for entry into the TCA cycle and production of ATP. Secondarily, L-carnitine is involved in processes that prevent accumulation of toxic metabolites inside the mitochondrion. (Adapted from Neu H. Kleintierpraxis; 40: 197-220.)

related to heart rate and stroke volume (CO = HR x SV). Diseases associated with hypertension that increase heart rate include: 1) hyperthyroidism, 2) anemia, 3) hyperviscosity, 4) polycythemia and 5) pheochromocytoma. Increased stroke volume may occur during hypervolemic states, but is usually due to increased retention of sodium, chloride and water. Renal failure, hyperadrenocorticism and hyperaldosteronism may cause increased total body sodium, chloride and water.

Activation of the RAA pathway may elevate blood pressure by increasing stroke volume and total peripheral resistance. Angiotensin II is a potent vasoconstrictor, and angiotensin II and aldosterone stimulate renal sodium and chloride retention. Increased arteriolar tone, sensitivity to circulating vasopressors and levels of circulating catecholamines and decreased arteriolar elasticity may also increase total peripheral resistance.

Common causes of secondary hypertension include: 1) chronic progressive renal disease in dogs and cats (glomerulonephritis, amyloidosis, chronic interstitial nephritis, pyelonephritis and polycystic renal disease), 2) hyperadrenocorticism in dogs and 3) hyperthyroidism in cats. The "target organs" or end organs or systems that appear most sensitive to increased blood pressure include the eyes, kidneys, cardiovascular system and cerebrovascular system (Littman and Drobatz, 1995). Clinical signs related to end-organ damage are usually the reason an animal with hypertension is brought to a veterinarian for examination.

Pleural Effusion

Hydrostatic and oncotic forces (Starling's forces) are balanced within the pleurae and pleural space. Hydrostatic and oncotic pressures within the systemic circulation, pulmonary circulation and intrapleural space favor transudation of pleural fluid from the parietal pleura (pleura covering the inner chest wall) into the pleural space with subsequent absorption of the fluid into the visceral pleura's vasculature (Bauer and Woodfield, 1995). The result is a continuous flow of fluid through the pleural space. This delicate balance can be disrupted by any disorder that alters oncotic pressure, systemic or pulmonary capillary pressure, lymphatic compliance, capillary permeability or effective pleural surface area.

Biventricular CHF with systemic and pulmonary venous hypertension is a primary cause of pleural effusion. However, other causes of pleural effusion can masquerade as heart failure and may occur in patients with known heart disease, especially older dogs and cats. Other common causes of pleural effusion include diseases that increase capillary permeability and alter the normal flow and absorption of pleural fluid (e.g., primary intrathoracic or metastatic malignancy, pleural space infection, traumatic diaphragmatic hernia with incarceration of abdominal viscera).

Chylothorax is the accumulation of intestinal lymph (chyle) in the pleural space. This milky fluid has a high concentration of chylomicrons and triglycerides (the triglyceride concentration usually exceeds 100 mg/dl) and is low in cholesterol (the triglyceride-cholesterol ratio is greater than 1) (Fossum et al, 1986). The etiology of chylothorax is poorly understood, but has been associated with: 1) traumatic leakage, 2) diaphragmatic hernia, 3) lymphosarcoma, 4) cranial mediastinal masses, 5) pulmonary neoplasia, 6) dirofilariasis, 7) congenital abnormalities of the thoracic duct and 8) CHF. Experimental and clini-

Table 36-4. Key nutritional factors for foods for dogs and cats with cardiovascular disease.*

Factors	Recommended levels
Sodium	Dogs: Class Ia = 0.15 to 0.25%** Class Ib, II and III = 0.08 to 0.15% Cats: 0.07 to 0.30%
Chloride	Dogs: Class Ia = 1.5 x sodium levels** Class Ib, II and III = 1.5 x sodium levels Cats: 1.5 x sodium levels
Taurine	Dogs: ≥0.1% Cats: ≥0.3%
L-Carnitine	Dogs: ≥0.02%
Phosphorus	Dogs: 0.2 to 0.7% Cats: 0.3 to 0.7%
Potassium	Dogs: ≥0.4% Cats: ≥0.52%
Magnesium	Dogs: ≥0.06% Cats: ≥0.04%

*All values are expressed on a dry matter basis.
**Also appropriate in Class Ib, II and III patients when ACE inhibitors are used, especially when used in combination with diuretics.

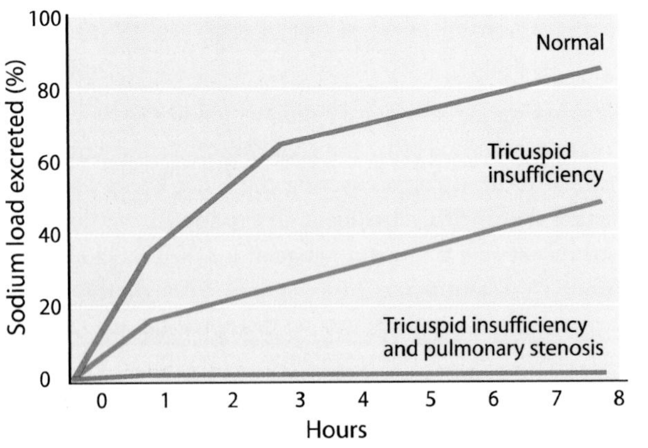

Figure 36-6. The cumulative excretion of sodium after a sodium load in a normal dog (top curve), the same dog with tricuspid insufficiency (middle curve) and the same dog with combined tricuspid insufficiency and pulmonary stenosis with the development of CHF (bottom curve). The inability of the dog to excrete excess sodium is the result of compensatory mechanisms that occur with advanced heart disease. (Adapted from Barger AC, et al. American Journal of Physiology 1955; 180: 249-260.)

cal evidence suggests that cranial mediastinal lymphangiectasia in cats is produced by either a functional or mechanical obstruction to thoracic duct flow. Obstruction of blood flow to the heart via the cranial vena cava, increased lymph flow from biventricular heart failure, elevated central venous pressure and direct duct obstruction may also contribute to lymphangiectasia and chyle accumulation in the pleural space (Smeak and Kerpsack, 1995).

Removal of large volumes of chyle via thoracentesis or chest drains may cause dehydration, electrolyte imbalances and protein-calorie malnutrition. A balance must be established between adequately evacuating the pleural space to prevent respiratory distress and meeting the animal's nutritional, fluid and electrolyte needs.

Key Nutritional Factors

The key nutritional factors for dogs and cats with cardiovascular disease are listed in **Table 36-4** and described in more detail below.

Sodium and Chloride

Because CHF is associated with retention of sodium, chloride and water, these nutrients are of primary importance in patients with cardiovascular disease. Within a few hours of ingesting high levels of sodium, normal dogs and cats easily excrete the excess in their urine. Early in the course of cardiac disease, patients may lose this ability to excrete excess sodium because of compensatory mechanisms described previously. In one experimental model, creation of valvular insufficiency in a dog reduced the excretion of excess sodium by almost 50% (**Figure 36-6**) (Barger et al, 1955). As heart disease worsens and CHF ensues, the ability to excrete excess sodium is severely depressed (**Figure 36-6**).

In the past, retention of sodium was primarily implicated in the pathogenesis of CHF and some forms of hypertension. A number of studies have examined the interaction of sodium with other ions, including chloride. The full expression of sodium chloride-sensitive hypertension in people depends on the concomitant administration of both sodium and chloride (Kurtz et al, 1987; Boegehold and Kotchen, 1989; Luft et al, 1990). In experimental models of sodium chloride-sensitive hypertension in rodents and in clinical studies with small numbers of hypertensive people, blood pressure or volume was not increased by a high sodium intake provided with anions other than chloride, and high chloride intake without sodium affected blood pressure less than the intake of sodium chloride (**Figure 36-7**) (Kurtz et al, 1987; Boegehold and Kotchen, 1989; Kotchen et al, 1981). The failure of nonchloride sodium salts to produce hypertension or hypervolemia may be related to their failure to expand plasma volume; renin release occurs in response to renal tubular chloride concentration (Boegehold and Kotchen, 1989; Luft et al, 1990; Kotchen et al, 1981, 1987). Chloride may also act as a direct renal vasoconstrictor (Boegehold and Kotchen, 1989). These findings suggest that both sodium and chloride are nutrients of concern in patients with hypertension and heart disease.

The minimum recommended allowance for sodium and chloride in foods for adult dogs is 0.08 and 0.12% dry matter (DM), respectively (NRC, 2006); for foods for cats it is 0.068 for sodium and 0.096% for chloride DM (NRC, 2006). In general, sodium levels for foods for cardiovascular disease should be restricted to 0.08 to 0.25% DM for dogs and 0.07 to 0.3% DM for cats. Recommended chloride levels are typically 1.5 times sodium levels. Avoiding excess sodium chloride in cat foods is more difficult than in dog foods because ingredients used to meet the higher protein requirement of cats also contain sodium and chloride and thus increase the sodium chloride content of cat food.

Specific evidence is not available to support the idea that foods low in sodium chloride fed to dogs in the early stages of heart disease will delay disease progression. However, a prudent recommendation for these patients is to begin avoiding excess sodium chloride early in the disease process. Thus, at the first sign of heart disease without cardiac dilatation (Class Ia), foods with levels of sodium and chloride in the upper part of the recommended range (0.15 to 0.25% DM sodium) should be introduced. Cardiac dilatation implies abnormal sodium chloride handling and intravascular volume expansion and, thus, dilatation is a prelude to venous congestion. When cardiac dilatation becomes evident on radiographs or echocardiograms (Class Ib), then foods that are even more sodium chloride restricted (sodium = 0.08 to 0.15% DM) are advised (Roudebush et al, 1994; Rush et al, 2000). As might be expected, moderate to severe cardiac dilatation, congestion or both conditions (Class II or III) also require foods with sodium chloride levels in the lower end of the range.

Water can be a potential source of sodium and chloride. Distilled water or water with less than 150 ppm sodium should be considered for patients with advanced CHF in whom more strictly limited sodium intake is desirable.

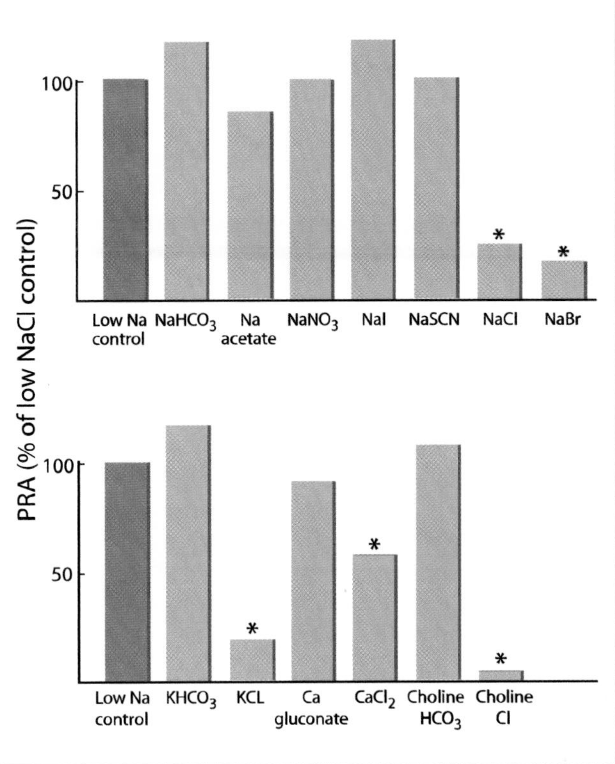

Figure 36-7. Effect of nutritional loading with different sodium and chloride salts on plasma renin activity (PRA) in sodium chloride-deprived rats. Bars marked with * are significantly different ($p < 0.05$) compared with the low-sodium control. These data suggest that chloride is an important determinant of renin secretion by the kidneys. (Adapted from Kotchen TA, et al. Journal of Laboratory Clinical Medicine 1987; 110: 533-539.)

Taurine

Taurine can be important in dogs and cats with myocardial failure. The mechanism of heart failure in taurine-deficient cats and dogs is not well understood. Taurine may function in inactivation of free radicals, osmoregulation and calcium modulation (Pion et al, 1998). Taurine also has direct effects on contractile proteins and is a natural antagonist to angiotensin II (Lake, 1993; Gentile et al, 1994). Other unidentified factors may be involved in the development of myocardial failure in patients with taurine deficiency. Dilated cardiomyopathy and heart failure may result from an inciting or contributing factor, or factors, in combination with taurine deficiency (Fox and Sturman, 1992). For example, studies have demonstrated an association between taurine and potassium balance in cats (Dow et al, 1992). Inadequate potassium intake may be sufficient to induce significant taurine depletion and cardiovascular disease in healthy cats (Dow et al, 1992).

Because taurine is an essential amino acid in cats, there is a minimum recommended allowance for taurine in highly digestible purified foods for healthy adult cats, which is 0.04% DM; the minimum recommended allowances for dry expanded and moist foods for adult cats are 0.10 and 0.17% DM, respectively (NRC, 2006). Taurine content of foods for cats with cardiovascular disease should probably contain at least 0.3% DM. Levels of taurine typically recommended for supplementation of feline cardiovascular patients (250 to 500 mg taurine/day) (Pion et al, 1989) provide approximately twice that much. There are no reports of acute or chronic toxicity related to feeding large quantities of free taurine to cats. In one study, foods containing up to 1.0% DM taurine were fed for up to three years and no adverse effects were noted (Sturman and Messing, 1992). The safe upper limit of taurine in foods for kittens is more than 0.89% DM (NRC, 2006).

Taurine is not an essential amino acid for dogs. However, dilated cardiomyopathy has been associated with plasma taurine deficiency and low myocardial taurine concentrations in captive foxes and a small number of dogs (Moise et al, 1991; Kramer et al, 1995; Kittleson et al, 1997; Pion et al, 1998; Freeman et al, 2001). In dogs, the association between taurine deficiency and dilated cardiomyopathy is strongest in American cocker spaniels and golden retrievers (Kramer et al, 1995; Kittleson et al, 1997, 1991; Pion et al, 1998). An association between taurine deficiency and dilated cardiomyopathy has also been shown in Newfoundlands, Labrador retrievers, Dalmatians, English bulldogs, Portuguese water dogs and Irish wolfhounds (Sanderson, 2006; Vollmar and Biourge, 2004). Even if plasma and whole blood taurine levels are normal in canine dilated cardiomyopathy patients, additional taurine may still be beneficial. Thus, it is reasonable that foods for dogs with cardiovascular disease contain added taurine. Because dogs can synthesize taurine, the level for foods for canine patients can be lower than for cats. The recommendation for taurine in foods for canine cardiovascular disease patients is at least 0.1% DM. This is somewhat lower than would be supplied by the typical recommendation for taurine supplementation of foods for dogs with dilated cardiomyopathy (500 to 1,000 mg taurine/day) (Pion et al, 1998). In dogs, as in cats, taurine is safe. No reports could be found on acute or chronic toxicity related to feeding large quantities of taurine to dogs and no safe upper limit has been established (NRC, 2006).

L-Carnitine

L-carnitine deficiency has been associated with dilated cardiomyopathy in dogs. Carnitine is important to cardiac muscle function because it is a critical component of the mitochondrial membrane enzymes that transport activated fatty acids in the form of acyl-carnitine esters across the mitochondrial membranes to the matrix, where β-oxidation and subsequent high-energy phosphate generation occur. Also, free L-carnitine serves as a mitochondrial detoxifying agent by scavenging acyl groups and other potentially toxic metabolites and transporting them out of the mitochondria as carnitine esters (Pion et al, 1998).

A subset of dogs with dilated cardiomyopathy apparently suffers from myopathic L-carnitine deficiency and may respond to L-carnitine supplementation (Keene, 1992; Pion et al, 1998). Plasma L-carnitine deficiency appears to be a specific but insensitive marker for myocardial L-carnitine deficiency in dogs with dilated cardiomyopathy (Keene, 1992; Pion et al, 1998). Thus, dogs with myocardial L-carnitine deficiency do not always have low plasma L-carnitine concentrations. Most dogs in which myocardial L-carnitine deficiency has been associated with dilated cardiomyopathy fall into the classification of myopathic L-carnitine deficiency (i.e., decreased myocardial L-carnitine concentrations in the presence of normal or elevated plasma L-carnitine concentrations). Many of these patients suffer from a membrane transport defect that prevents adequate amounts of L-carnitine from moving into the myocardium from the plasma at plasma L-carnitine concentrations found in dogs fed most commercial foods. Systemic L-carnitine deficiency (decreased plasma and myocardial L-carnitine concentrations) accounts for approximately 20% of the cases.

Most authors recommend supplementing canine dilated cardiomyopathy patients with 50- to 100-mg L-carnitine/kg body weight three times daily. One report suggests that in dogs with systemic carnitine deficiency, a much lower dose generated a better response than the effective dose for myopathic cardiomyopathy (Sanderson, 2006). Even if carnitine deficiency was not the cause of cardiomyopathy in a heart disease patient, supplementing dogs with carnitine does no harm and may be beneficial. Because carnitine is expensive, foods for canine patients with cardiovascular disease do not contain the higher levels recommended for supplementation. Foods for heart disease patients should provide at least 0.02% DM. For a point of reference, this inclusion level provides approximately 1/20th of the amount that would be achieved by supplementing at 50- to 100-mg carnitine/kg body weight.

Phosphorus

Phosphorus is a nutrient of concern in patients with concurrent chronic kidney disease (Chapter 37). To avoid excess phosphorus in patients with concurrent chronic kidney disease, restrict phosphorus to 0.2 to 0.7% DM in dogs and 0.3 to 0.7% DM in cats.

Potassium and Magnesium

Potassium and magnesium metabolism is a concern in patients with cardiovascular disease. Hypokalemia, hyperkalemia and hypomagnesemia, are potential complications of drug therapy in patients with cardiovascular disease. Abnormalities in potassium or magnesium homeostasis can: 1) cause cardiac dysrhythmias, 2) decrease myocardial contractility, 3) produce profound muscle weakness and 4) potentiate adverse effects from cardiac glycosides and other cardiac drugs.

Foods for dogs and cats with CHF should contain at least the amounts of potassium and magnesium recommended for adult maintenance (0.4 and 0.52% DM potassium, respectively, and 0.06 and 0.04% DM magnesium) (NRC, 2006). If abnormalities in these electrolytes occur, supplementation or switching to a different food may be necessary.

Other Nutritional Factors

Protein

The protein requirements of patients with cardiac cachexia have not been investigated and it is unknown how the metabolic changes associated with cachexia affect overall nutrient requirements. Many patients with cachexia have concomitant disease, such as chronic kidney disease, which affects nutrient requirements. Profound anorexia enhances protein-energy malnutrition in patients with cachexia. Patients with cachexia should be encouraged to eat a complete and balanced food that contains adequate calories and adequate high-quality protein.

Omega-3 Fatty Acids

The cytokines TNF and IL-1 have been implicated as pathogenic mediators in cardiac cachexia. Fish oil, which is high in omega-3 (n-3) fatty acids, alters cytokine production. Preliminary results suggest that fish-oil-mediated alterations in cytokine production may benefit dogs with CHF (Freeman et al, 1995). Circulating TNF and IL-1 concentrations decreased significantly in a group of dogs with CHF secondary to idiopathic dilated cardiomyopathy when they were treated with fish oil supplements. Dogs receiving fish oil tended to be judged as less cachectic when compared with those in the placebo group. Ventricular function also improved significantly in the group treated with fish oil when compared with dogs receiving a placebo. These findings suggest that heart failure patients with cachexia may benefit from the alterations of cytokine production brought about by omega-3 fatty acid supplementation or other methods.

Parenteral administration of omega-3 fatty acids (α-linolenic acid, eicosapentaenoic acid [EPA], docosahexaenoic acid [DHA]) was shown to prevent sudden cardiac death in an experimental model of myocardial infarction in dogs (Billman et al, 1999; Leaf et al, 2005). Omega-3 fatty acids appear to electrically stabilize heart cells through modulation of the fast voltage-dependent $Na^{(+)}$ currents and the L-type $Ca^{(2+)}$ channels in a manner that makes the heart cells resistant to dysrhythmias (Leaf et al, 2005a). Clinical studies have also confirmed that fish oil as a source of long-chain omega-3 fatty acids will reduce the frequency of ventricular arrhythmia in boxer dogs with arrhythmogenic right ventricular cardiomyopathy (Smith et al, 2007). These data suggest that fish oil supplementation may be useful to help reduce cardiac arrhythmias in dogs. Further studies are needed to determine optimal dose and duration of treatment.

FEEDING PLAN

Assess and Select the Food

The food for patients with cardiovascular disease should be evaluated for all the key nutritional factors mentioned in **Table 36-4**. **Tables 36-5** and **36-6** list key nutritional factor content of selected veterinary therapeutic and other commercial foods marketed for dogs and cats with cardiovascular disease, respectively, and compares them to the recommended levels. Key nutritional factor amounts for foods not listed in these tables must be obtained by contacting the manufacturer or consulting published product information. The levels of the key nutritional factors for regular commercial dog and cat foods typically are considerably outside the recommendations for patients with cardiovascular disease. Some commercial foods greatly exceed the minimum recommended allowance for sodium chloride (Roudebush et al, 2000). Nutrient sources other than commercial pet foods should be investigated. Water quality varies considerably, even within the same community. Water can be a significant source of sodium, chloride and other minerals. Veterinarians should be familiar with the mineral levels in their local water supply. Water samples can be submitted to state or other government laboratories for analysis; municipal water companies can be contacted or private companies that market water conditioning systems can be asked about mineral levels in local water supplies. Distilled water or water with less than 150 ppm sodium is recommended for patients with advanced heart disease and failure (Morris et al, 1976).

Other sources of nutrients include commercial treats and snacks for pets, and human foods offered as snacks or part of the pet's food. Processed human foods are often high in sodium (**Table 36-7**). Some commercial rawhide chews do not contain excessive levels of sodium (Morris and Ettinger, 1995). **Table 36-8** lists selected commercial low sodium canine treats.

Although there is currently little or no evidence that proves foods low in sodium chloride delay disease progression in the initial stages of heart disease in dogs, a prudent recommendation is to begin avoiding excess sodium chloride early in the disease process. Thus, at the first sign of heart disease without cardiac dilatation (Class Ia), foods with levels of sodium in the upper part of the recommended range (0.15 to 0.25% DM) should be introduced. Early intervention may help the patient accept foods if more restricted sodium chloride levels are necessary later, and reminds the owners to remain vigilant for signs of disease progression. Furthermore, avoiding excessive amounts of sodium chloride early in heart disease has not been shown to be harmful.

When cardiac dilatation becomes evident on radiographs or echocardiograms (Class Ib), then sodium chloride-restricted foods are appropriate (Roudebush et al, 1994; Rush et al, 2000). Cardiac dilatation implies abnormal sodium chloride handling and intravascular volume expansion, and it is a prelude to venous congestion. The presence of moderate to severe cardiac dilatation, congestion or both conditions (Class II or III) indicates that foods lower in sodium chloride are appropriate. Many veterinary cardiologists prescribe foods with levels of sodium in the upper part of the recommended range (0.15 to 0.25% DM) when ACE inhibitors are used, especially when used in combination with diuretics. **Table 36-9** outlines the daily sodium intake of a 15-kg dog and a 4-kg cat fed different foods, including grocery, specialty and veterinary therapeutic foods. Normal dogs and cats are able to eliminate the excess levels of sodium found in many commercial foods, but patients with heart disease and failure have an impaired ability to handle these sodium levels. There is often concern about the palatability of low-salt foods compared to that of a patient's current food. Low-salt foods can be even more palatable than maintenance foods with higher salt content (**Box 36-1**). However, a few patients might not eat low-salt foods. A common mistake is to insist that an owner feed only a salt-restricted food even if caloric intake is inadequate. Although avoiding excess sodium chloride is important in CHF patients, offering only a salt-restricted food should not be imposed to the detriment of overall nutrient intake. Changing to a different commercial food or homemade food may be a more beneficial solution in some patients. Appetite may be cyclical in patients with advanced heart failure, both in respect to overall appetite and food preferences. A dedicated owner is often required and a trial-and-error approach should be used with different foods and feeding methods.

Low-salt foods may also be of value in the management of respiratory diseases (**Box 36-2**). Another criterion for selecting a food that may become increasingly important in the future is evidence-based clinical nutrition. Practitioners should know how to determine risks and benefits of nutritional regimens and counsel pet owners accordingly. Currently, veterinary medical education and continuing education are not always based on rigorous assessment of evidence for or against particular management options. Still, studies have been published to establish the nutritional benefits of certain pet foods. Chapter 2 describes evidence-based clinical nutrition in detail and applies its concepts to various veterinary therapeutic foods.

Adjunctive Management: Drugs and Supplements

Most patients with cardiovascular disease in which nutritional management is used also receive drug therapy. In the past, drug-drug interactions received considerable attention but few investigators evaluated or discussed how nutrient levels might affect drug availability and pharmacokinetics and vice versa (Chapter 69). Because many cardiovascular patients are treated with a combination of veterinary therapeutic foods and drugs, potential food-drug or nutrient-drug interactions are important.

Table 36-5. Levels of key nutrients in selected commercial foods for dogs with cardiovascular disease compared to the recommended levels.*

Dry foods for Class Ia patients**	Energy density (kcal/cup)***	Na (%)	Taurine (%)†	Carnitine (%)†	P (%)	K (%)†	Mg (%)†
Recommended levels	–	**0.15-0.25**	**≥0.1**	**≥0.02**	**0.2-0.7**	**≥0.4**	**≥0.06**
Hill's Prescription Diet g/d Canine	358	0.21	0.1	na	0.41	0.61	0.068
Hill's Prescription Diet j/d Canine	356	0.17	0.13	0.04	0.54	0.83	0.139
Hill's Prescription Diet k/d Canine	396	0.23	0.12	na	0.24	0.67	0.107
Hill's Science Diet Mature Adult Active Longevity Original	363	0.18	0.13	na	0.58	0.83	0.109
Hill's Science Diet Mature Adult Large Breed	357	0.17	0.13	0.03	0.59	0.82	0.108
Hill's Science Diet Mature Adult Small Bites	363	0.18	0.13	na	0.58	0.83	0.109
Medi-Cal Early Cardiac	300	0.3	0.2	0.1	0.8	0.8	0.1
Purina Veterinary Diets NF KidNey Function	459	0.22	na	na	0.29	0.86	0.070
Royal Canin Veterinary Diet Early Cardiac EC 22	291	0.19	0.22	na	0.77	0.82	0.077
Moist foods for Class Ia patients**	**Energy density (kcal/can)*****	**Na (%)**	**Taurine (%)†**	**Carnitine (%)†**	**P (%)**	**K (%)†**	**Mg (%)†**
Recommended levels	–	**0.15-0.25**	**≥0.1**	**≥0.02**	**0.2-0.7**	**≥0.4**	**≥0.06**
Hill's Prescription Diet g/d Canine	377/13 oz.	0.22	0.11	na	0.41	0.78	0.067
Hill's Prescription Diet j/d Canine	498/13 oz.	0.19	0.12	0.03	0.56	0.81	0.112
Hill's Prescription Diet k/d Canine	458/13 oz.	0.19	0.11	na	0.22	0.37	0.141
Hill's Science Diet Mature Adult Active Longevity Gourmet Beef Entrée	164/5.8 oz. 368/13 oz.	0.16	0.12	0.02	0.52	0.76	0.104
Hill's Science Diet Mature Adult Active Longevity Savory Chicken Entrée	155/5.8 oz. 347/13 oz.	0.16	0.12	na	0.57	0.7	0.111
Hills Science Diet Mature Adult Active Longevity Gourmet Turkey Entrée	369/13 oz.	0.17	0.12	na	0.62	0.83	0.107
Iams Veterinary Formula Stress/Weight Gain Formula Maximum-Calorie	333/6 oz.	0.24	0.33	na	0.83	1.01	0.089
Medi-Cal Renal MP	532/380 g	0.2	na	na	0.4	1.5	na
Purina Veterinary Diet NF KidNey Function Formula	498/12.5 oz.	0.24	na	na	0.30	0.72	0.080
Dry foods for Class Ib, II and III patients	**Energy density (kcal/cup)*****	**Na (%)**	**Taurine (%)†**	**Carnitine (%)†**	**P (%)**	**K (%)†**	**Mg (%)†**
Recommended levels	–	**0.08-0.15**	**≥0.1**	**≥0.02**	**0.2-0.7**	**≥0.4**	**≥0.06**
Hill's Prescription Diet h/d Canine	407	0.08	0.14	0.03	0.54	0.8	0.122
Medi-Cal Renal LP	283	0.1	na	na	0.3	0.7	na
Medi-Cal Renal MP	336	0.1	na	na	0.4	0.7	na
Moist foods for Class Ib, II and III patients	**Energy density (kcal/can)*****	**Na (%)**	**Taurine (%)†**	**Carnitine (%)†**	**P (%)**	**K (%)†**	**Mg (%)†**
Recommended levels	–	**0.08-0.15**	**≥0.1**	**≥0.02**	**0.2-0.7**	**≥0.4**	**≥0.06**
Hill's Prescription Diet h/d Canine	480/13 oz.	0.11	0.21	0.03	0.57	0.81	0.131
Medi-Cal Renal LP	643/385 g	0.1	na	na	0.2	1.0	na
Purina Veterinary Diet CV Cardiovascular Formula	638/12.5 oz.	0.12	0.24	na	0.40	1.21	0.060

Key: Na = sodium, P = phosphorus, K = potassium, Mg = magnesium, na = information not available from the manufacturer, g = grams.

*Values are on a dry matter basis unless otherwise stated.

**Also recommended for Class Ib, II and III patients when ACE inhibitors are used, especially when used in combination with diuretics.

***As fed energy values (kcal/cup or can) are useful for determining the amount to feed; these values can be converted to an amount of food to feed by dividing the energy density of the food (as fed basis) by the patient's daily energy requirement (DER); cup = 8-oz. measuring cup; to convert kcal to kJ, multiply kcal by 4.184. Providing the right amount of food is vital for managing patients with cardiovascular disease. Overweight patients should be fed foods with reduced energy as part of a weight-reduction program (Chapter 27). Patients suffering from cardiac cachexia may need more energy than otherwise normal pets. Body condition scoring should be used frequently to determine the patient's response to the amount of food fed.

†See discussion under "Adjunctive Management: Drugs and Supplements" in the "Feeding Plan" section if additional supplementation is required beyond that present in foods in this table.

Table 36-6. Levels of key nutrients in selected commercial foods for cats with cardiovascular disease compared to the recommended levels.*

Dry foods	Energy density (kcal/cup)**	Na (%)	Taurine (%)***	P (%)	K (%)***	Mg (%)***
Recommended levels	**-**	**0.07-0.30**	**≥0.3**	**0.3-0.7**	**≥0.52**	**≥0.04**
Hill's Prescription Diet g/d Feline	297	0.32	0.14	0.54	0.77	0.049
Hill's Prescription Diet k/d Feline	477	0.24	0.16	0.46	0.75	0.058
Hill's Science Diet Mature Adult Active Longevity Original	475	0.32	0.2	0.69	0.88	0.069
Medi-Cal Mature Formula	355	0.4	0.4	0.8	1.0	na
Medi-Cal Reduced Protein	440	0.3	0.4	0.6	0.8	na
Medi-Cal Renal LP	409	0.2	0.2	0.5	1.0	na
Purina Veterinary Diets NF KidNey Function	398	0.2	0.18	0.41	0.88	0.10

Moist foods	Energy density (kcal/can)**	Na (%)	Taurine (%)***	P (%)	K (%)***	Mg (%)***
Recommended levels	**-**	**0.07-0.30**	**≥0.3**	**0.3-0.7**	**≥0.52**	**≥0.04**
Hill's Prescription Diet g/d Feline	165/5.5 oz.	0.32	0.44	0.52	0.72	0.088
Hill's Prescription Diet k/d with Chicken Feline	183/5.5 oz.	0.3	0.42	0.38	1.18	0.049
Hill's Science Diet Mature Adult Active Longevity	87/3 oz.					
Gourmet Turkey Entrée Minced	160/5.5 oz.	0.28	0.48	0.64	0.84	0.072
Iams Veterinary Formula Stress/Weight Gain Formula Maximum-Calorie	333/6 oz.	0.24	0.33	0.83	1.01	0.089
Medi-Cal Mature Formula	205/170 g	0.3	0.3	0.6	0.7	na
Medi-Cal Reduced Protein	265/170 g	0.2	0.3	0.5	0.7	na
Medi-Cal Renal LP	125/85 g pouch	0.6	0.8	0.5	1.1	na
Purina Veterinary Diets CV Cardiovascular Formula	223/5.5 oz.	0.2	0.31	0.92	1.33	0.07
Purina Veterinary Diets NF KidNey Function	234/5.5 oz.	0.16	0.45	0.52	0.96	0.10

Key: Na = sodium, P = phosphorus, K = potassium, Mg = magnesium, na = information not available from the manufacturer.
*Values are on a dry matter basis unless otherwise stated.
**As fed energy values (kcal/cup or can) are useful for determining amount to feed; These values can be converted to an amount of food to feed by dividing the energy density of the food (as fed basis) by the patient's daily energy requirement (DER); cup = 8-oz. measuring cup; to convert kcal to kJ, multiply kcal by 4.184. Providing the right amount of food is vital for managing patients with cardiovascular disease. Overweight patients should be fed foods with reduced energy as part of a weight-reduction program (Chapter 27). Patients suffering from cardiac cachexia may need more energy than otherwise normal pets. Body condition scoring should be used frequently to determine the patient's response to the amount of food fed.
***See discussion under "Adjunctive Management: Drugs and Supplements" in the "Feeding Plan" section if additional supplementation is required beyond that present in foods in this table.

Diuretics

Diuretics continue to be a pharmacologic mainstay of acute therapy for heart failure. Sodium restriction, ACE inhibition, venodilating drugs and diuretics represent the major available methods for preload reduction.

Sodium chloride restriction is a key component of CHF treatment even with the use of diuretics. Well-controlled studies have demonstrated that loop diuretics such as furosemide given once daily fail to achieve a negative sodium balance in people with high sodium intake (Wilcox et al, 1983). Although there is an impressive natriuresis for several hours after furosemide administration, a compensatory increase in sodium reabsorption in the next 24 hours exactly matches the earlier losses (Wilcox et al, 1983). Thus, it is essential to limit sodium intake to ensure negative sodium balance. Balance studies with normal people have demonstrated that significant negative sodium balance can be predictably obtained with loop diuretics if sodium intake is limited to 20 mEq/day (roughly equivalent to 460 mg sodium or 1.2 g sodium chloride per day) (Kokko, 1994). This level of sodium restriction in people is equivalent to that achieved with use of foods formulated for patients with cardiovascular disease (**Tables 36-5** and **36-6**).

Blood volume contraction and circulatory impairment are potential complications of aggressive diuretic therapy. These complications can exacerbate pre-existing renal disease, alter excretion of drugs dependent on renal elimination and reduce cardiac output by reducing cardiac filling pressures (Fox, 1992). Reduced levels of sodium in the food have been implicated, but have not been proven to contribute to volume depletion from excessive diuresis (Fox, 1992). Fractional excretion of sodium in urine actually decreases in normal dogs fed a sodium-restricted food (Navar et al, 1982). The influence of diuretics on sodium and chloride balance in dogs with heart disease and failure fed sodium- and chloride-restricted foods has not been evaluated.

Furosemide contributes to hypokalemia and hypomagnesemia because of increased urinary loss of potassium and mag-

Table 36-7. Sodium content of selected human foods.*

Food	Amount	Sodium (mg)
Bread, cereals and potatoes		
Recommended		
Macaroni	1 cup	1-10
Potato	1 (medium)	<5
Puffed wheat	1 oz.	1-10
Rice (polished)	1/2 cup	1-10
Spaghetti	1 cup	1-10
Not recommended		
Bread	1 slice	200
Corn chips	1 oz.	230
Potato chips	1 oz.	300
Pretzel	1	275
Margarine and oil		
Recommended		
Unsalted margarine	1 tsp	0-1
Vegetable shortening	1 tbs	0-1
Not recommended		
Mayonnaise	1 tbs	60-90
Dairy products		
Not recommended		
American cheese	1 oz.	200-300
Butter	1 tsp	50
Cottage cheese	3 oz.	200-300
Cream cheese	1 1/2 oz.	100-120
Milk (regular and skim)	1 cup	122
Meats, poultry, fish		
Recommended		
Beef (fresh)	3 1/2 oz.	50
Chicken (no skin)		
Light meat	3 1/2 oz.	64
Dark meat	3 1/2 oz.	86
Lamb (fresh)	3 1/2 oz.	84
Pork (fresh)	3 1/2 oz.	62
Turkey (no skin)		
Light meat	3 1/2 oz.	82
Dark meat	3 1/2 oz.	98
Not recommended		
Bacon	2 slices	385
Egg	1	70
Frankfurter	1	560
Ham (processed)	3 oz.	940
Tuna (canned)	1 can	320
Vegetables (fresh or dietetic canned)		
Recommended		
Corn	1/2 cup	<5
Cucumber	1/2 cup	<5
Green beans	1/2 cup	<5
Green pepper	1/4 cup	<5
Lettuce	1/4 cup	<5
Peas	1/2 cup	<5
Tomato	1	<5
Not recommended		
Most canned vegetables	1/2 cup	190-450
Fruits		
Most fresh and canned fruits are low in sodium and are permitted		
Other food items		
Not recommended		
Macaroni with cheese	1 cup	1,000
Peanut butter	1 tbs	81
Pizza (cheese)	1 slice	650
Desserts		
Recommended		
Sherbet	1/2 cup	15-25
Not recommended		
Cookies	1	35-100
Gelatins	1/2 cup	60-85
Ice cream	1/2 cup	60-85
Puddings	1/2 cup	100-200

*Sodium amounts are on an as fed basis; adapted from Morris ML Jr, Ettinger SJ. In: Ettinger SJ, Feldman EC, eds. Textbook of Veterinary Internal Medicine, 4th ed. Philadelphia, PA: WB Saunders Co, 1995; 237.

nesium (Fox, 1992). The role of magnesium and potassium in the development of cardiac dysrhythmias has not received attention beyond the recognition that digitalis toxicosis appears to be much more dysrhythmogenic in hypomagnesemic and hypokalemic patients (Edwards, 1991). Hypomagnesemia may potentiate cardiac dysrhythmias caused by catecholamine release and is also associated with increased vascular reactivity (Bean and Varghese, 1994).

Conflicting reports have been published about the serum electrolyte and magnesium concentrations of dogs with CHF. A study of 113 dogs with CHF identified only four dogs with hypomagnesemia (Edwards, 1991). Three of the four hypomagnesemic dogs received combined therapy with a commercial sodium-restricted veterinary therapeutic food, furosemide and either hydralazine or enalapril. In another study, furosemide-treated dogs with heart failure had significantly lower serum magnesium and potassium values than did age-matched healthy controls (Cobb and Mitchell, 1991). A third study showed no significant differences in serum magnesium concentrations between clinically normal dogs, dogs with heart failure before any treatment, heart-failure dogs treated only with furosemide and heart-failure dogs treated with furosemide and digoxin (O'Keefe and Sisson, 1993). The feeding history was not included in the last two studies; therefore, specific food-diuretic interactions could not be interpreted. Normal dogs treated with a commercial sodium-restricted veterinary therapeutic food and furosemide for four weeks had no significant change in serum potassium concentrations (Roudebush et al, 1994).

Several studies have shown that the RAA system is not activated in human patients with moderate heart failure in the absence of diuretic therapy (Kubo, 1990; Bayliss et al, 1987). The major increase in plasma renin activity and plasma aldosterone concentration occurs with the introduction of diuretic drugs into the treatment regimen rather than as a result of the disease process itself. Furosemide apparently stimulates renin release by inhibiting chloride transport in the ascending limb of the loop of Henle, even if blood volume contraction is prevented (Kotchen et al, 1981). Treatment of normal geriatric dogs with moderate doses of furosemide profoundly stimulates the RAA system, irrespective of the sodium level in the food (Roudebush and Allen, 1996; Lovern et al, 2001). Use of furosemide with either hydralazine or enalapril also stimulates the RAA system in dogs with heart failure due to acquired mitral valve regurgitation (Haggstrom et al, 1996).

Although diuretics will remain important first-line drugs for management of acute cardiogenic pulmonary edema, findings in people suggest that diuretics continue to stimulate the RAA system and may play a pivotal role in the progressive self-perpetuating cycle of heart failure (Kubo, 1990). Veterinary cardiologists now recommend against the use of diuretic monotherapy early in the management of symptomatic heart failure (Keene and Rush, 1995; Keene and Bonagura, 2009). Diuretics should be reserved for managing more advanced heart failure in patients already receiving moderately sodium chloride-restricted foods, ACE inhibitors, pimobendan or combination therapy. Feeding patients foods without excess sodium chloride may allow lower dosages of diuretics to be used for control of the clinical signs of CHF.

Sodium, chloride, potassium and magnesium levels vary in commercial veterinary therapeutic foods for dogs and cats with cardiovascular disease (**Tables 36-5** and **36-6**). These nutrients in regular commercial foods vary markedly. Mineral levels should be considered when using concurrent diuretic therapy.

Long-term furosemide therapy may be associated with clinically significant thiamin deficiency, due to excessive urinary loss of thiamin, and may contribute to impaired cardiac performance in patients with CHF (Seligman et al, 1991). Patients receiving long-term diuretic therapy should be given supplements containing thiamin and other water-soluble vitamins or be fed a commercial food with increased concentrations of these vitamins. Veterinary therapeutic foods for patients with cardiac and renal disease are often formulated with higher levels of water-soluble vitamins to offset excessive urinary losses.

ACE Inhibitors

Enalapril, benazepril, ramipril and lisinopril, all ACE inhibitors, are commonly used to treat dogs and cats with CHF. Inhibition of the conversion of angiotensin I to angiotensin II results in vascular dilatation and decreased circulating plasma aldosterone concentrations. Angiotensin II and aldosterone play important roles in the maintenance of vascular volume and potassium balance. Both increase the reabsorption of sodium and chloride, and aldosterone promotes the excretion of potassium.

The use of ACE inhibitors in human patients with severe renal insufficiency or in patients given potassium supplements may increase the risk for hyperkalemia (Warren and O'Connor, 1980; Dzau et al, 1980; Rotmensch et al, 1988). In a study, more than half the dogs with CHF developed mild serum potassium elevations when treated with a commercial sodium-restricted veterinary therapeutic food, furosemide and captopril (Roudebush et al, 1994). Another study confirmed that heart-failure dogs treated with furosemide, digoxin and an ACE inhibitor had significantly higher mean serum potassium concentrations when compared with clinically normal dogs, dogs with heart failure before any treatment, heart-failure dogs treated only with furosemide and heart-failure dogs treated with furosemide and digoxin (O'Keefe and Sisson, 1993). Mild elevations in serum potassium concentrations have also been observed in dogs treated with enalapril (COVE, 1995). In another study, serum potassium concentration decreased in a subset of heart-failure dogs treated with ACE inhibitors and furosemide, although the specific feeding history was not reported (Cobb and Mitchell, 1991).

When mild hyperkalemia occurs in people with heart failure, reducing oral potassium intake and discontinuing potassium-sparing diuretics is recommended (Rotmensch et al, 1988). Although clinically significant hyperkalemia (serum potassium 6.5 mEq/l) is uncommon, the use of ACE inhibitors in dogs with CHF or renal insufficiency fed commercial or veterinary therapeutic foods with high potassium content may increase the risk for hyperkalemia (Roudebush et al, 1994).

Table 36-8. Low sodium commercial treats for dogs with cardiovascular disease.

Treats	Sodium (%DM)
Recommended sodium range for dogs with cardiac disease	**0.08 to 0.25**
Hill's Science Diet Adult Treats Medium/Large Bone with Real Chicken	0.23
Hill's Science Diet Adult Light Treats Medium/Large Bone with Real Chicken	0.24
Hill's Science Diet Jerky Plus with Real Beef and Vegetables	0.29
Medi-Cal Medi-Treats	0.1
Purina Veterinary Diets Lite Snackers Canine Formula	0.21
Royal Canin Veterinary Diet Treats for Dogs	0.21

Key: DM = dry matter.

Table 36-9. Daily sodium intake for a dog and a cat eating various foods.

Daily sodium consumption for a 15-kg dog eating 935 kcal/day

Food	Sodium intake (mg/day)
Grocery moist food[a]	2,338
Grocery dry food[b]	944
Specialty dry food[c]	552
Geriatric dry food[d]	430
Renal moist food[e]	468
Cardiac dry food[f]	159
Cardiac dry food and 1 slice bread	370
Renal moist food and 30 g cheese	700

[a]Pedigree with Chopped Beef
[b]Purina Dog Chow
[c]Hill's Science Diet Adult Original Dog Food
[d]Hill's Science Diet Mature Adult 7+ Original Dog Food
[e]Purina Veterinary Diets NF KidNey Function Canine Formula
[f]Hill's Prescription Diet h/d Canine

Daily sodium consumption for a 4-kg cat eating 270 kcal/day

Food	Sodium intake (mg/day)
Grocery moist food[g]	823
Grocery dry food[h]	405
Specialty dry food[i]	232
Geriatric moist food[j]	184
Renal moist food[k]	135
Renal dry food[l]	151
Renal dry food and 1/2 can tuna	295

[g]Fancy Feast Elegant Medleys White Meat Chicken Florentine
[h]Purina Cat Chow Complete Formula
[i]Hill's Science Diet Adult Original Cat Food
[j]Hill's Science Diet Turkey Entrée Mature Adult 7+ Cat Food
[k]Purina Veterinary Diets NF KidNey Function Feline Formula
[l]Hills Prescription Diet k/d Feline

Functional renal insufficiency occurs in up to one-third of human patients with severe CHF treated with sodium chloride restriction, ACE inhibitors and diuretics (Parker et al, 1987). This decline in renal function has been attributed to loss of angiotensin II-mediated systemic and intrarenal vasoconstrictor effects, which maintain renal perfusion pressure and glomerular filtration rate in low-output heart failure. Functional renal insufficiency appears to be alleviated in human patients when efforts are made to replenish total body stores of

Box 36-1. Palatability of Low-Salt Foods.

The question often arises whether sodium chloride enhances palatability of foods for dogs and cats. Sodium chloride and other inorganic salts stimulate specific taste chemosensory neural groups in these species. This finding suggests that dogs and cats can indeed taste sodium chloride and other inorganic salts. These "taste" groups are also stimulated by simple sugars in dogs and specific amino acids in dogs and cats. Standard palatability testing indicates that dogs prefer the taste of a moist food as the level of sodium chloride is increased, whereas increasing levels of salt in a dry food have no effect on palatability of the food. Palatability enhancers added topically to dry pet foods probably mask any taste effects of sodium chloride or other salts. Many foods with reduced sodium chloride levels for use in patients with cardiovascular disease have comparable or better palatability than grocery or specialty brand pet foods.

The Bibliography for **Box 36-1** can be found at www.markmorris.org.

Box 36-2. Use of Low-Salt Foods in Chronic Respiratory Diseases.

Avoiding excess sodium chloride may also be important in patients with some forms of chronic respiratory disease such as chronic bronchitis or asthma. Both epidemiologic and experimental evidence in people suggest that high sodium chloride intake may increase airway responsiveness and exacerbate clinical signs associated with asthma. When some people with asthma are subjected to salt loading, clinical signs worsen, lung function deteriorates and the need for antiasthmatic drugs increases. However, not all studies in people with asthma show benefits of avoiding excess dietary sodium. A serum-borne factor in human patients with airway hyperresponsiveness stimulates increased sodium influx into cells. Reduced sodium levels in food also result in increased levels of vasoactive intestinal peptide (VIP) in the plasma and lung; VIP acts as a bronchodilator. Although similar canine and feline studies have not been completed, foods that avoid excess salt may be helpful in conjunction with other forms of therapy in animals with chronic bronchitis or asthma-like clinical signs.

The Bibliography for **Box 36-2** can be found at www.markmorris.org.

sodium by reducing the diuretic dosage and liberalizing sodium intake (Parker et al, 1987). Renal insufficiency is a potential complication of ACE inhibitor therapy in dogs with CHF, but the role of sodium restriction is unknown (Roudebush et al, 1994; Longhofer et al, 1993; DeLillis and Kittleson, 1992). Four of 10 heart-failure dogs treated with captopril, furosemide and a sodium-restricted veterinary therapeutic food developed azotemia during the first five weeks of treatment; one of these dogs developed clinical signs of uremia (Roudebush et al, 1994). Two of the dogs that developed severe azotemia had isosthenuria on the initial urinalysis, which suggested some degree of pre-existing renal insufficiency. Azotemia is a more frequent complication when canine heart failure is treated with furosemide and enalapril rather than with furosemide alone (DeLillis and Kittleson, 1992).

Drug-induced azotemia in heart failure patients is treated by reducing the diuretic dose (usually at least by half–skip a dose if there is not active pulmonary edema); if that fails to resolve the problem, the ACE inhibitor dose can be reduced by half, the sodium intake can be increased to the next level (**Tables 36-5** and **36-6**) or a combination of these tactics may be used.

Management of Hyponatremia

The correction of hyponatremia associated with CHF has been evaluated in people but not in domestic animals. The combined administration of an ACE inhibitor and furosemide (but usually not of either agent alone) usually reverses CHF-associated hyponatremia in people, at least in part (Oster et al, 1994). The reversal of hyponatremia probably results from the combined effects of the ACE inhibitor (i.e., decreased thirst, decreased proximal tubular reabsorption of sodium chloride, interference with the hydro-osmotic effect of AVP) and the loop diuretic (i.e., increased distal delivery of glomerular filtrate, reduction in urine osmolality) acting to offset the pathophysiologic factors that impair excretion of water (Oster et al, 1994; Packer et al, 1984). Studies are needed to determine whether similar measures are effective in reversing CHF-associated hyponatremia in animals. Hyponatremia secondary to severely decreased cardiac output and inappropriate secretion of ADH would not be expected to resolve with either further diuretic therapy, or with ACE inhibition. In this case, increasing cardiac output (generally accomplished by inotropic stimulation, afterload reduction or a combination of the two) would be needed, and pimobendan would be the most easily available potentially effective therapy.

Pimobendan

Pimobendan is an inodilator drug (combination positive inotrope and vasodilator) approved by the FDA for the treatment of heart failure in dogs in 2007 in the United States.[d] This drug, used at an oral dose of 0.3 mg/kg twice daily in combination with an ACE inhibitor and furosemide, is now part of the standard medical therapy for dogs in heart failure from either chronic valvular heart disease or dilated cardiomyopathy. There are no known dietary considerations that influence the pharmacodynamic effects of pimobendan. The drug appears to be associated with a dramatic and helpful appetite stimulating effect in many patients. It is not approved by the FDA for use in cats.

Cardiac Glycosides

Pimobendan has largely supplanted the routine use of digoxin in dogs and cats in sinus rhythm, at least until their heart failure becomes refractory to standard treatment with pimobendan, furosemide, an ACE inhibitor and moderate dietary salt restriction. Cardiac glycosides have been used for more than two centuries and are still widely prescribed to manage cardiac disorders in dogs and cats when atrial fibrillation is present. Appropriate use of cardiac glycosides is based on an appreciation of the nutritional factors that influence the pharmacokinetic properties of these drugs.

Absorption of cardiac glycosides is influenced by the formulation of the drug and its administration in relation to meals (Chapter 69). Because administering digoxin or digitoxin with food may result in up to a 50% reduction in serum concentrations, these drugs are best given between meals (Snyder and Atkins, 1992). The body condition of the patient can also influence the pharmacokinetics of these drugs. Digoxin is minimally distributed in adipose tissue; the dosage of the drug should be based on lean body weight even for obese patients. Digitoxin is more lipid soluble than digoxin; so its dosage need not be adjusted for overweight animals.

The dosage of digoxin for cats is influenced by concurrent drug and nutritional therapy. The digoxin dose should be reduced by one-third if the cat is receiving concomitant furosemide, aspirin and a sodium-restricted veterinary therapeutic food (Atkins et al, 1988).

Metabolic derangements associated with increased risk of digoxin toxicosis include hypokalemia, hypomagnesemia, hypercalcemia, renal insufficiency, hypothyroidism and obesity (Snyder and Atkins, 1992). Serum electrolyte and magnesium concentrations should be measured and corrections made before starting cardiac glycoside therapy.

Potassium and/or Magnesium Supplementation

Electrolyte abnormalities, including hypokalemia, hyperkalemia and hypomagnesemia, are potential complications of drug therapy in patients with cardiovascular disease. Patients receiving diuretic therapy should receive adequate amounts of potassium and magnesium. Patients treated with ACE inhibitors may be predisposed to mild hyperkalemia; so their food should not contain excess levels of potassium. If hyperkalemia develops, switch to a food with a lower potassium level and discontinue any potassium supplementation. Loop or thiazide diuretics should be considered instead of potassium-sparing ones. Chronic kidney disease is often a concomitant disease of patients with cardiovascular disorders. If hypokalemia develops, feed a food with a higher potassium level or supplement the existing food with 3 to 5 mEq or mmol of potassium/kg body weight per day. If hypomagnesemia develops, feed a food with a higher magnesium content or provide oral magnesium supplementation (magnesium oxide, 20 to 40 mg/kg body weight per day).

Taurine Supplementation

Cats and dogs with myocardial failure may benefit from taurine supplementation to their regular food or use of foods that already contain increased levels of taurine. Patients with documented taurine deficiency are more likely to respond favorably to taurine supplementation. In dogs, the association between taurine deficiency and dilated cardiomyopathy is strongest in American cocker spaniels and golden retrievers (Kramer et al, 1995; Kittleson et al, 1997, 1991; Pion et al, 1998). Cats should receive 250- to 500-mg taurine per os daily (Pion et al, 1989), whereas dogs should receive 500- to 1,000-mg taurine per os three times daily (Pion et al, 1998). Some foods formulated for nutritional management of cardiovascular disease usually already contain increased levels of taurine (**Tables 36-5** and **36-6**). Patients eating these foods usually do not need additional taurine supplementation. **Table 36-10** lists levels of taurine found in various types of natural foods.

Table 36-10. Taurine concentrations (mg/kg dry matter) in selected natural food sources.

Source	Concentration
Beef muscle, uncooked	1,200
Chicken muscle, uncooked	1,100
Cod fish, uncooked	1,000
Lamb muscle, uncooked	1,600
Mouse carcass	7,000
Pork muscle, uncooked	1,600
Tuna, canned	2,500

Taurine supplementation of feline foods can be discontinued within 12 to 16 weeks if: 1) clinical signs of heart failure have resolved, 2) echocardiographic values are near normal and 3) the cat will eat a food known to support normal whole blood taurine concentrations. The length of time needed for taurine supplementation of canine foods is currently unknown.

L-Carnitine Supplementation

The recommended oral dosage for dogs with myocardial L-carnitine deficiency is 50- to 100-mg L-carnitine/kg body weight three times daily (Keene, 1992). Dogs weighing 25 to 40 kg are most often affected and should receive 2 g of L-carnitine mixed with food three times daily. This high oral dosage will elevate plasma L-carnitine concentration 10 to 20 times above usual pretreatment values (Keene et al, 1991). These high plasma L-carnitine levels will usually, but not always, raise myocardial L-carnitine concentrations into the normal range. The cost of this level of L-carnitine supplementation is approximately $80 (U.S.) per month for a large-breed dog. L-carnitine is usually available in human health food stores.

Dogs that respond dramatically to L-carnitine therapy do so in a reasonably predictable manner. Owners often report generalized improvement in clinical signs within one to four weeks and echocardiographic improvement is noted after eight to 12 weeks of supplementation. Improvement may continue for about six to eight months, at which time patients often reach a plateau and though they appear clinically normal they have depressed ventricular function as determined by echocardiography (Keene, 1992).

Assess and Determine the Feeding Method

The method of feeding is often not altered in the nutritional management of cardiovascular disease. If a new food is fed, the amount to feed can be determined from the product label or other supporting materials. The food dosage may need to be changed if the caloric density of the new food differs from that of the previous food. The food dosage is usually divided into two or more meals per day. The food dosage and feeding method should be altered if the patient's body weight and condition are not optimal. If the patient has a normal body condition score (2.5/5 to 3.5/5), the amount of food it was fed previously (energy basis) was probably appropriate. To determine the starting point for the amount of new food to feed, if the patient's body condition score is within the normal range (2.5/5 to 3.5/5), the amount of calories were appropriate. If the energy density of the previous food is available, the number of calories consumed per day (daily energy requirement [DER]) can be determined by multiplying the energy density of the food (kcal/cup and/or can) by the number of cups and/or cans fed. Then the amount of new food to feed can be obtained by dividing the DER value by the energy density of the new food. The energy densities of foods for heart disease are included in **Tables 36-5** and **36-6**. Manufacturers' feeding information can also be used to determine an initial amount of new food to feed. Body weight should be monitored for a few weeks after the food change is accomplished.

Food dosage should be modified for patients with obesity or cachexia. A diary maintained by the client is helpful for documenting what types and quantities of foods and supplements are being offered and eaten by the patient. This caloric intake can be compared with the number of calories that are usually needed to maintain ideal body weight and condition in that patient.

Obesity causes profound changes that can complicate cardiovascular disorders. Obese patients should undergo management with a calorie-restricted food and client education should focus on the importance of the pet achieving an ideal body weight and condition (Chapter 27). The veterinary health care team should emphasize the potentially damaging effects of obesity in patients with heart disease to clients to enlist their active participation in a successful weight-management program.

For clinical nutrition to be effective, there needs to be good compliance. Enabling compliance includes limiting access to other foods and knowing who feeds the patient. If the patient comes from a household with multiple pets, it should be determined whether the pet with cardiovascular disease has access to other pets' food. Access to other food (table food, other pets' food, etc.) may contribute to cardiovascular disease and thus should be denied (Chapter 1).

Occasionally, it is difficult to get a patient to accept a change to a lower salt commercial food. This can occur because of: 1) advanced illness associated with heart failure, 2) established feeding habits of older patients and their owners, 3) anorexia associated with concurrent renal failure and some cardiac drugs and 4) the "all or nothing" approach to feeding, rather than slowly changing to the new food. Changing the eating habits of most dogs is relatively easy, but changing the feeding habits and preconceptions (e.g., "low-salt food is always unpalatable") of some pet owners and veterinarians is often much more difficult. Results of feeding studies using hospitalized dogs have shown that most dogs will readily accept a food that is very low in sodium chloride by the third day (Ross, 1987). For individual dogs, these foods can be made more palatable by warming the food or adding flavor enhancers (low-sodium soup or tomato sauce; sweeteners such as honey or syrup). Use of foods that are very low in sodium chloride in advanced heart disease and failure will be much easier if the dog has already been fed a low-sodium food (Tables 13-4 and 14-3 for dogs and Tables 20-4 and 21-4 for cats).

REASSESSMENT

In general, the survival of patients with heart failure is related to the degree of myocardial failure, whereas their clinical signs are related more to CHF and its compensatory mechanisms. The overall objectives of treatment for chronic heart failure, as for almost any cardiovascular disease, are threefold: 1) prevention (prevent myocardial damage, prevent recurrence of heart failure), 2) relief of clinical signs (eliminate edema and fluid retention, increase exercise capacity, reduce fatigue and respiratory compromise) and 3) improvement of prognosis (reduce mortality).

Dogs and cats with suspected cardiovascular disease should undergo a routine serum biochemistry profile and urinalysis before any nutritional or drug therapy is initiated. Dogs and cats with heart failure and evidence of preexisting renal disease, including isosthenuria, may be at increased risk for developing azotemia during combined food-drug therapy. There are no universal recommendations for controlling: levels of sodium, chloride and potassium; fluid intake; ACE inhibition and diuretic administration for patients with cardiovascular disease. Rather, each patient should be monitored frequently (weekly for the first four to six weeks). Reassessment should include: 1) measurement of body weight, 2) assessment of body condition, 3) determination of serum electrolyte and magnesium concentrations and 4) evaluation of renal function.

FEEDING PLANS FOR PATIENTS WITH CHYLOTHORAX

Depending on the chronicity of the disease, amount of pleural effusion and prior treatment attempts, dogs and cats with chylothorax may be emaciated and dehydrated. The goal of medical management is to support the metabolic and nutritional needs of the patient until the effusion spontaneously resolves, specific therapy for an underlying disease is instituted (e.g., chemotherapy, radiation therapy or both for a mediastinal mass; surgical correction of diaphragmatic hernia) or the patient's thoracic duct is ligated.

Dehydration and electrolyte abnormalities should be corrected before initiating nutritional support. Serious hyponatremia and hyperkalemia occur in dogs with chylothorax and should be corrected, especially if anesthesia is planned for placement of a thoracic tube or exploratory thoracotomy (Willard et al, 1991). Parenteral nutrition is a proven way to reduce the quantity of lymph flow through the thoracic duct in human patients with chylothorax and can be used in feline and canine patients (Chapter 26). No clinical trials to evaluate the efficacy of parenteral nutrition in patients with chylothorax have been reported.

In the past, feeding a low-fat homemade or commercial food supplemented with medium-chain triglycerides was recommended for patients with chylothorax because it was thought to minimize thoracic duct flow. However, newer information challenged this concept and showed that thoracic duct flow may not be altered significantly by nutritional changes in dogs (Sikkema et al, 1993). Until more information is available, the primary management goals for chylothorax should be to meet the overall nutritional needs of the patient rather than focusing on nutritional changes designed to reduce chyle production. In most patients, medical and nutritional management are usually temporary means to support the patient until surgery (Birchard et al, 1988; Fossum et al, 1991). Fewer than 20% of cats with idiopathic chylothorax respond to long-term medical and nutritional management alone (Fossum et al, 1991).

ENDNOTES

a. Pipers F. Merial U.S. Personal communication. 2002.
b. Metabolic Analysis Lab, Inc., 1202 Ann Street, Madison, WI, USA.
c. Shelton GD. Director, Comparative Neuromuscular Laboratory, School of Medicine, University of California-San Diego, LaJolla, CA, USA.
d. Pimobendan. (Vetmedin). Boehringer Ingelheim, USA.

REFERENCES

The references for **Chapter 36** can be found at www.markmorris.org.

CASE 36-1

Congestive Heart Failure in a Beagle Crossbred Dog

Bruce W. Keene, DVM, Dipl. ACVIM (Cardiology)
College of Veterinary Medicine
North Carolina State University
Raleigh, North Carolina, USA

Patient Assessment

An 11-year-old, neutered female beagle crossbred dog weighing 10 kg was admitted to the hospital with a three-month history of weight loss and reduced appetite. The patient had been short of breath for the past 24 hours and would not lie down the previous night. The dog had been examined by a veterinarian two months earlier for coughing and exercise intolerance. At that time a tentative diagnosis of tracheobronchitis was made and the patient was treated with a trimethoprim-sulfadiazine combination for seven days and a sustained-release theophylline compound for three weeks. Clinical signs improved some during the first week of therapy.

The dog's vaccinations were current. Yearly heartworm antigen tests were negative for the past five years. The patient received ivermectin monthly for heartworm prevention, and except for intermittent flea problems and mild periodontal disease, had been exceptionally healthy its entire life.

On presentation, the dog's rectal temperature was 38.9°C (102.1°F), the pulse 160/min. and the respiratory rate 70/min. The patient appeared alert and anxious, with rapid, labored breathing. Mucous membranes were pale pink and the capillary refill time was slightly slow. A modest amount of periodontal disease and dental calculus was noted.

The bronchovesicular sounds were louder than normal and end-inspiratory crackles were heard diffusely over the lung fields bilaterally, accompanied by some expiratory wheezes. The precordial impulse was normally located and the arterial pulses were rapid but regular. A 3/6 holosystolic (regurgitant quality) murmur heard best at the left cardiac apex and radiating somewhat to the heart base was auscultated. A softer, regurgitant quality systolic murmur was audible at the right hemithorax. The jugular veins were modestly distended and a systolic jugular venous pulse was present. The abdomen was nonpainful. The liver was descended about 2 cm below the costal arch. Body condition score was 2/5. The rest of the physical examination was unremarkable.

Results of the initial laboratory tests included: complete blood count (normal); urinalysis (urine specific gravity = 1.022 [reference range = 1.001 to 1.070], dipstick and sediment examination were normal); and serum biochemistry profile (normal, except for a mild elevation in serum creatinine concentration). Generalized cardiomegaly with especially prominent left atrial and left ventricular enlargement was evident radiographically. Pulmonary venous distention and air bronchograms typical of cardiogenic pulmonary edema were also visualized (**Figures 1A** and **1B**).

The clinical diagnosis was congestive heart failure (CHF) secondary to chronic valvular heart disease (endocardiosis) and mitral/tricuspid regurgitation.

Assess the Food and Feeding Method

The dog was fed a mixture of commercial moist and dry dog food, with 10 to 20% of the intake from lean meat and vegetable table foods.

Questions

1. What are nutrients of concern and general nutritional recommendations for patients with cardiac disease and CHF?
2. What are the potential interactions between pharmacologic and nutritional prescriptions that might be made for this patient?
3. What is the patient's daily energy requirement (DER)?

Answers and Discussion

1. General nutritional recommendations for patients with cardiac disease and CHF include: avoid excess sodium and chloride; ensure adequate magnesium intake; ensure adequate potassium intake, if using diuretics; avoid excess potassium intake, if using angiotensin-converting enzyme (ACE) inhibitor drugs; ensure adequate energy and protein intake; avoid excess phosphorus and protein intake, especially when renal disease is present; and provide additional taurine and carnitine, if myocardial failure is present.
2. Most patients with advanced heart disease and failure are treated with a combination of nutritional management and drug therapy. The interaction between drugs and nutrient levels in foods used in cardiovascular patients is an important consideration.

   Furosemide may contribute to hypokalemia and hypomagnesemia (especially in patients with anorexia) by increasing urinary loss of potassium and magnesium. Hypokalemia and hypomagnesemia may potentiate cardiac dysrhythmias. Patients receiving diuretic therapy should be encouraged to eat a food that provides moderate, but not excessive, intake of these nutrients (0.10 to 0.15% magnesium on a dry matter basis; 0.6 to 0.9% potassium on a dry matter basis).

   Mild elevations in serum potassium concentrations have been noted in some dogs treated with ACE inhibitors such as captopril and enalapril. Although clinically significant hyperkalemia (serum potassium >6.5 mEq/l) is uncommon, the use of ACE inhibitors in dogs with CHF or renal insufficiency fed commercial or veterinary therapeutic foods with high potassium content may increase the risk for hyperkalemia.

   Hypotension and renal insufficiency are two common complications of ACE inhibitor therapy. When these complications occur, the dosage of the ACE inhibitor drug is often reduced. An alternative method is to replete total body sodium concentrations by reducing the dosage of diuretic and increasing the daily sodium intake of the animal. This may be successful in reversing hypotension or renal insufficiency without having to change the ACE inhibitor drug dosage.
3. This patient's calculated resting energy requirement (RER), based on a body weight of 10 kg, is approximately 370 kcal/day (1,548 kJ/day). However, the RER is probably higher because of the patient's increased heart and respiratory rates. Calculation of RER based on an estimated ideal body weight of 12 kg can be used and would result in an RER of 430 kcal/day (1,799 kJ/day). The dog's DER would be 520 to 600 kcal/day (2,176 to 2,510 kJ/day). Frequent monitoring of body condition is important so that appropriate adjustments to energy intake can be made.

Therapy Including Feeding Plan

The patient was treated initially with a diuretic (furosemide, 3 mg/kg body weight subcutaneously) and nitroglycerine (5 mg/24-hr transdermal patch), and was placed in an oxygen-enriched environment. Within four hours, breathing was less labored and oxygen supplementation was discontinued. A second dose of furosemide (2 mg/kg body weight orally) was administered and water was offered free choice. The dog spent a quiet night.

The next day, an electrocardiogram confirmed the presence of a sinus rhythm with evidence of left atrial and ventricular enlargement. An echocardiogram disclosed thickened mitral and tricuspid valve leaflets typical of endocardiosis (**Figure 2**). Also, severe mitral and tricuspid regurgitation was seen on color flow Doppler. Enalapril was initiated (0.5 mg/kg body weight per os, twice daily), furosemide was continued (1 mg/kg body weight per os, twice daily) and digoxin was begun (0.006 mg/kg body weight per os, twice daily).

The dog was fed one can of Prescription Diet k/d Canine[a] (570 kcal/can; 2,384 kJ/can) per day and discharged from the hospital. The owners were instructed to return with the dog in five days for further evaluation.

Progress Notes

During the recheck examination, the owners reported that the dog was doing well. The body weight remained stable at 10 kg, the serum digoxin concentration was 1.4 ng/ml (therapeutic range = 1.0 to 2.0 ng/ml) and serum electrolyte, urea nitrogen and creatinine concentrations were within normal ranges. Rechecks were scheduled at three-month intervals, or sooner if clinical problems arose. The owners were instructed to adjust the furosemide dosage as needed to keep the dog comfortable, within a range of 0.5 to 2.0 mg/kg body weight once to twice daily.

The patient remained well for about eight months, when it was admitted to the hospital for evaluation of mild dyspnea. The owners reported that they had been gradually increasing the furosemide dosage, which was now consistently at 2 mg/kg body weight per os, twice daily. Houseguests had fed the dog pretzels and potato chips several hours before presentation. Auscultation revealed

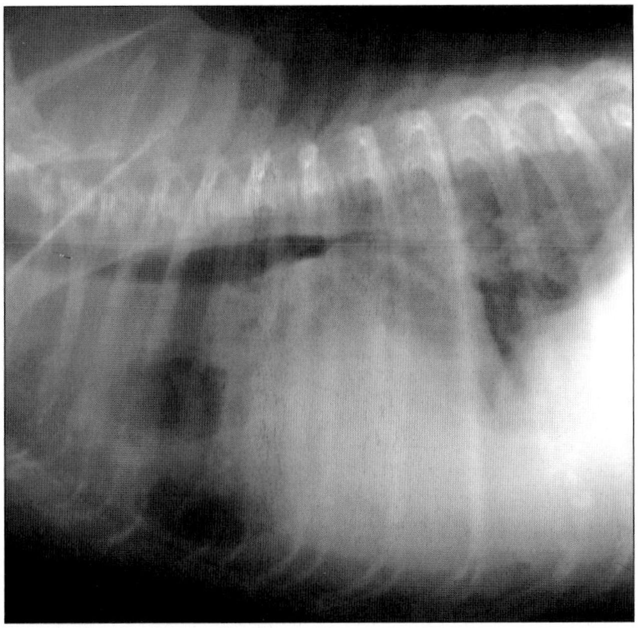

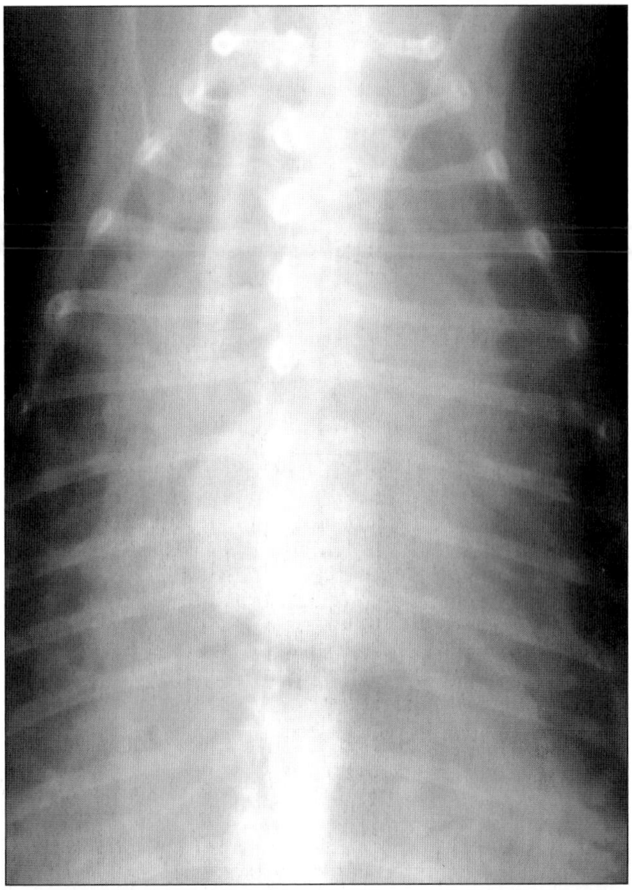

Figures 1A (above) and 1B (right). Lateral and ventrodorsal thoracic radiographs taken on the day of admission to the hospital. Generalized cardiomegaly with prominent left atrial and ventricular enlargement is present. Pulmonary venous distention and air bronchograms typical of cardiogenic pulmonary edema are also visualized.

some end-inspiratory crackles over the lung fields. An additional dose of 2 mg/kg body weight of furosemide was administered subcutaneously. Serum urea nitrogen, creatinine and electrolyte concentrations were within normal limits. The serum digoxin concentration was 1.2 ng/ml.

The food was changed to moist Prescription Diet h/d Canine[a] (583 kcal/can; 2,439 kJ/can), which is lower in sodium than the food fed previously. Three days later, the owners reported that the dog was feeling well. Its serum biochemistry values continued to be normal.

Approximately 10 months later, another episode of severe pulmonary edema occurred that was unassociated with any known nutritional indiscretion. This condition was unresponsive to 12 hours of intensive preload and afterload reducing therapy (increasing doses of furosemide, the arterial dilator hydralazine and nitroglycerine). The dog was euthanatized at an emergency clinic at the owner's request. Postmortem examination revealed a ruptured primary chorda tendinea to be the cause of the dramatically worsened mitral regurgitation and unresponsive pulmonary edema.

Endnote

a. Hill's Pet Nutrition Inc., Topeka, KS, USA.

Bibliography

Keene BW, Bonagura JB. Management of heart failure in dogs. In: Bonagura JD, Twedt DC, eds. Current Veterinary Therapy XIV. Philadelphia, PA: Saunders Elsevier, 2009; 769-780.

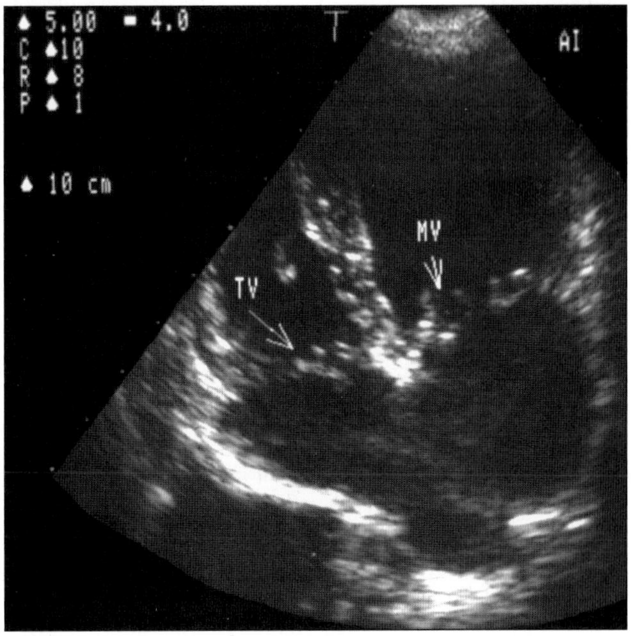

Figure 2. An echocardiogram obtained on the second day of hospitalization shows thickened mitral (MV) and tricuspid (TV) valve leaflets typical of endocardiosis.

CASE 36-2

Dilated Cardiomyopathy in an American Cocker Spaniel Dog

Bruce W. Keene, DVM, Dipl. ACVIM (Cardiology)
College of Veterinary Medicine
North Carolina State University
Raleigh, North Carolina, USA

Patient Assessment

A nine-year-old, male black American cocker spaniel dog was examined for dyspnea and lethargy that began two days after a routine elective surgical procedure (removal of a subcutaneous mass). The dog was thin (body condition score 2/5) and weighed 12 kg. Vaccinations were current and the dog received heartworm preventive medication. The dog had not had any major health problems in the past.

The heart rate was 180 beats/min. and regular, the respiratory rate 76 breaths/min. and the rectal temperature 39.9°C (103.8°F). The mucous membranes were dusky pink, with slow capillary refill. A soft (1/6 to 2/6) holosystolic murmur was heard best at the left cardiac apex, accompanied by a diastolic gallop sound (felt to be S3). The lung sounds were loud with some inspiratory crackles heard bilaterally. Otitis externa was noted bilaterally. An incision behind the right shoulder oozed slightly on palpation.

Thoracic radiographs revealed generalized, severe cardiomegaly with alveolar pulmonary edema (**Figures 1A** and **1B**). An echocardiogram revealed a left ventricular diameter of 5.68 cm in diastole (extremely dilated), with only an 8% shortening fraction (normal = 30 to 45%), but no major structural lesions were found on any valves (**Figure 2**). The echocardiographic findings were consistent with a diagnosis of dilated cardiomyopathy.

Results of an arterial blood gas analysis revealed hypoxemia and hyperventilation (PaO_2 = 71 mm Hg [reference range = 92.1 ± 5.6], pH = 7.4 [7.4], $PaCO_2$ = 30.8 mm Hg [36.8 ± 3.0]). Results of a complete blood count included normal red cell indices (packed cell volume = 39% [reference range = 38 to 57]), with an elevated leukocyte count (23,900/µl [reference range = 6.1 to 17.4]) consisting of a neutrophilia with a left shift (2,868 bands/µl [reference range = 0 to 300]). The platelet count was normal. Results of a serum biochemistry profile (including albumin, creatinine, urea nitrogen, electrolytes and liver enzymes) were within normal limits. Urinalysis disclosed an inactive sediment with a urine specific gravity of 1.024 (reference range = 1.001 to 1.070). The taurine concentration in a sample of whole blood was decreased (28.6 µmol/l; normal = 40.0 to 120.0), as was the plasma concentration of L-carnitine (plasma free carnitine 4.2 µmol/l; normal = 8.0 to 36.0).

Assess the Food and Feeding Method

The dog was fed a variety of dry commercial dog foods, free choice.

Questions

1. What is the feeding plan for this patient?
2. Should this dog be given nutritional supplementation?

Answers and Discussion

1. General nutritional recommendations for patients with cardiac disease and congestive heart failure (CHF) include the following: avoid excess sodium and chloride; ensure adequate magnesium intake; ensure adequate potassium intake, if using diuretics; avoid excess potassium intake, if using angiotensin-converting enzyme (ACE) inhibitor drugs; ensure adequate energy and protein intake; avoid excess phosphorus and protein intake, especially with evidence of concurrent renal disease; and provide additional taurine and carnitine, if myocardial failure is present. This patient's calculated resting energy requirement (RER), based on the current body weight of 12 kg, is approximately 430 kcal/day (1,806 kJ/day). However, the RER is probably higher because of the patient's increased heart and respiratory rates. The dog's daily energy requirement (DER) would be 600 to 700 kcal/day (2,510 to 2,928 kJ/ day). Frequent monitoring of body condition helps guide appropriate adjustments to this energy calculation.
2. Because of the suspected association of carnitine and taurine deficiency with dilated cardiomyopathy in American cocker spaniel dogs, supplementation with L-carnitine (1 g per os, three times daily) and taurine (500 mg per os, twice daily) was also begun. In this case, the whole blood taurine and plasma carnitine concentrations were depressed, justifying use of these supplements. In many cases of L-carnitine deficiency, the plasma carnitine concentration is "normal" (for dogs fed commercial dry foods), although endomyocardial biopsy may disclose myocardial carnitine deficiency. The relationship between blood and myocardial taurine concentrations is less well defined, but it seems prudent to supplement the food of American cocker spaniels with both taurine and L-carnitine.

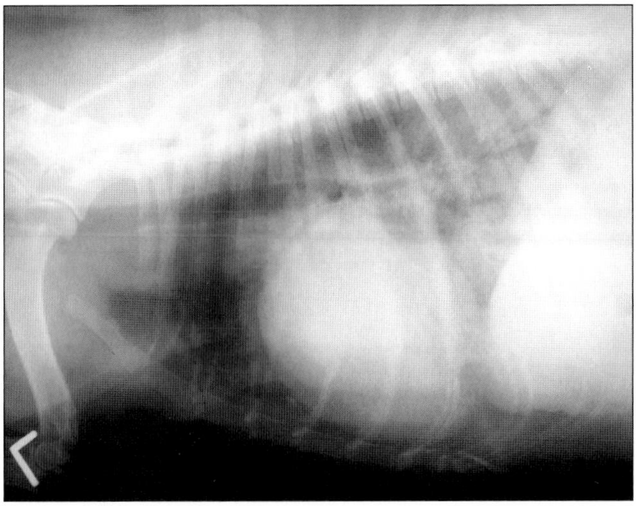

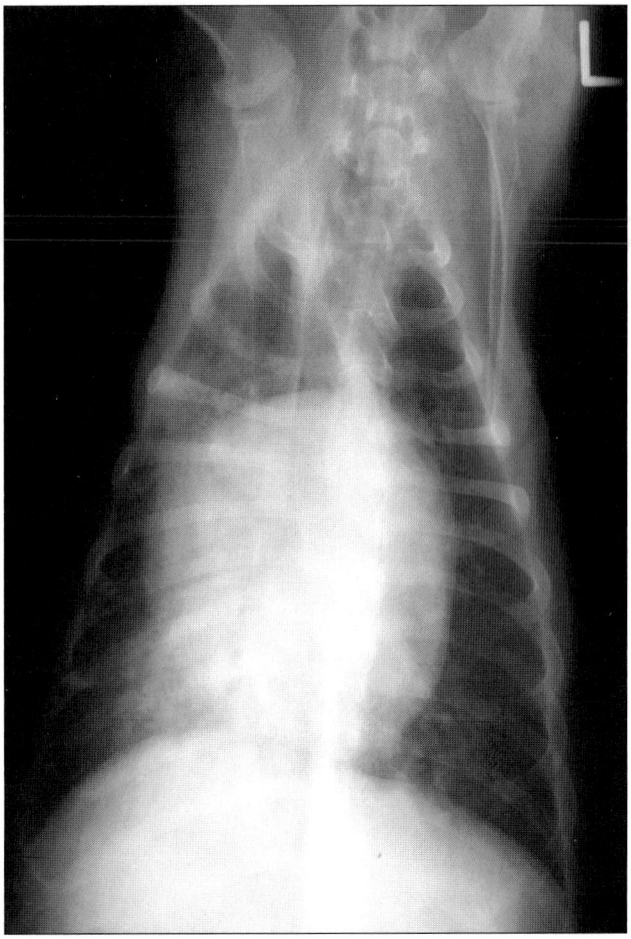

Figures 1A (above) and 1B (right). Lateral and ventrodorsal radiographs taken at the time of admission. Generalized cardiomegaly and pulmonary edema consistent with CHF are present.

Therapy Including Feeding Plan

Therapy was initiated with furosemide (2 mg/kg body weight subcutaneously, twice daily), enalapril (0.5 mg/kg body weight per os, twice daily), digoxin (0.006 mg/kg body weight per os, twice daily) and nitroglycerine (0.2 mg/hr transdermal patch, applied for the initial 12 hours of hospitalization). After culture of the surgical wound, a first-generation cephalosporin was given orally. The dog was maintained in an oxygen-enriched environment (40% oxygen) and its respiratory rate was monitored hourly.

A commercial veterinary therapeutic food designed for patients with cardiovascular disease (Prescription Diet h/d Canine[a]) was initially offered free choice, but was refused by the dog. A different commercial veterinary therapeutic food (Prescription Diet k/d Canine) was offered two days later when the azotemia was beginning to resolve; this food was readily accepted. This food avoids excess sodium, chloride, phosphorus, potassium and protein found in regular commercial dog foods (**Table 36-5**).

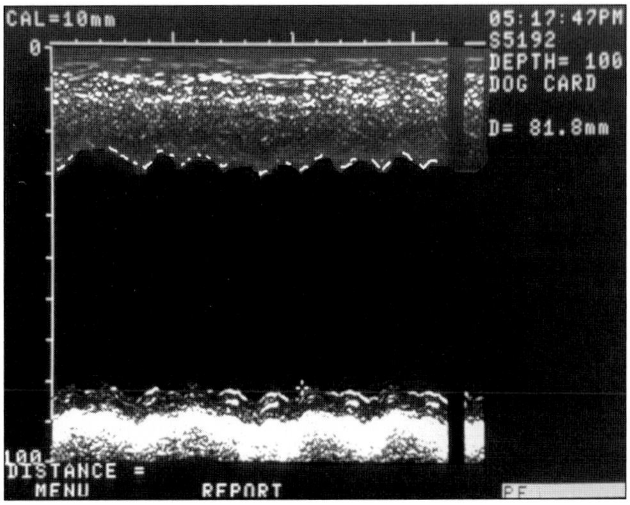

Figure 2. M-mode echocardiography reveals a marked increase in ventricular volume due to myocardial failure.

Progress Notes

The next day, the dog weighed 0.5 kg less, was afebrile, depressed and refused food, but was breathing much easier. Oxygen supplementation and nitroglycerine were discontinued. A serum biochemistry profile revealed that the serum urea nitrogen and creatinine concentrations had risen dramatically. An intravenous catheter was placed and maintenance fluid therapy was initiated with a relatively low-sodium physiologic electrolyte solution. Digoxin was withheld for 24 hours, and furosemide and enalapril were discontinued for 12 hours. Dobutamine (2.5 µg/kg body weight/min., increased to 5 µg/kg body weight/min. four hours later) was begun by continuous intravenous infusion to improve cardiac and renal function. An electrocardiogram was monitored continuously during dobutamine therapy for ventricular ectopic activity or other tachyarrhythmias.

The patient was much brighter and more active the following day. The serum urea nitrogen and creatinine concentrations had decreased. Fluid therapy and enalapril were continued, and the dobutamine drip was tapered over 12 hours. That evening, furosemide and enalapril were administered. The serum urea nitrogen and creatinine concentrations were normal the next day. The

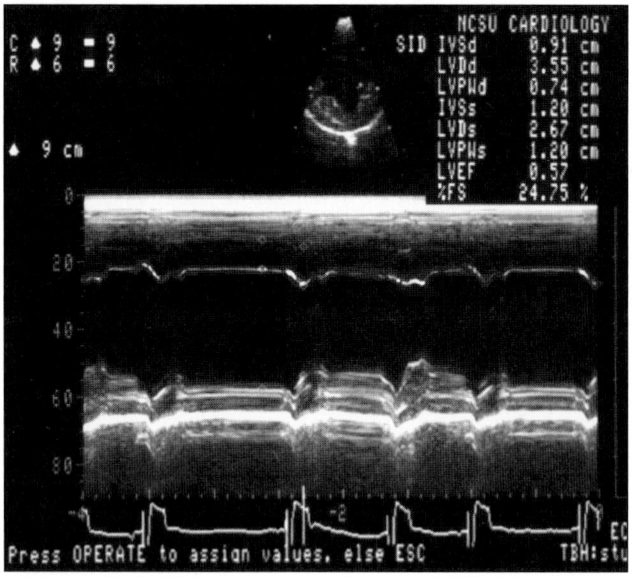

Figure 3. M-mode echocardiography one year after the initial admission for heart failure reveals normal left ventricular volume and function.

dog was now drinking and ate the veterinary therapeutic food that was offered (Prescription Diet k/d, one can). Fluid therapy was discontinued and digoxin (0.006 mg/kg body weight per os, twice daily), enalapril (0.5 mg/kg body weight per os, twice daily) and furosemide (1 mg/kg body weight per os, twice daily) were administered.

The dog improved and was able to go home four days after entering the hospital. Five days later, the owner reported that the patient was feeling better than it had in months. One and one-third cans of the veterinary therapeutic food were fed to meet the increased DER expected in the home environment. Three months postadmission, an echocardiogram and chest radiographs showed some improvement in fractional shortening, and complete resolution of pulmonary edema and pulmonary venous distention. Results of a serum biochemistry profile were normal. Furosemide was discontinued at that time. Body weight was now 13.2 kg. Digoxin, enalapril, k/d Canine and taurine and L-carnitine supplementation were continued. The food was fed in the same amount.

One year after the initial admission, an echocardiogram (**Figure 3**) disclosed remarkable reduction in left ventricular size and improved left ventricular systolic function (left ventricular diastolic diameter 3.55 cm; left ventricular shortening fraction 24.75%). Thoracic radiographs revealed no cardiomegaly or pulmonary edema (**Figures 4A** and **4B**). The owner had discontinued digoxin and enalapril approximately 10 months after the first admission (he had gone out of town and not started therapy again when he returned), although he continued to feed Prescription Diet k/d Canine and administer the taurine and L-carnitine supplements. The dog weighed 13.6 kg and had a body condition score of 3/5. The dog did well for three additional years, maintaining its improved ventricular function.

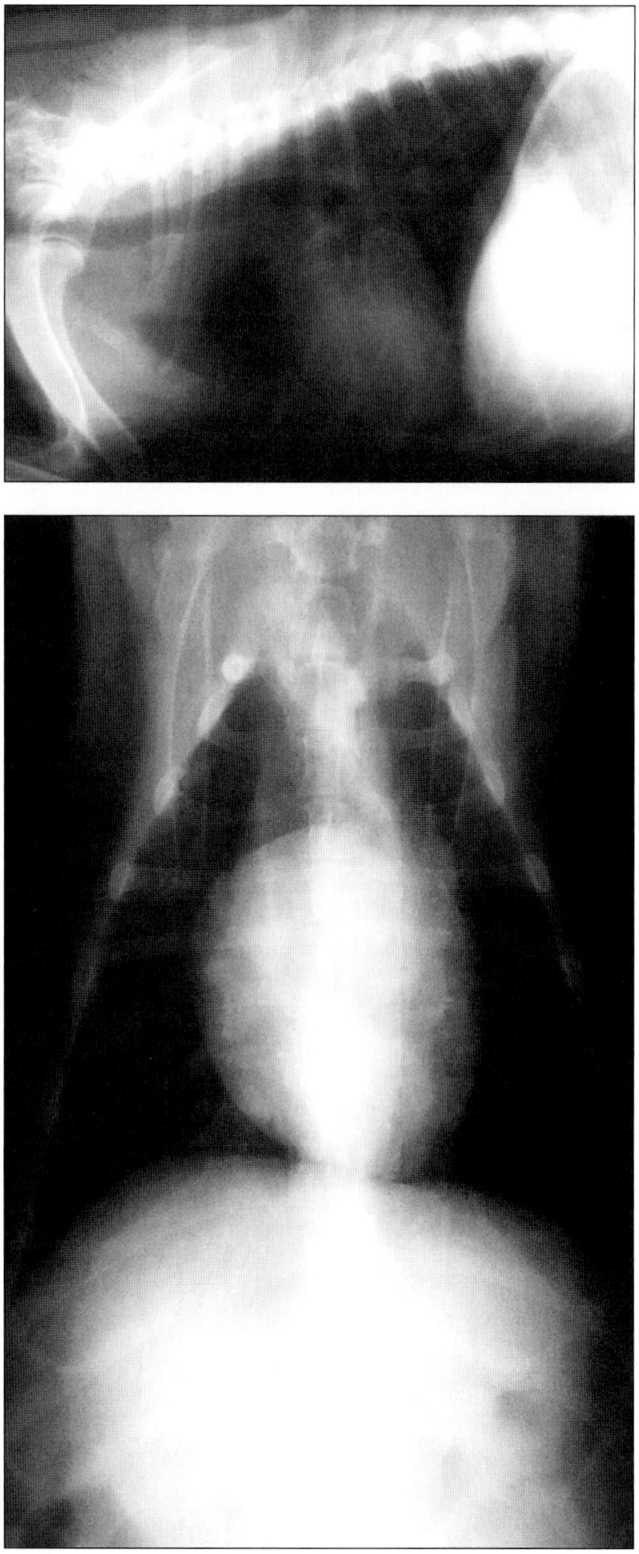

Figures 4A (top) and 4B (above). Lateral and ventrodorsal radiographs taken one year after the initial admission for heart failure reveal normal cardiac size and no evidence of pulmonary edema.

Four years after the initial diagnosis, the patient developed ascites. The heart and lungs were unchanged and the central venous pressure was normal. Ultrasonographic evaluation of the abdomen revealed a mass originating in the left adrenal gland, with intravascular invasion and extension into the right adrenal gland and obstruction of the caudal vena cava. Body weight was 10.5 kg with cachexia (body condition score of 1/5). A pheochromocytoma was diagnosed at postmortem examination.

Endnote

a. Hill's Pet Nutrition Inc., Topeka, KS, USA.

Bibliography

Freeman LM, Rush JE, Brown DJ, et al. Relationship between circulating and dietary taurine concentrations in dogs with dilated cardiomyopathy. Veterinary Therapeutics 2001; 2: 370-378.

Keene BW, Bonagura JB. Management of heart failure in dogs. In: Bonagura JD, Twedt DC, eds. Current Veterinary Therapy XIV. Philadelphia, PA: Saunders Elsevier, 2009; 769-780.

Kittleson MD, Keene BW, Pion PD, et al. Results of the Multicenter Spaniel Trial (MUST): Taurine- and carnitine-responsive dilated cardiomyopathy in American Cocker spaniels with decreased plasma taurine concentration. Journal of Veterinary Internal Medicine 1997; 11: 204-211.

Kramer GA, Kittleson MD, Fox PR, et al. Plasma taurine concentrations in normal dogs and dogs with heart disease. Journal of Veterinary Internal Medicine 1995; 9: 252-258.

Section 14

Renal Disorders

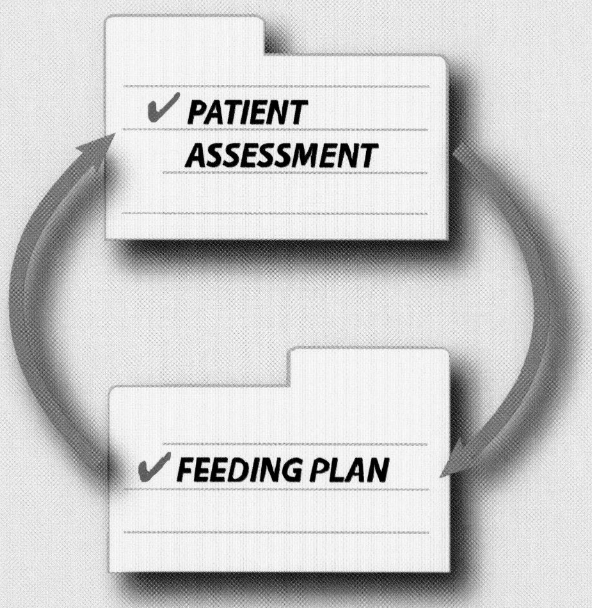

Chapter 37

Chronic Kidney Disease

S. Dru Forrester
Larry G. Adams
Timothy A. Allen

"When things are investigated, then true knowledge is achieved."
Confucius

INTRODUCTION

Chronic kidney disease (CKD) is the most common disease affecting the kidneys of dogs and cats. It may be recognized by reduced kidney function or the presence of kidney damage. CKD is defined as kidney damage present for at least three months, with or without decreased glomerular filtration rate (GFR) or greater than 50% reduction in GFR persisting for at least three months (Polzin et al, 2005). Kidney damage is further defined as either 1) microscopic or macroscopic pathologic changes detected by histologic or direct visualization of the kidneys or 2) markers of damage detected by blood or urine tests or imaging studies. In the past, multiple terms were used to define the severity of renal functional abnormalities including renal insufficiency, renal failure and uremia. However, there has not been uniform agreement on the specific definition of renal insufficiency vs. renal failure. Therefore, it has been recently proposed by the International Renal Interest Society (IRIS) to replace these terms with a scheme to classify severity of CKD into four stages based on stable serum creatinine concentrations (**Table 37-1**). Two of the foundational assumptions inherent in this classification scheme are that the presence of CKD has been confirmed and that azotemia, if present, has been localized as renal in origin. This classification scheme emphasizes the continuum of severity of renal injury of dogs and cats with documented presence of kidney damage without evidence of azotemia in stage 1 CKD, to progressively more severe CKD with resultant increasing serum creatinine concentration for stages 2 to 4. Furthermore, by using the term "kidney disease" and staging the severity of disease, it is possible to facilitate understanding, communication and application of management guidelines for patients in each stage.

The goals of this chapter are to provide pathophysiologic concepts and practical nutritional management recommendations for dogs and cats with CKD. Nutritional management of patients with CKD includes measures to reduce signs of uremia and slow progression to later stages of disease. There is general agreement regarding nutritional management of CKD when overt signs exist; however, the role of nutritional intervention during earlier stages of CKD is less well defined. Thus, in a sense, the question is not whether to use nutritional management but when should it be initiated. Because detection of CKD in its early stages is difficult and there appears to be no harm in avoiding nutrient excess (e.g., phosphorus) during earlier stages, nutritional management should be considered by stage 2 CKD and is clearly indicated when serum creatinine exceeds 2 mg/dl (179 µmol/l) (Jacob et al, 2002; Ross et al, 2006). Similarly, significant and persistent renal proteinuria,

Table 37-1. International Renal Interest Society (IRIS) Staging System for Chronic Kidney Disease in Dogs and Cats.

Stage	Serum creatinine (dogs)	Serum creatinine (cats)	Substage based on proteinuria and hypertension	Comments
1	<1.4 mg/dl (<125 µmol/l)	<1.6 mg/dl (<140 µmol/l)	Proteinuria: NP/BP/P* Hypertension: N/L/M/H/nc/c/RND**	Non-azotemic CKD Clinical signs (other than PU/PD) usually absent
2	1.4-2.0 mg/dl (125-179 µmol/l)	1.6-2.8 mg/dl (140-249 µmol/l)	Proteinuria: NP/BP/P* Hypertension: N/L/M/H/nc/c/RND**	Mild renal azotemia (overlaps with reference range) Clinical signs (other than PU/PD) usually mild or absent
3	2.1-5.0 mg/dl (180-439 µmol/l)	2.9-5.0 mg/dl (250-439 µmol/l)	Proteinuria: NP/BP/P* Hypertension: N/L/M/H/nc/c/RND**	Moderate renal azotemia Extrarenal clinical signs usually begin in this stage
4	>5.0 mg/dl (>440 µmol/l)	>5.0 mg/dl (>440 µmol/l)	Proteinuria: NP/BP/P* Hypertension: N/L/M/H/nc/c/RND**	Severe renal azotemia Many extrarenal clinical signs usually present

Key: PU/PD = polyuria/polydipsia, UPC = urine protein-creatinine ratio, BP = blood pressure.
*NP = non-proteinuric (UPC <0.2), BP = borderline proteinuric (UPC = 0.2 to 0.4 in cats and 0.2 to 0.5 in dogs), P = proteinuric (UPC >0.4 in cats and >0.5 in dogs).
**N = minimal risk of complications (systolic BP <150 mm Hg), L = low risk of complications (systolic BP 150 to 159 mm Hg), M = moderate risk of complications (systolic BP 160 to 179 mm Hg), H = high risk of complications (systolic BP >180 mm Hg), nc = no evidence of hypertensive complications, c = hypertensive complications present, RND = risk not determined (blood pressure not measured).
Adapted from www.iris-kidney.com.

even in the absence of azotemia, reflects marked renal damage and signals the need for nutritional management regardless of the CKD stage.

CLINICAL IMPORTANCE

Prevalence of Chronic Kidney Disease

CKD is a common cause of morbidity and mortality in dogs and cats. In a survey of 1,600 pet dogs over five years of age examined at a European veterinary college for a variety of reasons, approximately 20% had abnormally increased markers of renal function. It is not known how many of these dogs had kidney disease (Leibetseder and Neufeld, 1991). In a cross-sectional study of 31,484 dogs and 15,226 cats evaluated in private practices across the United States in 1995, the prevalence of kidney disease was 2.2% in cats and 0.8% in dogs (Kirk et al, 2001). During 1990, the diagnosis of CKD in cats of all ages reported to the Veterinary Medical Data Base was 16 cases/1,000 cats examined. By 2000, diagnosis of CKD in cats of all ages was 96 cases/1,000 cats examined (Ross et al, 2006). Increased diagnosis of CKD in cats may be due to their living longer, more of them being screened for CKD and/or increased awareness of CKD by veterinarians. CKD appears to be a common cause of death in dogs and cats. In a retrospective study of dogs, 2% died from chronic nephritis, 2% from pyelonephritis and 1% from glomerulonephritis (Bronson, 1982). Thus, the overall mortality from kidney diseases was 5%. With the exception of cancer, kidney disease was the most common cause of death in this study. In a 1991 survey by the Morris Animal Foundation of readers of *Companion Animal News,* respondents indicated that of 325 cats that had died, 94 succumbed to kidney disease (MAF, 1991). By comparison, 39 of the 325 died of feline leukemia and 45 died due to other causes.

Relationship Between Age and Kidney Disease

CKD occurs in dogs and cats of all ages, but it is frequently a disease of older pets. In a retrospective study of 70 cats with CKD, diagnosed from 1973 to 1984, ages ranged from nine months to 22 years (mean, 9.2 ± 5.5 years). Nine cats (12.8%) were less than three years old, 24 (34.3%) were four to seven years old and 37 (52.9%) were more than seven years old (DiBartola et al, 1987). In a study of 175 cats diagnosed with CKD in Australia from 2000 to 2003, ages ranged from two to 21 years (mean, 13.2 ± 3.7 years). However, the majority (69%) were 12 to 18 years old (White et al, 2006). The mean age for cats diagnosed with CKD at the Animal Medical Center in New York from 2000 to 2002 was 12.8 ± 4.4 years (Boyd et al, 2008). Analysis of data from university teaching hospitals contributed to the Veterinary Medical Data Base from 1980 to 1990 indicated that 37% of cats with CKD were less than 10 years old, 31% of cats were between 10 and 15 years old and 32% of cats were older than 15 years (Lulich et al, 1992). In a 1995 survey of private practices, the mean ages of dogs and cats with kidney disease were 10.2 and 13.2 years, respectively (Kirk et al, 2001). Another study in dogs showed a similar relationship between aging and occurrence of CKD. Prevalence of CKD was reported to be nine cases/1,000 dogs of all ages examined, 12.5 cases/1,000 in dogs between seven and 10 years old, 24 cases/1,000 in dogs between 10 and 15 years old and 57 cases/1,000 in dogs over 15 years old (Polzin et al, 1995).

Causes of Kidney Disease

Familial Kidney Diseases

Juvenile kidney disease increases suspicion of a familial

Table 37-2. Kidney diseases suspected or confirmed to be inherited in dogs and cats.

Kidney disease	Canine breeds	Feline breeds
Amyloidosis	Beagle, collie, foxhound, Chinese Shar-Pei, Walker hound	Abyssinian, Siamese, Oriental
Atrophic glomerulopathy	Rottweiler	–
Fanconi syndrome	Basenji, border terrier, miniature schnauzer, Norwegian elkhound, Shetland sheepdog	–
Glomerulonephropathy	Beagle, Bernese mountain dog, bull mastiff, Dalmatian, Doberman pinscher, soft-coated wheaten terrier	–
Glomerulosclerosis	Newfoundland	–
Hereditary nephritis	Bull terrier, English cocker spaniel, Samoyed	–
Medullary cystic disease	Miniature schnauzer	–
Polycystic kidney disease	Beagle, cairn terrier, collie, foxhound, miniature poodle	Domestic longhair cat, Himalayan, Persian
Primary renal glucosuria	Norwegian elkhound, Scottish terrier	–
Renal cystadenocarcinoma	German shepherd dog	–
Renal dysplasia	Alaskan malamute, beagle, boxer, bulldog, cavalier King Charles spaniel, chow chow, cocker spaniel, Dutch kookier, Great Dane, Great Pyrenees, golden retriever, Irish wolfhound, keeshond, Lhasa apso, Samoyed, Shih Tzu, soft-coated wheaten terrier, standard poodle, Yorkshire terrier	Persian
Renal telangiectasia	Pembroke Welsh corgi	–
Tubulointerstitial nephropathy	Norwegian elkhound	–
Unilateral renal agenesis	Beagle, Doberman pinscher	Domestic shorthair cat, Himalayan

nephropathy; however, juvenile kidney disease may be due to non-genetic causes. The specific term juvenile nephropathy has been used to describe disorganized nephrogenesis including kidney failure in young dogs. The term renal dysplasia describes abnormal differentiation of the kidneys. Specific histologic findings in renal dysplasia include fetal glomeruli, atypical tubular epithelia and persistent mesenchyme. Although renal dysplasia occurs most often as an inherited disorder, it can also be an isolated congenital abnormality that is not inherited. Juvenile nephropathy has been reported to occur in Alaskan malamutes, boxers and golden retrievers. Both males and females were affected. The lesions included moderate to severe interstitial fibrosis and mild to moderate lymphoplasmacytic interstitial inflammation. Mild to moderate tubular dilatation and atrophy were also present. Cystic glomerular atrophy and periglomerular fibrosis were prominent findings in most dogs (de Morais and DiBartola, 1995; de Morias et al, 1996; Chandler et al, 2007).

Familial disorders resulting in CKD have been documented or suspected to occur in a number of breeds (**Table 37-2**) (Lees, 1996). Familial nephropathies should be suspected when CKD is diagnosed in related pets with a higher frequency than would be expected by chance and there is no apparent underlying cause. Age of cats and dogs with familial nephropathies at presentation often is less than that of most pets presenting with CKD. In some familial nephropathies, the kidneys are seemingly normal at birth but because of an inborn metabolic defect, progressive structural and functional deterioration develops in the first few years of life. The term hereditary nephropathy is reserved for conditions in which an inherited basis has been documented by pedigree analysis or test breeding.

Hereditary nephropathy has been reported to occur in several breeds of dogs including Samoyeds, English cocker spaniels and bull terriers. Affected male Samoyed dogs with X-linked hereditary nephritis have splitting of glomerular basement membranes and develop overt CKD within the first year of life (Valli et al, 1991; Grodecki et al, 1997). The underlying inborn error is a defect in the formation of Type IV collagen. Carrier females with X-linked nephritis have isolated splitting of glomerular basement membranes although advanced CKD is not observed until later in life (Valli et al, 1991). In English cocker spaniels, a Type IV collagen defect is transmitted as an autosomal recessive trait (Davidson et al, 2007). Proteinuria is the initial finding and affected dogs typically die of terminal CKD between six and 24 months of age (Nash, 1989). Light microscopic renal lesions are mild and nonspecific but distinctive electron microscopic changes are observed in the glomerular basement membrane (Lees et al, 1998). The defect in bull terriers appears to be an autosomal dominant disorder (Hood and Savige, 1995). The rate of progression in bull terriers is quite variable with dogs dying of terminal CKD from a few months to 10 years of age. Hematuria is observed in many affected bull terriers.

Two distinct familial nephropathies have been reported to occur in soft-coated wheaten terriers (Littman et al, 2000; Ericksen and Grondalen, 1984). One nephropathy is a form of renal dysplasia. Kidneys from affected dogs are small, irregular and fibrous. Glomeruli are small and hypercellular and there are increased numbers of fetal glomeruli. The second form of nephropathy in soft-coated wheaten terriers is characterized by protein-losing enteropathy and concomitant nephropathy. Although a genetic basis for this syndrome has not been proven, dogs become symptomatic between two and five years of age. Membranoproliferative glomerulonephritis, glomerulosclerosis, or both, are present microscopically.

Renal amyloidosis has been recognized in related dogs of two

Table 37-3. Elements of the physical examination that should be emphasized in patients with suspected chronic kidney disease.

Body weight and body condition score
Cardiovascular system: Abnormal heart sounds? Increased tortuosity of superficial veins? Systemic blood pressure (direct or indirect measurement) abnormalities? Pulse rate and character?
Cervical region: Thyroid masses (cats)?
Fundus: Retinal detachment? Hemorrhage? Increased tortuosity of arteries? Retinal edema? Lipemia retinalis?
Genitourinary tract (urethra, prostate gland, penis, prepuce, vulva): Shape? Position? Pain? Discharge?
Hydration status
Kidneys: Both palpable? Size? Shape? Position? Surface contours? Pain? Bilaterally symmetrical?
Musculoskeletal: Muscle masses? Evidence of osteodystrophy?
Oral examination: Mucosal ulcers? Pallor? Necrosis or discoloration of tongue?
Temperature, pulse, heart and respiratory rates
Urinary bladder: Size? Position? Shape? Pain? Thickness of wall? Intraluminal masses? Grating sensation?

Table 37-4. Diagnostic tests for evaluating patients with suspected chronic kidney disease.

Bacterial urine culture
Complete blood cell count
Diagnostic imaging (abdominal radiography and/or ultrasonography)
Excretory urography, if indicated for obstructive uropathy
Renal biopsy, if indicated for evaluation of persistent proteinuria or suspected renal neoplasia
Serum biochemistry profile
Systemic blood pressure measurement
Urinalysis, including microscopic examination of urine sediment
Urine protein-creatinine ratio

breeds (beagles, Chinese Shar-Peis) and related Abyssinian cats (Chew et al, 1982; Boyce et al, 1984; Bowles and Mosier, 1992; DiBartola et al, 1986, 1990). Histologic findings in renal tissue from beagles include moderate to severe glomerular amyloidosis with inconsistent mild medullary interstitial amyloidosis (Bowles and Mosier, 1992). Medullary amyloid was identified in all Chinese Shar-Pei dogs and nine dogs (64%) had glomerular involvement (DiBartola et al, 1990). In 15 Abyssinian cats involved in one study, amyloid was deposited in the medullary interstitium of all cats and 11 cats had glomerular involvement (DiBartola et al, 1986).

Acquired Kidney Diseases

CKD may result from a variety of systemic conditions that cause kidney damage or there may be no apparent underlying cause. Infectious, inflammatory and immune-mediated diseases (e.g., leptospirosis, rickettsial diseases, pyelonephritis, amyloidosis) may cause inflammation of the renal interstitium or glomeruli. Glomerulonephritis secondary to systemic infectious, inflammatory or neoplastic diseases may be a common cause of CKD, especially in dogs. Renal neoplasia, particularly lymphoma in cats, may be a cause of CKD. Drugs that may cause nephrotoxicosis include antimicrobials (aminoglycosides), antifungals (amphotericin B), analgesics (aspirin, ibuprofen and phenylbutazone), immunosuppressive agents (penicillamine) and chemotherapeutic drugs (cisplatin, methotrexate and daunorubicin) (Grauer, 1996). Geriatric patients may be at greater risk for drug-induced nephrotoxicity because of a decline in kidney function associated with aging, use of multiple drugs with nephrotoxic potential and altered metabolism and excretion that occurs in older patients.

PATIENT ASSESSMENT

History

Historical findings in patients with CKD may include polyuria/polydipsia (less frequent in cats than dogs), lethargy, inappetence, vomiting, weight loss, nocturia, constipation, diarrhea, acute blindness (associated with hypertension) and seizures or coma (terminal uremia). Cats also may have ptyalism and muscle weakness with cervical ventriflexion due to hypokalemic myopathy. In a retrospective study of cats with CKD, polyuria and polydipsia were observed in 40%, vomiting in 52%, inappropriate urination in less than 10% and diarrhea in 3% (Lulich et al, 1992). Nonspecific signs such as inappetence and weight loss also are common in dogs and cats with CKD. Rarely, signs of thromboembolic disease (e.g., severe respiratory distress, posterior paresis) may be present in patients with nephrotic syndrome (i.e., proteinuria, hypoalbuminemia, hypercholesterolemia and ascites/peripheral edema). Occurrence of clinical signs may depend on the stage of CKD at diagnosis. Dogs and cats with stage 1 CKD generally have no or minimal clinical signs. However, polyuria/polydipsia may occur in some patients during this stage. Systemic clinical signs become more obvious in stages 3 and 4.

Physical Examination

A thorough physical examination is indicated for patients with suspected CKD, with emphasis on those items listed in **Table 37-3**. Dehydration (70%) and decreased body condition (58%) were the most common abnormal physical examination findings in a clinical series of cats with CKD (Lulich et al, 1992). An abnormally large kidney was detected by palpation in 25% of cases and an abnormally small kidney in 16% of cases in this series. Gingivitis, halitosis and oral ulcers were occasionally reported. Firm swellings in the nasomaxillary region, including the maxillary and mandibular gingival surfaces and extending to frontal sites, may be present in young dogs with stage 4 CKD. These changes result from renal osteodystrophy. Ascites or peripheral edema may be identified in patients with nephrotic syndrome; this finding is more common in dogs than cats.

The primary abnormal findings in some patients with CKD are due to ocular changes (e.g., retinal hemorrhage and detachment) associated with hypertension. In one study, 15 of 23 cats (65%) with CKD had indirect blood pressure measurements consistent with systemic hypertension (Stiles et al, 1994). Twelve of the 15 cats (80%) with hypertension had active hypertensive retinopathy including increased tortuosity of arteries, retinal edema and focal detachments. In a larger study of cats with CKD in a primary care practice setting, prevalence of hypertension in cats with CKD was about 20% (Syme et al, 2002). Hypertensive retinopathy has been reported to occur in dogs with CKD, but it appears to be less common than in cats (Jacob et al, 2003).

Routine Laboratory Evaluation

Most major renal functions can be evaluated diagnostically by routine laboratory tests including complete blood counts (CBC), serum biochemistry profiles and urinalyses (DiBartola, 2005). **Table 37-4** lists diagnostic tests that are recommended for patients with suspected CKD. CBC results are useful in dogs and cats with CKD to evaluate the presence of anemia and concurrent disorders such inflammation from systemic infection. Azotemia is increased serum urea nitrogen or creatinine concentrations. Increased serum concentrations of urea nitrogen or creatinine may result from prerenal, renal or postrenal disorders. (See Glomerular Filtration and Localization of Azotemia below.) Results of serum biochemistry profiles reveal renal azotemia from reduced GFR in patients in stages 2 to 4 CKD. Dogs and cats with stage 1 CKD do not have azotemia. Dogs and cats with CKD have impaired urine concentrating ability and usually have urine specific gravity values <1.030 (dogs) or <1.040 (cats), with concurrent clinical dehydration or azotemia. Some cats with stage 2 CKD may retain urine concentrating ability (urine specific gravity values >1.040). However, these patients have gradually decreasing urine specific gravity values as CKD progresses (e.g., over a period of 18 months) (Polzin et al, 2005). Additional notable urinalysis findings may include proteinuria (See Altered Membrane Permselectivity below.), glucosuria from tubular dysfunction or pyuria associated with urinary tract infection.

Diagnostic Imaging

Radiography and ultrasonography are complementary imaging modalities that help assess renal structure and localize disease within the urinary tract (Rivers and Johnston, 1996). Survey radiographs can assess renal size by comparing the length of the kidneys with the length of the second lumbar vertebral body on the ventrodorsal view. In a retrospective series of cats with CKD, 33% had small kidneys, 40% had kidneys of normal size and 27% had larger than normal kidneys as determined by imaging procedures (Dibartola et al, 1987). Polycystic kidney disease and lymphoma were the most common causes of renomegaly in cats. Feline polycystic kidney disease can be diagnosed ultrasonographically with a high level of confidence, although extensive polycystic disease must be differentiated from severe hydronephrosis and perirenal pseudocysts (Walter et al, 1988). Excretory urography can be used to qualitatively assess renal function and detect evidence of upper urinary tract obstruction.

Ultrasonography provides information about intrarenal architecture even when reduced renal function makes excretory urography impractical (Walter et al, 1987, 1988). It also can provide images of the kidneys when abdominal effusion or loss of abdominal fat reduces radiographic contrast. Ultrasonographic patterns are not specific for histologic lesions. However, it is possible to differentiate solid lesions from fluid-filled lesions and to assess distribution patterns. Ultrasonography also may be used to detect renal pelvic dilatation secondary to obstruction of the ureter by ureteroliths or nephroliths.

Radiography also is useful in the diagnosis of renal osteodystrophy. In young dogs with advanced CKD, radiographs of the skull reveal generalized osteopenia, irregular mineralization and dense soft-tissue swelling of the mandibles, maxillae and zygomatic arches. The most striking radiographic finding is demineralization of lamina dura dentes (i.e., bone surrounding the teeth). Radiographs of long bones reveal normal-appearing cortices with a coarse trabecular pattern of the metaphyseal and epiphyseal regions, suggesting demineralization. Spontaneous fractures may be evident. The radiographic diagnosis of fibrous osteodystrophy is applied to this constellation of findings.

Blood Pressure Measurement

Systemic blood pressure varies markedly in healthy pets and may be compounded further by effects of anxiety associated with blood pressure measurement in a hospital environment, and other factors (Bodey and Michell, 1996; Remillard et al, 1991; Brown et al, 2007). Several studies have evaluated different techniques for measuring blood pressure in dogs and cats. In the clinical setting, however, blood pressure is most often measured indirectly (e.g., Doppler ultrasonography, oscillometry). Follow a standard protocol to obtain reliable blood pressure values (**Table 37-5**) (Brown et al, 2007).

About 10% of apparently healthy dogs (Remillard et al, 1991) and 9 to 93% of dogs with CKD are hypertensive (Brown et al, 2007); whereas, 19 to 65% of cats with CKD are hypertensive (Syme et al, 2002; Brown et al, 2007). Depending on measurement techniques and methods used to determine reference ranges, indirect systolic arterial blood pressures greater than 141, 160, 170 or 185 mm Hg have been used to indicate systemic hypertension. Despite difficulties measuring blood pressure and confusion regarding diagnostic criteria, hypertension is a clinically important problem because of its apparent prevalence and potential for associated end-organ damage (e.g., retinal hemorrhage and left ventricular hypertrophy) (Morgan, 1986; Littman, 1994; Elliott et al, 2006a; Brown et al, 2007).

The IRIS has proposed that dogs and cats with CKD should be substaged on the basis of risk of hypertensive injury as determined by serial blood pressure measurements (**Table 37-1**). Dogs and cats with CKD with indirect systolic blood pressures less than 150 mm Hg are considered to have minimal risk of hypertensive injury. Patients with CKD and moderate or high risk of hypertensive injury or with overt evidence of hypertensive injury (e.g., hypertensive retinopathy) should be treated with appropriate antihypertensive medications.

Table 37-5. Standard protocol for measuring blood pressure in dogs and cats.*

Calibrate the blood pressure measurement device twice yearly.
Standardize the procedure used.

- Obtain measurements in an environment that is quiet, located away from distractions (e.g., other patients) and with the owner present.
- Restrain patients in a comfortable position, ideally in ventral or lateral recumbency to limit the distance from the base of the heart to the measurement cuff. Patients should be calm and motionless during the procedure.
- Use a cuff that is approximately 30 to 40% of the circumference of the measurement site in cats and 40% in dogs.
- Have the same trained individual, ideally a technician, perform blood pressure measurements each time.
- Determine and record five to seven consecutive and consistent (<20% variability) values.
- Discard the first measurement and determine the mean of all remaining values to obtain the patient's blood pressure measurement.
- Record the cuff size and site of placement (e.g., limb, tail), values for all measurements obtained, final (mean) value, details of any additional information (e.g., nervous patient) and interpretation of results by a veterinarian.

*Adapted from Brown S, Atkins C, Bagley R, et al. Guidelines for the identification, evaluation, and management of systemic hypertension in dogs and cats. Journal of Veterinary Internal Medicine 2007; 21: 542-558.

Evaluation of Renal Function

The primary functions of the kidneys are to excrete metabolic wastes (e.g., urea, creatinine), regulate fluid, electrolyte and acid-base balance and produce or activate several hormones including erythropoietin, calcitriol and renin. Anatomically, these functions occur in glomeruli (i.e., glomerular filtration and membrane permselectivity), renal tubules (i.e., urine concentration and tubular resorption) and other areas of the kidney (i.e., erythropoietin, calcitriol, renin). CKD may be associated with generalized renal dysfunction or it may involve only one function (e.g., tubular resorptive defect in Fanconi syndrome).

Glomerular Filtration

The most commonly evaluated renal function is glomerular filtration, which is determined by estimating or measuring GFR. Under steady state conditions, serum concentrations of urea nitrogen and creatinine are the time-honored methods for indirectly estimating GFR. These tests are useful for detecting large decreases in GFR (75% or greater), but lack sensitivity for detecting smaller decreases in glomerular filtration (**Figure 37-1**). In addition, serum urea nitrogen and creatinine values are affected by nonrenal factors, which contribute to the broad ranges for normal values.

Urea is produced in the liver from ammonia derived from the ornithine cycle, which catabolizes amino acids. The catabolized amino acids come from exogenous (dietary) and endogenous proteins. Urea is distributed throughout intracellular and extracellular water and is freely diffusible; therefore, it is common to use the terms blood urea nitrogen, serum urea nitrogen and plasma urea nitrogen interchangeably. The kidneys excrete urea by glomerular filtration, and serum urea nitrogen concentrations are inversely proportional to GFR. However, because urea is passively reabsorbed in the tubules, especially at reduced tubular flow rates, urea clearance is not an accurate measure of GFR. Clinical conditions that can increase serum urea nitrogen concentration include gastrointestinal hemorrhage, consumption of high-protein foods and catabolic drugs (e.g., glucocorticoids). Severe hepatic disease (e.g., portosystemic vascular shunts), feeding a low-protein food and conditions causing increased urine volume (e.g., intravenous fluid therapy) can decrease serum urea nitrogen concentrations independent of renal function.

Creatinine results from the nonenzymatic breakdown of muscle phosphocreatine. During steady states, creatinine production is constant and related to muscle mass. Serum creatinine concentration is less influenced by feeding than serum urea nitrogen concentration. However, it may be affected by breed and body size (Gleadhill, 1995). In a study of retired racing greyhounds, mean values for serum creatinine concentration (1.8 ± 0.1 mg/dl) and GFR (3.0 ± 0.1 ml/min./kg) were significantly greater than values from control dogs. However, blood urea nitrogen values were not different (Drost et al, 2006). Increased serum creatinine levels in greyhounds may be due to increased muscle mass in this breed. In contrast, it is possible for serum creatinine concentration to remain lower than expected or to not be increased in proportion to the decrease in GFR in older patients with decreased muscle mass and kidney disease.

When considering the magnitude of azotemia it's important to recognize that the relationship between serum urea nitrogen and creatinine concentrations and GFR is not linear (**Figure 37-1**). Thus, very large changes in GFR early in the natural course of CKD cause only small changes in serum urea nitrogen and creatinine concentrations. These small changes may not exceed the upper limit of the laboratory reference range and thus may go unrecognized throughout most of stage 1 CKD. Small decreases in GFR cause disproportionately large increases in serum urea nitrogen and creatinine concentrations in more advanced CKD (stages 3 and 4).

Evaluation of serum urea nitrogen and creatinine is used to indirectly assess GFR in most patients; however, measuring GFR is helpful for identifying kidney dysfunction that occurs before the onset of azotemia (e.g., breeds known to have familial kidney disease, patients with polyuria/polydipsia due to kidney disease, when potentially nephrotoxic treatment will be used). Urinary clearance of infused inulin is the gold standard for measuring GFR. However, this technique is limited to research settings because it requires collection of multiple, timed blood and urine samples and a constant rate infusion of inulin. Other methods have been used to estimate GFR but each has disadvantages. Endogenous creatinine clearance underestimates GFR because non-creatinine chromogens are present in plasma. Exogenous administration of creatinine reduces this potential problem by decreasing the proportion of non-creatinine chromogens in plasma. A newer creatinine-specific enzymatic analytical method eliminates the problem

(Finco et al, 1993). However, in cats, exogenous creatinine clearance does not accurately estimate GFR (Finco et al, 1996). In addition, factors other than GFR (e.g., hydration status) can affect creatinine clearance and serum creatinine concentration. Clearance of iohexol, a readily available radiographic contrast medium, has been used to reliably estimate GFR in dogs and cats and is a convenient method that can be used in clinical practice (Finco et al, 2001; Miyamoto 2001, 2001a; Goy-Thollot et al, 2006; Sanderson, 2009).

Altered Membrane Permselectivity

Proteinuria is the hallmark of altered glomerular membrane permselectivity. In patients with glomerular disease, permselective properties of the glomerular capillary wall are altered and increased amounts of protein are present in urine. Glomerulopathies are the most common cause of severe (heavy) proteinuria in dogs and cats although they appear to be more common in dogs than cats. Glomerulopathies can be primary (e.g., renal amyloidosis in dogs or idiopathic membranous nephropathy) or secondary to systemic infectious, inflammatory or neoplastic diseases (e.g., lupus erythematosus, heartworm disease, ehrlichiosis, lymphoma).

Proteinuria is defined as excretion of greater than normal amounts of protein in urine. Potential causes include urinary tract hemorrhage or inflammation, tubular resorptive defects, "overflow" proteinuria and altered glomerular permselectivity. Clinical significance of proteinuria depends on its severity and persistence. In the absence of hyperproteinemia, hematuria and urinary tract inflammation, persistent proteinuria usually indicates kidney disease and severe proteinuria (urine protein-creatinine ratio [UPC] ≥2) is generally associated with glomerular disease. The magnitude of proteinuria does not predict reversibility of the underlying disease, however. Serial quantitative evaluation of proteinuria is necessary for prognosis and assessment of response to treatment. Clinicians should confirm the persistence of proteinuria and attempt to localize its source before performing invasive and expensive diagnostic tests such as renal biopsy. Significance of proteinuria should always be interpreted in context of other laboratory and clinical findings (e.g., microscopic urine sediment examination).

Qualitative techniques for measurement of proteinuria include dipstick methods and precipitation techniques such as the sulfosalicylic acid (SSA) test. Urine concentration (refractive index, specific gravity) should be considered when interpreting results of these qualitative techniques (Finco, 1995). The most commonly used qualitative test is the colorimetric dipstick test. The test depends on ability of proteins, especially albumin, to alter the color reaction in paper impregnated with a pH-sensitive dye, tetrabromophenol blue. The test pad is buffered so that color changes reflect changes in protein concentration. In one study, sensitivity of the urine protein test strip for albuminuria in canine and feline urine was 54 and 60%, respectively. This means that 46 and 40% of dogs and cats, respectively, had proteinuria that was not detected by the dipstick (Grauer et al, 2004). Urine protein test strip specificity for canine and feline albuminuria was 69 and 31%, respectively. Therefore, 31 and 69% of dogs and cats, respectively, with a positive dipstick reaction for protein did not have proteinuria. Based on this, false positive reactions are common, especially in cats, and may occur with concentrated or alkaline urine, hematuria, pyuria, urine contaminated with quaternary ammonium compounds or with excessive urine contact time with the dipstick pad (Grauer et al, 2004). Observer variation is a documented and unavoidable source of error with dipstick tests. All positive dipstick reactions for proteinuria should be followed up with additional testing such as the SSA test or testing for microalbuminuria (Lees et al, 2005). The SSA test is used by most commercial laboratories and can be performed in-house by mixing equal volumes of centrifuged urine and 5% SSA,[a] available from chemical supply companies. Resulting turbidity of urine is graded on a scale of 0 (no turbidity) to 4+ (completely opaque). Microalbuminuria can be detected in-house using a species-specific point-of-care test.[b]

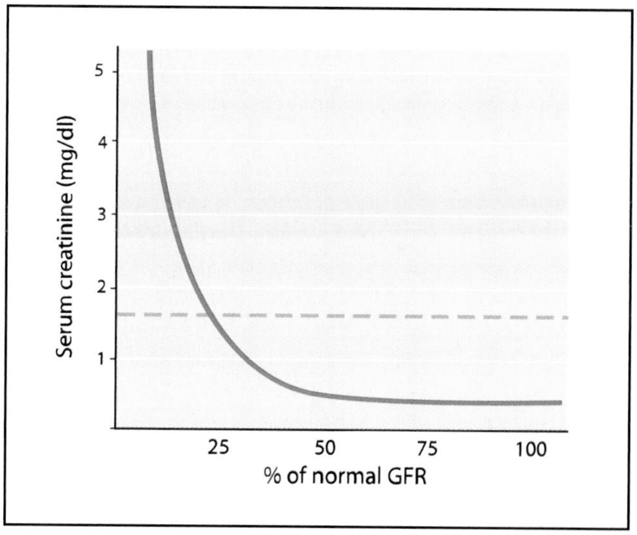

Figure 37-1. The relationship between serum creatinine concentration and % of normal glomerular filtration rate (GFR) or % of remaining functional nephrons is not linear. Therefore, small changes in GFR during early chronic kidney disease do not result in increased serum creatinine concentrations. Notice that values for serum creatinine do not exceed the upper reference range (broken line) until kidney dysfunction is marked (i.e., when 75% of nephrons are nonfunctional).

In patients with stable renal function, the UPC ratio is a semiquantitative method for assessing proteinuria. The UPC ratio is calculated by dividing urinary protein concentration by urinary creatinine concentration. Urinary protein is measured by a quantitative analytical technique rather than by dipstick. It may be determined in commercial laboratories or by using an in-house kit.[c] Because urinary excretion of creatinine and protein is presumed constant in the presence of stable GFR, the UPC ratio in a single urine sample can be used to estimate 24-hour urinary protein loss. The time of day and method of urine sample collection are not critical. The UPC ratio eliminates the potentially confounding effect of urine concentration on interpretation of urinary protein concentration. A UPC ratio less than 0.5 was found in the majority of non-proteinuric dogs studied (Grauer et al, 1985; White et al, 1984; Center et al, 1985). The upper limit of the reference range for UPC ratios in cats is 0.2 (Monroe et al, 1989; Adams et al, 1994). However, in one study of healthy male cats, the 24-hour urinary protein loss was greater in males than females and UPC values up to 0.6 were observed. This difference may be attributable to secretions of secondary sex glands in male cats (Monroe et al, 1989). Dietary protein intake significantly affected UPC values in normal cats and cats with surgically induced CKD (Adams et al, 1994). Consequently, dietary protein levels should be considered when interpreting UPC values because high protein intake may increase proteinuria.

UPC ratios should be performed on all dogs and cats with CKD to allow for substaging based on severity of proteinuria (**Table 37-1**). Studies in dogs and cats with CKD indicate that proteinuria is an important predictor of survival (Syme et al, 2006; Jepson et al, 2007; Jacob et al, 2005). Cats with UPC values consistently less than 0.2 have significantly longer survival than cats with UPC values greater than 0.4 (Syme et al, 2006; Jepson et al, 2007). Similarly, dogs with CKD and UPC values above 1.0 had significantly shorter survival than dogs with UPC values less than 1.0 (Jacob et al, 2005). Despite correlation of survival with proteinuria in cats with CKD, there is considerable overlap of survival times across the severity range of proteinuria. Accurate prediction of survival time for individual patients is not possible based on severity of proteinuria (Syme et al, 2006).

Urine Concentration

Disorders of urine concentrating ability generally involve abnormalities in the secretion of, or response to, antidiuretic hormone. Loss of concentrating ability can be one of the earliest indicators of kidney dysfunction, which is generally recognized when two-thirds of nephrons are nonfunctional. In CKD, the renal interstitial osmolality gradient is decreased because of increased urine flow per nephron or because of inability to establish and maintain the medullary concentration gradient. The resultant decrease in responsiveness to antidiuretic hormone leads to excretion of urine with osmolality or specific gravity values similar to those of plasma (i.e., isosthenuria).

Estimation of urine concentrating ability from urine specific gravity or refractive index is most often used for clinical purposes. The physiologic range for urine specific gravity is 1.001 to 1.070 in dogs and 1.001 to 1.080 in cats. Any urine specific gravity value may be normal; therefore, it's important to interpret specific gravity in the context of clinical findings including hydration status, concurrent disease and medications. (See Diagnosis of Chronic Kidney Disease.) In a retrospective series of cats with CKD, 37% had urine specific gravity values between 1.008 to 1.012 and 60% were between 1.013 and 1.034 (Lulich et al, 1992). However, some cats with CKD may have urine specific gravity values greater than 1.040 and remain persistently azotemic (up to 18 months) before losing concentrating ability (Polzin et al, 2005). In a study of cats with induced kidney disease (5/6 reduction of renal mass), mean urine specific gravity was 1.050 ± 0.015 in cats fed a 27.6% protein food and 1.038 ± 0.013 in a group fed a 51.7% protein food (Adams et al, 1994). However, the majority of cats with spontaneously occurring CKD have urine specific gravity values less than 1.035 (Polzin et al, 2005). Although it has not been reported, it is generally accepted that urine specific gravity in dogs with naturally occurring CKD is less than 1.030.

Tubular Resorption

Water and many solutes are reabsorbed from the tubular lumen into the peritubular interstitial fluid and ultimately the blood. In general, tubular resorption conserves substances that are essential for normal function (e.g., electrolytes, water, glucose and amino acids). Alterations in the renal handling of solutes may indicate kidney dysfunction. Abnormalities in tubular resorption may be generalized or limited to one or more tubular transport processes. Clinical syndromes are defined by the particular transport process involved. These syndromes include diverse disorders such as nephrogenic diabetes insipidus, renal tubular acidosis, renal glucosuria and aminoaciduria (e.g., cystinuria). Diagnosis is based on urinalysis findings (e.g., cystine crystalluria) or other tests such as quantitation of urinary amino acid concentrations.

Endocrine Function

Renal endocrine function can be evaluated by directly measuring the plasma concentration of the hormone or by indirectly assessing the action of that hormone. Erythropoietin concentration can be measured, but it is more practically assessed by serial monitoring of CBCs to detect progressive non-regenerative anemia that may occur in patients with stages 2 to 4 CKD. In CKD, reduced renal excretion of phosphorus causes phosphorus retention, which in turn stimulates increased parathyroid hormone (PTH) production and secretion. Phosphorus retention and hyperphosphatemia also inhibit renal tubular activity of 1-α hydroxylase, the enzyme responsible for renal conversion of inactive vitamin D to its active form, calcitriol. Decreased calcitriol concentrations, along with hypocalcemia (decreased ionized calcium) and hyperphosphatemia, contributes to development of hyperparathyroidism. Diagnosis of hyperparathyroidism is based on increased plasma concentrations of intact PTH. Although measurement of PTH is not routinely performed for patients with CKD, it should be measured (with serum calcium, phosphorus and ionized calcium) when calcitriol is administered for management of CKD. In the future, it may be recommended to monitor serum PTH concentrations in all patients with CKD, before the onset of hyperphosphatemia, so that treatment (e.g., dietary phosphorus restriction) can be adjusted to control secondary renal hyperparathyroidism earlier.

Diagnosis of Chronic Kidney Disease

Most routine tests used to diagnose CKD do not identify abnormal findings until there is advanced disease (stage 2 or higher). At present, the most common way to diagnose CKD is by first detecting evidence of changes in renal function (e.g., azotemia, proteinuria) that arise as a result of renal lesions (Lees, 2004). Looking for subtle changes (e.g., gradually increasing serum creatinine over time, progressive decline in urine concentrating ability or presence of mild proteinuria) is helpful for identifying CKD at earlier stages (Lees, 2004). Earlier diagnosis of CKD allows earlier therapeutic intervention, which could slow or halt disease progression.

Localizing Azotemia

Azotemia is present by the time CKD is diagnosed in most dogs or cats. Increased serum concentrations of urea nitrogen or creatinine may result from prerenal, renal or postrenal disorders. Prerenal azotemia may be caused by catabolic states (e.g., treatment with corticosteroids), consumption of a high-protein food, gastrointestinal hemorrhage, dehydration, hypovolemia or decreased cardiac output. Renal structure remains normal and the kidneys are capable of normal function if the prerenal insult is corrected before permanent damage occurs. Renal azotemia is caused by kidney disease and generally occurs when 75% of nephrons are nonfunctional. Renal azotemia should be further classified as either acute or chronic because of differences in treatment and prognosis. Postrenal azotemia is caused by disorders that impair elimination of urine from the body (e.g., urinary tract obstruction or rupture). Sites most often affected are the urethra and urinary bladder, and less often, ureters and kidneys. For upper urinary tract disease to cause postrenal azotemia, bilateral renal or ureteral disease must be present (unless the patient has concomitant kidney disease). As with prerenal disorders, renal function in patients with postrenal azotemia is normal initially; development of irreversible renal injury depends on severity, duration and nature of the disorder impairing urine outflow.

One of the most useful tests for distinguishing between prerenal and renal azotemia is analysis of urine obtained before any treatment, especially fluid therapy. Patients with azotemia and evidence of adequate urine concentration (i.e., specific gravity >1.030 in dogs and >1.040 in cats) usually have prerenal disorders. There are two exceptions to this rule: 1) some cats with CKD may have renal azotemia and still retain urine concentrating ability (specific gravity >1.040); it may be many months before they finally develop concurrent azotemia and inadequate concentrating ability, 2) some dogs with glomerular disease may develop azotemia initially and then lose concentrating ability; this "glomerulotubular imbalance" should be suspected in dogs that have significant proteinuria, azotemia and urine specific gravity values greater than 1.030. When azotemia is initially identified, it's important to determine if the patient has received any treatment that may interfere with urine concentrating ability such as intravenous fluids, diuretics or corticosteroids. Also, disorders that may cause prerenal azotemia but concomitantly decrease urine specific gravity must be excluded; examples include hypoadrenocorticism, diabetic ketoacidosis, hypercalcemia, hepatic disease and pyometra. Hypoadrenocorticism may be easily misdiagnosed as acute kidney failure because of similar clinical and laboratory findings. Dogs and cats with renal azotemia usually have either isosthenuria (urine specific gravity of 1.008 to 1.013) or minimally concentrated urine (specific gravity <1.025). However, as previously noted, some patients with CKD may retain the ability to produce concentrated urine.

Postrenal azotemia should be suspected in patients with stranguria, dysuria, pollakiuria, abdominal pain, ascites, firm/painful urinary bladder, subcutaneous swelling or discoloration of the perineum or a history of recent abdominal trauma. Palpable urethroliths or masses in the urethra, urinary bladder or prostate gland also suggest a postrenal cause of azotemia. Complete absence of urine production (i.e., anuria) most often is caused by lower urinary tract obstruction, although it may occur in some cases of acute kidney disease (e.g., ethylene glycol toxicosis). An attempt should be made to pass a urinary catheter if there is any question regarding patency of the lower urinary tract. However, the ability to pass a urinary catheter does not definitively exclude urethral obstruction. Urine specific gravity often is not helpful for distinguishing between renal and postrenal azotemia because urinary tract obstruction may cause renal tubular dysfunction and interfere with urine concentrating ability. Abdominal ultrasonography is helpful for detecting masses and accumulation of fluid when urinary tract obstruction or rupture is suspected. Abdominal fluid analysis in patients with uroabdomen reveals a modified transudate or exudate characterized cytologically by neutrophils, macrophages and mesothelial cells; bacteria may be seen if there is urinary tract infection. If uroabdomen is suspected, a sample of abdominal fluid should be submitted for measurement of creatinine and potassium concentrations so these values can be compared to concomitant serum concentrations. Measurement of urea nitrogen concentration in abdominal fluid often equals that of serum or blood and is therefore not helpful in patients with uroabdomen. Contrast urethrocystography is indicated when rupture or obstruction of the urethra or urinary bladder is likely; whereas, excretory urography is indicated when rupture of the upper urinary tract is suspected. If available, urethrocystoscopy may also be used to confirm rupture of the bladder or urethra.

Response to treatment may help localize azotemia. In general, pre- and postrenal azotemia resolve rapidly within one to three days after the underlying cause is corrected. In contrast, renal azotemia usually decreases more slowly, persists after appropriate treatment or recurs soon after discontinuation of treatment. Note that severe or prolonged pre- or postrenal azotemia may cause renal injury, which eventually leads to permanent kidney disease. It is also possible for renal azotemia to exist concomitantly with either pre- or postrenal disorders; this possibility should be suspected in patients that do not respond to treatment as expected.

Differentiating Between Acute and Chronic Kidney Disease

After renal azotemia is confirmed, additional evaluation is indicated to distinguish between acute and CKD (Vaden, 2000). Careful review of history, physical examination findings and laboratory evaluation results usually distinguishes between acute and CKD (**Table 37-6**). Acute kidney disease is a rapid

Table 37-6. Distinguishing between acute and chronic kidney disease in dogs and cats on the basis of clinical and laboratory findings.*

Findings	Acute kidney disease	Chronic kidney disease
Clinical findings	Acute onset of clinical signs (usually <seven days)	Vague onset of clinical signs (often over weeks to months)
	Usually moderately to severely depressed	Alert, responsive or only slightly depressed
	Urine volume often decreased	Polyuria/polydipsia more likely
	Often good body condition	May be thin
	Kidneys enlarged, painful or may be normal	Kidneys small, irregular or may be normal
Laboratory and diagnostic imaging findings	Normal or increased hematocrit; anemia may result from blood loss (e.g., gastrointestinal hemorrhage)	Nonregenerative anemia typical; hematocrit decreases progressively over time
	Serum urea nitrogen and creatinine previously normal but increase progressively	Serum urea nitrogen and creatinine previously increased and typically remain stable
	Normal to increased serum potassium	Normal to decreased serum potassium, especially in cats
	Moderate to severe metabolic acidosis	Mild to moderate metabolic acidosis
	Urinary casts in some patients	Usually no urinary casts
	Proteinuria or glucosuria may result from acute tubular necrosis	Proteinuria often present, more likely due to glomerular disease
	Bone density normal	Bone density may be decreased

*Modified from Vaden SL. Differentiation of acute from chronic renal failure. In: Bonagura JD. Kirk's Current Veterinary Therapy XIII. Philadelphia, PA: WB Saunders Co, 2000; 856-858.

Table 37-7. Potential mechanisms in the pathogenesis of chronic kidney disease.

Altered lipid metabolism
Amyloidosis
Compensatory renal growth (hypertrophy)
Effects of renal aging
Glomerular hyperfiltration
Glomerular hypertension
Hyperphosphatemia and secondary renal hyperparathyroidism
Inadequate urinary concentration
Increased renal ammoniagenesis
Metabolic acidosis
Renal oxidative stress
Systemic hypertension
Tubulointerstitial changes

deterioration of renal function that occurs over a period of hours to days, whereas CKD occurs over a period of months to years. A careful medical history may reveal causes of acute kidney disease (e.g., ingestion of a nephrotoxin such as ethylene glycol). Patients with acute kidney disease generally are healthy before sudden onset of lethargy, depression and vomiting, whereas clinical signs in CKD such as inappetence, weight loss and polyuria/polydipsia occur more gradually. Patients with acute exacerbation of CKD are common and may present a diagnostic challenge. However, careful questioning of owners in these cases usually establishes a more chronic history. If it is still not possible to distinguish between acute and chronic disease, renal biopsy may be helpful, particularly if results will alter treatment or provide prognostic information that would help owners decide on a course of action.

Etiopathogenesis of Chronic Kidney Disease

A variety of compensatory and adaptive responses are likely involved in the pathogenesis and progression of naturally occurring CKD (**Table 37-7**). In addition, sequelae of CKD (e.g., hypertension, proteinuria, metabolic acidosis and tubulointerstitial injury), changes in lipid metabolism and coagulation and normal renal aging may contribute to progression. Although some of these mechanisms initially are adaptive when renal function declines, they may ultimately lead to progressive renal injury (**Figure 37-2**). In addition, these etiopathogenic mechanisms are not mutually exclusive and in some instances may act synergistically. Understanding these mechanisms helps guide selection of treatment for patients with CKD.

Much of what we currently know about etiopathogenic mechanisms in CKD comes from studies in which kidney disease was induced by reduction or ablation of renal mass. This "remnant kidney model" causes progressive azotemia, mild proteinuria and arterial hypertension. In rats, this model is characterized by relentless progression to endstage kidney disease following the loss of a critical number of functioning nephrons (i.e., approximately three-fourths of the functional renal mass). Similarly, in human patients, progression from early to late stages of CKD has been reported regardless of the inciting renal injury and whether the initiating cause is present or not (Ihle et al, 1989).

Some controversy has existed about whether similar progressive renal injury occurs in other species, because the remnant kidney model has not been uniformly progressive in dogs and cats. Reduction of renal mass by 7/8 or less did not result in a consistently progressive decline in GFR in studies in dogs and cats (Polzin et al, 1991; Adams et al, 1994; Finco et al, 1998). It is possible that progression was not observed in these studies because the extent of the induced renal injury was insufficient to alter glomerular hypertension or renal autoregulation or perhaps because only mild proteinuria occurred. In experimental studies in dogs, reduction of renal mass resulted in glomerular changes and proteinuria; the severity of these changes appeared to correlate with the amount of renal tissue ablated (Bourgoignie et al, 1987). In a remnant kidney model in which renal mass was reduced by 15/16 in dogs, GFR progressively declined, providing evidence that progressive kidney disease occurs in dogs if adequate renal tissue is ablated (Brown et al, 1991; Finco et al, 1992). It is generally accepted that naturally occurring CKD (stages 2 through 4) in dogs and cats tends to be progressive (Allen et al, 1987; Jacob et al, 2002; Ross et al, 2006; Polzin et al, 2005). Therefore, it appears that after a critical mass of nephrons becomes nonfunctional in dogs and cats, either due to renal ablation or natural causes, disease characterized by several pathophysiologic adaptations progresses. See sections below for more detailed information about specific mechanisms and how they may contribute to progression of CKD in dogs and cats.

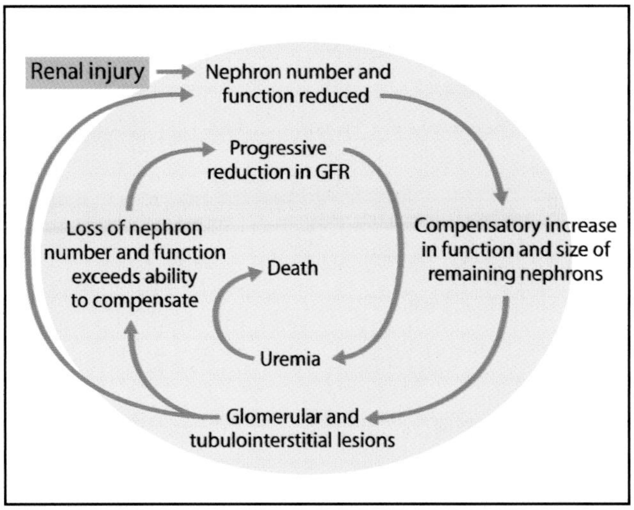

Figure 37-2. Vicious cycle of relentless progression of chronic kidney disease. After a critical amount of damage has occurred, compensatory mechanisms, which are initially beneficial, are activated and ultimately contribute to progressive injury. The amount of damage required to trigger progression probably varies from species to species and from individual to individual. (Adapted from Churchill J, Polzin DJ, Osborne CA, et al. The influence of dietary protein intake on progression of chronic renal failure in dogs. Seminars in Veterinary Medicine and Surgery: Small Animal 1992; 7: 246.)

Glomerular Hypertension and Hyperfiltration

In normal kidneys, single-nephron GFR and single-nephron plasma flow are submaximal under basal conditions. Reduction of nephron mass leads to hypertrophy of the residual nephrons with increases in filtration and perfusion of surviving nephrons to maintain total GFR (Polzin et al, 2005). Although these compensatory increases in single-nephron GFR and renal plasma flow initially help maintain homeostasis, eventually they contribute to progressive kidney damage. Single-nephron GFR increases are accompanied by glomerular hyperfiltration and intraglomerular hemodynamic changes, which increase flux of plasma proteins through the glomerular mesangium. These proteins stimulate mesangial cell proliferation and matrix production and eventually lead to glomerulosclerosis (**Figure 37-3**). Glomerular capillary hypertension is the critical intraglomerular hemodynamic factor responsible for promoting glomerular injury, perhaps through increasing proteinuria. Decreased dietary protein intake prevents these hemodynamic changes and preserves normal glomerular structure in rats (Brenner et al, 1982). The impact of dietary protein intake on glomerular hemodynamics and structure in dogs and cats is less certain.

As kidney disease develops, the afferent renal arterioles dilate, directly exposing glomeruli to systemic blood pressure; this causes glomerular hypertension, which distends the capillaries. The resultant mesangial stretch stimulates accumulation of collagen and progressive loss of glomerular function (**Figure 37-4**) (Riser et al, 1992). Continued strain on mesangial cells is a stimulus for cytokine release and extracellular matrix production (Polzin et al, 2005). Mesangial cells are stretched because of their relationship to capillaries and their attachment to the glomerular basement membrane. When mesangial cells in culture are stretched and relaxed repeatedly, stretch-induced release of transforming growth factor-β mediates production of collagen (Cortes et al, 1994). Intraglomerular hypertension also may lead to decreased glomerular permselectivity with resultant proteinuria (Polzin et al, 2005). Proteinuria, in turn, may mediate progressive injury of glomeruli and the renal tubulointerstitium (Lees et al, 2005; Polzin et al, 2005). Proteinuria has been associated with more rapid progression of CKD in dogs (Jacob et al, 2005) and cats (Syme et al, 2006).

Proteinuria

Proteinuria may mediate progressive renal injury through several mechanisms (Polzin et al, 2005; Elliott and Syme, 2006). Impaired glomerular permselectivity allows passage of proteins that are not normally filtered including albumin, transferrin and complement (Polzin et al, 2005). Proteinuria may result in direct mesangial cell toxicity, fibrosis of glomeruli and subsequent glomerulosclerosis. Progression of CKD in experimental models more closely relates to the degree of tubulointerstitial disease than to the severity of glomerular lesions. Proteinuria may injure tubular cells through overloading tubular reabsorptive mechanisms or by receptor-mediated mechanisms (Polzin et al, 2005). Proximal tubular cells reabsorb abnormally filtered proteins such as albumin through endocytosis and lysosomal degradation. Excessive albuminuria can overload this resorptive capacity, causing lysosomal swelling and rupture, leading to lysosomal enzyme-mediated injury of tubular cells. Excessive albuminuria also increases oxidative stress, which appears to be an important mechanism of progressive renal injury. (See Renal Oxidative Stress.)

Abnormally filtered transferrin, a plasma protein that transports iron, increases absorption of iron by proximal tubular cells. Increased intracellular iron concentration of tubular cells produces reactive oxygen species (ROS) leading to oxidative injury. Complement binds to the luminal membrane of tubular cells and activates the membrane attack complex, culminating in cellular injury and lysis. These mechanisms contribute to loss of tubular cells and ultimately loss of nephrons. Cellular activation of inflammatory genes also stimulates secretion of inflammatory mediators into the interstitium, which promotes inter-

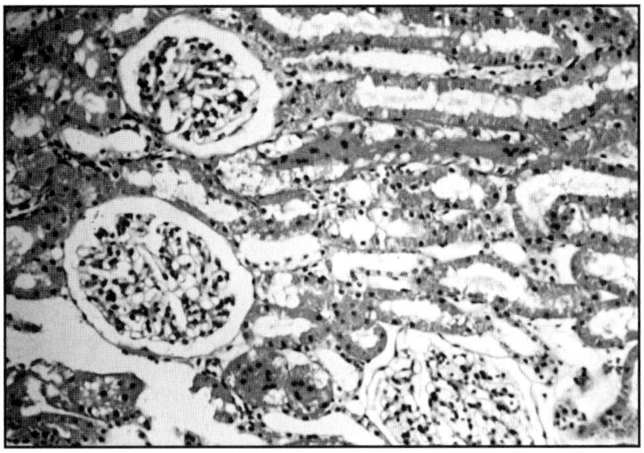

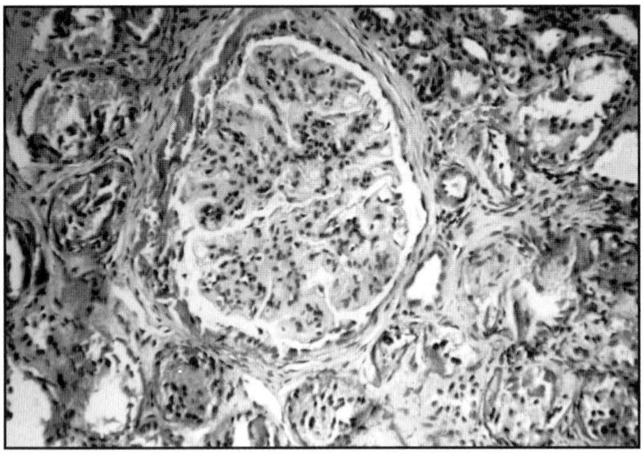

Figure 37-3. Microscopic view of early stages of kidney disease. (Above) Photomicrograph (hematoxylin-eosin stain) showing normal glomeruli, tubules and interstitium. (Below) Early progressive chronic kidney disease. Photomicrograph (hematoxylin-eosin stain) showing increased mesangial matrix, increased glomerular cellularity and increased interstitial infiltrates.

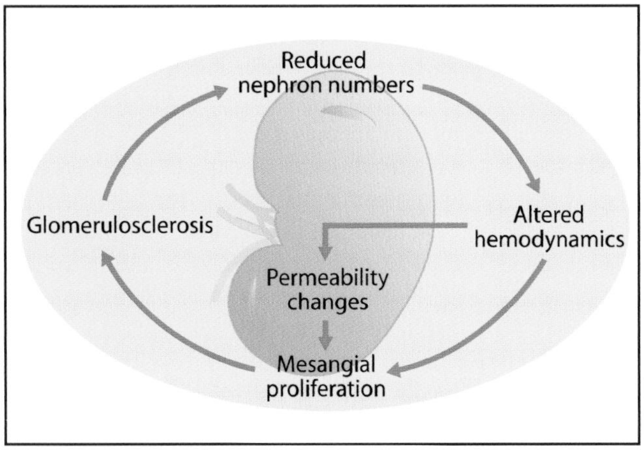

Figure 37-4. Schematic showing the progressive effect of glomerular capillary hypertension.

stitial fibrosis. These mechanisms of glomerular and tubular injury explain why even modest levels of proteinuria are associated with more rapid progression of CKD in dogs (Jacob et al, 2005) and cats (Syme et al, 2006).

Systemic Hypertension

In dogs and cats, hypertension usually occurs secondary to other diseases including kidney disease, obesity, hyperadrenocorticism, hyperthyroidism, pheochromocytoma and diabetes mellitus (Kobayashi et al, 1990; Rocchini et al, 1987; Brown et al, 2007). However, CKD appears to be the disease most commonly associated with systemic hypertension (Brown et al, 2007). When considering hypertension in CKD, it is important to note that CKD may cause hypertension and hypertension can promote progression of CKD. Systemic hypertension can also damage a number of other end organs, including the eyes, central nervous system and cardiovascular system (Morgan, 1986). The IRIS scheme for staging CKD in dogs and cats identifies substages based on magnitude of systemic blood pressure and risk of end-organ damage (**Table 37-1**).

Impaired autoregulation occurs in dogs with ischemic acute kidney failure and reduced renal mass. In normal dogs, the renal autoregulatory mechanism limits the effect of systemic blood pressure changes on renal blood flow and GFR. This protection is achieved by adjusting preglomerular resistance so that renal hemodynamics remain stable between mean systemic arterial blood pressures of 70 to 150 mm Hg. Dogs with severe reductions in functional mass have impaired renal autoregulation with elevations in renal arterial pressure. Impaired autoregulation may lead to renal injury during systemic hypertensive episodes and contribute to a progressive decline in kidney function (Brown et al, 1995; Polzin et al, 2005). Hypertension has been associated with increased risk of uremic crisis and death in dogs with CKD (Jacob et al, 2003).

Hyperphosphatemia and Secondary Renal Hyperparathyroidism

Hyperphosphatemia and secondary renal hyperparathyroidism have been incriminated as causes of progressive renal injury (Felsenfeld and Llach, 1993; Lumlertgul et al, 1986). Secondary renal hyperparathyroidism, characterized by increased PTH concentration, is an inevitable consequence of CKD (Nagode and Chew, 1992; Nagode et al, 1996; Barber and Elliott, 1998; Barber et al, 1999) (**Figure 37-5**). A study of cats with spontaneous CKD found an overall prevalence of secondary renal hyperparathyroidism of 84% (Barber and Elliott, 1998). Hyperparathyroidism was present in 100% of cats with endstage CKD and 47% of cats with biochemical evidence of CKD, but no clinical signs. Secondary renal hyperparathyroidism may be present based on increased PTH concentrations, even if serum phosphorus concentrations are within the reference range.

The inciting event in the pathogenesis of secondary renal hyperparathyroidism is phosphate retention (**Figure 37-6**). Destruction of nephrons decreases phosphorus filtration with a subsequent increase in serum phosphate, which stimulates PTH release from the parathyroid gland (Burkholder, 2000; Polzin et al, 2005). Hyperphosphatemia also decreases ionized calcium concentration, which stimulates PTH secretion. In a normal kidney and in early CKD, one effect of PTH is to decrease phosphate resorption in the proximal tubules so that more phosphate is excreted and serum phosphorus concentration is maintained within the normal range. However, as CKD progresses and more nephrons become nonfunctional, a greater concentration of PTH is required to maintain serum phosphorus concentration and eventually hyperphosphatemia develops. The primary consequence of hyperphosphatemia is development and progression of hyperparathyroidism. Although hyperparathyroidism helps maintain serum phosphorus concentrations initially, it has other effects that may be harmful. PTH stimulates resorption and release of minerals (e.g., phosphate) from bone, which increases the amount of phosphate that remaining nephrons must excrete. Increased PTH concentration correlates with histologic evidence of renal tissue inflammation and mineralization; therefore, hyperparathyroidism may damage the kidneys (Finco et al, 1992, 1992a; Ross et al, 1982; Brown et al, 1991).

Chronic Renal Hypoxia

The kidney has a very high rate of oxygen consumption, the majority of which is expended reabsorbing sodium. With kidney damage, surviving nephrons increase sodium resorption and correspondingly increase oxygen consumption. The renal medulla concentrates urine by means of the countercurrent system of blood vessels and tubules that actively absorb sodium. The major determinant of medullary oxygen demand is the rate of active absorption in the medullary thick ascending loop, which is a relatively hypoxic environment. Hypoxia of the renal medulla can predispose to acute and chronic renal injury because the kidneys are extremely susceptible to hypoxic injury (O'Connor, 2006; Eckardt et al, 2005; Brezia and Rosen, 1995).

In CKD, increased fibrosis in the kidneys may result from intrarenal hypoxia due to increased oxygen consumption by surviving nephrons. Acute kidney injury often is associated with altered intrarenal microcirculation and oxygenation (Rosenberger et al, 2006). Hypoxia deprives tissues of energy and induces various regulatory mechanisms. The transcription factor, hypoxia-inducible factor, is involved in cellular regulation of development of new blood vessels, blood vessel tone, glucose metabolism and cell death. Kidney disease activates hypoxia-inducible factor, which presumably is renoprotective during oxygen deprivation (Eckardt et al, 2005). Hypoxia induces profibrogenic changes in proximal tubular epithelial cells and interstitial fibrosis (Norman and Fine, 2006). Hypoxia causes release of cytokines such as TGF-β and platelet derived growth factor, which stimulate intrarenal production of collagen. Furthermore, anemia may contribute to progression of CKD because anemia reduces oxygen delivery within the kidney, further promoting hypoxia and progressive renal damage (Rossert and Froissart, 2006).

A variety of mechanisms regulate medullary oxygen homeostasis; these include medullary vasodilators (e.g., nitric oxide, prostaglandin E_2, adenosine, dopamine and urodilatin) and vasoconstrictors (e.g., endothelin, angiotensin II and vasopressin). Tubuloglomerular feedback controls glomerular filtration and, indirectly, medullary oxygen demand. Reduced resorption of sodium activates signals that constrict the

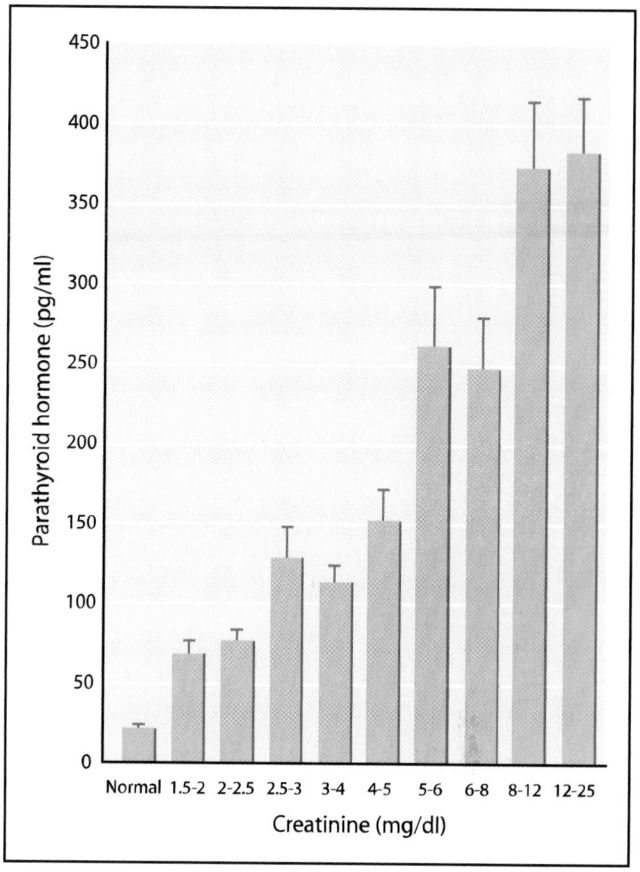

Figure 37-5. Relationship of serum parathyroid hormone concentrations to serum creatinine concentrations in 35 normal dogs and 333 dogs with uremia. (Adapted from Nagode LA, Chew DJ. Nephrocalcinosis caused by hyperparathyroidism in progression of renal failure: Treatment with calcitriol. Seminars in Veterinary Medicine and Surgery: Small Animal 1992; 7: 206.)

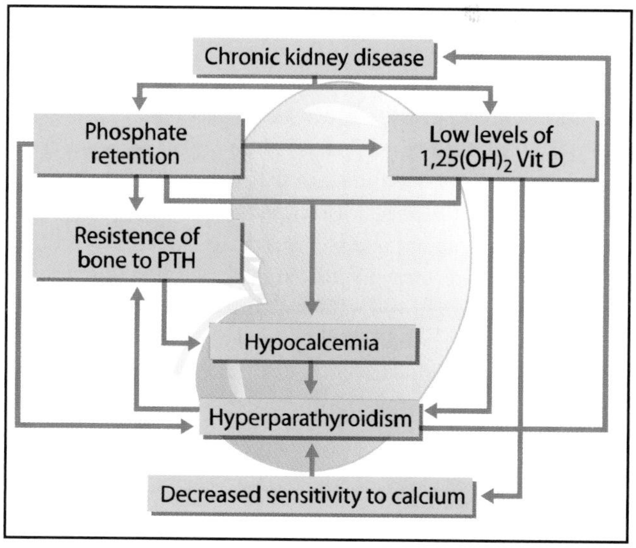

Figure 37-6. The pathogenesis of secondary renal hyperparathyroidism. Key: PTH = parathyroid hormone, $1,25(OH)_2$ Vit. D = 1,25-dihydroxycholecalciferol.

glomerulus, reducing glomerular filtration and subsequent delivery and resorption of sodium from the tubule. A related

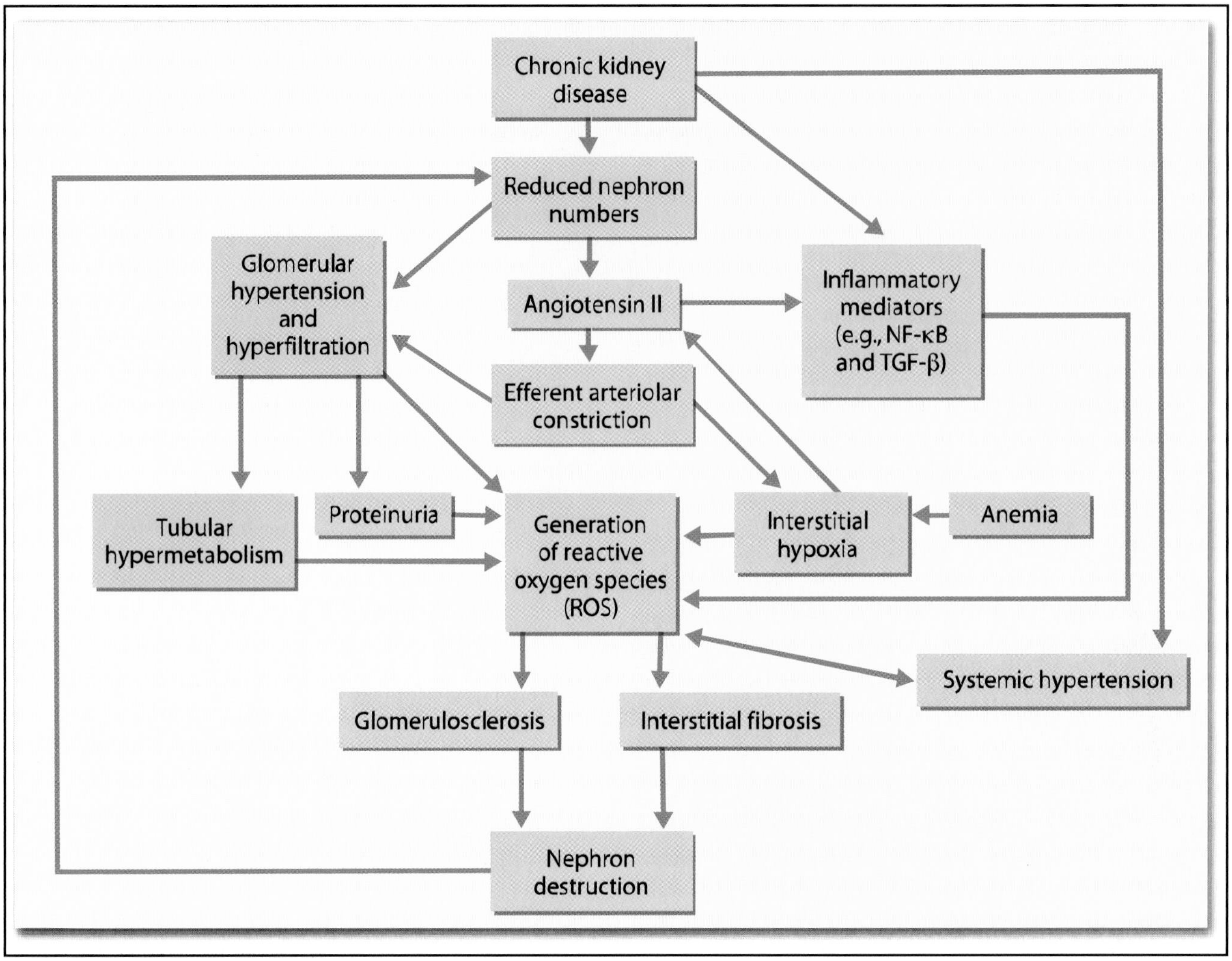

Figure 37-7. Increased generation of reactive oxygen species (ROS) occurs in chronic kidney disease and may play a role in disease progression. (Adapted from Brown SA. Oxidative stress and chronic kidney disease. Veterinary Clinics of North America: Small Animal Practice 2008; 38: 157-166).

reaction is shifting of the corticomedullary blood flow to the medulla when renal blood flow is reduced. Because the work of concentrating urine predisposes a patient to medullary hypoxic injury, reducing the need for concentration of urine may prevent medullary injury. Reducing transport activity protects medullary tubules from hypoxic injury. Dehydration, volume depletion and renal hypoperfusion stimulate urine concentration; avoiding these conditions reduces the work of urine concentration and stimulates intrarenal protective mechanisms, such as prostaglandin and dopamine production.

Renal Oxidative Stress

ROS are examples of free radicals that are produced at low levels by normal aerobic metabolism in the kidney (Brown, 2008). Examples of ROS produced in the kidney include hydrogen peroxide (H_2O_2), hydroxyl radical (OH), superoxide anion (O_2^-), lipid peroxy radicals, lipid and DNA hydroperoxides, hypochlorous acid and peroxynitrite. These ROS may damage proteins, lipids, DNA and carbohydrates, resulting in structural and functional abnormalities and progressive renal injury. Antioxidant defense mechanisms are designed to minimize damage by ROS including superoxide dismutase, catalase, nitric oxide synthase, glutathione peroxidase, vitamins E and C and carotenoids (Brown, 2008). Erythrocytes and albumin may also play important roles in minimizing oxidative injury to tissues (Agarwal, 2003; Brown, 2008; Rossert and Froissart, 2006). Erythrocytes represent a major antioxidant component of blood through enzymes such as superoxide dismutase, catalase and glutathione peroxidase. Also, erythrocyte glutathione reductase can regenerate reduced glutathione from its oxidized form (Rossert and Froissart, 2006).

Renal tissue damage occurs when production of ROS exceeds capacity of antioxidant defense mechanisms and is called renal oxidative stress (Brown, 2008). Oxidative damage has been incriminated as a cause of progressive renal injury in several types of kidney disease (Diamond et al, 1986; Agarwal, 2003; Vasavada and Agarwal, 2005; Brown, 2008) (**Figure 37-7**). In rats with remnant kidneys, increased oxygen consumption associated with increased dietary protein is accompanied by increased urinary clearance of oxidative products (Nath et al,

1994). The role of ROS in progressive renal injury has also been evaluated in studies using vitamin E and selenium-deficient diets (Nath et al, 1994). Vitamin E is a major scavenger of ROS in lipid bilayers and selenium is required for glutathione peroxidase activity. Glutathione peroxidase is the enzyme that degrades hydrogen peroxide. Deficiency of vitamin E or selenium favors hydrogen peroxide accumulation and its associated oxidative effects. Increased renal oxidative stress has been linked to proteinuria as a potential mediator of tubulointerstitial damage and to progression of CKD (Brown, 2008; Agarwal, 2003; Agarwal et al, 2004; Vasavada and Agarwal, 2005). Overloading tubular mechanisms for resorption of filtered albumin by proximal tubular cells can stimulate production of proinflammatory and profibrotic cytokines by activation of the redox-sensitive gene nuclear factor-κB thereby contributing to tubulointerstitial damage (Agarwal, 2003; Rossert and Froissart, 2006).

Hypokalemia

Several investigators have recognized an association between CKD and hypokalemia in cats (Lulich et al, 1992; Dow and Fettman, 1992; DiBartola, 1994). Hypokalemia occurred in 19% of cats with spontaneous CKD in one study and was moderate to severe in more than half (DiBartola et al, 1987). In cats with CKD and hypokalemia, renal function may improve after potassium supplementation and restoration of normokalemia, suggesting that hypokalemia may be associated with a reversible, functional decline in GFR. Renal function adversely affected normal cats when an acidified, low-potassium food was fed (Dow et al, 1990). In this study, potassium depletion and acidosis appeared to have additive effects on impairing renal function.

Limited evidence suggests; however, that hypokalemia is a cause of, and contributing factor to, CKD in cats rather than simply a consequence of the disease. In an uncontrolled study, renal lesions and dysfunction developed in three of nine cats fed a potassium-restricted, acidifying food for several months (DiBartola et al, 1993). However, it was not clear whether potassium depletion or hypokalemia preceded the onset of kidney disease. In another study, four of seven cats with induced CKD fed a food containing 0.3% dry matter (DM) potassium developed hypokalemia, but four cats with normal renal function fed the same food did not develop hypokalemia (Adams et al, 1993). Muscle potassium content is decreased in normokalemic cats with spontaneous CKD, indicating that a total body deficit of potassium may develop well before the onset of hypokalemia (Theisen et al, 1997). The latter findings support the concept that reduced renal function precedes the development of hypokalemia.

Metabolic Acidosis and Renal Ammoniagenesis

Metabolic acidosis appears to be a common complication of CKD in dogs and cats (DiBartola et al, 1987; Lulich et al, 1992; Jacob et al, 2002). In one report, six of 38 dogs with CKD had metabolic acidosis of sufficient severity to warrant treatment (Jacob et al, 2002). A cross-sectional study involving 59 cats with CKD showed that more than half of patients with severe CKD had acidemia and low plasma bicarbonate concentrations (Elliott et al, 2003, 2003a). These data also suggested that biochemical evidence of severe metabolic acidosis does not generally occur in cats until late in the course of CKD (Elliott et al, 2003). Patients with CKD tend to develop metabolic acidosis because of impaired ability of the failing kidneys to excrete the daily net acid load. The kidney eliminates hydrogen ions by three major mechanisms: reclaiming filtered bicarbonate, buffering secreted hydrogen ions with filtered phosphate and sulfate (titratable acidity) and renal ammoniagenesis. Of these three mechanisms, renal ammoniagenesis can be markedly upregulated to increase net acid secretion by the kidneys. As functional renal mass decreases in CKD, ammonia production per surviving nephron is increased several-fold, although total ammonia production is still reduced. Because ammonia is nonpolar, it diffuses into the tubular lumen and the surrounding interstitium.

Ammonia activates the alternate complement cascade, which may lead to renal injury by several mechanisms including: release of cytokines, prostanoids and ROS, cell lysis and stimulation of collagen synthesis. In studies involving rats, supplementation with bicarbonate reduced concentrations of complement components (i.e., C_3 and C_{5b-9}) (Nath et al, 1985). Bicarbonate administration also reduced cortical levels of ammonia, decreased proteinuria, reduced structural damage and improved tubular function. The interaction of ammonia and complement in the etiopathogenesis of tubulointerstitial disease has also been demonstrated in studies of hypokalemic nephropathy in rats (Nath et al, 1985). Studies in rats, however, failed to demonstrate a role for acidemia and increased renal ammoniagenesis as a cause of renal injury and progression of kidney disease (Throssell et al, 1995). In an investigation of cats with induced CKD, those fed an acidifying food for six months did not develop progressive glomerular dysfunction or renal tubulointerstitial injury vs. cats fed a non-acidifying food (James, 2001). Therefore the relative importance of renal ammoniagenesis in progressive renal injury in dogs and cats with CKD is unknown.

Lipid Disorders

Cholesterol, triglycerides and possibly some classes of lipoproteins are cytotoxic to endothelial cells and stimulate glomerular mesangial cell proliferation and production of excess mesangial matrix. Abnormalities of lipid metabolism in dogs with kidney disease generally include increased serum concentrations of total cholesterol, low-density lipoproteins and triglycerides (Brown et al, 1991). Cats with experimentally induced renal dysfunction demonstrate hypercholesterolemia compared with normal cats. Despite occurrence of lipid abnormalities in dogs and cats with CKD, there is little evidence to show they play a role in causing progression of disease.

Tubulointerstitial Changes

Endstage kidney disease is characterized by glomerulosclerosis, tubulointerstitial fibrosis and tubular atrophy (Wolf, 2006; Polzin et al, 2005). Tubulointerstitial changes are a consistent feature in CKD, irrespective of the cause or initial structure

Table 37-8. Potential etiopathogenic mechanisms in chronic kidney disease and therapeutic approaches for each.

Factors	Therapeutic approaches
Chronic renal hypoxia	Maintain hydration (increased water intake) Avoid excessive sodium intake ACE inhibitors Control anemia (erythropoietin)
Glomerular hypertension and hyperfiltration	Avoid excessive dietary protein and sodium Increased dietary omega-3 fatty acids ACE inhibitors
Hyperphosphatemia and secondary renal hyperparathyroidism	Limit dietary phosphorus Intestinal phosphate binders Calcitriol (after normophosphatemia is achieved)
Hypokalemia	Potassium supplementation
Metabolic acidosis	Avoid excessive dietary protein Alkalinizing foods (therapeutic renal foods) Alkalinizing agents (bicarbonate, potassium citrate)
Proteinuria	Avoid excessive dietary protein Increased dietary omega-3 fatty acids ACE inhibitors
Renal oxidative stress	Avoid excessive dietary protein, phosphorus and sodium Increased dietary antioxidants Omega-3 fatty acid supplementation
Systemic hypertension	Avoid excessive dietary sodium ACE inhibitors Calcium-channel antagonists (amlodipine)
Tubulointerstitial inflammation/fibrosis	Increased dietary omega-3 fatty acids Avoid excessive dietary phosphorus and protein

Key: ACE = angiotensin-converting enzyme.

involved (Eddy, 1994). The extent of tubulointerstitial injury correlates with the decline in renal function, whereas the severity of glomerular injury does not correlate well with progression of CKD models. It appears that GFR is influenced to a greater degree by interstitial fibrosis than by glomerulosclerosis (Nath, 1992).

Although chronic, progressive tubulointerstitial disease plays a critical role in progression of renal lesions, the basic mechanisms that generate the tubulointerstitial damage remain unclear. There appears to be a clinically silent acute phase that is characterized by inflammation and tubular cell injury. Possible mediators of tubular injury include antibodies, ROS, obstruction, complement and lysosomal enzymes (Eddy, 1994). Damaged tubular cells can regenerate or die. Factors responsible for recruitment of mononuclear cells to the interstitium are important because of evidence that monocytes and macrophages play a key role in interstitial fibrosis (Eddy et al, 1991). Recruitment is probably mediated by the release of fibrosis-promoting cytokines, such as TGF-β (Wolf, 2006). TGF-β directly stimulates transcription of many extracellular matrix genes in renal cells including mesangial, endothelial and tubular cells. TGF-β also appears to trigger increased matrix production by perivascular and interstitial fibroblasts. Dietary protein restriction inhibits secretion of TGF-β and glomerular scarring in rats with glomerulonephritis (Fukui et al, 1993). Furthermore, the renin-angiotensin-aldosterone system is linked to activation of the TGF-β pathway, which in turn promotes interstitial fibrosis (**Figure 37-7**) (Wolf, 2006).

Tubulointerstitial injury can impair renal function by a number of mechanisms: 1) vascular effects, 2) glomerular injury, 3) interstitial and tubuloepithelial processes, 4) nephron obstruction and 5) deposition of crystals (Nath, 1992). Postglomerular blood flow is decreased when the cortical interstitium expands due to fibrosis and mononuclear infiltration. Decreased blood supply also results from release of vasoactive cytokines, growth factors and ROS produced by the interstitial infiltrate and damaged tubules. Decreased postglomerular blood flow decreases tubular blood flow and changes glomerular size and pressure. Decreased tubular blood flow may impair tubular function and glomerular size and pressure changes may lead to glomerular injury (Nath, 1992).

As discussed above, abnormal glomerular function can incite tubulointerstitial injury (Diamond and Anderson, 1990). Loss of glomerular permselectivity and resultant proteinuria are accompanied by tubulointerstitial damage. Increased trafficking of protein in the proximal tubules may cause cellular damage. Filtered protein is endocytosed in the proximal tubules and subsequently degraded by lysosomal action. Excessive release of lysosomal enzymes may be one of the pathways for tubular damage. Tubular damage may also be induced by plasma proteins that have escaped into the urine. Incriminated plasma proteins include albumin, lipoproteins, complement components and transferrin. Studies in cats with spontaneously occurring CKD demonstrated that progression of CKD is most closely linked to severity of proteinuria, which may be explained by tubular damage during tubular resorption of leaked proteins (Syme et al, 2006; Jepson et al, 2007). Progression of spontaneously occurring CKD in dogs is also related to severity of proteinuria (Jacob et al, 2005).

Effects of Renal Aging

The kidney is one of the most vulnerable organs to age-associated changes. Renal changes associated with aging are manifested by significant structural and functional alterations. Functional changes include decreased GFR, decreased renal blood flow, decreased urine concentrating ability and decreased ability to maintain sodium, water, endocrine and acid-base homeostasis. Structural changes include alterations in renal weight, volume and histologic appearance. Fibroconnective tissue replaces functionally active parenchyma in aging kidneys. In a study of dogs with spontaneous glomerulonephritis, the incidence of interstitial nephritis increased with increasing age. Interstitial nephritis was present in 10% of dogs less than one year of age, in 60% of dogs between one and five years of age and in 85% of dogs more than five years of age (Muller-Peddinghaus and Trautwein, 1977). In another study, 59% of the dogs older than four years had evidence of interstitial nephritis (Shirota et al, 1979). Glomerular lesions were noted in 43 to 78% of these dogs. Based on these reports, interstitial nephritis and glomerulosclerosis apparently are common and occur with increased frequency in aging dogs.

It is possible that CKD occurs as a consequence of life-preserving adaptive mechanisms that accompany the aging process (Lawler et al, 2006). A study of postmortem data collected from 1979 to 2001 revealed that of 676 cats living in a research colony, cats that died from kidney disease most often had renal histologic changes (i.e., progressive tubular deletion and peritubular interstitial fibrosis); however, their mean lifespan was longer than cats that died from other causes (Lawler et al, 2006). In addition, among cats that died from causes other than kidney disease, those with renal histologic changes had a longer mean lifespan compared with cats that had no changes in their kidneys. It was hypothesized that these renal changes may represent an intrinsic mechanism that is protective until the point of failure. Regardless of the initiating cause, CKD often is characterized by irreversible loss of renal functional mass. After a critical amount of kidney damage occurs, CKD tends to be a progressive condition that often terminates with uremia-associated death.

Key Nutritional Factors

The goals of managing patients with CKD are to: 1) control clinical signs of uremia, 2) minimize disturbances associated with fluid, electrolyte and acid-base balance, 3) support adequate nutrition and 4) modify progression of CKD (Polzin et al, 2005). Nutritional management plays a role in all of these goals and is indicated to address the etiopathogenic mechanisms that occur in CKD (**Table 37-8**). In addition, the use of an appropriately formulated commercial veterinary therapeutic renal food is the only treatment that has been shown in randomized, controlled clinical studies to prolong survival time and improve quality of life in dogs and cats with CKD (Polzin et al, 2009; Roudebush et al, 2009; Jacob et al, 2002, 2004; Ross et al, 2006). Therefore, nutritional intervention should be considered a critical component of managing patients with CKD.

When designing a therapeutic regimen for dogs and cats with CKD, it is helpful to consider a food's key nutritional factors. Recommended ranges of these key nutritional factors were determined by considering nutrient levels in foods evaluated in dogs and cats with naturally occurring CKD and experimentally induced kidney disease (**Table 37-9**). Although numerous studies have been published about dogs and cats regarding the benefits of various combinations of these factors, little work has been done to isolate effects of individual nutrients (Adams et al, 1993; Barber et al, 1999; Bovee, 1991; Brown et al, 1991, 1998, 2000; Burkholder, 2000; Burkholder et al, 2004; Elliott et al, 2000; Finco et al, 1985, 1992, 1992a, 1998; Jacob et al, 2002; McCarthy et al, 2001; Polzin et al, 1982, 1983, 1983a, 1984, 1991, 1991a, 2000; Robertson et al, 1986; Ross et al, 1982, 2006; Valli et al, 1991). Commercially available veterinary therapeutic foods for dogs and cats with CKD are usually designed with these key nutritional factors in mind. Compared with typical maintenance pet foods, appropriately formulated veterinary therapeutic foods for dogs and cats with CKD generally contain less protein, phosphorus and sodium and have increased fat, omega-3 fatty acids and buffering capacity. Feline renal foods contain increased potassium to help prevent hypokalemia. In addition to key nutritional factors, it is important to consider available evidence supporting effectiveness of specific veterinary therapeutic renal foods and other treatments for CKD (**Table 37-10**). Finally, individual patient needs and responses and owner preferences must be considered to design an optimal therapeutic regimen.

Table 37-9. Key nutritional factors for dogs and cats with chronic kidney disease.*

Factors	Dietary recommendations
Water	Parenteral fluid therapy if dehydration, blood volume contraction or renal hypoperfusion is clinically significant Offer water free choice at all times Recommend moist foods
Protein	14 to 20% in foods for dogs 28 to 35% in foods for cats
Phosphorus	0.2 to 0.5% in foods for dogs 0.3 to 0.6% in foods for cats
Sodium	≤0.3% in foods for dogs ≤0.4% in foods for cats
Chloride	1.5 x sodium levels in foods for dogs 1.5 x sodium levels in foods for cats
Potassium	0.4 to 0.8% in foods for dogs 0.7 to 1.2% in foods for cats If patient becomes hyperkalemic, switch to a lower potassium food
Omega-3 fatty acids	0.4 to 2.5% in foods for dogs and cats Omega-6:omega-3 fatty acid ratio of 1:1 to 7:1
Antioxidants	
Vitamin E	≥400 IU vitamin E/kg of food for dogs ≥500 IU vitamin E/kg of food for cats
Vitamin C	≥100 mg vitamin C/kg of food for dogs 100 to 200 mg vitamin C/kg of food for cats

*All values expressed on a dry matter basis, unless otherwise indicated.

Water

Kidney disease causes a progressive decline in urine concentrating ability, and maximal urine osmolality approaches that of plasma (300 mOsm/kg) (i.e., isosthenuria). As CKD progresses; these changes may be observed in patients with stage 1 CKD. If total solute excretion remains normal, but the maximal achievable urine osmolality decreases, obligatory water loss occurs to eliminate the osmolar load. This obligatory water loss may lead to development of polyuria. Compensatory polydipsia occurs to maintain fluid balance. Dehydration, volume depletion, renal hypoperfusion and dietary salt (sodium) intake stimulate urine concentration. Concentrating urine solutes represents "osmotic work" for the kidneys and represents a burden for diseased kidneys. Reducing the amount of solutes to be concentrated by decreasing dietary protein and sodium intake or by providing more water for the excretion of the same amount of solutes independently reduces the amount of osmotic work. Patients with CKD should have unlimited access to fresh water for free-choice consumption. If readily consumed by the patient, moist foods are preferred because their consumption gen-

Table 37-10. Summary of evidence for treatments of chronic kidney disease.

	Dogs	Cats
Grade I	Some therapeutic renal foods (for prolonging survival time and increasing quality of life when serum creatinine [SCr] >2 mg/dl) Calcitriol (for prolonging survival) ACE inhibitor (enalapril) (for reducing proteinuria)*	Some therapeutic renal foods (for prolonging survival time and increasing quality of life when SCr >2 mg/dl) ACE inhibitor (benazepril) (for reducing proteinuria; increasing appetite in cats with urine protein-creatinine ratios ≥1)*
Grade II	ACE inhibitor (enalapril) (for delaying progression)*	–
Grade III	Recombinant human erythropoietin (for correcting anemia) Dietary phosphorus restriction (IRIS stages 3 and 4) Omega-3 fatty acid supplementation (IRIS stages 3 and 4)	Some therapeutic renal foods (for prolonging survival time) Dietary phosphorus restriction (IRIS stages 3 and 4) Recombinant human erythropoietin (for correcting anemia) Amlodipine (for controlling hypertension) Potassium supplementation (for correcting hypokalemia)
Grade IV	Therapeutic renal foods (for delaying progression when SCr is <2 mg/dl) Subcutaneous fluid therapy (for maintaining hydration) ACE inhibitors (non-proteinuric) (for delaying progression) Antihypertensive therapy (confirmed hypertension) Alkalinizing therapy (acidemia) Assisted feeding (anorexia and malnutrition) Phosphate binders (for hyperphosphatemia) Others (e.g., enteric dialysis)	Therapeutic renal foods (for delaying progression when SCr is <2 mg/dl) Subcutaneous fluid therapy (for maintaining hydration) ACE inhibitor (benazepril) (for cats without proteinuria) Alkalinizing therapy (acidemia) Assisted feeding (anorexia and malnutrition) Calcitriol therapy Phosphate binders (for hyperphosphatemia) Potassium supplementation (for cats with normokalemia)

Others (e.g., enteric dialysis)

Key: ACE = angiotensin-converting enzyme, IRIS = International Renal Interest Society, SCr = serum creatinine.
*Combined with feeding a veterinary therapeutic renal food. See Chapter 2 and Table 46-20 for more information about evidence grades I through IV.

erally results in increased total water intake compared with dry food consumption.

Protein

There is general consensus that avoiding excessive dietary protein intake is indicated to control clinical signs of uremia in dogs and cats with CKD; uremic signs most often occur in stage 4 disease but may be observed earlier (Polzin et al, 2005; Elliott et al, 2006). Many of the extrarenal clinical and metabolic disturbances associated with uremia are direct results of the accumulated waste products derived from protein catabolism. Early studies in laboratory animals showed rapid improvement when dietary protein was reduced (Klahr et al, 1983; Brenner, 1983). However, urea by itself does not account for all, if any, of the clinical signs of uremia. Serum urea nitrogen generally is considered to simply be a marker for other more important uremic toxins. Excessive dietary protein is catabolized to urea and other nitrogenous compounds that normally are excreted by the kidneys. And, as mentioned above, endogenous proteins will be degraded if amino acid intake is insufficient to maintain nitrogen balance. The goal of managing patients with CKD is to achieve nitrogen balance and limit accumulation of nitrogenous waste products by proportionally decreasing protein intake as renal function declines.

The role of decreased dietary protein intake is less clear in patients with CKD that do not have clinical signs of uremia (Polzin et al, 2005). Limiting protein intake has been advocated to slow progression of CKD on the basis of studies in rats, which revealed that excessive dietary protein consumption was associated with glomerular capillary hypertension and hyperfiltration (Brenner et al, 1982). Decreased dietary protein intake prevents these hemodynamic changes and preserves normal glomerular structure in rats (Brenner et al, 1982). The role of decreased dietary protein in delaying progression of CKD in dogs and cats is less clear and has been the subject of numerous studies and a topic of considerable debate (Polzin et al, 2000; Finco et al, 1998a) (**Box 37-1**).

Despite the lack of clarity about the effects of dietary protein on progression of CKD in dogs and cats, potential benefits should be considered. Decreased dietary protein intake inhibits secretion of TGF-β, a cytokine that may be involved in progression of kidney disease (Fukui et al, 1993). (See Etiopathogenesis of Chronic Kidney Disease, Tubulointerstitial Changes.) Decreased protein intake potentially reduces tubular hyperfunction by decreasing the renal acid load and decreasing renal ammoniagenesis. In general, protein metabolism is the major source of hydrogen ions. Consequently, avoiding excess dietary protein and decreasing endogenous protein catabolism for energy contribute markedly to the maintenance of acid-base balance (Relman et al, 1961). Primary dietary protein contributions to the renal acid load are from the sulfur-containing amino acids (methionine and cysteine). Animal proteins tend to be higher in sulfur-containing amino acids than plant protein sources. This is true whether the source of the animal pro-

Box 37-1. Role of Dietary Protein in Progression of Chronic Kidney Disease.

There has been considerable debate about the effects of dietary protein on the progression of chronic kidney disease (CKD) in dogs and cats. Studies that have attempted to evaluate the role of protein intake alone (vs. other nutrients such as phosphorus) have been conducted in dogs and cats with experimentally induced CKD (i.e., remnant kidney model or renal ablation); however, none have been performed in patients with naturally occurring disease. Feeding a veterinary therapeutic renal food, with decreased protein, significantly prolongs survival time, decreases uremic episodes and delays disease progression in dogs and cats with naturally occurring CKD. However, compared with typical maintenance pet foods, veterinary therapeutic renal foods have other features in addition to less protein (i.e., decreased phosphorus, increased fat, increased omega-3 fatty acids), which likely contribute to their effectiveness. When evaluating the evidence for or against limiting dietary protein intake, factors to consider include mechanism(s) by which protein may exert its effect(s), experimental design of previously conducted studies and appropriateness of the remnant kidney model as a predictor of what occurs in dogs and cats with naturally occurring CKD. Practically speaking, it's also important to consider what foods are readily available for patients with CKD.

When evaluating conclusions from reported studies, it is necessary to critically evaluate the research methods and results, which could affect interpretation of data. For example, in a study widely cited to support the position that feeding less protein is ineffective in slowing progression of kidney disease, some dogs in the high-protein groups, but not the low-protein groups, were supplemented with potassium citrate to correct metabolic acidosis observed with high dietary protein intake. Metabolic acidosis may contribute to renal injury by increasing renal ammoniagenesis and may increase renal oxygen consumption. Thus, conclusions regarding the effect of dietary protein on progression based on this study may be invalid because the study neutralized one mechanism by which protein may exert its beneficial effect. In the same study, some dogs developed "diet-related uremia" when they were abruptly switched to the high-protein food following renal ablation. Those dogs were removed from the study, which could have resulted in selecting for study dogs that were "resistant" to the effects of protein.

Another question that is not typically addressed in the debate on the effect of dietary protein intake on progressive renal injury is whether studies had sufficient statistical power. Before declaring that there is no treatment effect, it is useful to consider whether the group size studied was sufficient to detect an effect if one truly existed. At the conclusion of one frequently cited study, there were four dogs evaluated in the high-protein group, three dogs in the moderate-protein group and four dogs in the low-protein group. However, this study did not address the question of whether group sizes were adequate to support the conclusions made. Another study that did not show an effect of dietary protein levels on glomerular lesions in uninephrectomized dogs did mention low power in their study (i.e., power calculations of 15 and 20%). The authors indicated that factors responsible for the low power included small sample size and large inter-dog differences.

Finally, in evaluating the role of protein in CKD most veterinary investigators have used the remnant kidney model. Although this model eliminates some of the variability associated with clinical trials, it does not exactly mimic naturally occurring kidney disease and all conclusions drawn from this model may not be applicable to clinical patients. For example, in a study evaluating effects of different dietary protein levels in dogs with 75% nephrectomy, mean plasma creatinine concentrations during the four-year study ranged from 0.8 to 0.9 mg/dl in all diet groups; these values are much lower than expected in clinical patients with progressive CKD. Although it may be appropriate to conclude that feeding high levels of protein to dogs with 75% reduction in renal mass was not associated with a progressive decline in renal function, it would not be valid to state that similar dietary protein levels have the same effect in dogs with naturally occurring CKD. Several studies evaluating the role of dietary protein in limiting progression of CKD have been performed in dogs and cats that maintained stable renal function throughout the entire study period; the stable nature of renal dysfunction in such studies does not permit assessment of the role of dietary protein in limiting progression of CKD.

The Bibliography for **Box 37-1** can be found at www.markmorris.org.

tein is from food or catabolism of a patient's body tissue. Catabolism of a patient's protein stores can occur if insufficient energy (carbohydrates and fats) and/or protein are consumed. In the case of inadequate energy intake, the body's amino acids stores (tissue protein) are used for gluconeogenesis to meet glucose needs. Avoiding dietary protein excess, without imposing dietary protein deficiency can help limit the acid load imposed on patients with CKD (Burkholder, 2000).

Another potential benefit of limiting dietary protein is its effects on proteinuria. Results of studies in rats with experimentally induced nephrotic syndrome suggest that the permselective properties of the filtration barrier are altered as a consequence of increasing dietary protein intake, permitting albumin to cross the capillary wall more readily (Kaysen et al, 1984; Hutchison et al, 1987, 1990). In healthy dogs and in dogs with kidney disease, increasing dietary protein intake increases renal blood flow and GFR, which may increase filtration of plasma proteins through the glomerular membrane, resulting in proteinuria (Polzin et al, 1983a, 1984; Devaux et al, 1996; Bovee, 1991; Brown et al, 1992; Bovee et al, 1981). Proteinuria may result in direct mesangial cell toxicity, glomerular fibrosis and eventual glomerulosclerosis (**Figure 37-3**). Excessive albuminuria and abnormally filtered transferrin may lead to increased oxidative stress, which appears to be an important mechanism of progressive renal injury (**Figure 37-7**). (See Renal Oxidative Stress.) The end result of proteinuric-induced glomerulosclerosis and tubular damage is further loss of nephrons. This reduction of functional renal mass and subsequent increase in single-nephron GFR further increase proteinuria and progression of renal damage. The impact of varying dietary protein intake on glomerular hemodynamics and structure in dogs and cats with CKD is less certain; however, studies in dogs have shown that feeding a vet-

Box 37-2. Nutritional Management of Patients with Proteinuria.

Previously, it was recommended to estimate urinary protein loss and replace a similar amount by increasing dietary protein intake (e.g., supplementing with hard-boiled eggs) in patients with glomerular disease. This recommendation seemed prudent based on pathophysiologic rationale, but was not validated. Investigations in people and laboratory animals with protein-losing glomerulonephropathy indicate that reductions in dietary protein limit proteinuria and preserve serum albumin concentrations without impairing protein nutriture. The advisability of replacing persistent, severe renal protein loss has therefore been questioned.

Two studies have evaluated the effects of limiting dietary protein intake in dogs with X-linked hereditary nephritis, a glomerular disease that causes proteinuria. Male dogs have rapid progression of disease during the first year of life whereas females typically have stable disease characterized by proteinuria that may progress to advanced stages of CKD after five years of age.

In one study, effects of feeding a veterinary therapeutic renal food[a] were evaluated in male and female dogs with X-linked hereditary nephritis. One group of dogs was fed the therapeutic food with reduced protein (13.5% dry matter [DM]), phosphorus and sodium and the other group was fed a maintenance food (23% DM protein). Onset and progression of kidney disease were delayed and severity of glomerular basement membrane splitting was reduced in affected male dogs eating the commercial veterinary therapeutic renal food. In addition, these dogs lived 53% longer (362 ± 17 days vs. 239 ± 14 days) than dogs fed the regular maintenance food.

Effects of decreased dietary protein intake on proteinuria have also been studied in female dogs with heterozygous X-linked hereditary nephropathy. Dogs were blocked by urine protein-creatinine (UPC) ratios and randomly assigned to receive either a high-protein food (HP) (34.6% DM) or a veterinary therapeutic renal food[b] with less protein (LP) (14.1% DM). Phosphorus, sodium, chloride and potassium levels were essentially the same in both foods; the first three of these nutrients were decreased, relative to typical amounts in regular maintenance foods. The study was conducted using a three-period double-crossover design in which each dog served as its own control. Treatment periods 1 and 2 lasted 28 days each and treatment period 3 lasted 42 days. The groups were fed in HP-LP-HP or LP-HP-LP sequence. Proteinuria, as indicated by UPC ratios, was significantly decreased whenever the LP food was fed vs. when the HP food was fed (UPC 1.8 ± 1.1 vs. 4.7 ± 2.2; [p <0.0001]). However, an unexpected result was that the dogs lost body weight when fed the LP food. Unfortunately, the energy content of the LP food was approximately 13 to 14% lower than that of the HP food due to energy digestibility differences between the two foods that were not determined until study completion. Whether or not the body weight loss was due to excessively low amounts of dietary protein or inadequate energy intake could not be determined.

On the basis of current evidence, dogs with protein-losing glomerulonephropathy should be fed reduced-protein foods designed for patients with kidney disease. Patients should be monitored periodically (e.g., every two to four weeks initially) to determine the optimal quantity of dietary protein. The food with reduced levels of dietary protein should continue to be fed if the magnitude of proteinuria declines (as measured by UPC ratios) without substantial evidence of protein malnutrition (i.e., stable or increasing serum albumin and total protein concentrations, stable body weight and body condition score). If evidence of protein malnutrition develops, dietary protein intake should be gradually increased in stepwise fashion while closely monitoring the patient.

Although proteinuria occurs in cats with CKD, glomerular disease is infrequently diagnosed. Feeding a veterinary therapeutic renal food may benefit cats with glomerular disease or proteinuria; however, this has not been studied.

ENDNOTES

a. Prescription Diet k/d Canine. Hill's Pet Nutrition, Inc., Topeka, KS, USA.

b. Purina Veterinary Diets NF KidNey Function Canine Formula. Néstle Purina PetCare Co., St. Louis, MO. USA.

The Bibliography for **Box 37-2** can be found at www.markmorris.org.

erinary therapeutic renal food with decreased protein, before the onset of azotemia, has beneficial effects in dogs with proteinuria (Valli et al, 1991; Burkholder et al, 2004) (**Box 37-2**).

Effects of decreased dietary protein intake have been studied in dogs with induced CKD (Polzin et al, 1983; Finco et al, 1992a). In a 40-week study, dogs were fed a commercial veterinary therapeutic food[d] containing 8.2% DM protein, a commercial food[e] with 17.2% DM protein or a control food with 44.4% DM protein (Polzin et al, 1983). Feeding the lower protein foods was associated with reduced mortality, serum urea nitrogen concentrations and clinical signs of uremia. Throughout the study, all dogs fed the highest protein food had reduced physical activity and poorer hair quality compared with those parameters in dogs fed the lower protein foods. There were other nutrient differences between foods, which may have contributed to the beneficial effects observed. In another study conducted for two years, reduced dietary protein (16% DM) was not associated with a significant effect on mortality compared with feeding a food containing 32% DM protein (Finco et al, 1992a). Some differences in treatment in addition to nutritional management could have affected study outcome, however (**Box 37-1**).

Two studies evaluated effects of dietary protein on progression of induced CKD for one year in cats (Adams et al, 1993; Finco et al, 1998). In one study, renal function did not progressively decrease, regardless of dietary protein amount and caloric intake (Adams et al, 1993). However, remnant kidneys of cats with induced CKD that were fed a food containing 52% DM protein had significantly more severe glomerular and tubulointerstitial damage than cats with CKD that were fed a food containing 28% DM protein (Adams et al, 1993). Phosphorus amounts were similar between study groups (0.54% DM in the high-protein group and 0.61% DM in the low-protein group); however, cats in the high-protein group consumed significantly more calories. Therefore, changes in renal morphology could have resulted from differences in protein and/or caloric intake. In the other study, no difference in renal function or glomerular lesions were found in cats consuming high-protein foods (52% DM) compared with lower protein foods (28% DM) (Finco et al, 1998). Phosphorus amounts were similar for all study groups (0.87 to 0.96% DM). There were mild and significant increases in cellular infiltrate and tubular lesions in cats that consumed more calories, but no differences were detected based on amount of dietary protein. The authors concluded that protein intake was not a risk factor for progression of renal lesions and that the practice of severe protein restriction was questionable. However, because renal function remained stable throughout both studies, it was not possible to assess the role of limiting dietary protein in decreasing progression of CKD.

Four clinical studies of cats or dogs with naturally occurring CKD compared effects of feeding a commercial veterinary therapeutic renal food with either a control or regular maintenance food that contained more protein (Harte et al, 1994; Elliott et al, 2000; Jacob et al, 2002; Ross et al, 2006). In a six-month study, mean serum creatinine and urea nitrogen concentrations progressively increased in 10 cats receiving more dietary protein (39.4% DM) and declined or remained stable in 25 cats that were fed a lower protein food[f] (25.2% DM) (Harte et al, 1994). In a non-randomized, prospective study, cats receiving a lower protein food[g] (22 to 24% protein) had significantly prolonged median survival time compared with cats that continued eating different maintenance cat foods with higher protein (48% DM) (Elliott et al, 2000). In a two-year study, cats eating a commercial veterinary therapeutic renal food[h] with 28 to 29% DM protein had no uremic episodes or renal-related deaths whereas 26% of cats in the control group consuming a food with higher protein (46 to 48% DM protein) had a uremic crisis and 22% died as a result of CKD (Ross et al, 2006). Finally, dogs receiving a commercial veterinary therapeutic renal food[e] with 14% DM protein had delayed time to onset of uremic crisis, slower decline in renal function and improved survival compared to parameters in dogs receiving a control food that contained 25% DM protein (Jacob et al, 2002). Based on these findings, it is clear that foods with less protein in these studies were associated with significantly improved quality and quantity of life in dogs and cats with naturally occurring CKD. However, because the protein amount was not the only nutrient difference between the veterinary therapeutic renal foods and comparison foods, it is not possible to conclude that limiting dietary protein alone was the sole reason for beneficial effects. **Box 37-3** provides detailed information about long-term studies that evaluated effects of veterinary therapeutic renal foods on survival time of dogs and cats with CKD.

In summary, limiting dietary protein intake is indicated to control clinical signs of uremia in dogs and cats with CKD. Although currently available evidence fails to support a recommendation for or against limiting dietary protein intake alone in non-uremic patients with CKD, there are potential benefits, assuming that patients maintain adequate caloric intake and body condition. Patients may be more likely to accept a change to a new food if it is offered before clinical signs of uremia occur and it may delay onset of uremic signs as CKD progresses (Polzin et al, 2005). On a practical note, it is difficult to achieve the degree of phosphorus restriction desired in veterinary therapeutic renal foods using typical ingredients without limiting the amount of dietary protein (Burkholder, 2000).

In regards to determining how much protein to recommend for dogs and cats with CKD, all patients should be monitored for signs of protein insufficiency and nutritional management adjusted to maintain ideal body condition (**Box 37-4**). For cats with CKD, the minimum dietary protein requirement identified in one study was 20% of calories (Kirk and Hickman, 2001); this translates to approximately 24% DM protein. Similar studies have not been reported for dogs. The minimum recommended allowances for DM dietary protein in foods for healthy adult dogs and cats are 10 and 20%, respectively (NRC, 2006). The minimum DM levels recommended by the Association of American Feed Control Officials are 18% for dog foods and 26% for cat foods (AAFCO, 2007). A report of the mean DM protein content of several popular U.S. grocery brand dog foods was 41.7% for moist foods and 25% for dry foods. For grocery brand cat foods it was 51.5% for moist foods and 35.1% for dry foods (Allen et al, 2000). The recommended range for DM protein levels in foods intended for most patients with CKD is 14 to 20% for dogs and 28 to 35% for cats. Foods with less protein may be needed to control signs of uremia in patients with more advanced CKD; in these patients, it's important to monitor for signs of protein deficiency. In addition to the amount of protein, patients with CKD should receive protein of high biologic value. The concept of ideal protein is useful when considering biologic value (Baker and Czarnecki-Maulden, 1991). Lysine is the limiting amino acid in practical foods for dogs and cats (Baker and Czarnecki-Maulden, 1991). However, experience with typical ingredients used in commercial veterinary therapeutic foods suggests that tryptophan is more frequently limiting. Therefore, based on the concept of ideal protein, foods that meet the requirement for lysine and tryptophan can be assumed to meet the requirement for all indispensable amino acids.

Phosphorus

Decreased dietary phosphorus intake is indicated in dogs and cats with CKD to limit phosphorus retention, hyperphosphatemia, secondary renal hyperparathyroidism (**Figures 37-8** and **37-9**) and progression of kidney disease (Polzin et al, 2005; Rutherford et al, 1977; Barber at al, 1999). The mechanism for the protective effect of limiting phosphorus intake is unknown. Possible factors include reduced nephrocalcinosis, suppression of hyperparathyroidism, reduced cellular energy metabolism and altered renal hemodynamics. It is possible that these mechanisms may synergistically contribute to the beneficial effects of lowering phosphorus intake.

Several studies evaluated effects of limiting dietary phosphorus intake in cats and dogs with induced kidney disease. In cats, high dietary phosphorus intake (1.56% DM phosphorus) for 65 to 343 days was associated with renal mineralization, fibrosis

Box 37-3. Summary of Studies Evaluating Effects of Veterinary Therapeutic Renal Foods on Survival in Dogs and Cats with Naturally Occurring Chronic Kidney Disease.

Numerous studies have evaluated effects of nutritional management of chronic kidney disease (CKD) in dogs and cats. Most were conducted using the remnant kidney model. Although we have learned valuable information from these studies, their findings may not be directly transferable to patients with naturally occurring disease. Three clinical studies evaluated the effects of commercial veterinary therapeutic renal foods on survival and quality of life in cats and dogs with CKD. Those studies are summarized below.

STUDY 1

Fifty cats with naturally occurring stable CKD were evaluated in a prospective study of the effects of feeding a dry or moist veterinary therapeutic renal food[a] compared with a maintenance food. The renal food contained 22 to 24% dry matter (DM) protein and 0.27 to 0.42% DM phosphorus whereas the maintenance food contained 48% DM protein and 1.9% DM phosphorus. Twenty-nine cats accepted the renal food and were assigned to the renal food group, whereas compliance (due to limited intake by the cats or owner resistance to diet change) was not achieved in the remaining 21 cats, which were assigned to the maintenance food group. Cats in the maintenance food group were fed commercial maintenance cat foods with varying amounts of fresh meat or fish. In all cases, the dietary regimens were considered appropriate for maintenance. At diagnosis, both groups of cats were matched in terms of age, body weight, plasma creatinine, phosphate, potassium and parathyroid hormone (PTH) concentrations, packed cell volume and urine specific gravity. Cats in the renal food group received their assigned food for an average of 86.6% of their survival time. Feeding the renal food was associated with a reduction in plasma phosphorus and urea nitrogen concentrations and prevented the increase in plasma PTH concentrations that occurred in the maintenance food group. Median survival time was significantly longer in the renal food group (633 days) compared with the maintenance food group (264 days). *Results of this study provide Grade III evidence for using this commercial veterinary therapeutic renal food to control secondary renal hyperparathyroidism and prolong survival time in cats with naturally occurring CKD.*

STUDY 2

Thirty-eight dogs with stable CKD (serum creatinine values between 2 and 8 mg/dl) were evaluated in a double-blinded, randomized, controlled prospective study to determine effects of feeding a commercial dry veterinary therapeutic renal food[b] compared with a control food formulated to represent the nutrient content of the 10 most popular selling grocery brand maintenance foods. The renal food contained 14% DM protein, 0.28% DM phosphorus and 1.6% DM omega-3 fatty acids, whereas the control food contained 25% DM protein, 1% DM phosphorus and 0.22% DM omega-3 fatty acids. At baseline, clinical and laboratory findings were similar between groups. At the end of the two-year study there were 17 dogs in the control group and 21 dogs in the renal food group. By the end of the study, 33% of dogs in the renal food group had developed uremic crises vs. 65% of dogs in the control group. Time to onset of uremic crises was significantly longer in the renal food group (615 days) compared with the control group (252 days). Feeding the renal food was associated with decreased progression of kidney disease and significantly prolonged median survival time (594 days) vs. the control group (188 days). As described elsewhere, feeding the renal food was associated with significantly improved health-related quality of life. *Results of this study provide Grade I evidence for using this commercial veterinary therapeutic renal food to decrease uremic episodes, delay onset of uremia and progression of kidney disease, increase survival time and improve quality of life in dogs with CKD.*

STUDY 3

Forty-five cats with stable CKD (serum creatinine values of 2.1 to 4.5 mg/dl) were evaluated in a double-blinded, randomized, controlled prospective study to determine effects of feeding a commercial dry and/or moist veterinary therapeutic renal food[c] compared with a control food that was similar to a typical adult maintenance cat food. The renal food contained 28 to 29% DM protein, 0.5% DM phosphorus, and 0.2 to 0.6% DM omega-3 fatty acids, whereas the control food contained 46 to 48% DM protein, 0.9 to 1% DM phosphorus and 0.2% DM omega-3 fatty acids. Cats were fed a combination diet (half renal food, half control food) for six weeks before random assignment to treatment groups; this was done to gradually transition cats to a new food. At the end of the two-year study there were 23 cats in the control group and 22 cats in the renal food group. Dietary compliance (defined as receiving >85% of daily caloric requirement from the assigned food) was excellent throughout the study; 91% of cats continued eating their assigned food. Four cats (two in each group) stopped eating due to nonrenal diseases. A significantly greater percentage of cats in the control group had uremic episodes (26%) compared with the renal food group (0%). There was significant reduction in deaths due to CKD in the renal food group; none of the cats receiving the renal food died during the study whereas 22% of cats in the control group died. *Results of this study provide Grade I evidence for using this commercial veterinary therapeutic renal food to decrease occurrence of uremic episodes and mortality in cats with CKD.*

ENDNOTES

a. Waltham Veterinary Diet, Whiskas Low Phosphorus Low Protein. Masterfoods, Bruck, Austria.
b. Prescription Diet k/d Canine. Hill's Pet Nutrition, Inc., Topeka, KS, USA.
c. Prescription Diet k/d Feline. Hill's Pet Nutrition, Inc., Topeka, KS, USA.

The Bibliography for **Box 37-3** can be found at www.markmorris.org.

Box 37-4. Dietary Protein Needs in Dogs and Cats with Chronic Kidney Disease and Maintenance of Lean Body Mass.

Minimum protein requirements for patients with chronic kidney disease (CKD) are assumed to be similar to those for healthy dogs and cats; however, this has not been well evaluated. Ten cats with CKD and nine healthy cats were fed foods (free choice) with different amounts of protein (16, 20 or 24% of calories as metabolizable energy [ME]) for four months. Body weight, lean body mass, nitrogen balance and laboratory parameters (hematocrit and serum concentrations of urea nitrogen, albumin and total protein) were measured to assess adequacy of dietary protein intake. Based on study findings, the authors concluded that the protein requirement for cats with CKD and healthy controls appeared to be approximately 20% ME, which is similar to results from previous studies that evaluated protein requirement in healthy cats.

The amount of protein contained in most commercially available veterinary therapeutic renal foods is more than adequate to meet minimum protein requirements of dogs and cats with CKD; however, there is a common perception that these foods are protein deficient. The terminology used to describe therapeutic foods formulated for management of kidney disease may encourage this perception. It may be more appropriate to refer to these foods as "formulated to avoid excessive protein" or "modified protein foods" instead of being "protein restricted", which may incorrectly be interpreted as protein-deficient by pet owners and health care team members.

Loss of lean body mass occurs in patients with kidney disease and may contribute to the perception that veterinary therapeutic renal foods do not contain adequate amounts of protein. Potential mechanisms for decreased lean body mass in dogs and cats with CKD include inadequate dietary protein or caloric intake, altered response to decreased protein intake, increased protein loss (e.g., proteinuria), metabolic acidosis and activation of cytokines by chronic inflammation. Failure to consume an adequate amount of calories may result in catabolism of muscle protein as a source of energy; this is one reason why veterinary therapeutic renal foods have relatively higher amounts of dietary fat. It is important to ensure adequate dietary protein intake; however, protein that is consumed in excess of the patient's needs is metabolized and used for energy, which could worsen clinical signs of uremia. Metabolic acidosis, a common complication of uremia, stimulates the degradation of branched-chain amino acids and proteins and blocks the ability of the patient to respond appropriately to lower protein intake. The specific mechanisms involve increased activity of branched-chain ketoacid dehydrogenase and the ubiquitin-proteasome proteolytic pathway. Besides acidosis, cytokines activate the ubiquitin-proteasome proteolytic pathway and cytokine release occurs with chronic inflammation. These potential mechanisms for loss of muscle mass emphasize the importance of controlling metabolic acidosis, infection and other stressors in patients with CKD.

Although some patients with CKD lose lean body mass, evidence supports that these patients can maintain body condition and weight while eating a veterinary therapeutic renal food. In a study of cats with induced CKD, those that consumed adequate calories of a low-protein food (28% dry matter protein; 20% protein as calories) maintained stable or increasing body weights, hematocrit values and serum albumin concentrations and had no clinical signs of protein-calorie malnutrition. In the absence of metabolic acidosis, dietary protein requirements did not appear to be different between cats with CKD and control cats with normal renal function. In another study of cats with naturally occurring CKD, mean body weight of the control group that received the higher protein food continued to decline, with most of the cats experiencing weight loss, compared with a mean weight gain in the group receiving a commercial veterinary therapeutic renal food with less protein. Although clinical condition (halitosis, gingivitis, appetite and body condition) deteriorated in both groups of cats, it was less apparent in the lower protein group based on observations by pet owners and veterinary clinical evaluations. The methods for assessing these observations were not indicated. In addition, packed cell volume, serum albumin and total protein increased in the lower protein group and decreased in the higher protein group. In another clinical study of cats with CKD that received either a veterinary therapeutic renal food or a typical maintenance food, no significant differences in body weights or hematocrit values were noted between groups at the midpoint of the study. In a randomized, double-blinded clinical study of cats with CKD managed by feeding either a veterinary therapeutic renal food or a control food (with higher protein), there were no significant differences in body weights or body condition scores at the midpoint and end of the two-year study.

In a double-blinded clinical study of dogs with naturally occurring CKD that received either a veterinary therapeutic renal food or a control food (with higher protein), health-related quality of life was determined using a content-validated questionnaire to obtain owner assessments. Nutritional status was assessed by periodic physical examinations and measurement of laboratory parameters. The renal food was superior to the control food for maintaining health-related quality of life and nutritional status; the renal food group remained stable based on body weights, body condition scores, hematocrit values and serum albumin concentrations.

It is highly likely that beneficial effects of feeding a veterinary therapeutic renal food are due to a combination of key nutritional factors (in addition to limited dietary protein). However, results of studies described above demonstrate that nutritional status can be maintained and quality of life improved in dogs and cats with CKD when fed a commercial veterinary therapeutic renal food containing less protein than typical adult maintenance pet foods. Regardless, all patients with CKD should be monitored for signs of protein-calorie malnutrition so that treatment can be adjusted to maintain body condition and improved quality of life.

The Bibliography for **Box 37-4** can be found at www.markmorris.org.

and mononuclear cell infiltration whereas lower phosphorus intake (0.42% DM phosphorus) was not (Ross et al, 1982) (**Figure 37-10**). Progressive changes in GFR were not detected; however, in either the high- or low-phosphorus group. Effects of dietary phosphorus restriction were studied in dogs that were fed either a low-phosphorus (0.44% DM) food or a high-phosphorus (1.44% DM) food for 24 months (Brown et al, 1991). Both foods provided reduced amounts of protein (17% DM).

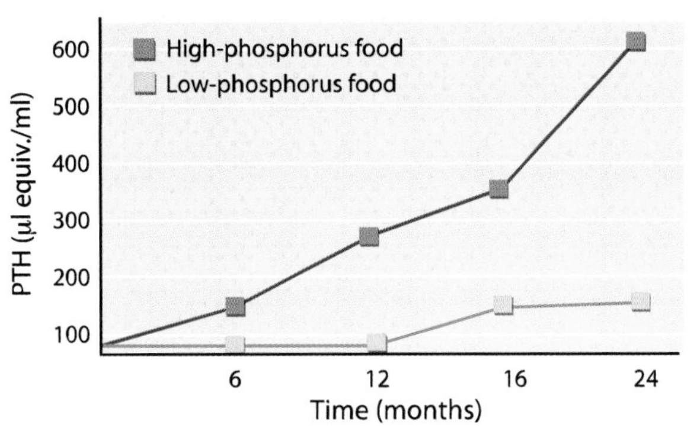

Figure 37-8. The effect of dietary phosphorus on serum parathyroid hormone (PTH) concentrations in dogs with experimentally induced kidney disease. Note that consumption of higher levels of phosphorus resulted in excessive PTH secretion. High phosphorus means dogs ingested 60 to 80 mg phosphorus/kg body weight/day, Low phosphorus means dogs ingested 15 to 40 mg phosphorus/kg body weight/day. (Adapted from Rutherford WE, Bordier P, Marie P, et al. Phosphate control and 25-hydroxycholecalciferol administration in preventing experimental renal osteodystrophy in the dog. Journal of Clinical Investigation 1977; 60: 332-341.)

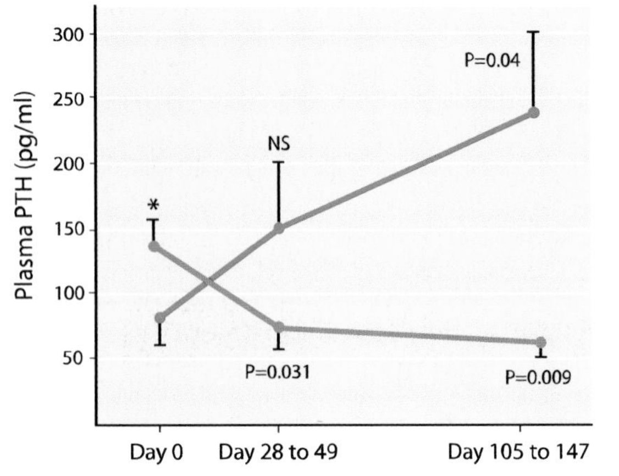

Figure 37-9. Plasma parathyroid hormone (PTH) concentrations in cats with chronic kidney disease that were fed either a veterinary therapeutic renal food with decreased phosphorus (blue line) (n=14) or a maintenance food with higher phosphorus (red line) (n=8). Results expressed as mean ± SEM. NS = not significant.
P values represent statistical significance of each value compared with pre-treatment value (Day 0).
*No significant difference between groups at baseline (Day 0).
(Adapted from Barber PJ, Rawlings JM, Markwell PJ, et al. Effect of dietary phosphate restriction on renal secondary hyperparathyroidism in the cat. Journal of Small Animal Practice 1999; 40: 62-70.)

Survival rate was significantly higher in the low-phosphorus group (75%) compared with the high-phosphorus group (33%) (**Figure 37-11**). Kidney function also deteriorated at a more rapid rate in the high-phosphorus group. Decrements of renal function were more closely related to nephrocalcinosis and tubulointerstitial lesions than to glomerular abnormalities (Brown et al, 1991). Specifically, in this study, progression and death were associated with interstitial fibrosis, tubular atrophy and dilatation and mineralization of cortical basement membranes, tubular epithelia and vascular and tubular lumina. The association of progression with tubulointerstitial lesions and nephrocalcinosis, however, does not necessarily establish a causal role for nephrocalcinosis. A similar study was conducted by investigators in the same laboratory to evaluate effects of dietary phosphorus restriction (0.48 vs. 1.46% DM) when a higher protein food (32% DM) was fed (Finco et al, 1992). In contrast to the previous study, improved survival was not observed in the group fed low-phosphorus food. An additional study compared the effects of feeding four foods of varying phosphorus and protein content (low phosphorus/low protein; high phosphorus/low protein; low phosphorus/high protein; high phosphorus/high protein) to four groups of dogs with CKD (remnant kidney model). In this study, survival was significantly increased by feeding either of the low-phosphorus foods (0.44 to 0.49% DM phosphorus) and was not affected by the amount of dietary protein (16.7 to 32% DM) (Finco et al, 1992a).

Beneficial effects of limiting dietary phosphorus intake, by feeding a veterinary therapeutic renal food, have also been demonstrated in cats and dogs with naturally occurring CKD (Elliott et al, 2000; Barber et al, 1999; Jacob et al, 2002; Ross et al, 2006). In one study, feeding a dry or moist veterinary therapeutic renal food[e] with low phosphorus (0.29 or 0.41% DM) was associated with significantly decreased plasma phosphorus and PTH concentrations compared with results from cats fed a typical maintenance food with higher phosphorus (1.9% DM) (Barber et al, 1999). In three additional studies, dogs and cats managed by feeding a veterinary therapeutic renal food with decreased phosphorus had significantly prolonged survival times compared with patients that were fed a higher phosphorus maintenance food (Elliott et al, 2000; Jacob et al, 2002; Ross et al, 2006) (**Box 37-3**).

The minimum recommended allowance for dietary phosphorus is 0.3% DM in foods for healthy adult dogs and 0.26% DM for healthy adult cats (NRC, 2006). The mean DM phosphorus contents of several grocery brand dog and cat foods were 1.39 and 1.54%, respectively (Allen et al, 2000). To achieve beneficial effects, the recommended phosphorus levels for foods used to manage CKD are 0.2 to 0.5% DM for dogs and 0.3 to 0.6% DM for cats.

Sodium and Chloride

As renal function deteriorates, fractional sodium excretion increases to maintain sodium balance and preserve extracellular fluid volume. The fractional excretion of sodium must change markedly to maintain sodium balance when dietary sodium intake changes (Klahr and Slatopolsky, 1973). Patients with decreased renal function can only vary sodium excretion over a limited range, which narrows progressively as GFR declines. Thus, patients with CKD may not tolerate excessively high or low dietary sodium levels. If excessive sodium is ingested, sodium retention with expansion of extracellular fluid volume can occur and produce or worsen preexisting hypertension, fluid overload and edema. If sodium intake is inadequate, negative sodium balance develops with resultant declines in extracellular fluid volume, plasma volume and GFR. Also, excessive dietary sodium intake may increase the absorptive workload on surviving nephrons, increasing oxygen consumption and contributing to hypoxia and increased production of damaging ROS. (See Antioxidants below.)

Limiting dietary sodium intake has been recommended for patients with CKD because of its potential to help manage concomitant hypertension; however, this has not been critically evaluated in dogs and cats with CKD. Systemic hypertension has been reported in 9 to 93% of dogs and 19 to 65% of cats with CKD (Elliott et al, 2001; Syme et al, 2002; Brown et al, 2007). The mechanism for hypertension in renal parenchymal disease is not well understood. It has been postulated that reduced intrarenal blood flow activates the renin-angiotensin-aldosterone system, which leads to chronic expansion of the extracellular fluid and elevations in blood pressure. Other possible mechanisms include secondary renal hyperparathyroidism and reduced levels of renal vasodilators such as prostaglandins.

Kidney disease may cause hypertension, and the kidneys may suffer the consequences of uncontrolled hypertension. The mechanism by which hypertension damages the kidney is not completely understood (Klahr, 1989). Canine CKD patients with major reduction of functional renal mass have impaired renal autoregulation as evidenced by increased renal arterial pressure. Dysfunctional autoregulation may result in further renal damage during hypertensive episodes, which contribute to a progressive decline in kidney function (Brown et al, 1995). Dogs with surgically induced CKD with more pronounced hypertension had significantly lower GFR values, higher UPC ratios and increased renal lesions (Finco, 2004). Hypertension has been associated with increased risk of uremic crisis and death in dogs with naturally occurring CKD (Jacob et al, 2003). In cats with CKD, however, hypertension has not been associated with decreased survival (Elliott et al, 2001; Syme et al, 2006; Jepson et al, 2007). Based on other studies, increased dietary sodium intake has not been associated with increased blood pressure in healthy cats, dogs, cats with induced kidney disease, or cats with naturally occurring CKD (Buranakarl et al, 2004; Greco et al, 1994; Luckschander et al, 2004; Kirk et al, 2006).

Currently, the role of sodium intake in progression of CKD is a topic of considerable interest in human medicine and has been mentioned in dogs and cats with CKD (Polzin, 2007; Chandler, 2008). Sodium may be directly nephrotoxic and restricting sodium intake may be beneficial in CKD, independent of its effect on blood pressure (Cianciaruso et al, 1998; Ritz et al, 2006; Jones-Burton et al, 2006; Sanders, 2004; Weir and Fink, 2005; Verhave et al, 2004). Potential mechanisms for the negative effects of salt in patients with CKD include: 1) increased TGF-β expression in renal endothelial cells, which may lead to renal fibrosis, 2) increased oxidative stress and 3) increased proteinuria. Angiotensin II or increased dietary salt intake may independently increase production of TGF-β (Sanders, 2004). Increased production of TGF-β, in turn, results in increased renal oxidative stress by production of ROS

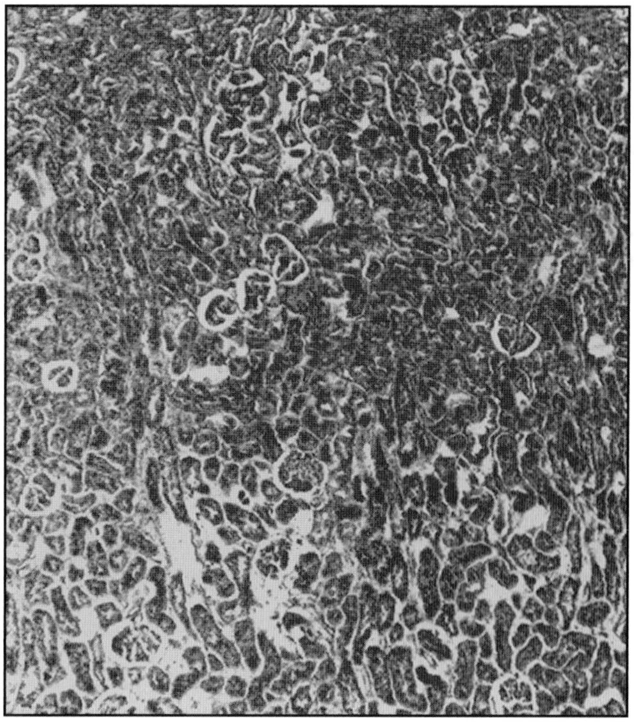

Figure 37-10. Photomicrographs of the renal cortex from cats with experimentally induced chronic kidney disease. (Above) Renal tissue from a cat fed a low-phosphorus food (0.42% DM phosphorus). Mineralized foci are not seen in this kidney (hematoxylin-eosin stain). (Below) Renal tissue from a cat fed a food with normal phosphorus levels (1.56% DM phosphorus). Mineralization (black foci), fibrosis and mononuclear cell infiltrates are extensive compared with that seen on a renal photomicrograph from a cat eating the lower phosphorus food (von Kossa's stain). (Reprinted with permission from Ross LA, Finco DR, Crowell WA. Effect of dietary phosphorus restriction on the kidneys of cats with reduced renal mass. American Journal of Veterinary Research 1982; 43: 1023-1026.)

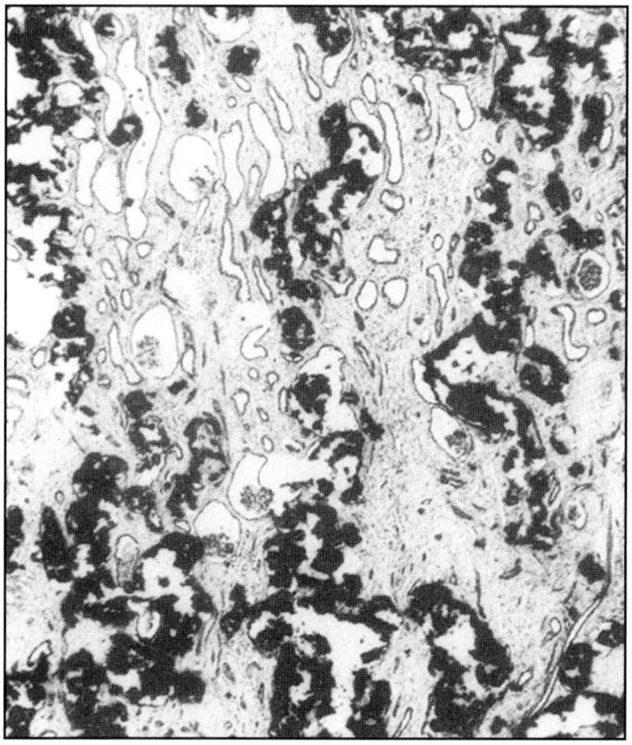

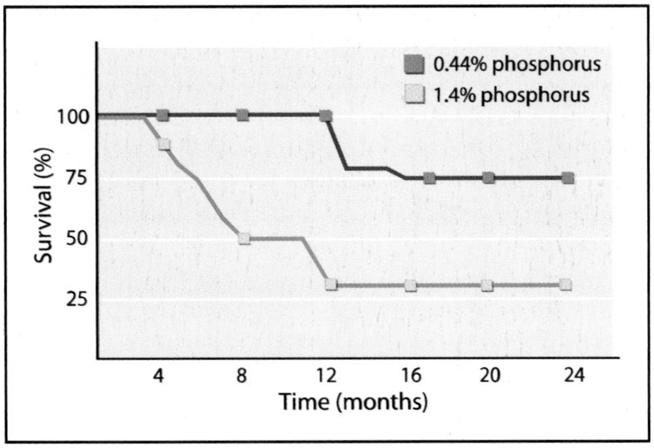

Figure 37-11. Survival of dogs with experimentally induced chronic kidney disease fed low-protein foods with different levels of phosphorus. Note that survival was much improved in dogs consuming the low-phosphorus food. (Adapted from Brown SA, Crowell WA, Barsanti JA, et al. Beneficial effects of dietary mineral restriction in dogs with marked reduction of functional renal mass. Journal of the American Society of Nephrology 1991; 1: 1169-1179.)

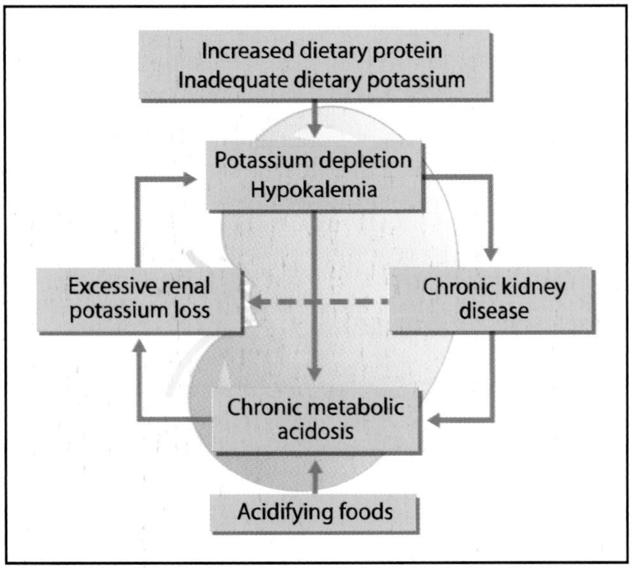

Figure 37-12. Proposed relationship between dietary potassium intake, excessively acidifying foods and feline chronic kidney disease.

(**Figure 37-7**). In human patients with CKD, the anti-proteinuric effect of angiotensin-converting enzyme (ACE) inhibition was strongly dependent on dietary sodium restriction; increased sodium intake virtually abolished the anti-proteinuric effect of the ACE inhibitor lisinopril (Heeg et al, 1989). Administration of ACE inhibitors has been associated with decreased proteinuria in dogs and cats (Grauer et al, 2000; King et al, 2006; Mizutani et al, 2006). The role of dietary sodium on beneficial effects of ACE inhibition has not been evaluated in dogs and cats; however, most patients in these studies were also fed veterinary therapeutic renal foods, which likely contained decreased amounts of sodium. Additional clinical studies are needed to evaluate the role of salt in progression of CKD; however, until results of such studies are available, it has been recommended that modest dietary avoidance of salt be encouraged in human patients with CKD, especially if they have hypertension and/or proteinuria (Jones-Burton et al, 2006).

The long-term effects of altering dietary sodium intake alone in cats and dogs with naturally occurring CKD have not been reported. Feeding veterinary therapeutic renal foods with decreased sodium (0.18 to 0.3% DM sodium in cats and 0.17% DM sodium in dogs) has been associated with increased survival time compared with feeding maintenance foods that contain more sodium (0.4 to 1.1% DM sodium in cats and 0.4% DM sodium in dogs) (Ross et al, 2006; Jacob et al, 2002; Elliott et al, 2000). Several reports describe short-term effects (seven days to six months) of feeding differing amounts of sodium on renal function in dogs and cats (Buranakarl et al, 2004; Greco et al, 1994; Luckschander et al, 2004; Kirk et al, 2006; Xu et al, 2009). In healthy adult cats (mean age = seven years), feeding foods containing 1.11% DM sodium was not associated with increased serum concentrations of urea nitrogen, creatinine or phosphorus, compared with feeding foods containing 0.55% DM sodium for six months (Xu et al, 2009). In this study, data from nine cats with serum creatinine values >1.5 mg/dl were evaluated; there were no significant differences between groups based on dietary sodium intake. Urine concentrating ability for these nine cats was not reported; however, mean urine specific gravity for all cats at the beginning of the study ranged from 1.049 to 1.053. In a study in cats with induced kidney disease, three different amounts of sodium (0.34, 0.68 and 1.35% DM) were fed for seven days (Buranakarl et al, 2004). Feeding the lowest amount of sodium was associated with increased urinary potassium loss and reduced GFR (Buranakarl et al, 2004). The effects of high salt intake (1.19% DM sodium) for three months were evaluated in six cats with naturally occurring CKD (azotemia with urine specific gravity <1.035) (Kirk et al, 2006). The CKD cats fed the high-salt food had significant and progressive increases in blood urea nitrogen, serum creatinine and serum phosphorus compared with results from cats consuming food with 0.37% DM sodium (Kirk et al, 2006). Two of the cats were removed from the study after beginning the high-sodium food due to decreased food intake; this did not affect results of statistical analysis or study conclusions.

A number of studies examined the interaction of dietary sodium with other ions, including chloride. The full expression of sodium chloride-sensitive hypertension in people depends on the concomitant administration of both sodium and chloride (Kurtz et al, 1987; Boegehold and Kotchen, 1989; Luft et al, 1990). In experimental models using rodents with sodium chloride-sensitive hypertension and in clinical studies with small numbers of hypertensive people, blood pressure and volume were not increased by a high dietary sodium intake provided with anions other than chloride. Furthermore, high chloride intake without sodium has less effect on blood pressure than does sodium chloride intake (Kurtz et al, 1987; Boegehold and Kotchen, 1989; Kotchen et al, 1981). The failure of non-chloride sodium salts to produce hypertension or hypervolemia may be related to their failure to expand plasma volume because the renal tubular signal for renin release is responsive to renal tubular chloride (Boegehold and Kotchen, 1989; Luft et al, 1990; Kotchen et al, 1981, 1987). Chloride may also act as a direct renal vasoconstrictor (Boegehold and Kotchen, 1989). These findings suggest that both sodium and chloride are nutrients of concern in patients with hypertension and CKD.

Based on current information, dietary DM sodium intakes for patients with CKD are 0.3% or less for dogs and no more than 0.4% for cats. For comparison, the minimum recommended DM allowances for sodium in foods for healthy adult dogs and cats are 0.08 and 0.096%, respectively (NRC, 2006). The mean sodium levels in several moist grocery brand dog foods were 0.87% DM and 0.9% DM in moist cat foods, although some moist foods contain more sodium. In contrast, dry foods contained approximately half those amounts (Allen et al, 2000). The minimum recommended allowances for chloride for foods for healthy adult dogs and cats are 1.5 times the recommended sodium levels (NRC, 2006). That same factor is suggested for chloride content of foods for canine and feline CKD patients. Some patients may have obligatory urinary sodium losses and abruptly changing these patients to a low-sodium food may result in dangerous contraction of the extracellular fluid volume. Therefore, it is recommended that dogs and cats with CKD be gradually transitioned to foods with reduced amounts of sodium.

Potassium

Cats with CKD appear to be particularly predisposed to disorders in potassium homeostasis (**Figure 37-12** and **Case 37-3**). Decreased dietary potassium intake due to inappetence or vomiting and increased urinary losses due to polyuria can contribute to hypokalemia in CKD. Hypokalemia (potassium values <3.5 mEq/l) has been reported to occur in 19 to 20% of cats with CKD and was moderate to severe (potassium <3.1 mEq/l) in more than half of the cases in one study (DiBartola et al, 1987; Elliott and Barber, 1998). Conversely, hyperkalemia was observed in 9 to 13% of these cats. Hyperkalemia was observed in oliguric and polyuric kidney disease and was most common (22%) in cats with endstage CKD.

Potassium depletion leads to functional and morphologic changes in the kidneys of dogs and cats. Functional changes include reduced GFR and urine concentrating ability. Chronic potassium depletion stimulates renal ammonia synthesis. In hypokalemic rats, increased renal ammoniagenesis contributed to chronic lymphoplasmacytic tubulointerstitial nephritis (Nath et al, 1985). Studies in cats demonstrated that potassium depletion may result from feeding acidifying foods that are high in protein and low in potassium. CKD was observed in three of nine adult cats fed a food high in protein (40% DM) and low in potassium (0.32% DM) content for two years. Lymphoplasmacytic interstitial nephritis and interstitial fibrosis were detected in these cats and in two other cats without laboratory abnormalities (DiBartola et al, 1993).

The minimum recommended allowances for foods for healthy adult dogs and cats are 0.4% DM, and 0.52% DM, respectively (NRC, 2006). The potassium requirement for cats is proportional to the protein content of the food. Using purified foods, 0.3% potassium was required for growth in kittens fed a 33% protein food; however, 0.5% potassium was required with a 68% protein food (Hills et al, 1982). Acidifying foods and chronic metabolic acidosis may contribute to hypokalemia (**Figure 37-12**) (Dow et al, 1990).

The recommended range for potassium for foods for dogs with CKD is 0.4 to 0.8% DM and for cats 0.7 to 1.2% DM. For cats with hypokalemia, oral supplementation with potassium gluconate should be considered if diet alone does not maintain serum potassium concentration above 4.0 mEq/l (Polzin, 2007). Oral administration is safest and is the preferred route unless a critical emergency exists or if oral administration is impossible or contraindicated. Oral potassium gluconate appears to be tolerated well; the initial recommended dose is 2 to 6 mEq potassium gluconate/cat/day, depending on the size of the cat and severity of clinical signs. The potassium gluconate dose should be adjusted based on clinical response and serial analyses of serum potassium concentration. During initial treatment, serum potassium concentration should be checked every two to four days. Later, serum potassium should be checked every two to four weeks. Additional studies are needed to determine whether routine potassium supplementation is indicated in all cats with CKD, regardless of serum potassium concentration (Polzin et al, 2000).

Omega-3 Fatty Acids

The specific dietary fatty acid content of a food can influence progression of CKD by affecting: 1) renal hemodynamics, 2) platelet aggregation, 3) lipid peroxidation, 4) systemic blood pressure, 5) proliferation of glomerular mesangial cells and 6) plasma lipid concentration. Appropriate levels of omega-3 (n-3) fatty acids (e.g., eicosapentaenoic acid [EPA] and docosahexaenoic acid) in foods compete with arachidonic acid in several ways to alter eicosanoid production. These alterations are considered to be renoprotective (Brown et al, 1998).

Specific ingredients (e.g., menhaden fish oil) contain increased levels of omega-3 fatty acids; therefore, animals fed menhaden fish oil have decreased levels of 2-series eicosanoids, which are normally derived from arachidonic acid, and increased levels of 3-series eicosanoids, derived from omega-3 fatty acids. The 3-series eicosanoids are less potent at inducing vasoconstriction and platelet aggregation than the 2-series eicosanoids. Saturated fatty acids found in animal fat do not serve as precursors for eicosanoid production.

In dogs with a remnant kidney model of CKD, dietary omega-3 fatty acid supplementation reduced proteinuria, prevented glomerular hypertension and decreased production of proinflammatory eicosanoids (Brown et al, 1998, 2000). Dietary fat composition altered the rate of CKD progression in dogs following 15/16 nephrectomy (**Figure 37-13**). A low-fat food (<1% DM fat) was supplemented with one of three different fat sources (menhaden fish oil, beef tallow or safflower oil) to achieve a total DM fat concentration in the food of 15%. Dogs were assigned to dietary treatment two months following nephrectomies and followed for 20 months. Compared with

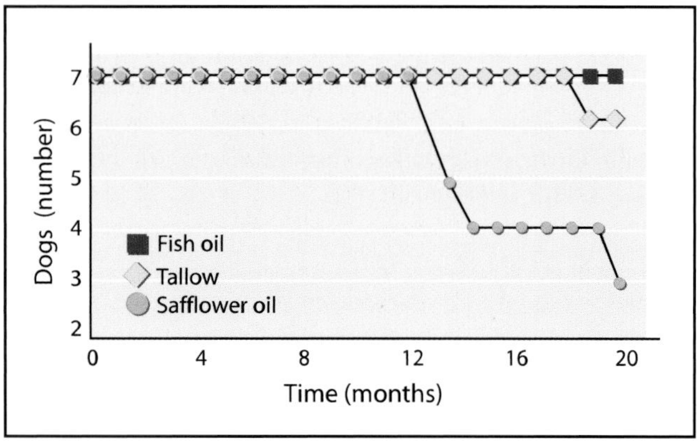

Figure 37-13. Survival of dogs with experimentally induced chronic kidney disease fed foods with three different fat sources (fish oil, tallow, safflower oil). Note that survival was increased in those dogs consuming foods with either tallow or fish oil compared to safflower oil. Dietary fatty acid composition appears to affect hemodynamic adaptations to renal disease in dogs. (Adapted from Brown SA, Brown CA, Crowell WA, et al. Dietary lipid composition alters chronic course of canine renal disease (abstract). Journal of Veterinary Internal Medicine 1996; 10: 168.)

the other two groups, the group receiving the food supplemented with safflower oil had greater glomerular enlargement and mean glomerular capillary pressure. Dietary fatty acid composition appeared to alter hemodynamic responses to renal insufficiency. Final mean exogenous creatinine clearance was 1.3 ml/min./kg body weight for the menhaden fish oil group, 0.9 ml/min./kg body weight for the beef tallow group and 0.5 ml/min./kg body weight for the safflower oil group. Mean UPC ratios were 0.6 in the menhaden fish oil group, 1.5 in the beef tallow group and 2.1 in the safflower oil group. Survival was similar in groups receiving menhaden oil and beef tallow; however, four of seven dogs in the safflower oil group were euthanized. In other studies in dogs with a remnant kidney model of CKD, dietary supplementation with either omega-3 fatty acids or antioxidants was renoprotective and their effects were additive when used together (Brown, 2008).

However, in normal and CKD dogs fed foods supplemented with safflower and menhaden fish oil, the oil supplement had no significant effect on the ratio of urinary eicosanoids (Crocker et al, 1996). The ratio of the urinary eicosanoids thromboxane B_2 (a stable urinary metabolite of thromboxane A_2) and prostaglandin E_2 has been used as an index of renal vascular tone in normal and CKD dogs. Failure to demonstrate a change in the ratio may be related to the length of the washout period (three weeks) and uncertain stability of lipid supplements in this study.

A retrospective CKD study was conducted to evaluate survival times in 146 cats fed one of seven commercial veterinary therapeutic renal foods, compared with survival times in 175 cats fed regular maintenance foods (Plantinga et al, 2005). The median survival time for cats fed maintenance foods was seven months whereas the median survival time for cats fed veterinary therapeutic renal foods was 16 months. The group with the longest median survival time (23 months) was fed the food with the highest reported content of EPA. However, because of study design and differences between groups (e.g., age of cats, plasma creatinine concentrations) and foods (e.g., potassium, phosphorus) used, it is not possible to conclude that differences in survival times were due to increased amounts of EPA. In addition, EPA content was not determined for all foods used in the study.

Although the recommended amount of omega-3 fatty acids for foods for CKD patients has not been definitively determined, the amounts in the aforementioned studies in dogs (Brown et al, 1998, 2000; Brown, 2008) ranged from 0.41 to 4.37% DM. With a 5:1 omega-6:omega-3 fatty acid ratio, the lower end of the range (0.41%) was effective in reducing the magnitude of glomerular hypertension and renal generation of inflammatory eicosanoids (Brown, 2008). The omega-6:omega-3 ratio was not reported in the earlier studies (Brown et al, 1998, 2000). To date, studies like these have not been done in cats but it seems likely that similar levels would be effective. Based on results of canine studies described above, the recommended range for total omega-3 fatty acid content in foods for canine and feline CKD patients is 0.4 to 2.5% DM. Until there is definitive work, a somewhat broad range for the omega-6:omega-3 fatty acid ratio is recommended (1:1 to 7:1). These recommendations are similar to omega-3 fatty acid content and omega-6:omega-3 ratios recommended for dogs and cats with cancer, osteoarthritis and inflammatory skin diseases.

Dietary omega-3 fatty acid supplementation in combination with antioxidants (See Antioxidants below.) can further reduce renal oxidant injury. In a study in dogs with the remnant model of CKD, dietary supplementation with omega-3 fatty acids and antioxidants (vitamin E, carotenoids and lutein), both were independently renoprotective; when combined, their effects were additive (Brown, 2008). In this model, addition of antioxidants reduced proteinuria, glomerulosclerosis and interstitial fibrosis independent of the ratio of dietary omega-6 to omega-3 fatty acids (Brown, 2008).

Antioxidants: Vitamins E and C

Oxidative damage is a component in the progression of renal injury in several types of kidney disease (**Figure 37-7**) (Diamond et al, 1986; Agarwal, 2003; Vasavada and Agarwal, 2005). Unquenched ROS may damage proteins, lipids, DNA and carbohydrates, resulting in structural and functional abnormalities and progressive renal injury. Renal oxidative stress occurs when production of ROS exceeds quenching capacity of antioxidant defense mechanisms (Brown, 2008). As previously discussed (See Etiopathogenesis above.), increased renal oxidative stress has been linked to proteinuria as a potential mediator of tubulointerstitial damage and to progression of CKD (Brown, 2008; Agarwal, 2003; Agarwal et al, 2004; Vasavada and Agarwal, 2005). Specifically, overloading tubular mechanisms for resorption of filtered albumin by proximal tubular cells can stimulate production of proinflammatory and profibrotic cytokines by activation of the redox-sensitive gene nuclear factor-κB thereby contributing to tubulointerstitial damage (Agarwal, 2003; Rossert and Froissart, 2006).

Numerous antioxidant defense mechanisms are designed to

minimize damage by ROS including several nutritional antioxidants: vitamins E and C and carotenoids (Brown, 2008). Supplementation of foods with these antioxidants has been evaluated in dogs and cats with naturally occurring CKD. In a canine study, 10 patients with CKD (IRIS stage 2 to 3) and 10 healthy dogs were evaluated to determine effects of supplementation of vitamins E (1,200 IU/kg DM) and C (150 mg/kg DM), and β-carotene (1.6 mg/kg DM) in a dry veterinary therapeutic renal food (Yu et al, 2006). Levels of vitamins E and C and β-carotene in the control food were not reported. The antioxidant supplementation reduced oxidative stress as measured by significantly reduced plasma malondialdehyde concentration. The antioxidant-supplemented renal food significantly reduced serum creatinine concentration and resulted in increased body weight and activity (eight of 10 dogs) in the CKD dogs compared with dogs receiving the unsupplemented commercial maintenance-type food (Yu et al, 2006).

Similarly, effects of antioxidants on renal oxidative stress were studied in 10 cats with CKD compared with healthy cats (Yu and Paetau-Robinson, 2006). Supplementation of vitamins E (742 mg/kg DM) and C (84 mg/kg DM) and β-carotene (2.1 mg/kg DM), compared with the control food containing 166 mg/kg DM vitamin E, less than 5 mg/kg DM vitamin C and 1.4 mg/kg DM β-carotene, resulted in reduced markers of oxidative injury. Antioxidant supplementation significantly reduced DNA damage in cats with CKD as evidenced by reduced serum 8-hydroxy-2'-deoxyguanosine (8-OHdG) and comet assay parameters (Yu and Paetau-Robinson, 2006). Based on these studies, supplementation with vitamins E and C and β-carotene as antioxidants may benefit dogs and cats with CKD.

Dietary supplementation with antioxidants in combination with increased omega-3 fatty acids (discussed above) reduces renal oxidant injury. Supplementation with vitamin E suppressed renal oxidative stress in rats with 5/6 nephrectomy (Tain et al, 2007). Also, as mentioned above in dogs with a remnant kidney model of CKD, dietary omega-3 fatty acid supplementation reduced proteinuria, prevented glomerular hypertension and decreased production of proinflammatory eicosanoids (Brown et al, 1998, 2000). In other studies in dogs with a remnant kidney model of CKD, dietary supplementation with omega-3 fatty acids and antioxidants (vitamin E, carotenoids and lutein) both independently were renoprotective and their effects were additive when used together (Brown, 2008). In this model, addition of antioxidants reduced proteinuria, glomerulosclerosis and interstitial fibrosis independent of the ratio of dietary omega-6 polyunsaturated fatty acids to omega-3 polyunsaturated fatty acids (Brown, 2008).

The DM requirement of vitamin E in foods for adult dogs is 30 IU/kg (NRC, 2006). An upper limit of 1,000 to 2,000 IU/kg food DM has been suggested for dogs (AAFCO, 2007). One antioxidant biomarker study in dogs indicated that for improved antioxidant performance, foods should contain at least 500 IU vitamin E/kg DM (Jewell et al, 2000). Besides helping to prevent chronic diseases associated with oxidative stress, increasing dietary intake of vitamin E, up to 2,010 mg/kg food DM in older dogs improved immune function (Hayes et al, 1969; Hall et al, 2003; Meydani et al, 1998). Based on the above studies, foods for canine CKD patients should contain at least 400 IU vitamin E/kg DM and higher levels are probably better. In one report, dietary supplementation of food for dogs with induced CKD, 5 IU/kg body weight was effective; this amount translates to approximately 450 IU/kg food DM (Brown, 2008).

The minimum recommended allowance of vitamin E in foods for healthy adult cats is 38 IU/kg DM (NRC, 2006). No safe upper limit has been established for cats. One antioxidant biomarker study suggested that cat foods should contain 600 IU/kg DM for improved antioxidant function (Jewell et al, 2000). A study in aged cats showed that increasing dietary intake of vitamin E to 272 and 552 IU/kg of food DM improved immune function (Hayes et al, 1969; Hall et al, 2003). Based on these data and studies in cats with CKD discussed above, foods for cats with CKD should contain at least 500 IU/kg DM and, as with dogs, higher levels are probably better. Foods high in polyunsaturated fatty acids (e.g., those containing fish oils), may require increased amounts of vitamin E (four or more times levels in typical foods) to prevent steatitis (NRC, 2006).

Healthy dogs can synthesize required amounts of vitamin C for normal maintenance conditions (Innes, 1931; Naismith, 1958; Chatterjee et al, 1975) and they can rapidly absorb supplemental vitamin C (Wang et al, 2001). However, in vitro studies indicate that dogs and cats have from one-quarter to one-tenth the ability to synthesize vitamin C as other mammals (Chatterjee et al, 1975). Foods for canine and feline CKD patients should contain at least 100 and 100 to 200 mg vitamin C/kg DM, respectively. This recommendation is based on the aforementioned vitamin E levels in foods for dogs and cats with CKD and data indicating that vitamin C regenerates vitamin E at about a 1:1 molar ratio (Barclay et al, 1985). This range is not a risk factor for urinary oxalate production in cats (Yu and Gross, 2005).

Other Nutritional Factors

β-carotene

β-carotene is a carotenoid like lutein and lycopene. As mentioned above, the carotenoids have antioxidant properties. β-carotene can be absorbed by dogs and cats. β-carotene is also a precursor for vitamin A. Dogs, but not cats, are able to convert β-carotene to vitamin A. β-carotene can be pro-oxidant at high levels in people and laboratory animals (Alpha-Tocopherol, Beta-Carotene Cancer Prevention Study Group, 1994). β-carotene values in foods typically are difficult to obtain from manufacturers. For these reasons, at this time, β-carotene is not considered a key nutritional factor for foods for dogs or cats with CKD.

Acidifiers and Buffers

Metabolic acidosis is a common finding in patients with CKD. Decreased venous blood pH and plasma bicarbonate or total CO_2 concentrations are common, particularly in cats with uremic signs or endstage disease (Lulich et al, 1992; Elliott and Barber, 1998; Elliott et al, 2003, 2003a). The kidneys play an important role in regenerating bicarbonate and excreting dietary acids, which may be derived from several sources. Sulfuric acid is formed when sulfur-containing amino acids (i.e., methionine and cysteine) are oxidized to sulfate. In general, animal-source proteins are higher in sulfur-containing amino acids than are plant-source proteins. Exogenous- and endogenous-source proteins are equally important. Insufficient energy intake results in protein catabolism and increased hydrogen ion production. Urinary urea production and total urinary hydrogen ion excretion are directly proportional. Organic acids are produced from partial oxidation of carbohydrates, fats, proteins and nucleic acids. Phosphoric acid can be ingested in the food or it can be produced endogenously. Phosphoric acid is used in some cat foods as a palatability enhancer, either separately or as a component of topically applied animal digests. Phosphoric acid can be derived from hydrolysis of phosphate esters in proteins and nucleic acids, if they are not neutralized by mineral cations (e.g., sodium, potassium and magnesium). The contribution of dietary phosphate to acid production depends on the type of protein ingested. Some proteins generate phosphoric acid, whereas others generate only neutral phosphate salts. Hydrochloric acid is generated when positively charged cationic amino acids (e.g., lysine and arginine) are broken down into neutral products.

Some commercial veterinary therapeutic renal foods are formulated with combinations of ingredients that will alkalinize the urine and blood, which minimizes dietary acid load (Burkholder et al, 2000). These foods are limited in protein ingredients, particularly those that are high in sulfur-containing amino acids. For patients with CKD, the serum total CO_2 should be maintained within the reference range for healthy patients. Ideally, blood gas analysis should be done to more accurately confirm the presence of metabolic acidosis. As CKD progresses and acidosis becomes more severe, alkali therapy (e.g., sodium bicarbonate, potassium citrate) should be considered in addition to nutritional management. Although urinary pH may be used as an indirect assessment of acid/base status, monitoring venous blood gases is a more sensitive method to evaluate effectiveness of alkalinization therapy.

Vitamin D
Calcitriol (1,25-dihydroxyvitamin D) plays an important role in the pathogenesis of secondary renal hyperparathyroidism. Patients with severe CKD have decreased circulating levels of 1,25-dihydroxyvitamin D because of decreased synthesis by the kidney. Hyperphosphatemia and the progressive loss of renal epithelial cells inhibit conversion of 25-hydroxyvitamin D to calcitriol by renal 1-α-hydroxylase. At earlier stages of CKD, circulating levels of 1,25-dihydroxyvitamin D may be normal due to the compensatory effect of increased concentrations of PTH on renal 1-α-hydroxylase activity and tubular synthesis of 1,25-dihydroxyvitamin D.

Calcitriol is an important regulator of parathyroid chief-cell function. Calcitriol acts by decreasing PTH messenger RNA expression, increasing expression of vitamin D receptors and controlling the "set point" of chief cells, which determines responsiveness to negative feedback by ionized serum calcium concentrations. Decreased circulating calcitriol levels in CKD lead to chief-cell hyperplasia and increased secretion of PTH. Increased PTH levels have been suggested to play a role in the severity of clinical signs and progression of CKD (Nagode and Chew, 1992).

Avoiding excessive dietary phosphorus and using phosphate binders reduce the inhibitory effects of hyperphosphatemia on renal 1-α-hydroxylase activity, thereby increasing calcitriol production by tubular cells. Oral administration of low doses of calcitriol is associated with decreased serum PTH concentrations. Strong evidence supports the use of calcitriol therapy for slowing progression of CKD in dogs but not in cats (Polzin et al, 2005a; Polzin, 2007). The effect of varying vitamin D levels in foods has not been studied; therefore, it is not included as a key nutritional factor.

B Vitamins
Limited information exists concerning vitamin nutrition in dogs and cats with CKD; however, these patients are at risk for B-vitamin deficiency because of decreased appetite, vomiting, diarrhea and polyuria. Human patients with CKD apparently are especially prone to pyridoxine and folate deficiency (Gilmour et al, 1993). Thiamin and niacin deficiency may contribute to anorexia associated with renal failure. Empirical administration of vitamins seems appropriate in anorectic patients with CKD. However, care must be taken to avoid excessive amounts of fat-soluble vitamins. Patients eating adequate amounts of commercial veterinary therapeutic renal foods are unlikely to need B-vitamin supplementation.

Trace Minerals
Presumably, CKD alters metabolism of trace minerals. For example, nutrients such as copper and zinc that are highly bound to protein may be lost with severe proteinuria. Aluminum may accumulate in human patients with CKD who are treated with aluminum-containing phosphate binders. Aluminum toxicity can cause metabolic bone disease, encephalopathy and anemia. However, exact data are not available to support making a routine recommendation for dietary trace mineral modification for dogs and cats with CKD. There are no reports of trace mineral problems in dogs and cats with CKD that eat commercial veterinary therapeutic renal foods.

Soluble Fiber
It is well established that soluble fiber causes bacterial proliferation in the colon. Bacterial growth requires a source of nitrogen. Although dietary protein provides some nitrogen, blood urea is the largest and most available source of nitrogen for bacterial protein synthesis in the colon (Younes et al, 1995). Urea is the major end product of protein catabolism in mammals. When blood urea diffuses into the large bowel it is broken

down by bacterial ureases and used for bacterial protein synthesis. These bacterial proteins are excreted in the feces. The net effect is increased fecal urea excretion, reduced serum urea nitrogen concentration and reduced urinary urea excretion in rats and people (Younes et al, 1995, 1996; Bliss et al, 1996). Whether soluble fiber is effective in foods for dogs and cats with CKD has not been studied.

FEEDING PLAN

Based on current evidence, nutritional management with an appropriately formulated commercial veterinary therapeutic renal food should begin when serum creatinine exceeds 2 mg/dl in dogs and cats with CKD (stage 2 CKD and higher). Although not evaluated in controlled studies, recommending a veterinary therapeutic renal food seems logical when earlier stages of CKD are documented (e.g., persistent renal proteinuria, loss of urine concentrating ability or mild azotemia). Nutritional management is the cornerstone of treatment for dogs and cats with CKD; however, inappetence, vomiting and diarrhea may be prominent in patients with moderate to severe CKD and evidence of systemic illness (uremia). These patients should receive aggressive fluid and electrolyte therapy in an attempt to ameliorate azotemia, uremia, electrolyte abnormalities and acidosis before initiating a traditional feeding plan.

Assess and Select the Food

Foods for dogs and cats with CKD should be evaluated for all the key nutritional factors previously discussed (**Table 37-9**). **Tables 37-11** and **37-12** list commercial veterinary therapeutic foods designed for CKD patients (dogs and cats, respectively), including comparisons to recommended levels of key nutritional factors. These comparisons will help determine the best food to consider for initial feeding. Although commercial veterinary therapeutic renal foods share some features in common, they are not the same. It is important to consider the evidence supporting effectiveness of individual foods when making nutritional recommendations for patients with CKD (**Table 37-10** and **Box 37-3**). In addition, it may be necessary to consider nutrients that may affect concomitant diseases (e.g., dogs with CKD and pancreatitis or cats with CKD and diabetes mellitus) (**Case 37-4**).

All possible sources of nutrients that patients with CKD will receive should be evaluated and discussed with pet owners. It may be easy to simply recommend that owners not give any treats; however, the reality is that most owners give their pet treats. When asked how they showed affection to their pets, 71% of 1,212 dog owners and 44% of 820 cat owners said they give their pets treats and 42 and 25% of dog and cat owners, respectively, said they give their pets people food (Habits and Practices Study, 2002). Therefore, when communicating feeding plan recommendations for dogs and cats with CKD, it's important to discuss treats with pet owners. One option is to recommend that the owner keep kibbles of dry veterinary therapeutic renal food in a separate container located in a different area from where the pet is normally fed and use these as treats. Small amounts of moist veterinary therapeutic renal food formed into balls could also be offered. If an owner insists on feeding other treats, the amount of treats and snacks fed should be less than 5% of the volume or weight of the total food intake. Many commercial pet treats and processed human foods contain excess sodium, chloride and phosphorus and should be avoided in CKD patients. However, some commercial treats contain moderate amounts of these nutrients. High-phosphorus human foods (e.g., milk, milk products, cheese, fish, beef liver, chocolate, nuts and legumes) should be avoided. In addition to treats, it's important to discuss with owners what forms of food they prefer to feed and to offer them the same forms (dry and moist) of the veterinary therapeutic renal food. In a survey of more than 800 cat owners, 66% preferred to feed both moist and dry food to their cats (Habits and Practices Study, 2002). In this situation, if the owners purchased a dry veterinary therapeutic renal food from their veterinarian for a cat with CKD, it is highly likely they would buy a moist food elsewhere and use it with the dry food. Feeding a typical over-the-counter moist cat food that contains increased amounts of sodium, chloride and phosphorus could decrease or negate effectiveness of the veterinary therapeutic renal food.

Assess and Determine the Feeding Method

Changing the feeding method in the management of CKD may not be necessary, especially in patients with early or uncomplicated CKD. It is important, however, to verify that an appropriate feeding method is being used. Items to consider include access to water, amount fed, how food is offered, access to other foods and who feeds the pet. Patients with uremia and other signs of systemic disease may be partially or completely anorectic and require alternate feeding methods (Chapters 25 and 26).

How the previous food was offered (e.g., free-choice feeding or multiple offerings per day of a prescribed amount) can be continued if the form of the food is unchanged.

The amount to feed is based on the patient's energy requirement. The energy needs of patients with kidney disease are presumed to be similar to those of normal pets having the same level of activity. In general, energy intake tends to decrease as renal function declines because of progressive anorexia. In addition, numerous factors (e.g., gender, changes in environment and activity) influence the energy requirement for an individual patient. The starting point for estimating daily energy requirement (DER) for an individual patient is to calculate the resting energy requirement (RER) and multiply this number by a factor that varies based on the severity of chronic metabolic disease. The formula for calculating RER in kcal/day is $70(BW_{kg})^{0.75}$. Table 5-2 also provides RER estimates for dogs and cats. The recommended DER range for most canine patients with CKD is 1.1 to 1.6 x RER. The DER range for most feline patients with CKD is 1.1 to 1.4 x RER. After the DER is estimated, it is divided by the energy density of the food on an as fed basis to determine the amount to feed. Feeding recommendations from the manufacturer of the select-

Table 37-11. Key nutritional factors in selected commercial veterinary therapeutic foods for dogs with chronic kidney disease compared to recommended levels.*

Moist foods	Energy density (kcal/can)**	Protein (%)	P (%)	Na (%)	K (%)	Omega-3 fatty acids (%)	Omega-6: omega-3	Vit. E (IU/kg)	Vit. C (mg/kg)
Recommended levels	**–**	**14-20**	**0.2-0.5**	**≤0.3**	**0.4-0.8**	**0.4-2.5**	**1:1-7:1**	**≥400**	**≥100**
Hill's Prescription Diet g/d Canine	377 kcal/13 oz.	18.1	0.41	0.22	0.78	0.67	3.7:1	719	107
Hill's Prescription Diet k/d Canine	458 kcal/13 oz.	14.8	0.22	0.19	0.37	1.93	2.3:1	844	130
Hill's Prescription Diet u/d Canine	489 kcal/13 oz.	13.3	0.17	0.28	0.45	0.38	13.5:1	643	na
Medi-Cal Reduced Protein	525 kcal/396 g	16.5	0.5	0.2	0.5	na	na	na	na
Medi-Cal Renal LP	643 kcal/385 g	16.8	0.2	0.1	1.0	na	na	na	na
Medi-Cal Renal MP	532 kcal/380 g	28.2	0.4	0.2	1.5	na	na	na	na
Medi-Cal Weight Control/Mature	370 kcal/396 g	21.5	0.6	0.3	0.6	na	na	na	na
Purina Veterinary Diets NF KidNey Function Canine Formula	498 kcal/12.5 oz.	16.5	0.30	0.24	0.72	0.59	6.9:1	na	na
Royal Canin Veterinary Diet Renal LP	785 kcal/13.6 oz.	16.1	0.24	0.08	0.84	na	na	1,034	na
Royal Canin Veterinary Diet Renal MP	670 kcal/13.4 oz.	26.2	0.42	0.19	1.17	na	na	552	na
Dry foods	**Energy density (kcal/cup)****	**Protein (%)**	**P (%)**	**Na (%)**	**K (%)**	**Omega-3 fatty acids (%)**	**Omega-6: omega-3**	**Vit. E (IU/kg)**	**Vit. C (mg/kg)**
Recommended levels	**–**	**14-20**	**0.2-0.5**	**≤0.3**	**0.4-0.8**	**0.4-2.5**	**1:1-7:1**	**≥400**	**≥100**
Hill's Prescription Diet g/d Canine	358	18.7	0.41	0.21	0.61	0.78	3.5:1	263	na
Hill's Prescription Diet k/d Canine	396	14.7	0.24	0.23	0.67	1.54	1.9:1	679	344
Hill's Prescription Diet u/d Canine	396	11.2	0.15	0.23	0.54	0.74	4.4:1	856	na
Iams Veterinary Formula Renal Early Stage	245	21.0	0.46	0.41	0.63	na	5:1	na	na
Medi-Cal Reduced Protein	360	13.7	0.4	0.2	0.7	na	na	na	na
Medi-Cal Renal LP	283	14.7	0.3	0.1	0.7	na	na	na	na
Medi-Cal Renal MP	336	18.4	0.4	0.1	0.7	na	na	na	na
Medi-Cal Weight Control/Mature	320	19.5	0.8	0.2	0.8	na	na	na	na
Purina Veterinary Diets NF KidNey Function Canine Formula	459	15.9	0.29	0.22	0.86	0.30	9.3:1	na	na
Royal Canin Veterinary Diet Renal LP 11	275	14.7	0.30	0.08	0.66	na	na	302	na
Royal Canin Veterinary Diet Renal MP 14	327	18.4	0.40	0.10	0.66	na	na	302	na

Key: P = phosphorus, Na = sodium, K = potassium, omega-6:omega-3 = omega-6 to omega-3 fatty acid ratio, Vit. E = vitamin E, Vit. C = vitamin C, na = information not available from manufacturer, g = grams.

*All values are reported on a dry matter basis unless otherwise indicated. Moist foods are best. All values were obtained from manufacturers' published information.

**Energy density as fed (per can or cup) is useful for determining the amount to feed; cup = 8-oz. measuring cup; to convert kcal to kJ, multiply kcal by 4.184.

ed food can also be used as a starting point. Also, feeding a similar amount to the amount of maintenance food that was previously fed is another starting point. The initial food dose should be adjusted from these starting points to maintain optimal body weight and condition. Gradual transition to a new food improves acceptance and also decreases the likelihood of problems in those patients that cannot rapidly adjust urinary sodium levels because of their renal dysfunction. Dogs with CKD usually tolerate a dietary change over seven to 10 days, whereas, cats may need three to four weeks or longer to make a successful transition. This requires patience and persistence by the pet owner and veterinary health care team. However, the end result is worth it because feeding a commercial veterinary therapeutic renal food is the only treatment that has been shown to prolong survival time in dogs and cats with CKD. Unfortunately, the "cold turkey" approach to feeding (i.e., own-

Table 37-12. Key nutritional factors in selected commercial veterinary therapeutic foods for cats with chronic kidney disease compared to recommended levels.*

Moist foods	Energy density (kcal/can)**	Protein (%)	P (%)	Na (%)	K (%)	Omega-3 fatty acids (%)	Omega-6: omega-3	Vit. E (IU/kg)	Vit. C (mg/kg)
Recommended levels	**–**	**28-35**	**0.3-0.6**	**≤0.4**	**0.7-1.2**	**0.4-2.5**	**1:1-7:1**	**≥500**	**100-200**
Hill's Prescription Diet g/d Feline	165 kcal/5.5 oz.	34.3	0.52	0.32	0.72	0.64	6.1:1	817	104
Hill's Prescription Diet k/d with Chicken Feline	183 kcal/5.5 oz.	28.9	0.38	0.30	1.18	0.72	6.1:1	814	103
Iams Veterinary Formula Multi Stage Renal	199 kcal/6 oz.	33.6	0.60	0.40	1.03	na	5:1	na	na
Medi-Cal Reduced Protein	265 kcal/170 g	33.9	0.5	0.2	0.7	na	na	na	na
Medi-Cal Renal LP	125 kcal/85-g pouch	29.3	0.5	0.6	1.1	na	na	na	na
Purina Veterinary Diets NF KidNey Function	234 kcal/5.5 oz.	31.1	0.52	0.16	0.96	0.85	3.7:1	na	na
Royal Canin Veterinary Diet Modified Formula	256 kcal/6 oz.	34.7	0.65	0.28	0.81	na	na	178	na
Royal Canin Veterinary Diet Renal LP	126 kcal/3-oz. pouch	34.1	0.55	0.47	1.10	na	na	437	na
Dry foods	**Energy density (kcal/cup)****	**Protein (%)**	**P (%)**	**Na (%)**	**K (%)**	**Omega-3 fatty acids (%)**	**Omega-6: omega-3**	**Vit. E (IU/kg)**	**Vit. C (mg/kg)**
Recommended levels	**–**	**28-35**	**0.3-0.6**	**≤0.4**	**0.7-1.2**	**0.4-2.5**	**1:1-7:1**	**≥500**	**100-200**
Hill's Prescription Diet g/d Feline	297	33.5	0.54	0.32	0.77	0.19	15.5:1	232	na
Hill's Prescription Diet k/d Feline	477	28.8	0.46	0.24	0.75	0.25	15.1:1	952	229
Iams Veterinary Formula Multi Stage Renal	514	32.1	0.42	0.39	0.65	na	5:1	na	na
Medi-Cal Reduced Protein	440	28.1	0.6	0.3	0.8	na	na	na	na
Medi-Cal Renal LP	409	24.7	0.5	0.2	1.0	na	na	na	na
Purina Veterinary Diets NF KidNey Function	398	30.8	0.41	0.20	0.88	0.31	6.4:1	na	na
Royal Canin Veterinary Diet Modified Formula	432	27.1	0.49	0.23	1.07	na	na	380	na
Royal Canin Veterinary Diet Renal LP 21	395	24.7	0.49	0.16	1.02	na	na	355	na

Key: P = phosphorus, Na = sodium, K = potassium, omega-6:omega-3 = omega-6 to omega-3 fatty acid ratio, Vit. E = vitamin E, Vit. C = vitamin C, na = information not available from manufacturer, g = grams.

*All values are reported on a dry matter basis unless otherwise indicated. Moist foods are best. All values were obtained from manufacturers' published information.

**Energy density as fed (per can or cup) is useful for determining the amount to feed; cup = 8-oz. measuring cup; to convert kcal to kJ, multiply kcal by 4.184.

ers returns home with their pet and immediately switch to the new food), rather than transitioning to the new food over several days to weeks is common. In this scenario, the outcome often results in failure to implement the nutritional recommendation. Changing the eating habits of most dogs and cats is relatively easy, but changing the feeding habits of some pet owners and veterinarians is often more difficult. Some veterinarians are still unaware that commercial veterinary therapeutic renal foods are as palatable, or more so, than regular maintenance foods. The feeding plan is more likely to be successful if the owner is told that the veterinary therapeutic renal foods are highly palatable (positive bias). **Box 37-5** provides additional tips to aid in increasing acceptance of veterinary therapeutic renal foods by dogs and cats with CKD.

When switching to a veterinary therapeutic food, it may help to use a familiar form of food initially (e.g., moist or dry or a combination). However, some patients may switch their preferences after CKD develops and prefer different forms of foods. Moist veterinary therapeutic renal foods can be made more palatable by warming (not above body temperature). Palatability of dry foods can often be increased by adding water or flavoring agents such as tuna juice, clam juice, chicken broth, low-sodium soups, garlic, brewer's yeast or sweeteners (dogs only) such as honey or syrup. Uneaten moistened foods should not be allowed to remain at room temperature for more than a few hours (Chapter 11). Some of the aforementioned supple-

Box 37-5. Tips for Encouraging Acceptance of Veterinary Therapeutic Renal Foods in Patients with Chronic Kidney Disease.

Educate pet owners about the effectiveness of nutritional management for prolonging survival time and improving quality of life in patients with kidney disease. For treatment to succeed, owners must commit their time and money, which is more likely to occur if they understand the benefits of their efforts.

Begin nutritional management sooner rather than later. Current evidence supports feeding a veterinary therapeutic renal food when serum creatinine is ≥2 mg/dl. Waiting until later (e.g., when there are signs of uremia) is not advised because patients with more advanced disease may be less likely to accept a change in treatment and therefore will not receive optimal benefits of a renal therapeutic food.

Probably the single most important thing you can do to increase patient acceptance of a veterinary therapeutic renal food is gradually transition to the new food. The transition period should be a minimum of seven days; however, some patients (especially cats) need a transition of three to four weeks or longer. It is critical to discuss the need for this transition with pet owners, otherwise, they are likely to buy a new food, go home and switch from the old food to the new food at the next meal. In this scenario, many patients will refuse to eat the new food, which results in an unhappy owner and a patient that will likely not receive the benefits of nutritional management.

One option for transitioning to a renal food is to mix the old and new food, gradually adding more of the new food over time. Another approach is to provide both foods (old and new) in side-by-side food dishes. This technique assists with gradual transition and also allows cats to express their preferences. For more information, visit www.vet.osu.edu/indoorcat for The Indoor Cat Initiative.

If transitioning cats from dry to moist food, use a flat food dish (e.g., saucer) instead of a bowl. This avoids rubbing the cat's whiskers on the food dish, which could affect acceptance of new food.

Avoid offering veterinary therapeutic renal foods in stressful environments (e.g., sick and/or hospitalization, during force-feeding); a food aversion may develop causing decreased acceptance of the food when the patient is feeling better. Stated another way, while patients are hospitalized, do not feed them (especially cats) the food you want them to eat for the rest of their lives. In this situation, one option would be to feed a maintenance food that avoids excessive protein, phosphorus and sodium until the patient is feeling better and then gradually transition to a therapeutic renal food.

Use fresh food at room temperature. Some patients may eat refrigerated food that is warmed, but others will only eat food from a newly opened container. Some patients may eat food that has been refrigerated and stored in a plastic container vs. food stored in the original can.

Offer foods with different textures (e.g., minced formulas) or form (dry vs. moist). Some pets may prefer dry or moist food all their lives and when they develop kidney disease, their preferences may switch (e.g., a cat that has eaten dry food all its life may eat moist food after kidney disease occurs and vice versa).

Add flavor enhancers (low-sodium chicken broth or tuna juice) or a small amount of maintenance food to encourage the patient to eat all the veterinary therapeutic food. Excessive use of other foods will likely decrease the beneficial effects of the veterinary therapeutic renal food; therefore, the smallest amount possible should be used.

If you have followed the steps above and there is still reluctance to eat a veterinary therapeutic renal food, switch to a different brand. Although commercially available renal foods have general features in common, they are not the same. In addition, individual pets may express a preference for one brand over another. Avoid giving the owner samples of several different brands of foods at once; this could result in a food aversion to all veterinary therapeutic renal foods, especially if owners offer each sample at successive meals or on consecutive days. **Tables 37-11** and **37-12** can be used to select foods with the best key nutritional factor profiles for dogs and cats, respectively.

ments are high in sodium content (e.g., clam and tuna juice); however, and should not be used long-term due to excessive sodium intake above the amount in the veterinary therapeutic food. Environmental factors should also receive consideration when transitioning pets to a veterinary therapeutic renal food. Owner compliance and pet acceptance of the food must be adequate for nutritional management to be effective. Knowing who feeds the patient is important for compliance, and limiting the patient's access to other foods improves acceptability (e.g., a dog having access to cat food or a cat living in a multi-cat household). Feeding location and presentation are important. Timid animals should be fed in a quiet place. Cats should be fed away from loud, persistent barking or other distracting noises. Food bowls should not be kept in close proximity to litter boxes and noisy areas. Food for cats should be offered in wide bowls or on a plate to avoid stimulation of tactile whiskers. Placing small quantities of palatable food in a patient's mouth or on its paws (moist food) to stimulate licking or swallowing (i.e., hand feeding) may facilitate eating. Patients' appetite can be influenced by the person feeding the patient (server). The likelihood of eating increases in direct proportion to the time the patient has spent with the server in a nonstressful situation (Delaney, 2006). For hospitalized pets, the ideal server is likely the pet owner followed by either a technician or kennel assistant who has not restrained or otherwise antagonized the patient.

Food aversion is possible if a nauseated pet is force-fed or if a painful or unpleasant experience is associated with feeding. Unpalatable medications (e.g., some phosphate binders) should not be mixed with veterinary therapeutic foods. Managing underlying abnormalities in fluid, electrolyte and acid-base balance will help minimize nausea and vomiting. Pharmacologic agents (e.g., ranitidine, famotidine, metoclopramide and sucralfate) can be used to limit uremic gastritis, nausea and vomiting. Veterinary therapeutic foods intended for long-term management of patients with CKD should not be offered during periods of nausea and vomiting to prevent possible food aversions. Consider using an appropriate, alternative food temporarily during hospitalization for dogs and cats with uremic signs.

Finally, a common approach that is used for "picky" eaters is to offer samples of several different foods and then recommend the food they will eat. This may be effective in some patients but there is a major disadvantage of using this approach in patients with CKD. The "cafeteria" approach should not be used in patients with diseases that commonly have a learned food aversion or that have limited commercial veterinary therapeutic food options (Delaney, 2006). Offering samples of all the commercially available veterinary therapeutic renal foods to a CKD patient that is not eating well or has uremic signs should be avoided to minimize the likelihood of a learned food aversion to all the foods the patient may need to be fed long-term (Delaney, 2006).

REASSESSMENT

Frequency of reassessment depends on the stage of CKD and presence of concurrent conditions. Patients with azotemia should be rechecked every two to three months and uremic patients should be rechecked as often as every two to four weeks. Duration between evaluations may be longer in patients with stable disease. Parameters included in the reassessment are listed in **Table 37-13**. Serial evaluation of appropriate laboratory tests, including UPC ratios, is a good means of reassessment. Because of daily variation in UPC ratios, minor changes in UPC ratio may or may not be clinically important. It is important to monitor trends on multiple UPC ratios over time rather than rely on individual measurements. Increasing UPC ratios over time can indicate worsening glomerular disease, whereas serial declining UPC ratios are consistent with clinical improvement. Decreases in urine protein concentrations, however, may not always be associated with improved glomerular function. If accompanied by increases in serum creatinine concentrations, declining UPC ratios may reflect progressive glomerular sclerosis and obsolescence. As glomeruli become obsolescent, they no longer lose protein; however, these same glomeruli also lose their functional ability, potentially resulting in azotemia.

After nutritional management has been implemented for patients with CKD, it is very important to monitor for signs of malnutrition (e.g., accurate body weights over time, body condition score, hematocrit, serum albumin) so that food offerings can be adjusted as needed. Unfortunately, it is common to see gradual weight loss over time and increasing the amount of food offered does not help if the patient has anorexia. A common mistake is to insist that an owner feed only a veterinary therapeutic renal food, even if caloric intake is inadequate. Although avoiding excess dietary protein and minerals is important in patients with CKD, offering only such a food should not be imposed to the detriment of overall nutrient intake. Changing to a different commercial food or homemade food may be a more beneficial solution for some patients. Appetite may be cyclical in patients with advanced CKD, both in respect to overall appetite and food preferences. A dedicated owner is often required and a trial-and-error approach must be used with different foods, food forms (dry vs. moist) and feeding methods (**Box 37-5**).

If caloric intake is insufficient to maintain body weight, clinical recommendations often include a stepwise approach designed to facilitate adequate food intake (Polzin et al, 2005; Polzin, 2007). The first step is to ensure that metabolic and other medical causes of decreased appetite have been corrected including dehydration, gastrointestinal hemorrhage, metabolic acidosis, hypokalemia, anemia, urinary tract infection, dental disease and drug-associated anorexia. Recombinant human erythropoietin[i] has been used successfully to improve clinical well-being of dogs and cats with CKD; improved appetite may precede improvement in hematocrit values in some CKD patients managed with erythropoietin (Cowgill et al, 1998). Significantly improved appetite also has been noted in cats with proteinuria (UPC ≥1), when managed with the ACE inhibitor benazepril[j] (King et al, 2006). When metabolic and other medical causes of anorexia have been excluded or corrected, therapy for uremic gastroenteritis should be initiated with an H_2-antagonist such as ranitidine or famotidine. If inappetence still persists, appetite stimulants such as cyproheptadine or mirtazapine[k] can be attempted; however, results are unpredictable, intermittent and tend to be short-lived (Delaney, 2006). Regardless of the effects of the above treatments on appetite, it is important to confirm that any apparent response to such therapy sufficiently enhances food intake to meet nutritional goals.

If food intake remains inadequate to meet caloric needs for more than three to five days with no trend toward improving, assisted feeding is indicated (Delaney, 2006). Long-term use of percutaneous gastrostomy or esophagostomy tubes has been successful for delivering food, extra water and medications to patients with CKD (Elliott et al, 2000a; Elliott, 2009) (Chapter 25). Anecdotal reports suggest that tube feeding can reverse the progressive weight loss associated with CKD and patients can have extended periods of improved quality of life (Polzin et al, 2005; Polzin, 2007).

SUMMARY

CKD is commonly diagnosed in dogs and cats and increases in frequency with age. A variety of compensatory and adaptive responses are likely involved in the pathogenesis and progression of naturally occurring CKD. The goals of managing patients with CKD are to improve quality and quantity of life. Nutritional management plays a key role in both of these goals. Although there are many available treatments, veterinary therapeutic renal food is the only one that has been shown to prolong survival time and improve quality of life for dogs and cats with CKD. Therefore, nutritional intervention is a critical component of managing patients with CKD. When designing a therapeutic regimen for dogs and cats with CKD, it is helpful to consider key nutritional factors (water, protein, phosphorus, omega-3 fatty acids, antioxidants, sodium, chloride and potas-

Table 37-13. Reassessment of patients with chronic kidney disease.

Physical examination
Abdominal palpation (size and contour of kidneys, presence of ascites)
Blood pressure measurement
Body condition/muscle mass
Body weight
Fundic examination (retinal hemorrhage, detached retina)
Hair and coat quality
Hydration status
Oral examination (uremic odor, ulcers, mucous membrane color)
Laboratory evaluation
Serum biochemistries (urea nitrogen, creatinine, albumin, phosphorus)
Serum electrolytes (calcium, potassium, chloride, sodium, magnesium)
Total serum carbon dioxide or venous blood gases (blood pH, bicarbonate, base excess) to evaluate acid-base status
Urinalysis
Microscopic sediment exam (pyuria or bacteriuria may indicate urinary tract infection)
Urine specific gravity (crude index of tubulointerstitial function)
pH (very crude index of acid-base status)
Urine protein-creatinine ratio (assess proteinuria and response to treatment)
Diagnostic imaging
Abdominal radiographs (assess kidney shape and size, reference L_2 vertebra on ventrodorsal view)
Excretory urogram (assess obstruction due to nephroliths)
Ultrasound (assess kidney and prostate gland, presence of hydronephrosis, hydroureter, uroliths)

sium). In addition to key nutritional factors, it is important to consider available evidence supporting effectiveness of specific veterinary therapeutic renal foods as well as other treatments for CKD. Individual patient needs and responses and owner preferences must also be considered to design an optimal therapeutic regimen. Transitioning to a therapeutic renal food often requires a team approach and effective communication involving the owner and health care team. There are many strategies that can be used to increase therapeutic success and thus improve the lifespan and quality of life for dogs and cats with CKD.

ACKNOWLEDGMENT

The authors and editors thank Dr. David J. Polzin for his contribution to this chapter in the previous edition.

ENDNOTES

a. Sulfosalicylic acid (5%). Ricca Chemical Company, Arlington, TX, USA.
b. E.R.D.-HealthScreen. Heska Corporation, Loveland, CO, USA.
c. VetTest Urine P:C ratio. IDEXX Laboratories, Inc., Westbrook, ME, USA.
d. Prescription Diet u/d Canine. Hill's Pet Nutrition, Inc., Topeka, KS, USA.
e. Prescription Diet k/d Canine. Hill's Pet Nutrition, Inc., Topeka, KS, USA.
f. Whiskas Feline Low Protein Diet. Waltham, Effem, Austria.
g. Whiskas Feline Low Phosphorus, Low Protein. Waltham Veterinary Diet, Masterfoods, Bruck, Austria.
h. Prescription Diet k/d Feline. Hill's Pet Nutrition, Inc., Topeka, KS, USA.
i. Epogen. Amgen Inc., Thousand Oaks, CA, USA.
j. Fortekor. Norvartis Animal Health, Basel, Switzerland.
k. Remeron. Organon, West Orange, NJ, USA.

REFERENCES

The references for **Chapter 37** can be found at www.markmorris.org.

CASE 37-1

Hematemesis in a Shih Tzu

Larry G. Adams, DVM, PhD, Dipl. ACVIM (Small Animal Internal Medicine)
Purdue University
School of Veterinary Medicine
West Lafayette, Indiana, USA

Patient Assessment

The referring veterinarian initially evaluated a four-year-old intact male Shih Tzu for hematuria, anorexia and vomiting. The dog had been diagnosed with chronic kidney disease (CKD) and a possible urinary tract infection. The suspected urinary tract infection had been treated with a combination of trimethoprim and sulfamethoxazole. The dog had also developed thrombocytopenia (platelet count 11 x 10^3/µl [reference range 300 to 900 x 10^3/µl]) and progressive anemia in the month before referral. The trimethoprim-sulfamethoxazole combination was discontinued and the dog was treated with prednisone for thrombocytopenia and suspected immune-mediated hemolytic anemia. The current history included vomiting, hematemesis, hematochezia and decreased appetite. The dog also had a lifelong history of polydipsia and polyuria.

Physical examination revealed 5% dehydration, thin body condition (body condition score 2/5, body weight 5.9 kg), pale mucous membranes, poor coat quality, blood dripping from the penis and a small, irregular left kidney. Rectal examination revealed symmetric, nonpainful prostatomegaly and hematochezia.

Clinicopathologic abnormalities included nonregenerative anemia (hematocrit 15% [reference range 37 to 55%]), azotemia (urea nitrogen 139 mg/dl [reference range 7 to 32 mg/dl], creatinine 3.3 mg/dl [reference range 0.5 to 1.5 mg/dl]) and hyperphosphatemia (8.3 mg/dl [reference range 2.2 to 7.9 mg/dl]). Examination of the blood smear revealed acanthocytosis (1+), poikilocytosis (1+) and occasional schistocytes; spherocytes were not present. The platelet count was within normal limits (341 x 10^3/µl). Urinalysis revealed isosthenuria (specific gravity 1.012) and hematuria (too numerous to count red blood cells per high-power field).

Problems identified included CKD, nonregenerative anemia, prostatomegaly, hematemesis and hematochezia. Additional diagnostic procedures performed included fecal flotation, urine culture, bone marrow aspiration, indirect blood pressure measurement, fundic examination, abdominal radiographs and ultrasound and ultrasound-guided fine-needle aspiration of the prostate gland. Fecal flotation was negative for intestinal parasites. Aerobic urine culture yielded no bacterial growth. Cytologic examination of the bone marrow aspirate revealed erythroid hypoplasia with adequate iron stores. Abdominal radiographs revealed prostatomegaly and small irregular renal margins. Abdominal ultrasonography revealed that the kidneys were bilaterally hyperechoic with very thin renal cortices (3 cm width). Considering the dog's age and breed, these findings were consistent with congenital renal dysplasia. Ultrasonography of the prostate gland revealed diffuse prostatomegaly with multiple small intraprostatic cysts. Cytologic examination of the prostatic aspirates revealed normal prostatic epithelial cells, numerous RBCs and small numbers of neutrophils and macrophages. The ultrasonographic and cytologic findings were consistent with benign prostatic hyperplasia with intraprostatic cyst formation. Aerobic culture of the prostatic aspirate yielded no bacterial growth. Results of indirect measurements of systemic blood pressure were within normal limits. The fundic examination was normal.

Assess the Food and Feeding Method

Originally the dog had been fed a commercial dry dog food; after the diagnosis of CKD was made, a commercial veterinary therapeutic renal food[a] with controlled levels of protein, phosphorus and sodium was recommended. The dog continued to vomit and refused to eat the food, however. The owner had switched to a moist commercial grocery brand dog food supplemented with commercial treats. The moist food was fed twice daily and treats were given multiple times throughout the day to encourage the dog to eat. The dog only ate small amounts of the moist food and some treats during the week before admission.

Questions

1. What are the most likely reasons for this dog's anemia?
2. Why was the magnitude of increase in serum creatinine and urea nitrogen concentrations markedly different?
3. What nutritional recommendations should be made to optimize management of this dog's problems?
4. What other therapies might improve nutritional management of this patient?

Answers and Discussion

1. There were multiple reasons for this dog's anemia. Although the anemia was initially presumed to be an immune-mediated hemolytic anemia, this diagnosis was unlikely at this time. The referring veterinarian submitted a sample to a commercial laboratory for a Coombs test, and results were negative. Red blood cell morphologic examination revealed evidence of fragmentation (which occurs with uremia) and no spherocytes. Likewise, the serum bilirubin concentration remained normal and bilirubinuria was not present. The presumption of an immune-mediated process was based on the concurrent thrombocytopenia and progressive anemia following trimethoprim-sulfamethoxazole therapy. The thrombocytopenia quickly resolved with discontinuation of trimethoprim-sulfamethoxazole therapy and treatment with prednisone. However, anemia worsened progressively. Thrombocytopenia was likely immune-mediated secondary to trimethoprim-sulfamethoxazole therapy; however, there was no evidence of immune-mediated hemolytic anemia.

   Results of bone marrow examination were interpreted to be consistent with a hypoproliferative anemia secondary to relative erythropoietin deficiency. Dogs with moderate to severe CKD consistently have low erythropoietin concentrations relative to the degree of anemia. Therefore, based on the bone marrow findings and concurrent diagnosis of CKD, it was likely that erythropoietin deficiency secondary to CKD was responsible for a major component of the anemia.

   Another contributing factor to the anemia was gastrointestinal (GI) blood loss from uremic gastritis and concurrent prednisone therapy. The dog had a history of hematemesis (fresh blood and vomitus that appeared like "coffee grounds") and hematochezia. Additionally, during hospitalization the dog had marked melena. Uremic gastritis may contribute to GI bleeding, vomiting and anorexia as seen in this dog. Prednisone therapy probably contributed to some of the GI ulceration presumed to be present.
2. There are multiple reasons for the discrepancy in the magnitude of serum creatinine and urea nitrogen concentrations in this dog. Creatinine enters the blood as a result of the nonenzymatic breakdown of phosphocreatine in skeletal muscle. Therefore, the rate of entry of creatinine into the blood depends on muscle mass. Serum creatinine concentration will be lower than would be expected from the glomerular filtration rate (GFR) in a dog with decreased muscle mass. Therefore, the serum creatinine concentra-

tion was probably low in this dog relative to serum urea nitrogen concentration, thereby overestimating relative GFR and underestimating the severity of renal dysfunction.

The urea nitrogen concentration was probably higher relative to the GFR in this dog. The rate of urea production depends on dietary protein intake, rate of production by the liver and catabolism of endogenous body protein stores. This dog was currently being fed relatively high levels of dietary protein, which would contribute to greater production of nitrogenous waste products such as urea. GI hemorrhage mimics a high-protein meal resulting in an increased rate of urea synthesis by the liver. Also, administration of corticosteroids results in catabolism of body proteins, which releases nitrogen-containing amino acids. Urea is produced when these amino acids are catabolized for energy. Therefore, the rate of urea production in this dog was probably increased from GI bleeding and catabolism induced by prednisone therapy. The net result is that the urea nitrogen concentration was increased relative to the serum creatinine concentration and actual GFR. Increased production of potentially toxic nitrogenous breakdown products (represented by urea) probably worsened uremic signs in this dog.

3. This dog was classified as having CKD, most likely stage 3; however, final staging should be based on a stable serum creatinine concentration obtained after correction of dehydration. Feeding a veterinary therapeutic renal food[a] to dogs with stage 2 to 3 CKD has been associated with prolonged survival time, decreased uremic episodes and improved quality of life compared with feeding a maintenance food that contains higher amounts of protein, phosphorus and sodium. Avoiding excessive protein intake is important in advanced stages of CKD to control clinical signs of uremia. However, attempting to immediately feed any food to a patient with anorexia and vomiting from severe uremic gastritis is likely to fail. Therefore, our recommendation was to treat the uremic crisis first, and then reintroduce an appropriate food after the GI signs were controlled. To avoid food aversion associated with hospitalization or nausea in some patients (especially cats and small dogs), it may be more appropriate to feed a food for mature adult dogs during hospitalization and then have the owner gradually transition to the therapeutic renal food at home.
4. Other therapies to treat the consequences of the uremic syndrome are indicated when a dog has moderate to advanced CKD (late stage 3 and stage 4). Therapy should be aimed at controlling uremic gastritis, secondary renal hyperparathyroidism, anemia and hypertension (if present). Uremic gastritis is thought to occur secondary to hypergastrinemia in dogs with advanced stages of CKD. Therapy designed to minimize uremic gastritis and gastric and duodenal ulceration includes H_2-receptor antagonists (i.e., cimetidine, famotidine, etc.), misoprostol, omeprazole and sucralfate. Therapy designed to minimize secondary renal hyperparathyroidism includes avoiding excessive phosphorus intake, intestinal phosphate-binding agents and potentially low-dose calcitriol therapy after correction of hyperphosphatemia. The most effective method of treating the anemia of CKD is to administer recombinant human erythropoietin (r-HuEPO). Therapy with r-HuEPO is reserved for patients with moderately severe anemia (i.e., hematocrit values <20 to 25% in dogs).

Therapy Including Feeding Plan

The dog was initially treated with intravenous fluid therapy, intravenous cimetidine[b] and oral misoprostol[c] and sucralfate.[d] Food was withheld for 48 hours until the vomiting ceased. The dog was then offered a food for mature adults with controlled levels of protein, phosphorus and sodium, divided into four small meals per day. The amount of food was initially calculated to meet the resting energy requirement for an ideal body weight of 7.5 kg.

Progress Notes

The vomiting, hematemesis, hematochezia and melena resolved. Azotemia improved with intravenous fluid therapy; serum urea nitrogen concentration decreased to 58 mg/dl and serum creatinine decreased to 2.1 mg/dl. However, hematocrit decreased to 11%. These findings are consistent with stage 3 CKD. The dog was discharged after five days of hospitalization while the owners considered castration. Nutritional recommendations were to gradually transition to a veterinary therapeutic renal food[a] or a homemade food that avoided excessive levels of protein and phosphorus. Therapy was continued at home including oral famotidine, oral aluminum hydroxide and subcutaneous injections of r-HuEPO[e] three times per week.

Reevaluation nine days after discharge from the hospital revealed the dog's attitude and appetite had improved. The dog had been chewing its tail for two days; however, and the distal 4 cm of the tail were dark blue to black, had several scabs and lacked pain sensation. The tail lesions were thought to be due to ischemic necrosis related to uremic vasculitis. Serum creatinine concentration was 3.1 mg/dl and urea nitrogen concentration was 111 mg/dl. Hematocrit had improved to 19%. The dog was given intravenous fluid therapy in preparation for surgical amputation of the distal tail. Castration was also recommended to treat the benign prostatic hyperplasia with intraprostatic cysts. The serum urea nitrogen and creatinine concentrations decreased with fluid therapy and surgery was performed for tail amputation and castration (**Figure 1**). The dog was discharged with similar treatment recommendations to those listed above. In addition, a combination of amoxicillin and clavulanic acid[f] was administered for two weeks as a prophylactic antibiotic for the tail amputation, and low-dose calcitriol[g] therapy was initiated. Calcitriol was administered to decrease serum parathyroid hormone concentration associated with renal secondary hyperparathyroidism.

The dog's condition remained stable with this combination of nutritional and medical therapy for several months. The dog continued to eat the veterinary therapeutic renal food well and gained weight (body weight 7.5 kg). The coat returned to normal quality (**Figure 2**). The anemia resolved and the r-HuEPO was decreased to a maintenance dose twice weekly. The magnitude of

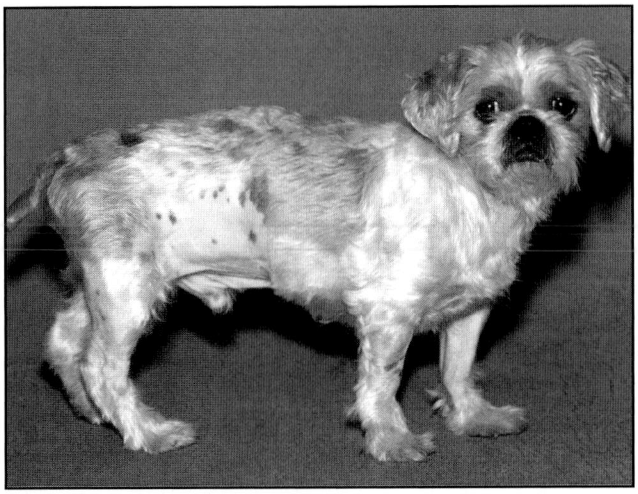

Figure 1. Postoperative picture of a four-year-old male Shih Tzu with CKD and probable uremic vasculitis involving the tail. The tail was amputated and a castration was performed to manage concurrent prostatic disease.

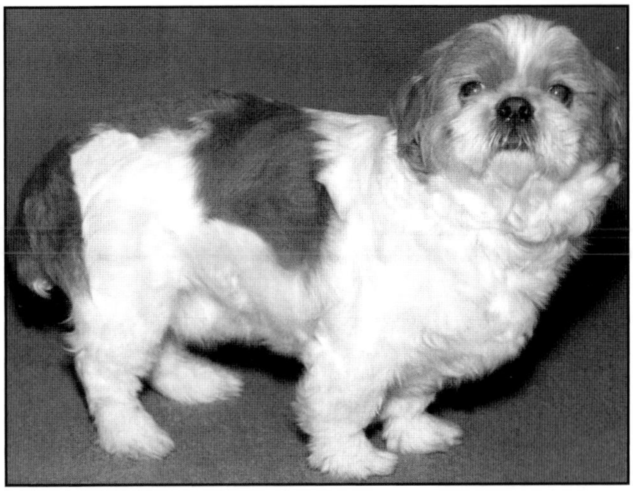

Figure 2. A four-year-old castrated male Shih Tzu two months after therapy was instituted for CKD. The dog's coat quality had returned to normal and overall clinical condition was improved.

azotemia progressively increased over the next six months. Subcutaneous fluid therapy (100 ml every other day) was added when serum creatinine concentration exceeded 5 mg/dl. The dog died of progressive CKD 11 months after initial evaluation.

Endnotes

a. Prescription Diet k/d Canine. Hill's Pet Nutrition, Inc., Topeka, KS, USA.
b. Tagamet. SmithKline Beecham Pharmaceuticals, Philadelphia, PA, USA.
c. Cytotec. GD Searle & Co, Chicago, IL, USA.
d. Carafate. Marion Merrell Dow, Kansas City, MO, USA.
e. Epogen. Amgen Inc., Thousand Oaks, CA, USA.
f. Clavamox. Pfizer Animal Health, Exton, PA, USA.
g. Rocaltrol. Roche Laboratories, Nutley, NJ, USA.

Bibliography

Brown SA. Management of chronic kidney disease. In: Elliot JA, Grauer GF, eds. BSAVA Manual of Canine and Feline Nephrology and Urology, 2nd ed. Gloucester, UK: British Small Animal Veterinary Association, 2007; 223-230.

Kerl ME, Langston CE. Treatment of anemia in renal failure. In: Bogaura JD, Twedt DC, eds. Kirk's Current Veterinary Therapy XIV. St. Louis, MO: Saunders Elsevier, 2009; 914-918.

Polzin DJ, Osborne CA, Ross S. Evidence-based management of chronic kidney disease. In: Bogaura JD, Twedt DC, eds. Kirk's Current Veterinary Therapy XIV. St. Louis, MO; Saunders Elsevier, 2009; 872-879.

Polzin DJ, Ross S, Osborne CA. Calcitriol. In: Bogaura JD, Twedt DC, eds. Kirk's Current Veterinary Therapy XIV. St. Louis, MO: Saunders Elsevier, 2009; 892- 895.

Ross S, Osborne CA, Kirk CA, et al. Clinical evaluation of dietary modification for treatment of spontaneous chronic kidney disease in cats. Journal of the American Veterinary Medical Association 2006; 229: 949-957.

CASE 37-2

Weight Loss in a Cat

David J. Polzin, DVM, PhD, Dipl. ACVIM (Small Animal Internal Medicine)
College of Veterinary Medicine
University of Minnesota
St Paul, Minnesota, USA

Patient Assessment

A 13-year-old spayed female domestic shorthair cat was examined for weight loss of several months' duration. The owners had also noticed increased water intake and urine volume, decreased appetite and a few episodes of vomiting in the last month. The cat also seemed weak. Characteristics of the feces were unknown because the family dog often consumed any fecal material deposited in the litter box. The cat usually remained indoors but did spend some time outdoors during the summer.

Physical examination revealed a very thin cat, with a body weight of 2.4 kg and a body condition score of 1/5. According to the medical record, the cat weighed 5 kg four years earlier. Moderate accumulation of dental calculus was noted. Abdominal palpation revealed excess accumulation of gas in the intestines and a small left kidney; the right kidney could not be palpated.

Results of a complete blood count revealed anemia (i.e., decreased total erythrocyte count, hemoglobin and hematocrit). Significant serum biochemistry profile findings included azotemia, hyperphosphatemia, low normal serum potassium concentration and metabolic acidosis (**Table 1**). Serum thyroxine (T_4) concentration was normal. Urinalysis was normal except for a urine specific gravity of 1.009. The tentative diagnosis was stage 4 chronic kidney disease (CKD).

Assess the Food and Feeding Method

The cat was normally fed a mixture of two different commercial specialty brand dry foods; one was a "light" food and the other was a food formulated for older cats (mature adult food). The combination of dry foods was offered free choice. The owners noted that the cat was still eating but overall appetite had decreased.

Questions

1. What are the key nutritional factors to consider in cats with CKD?
2. Prepare a treatment and feeding plan for this cat.
3. What parameters should be monitored if this patient goes home with conservative management?

Answers and Discussion

1. Key nutritional factors to consider in cats with CKD include water, protein, phosphorus, sodium, chloride, potassium, omega-3 fatty acids and antioxidants. Adequate water intake is important to maintain hydration, blood volume and renal perfusion in a patient with polyuria. Parenteral fluids are indicated if vomiting, diarrhea, dehydration, blood volume contraction and renal hypoperfusion are clinically important. Avoiding excess dietary phosphorus and protein will help reduce clinical signs of uremia and may slow progression of kidney disease. Compared with feeding a maintenance food, feeding a therapeutic renal food[a] has been associated with prolonged survival time and decreased occurrence of uremic episodes in cats with CKD. Increased intake of omega-3 fatty acids and antioxidants has beneficial effects in CKD. Avoiding excess dietary sodium and chloride may help control systemic hypertension, which is a common sequela to CKD in cats. Potassium is also an important nutrient because hypokalemia is common in cats with CKD and may lead directly to clinical signs in some cats. Adequate energy intake in the form of non-protein calories is important in this cat to promote weight gain and minimize further catabolism of lean body mass.
2. Parenteral fluid therapy is indicated to promote excretion of nitrogenous wastes and improve overall hydration status. Water should be available free choice at all times. The food offered to this cat should avoid excessive phosphorus, protein, sodium and chloride while providing adequate amounts of potassium and increased omega-3 fatty acids and antioxidants. A commercial veterinary therapeutic food or homemade food designed for cats with CKD should meet these nutritional goals. Because of nausea associated with uremia, the food should be offered in small, frequent meals. The daily energy requirement (DER) should be calculated to promote weight gain (i.e., 1.2 x resting energy requirement [RER] for an ideal body weight of 4.5 kg) after a normal appetite has returned. Enteral or parenteral nutritional support may be necessary if the cat is eating less than its calculated RER per day. Adjunctive medical therapy including antiemetics and H_2-receptor antagonists for uremic gastropathy and erythropoietin for anemia is indicated to improve the overall well being of the patient.
3. Clinical and biochemical parameters should be monitored two to four weeks after implementing nutritional recommendations. A good response to conservative management includes decreased vomiting, increased appetite and activity level, weight gain, decreased serum urea nitrogen and phosphorus concentrations and increased plasma bicarbonate concentration (or total CO_2). Plasma bicarbonate concentration should be maintained within the laboratory reference range. Alkalinization therapy should be

considered if the plasma bicarbonate or total CO_2 concentration remains below the recommended range. Phosphorus binders should be considered if hyperphosphatemia persists despite avoiding excessive dietary phosphorus. Retinal examinations are important to evaluate for end-organ changes associated with systemic hypertension. The owner should be encouraged to closely monitor the cat's daily food intake to ensure that adequate energy is being consumed.

Table 1. Selected serum biochemistry values from a cat with vomiting and weight loss.

Parameters	Day 1	Day 57	Day 160	Reference values
Urea nitrogen (mg/dl)	104	78	66	10-32
Creatinine (mg/dl)	7.4	5.4	5.0	0.1-2.1
Phosphorus (mg/dl)	8.2	5.4	5.2	2.4-6.1
Potassium (mg/dl)	3.4	4.7	4.8	3.2-6.2
Total CO_2 (mmol/l)	12.8	20.0	18.5	18-21

Progress Notes

The cat was stabilized with parenteral fluid therapy and was discharged from the hospital. The owner was instructed to gradually transition to a commercially available veterinary therapeutic renal food.[a] The DER was calculated at 1.2 x RER for an ideal body weight of 4.5 kg to promote weight gain. This was approximately 250 kcal (1,046 kJ) or one-half cup of dry food daily. Subcutaneous fluids (120 ml/24 hours) and oral famotidine were administered at home.

Two months later (Day 57), the cat was examined and found to have gained weight (body weight 3.1 kg). Serum urea nitrogen, creatinine and phosphorus concentrations were decreased and serum potassium and total CO_2 concentrations were increased (**Table 1**). These serum biochemistry changes persisted when the cat was reevaluated on Day 160; however, body weight was not recorded at that time. The owners reported that the cat was active, maintained a good appetite and had no evidence of vomiting when the combination of dietary therapy and subcutaneous fluids was used.

The owners did not return with the cat again until one year later. The cat was experiencing an acute uremic crisis and was euthanatized at the owners' request without further diagnostic or postmortem evaluation.

Endnote

a. Prescription Diet k/d Feline. Hill's Pet Nutrition, Inc., Topeka, KS, USA.

Bibliography

Elliott DA. Gastrostomy tube feeding in kidney disease. In: Bogaura JD, Twedt DC, eds. Kirk's Current Veterinary Therapy XIV. St. Louis, MO: Saunders Elsevier, 2009; 906-910.

Jacob F, Polzin DJ, Osborne CA, et al. Clinical evaluation of dietary modification for treatment of spontaneous chronic renal failure in dogs. Journal of the American Veterinary Medical Association 2002; 220: 1163-1170.

Polzin DJ, Osborne CA, Ross S. Evidence-based management of chronic kidney disease. In: Bogaura JD, Twedt DC, eds. Kirk's Current Veterinary Therapy XIV. St. Louis, MO: Saunders Elsevier, 2009; 872-879

CASE 37-3

Generalized Weakness in a Cat

Timothy A. Allen, DVM, Dipl. ACVIM (Small Animal Internal Medicine)
Lawrence, Kansas, USA

Patient Assessment

A 13.5-year-old spayed female domestic shorthair cat was examined for lethargy, weakness and anorexia of two days' duration. The owner reported that the cat was so weak that it could not lift its head. Physical examination revealed a thin cat (body condition score [BCS] 1/5) weighing 2.2 kg. The coat was dull and unkempt. Generalized weakness, cervical ventriflexion and ataxia were noted. Small, irregular kidneys were evident during abdominal palpation. Dehydration was suspected on the basis of dry mucous membranes.

The cat was hospitalized and a blood sample obtained for a complete blood count and serum biochemistry profile. Urine was obtained by cystocentesis for urinalysis. The complete blood count was normal except for a low hematocrit. Serum biochemistry profile abnormalities included azotemia, hypernatremia, hyperchloremia, hypokalemia, decreased total CO_2 and increased total protein concentration (**Table 1**). Urinalysis results included a urine specific gravity of 1.013, 2+ protein on the dipstick and normal sediment examination.

On the basis of renal azotemia (i.e., increased urea nitrogen and creatinine values with low urine specific gravity and small, irregular kidneys) with associated dehydration and evidence of blood volume contraction (i.e., tacky mucous membranes and increased total protein, sodium and chloride concentrations), anemia (i.e., low hematocrit with dehydration), metabolic acidosis (i.e., decreased TCO_2) and hypokalemia, the cat was diagnosed with chronic kidney disease (CKD).

Assess the Food and Feeding Method

The cat was fed a mixture of commercial semi-moist and dry foods. These foods and water were always available.

Questions

1. What is the cause of this cat's generalized weakness and cervical ventriflexion?
2. What is the likely cause of the hypokalemia?
3. Outline a treatment and feeding plan for this cat.
4. What parameters should be monitored to assess response to treatment?
5. How would you classify the stage of CKD in this cat using the International Renal Interest Society staging scheme (**Table 37-1**)?

Answers and Discussion

1. Potassium depletion results in morphologic and functional changes in muscle and kidney, alterations in carbohydrate metabolism and protein synthesis and disturbances in acid-base balance. Muscle weakness develops when the serum potassium concentration falls below 3.0 mEq (mmol)/l and frank rhabdomyolysis or life-threatening respiratory muscle paralysis may occur when the serum potassium concentration is less than 2.0 mEq/l.

   Clinical signs of hypokalemic polymyopathy include appendicular muscle weakness, reluctance to walk or a stiff stilted gait with forelimb hypermetria and a broad-based hind-limb stance and apparent pain on palpation of muscles. The most dramatic myopathic finding is a characteristic cervical ventriflexion due to weakness of the extensor muscles of the neck. Similar ventriflexion has been observed in cats with thiamin deficiency and myasthenia gravis. Other neuromuscular signs may be observed in some cats, including bilateral mydriasis, disorientation, staggering and falling.
2. In retrospective studies, hypokalemia was found in approximately 20% of cats with CKD and CKD was the most common associated disorder in cats with hypokalemia. The hypokalemia observed in cats with CKD presumably is caused by a combination of inappetence, weight loss with muscle wasting and polyuria. A clinically distinct syndrome of polymyopathy and nephropathy characterized by hypokalemia, azotemia, impaired renal concentrating ability and lymphoplasmacytic tubulointerstitial nephritis has been documented to occur in cats fed a food low in potassium and high in acid content; however, the role of hypokalemia as a cause of CKD is uncertain.
3. The initial management of cats with clinically apparent potassium-depletion requires diligent potassium supplementation by oral and intravenous routes. Potassium chloride usually is added to parenteral fluids for intravenous administration. Infusion of potassium-containing fluids initially may be associated with a further decrease in serum potassium concentration as a result of dilution, increased distal renal tubular flow and cellular uptake of potassium, especially if the fluid contains glucose. Selecting a fluid that does not contain glucose, administering fluids at an appropriate rate and beginning oral potassium supplementation as soon as possible can minimize this complication.

   Potassium gluconate is recommended for oral supplementation of hypokalemic cats because potassium chloride and potassium bicarbonate are often unpalatable. The recommended initial oral dosage of potassium gluconate is 2 to 6 mEq potassium gluconate/day divided into two or three doses; the dose should be adjusted based on clinical response and serial analyses of serum potassium concentration. Clinical improvement is usually seen after one to three days of treatment. Feeding a commercial veterinary therapeutic renal food, which contains increased amounts of potassium, may be all that is need to maintain normokalemia. However, oral supplementation with potassium gluconate should be considered if food alone does not maintain serum potassium concentration above 4.0 mEq/l. Additional studies are needed to determine whether routine potassium supplementation is indicated in all cats with CKD, regardless of serum potassium concentration.
4. It is difficult to estimate the amount of potassium required to reestablish normal potassium balance in a given patient. Thus, the amount of potassium required must be determined by judicious supplementation and serial measurement of serum potassium concentrations during treatment and recovery. Treatment usually results in resolution of muscle weakness within one to two weeks, weight gain and an improved coat. During recovery, renal function (i.e., urea nitrogen and creatinine concentrations) and anemia (i.e., hematocrit values and red blood cell count) may stabilize and improve in some cats. Persistent CKD is managed using conservative medical and nutritional management.
5. Staging of CKD should be performed on the basis of stable serum creatinine concentrations (at least two measurements approximately two weeks apart) obtained while the patient is well hydrated. Because the initial serum biochemistry profile was obtained while the cat was clinically dehydrated, the serum creatinine may be higher because of an additional prerenal component of the azotemia. Therefore staging should be determined after rehydration and measurement of stable serum creatinine concentrations. The cat was eventually classified as having stage 2 CKD (**Table 1**).

Progress Notes

An intravenous catheter was inserted in the cat's jugular vein and 20 ml of lactated Ringer's solution was administered per hour during the first eight hours. After eight hours, the rate was reduced to 12 ml/hour. Sixteen mEq of potassium chloride were added to each liter of lactated Ringer's solution to produce a final potassium concentration of 20 mEq/l. During the first day of hospitalization, 4 mEq of potassium gluconate gel (Tumil-K[a]) were administered per os every 12 hours. Water was offered free choice. Body weight was measured daily using the same pediatric scale, and urine output was estimated by weighing the litter box before and after voiding.

Table 1. Selected serum biochemistry values from a cat with generalized weakness.

Parameters	Day 1	Day 2	Day 3	Day 4	Day 6	Day 25	Reference values
Hematocrit (%)	31	20.3	ND	ND	ND	ND	30-45
Hemoglobin (g/dl)	9.9	6.7	ND	ND	ND	ND	8-15
Total protein (g/dl)	7.9	7.1	6.1	6.3	6.5	ND	6.1-7.7
Urea nitrogen (mg/dl)	53	58	47	48	51	36	15-25
Creatinine (mg/dl)	3.0	3.1	2.0	1.9	2.1	2.3	0.8-1.8
Sodium (mmol/l)	165	167	160	158	153	152	140-157
Potassium (mmol/l)	3.0	3.4	4.2	5.5	4.6	5.2	3.8-5.3
Chloride (mmol/l)	137	134	124	122	116	118	115-128
Total CO_2 (mmol/l)	11	17	23	29	28	23	18-23

Key: ND = not done.

The cat's weakness was noticeably improved by Day 2. The cat's resting energy requirement (RER) was calculated at its estimated ideal body weight of 3.5 kg (RER at 3.5 kg = 175 kcal [732 kJ]). The cat was offered small quantities of dry and moist forms of a commercial food for mature adult cats with controlled amounts of protein and phosphorus, every three to four hours. The cat was consuming sufficient food to meet its RER by Day 4.

The azotemia, hypokalemia, acidosis and muscle strength progressively improved over the next three days (**Table 1**). Six days after initial hospitalization, the patient was discharged to the owner's care with instructions to gradually transition to feeding a dry veterinary therapeutic renal food[b] and to administer 4 mEq potassium gluconate gel every 12 hours. The quantity of food was increased to a daily energy requirement of 1.4 x RER.

The owner reported that the cat was bright, alert, active and eating well with normal muscle strength 25 days after initial examination. Physical examination was normal except the patient was still underweight (body weight 2.8 kg, BCS 2/5) and the kidneys were still palpably small and irregular. Results of a serum biochemistry profile included mild azotemia, normal serum electrolyte concentrations and normal acid-base status (**Table 1**). Oral potassium gluconate was discontinued and the dry veterinary therapeutic renal food was continued. The owners asked about purchasing moist food from the grocery store to add to the dry veterinary therapeutic renal food. Because most grocery brand foods contain excessive phosphorus and protein compared with therapeutic renal foods, this was not recommended. Instead, several cans of the veterinary therapeutic renal food were dispensed so the owners could determine if the cat preferred moist food in addition to the dry food.

Endnotes

a. Daniels Pharmaceuticals Inc., St. Petersburg, FL, USA.
b. Prescription Diet k/d Feline. Hill's Pet Nutrition, Inc., Topeka, KS, USA.

Bibliography

DiBartola SP, Buffington CA, Chew DJ, et al. Development of chronic renal failure in cats fed a commercial diet. Journal of the American Veterinary Medical Association 1993; 202: 744-751.

Dow SW, LeCouteur RA, Fettman MJ, et al. Hypokalemia in cats: 186 cases (1984-1987). Journal of the American Veterinary Medical Association 1989; 194: 1604-1608.

Dow SW, LeCouteur RA, Fettman MJ, et al. Potassium depletion in cats: Hypokalemic polymyopathy. Journal of the American Veterinary Medical Association 1987; 191: 1569-1575.

Elliott J, Barber PJ. Feline chronic renal failure: Clinical findings in 80 cases diagnosed between 1992 and 1995. Journal of Small Animal Practice 1998; 39: 78-85.

Theisen SK, DiBartola SP, Radin J, et al. Muscle potassium content and potassium gluconate supplementation in normokalemic cats with naturally occurring chronic renal failure. Journal of Veterinary Internal Medicine 1997; 11: 212-217.

CASE 37-4

Chronic Kidney Disease in a Miniature Schnauzer with Multiple Problems

S. Dru Forrester, DVM, MS, Dipl. ACVIM (Small Animal Internal Medicine)
Hill's Scientific Affairs
Topeka, Kansas, USA

Patient Assessment

A 12-year-old spayed female miniature schnauzer was presented for evaluation of vulvar discharge, possible polydipsia and occasional vomiting that began within the past month. Laboratory evaluation performed by the referring veterinarian revealed mild azotemia. The dog was currently receiving a low dose of enrofloxacin[a] once daily. The dog's appetite was normal. However, the owner thought it was losing weight. Physical examination abnormalities included a grade III/VI holosystolic murmur (left side), purulent vulvar discharge and vulvar erythema, malodorous breath and markedly decreased body condition (body condition score = 1.5/5); body weight was 5.5 kg (**Figure 1**).

Initial diagnostic evaluation included a CBC, serum biochemistry profile, urinalysis and diagnostic imaging (**Table 1**). Significant abnormal laboratory findings included leukocytosis characterized by mature neutrophilia, azotemia, low-normal serum albumin, inappropriately concentrated urine (specific gravity = 1.028), proteinuria (3+ dipstick) and hematuria (60 to 70 RBCs/hpf). Thoracic radiographs revealed no significant abnormal findings. Abdominal ultrasound revealed a mildly enlarged left renal pelvis. Additional diagnostic tests were performed to further evaluate initial abnormal findings. Urine culture revealed growth of *Escherichia coli* (800 colony forming units/ml of urine) and the urine protein-creatinine (UPC) ratio was 4.3. Systolic blood pressure measured indirectly by Doppler technique was 180 mm Hg. Results of an assay for canine pancreatic lipase immunoreactivity were normal.

On the basis of all findings, CKD, hypertension and urinary tract infection (UTI) were diagnosed. Mitral valvular disease was also considered likely. CKD was determined to be stage 2, P, Hnc (P = proteinuric, Hnc = high risk for target organ damage due to hypertension but no current evidence of complications [**Table 37-1**]). Pyelonephritis was suspected because of renal ultrasound findings and presence of leukocytosis. There was no evidence of cardiac decompensation on thoracic radiographs. Active pancreatitis was considered unlikely.

Assess the Food and Feeding Method

Because of several episodes of apparent pancreatitis in the past, the patient was eating a commercial dry, low-fat veterinary therapeutic weight-reduction food.[b] Water was available free choice at all times.

Questions

1. What treatment is indicated for UTI and hypertension in this dog?
2. What treatment recommendations are appropriate for managing CKD in this patient?
3. What key nutritional factors should be considered in a dog with a history of pancreatitis?
4. What are some guidelines for managing patients with concurrent disorders such as CKD and pancreatitis?

Answers and Discussion

1. Because this dog has CKD, UTI and a dilated left renal pelvis, treatment for pyelonephritis is indicated. An extended course of treatment is needed; therefore, an appropriate antimicrobial should be selected based on susceptibility testing. In addition, urine cultures should be done periodically during and after treatment to confirm therapeutic success.

   Controlling hypertension is indicated because this patient is at severe risk for target organ damage because systolic blood pressure is ≥180 mm Hg. Hypertension may worsen progression of CKD in dogs and has been associated with increased risk of uremic crisis and death in dogs with naturally occurring CKD. Treatment of hypertension also is indicated to avoid worsening of mitral valve disease. Excessive dietary intake of sodium should be avoided; however, selection of an appropriate food should be based on

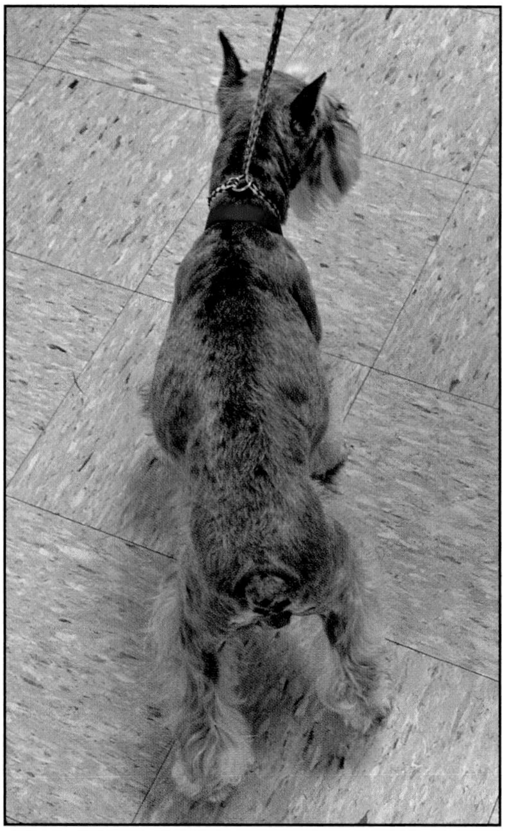

Figure 1. A 12-year-old miniature schnauzer that presented for evaluation of multiple problems.

other patient factors such as presence of CKD in this case. In dogs, administration of an angiotensin-converting enzyme (ACE) inhibitor usually is the initial treatment of choice for hypertension. Because ACE inhibitors preferentially dilate the efferent arteriole, they have the potential to decrease glomerular filtration rate and worsen azotemia. Therefore starting at a lower dose and gradually increasing it over time while monitoring renal function may be helpful.

2. It is difficult to definitively localize the proteinuria as of renal origin from CKD vs. postrenal from the UTI. UTIs add plasma proteins to the urine after glomerular filtration, thus postrenal proteinuria is recognized by the presence of proteinuria with hematuria and pyuria. The urine sediment examination only revealed hematuria without pyuria, most likely because of current antibiotic administration. Therefore, postrenal proteinuria was less likely. The proteinuria was confirmed to be of renal origin by follow-up urinalyses that showed persistence of proteinuria despite resolution of the UTI.

Table 1. Results of initial laboratory evaluation including CBC, serum biochemistries and urinalysis.

Parameters	Day 1	Reference ranges
Hematocrit (%)	46	37-62
Total white blood cell count (x 1,000/µl)	21.5	5.4-16.6
Segmented neutrophils (x 1,000/µl)	18.92	3.24-10.7
Bands (x 1,000/µl)	0.215	0.0-0.25
Lymphocytes (x 1,000/µl)	1.29	0.75-5.65
Monocytes (x 1,000/µl)	1.075	0.1-1.19
Glucose (mg/dl)	119	89-135
Urea nitrogen (mg/dl)	67	8-27
Creatinine (mg/dl)	1.6	0.6-1.4
Phosphorus (mg/dl)	5.2	2.6-6.0
Calcium (mg/dl)	10.1	9.5-11.6
Total protein (g/dl)	6.5	5.4-7.2
Albumin (g/dl)	2.8	2.7-3.8
Total CO_2 (mmol/l)	19	18-24
Potassium (mg/dl)	4.6	3.5-5.5
Amylase (IU/l)	985	338-1,007
Lipase (IU/l)	1,245	268-1,796

Proteinuria occurs as a result of CKD; however, it may also play a role in the pathogenesis of progressive CKD. In one study, an initial UPC ≥1 in dogs with CKD was associated with greater risk of having a uremic crisis or dying compared with dogs that had a UPC <1. Dogs with proteinuria should be fed a reduced-protein food designed for patients with CKD, whether azotemia exists or not (**Box 37-2**). Patients should be monitored periodically (e.g., every two to four weeks initially) to determine the optimal quantity of dietary protein that maintains lean body mass and decreases magnitude of proteinuria, as measured by UPC ratios. Patients should receive enough calories to achieve and maintain ideal body weight and condition. Administration of an ACE inhibitor also is indicated for dogs with proteinuria due to glomerular disease. In a study of dogs with naturally occurring idiopathic glomerulonephritis, treatment with enalapril was associated with significant improvement compared with dogs that received a placebo. Both groups also received low-dose aspirin and a veterinary therapeutic renal food.[c] Resorption of excessive amounts of protein from the tubular filtrate in dogs with CKD and proteinuria may damage the tubules resulting in progressive tubulointerstitial injury. (See Renal Oxidative Stress in the Etiopathogenesis section.)

3. This dog does not have active pancreatitis. However, long-term management should include feeding foods with relatively less fat that avoid excessive protein because both are stimuli for pancreatic secretion. Feeding a moderate-fat food (≤15% dry matter [DM]) has been recommended for patients recovering from pancreatitis, whereas a low-fat food (≤10% DM) may be more appropriate for those with concurrent obesity or hypertriglyceridemia. Clinical studies have not evaluated effects of feeding different amounts of fat on recurrence of pancreatitis. One approach is to feed less fat than the patient was eating when the most recent episode of pancreatitis occurred.
4. Patients with multiple disorders can be challenging to manage, especially when treatment for one condition may not be ideal for a concurrent disease. Feeding a veterinary therapeutic renal food is indicated for this patient. These foods often contain increased amounts of fat, which would not be ideal for a patient at risk for pancreatitis. One approach for this patient would be to recommend a renal food with the lowest fat content. In general, dry foods contain less fat; therefore, feeding a dry food may be preferable as long as the dog is able to maintain hydration. If the patient does not respond well to a commercially available food, an alternative would be to formulate a homemade food. In these cases, it is recommended to seek input from a board-certified clinical nutritionist who can help design a nutritionally balanced maintenance food tailored for that patients' particular needs.

Progress Notes

Enrofloxacin (5 to 7 mg/kg per os twice daily for six to eight weeks) was recommended to treat possible pyelonephritis. This antimicrobial was selected because the organism was susceptible based on urine culture and sensitivity results. A low number of organisms most likely grew on the initial urine culture because the dog was receiving a low dose of antimicrobial at the time urine was collected. A follow-up urine culture was recommended one week after beginning treatment, one week after completing antimicrobial treatment and once monthly for three months thereafter to ensure eradication of infection.

Additional treatment included administration of an ACE inhibitor, H_2-receptor antagonist and a veterinary therapeutic renal food. Benazepril[d] (0.25 to 0.5 mg/kg orally once or twice daily) was begun to manage hypertension and proteinuria. To avoid potential for worsening azotemia, it was recommended to begin at the lowest dose once daily and gradually increase while monitoring serum creatinine and urea nitrogen concentrations. Cimetidine[e] (5 to 10 mg/kg orally, twice daily) was prescribed to help manage possible uremic gastritis. All dry versions of commercially available veterinary therapeutic renal foods from major companies contain <20% DM fat, which would be appropriate for a dog with a history of pancreatitis (**Table 2**). The dog's current food contained approximately 9% DM fat; therefore, it was recommended to initially transition to a veterinary therapeutic renal food[f] formulated for early kidney disease that contained a similar amount of fat.

The amount of new food to feed was based on an estimate of the patient's resting energy requirement (RER) at its ideal weight (7.3 kg) and multiplying it by a factor of 1.2 (assumes a small amount of physical activity) to determine the daily energy requirement (DER). RER at 7.3 kg = 311 kcal (1,300 kJ); DER = RER x 1.2 = 373 kcal (1,561 kJ). The as fed energy density of the food was 358 kcal/8-oz. measuring cup. The daily amount to feed is estimated by dividing the DER (373 kcal) by the as fed energy density (358 kcal/cup), which equals slightly more than one cup of food daily. The patient was offered small quantities of the food every three to four hours.

The owners were instructed to return the dog to their primary care veterinarian seven to 10 days after discharge for physical examination, urine culture, blood pressure evaluation and measurement of serum biochemistries and UPC ratio. Long-term monitoring was recommended every one to four months indefinitely to assess effectiveness of treatment and make adjustments as needed. The dog's condition continued to decline over the next six months and the patient was euthanized after it began having seizures; a postmortem examination was not done.

Table 2. Fat content of canine therapeutic renal foods.

Foods	Form	Fat (%)*
Hill's Prescription Diet g/d Canine	Can	10.8
Hill's Prescription Diet g/d Canine	Dry	11.0
Hill's Prescription Diet k/d Canine	Dry	19.4
Hill's Prescription Diet k/d Canine	Can	26.7
Iams Eukanuba Veterinary Formula Renal Early Stage	Dry	13.7
Purina Veterinary Diets NF KidNey Function Canine Formula	Dry	15.7
Purina Veterinary Diets NF KidNey Function Canine Formula	Can	27.4
Royal Canin Veterinary Diet Renal LP	Can	29.9
Royal Canin Veterinary Diet Renal LP 11	Dry	14.0
Royal Canin Veterinary Diet Renal MP 14	Dry	16.5

*Dry matter basis.

Endnotes

a. Baytril. Bayer HealthCare, Shawnee Mission, KS, USA.
b. Prescription Diet r/d Canine. Hill's Pet Nutrition, Inc., Topeka, KS, USA.
c. Prescription Diet k/d Canine. Hill's Pet Nutrition, Inc., Topeka, KS, USA.
d. Fortekor. Norvartis Animal Health, Basel, Switzerland.
e. Tagamet. SmithKline Beecham Pharmaceuticals, Philadelphia, PA, USA.
f. Prescription Diet g/d Canine. Hill's Pet Nutrition, Inc., Topeka, KS, USA.

Bibliography

Brown S, Atkins C, Bagley R, et al. Guidelines for the identification, evaluation, and management of systemic hypertension in dogs and cats. Journal of Veterinary Internal Medicine 2007; 21: 542-558. (Article can be downloaded from www.acvim.org. See Journal of Veterinary Internal Medicine, Consensus Statements).

Grauer GF, Greco DS, Getzy DM, et al. Effects of enalapril versus placebo as a treatment for canine idiopathic glomerulonephritis. Journal of Veterinary Internal Medicine 2000; 14: 526-533.

Jacob F, Osborne CA, Polzin DJ, et al. Effect of dietary modification on health-related quality of life in dogs with spontaneous chronic renal failure (abstract). Journal of Veterinary Internal Medicine 2004; 18: 417.

Jacob F, Polzin DJ, Osborne CA, et al. Association between initial systolic blood pressure and risk of developing a uremic crisis or of dying in dogs with chronic renal failure. Journal of the American Veterinary Medical Association 2003; 222: 322-329.

Jacob F, Polzin DJ, Osborne CA, et al. Clinical evaluation of dietary modification for treatment of spontaneous chronic renal failure in dogs. Journal of the American Veterinary Medical Association 2002; 220: 1163-1170.

Jacob F, Polzin DJ, Osborne CA, et al. Evaluation of the association between initial proteinuria and morbidity rate or death in dogs with naturally occurring chronic renal failure. Journal of the American Veterinary Medical Association 2005; 226: 393-400.

Section 15

Canine Urolithiasis

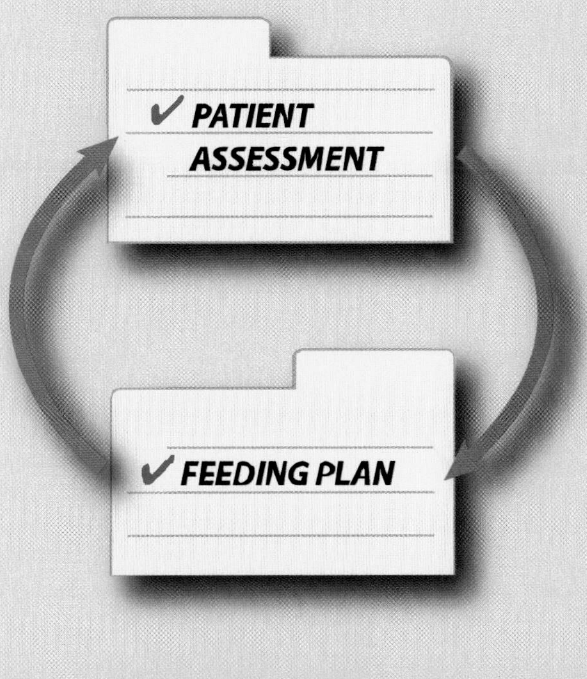

Canine Urolithiasis

Chapter 38

Canine Urolithiasis: Definitions, Pathophysiology and Clinical Manifestations

Carl A. Osborne
Jody P. Lulich
Lisa K. Ulrich

"If the patient you treat is harmed more than helped, then best leave the stones alone. But by taking a look at the thoughts in this book, ways to treat stones by how patients eat you'll be shown."
Carl A. Osborne, 1999

CLINICAL IMPORTANCE

Urolithiasis is a common disorder of the urinary tract in dogs. However, the incidence (annual rate of appearance of new cases among the entire population at risk for the disease) of canine urolithiasis has not been established. Urolithiasis was diagnosed in 3,628 of 676,668 dogs (0.53%) admitted to veterinary teaching hospitals in North America between 1980 and 1993. The proportion of dogs with urolithiasis admitted to veterinary hospitals in Germany was similar (Lulich et al, 1995).

Clinical signs of urolithiasis may be the first indication of underlying systemic disorders, or defects in the structure or function of the urinary tract (**Table 38-1**). Uroliths may pass through various parts of the excretory pathway of the urinary tract, they may dissolve, they may become inactive or they may continue to form and grow. If uroliths associated with clinical signs are allowed to remain untreated, they may result in serious sequelae. Despite urolith removal by voiding, dissolution protocols, or surgery, uroliths frequently recur if risk factors associated with their formation are not suppressed or corrected.

Urolithiasis should not be viewed as a single disease, but rather as a sequela of one or more underlying abnormalities. The fact that urolith formation is often erratic and unpredictable indicates that several interrelated complex physiologic and pathologic factors are involved. Therefore, detection of uroliths is only the beginning of the diagnostic process. Determination of urolith composition narrows etiologic possibilities. Knowledge of the patient's food and how it is fed and serum and urine concentrations of lithogenic minerals, crystallization promoters, crystallization inhibitors and their interactions aids in the diagnosis, treatment and prevention of urolithiasis (**Box 38-1**).

FORMATION OF UROLITHS

Initiation and Growth

Urolith formation is associated with two complementary but separate phases: initiation and growth. It appears that initiating events are not the same for all types of uroliths. In addition, factors that initiate urolith formation may be different from those that allow urolith growth.

The initial step in urolith formation is formation of a crystal nidus (or crystal embryo). This initiation phase of urolith for-

Table 38-1. Clinical importance of urolithiasis.

- **First evidence of an underlying systemic disorder**
  - Hypercalcemia
    - Calcium oxalate uroliths
    - Calcium phosphate uroliths
  - Cushing's syndrome
    - Calcium oxalate uroliths
    - Calcium phosphate uroliths
    - Struvite uroliths
  - Defects in purine metabolism
    - Portal vascular anomalies
      - Ammonium urate uroliths
    - Enzyme defects
      - Xanthine uroliths
- **First evidence of an underlying urinary tract disorder**
  - Renal tubular transport defect
    - Cystinuria
      - Cystine uroliths
    - Renal tubular acidosis
      - Calcium oxalate uroliths
      - Calcium phosphate uroliths
  - Defects in local host defenses against urease-producing microbes
    - Struvite uroliths
  - Foreign bodies in urinary tract
    - Suture material
      - Usually struvite uroliths
    - Catheters
      - Usually struvite and sometimes calcium oxalate uroliths
- **Sequelae to urolithiasis**
  - Dysuria, pollakiuria, urge incontinence
  - Secondary microbial urinary tract infection
  - Partial or total obstruction to urine outflow
    - Bacterial urinary tract infection that may progress
    - Impaired renal function and postrenal azotemia
    - Rupture of the outflow tract
      - Uroperitoneum
      - Inflammation of tissues adjacent to various portions of the urinary tract
  - Formation of inflammatory bladder polyps

mation, called nucleation, is dependent on supersaturation of urine with lithogenic crystalloids. The inciting factor and the precise sequence of events that lead to the formation of most types of stones are still unknown. The degree of urine supersaturation may be influenced by the magnitude of renal excretion of crystalloids, urinary pH and/or crystallization inhibitors or promoters in urine. Noncrystalline proteinaceous matrix substances may also play a role in nucleation in some instances.

Three theories have been proposed to explain initiation of lithogenesis: 1) supersaturation-crystallization theory, 2) matrix-nucleation theory and 3) crystallization-inhibition theory (Osborne and Kruger, 1984). Each theory emphasizes a single factor. The supersaturation-crystallization theory incriminates excessive supersaturation of urine with urolith-forming crystalloids as the primary event in lithogenesis. In this hypothesis, crystal nucleation is considered to be a physiochemical process involving precipitation of crystalloids from a supersaturated solution. Urolith formation is thought to occur independently of preformed matrix or crystallization inhibitors.

The matrix-nucleation theory incriminates preformed organic matrix (thought to be a mucoprotein with mineral-binding properties) as the primary determinant in lithogenesis. This theory is based on the assumption that preformed organic matrix forms an initial nucleus that subsequently permits urolith formation by precipitation of crystalloids. The role of organic matrix in lithogenesis has not been defined with certainty; however, the similarity of the overall composition of matrix from human uroliths of various mineral composition supports this hypothesis.

The crystallization-inhibition theory proposes that reduction or absence of organic and inorganic inhibitors of crystallization is the primary determinant of calcium oxalate and calcium phosphate lithogenesis. This theory is based on the fact that several lithogenic substances in urine are maintained in solution at concentrations significantly higher than is possible in water (i.e., driving forces for crystal precipitation of normally saturated urine are minimized by crystallization inhibitors). Similarly, inhibitors are important in minimizing crystal growth and aggregation. These three theories are not mutually exclusive. In fact, supersaturation of urine with the crystal's components is a prerequisite for each theory of nucleation.

Further growth of the crystal nidus depends on: 1) whether or not it remains in the lumen of the excretory pathway of the urinary system, 2) the degree and duration of supersaturation of urine with crystalloids identical or different from those in the nidus and 3) physical characteristics of the crystal nidus. Crystals that are compatible with other crystalloids may align themselves and grow on the surface of other crystals. This is called epitaxial growth. Epitaxy may represent a heterogeneous form of nucleation, and may account for some mixed and compound uroliths. For example, in people, the structural similarities of uric acid and calcium oxalate permit urolith growth by epitaxy (Coe, 1977).

Nucleation

Nucleation refers to the initial event in the formation (or precipitation) of uroliths and is characterized by the appearance of submicroscopic molecular aggregates of crystalloids. Initially, the aggregates are approximately 100 molecules in size and represent potential crystal embryos (or a nidus). Crystals represent an orderly arrangement of atoms in a periodic pattern or lattice. To become a urolith, crystal embryos must have a lattice arrangement that allows continued growth. They must also be large enough to prevent dispersion back into the dissolved phase (Pak, 1976).

Nucleation has been classified as homogeneous (also called self nucleation or generalized nucleation) or heterogeneous (also called localized nucleation) (Lyon and Vermeulen, 1965). Homogeneous nucleation occurs spontaneously in highly supersaturated urine in the absence of foreign substances (**Figure 38-1**). Therefore, the nidus is composed of identical crystalloids. Heterogeneous nucleation is catalyzed by foreign material such as suture material, indwelling catheters, tissue debris, crystal embryos of different composition, etc. (**Figure 38-2**). Urine contains many impurities that might promote heterogeneous nucleation and initiate crystal formation at a concentration of crystalloids below the formation concentration.

Box 38-1. Urolithiasis Terms and Concepts.

UROLITHIASIS

The urinary system is designed to dispose of waste products in soluble form. However, some waste products are sparingly soluble and occasionally precipitate out of solution to form crystals. Growth or aggregation of microscopic crystals may lead to formation of macroscopic uroliths. Urolithiasis may be conceptually defined as the formation of uroliths anywhere in the urinary tract from less soluble crystalloids of urine as a result of multiple congenital and/or acquired physiologic and pathologic processes. If such crystalloids become trapped in the urinary system, they may grow to sufficient size to cause clinical signs.

Urolithiasis should not be thought of as a single disease, but rather as a sequela of one or more underlying abnormalities. The fact that urolith formation is often erratic and unpredictable indicates that several interrelated complex physiologic and pathologic factors are involved. Therefore, detection of uroliths is only the beginning of the diagnostic process. Determination of urolith composition narrows etiologic possibilities. Knowledge of the patient's food, and serum and urine concentrations of lithogenic minerals, crystallization promoters, crystallization inhibitors and their interactions aids in the diagnosis, treatment and prevention of urolithiasis.

UROLITHS

Uroliths are polycrystalline concretions that typically contain more than 95% organic or inorganic crystalloids, and less than 5% organic matrices (weight vs. weight ratio). (The exception to this generality is infection-induced uroliths which contain as much as 50% matrix). Uroliths may also contain a number of minor constituents. A variety of different types of uroliths may occur in dogs (**Figure 1**). Uroliths are typically composed of organized crystal aggregates with a complex internal structure. Cross sections of uroliths frequently reveal nuclei and laminations, and less frequently radial striations. Urine that bathes uroliths varies in composition (and probably in degree of saturation with lithogenic crystalloids) from day to day and perhaps from hour to hour. This phenomenon is of conceptual importance in understanding the physical characteristics of uroliths.

The incidence and composition of uroliths may be influenced by a variety of factors including: 1) species, 2) breed, 3) gender, 4) age, 5) geography, 6) food, 7) anatomic abnormalities, 8) physiologic abnormalities, 9) urinary tract infection and 10) urinary pH. Uroliths may be named according to mineral composition, location (i.e., nephroliths, ureteroliths, cystoliths, vesical calculi, urethroliths) or shape (i.e., smooth, faceted, pyramidal, laminated, mulberry, jackstone, staghorn or branched). Characteristic shapes of crystals and uroliths are influenced primarily by the internal structure of crystals and the environment in which they form. Crystals of calcium oxalate monohydrate tend to fuse, producing smoothly rounded or mammillated uroliths. Local factors that influence the size and shape of uroliths include: 1) number of uroliths present, 2) mobility or fixation of uroliths, 3) flow characteristics of urine and 4) anatomic configuration of the structure in which uroliths grow.

MINERAL

A mineral is a naturally occurring, inorganically formed substance that has a characteristic chemical composition and usually has an ordered atomic arrangement that may influence its external geometric form. Minerals commonly found in uroliths often have a chemical name and a crystal (or mineral) name. Even though a particular mineral usually predominates, the mineral composition of many uroliths may be mixed. Occasionally, the center of a urolith may be composed of one type of crystalloid (e.g., silica), whereas outer layers are composed of a different crystalloid (especially struvite). Detection, treatment and prevention of the underlying causes of urolithiasis depend on knowledge of the composition and structure of all portions of uroliths.

MATRIX

The nondialyzable portion of uroliths that remains after crystalline components have been dissolved with mild solvents is organic matrix. Uroliths consistently contain variable quantities of organic matrix substances in addition to crystalloids. Organic matrix substances identified in human uroliths and experimentally produced in animals include matrix substances A, Tamm-Horsfall glycoprotein, uromucoid, serum albumin and alpha and gamma globulins. Of these, matrix substance A, Tamm-Horsfall glycoprotein and uromucoid appear to be quantitatively more significant than alpha and gamma globulins.

The complex of diverse mucoprotein compounds composing matrix substances may represent the skeleton of uroliths. Although the physical characteristics of uroliths suggest organized relationships between the matrix skeleton and crystalline building blocks, the role of each of these components in formation, retention and growth of uroliths is still poorly understood.

Organic matrix may affect urolith formation by one or more of several mechanisms including: 1) sites of heterogeneous nucleation, 2) templates for organizing and modifying growth of crystals 3) binding agents that cement urolith particles together and promote retention of crystals and 4) protective colloids that prevent further growth of uroliths. Organic matrix may also be composed of passive substances that have no effect on urolith formation or growth.

NUCLEI AND LAMINATIONS

Examination of cross sections of uroliths often reveals a nucleus and adjacent peripheral laminations. Laminated uroliths may be detected by radiography. Nuclei are focal points (or cores) that differ in appearance from more peripheral portions of the urolith. Nuclei are usually but not invariably located in the center of uroliths. Nuclei may be of crystalline composition or they may be composed of foreign material, tissue debris, blood clots, bacteria, etc. The mineral composition of crystalline nuclei may be identical or different from the remainder of the urolith. Nuclei surrounded by well-defined layers (or lamellae) of solid material suggest an early phase of urolith evolution. However, crystalline nuclei large enough to be detected visually are too large to represent an initial crystalline nidus for crystal nucleation in the physiochemical sense. Centrally located nuclei imply that the urolith was freely accessible to urine from all sides and that growth proceeded at a similar rate on all sides.

Laminated uroliths are common and may represent: 1) alternating bands of different mineral types, 2) periods during which urolith

Box 38-1 continued

growth occurred without interruption or 3) alternating periods of precipitation of minerals and gel. Although a difference in appearance between two consecutive layers should prompt suspicion of differences in composition, this is not always the case.

MATRIX CONCRETIONS

By definition, a urolith must contain some minerals. However, concretions composed primarily (more than 65%) of matrix may occur. These concretions, commonly called matrix stones, often occur in the urethra of male cats and sheep, and sometimes occur in dogs and people. They may form a cast of that portion of the excretory pathway in which they are formed (e.g., urethral plugs), implying a rapid rate of formation. In dogs, matrix concretions usually occur secondary to bacterial infections.

COMPOUND UROLITHS

Compound uroliths have one or more layers of mineral composition (e.g., struvite) different from minerals identified in the nucleus (e.g., calcium oxalate).

MIXED UROLITHS

Mixed uroliths contain more than one mineral, neither of which composes at least 70% of the urolith, but without a nucleus or well-defined laminations.

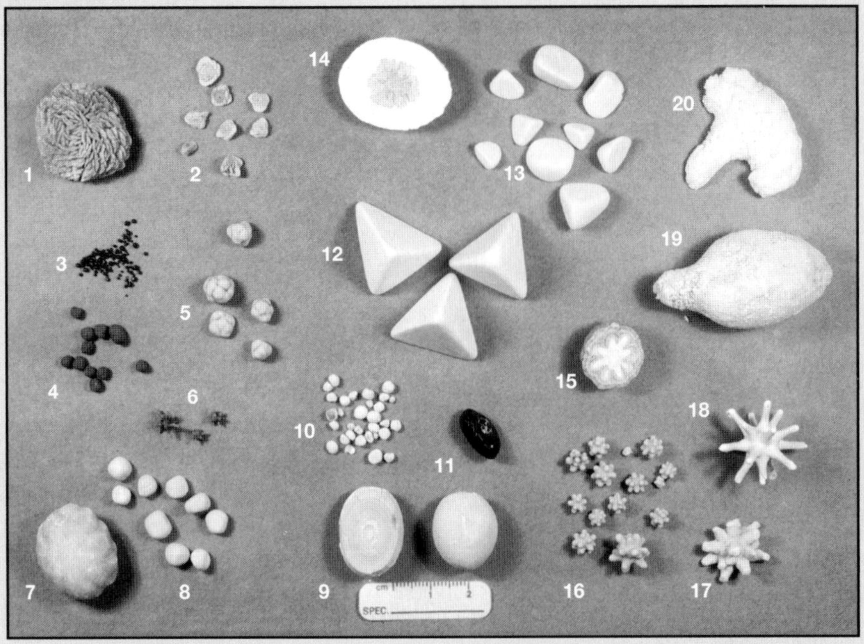

Figure 1. Different mineral types of canine uroliths illustrating common sizes, shapes and surface characteristics. 1) Calcium oxalate dihydrate; 2) Calcium oxalate dihydrate; 3) Calcium oxalate monohydrate; 4) Calcium oxalate monohydrate; 5) Calcium oxalate monohydrate; 6) Calcium oxalate dihydrate; 7) Cystine; 8) Cystine; 9) Ammonium urate (left urolith has been bisected to illustrate laminations); 10) Ammonium urate; 11) Ammonium urate; 12) Struvite; 13) Struvite; 14) Compound urolith with a nidus of calcium oxalate monohydrate surrounded by a shell of struvite and calcium carbonate apatite; 15) Compound urolith with a nidus of silica surrounded by shells containing a mixture of calcium oxalate, silica and ammonium urate; 16) Silica; 17) Silica; 18) Silica; 19) Struvite that has the shape of the urinary bladder and proximal urethra; 20) Struvite that has the shape of the renal pelvis and proximal ureter.

The Bibliography for **Box 38-1** can be found at www.markmorris.org.

These substances may be thought of as facilitators or potentiators of crystallization. Any crystal type may be a potential nidus for nucleation of another crystal type. A greater degree of supersaturation (i.e., a higher formation product) is required for homogeneous nucleation than for heterogeneous nucleation. Once nucleation has occurred, however, crystal growth can occur at any degree of supersaturation (even at metastability).

Undersaturated Solutions

An undersaturated solution contains a sufficiently low concentration of a crystalloid to permit dissolution of additional quantities of the crystalloid. Urine is undersaturated when the solute concentration (or activity product) is less than the solubility of the solute in question. Formation of urine that is undersaturated with lithogenic crystalloids may permit varying degrees of urolith dissolution.

Saturated Solutions

Saturated solutions are in equilibrium with undissolved solute at a given temperature. Saturated solutions contain so much dissolved substances that no more can be dissolved at a given temperature. With respect to urine, the saturation concentration is that concentration of a crystalloid that remains unchanged when the urine is mixed with uroliths (or the solid phase) containing that crystalloid. The saturation of salts in urine is influenced by several variables including pH, ionic strength and temperature.

Supersaturated Solutions

A supersaturated solution is more saturated with a substance at a given temperature than would be normally expected (i.e., it is any concentration greater than the saturation concentration). Supersaturated urine contains a greater concentration of a crystalloid (cystine, phosphate, calcium, ammonium, etc.) than the associated solvent (water) would be predicted to be able to normally hold in solution. Supersaturation can vary in degree. Urine is metastable at lower levels of supersaturation. At higher levels of supersaturation, however, urine becomes unstable with regard to its capacity to keep lithogenic substances in solution (**Figure 38-3**). Factors that increase the saturation of crystalloids in urine predispose patients to precipitation of crystals and thus urolith formation. Spontaneous precipitation will occur if the concentration of the crystalloid is greater than its formation product.

Metastable Region

The metastable region refers to the degree of supersaturation of a crystalloid that lies between the solubility product and the formation product. Metastability applies to those liquids (e.g., urine) that have the capacity to retain more of a compound in solution than would be predicted by knowledge of its true solubility in water. The term "metastable" is appropriate because it implies a condition subject to change. A metastable solution is thermodynamically unstable, but does not contain enough energy to initiate crystal formation. However, crystals already present may grow. The region of metastability varies with the type of lithogenic crystalloid. For example, in people, it has been estimated that the difference between the solubility product and the formation product of calcium oxalate in urine is a multiple of about 8.5 to 10.0 (Coe, 1978).

Oversaturated Solutions

An oversaturated solution is one in which the degree of supersaturation of a crystalloid is greater than the formation product (**Figure 38-3**). Recall that supersaturated urine exceeds the solubility product, but does not exceed the formation product. Oversaturated urine is no longer metastable. Nucleation will take place in the absence of heterogeneous factors. Oversaturation of urine is thought to cause crystals observed by microscopic examination of urine sediment.

Inhibitors and Promoters of Crystal Formation

Urine is a complex solution containing a variety of substances that can inhibit or promote crystal formation and growth. Inhibitors include molecules that reduce calcium oxalate and calcium phosphate supersaturation. Some inhibitors (e.g., citrate, magnesium, pyrophosphate) form soluble salts with calcium, oxalic acid or phosphoric acid, thereby reducing the quantity of these metabolites available for precipitation. Other inhibitors (e.g., nephrocalcin, uropontin, glycosaminoglycans, Tamm-Horsfall glycoprotein, other inert ions) interfere with the ability of calcium and oxalic acid to combine, thereby minimizing crystal formation and growth. Also, glycosaminoglycans act as protectors by preventing crystals from adhering to the urinary tract mucosa.

Clinical Concepts of Urine Supersaturation

Salts (crystals) are neutral compounds derived from the reversible interaction of a cation (e.g., calcium) and an anion (e.g., oxalic acid). The ability of a salt to dissolve in solution depends on the concentration of its ions in solution, and its interaction with other ions and neutral molecules in the same solution. For example, the state of urine saturation for any specific crystal system is the product of urine solute concentration, pH, ionic strength, tem-

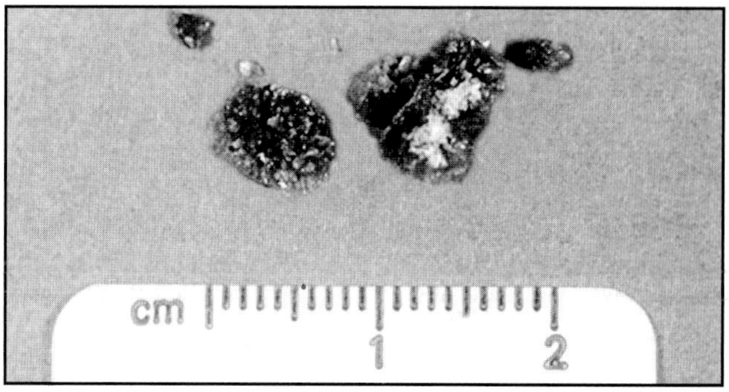

Figure 38-1. Layered urocystolith composed of 100% calcium oxalate dihydrate removed from an adult male miniature schnauzer. The difference in color of the center of the urolith vs. the outer layer is due to the large quantity of blood in the matrix of the outer layer.

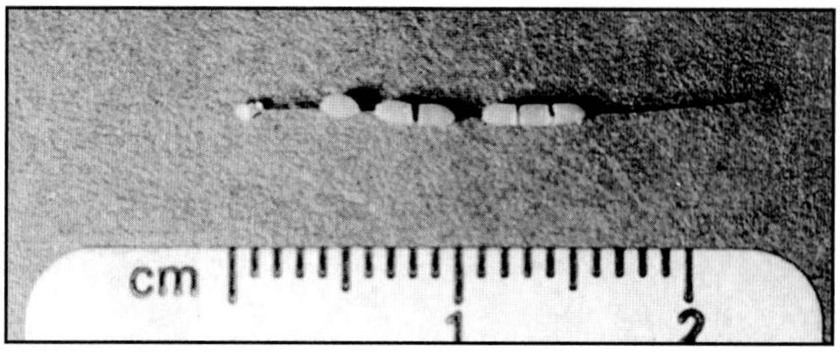

Figure 38-2. Struvite uroliths that have formed on a hair shaft.

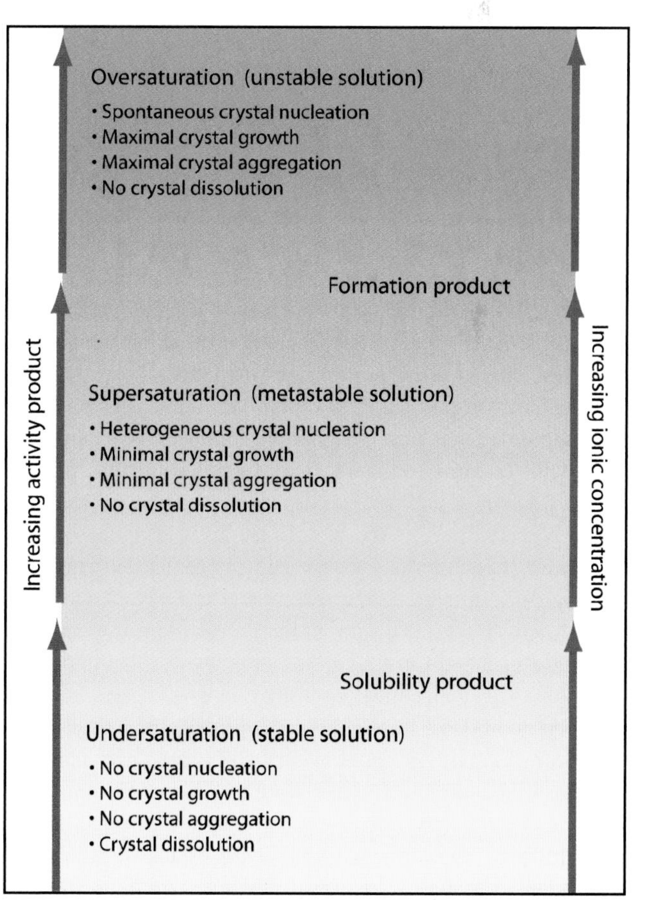

Figure 38-3. Probable events in formation of crystals in urine. A variety of factors influence the solubility of minerals in urine including concentration of lithogenic and non-lithogenic minerals, the concentration of crystallization inhibitors and crystallization promoters, urine temperature, urinary pH and urine ionic strength.

perature and preformed chemical complexes.

To illustrate these principles, consider pure water as a solution and calcium oxalate as a salt. Small amounts of calcium oxalate added to water dissolve completely because water is undersaturated with calcium and oxalic acid ions. As more calcium oxalate is added, the water's capacity to dissolve additional calcium oxalate is decreased until the solution becomes saturated. In this context, saturation of the solution with calcium and oxalic acid ions occurs when no additional calcium oxalate can be dissolved at a given pH and temperature of the solution. If additional calcium oxalate is added, it will appear as a solid.

As in water, calcium oxalate can also be dissolved in undersaturated urine. However, unlike water, urine is a complex solution containing a unique combination of ionic and nonionic molecules that may increase the solubility of calcium oxalate. Therefore, calcium oxalate added beyond the point of saturation will remain in solution. Thus, the solution becomes supersaturated with calcium and oxalic acid ions. Supersaturation is conceptually significant because the solution contains enough energy to form solids from dissolved ions (i.e., it is thermodynamically unstable). When supersaturated, the solution must "struggle" to maintain the homogeneous nature between the ions it contains. One method by which the solution returns to thermodynamic stability is by concentrating excess calcium and oxalic acid ions as solids or crystals on pre-existing surfaces or templates (e.g., other crystals or foreign material). This phenomenon is called heterogeneous nucleation. However, if the solution becomes oversaturated by addition of more calcium and oxalic acid ions, calcium oxalate crystals will form without an existing template (so-called homogeneous nucleation). After crystals have formed, available thermodynamic energy favors crystal growth whereby free ions become incorporated into the crystals. Crystal growth continues until ions in solution become depleted, allowing the solution to return to thermodynamic stability (or saturation). Crystals retained in the urinary tract may grow (the second phase of urolith formation).

Urine is a complex solution containing "inert" ions (i.e., sulfate, sodium, potassium, magnesium) unlikely to chemically bond with calcium and oxalic acid. In this way, they increase calcium oxalate solubility. The negative ions (e.g., sulfate) surround positive calcium ions, and the positive ions (e.g., sodium, potassium, magnesium) surround negative oxalic acid ions. The net effect is a decrease in attraction between calcium and oxalic acid ions. Because calcium and oxalic acid ion interaction is required for crystal formation, the solubility of calcium oxalate increases as the concentration of "inert" ions increases.

Supersaturation of urine with certain lithogenic ions also depends on another group of substances called "crystallization inhibitors." These include citric acid and pyrophosphates that chelate calcium but remain dissolved in solution. Likewise, certain mucoproteins, glycosaminoglycans, glycoproteins (e.g., nephrocalcin) and other poorly identified substances may interact with calcium. The result is a decrease in the amount of calcium available to bind with oxalic acid (and phosphoric acid). It is of significance that these inhibitors have been found to be deficient or abnormal in some calcium oxalate urolith-forming patients.

Activity Product

The product of the chemical activities of two ionic materials is called the activity product. It is a mathematical expression used to estimate the degrees of saturation (i.e., undersaturation, supersaturation or oversaturation) of a dog's urine with lithogenic minerals (**Figure 38-3**). In addition to concentration of minerals, it encompasses other variables including urinary pH and ionic strength of the solution (Pak et al, 1977). Activity product encompasses solubility product and formation product. Activity products are calculated by measuring total concentrations of major ionizable solutes in urine. For efficiency, computer programs are commonly used to aid calculation of ion concentrations and activity products (Brown et al, 1994).

Solubility Product

The solubility product is a type of activity product reflecting the urine's ability to dissolve a known concentration of lithogenic ions at variable but known pH and temperature. It is constant for each mineral component at a given temperature and pH. Urine is saturated when the solubility product value is reached. Below this value, urine is undersaturated with lithogenic ions; above this value urine is supersaturated. When devising dietary and medical protocols to dissolve or prevent urolith formation, the goal is to achieve an activity product less than the solubility product (or a state of undersaturation) (**Figure 38-3**).

Formation Product

The formation product is a type of activity product reflecting the concentration of ions at which precipitation of solute (homogeneous nucleation and eventually crystal formation) occurs at a given pH and temperature. It is the upper limit of metastability. Urinary pH may affect the ionization of some urine constituents and thus their solubility. If urinary pH varies during the day, urine may be intermittently supersaturated or oversaturated. Ion activities above the formation product are associated with an unstable state of oversaturation resulting in spontaneous crystal formation and rapid crystal growth. Because this condition may be influenced by the product of several factors (including the time of incubation, a crystallizable matrix and inhibitors of nucleation) in addition to the concentration of lithogenic crystalloids, it is commonly called the formation product. In people, as mentioned above, the formation product for calcium oxalate is approximately 8.5 to 10 times greater than its solubility product (Coe, 1978). This indicates that urine, because of the addition of a variety of crystallization inhibitors, must be saturated at least eight times above the solubility product before crystals will form. In general, urine of urolith formers is more supersaturated with respect to the constituents of their uroliths than is the urine of normal subjects.

PATIENT ASSESSMENT

History and Physical Examination

The history of dogs with urolithiasis depends on: 1) anatomic location(s) of uroliths, 2) duration of uroliths in specific location(s), 3) physical characteristics of uroliths (size, shape, number), 4) secondary urinary tract infection (UTI) and virulence of infecting organism(s) and 5) presence of concomitant diseases in the urinary tract and other body systems. After a diagnosis of urolithiasis has been confirmed, the history and physical examination should focus on detection of any underlying illness that may predispose the dog to urolith formation.

A dietary history should also be obtained for all patients with urolithiasis, with the objective of identifying risk factors that predispose the patient to specific mineral types. Likewise, owners should be questioned about vitamin-mineral supplements, previous illnesses and medications that may predispose the patient to various types of uroliths.

Signs typical of lower urinary tract disease include dysuria, pollakiuria, hematuria, urge incontinence, paradoxical incontinence and voiding small uroliths during micturition. Signs of uremia may occur if urine flow has been obstructed for a sufficient period, or if there is extravasation of urine into the peritoneal cavity due to rupture of the excretory pathways.

Signs of upper tract disease include painless hematuria and polyuria if sufficient nephrons have impaired function. Abdominal pain may occur if there is overdistention of the renal pelvis with urine due to outflow obstruction (**Table 38-2**). Many patients with uroliths have no clinical signs. Absence of signs is especially common in patients with nephroliths.

If gross hematuria is present, determining when during the process of micturition it is most severe may be of value in localizing its source. If hematuria occurs throughout micturition, lesions (including uroliths) may be present in the kidneys, ureters, urinary bladder, prostate gland and/or urethra. If hematuria occurs primarily at the end of micturition, lesions of the ventral bladder wall or intermittent renal hematuria should be suspected. If hematuria occurs at the beginning or is independent of micturition, lesions in the urethra or genital tract should be suspected.

Digital palpation of the entire urethra, including evaluation by rectal examination, may reveal urethroliths or uroliths lodged in the bladder neck. A firm, non-yielding mass may be palpated in the urinary bladder if a solitary urolith is present; a grating sensation confined to the bladder may be detected if multiple uroliths are present. It may be impossible to palpate small or solitary urocystoliths if the bladder wall is contracted and/or thickened due to inflammation. Likewise, it may be impossible to palpate uroliths in a distended or overdistended bladder. In this situation, the bladder should be repalpated after urine has been eliminated by voiding, manual compression of the bladder, cystocentesis or catheterization. One should suspect urethroliths when urethral catheters cannot be advanced into the bladder. However, inability to advance a catheter through the urethra may also be associated with urethral strictures or space occupying lesions that partially or totally occlude the urethral lumen.

In the absence of infection or outflow obstruction, abnormalities are usually not associated with nephroliths unless bilateral nephroliths are associated with sufficient renal damage to cause uremia. If infection or obstruction is present, there may be pain in the area of the kidneys and/or palpable enlargement of the affected kidney(s). Concomitant bacterial pyelonephritis may be associated with polysystemic signs due to sepsis.

Table 38-2. Clinical signs of uroliths that may be associated with urinary system dysfunction.

Urethroliths
- Asymptomatic
- Dysuria, pollakiuria, urge incontinence and/or periuria
- Gross hematuria
- Palpable urethral uroliths
- Spontaneous voiding of small uroliths
- Partial or complete urine outflow obstruction
  - Overflow incontinence
  - Anuria
  - Palpation of an overdistended and painful urinary bladder
  - Urinary bladder rupture, abdominal distention and abdominal pain
  - Signs of postrenal azotemia (anorexia, depression, vomiting and diarrhea)
  - Signs associated with concurrent urocystoliths, ureteroliths and/or renoliths

Urocystoliths
- Asymptomatic
- Dysuria, pollakiuria and urge incontinence
- Gross hematuria
- Palpable bladder uroliths
- Palpably thickened urinary bladder wall
- Partial or complete urine outflow obstruction of bladder neck (See Urethroliths.)
- Other signs associated with concurrent urethroliths, ureteroliths and/or renoliths

Ureteroliths
- Asymptomatic
- Gross hematuria
- Constant abdominal pain
- Unilateral or bilateral urine outflow obstruction
  - Palpably enlarged kidney(s)
  - Signs of postrenal azotemia (See Urethroliths.)
- May have other signs associated with concurrent urethroliths, urocystoliths and/or nephroliths

Nephroliths
- Asymptomatic
- Gross hematuria
- Constant abdominal pain
- Signs of systemic illness if generalized renal infection is present (anorexia, depression, fever and polyuria)
- Palpably enlarged kidney(s)
- Signs of postrenal azotemia (See Urethroliths.)
- Other signs associated with concurrent urethroliths, urocystoliths and/or ureteroliths

Diagnostic Studies

Urinalysis

Results of urinalysis are usually characterized by abnormalities typical of inflammation (pyuria, proteinuria, hematuria and increased numbers of epithelial cells), which may or may not be associated with infection. Whereas urease-producing microbes (staphylococci, *Proteus* spp., ureaplasmas) may cause infection-induced struvite (magnesium ammonium phosphate) uroliths to form, opportunistic bacteria that are not lithogenic (e.g., *Escherichia coli* and streptococci) may colonize the urinary tract as a result of urolith-induced alterations in local host defenses. Quantitative urine culture of all patients with uroliths is recommended because knowledge of bacterial type is important in predicting the mineral composition of uroliths, and in selecting an appropriate antimicrobial agent for treatment.

The pH of urine obtained from patients with uroliths is variable; however, it may become persistently alkaline if secondary infection with urease-producing bacteria occurs. The significance of a single urinary pH measurement should be interpreted cautiously because there are significant fluctuations throughout the day, especially with respect to the time, amount and types of food consumption. In general, magnesium ammonium phosphate and calcium phosphate uroliths are associated with alkaline urine, whereas ammonium urate, sodium urate, uric acid, calcium oxalate, cystine and silica uroliths tend to be associated with acidic urine.

The advent of effective dietary and medical protocols to dissolve and prevent uroliths in dogs and cats has resulted in renewed interest in detection and interpretation of crystalluria. Evaluation of urine crystals may aid in: 1) detection of disorders predisposing animals to urolith formation, 2) estimation of the mineral composition of uroliths and 3) evaluation of the effectiveness of dietary and medical protocols initiated to dissolve or prevent uroliths.

Crystals form only in urine that is or recently has been supersaturated with lithogenic substances. Therefore, crystalluria represents a risk factor for urolithiasis. However, detection of urine crystals is not synonymous with urolithiasis and clinical signs associated with uroliths. Nor are urine crystals irrefutable evidence of a urolith-forming tendency. For example, crystalluria that occurs in individuals with anatomically and functionally normal urinary tracts is usually harmless because the crystals are eliminated before they aggregate or grow to sufficient size to interfere with normal urinary function. In addition, crystals that form after elimination or removal of urine from the patient often are of no clinical importance. Identification of crystals that have formed in vitro does not justify therapy.

Detection of some types of crystals (e.g., cystine and ammonium urate) in clinically asymptomatic patients, frequent detection of large aggregates of crystals (e.g., calcium oxalate or magnesium ammonium phosphate) in apparently normal individuals, or detection of any form of crystals in fresh urine collected from patients with confirmed urolithiasis may be of diagnostic, prognostic and therapeutic importance. Large crystals and aggregates of crystals are more likely to be retained in the urinary tract, and therefore may be of greater clinical significance than small or single crystals.

Although there is not a direct relationship between crystalluria and urolithiasis, detection of crystals in urine is proof that the urine sample is oversaturated with lithogenic substances. However, oversaturation may occur as a result of in vitro events in addition to or instead of in vivo events. Therefore, care must be used not to overinterpret the significance of crystalluria. In vivo variables that influence crystalluria include: 1) the concentration of lithogenic substances in urine (which in turn is influenced by their rate of excretion and the volume of water in which they are excreted), 2) urinary pH (**Table 38-3**), 3) the solubility of lithogenic substances and 4) excretion of diagnostic agents (e.g., radiopaque contrast media) and medications (e.g., sulfonamides).

In vitro variables that influence crystalluria include: 1) temperature, 2) evaporation, 3) urinary pH and 4) the technique of

Table 38-3. Common characteristics of selected urine crystals.

		Urinary pH at which crystals commonly form		
Crystal types	**Appearances**	**Acidic**	**Neutral**	**Alkaline**
Ammonium urate	Yellow-brown spherulites, thorn apples	+	+	+
Amorphous urates	Amorphous or spheroidal yellow-brown structures	+	±	-
Bilirubin	Reddish-brown needles or granules	+	-	-
Calcium carbonate	Large yellow-brown spheroids with radial striations, or small crystals with spheroidal or dumbbell shapes	-	±	+
Calcium oxalate dihydrate	Small colorless envelopes (octahedral form)	+	+	±
Calcium oxalate monohydrate	Small spindles "hempseed" or dumbbells	+	+	±
Calcium phosphate	Amorphous or long thin prisms	±	+	+
Cholesterol	Flat colorless plates with corner notch	+	+	-
Cystine	Flat colorless hexagonal plates	+	+	±
Hippuric acid	Four- to six-sided colorless elongated plates or prisms with rounded corners	+	+	±
Leucine	Yellow-brown spheroids with radial and concentric laminations	+	+	-
Magnesium ammonium phosphate	Three- to six-sided colorless prisms	±	+	+
Sodium urate	Colorless or yellow-brown needles or slender prisms, sometimes in clusters or sheaves	+	±	-
Sulfa metabolites	Sheaves of needles with central or eccentric binding, sometimes fan-shaped clusters	+	±	-
Tyrosine	Fine colorless or yellow needles arranged in sheaves or rosettes	+	-	-
Uric acid	Diamond or rhombic rosettes, or oval plates, structures with pointed ends, occasionally six-sided plates	+	-	-
Xanthine	Yellow-brown amorphous, spheroidal or ovoid structures	+	±	-

Key: + = crystals commonly occur at this pH, ± = crystals may occur at this pH, but are more common at the other pH, - = crystals are uncommon at this pH.

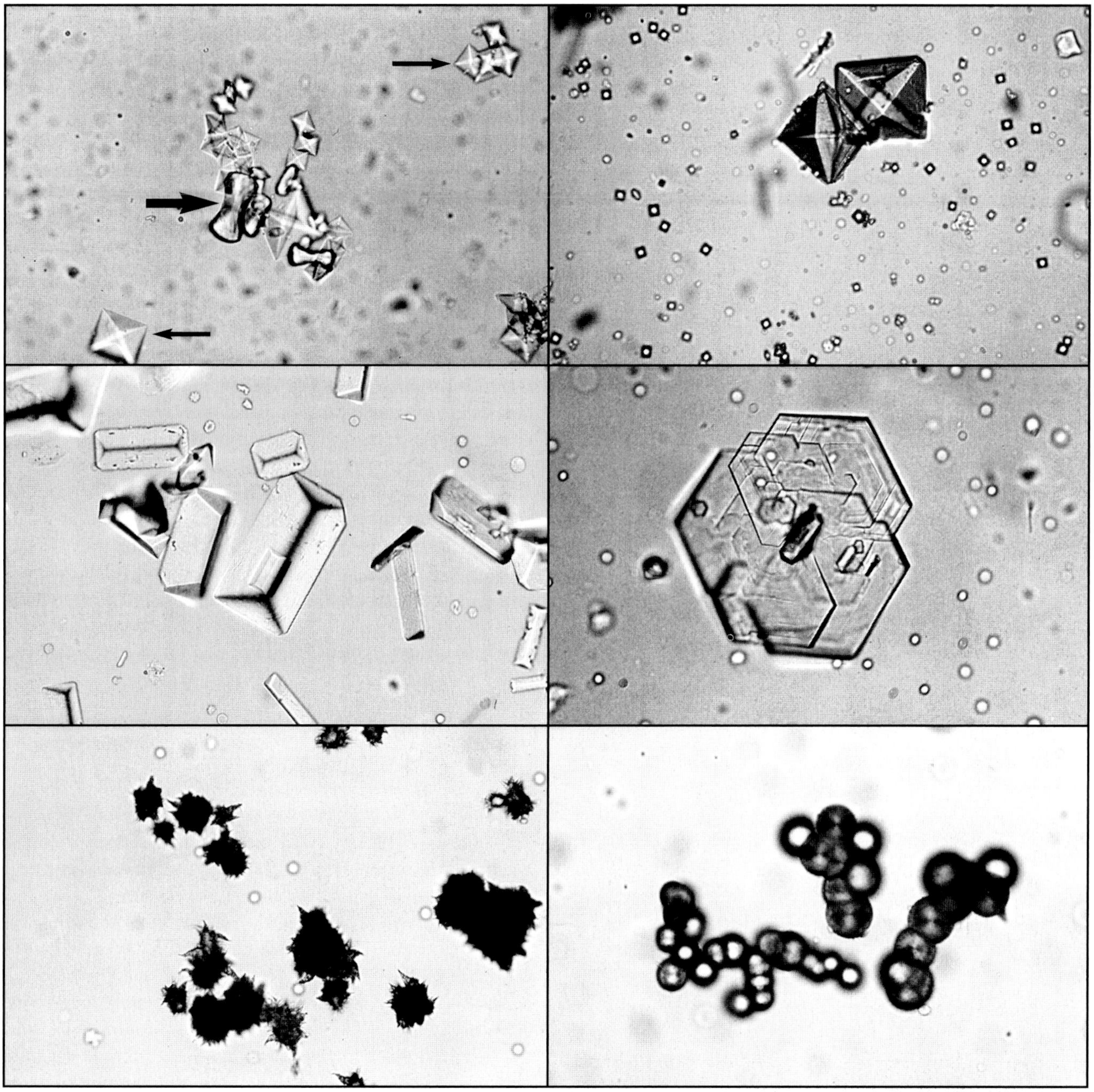

Figure 38-4. Photomicrographs of common crystals found in urine sediment. Calcium oxalate monohydrate (dumbbell form, large arrow) and calcium oxalate dihydrate (octahedral form, small arrows) (Top, Left). Calcium oxalate dihydrate; octahedral form (Top, Right). Magnesium ammonium phosphate (struvite); prisms (Middle, Left). Cystine; flat, colorless hexagonal plates (Middle, Right). Ammonium urate; thorn apple form (Bottom, Left). Amorphous xanthine; spheroids (Bottom, Right).

specimen preparation (e.g., centrifugation vs. noncentrifugation and volume of urine examined) and preservation. As mentioned above, in vitro changes that occur after urine collection may enhance formation or dissolution of crystals. Although in vitro changes may be used to enhance detection of certain types of crystals (e.g., acidification to cause precipitation of cystine), in vitro crystal formation may have no clinical relevance to in vivo formation of crystals in urine. When knowledge of in vivo urine crystal type is especially important, fresh, warm specimens should be serially examined. The number, size and structure of crystals should be evaluated, as well as their tendency to aggregate.

Urinary pH influences the formation and persistence of several types of crystals. Therefore, it is often useful to consider pH when interpreting crystalluria (**Table 38-3**). Different crystals tend to form and persist in certain urinary pH ranges, although there are exceptions. Exceptions may be related to large concentrations of lithogenic substances in urine or recent in vivo or in vitro changes in urinary pH.

Refrigeration is an excellent method to preserve many phys-

Table 38-4. Advantages and disadvantages of survey radiography, double-contrast radiography and ultrasonography in assessing uroliths.

Parameters	Survey radiography	Double-contrast radiography	Ultrasonography
Assessment of urethroliths	Yes, if radiodense	Indirectly*	Poor
Assessment of radiolucent urocystoliths	Unreliable	Yes	Yes
Distinguishing blood clots from urocystoliths	No	Probably	Yes
Assessment of laminated urocystoliths	Best of the three methods	Probably	No
Assessment of other bladder disorders	Unreliable	Yes	Sometimes
Assessment of urocystolith number	Yes (>3 mm)	Yes (>1 mm)	Equipment and observer dependent
Assessment of urocystolith size	Yes (>3 mm)	Yes (>1 mm)	Equipment and observer dependent
Assessment of urocystolith density	Yes (>3 mm)	No	No
Assessment of urocystolith shape	Yes (>3 mm)	Yes (>1 mm)	No
Immediate postsurgical assessment for uroliths	Yes	Not recommended**	No (air artifacts)
Risk of air artifact in bladder	No	Yes	No
Risk of iatrogenic bacterial urinary tract infection	No	Yes	No
Exposure to ionizing radiation	Yes	Yes	No
Necessary to remove hair	No	No	Often
Authors' overall choice	**Screening**	**Investigation**	**Third choice**

*During transurethral catheterization.
**Due to risk of iatrogenic bacterial urinary tract infection.

Table 38-5. Comparison of relative densities of common uroliths detected by survey radiography.*

Mineral types	Relative atomic number**
Water	**7.7**
Urate	6.9-7.7
Struvite	9.81
Cystine	10
Silica	11.6
Calcium oxalate dihydrate	13
Calcium oxalate monohydrate	13.6
Cortical bone	**15**
Calcium phosphate	15.9

*Adapted from Feeney DA, Weichselbaum RC, Jessen CR, et al. Imaging canine urocystoliths: Detection and prediction of mineral content. Veterinary Clinics of North America: Small Animal Practice 1999; 29: 59-72.
**Effective atomic numbers (Zeff), which is the sum of different elements in the urocystolith and is related to its mass.

ical, chemical and morphologic properties of urine sediment. However, refrigeration must be used with caution when evaluating crystalluria from qualitative and quantitative standpoints. Although refrigeration of urine samples is likely to enhance formation of various types of crystals, this phenomenon may have no relationship to events occurring in the patient's body.

Crystalluria may also be influenced by food, including water intake. Dietary influence on crystalluria is of diagnostic importance because urine crystal formation that occurs while patients are consuming hospital foods may be dissimilar to urine crystal formation that occurs when patients are consuming foods fed at home.

Microscopic evaluation of urine crystals should not be used as the sole criterion to predict the mineral composition of macroliths in patients with confirmed urolithiasis (**Table 38-3** and **Figure 38-4**). Only quantitative analysis can provide definitive information about the mineral composition of the entire urolith. However, interpretation of crystalluria in light of other clinical findings often allows the clinician to tentatively identify the mineral composition of uroliths, especially their outermost layers. Subsequent reduction or elimination of crystals by therapy provides a useful index of the efficacy of medical and dietary protocols designed to dissolve or prevent uroliths.

Radiography and Ultrasonography

The primary objective of radiographic or ultrasonographic evaluation of patients suspected of having uroliths is to determine the site(s), number, density and shape of uroliths. However, the size and number of uroliths are not a reliable index of the probable efficacy of therapy. After urolithiasis has been confirmed, radiographic or ultrasonographic evaluation also aids in detection of predisposing abnormalities (**Table 38-4**).

The size, number, location and mineral composition of uroliths influence their radiographic and ultrasonographic appearance. Most uroliths greater than 3 mm in diameter have varying degrees of radiodensity, and therefore can be detected by survey abdominal radiography or ultrasonography (Osborne et al, 1995). Very small uroliths (<3 mm in diameter) may not be visualized by survey radiography or ultrasonography. Uroliths greater than 1 mm in diameter can usually be detected by double-contrast cystography, provided excessive contrast medium is not used (Feeney et al, 1999). **Table 38-5** lists relative densities of common uroliths based on survey radiography (Feeney et al, 1999). Because of significant variation, the radiodensity of uroliths is not by itself a reliable index of mineral composition.

Uroliths greater than 3 mm in diameter are not commonly radiolucent. An exception to this generality is uroliths composed of 100% ammonium or sodium urate or uric acid. However, in our experience many ammonium urate uroliths of dogs are marginally radiodense. This finding may be related to a variable quantity of phosphates and other minerals in urate uroliths of dogs.

Matrix uroliths may be radiolucent or have some radiodensity. Blood clots are radiolucent and may be mistaken for radiolucent uroliths. Radiolucent uroliths may be readily distinguished from blood clots when evaluated by two-dimensional, gray-scale ultrasonography. Uroliths are usually in the dependent portion of the bladder lumen, produce sharply marginated shadows containing few echoes and are associated with acoustic shadowing. Blood clots may be located anywhere in the bladder lumen, typically have an irregular outline and indistinct margins and are not associated with acoustic shadowing.

Uroliths that are radiodense on survey radiographs may appear to be radiolucent when evaluated by positive-contrast radiography. This finding is related to the fact that many uroliths are more radiodense than body tissue, but less radiodense than the contrast material. A diagnosis of radiolucent uroliths should be based on their radiodensity compared with soft tissues, and not their radiodensity compared with positive-contrast medium.

A urolith may be larger than that depicted by its radiodensity if only a portion of it contains radiodense minerals. This phenomenon is most likely to occur with rapidly growing struvite uroliths that contain large quantities of matrix.

Hematology and Serum Chemistry

Hemograms of dogs with uroliths are usually normal unless there is concomitant generalized infection of the kidneys or prostate gland associated with leukocytosis. Microcytosis, anemia, target cells and leukocytosis have occasionally been associated with portal vascular anomalies in dogs with and without urate uroliths (Cornelius et al, 1975; Ewing et al, 1974; Griffiths et al, 1981; Rothuizen and van den Ingh, 1980).

Serum chemistry values are usually normal in patients with infection-induced magnesium ammonium phosphate, cystine and silica uroliths unless obstruction of urine outflow or generalized renal infection leads to changes characteristic of renal failure. Although most patients with calcium oxalate and calcium phosphate uroliths are normocalcemic, some are hypercalcemic.

Calcium phosphate and sterile struvite uroliths may be associated with distal renal tubular acidosis characterized by hyperchloremic (normal anion gap) metabolic acidosis, urinary pH values consistently greater than approximately 6 and hypokalemia.

A variety of biochemical alterations may exist in patients with urate urolithiasis. The following changes may be observed in patients with urate uroliths due to congenital or acquired hepatic disorders (Rothuizen and van den Ingh, 1980; Barrett et al, 1976; Marretta et al, 1981): 1) decreased urea nitrogen concentrations, 2) decreased total protein and albumin concentrations, 3) abnormal bile acid concentrations, 4) increased concentrations of total bilirubin and fasting blood ammonia and 5) increased serum alanine aminotransferase and serum alkaline phosphatase enzyme activities. Dogs with portal vascular anomalies typically have reduced hepatic functional mass and altered portal blood flow evidenced by abnormally elevated bile acid concentrations, prolonged sulfobromophthalein retention times and abnormal ammonia tolerance tests (Griffiths et al, 1981; Rothuizen and van den Ingh, 1980; Barrett et al, 1976; Marretta et al, 1981; Center et al, 1985).

Urine Chemistry

Detection of the underlying causes of specific types of urolithiasis is often linked to evaluation of the biochemical composition of urine. For best results, at least one and preferably two consecutive 24-hour urine samples should be collected because determination of fractional excretion of many metabolites in "spot" urine samples does not accurately reflect 24-hour metabolite excretion (**Table 38-6**).

Water consumption and hydration status must be considered when interpreting laboratory results. Decreased water consumption and dehydration are associated with several alterations, including decreased renal clearance of metabolites and increased urine specific gravity and urine solute concentrations (Taburu et al, 1993). Caution must be used in interpreting 24-hour excretion of solutes in the diagnosis and therapy of urolithiasis if hospitalized animals consume less water than in the home environment.

Urine concentrations of potentially lithogenic metabolites are also influenced by the amount and composition of food consumed, and whether urine was collected during conditions of fasting or food consumption (Lulich et al, 1991, 1991a). Aldosterone secretion increases following food deprivation. Increased aldosterone secretion promotes renal tubular sodium reabsorption and potassium excretion. As a consequence, plasma potassium concentration decreases, urinary potassium excretion increases and urinary sodium and chloride excretion decrease (Lulich et al, 1991a). Urinary calcium, magnesium and uric acid excretions are reduced during fasting. However, urinary excretion of phosphorus, oxalate and citrate are apparently unaffected by fasting (Lulich et al, 1991a). In dogs, urinary ammonia, titratable acid and hydrogen ion excretion decrease and urinary pH values increase when food is withheld (Lulich et al, 1991a; Lemieux and Plante, 1968). Therefore, values for 24-hour urinary solute excretion may differ when measured following food consumption vs. values obtained when food is withheld.

Consumption of food stimulates gastric secretion of hydrochloric acid. As a result, concentrations of chloride decrease and bicarbonate increase in venous blood draining the stomach. Total serum concentration of carbon dioxide increases. The resulting metabolic alkalosis is commonly called the postprandial alkaline tide. Urinary pH will increase unless acidifying substances are contained in the food. In a study of healthy beagles, eating was associated with increased urinary excretion of hydrogen ions, ammonia, sodium, potassium, calcium, magnesium and uric acid (Lulich et al, 1991a).

Laboratory results may be markedly affected by changes in foods fed in a home environment vs. different foods fed in a hospital environment. For example, urinary excretion of potentially lithogenic metabolites while animals consume foods fed in the hospital may be different from those excreted by animals eating at home. To determine the influence of home-fed foods on laboratory test results, consider asking clients to bring

Table 38-6. Protocol for measuring 24-hour urinary excretion of various substances associated with urolithiasis.

Technique

1. To allow for food acclimation, feed the patient either the food it was consuming just before urolith formation or a standard food at home for 10 to 14 days. We commonly use Prescription Diet k/d Canine* as the standard food.
2. If possible, house and feed the dog in the urine collection cage for at least one day before urine collection. As dogs become acclimated to their new environment, they are more likely to consume quantities of food and water similar to that consumed in their home environment.
3. Begin each 24-hour urine collection period by removing urine from the urinary bladder by transurethral catheterization. This urine is discarded. Record the actual time that urine collection is initiated.
4. Weigh the dog.
5. Then feed the dog its food as if at home. Water should be continuously available for consumption.
6. Begin administering a broad-spectrum antibiotic that achieves high concentrations in urine to prevent catheter-induced urinary tract infection. The dosage, dosing interval and route of administration should be based on manufacturer recommendations.
7. Keep the patient in the collection cage during urine collection. When using metabolism cages designed for urine collection, catheterization of the urinary tract is unnecessary except at the end of the 24 hours. House-trained dogs may not voluntarily void in their cage. Bladder catheterization may be necessary to obtain urine from these dogs. Dogs may be catheterized as often as necessary to keep them comfortable (usually every six to eight hours).
8. Catheterize the urinary bladder at the end of 24 hours to remove all urine. Save this urine.
9. Record the exact time of collection termination.
10. Pool all urine collected during the 24-hour period in a single container and measure its volume.
11. Thoroughly mix the pooled urine before removing aliquots for analysis.

Preservation

1. Preservatives have different roles, but are often used to minimize bacterial growth, reduce chemical decomposition, solubilize constituents that might otherwise precipitate out of solution, or decrease atmospheric oxidation of unstable compounds.
2. The method of preservation may vary depending on the substances being measured and the tests used to measure them. Consult the laboratory to determine the recommended method of preservation.
3. Preservatives should not be added to some specimens because of possible interference with analytical methods.
4. Refrigeration is a common method for preserving urine collected for analysis. Urine removed by intermittent catheterization can be stored in a refrigerator in clean containers with screw top lids. Containers used for continuous collection beneath metabolism cages can be surrounded by ice packs and then insulated. Refrigeration causes some minerals to precipitate out of solution.
5. Specimens can be acidified (add 10 ml of 1 N hydrochloric acid per liter to achieve a pH of 3 or less) to preserve oxalate and calcium for analysis. However, acidified urine is unsuitable for measuring uric acid because it precipitates in acidic solutions.

Storage of selected analytes in urine

1. No single preservative is ideal if multiple substances in urine are to be analyzed. To minimize degradation, we routinely collect urine under conditions of refrigeration. Immediately following urine collection, preservatives are added to appropriate aliquots of urine for storage until analysis.
2. Uric acid and xanthine: Aliquots of urine should be diluted (1 ml of urine with 19 ml of distilled water) to preserve uric acid and xanthine. This mixture can then be frozen.
3. Ammonia: Aliquots of urine (3 to 5 ml) may be frozen for up to 30 days.
4. Oxalate: Aliquots of urine (2 ml) are diluted with 1 N hydrochloric acid (1.66 ml) and then frozen.

Calculations

1. Calculating 24-hour urine volume
   a. Although 24-hour urine specimens are recommended to minimize the effects of short-term biologic variations in mineral excretion, collecting perfectly timed 24-hour samples may be difficult. The following formula can be used to adjust actual urine volume to a 24-hour period: 1,440 ÷ actual time interval (minutes) x urine volume (1,440 = number of minutes in 24 hours).
   b. Example: A 24-hour urine collection was started at 9:30 a.m. and ended the following day at 8:30 a.m. A total of 350 ml of urine were collected during this period. What is the 24-hour urine volume? 1,440 ÷ 1,380 x 350 = 356.2 ml.
2. Converting mmol/l to mg/dl
   a. Scientists are striving to adopt a uniform system of measurement termed the *System International d 'Unites* to standardize measurements. In this system, concentration is often expressed as moles, millimoles or micromoles of a substance per liter of fluid. Most normal values in the United States are expressed as mg/dl. The following formula can be used to convert mmol/l to mg/dl: mmol/l x atomic weight of substance ÷ 10. The atomic weights of elements can be found in the periodic tables of general chemistry books.
   b. Example: The concentration of calcium from a 24-hour urine sample was 1.35 mmol/l. Convert this value to mg/dl for comparison with normal values. The atomic weight of calcium is 40.08. 1.35 mmol/l x 40.08 ÷ 10 = 5.4 mg/dl.
3. Calculating mg/kg/24-hour or mEq/kg/24-hour excretion
   a. Excretion of metabolites is often expressed on a per kg basis to standardize excretion for dogs of different weights. The following formula can be used to standardize excretion rates: Concentration of substance x 24-hour urine volume ÷ body weight in kg. The units used to express the volume of urine and the concentration of the substance evaluated must be the same.
   b. Example: The concentration of calcium in a 24-hour urine sample was 5.4 mg/dl. A total of 356.2 ml of urine was collected. The dog weighed 10 kg. What is the daily calcium excretion on a per kg basis? First, express the volume of urine collected in the same units as the concentration of the substance measured. The 356.2 ml = 3.562 dl; therefore, 5.4 mg/dl x 3.562 dl ÷ 10 kg = 1.92 mg/kg/24 hours.

Additional considerations

1. Midpoint blood samples. Evaluation of blood during the midpoint of a 24-hour urine collection may help determine if changes in urine concentration reflect changes in serum or plasma concentration of analytes. This information can help detect underlying causes and mechanisms of abnormal mineral excretion. Likewise, evaluation of blood concentrations of some hormones (i.e., parathyroid hormone, calcitriol, etc.) may be helpful in determining the role of hormones in the regulation of mineral excretion.

Table 36-6 continued

2. Antimicrobials
   a. Antimicrobials are administered to prevent iatrogenic urinary tract infection during catheterization of the urinary bladder. The dosage, dosing interval and route should be based on the recommendations of the manufacturer. We recommend that antimicrobial administration be continued for three to five days after urine collection. This represents the time required for normal urothelial repair and replacement.
   b. Select antimicrobials that are primarily excreted in the urine and that minimally affect urine concentrations of minerals, promoters and inhibitors associated with urolith formation. Because some antimicrobials are formulated as salts of sodium or potassium, high concentrations of sodium or potassium may be excreted in urine. We routinely use cephalosporins when collecting urine for amino acid evaluation (i.e., cystine urolithiasis), and ampicillin when collecting urine from dogs with calcium oxalate or urate uroliths.
3. Fasting urine collection
   a. Fasting urine collections have been evaluated to characterize the pathophysiologic mechanism of hypercalciuria in dogs with calcium oxalate uroliths. Dogs that absorb excessive amounts of calcium from their food and subsequently excrete large quantities of calcium in their urine have intestinal hypercalciuria. Hypercalciuria primarily occurs during food consumption; normal or lower quantities of urine calcium are excreted when food is withheld. In addition, dogs with intestinal hypercalciuria have normal serum concentrations of calcium and normal or low serum concentrations of parathyroid hormone. In contrast, urinary calcium excretion during fed and nonfed conditions is similar in dogs with primary hyperparathyroidism (resorptive hypercalciuria) or impaired renal tubular absorption of calcium (renal-leak hypercalciuria).
   b. Fasting urine collections are initiated immediately following collection of urine during standard feeding.
4. Urinary pH. The solubility of mineral salts is influenced by urinary pH. Determination of urinary pH from 24-hour urine samples may be helpful in understanding crystal formation, and can also be used to calculate activity products for several mineral salts commonly found in uroliths. We use an ion selective electrode and pH meter to accurately measure urinary pH.
5. Activity products
   a. The activity product of urine is a mathematical expression used to estimate the degree of saturation of urine with mineral salts. Activity products are calculated by measuring concentrations of major ionizable solutes in urine. For efficiency, computer programs are commonly used to aid in calculating activity products.
   b. Urine in which the activity product exceeds the solubility product is saturated for that particular mineral salt. Although crystals may not form at this degree of saturation, uroliths already present are likely to grow.
   c. Urine in which the activity product exceeds the formation product for a particular mineral salt is associated with an unstable state of oversaturation. Crystal nucleation and rapid crystal growth are likely at this urine concentration.

*Hill's Pet Nutrition, Inc., Topeka, KS, USA.

home-fed foods for use during periods of diagnostic hospitalization (Osborne et al, 1990).

Urolith Analysis

Small uroliths in the urinary bladder or urethra are commonly voided during micturition by female dogs and occasionally by male dogs. Uroliths with a smooth surface (e.g., those composed of ammonium urate or calcium oxalate monohydrate) are more likely to pass through the urethra than uroliths with a rough surface (e.g., those composed of calcium oxalate dihydrate or silica). Commercially manufactured tropical fish nets designed for household aquariums facilitate retrieval of uroliths during voiding (Osborne et al, 1992). They are much less expensive than collection cups with wire mesh bottoms designed for people and available from medical supply houses. Urocystoliths may also be obtained by voiding urohydropropulsion (**Figure 38-5** and **Table 38-7**). If the unaided eye can detect a urolith, it will usually be sufficient size for quantitative analysis.

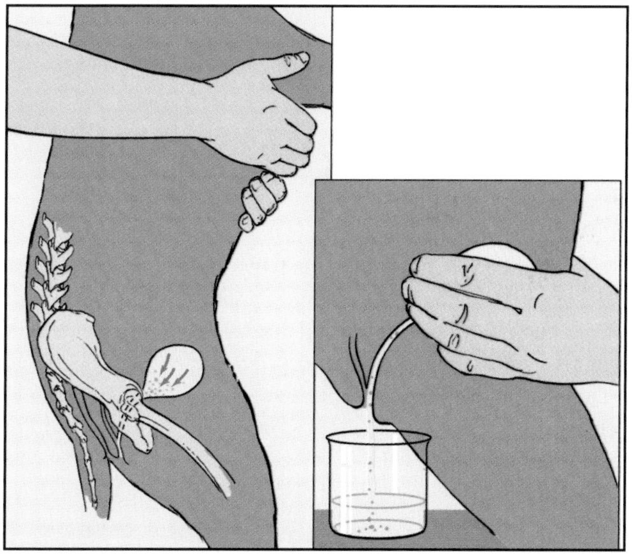

Figure 38-5. To remove urocystoliths by voiding urohydropropulsion, position the patient so that its vertebral column is approximately vertical (Left). The urinary bladder is then gently agitated to promote gravitational movement of urocystoliths into the bladder neck. To expel urocystoliths (Right), voiding is induced by applying steady digital pressure to the urinary bladder. (Adapted from Lulich JP, Osborne CA, Carlson M, et al. Nonsurgical removal of uroliths from dogs and cats by voiding urohydropropulsion. Journal of the American Veterinary Medical Association 1993; 203: 660-663.)

CATHETER-ASSISTED RETRIEVAL OF UROCYSTOLITHS

Small urocystoliths may be retrieved for analysis by aspirating them through a urethral catheter into a syringe (Osborne et al, 1992; Lulich and Osborne, 1992). Urocystoliths detected by survey radiography may be too large to be removed with the aid of a urethral catheter. However, large urocystoliths are often associated with small ones that may be detected by double-contrast cystography. The diameter of uroliths retrieved is limited by the size of openings or "eyes" in the proximal portion of the catheter and by the diameter of the catheter lumen. It is best to select the largest-diameter catheter that can be advanced into the bladder lumen without traumatizing the urethral mucosa.

Table 38-7. Voiding urohydropropulsion: A nonsurgical technique for removing small urocystoliths.

1. Perform appropriate diagnostic studies, including complete urinalysis, quantitative urine culture and diagnostic radiography. Determine the location, size, surface contour and number of urocystoliths.
2. Anesthetize the patient, if needed.
3. If the urinary bladder is not distended with urine, moderately distend it with a physiologic solution (e.g., saline, Ringer's, etc.) injected through a transurethral catheter. To prevent overdistention, palpate the bladder per abdomen during infusion. Remove the catheter.
4. Position the patient such that the vertebral spine is approximately vertical.
5. Gently agitate the urinary bladder, with the objective of promoting gravitational movement of urocystoliths into the bladder neck.
6. Induce voiding by manually expressing the urinary bladder. Use steady digital pressure rather than an intermittent squeezing motion.
7. Collect urine and uroliths in a cup. Compare urolith number and size to those detected by radiography and submit them for quantitative analysis.
8. If needed, repeat Steps 3 through 7 until the number of uroliths detected by radiography are removed or until uroliths are no longer voided.
9. Perform double-contrast cystography to ensure that no uroliths remain in the urinary bladder. Repeat voiding urohydropropulsion if small urocystoliths remain.
10. Administer prophylactic antimicrobials for three to five days, or longer if needed.
11. Monitor the patient for adverse complications (i.e., hematuria, dysuria, bacterial urinary tract infection and urethral obstruction with uroliths).
12. Formulate appropriate recommendations to minimize urolith recurrence or to manage uroliths remaining in the urinary tract on the basis of quantitative mineral analysis of voided urocystoliths.

Well-lubricated, soft, flexible catheters are preferable to less flexible ones. The size of openings in the proximal portion of the catheter may be enlarged with a scalpel, razor blade or scissors to facilitate retrieval of urocystoliths. However, care must be used not to weaken the catheter to the point where it could break while being inserted into or removed from the urethra and urinary bladder.

Uroliths may be retrieved by catheter aspiration as follows (**Figure 38-6**). With the patient in lateral recumbency, a well-lubricated catheter should be advanced through the urethra into the bladder lumen. The tip of the catheter should be positioned so that it will not interfere with movement of the bladder wall as fluid is aspirated from the bladder lumen. If the urinary bladder is not distended with urine, it should be partially distended with physiologic (0.9%) saline solution. As a rule of thumb, a normal, empty canine or feline urinary bladder can be partially distended by injecting 3 to 4 ml of fluid per kg body weight. However, the urinary bladder should be palpated per abdomen during the time it is distended with saline solution to ensure that it is not overdistended.

The next step is crucial to successful retrieval of urocystoliths. While urine (and saline solution) is aspirated into the syringe,

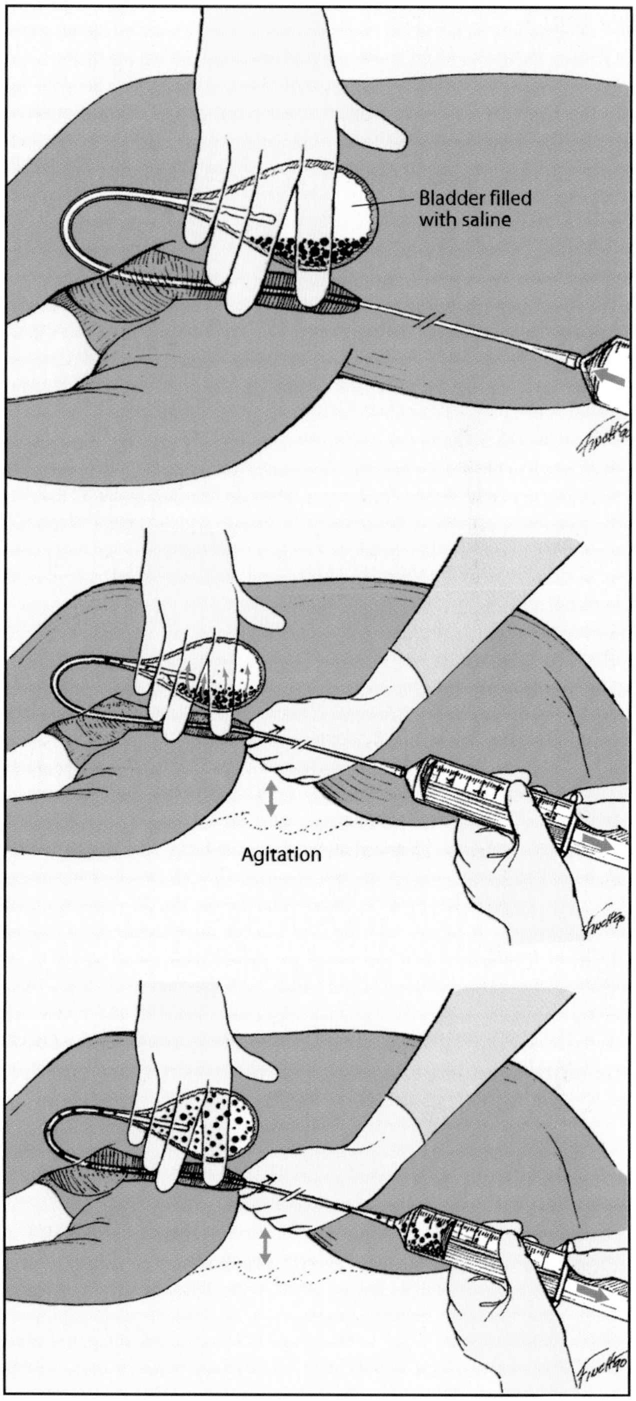

Figure 38-6. Illustration of catheter-assisted retrieval of urocystoliths. With the patient in lateral recumbency, uroliths have gravitated to the dependent portion of the urinary bladder (Top). The bladder lumen has been distended by injection of 0.9% saline solution. Vigorous movement of the abdomen in an up-and-down motion disperses uroliths throughout fluid in the bladder lumen (Middle). Aspiration of fluid from the urinary bladder during movement of the abdominal wall (Bottom) may result in movement of one or more small uroliths into the catheter and syringe. (Adapted from Lulich JP, Osborne CA. Catheter assisted retrieval of canine and feline urocystoliths. Journal of the American Veterinary Medical Association 1992; 201: 111-113.)

an assistant should vigorously and repeatedly move the patient's abdomen in an up-and-down motion. This maneuver disperses uroliths located in the dependent portion of the bladder throughout fluid in the bladder lumen. Small uroliths in the vicinity of the catheter tip may then be aspirated into the catheter along with the urine-saline mixture. It may be necessary to repeat this sequence of steps several times before a sufficient number of uroliths are retrieved. The bladder lumen should be redistended with saline solution each time. Difficulty in aspirating urine and saline solution into the syringe may be caused by poor positioning of the catheter tip or by partial occlusion of the catheter lumen with one or more uroliths. Flushing saline solution through the catheter after it has been removed from the patient often results in the retrieval of uroliths that occlude the catheter lumen.

Care must be used not to overdistend the urinary bladder with saline solution because this will increase the space in which the uroliths are suspended. Because patients with uroliths are predisposed to catheter-induced bacterial UTIs, antimicrobial therapy should be considered immediately before this procedure and for an appropriate period afterward. Proper selection, insertion and positioning of urethral catheters minimize iatrogenic trauma to the lower urinary tract.

COLLECTION AND QUANTITATIVE ANALYSIS OF URINE CRYSTALS

If available data do not indicate the probable mineral composition of uroliths and if uroliths cannot be retrieved with the aid of a urethral catheter, consider preparing a large pellet of urine crystals by centrifugation of urine in a conical-tip centrifuge tube (Osborne et al, 1992, 1995). The quantity of crystalline sediment available for analysis may be increased by repeatedly removing the supernatant after centrifugation, adding additional noncentrifuged urine to the tube containing sediment and again centrifuging the preparation. If the conditions that caused urolith formation are still present, evaluation of the pellet formed from crystalline sediment by quantitative methods designed for urolith analysis may provide meaningful information about the mineral composition of a patient's uroliths. However, crystals identified by this method may only reflect the outer portions of compound uroliths. Therefore, results of quantitative urine crystal analysis should be interpreted in conjunction with other pertinent clinical data.

QUANTITATIVE ANALYSIS OF UROLITHS

The location, number, size, shape, color and consistency of uroliths removed from the urinary tract should be recorded. All uroliths should be saved in a container (preferably a sterile one) and submitted for analysis. Do not give uroliths to owners before analysis. If multiple uroliths are present, one may be placed into a container of 10% buffered formalin for demineralization and microscopic examination. However, formalin should not be used to preserve uroliths for mineral analysis because formalin may alter the results. Because many uroliths contain two or more mineral components, it is important to examine representative portions. The mineral composition of

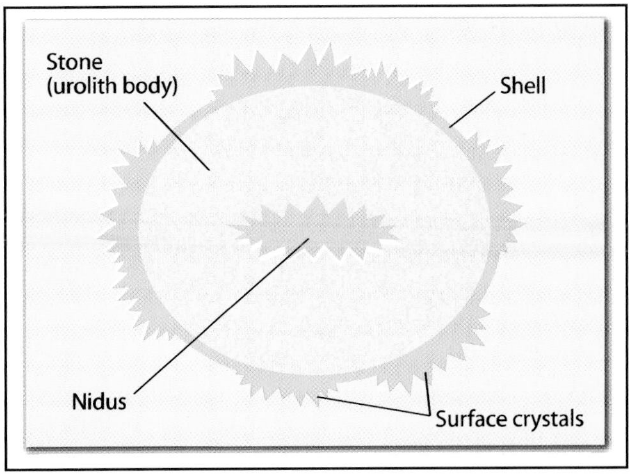

Figure 38-7. Schematic demonstrating the different components that may be observed on the cut surface of a bisected urolith. (Adapted from Osborne CA, Lulich JP, Polzin DJ, et al. Analysis of 77,000 canine uroliths: Perspectives from the Minnesota Urolith Center. Veterinary Clinics of North America: Small Animal Practice 1999; 29: 23.)

crystalline nuclei may be identical or different from outer layers of uroliths (**Figure 38-7**). The nuclei of uroliths should be analyzed separately from outer layers because knowledge of the mineral composition of the nuclei may suggest the initiating cause of the urolith. Uroliths should not be broken before submission because the central core may be distorted or lost.

Routine analysis of uroliths by qualitative methods of chemical analysis is not recommended. The major disadvantage of this procedure is that only some of the chemical radicals and ions can be detected. In addition, the proportion of the different chemical constituents in the urolith cannot be quantified. In contrast to chemical methods of analysis, physical methods have proved to be far superior in identification of crystalline substances. Physical methods also permit detection of silica and drugs and drug metabolites. They also permit differentiation of various subgroups of minerals (e.g., calcium oxalate monohydrate and calcium oxalate dihydrate, or uric acid, ammonium acid urate and xanthine) and allow semiquantitative determination of various mineral components. Physical methods commonly used by laboratories that specialize in quantitative urolith analysis include a combination of polarizing light microscopy, x-ray diffractometry and infrared spectroscopy (Osborne et al, 1983; Zinn et al, 1986; Ulrich et al, 1996). Some laboratories also are equipped to perform elemental analysis with an energy dispersive x-ray microanalyzer or by neutron activation. Occasionally, chemical methods of analysis and paper chromatography may be used to supplement information provided by physical methods. Chapter 46 lists selected laboratories that perform quantitative urolith analysis.

UROLITH CULTURE

Bacterial culture of the interior of uroliths is indicated if: 1) urine obtained from the patient has not been previously cultured, 2) culture of urine obtained from patients suspected of having struvite uroliths yields no growth or 3) the patient has a

Table 38-8. Mineral composition of 350,803 canine uroliths evaluated at the Minnesota Urolith Center by quantitative methods: 1981 to 2007.

Predominant mineral type	Proportion of predominant mineral (%)	Number	Percent
Magnesium ammonium phosphate•6H_2O	-	**149,199**	**42.53**
	100	(66,481)	-
	70-99*	(82,718)	-
Magnesium hydrogen phosphate•3H_2O	-	**52**	**0.01**
	100	(19)	-
	70-99*	(33)	-
Magnesium phosphate hydrate	70-100	**4**	**<0.01**
Calcium oxalate	-	**133,338**	**38.01**
Calcium oxalate monohydrate	100	(69,863)	-
	70-99*	(31,677)	-
Calcium oxalate dihydrate	100	(8,341)	-
	70-99*	(13,896)	-
Calcium oxalate monohydrate and dihydrate	100	(8,004)	-
	70-99*	(1,557)	-
Calcium phosphate	-	**1,801**	**0.51**
Calcium phosphate	100	(413)	-
	70-99*	(694)	-
Calcium hydrogen phosphate•2H_2O	100	(233)	-
	70-99*	(460)	-
Tricalcium phosphate	70-99*	(1)	-
Purines	-	**22,412**	**6.39**
Ammonium urate	100	(15,607)	-
	70-99*	(2,820)	-
Sodium urate	100	(1,577)	-
	70-99*	(118)	-
Sodium calcium urate (salts of uric acid)	100	(1,153)	-
	70-99*	(117)	-
Ammonium calcium urate	70-99*	(1)	-
Uric acid	100	(464)	-
	70-99*	(32)	-
Xanthine	100	(197)	-
	70-99*	(72)	-
Uric acid monohydrate (formerly unidentified uric acid)	100	(251)	-
	70-99*	(3)	-
Cystine	-	**3,402**	**0.97**
	100	(3,275)	-
	70-99*	(127)	-
Silica	-	**1,414**	**0.4**
	100	(982)	-
	70-99*	(432)	-
Other	-	**24**	**0.01**
Calcium carbonate	**70-100**	**6**	**<0.01**
Dolomite	**100**	**1**	**<0.01**
Mixed**	-	**8,146**	**2.32**
Compound***	-	**30,832**	**8.79**
Matrix	-	**153**	**0.04**
Drug metabolite	-	**19**	**0.01**

*Urolith composed of 70 to 99% of mineral type listed; no nucleus and shell detected.
**Uroliths did not contain at least 70% of mineral type listed; no nucleus or shell detected.
***Uroliths contained an identifiable nucleus and one or more surrounding layers of a different mineral type.

UTI with bacteria that do not produce urease. Bacteria harbored inside uroliths are not always the same as those present in urine. Bacteria detected within uroliths probably represent those present at the time they were formed, and may serve as a source of recurrent UTI. Bacteria may remain viable within uroliths for long periods. In a pilot study, we cultured viable staphylococci from struvite uroliths removed from a miniature schnauzer up to three months following surgery. If all the uroliths have not been removed from the patient, knowledge of the type and antimicrobic susceptibility of bacteria inside uroliths that have been voided or removed may be of therapeutic significance. Procedures for culture of microbes from the inner portions of uroliths have been developed and can be performed by most veterinary diagnostic laboratories (Osborne et al, 1983; Ruby and Ling, 1986).

GUESSTIMATION OF UROLITH COMPOSITION

Formulation of effective dietary and medical protocols for urolith dissolution depends on knowledge of the mineral com-

Table 38-9. Mineral composition of 5,050 canine nephroliths and ureteroliths evaluated at the Minnesota Urolith Center by quantitative methods: 1991 to 2006.

Predominate mineral type	Proportion of predominant mineral (%)	Number	Percent
Calcium oxalate	**-**	**2,174**	**43.1**
Calcium oxalate monohydrate	100	(1,168)	-
	70-99	(511)	-
Calcium oxalate dihydrate	70-100*	(234)	-
Calcium oxalate monohydrate and dihydrate	70-100	(161)	-
Calcium phosphate	**-**	**81**	**1.6**
Calcium apatite	70-100	(67)	-
Calcium hydrogen phosphate•$2H_2O$	70-100	(14)	-
Magnesium ammonium phosphate•$6H_2O$	**70-100**	**1,299**	**25.7**
Purines	**-**	**671**	**13.3**
Ammonium acid urate	70-100	(476)	-
Sodium acid urate	70-100	(47)	-
Sodium calcium urate	70-100	(17)	-
Uric acid	70-100	104	-
Xanthine	70-100	(24)	-
Cystine	**70-100**	**77**	**-**
Silica	**70-100**	**18**	**0.4**
Mixed**	**-**	**132**	**2.6**
Compound***	**-**	**575**	**11.4**
Matrix	**-**	**13**	**0.3**
Drug metabolite	**na**	**1**	**0.02**
Other	**na**	**7**	**0.1**

Key: na = not applicable.
*Uroliths composed of 70 to 100% of mineral type listed; no nucleus and shell detected.
**Uroliths contained less than 70% of predominant mineral; no nucleus or shell detected.
***Uroliths contained an identifiable nucleus and one or more surrounding layers of a different mineral type.

Table 38-10. Problem-specific and therapeutic-specific database for diagnosis and management of urolithiasis.

1. Obtain appropriate history and perform physical examination, including a rectal examination of the urethra.
2. Perform complete urinalysis; save aliquots of urine for possible determination of mineral concentration.
3. Obtain quantitative urine culture and determine urease activity; test for antimicrobial susceptibility if bacterial pathogens are identified. Consider attempts to isolate ureaplasmas if urease-positive urine is bacteriologically sterile.
4. Perform a complete blood cell count.
5. Freeze an aliquot of serum collected at the time the sample was obtained for the complete blood cell count for possible determination of urea nitrogen, creatinine, calcium and/or uric acid concentrations.
6. Obtain radiographs.
   a. Take survey radiographs of the entire urinary system.
   b. Consider intravenous urography for patients with renal or ureteral uroliths.
   c. Consider intravenous urography or contrast cystography for patients with bladder uroliths.
   d. Consider contrast urethrography for patients with urethral uroliths.
   e. Ultrasonography is recommended if equipment is available.
7. Determine mineral composition of uroliths.
   a. Submit uroliths passed during micturition or retrieved during diagnostic procedures for quantitative analysis.
   b. Use results obtained from the history, physical examination, laboratory examination and radiography to determine probable mineral composition of uroliths.
8. Initiate therapy to eradicate urinary tract infection, if present.
9. Initiate therapy for urolithiasis.
   a. Initiate therapy to promote dissolution of uroliths if amenable to dietary and medical therapy.
      Formulate followup protocol to monitor dissolution of uroliths.
      Formulate alternative treatment options if uroliths do not dissolve or if problems such as recurrent outflow obstruction occur.
   b. Remove uroliths by voiding urohydropropulsion.
   c. Remove uroliths by nephrotomy or cystotomy.
      Obtain bladder or kidney biopsy specimens for microscopic examination during surgical procedure.
      Correct any anatomic defects, if present.
      Compare number of uroliths removed during surgery with the number identified by radiography.
      Obtain postsurgical radiographs to evaluate completeness of urolith removal.
      Submit uroliths for quantitative analysis.
10. After uroliths are surgically removed or medically dissolved, initiate therapy to prevent recurrence.
11. Formulate followup protocol with clients.

Box 38-2. Principles of Urolith Treatment and Prevention.

OVERVIEW

Surgery has been the time-honored method of managing all types of urolithiasis in dogs. Although surgery has been an effective method that provides immediate elimination of uroliths, it is associated with several limitations, including: 1) persistence of underlying causes and a high rate of recurrence of uroliths despite surgery, 2) patient factors that enhance adverse consequences of general anesthesia or surgery and 3) inability to remove all uroliths or fragments of uroliths during surgery. In addition, situations occasionally arise in which owners of companion animals will not consent to surgical therapy but will consider dietary and medical therapy. Dietary and medical dissolution of uroliths may be considered for these and other reasons (i.e., the urolith is asymptomatic).

Results of several experimental and clinical investigations have confirmed the efficacy of dietary and medical dissolution of canine uroliths. Despite the feasibility of dissolution of uroliths, however, this form of therapy is associated with potential hazards. Uroliths always predispose patients to urinary tract infection (UTI) and obstructive uropathy. Risks and benefits of dietary and medical vs. surgical and dietary and medical therapy must be considered for each patient.

Detailed descriptions of nonsurgical and surgical methods for reestablishing urine outflow are beyond the scope of the discussion but are available elsewhere. Likewise, details pertaining to surgical removal of uroliths, endoscopic and percutaneous manipulation of uroliths, chemolysis via nephrostomy, disintegration of renal and ureteral uroliths via ultrasound and shockwave lithotripsy have been reviewed.

DIETARY AND MEDICAL DISSOLUTION OF UROLITHS

Therapy should not be initiated before appropriate samples have been collected for diagnosis. The objectives of dietary and medical management of uroliths are to arrest further growth and to promote urolith dissolution by correcting or controlling underlying abnormalities. For therapy to be effective, it must induce undersaturation of urine with lithogenic crystalloids by: 1) increasing the solubility of crystalloids in urine, 2) increasing the volume of urine in which crystalloids are dissolved or suspended and 3) reducing the quantity of lithogenic crystalloids in urine. For example, attempts to increase the solubility of crystalloids in urine often include administration of medications designed to change urinary pH to create a less favorable environment for crystallization. Likewise, diuresis is commonly induced to increase the volume of urine in which crystalloids are dissolved or suspended. A dietary change is an example of a method to reduce the quantity of lithogenic crystalloids in urine.

In general, dietary and medical treatment should be formulated in stepwise fashion, with the initial goal of reducing the urine concentration of lithogenic substances. Medications that have the potential to induce a sustained alteration in body composition of metabolites, in addition to urine concentration of metabolites, should be reserved for patients with active or frequently recurrent uroliths. Caution must be used so that the side effects of treatment are not more detrimental than the effects of the uroliths.

Results of experimental and clinical studies have revealed that the size and number of uroliths do not dictate the likelihood of response to therapy. We have had success in dissolving uroliths that are small and large, single and multiple. However the rate of dissolution is related to size and surface area of the urolith exposed to urine. Just as one large ice cube dissolves more slowly than an equal volume of crushed ice, one large urolith will dissolve more slowly than an equal volume of many smaller uroliths. Rate of dissolution is influenced by surface area of the urolith exposed to undersaturated urine.

Difficulty in inducing complete dissolution of uroliths by creating urine that is undersaturated with the suspected lithogenic crystalloid should prompt consideration that: 1) the wrong mineral component was identified, 2) the nucleus of the urolith is of different mineral composition than outer portions and/or 3) the owner or the patient is not complying with therapy.

SURGICAL REMOVAL OF UROLITHS

Detection of uroliths is not in itself an indication for surgery. However, along with dietary and medical management, surgical intervention may play an important role in therapy of urolithiasis.

position of uroliths. Because a variety of different types of uroliths and nephroliths occur in dogs (**Tables 38-8** and **38-9**), veterinarians should use a protocol that facilitates determination of the mineral composition of uroliths based on probability (**Tables 38-10** and **38-11**). Formulation of dietary and medical therapy based on the mineral composition of uroliths determined by this protocol is usually associated with a high degree of success in dissolving uroliths or arresting their growth.

Attempts to induce dissolution of uroliths may be hampered if the uroliths are heterogeneous in composition. This has not been a significant problem in dogs with uroliths composed primarily of magnesium ammonium phosphate with small quantities of calcium apatite because the solubility characteristics of the two minerals are similar. Veterinarians have encountered difficulty in dissolving uroliths composed primarily of struvite with an outer shell composed primarily of calcium apatite. Difficulty will also be encountered in attempting to induce complete dissolution of a urolith with a nucleus of calcium oxalate, calcium phosphate, ammonium urate or silica and a shell of struvite because the solubility characteristics of this combination of minerals are dissimilar. These phenomena should be considered if dietary and medical therapy seems to be ineffective after initially reducing the size of uroliths (**Box 38-2**).

REFERENCES

The references for **Chapter 38** can be found at www.markmorris.org.

Surgical candidates include patients: 1) with urolith-induced obstruction to urine outflow that cannot be corrected by nonsurgical techniques, especially in patients with concomitant UTI, 2) with uroliths that are refractory to current methods of dietary and medical dissolution (e.g., silica, calcium oxalate and calcium phosphate uroliths), 3) with uroliths that are increasing in size or number despite dietary and medical therapy designed to inhibit their growth or cause their dissolution (especially if they are obstructing urine outflow or causing progressive deterioration in renal function), 4) with nephroliths and renal dysfunction of such a nature that the time required to induce dietary and medical dissolution is likely to be associated with more renal dysfunction than that associated with surgical procedures, 5) with anatomic defects of the urogenital tract that predispose patients to recurrent UTI and urolithiasis and are amenable to surgical correction at the time uroliths are removed and 6) unable to respond to dietary and medical management because of poor client compliance with therapeutic recommendations.

Complete obstruction to urine outflow caused by uroliths in patients with concomitant UTI should be regarded as a surgical emergency. In this situation, rapid spread of infection and associated damage to the urinary tract, especially the kidneys, are likely to induce septicemia and peracute renal failure caused by a combination of obstruction and pyelonephritis.

Unilateral nephroliths and ureteroliths that cause outflow obstruction and markedly impair function of the associated kidney should be managed by surgical intervention or (if possible) percutaneous nephropyelolithotomy. Dietary and medical therapy designed to induce urolith dissolution over several weeks in patients with poorly draining kidneys is unlikely to be effective because the urolith(s) will not be continuously bathed with newly formed urine modified to induce litholysis. The same concept applies to urethroliths that cannot be removed by nonsurgical methods.

Surgical removal of uroliths followed by dietary and medical litholytic protocols may be of value in some patients. Examples include patients in which uroliths or fragments of uroliths remain after surgery, and patients with crystalluria of a character and magnitude that indicate rapid recurrence is likely. Surgical incisions should be repaired using meticulous technique if protein-restricted canine litholytic foods are used.

PREVENTION OF UROLITH RECURRENCE

Uroliths tend to recur. Prevention of recurrent uroliths, which reduces the need for dietary and medical therapy and surgery, is therefore cost effective. In general, preventive strategies are designed to eliminate or control the underlying causes of various types of uroliths. When causes cannot be identified, preventive strategies encompass efforts to minimize risk factors associated with lithogenesis. These strategies commonly include dietary modification.

The Bibliography for **Box 38-2** can be found at www.markmorris.com

Table 38-11. Predicting mineral composition of common canine uroliths.

Mineral types	Predictors								
	Urinary pH	**Crystal appearance**	**Urine culture**	**Radiographic density**	**Radiographic contour**	**Serum abnormalities**	**Breed predisposition**	**Gender predisposition**	**Common ages**
Magnesium ammonium phosphate	Neutral to alkaline	Three- to eight-sided colorless prisms	Urease-producing bacteria (staphylococci, *Proteus* spp., *Ureaplasma* spp.)	1+ to 4+ (sometimes laminated)	Smooth, round or faceted May assume shape of renal pelvis, ureter, bladder or urethra	None	Miniature schnauzer, miniature poodle, Bichon Frise, cocker spaniel	Females (>80%)	2 to 9 years
Calcium oxalate	Acidic to neutral	Colorless envelope or octahedral shape (dihydrate salt) Spindles or dumbbell shape (monohydrate salt)	Negative	2+ to 4+	Rough or speculated (dihydrate salt) Small, smooth, round (monohydrate salt) Sometimes jackstone	Usually normocalcemic, occasionally hypercalcemic	Miniature schnauzer, standard schnauzer, Lhasa apso, Yorkshire terrier, miniature poodle, Shih Tzu, Bichon Frise	Males (>70%)	5 to 12 years
Urate	Acidic to neutral	Yellow-brown amorphous shapes (ammonium urate)	Negative	0 to 2+	Smooth (occasionally irregular) round or oval	Low serum urea nitrogen and albumin values In dogs with hepatic portosystemic shunts	Dalmatian, English bulldog, miniature schnauzer, Yorkshire terrier, Shih Tzu	Males (>90%)	1 to 5 years
Calcium phosphate	Alkaline to neutral (brushite forms in acidic urine)	Amorphous or long thin prisms	Negative	2+ to 4+	Smooth or irregular, round or faceted	Occasionally hypercalcemic	Yorkshire terrier, miniature schnauzer, Shih Tzu	Males (>55%)	<1 year, 6 to 10 years
Cystine	Acidic to neutral	Flat colorless hexagonal plates	Negative	1+ to 2+	Smooth (occasionally irregular) round or oval	None	English bulldog, dachshund, basset hound, Newfoundland	Males (>98%)	1 to 7 years
Silica	Acidic to neutral	None observed	Negative	2+ to 3+	Round center with radial spoke-like projections (jackstone)	None	German shepherd, golden retriever, Labrador retriever, miniature schnauzer, cavalier King Charles spaniel	Males (95%)	3 to 10 years

Chapter 39

Canine Purine Urolithiasis: Causes, Detection, Management and Prevention

Carl A. Osborne
Joseph W. Bartges
Jody P. Lulich
Hasan Albasan
Carroll Weiss

"We should provide the type of medical care that we would desire if we were the patient rather than the doctor."
Carl A. Osborne

TERMINOLOGY

Purines are catabolites derived from DNA and RNA. They include adenine, guanine, hypoxanthine, xanthine, anhydrous uric acid, uric acid monohydrate, uric acid dihydrate, salts of uric acid (e.g., ammonium urate, sodium urate, calcium sodium urate) and in most mammals, allantoin. Each of these catabolites may behave differently.

PREVALENCE AND MINERAL COMPOSITION

Purine uroliths (ammonium urate, sodium urate, calcium urate, uric acid, xanthine, etc.) accounted for 6.4% (22,412 of 350,803) of all canine uroliths submitted to the Minnesota Urolith Center from 1981 to 2007 (Table 38-8), and 4.97% (2,020 of 40,612) of all canine uroliths analyzed in 2007. Purines accounted for 13.3% of all upper tract uroliths analyzed at the Minnesota Urolith Center from 1981 to 2006 (Table 38-9). Most dogs with xanthine uroliths had a history of treatment with allopurinol. Purines composed 23% of uroliths retrieved from dogs less than 12 months old. The mean age of dogs at the time of ammonium urate urolith retrieval was approximately four years (range one month to 17 years). The mean age of dogs at the time of sodium urate and calcium urate urolith retrieval was also approximately four years (range six months to 14 years). The mean age of dogs at the time of uric acid urolith retrieval was three years (range one month to 12 years). The mean age at the time of xanthine urolith retrieval was approximately five years (range one and one-half to nine years). Males were affected more often than females with ammonium urate (90 vs. 10%), sodium and calcium urate (99 vs. 1%), uric acid (88 vs. 12%) and xanthine (81 vs. 19%) uroliths.

In our series, 66 different breeds were affected with ammonium urate uroliths including Dalmatians (61%), miniature schnauzers (7%), Yorkshire terriers (5%), Shih Tzus (4%) and English bulldogs (4%). Twelve different breeds had sodium and

Table 39-1. Common characteristics of canine purine uroliths.

Chemical names	**Formulas**
Ammonium acid urate	$C_5H_3N_4O_3NH_4 \cdot H_2O$
Sodium acid urate	$C_5H_3N_4O_3Na \cdot H_2O$
Uric acid	$C_5H_4N_4O_3 \cdot 2H_2O$
Xanthine	$C_5H_4N_4O_2$

Some variations in mineral composition
Ammonium urate only
Sodium calcium urate
Sodium urate only
Uric acid only
Xanthine only
Ammonium urate mixed with variable quantities of sodium urate, or sodium and calcium urate, magnesium ammonium phosphate and/or calcium oxalate
Sodium and calcium oxalate
Xanthine and uric acid
Physical characteristics
Color: Light or dark brown, brown-green
Shape: Variable. Usually round or ovoid in urinary bladder, may assume shape of renal pelvis (funnel shaped), may assume jackstone appearance. Usually smooth, occasionally irregular or rough.
Nuclei: Nuclei and concentric laminations are common.
Density: Usually dense and brittle. Radiographically, purine uroliths have marginal radiodensity compared with soft tissue. Some may be radiolucent.
Number: Single or multiple
Location: May be located in kidneys, ureters, urinary bladder (most common) and/or urethra.
Size: Usually small (1 mm to 1 cm in diameter), occasionally large (more than 1 cm)
Prevalence
Approximately 5 to 6% of all canine uroliths. Approximately 13% of canine nephroliths.
May be recurrent.
Characteristics of affected canine patients
In Dalmatian dogs, most common in males.
Mean age at diagnosis is four years (range <1 to >17 years).
Most commonly observed in Dalmatian dogs, English bulldogs, miniature schnauzers, Yorkshire terriers and Shih Tzus.

calcium urate uroliths; however, these uroliths were primarily encountered in Dalmatians (92%) and English bulldogs (4%). Six different breeds had uric acid uroliths; Dalmatians were affected most commonly (80%). Five different breeds had xanthine uroliths, including Dalmatians (56%) and English bulldogs (35%). Ammonium urate (97%), sodium and calcium urate (96%), uric acid (100%) and xanthine (94%) uroliths were more commonly removed from the lower urinary tract than the upper urinary tract.

Ammonium urate, sodium and calcium urate and uric acid uroliths typically appear as multiple, small, smooth, hard, round or ovoid structures with a characteristic brown-green color (**Table 39-1**). However, the physical appearance of urate uroliths may vary depending on the presence and quantity of different mineral components, the quantity of matrix they contain, the site(s) of their formation and growth and whether or not they are associated with concurrent urinary tract disorders. Rarely, they form jackstones. Examination of cross sections of urate uroliths frequently reveals concentric laminations and nuclei located in the geographic center of the urolith.

ETIOPATHOGENESIS AND RISK FACTORS

Applied Biochemistry: Uric Acid Metabolism

Uric acid is one of several biodegradation products of purine nucleotide metabolism (**Figure 39-1**) (Foreman, 1984; Gutman, 1964; Greene et al, 1969; Williams and Wilson, 1990; Wyngaarden and Holmes, 1978). Purines are made up of three groups of compounds: 1) oxypurines (hypoxanthine, xanthine, uric acid and allantoin), 2) aminopurines (adenine, guanine) and 3) methylpurines (caffeine, theophylline and theobromine). In most dogs and cats, allantoin is the major metabolic end product, and it is the most soluble of the purine metabolic products excreted in urine (Bartges et al, 1992; Cohen et al, 1965; Giesecke and Stangassinger, 1990; Roch-Ramel and Peters, 1978). Whereas uric acid provides a means for nitrogen excretion in some animals (reptiles, birds, etc.), mammals excrete nitrogen in the form of urea (ureotelics). Because people and apes lack the enzyme uricase (urate oxidase), they cannot metabolize uric acid into allantoin. It has been estimated that the serum uric acid level of people is up to 100 times greater than serum creatinine concentrations in other mammals (Rafey et al, 2003).

The serum concentration of uric acid is derived from two sources: 1) exogenously from food and 2) endogenously from de novo purine biosynthesis, involving nucleic acid turnover and production from non-purine precursors. Purine synthesis occurs in the liver and involves recycling of guanine and hypoxanthine. In people, excess nucleotides are converted to xanthine and then uric acid via xanthine oxidase (Asplin, 1996). In most dogs and cats, excess uric acid is converted to allantoin via the hepatic enzyme uricase. Allantoin is highly soluble in urine, whereas uric acid and xanthine are not. Therefore, people are at greater risk for uric acid urolithiasis than most dogs and cats (Cameron and Sakhaee, 2007). Tissue catabolism or consumption of foods high in purine content may increase purine catabolism. In people, consumption of high-purine foods can cause as much as a 50% increase in urinary excretion of uric acid compared to consumption of a purine-free diet (Fellstrom et al, 1983).

In people, it has been estimated that approximately one-third of excess uric acid is eliminated by way of the intestinal tract (Sorensen, 1965). The kidneys eliminate the remainder. Although the mechanisms involved in glomerular filtration, renal tubular absorption and renal tubular secretion of uric acid have not yet been completely defined, it appears that all three mechanisms are involved (Cameron and Sakhaee, 2007). It has been proposed that glomeruli freely filter uric acid. The proximal tubules actively reabsorb approximately 99% of filtered uric acid. Subsequently, the renal tubules secrete approximately 50% of the filtered uric acid, followed by 40% postsecretory reabsorption. The final uric acid excretion is approximately 10% (Cameron and Sakhaee, 2007).

Uric acid is a weak organic acid with an ionization constant (pKa) of 5.5. At a temperature of 37°C (98.6°F), human urine has a pKa of 5.35. Uric acid is less soluble than its base (urate) (Cameron and Sakhaee, 2007).

Uroliths composed of uric acid (anhydrous uric acid, uric acid dihydrate, sodium urate, ammonium urate) or xanthine form because urine is oversaturated with these substances (Brown and Purich, 1992; Finlayson, 1978; Porter, 1963; Smith, 1990). Ammonium urate (also known as ammonium acid urate and ammonium biurate) is the monobasic ammonium salt of uric acid. It is the most common naturally occurring purine urolith form observed in dogs (Osborne et al, 1995). Other naturally occurring purine uroliths include sodium urate (also known as sodium acid urate or monosodium urate), sodium calcium urate, potassium urate and uric acid dihydrate (Osborne et al, 1995).

Uric Acid, Sodium Urate and Ammonium Urate

Risk factors for urate lithogenesis in dogs include: 1) increased renal excretion and urine concentration of uric acid, 2) increased renal excretion or renal production of ammonium ions, 3) increased microbial production of ammonium ions, 4) aciduria, 5) formation of highly concentrated urine and 6) presence of promoters or absence of inhibitors of urate urolith formation (Kruger and Osborne, 1986). Genetic factors may be important because urate uroliths are common in certain breeds of dogs. For example, Dalmatian dogs and English bulldogs have an inherent predisposition to forming urate uroliths (See sections about Dalmatian and non-Dalmatian dogs below.) (Case et al, 1993; Sorenson and Ling, 1993). Dietary components may promote urate urolith formation in predisposed dogs because dietary purines may be digested, absorbed, incorporated into the body's purine pool and eventually excreted in urine (**Tables 39-2** and **39-3**). Thus, metabolism of dietary purines may result in oversaturation of urine with urate lithogenic substances (e.g., other related metabolites of uric acid). In studies of normal dogs, consumption of high-protein foods was associated with greater urine uric acid excretion and increased urine saturation with uric acid, sodium urate and ammonium urate, when compared with consumption of low-protein foods (Bartges et al, 1995, 1995a, 1995b). The same association was found in Dalmatian dogs (Giesecke and Tiemeyer, 1984; Lulich et al, 1995).

Xanthine

Xanthine is a product of purine metabolism and is converted to uric acid by the enzyme xanthine oxidase (Bartges et al, 1992; Parks and Granger, 1986). Hereditary xanthinuria is a rarely recognized disorder of people characterized by a deficiency of xanthine oxidase (Fildes, 1989; Holmes et al, 1974; Kario et al, 1991; Kawachi et al, 1990; Landas et al, 1989; Mateos, 1987). Consequently, abnormal quantities of xanthine are excreted in urine as a major end product of purine metabolism. Because xanthine is the least soluble of the purines naturally excreted in urine, xanthinuria may be associated with formation of uroliths (Bartges et al, 1992; Fildes, 1989; Kario et al, 1991; Ling et al, 1991; Pyrah, 1979).

Naturally occurring xanthinuria and xanthine urolithiasis have been reported to occur in a few dogs (Kidder and Chivers, 1968; Kucera et al, 1997). Xanthine urolithiasis was reported in a family of cavalier King Charles spaniels (van Zuilen et al, 1997).

Uroliths whose composition was at least 70% xanthine

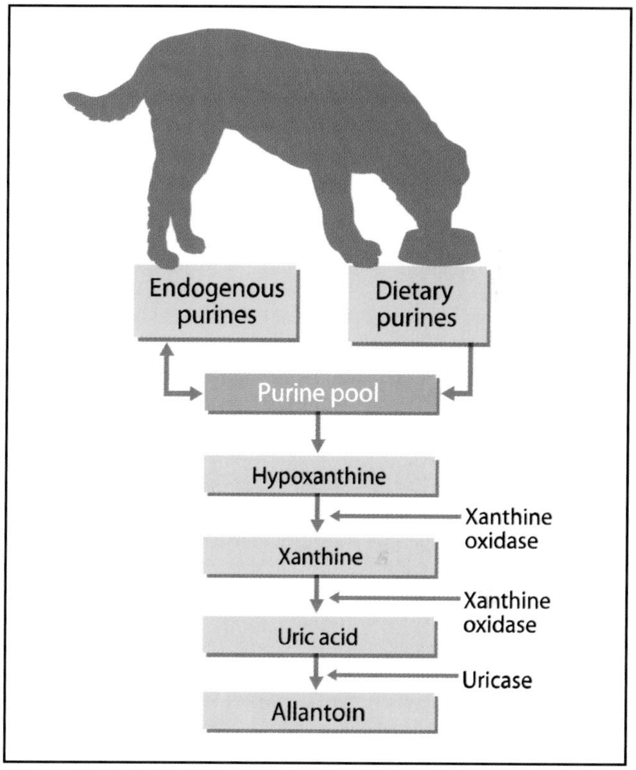

Figure 39-1. Diagram of normal canine purine degradation.

Table 39-2. Some potential risk factors for canine purine uroliths.

Food	Urine	Metabolic	Drugs
High purine content (**Table 39-3.**)	Hyperuricuria	Males	Urine acidifiers
Acidifying potential	Hyperammonuria	Breed	Salicylates
Low moisture content	Acidic pH	Dalmatians	Chemotherapeutic agents (especially 6-mercaptopurine)
Ascorbic acid?	Urine concentration	English bulldogs	
	Urine retention	Miniature schnauzers	
	Urease-producing microburia	Yorkshire terriers	
	Increased promoters?	Shih Tzus	
	Decreased inhibitors?	Hyperuricemia	
		Hyperammonuria	
		Hepatic dysfunction	
		Neoplasia with rapid cell destruction	

Table 39-3. Purine content of selected foods.

Foods to avoid (high purine concentration)	Foods to use sparingly (moderately high purine concentration)	Foods that can be fed (negligible purine concentration)
Anchovies	Asparagus	Breads (whole grain cereal products)
Brain	Cauliflower	Butter and fats
Clams	Fish*	Cheese
Goose	Legumes (beans and peas)	Eggs
Gravies	Lentils	Fruits and fruit juices
Heart	Meats	Gelatin
Kidney	Mushrooms	Milk
Liver	Spinach	Nuts
Mackerel		Refined cereals
Meat extracts including bouillon		Sugars
Mussels		Vegetable soups
Oysters		Cream soups
Salmon		Vegetables**
Sardines		Water
Scallops		
Shrimp		
Sweetbreads		
Tuna		
Yeast (baker's and brewer's)		

*Except those listed in the first column.
**Except those listed in the second column.

accounted for less than 0.1% (362 of 373,612) of all canine uroliths submitted to the Minnesota Urolith Center from 1998 to 2007. Almost all canine xanthine uroliths in our series were obtained from dogs treated with varying doses of allopurinol given orally.

At the Minnesota Urolith Center, the mean age of dogs at the time of xanthine urolith retrieval was five years (range = three to 168 months). In this regard, the cavalier King Charles spaniel breed is an exception inasmuch that naturally occurring xanthine uroliths have been recognized when these dogs were less than one year of age.

Male dogs (86%) were affected more often than females (9%) in our series (5% were of unknown gender). Of these dogs, 190 were castrated males (53%), 122 were intact males (34%), 23 were spayed females (6%), 11 were intact females (3%) and 16 were of unknown gender (4%). With the apparent exception of cavalier King Charles spaniels (six dogs in our series), the predominance of allopurinol-induced xanthine uroliths in males has also been observed by others (Bartges et al, 1993; Ling et al, 1991). In a report of 38 xanthine-containing uroliths, 36 occurred in males and two occurred in females (Ling et al, 1991).

At our center, 40 different breeds were affected including Dalmatians (50%), mixed breed (12%), English bulldogs (4%), miniature schnauzers (4%), German shepherd dogs (2%), boxers (2%) and cavalier King Charles spaniels (six dogs = 2%). Similar observations have been made by others (Ling et al, 1991). In one report, of 38 xanthine-containing uroliths, 30 were found in Dalmatians, two were found in miniature/toy poodles and one was retrieved from a Shih Tzu (Ling et al, 1991). The affected breeds for five xanthine specimens were apparently unknown. Of the 362 uroliths composed of xanthine in our series, 316 dogs were given allopurinol, 10 were given fluoroquinolones and two received sulfadiazine (34 uroliths were submitted without a drug history).

The most common cause of xanthine uroliths in dogs is formation secondary to therapy with allopurinol. Allopurinol rapidly binds to and inhibits the action of xanthine oxidase, thereby decreasing conversion of hypoxanthine to xanthine and xanthine to uric acid. The result is a reduction of serum and urine concentrations of uric acid with a reciprocal increase in serum and urine concentrations of xanthine (**Figure 39-2**). Administration of allopurinol at high doses, especially with concurrent consumption of high purine foods, will result in formation of xanthine uroliths (**Figure 39-3**).

Dalmatian Dogs

Dalmatian dogs are predisposed to urate uroliths because their ability to oxidize uric acid to allantoin is intermediate between that of people and many non-Dalmatian dogs (Bartges et al, 1994; Duncan and Curtiss, 1971; Friedman and Byers, 1948). This characteristic is due to an autosomal recessive trait (Safra et al, 2005). People normally have a serum uric acid concentration of approximately 3 to 7 mg/dl, and excrete approximately 500 to 700 mg of uric acid in their urine per day (Williams and Wilson, 1990). Of all non-Dalmatian dogs studied to date, most have a serum uric acid concentration of less than 0.5 mg/dl, and excrete approximately 10 to 60 mg of uric acid in their urine per day. Dalmatian dogs have a serum uric acid concentration that is two to four times that of non-Dalmatian dogs and excrete more than 400 to 600 mg of uric acid in their urine per day (Bovee, 1984; Ling et al, 1997).

Studies of the fate of uric acid in Dalmatian dogs have revealed unique hepatic and renal pathways of metabolism (Friedman and Byers, 1948; Duncan and Curtiss, 1971). Of these two metabolic sites, reciprocal allogenic renal and hepatic transplantations between Dalmatian and non-Dalmatian dogs indicate that the hepatic mechanism is quantitatively the more significant (Cohn et al, 1965; Kuster et al, 1972). The liver of Dalmatian dogs does not completely oxidize available uric acid, even though it contains sufficient concentrations of uricase. Compared with non-Dalmatian dogs, Dalmatian dogs convert uric acid to allantoin at a reduced rate (Benedetti et al, 1997; Kocken et al, 1996; Kuster et al, 1972). It has been hypothesized that their hepatic cellular membranes are partially impermeable to uric acid (Harvey and Christensen, 1964; Tiemeyer et al, 1986).

The proximal renal tubules of Dalmatian dogs reabsorb less uric acid than those of non-Dalmatian dogs; a small amount is secreted by the distal tubules (Kessler et al, 1959). In non-Dalmatian dogs, 98 to 100% of the uric acid in the glomerular filtrate is reabsorbed by the proximal tubules and returned to the liver for further metabolism (Kessler et al, 1959; Roch-Ramel et al, 1978). The distal tubules are thought to secrete uric acid in the urine of non-Dalmatian dogs (Foreman, 1984; Mudge et al, 1968; Nolan and Foulkes, 1971; Tiemeyer et al, 1986).

The definitive mechanism(s) of urate urolith formation in Dalmatian dogs is unknown. Increased urinary excretion of uric acid is a risk factor rather than a primary cause. Urate uroliths are recognized 13 times more commonly in males than females; the average age of dogs when uroliths are diagnosed is 4.5 years (Albasan et al, 2005; Case et al, 1993). Although all Dalmatian dogs excrete relatively high quantities of uric acid in their urine, apparently only a small percentage forms urate uroliths (Case et al, 1993; Albasan et al, 2005). At one time, it was thought that urolith-forming Dalmatian dogs did not excrete greater quantities of uric acid in their urine than non-urolith-forming Dalmatian dogs. However, further studies revealed that insensitive methods for measuring urine uric acid concentration were responsible for this erroneous conclusion. When steps are taken to ensure that urine uric acid remains in solution, differences in urine uric acid concentrations between non-urolith-forming Dalmatian and urolith-forming Dalmatian dogs may be expected (Felice et al, 1990; Schaible, 1986).

Urate uroliths commonly affect Dalmatian dogs; however, not all uroliths formed by Dalmatian dogs are composed of ammonium urate. For example, of 2,020 uroliths formed by Dalmatian dogs, 93% were composed of purines (ammonium urate, sodium urate, uric acid and xanthine), 3% were of mixed composition, 1% were struvite, 1% were calcium oxalate, 2% were compound uroliths and less than 1% were cystine.

Non-Dalmatian Dogs

Comparatively little is known about urate lithogenesis in non-Dalmatian dogs that do not have portal vascular anomalies. Many breeds of dogs are affected with urate urolithiasis. Although urate uroliths are commonly encountered in Dalmatian dogs, approximately 30 to 60% of all canine urate uroliths analyzed by quantitative methods are found in other breeds (Bovee and Mcquire, 1984; Kruger and Osborne, 1986; Osborne et al, 1995). English bulldogs have a significantly higher incidence of urate urolithiasis compared with other breeds (Bartges et al, 1994). Clinical evaluation of eight male English bulldogs with confirmed ammonium urate urocystoliths revealed mild elevations in serum uric acid concentration. The size of their livers was normal, as was the serum concentration of hepatic enzymes, blood concentration of ammo-

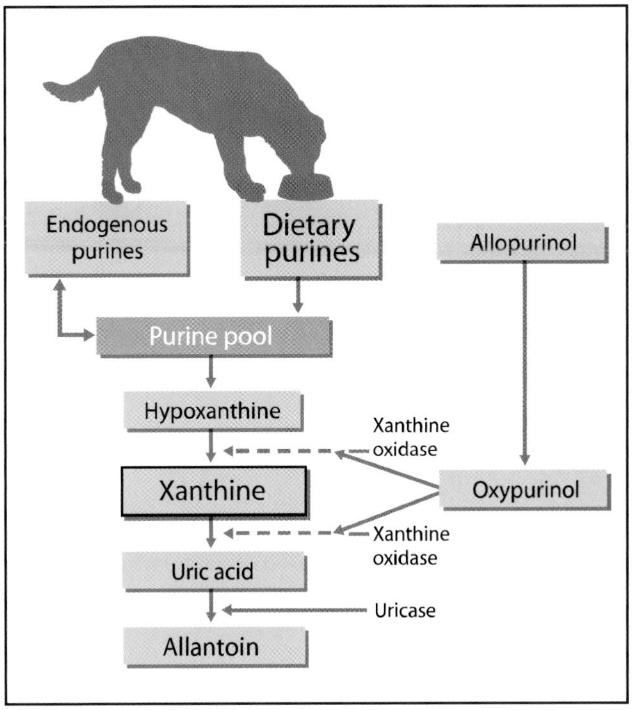

Figure 39-2. Diagram of purine degradation in dogs fed a maintenance food and given allopurinol.

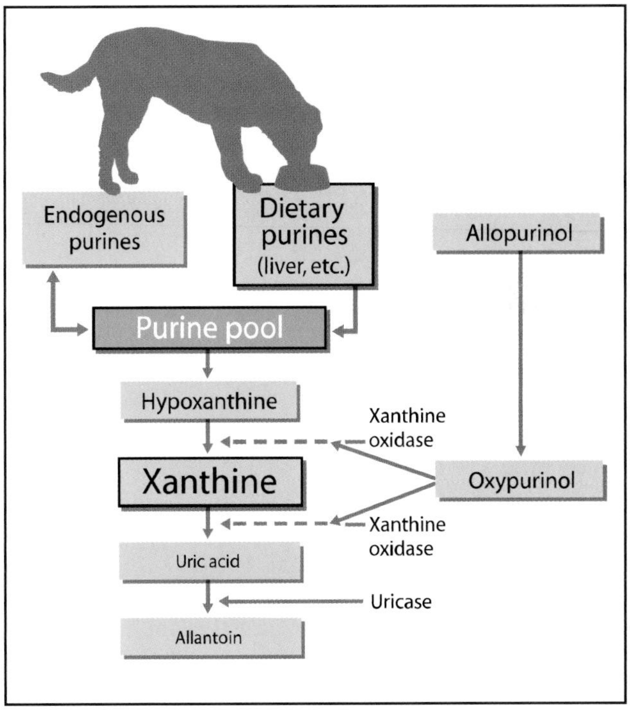

Figure 39-3. Diagram of purine metabolism in dogs that consume a purine-rich food and are given allopurinol.

nia and bromsulphalein retention. Other non-Dalmatian breeds that appear to have a significantly higher incidence of urate urolithiasis based on quantitative urolith analyses are miniature schnauzers, Shih Tzus and Yorkshire terriers (Osborne et al, 1995).

Urate uroliths from non-Dalmatian dogs have been recognized most frequently in males. Uroliths have been detected throughout the lifespan of affected dogs; however, they were most frequently detected in dogs three to six years of age.

Regardless of cause, severe hepatic dysfunction may predispose dogs to urate lithogenesis, especially ammonium urate uroliths. Observations and evidence derived from experimental models suggest that prolonged consumption of foods with markedly restricted levels of protein may be associated with formation of urate uroliths in dogs (Kruger and Osborne, 1986). Biochemical and histologic evaluation of these dogs suggests that long-term consumption of foods severely restricted in protein may induce hepatocellular dysfunction and concomitant hyperuricemia. Hepatic cirrhosis has also been associated with urate uroliths in dogs and other species (Rothuizen and van den Ingh, 1980). However, foods with severely restricted protein levels and other causes of hepatic dysfunction have been uncommon causes of ammonium urate urolithiasis. Nonetheless, their significance relative to ammonium urate lithogenesis deserves further study.

Dogs with Portal Vascular Anomalies or Hepatic Microvascular Dysplasia

Ammonium urate uroliths have frequently been observed in dogs with portal vascular anomalies. These uroliths occur in males and females and usually have been detected before dogs reach three years of age (Rothuizen and van den Ingh, 1980; Marretta et al, 1981; Hardy and Klausner, 1983; Kruger and Osborne, 1986).

Direct communication between the portal and systemic vasculature shunts blood around the liver. Severe hepatic atrophy and diminished hepatic function may occur as a result. Hepatic dysfunction in turn is associated with reduced hepatic conversion of uric acid to allantoin and reduced conversion of ammonia to urea. The predisposition of dogs with portal vascular anomalies to urate urolithiasis is probably associated with concomitant hyperuricemia, hyperammonemia, hyperuricuria and hyperammonuria (Kruger and Osborne, 1986; Hardy and Klausner, 1983). Serum uric acid concentrations in 15 dogs with portal vascular anomalies evaluated at the University of Minnesota Veterinary Teaching Hospital were increased (values ranged from 1.2 to 4.0 mg/dl) (Hardy and Klausner, 1983). Concurrent hyperuricuria, hyperammonuria, hyperuricemia and hyperammonemia were observed in an 18-month-old Bernese mountain dog with recurrent ammonium urate uroliths associated with a portal vascular anomaly (Kruger and Osborne, 1986). This dog had a urine uric acid concentration of 42 mg/kg body weight/day and a urine ammonia concentration of 3.2 mM/kg body weight/day while the dog was fed a protein-restricted food. Hyperuricuria, hyperammonuria, hyperuricemia and hyperammonemia were observed in three miniature schnauzers with ammonium urate uroliths associated with portal vascular anomalies. In these dogs, urine uric acid concentrations were approximately 50 mg/kg body weight/day and urine ammonia concentrations were approximately 1.5 mM/kg body weight/day while the dogs consumed a growth-type food. When two of these dogs consumed a purine-restricted food, urine uric acid concentrations were approximately 17 mg/kg body weight/day and urine ammonia concentrations were approximately 0.6 mM/kg body weight/day.

Not all dogs with portal systemic anomalies develop concurrent ammonium urate urolithiasis. Definition and characterization of other factors responsible for promoting or inhibiting urate lithogenesis in affected dogs require further investigation.

We have observed urate urocystolith formation in miniature schnauzers and Yorkshire terriers with hepatic microvascular dysplasia. Dogs with this disorder do not have macrovascular shunts. Rather, intrahepatic microvascular shunting apparently occurs. Clinical signs and biochemical abnormalities are similar to those seen in dogs with macroscopic vascular shunts. When affected dogs consumed a growth-type food, urinary uric acid excretion was approximately 30 mg/kg body weight/24 hours, urinary ammonia excretion was approximately 1.25 mmol/kg body weight/24 hours and urinary pH was less than 6.5 pH units. When dogs were fed a purine-restricted food, urinary uric acid excretion was approximately 16 mg/kg body weight/24 hours, urinary ammonia excretion was approximately 0.5 mmol/kg body weight/24 hours and urinary pH was greater than 7.0 pH units.

Not all dogs with portal systemic anomalies or hepatic microvascular dysplasia develop concurrent ammonium urate urolithiasis. Definition and characterization of other factors responsible for promoting or inhibiting urate lithogenesis in affected dogs require further investigation.

Dietary Risk Factors

Concentrations of lithogenic substances in urine depend on urine volume. Because commercial dry foods are associated with production of less urine compared with moist foods, consumption of dry foods is likely a risk factor for urate urolith formation.

Dalmatian dogs consuming foods containing more than 20% dry matter (DM) protein, and protein sources high in purines and purine precursors (**Table 39-3**) are at increased risk for urate lithogenesis. Because urate uroliths associated with portal vascular anomalies are often diagnosed in dogs less than one year of age, it is probable that they were consuming foods with increased protein content.

Urine acidity is a risk factor for urate lithogenesis because the solubility of most purines, especially ammonium urate, is pH-dependent. Therefore, consumption of foods that promote aciduria (e.g., high-protein foods or those with other acidifying ingredients) may be a risk factor.

BIOLOGIC BEHAVIOR

Purine uroliths have the potential to undergo spontaneous dissolution, remain active (grow) or become inactive (remain unchanged). Although spontaneous dissolution of non-urate-containing uroliths has occasionally been observed, spontaneous dissolution of urate uroliths has apparently not been reported.

Recurrence of urate uroliths may be influenced by several factors including: 1) persistence of underlying causes, 2) incomplete removal of all uroliths from the urinary tract at the time of lithotripsy or surgery, 3) persistence or recurrence of urinary tract infections (UTIs) with urease-producing bacteria and/or 4) failure to comply with therapeutic or prophylactic recommendations. Frequent recurrence of urate uroliths is not surprising considering the persistence of disorders associated with urate urolithiasis.

A relatively high incidence of recurrence following surgical removal is a unique characteristic of urate urolithiasis in Dalmatian and non-Dalmatian dogs. In several studies using qualitative methods of urolith analysis, recurrence was reported in 33 to 50% of dogs with urate uroliths (Brown et al, 1977; Finco et al, 1970; Weaver, 1970). In these dogs, uroliths generally recurred within one year after diagnosis and treatment. Recurrence of urate urolithiasis in non-Dalmatian dogs with portal vascular anomalies also appears to be similar (Marretta et al, 1981; Hardy and Klausner, 1983). In dogs, recurrence of urolithiasis with uroliths composed of minerals other than those present during the initial episode is uncommon. However, uroliths predominantly composed of minerals other than ammonium urate, sodium urate or uric acid may form in canine patients originally affected with urate uroliths (Porter, 1963; Brown et al, 1977).

KEY NUTRITIONAL FACTORS

The key nutritional factors for foods intended for dissolution and prevention of urate uroliths in dogs are discussed below and summarized in **Table 39-4**.

Water

Concentrations of lithogenic substances in urine depend on urine volume. Augmenting urine volume with the goal of decreasing urine uric acid and ammonium concentrations and enhancing urine flow through the excretory pathway is an important strategy. Feeding moist foods is recommended because commercial dry foods are associated with production of a smaller volume of more concentrated urine. Clients should encourage water intake to achieve a urine specific gravity less than 1.020. (See Assess and Determine the Feeding Method: Urate Urolith Dissolution below.)

Sodium chloride supplementation is sometimes recommended to increase urine volume. However, increased sodium intake poses other risks to urate urolithiasis patients. (See Sodium below.) It is noteworthy that sodium chloride given orally to normal human volunteers for 10 days did not alter urine uric acid concentration (Breslau and Pak, 1983).

Attempts at increasing urine volume through administration of diuretic drugs have been reported in people. Long-term administration (up to three years) of hydrochlorothiazide to human patients with uroliths containing calcium salts resulted in increased serum and urine uric acid concentrations (Pak et al, 1978).

Table 39-4. Key nutritional factors for foods for dissolution and prevention of canine purine uroliths.

Factors	Dietary recommendations
Water	Water intake should be encouraged to achieve a urine specific gravity <1.020
Protein and purines	Restrict dietary protein to 10 to 18% dry matter (DM) Restrict dietary purine: the first three non-water ingredients on product label ingredient panel should be low in purines (**Table 39-3**)
Sodium	Moderate sodium restriction (<0.3% DM) Avoid sodium supplements
Urinary pH	Feed a food that maintains an alkaline urine (urinary pH = 7.1 to 7.5)

Protein and Purines

Dalmatian dogs consuming foods containing more than 20% DM protein and protein sources high in purines and purine precursors (**Table 39-3**) are at increased risk for urate lithogenesis. We have observed formation of purine uroliths in some dogs consuming lesser amounts of dietary purines; therefore, other factors are apparently involved.

The range of dietary protein associated with urate urolith formation in dogs with portal vascular anomalies is unknown. In these dogs, the degree of urine saturation with purines is probably related, at least in part, to the degree of vascular shunting and to dietary protein consumption. Because urate uroliths associated with portal vascular anomalies are often diagnosed in dogs less than one year of age, it is probable that these dogs were consuming foods with increased protein content. Growth-type foods are typically higher in protein than foods formulated for adult maintenance.

High-protein foods, besides being potential sources of urine ammonium, purines and purine precursors, can also induce aciduria. Urine acidity is a risk factor for urate lithogenesis because the solubility of most purines, especially ammonium urate, is pH-dependent. On the other hand, protein restriction, to the degree that would be found in a restricted-protein, urate-litholytic food, can impair urine concentrating ability (by decreasing renal medullary urea concentration), making use of additional diuretic agents unnecessary. Furthermore, feeding low-protein, low-purine foods to patients with ammonium urate uroliths, in combination with appropriate allopurinol therapy, has resulted in urolith dissolution (Bartges et al, 1994; Osborne et al, 1986, 1995). Therefore, for urate litholytic foods, or to aid in the prevention of purine lithogenesis, recommend foods that restrict dietary protein to 10 to 18% DM. The minimum recommended allowance for protein in foods for healthy adult dogs is 10% DM (NRC, 2006). Also, if possible, clients should avoid feeding foods with a high purine content. Ideally, at least the first three non-water ingredients in the ingredient panel on a food label should be low in purines (**Table 39-3**).

Sodium

Sodium chloride can be added to food to increase thirst and urine volume. However, excess sodium increases urine calcium excretion and therefore is a risk factor for calcium oxalate and calcium phosphate urolithiasis, particularly if the urinary pH is high. Also, for the same reason, if oral urine alkalinizing agents are used, potassium citrate may be a better choice than sodium bicarbonate. Besides these risks, supplemental sodium sources may contribute to hypertension in salt-sensitive dogs.

Moderate restriction of dietary sodium (<0.3% DM) in urate litholytic and prevention foods is unlikely to be harmful and may be helpful. Typically, commercial dog foods contain two to three times this amount. The minimum recommended allowance for sodium in foods for healthy adult dogs is 0.08% DM (NRC, 2006).

Urinary pH

Under physiologic conditions associated with alkaluria, urine contains low concentrations of ammonia and ammonium ions (Hande et al, 1984). The specific goal of treatment with a urate litholytic food or an oral urine alkalinizing agent (e.g., potassium citrate) is to maintain a urinary pH within a range of 7.1 to 7.5. Urinary pH values greater than 7.5 should be avoided until it is determined whether or not they provide a significant risk factor for formation of calcium phosphate uroliths. Deposition of a layer of calcium phosphate crystals around existing urate uroliths may impede urolith dissolution. Potassium citrate apparently prevents acid metabolites from increasing renal tubular production of ammonia.

FEEDING PLAN

Current recommendations for dissolution of canine ammonium urate uroliths include a combination of: 1) feeding a litholytic food, 2) formation of an increased quantity of less concentrated urine, 3) alkalinization of urine, 4) administration of xanthine oxidase inhibitors (i.e., allopurinol) and 5) eradication or control of UTIs (Bartges et al, 1992, 1994; Ling, 1995; Lulich et al, 1995; Osborne et al, 1986). **Table 39-5** summarizes the recommendations for dietary and medical dissolution and prevention of canine ammonium acid urate uroliths.

Assess and Select the Food: Urate Urolith Dissolution

Urate litholytic foods have been used most successfully in patients with normal portal vasculature. However, occasional successes have been reported to occur in patients with portal vascular anomalies (Bartges et al, 1994; Osborne et al, 2000). Consumption of a properly formulated urate litholytic food by healthy and urate urolith forming dogs resulted in marked reductions in urine uric acid and ammonia excretion (Lulich et al, 1995; Bartges et al, 1995). **Table 39-6** lists selected commercial veterinary therapeutic foods used for urate urolith dissolution (and prevention) and compares their key nutritional factor content with recommended levels. Select a food that most closely matches the recommended levels of key nutritional factors. Recommend that clients avoid feeding inappropriate amounts of treats or vitamin-mineral supplements. Check the product label or contact the manufacturer to see if the product is approved by the Association of American Feed Control Officials (AAFCO) or some other credible regulatory agency for long-term feeding to adult dogs (**Box 39-1**).

Encourage clients to increase water consumption of patients with urate urolithiasis. When possible, recommend they feed a moist food. Although understandably difficult in some patients, fluid intake should be encouraged throughout the day to help promote a constantly high urine volume. Clients should ensure water is readily available and is not too cold or warm.

Another criterion for selecting a food that may become increasingly important in the future is evidence-based clinical nutrition. Practitioners should know how to determine risks and benefits of nutritional regimens and counsel pet owners accordingly. Currently, veterinary medical education and continuing education are not always based on rigorous assessment of evidence for or against particular management options. Still, studies have been published to establish the nutritional benefits of certain pet foods. Chapter 2 describes evidence-based clinical nutrition in detail and applies its concepts to various veterinary therapeutic foods.

Dogs Without Portal Vascular Anomalies

At the Minnesota Urolith Center, 25 dogs with ammonium urate uroliths were treated with dietary (urate litholytic food) and allopurinol therapy. Complete dissolution occurred in nine dogs (36%), partial dissolution in eight dogs (32%) and no dissolution in eight dogs (32%). A similar dissolution protocol in seven dogs with sodium urate uroliths resulted in complete dissolution in two dogs (29%), partial dissolution in three dogs (42%) and no dissolution in two dogs (29%) (Bartges et al, 1994). Inability to dissolve urate uroliths was usually associated with formation of xanthine. In some dogs with partial urolith dissolution, the remaining uroliths were completely retrieved using voiding urohydropropulsion (Figure 38-5 and Table 38-7) (Lulich et al, 1993) or catheter-assisted retrieval (Figure 38-6) (Lulich and Osborne, 1992). The mean time for urate urolith dissolution in 11 dogs was 3.5 months (median one month, range one to 18 months). Using the above protocol, a nephrolith presumed to be composed of urate was dissolved in nine months in a six-year-old, neutered female English bulldog.

Dogs with Portal Vascular Anomalies

Few studies have been reported about the biologic behavior of ammonium urate uroliths in dogs with portal vascular anomalies. It is logical to hypothesize that elimination of hyperuricuria and reduction of urine ammonium concentration following surgical correction of anomalous shunts would result in sponta-

Table 39-5. Summary of recommendations for dietary and medical dissolution and prevention of canine purine uroliths.

1. Perform appropriate diagnostic studies, including complete urinalysis, quantitative urine culture and diagnostic radiography. Determine precise location, size and number of uroliths. The size and number of uroliths are not a reliable index of probable therapeutic efficacy.
2. If uroliths are available, determine their mineral composition. If unavailable, determine their composition by evaluating appropriate clinical data.
3. Consider surgical correction if uroliths obstruct urine outflow. Small urocystoliths may be removed by voiding urohydropropulsion (Figure 38-5 and Table 38-7) or lithotripsy.
4. Determine baseline pretreatment serum uric acid concentrations and (if possible) 24-hour excretion of urine uric acid.
5. Initiate therapy with a purine litholytic food (**Table 39-6**). Other foods or supplements should not be fed to the patient. Reduction in serum urea nitrogen concentration (usually <10 mg/dl) suggests compliance with dietary recommendations.
6. Initiate therapy with allopurinol at a dosage of 30 mg/kg body weight/day divided into two equal subdoses (azotemic patients require a lesser dose). Xanthine uroliths may form if foods containing excessive purines are fed or if excessive allopurinol is given.
7. If necessary, administer potassium citrate orally to eliminate aciduria. Strive for a urinary pH of approximately 7.1 to 7.5.
8. If necessary, eradicate or control urinary tract infections with appropriate antimicrobial agents. Maintain antimicrobial therapy during and for an appropriate period after purine urolith dissolution.
9. Devise a protocol to monitor efficacy of therapy.
   a. Try to avoid diagnostic followup studies that require urinary tract catheterization. If they are required, give appropriate pericatheterization antimicrobial agents to prevent iatrogenic urinary tract infection.
   b. Perform serial urinalyses. Determination of urinary pH, urine specific gravity and microscopic examination of sediment for urate crystals are especially important. Remember, crystals formed in urine stored at room or refrigeration temperatures may represent in vitro artifacts.
   c. Serially evaluate serum uric acid concentrations and (if possible) fractional excretion of urine uric acid.
   d. Evaluate the location(s), number, size, density and shape of uroliths at monthly intervals. Intravenous urography or ultrasonography may be used for radiolucent uroliths located in the kidneys, ureters or urinary bladder. Retrograde contrast urethrocystography may be required for radiolucent uroliths in the bladder and urethra.
   e. If necessary, perform quantitative urine cultures. They are especially important in patients that are infected before therapy and in patients that are catheterized during therapy.
10. Continue the litholytic food, allopurinol and alkalinizing therapy for approximately one month following the disappearance of uroliths as detected by radiography.
11. Prevention. Purine uroliths are highly recurrent. Preventive therapy should be directed at minimizing urine concentrations of ammonia and uric acid. This may be achieved by feeding a food low in protein that also promotes an alkaline urine (**Table 39-6**). The effectiveness of dietary management for the prevention of purine uroliths in dogs with portosystemic shunts is unknown. The long-term use of allopurinol is discouraged because of the potential for development of xanthine uroliths.

Table 39-6. Levels of key nutritional factors in selected veterinary therapeutic foods used for dissolution and to minimize recurrence of urate urolithiasis in dogs compared to recommended levels.*

Dry foods	Protein (%)	Restricted purines (Yes/No)**	Sodium (%)	Urinary pH***
Recommended levels	**10-18**	**Yes**	**<0.3**	**7.1-7.5**
Hill's Prescription Diet u/d Canine	11.2	Yes	0.23	7.70
Medi-Cal Reduced Protein	13.7	Yes	0.2	na
Medi-Cal Renal LP	14.7	Yes	0.1	na
Medi-Cal Renal MP	18.4	Yes	0.1	na
Medi-Cal Vegetarian Formula	20.9	Yes	0.4	na
Purina Veterinary Diets NF KidNey Function	15.9	Yes	0.22	6.7-7.5
Purina Veterinary Diets HA HypoAllergenic	21.3	Yes	0.24	na
Royal Canin Veterinary Diets Vegetarian Formula	19.1	Yes	0.15	6.78
Moist foods	**Protein (%)**	**Restricted purines (Yes/No)****	**Sodium (%)**	**Urinary pH*****
Recommended levels	**10-18**	**Yes**	**<0.3**	**7.1-7.5**
Hill's Prescription Diet u/d Canine	13.3	Yes	0.28	7.4
Medi-Cal Reduced Protein	16.5	No	0.2	na
Medi-Cal Renal LP	16.8	No	0.1	na
Medi-Cal Renal MP	28.2	No	0.2	na
Medi-Cal Vegetarian Formula	26.4	Yes	0.5	na
Purina Veterinary Diets NF KidNey Function	16.5	No	0.24	6.7-7.5

Key: na = information not available from manufacturer.
*Manufacturers' published values; nutrients expressed as % dry matter; moist foods are best.
Restricted purines = products having low-purine ingredients (Table 39-3**) as the first three non-water ingredients on the ingredient panel of the product label.
***Protocols for measuring urinary pH may vary.

neous dissolution of uroliths composed primarily of ammonium urate. Appropriate clinical trials are needed to prove or disprove this hypothesis (Kruger and Osborne, 1986). Occasionally, success has been reported in dissolving urate uroliths in dogs with portal vascular anomalies. For example, dissolution of a urolith presumed to be composed of ammonium urate

Box 39-1. Nutritional Adequacy of Low-Protein Foods Recommended for Canine Patients with Urolithiasis.

A commercial veterinary therapeutic food that reduces urine concentration, produces alkaline urine and avoids excess levels of dietary protein, purines, calcium and phosphorus[a] is frequently recommended for management of several different types of canine uroliths. Some of these foods have very low protein content (10 to 11% [dry matter, DM]). This level of dietary protein is a concern for some veterinarians and their health care teams because it is less than the recommended dietary allowance for protein established by the Association of American Feed Control Officials (AAFCO) (minimum 18% DM for adult maintenance).

However, based on several criteria, these foods are nutritionally adequate for maintenance of adult, non-reproducing dogs. First, the National Research Council's minimum recommended allowance for foods for maintenance of healthy adult dogs is 10% DM. Second, many of these veterinary therapeutic foods have successfully completed AAFCO adult maintenance feeding trials (see product labels and published product information). In addition, protein digestibility in some of these low-protein foods approaches 100%, which means their essential amino acids are readily available to dogs. The final criterion is practical experience with these foods; some have been used successfully for long-term feeding of thousands of canine patients with urolithiasis.

ENDNOTE

a. Hill's Prescription Diet u/d Canine dry. Hill's Pet Nutrition, Inc., Topeka, KS, USA.

The Bibliography for **Box 39-1** can be found at www.markmorris.org.

occurred in a two-year-old female miniature schnauzer with a portal vascular anomaly. The dog was consuming a veterinary therapeutic food designed for treatment of renal failure.[a] The mechanisms involved were presumably decreased production of ammonium ions from urea and reduced formation of uric acid from dietary protein.

Likewise, a nephrolith in the right renal pelvis of a seven-year-old female malamute with a portal vascular anomaly disappeared while the dog consumed the same veterinary therapeutic food designed for treatment of renal failure.[a] A marked reduction of urine uric acid concentration was observed in a three-month-old female miniature schnauzer following surgical correction of an extrahepatic portacaval shunt. Furthermore, undersaturation of urine with ammonium urate and no recurrence of urolith formation were observed in two dogs with surgically uncorrectable portal vascular anomalies and ammonium urate uroliths. The dogs were fed a urate litholytic[b] food for prevention of recurrence of the uroliths and for management of hepatic encephalopathy.

Additional clinical studies are needed to evaluate the relative value of litholytic foods, allopurinol and/or alkalinization of urine in dissolving ammonium urate uroliths in dogs with portal vascular anomalies. The efficacy of allopurinol may be altered in such dogs because biotransformation of this drug, which has a very short half-life, to oxypurinol, which has a longer half-life, requires adequate hepatic function (Osborne et al, 1986).

Immature Dogs with Urate Uroliths

Providing safe and effective therapy for urate uroliths in immature dogs presents a challenge. Formation of urate uroliths associated with portal vascular anomalies and their management are discussed above. Growing dogs usually consume greater quantities of protein and, thus, greater quantities of purines than adult dogs. The safety and efficacy of litholytic foods in young dogs with urate uroliths are unknown. Adding non-purine-containing protein to the litholytic food may be effective (**Box 39-2**); however, no studies have yet been performed to confirm this hypothesis. The metabolism of allopurinol in young dogs has not been evaluated. Surgical removal of large uroliths remains the option with the most predictable short-term outcome.

Assess and Determine the Feeding Method: Urate Urolith Dissolution

Transitioning patients from their current food to a urate litholytic food should be done gradually (i.e., over a period of a few days). Begin the transition by feeding 75% of the current food and 25% of the litholytic food on Day 1. On Day 2, feed half of each food. On Day 3, feed 75% as the litholytic food. By Day 4 or 5, feed only the litholytic food.

As discussed above, modification of urinary pH is a significant part of overall dietary management of urate urolithiasis. Free-choice feeding is often associated with more persistent aciduria compared to meal feeding. However, if moist foods are fed, as is recommended, free-choice feeding can result in spoilage if the food is left uneaten for several hours at room temperature (Chapter 11). Opened containers of moist foods should be refrigerated and the feeding bowl should be kept clean. Ideally, moist foods should be meal fed several times per day. If that is not possible, clients should meal feed moist food as often as practical.

Besides offering moist foods, there are several additional ways to facilitate increased water intake. These include: 1) Ensuring multiple water bowls are available in prominent locations in the dog's environment; this may mean providing several bowls outside in a large enclosure or a bowl on each level of the house. 2) Providing clean water bowls that are always filled with fresh water. 3) Offering ice cubes as treats or snacks. 4) Adding liberal quantities of water to dry foods. However, potential food safety issues might arise from leaving moistened dry foods out for prolonged intervals (Chapter 11). Using small amounts of salt-free bouillon as a flavoring substance in drinking water to encourage more water consumption is not recommended for management of urate uroliths because meat extracts such as bouillon contain increased levels of purines (**Table 39-3**).

If the patient has a normal body condition score (BCS 2.5/5 to 3.5/5), the amount of food fed previously was probably appropriate. On an energy basis, a similar amount of the new

Box 39-2. Recipes for Supplementing a Low-Protein Urate Litholytic Canine Adult Food for Use in Immature Canine Patients with Urate Urolithiasis.

Providing a safe and effective urate litholytic food for immature dogs presents a challenge. Growing dogs usually consume greater quantities of protein and, thus, purines than adult dogs. The safety and efficacy of low-protein litholytic foods in young dogs with urate uroliths are unknown. Adding non-purine-containing protein to the litholytic food may be effective; however, no studies have yet been performed to confirm this hypothesis. Also, the metabolism of allopurinol in puppies has not been evaluated. Therefore, surgical removal of large uroliths remains the option with the most predictable short-term outcome.

The dry formulation of a low-protein veterinary therapeutic food[a] often recommended for dogs with urate urolithiasis can be modified for growing dogs (**Table 1**). However, the long-term safety and efficacy of this modified food in young dogs with urate or other uroliths are unknown. Therefore, growing dogs should be appropriately monitored for protein-calorie malnutrition if fed foods based on these recipes.

Table 1. Modified recipes for growing dogs based on the dry formulation of a low-protein, low-purine veterinary therapeutic food.

Recipe A
1 cup dry Prescription Diet u/d Canine
1 tsp dicalcium phosphate
1 cup cottage cheese
Multivitamin-mineral supplement for dogs

Nutrient levels (% dry matter)	
Protein	30.5
Fat	19.5
Calcium	1.0
Phosphorus	1.0
Magnesium	0.02
Sodium	0.6
Potassium	0.5

Recipe B
1 cup dry Prescription Diet u/d Canine
3/4 tsp dicalcium
2 cooked eggs
Multivitamin-mineral supplement for dogs

Nutrient levels (% dry matter)	
Protein	17.6
Fat	27.1
Calcium	1.1
Phosphorus	1.0
Magnesium	0.02
Sodium	0.4
Potassium	0.6

ENDNOTE

a. Hill's Prescription Diet u/d Canine dry. Hill's Pet Nutrition, Inc., Topeka, KS, USA.

food would be a good starting place.

ADJUNCTIVE MEDICAL AND SURGICAL MANAGEMENT

Diuretics

Because a properly formulated low-protein urate litholytic food impairs urine-concentrating capacity by decreasing renal medullary urea concentration, additional diuretic agents are unnecessary.

Xanthine Oxidase Inhibitors

Allopurinol is a synthetic isomer of hypoxanthine (Hande et al, 1978). It rapidly binds to and inhibits the action of xanthine oxidase, and thereby decreases production of uric acid by inhibiting the conversion of hypoxanthine to xanthine, and xanthine to uric acid. The result is a reduction in serum and urine uric acid concentration within approximately two days, and a concomitant but lesser increase in the serum concentrations of hypoxanthine and xanthine (Foreman, 1984; Osborne et al, 1986). Although allopurinol has a short half-life in people with normal renal function (approximately 90 minutes), its metabolic derivative oxypurinol is also a xanthine oxidase inhibitor and has a half-life of 12 to 16 hours (Elion et al, 1966). In mongrel dogs and beagles, the half-life of allopurinol is dose dependent (approximately 2.5 hours following a 5 mg/kg body weight dose and three hours following a 10 mg/kg body weight dose). The half-life of oxypurinol is three to five hours (Bartges et al, 1993; Elion, 1966). Food does not affect availability of allopurinol; therefore, it can be administered with meals.

The dosage of allopurinol for dissolution of ammonium urate uroliths in dogs is 15 mg/kg body weight q12h (Lulich et al, 1995; Bartges et al, 1992; Osborne et al, 1986). According to the manufacturer, the drug has been given to normal dogs at this dosage for one year without causing significant abnormalities.[c] This dosage has been given to nonazotemic, urate urolith-forming dogs for up to six months without detectable consequences. However, when owners supplemented a therapeutic food with foods containing purine precursors, a layer of xanthine formed around ammonium urate uroliths (**Figures 39-2** and **39-3**). Therefore, to minimize xanthine formation, allopurinol should only be administered to patients consuming purine-restricted foods (**Figure 39-4**) (Bartges et al, 1995c; Osborne et al, 2000).

The efficacy of allopurinol may be altered in dogs with portal vascular anomalies because biotransformation of this drug, which, as mentioned above, has a very short half-life, to oxypurinol, which has a longer half-life, requires adequate hepatic function (Osborne et al, 1986). Pending further studies, we do not recommend allopurinol for treatment or prevention of urate uroliths formed by dogs as a result of portal vascular shunts or hepatic microvascular dysplasia.

Reported adverse effects of allopurinol in people include gastrointestinal disturbances, skin rashes, leukopenia, thrombocytopenia, vasculitis and hepatitis (Al-Kawas et al, 1981; Medline et al, 1978). We found only one report of a possible immune-mediated reaction (hemolytic anemia, trigeminal neuropathy) to allopurinol administration in a dog (Pedroia, 1981). Because allopurinol and its metabolites are excreted by the kidneys, the

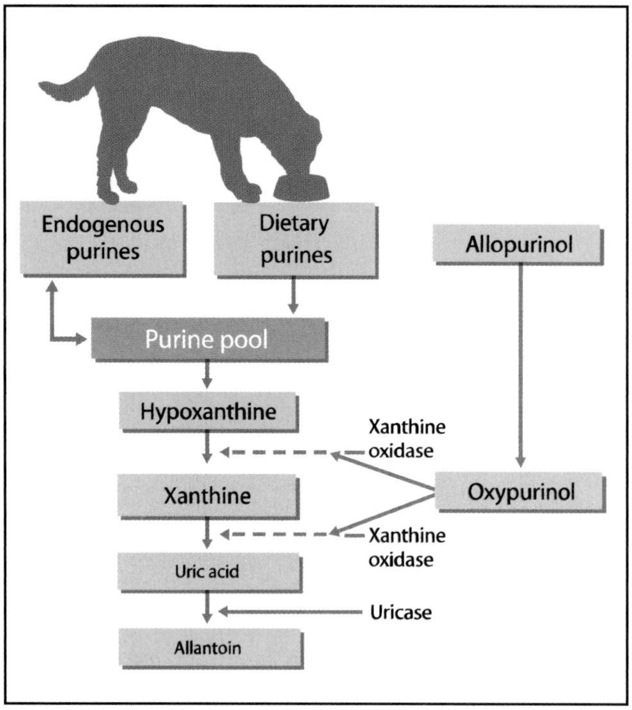

Figure 39-4. Diagram of purine metabolism in dogs that consume a purine-restricted food and are given allopurinol.

dosage is commonly reduced in people with renal dysfunction. Allopurinol has been reported to cause life-threatening erythematous desquamative skin rashes, fever, hepatitis, eosinopenia and further decline in renal function when given to people with renal insufficiency (Hande et al, 1978). Pending further studies, appropriate precautions including informed consent, should be used when considering use of allopurinol in dogs with primary renal failure.

Urine Alkalinizing Agents

Because ammonium ions and hydrogen ions appear to precipitate urates in dog urine, oral administration of alkalinizing agents (e.g., potassium citrate) may be of value in preventing acid metabolites from increasing renal tubular production of ammonia. Under physiologic conditions associated with alkaluria, urine contains low concentrations of ammonia and ammonium ions (Hande et al, 1984).

Dosage of urine alkalinizing agents should be individualized for each patient, depending on the status of the patient and pretreatment urinary pH values. Although sodium bicarbonate is a readily available urine alkalinizing agent, effective doses, (25 to 50 mg/kg body weight q12h) result in a significant increase in sodium intake. Also, sodium may combine with uric acid to form sodium urate. Alternatively, potassium citrate in wax matrix tablets (Urocit-K[d]) or as a liquid (Polycitra-K[e]) (40 to 75 mg/kg body weight q12h) may be given. Divided doses should be administered to maintain a consistently nonacidic environment in the urinary tract. A properly formulated urate dissolution food should contain potassium citrate (check ingredient label). Consumption of potassium citrate typically results in alkaluria in dogs (Bartges et al, 1995, 1995a).

The goal of treatment with urine alkalinizing agents or the urate litholytic food is to maintain a urinary pH between 7.1 to 7.5. Higher values (>7.5) should be avoided until it is determined whether or not they provide a significant risk factor for formation of calcium phosphate uroliths. Deposition of a layer of calcium phosphate crystals around existing urate uroliths may impede urolith dissolution. Owners may monitor urinary pH with pH paper or handheld "pocket" pH meters.

Eradication or Control of UTIs

Clinical studies indicate that UTIs in dogs with ammonium urate uroliths usually occur as a consequence of altered local host defenses. These alterations may be caused by urolith-induced trauma to the urothelium, or they may occur as a consequence of catheterization or other invasive diagnostic procedures. Efforts should be made to prevent, eradicate or control infections because they may cause problems of equal or greater severity as the uroliths.

Studies of ammonium urate uroliths in people have been interpreted to suggest that UTIs caused by urease-producing microbes may be a causative factor (Garcia and Cifuentes Dellate, 1981). In this circumstance, formation of ammonium ions as a consequence of urease-mediated hydrolysis of urea may result in formation of insoluble ammonium urate crystals. If a similar phenomenon occurs in dogs, eradication or control of potent urease-producing microbes (staphylococci, *Proteus* spp. and ureaplasmas) would be especially important.

Appropriate antimicrobial agents selected on the basis of susceptibility or minimum inhibitory concentration tests should be used at therapeutic dosages. The fact that diuresis reduces the urine concentration of the antimicrobial agent should be considered when formulating antimicrobial dosages.

Surgery

There are several situations in which a combination of surgical removal of urate uroliths followed by combined dietary and medical dissolution protocols might be beneficial. One involves the inability to remove all uroliths by surgery. This occasionally occurs because ammonium urate uroliths are frequently multiple and small. The fact that they may be radiolucent creates an additional problem by interfering with their radiographic detection immediately after surgery.

In some patients, immediate surgery may be required to remove uroliths obstructing the renal pelvis, ureter(s) or urethra. Lithotripsy has proved to be highly effective in removing uroliths that obstruct the urethra. Initiation of dietary and medical dissolution protocols may prove advantageous if such patients have multiple uroliths in several locations, and if circumstances preclude their surgical removal at the time the obstructing urolith is removed.

Techniques have been devised to correct some types of intrahepatic and extrahepatic shunts in dogs. Certain patients with portal vascular anomalies and urate uroliths may benefit from a combination of surgical, dietary and medical urolith dissolution protocols. Surgical correction, by itself, of an extrahepatic portacaval shunt in a three-month-old female miniature schnauzer resulted in a marked reduction of urine uric acid concentration (Osborne et al, 2000). However, the condition of the patient and factors related to anesthesia and surgery may preclude urolith removal at the time the anomalous portal vessels are corrected. In this situation, postsurgical dietary and medical therapy designed to dissolve uroliths should be considered. Also, some types of portal vascular anomalies are not amenable to surgical correction. If the uroliths cause unacceptable signs of urinary tract disease, they should be surgically removed and postsurgical preventive measures should be initiated. Voiding urohydropropulsion may be used to remove small urocystoliths (Figure 38-5 and Table 38-7) (Lulich et al, 1993).

REASSESSMENT

Ammonium urate urocystoliths have a propensity to move into the urethra of dogs. This finding may be related to their small size, round to ovoid shape and smooth surface. If small enough, they readily pass through the urethra. However, they often become lodged behind the os penis of male dogs. Owners should be informed of this likelihood and given a written summary of associated clinical signs. Urethroliths causing clinical signs may be easily returned to the bladder lumen by urohydropropulsion (Figure 38-5 and Table 38-7) (Lulich et al, 1993), or removed by lithotripsy. The physical characteristics that permit passage of these uroliths into the urethra also facilitate their removal from the urethra.

When attempting dietary and medical dissolution of urate uroliths, owners should be counseled to adhere strictly to feeding the low-purine urate litholytic food. Consumption of a high-purine food by dogs, while receiving allopurinol, will result in formation of a xanthine shell around urate uroliths or formation of xanthine uroliths (**Figure 39-3**) (Bartges et al, 1992; Ling et al, 1991; Osborne et al, 1986a). Xanthine uroliths may not dissolve. However, spontaneous dissolution of xanthine shells and underlying uroliths may occur by discontinuing allopurinol and continuing the low-purine litholytic food (Bartges et al, 1994). Alternatively, dissolution of urate uroliths may occur as a result of feeding a low-purine litholytic food and administering a lower dose of allopurinol than that associated with formation of xanthine shells.

Because allopurinol and its metabolites are excreted from the body primarily in urine, the drug should be used cautiously in patients with renal dysfunction (Bartges, 1993; Hande et al, 1984). Reduction in the dosage of allopurinol is recommended for human patients with primary renal failure. Pending further studies, a similar recommendation should be applied to dogs with primary renal failure.

The size of uroliths should be periodically monitored by survey and (if necessary) double-contrast radiography or ultrasonography (**Table 39-7**). It is more difficult to monitor changes in size and number if the uroliths are radiolucent. Double-contrast cystography is superior to ultrasonography because: 1) it is minimally invasive, 2) sedation is usually not

Table 39-7. Expected changes associated with dietary and medical therapy of purine uroliths.

Factors	Pre-therapy	During therapy	Prevention therapy
Polyuria	±	1+ to 3+	1+ to 3+
Pollakiuria	0 to 4+	↑ then ↓	0
Hematuria	0 to 4+	↓	0
Urine specific gravity	Variable	1.004 to 1.015	1.004 to 1.015
Urinary pH	<7.0	>7.0	>7.0
Pyuria	0 to 4+	↓	0
Purine (urate) crystals	0 to 4+	0	Variable
Bacteriuria	0 to 4+	0	0
Bacterial culture of urine	0 to 4+	0	0
Urea nitrogen (mg/dl)	Variable	≤15	≤15
Urolith size and number	Small to large	↓	0

required to perform the procedure, 3) virtually all uroliths can be visualized, including their size, shape and number and 4) uroliths may be retrieved through the catheter and submitted for quantitative analysis. If retrograde double-contrast urethrocystography is used to monitor dissolution of radiolucent urethrocystoliths, appropriate prophylactic antibiotics should be administered around the time of urinary tract catheterization to minimize iatrogenic UTIs. Excretory urography or ultrasonography may be used to monitor dissolution or recurrence of urate nephroliths.

Urinary pH should be monitored at appropriate intervals (**Table 39-7**). Periodic evaluation of urine sediment for crystalluria should also be considered. Ammonium urate crystals should not form in fresh urine if therapy has been effective in promoting formation of urine that is undersaturated with ammonium ions and uric acid. Periodic evaluation of serum urea nitrogen concentration, serum uric acid concentration and (if possible) urine uric acid concentration is recommended. Reduction of serum urea nitrogen concentration below pretreatment values (usually <10 mg/dl in previously nonazotemic patients), reduction of urine specific gravity (usually <1.020) and an increase in urinary pH (usually >7.0) indicate owner and patient compliance with dietary therapy (**Table 39-7**). Reductions in serum and urine uric acid concentrations also indicate compliance with recommendations for dietary and allopurinol therapy.

Determination of urine urate-to-creatinine ratios in randomly collected single urine samples has been recommended to aid in diagnosis and to monitor medical and dietary therapy of dogs with urate uroliths (Schaible, 1986; Senior, 1989). However, in a controlled study, spot urine urate-to-creatinine ratios correlated poorly with 24-hour urine uric acid excretion in healthy non-urolith-forming beagles (Bartges et al, 1994a). Although urine urate-to-creatinine ratios decrease significantly in dogs with urate uroliths given allopurinol (Moentk et al, 1994), they do not correlate with 24-hour urine uric acid excretions in these dogs, nor are they useful in predicting urolith dis-

Table 39-8. Managing purine uroliths refractory to complete dissolution.

Cause	Identification	Therapeutic goal
Client and patient factors		
Inadequate dietary compliance	Question owner Persistent purine crystalluria Urea nitrogen >10-17 mg/dl Urine specific gravity >1.010-1.020 Urinary pH <7.1-7.5 during dietary management with appropriate litholytic food (**Table 39-6**) (use lower values for moist food)	Emphasize need to exclusively feed dissolution food
Inadequate allopurinol administration	Question owner Count remaining pills	Emphasize need to administer allopurinol Determine if owner is capable and willing to administer medication Demonstrate a variety of methods to administer medication
Clinician factors		
Incorrect prediction of mineral type	Analysis of retrieved urolith	Alter therapy based on identification of mineral type
Excessive allopurinol administration	Xanthine urolith formation	Reduce allopurinol administration in conjunction with appropriate dietary therapy to minimize purine consumption Clinically active uroliths may require surgical removal Remove small uroliths by voiding urohydropropulsion (Figure 38-5 and Table 38-7)
Disease factors		
Xanthine urolith formation	Analysis of retrieved urolith Allopurinol administration without concomitant reduction in dietary protein consumption Excessive allopurinol dose	Clinically active uroliths may require surgical removal Remove small uroliths by voiding urohydropropulsion (Figure 38-5 and Table 38-7)
Inadequate hepatic function	Suspect hepatic portosystemic shunts or hepatic microvascular dysplasia in breeds other than Dalmatians and English bulldogs Elevated postprandial serum bile acid concentration Microhepatica	Clinically active uroliths may require surgical removal Remove small uroliths by voiding urohydropropulsion (Figure 38-5 and Table 38-7) Repair vascular anomaly
Compound urolith	Radiographic density of nucleus and outer layer(s) of urolith is different Analysis of retrieved urolith	Alter therapy based on identification of a new mineral type Uroliths not causing clinical signs should be monitored for potentially adverse consequences (obstruction, urinary tract infection, etc.) Clinically active uroliths may require surgical removal Remove small uroliths by voiding urohydropropulsion (Figure 38-5 and Table 38-7)

solution. Furthermore, urine xanthine-to-creatinine ratios in these dogs did not correlate with 24-hour urine xanthine excretions, nor were they predictive for urate urolith dissolution or xanthine formation.

There is no rigid time interval after which response to dissolution therapy is unlikely. The fact that current medical and dietary protocols are not designed to induce dissolution of urolith matrix may be a factor that influences dissolution rate. The time required to induce dissolution of nine episodes of urate urolithiasis in a clinical study ranged from four to 40 weeks (mean 14.2 weeks). Reevaluation of the diagnosis and/or alternate methods of management should be considered if uroliths enlarge during therapy or do not begin to decrease in size after approximately eight weeks of appropriate medical and dietary therapy (**Table 39-8**).

If it is difficult to completely dissolve urate uroliths by creating urine that is undersaturated with uric acid and ammonium ions, consider that: 1) the wrong mineral component was identified, 2) the nucleus of the urolith was of different mineral composition than the outer portions of the urolith, 3) a xanthine shell or xanthine uroliths had formed or 4) the owner or patient was not complying with therapeutic recommendations.

PREVENTION OF URATE UROLITHIASIS

Dalmatian Dogs

Prophylactic therapy should be considered for urate-forming Dalmatian dogs because of the high risk for recurrent urate uroliths. As a first choice, urate litholytic foods that are restricted in purines and that promote formation of less concentrated alkaline urine should be considered (**Table 39-6**). In one study of naturally occurring ammonium urate urocystoliths in Dalmatian dogs, a low-protein, nonacidifying moist commercial veterinary therapeutic food[b] reduced urolith recurrence by 50% compared with an adult moist maintenance food (Lulich et al, 1998). If dry foods are fed, water should be added with the goal of maintaining a urine specific gravity less than approximately 1.025.

If urate crystalluria or hyperuricuria persists, serial urinary pH measurements are indicated to ensure appropriate alkalinization. If necessary, urine alkalinizing agents may be added to the protocol. If difficulties persist, low doses of allopurinol (approximately 10 to 20 mg/kg body weight/day) may be given cautiously. Prolonged administration of high doses (30 mg/kg body weight/day) of allopurinol may result in formation of xanthine uroliths (Bartges et al, 1992; Ling, 1995). The risk of xanthine urolithiasis is enhanced if dietary purines are not restricted during allopurinol therapy. Therefore, appropriate caution in long-term administration of this drug is indicated. Because it is possible to induce dissolution of recurrent ammonium urate uroliths, it is unnecessary to risk the use of prophylactic protocols that may themselves cause disorders.

When considering use of foods to minimize occurrence of urolithiasis, avoid an "always" or "never" approach. The final decision should be based on the overall balance of benefits to the patient and associated risks.

Non-Dalmatian Dogs

We did not find any published information concerning recurrence rates of urate uroliths in non-Dalmatian dogs; however, recurrence of urate uroliths was observed in three of five English bulldogs. Therefore, preventive measures should also be considered for non-Dalmatian dogs.

There have been few studies of the biologic behavior of ammonium urate uroliths in dogs and cats with portal vascular anomalies and/or microvascular dysplasia. It is logical to hypothesize that elimination of hyperuricuria and reduction of urine ammonium concentration following surgical correction of anomalous shunts would result in spontaneous dissolution of uroliths composed primarily of ammonium urate.

Additional clinical studies are needed to evaluate the relative value of litholytic foods, allopurinol and/or alkalinization of urine in dissolving ammonium urate uroliths in dogs and cats with portal vascular anomalies. The likelihood of adverse side effects or further deterioration in hepatic function following administration of allopurinol to dogs with portal vascular anomalies has apparently not been determined. Reversible hepatitis has been reported to be an uncommon reaction to allopurinol given to people (Al-Kawas et al, 1981; Murrell and Rapeport, 1986; Nelson and Elion, 1984). Pending further study, appropriate precautions should be taken to monitor patients for adverse reactions if allopurinol is given to dogs with portal vascular anomalies. Because tetracycline exacerbates hepatic and renal dysfunction in dogs with experimentally produced portal vascular anomalies, it should not be routinely used to treat UTIs in dogs with naturally occurring portal vascular anomalies (Faraj et al, 1982).

ENDNOTES

a. Prescription Diet k/d Canine. Hill's Pet Nutrition, Inc., Topeka, KS, USA.
b. Prescription Diet u/d Canine. Hill's Pet Nutrition, Inc., Topeka, KS, USA.
c. Zyloprim. Glaxo Wellcome, Research Triangle Park, NC, USA.
d. Urocit-K. Mission Pharmacal, San Antonio, TX, USA.
e. Polycitra-K. Willen Drug Co., Baltimore, MD, USA.

REFERENCES

The references for **Chapter 39** can be found at www.markmorris.org.

CASE 39-1

Stranguria in a Dalmatian Dog

Joseph W. Bartges, DVM, PhD, Dipl. ACVN and ACVIM (Internal Medicine)
College of Veterinary Medicine
University of Tennessee
Knoxville, Tennessee, USA

Patient Assessment

A three-year-old, neutered male Dalmatian dog was referred to the University of Minnesota Veterinary Teaching Hospital for inability to urinate and straining to urinate during the past 24 hours (**Figure 1**). The dog had received an antibiotic (unknown type and dosage) for the past month because of bacterial folliculitis (**Figure 2**).

Physical examination revealed a depressed dog with patchy areas of alopecia and erythema, and a distended, tense, painful urinary bladder. The dog weighed 34.2 kg and had a normal body condition score (BCS 3/5). No other abnormalities were noted.

Blood samples were submitted for a complete blood count (**Table 1**) and a serum biochemistry profile (**Table 2**). These tests revealed leukocytosis due to mature neutrophilia and an elevated serum uric acid concentration. Survey radiographs revealed three slightly radiopaque round densities in the region of the urinary bladder (**Figure 3**) and multiple urethroliths. A urine sample was collected for a complete urinalysis and aerobic bacterial culture (**Table 3**).

An 8-Fr. urinary catheter was advanced into the urinary bladder without difficulty. The catheter and many small round, smooth, green uroliths were voided. The urinary catheter was reinserted, all of the urine removed and a double-contrast cystogram was performed (**Figure 4**).

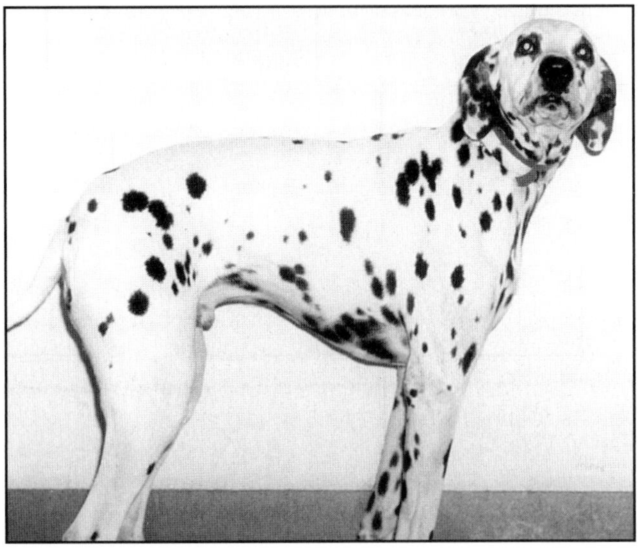

Figure 1. A three-year-old, neutered male Dalmatian dog with dysuria and inability to void urine.

Assess the Food and Feeding Method

At the time of admission, the dog was being fed a dry veterinary therapeutic food[a] that avoids excess levels of phosphorus, sodium and protein. The food was offered free choice.

Questions

1. What is the probable mineral composition of the uroliths in this dog?
2. What are the advantages and disadvantages of surgical vs. dietary and medical management of these uroliths?
3. If dietary and medical dissolution is chosen as the treatment plan, what parameters should be monitored?

Answers and Discussion

1. The most likely mineral composition of the uroliths is ammonium urate based on the physical and radiographic characteristics of the uroliths, the presence of ammonium urate crystalluria and the breed of dog. Dalmatian dogs are predisposed to formation of purine uroliths, primarily ammonium urate, because of unique purine metabolism that results in greater urinary excretion and concentration of uric acid compared with most non-Dalmatian dogs.
2. Although surgery may be effective, dietary and medical protocols have been developed to dissolve ammonium urate uroliths. Surgical removal of urocystoliths has the obvious advantage of rapid correction of the disease process. Combined dietary and medical therapy is also often effective and includes using a moist low-purine commercial veterinary therapeutic food[b] and allopurinol, a xanthine oxidase inhibitor. In a prospective controlled study of canine ammonium urate urocystoliths, complete dissolution was achieved in approximately 40% of the cases and reduction of urolith size

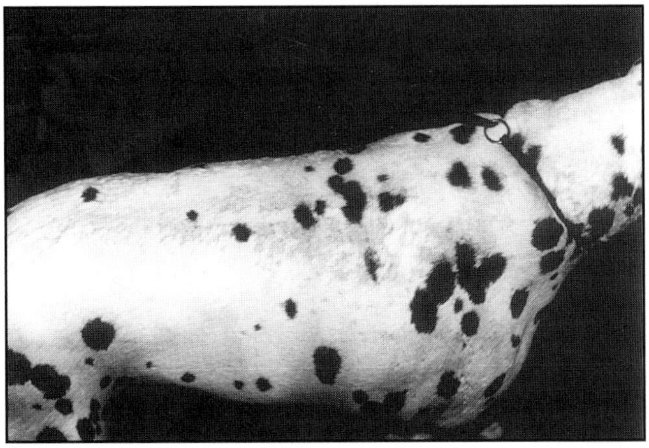

Figure 2. Photograph of the dog described in Figure 1 demonstrating patchy alopecia due to folliculitis.

Table 1. Hemograms of a three-year-old, neutered male Dalmatian dog with urocystoliths.

Factors	Reference values	Day 1*	25	59	88	123	157	186	214	247	275
Hct (%)	30-58	49.6	47.6	46.1	47.6	46.0	48.6	46.5	48.7	48.0	46.2
RBC (10^6/µl)	5.2-8.1	6.95	6.77	6.48	6.74	6.53	6.80	6.65	6.92	6.82	6.53
Hemoglobin (g/dl)	10.2-16.9	17.3	16.7	15.9	16.5	16.1	16.0	19.1	16.9	16.9	19.8
MCV (fl)	63-72	71	70	71	71	70	71	70	70	70	71
MCH (pg)	22-25	25	25	25	35	25	24	29	24	25	30
MCHC (%)	34-37	35	35	35	35	35	33	41	35	35	43
Nucleated RBC (/µl)	-	0	0	0	1	0	1	1	1	0	0
WBC (10^3/µl)	5.4-15.3	23.4	11.5	11.5	11.2	13.7	12.8	12.8	13.1	10.7	13.6
Segmented neutrophils (10^3/µl)	2.75-12.85	21.18	6.56	8.34	7.49	9.86	10.6	9.02	8.06	7.92	10.0
Band neutrophils (10^3/µl)	0-150	0	0	0	0	0	0	0	0	50	70
Metamyelocytes (10^3/µl)	0	0	0	0	0	0	0	0	0	0	2,040
Lymphocytes (10^3/µl)	430-5,800	820	3,050	1,440	2,220	2,400	1,400	2,600	3,770	1,870	200
Monocytes (10^3/µl)	50-1,400	1,290	400	350	170	340	320	440	460	160	1,290
Eosinophils (10^3/µl)	0-1,400	120	1,500	1,380	1,220	1,100	380	570	720	700	0
Basophils (10^3/µl)	Rare	0	0	0	0	0	0	60	0	0	0
Platelets (10^3/µl)	160-525	378	378	381	352	395	406	644	369	358	Normal**
Total solids (g/dl)	5.8-7.5	7.3	6.6	6.5	6.8	6.7	7.0	9.3	7.1	7.3	9.1
Comments	-	-	-	-	-	-	-	Lipemic	-	-	Lipemic

Key: Hct = hematocrit, RBC = red blood cells, MCV = mean corpuscular volume, MCH = mean corpuscular hemoglobin, MCHC = mean corpuscular hemoglobin concentration, WBC = white blood cells.
*Therapy consisting of a urate litholytic food and allopurinol was initiated on Day 2; allopurinol therapy was discontinued on Day 186.
**Platelets were estimated on a blood film and considered adequate.

Table 2. Serum biochemistry values of a three-year-old, neutered male Dalmatian dog with urocystoliths.

Factors	Reference values	Day 1*	25	59	88	123	157	186	214	247	275	924	1,268
Urea nitrogen (mg/dl)	7-26	17	9	7	7	5	6	5	4	4	3	5	4
Creatinine (mg/dl)	0.6-1.4	1.0	1.3	1.1	1.2	1.0	1.0	0.9	1.0	1.1	1.0	0.9	0.9
Alk phos activity (U/l)	3-60	53	83	66	94	142	212	258	239	335	490	854	760
ALT activity (U/l)	4-91	28	22	27	26	25	26	24	25	26	27	21	21
Total bilirubin (mg/dl)	0-0.7	0.6	0.4	0.4	0.3	0.7	0.8	1.5	0.9	0.9	1.3	0.4	0.6
Glucose (mg/dl)	79-140	136	122	123	113	127	133	113	116	125	132	129	115
Total protein (g/dl)	5.8-7.9	7.4	6.3	6.3	6.5	5.9	5.5	5.7	6.1	6.1	6.0	6.4	6.7
Albumin (g/dl)	2.6-4.0	3.8	3.3	3.2	3.3	3.1	3.3	3.4	3.1	3.3	3.3	2.6	2.7
Globulin (g/dl)	2.2-4.0	3.6	3.0	3.1	3.2	2.8	2.2	2.3	3.0	2.8	2.7	3.8	4.0
Uric acid (mg/dl)	0-0.6	1.5	0.3	0.4	0.3	0.4	0.4	0.5	0.7	2.0	1.7	0.9	0.8
CK (U/l)	36-155	394	79	70	76	57	66	90	90	57	67	50	-
Amylase activity (U/l)	220-1,400	976	779	742	997	715	805	786	851	795	963	856	912
Sodium (mEq/l)	146-156	148	150	150	140	150	151	150	150	150	151	147	148
Potassium (mEq/l)	3.8-5.1	3.6	4.5	4.0	3.6	4.4	4.4	4.0	4.3	4.0	4.3	4.5	4.5
Chloride (mEq/l)	109-122	110	114	116	112	114	111	112	113	114	111	111	110
Total CO_2 (mEq/l)	17-27	21	23	21	18	23	23	23	22	22	24	22	23
Anion gap	8-20	17	13	13	10	13	17	15	15	14	16	14	15
Osmolality (mOsm/l)	289-313	298	298	297	278	297	299	296	296	296	298	291	292
Calcium (mg/dl)	9.6-11.6	9.9	9.9	9.7	9.7	9.8	9.9	9.6	10.1	10.0	10.1	9.6	10.4
Phosphorus (mg/dl)	2.5-6.2	3.9	2.4	4.2	2.5	3.9	4.1	3.5	3.2	2.1	3.1	4.2	5.2

Key: ALT = alanine aminotransferase, Alk phos = alkaline phosphatase, CK = creatine kinase.
*Therapy consisting of a urate litholytic food and allopurinol was initiated on Day 2; allopurinol therapy was discontinued on Day 186.

and/or number occurred in another 30% of cases. With combined dietary and medical therapy, the average time for dissolution of ammonium urate uroliths is three and one-half months; however, the median time is approximately one month. Thus, most ammonium urate uroliths dissolve in approximately one month.

3. Clinical signs often resolve within three to five days of initiating therapy. Clients should be advised that urethral obstruction may occur at any time when uroliths are present in the bladder. If urethral obstruction with uroliths recurs, the urolith(s) can be retropulsed back into the bladder. Urocystoliths (bladder stones) can be dissolved but urethroliths (urethral stones) cannot. However, when necessary, urethroliths can be removed by lithotripsy. Initially, the dog should be reexamined every four weeks (urinalysis and double-contract cystography). With good compliance, the urine specific gravity should be reduced (<1.015), the

Table 3. Urinalyses of a three-year-old, neutered male Dalmatian dog with urocystoliths.

	Day									
Factors*	**1****	**25**	**59**	**88**	**123**	**157**	**186**	**214**	**247**	**275**
Method of collection	Voided	Midstream	Cysto	Cath	Cath	Cath	Cysto	Cath	Cath	Cysto
Specific gravity	1.028	1.018	1.014	1.022	1.019	1.013	1.018	1.017	1.010	1.008
pH	7.0	8.0	7.5	8.5	8.0	8.0	8.0	8.0	8.5	8.5
Protein***	1+	Trace	0	1+	1+	Trace	Trace	2+	Trace	Trace
Epithelial cells†	Rare	Few	0	Mod	0	Few	Few	Few	0	Few
WBC†	0	0	0	0	0	0	0	0	0	0
RBC†	1-2	120-150	Rare	Rare	Occ	20-24	0	0	0	0
Crystals††	Many urate	Few urate	0	0	Rare urate	Rare urate	0	Few amorphous	0	0

(Continued from above)

Factors*	**598**	**654**	**728**	**924**	**1,046**	**1,254**	**1,268**	**1,580**	**1,640**
Method of collection	Cath	Cath	Cysto	Cysto	Cath	Cath	Cath	Cath	Cath
Specific gravity	1.012	1.013	1.006	1.006	1.010	1.006	1.008	1.005	1.011
pH	8.5	8.5	7.0	7.5	8.0	8.0	7.5	7.0	8.5
Protein***	1+	3+	Trace	0	1+	1+	1+	Trace	1+
Epithelial cells†	Mod	Mod	0	Occ	Occ	Few	Few	Rare	Rare
WBC†	0	0	0	0	0	0	0	0	0
RBC†	Rare	0-2	25-30	0	0	0	Rare	0-1	0
Crystals††	0	0	0	0	0	0	0	0	0

Key: Cysto = cystocentesis, Cath = catheterization, Mod = moderate, WBC = white blood cells, RBC = red blood cells, Occ = occasional.
*Glucose, bilirubin, acetone and bacteria were not detected in any specimen.
**Therapy consisting of a urate litholytic food and allopurinol was initiated on Day 2; allopurinol therapy was discontinued on Day 186.
***Values represent semiquantitative evaluations based on a scale of 0 to 4; urine volume was not considered.
†Number per high power field (x450).
††Number per low power field (x100).

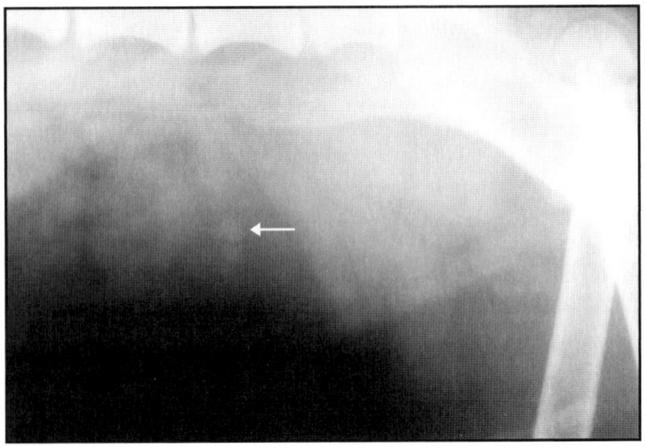

Figure 3. Survey abdominal radiograph of the dog described in Figure 1. Note the radiodense urocystoliths in the urinary bladder (arrow). Several uroliths of marginal density were also located near the os penis.

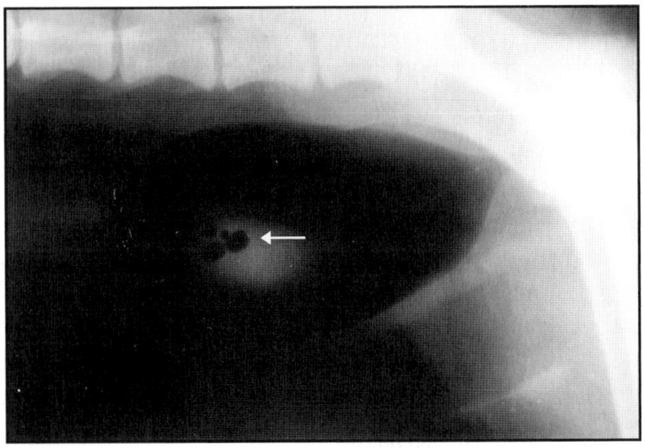

Figure 4. Double-contrast cystogram revealing urocystoliths (arrow).

urinary pH should be alkaline, no ammonium urate crystalluria should be detected and uroliths should be smaller and/or fewer as detected by double-contrast radiography. The serum urea nitrogen concentration should be low (<15 mg/dl) if additional blood work is performed.

Progress Notes

Uroliths retrieved on Day 1 were analyzed and found to be composed of 100% ammonium urate. Medical and dietary therapy was initiated with moist Prescription Diet u/d Canine and allopurinol (15 mg/kg body weight, per os, q12h). The dog's daily energy requirement was estimated to be 1,745 kcal/day (7.3 MJ) (1.5 cans twice daily). Amoxicillin-clavulanic acid (22 mg/kg, per os, q12h) was also used because of suspected superficial staphylococcal pyoderma. Twenty-five days later, the owners reported that the patient's urination was normal although an increased urine volume was noticed. Physical examination was normal and the folliculitis had resolved. The urine specific gravity and serum concentrations of urea nitrogen and uric acid were predictably decreased (**Tables 2** and **3**) and the urinary pH was alkaline. Double-contrast cystography revealed that the urocystoliths were approximately 50% smaller.

Thereafter, the dog was evaluated approximately every four weeks. Uroliths progressively decreased in size and number until they were no longer visible by double-contrast cystography (**Figure 5**, Day 186). Medical therapy was continued for an additional month at which time allopurinol was discontinued. Prophylactic therapy consisted of continuing the veterinary therapeutic food. Uroliths did not recur over the next four years (**Tables 2** and **3**). Superficial pyoderma recurred seasonally and was treated with appropriate antibiotics.

Further Discussion

Ammonium urate uroliths are highly recurrent, so prophylactic therapy should always be considered. Use of a food that avoids excessive levels of dietary purines and promotes formation of dilute, alkaline urine is effective in preventing recurrence of ammonium urate uroliths approximately 80% of the time. Allopurinol has been recommended for preventive therapy; however, recent studies indicate that prolonged administration of high doses of allopurinol may result in formation of xanthine uroliths. The risk of xanthine urolith formation is enhanced if dietary purines are not restricted during allopurinol administration.

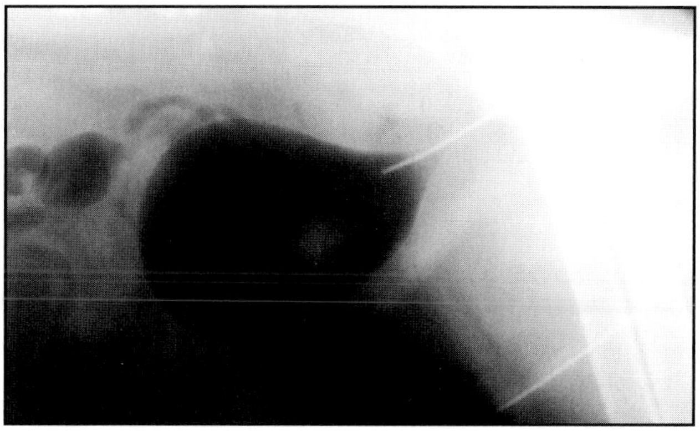

Figure 5. Double-contrast cystogram 186 days after initiating medical and dietary therapy to dissolve ammonium urate uroliths. No uroliths are detectable in the urinary bladder.

Endnotes

a. Prescription Diet k/d Canine. Hill's Pet Nutrition Inc., Topeka, KS, USA.

b. Prescription Diet u/d Canine. Hill's Pet Nutrition Inc., Topeka, KS, USA.

Bibliography

Osborne CA, Lulich JP, Bartges JW, et al. Canine and feline urolithiasis: Relationship of etiopathogenesis to treatment and prevention. In: Osborne CA, Finco DR, eds. Canine and Feline Nephrology and Urology. Baltimore, MD: Williams & Wilkins, 1995; 798-888.

CASE 39-2

Recurrent Urolithiasis in an English Bulldog

Carl A. Osborne, DVM, PhD, Dipl. ACVIM (Internal Medicine)
College of Veterinary Medicine
University of Minnesota
St. Paul, Minnesota, USA

Patient Assessment

A two-year-old, intact male English bulldog with normal body condition (body condition score 3/5) and weight (24 kg) was evaluated for recurrent urolithiasis. The dog had voided uroliths since it was a puppy. A cystotomy was performed six months earlier to remove urocystoliths, which were not submitted for quantitative mineral analysis. Urethral obstruction occurred three months ago. Urethral patency was reestablished by retrograde urohydropropulsion but the uroliths had again not been analyzed. The dog was voiding small uroliths again (**Figure 1**). Physical examination was normal; uroliths were not palpable in the bladder or urethra.

Results of a complete blood count and serum biochemistry profile were normal, except for a mildly elevated uric acid concentration. Analysis of a urine specimen obtained by cystocentesis revealed the following: specific gravity = 1.035, pH = 6.0, proteinuria, numerous urate crystals and no erythrocytes, leukocytes or bacteria (**Table 1**). Aerobic bacterial culture of an aliquot of urine was negative.

Uroliths were not detected by survey abdominal radiography (**Figure 2**). However, numerous small urocystoliths were detected by double-contrast cystography (**Figure 3**).

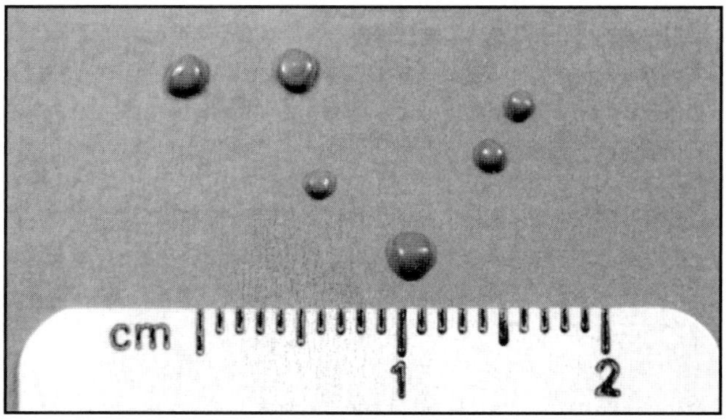

Figure 1. Photograph of ammonium urate uroliths voided by a two-year-old intact male English bulldog.

Table 1. Results of selected urinalysis and serum biochemistry parameters of a two-year-old male English bulldog with recurrent urocystoliths.

Factors	Reference values	Day 1*	35	78	114
Urine specific gravity	-	1.035	1.005	1.006	1.027
Urinary pH	-	6	6	7.5	6
Hematuria	-	0	0	+	+
Pyuria	-	0	0	0	+
Crystals	-	Urate	0	0	Urate
Urine culture	-	Neg	Neg	Neg	Neg
SUN (mg/dl)	7-28	13	4	4	8
Creatinine (mg/dl)	0.5-1.5	1.1	0.7	0.7	0.9
Albumin (mg/dl)	2.4-3.8	3.3	3.0	3.1	3.5

Key: 0 = absent, + = present, Neg = negative, SUN = serum urea nitrogen.
*Therapy consisting of a moist urate litholytic food and allopurinol was initiated on Day 1 and discontinued on Day 78.

Assess the Food and Feeding Method

The dog was fed a commercial dry grocery brand food[a] free choice.

Questions

1. Based on the available information, what is the most likely mineral composition of the uroliths in this patient?
2. Outline a treatment and feeding plan for this dog.
3. How should response to therapy be monitored?

Answers and Discussion

1. The mineral composition of the uroliths in this dog is most likely ammonium urate based on the following: 1) multiple radiolucent uroliths, 2) urinary pH = 6.0, 3) ammonium urate crystalluria, 4) sterile urine, 5) a slight increase in serum uric acid concentration and 6) English bulldog breed. Quantitative mineral analysis of a voided urolith would be important to confirm this diagnostic assessment.
2. Dissolution of ammonium urate uroliths can be induced using a combination of a commercial veterinary therapeutic urate litholytic food[b] and allopurinol.[c] Secondary urinary tract infections should also be eradicated or controlled with appropriate antimicrobial therapy. The urate litholytic food contains low levels of dietary purines, which are the precursors of uric acid, and results in production of less concentrated, alkaline urine that enhances urate crystal solubility. Allopurinol is a xanthine oxidase inhibitor that decreases production of uric acid, and thus the quantity of uric acid in the urine.
3. Therapeutic efficacy should be monitored by physical examination and serial evaluation of radiographs, urinalyses and quantitative urine cultures, if necessary. Dietary therapy and allopurinol should be continued for one month following radiographic disappearance of uroliths. Compliance with the feeding plan is indicated by a reduction in the serum urea nitrogen concentration and formation of less concentrated, alkaline urine.

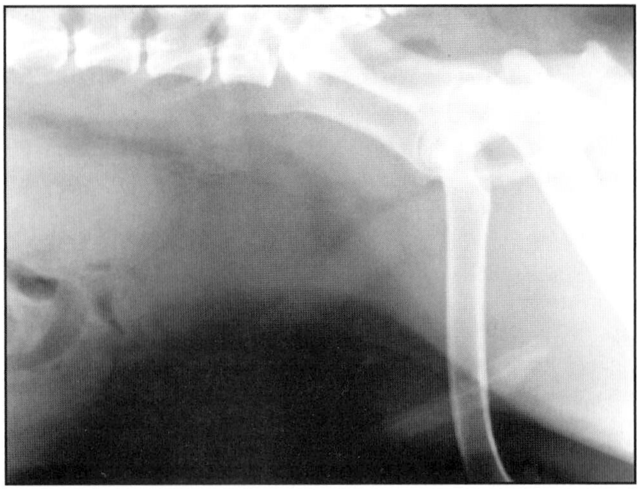

Figure 2. Survey abdominal radiograph of the same dog described in Figure 1. The dog voided small ammonium urate uroliths during micturition. Note that radiodense uroliths are not detectable in the bladder.

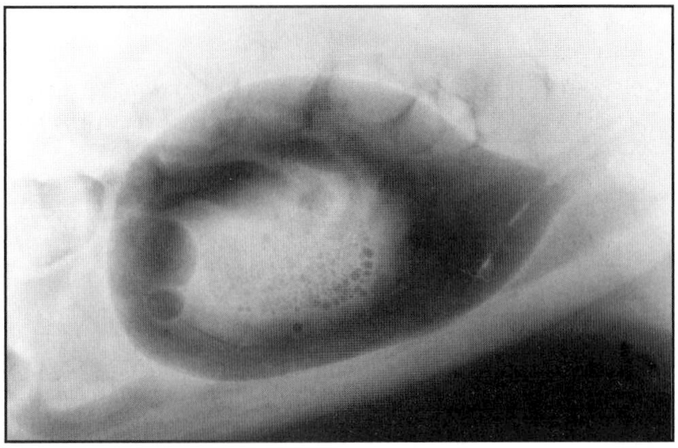

Figure 3. Double-contrast cystogram of the same dog described in Figure 1 demonstrating numerous ammonium urate urocystoliths.

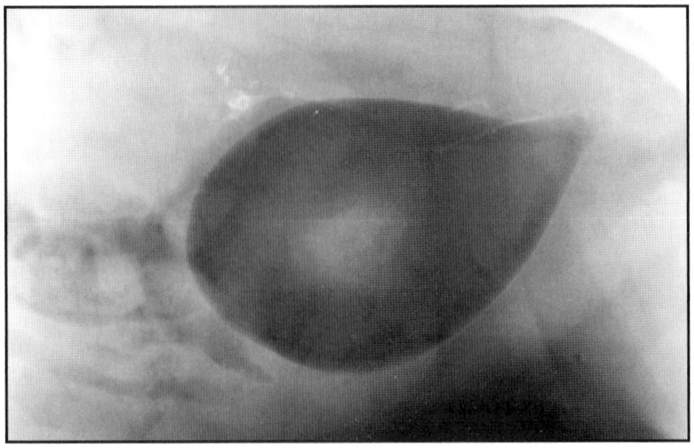

Figure 4. Double-contrast cystogram of the same dog described in Figure 1 obtained 35 days after initiating therapy. There is no evidence of urocystoliths.

Progress Notes

Quantitative analysis of a voided urolith confirmed it was composed of 100% ammonium urate. Combination therapy with the moist urate litholytic food and allopurinol (15 mg/kg body weight, per os, twice daily) was initiated. The daily energy requirement was estimated to be approximately 1,265 kcal (5.29 MJ) (1.6 x resting energy requirement) or one can of the urate litholytic food twice daily. By Day 35 following initiation of therapy, there was no radiographic evidence of uroliths (**Figure 4**). Urinalysis revealed less concentrated urine with no evidence of crystalluria. The serum urea nitrogen concentration was decreased, which implied good compliance with the feeding plan (**Table 1**). The dietary and drug therapy were continued for another month. Similar clinical findings were observed (**Table 1**, Day 78).

The owner elected to discontinue both the dietary and drug therapy. By Day 114 after the original diagnosis, urine specific gravity was increased and pyuria and urate crystalluria were evident (**Table 1**). The dog was voiding uroliths again three months later. These uroliths were found to be composed of 100% ammonium acid urate. Multiple urocystoliths were confirmed by double-contrast cystography. Combination dietary and drug therapy was used again for dissolution of the uroliths. Prevention of recurrence included continued feeding of the moist urate litholytic food and using allopurinol only as necessary to help control urate crystalluria. Monitoring over the next nine months documented one episode of bacterial urinary tract infection; however, the dog had been asymptomatic and no uroliths were detected by contrast radiography.

Endnotes

a. Purina Dog Chow. Purina Pet Care Co., St. Louis, MO, USA.
b. Prescription Diet u/d Canine. Hill's Pet Nutrition, Inc., Topeka, KS, USA.
c. Zyloprim. Glaxo Welcome Inc., Research Triangle Park, NC, USA.

Bibliography

Osborne CA, Lulich JP, Bartges JW, eds. The Rocket Science of Canine Urolithiasis. Veterinary Clinics of North America: Small Animal Practice; 28: 1-306.

Osborne CA, Lulich JP, Bartges JW, et al. Canine and feline urolithiasis: Relationship of etiopathogenesis to treatment and prevention. In: Osborne CA, Finco DR, eds. Canine and Feline Nephrology and Urology. Baltimore, MD: Williams & Wilkins, 1995; 798-888.

Chapter 40

Canine Calcium Oxalate Urolithiasis: Changing Paradigms in Detection, Management and Prevention

Jody P. Lulich
Carl A. Osborne
Lori A. Koehler

"A well-defined problem is half solved."
Carl A. Osborne

OVERVIEW

Uroliths composed of calcium oxalate monohydrate and calcium oxalate dihydrate form as a result of the interaction of several different environmental and demographic risk factors, and several different metabolic disturbances. That is, not all calcium oxalate uroliths are "created in the same way." Some of these factors are primary and some are compensatory. Identification of primary and secondary abnormalities associated with calcium oxalate urolithiasis is essential if therapy is to be consistently safe and effective.

Of the biogenic uroliths that affect dogs, cats and people, those composed of calcium oxalate have been the most problematic. However, substantial progress has been made in the last 10 years. We predict that within the next 10 years, we will understand how to identify and safely modify the underlying mechanisms involved with calcium oxalate urolithiasis. That is, within the next decade we will have reached our goal of making the surgical removal of uroliths a treatment of historical interest.

PREVALENCE AND MINERAL COMPOSITION

Calcium oxalate accounted for 38% of all canine uroliths submitted to the Minnesota Urolith Center from 1981 to 2007 (Table 38-8) and 41% (16,761 of 40,612) of all canine uroliths submitted in 2007 (**Figure 40-1**) (Osborne and Lulich, 2007). Calcium oxalate also accounted for 43% of all upper urinary tract uroliths analyzed at our Center from 1981 to 2006 (Table 38-9). From 2000 to 2006 calcium oxalate composed only 1% of uroliths retrieved from dogs less than 12 months old. The mean age of dogs at the time of calcium oxalate urolith retrieval was approximately 8.5 years (range = one to 25 years; median = 8.7 years). Males (74%) were affected more often than females (22%); the age of approximately 4% of affected dogs was not specified. A total of 214 different breeds were affected including miniature schnauzers (18%), mixed breeds (14%), Yorkshire terriers (9%), Bichon Frises (8%), Shih Tzus (7%), Lhasa apsos (5%), Pomeranians (4%), dachshunds (3%), Maltese (3%),

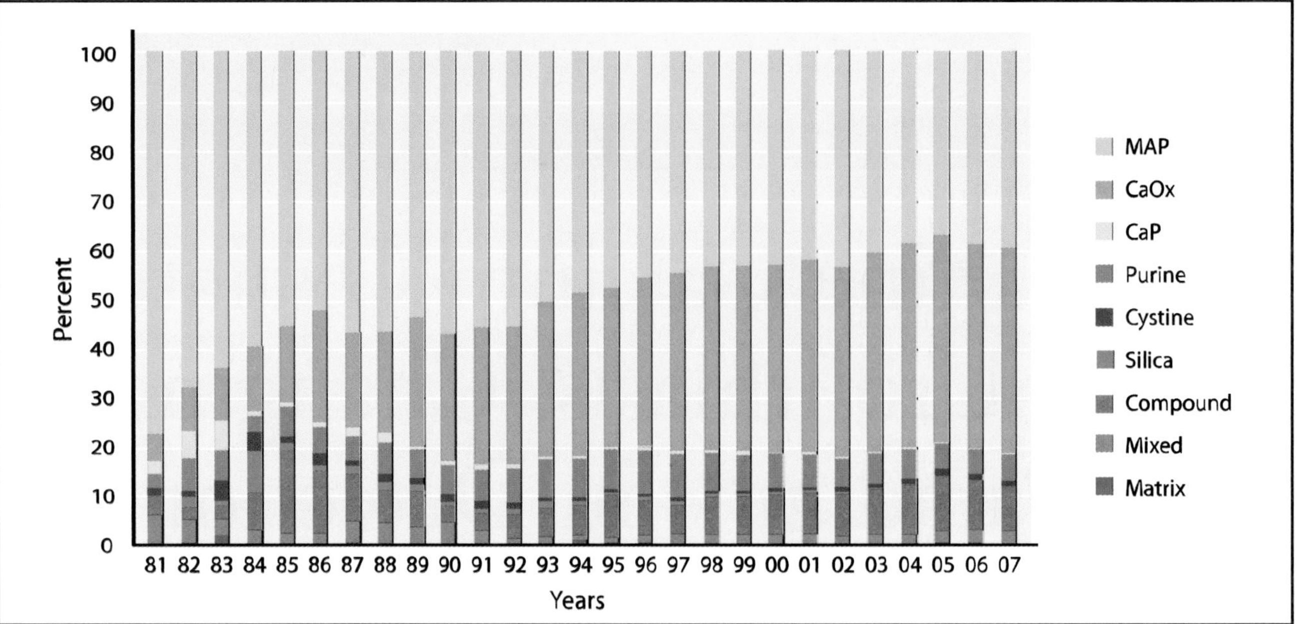

Figure 40-1. Bar graph illustrating increased occurrence of canine calcium oxalate uroliths submitted to the Minnesota Urolith Center from 1981 to 2007. Note the overall decline in struvite urolith submissions and the increase in calcium oxalate submissions. Key: MAP = magnesium ammonium phosphate (struvite), CaOx = calcium oxalate, CaP = calcium phosphate.

miniature poodles (3%), Chihuahuas (2%) and Jack Russell terriers (2%). Calcium oxalate uroliths were more commonly removed from the lower urinary tract (97%) than the upper urinary tract (3%).

Although different combinations of calcium oxalate salts have been identified in canine uroliths, the predominant form encountered has been calcium oxalate monohydrate (whewellite; Table 38-8). Pure calcium oxalate monohydrate has been observed in dogs more frequently than pure calcium oxalate dihydrate (weddelite). A similar observation has been made in cats and people with calcium oxalate uroliths. When calcium oxalate salts occur in combination in human, feline and canine uroliths, the dihydrate salt is usually found surrounding a nucleus of the monohydrate salt (Koide et al, 1982). The significance of this observation has not yet been confirmed, although it has been suggested that calcium oxalate dihydrate may form initially and then be converted to calcium oxalate monohydrate (Leusmann et al, 1984; Otnes, 1983; Schubert and Brien, 1981; Tomazic and Nancollas, 1982). In people, detection of calcium oxalate dihydrate on the outside of a urolith may indicate recent formation, whereas detection of external layers of calcium oxalate monohydrate indicates lack of recent urolith formation (Berenyl et al, 1972). If valid in dogs, this hypothesis would be of clinical significance because it would help to determine if the disorders underlying calcium oxalate urolithiasis were persistent. This in turn would provide evidence of the need for continuous therapy to minimize urolith recurrence. In one study, human patients with calcium oxalate dihydrate uroliths had more recurrences of uroliths than did patients with calcium oxalate monohydrate uroliths (Leusmann et al, 1984).

Calcium oxalate monohydrate and dihydrate uroliths are typically dense and brittle; they have relatively small quantities (~3%) of matrix. Pure calcium oxalate monohydrate and calcium oxalate dihydrate have different colors and shapes (**Table 40-1**). In people, uroliths composed of calcium oxalate monohydrate frequently assume the shape of mulberries or jackstones (Otnes, 1983). To date, only a few canine calcium oxalate jackstones have been observed at the Minnesota Urolith Center.

ETIOPATHOGENESIS AND RISK FACTORS

In order for calcium oxalate uroliths to form, urine must be supersaturated with calcium and oxalic acid. Therefore, increasing the urine concentration of calcium and/or oxalic acid promotes calcium oxalate crystal formation. Hypercalciuria has been documented to occur in dogs with calcium oxalate uroliths (Lulich et al, 1991).

At one time it was thought that increases in urine oxalic acid concentration promoted calcium oxalate urolith formation in people to a greater degree than comparable increases in urine calcium concentration (Smith, 1991). Results of more recent studies, however, indicate that oxalic acid and calcium contribute equally to urine supersaturation with calcium oxalate (Pak et al, 2004). Although hyperoxaluria apparently has not been documented to occur in dogs with calcium oxalate uroliths, the relationship between the concentrations of calcium and oxalic acid within the digestive and urinary tracts is fundamental to understanding calcium oxalate urolithiasis.

Dietary Risk Factors

Dietary ingredients that promote hypercalciuria or hyperoxaluria represent nutritional risk factors for calcium oxalate urolith formation (**Tables 40-2** and **40-3**). Therefore, reduction of dietary calcium and oxalate appears to be a logical therapeutic goal. However, it is not necessarily harmless. Reducing consumption of only one of these substances (calcium) may increase the availability of the other (oxalic acid) for intestinal absorption and subsequent urinary excretion. To minimize this undesirable shift in the modulation of oxalic acid absorption from the intestine, reduction in dietary calcium should be accompanied by an appropriate reduction in dietary oxalic acid.

Dogs with calcium oxalate urolithiasis frequently consume human food. Calcium oxalate is the most common urolith type recognized in people living in developed countries. As people feed their dogs the same dietary proportions and ingredients they feed themselves, it is logical to postulate that dogs would be exposed to similar nutritional risk factors for urolith formation (**Table 40-2**). Results of epidemiologic studies performed at the Minnesota Urolith Center support this hypothesis.

In addition to human food consumption, an association between calcium oxalate urolithiasis and consumption of commercially available treats has also been recognized. The high sodium content of some commercial dog treats may help explain this association because sodium consumption promotes hypercalciuria (Lulich et al, 1992).

Certain dietary excesses and deficiencies have also been recognized as potential risk factors. Excessive administration of vitamin D, sodium or magnesium promotes hypercalciuria. Because ascorbic acid is a precursor of oxalate, excessive quantities of vitamin C should be avoided. Although dogs with calcium oxalate uroliths have not been evaluated for pyridoxine deficiency, kittens fed pyridoxine-deficient foods exhibited hyperoxaluria (Bai et al, 1989).

Table 40-1. Common characteristics of canine calcium oxalate uroliths.

Chemical names	Formulas	Crystal names
Calcium oxalate monohydrate	$CaC_2O_4 \bullet H_2O$	Whewellite
Calcium oxalate dihydrate	$CaC_2O_4 \bullet 2H_2O$	Weddellite

Variations in mineral composition
Calcium oxalate monohydrate only
Calcium oxalate dihydrate only
Combinations of calcium oxalate monohydrate and dihydrate
Calcium oxalate (monohydrate and/or dihydrate) mixed with variable quantities of calcium phosphate. Variable quantities of struvite or ammonium acid urate may also be present.
Calcium oxalate (monohydrate and/or dihydrate) nucleus surrounded by other minerals especially infection-induced struvite

Physical characteristics
Color: Calcium oxalate monohydrate uroliths are usually tan or brown. Calcium oxalate dihydrate uroliths are usually white or cream colored. Surfaces may be red to black if uroliths are coated with blood.
Shape: Variable. Calcium oxalate monohydrate uroliths are usually round or elliptical and have a smooth, polished surface. Occasionally, they may develop a jackstone or mulberry shape. Calcium oxalate dihydrate uroliths and mixed calcium oxalate monohydrate/calcium oxalate dihydrate uroliths are usually round to ovoid and have an irregular surface caused by protrusion of sharp-edged crystals. Occasionally, they may develop a jackstone shape.
Nuclei: Radial striations and concentric laminations may occur.
Density: Very dense and brittle. Survey radiographs reveal that calcium-containing uroliths are radiodense compared with soft tissue.
Number: Single or multiple
Location: May be located in renal pelves, ureters, urinary bladder (most common) and/or urethra.
Size: Sub-visual to several centimeters

Prevalence
Approximately 41% of all canine uroliths. More than 43% of canine upper tract uroliths.
May be recurrent (more than 50% recur by three years after removal)

Characteristics of affected canine patients
More common in males (73%) than females (22%)
Mean age at diagnosis is about eight years (range <1 to >25 years)
Most commonly observed in miniature schnauzers, Lhasa apsos, Yorkshire terriers, Shih Tzus and Bichon Frises

Other Risk Factors

Calcium oxalate uroliths have been recognized in many breeds of dogs (see Prevalence and Mineral Composition above). Infrequently encountered breeds include boxers, bloodhounds, coonhounds, Dalmatians, English bulldogs, Newfoundlands, German shorthaired pointers, Skye terriers, wirehaired terriers, golden retrievers, Labrador retrievers and St. Bernards. Approximately 74% of calcium oxalate uroliths have affected male dogs. Most were detected in adults (mean and median age was eight to nine years).

Geographic location has been identified as a risk factor for calcium oxalate urolith formation in people living in the United States (Mandel and Mandel, 1989). In a study of approximately one million people, investigators observed a north-south and west-east gradient such that people living in the southeastern U.S. (Alabama, Arkansas, Florida, Georgia, Louisiana, Mississippi, North and South Carolina, Tennessee and Virginia) had the highest rate of urolith formation (Soucie et al, 1996). Studies evaluating geographic location as a risk factor for calcium oxalate urolith formation in dogs have apparently not yet been reported.

Certain clinical conditions also represent potential risk factors for calcium oxalate urolith formation. Hyperparathyroidism, hyperadrenocorticism, hypervitaminosis D, paraneoplastic hypercalcemia and furosemide administration promote hypercalciuria. In people, intestinal resection, hereditary hyperoxaluria and excessive ascorbic acid administration promote hyperoxaluria (Park and Pearle, 2007).

Hypercalciuria

Hypercalciuria can be localized into at least three subtypes according to the primary site of the underlying cause (i.e., intestine, kidney or skeleton): 1) absorptive hypercalciuria is characterized by intestinal hyperabsorption of calcium, 2) renal hypercalciuria is characterized by impaired renal tubular reabsorption of calcium and 3) resorptive hypercalciuria is characterized by bone demineralization.

Available evidence indicates that calcium homeostasis is principally achieved through the actions of parathyroid hormone (PTH) and 1,25-dicholecalciferol (1,25-vitamin D) on the intestines, kidneys and skeleton. For example, states of low

Table 40-2. Some potential risk factors for canine calcium oxalate uroliths.

Diet	Urine	Metabolic status	Drugs
Acidifying potential	Hypercalciuria	Chronic metabolic acidosis	Urine acidifiers
High protein content	Hyperoxaluria	Males	Furosemide
High sodium content	Hypocitraturia?	Breed	Glucocorticoids
Excessive calcium content	Hypomagnesuria?	Miniature schnauzers	Sodium chloride
Excessive restriction of calcium	Hyperuricuria?	Miniature poodles	Vitamin D
Low moisture content	Increased crystal promoters	Lhasa apsos	Ascorbic acid
Excessive phosphorus restriction	Decreased crystal inhibitors	Yorkshire terriers	
Excessive magnesium content	Urine concentration	Shih Tzus	
Excessive magnesium restriction	Urine retention	Bichon Frises	
Excessive vitamin D content		Older age	
Excessive vitamin C content		Hypercalcemia	
Deficient pyridoxine?		Glucocorticoid excess	
High oxalate content		Hypophosphatemia	
		Hyperoxalemia?	
		Osteolysis?	

Table 40-3. Selected human foods to limit or avoid feeding to dogs with calcium oxalate uroliths.*

Moderate/high-calcium foods	Moderate/high-oxalate foods	
Food items	**Food items**	
Meats	**Meats**	
Bologna (M)	Sardines (M)	Oranges (M)
Herring (M)	**Vegetables**	Peaches (M)
Oysters (M)	Asparagus (M)	Pears (M)
Salmon (H)	Broccoli (M)	Peel of lemon, lime or orange (H)
Sardines (H)	Carrots (M)	Pineapple (M)
Vegetables	Celery (H)	Tangerine (H)
Baked beans (M)	Corn (M)	**Breads, grains, nuts**
Broccoli (H)	Cucumber (H)	Cornbread (M)
Collards (H)	Eggplant (H)	Fruitcake (H)
Lima beans (M)	Green beans (H)	Grits (H)
Spinach (M)	Green peppers (H)	Peanuts (H)
Tofu (soybean curd) (M)	Lettuce (M)	Pecans (H)
Milk and dairy products	Spinach (H)	Soybeans (H)
Cheese (H)	Summer squash (H)	Wheat germ (H)
Ice cream (H)	Sweet potatoes (H)	**Miscellaneous**
Milk (H)	Tofu (H)	Beer (H)
Yogurt (H)	Tomatoes (M)	Chocolate (H)
Breads, grains, nuts	**Fruits**	Cocoa (H)
Brazil nuts (M)	Apples (H)	Coffee (M)
Miscellaneous	Apricots (H)	Tea (H)
Cocoa (M)	Cherries (M)	Tomato soup (H)
Hot chocolate (M)	Most berries (H)	Vegetable soup (H)

Key: M = moderate; feed in limited amounts. H = high; avoid feeding.
*Adapted from Wainer L, Resnick VA, Resnick MI. Nutritional aspects of stone disease. In: Pak CYC, ed. Renal Stone Disease, Pathogenesis, Prevention, and Treatment. Boston, MA: Martinus Nihoff Publishing, 1987; 85-120. Burroughs M. Renal diseases and disorders. In: Nelson JK, Moxness KE, Jensen MD, et al, eds. Mayo Clinic Diet Manual, 7th ed. St. Louis, MO: Mosby, 1994; 208-209.

serum ionized calcium concentration result in compensatory PTH- and 1,25-vitamin D-mediated mobilization of calcium from the skeleton, absorption of calcium from the intestine and conservation of calcium by the kidneys. High serum ionized calcium concentrations suppress release of PTH and production of 1,25-vitamin D. The result is decreased skeletal mobilization and intestinal absorption of calcium and enhanced renal calcium excretion. Thus, it is apparent that hypercalciuria can result from increased renal clearance of calcium due to: 1) excessive intestinal absorption of calcium, 2) impaired renal conservation of calcium and/or 3) excessive skeletal mobilization of calcium. Although hypercalciuria can be localized according to the site of the apparent primary defect in calcium transport, compensatory changes typically occur that involve other sites. For example, renal-leak hypercalciuria is associated with secondary hyperparathyroidism, which in turn is associated with varying degrees of bone resorption of calcium and phosphorus and varying degrees of intestinal calcium absorption. Absorptive hypercalciuria results in a positive calcium balance, which in turn suppresses production and release of PTH, decreasing renal tubular reabsorption of calcium.

Hypercalcemic hypercalciuria results from increased glo-

Table 40-4. Summary of distinguishing clinical manifestations for different types of hypercalciuria.

Features	Absorptive hypercalciuria	Renal-leak hypercalciuria	Resorptive hypercalciuria
Serum calcium	Normal	Normal	Increased
Serum parathyroid hormone	Decreased/normal	Increased	Increased
Serum phosphorus	Normal/increased	Normal	Decreased/increased*
Urine calcium			
Fasting	Normal	Increased	Increased
Dx food**	Increased	Increased	Increased
Urine oxalic acid	Normal	Normal	Normal
Urine uric acid	Normal	Normal	Normal
Bone density	Normal	Decreased	Decreased
Calcium balance (total body)	Positive	Negative	Negative

*Phosphorus is retained in serum as glomerular filtration rate declines.
**Dx food = diagnostic food used in the evaluation of normal dogs and those with calcium oxalate uroliths.

merular filtration of mobilized calcium, which overwhelms normal renal tubular reabsorptive mechanisms. This phenomenon is called resorptive hypercalciuria because excessive bone resorption is associated with increased serum calcium concentrations. In dogs, normocalcemic hypercalciuria is thought to result from either intestinal hyperabsorption of calcium (so-called absorptive hypercalciuria), or decreased renal tubular reabsorption of calcium (so-called renal-leak hypercalciuria) (**Table 40-4**). Absorptive hypercalciuria is characterized by increased urine calcium excretion and urine calcium concentration, normal serum calcium concentration and normal or low serum PTH concentration. Because absorptive hypercalciuria depends on dietary calcium, urine calcium excretion and urine calcium concentration are normal or significantly reduced during the fasting state. However, urine calcium excretion and urine calcium concentration typically increase during non-fasting conditions. Mean 24-hour urine calcium excretion in 33 normal beagles was 0.32 ± 0.2 mg/kg body weight/day during fasting and 0.51 ± 0.3 mg/kg body weight/day when dogs consumed a standard food[a] (Lulich et al, 1991a). By comparison, mean urine calcium excretion in five miniature schnauzers with calcium oxalate urolithiasis and absorptive hypercalciuria was 1.0 ± 0.5 mg/kg body weight/day during fasting and 2.84 ± 0.9 mg/kg body weight/day during non-fasting urine collections (Lulich et al, 1991).

A primary defect observed in people with absorptive hypercalciuria is apparent intestinal hyperabsorption of calcium, which results in increased excretion of excess calcium in urine. In addition to enhanced glomerular filtration of absorbed dietary calcium, decreased PTH secretion results in decreased renal tubular reabsorption of filtered calcium. The same phenomenon appears to occur in dogs with absorptive hypercalciuria.

Primary intestinal abnormalities of calcium absorption, disorders of 1,25-vitamin D production and hypophosphatemia-induced hypervitaminosis D have been recognized as causes of hypercalciuria in people (Park and Pearle, 2007). Absorptive hypercalciuria in people has recently been further subclassified as to whether increased calcium excretion is food unresponsive (Type 1) or food responsive (Type II). The underlying mechanism(s) of absorptive hypercalciuria has not been identified in dogs. However, hypophosphatemia or elevated levels of 1,25-vitamin D were not observed in five dogs with absorptive hypercalciuria.

In human studies, renal-leak hypercalciuria and resorptive hypercalciuria have been documented, but have been recognized less frequently than excessive intestinal absorption of calcium. The defect with renal-leak hypercalciuria is impaired tubular reabsorption of calcium. Patients with renal-leak hypercalciuria have high serum PTH concentrations. Increasing PTH secretion counters the effect of additional calcium lost in urine and maintains normal blood calcium levels. Hypercalcemia associated with calcium oxalate urolithiasis is the hallmark of patients with resorptive hypercalciuria. Hypercalcemia is not a characteristic of patients with excessive intestinal absorption of calcium or renal-leak hypercalciuria. An in-depth review of the pathophysiology of hypercalciuria has recently been published (Park and Pearle, 2007).

Hyperoxaluria

As described above in the discussion about dietary risk factors influencing calcium oxalate urolithiasis, the effect of oxalic acid on calcium oxalate urolithiasis depends on the interactions of calcium and oxalic acid that occur in the lumen of the intestine and in urine. Intestinal hyperabsorption or accelerated endogenous synthesis of oxalic acid can result in hyperoxaluria. In healthy people, the majority of urine oxalic acid is derived from the endogenous metabolism of ascorbic acid, glycine, glyoxylate and tryptophan. The daily quantity of endogenously produced oxalic acid is apparently minimal. In people, hyperoxaluria has been associated with inherited abnormalities of excessive oxalic acid synthesis (primary hyperoxaluria), increased consumption of foods containing high quantities of oxalic acid or oxalic acid precursors (**Table 40-3**), pyridoxine deficiency and disorders associated with fat absorption (Williams and Smith, 1983). We could not find any reports of inherited hyperoxaluria or hyperoxaluria associated with intestinal resection and fat malabsorption in dogs. However, increases in urine oxalic acid excretion have been recognized in kittens fed pyridoxine-deficient foods (Bai et al, 1989).

In people, approximately 10 to 20% of urine oxalic acid is

absorbed from dietary ingredients. Urine oxalic acid excretion is inversely related to dietary intake of calcium. In the intestinal tract, oxalic acid complexes with calcium and is excreted in feces as an insoluble salt. A decrease in the combination of oxalic acid with calcium to form calcium oxalate results in an increased quantity of soluble oxalic acid available for intestinal absorption. Therefore, it is logical to assume that urolith-forming patients with intestinal hyperabsorption of calcium, or those consuming foods with inappropriately low calcium compared with oxalic acid, would be at risk for increased intestinal absorption of dietary oxalic acid, hyperoxaluria and subsequent calcium oxalate urolith formation.

Hypocitraturia

Hypocitraturia is a common physiologic disturbance in people with calcium oxalate urolithiasis. It has been reported to affect 20 to 60% of calcium stone formers (Hamm and Hering-Smith, 2002). Urine citric acid is a negative anion that combines with cationic calcium, thus reducing the quantity of calcium available to complex with oxalic acid. Calcium citrate is more soluble than calcium oxalate. Citrate is also a buffer, and as such, minimizes the formation of calcium phosphate. Citrate also directly inhibits crystallization and aggregation of calcium oxalate and calcium phosphate (Park and Pearle, 2007).

The role of low urine citric acid concentration in the etiology of canine calcium oxalate urolithiasis is not completely resolved. Hypocitraturia has been observed in dogs with calcium oxalate uroliths; however, mechanisms responsible for decreased urine citric acid excretion in dogs are as yet unknown. It is known that acid-base homeostasis influences the quantity of citric acid excreted in urine (Simpson, 1983). In normal dogs, acidosis is associated with decreased urine citric acid formation and excretion, whereas alkalosis promotes urine citric acid formation and excretion.

Several abnormalities associated with acidosis may lead to hypocitraturia. Examples include distal renal tubular acidosis, chronic diarrhea associated with systemic acidosis and excessive consumption of animal protein, which produces excess acid and promotes bone demineralization. A recent study of a high-protein, low-carbohydrate diet typified by the so-called Atkins diet revealed a significant reduction in urinary pH and citrate during the induction and maintenance phases of the diet (Reddy et al, 2002). Hypocitraturia may also occur in association with thiazide-induced hypokalemia, which produces intracellular acidosis. Idiopathic hypocitraturia may also occur independent of acidosis.

The Role of Oxalate-Degrading Bacteria

Recent studies have revealed a correlation between enteric colonization of oxalate-degrading bacteria (ODB), mainly *Oxalobacter formigenes*, and the absence of hyperoxaluria and/or calcium oxalate formation in rats and people (Sidhu et al, 1999; Troxel et al, 2003). Consider the following evidence: 1) Using a rat model, one group of investigators demonstrated a rapid reversal of hyperoxaluria after probiotic administration of *O. formigenes* (Sidhu et al, 2001). 2) Oral administration of *O. formigenes* to people with Type 1 hyperoxaluria reduced the oxalate concentration in plasma and urine (Hoppe et al, 2006). 3) In rats, *O. formigenes* colonization induced colonic secretion/excretion of endogenous oxalate and was associated with reduced oxalate levels in plasma (Hatch et al, 2006). These studies indicate that colonization of ODB in the gastrointestinal (GI) tract can prevent enteric absorption of oxalic acid and increase fecal excretion of endogenously produced oxalate. ODB possess two enzymes, formyl CoA transferase and oxalate CoA decarboxylase, that metabolize oxalic acid to formate and CO_2 (Lung et al, 1994; Sidhu et al, 1997). In addition, *O. formigenes* carries a specialized membrane transporter, oxalate/formate antiporter, to transport the substrate and product across the membrane (Ruan et al, 1992). *O. formigenes*, *Lactobacillus* spp., *Bifidobacterium lactis*, *Enterococcus faecalis* and *Eubacterium lentum* are major ODB found in mammalian GI tracts (Allison et al, 1986; Federici et al, 2004; Hokama et al, 2000; Ito et al, 1996; Weese et al, 2004). *O. formigenes,* an anaerobe, is solely dependent on oxalate as an energy source. It is considered to efficiently degrade oxalate in the GI tract of rats, sheep, pigs and people (Allison et al, 1985, 1986; Daniel et al, 1987).

There have been few studies reported in which ODB have been evaluated in dogs in context of calcium oxalate uroliths. Oxalate-degrading *Lactobacillus* spp. are present in healthy dogs and cats (Weese et al, 2004). However, the effect of intestinal colonization with ODB on urine oxalate excretion has apparently not been investigated. Oxalate-degrading bacterial activity in canine feces has been demonstrated (Daniel et al, 1987). However, the role of ODB in the pathogenesis of canine and feline calcium oxalate urolithiasis apparently has not been reported.

Considering the current evidence derived from human and rodent models, we hypothesize that decreased concentrations of intestinal ODB are a likely risk factor for calcium oxalate urolith formation in dogs and cats (Lulich et al, 2008). We also hypothesize that the prevalence of ODB in the intestine of dogs with calcium oxalate uroliths is lower than in clinically healthy dogs without uroliths. If our hypothesis is correct, administration of novel probiotics that deliver viable ODB to the intestine and subsequent colonization of the intestinal mucosa with *O. formigenes* should minimize calcium oxalate urolith recurrence.

Macromolecular Crystal Growth Inhibitors

In addition to urine concentration of lithogenic minerals and other ions, large molecular weight glycoproteins in urine profoundly enhance solubility of calcium oxalate. One such protein called nephrocalcin minimizes calcium oxalate crystal growth in human urine (Nakagawa et al, 1983). In studies of nephrocalcin obtained from urolith-forming patients, this crystallization inhibitor lacked appropriate quantities of carboxyglutamic acid residues and was unable to prevent crystal growth. Preliminary studies of urine obtained from dogs with calcium oxalate uroliths have revealed that nephrocalcin also lacks appropriate numbers of carboxyglutamic acid residues compared with nephrocalcin isolated from normal canine urine (Carvalho et al, 2006).

Tamm-Horsfall glycoprotein and glycosaminoglycans inhibit calcium oxalate crystal aggregation. One hypothesis is that the mechanism of action of these proteins is to block growth sites on crystals, thereby inhibiting formation of calcium oxalate uroliths (Deganello, 1993).

BIOLOGIC BEHAVIOR

Calcium oxalate uroliths may be voided in the urine or become lodged in any portion of the urinary tract. Uroliths that remain in the urinary tract may continue to grow slowly or may become inactive (no further growth). Not all persistent uroliths are associated with clinical signs. Unlike infection-induced struvite uroliths, most calcium oxalate uroliths are not associated with urinary tract infection (UTI). Uroliths composed of the dihydrate salt of calcium oxalate appear to be less likely to cause complete urinary obstruction because of their irregular surface contour. Their jagged surface may prevent them from forming a continuous seal within the lumen of the urethra. However, if uroliths remain in the urinary tract, dysuria, UTI, partial or total urinary obstruction and polyp formation are potential sequelae. Spontaneous dissolution of calcium oxalate uroliths in dogs has apparently not been reported.

In a retrospective clinical survey of 438 dogs surgically treated for urolithiasis, 111 patients had 155 known recurrences (Brown et al, 1977). Recurrence was observed in 25% of dogs with calcium oxalate uroliths. We performed two retrospective studies and found that the rate of recurrence of calcium oxalate uroliths increased with the length of time that dogs were evaluated: 3% recurred after three months, 9% after six months, 36% after one year, 42% after two years and 48% after three years (Lulich et al, 1992a). The second study evaluated urolith recurrence in Bichon Frise dogs. After one year, 37% had their first recurrence; after two years, 64% had their first recurrence and 8% had their second recurrence; after three years, 90% had their first recurrence, 15% had their second recurrence and 4% had their third recurrence. Urolith recurrence was detected in 100% of dogs evaluated at or after four years (Lulich et al, 2004). Owner and patient compliance with therapy and persistence of factors responsible for urolith initiation at the time of urolith eradication influence the frequency of urolith recurrence.

KEY NUTRITIONAL FACTORS

Because dissolution of calcium oxalate uroliths in dogs has not been reported, the focus of dietary management is to prevent calcium oxalate urolith recurrence. The goals of dietary prevention include: 1) reducing calcium concentration in urine, 2) reducing oxalic acid concentration in urine, 3) promoting high concentration and activity of inhibitors of calcium oxalate crystal growth and aggregation in urine and 4) reducing concentration of urine.

Certain dietary excesses and deficiencies have been recognized as potential risk factors for calcium oxalate urolithiasis and are the basis of key nutritional factors. **Table 40-5** summarizes the key nutritional factors for calcium oxalate prevention.

Table 40-5. Key nutritional factors for foods for prevention of calcium oxalate uroliths.

Factors	Recommended levels
Water	Water intake should be encouraged to achieve a urine specific gravity <1.020 Moist food will increase water consumption and formation of less concentrated urine
Protein	Avoid excess dietary protein Restrict dietary protein to 10 to 18% dry matter (DM)
Calcium	Avoid excess dietary calcium, especially dietary supplements given independent of diet Restrict dietary calcium to 0.4 to 0.7% DM
Oxalate	Avoid foods high in oxalic acid (**Table 40-3**)
Phosphorus	Avoid phosphorus deficiency and maintain a normal Ca:P ratio (1.1:1 to 2:1) Dietary phosphorus should be in the range of 0.3 to 0.6% DM
Sodium	Recommend moderate dietary sodium restriction Dietary sodium should be <0.3% DM
Magnesium	Avoid excess or deficient dietary magnesium Dietary magnesium should be in the range of 0.04 to 0.15% DM
Ascorbic acid (vitamin C)	Avoid pet foods, supplements or human foods that contain ascorbic acid
Urinary pH	Avoid acidifying foods Foods should produce a urinary pH 7.1-7.5

Water

Dogs consuming dry commercial foods may be at greater risk for urolithiasis than dogs consuming moist foods because dry foods are often associated with higher urine concentrations of calcium and oxalic acid and more concentrated urine. Therefore, consider moist foods, rather than dry foods, to aid in the prevention of recurrence of calcium oxalate uroliths. Water intake should be encouraged to achieve a urine specific gravity less than 1.020. In addition to decreasing urine specific gravity, increased water intake is likely to be associated with increased voiding frequency. Frequent voiding reduces crystal retention time thereby minimizing crystal growth.

Protein

Ingestion of foods that contain high quantities of animal protein may contribute to calcium oxalate urolithiasis by increasing urine calcium excretion and decreasing urine citrate excretion (Breslau et al, 1988; Lekcharoensuk et al, 2002, 2002a). Some of these consequences result from obligatory acid excretion associated with protein metabolism. Hypercalciuria occurs in normal dogs fed high-protein foods (40% dry matter [DM]). Therefore, excessive dietary protein consumption should be avoided in dogs with active calcium oxalate urolithiasis. The recommended range for dietary protein is 10 to 18% DM. The

Table 40-6. Selected human foods with minimal calcium or oxalate content.

Food items	Low-calcium foods	Low-oxalate foods
Meats and eggs	Eggs Poultry	Beef Eggs Fish and shellfish* Lamb Pork Poultry
Vegetables		Cabbage Cauliflower Mushrooms Peas, green Radishes Potatoes, white
Milk and dairy products		Cheese* Milk* Yogurt*
Fruits		Apple Avocado Banana Bing cherries Grapefruit Grapes, green Mangos Melons Cantaloupe Casaba Honeydew Watermelon Plums, green or yellow
Breads, grains, nuts	Almonds Macaroni Pretzels Rice Spaghetti Walnuts	Bread, white Macaroni Noodles Rice Spaghetti
Miscellaneous	Popcorn	Jellies Preserves Soups with allowed ingredients

*Low in oxalate, but not low in calcium content.

minimum recommended allowance for protein in foods for healthy adult dogs is 10% DM (NRC, 2006).

Calcium and Oxalic Acid

Reduction of dietary calcium appears to be a logical therapeutic goal because intestinal hyperabsorption of calcium has been identified as one mechanism promoting hypercalciuria in dogs with calcium oxalate uroliths. However, reducing consumption of calcium may increase the availability of oxalic acid for intestinal absorption and subsequent urinary excretion. As in the urinary bladder, calcium and oxalic acid in the intestinal lumen form a relatively insoluble complex, thereby preventing the absorption of one another. This provides a plausible explanation as to why an epidemiologic study evaluating risk factors for calcium oxalate urolith formation in people unexpectedly discovered that foods with higher calcium levels were associated with reduced risk for urolith formation (Curhan et al, 1993, 1997; Curhan, 2007). Therefore, in hypercalciuric patients, reduction in dietary calcium should be accompanied by an appropriate reduction in dietary oxalic acid (**Tables 40-3** and **40-6**) (Lulich et al, 2001). The increase in the urine concentration of oxalic acid can be prevented by concomitantly reducing calcium and oxalic acid in the food. Caution: severe calcium restriction should be avoided to prevent negative calcium balance. The minimum requirement for calcium in foods for healthy dogs is 0.2% DM and the minimum recommended allowance is 0.4% DM (NRC, 2006). For prevention of recurrence of calcium oxalate uroliths, reduce dietary calcium to 0.4 to 0.7% DM.

People with calcium oxalate uroliths are often cautioned to avoid milk and milk products because the carbohydrate component (lactose) of these products may augment intestinal absorption of calcium from any dietary source (Leman et al, 1969). Likewise, they are often discouraged from consuming foods containing relatively high quantities of oxalic acid (**Table 40-3**). Although there is agreement that excessive consumption of calcium and oxalic acid should be avoided, the consensus of urologists is that it is inadvisable to restrict dietary calcium unless persistent absorptive hypercalciuria has been documented. Even then, only moderate restriction is advocated to minimize development of negative calcium balance.

Phosphorus

Studies of laboratory animals, dogs and people suggest that dietary phosphorus should not be overly restricted in patients with calcium oxalate urolithiasis because reduction in dietary phosphorus is often associated with augmentation of intestinal calcium absorption and hypercalciuria (Brautbar et al, 1979). If calcium oxalate urolithiasis is associated with hypophosphatemia and normal serum calcium concentration, oral phosphorus supplementation should be considered. However, caution must be used because excessive dietary phosphorus may predispose hypercalciuric patients to formation of calcium phosphate uroliths.

Based on a recommended range for calcium (0.4 to 0.7% DM) in foods for calcium oxalate urolith prevention in canine patients, dietary phosphorus levels should be in the range of 0.3 to 0.6% DM with a calcium-phosphorus ratio range of 1.1:1 to 2:1. The minimum recommended allowance for phosphorus in foods for healthy adult dogs is 0.3% DM (NRC, 2006).

Sodium

Sodium chloride can be added to food to increase thirst and urine volume. However, excess sodium increases urine calcium excretion and therefore is a risk factor for calcium oxalate and calcium phosphate urolithiasis, particularly if the urinary pH is high. For the same reason, if oral urinary alkalinizing agents are used, potassium citrate may be a better choice than sodium bicarbonate. Supplemental sodium sources may also contribute to hypertension in salt-sensitive dogs.

In people, high dietary sodium consumption also reduces urine citrate concentration via sodium-induced bicarbonate loss. Daily urine calcium excretion of normal dogs consuming foods with 0.8% DM sodium was comparable to calcium excretion observed in dogs with calcium oxalate uroliths (Lulich, 1991). Based on this evidence, we recommend moderate dietary restriction of sodium (<0.3% DM sodium) for active calcium oxalate urolith formers (Lulich et al, 2001). Typically, commercial dog foods contain two to three times this amount. The minimum recommended allowance for sodium in foods for healthy adult dogs is 0.08% DM (NRC, 2006).

Magnesium

Although supplemental dietary magnesium contributes to formation of magnesium ammonium phosphate uroliths in some species (cats and ruminants), urine magnesium apparently impairs formation of calcium oxalate crystals (Finco et al, 1985; Kallfez et al, 1986; Meyer and Smith, 1969). Therefore, supplemental magnesium has been used in human patients in an attempt to minimize recurrence of calcium oxalate uroliths (Melnick et al, 1971). However, increased urine excretion of calcium by normal dogs given supplemental magnesium has been observed. Urine calcium excretion was 0.5 ± 0.2 mg/kg body weight/day in six normal dogs consuming a food containing 0.03% DM magnesium vs. 2.65 ± 1.7 mg/kg body weight/day when the same dogs consumed a food containing 0.38% DM magnesium (Lulich, 1991a). Pending further studies, dietary magnesium restriction or supplementation is not recommended for treatment of canine calcium oxalate uroliths. A range of 0.04 to 0.15% DM is recommended. The minimum recommended allowance for magnesium content of foods for healthy adult dogs is 0.06% DM (NRC, 2006).

Ascorbic Acid (Vitamin C)

Supplemental ascorbic acid (a precursor of oxalate) should be avoided.

Urinary pH

Urinary pH in healthy subjects reflects the acid load (acidifying effects) of a food. Although formation of acidic urine is desirable for management of struvite uroliths, foods that promote acidic urine promote hypercalciuria and hypocitraturia. Therefore, consumption of foods that result in formation of acidic urine enhances the risk of calcium oxalate urolithiasis in susceptible dogs. Thus, for prevention of calcium oxalate uroliths, the urinary pH should not be less than 7.0.

A recent study of a high-protein, low-carbohydrate food typified by the so-called Atkins diet revealed a significant reduction in urinary pH and citrate during the induction and maintenance phases of the diet (Reddy et al, 2002).

Urine Alkalinizing Agents

Dosage of urine alkalinizing agents should be individualized for each patient, depending on the status of the patient and pretreatment urinary pH values. Although sodium bicarbonate is a readily available urine alkalinizer, at recommended doses, (25 to 50 mg/kg body weight q12h), it provides a significant increase in sodium intake. Also, sodium may combine with uric acid to form sodium urate. In people, urate salts may serve as a nidus for calcium oxalate urolith formation. For these reasons, we prefer potassium citrate. Potassium citrate in wax matrix tablets (Urocit-K[b]), as a liquid (Polycitra-K[c]) or as chewable tablets (K-CIT-V[d]) may be given. An initial dose of 40 to 75 mg/kg body weight q12h is recommended. The final dose should be individualized based on patient response. Potassium citrate should be administered with meals to reduce gastric irritation. Divided doses should be administered to maintain a consistently nonacidic environment in the urinary tract. Additional supplementation is usually unnecessary when feeding foods (e.g., Prescription Diet u/d Canine canned) containing adequate quantities of potassium citrate.

The goal of treatment with urine alkalinizing agents is to maintain a urinary pH between 7.1 to 7.5. Higher values (>7.5) should be avoided until it is determined whether or not high urinary pH is a significant risk factor for formation of calcium phosphate uroliths. Owners may monitor urinary pH with pH paper or handheld "pocket" pH meters.

OTHER NUTRITIONAL FACTORS

Pyridoxine (Vitamin B_6)

A deficiency of pyridoxine should be avoided because vitamin B_6 promotes endogenous production of oxalic acid (Smith, 1992). Pyridoxine increases the transamination of glyoxylate, an important precursor of oxalic acid, to glycine. Experimentally induced pyridoxine deficiency resulted in renal precipitation of calcium oxalate and hyperoxaluria in kittens (Bai et al, 1989). Commercial foods routinely fortified with vitamin supplements would not be deficient in pyridoxine or other vitamins. However, a homemade food might be deficient in pyridoxine if a multivitamin supplement is not added. Because the ability of supplemental pyridoxine (above nutritional requirements) to reduce urine oxalic acid excretion in dogs is unknown, there is insufficient evidence to recommend or abandon this practice. The minimum recommended allowance for pyridoxine in foods for healthy dogs is 1.5 mg/kg DM (NRC, 2006).

Vitamin D

Excessive levels of vitamin D (which promote intestinal absorption of calcium) in foods for patients at risk for calcium oxalate urolithiasis should be avoided. Commercial foods are typically replete with vitamin D and should not be further supplemented. Excessive supplementation of homemade foods with vitamin D could also pose a risk. For prevention of calcium oxalate urolithiasis, restrict vitamin D in foods to between 500 to 1,500 IU/kg DM. The recommended minimum allowance for foods for healthy adult dogs is 552 IU/kg DM (NRC, 2006).

FEEDING PLAN

Although struvite, urate and cystine uroliths dissolve when urine is no longer supersaturated with lithogenic substances, dissolution of calcium oxalate uroliths in dogs has not been

Table 40-7. Recommendations for the management of calcium oxalate urolithiasis in dogs.

1. Obtain data (postsurgical radiography, complete urinalysis, serum concentrations of calcium, urea nitrogen and creatinine) to evaluate effectiveness of renal function, calcium homeostasis, surgery, voiding urohydropropulsion or lithotripsy.
2. If the dog is hypercalcemic, correct underlying cause.
3. If the dog is normocalcemic, consider foods with reduced calcium, oxalate, sodium and protein that do not promote formation of acidic urine. Ideally foods should contain additional water and citrate and have adequate phosphorus and magnesium. Avoid excess and/or supplemental vitamins C and D. Prescription Diet u/d Canine or w/d Canine* is often recommended.
4. Reevaluate patient in two to four weeks to verify dietary compliance (urine specific gravity and pH and serum urea nitrogen concentration) and amelioration of crystalluria (urine sediment examination).
5. Consider additional potassium citrate if calcium oxalate crystals and aciduria persist.
6. Reevaluate patient in two to four weeks to verify dietary compliance (urine specific gravity and pH and serum urea nitrogen concentration) and amelioration of crystalluria (urine sediment examination). Consider vitamin B_6 supplementation (2 to 4 mg/kg body weight q24 to 48 hours) if calcium oxalate crystalluria persists.
7. Again, reevaluate patient in two to four weeks to verify dietary compliance and amelioration of crystalluria. Consider administration of hydrochlorothiazide (2 mg/kg body weight q24 to 48 hours) if calcium oxalate crystalluria persists. Adverse effects of hydrochlorothiazide administration include dehydration, hypokalemia and hypercalcemia.
8. After three to six months, reevaluate patient to verify dietary compliance and amelioration of crystalluria. Check for urolith recurrence by abdominal radiography. If no uroliths are present, continue current therapy and reevaluate in three to six months. If uroliths have recurred, consider voiding urohydropropulsion (Figure 38-5 and Table 38-7), or lithotripsy. If unsuccessful and clinical signs referable to urocystoliths are persistent, consider surgery. Continue therapy to minimize urolith growth if clinical signs are not present.

*Hill's Pet Nutrition, Inc., Topeka, KS, USA.

reported. Therefore, only physical methods are currently available for removing clinically active calcium oxalate uroliths. Surgery is the time-honored method to remove calcium oxalate uroliths from the urinary tract; however, complete surgical removal of all visible uroliths may be difficult because of their small size and irregular contour. Small urocystoliths may be aspirated through a transurethral catheter (Figure 38-6) (Lulich and Osborne, 1992) or removed by voiding urohydropropulsion (Figure 38-5 and Table 38-7) (Lulich et al, 1993). Extracorporeal lithotripsy also provides a nonsurgical means of treating some dogs with calcium oxalate nephroliths and/or ureteroliths (Adams and Senior, 1999). We have had success fragmenting calcium oxalate urocystoliths and urethroliths with intracorporeal laser lithotripsy.

In some patients, calcium oxalate uroliths are clinically silent, obviating the need for intervention. For patients in which intervention is not warranted, the status of uroliths should be periodically assessed by urinalyses, renal function tests and radiography or ultrasonography. (See Reassessment below.)

Dietary and medical dissolution of calcium oxalate uroliths in dogs has not been reported. However, there is a role for dietary management in prevention of calcium oxalate urolith recurrence. In general, dietary and medical therapy should be implemented in stepwise fashion, with the initial goal of reducing the urine concentration of lithogenic substances (**Table 40-7**). Medications that have the potential to induce unwanted, sustained, detrimental alterations in the composition of metabolites should be reserved for patients with active or frequently recurring calcium oxalate uroliths. Caution should be used to ensure that side effects of treatment are not more detrimental than the effects of uroliths. The cause of hypercalcemia (e.g., primary hyperparathyroidism) should be corrected in patients with hypercalcemia and resorptive hypercalciuria. An attempt should be made to identify risk factors for urolith formation in patients with normal serum calcium concentrations (**Table 40-2**). Amelioration or control of the consequences of risk factors (e.g., urine oversaturation with lithogenic minerals) should minimize urolith growth and recurrence.

The feeding plan includes assessing and selecting the best food and assessing and determining the feeding method.

Assess and Select the Food

Table 40-8 compares the recommended levels of key nutritional factors to the key nutritional factor content of selected commercial veterinary therapeutic foods for calcium oxalate urolith prevention. Select the food that most closely matches the recommended levels of key nutritional factors for preventing the recurrence of calcium oxalate uroliths. Because these foods are intended for long-term feeding, they should also be approved by the Association of American Feed Control Officials (AAFCO), or some other credible regulatory agency. Dogs consuming dry commercial foods may be at greater risk for urolithiasis than those consuming moist foods because dry foods are often associated with higher urine concentrations of calcium and oxalic acid and more concentrated urine. When possible, moist foods should be selected.

Dogs with calcium oxalate urolithiasis frequently consume human food. Calcium oxalate is the most common urolith type recognized in people living in developed countries. As people feed their dogs the same dietary proportions and ingredients they feed themselves, it is logical to assume that dogs would be exposed to the same nutritional risk factors for urolith formation (**Tables 40-2** and **40-3**). Therefore, feeding human foods with high levels of calcium and oxalic acid should be avoided.

In addition to consumption of human food, an association between calcium oxalate urolithiasis and consumption of commercially available treats has been noted. The high sodium content of some commercial dog treats may help explain this association because sodium consumption promotes hypercalciuria (Lulich et al, 1992). Like foods, treats should not contain more than 0.3% DM sodium and they should be limited to less than 10% of the total food regimen (volume or weight basis).

Feeding foods designed to dissolve struvite uroliths provides

Table 40-8. Levels of key nutritional factors in selected veterinary therapeutic foods used to minimize recurrence of calcium oxalate urolithiasis in dogs compared to recommended levels.*

Dry foods	Protein (%)	Calcium (%)**	Phosphorus (%)**	Sodium (%)	Magnesium (%)	Urinary pH***
Recommended levels	**10-18**	**0.4-0.7**	**0.3-0.6**	**<0.3**	**0.04-0.15**	**7.1-7.5**
Hill's Prescription Diet u/d Canine	11.2	0.34	0.15	0.23	0.046	7.70
Medi-Cal Urinary SO 13	16.7	1.0	0.6	1.3	0.2	5.5-6.0
Purina Veterinary Diets NF KidNey Function	15.9	0.76	0.29	0.22	0.07	6.7-7.5
Royal Canin Veterinary Diet Urinary SO 14	17.0	0.80	0.63	1.38	0.066	5.5-6.0
Moist foods	**Protein (%)**	**Calcium (%)****	**Phosphorus (%)****	**Sodium (%)**	**Magnesium (%)**	**Urinary pH*****
Recommended levels	**10-18**	**0.4-0.7**	**0.3-0.6**	**<0.3**	**0.04-0.15**	**7.1-7.5**
Hill's Prescription Diet u/d Canine	13.3	0.35	0.17	0.28	0.049	7.4
Medi-Cal Urinary SO	18.7	1.0	0.8	1.1	0.10	5.5-6.0
Purina Veterinary Diets NF KidNey Function	16.5	0.50	0.30	0.24	0.08	6.7-7.5
Royal Canin Veterinary Diet Urinary SO	18.5	0.97	0.86	1.45	0.059	5.5-6.0

*Manufacturers' published values. Nutrients expressed as % dry matter, unless otherwise stated; moist foods are best; avoid foods with added vitamin C (ascorbic acid); avoid foods with high oxalate ingredients (**Table 40-3**).
**Calcium-phosphorus ratio should be in the range of 1.1:1 to 2:1.
***Protocols for measuring urinary pH may vary.

some benefits, but also presents several risks to patients with calcium oxalate uroliths (**Table 40-2**). The lower protein content and potential to enhance formation of less concentrated urine promote reduction of calcium and oxalic acid concentrations in urine. Although formation of acidic urine is desirable for management of struvite uroliths, foods that promote acidic urine promote hypercalciuria and hypocitraturia. Therefore, consumption of struvite litholytic foods that result in formation of acidic urine enhances the risk of calcium oxalate urolithiasis in susceptible dogs. Likewise, aggressive reduction of dietary phosphorus may also promote hypercalciuria. If struvite uroliths occur in breeds of dogs commonly affected with calcium oxalate uroliths, patients should be evaluated for calcium oxalate crystalluria after initiating dietary therapy designed to prevent struvite urolith formation. If calcium oxalate crystalluria persists, alternate methods of preventing struvite uroliths should be considered.

Another criterion for selecting a food that may become increasingly important in the future is evidence-based clinical nutrition. Practitioners should know how to determine risks and benefits of nutritional regimens and counsel pet owners accordingly. Currently, veterinary medical education and continuing education are not always based on rigorous assessment of evidence for or against particular management options. Still, studies have been published to establish the nutritional benefits of certain pet foods. Chapter 2 describes evidence-based clinical nutrition in detail and applies its concepts to various veterinary therapeutic foods.

Assess and Determine the Feeding Method

Transitioning the patient from its current food to a calcium oxalate urolith preventive food should be done gradually over several days. Begin the transition by feeding 75% of the current food and 25% of the new food on Day 1. On Day 2 feed half of each food. On Day 3 feed 75% as the new food. By Day 4 or 5, feed only the new food.

Because moist foods are recommended to increase water intake and production of less concentrated urine, specific amounts (meal fed) should be fed two to three times per day rather than free-choice feeding. Moist foods can spoil if left uneaten at room temperature for several hours (Chapter 11). Opened containers of moist foods should be refrigerated and the feeding bowl should be kept clean.

Table 40-9. Expected changes associated with dietary and medical therapy to minimize recurrence of calcium oxalate uroliths.

Factors	Pre-therapy	Prevention therapy
Polyuria	±	Variable
Pollakiuria	0 to 4+	0
Hematuria	0 to 4+	0
Urine specific gravity	Variable	1.004-1.015
Urinary pH	<7.0	>7.0
Pyuria	0 to 4+	0
Calcium oxalate crystals	0 to 4+	0
Bacteriuria	0 to 4+	0
Bacterial culture of urine	0 to 4+	0
Urea nitrogen (mg/dl)	>15	<15
Urolith size and number	Small to large	0

Besides offering moist foods, several additional approaches may facilitate increased water intake. First, ensure multiple bowls are available in prominent locations in the dog's environment; this may mean providing several bowls outside in a large enclosure or a bowl on each level of the house. Second, bowls should be clean and always be filled with fresh water. Third, small amounts of flavoring substances (e.g., salt-free bouillon) can be added to water sources. Fourth, ice cubes can be offered. Fifth, if a dry food is selected, add liberal quantities of water; however, as with moist foods, be aware that potential food safety issues might arise if moistened dry foods are left uneaten for prolonged intervals at room temperature (Chapter 11).

If the patient has a normal body condition score (2.5/5 to 3.5/5), the amount of the previous food being fed was probably appropriate. On an energy basis, a similar amount of the new food would be a good starting place.

Table 40-10. Managing highly recurrent calcium oxalate uroliths.

Causes	Identification	Therapeutic goal
Client and patient causes		
Inadequate dietary compliance	Question owner Persistent calcium oxalate crystalluria Urea nitrogen >10-15 mg/dl Urine specific gravity >1.010-1.020 Urinary pH <7.0-7.5 during treatment with Prescription Diet u/d Canine* (use lower values for the canned food)	Emphasize need to feed dissolution food exclusively
Administration of vitamin-mineral supplements	Question owner	Discontinue vitamin-mineral supplements containing calcium and vitamins C and D
Clinician factors		
Incomplete surgical removal of uroliths	Postsurgical radiography revealing uroliths Persistence of clinical signs after cystotomy or recurrence of clinical signs soon after cystotomy (within one to three months)	Uroliths not causing clinical signs should be monitored for potentially adverse consequences (obstruction, urinary tract infection, etc.) Clinically active uroliths may require surgical removal Remove small uroliths by voiding urohydropropulsion or lithotripsy
Inappropriate food choice	Persistent calcium oxalate crystalluria	Choose foods with reduced levels of calcium, oxalic acid, protein and sodium that do not promote formation of acidic urine Consider adding potassium citrate if aciduria persists
Inadequate monitoring	Postsurgical radiography to verify complete urolith removal was not performed Urinalysis or urine sediment examinations were not performed within three to six months of initiation of therapy	Perform postsurgical radiography to evaluate success of surgery Perform complete urinalysis within one to three months of initiation of therapy Once stable, urinalysis should be performed every four to six months Perform survey lateral abdominal radiography every four to six months to assess recurrence
Corticosteroid administration	Corticosteroids were prescribed to manage other disease conditions	If possible, discontinue corticosteroid administration
Disease factors		
Hypercalcemia	Elevated serum calcium concentration	Identify and, if possible, eliminate underlying cause for hypercalcemia (hyperparathyroidism, neoplasia, hypervitaminosis D, etc.)
Recurrence of uroliths despite appropriate management	Lateral radiograph of abdomen	Uroliths not causing clinical signs should be monitored for potentially adverse consequences (obstruction, urinary tract infection, etc.) Clinically active uroliths may require surgical removal Remove small uroliths by voiding urohydropropulsion or lithotripsy

*Hill's Pet Nutrition, Inc., Topeka, KS, USA.

ADJUNCTIVE MEDICAL MANAGEMENT

Citric Acid

Citric acid forms soluble salts with calcium thereby minimizing calcium oxalate crystal formation (Nicar et al, 1987). Citric acid is also beneficial because it is metabolized to bicarbonate and promotes formation of alkaline urine (Baruch et al, 1975). In dogs, chronic metabolic acidosis inhibits renal tubular reabsorption of calcium, whereas metabolic alkalosis enhances tubular reabsorption of calcium (Sutton et al, 1979). Potassium citrate is preferred to sodium bicarbonate as an alkalinizing agent because oral administration of sodium enhances urine calcium excretion. If persistent aciduria or hypocitraturia is recognized (mean urine citrate excretion of 33 normal beagles was 2.57 ± 2.31 mg/kg body weight/day), therapy with wax matrix tablets of potassium citrate (Urocit-K) should be considered. Alternatively, a liquid product (Polycitra-K) may be given to small dogs. Chewable treats containing potassium citrate (K-CIT-V) are also available. An initial dose of 40 to 75 mg/kg body weight q12h is recommended. The final dose should be based on patient response. Potassium citrate should be administered with meals to reduce gastric irritation. When feeding foods with adequate quantities of potassium citrate, additional supplementation is often not needed.

Thiazide Diuretics

Thiazide diuretics have been recommended to reduce recurrence of calcium-containing uroliths in people because of their

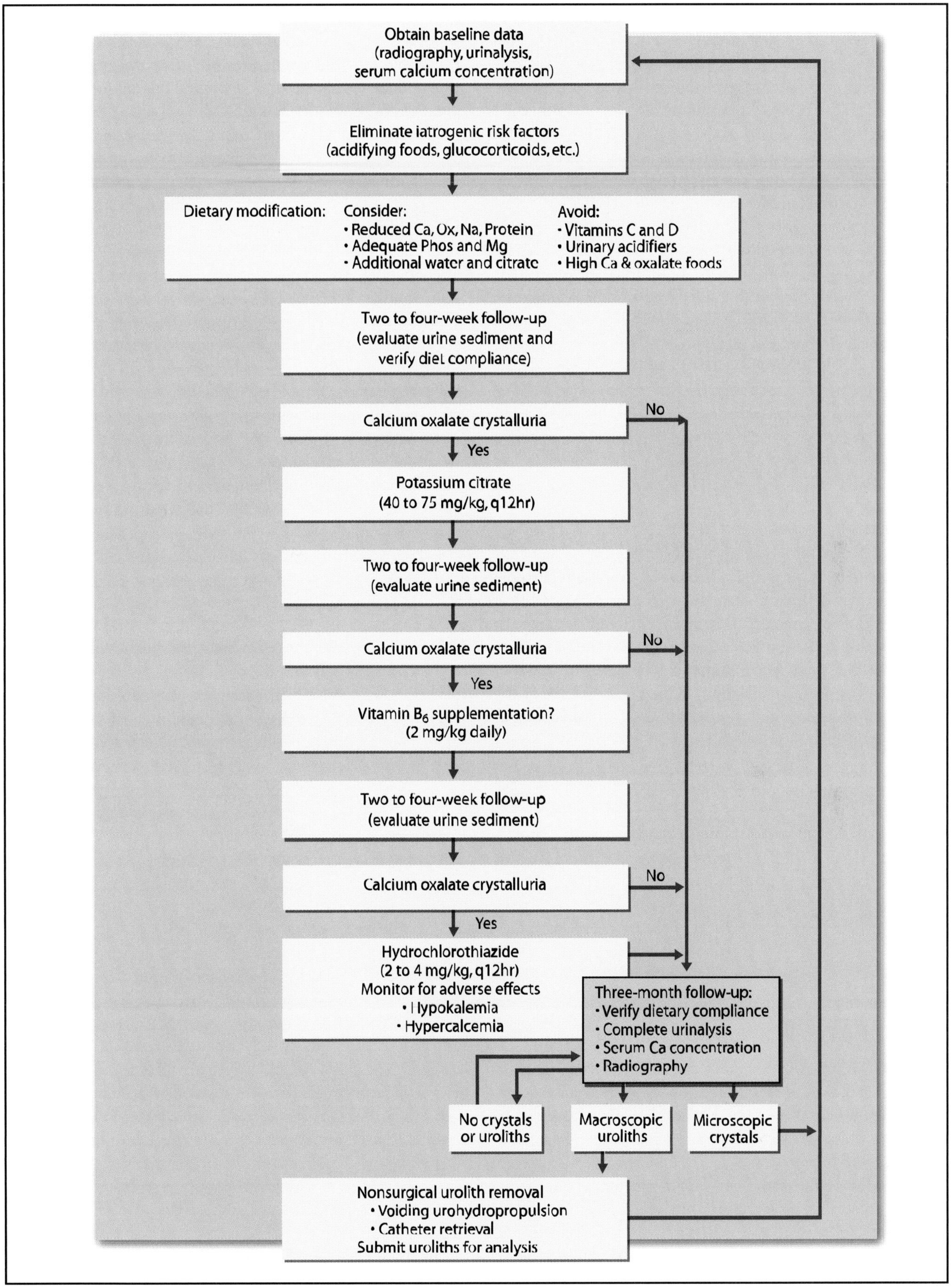

Figure 40-2. Algorithm for dietary and medical management of calcium oxalate uroliths in dogs.

ability to reduce urine calcium excretion (Churchill and Taylor, 1985). However, they should only be considered for patients with severe hypercalciuria. A beneficial reduction in urine calcium excretion in dogs with calcium oxalate urolithiasis has been observed following administration of hydrochlorothiazide (2 to 4 mg/kg body weight q12h) for two weeks. However, a reduction in urine calcium excretion was not detected following hydrochlorothiazide administration (20 to 65 mg/kg body weight q12h) to clinically healthy beagles (Lulich, 1991b). Results of a short-term study of the effects of hydrochlorothiazide on calcium excretion in the urine of adult dogs with naturally occurring calcium oxalate urolithiasis revealed that hydrochlorothiazide significantly reduced urine calcium concentration (Lulich et al, 2001). The greatest reduction in urine calcium concentration and excretion was achieved when dogs received hydrochlorothiazide and a urolith prevention diet. Thiazide diuretic administration is not recommended as first-line therapy at this time. The decision to use thiazides should be accompanied by owner informed consent and appropriate clinical and laboratory monitoring for early detection of adverse effects (dehydration, hypokalemia, hypercalcemia).

Allopurinol

Some people who form calcium oxalate uroliths associated with marked hyperuricosuria have benefited from allopurinol-induced reductions in the magnitude of hyperuricosuria. We are unaware of any counterpart of this phenomenon in dogs. In context of this discussion, it is relevant that the end product of purine metabolism in people is uric acid. However in dogs, the end product of purine metabolism is the highly soluble allantoin. Therefore, we do not recommend that allopurinol be considered for dogs that form calcium oxalate uroliths.

REASSESSMENT

The goal of therapy is to minimize calcium oxalate urolith recurrence (**Figure 40-2**). However, this expectation may be unrealistic because the primary causes responsible for urolith formation are multifactorial and incompletely understood. With the information and techniques currently available, however, veterinarians can minimize urolith recurrence and prevent the need for additional surgical removal of uroliths by appropriate monitoring and intervention.

Therapy should be initiated in a stepwise fashion (**Table 40-7**). If therapy is effective and clients remain compliant, dietary and pharmacologic management should result in formation of less concentrated urine without calcium oxalate crystalluria (**Table 40-9**). Strive to achieve urine specific gravity values less than 1.020. After this is achieved, a urinalysis and survey lateral abdominal radiographs should be performed every two to four months. Dietary and pharmacologic changes should be considered if crystalluria or concentrated urine persist (**Table 40-10**). These recommendations should facilitate detection of recurrent urocystoliths by radiography when they are small enough to remove by voiding urohydropropulsion (Figure 38-5 and Table 38-7). Likewise, urethroliths may be fragmented by intracorporeal laser lithotripsy. Nephroliths may be fragmented by extracorporeal shockwave lithotripsy. After the frequency of urolith recurrence has been established, the frequency of evaluation can be modified such that predicted recurrences can be diagnosed and managed accordingly.

ENDNOTES

a. Prescription Diet k/d Canine. Hill's Pet Nutrition, Inc., Topeka, KS, USA.
b. Urocit-K. Mission Pharmacal, San Antonio, TX, USA.
c. Polycitra-K. Willen Drug Co., Baltimore, MD, USA.
d. K-CIT-V. V.E.T. Pharmaceuticals, Inc., Fenton, MO, USA.

REFERENCES

The references for **Chapter 40** can be found at www.markmorris.org.

CASE 40-1

Urine Dribbling in a Yorkshire Terrier

Jody P. Lulich, DVM, PhD, Dipl. ACVIM (Internal Medicine)

Carl A. Osborne, DVM, PhD, Dipl. ACVIM (Internal Medicine)
College of Veterinary Medicine
University of Minnesota
St. Paul, Minnesota, USA

Patient Assessment

A nine-year-old, neutered male Yorkshire terrier was examined for urine dribbling and depression of two days' duration. Physical examination revealed that the dog was 8 to 10% dehydrated; capillary refill time was slightly delayed. The dog voided small spurts of reddish-brown urine onto the examination table when its abdomen was palpated. The physical examination was otherwise normal. Body weight was 5 kg; the dog had a normal body condition score (3/5). Survey radiographs revealed a large urinary bladder and a radiodense urolith in the urethra at the proximal end of the os penis and several uroliths in the urinary bladder (**Figure 1**).

The diagnosis was urolithiasis of the lower urinary tract associated with urethral obstruction. The depression was probably a consequence of postrenal azotemia.

Assess the Food and Feeding Method

The dog was fed a commercial moist adult maintenance food twice daily and various table foods.

Questions

1. What additional assessments should be performed?
2. What should be the patient's initial treatment plan?

Answers and Discussion

1. A blood sample should be submitted for biochemical analysis to evaluate the degree of azotemia and detect concurrent electrolyte abnormalities. A urinalysis and aerobic bacterial culture of the urine will help predict the mineral composition of the uroliths.
2. Replacement of the patient's fluid deficits with an appropriate fluid given intravenously is important. The urinary bladder can be evacuated by decompressive cystocentesis to enhance renal elimination of waste products. Reducing pressure in the urinary bladder also would facilitate retrograde urohydropropulsion of the urethrolith.

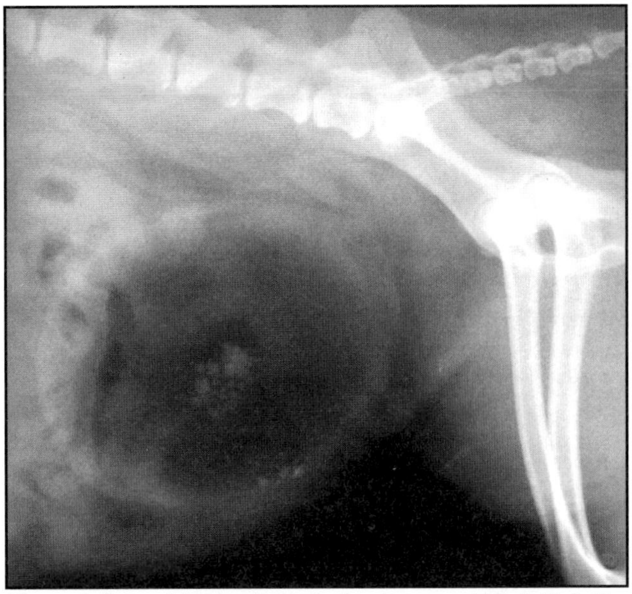

Figure 1. Survey lateral radiograph of a nine-year-old male Yorkshire terrier revealing multiple radiodense uroliths in the urinary bladder and a radiodense urolith at the proximal end of the os penis.

Further Assessment

Results of laboratory tests revealed azotemia, hyperphosphatemia and hypobicarbonatemia (**Table 1**). Serum alkaline phosphatase activity was also increased. Crystals were not observed by urine sediment examination and the urine culture was negative (**Table 2**). The urethrolith was successfully flushed into the urinary bladder by retrograde urohydropropulsion. Prophylactic antimicrobials were administered (amoxicillin-clavulanic acid, 14 mg/kg, q12h) to prevent iatrogenic bacterial urinary tract infection associated with transurethral catheterization.

Table 1. Serum biochemistry values of a nine-year-old male Yorkshire terrier with radiodense urocystoliths.*

Factors	Reference values	Day 1	Day 2	Day 3
SUN (mg/dl)	7-28	186	141	16
Creatinine (mg/dl)	0.5-1.5	6.5	1.2	0.9
Calcium (mg/dl)	9.3-11.4	8.7	8.2	8.7
Phosphorus (mg/dl)	1.9-7.0	19.2	3.5	3.2
Sodium (mEq/l)	143-150	144	149	149
Potassium (mEq/l)	3.2-5.6	4.7	3.6	3.3
ALT activity (U/l)	5-62	78	ND	ND
Alk phos activity (U/l)	10-149	223	ND	ND
Total CO_2 (mEq/l)	17-26	14.5	ND	ND

Key: SUN = serum urea nitrogen, ALT = alanine aminotransferase, Alk phos = alkaline phosphatase, ND = not done.
*Dietary therapy was initiated on Day 14.

Additional Question

What is the most likely mineral composition of these radiodense uroliths?

Answer and Discussion

The advantages and disadvantages of medical urolith dissolution and surgical urolith removal can be more accurately assessed by predicting the mineral composition of uroliths. Magnesium ammonium phosphate (struvite), calcium oxalate, calcium phosphate, silica and cystine uroliths can all be radiodense (**Table 3**). It was surmised that this patient's uroliths were probably not composed of magnesium ammonium phosphate because of the breed and gender of the dog along with findings of aciduria and a negative bacterial culture. These findings suggested that the uroliths were not composed of struvite and therefore were not amenable to medical dissolution.

Treatment and Further Assessment

The uroliths were surgically removed following resolution of azotemia on the third day of hospitalization (**Table 1**). Postsurgical radiographs verified that all uroliths were removed. Quantitative analysis revealed that the uroliths were composed of 100% calcium oxalate monohydrate.

Further Questions

1. Outline an appropriate feeding plan (food and feeding method) for this dog.

Table 2. Urinalyses of a nine-year-old male Yorkshire terrier with radiodense urocystoliths.*

Factors**	Day 1	Day 14***	Day 28	Day 60
Specific gravity	1.015	1.025	1.008	1.015
pH	6.0	6.5	7.5	7.5
Protein†	1+	1+	Trace	Trace
RBC††	100-150	8-12	0	1-3
WBC††	12-16	2-4	1-2	0
Crystals†††	None	None	None	None
Aerobic bacterial culture	Neg	Neg	Neg	Neg

Key: RBC = red blood cells, WBC = white blood cells, Neg = negative.
*Samples collected by cystocentesis.
**Glucose, bilirubin and acetone were not detected in any specimen.
***Dietary therapy was initiated on Day 14.
†Values represent semiquantitative evaluations based on a scale of 0 to 4; urine volume was not considered.
††Per high power field (x450).
†††Per low power field (x100).

Table 3. The advantages and disadvantages of medical urolith dissolution and surgical urolith removal can be accurately assessed after the mineral composition of the urolith is known or predicted. This table lists factors used to predict mineral composition of radiodense uroliths when no uroliths are available for quantitative analysis vs. clinical findings in the patient described in this case.*

Factors	MAP	CaOx	CaP	Silica	Cystine
Typical urinary pH	No	Yes	Possible	Yes	Yes
Typical crystalluria	Possible	Possible	Possible	Possible	Possible
Typical urine culture	No	Yes	Yes	Yes	Yes
Typical radiographic density	Yes	Yes	Yes	Yes	Yes
Typical radiographic contour	Yes	Yes	Yes	No	No
Typical serum biochemistry values	Yes	Yes	Possible	Yes	Yes
Typical breed	No	Yes	Yes	No	No
Typical gender	No	Yes	Yes	Yes	Yes
Typical age	No	Yes	Yes	Yes	No

Key: MAP = magnesium ammonium phosphate, CaOx = calcium oxalate, CaP = calcium phosphate.
*Characteristics of urate uroliths were not considered because they are typically radiolucent.

2. Is reassessment important for this patient?

Answers and Discussion

1. Dietary therapy to prevent urolith recurrence was initiated at the time of suture removal. Dietary recommendations included reducing calcium, oxalic acid, protein and sodium, providing additional water and citrate and maintaining adequate phosphorus and magnesium. A moist veterinary therapeutic food (Prescription Diet u/d Canine[a]) was chosen because its nutrient content matches this nutrient profile. This food avoids excess dietary protein, oxalic acid and calcium, and promotes formation of less concentrated, alkaline urine. These dietary characteristics are helpful in preventing recurrence of calcium oxalate uroliths. The food was offered in two separate meals each day (one-fourth can twice daily, total 375 kcal [1.57 MJ]). The owners were also instructed to avoid feeding the dog any human foods, commercial dog treats and vitamin-mineral supplements (especially those containing vitamins C and D and calcium).
2. Regular reassessment is important because calcium oxalate uroliths commonly recur. Results of a retrospective study on the recurrence rate of calcium oxalate uroliths in dogs indicated that the rate of recurrence increased with the length of time that dogs were evaluated: 3% recurred after three months, 9% after six months, 35% after one year, 42% after two years and 48% after three years. This dog should be examined (i.e., urinalysis, survey abdominal radiography) at regular intervals to evaluate efficacy of medical therapy and to detect uroliths while they are small enough to remove with nonsurgical techniques. This patient should also be evaluated for hyperadrenocorticism because of the increased serum alkaline phosphatase activity. Glucocorticoid administration and hyperadrenocorticism are associated with hypercalciuria and increase the risk for calcium oxalate urolith formation.

Progress Notes

Table 2 summarizes the urinalysis results following six weeks of dietary management. Prescription Diet u/d Canine was successful in promoting less concentrated, alkaline urine in this dog. Reassessment every three to six months was recommended to the owner.

Endnote

a. Hill's Pet Nutrition Inc., Topeka, KS, USA.

Bibliography

Osborne CA, Lulich JP, Bartges JW, et al. Canine and feline urolithiasis: Relationship of etiopathogenesis to treatment and prevention. In: Osborne CA, Finco DR, eds. Canine and Feline Nephrology and Urology. Baltimore, MD: Williams & Wilkins, 1995; 798-888.

Chapter 41

Canine Calcium Phosphate Urolithiasis: Causes, Detection and Prevention

Carl A. Osborne
Jody P. Lulich
John M. Kruger
Amy Cokley

"If misinterpreted observations are accepted as facts, the result may be misdiagnosis leading to ineffective or even contraindicated treatment."
Carl A. Osborne

PREVALENCE AND MINERAL COMPOSITION

Uroliths composed predominantly of calcium phosphate have been infrequently identified in dogs and cats. However, calcium phosphate is commonly found as a minor component in naturally occurring struvite and calcium oxalate uroliths. Occasionally a shell of calcium phosphate will form around a urolith composed primarily of struvite.

At least four mineral types have been identified in calcium phosphate uroliths **(Table 41-1)**. The most common form identified in calcium phosphate uroliths from dogs and cats is hydroxyapatite, followed by brushite. Calcium carbonate uncommonly exists as a pure compound in canine and feline uroliths. Calcium carbonate often occurs in equine, rabbit, guinea pig and caprine uroliths (Osborne et al, 1989). In the presence of conditions associated with urinary tract infections (UTIs) caused by urease-positive bacteria, carbonate radicals may be generated that associate with the complex apatite structure to form a carbonate apatite lattice (Osborne et al, 1985). Uncommonly identified crystalline forms of calcium phosphate in uroliths include whitlockite and octacalcium phosphate.

More than one crystalline form of calcium phosphate may be present in a single urolith. In alkaline urine, brushite is readily transformed to apatite; it is possible that some apatite identified in uroliths originated from brushite (Pak et al, 1971). In addition, mixtures of calcium phosphate and calcium oxalate often occur. With the exception of brushite, canine calcium phosphate uroliths do not appear to have a characteristic shape.

Calcium phosphate accounted for 0.51% (1,801) of all (350,803) canine uroliths submitted to the Minnesota Urolith Center from 1981 to 2007 (Table 38-8), and 0.67% (273 of 40,612) of the uroliths submitted in the year 2007. Calcium phosphate accounted for 1.6% of canine upper tract uroliths analyzed at the Minnesota Urolith Center from 2000 to 2006 (Table 38-9). Calcium phosphate accounted for 2.8% of uroliths retrieved from dogs less than 12 months old. Of 1,801 canine

Table 41-1. Common characteristics of canine calcium phosphate uroliths.

Variations in mineral composition
Calcium apatite only
Brushite only
Calcium apatite mixed with calcium oxalate
Brushite mixed with calcium oxalate
In dogs, the carbonate apatite form of calcium phosphate is most commonly detected as a minor component of infection-induced struvite
Physical characteristics
Color: Calcium phosphate uroliths are usually cream or tan. Blood clots mineralized with calcium phosphate are typically black.
Shape: Variable. With the exception of brushite, calcium phosphate uroliths do not have a characteristic shape. The external surface of brushite uroliths is typically round and smooth.
Nuclei: Brushite uroliths are often laminated.
Density: Generally dense and brittle, sometimes chalk-like. Mineralized blood clots may be softer. All forms of calcium phosphate are radiodense compared to soft tissue.
Number: Single or multiple
Location: Kidneys, ureters, urinary bladder (most common) and/or urethra
Size: Variable, with smaller sizes more common
Prevalence
Approximately 0.5% of all canine uroliths. Approximately 1.6% of canine upper tract uroliths.
Characteristics of affected canine patients
No gender prevalence for calcium apatite. Brushite is more common in males. Mean age at diagnosis is seven years (range <1 to >16 years).

hydroxyapatite and carbonate apatite uroliths, 473 were composed entirely (100%) of calcium phosphate, and 694 were composed of at least 70% of these minerals. Of 693 canine brushite uroliths, 233 were composed entirely (100%) of calcium phosphate, and 460 were composed of at least 70% of this mineral. The mean age of dogs at the time of urolith retrieval was approximately nine years (range one month to 19 years). Calcium phosphate accounted for less than 2.3% of calcium phosphate uroliths formed by dogs less than 12 months old. Males were affected (57%) more commonly than females (43%). Forty different breeds were affected including cocker spaniels (10%), mixed breeds (20%), miniature schnauzers (10%), Yorkshire terriers (7%), Shih Tzus (6%) and springer spaniels (5%). Hydroxyapatite uroliths were more commonly removed from the lower urinary tract (81%) than the upper urinary tract (8%). The location of 11% of the hydroxyapatite uroliths was not specified.

ETIOPATHOGENESIS AND RISK FACTORS

Solubility of Calcium Phosphates in Urine

Overview

The solubility of calcium phosphates in urine depends on: 1) urinary pH, 2) urine calcium ion concentration, 3) total urine inorganic phosphate concentration, 4) urine concentration of inhibitors of calcium crystallization and 5) urine concentration of potentiators of crystallization. Factors that decrease calcium phosphate solubility predispose patients to urolith formation.

Urinary pH

Urinary pH has a profound effect on the solubility of some forms of calcium phosphate (Elliot, 1957). With the exception of brushite, calcium phosphate solubility markedly decreases in alkaline urine and increases in acidic urine. Increased urinary pH increases the availability of ionic PO_4^{3-} and HPO_4^{2-}, which are available for incorporation into calcium phosphates (Asplin et al, 1996). Apatite will not crystallize from human urine unless the pH is 6.6 or greater (Elliot, 1968). Approximately 400 mg of calcium phosphate/l can be held in solution at a pH of 5.5, whereas only 32 mg of calcium phosphate/l will be held in solution at a pH of 7.8 (Elliot, 1965). Therefore, people with disorders associated with persistent elevation of urinary pH (e.g., distal renal tubular acidosis [RTA]) are predisposed to calcium phosphate urolith formation. In contrast to carbonate apatite and hydroxyapatite, the solubility of brushite decreases in acidic urine.

Hypercalciuria

Hypercalciuria decreases calcium phosphate solubility and may result in oversaturation with calcium phosphate (Pak, 1978). Hypercalciuria may result from: 1) excessive resorption of calcium from bone, 2) enhanced intestinal absorption of calcium, 3) impaired renal tubular reabsorption of calcium and/or 4) combinations of these factors. Urine specimens obtained from human patients with hypercalciuria and calcium uroliths are usually supersaturated with brushite.

Controversy exists as to the relative importance of urinary pH and hypercalciuria as determinants of calcium phosphate solubility in vivo. Some investigators believe that calcium phosphate crystallization is primarily governed by changes in urinary pH; they minimize the importance of hypercalciuria (Elliot, 1968). However, other investigators suggest that persistent hypercalciuria tends to increase the calcium phosphate saturation of urine so that small increases in urinary pH will result in calcium phosphate crystalluria. Apparently, there have been no studies reported on the relative effect of hypercalciuria and urinary pH on the solubility of different types of calcium phosphate in canine urine.

Crystallization Inhibitors

Normally, urine contains calcium phosphate crystal inhibitors. One mechanism by which inhibitors prevent urolith formation is by chelating urolith constituents, making them unavailable for nidus formation or crystal growth. In addition, crystallization inhibitors may alter crystalline structure in such a way that crystal growth and aggregation are prevented. Inhibitors of calcium phosphate crystallization include inorganic pyrophosphates, citric acid ions, magnesium ions and nephrocalcin (Bisaz et al, 1978; Ito and Coe, 1977). In healthy human urine, these inhibitors provide 70 to 80% of the inhibitory capacity to calcium phosphate crystallization (Asplin et al, 1996). As yet unidentified low-molecular-weight inhibitors provide the remaining 20 to 30%.

Pyrophosphates increase the upper limit of urine calcium phosphate saturation at which spontaneous precipitation occurs. Pyrophosphates also retard growth of hydroxyapatite crystals by adsorbing to their surfaces and blocking active growth sites. In addition, pyrophosphates inhibit transformation of amorphous calcium phosphate into a crystalline form (Fleisch, 1978). Citrate forms soluble complexes with calcium, thereby decreasing the availability of calcium for incorporation into crystals. Magnesium may replace calcium on the surface of growing crystals and thus block epitaxial growth.

Crystallization Promoters

Formation of calcium phosphate uroliths may be promoted by epitaxy. Epitaxy is the process by which crystals of one salt induce the formation of crystals of another salt. Epitaxic induction occurs between crystals having similar lattice dimensions. Calcium phosphate precipitation has been reported to be stimulated by calcium oxalate and monosodium urate crystals (Fleisch, 1978).

Disorders Associated with Formation of Calcium Phosphate Uroliths

Overview

Calcium phosphate uroliths may occur in patients with: 1) primary hyperparathyroidism, 2) other hypercalcemic disorders, 3) distal RTA and 4) idiopathic hypercalciuria (**Table 41-2**) (Asplin et al, 1996; Curhan et al, 1997; Menon et al, 1998). Because the prevalence of calcium phosphate uroliths in dogs is low, and because appropriate metabolic studies have rarely been performed in affected cases, the association of calcium phosphate uroliths with other canine metabolic disorders has not been as well established.

Primary Hyperparathyroidism

Between 18 to 20% of human patients with primary hyperparathyroidism have uroliths at the time of diagnosis (Nikkila et al, 1989). In one series of 72 dogs with primary hyperparathyroidism, 22 (31%) had uroliths (Feldman and Nelson, 1996). Uroliths from patients with primary hyperparathyroidism are typically composed of calcium phosphate, calcium oxalate or a mixture of the two. Uroliths composed predominantly of calcium phosphate are more commonly identified in people and dogs with primary hyperparathyroidism; uroliths composed primarily of calcium oxalate are more commonly identified in people and dogs with normocalcemic hypercalciuria (Klausner and Osborne, 1986). Bladder uroliths composed primarily of calcium phosphate have been experimentally induced in dogs following injections of parathyroid hormone (PTH) (Leberman, 1940).

Factors that predispose patients with primary hyperparathyroidism to calcium phosphate urolith formation include: hypercalciuria, increased urinary pH and increased renal excretion of metabolites that promote spontaneous precipitation of calcium salts (**Table 41-3**). Hypercalcemia results from PTH-induced bone resorption and renal tubular reabsorption of calcium. In addition, increased intestinal absorption of calcium results from PTH-stimulated conversion of 25-hydroxycholecalciferol to 1,25-dihydroxycholecalciferol (1,25-vitamin D) (Pak, 1978).

Table 41-2. Comparison of disorders that may predispose dogs, people and cats to formation of calcium phosphate uroliths.

Disorders	Dogs	People	Cats
Primary hyperparathyroidism*	Yes	Yes	NR
Other hypercalcemic disorders			
Hypercalcemia of malignancy**	–	Yes	NR
Vitamin D intoxication**	NR	Yes	NR
Excessive calcium consumption**	NR	Yes	NR
Thyrotoxicosis**	NR	Yes	NR
Hyperadrenocorticism***	Yes	Yes	NR
Granulomatous disease**	NR	Yes	NR
Immobilization**	NR	Yes	NR
Distal renal tubular acidosis†	NR	Yes	NR
Normocalcemic hypercalciuria			
Intestinal hyperabsorption**	NR	Yes	NR
Renal leak	Yes	Yes	NR

Key: NR = not reported.
*Adapted from Broadus A. Nephrolithiasis in primary hyperparathyroidism. In: Coe F, Brenner B, Stein J, eds. Nephrolithiasis. New York, NY: Churchill Livingstone, 1980; 59. Goulden BE, MacKenzie CP. Suspected primary hyperparathyroidism in the dog. New Zealand Veterinary Journal 1968; 16: 13. Klausner JS, Osborne CA. Canine calcium phosphate uroliths. Veterinary Clinics of North America: Small Animal Practice 1986; 16: 171. Krook L. Spontaneous hyperparathyroidism in the dog. A pathological-anatomical study. Acta Pathology and Microbiology Scandinavia 1957; Suppl. 122: 27.
**Adapted from Menon M, Bhalchondra GP, Drach GW. Urinary lithiasis: Etiology, diagnosis, and medical management. In: Walsh PC, Retik AB, Vaughan ED, et al, eds. Campbell's Urology, 7th ed. Philadelphia, PA: WB Saunders Co, 1998; 2661.
***Adapted from Hess RS, Kass PH, Ward CR. Association between hyperadrenocorticism and development of calcium-containing uroliths in dogs with urolithiasis. Journal of the American Veterinary Medical Association 1998; 212: 1889. Menon M, Bhalchondra GP, Drach GW. Urinary lithiasis: Etiology, diagnosis, and medical management. In: Walsh PC, Retik AB, Vaughan ED, et al, eds. Campbell's Urology, 7th ed. Philadelphia, PA: WB Saunders Co, 1998; 2661.
†Adapted from Caruana RJ, Buckalew VM. The syndrome of distal (type 1) renal tubular acidosis: Clinical and laboratory findings in 58 cases. Medicine 1988; 67: 84.

Hypercalcemia results in increased glomerular filtration of calcium and hypercalciuria, which in turn enhances the likelihood of urolith formation by increasing urine saturation with brushite and calcium oxalate (Pak, 1978). The urine of most hypercalciuric people with primary hyperparathyroidism is supersaturated with brushite and calcium oxalate. Hypercalciuria and hyperphosphaturia have been documented to occur in dogs with primary hyperparathyroidism and calcium uroliths (Klausner and Osborne, 1986; Klausner et al, 1987).

Persistent elevation in urinary pH may predispose some patients with primary hyperparathyroidism to calcium phosphate urolithiasis. Urinary pH is elevated in these patients because of impaired renal tubular reabsorption of bicarbonate (Broadus, 1980). This abnormality may explain, at least in part, the increased occurrence of calcium phosphate uroliths in patients with primary hyperparathyroidism compared with patients with other hypercalciuric diseases.

It has been suggested that some human patients with pri-

Table 41-3. Some potential risk factors for canine calcium phosphate uroliths.

Food	Urine	Metabolic	Drugs
Alkalinizing potential	Alkaline pH	Hypercalcemia	Urine alkalinizing drugs
High calcium content	Hypercalciuria	Distal renal tubular acidosis	Furosemide
High sodium content	High phosphate ion concentration		Glucocorticoids
High phosphorus content?	Increased concentration of promoters		Sodium chloride
Low-moisture content	Decreased concentration of inhibitors		Vitamin D
Excessive vitamin D content	Hypocitraturia		
High protein content	Hypomagnesuria		
Low magnesium content	Blood clots in renal pelvis or bladder lumen		
	Urine concentration		
	Urine retention		

Table 41-4. Diagnostic characteristics of disorders that predispose to calcium phosphate uroliths.

Test	Absorptive hypercalciuria	Renal-leak hypercalciuria	Primary hyperparathyroidism	Distal renal tubular acidosis
Serum				
Calcium concentration	Normal	Normal	Increased	Normal to decreased
PO_4 concentration	Normal to decreased	Normal	Normal to decreased	Normal to decreased
HCO_3 concentration	Normal	Increased	Normal to decreased	Decreased
PTH concentration	Normal to decreased	Increased	Normal to increased	Normal to increased
1,25-vitamin D concentration	Variable	Increased	Increased	Normal
Urine				
Fasting 24-hour calcium excretion	Normal	Increased	Increased	Normal to increased
Fed 24-hour calcium excretion?	Increased	Increased	Increased	Normal to increased
pH	Variable	Variable	Variable	>6.0

Key: PTH = parathyroid hormone.

mary hyperparathyroidism excrete a substance in their urine that facilitates calcium phosphate and calcium oxalate precipitation (Pak, 1978). The specific nature of this urolithiasis-promoting factor has not been determined.

Other Hypercalcemic Disorders

In addition to primary hyperparathyroidism, other hypercalcemic disorders may predispose patients to formation of calcium phosphate uroliths. Uroliths have been identified in human patients with hypervitaminosis D, neoplastic disorders, Cushing's syndrome and in some patients who are immobilized for long periods (**Table 41-2**) (Menon et al, 1998). Although calcium phosphate is the most frequently identified mineral in uroliths obtained from these patients, calcium oxalate may also be present. Because the frequency of occurrence of uroliths in patients with these hypercalcemic disorders is low, it is likely that factors in addition to hypercalcemia are involved.

Distal Renal Tubular Acidosis

Nephrolithiasis is a common manifestation of hereditary, acquired and idiopathic forms of RTA (Type I) in people (Caruana and Buckalew, 1988). Uroliths are typically composed entirely of calcium phosphate, calcium oxalate and struvite (Backman et al, 1980). Urolith formation has also been observed occasionally in patients with proximal RTA (Type II) (Menon et al, 1998). To the best of our knowledge, struvite uroliths are the only urolith type observed in canine patients with RTA (Bovee et al, 1979; Polzin et al, 1986).

Distal RTA results from functional inability of the distal nephron to establish a hydrogen ion gradient between blood and tubular fluid, regardless of the severity of acidemia. The disorder in people is characterized by the inability to decrease urinary pH below 5.4, hypokalemia, hyperchloremia, hypophosphatemia, hypocalcemia, metabolic acidosis, osteomalacia, nephrocalcinosis and urolithiasis (Caruana and Buckalew, 1988; Menon et al, 1998).

Hypercalciuria, alkaline urine, low urine citrate concentration and excessive urine phosphate excretion contribute to formation of calcium phosphate uroliths observed in patients with distal RTA (**Table 41-4**) (Caruana and Buckalew, 1988; Menon et al, 1998). Hypercalciuria and hyperphosphaturia tend to increase urine saturation with calcium phosphate. Acidosis increases calcium mobilization from bone, causing an increase in the quantity of calcium excreted in urine (Klausner and Osborne, 1986). In addition, acidosis decreases renal tubular reabsorption of calcium, further increasing calcium excretion. Acidosis may alter renal tubular calcium transport, the response of the tubules to PTH or both.

Elevated urinary pH increases the availability of PO_4^{3-} and HPO_4^{2-}, which may be incorporated into ionic octacalcium phosphate and brushite, respectively (Asplin et al, 1996). Increased urinary pH is considered more important than hypercalciuria in predisposing patients with distal RTA to calcium phosphate urolith formation (Asplin et al, 1996).

Patients with distal RTA consistently excrete decreased amounts of citrate in their urine (Caruana and Buckalew, 1988). Hypocitratemia in patients with distal RTA has been attributed to: 1) increased proximal tubule reabsorption of citrate as a consequence of intracellular acidosis, 2) a primary defect in tubular function and 3) the effects of hypokalemia (Caruana and Buckalew, 1988). Because citrate is a major chelator of calcium, hypocitraturia decreases calcium solubility and may represent an important risk factor in the pathogenesis of calcium phosphate and calcium oxalate uroliths associated with RTA (Menon et al, 1998).

In human patients, distal RTA sometimes occurs as an incomplete form in which urolith formation occurs without systemic acidosis. Urolithiasis may be the only clinical manifestation of this disorder (Konnak et al, 1982). The tubular defect can be recognized by an abnormal response to an ammonium chloride loading test.

Normocalcemic Hypercalciuria

Normocalcemic hypercalciuria is a syndrome characterized by normal serum calcium concentration, increased urinary excretion of calcium, absence of systemic disease and increased tendency for formation of calcium phosphate or calcium oxalate uroliths (Curhan et al, 2007). Approximately 33% of human calcium urolith formers have normocalcemic hypercalciuria (Menon et al, 1998). Normocalcemic hypercalciuria has also been recognized in dogs (Lulich et al, 1991). It has not been documented to occur in cats, likely due to little effort to detect it.

Two types of normocalcemic hypercalciuria have been recognized in dogs (Lulich et al, 1991). One type, called absorptive hypercalciuria, is associated with increased intestinal absorption of calcium. The subsequent increase in serum calcium concentration suppresses PTH secretion, resulting in decreased tubular reabsorption of calcium and hypercalciuria. Hyperabsorption of calcium from the intestinal tract may result from a primary intestinal disturbance in calcium transport. It is also possible that increased calcium absorption results from increased synthesis of 1,25-vitamin D. Absorptive hypercalciuria has been divided into subtypes based on urinary calcium excretion following consumption of different levels of dietary calcium (Menon et al, 1998).

The second type of normocalcemic hypercalciuria, termed renal-leak hypercalciuria, is thought to result from impaired ability of the proximal tubules to reabsorb filtered calcium (Lulich et al, 1991a; Menon et al, 1998). A defect in reabsorption of magnesium may also be present. Renal calcium loss stimulates 1,25-vitamin D and PTH synthesis, resulting in an increase in intestinal absorption of calcium.

Hypercalciuria is probably not the only factor involved in urolith formation in patients with normocalcemic hypercalciuria because many hypercalciuric patients do not form uroliths. Crystallization inhibitor and promoter interaction are also important contributing factors.

The diagnosis of idiopathic hypercalciuria is established by demonstrating an increase in 24-hour urinary calcium excretion and by eliminating other nonhypercalcemic, hypercalciuric disorders such as RTA (**Table 41-4**) (Lulich et al, 1991a, 1991; Menon et al, 1998). Unlike absorptive hypercalciuria, renal-leak hypercalciuria is not affected by withholding food. **Table 41-5** presents a problem-specific database for dogs suspected of having calcium phosphate uroliths, and is a useful clinical tool.

Mineralization of Blood Clots

Nephroliths, urocystoliths and urethroliths composed of blood clots mineralized with calcium phosphate have been observed on numerous occasions in dogs (and cats). Formation of highly concentrated urine in patients with gross hematuria may favor formation of mineralized blood clots. Contrary to one theory, these black-colored uroliths are not composed of bile metabolites.

BIOLOGIC BEHAVIOR

Calcium phosphate uroliths may increase in size and number if underlying causes persist. In our experience, blood clots within the urinary tract that have become mineralized with calcium phosphate often remain inactive for years.

KEY NUTRITIONAL FACTORS

The determination of key nutritional factors for prevention of calcium phosphate uroliths is complicated because these uroliths occur relatively infrequently and there are several different potentially underlying causes. Dietary dissolution of calcium phosphate uroliths has not been successful. Depending on the size, calcium phosphate uroliths are readily removed by surgery, lithotripsy, voiding urohydropropulsion (Figure 38-5 and Table 38-7) (Lulich et al, 1993) or aspiration through a urinary catheter (Figure 38-6) (Lulich and Osborne, 1992). Thus, dietary therapy of patients with recurring calcium phosphate uroliths is limited to removing or minimizing risk factors that contribute to supersaturation of urine with calcium phosphate.

The solubility of calcium phosphates in urine depends on: 1) urinary pH, 2) urine calcium ion concentration, 3) total urine inorganic phosphate concentration, 4) urine concentration of inhibitors of calcium crystallization and 5) urine concentration of potentiators of crystallization. The key nutritional factors that are thought to increase calcium phosphate solubility to help prevent recurrence of uroliths are summarized in **Table 41-6** and are discussed in more detail below.

Water

Dogs eating dry commercial foods are probably at greater risk for urolith formation than dogs consuming moist foods because dry foods tend to be associated with production of a reduced volume of more concentrated urine. Low urine volume is a risk factor for all types of uroliths because it increases the relative urine saturation of lithogenic constituents. However, it is highly improbable that low urine volume alone would create an environment conducive to calcium phosphate urolith formation.

Although understandably difficult in some patients, encouraging fluid consumption throughout the day with the goal of promoting a consistently large volume of urine is likely to be of benefit. Enhancing urine volume by feeding a moist food may

Table 41-5. Problem-specific database for dogs suspected of having calcium phosphate uroliths.

Blood, serum and plasma tests	
Urea nitrogen and creatinine	Calcium
Phosphorus	Sodium
Chloride	Potassium
Blood gases or total CO_2	Intact parathyroid hormone
25-hydroxy-vitamin D	Magnesium
	Low dose dexamethasone suppression or corticotrophin stimulation test
Urine tests	
Complete urinalysis, including careful evaluation of pH and crystals	
Quantitative urine culture	
Consider 24-hour urine collection for:	
Volume	Creatinine
Calcium	Phosphorus
Magnesium	Citric acid
Oxalic acid	

Table 41-6. Key nutritional factors for foods for the prevention of recurrence of calcium phosphate urolithiasis in dogs.*

Factors	Recommended levels
Water	Water intake should be encouraged to achieve a urine specific gravity <1.020 Moist food will increase water consumption and formation of less concentrated urine
Protein	10 to 25%
Calcium	0.4 to 0.7%
Phosphorus	0.3 to 0.6%
Ca:P ratio	1.1:1 to 2:1
Sodium	<0.3%
Magnesium	0.06 to 0.15%
Vitamin D	500 to 1,500 IU/kg
Urinary pH	6.2 to 6.6**

Key: Ca:P ratio = calcium-phosphorus ratio.
*Nutrients expressed on a dry matter basis.
**Alkaline urine is recommended for patients with distal renal tubular acidosis.

be helpful. Water intake should be encouraged to achieve a urine specific gravity <1.020.

Protein

Foods with a high protein content tend to contribute to hypocitraturia. Citric acid ions inhibit calcium phosphate crystallization. Citrate forms soluble complexes with calcium, thereby decreasing the availability of calcium for incorporation into crystals.

High-protein foods also contribute to hypercalciuria and hyperphosphaturia. Some of the consequences of eating high-protein foods result from obligatory acid excretion associated with protein metabolism. Hypercalciuria occurs in normal dogs fed high-protein foods (40% dry matter [DM]). Therefore, excessive dietary protein consumption should be avoided in dogs at risk for recurrence of calcium phosphate urolithiasis. The recommended range for dietary protein is 10 to 25% DM; the lower end of this range is probably better. The minimum recommended allowance for protein in foods for healthy adult dogs is 10% DM (NRC, 2006).

Calcium and Phosphorus

Hypercalciuria decreases calcium phosphate solubility and may result in oversaturation with calcium phosphate (Pak, 1978). Reduction of dietary calcium appears to be a logical goal for prevention of calcium phosphate urolithiasis because intestinal hyperabsorption of calcium has been identified as one mechanism promoting hypercalciuria in dogs with calcium oxalate uroliths.

Foods with higher levels of phosphorus tend to augment hyperphosphaturia and may predispose hypercalciuric patients to form calcium phosphate uroliths. However, excessive restriction of dietary phosphorus may enhance the availability of dietary calcium for intestinal absorption. It may also enhance production of 1,25-vitamin D by the kidneys, thereby promoting hypercalciuria.

The optimal levels of dietary calcium and phosphorus for dogs with calcium phosphate urolithiasis have not been determined. The following recommendations are the same as for prevention of recurrence of calcium oxalate uroliths (Chapter 40): foods for prevention of calcium phosphate urolith recurrence should contain 0.4 to 0.7% DM calcium and 0.3 to 0.6% DM phosphorus with a calcium-phosphorus ratio range of 1.1:1 to 2:1. The minimum recommended allowances for calcium and phosphorus in foods for healthy adult dogs are 0.4 and 0.3% DM, respectively (NRC, 2006). One survey of the average calcium content of numerous dry grocery brand dog foods was shown to be 1.36% DM and for moist foods 1.73% DM (Debraekeleer, 2000).

In people, some high-fiber foods have been shown to reduce intestinal absorption and urinary excretion of calcium (Menon et al, 1998).

Sodium

Foods with higher quantities of sodium and/or oral administration of sodium chloride are often empirically recommended for prevention of all forms of urolithiasis. However, such excess sodium intake may promote hypercalciuria and enhance the risk of calcium phosphate urolith formation. Therefore, oral sodium chloride therapy is not recommended to promote diuresis in dogs with uroliths containing calcium salts.

Sodium content of foods for canine patients at risk for recurrence of calcium phosphate uroliths should be moderately restricted (<0.3% DM sodium). Typically, commercial dog foods contain two to three times this amount. The minimum recommended allowance for sodium in foods for healthy adult dogs is 0.08% DM (NRC, 2006).

Magnesium

Normally, urine contains calcium phosphate crystal inhibitors. One mechanism by which inhibitors prevent urolith formation is by chelating urolith constituents, making them unavailable for nidus formation or crystal growth. In addition, crystallization inhibitors may alter crystalline structure in such a way that crystal growth and aggregation are prevented. Magnesium ions are inhibitors of calcium phosphate crystallization (Bisaz et al, 1978; Ito and Coe, 1977).

However, increased urinary excretion of calcium by normal dogs given supplemental magnesium has been observed. Urinary calcium excretion was 0.5 ± 0.2 mg/kg body weight/day in six normal dogs consuming a food containing 0.03% DM magnesium vs. 2.65 ± 1.7 mg/kg body weight/day when the same dogs consumed a food containing 0.38% DM magnesium (Lulich, 1991b). Pending further studies, dietary magnesium restriction or supplementation is not recommended for treatment of canine calcium phosphate uroliths. A moderate range of 0.06 to 0.15% DM is recommended. The minimum recommended allowance for magnesium content of foods for healthy adult dogs is 0.06% DM (NRC, 2006).

Vitamin D

Foods with higher quantities of vitamin D or excessive supplementation with vitamin D may promote hypercalciuria (**Table 41-4**). Vitamin D promotes intestinal absorption of calcium. Commercial foods typically have adequate vitamin D content and should not be further supplemented. Excessive supplementation of homemade foods with vitamin D could also pose a risk. For prevention of calcium phosphate urolithiasis, restrict vitamin D in foods to between 500 to 1,500 IU/kg DM. The recommended minimum allowance for foods for healthy adult dogs is 552 IU/kg DM (NRC, 2006).

Urinary pH

Urinary pH profoundly affects the solubility of some forms of calcium phosphate (Elliot, 1957). With the exception of brushite, calcium phosphate solubility markedly decreases in alkaline urine and increases in acidic urine. Increased urinary pH increases the availability of ionic PO_4^{3-} and HPO_4^{2-}, which are available for incorporation into calcium phosphates (Asplin et al, 1996). Apatite will not crystallize from human urine unless the pH is 6.6 or greater (Elliot, 1968). As mentioned above, approximately 400 mg of calcium phosphate/l can be held in solution at a pH of 5.5, whereas only 32 mg of calcium phosphate/l will be held in solution at a pH of 7.8 (Elliot, 1965). Therefore, people with disorders associated with persistent elevation of urinary pH (e.g., distal RTA) are predisposed to calcium phosphate urolith formation. In contrast to carbonate apatite and hydroxyapatite, the solubility of brushite decreases in acidic urine. Acidification to the degree that induces acidosis should be avoided because it promotes hypercalciuria and hypocitraturia.

For prevention of recurrence of calcium phosphate uroliths in most patients (non-distal RTA patients and non-brushite urolith patients), the food should produce a urinary pH of 6.2 to 6.6.

Long-term alkalinization therapy appears to be beneficial in preventing calcium phosphate urolith formation in people with distal RTA (Caruana and Buckalew, 1988; Menon et al, 1998). Such therapy has been advocated for patients with complete or incomplete forms of distal RTA because it decreases urolith formation and nephrocalcinosis, and it increases urine citrate concentration.

FEEDING PLAN

Patients with primary hyperparathyroidism usually require surgery (Feldman and Nelson, 1996). Parathyroidectomy may result in dissolution of uroliths and generally prevents their recurrence. Parathyroidectomy in a dog with primary hyperparathyroidism and recurrent calcium phosphate uroliths resulted in decreased urinary calcium excretion and prevention of new urolith formation (Klausner et al, 1987).

Surgery and/or lithotripsy are the most reliable ways to remove active calcium phosphate uroliths from the urinary tract. However, surgery may be unnecessary for clinically inactive calcium phosphate uroliths. Voiding urohydropropulsion may be used to remove small urocystoliths (Figure 38-5 and Table 38-7) (Lulich et al, 1993). Although calcium-chelating agents have been reported to be of value in dissolving calcium phosphate uroliths in people, the feasibility of this type of therapy has not yet been reported in dogs and cats.

The frequency of recurrence of calcium phosphate uroliths following removal is not well established. However, unless the underlying cause(s) have been eliminated or controlled, recurrence is likely. Therefore, patients should be periodically monitored by urinalysis, radiographic procedures, and, if indicated, blood and urine tests (**Table 41-7**). If recurrent urocystoliths are detected when they are small, they may be removed by nonsurgical means as described above. Dietary or combined dietary and medical therapy of patients with recurring calcium phosphate uroliths should then be directed at removing or minimizing risk factors that contribute to supersaturation of urine with calcium phosphate.

Assess and Select the Food

Formulation of an optimal food remains a goal for the future. Until such a food becomes available, it is reasonable to recommend trial therapy with foods that most nearly match the key nutritional factor recommendations. **Table 41-8** lists selected veterinary therapeutic foods that can be considered for prevention of calcium phosphate urolith recurrence and compares their key nutritional factor content to the recommended levels. Select the food that most closely matches the key nutritional factor levels described above for preventing the recurrence of calcium phosphate uroliths. Because these foods are intended for long-term feeding, they should also be approved by the Association of American Feed Control Officials (AAFCO), or some other credible regulatory agency. Dogs consuming dry foods may be at greater risk for urolithiasis than dogs consuming moist foods. Dry foods are often associated with higher urine concentrations of urolith constituents and more concentrated urine. Therefore, when possible, moist foods should be selected.

The sodium content of treats should be checked. Treats should not contain more than 0.3% DM sodium and they should be limited to less than 10% of the total food regimen

Table 41-7. Summary of recommendations for managing canine calcium phosphate uroliths.

1. Surgery remains the most reliable way to remove active calcium phosphate uroliths from the urinary tract. However, surgery may be unnecessary for clinically inactive calcium phosphate uroliths. Small urocystoliths may be nonsurgically removed by lithotripsy, voiding urohydropropulsion (Figure 38-5 and Table 38-7) or by aspiration through a urinary catheter (Figure 38-6). Medical therapy of patients with recurrent calcium phosphate uroliths should then be directed at removing or minimizing risk factors that contribute to supersaturation of urine with calcium phosphate.
2. Patients with hypercalcemia and primary hyperparathyroidism usually require surgery. Parathyroidectomy may result in dissolution of uroliths and prevent recurrence in cases that have been properly managed.
3. Several different medical protocols have been reported to be of value in people with normocalcemic hypercalciuria. Ideally, the choice of therapy should be based on the cause of idiopathic hypercalciuria.
   a. There has been little clinical experience with the use of drugs in dogs and cats with calcium phosphate uroliths. However, medications that can enhance urine calcium excretion such as glucocorticoids, furosemide and those containing large quantities of sodium should be avoided (if possible).
   b. Foods designed to avoid excessive protein, sodium, calcium and vitamin D may be of benefit. Excessive restriction or supplementation of dietary phosphorus should probably be avoided. Enhancing urine volume by feeding a moist food (and/or a protein-restricted food to dogs to reduce renal medullary urea concentrations) and encouraging water consumption may be of benefit. Although understandably difficult to accomplish in some patients, fluid intake should be encouraged throughout the day to promote a constantly high urine volume. In people, some high-fiber diets reduce intestinal absorption and urinary excretion of calcium.
   c. With the exception of brushite, calcium phosphates tend to be less soluble in alkaline urine. Whether or not patients with such mineral types would benefit from appropriate dosages of urine acidifiers is unknown. Acidification tends to enhance urine calcium excretion and is a risk factor for calcium oxalate urolith formation. Pending further studies, routine use of urine acidifiers for patients with calcium phosphate urolithiasis is not recommended.
4. Medical dissolution of calcium phosphate uroliths has not been attempted in dogs with distal renal tubular acidosis (RTA). Foods designed to dissolve struvite uroliths would generally not be expected to promote dissolution of calcium phosphate uroliths, in part because they may tend to promote acidemia and aciduria, thus potentially enhancing hypercalciuria and hypocitraturia. However, correction of hypercalciuria, hyperphosphaturia and hypocitraturia by alkalinization therapy with potassium citrate might promote dissolution of these uroliths in patients with complete or incomplete distal RTA. Long-term alkalinization therapy appears to be beneficial in preventing calcium phosphate urolith formation in people with distal RTA. Alkalinization of urine has been advocated for human patients with complete or incomplete forms of distal RTA because it decreases urolith formation and nephrocalcinosis and increases urine citrate concentration. Oral administration of sodium chloride, long recommended for all forms of urolithiasis, may promote hypercalciuria and calcium phosphate urolith formation. Therefore, oral salt therapy is not recommended to promote diuresis in dogs with uroliths containing calcium salts.

(volume or weight basis).

Moderate urinary acidification is recommended for prevention of recurrent calcium phosphate uroliths in most patients. However, for distal RTA patients, long-term alkalinization therapy appears to be beneficial.

Another criterion for selecting a food that may become increasingly important in the future is evidence-based clinical nutrition. Practitioners should know how to determine risks and benefits of nutritional regimens and counsel pet owners accordingly. Currently, veterinary medical education and continuing education are not always based on rigorous assessment of evidence for or against particular management options. Still, studies have been published to establish the nutritional benefits of certain pet foods. Chapter 2 describes evidence-based clinical nutrition in detail and applies its concepts to various veterinary therapeutic foods.

Assess and Determine the Feeding Method

Transitioning a patient from the current food to a new food to help prevent recurrence of calcium phosphate uroliths should be done gradually. Begin the transition by feeding 75% of the current food and 25% of the new food on Day 1. On Day 2, feed half of each food. On Day 3, feed 75% of the new food and 25% of the old food. Feed only the new food beginning on Day 4.

Because moist foods increase water intake and produce a more dilute urine, feeding specific amounts (meal fed) of food two to three times per day is preferred to free-choice feeding. Moist foods can spoil if left at room temperature for several hours (Chapter 11). Opened containers of moist foods should be refrigerated and the feeding bowl should be kept clean.

Besides offering moist foods, several additional ways can facilitate increased water intake. These include: 1) Ensuring multiple bowls are available in prominent locations in the dog's environment; this may mean providing several bowls outside in a large enclosure or a bowl on each level of the house. 2) Bowls should be clean and always be filled with fresh water. 3) Small amounts of flavoring substances (e.g., salt-free bouillon) can be added to water sources. 4) Ice cubes can be offered as treats or snacks. 5) If a dry food is selected, add liberal quantities of water; however, potential food safety issues might arise from leaving moistened dry foods out for prolonged intervals (Chapter 11).

If the patient has a normal body condition score (BCS 2.5/5 to 3.5/5), the amount fed previously was probably appropriate. On an energy basis, a similar amount of the new food would be a good starting place.

ADJUNCTIVE MEDICAL AND SURGICAL MANAGEMENT

Urine Acidifying and Alkalinizing Agents

With the exception of brushite, calcium phosphates tend to be less soluble in alkaline urine. Acidification reduces urine concentrations of ionic phosphate (PO_4^{3-}) and hydroxyl ions (OH^-). However, whether or not patients with calcium phos-

Table 41-8. Levels of key nutritional factors in selected commercial veterinary therapeutic foods used to minimize recurrence of calcium phosphate urolithiasis in dogs compared to recommended levels.*

Dry foods	Protein (%)	Calcium (%)	Phosphorus (%)	Ca:P ratio	Sodium (%)	Magnesium (%)	Vitamin D (IU/kg)	Urinary pH
Recommended levels	**10-25**	**0.4-0.7**	**0.3-0.6**	**1.1:1-2:1**	**<0.3**	**0.06-0.15**	**500-1,500**	**6.2-6.6****
Hill's Prescription Diet c/d Canine	22.3	0.82	0.59	1.4:1	0.28	0.111	618	6.22
Hill's Prescription Diet w/d Canine	18.9	0.66	0.56	1.2:1	0.22	0.088	632	6.40
Hill's Prescription Diet w/d with Chicken Canine	19.1	0.66	0.56	1.2:1	0.27	0.080	677	6.30
Medi-Cal Urinary SO 13	16.7	1.0	**0.6**	na	1.3	0.2	na	5.5-6.0

Moist foods	Protein (%)	Calcium (%)	Phosphorus (%)	Ca:P ratio	Sodium (%)	Magnesium (%)	Vitamin D (IU/kg)	Urinary pH
Recommended levels	**10-25**	**0.4-0.7**	**0.3-0.6**	**1.1:1-2:1**	**<0.3**	**0.06-0.15**	**500-1,500**	**6.2-6.6****
Hill's Prescription Diet c/d Canine	23.6	0.68	0.51	1.3:3	0.27	0.079	1,370	6.16
Hill's Prescription Diet w/d Canine	17.9	0.64	0.52	1.2:1	0.24	0.088	1,745	6.40
Medi-Cal Urinary SO	18.7	1.0	0.8	na	1.1	0.1	na	5.5-6.0

Key: na = information not available from the manufacturer.
*This list represents products with the largest market share for which published information is available. Nutrient levels expressed on a dry matter basis. Moist foods are best.
**Alkaline urine recommended for patients with distal renal tubular acidosis.

phate uroliths would benefit from appropriate dosages of urine acidifiers is unknown. Overacidification tends to enhance urine calcium excretion and is a risk factor for calcium oxalate urolith formation. Pending further studies, we do not recommend routine use of urine acidifiers with urine acidifying foods for patients with calcium phosphate urolithiasis.

Because calcium hydrogen phosphate dihydrate (brushite) is less soluble in acidic urine, it might seem logical to promote formation of alkaline urine in patients with brushite uroliths. However, brushite may be converted to other insoluble forms of calcium phosphate in alkaline urine (Pak et al, 1971). Use of potassium citrate, an alkalinizing agent, might be rationalized on the basis of minimizing acidosis-induced hypercalciuria, and formation of soluble calcium citrate rather than insoluble calcium phosphate in urine. The benefits or detrimental effects of orally administered potassium citrate to dogs and cats with calcium phosphate urolithiasis, however, have not been carefully evaluated. Consult Chapter 40 (canine calcium oxalate urolithiasis) for additional therapeutic information about potassium citrate.

Thiazide Diuretics

Because thiazide diuretics decrease renal calcium excretion, they may be considered to minimize renal-leak hypercalciuria (Pak, 1982). However, because the long-term effects of thiazide diuretics have not been reported, appropriate caution should be used when giving them to prevent recurrence of calcium-containing uroliths. Patients should be monitored for dehydration, hypercalcemia, hypokalemia and magnesium depletion. Hydrochlorothiazide may be given on a trial basis at a dosage of 2 to 4 mg/kg body weight q12h. Thiazide diuretic therapy is not recommended to treat absorptive hypercalciuria because it does not correct the hyperabsorptive state and may promote positive systemic calcium balance that in turn would predispose the patient to soft-tissue calcification.

Other Drugs

Other drugs have been used in an attempt to minimize hypercalciuria in people (Asplin et al, 1996). Sodium cellulose phosphate, the sodium salt of the phosphoric ester of cellulose, is an ion-exchange cellulose with special affinity for divalent ions. In the gastrointestinal tract it exchanges sodium for dietary calcium, which is then eliminated in the feces. It also binds calcium secreted into the gastrointestinal tract, minimizing its reabsorption. Oral administration of orthophosphates to people with normocalcemic hypercalciuria reduces urine excretion of calcium and increases urine crystal inhibitory activity by increasing the urine concentration of pyrophosphates (Pak, 1982). We have had minimal experience with the use of sodium cellulose phosphate.

REASSESSMENT

Therapy should be initiated in a stepwise fashion (**Table 41-7**). The likelihood of recurrence of calcium phosphate uroliths following removal is not well established. Therefore, patients should be periodically monitored by urinalysis, radiographic or ultrasonographic procedures and other hematologic and urologic laboratory tests, as indicated (**Table 41-7**). Small, recurrent urocystoliths may be removed by voiding urohydropropulsion (Figure 38-5 and Table 38-7) (Lulich et al, 1993), by aspiration through a urinary catheter (Figure 38-6) (Lulich and Osborne, 1992) or by lithotripsy. Dietary and combined dietary and medical therapy of patients with recurring calcium phosphate uroliths should be directed at removing or minimizing risk factors that contribute to supersaturation of urine with calcium phosphate.

REFERENCES

The references for **Chapter 41** can be found at www.markmorris.org.

Chapter 42

Canine Cystine Urolithiasis: Causes, Detection, Dissolution and Prevention

Carl A. Osborne
Jody P. Lulich
Michelle Buettner

"If in doubt whether or not to give a drug, DON'T."
D.R. Lawrence

INTRODUCTION

Cystine (also called dicysteine) is a nonessential sulfur-containing amino acid composed of two molecules of the amino acid cysteine. What is the etymology of the name cystine? A report published in 1810 described some unusual bladder stones in people as "cystic oxide" (Wollenstan). The etymology of the name cystic oxide was based on the location of the stones in the urinary bladder ("kystis," the Greek term for bladder, is spelled "cystic" in English) and "oxide" for what was thought to be these unique stone's chemical nature. A few decades later, the fact that these stones were not an "oxide" was recognized; however, they were still considered to be composed of material that originated from the urinary bladder (or urocyst). The authors renamed the stones "cystine" (Berzelius, 1833). Subsequently, it was discovered that the stones were composed of a nonessential sulfur-containing amino acid, some of which is eliminated from the body by the urinary system (Segal and Thier, 1989). However, this amino acid is still called cystine (Rogers et al, 2007).

PREVALENCE

The prevalence of cystine uroliths in dogs varies geographically. The prevalence is 1 to 3% of the uroliths removed from dogs in the United States (Bovee and McGuire, 1984; Ling and Ruby, 1986; Osborne et al, 1986, 1999) and as high as 39% in some European centers (Hicking et al, 1981). Cystine accounted for 0.97% (3,402 of 350,803) of all canine uroliths submitted to the Minnesota Urolith Center from 1981 to 2007 (Table 38-8) and 1.1% (447 of 40,612) of canine uroliths submitted in 2007. Cystine accounted for 0.4 to 1.5% (77 of 5,050) of upper tract canine uroliths analyzed at the Minnesota Urolith Center from 1981 to 2006 (Table 38-9). The mean age of dogs at the time of cystine urolith retrieval was approximately 6.0 years (range three months to 16 years). Only 1.4% of uroliths retrieved from dogs less than 12 months of age were cystine. Our epidemiologic data indicate that Newfoundlands appear to be an exception to this generality inasmuch as cystine uroliths were commonly detected before one year of age.

Males (98%) were affected more often than females (2%). With

Table 42-1. Key nutritional factors for foods for canine cystine urolith dissolution and prevention.

Factors	Dietary recommendations
Water	Water intake should be encouraged to achieve a urine specific gravity <1.020 Moist food will increase water consumption and formation of less concentrated urine
Protein	Avoid excess dietary protein Restrict high quality dietary protein to 10 to 18% dry matter
Sodium	Restrict sodium to less than 0.3% dry matter
Urinary pH	Feed a food that maintains an alkaline urine (urinary pH = 7.1 to 7.7)

few exceptions, notably Newfoundlands, other investigators have reported the predominance of cystine uroliths in male dogs. From 2000 to 2006, 146 different breeds were affected including English bulldogs (18%), mixed breeds (16%), dachshunds (6%), mastiffs (6%), basset hounds (3%) and Newfoundlands (2%). At the University of Minnesota Veterinary Medical Center, English bulldogs have surpassed dachshunds in frequency of admissions for evaluation of cystine urolithiasis.

MINERAL COMPOSITION AND ARCHITECTURE

Quantitative analysis of canine cystine uroliths submitted to our center has revealed that most (3,275 of 3,402) are pure; however, a few contain ammonium urate, calcium oxalate and/or silica. Like cystine uroliths, ammonium urate and calcium oxalate uroliths tend to form in acidic urine. It is also of interest that in vitro studies have demonstrated that cystine is a promoter of calcium oxalate crystal growth and aggregation (Martins et al, 2002). Secondary urinary tract infections (UTIs) with urease-producing microbes may result in a nucleus of cystine surrounded by layers of struvite. However, this scenario is uncommon in our experience.

Pure cystine uroliths are usually multiple, ovoid and smooth. They are light yellow and vary from 0.5 mm to several cm in diameter. Some have a rough exterior, but this feature is unusual.

LOCATION

As mentioned above, cystine uroliths were more commonly removed from the lower urinary tract of dogs (98%) than the upper urinary tract (2%). The number of uroliths in each patient varied from one to more than 100. It is noteworthy that, compared to other affected breeds, a relatively high incidence of cystine nephroliths have been observed in Newfoundlands (Casal et al, 1995). Some of them may fill the renal pelvis, although this finding is uncommon. Whereas, cystine uroliths primarily affect the lower urinary tract of other breeds, the upper and lower urinary tracts of Newfoundlands may contain cystine uroliths.

ETIOPATHOGENESIS AND RISK FACTORS

Overview

Cystine is absorbed through the wall of the small intestine. It is normally present in low concentrations in plasma, and is freely filtered by glomeruli. Most filtered cystine is actively reabsorbed in the proximal tubules. The solubility of cystine in urine is pH dependent. It is relatively insoluble in acidic urine, but becomes more soluble in alkaline urine (Rogers et al, 2007). In dogs, the solubility of cystine at a urinary pH of 7.8 has been reported to be approximately double that at a urinary pH of 5.0 (Treacher, 1966).

Genetics

Cystinuria is an inborn error of metabolism characterized by impaired absorption of dibasic amino acids including cystine, ornithine, lysine and arginine by both the intestine and the proximal tubules of the kidneys. The amino acids other than cystine are soluble at the normal physiologic range of urinary pH, and therefore are not lithogenic. The intestinal defect in amino acid absorption is apparently harmless inasmuch as these amino acids are classified as nonessential, and their dipeptide forms are still absorbed. The precise genetic mode of inheritance of canine cystinuria in most breeds is unknown. Although in past years this genetic disorder was thought to be sex-linked in all affected breeds, cystinuria in Newfoundlands (and probably Labrador retrievers) has been recently confirmed to be a mutation in the rBAT gene (renal Basic Amino Acid Transporter) transmitted in a simple autosomal recessive pattern (Calonge et al, 1995; Henthorn, 2007; Segal et al, 1989). In Newfoundlands, the parents of cystinuric dogs are either cystinuric or are carriers, whereas littermates may be: 1) cystinuric, 2) cystinuric carriers or 3) normal. Evaluation of DNA and nitroprusside test results indicates that equal proportions of males and females are affected. However, as will be discussed, male Newfoundlands develop clinical signs referable to uroliths much more frequently than females.

Evaluation of the rBAT gene in several other breeds with cystinuria and with and without cystine uroliths (mastiffs, English bulldogs and Scottish deerhounds) has revealed no mutations.

Aminoaciduria

Cystinuria is characterized by abnormal transport of cystine and other dibasic amino acids by the renal tubules and intestines. Unlike normal dogs, some cystinuric dogs reabsorb a much smaller proportion of the amino acid from the glomerular filtrate (Bovee, 1984). Some may even have net cystine secretion.

The exact mechanism of abnormal renal tubular transport of cystine in most dogs is unknown. When measured, plasma concentrations of cystine in affected dogs were normal, indicating faulty tubular reabsorption and/or tubular secretion rather than hyperexcretion through glomeruli (Bovee, 1984, 1984a; Bovee and McGuire, 1984). Levels of plasma methionine, a precursor of cystine, have been found to be elevated in some cystinuric

Table 42-2. Levels of key nutritional factors in selected commercial veterinary therapeutic foods used for dissolution and to minimize recurrence of cystine uroliths in dogs compared to recommended levels.*

Dry foods	Protein (%)	Sodium (%)	Urinary pH**
Recommended levels	**10-18**	**<0.3**	**7.1-7.7**
Hill's Prescription Diet u/d Canine	11.2	0.23	7.70
Medi-Cal Reduced Protein	13.7	0.2	na
Medi-Cal Renal LP 11	14.7	0.1	na
Medi-Cal Renal MP 14	18.4	0.1	na
Medi-Cal Vegetarian Formula	20.9	0.4	na
Royal Canin Veterinary Diet Hypoallergenic HP 19	23.1	0.44	na
Royal Canin Veterinary Diet Vegetarian Formula	19.1	0.15	6.78
Moist foods	**Protein (%)**	**Sodium (%)**	**Urinary pH****
Recommended levels	**10-18**	**<0.3**	**7.1-7.7**
Hill's Prescription Diet u/d Canine	13.3	0.28	7.40
Medi-Cal Reduced Protein	16.5	0.2	na
Medi-Cal Renal LP	16.8	0.1	na
Medi-Cal Renal MP	28.2	0.2	na
Medi-Cal Vegetarian Formula	26.4	0.5	na

Key: na = information not available from the manufacturer.
*Manufacturers' published values; protein and sodium expressed as % dry matter; when possible chose moist foods.
**Protocols for measuring urinary pH may vary.

dogs. Results of some studies in people suggest that tubular reabsorption of cysteine, the immediate precursor of cystine, may be abnormal (Segal and Thier, 1989). In this situation, the increase in urinary cystine concentration may result from dimerization of two cysteine molecules in tubular urine.

In dogs with cystinuria, the pattern of dibasic aminoaciduria reported by various investigators has been variable (Bovee, 1984; Clark and Cuddeford, 1971; Cornelius et al, 1967; Crane and Turner, 1956). Apparently there are several different populations of cystinuric dogs (Bovee, 1984; Casal et al, 1995). One group had cystinuria without significant loss of other amino acids. Another group had cystinuria and a lesser degree of lysinuria. Our studies indicate that cystine urolith-forming English bulldogs have cystinuria and lysinuria. Another group had cystinuria, glutaminuria, threoninuria and citrullinuria (Hoppe et al, 1993). A fourth group had cystinuria, ornithinuria, lysinuria and arginuria, a pattern commonly encountered in people with this disorder (Bovee, 1984; Sanderson et al, 1995). This pattern of aminoaciduria may be remembered with the acronym COLA (cystine, ornithine, lysine, arginine).

Unless protein intake is severely restricted, abnormalities associated with loss of amino acids have not resulted in recognizable disorders, with the exception of formation of cystine uroliths. One general exception to this is cystinuric dogs with concomitant carnitinuria. Carnituric dogs consuming foods with reduced quantities of carnitine are predisposed to dilated cardiomyopathy (Sanderson et al, 1995). We have observed a cystinuric dachshund with carnitinuria.

The magnitude of cystinuria varies widely between cystinuric dogs, between serial measurements of the same dog and may decline in older dogs. In one study, four of 14 dogs with a history of cystine urolith formation had urine cystine concentrations that fell within the normal range of those found in control dogs (Bovee, 1984). One explanation that may be related, at least in part, to these differences is diurnal variations in urinary cystine excretion. Some variability may also be related to differences in diets consumed by cystinuric dogs, and differences related to urine collections during fasting and postprandial states. In a study of human cystinuric patients, analysis of six-hour urine samples revealed transient episodes of cystine saturation that were not observed in corresponding 24-hour urine samples.

The major causes of morbidity and mortality recognized in association with this disorder are sequelae of urolith formation. Unfortunately, the exact mechanisms of cystine urolith formation are unknown. Because not all cystinuric dogs form uroliths, and because not all dogs with cystine crystalluria form uroliths, cystinuria is a predisposing rather than the sole cause of cystine urolith formation.

Cystine is sparingly soluble at the usual urinary pH range of 5.5 to 7.5. However, a substantial increase in cystine solubility occurs at urinary pHs above 7.5.

On the basis of observations to date, it is possible to formulate the following working hypothesis. Newfoundlands and possibly other breeds of dogs (excluding mastiffs and English bulldogs) that form cystine uroliths before the age of one year have a severe form of cystinuria caused by homozygous mutation of the rBAT gene. To date, breeds in which cystine uroliths are recognized after the first year of life do not have a mutation in the rBAT gene. The quantity of cystine and other amino acids excreted in the urine of these dogs is highly variable, but is not as severe as the magnitude observed in Newfoundlands. It appears that the genetic abnormality in these dogs can be explained as an x-linked recessive inheritance with incomplete penetrance.

BIOLOGIC BEHAVIOR

Cystine uroliths are not recognized in most affected dogs until after they reach maturity. The average age at detection in many breeds is approximately two to five years. This is surprising inasmuch as one might expect an earlier onset of clinical manifestations of an inherited disorder. It is notable that cystinuria

Table 42-3. Summary of recommendations for combined dietary and medical/surgical treatment and prevention of canine cystine uroliths.

1. Perform appropriate diagnostic studies including complete urinalysis, quantitative urine culture and diagnostic radiography and/or ultrasonography. Determine precise location, size and number of uroliths. The size and number of uroliths are not a reliable index of probable therapeutic efficacy.
2. If uroliths are available, determine their mineral composition. If they are unavailable, determine their composition by evaluation of appropriate clinical data.
3. Consider surgical correction if uroliths obstruct urine outflow and/or if correctable abnormalities predisposing the patient to recurrent urinary tract infection are identified by radiography or other means. Small urocystoliths may be removed by voiding urohydropropulsion (Figure 38-5 and Table 38-7). Urethroliths may be removed by lithotripsy.
4. Initiate therapy with an appropriate litholytic food (**Table 42-2**). For optimal results, no other food or mineral supplements should be fed to the patient. Compliance with dietary recommendation is suggested by a reduction in urea nitrogen concentration (usually <10 mg/dl).
5. Initiate therapy with N-(2-mercaptopropionyl)-glycine (2-MPG)* at a daily dosage of approximately 30 mg/kg body weight, divided into two equal subdoses.
6. If necessary, administer potassium citrate orally to eliminate aciduria. Strive for a urinary pH of approximately 7.5 (range = 7.1 to 7.7).
7. If necessary, eradicate or control urinary tract infections with appropriate antimicrobial agents.
8. Devise a protocol for followup therapy.
   a. Try to avoid diagnostic followup studies that require urinary catheterization. If they are required, give appropriate peri-catheterization antimicrobial agents to prevent iatrogenic urinary tract infection.
   b. Perform serial urinalyses. Urinary pH, specific gravity and microscopic examination of sediment for crystals are especially important. Remember, crystals formed in urine stored at room or refrigeration temperatures may represent in vitro artifacts.
   c. Perform serial radiography monthly to evaluate urolith location(s), number, size, density and shape. Intravenous urography may be used to identify radiolucent uroliths in the kidneys, ureters and urinary bladder. Antegrade contrast cystourethrography may be required for radiolucent uroliths located in the bladder and urethra.
9. Continue litholytic food, 2-MPG and alkalinizing therapy for approximately one month after disappearance of uroliths as detected by radiography.
10. Prevention. Feeding a low-protein food that promotes alkaline urine (**Table 42-2**) has been effective in minimizing cystine urolith recurrence. If necessary, low doses of 2-MPG may also be given.

*Thiola, Mission Pharmacal, San Antonio, TX, USA.

and cystine uroliths have been detected in male and female Newfoundlands less than one year of age (Casal et al, 1995).

Compared to other breeds, the magnitude of the tubular transport defect for cystine in Newfoundlands is more severe. This provides a plausible explanation for the earlier onset of detectable cystine urolith formation in this breed and for the involvement of the kidneys in addition to the urinary bladder in female as well as male dogs (Casal et al, 1995). Because cystinuria is an inherited defect, uroliths commonly recur in two to 12 months unless prophylactic therapy has been initiated. Recurrence in Newfoundlands appears to be more rapid than in other breeds. In some older dogs, the rate of recurrence declines as a consequence of a reduction in magnitude of cystinuria. Spontaneous partial dissolution of cystine uroliths occurred in a 10-year-old neutered male dachshund (adopted by and evaluated for years by CAO). This dachshund was eating a moist maintenance food because it would not eat foods designed to minimize some risk factors for cystine urolithiasis. The patient was not given N-(2-mercaptopropionyl)-glycine (2-MPG[a]) to manage its cystine uroliths because on a previous occasion it developed protein-losing glomerulonephropathy while being treated with this drug.

DIAGNOSIS

Urinalysis

Detection of flat colorless hexagonal cystine crystals provides strong support for a diagnosis of cystinuria. The six sides of cystine crystals may or may not be equal, and the crystals tend to aggregate and may appear layered. Caution: cystine crystals are not constantly present in dogs with cystinuria or cystine uroliths. However, acidification of urine with glacial acetic acid, refrigeration and centrifugation may foster cystine crystal formation. Cystine crystals are insoluble in acetic acid, alcohol, acetone, ether and boiling water. They are soluble in ammonia and hydrochloric acid (pH <2).

We have observed crystals from a cystinuric, leucinuric female Scottish terrier that appeared similar to leucine crystals. Leucine crystals are highly refractile yellow to brown spheres with concentric circles or radial striations.

Assessment of Aminoaciduria

If a sufficient quantity of cystine is present in urine (75 to 125 mg/g of creatinine; 10 mmol/mol creatinine), the colorimetric cyanide-nitroprusside test result will be positive. Sodium cyanide reduces cystine to cysteine, and the free sulfhydryl groups subsequently react with nitroprusside to form a characteristic purple color. Ampicillin and sulfur-containing drugs have been reported to cause false positive reactions to this test.

Screening patients for cystinuria with the nitroprusside test may be aided by submitting fresh urine samples, or urine allowed to dry on 3-mm filter paper, to the Metabolic Screening Laboratory, Section of Medical Genetics, Veterinary Hospital, University of Pennsylvania, Philadelphia 19104-6010 (fax number 215-573-2162). Contact this center for specific instructions about DNA testing, urine and blood sample preservation and sample submission. Their website address is www.vet.upenn.edu./penngen/research/ (Henthorn and Giger, 2007).

Evaluation of urine amino acid excretion rates may provide additional definitive information about cystinuria and associated aminoacidurias. The most commonly used techniques are high-pressure liquid chromatography, and automated amino acid analyzers.

In breeds, such as Newfoundlands, in which the mode of inheritance is simple autosomal recessive, cystinuria may occur in the offspring of phenotypically normal parents. Unfortunately from a diagnostic standpoint, obligate carriers of the disease have no clinical signs, normal cystine urine concentrations and normal renal absorption of amino acids. Ongoing studies at the University of Pennsylvania to identify the gene(s) responsible for cystinuria will likely result in development of diagnostic molecular markers that can be used to identify these genetic carriers.

Radiography and Ultrasonography

The size of cystine uroliths varies from that just detectable by the unaided eye to more than three centimeters. The number present in each patient may vary from one to more than 100. Most canine cystine uroliths are smooth and spherical.

The radiodensity of cystine uroliths compared to soft tissue is similar to struvite and silica, less than calcium oxalate and calcium phosphate and greater than ammonium and sodium urate. Thus, when of sufficient size, cystine uroliths can be detected by survey radiography.

In our experience, double-contrast cystography is more sensitive in detecting small cystine urocystoliths than survey radiography and most techniques of ultrasonography. Cystine uroliths appear radiolucent when surrounded by, but not completely submerged in, radiopaque contrast medium.

Survey radiography may be insensitive for detecting cystine urethroliths. Positive-contrast urethrography may be required to detect and localize cystine uroliths that have passed into the urethral lumen.

Although uroliths can be detected by ultrasonography, this method does not provide information about the degree of their radiodensity or shape. Evaluation of the density and shape of uroliths often provides useful information in predicting their mineral type.

Urolith Analysis

Quantitative analysis of uroliths provides a definitive diagnosis of cystinuria. Uroliths may be collected with a tropical fishnet during the voiding phase of micturition, by catheter-assisted retrieval (Figure 38-6) (Lulich and Osborne, 1992) or by voiding urohydropropulsion (Figure 38-5 and Table 38-7) (Lulich et al, 1993). Samples may be submitted to the Minnesota Urolith Center for quantitative analysis (fax number 612-624-0751).

KEY NUTRITIONAL FACTORS

The key nutritional factors for foods intended for dissolution and prevention of cystine uroliths in dogs are discussed below and summarized in **Table 42-1**.

Table 42-4. Expected changes associated with combined dietary and medical therapy of cystine uroliths.

Factors	Pre-therapy	During therapy	Prevention therapy
Polyuria	±	1+ to 3+	1+ to 3+
Pollakiuria	0 to 4+	↑ then ↓	0
Hematuria	0 to 4+	↓	0
Urine specific gravity	Variable	1.004-1.020	1.004-1.020
Urinary pH	<7.0	>7.0	>7.0
Pyuria	0 to 4+	↓	0
Cystine crystals	0 to 4+	0	Variable
Bacteriuria	0 to 4+	0	0
Bacterial culture of urine	0 to 4+	0	0
Urea nitrogen (mg/dl)	Variable	<15	≤15
Urolith size and number	Small to large	↓	0

Water

Increasing urine volume to reduce urine cystine concentration is likely to be of benefit. Feeding moist rather than dry foods is recommended. Strive to obtain a urine specific gravity value less than 1.020.

Protein

High-protein foods should be avoided in dogs at risk for cystine urolithiasis. These include high-protein dry diets, especially those rich in methionine (a precursor of cysteine). Besides most meats, other food ingredients high in methionine include eggs, wheat and peanuts.

Reduction of dietary protein has the potential of minimizing formation of cystine uroliths. Pilot studies performed on cystinuric dogs at the University of Minnesota revealed a 20 to 25% reduction in 24-hour urine cystine excretion when subjects consumed a low-protein, moist veterinary therapeutic food[b] vs. when they received a moist, canine adult maintenance food. Reducing the concentration of urea in the renal medulla associated with reduced consumption of protein, and the associated reduction in urine concentration is an important indirect effect (Osborne et al, 1985). Protein levels in foods for dogs with cystine urolithiasis should be between 10 to 18% dry matter (DM). The minimum recommended allowance for protein in foods for healthy adult dogs is 10% DM (NRC, 2006).

Sodium

Data derived from studies in cystinuric people suggest that dietary sodium may enhance cystinuria (Jaeger et al, 1986). In one study of cystinuric people, dietary restriction of sodium reduced the urinary excretion of cystine. Further studies are required to evaluate the effect of dietary sodium on urinary excretion of cystine in dogs. Until data indicate otherwise, dietary sodium should be limited to less than 0.3% DM in cystine litholytic and prevention foods. Typically, commercial dog foods contain two to three times this amount. The minimum recommended allowance for sodium in foods for healthy adult dogs is 0.08% DM (NRC, 2006).

Table 42-5. Managing cystine uroliths refractory to complete dissolution.

Causes	Identification	Therapeutic goal
Client and patient factors		
Inadequate dietary compliance	Question owner Persistent cystine crystalluria Urea nitrogen >10-17 mg/dl Urine specific gravity >1.010-1.020 Urinary pH <7.0-7.5 during treatment with Prescription Diet u/d Canine* (use lower values for the moist food)	Emphasize value of feeding dissolution food
Inadequate 2-MPG** administration	Question owner Count remaining pills	Emphasize value of giving the full dose of medication Determine if owner is capable and willing to administer medication If necessary, demonstrate a variety of methods to administer medication
Clinician factors		
Incorrect prediction of mineral type	Analysis of retrieved urolith	Adjust therapy based on correct identification of mineral type
Inadequate 2-MPG dose for degree of diuresis	No change in urolith size after two months of appropriate therapy	Increase 2-MPG dose to 20 mg/kg body weight q12h
Disease factors		
Compound urolith	Radiographic density of nucleus and outer layer(s) of urolith are different Analysis of retrieved urolith	Adjust therapy based on identification of new mineral type Uroliths not causing clinical signs should be monitored for potentially adverse consequences(obstruction, urinary tract infection, etc.) Clinically active uroliths may require surgical removal Remove small uroliths by voiding urohydropropulsion (Figure 38-5 and Table 38-7); consider removing urethroliths by lithotripsy

*Hill's Pet Nutrition, Inc., Topeka, KS, USA.
**2-MPG = N-(2-mercaptopropionyl)-glycine. Thiola. Mission Pharmacal, San Antonio, TX, USA.

Urinary pH

The solubility of cystine in urine is pH dependent. Foods that promote formation of acidic urine are risk factors for cystine urolithiasis in susceptible dogs. Cystine is relatively insoluble in acidic urine, but becomes more soluble in alkaline urine (Rogers et al, 2007). In dogs, the solubility of cystine at a urinary pH of 7.8 has been reported to be approximately double that at a urinary pH of 5.0 (Treacher, 1966). Changes in urinary pH that remain in the acidic range have minimal effect on cystine solubility. A protein-restricted alkalinizing food without other therapy,[b] was observed to have a beneficial effect in promoting reduction in cystine urocystolith size in a three-year-old male dachshund (Osborne et al, 1989). Urinary pH values greater than 7.7 should be avoided until it is determined whether or not they provide a significant risk factor for formation of calcium phosphate uroliths. Thus, a food that produces a urinary pH range of 7.1 to 7.7 is recommended for dogs with cystine urolithiasis.

FEEDING PLAN

Current recommendations for dissolution of cystine uroliths encompass reducing urine concentration of cystine and increasing the solubility of cystine in urine. This may be accomplished by various combinations of: 1) dietary modification, 2) administration of thiol-containing drugs and 3) alkalinization of urine, if necessary. Small cystine urocystoliths may be removed by voiding urohydropropulsion (Figure 38-5 and Table 38-7) (Lulich et al, 1993) or retrieval with a urinary catheter (Figure 38-6) (Lulich and Osborne, 1992). Urethroliths may be removed by lithotripsy.

Assess and Select the Food

Table 42-2 lists selected veterinary therapeutic foods that can be considered for dissolution and prevention of cystine uroliths and compares their key nutritional factor content to the recommended levels. Select the food that is most similar to the key nutritional factor targets. Because these foods are intended for long-term feeding, they should also be approved by the Association of American Feed Control Officials (AAFCO), or some other credible regulatory agency. Dogs consuming dry foods may be at greater risk for urolithiasis than dogs consuming moist foods. Dry foods are often associated with higher urine concentrations of urolith constituents and more concentrated urine. Therefore, when possible, moist foods should be selected.

If treats are fed, their sodium content should be checked.

Treats should contain no more than 0.3% DM sodium (the same as the food recommendation) and they should be limited to less than 10% of the daily total food regimen (volume or weight basis).

Another criterion for selecting a food that may become increasingly important in the future is evidence-based clinical nutrition. Practitioners should know how to determine risks and benefits of nutritional regimens and counsel pet owners accordingly. Currently, veterinary medical education and continuing education are not always based on rigorous assessment of evidence for or against particular management options. Still, studies have been published to establish the nutritional benefits of certain pet foods. Chapter 2 describes evidence-based clinical nutrition in detail and applies its concepts to various veterinary therapeutic foods.

Assess and Determine the Feeding Method

Transitioning a patient from its current food to a new food selected for the management of cystine uroliths should be done gradually over a period of a few days. Begin the transition by feeding 75% of the current food and 25% of the new food on Day 1. On Day 2, feed half of each food. On Day 3, feed 75% of the new food and 25% of the old. By Day 4 or 5, feed only the new food.

Moist foods increase water intake and produce less concentrated urine; therefore, encourage clients to feed specific amounts (meal fed) of moist food two to three times per day rather than free-choice feeding. Moist foods can spoil if left at room temperature for several hours (Chapter 11). Opened containers of moist foods should be refrigerated and the feeding bowl should be kept clean.

Besides offering moist foods, increased water intake can be facilitated by: 1) Ensuring multiple bowls are available in prominent locations in the dog's environment; this may mean providing several bowls outside in a large enclosure or a bowl on each level of the house. 2) Bowls should be clean and kept filled with fresh water. 3) Small amounts of flavoring substances (e.g., salt-free bouillon) can be added to water sources to encourage consumption. 4) Ice cubes can be offered as treats or snacks. 5) If a dry food is selected, ask the client to add liberal quantities of water; however, as with moist foods left at room temperature for prolonged intervals, potential food safety issues might arise (Chapter 11).

If the patient has a normal body condition score (BCS 2.5/5 to 3.5/5), the amount of the previous food being fed was appropriate. On an energy basis, a similar amount of the new food would probably be a good starting place.

ADJUNCTIVE MEDICAL MANAGEMENT

Thiol-Containing Drugs

2-MPG

Drugs that increase the solubility of cystine in urine contain a thiol group that can dissociate and then bind with the sulfide moiety of cysteine. The resulting complexes are more soluble in urine than cystine (dicysteine).

2-MPG is commonly called tiopronin.[a] Tiopronin is a second-generation cysteine chelating agent that decreases the concentration of cystine by a thiol-disulfide exchange reaction. Studies in people and dogs indicate that the drug is highly effective in reducing urine cystine concentration and has less toxicity than D-penicillamine[c] (Hoppe et al, 1988, 1993; Osborne et al, 1989).

Oral administration of 2-MPG at a daily dosage of approximately 30 to 40 mg/kg of body weight (divided in two equal doses) was effective in inducing dissolution of multiple cystine urocystoliths in nine of 17 dogs evaluated (Hoppe et al, 1993; Osborne et al, 1989). Dissolution required two to four months of therapy. One dog developed nonpruritic vesicular skin lesions following three months of therapy. One month following reduction of the daily dosage of 2-MPG from 30 to 25 mg/kg of body weight, the skin lesions healed. Thrombocytopenia, anemia and elevated hepatic enzyme activities have also occurred in a few cystinuric dogs treated with 2-MPG (Osborne et al, 1989). During therapy with 2-MPG, we encountered protein-losing glomerular disease in a cystinuric dachshund.

Unfortunately, dogs that become hypersensitive to D-penicillamine may also simultaneously become hypersensitive to 2-MPG. The beneficial action of both drugs is dose dependent as are the associated side effects. To avoid this predicament when thiol-containing drugs are needed, we discourage use of D-penicillamine and encourage use of the less toxic 2-MPG. Appropriate evaluations should be performed, especially if 2-MPG is used in dogs with a history of D-penicillamine hypersensitivity.

In our experience, a combination of a litholytic food and 2-MPG therapy is more effective in promoting dissolution of uroliths than either alone. We induced dissolution of 18 episodes of cystine urocystoliths affecting 14 dogs using this combination of diet and drug therapy (Osborne et al, 1989). The mean time required to dissolve the cystine uroliths was 78 days (range 11 to 211 days).

D-Penicillamine

D-penicillamine,[c] also called dimethylcysteine, is commonly referred to as a first-generation cysteine chelating drug. It is a nonmetabolizable degradation product of penicillin that may combine with cysteine to form cysteine-D-penicillamine disulfide (Bovee, 1984a). This disulfide exchange reaction is facilitated by an alkaline pH. The resulting compound has been reported to be 50 times more soluble than free cystine (Lotz et al, 1966). The cysteine-D-penicillamine complex does not react with nitroprusside as does cystine, providing a marker to aid in titrating dosage of the drug (Pahira, 1987).

Although D-penicillamine is effective in reducing urine cystine concentrations, drug-related adverse events limit its use. With the availability of 2-MPG, we have discontinued use of D-penicillamine.

The most commonly used dosage of D-penicillamine for dogs has been 30 mg/kg body weight/day given in two divided doses. Higher dosages frequently cause vomiting and may cause other undesirable reactions. If nausea and vomiting occur with the aforementioned dosage, the drug may be mixed with food or given at mealtimes. In some instances, it may be necessary to prevent gastrointestinal disturbances by initiating therapy with a low dose and gradually increasing it until a therapeutic dosage is reached.

D-penicillamine has been associated with a variety of adverse reactions in people, including immune complex glomerulonephropathy, fever, lymphadenopathy and skin hypersensitivity (Pahira, 1987). We observed fever and lymphadenopathy in a dachshund given D-penicillamine at a dosage of 30 mg/kg body weight/day (Osborne et al, 1995). The signs subsided following withdrawal of the drug and administration of a short course of glucocorticoids. To minimize such adverse drug events, we prefer to use 2-MPG rather than D-penicillamine.

Captopril

Captopril is a thiol-containing angiotensin-converting enzyme inhibitor that is primarily used as an antihypertensive agent. Captopril has been reported to form a thiol-cystine disulfide that is markedly more soluble than cystine; the mechanism of action is similar to that of 2-MPG and D-penicillamine.

Results of uncontrolled clinical trials of treatment of cystinuric people with captopril have been interpreted to suggest a beneficial effect. However, the clinical value of thiol-containing angiotensin-converting enzyme inhibitors in the management of cystinuria remains unproved by properly controlled clinical trials. Note: the angiotensin-converting enzyme inhibitor enalapril is not a thiol-containing drug.

Bucillamine

Bucillamine[d] is a third-generation cysteine chelating agent that may have greater affinity for cysteine than 2-MPG. Bucillamine has been used to treat human patients with rheumatoid arthritis and apparently has been well tolerated. We have not critically evaluated the efficacy and safety of this drug.

Urine Alkalinizing Agents

The solubility of cystine is pH dependent. In dogs, the solubility of cystine at a urinary pH of 7.8 has been reported to be approximately double that at a urinary pH of 5.0 (Treacher, 1966). Changes in urinary pH that remain in the acidic range have minimal effect on cystine solubility. Therefore, if lack of cystine urolith dissolution occurs in dogs whose urinary pH does not become sufficiently alkaline following compliant initiation of dietary therapy, a sufficient quantity of potassium citrate should be given orally in divided doses to sustain a urinary pH of approximately 7.5. Caution: recall that alkalinization of urine is a risk factor for calcium phosphate uroliths.

Data derived from studies in cystinuric people suggest that dietary sodium may enhance cystinuria (Jaeger et al, 1986). Therefore, potassium citrate may be preferable to sodium bicarbonate to alkalinize urine.

It is of interest that UTIs caused by urease-producing bacteria in an adult male human patient with cystine nephroliths resulted in extreme urine alkalinity and subsequent urolith dissolution (Gutierrez Millet et al, 1985).

REASSESSMENT

Therapy should be initiated in a stepwise fashion (**Table 42-3**). The goal of therapy is to promote cystine urolith dissolution. To be consistently effective, we have found that this requires careful and planned monitoring (**Tables 42-4** and **42-5**). Dietary management should result in formation of less concentrated urine without cystine crystalluria. Strive to achieve urine specific gravity values less than 1.020 (range of 1.015 to 1.020). If the urinary pH remains acidic despite dietary therapy in patients known to be compliant with dietary recommendations, orally administered potassium citrate may be considered.

We recommend that a urinalysis and survey abdominal radiographs be performed approximately every four weeks. Reduction in serum urea nitrogen concentration and urine specific gravity values provides supportive evidence that the client and patient are complying with recommendations to feed a moist food with reduced quantities of protein.

PREVENTION

Because cystinuria is an inherited metabolic defect, and because cystine uroliths recur in a high percentage of young to middle-aged dogs within two to 12 months after surgical removal, prophylactic therapy should be considered. Dietary therapy and if necessary, urine alkalinization may be initiated with the objective of minimizing cystine crystalluria and promoting a negative cyanide-nitroprusside test result. If necessary, 2-MPG may be added to the regimen in sufficient quantities to maintain a urine concentration of cystine less than approximately 200 mg/liter. If the dosage cannot be titrated by measurement of urine cystine concentration, 2-MPG may be given at a dosage of 15 mg/kg body weight q12h. Continuous therapy of urolith-free cystinuric dogs with 2-MPG has been effective in preventing formation of cystine uroliths in studies performed in Sweden and at the University of Minnesota (Hoppe et al, 1988, 1993a; Osborne et al, 1999a).

ENDNOTES

a. Thiola. Mission Pharmacal, San Antonio, TX, USA.
b. Prescription Diet u/d Canine. Hill's Pet Nutrition, Inc., Topeka, KS, USA.
c. Cuprimine. Merck and Co., Rahway, NJ, USA.
d. Rimatil. Santen Pharmaceutical Co., Ltd., Osaka, Japan.

REFERENCES

The references for **Chapter 42** can be found at www.markmorris.org.

CASE 42-1

Dysuria in a Dachshund

Carl A. Osborne, DVM, PhD, Dipl. ACVIM (Internal Medicine)
College of Veterinary Medicine
University of Minnesota
St. Paul, Minnesota, USA

Patient Assessment

A four-year-old, neutered male dachshund was examined for vomiting, depression, dysuria and anuria of two days' duration. Dysuria and pollakiuria were present for two weeks. Physical examination revealed a depressed, mildly dehydrated dog with a large urinary bladder. The dog weighed 6.5 kg and had a normal body condition score (3/5).

Survey radiographs confirmed obstructive uropathy due to multiple urethroliths with marginal radiodensity (**Figure 1**). Blood and urine were collected for routine diagnostic tests. The urethroliths were flushed back into the bladder lumen by urohydropropulsion after the bladder was decompressed via cystocentesis (**Figure 2**). Lactated Ringer's solution was given subcutaneously to correct the dehydration and oral amoxicillin-clavulanic acid (Clavamox[a]) was given to prevent urinary tract infection.

Results of the complete blood count were normal. The major serum biochemistry abnormalities were azotemia (urea nitrogen = 52 mg/dl, normal 4 to 26 mg/dl; creatinine = 3.1 mg/dl, normal 0.4 to 1.5 mg/dl) and hyperphosphatemia (phosphorus = 8.4 mg/dl, normal 2.9 to 6.4 mg/dl). Urinalysis results included the following: specific gravity = 1.025, pH = 6.5, hematuria, pyuria, proteinuria and numerous cystine crystals.

The diagnosis was obstructive uropathy due to urethroliths and postrenal azotemia.

Assess the Food and Feeding Method

The dog was fed a commercial dry adult maintenance food free choice and received a vitamin-mineral supplement each day.

Questions

1. What is the most likely mineral composition of this dog's uroliths?
2. Outline a treatment and feeding plan for this patient.

Answers and Discussion

1. The key diagnostic findings in this dog include: 1) multiple, smooth uroliths with marginal radiodensity, 2) urinary pH = 6.5, 3) cystine crystalluria, 4) sterile urine, 5) normal serum biochemistry profile results, other than azotemia and hyperphosphatemia and 6) dachshund breed. All these findings are consistent with cystine uroliths.
2. Fluid therapy should be continued if azotemia persists. Urohydropropulsion can be repeated if urethral obstruction occurs again. Combined dietary and medical dissolution of canine cystine uroliths is accomplished by a combination of N-(2-mercaptopropionyl)-glycine (2-MPG[b]) and dietary management with a food that reduces urinary excretion of cystine, promotes formation of alkaline urine and reduces urinary concentration. A veterinary therapeutic food that closely matches the key nutritional factor recommendations for cystine dissolution/prevention was selected (Prescription Diet u/d Canine[c]). 2-MPG reduces the urine concentration of cystine by combining with cysteine to form cysteine-2-MPG, which is more soluble than cystine. In studies conducted at the University of Minnesota, mean dissolution time with this combination of therapy was 10 weeks (range two to 30 weeks). Drug-induced adverse events associated with 2-MPG are uncommon in dogs, but when they occur they include Coombs positive spherocytic anemia, thrombocytopenia and

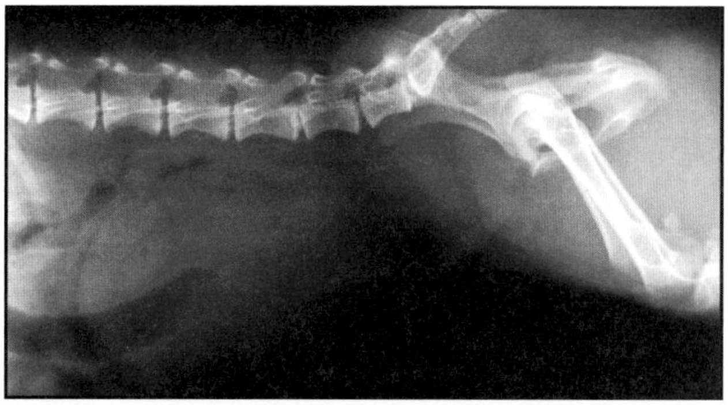

Figure 1. Survey abdominal radiograph of a four-year-old male dachshund illustrating marked distention of the urinary bladder. Two marginally radiodense urethroliths were located behind the os penis.

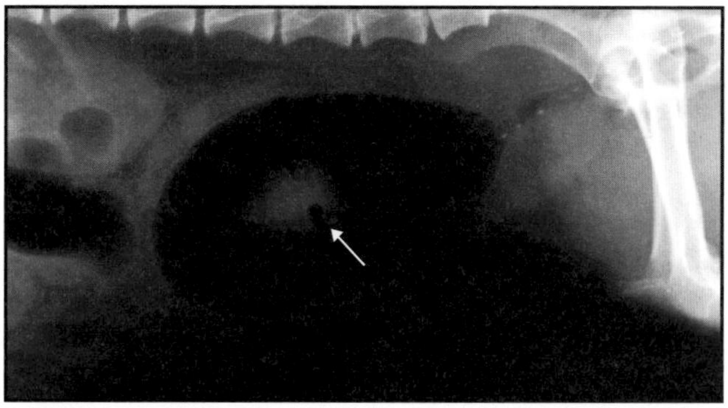

Figure 2. Double-contrast cystogram of the dog described in Figure 1. Three urocystoliths (arrow) can be seen surrounded by contrast media.

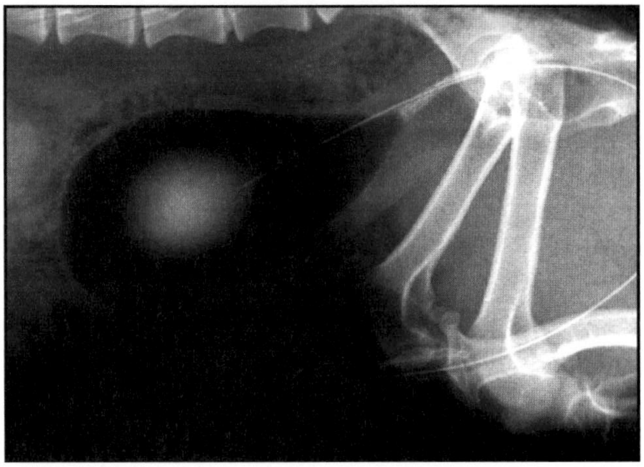

Figure 3. Double-contrast cystogram of the dog described in Figures 1 and 2 taken 40 days after initiation of therapy with 2-MPG and Prescription Diet u/d Canine. There are no uroliths in the bladder lumen. Contrast urethrography confirmed that there were no uroliths in the urethral lumen.

increased hepatic enzyme activity. Antibiotics should also be continued for at least 10 more days. The vitamin-mineral supplement is unnecessary and should be discontinued.

Progress Notes

The azotemia and hyperphosphatemia resolved by the second day of hospitalization, confirming their prerenal origin. The combination of amoxicillin and clavulanic acid was continued. The dog was released from the hospital with instructions for the owner to give 2-MPG at a dosage of 15 mg/kg body weight, per os, twice daily. The food was changed to moist Prescription Diet u/d Canine and the vitamin-mineral supplement was discontinued. Radiographs taken 40 days after initial hospitalization showed no evidence of uroliths (**Figure 3**). Urinalysis results included un-concentrated alkaline urine with amorphous crystals. The serum urea nitrogen concentration was 4 mg/dl, which confirmed that the low-protein food was being fed at home. 2-MPG was discontinued and Prescription Diet u/d Canine was continued. Examination 75 and 232 days after initial hospitalization revealed that the urine continued to be un-concentrated and alkaline with no evidence of crystalluria. The urea nitrogen concentration remained low (5 to 6 mg/dl), which indicated that the owner was compliant with the feeding plan.

Endnotes

a. Pfizer Animal Health, Exton, PA, USA.
b. Thiola. Mission Pharmacal, San Antonio, TX, USA.
c. Hill's Pet Nutrition, Inc., Topeka, KS, USA.

Bibliography

Osborne CA, Lulich JP, Bartges JW, et al. Canine and feline urolithiasis: Relationship of etiopathogenesis to treatment and prevention. In: Osborne CA, Finco DR, eds. Canine and Feline Nephrology and Urology. Baltimore, MD: Williams & Wilkins, 1995; 798-888.

Chapter 43

Canine Struvite Urolithiasis: Causes, Detection, Management and Prevention

Carl A. Osborne
Jody P. Lulich
Hasan Albasan
Laurie L. Swanson

"Diagnoses are often a matter of opinion rather than a matter of fact. It is one thing to make a diagnosis, and another thing to substantiate it."
Carl A. Osborne

PREVALENCE AND MINERAL COMPOSITION

Currently, the second most common type of mineral encountered in uroliths from dogs is magnesium ammonium phosphate (MAP) hexahydrate, also known as struvite (Figure 40-1 and Table 38-8). Struvite accounted for 43% of all canine uroliths submitted to the Minnesota Urolith Center from 2000 to 2006 and 39% (16,124 of 40,612) of all canine uroliths submitted during 2007. Struvite accounted for 26% of canine upper urinary tract uroliths analyzed at the Minnesota Urolith Center from 2000 to 2006 (Table 38-9).

Although urolithiasis is most commonly recognized in adult dogs, approximately 1.0% of the total canine uroliths analyzed at the Minnesota Urolith Center were obtained from dogs less than 12 months old. Of 800 uroliths retrieved from dogs less than one year of age, approximately 56% were struvite, 23% were purines (ammonium, sodium and calcium urate, uric acid), 8% were compound uroliths (minerals in the center of uroliths were different from minerals in outer layers), 5% were calcium oxalate, 4% were of mixed mineral composition, 2% were calcium phosphate, 2% were cystine and less than 1% were silica.

The mean age at the time of MAP retrieval from dogs was six years (range one month to 24 years). Females (85%) were affected more often than males (12%; 3% of affected breeds were of unknown gender). A total of 239 different breeds were affected, including mixed breeds (24%), Shih Tzus (11%), miniature schnauzers (9%), Bichon Frises (8%), pugs (4%), dachshunds (4%), Labrador retrievers (3%), miniature poodles (2%), Pekingese (2%), cocker spaniels (3%) and Lhasa apsos (2%). Struvite uroliths were more commonly removed from the lower urinary tract (99%) than the upper urinary tract (1%). They form in a variety of shapes and sizes (**Table 43-1**).

ETIOPATHOGENESIS AND RISK FACTORS

Infection-Induced Struvite Uroliths

Sequential Steps in Urolith Formation

Urine must be supersaturated with MAP hexahydrate for stru-

Table 43-1. Common characteristics of canine struvite uroliths.

Chemical name	Formula	Crystal name
Magnesium ammonium phosphate hexahydrate	$MgNH_4PO_4•6H_2O$	Struvite

Variations in mineral composition
Struvite only
Struvite mixed with lesser quantities of calcium apatite and/or ammonium acid urate
Nucleus of a different mineral surrounded by variable layers composed primarily of struvite. Small quantities of calcium apatite and/or ammonium acid urate also may be present.

Physical characteristics
Color: Struvite uroliths are usually white, cream or light brown. The surface of uroliths is commonly red because of concomitant hematuria and may be green due to bile pigments.
Shape: Variable. Solitary urocystoliths are commonly round or elliptic. Multiple urocystoliths may be any shape, but are often pyramidal. Rapidly growing uroliths with a large quantity of matrix may form a cast of the lumen (renal pelvis, ureter, bladder, urethra) in which they are formed.
Nuclei and laminations: Common in infection-induced uroliths
Density: Variable. Soft if they contain a large quantity of matrix. Dense and harder to cut if little matrix is present. A combination of hard and soft internal density may occur within the same urolith. Radiodense compared with non-skeletal tissue on survey radiographs. Degree of radiodensity is related to the quantity of matrix (inversely proportional) and other minerals, especially calcium apatite (more proportional).
Number: Single or multiple
Location: May be located in the kidney, ureter, urinary bladder and/or urethra. Most occur in the urinary bladder.
Size: Subvisual to a size limited by the capacity of the structure (kidney and urinary bladder) in which they form. Very large uroliths are often composed of struvite.

Predisposing factors
Urinary tract infections with urease-producing microbes in patients whose urine contains a large quantity of urea
Alkaline urinary pH
Unidentified factors

Characteristics of affected patients
Mean age: Six years (range = ≤1 to more than 24 years). Especially common in Shih Tzus, pugs, Bichon Frises, miniature schnauzers and dachshunds; however, any breed may be affected. More common in females (~85%) than males (~15%).

vite uroliths to form (Osborne et al, 1999). However, acidic urine from people and presumably dogs is normally undersaturated with respect to MAP (Elliot et al, 1958, 1959). Normally, physiologic concentrations of urine ammonium (NH_4^+) increase only when the kidneys excrete high concentrations of acid catabolites. The increase in urine concentration of ammonium in this situation represents a normal compensatory response by the renal tubular cells to secrete ammonia (NH_3) into the tubular lumen to reduce acidity by subsequent formation of ammonium.

Whereas ammonia is lipid soluble and can penetrate tubular cell walls, ammonium is lipid insoluble and cannot penetrate cell walls (so-called ion trapping). Likewise, excretion of alkaline urine under physiologic conditions is associated with reduced renal production of ammonia; thus the quantity of ammonium ions in urine is reduced. However, when urinary tract infections (UTIs) with urease-producing microbes occur in animals forming urine with a sufficient quantity of urea, the unique combination of concomitant elevation in the concentrations of ammonium and carbonate (CO_3^{2-}) in an alkaline en-

$$NH_2\text{-}\overset{O}{\overset{\|}{C}}\text{-}NH_2 + H_2O \xrightarrow{\text{urease}} 2NH_3 + CO_2$$

$$CO_2 + H_2O \leftrightarrow H_2CO_3 \leftrightarrow H^+ + HCO_3^- \leftrightarrow CO_3^{=}$$

$$NH_3 + H_2O \leftrightarrow NH_4^+ + OH^-$$

Figure 43-1. Illustration of factors leading to formation of struvite, calcium apatite and carbonate apatite as a consequence of degradation of urea by microbial urease. See text below for details.

vironment may develop. These conditions favor formation of uroliths containing struvite [$MgNH_4PO_4•6H_2O$], calcium apatite [$Ca_{10}(PO_4)_6(OH)_2$] and carbonate apatite [$Ca_{10}(PO_4CO_3OH_4)_6(OH)_2$] (**Figure 43-1**). The following mechanisms are involved (Osborne et al, 1999). First, urease (a metalloenzyme containing nickel) produced by some types of bacteria or ureaplasmas hydrolyze one molecule of urea to form two molecules of ammonia and one molecule of carbon dioxide. Second, the ammonia molecules react spontaneously with water to form ammonium and hydroxyl ions (pK of NH_3 = 9.03), which alkalinize urine by reducing hydrogen ion concentration. The solubility of struvite and calcium apatite decreases in alkaline urine (Hedelin et al, 1984). In addition to alkalinization of urine, the newly generated ammonium ions are available for formation of MAP crystals. Third, the newly generated molecules of carbon dioxide combine with water to form carbonic acid, which in turn dissociates to form bicarbonate (pK = 6.33) and hydrogen ions. In an extremely alkaline environment, bicarbonate may lose its proton to become carbonate (pK = 10.1). Carbonate anions may displace phosphate anions in calcium apatite crystals to form carbonate apatite crystals. Fourth, in the progressively alkaline environment induced by microbial hydrolysis of urea, dissociation of monobasic hydrogen phosphate (H_2PO^{4-}) results in an increased concentration of dibasic hydrogen phosphate ($H_2PO_4^{2-}$) and anionic phosphate (PO_4^{3-}). Given a constant concentration of total phosphate, a change in pH from 6.8 to 7.4 increases the PO_4^{3-} concentration by a factor of approximately 6 (Burns and Finlayson, 1982). Anionic phosphate is then available in increased quantities to combine with magnesium and ammonium to form struvite or with calcium to form calcium apatite. Fifth, ammonium ions may combine with urates to form ammonium urate (Garcia de la Pena and Cifuentes Delatte, 1981; He et al, 1984).

Both urea (molecular weight = 60 daltons) and urease (molecular weight = 483,000 daltons) are required for ammonia production, alkalinization, supersaturation and subsequent precipitation of struvite, calcium apatite and carbonate apatite crystals. The majority of urea in urine originates from dietary protein (Abdullahi et al, 1984), whereas the urease in vertebrates must be derived from microbes (some bacteria, some yeasts or ureaplasmas) (Delluva et al, 1968; Griffith and Klein, 1983; Kornberg et al, 1954; Levenson et al, 1959). The high

Table 43-2. Some potential risk factors for canine infection-induced struvite uroliths.

Diet	Urine	Patient/metabolic	Drugs
High protein content (source of urea)	Urease-positive UTI	Females	Glucocorticoid-associated bacterial UTI
Urine alkalinizing potential	High urea concentration	Breeds	
High phosphorus content	Hyperammonuria	Miniature schnauzers	
High magnesium content	High-ionic phosphorus concentration	Bichon Frises	
	High magnesium levels	Shih Tzus	
	High pH	Pugs	
	Urine retention	Dachshunds	
	Concentration of urine and thus lithogenic substances	Hyperadrenocorticism associated with bacterial UTI	

Key: UTI = urinary tract infection.

concentration of urea normally present in urine of individuals that consume dietary protein in excess of the daily requirement for protein anabolism makes urine an environment well suited to support the pathogenic effects of urease-producing microbes. Because of the importance of urease in the etiopathogenesis of struvite urolithiasis in people and many other animals, the name "urease stones" has been proposed (Griffith, 1978). Following a parallel line of reasoning in context of pathophysiologic events, the name "urea stones" would also be appropriate (Osborne et al, 1985).

Continued production of ammonia and perhaps other toxic reactants as a consequence of urease-induced ureolysis appears to induce an inflammatory response in the urothelium and adjacent structures (Griffith, 1978a; Krawiec et al, 1984, 1984a). In fact, urease production contributes to the virulence of uropathogens that produce this enzyme (Brande and Siemienski, 1960; MacLaren, 1968; Parsons et al, 1984; Rosenstein and Hamilton-Miller, 1984). The associated increase in urine concentration of proteinaceous inflammatory products acts as a form of matrix and contributes to lithogenesis.

Another mechanism that has been hypothesized to predispose patients with UTIs to urolithiasis is a bacteria-mediated reduction in the urine concentration of citrate (Conway et al, 1949; Robertson and Peacock, 1982; Scott et al, 1943). Citrate is often called a crystallization inhibitor because it can combine with cations such as calcium and magnesium to increase their solubility (Schwille et al, 1979). It has also been suggested that bacteria may produce lithogenic matrix substances (Stegmayr and Stegmayr, 1983).

Bacterial UTIs

Clinical and non-clinical studies involving dogs have repeatedly demonstrated a close relationship between formation of struvite uroliths and UTIs caused by urease-producing bacteria (Osborne et al, 1999). Bacterial UTIs have been such a common finding in dogs with struvite uroliths that they are sometimes called infection stones (Griffith, 1978; Osborne et al, 1981).

Several in vitro observations indicate that bacterial urease-induced supersaturation of urine with MAP is the primary (but not necessarily the only) cause of infection-induced struvite uroliths (Griffith, 1978; Griffith et al, 1976; Griffith and Musher, 1975). First, growth of urease-producing *Proteus* spp. in urea-free urine, or in urine containing a urease inhibitor, did not cause alkalinization, supersaturation or crystallization of struvite and apatite. Second, growth of weak urease-producing bacteria (*Klebsiella* spp. and *Pseudomonas* spp.) and non-urease-producing bacteria (*Escherichia* spp.) was not associated with alkalinization, supersaturation and subsequent precipitation of struvite and apatite crystals.

Staphylococcus and *Proteus* spp. are consistent and potent urease producers and have been commonly isolated from animals and people with infection-induced struvite uroliths (Griffith, 1978, 1978a; Osborne et al, 1981). For unexplained reasons, staphylococci have been more commonly associated with struvite uroliths in dogs than *Proteus* spp., whereas *Proteus* spp. are more commonly associated with struvite uroliths in people (Osborne et al, 1999; Griffith and Klein, 1983; Feit and Fair, 1979; Krajden et al, 1984; Lewis et al, 1984; Stamey, 1980). It appears that some strains of *Proteus mirabilis* have special affinity for the urinary tract of people (Senior, 1979). In pilot studies involving dogs at the University of Minnesota, better success occurred in inducing struvite uroliths with clinical isolates of staphylococci than with *Proteus* spp. Results of studies in rats were interpreted to indicate that different strains of staphylococci had different lithogenic potential (Vermeulen and Goetz, 1954).

Although other organisms such as *Klebsiella* and *Pseudomonas* spp. have potential to produce varying quantities of urease (Griffith, 1978), they have not been as commonly associated with initiation of struvite urolith formation in people or dogs. Likewise, *E. coli* and other non-urease-producing microbes have not been linked to naturally occurring struvite uroliths, presumably because they infrequently produce urease (Griffith, 1978; Lesher and Jones, 1978). However, it has been reported that urease activity may be transferred by bacterial plasmids (Grant et al, 1981).

The bacterial flora of urine may change after formation of struvite uroliths in dogs as a result of staphylococcal UTI. The change in bacterial flora may be associated with damage to local host defense mechanisms by uroliths, iatrogenic infection induced by urinary catheters or administration of antimicrobial agents.

A very small percentage of dogs with struvite uroliths have

Table 43-3. Key nutritional factors for dissolution and prevention of canine struvite uroliths.

Factors	Dietary recommendations
Water	Water intake should be encouraged to achieve urine specific gravity <1.020 Moist food will increase water consumption and formation of less concentrated urine
Protein	Avoid excess dietary protein Dissolution: restrict dietary protein to ≤8%, dry matter (DM) Prevention: restrict dietary protein to <25% DM
Phosphorus	Avoid excess dietary phosphorus Dissolution: restrict dietary phosphorus to ≤0.1% DM Prevention: restrict dietary phosphorus to <0.6% DM
Magnesium	Avoid excess dietary magnesium Dissolution: restrict dietary magnesium to <0.02% DM Prevention: restrict dietary magnesium to 0.04 to 0.1% DM
Urinary pH	Feed a food that maintains an acidic urine Dissolution: urinary pH = 5.9 to 6.1 Prevention: urinary pH = 6.2 to 6.4

sterile urine. In some of these cases, however, urease-forming bacteria have been isolated from the inside of uroliths even though the urine surrounding the uroliths was sterile. This observation indicates that bacterial infection of the urinary tract may undergo spontaneous remission after initiating urolith formation in some patients. Bacteria that become trapped within struvite uroliths may remain viable for long periods. Several studies have revealed that lithogenic bacteria harbored within uroliths are protected from the destructive effects of antimicrobial agents in urine by biofilms (Nikkila et al, 1989; Fowler, 1984; Nemoy and Stamey, 1971; Rocha and Santos, 1969; Takeuchi et al, 1984).

In contrast to struvite uroliths, bacterial infection of the urinary tract is not a consistent finding in dogs with non-struvite uroliths (ammonium urate, calcium oxalate, cystine, silica, etc.). When infection does occur in association with these so-called metabolic uroliths, it appears to be a sequela rather than a predisposing cause of urolith formation.

Ureaplasma UTIs

Ueaplasmas differ from all other mycoplasmas because they produce urease and, therefore, hydrolyze urea (Ford and MacDonald, 1967; Shepard and Lunceford, 1967). Urea is required for growth of these organisms. Ureaplasmas were recognized as etiologic agents in struvite urolithiasis when struvite uroliths were rapidly produced in male rat urinary bladders by intrarenal or intravesical injection of urease-producing ureaplasmas isolated from people (Friedlander and Braude, 1974; Lamm et al, 1977).

Ureaplasma urealyticum has been isolated from struvite uroliths removed from the renal pelves of people (Hedelin et al, 1984; Pettersson et al, 1983). However, ureaplasmas could not be isolated from nephroliths composed of calcium oxalate, calcium phosphate or uric acid. Large numbers of ureaplasmas were isolated from an adult female basset hound with uroliths presumed to be composed of struvite and located in the renal pelves and urinary bladder.[a] Although the urine from this dog contained urease, urease-producing bacteria could not be isolated from it.

Efforts at the University of Minnesota to isolate ureaplasmas from urine of other dogs with nonbacterial struvite uroliths have been unsuccessful. Further studies are necessary, however, because ureaplasmas are fastidious and cell associated. Factors reported to limit growth of ureaplasmas in broth cultures include pH values greater than 7.5 (Ford and MacDonald, 1967; Shepard and Lunceford, 1967), osmotic activity more than 600 mOsm/kg (Kenney and Cartwright, 1977) and a high ammonia concentration (Rosenstein and Hamilton-Miller, 1984; Ford and MacDonald, 1967).

Food

The quantity of dietary protein catabolized for energy influences formation and dissolution of infection-induced struvite uroliths. Consumption of dietary protein in quantities that exceed daily protein requirements for anabolism results in formation of urea from catabolism of amino acids. Hyperammonuria, hypercarbonaturia and alkaluria mediated by microbial urease are influenced by the quantity of urea (the substrate of urease) in urine (**Table 43-2**).

Abnormal urinary excretion of minerals as a result of enhanced glomerular filtration rate, reduced tubular reabsorption or enhanced tubular secretion is not required for initiation and growth of infection-induced uroliths.

Genetics

The high incidence of struvite urolithiasis in some breeds of dogs such as miniature schnauzers suggests a familial tendency (**Table 43-2**). Susceptible miniature schnauzers apparently inherit some abnormality of local host defenses of the urinary tract that increases their susceptibility to UTIs (Klausner et al, 1980, 1980a). Hereditary factors thought to be associated with inbreeding have been reported to increase the incidence of struvite uroliths in beagles (Kasper et al, 1978). The incidence of struvite uroliths was 10.7% in an inbred line vs. only 2.0% in an outbred line of beagles.

Sterile Struvite Uroliths

Clinical studies indicate that microbial urease is not involved in formation of struvite uroliths in some dogs (Bovee and McGuire, 1984; Osborne et al, 1985, 1999). Several observations suggest that dietary or metabolic factors may be involved in the genesis of sterile struvite uroliths. Pilot studies involving clinical cases of struvite uroliths in dogs at the University of Minnesota revealed a population of patients (nine of 20) whose urine was frequently alkaline but did not contain identifiable bacteria or detectable quantities of urease. Microscopic examination of demineralized, gram-stained sections of some struvite uroliths removed from dogs with bacteriologically sterile urine did not reveal gram-positive bacteria (Clark, 1974).[a] Whereas infection-induced struvite uroliths from people frequently contain calcium apatite or carbonate apatite, a substantial number of the canine sterile uroliths were 100% struvite.

Recurrent urocystoliths apparently composed of sterile struvite were encountered at the University of Minnesota in three related English cocker spaniels: a sire and two of its male offspring from different dams (Bartges et al, 1992). These dogs were followed for several years and had several episodes of struvite urocystolithiasis associated with alkaluria, but not with bacterial UTI, urinary urease enzyme activity or renal tubular acidosis (RTA). Since that time, other investigators have also observed sterile struvite urocystoliths in English cocker spaniel dogs (Lees et al, 1998).

Although struvite is less soluble in alkaline than acidic urine, the mechanism(s) of sterile struvite urolith formation in dogs is unclear. Under physiologic conditions associated with alkaluria, urine contains low concentrations of ammonia (and thus ammonium ions) (Tannen, 1983). Therefore, alkaline urine formed in the absence of ureolysis would not be expected to favor formation of crystals that contain ammonium ions (e.g., MAP hexahydrate). Clinical studies of naturally occurring urolithiasis in people support this generality (Griffith and Klein, 1983).

Formation of persistently alkaline urine in the absence of urease-mediated ureolysis may predispose patients to formation of uroliths containing hydroxyapatite [$Ca_{10}(PO_4)_6(OH)_2$] but not carbonate apatite. Pathologic conditions that may result in this sequence of events include distal RTA (Coe and Flavus, 1991), incomplete distal RTA (Backman et al, 1981) and perhaps primary hyperparathyroidism (Coe and Flavus, 1991; Klausner et al, 1987). Because alkaline urine favors dissociation of monobasic phosphate ($H_2PO_4^-$) to dibasic phosphate (HPO_4^{2-}) and phosphate ion (PO_4^{3-}), formation of calcium phosphate is enhanced. Patients with distal RTA have impaired ability to acidify urine associated with hypercalciuria and excretion of reduced concentration of urine citrate (Coe and Flavus, 1991; Dedmond and Wrong, 1962; Morrissey et al, 1963; Thornhill, 1977).

BIOLOGIC BEHAVIOR

Struvite uroliths can rapidly form (within two to eight weeks) after infection with urease-producing staphylococci (Klausner et al, 1980, 1980a). Struvite urocystoliths associated with UTI caused by staphylococci or *Proteus* spp. have been detected in puppies as young as five weeks of age (Hardy et al, 1972).

Spontaneous dissolution of uroliths appears to be uncommon. Five cases (two nephroliths and three urocystoliths) of struvite urolithiasis in dogs have been observed in which uroliths underwent spontaneous dissolution (Klausner and Osborne, 1979). Others have also reported spontaneous dissolution of canine nephroliths (Kirby et al, 1980). Bilateral nephroliths were reported to exist for about four years in a miniature schnauzer before causing death from renal failure (Pollack and Wagner, 1976). Urocystoliths frequently pass into the urethra. In male dogs, they commonly lodge behind the os penis, but in female dogs they are frequently voided. Small nephroliths may pass into the ureters. The rapid rates at which struvite uroliths form and the potential they have to migrate to lower portions of the urinary tract are of clinical importance. If several days have elapsed between the date of diagnostic imaging and the date scheduled to remove uroliths, the number and location of uroliths should be reevaluated by radiography or other suitable imaging technique.

Struvite uroliths have a tendency to recur after surgical removal or dietary and medical dissolution (Brown et al, 1977; Kasper et al, 1978; Brodey, 1955). Miniature schnauzers have been observed with at least seven known recurrences following surgery. However, many episodes of multiple recurrences have been associated with lack of removal of all uroliths at the time of surgery (pseudo-recurrence), and poor control of recurrent UTI with urease-producing microbes. With the advent of effective therapeutic and preventive antimicrobial protocols to control recurrent or persistent UTI, the frequency of recurrent infection-induced struvite urolithiasis in dogs has markedly declined. Multiple recurrences of sterile struvite uroliths have been observed in dogs, presumably because the underlying mechanisms causing their formation persisted following dietary and medical dissolution or surgical removal.

The rate of recurrence following dietary and medical dissolution of canine struvite uroliths is less frequent than that associated with surgery. In addition, time elapsed between recurrent episodes is longer following dietary and medical dissolution. The apparent higher rate of recurrence associated with surgical removal of uroliths may be associated with inability to remove all uroliths, especially those located in inaccessible sites or those that are subvisual. The tendency for uroliths to recur after surgery may also be associated with persistence of an environment that favors initiation and growth of struvite at the time of removal.

KEY NUTRITIONAL FACTORS

Urine must be saturated with magnesium, ammonium and phosphate for struvite uroliths to form (Osborne et al, 1999). However, as described above, the process is complex, including multiple interactions. Altering nutrient levels and specific food ingredients can modify several of these interactions, which are reflected in the following key nutritional factors for dissolution and prevention of struvite uroliths. **Table 43-3** summarizes these key nutritional factors.

Water

Increasing urine volume is an effective means of reducing the urinary concentration of urolith constituents. One way to increase urine volume is to increase the water content of the food. Total water intake increases as the moisture content of the food increases. Therefore, consumption of moist foods, which generally contain between 75 to 80% water, effectively increases urine volume. Foods can also be supplemented with sodium chloride to stimulate thirst and induce compensatory polyuria. However, the risks and benefits of adding sodium chloride should be considered in each individual patient, especially those with comorbid diseases that may be aggravated by excessive dietary sodium.

Dietary protein restriction can also increase urine volume by contributing to obligatory polyuria due to a decrease in renal medullary urea concentration resulting from a reduction of hepatic urea production. (See below.)

As a generality, as long as the struvite uroliths are present in the urinary tract, water intake should be encouraged with the goal of promoting a urine specific gravity <1.020.

Protein

The quantity of dietary protein catabolized for energy can influence formation and dissolution of infection-induced struvite uroliths. Consumption of dietary protein in quantities that exceed daily protein requirements results in increased formation of urea due to the deamination of the excess amino acids so that they can be used for energy. The majority of urea in urine originates from dietary protein (Abdullahi et al, 1984). Urease in vertebrates must be derived from microbes (some bacteria, some yeasts or ureaplasmas) (Delluva et al, 1968; Griffith and Klein, 1983; Kornberg et al, 1954; Levenson et al, 1959).

If patients have urinary tract infections caused by urease-producing microbes, and their urine contains a sufficient quantity of urea (the substrate of urease), the result is a unique combination of concomitant high urinary concentrations of ammonium and carbonate in an alkaline environment. These conditions favor formation of struvite (and calcium apatite and carbonate apatite) (**Table 43-2**). One goal of dietary management for patients with infected struvite uroliths is to reduce urinary concentration of urea.

Studies indicate that protein restriction is not essential for dissolution of canine sterile struvite uroliths (Boistelle et al, 1984). High ammonia concentrations were not necessary for formation of struvite crystals provided the concentration of (Mg) x (NH_4) x (PO_4) was of sufficient magnitude at a given pH. Corresponding in vivo studies in dogs have not been performed, but it is probable that similar observations would occur.

Acidification of urine to approximately 6.0 has been effective in promoting sterile struvite urolith dissolution (Osborne et al, 1987). In this respect, canine struvite uroliths are similar to feline sterile struvite uroliths. Dietary protein restriction has the additional advantage of contributing to obligatory polyuria by decreasing renal medullary urea concentration and thus enhancing the rate of sterile struvite urolith dissolution.

The minimum recommended allowance for protein in foods for adult dogs is 10% for foods providing 4 kcal/g dry matter (DM); the minimum requirement is 8% DM (NRC, 2006). For dissolution of struvite uroliths, high quality dietary protein should be restricted to 8% or less DM. For prevention of struvite uroliths, food protein content should be less than 25% DM.

Foods high in protein are generally high in phosphorus unless special ingredients are used in their formulation.

Phosphorus

Abnormal urinary excretion of minerals is not required for initiation and growth of infection-induced struvite uroliths. However, phosphate concentrations in dog urine relate directly to the amount of phosphorus consumed in food (Morris and Doering, 1978).

Although not validated by experimental or clinical studies in dogs, foods high in phosphorus (and magnesium) would be expected to predispose susceptible dogs to sterile struvite urolith formation. In vitro studies in which magnesium (in the form of $MgSO_4$), ammonium (in the form of ammonium of NH_4Cl) or phosphate (as $NH_4H_2PO_4$ or NaH_2PO_4) added to sterile human urine (ranging in pH from 5.0 to 9.6) revealed that struvite crystals could be induced to form in an acidic or an alkaline environment (Boistelle et al, 1984). It is probable that similar observations would occur in dog studies.

The minimum recommended allowance for phosphorus in foods for adult dogs is 0.3% DM (NRC, 2006). The recommended level for phosphorus in foods for dissolution of struvite uroliths should not exceed 0.1% DM. Patients consuming foods with this level of phosphorus could possibly be in negative phosphorus balance for the relatively short period of time they need to be fed a dissolution food. An older study noted that puppies fed a purified food containing 0.11% DM phosphorus from age two months through adulthood (age 34 months) had equivalent performance compared to dogs fed the same food with 0.63% DM phosphorus (Gershoff et al, 1958). Struvite dissolution using a food containing 0.1% DM phosphorus has been safely accomplished in puppies (Osborne et al, 1986; Lulich et al, 1989). For prevention of recurrence of struvite uroliths, phosphorus levels should be less than 0.6% DM.

As discussed above, urinary phosphate can exist in several states. Anionic phosphate is the important form in either the precipitation or dissolution of struvite. Furthermore, as discussed above, urinary concentration of anionic phosphate is reversibly influenced by pH.

Magnesium

Abnormal urinary excretion of minerals as a result of enhanced glomerular filtration rate, reduced tubular reabsorption or enhanced tubular secretion is not required for initiation and growth of infection-induced uroliths. Apparently, however, for sterile struvite precipitates to form, excess dietary magnesium would be required (Boistelle et al, 1984). Avoiding excessive dietary magnesium can reduce the urinary concentration of magnesium (Morris and Doering, 1978).

The minimum requirement for magnesium in foods for healthy adult dogs is 0.018% DM; whereas the minimum rec-

Table 43-4. Summary of recommendations for dietary and medical dissolution of canine struvite uroliths.

1. Adult dogs with urinary tract infection (UTI)
   a. Perform appropriate diagnostic studies including complete urinalysis, quantitative urine culture and diagnostic imaging. Determine precise location, size and number of uroliths. The size and number of uroliths are not a reliable index of probable therapeutic efficacy.
   b. If uroliths are available, determine their mineral composition. If unavailable, determine their composition by evaluation of appropriate clinical data.
   c. Consider lithotripsy or surgical correction if urethroliths obstruct urine outflow. Consider surgery if correctable abnormalities predisposing the patient to recurrent UTIs are identified by diagnostic imaging or other means. Small urocystoliths may be removed by voiding urohydropropulsion (Figure 38-5 and Table 38-7) or lithotripsy.
   d. Eradicate or control UTIs with appropriate antimicrobial agents. Maintain full-dose antimicrobial therapy during and for three to four weeks after urolith dissolution.
   e. Initiate therapy with litholytic foods. Other foods or mineral supplements should not be fed to the patient. Compliance with dietary recommendations is suggested by a reduction in urea nitrogen concentration (usually <10 mg/dl).
   f. Devise a protocol to monitor efficacy of therapy.
      1) Try to avoid diagnostic followup studies that require urinary tract catheterization. If they are required, give appropriate pericatheterization antimicrobial agents to prevent iatrogenic UTIs.
      2) Perform serial urinalyses. Determination of urinary pH and specific gravity and microscopic examination of sediment for crystals are especially important. Remember, crystals formed in urine stored at room or refrigeration temperatures may represent in vitro artifacts.
      3) Perform serial imaging monthly to evaluate urolith location(s), number, size, density and shape.
      4) If necessary, perform quantitative urine cultures. They are especially important in patients infected before therapy and in patients catheterized during therapy.
      5) Feed patients a litholytic food for one month following disappearance of uroliths as detected by survey radiography.
      6) Consider alternative methods if uroliths increase in size during dietary management, or do not begin to decrease in size after four to eight weeks of appropriate dietary and medical management. Difficulty in inducing complete dissolution of uroliths by creating urine that is undersaturated with the suspected lithogenic crystalloids should prompt consideration that: a) the wrong mineral component was identified, b) the nucleus of the uroliths is of different mineral composition than other portions of the urolith (i.e., a compound urolith) and/or c) the client or the patient is not complying with dietary and medical recommendations.
   g. Consider administration of acetohydroxamic acid (25 mg/kg body weight/day divided into two equal doses) to patients with persistent uroliths and persistent urease-producing microburia despite the use of antimicrobial agents and litholytic foods.
2. Adult dogs with persistently sterile urine
   a. Follow the protocol described above, but do not administer antimicrobial agents or acetohydroxamic acid.
   b. Periodically culture urine specimens obtained by cystocentesis to detect secondary UTIs. Initiate antimicrobial therapy if a UTI develops.
   c. Monitor urinary pH with a reliable pH meter. Monitor urine specific gravity with a reliable refractometer. Evaluate urine sediment for evidence of calcium oxalate, calcium phosphate and/or struvite crystalluria.
3. Immature dogs
   a. Use caution when feeding protein-restricted foods to growing dogs.
   b. Short-term therapy with litholytic foods has been effective in dissolving struvite urocystoliths. If initiated, monitor the patient for evidence of nutritional deficiencies (especially protein-calorie malnutrition).
   c. Acetohydroxamic acid has not been evaluated in growing dogs.
   d. Small urocystoliths may be removed by voiding urohydropropulsion (Figure 38-5 and Table 38-7) or lithotripsy. Pending further studies, surgery remains the safest means of removing large uroliths from immature dogs.

ommended allowance is 0.06% DM (NRC, 2006). For dissolution of struvite uroliths, the recommendation for magnesium in food is less than 0.02% DM. The recommendation for prevention of recurrence is 0.04 to 0.1% DM.

Urinary pH

Urinary pH can affect the concentration of important struvite constituents, including anionic phosphate (PO_4^{3-}). As discussed above, as urine becomes more acidic, anionic phosphate is converted to monobasic hydrogen phosphate (H_2PO^{4-}) and dibasic hydrogen phosphate ($H_2PO_4^{2-}$), thereby reducing the concentration of anionic phosphate for incorporation into struvite precipitates. Conversely, as urine becomes more alkaline, the reaction proceeds in the opposite direction and anionic phosphate is then available in increased quantities to combine with magnesium and ammonium to form struvite. Given a constant concentration of total phosphate, a change in pH from 6.8 to 7.4 increases the PO_4^{3-} concentration by a factor of approximately 6 (Burns and Finlayson, 1982).

Urinary tract infections caused by urease-producing microbes can modify urinary pH and anionic phosphate concentration. In the progressively alkaline environment induced by microbial hydrolysis of urea, dissociation of monobasic hydrogen phosphate results in an increased concentration of dibasic hydrogen phosphate and anionic phosphate.

In sterile urine, pH also influences the concentration of ammonium ions (NH_4^+), but in the opposite direction of anionic phosphate. In acidic urine, ammonia (NH_3) combines with hydrogen ions to form ammonium, a struvite constituent. The resolution of this seeming paradox results from the fact that the effect of acidic urine on anionic phosphate concentration is greater than its effect on ammonium; the net effect of urine acidification is a reduction in the likelihood of formation of struvite precipitates. Acidification of urine to approximately 6.0 has been effective in promoting sterile struvite urolith dissolution (Osborne et al, 1987). In this respect, canine sterile struvite uroliths are similar to feline sterile struvite uroliths.

However, if patients have UTIs caused by urease-producing

microbes, and their urine contains a sufficient quantity of urea (See Protein, above.), the result is a unique combination of concomitant high urinary concentrations of ammonium and carbonate in an alkaline environment, further contributing to the likelihood of formation of struvite precipitates.

Urinary pH can be modified by food ingredients and by feeding method. (See Feeding Methods, below.) The target urinary pH range for dissolution of struvite uroliths is 5.9 to 6.1. The target urinary pH range for prevention of recurrence of struvite is 6.2 to 6.4.

FEEDING PLAN

Current recommendations for dietary and medical dissolution of canine struvite uroliths include: 1) eradication or control of UTI (if present), 2) use of litholytic foods and 3) administration of urease inhibitors (acetohydroxamic acid) to patients if struvite uroliths persist because of persistent UTI caused by urease-producing microbes (**Table 43-4**). **Table 43-4** also summarizes the overall dietary/medical/surgical management of struvite urolithiasis in adult dogs with a UTI, adult dogs with sterile urine and immature dogs.

Assess and Select the Food: Struvite Dissolution

Table 43-5 lists commercially available litholytic foods and compares their key nutritional factor content with the recommended levels of key nutritional factors. Select a food that most closely matches the recommended key nutritional factors and/or has the best efficacy evidence. Avoid treats and vitamin-mineral supplements.

Encouraging water consumption is recommended. If possible, feed a moist food. Although understandably difficult to accomplish in some patients, fluid intake should be encouraged throughout the day to help promote a constantly high urine volume. Ensure water is readily available and is neither too cold nor too warm.

Certain nutrients in properly formulated canine litholytic foods are very restricted (See Key Nutritional Factors, above.); nutrient levels are near the minimum requirements for the majority of the dog population. For some patients, these foods may only be marginally adequate. As a result, serum biochemistry profiles of patients undergoing dietary dissolution of struvite uroliths may be altered. Consumption of a struvite litholytic food by dogs with induced staphylococcal UTIs and struvite uroliths was associated with a marked reduction in the serum concentration of urea nitrogen and mild reductions in the serum concentrations of magnesium, phosphorus and albumin (Abdullahi et al, 1984). A mild increase in the serum activity of hepatic alkaline phosphatase was also observed. These alterations in serum chemistry values were of no clinical consequence during six-month experimental studies or during clinical studies. However, they underscore the fact that struvite litholytic foods are designed for short-term (weeks to months) dissolution therapy rather than long-term (months to years) prophylactic therapy.

The anticipated reduction of serum urea nitrogen in such patients can be useful. Appropriate reduction in concentrations of serum urea nitrogen obtained while the patient is eating a properly formulated struvite litholytic food compared to values obtained while the patient was eating a maintenance food may be used as one index of client and patient compliance with dietary management (**Table 43-6**).

Another criterion for selecting a food that may become increasingly important in the future is evidence-based clinical nutrition. Practitioners should know how to determine risks and benefits of nutritional regimens and counsel pet owners accordingly. Currently, veterinary medical education and continuing education are not always based on rigorous assessment of evidence for or against particular management options. Still, studies have been published to establish the nutritional benefits of certain pet foods. Chapter 2 describes evidence-based clinical nutrition in detail and applies its concepts to various veterinary therapeutic foods.

Precautions with Litholytic Foods

There are several points to consider when feeding struvite litholytic foods. These include affected puppies and adult patients with certain medical conditions. Besides the benefits of feeding litholytic foods, there are also risks for certain patients. Not all patients are candidates for dietary dissolution. Included are patients with abnormal fluid retention, azotemic primary renal failure and patients at risk for pancreatitis. Benefits and risks of litholytic foods should be considered and discussed with the client if these health problems coexist in dogs with struvite uroliths, or if risk factors for their development are present. During such discussions with clients, avoid making "all or none" and "always or never" statements because risk factor associations are not synonymous with cause and effect relationships.

IMMATURE DOGS

Struvite urocystoliths can be successfully dissolved in immature dogs (**Table 43-4**). One such case involved a 12-week-old female miniature dachshund with a sterile struvite urocystolith (Osborne et al, 1986[a]). The urocystolith was dissolved within two weeks after feeding was begun with a struvite litholytic food. Another dog was a nine-week-old, male, mixed-breed puppy with a vesicourachal diverticulum, urethral stricture, *Staphylococcus intermedius* UTI and multiple struvite urocystoliths (Lulich et al, 1989). These urocystoliths dissolved within nine days of initiation of therapy with the litholytic food and a combination of amoxicillin and clavulanic acid. The food was discontinued on Day 10. Slight reductions in serum albumin concentration (from approximately 3.2 to 2.7 g/dl) were observed in both dogs during the two weeks of dietary therapy. Serum albumin concentrations returned to reference values soon after the puppies resumed eating a normal growth food.

Based on uncontrolled clinical experience, litholytic foods should not be fed to immature dogs with struvite uroliths for more than two weeks. If circumstances warrant that the food be fed for longer periods, serial monitoring of body weight,

Table 43-5. Key nutritional factors in selected commercial veterinary therapeutic foods used for dissolution of struvite uroliths in dogs compared to recommended levels.*

Dry foods	Protein (%)	Phosphorus (%)	Magnesium (%)	Urinary pH**
Recommended levels	**≤8**	**≤0.1**	**<0.02**	**5.9-6.1**
Royal Canin Veterinary Diet Control Formula	23.9	0.84	0.130	6.0-6.3
Royal Canin Veterinary Diet Urinary SO 14	17.0	0.63	0.066	5.5-6.0
Moist foods	**Protein (%)**	**Phosphorus (%)**	**Magnesium (%)**	**Urinary pH****
Recommended levels	**≤8**	**≤0.1**	**<0.02**	**5.9-6.1**
Hill's Prescription Diet s/d Canine	7.9	0.10	0.024	5.935
Royal Canin Veterinary Diet Control Formula	22.8	0.66	0.078	6.0-6.3
Royal Canin Veterinary Diet Urinary SO	18.5	0.86	0.059	5.5-6.0

*Manufacturers' published values; nutrients expressed on a dry matter basis; moist foods are best.
**Protocols for measuring urinary pH may vary.

Table 43-6. Characteristic clinical findings before and after initiation of dietary and medical therapy, or dietary therapy alone, to dissolve struvite uroliths in nonazotemic dogs.*

Factors	Pre-therapy	During therapy	After successful therapy**
Polyuria	±	1+ to 3+	Negative
Pollakiuria	1+ to 4+	Transient ↑; subsequent ↓	Negative
Gross hematuria	0 to 4+	↓ by 5 to 10 days	Negative
Abnormal urine odor	0 to 4+	↓ by 5 to 10 days	Negative
Small uroliths voided	±	Common in females	Negative
Urine specific gravity	Variable	1.004 to 1.014	Normal
Urinary pH	≥7	Decreased (usually acidic)	Variable
Urine protein	1+ to 4+	Decreased to absent	Negative
Urine RBC	1+ to 4+	Decreased to absent	Negative
Urine WBC	1+ to 4+	Decreased to absent	Negative
Struvite crystals	0 to 4+	Usually absent	Variable
Other crystals	Variable	May persist	May persist
Bacteriuria	0 to 4+	Decreased to absent	Negative
Quantitative bacterial urine culture	0 to 4+	Decreased to absent	Negative
Serum urea nitrogen	>15 mg/dl	<10 mg/dl	Dependent on food
Serum creatinine	Normal	Normal	Normal
Serum alkaline phosphatase	Normal	↑ by 2 to 5 times	Normal
Serum albumin	Normal	↓ by 0.5 to 1 g/dl	Normal
Serum phosphorus	Normal	Slight decrease	Normal
Urolith size (radiographic)	Small to large	Progressive decrease	Negative
Hemogram	Normal	Normal	Normal

*For dogs with urinary tract infection, therapy consists of a litholytic food and antimicrobial agents. For dogs without urinary tract infection, therapy consists of a litholytic food.
**All forms of therapy withdrawn.

body condition, serum albumin concentration and packed cell volume for evidence of protein-calorie malnutrition should be considered. Adjustments in dietary management should be made if marked reductions in these variables are observed. The urocystoliths may be removed by voiding urohydropropulsion (Figure 38-5 and Table 38-7) or lithotripsy, if their size has been reduced enough to permit their passage pass through a distended urethra (Lulich et al, 1993).

ABNORMAL FLUID RETENTION

Properly formulated struvite litholytic foods are restricted in protein and supplemented with sodium chloride. Both could affect fluid balance. Therefore, the food should not be routinely fed to patients with comorbid diseases associated with positive fluid balance (e.g., heart failure, nephrotic syndrome) or hypertension.

AZOTEMIC PRIMARY RENAL FAILURE

Complete obstruction of urine outflow caused by uroliths in patients with a concomitant UTI should be regarded as an emergency. In this situation, a combination of obstruction and pyelonephritis caused by a rapid spread of infection throughout the kidneys is likely to induce acute renal failure and then septicemia. Dietary dissolution of struvite uroliths located in the upper urinary tract should not be considered until adequate urine flow has been restored, and life-threatening deficits and excesses in fluid, electrolyte, acid-base and endocrine balance have been corrected.

Nonobstructing struvite nephroliths have been dissolved in patients with nonazotemic renal failure caused by ascending pyelonephritis (Osborne et al, 1985, 1986). But, protein-restricted litholytic foods should be used with caution in patients with azotemic primary renal failure. Such foods may induce protein malnutrition if fed for prolonged periods to dogs with moderate azotemic primary renal failure (Polzin et al, 1983).

To minimize adverse drug reactions/events, adjustments in doses and maintenance intervals of drugs excreted primarily by the kidneys should be considered in patients with azotemic primary renal failure.

PATIENTS AT RISK FOR PANCREATITIS

Approximately one in 250 dogs seen in private veterinary practices is affected by pancreatitis (0.4%). There appears to be no relationship between pancreatitis and gender, but there is a significant relationship between the disease and age. The mean age of dogs with pancreatitis in private veterinary practices is eight years (vs. 5.5 years for the general canine population). Breed is another strong risk factor for pancreatitis. For example, miniature schnauzers have a fivefold increase in risk for pancreatitis (i.e., about one in 50 miniature schnauzers can be expected to have pancreatitis). Other breeds at increased risk include Bichon Frises, Yorkshire terriers, Chihuahuas, Jack Russell terriers, Japanese spaniels, Labrador retrievers, Maltese and Shetland sheepdogs.

Investigators conducting an independent epidemiologic study asked veterinarians to ascertain the health of dogs fed a commercial veterinary therapeutic pet food.[b] This study disclosed an association between feeding a struvite litholytic food and acute pancreatitis. The risk of a dog developing pancreatitis when fed the struvite litholytic food was comparable to that of a miniature schnauzer developing acute pancreatitis, or about one in 40 (i.e., about one in 40 dogs fed the struvite litholytic food might develop pancreatitis).

The litholytic food that was tested is relatively high in fat, which increases the energy density of the food so that restriction of other specified nutrients is more readily accomplished. Because dietary fat is a risk factor for pancreatitis, the serum activity of pancreatic enzymes (amylase, lipase, trypsin-like immunoreactivity) should be monitored before initiating therapy with high-fat struvite litholytic foods in patients known to be at increased risk for pancreatitis. These tests should be repeated if signs of pancreatitis develop during treatment with the litholytic food. Because abnormal increases in activity of these enzymes are not pathognomonic for pancreatitis, other relevant findings should also be considered.

Female miniature schnauzers are at increased risk for infection-induced struvite uroliths and pancreatitis. Likewise, patients with hyperadrenocorticism are at increased risk for UTIs (which could include staphylococci) and pancreatitis. Although risk factors are not synonymous with cause and effect, clients should be informed of these associations and advised of how to respond to adverse events if they occur. They should be informed about adverse events that need medical attention and those that need medical attention only if they continue.

Assess and Determine the Feeding Method: Struvite Dissolution

Transitioning the patient from its current food to a litholytic food should be done gradually over a period of a few days. Begin the transition by feeding 75% of the current food and 25% of the litholytic food on Day 1. On Day 2, feed half of each food. On Day 3, feed 75% as the litholytic food. By Day 4 or 5, feed only the litholytic food.

As discussed above, modification of urinary pH is an important part of overall dietary management of struvite urolithiasis. Free-choice feeding is often associated with more persistent aciduria compared to meal feeding. Because moist foods are recommended to increase water intake and produce less concentrated urine, clients should be advised to feed specific amounts (meal feed) two to three times per day rather than free-choice feeding. More frequent feedings are desirable if the client can feed multiple meals per day. Moist foods often spoil if left uneaten at room temperature for several hours (Chapter 11). Opened containers of moist foods should be refrigerated and the feeding bowl should be kept clean.

Besides offering moist foods, several additional approaches may facilitate increased water intake. First, ensure multiple bowls are available in prominent locations in the dog's environment; this may mean providing several bowls outside in a large enclosure or a bowl on each level of the house. Second, bowls should be clean and always filled with fresh water. Third, small amounts of flavoring substances (e.g., salt-free bouillon) can be added to water sources. Fourth, ice cubes can be offered as treats or snacks. Fifth, if a dry food is selected, add liberal quantities of water; however, as with moist foods, be aware that potential food safety issues might arise if moistened dry foods are left uneaten for prolonged intervals at room temperature (Chapter 11).

If the patient has a normal body condition score (2.5/5 to 3.5/5), the amount of the previous food being fed was appropriate. On an energy basis, a similar amount of the new food would be a good starting place.

ADJUNCTIVE MEDICAL AND SURGICAL MANAGEMENT

Eradication or Control of UTIs

The importance of UTIs with urease-producing bacteria in the formation of many struvite uroliths in dogs emphasizes the need to eliminate or control infection. Because of the quantity of urease produced by bacterial pathogens, it may be impossible to consistently acidify urine with urine acidifiers administered at dosages that do not cause systemic acidosis (Musher et al, 1974). Therefore, sterilization of urine appears to be an important objective in creating a state of struvite undersaturation that would prevent further growth of uroliths or promote their dissolution.

Appropriate antimicrobial agents selected on the basis of susceptibility or minimum inhibitory concentrations should be used at therapeutic dosages. The fact that diuresis reduces the urine concentration of the antimicrobial agent should be considered when formulating antimicrobial dosages (Ling and Hirsch, 1983). Antimicrobial agents should be administered as long as uroliths can be identified by survey radiography. This recommendation is based on the fact that bacterial pathogens harbored inside uroliths may be protected from antimicrobial agents (Nickel et al, 1985). Although the urine and surface of uroliths may be sterilized following appropriate antimicrobial therapy, the original and secondary infecting microbes may remain viable below the surface of the urolith. Therefore, discontinuation of antimicrobial therapy may result in relapse of bacteriuria and infection.

Although use of antimicrobial agents alone may result in dissolution of struvite uroliths in some patients, studies in rats (Musher et al, 1974a) and dogs[a] and clinical studies in people (Feit and Fair, 1979; Lewis et al, 1983; Senior et al, 1984)[a] indicate that this phenomenon represents the exception rather than the rule. In one controlled study, six dogs with induced struvite uroliths were given therapeutic dosages of oral ampicillin (16 mg/kg body weight/day divided into three equal subdoses) and were fed a maintenance food. Only two uroliths dissolved; the remaining four uroliths increased in size.[a] In addition to the unpredictable response to this form of therapy, the time required to induce urolith dissolution with antimicrobial agents is usually measured in multiples of months rather than in multiples of weeks.

The litholytic effects of various combinations of antibiotics (ampicillin given orally at a dosage of 16 mg/kg body weight/day), acetohydroxamic acid and a struvite litholytic therapeutic food were studied in dogs with staphylococcal-induced struvite uroliths.[a] After five months of therapy, four uroliths increased in size and two dissolved in six dogs given ampicillin and an adult maintenance-type food. Four of six uroliths dissolved and two decreased in size in six dogs given ampicillin and the litholytic food over the same time frame. All uroliths in six dogs dissolved six weeks after initiation of therapy with a combination of the litholytic food, ampicillin and acetohydroxamic acid.

Similar results were obtained when a combination of the litholytic food and antimicrobial agents was given to 11 dogs with naturally occurring urease-positive UTIs and urocystoliths presumed to be composed of struvite (Osborne et al, 1984, 1985). The mean time required to induce urocystolith dissolution in these dogs was approximately three months (range two weeks to seven months).

Urease Inhibitors

Studies in dogs have revealed that administration of microbial urease inhibitors in pharmacologic doses is capable of inhibiting struvite urolith growth and promoting struvite urolith dissolution. Acetohydroxamic acid given orally to dogs at a dosage of 25 mg/kg body weight (divided into two daily subdoses) reduced urease activity, struvite crystalluria and urolith growth (Krawiec et al, 1984). By reducing the pathogenicity of staphylococci, acetohydroxamic acid may also result in less severe dysuria, bacteriuria, pyuria, hematuria and proteinuria.

Although higher dosages of acetohydroxamic acid may result in urolith dissolution, they are not recommended because they may cause a reversible hemolytic anemia and abnormalities in bilirubin metabolism (Krawiec et al, 1984; Kobashi et al, 1971). Likewise, acetohydroxamic acid should not be administered to pregnant dogs because it is teratogenic (Bailie et al, 1986).

Acetohydroxamic acid has not been used routinely in promoting dissolution of infection-induced struvite uroliths in dogs because of the efficacy of the litholytic food and antimicrobial therapy. However, acetohydroxamic acid has been used in combination with litholytic foods and antimicrobial agents in patients that have recalcitrant urease-producing UTIs associated with persistent struvite uroliths. Acetohydroxamic acid may be added to the therapeutic regimen if infection-induced struvite uroliths do not dissolve after an appropriate therapeutic trial with diet modification and antimicrobial agents.

INFECTION-INDUCED STRUVITE NEPHROLITHS

Nephroliths and ureteroliths causing outflow obstruction and marked impairment of renal function should be managed by surgical intervention or, if possible, by percutaneous nephropyelolithotomy, especially if associated with concomitant bacterial infection (Ross et al, 1999). Dietary and medical therapy designed to induce urolith dissolution over several weeks is unlikely to be effective in patients with poorly functioning kidneys because uroliths must be completely surrounded by urine that is undersaturated with struvite for prolonged periods to be dissolved. Intermittent passage of urine through a partially obstructed kidney or ureter would logically preclude dissolution of struvite nephroliths or ureteroliths.

Dissolution of nephroliths presumed to be composed of infection-induced struvite in six dogs has been reported. The mean time required for dissolution was 184 days (range 67 to 300 days). Although the dogs had varying degrees of impaired capacity to concentrate urine as a result of pyelonephritis, none had primary renal azotemia at the time therapy was initiated with the veterinary therapeutic struvite litholytic food and antimicrobial agents. This point is emphasized because dogs with moderate to severe primary renal failure require a greater quantity of protein for anabolism than normal. The litholytic food used could induce or aggravate protein malnutrition if given for prolonged periods to dogs with moderate azotemic primary renal failure, or other comorbid disorders associated with protein malnutrition (Polzin et al, 1983).

REASSESSMENT

Because litholytic foods stimulate thirst and promote diuresis, the magnitude of pollakiuria in dogs with urocystoliths may increase for a variable time following initiation of dietary therapy. However, pollakiuria and the abnormal urine odor caused by bacterial degradation of urea usually subside as infection is controlled and uroliths decrease in size (**Table 43-6**). Reduction in ammonia-induced chemical inflammation as a result of ureolysis may also be involved in remission of these clinical signs. **Table 43-7** summarizes mean times for struvite urolith dissolution.

The size of uroliths should be periodically monitored by survey radiography or ultrasonography (typically, monthly intervals are recommended). Survey radiography or ultrasonography is usually preferred to retrograde double-contrast urocystography because use of transurethral catheters during retrograde radiographic studies may result in iatrogenic UTI. Alternatively, intravenous urography may be considered.

Periodic evaluation of urine sediment for crystalluria also may be considered. Struvite crystals should not form in fresh uncontaminated urine if therapy has been effective in promoting formation of urine that is undersaturated with MAP.

UTIs may persist despite antimicrobial therapy in patients having infection-induced struvite uroliths and consuming the litholytic food. In most patients, however, the magnitude of bacteriuria is markedly reduced (i.e., from more than 100,000 to approximately 1,000 cfu (colony forming units)/ml of urine) and the associated inflammatory response progressively subsides. Difficulty in eradicating the infection while uroliths persist may be related to persistence of viable microbes within the uroliths (Nickel et al, 1985). Diet-induced diuresis should be considered when formulating dosages of antimicrobial agents that will achieve minimum inhibitory concentrations in urine. Excellent success may be achieved in inducing dissolution of struvite uroliths despite persistent bacteriuria during antimicrobial and dietary treatment. Even though the urine is not sterile, reduction in bacterial colony counts by logarithmic magnitudes (e.g., from 10^6 to 10^4 cfu/ml) has a marked effect in reducing the quantity of microbial urease in urine (Griffith and Osborne, 1987). Concomitant use of litholytic foods, antimicrobial agents and acetohydroxamic acid is the most effective method of inducing dissolution of uroliths when UTI complications persist.

Urine collected by cystocentesis should be quantitatively cultured during therapy and five to seven days after antimicrobial therapy is discontinued. Results of urine culture may not be the same as results obtained before therapy or from cultures of the interior of uroliths. Rapid recurrence of UTI caused by the same type of organism (relapse) or a different type of bacterial pathogen (reinfection) following withdrawal of antimicrobial therapy may indicate residual uroliths within the urinary tract or other abnormalities in local host defense mechanisms that predispose the patient to UTI and recurrent struvite urolithiasis (Osborne and Stevens, 1999a).

Because small uroliths may escape detection by survey radiography or ultrasonography, continue the struvite litholytic food and (if necessary) antimicrobial agents for at least one "insurance" month after radiographic or ultrasonographic documentation of urolith dissolution. Recall that survey radiography may not detect uroliths ≤0.3 mm in size. This protocol is likely to prevent recurrence of clinical signs from remaining uroliths that were missed by conventional survey radiography or ultrasonography. Alternate methods of management should be considered if uroliths increase in size during therapy or if urolith size remains unchanged after approximately eight weeks of appropriate dietary and medical therapy. Small uroliths that become lodged in the urethra of male or female dogs during therapy may be readily returned to the urinary bladder lumen by retrograde urohydropropulsion (Figure 38-5 and Table 38-7). They may also be removed by lithotripsy. Complete obstruction of a ureter or renal pelvis with a urolith, especially with concomitant UTI, is an indication for surgical intervention.

Attempts to induce dissolution of struvite uroliths may be hampered if the uroliths are heterogeneous in composition (**Table 43-8**). This has not been a significant problem in dogs with uroliths composed primarily of MAP with lesser quantities of calcium apatite because the solubility characteristics of the two minerals are similar. However, some clinicians have encountered difficulty in dissolving uroliths composed primarily of struvite with an outer shell composed primarily of calcium apatite. Difficulty will also be encountered in attempting to induce complete dissolution of a urolith with a nucleus of calcium oxalate or silica and a shell of struvite because the solubility characteristics of these minerals are dissimilar. This phenomenon should be considered if dietary and medical therapy seems to be ineffective after initially reducing the size of a urolith.

PREVENTION

Table 43-9 lists commercial veterinary therapeutic foods intended for the prevention of recurrence of struvite urolithiasis and compares them to the key nutritional factor targets. Because these foods are intended for long-term feeding, they should also be approved by the Association of American Feed Control Officials (AAFCO), or some other credible regulatory agency. However, recommendations for the use of these foods are not straightforward. Caveats regarding their use depend upon whether the struvite uroliths are infection-induced or form in sterile urine. Also, concurrent or alternative medical management must be considered.

Infection-Induced Struvite Uroliths

Eradication or control of UTIs due to urease-producing bacteria is the most important factor in preventing recurrence of most infection-induced struvite uroliths (Osborne and Stevens, 1999a). If UTI persists or is recurrent, indefinite therapy is indicated with prophylactic dosages of antimicrobial agents eliminated in high concentration in urine. These may include amoxicillin, nitrofurantoin and trimethoprim-sulfadiazine; however, the final choice is best determined by the results of the most recent antimicrobial susceptibility test. In light of the effectiveness of litholytic foods in inducing dissolution of struvite uroliths, use of these same foods (**Table 43-5**) to minimize recurrence of uroliths is logical and feasible. However, the long-term (measured in years) effects of low-protein litholytic foods in dogs that may be predisposed to urolith formation are not yet known. Litholytic foods induce polyuria, varying degrees of hypoalbuminemia and mild alterations in hepatic enzyme activities and morphology. Therefore, long-term use of litholytic foods with severely reduced protein levels should be recommended only if patients develop frequently recurrent urolithiasis despite attempts to control infection, augment fluid intake and urine acidification. In other words, the benefits of therapy should outweigh the risks.

Results of experimental and clinical studies to evaluate the effectiveness of acetohydroxamic acid indicate that this drug

Table 43-7. Mean times for struvite urolith dissolution.

Urolith location and infective status	Mean time for dissolution	Comments and precautions
Infection-induced urocystoliths	Approximately 2.5 months (range two weeks to seven months)	Use appropriate caution in dogs at increased risk for pancreatitis, dogs with renal failure and dogs with hypoalbuminemic edema
Sterile urocystoliths	Three to four weeks	If idiopathic, appropriately monitor for recurrence
Infection-induced struvite urocystoliths in immature dogs	Less than two weeks	If circumstances warrant feeding for a longer period, serial monitor body weight, body condition, serum albumin concentration and packed cell volume for evidence of protein-calorie malnutrition
Infection-induced nephroliths	Approximately 184 days (range 67 to 300 days)	Contraindicated in dogs with concomitant obstruction to urine outflow

Table 43-8. Managing magnesium ammonium phosphate uroliths refractory to complete dissolution.

Causes	Identification	Therapeutic goal
Client and patient factors		
Inadequate dietary compliance	Question owner Persistent struvite crystalluria Urea nitrogen >8-12 mg/dl Urine specific gravity >1.010-1.015 Urinary pH is alkaline during treatment with the litholytic food*	Emphasize need to feed dissolution food exclusively
Inadequate antibiotic administration	Question owner Count remaining antibiotic pills	Emphasize need to administer the full dose of antibiotics Determine if owner is capable and willing to administer medication Demonstrate a variety of methods to administer medication
Clinician factors		
Incorrect prediction of mineral type	Analysis of retrieved urolith	Alter therapy based on identification of mineral type
Inappropriate antibiotic choice	Positive urine culture with poor susceptibility for chosen antibiotic	Choose antibiotics based on susceptibility testing
Inappropriate antibiotic dose for degree of diuresis	Positive quantitative urine culture with same bacterial species and same susceptibility; number of bacteria may be lower (See text.)	Administer antibiotic at the higher recommended dose or consider a higher dose than recommended
Premature discontinuation of antibiotic	Discontinuing antibiotic before complete urolith dissolution Positive urine culture with same bacterial species and the same susceptibility (See text.)	Prescribe full antibiotic dose for the entire period of urolith dissolution
Disease factors		
Change in bacterial susceptibility	Positive urine culture with susceptibility results different from those of previous culture	Choose antibiotic based on susceptibility testing
New bacterial infection	Positive urine culture identifying new bacterial species	Choose antibiotic effective against both bacteria Avoid procedures requiring urinary tract catheterization
Compound urolith	Radiographic density of nucleus and outer layer(s) of urolith is different Analysis of retrieved urolith	Alter therapy based on identification of new mineral type Uroliths not causing clinical signs should be monitored for potentially adverse consequences (obstruction, urinary tract infection, etc.) Clinically active uroliths may require removal Remove small uroliths by voiding urohydropropulsion or lithotripsy

*See **Table 43-5**.

Table 43-9. Key nutritional factors in selected commercial veterinary therapeutic food used to minimize recurrence of struvite urolithiasis in dogs compared to recommended levels.*

Dry foods	Protein (%)	Phosphorus (%)	Magnesium (%)	Urinary pH**
Recommended levels	**<25**	**<0.6**	**0.04-0.1**	**6.2-6.4**
Hill's Prescription Diet c/d Canine	22.3	0.59	0.111	6.22
Hill's Prescription Diet w/d Canine	18.9	0.56	0.088	6.40
Hill's Prescription Diet w/d with Chicken Canine	19.1	0.56	0.080	6.30
Medi-Cal Preventive Formula	23.9	0.8	na	na
Medi-Cal Urinary SO	16.7	0.6	0.2	5.5-6.0
Medi-Cal Weight Control/Mature	19.5	0.8	na	6.4
Purina Veterinary Diet DCO Dual Fiber Control	25.3	0.93	0.130	6.0-6.2
Purina Veterinary Diet OM Overweight Management	31.1	0.89	0.130	6.2-6.4
Royal Canin Veterinary Diet Control Formula	23.9	0.84	0.130	6.0-6.3
Royal Canin Veterinary Diet Urinary SO 14	17.0	0.63	0.066	5.5-6.0
Moist foods	**Protein (%)**	**Phosphorus (%)**	**Magnesium (%)**	**Urinary pH****
Recommended levels	**<25**	**<0.6**	**0.04-0.1**	**6.2-6.4**
Hill's Prescription Diet c/d Canine	23.6	0.51	0.079	6.16
Hill's Prescription Diet w/d Canine	17.9	0.52	0.088	6.40
Medi-Cal Preventive Formula	23.8	0.7	na	na
Medi-Cal Urinary SO	18.7	0.8	0.1	5.5-6.0
Medi-Cal Weight Control/Mature	21.5	0.6	na	6.6
Purina Veterinary Diet OM Overweight Management	44.1	1.06	0.190	6.2-6.4
Royal Canin Veterinary Diet Control Formula	22.8	0.66	0.078	6.0-6.3
Royal Canin Veterinary Diet Urinary SO	18.5	0.86	0.059	5.5-6.0

Key: na = information not available from the manufacturer.
*Manufacturers' published values; nutrients expressed on a dry matter basis; moist foods are best.
**Protocols for measuring urinary pH may vary.

should be considered in an effort to minimize recurrence of infection-induced struvite urolithiasis in dogs with persistent UTI with urease-producing bacteria despite appropriate antimicrobial therapy. Administration of 25 mg of acetohydroxamic acid/kg body weight/day to dogs with urinary bladder foreign bodies (zinc disks) and induced urease-positive staphylococcal UTIs was effective in preventing formation of and minimizing the growth rate of uroliths (Krawiec et al, 1984a). Acetohydroxamic acid has also been reported to be effective in preventing struvite uroliths induced by ureaplasmas in rats.[a]

Previously, acidifying foods with mild to moderately reduced levels of protein, magnesium and phosphorus (**Table 43-9**) have been recommended as part of the therapeutic strategy to minimize recurrence of infection-induced struvite uroliths. However, clinical experience with use of such foods has prompted modification of this recommendation for two primary reasons. First, because infection-induced uroliths cannot form without an infection with urease-producing microbes, eradication of the UTI should be the first priority in context of the pathophysiology associated with this type of urolith. Infection-induced struvite will likely not recur in the absence of a urease-producing microbe. Second, prolonged use of this type of food has been associated with calcium oxalate crystalluria and/or calcium oxalate uroliths, especially in dogs predisposed to calcium oxalate uroliths. In addition, appropriate caution should be used in deciding whether or not to induce prophylactic diuresis in patients with a history of struvite uroliths induced by recurrent UTI. Although formation of less concentrated urine tends to minimize the supersaturation of urine with lithogenic crystalloids (a benefit), it tends to counteract innate antimicrobial properties of urine (a risk). Studies performed in rats and cats indicate that diuresis tends to minimize pyelonephritis, but enhance lower UTIs. This is not an "all or none; always or never" recommendation. However, pending the results of properly controlled clinical trials, this seems to be the safest and most effective ethical course of action.

Sterile Struvite Uroliths

Although apparently uncommon, sterile struvite uroliths have a greater tendency to recur than infection-induced struvite uroliths in which the UTI has been eradicated or controlled. Administration of urine acidifiers should be considered if the urinary pH of patients with sterile struvite uroliths remains persistently alkaline. The prophylactic value of concomitant restriction of dietary phosphorus, magnesium and urine acidification has not yet been conclusively determined primarily because of lack of clinical cases to perform double-blind controlled studies. Unfortunately, the infrequency with which dogs with sterile uroliths are encountered does not lend itself to such clinical studies. Nonetheless, it seems unreasonable and unethical to do nothing for patients with recurrent struvite uroliths until clinical trials are completed. Therefore, pending the availability of appropriate data, therapy should be designed to first do no harm. When considering dietary management (**Table 43-9**), emphasize minimizing recurrence of calcium oxalate and calcium phosphate uroliths, because these types of uroliths cannot be dissolved by dietary and medical management. Should struvite uroliths recur, they often can be dissolved by dietary management and antimicrobial agents (if necessary). When foods designed to produce acidic urine are used, urinary pH should be closely monitored with the aid of a reliable pH meter rather than commercially available reagent strips with a pH pad. Likewise, urine output should be estimated with the aid of a reliable refractometer designed to provide reproducible urine specific gravity values. Urine sediment should be evaluated for crystals and evidence of infection by microscopic examination of freshly voided urine.

Uncontrollable risk factors (i.e., defective inhibitors of crystal formation and/or defective inhibitors of crystal aggregation) may be present in those situations in which dogs have documented occurrences of either calcium oxalate or calcium phosphate followed by struvite urolithiasis. If struvite urolithiasis is associated with urease-positive UTIs, appropriate therapy should be devised to eradicate the UTI and minimize its recurrence.

ENDNOTES

a. Osborne CA. Unpublished data. 1987.
b. Hill's Pet Nutrition, Inc., Topeka, KS, USA.

REFERENCES

The references for **Chapter 43** can be found at www.markmorris.org.

CASE 43-1

Dysuria in a German Shepherd Crossbred Dog

Carl A. Osborne, DVM, PhD, Dipl. ACVIM (Internal Medicine)
College of Veterinary Medicine
University of Minnesota
St. Paul, Minnesota, USA

Patient Assessment

A 12-year-old neutered female German shepherd crossbred dog was examined for dysuria and pollakiuria of two months' duration. Other than nonspecific dermatitis and a perianal adenoma, the dog had no previous history of illness.

Physical examination revealed an alert, active, overweight dog (body weight 27 kg, body condition score 4/5). Multiple uroliths were palpated in the urinary bladder. No other abnormalities were detected. Results of a complete blood count and a serum biochemistry profile were normal except for a mild elevation in alkaline phosphatase activity (**Tables 1** and **2**). Analysis of a urine specimen collected by cystocentesis (**Table 3**) revealed an alkaline pH, struvite crystalluria and findings typical of inflammation (i.e., hematuria, pyuria, proteinuria). Quantitative culture of urine revealed more than 10^5 colony-forming units of urease-producing *Staphylococcus intermedius* organisms per ml of urine. The bacteria were susceptible to most antimicrobial drugs. Survey radiographs of the abdomen revealed three uroliths within the bladder lumen (**Figures 1** and **2**); the sizes of the kidneys and liver were normal.

Assess the Food and Feeding Method

A commercial dry adult maintenance food was offered free choice. Table foods were fed frequently.

Questions

1. What is the probable mineral composition of the uroliths in this dog?
2. What are the advantages and disadvantages of surgical vs. dietary and medical management of these uroliths?
3. How should therapeutic efficacy be monitored?

Answers and Discussion

1. The most likely mineral composition of the uroliths is struvite based on: 1) urease-positive staphylococcal urinary tract infection, 2) alkaline urinary pH, 3) struvite crystalluria (no oxalate, cystine or urate crystals) and 4) detection of radiodense uroliths.
2. Although surgery may be effective, dietary and medical protocols have been developed to dissolve struvite uroliths. Surgical removal of urocystoliths has the obvious advantage of rapid correction of the disease process. Dietary and medical therapy may also be effective and includes using a proven commercial veterinary therapeutic struvite litholytic food.[a] Concurrent treatment of the urinary tract infection with appropriate antimicrobials is an essential part of the treatment protocol. The litholytic food should be fed until radiographic evidence of urolith dissolution is obtained. The food is usually fed for one additional "insurance" month following dissolution because survey radiography is not sufficiently sensitive to detect small uroliths (≤3 mm).
3. Therapeutic efficacy should be monitored by monthly evaluation of clinical signs, radiographs, urinalyses and urine cultures. Clinical signs often resolve within three to five days of initiating therapy. Consumption of the litholytic food is usually associated with polyuria, formation of less concentrated acidic urine, marked reduction in serum urea nitrogen concentration, reduction

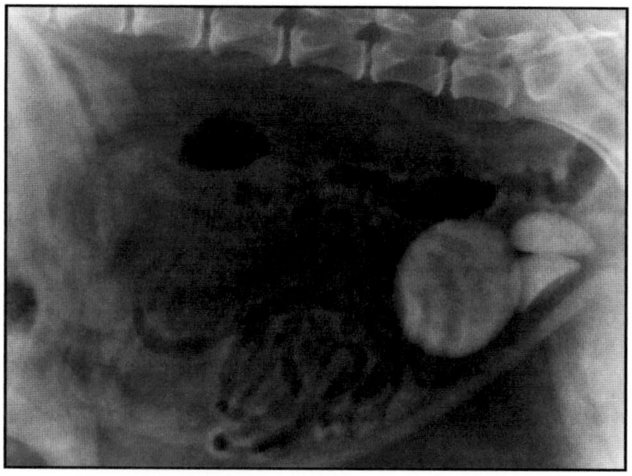

Figure 1. Survey lateral abdominal radiograph illustrating multiple radiodense uroliths in the urinary bladder of a 12-year-old spayed female German shepherd crossbred dog.

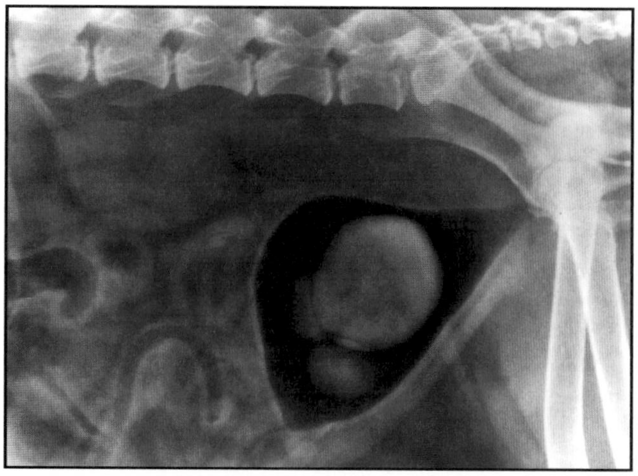

Figure 2. Pneumocystogram of the dog described in Figure 1. Note a diverticulum at the vertex of the urinary bladder.

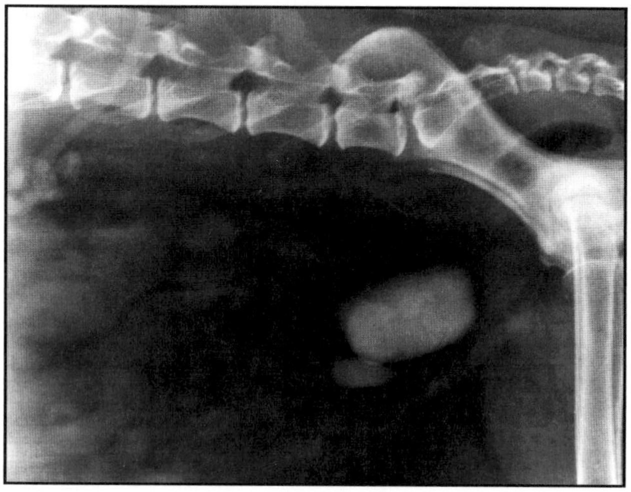

Figure 3. Survey lateral abdominal radiograph of the dog described in Figure 1. This radiograph was obtained 30 days after initiation of litholytic therapy. (Compare this Figure with Figures 4 through 6.)

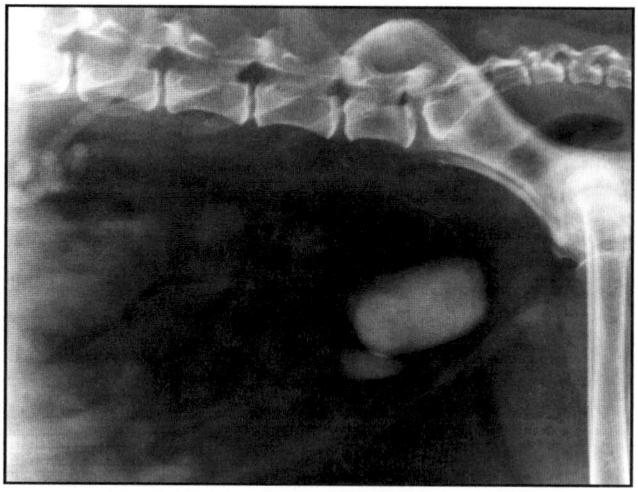

Figure 4. Survey lateral abdominal radiograph of the dog described in Figure 1. This radiograph was obtained 58 days after initiation of litholytic therapy. (Compare this Figure with Figures 5 and 6.)

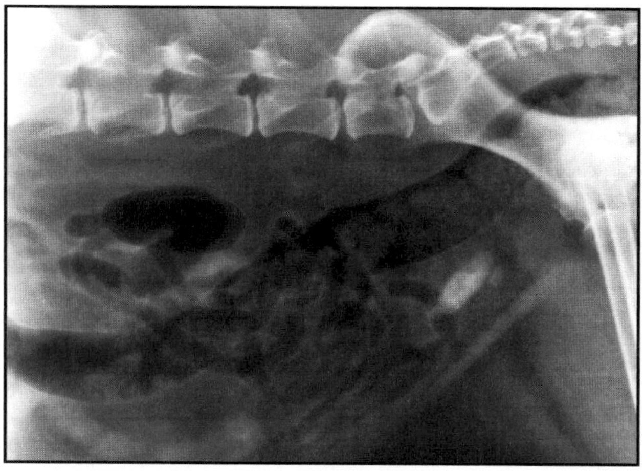

Figure 5. Survey lateral abdominal radiograph of the dog described in Figure 1. This radiograph was obtained 97 days after initiation of litholytic therapy. (Compare this Figure with Figure 6.)

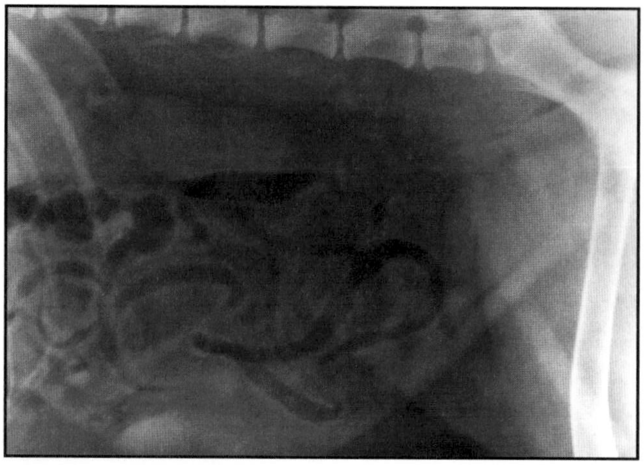

Figure 6. Survey lateral abdominal radiograph of the dog described in Figure 1. This radiograph was obtained 127 days after initiation of litholytic therapy.

Table 1. Hemograms of a 12-year-old spayed female German shepherd crossbred dog with urocystoliths.

Factors*	Reference values	Day 1**	Day 35	Day 63	Day 102	Day 132	Day 159	Day 196	Day 256
PCV (%)	38.5-56.7	41	40	41	39	38	38	38	40
Hb (g/dl)	13.5-19.9	15.6	15.3	15.1	15.8	15.2	14.7	15.0	16.4
WBC (10^3/µl)	4.1-13.3	16	8.9	7.3	6.2	8.9	9.4	7.4	4.7
Lymphocytes (10^3/µl)	0.3-5.1	1.6	2.6	3.4	2.3	4.2	3.4	2.6	4.6
Neutrophils (10^3/µl)	2.1-11.2	7.5	7.1	6.0	6.9	5.2	5.5	5.8	5.1
Eosinophils (10^3/µl)	0.0-1.2	1	0	2	2	3	5	9	2
Monocytes (10^3/µl)	0.0-1.2	8	3	4	6	3	4	6	1

Key: PCV = packed cell volume, Hb = hemoglobin, WBC = white blood cells.
*Platelets were estimated on a blood film and considered adequate in all specimens. Normoblasts and basophils were not observed.
**Therapy with a litholytic food and an antimicrobial agent was initiated on Day 5 and discontinued on Day 159.

Table 2. Serum biochemistry values of a 12-year-old spayed female German shepherd crossbred dog with urocystoliths.

Factors	Reference values	Day 1*	Day 35	Day 63	Day 102	Day 132	Day 159	Day 196	Day 256
SUN (mg/dl)	7-28	24	4	3	3	3	3	29	40
Creatinine (mg/dl)	0.5-1.5	1.3	1.4	1.4	1.4	1.4	1.3	1.7	1.5
Calcium (mg/dl)	9.3-11.4	10.2	9.7	10.0	10.1	10.4	10.0	10.7	10.3
Phosphorus (mg/dl)	1.9-7.0	3.5	3.5	4.3	3.0	3.6	3.1	3.6	4.7
Magnesium (mg/dl)	1.5-2.7	2.3	1.9	2.0	1.8	1.7	1.8	2.1	2.1
Sodium (mEq/l)	143-150	149	147	145	147	146	144	147	148
Potassium (mEq/l)	3.2-5.6	4.6	5.0	5.5	5.6	5.1	5.3	4.8	5.2
Chloride (mEq/l)	108-125	119	119	119	118	118	118	117	115
Albumin (g/dl)	2.4-3.8	2.4	2.2	2.2	2.3	2.3	2.1	2.8	-
ALT activity (U/l)	5-62	56	46	32	26	25	28	31	35
Alk phos activity (U/l)	10-149	238	1,270	1,580	1,920	1,470	695	337	208
Total bilirubin (mg/dl)	0.1-0.6	0.1	0.1	0.2	0.2	0.1	0.2	0.1	0.1

Key: SUN = serum urea nitrogen, ALT = alanine aminotransferase, Alk phos = alkaline phosphatase.
*Therapy with a litholytic food and an antimicrobial agent was initiated on Day 5 and discontinued on Day 159.

Table 3. Urinalyses of a 12-year-old spayed female German shepherd crossbred dog with urocystoliths.*

Factors**	Day 1***	Day 35	Day 63	Day 102	Day 132	Day 159	Day 196	Day 256
Specific gravity	1.019	1.008	1.007	1.008	1.007	1.006	1.019	1.018
pH	8.5	6.5	7.0	7.5	6.5	5.0	6.0	7.0
Protein†	4+	2+	2+	1+	1+	Trace	1+	2+
RBC††	TNTC	TNTC	TNTC	9-11	0	0	0	0
WBC††	75-85	1-2	0	1-3	0	0	0	0
Crystals†††	Struvite	Struvite	Struvite	Amorphous phosphate	0	0	0	0

Key: RBC = red blood cells, TNTC = too numerous to count, WBC = white blood cells.
*Samples collected by cystocentesis.
**Glucose, bilirubin and acetone were not detected in any specimen.
***Therapy with a litholytic food and an antimicrobial agent was initiated on Day 5 and discontinued on Day 159.
†Values represent semiquantitative evaluations based on a scale of 0 to 4; urine volume was not considered.
††Number per high power field (x450).
†††Number per low power field (x100).

in serum magnesium concentration and an increase in serum alkaline phosphatase activity. Hematuria, pyuria and bacteriuria should resolve with dietary and appropriate antimicrobial therapy.

Progress Notes

Therapy was initiated with Prescription Diet s/d Canine (1,150 kcal [4.8 MJ], one can fed twice daily) and ampicillin administered orally (7 mg/kg body weight q12h). Survey radiographs obtained monthly revealed progressive reduction in the size of the uroliths (**Figures 3** to **6**). Radiodense uroliths could not be detected by survey radiography on Day 132 (**Figure 6**).

Following initiation of antimicrobial therapy, bacteria could not be cultured from urine specimens obtained by cystocentesis. Urinalysis revealed acidification of urine and disappearance of pyuria and hematuria (**Table 2**). Consumption of the litholytic food was associated with formation of less concentrated urine, reduction in serum urea nitrogen concentration, reduction in serum magnesium concentration and an increase in serum alkaline phosphatase activity (**Tables 2** and **3**). Results of complete blood counts were normal over the treatment period. Most laboratory parameters returned to baseline values following withdrawal of antimicrobial therapy and a return to a commercial adult maintenance-type food on Day 159 (**Tables 2** and **3**).

Because the dog was overweight at the beginning of therapy, the owners fed a reduced amount of food to promote weight loss. The dog lost 1.6 kg during therapy.

Further Discussion

This case typifies dietary and medical dissolution of large urocystoliths. Reduction in the concentration of urea nitrogen, acidification of urine and formation of urine with a low specific gravity indicate that the owner and the dog were complying with therapy. Microbial sterilization of urine indicated that the proper antimicrobial agent was being given at the correct dosage and was being excreted in effective concentrations in urine. However, urine sterilization is not always achieved during medical therapy designed to induce urolith dissolution. Inability to sterilize urine during therapy may be related to: 1) release of bacteria from the urolith during dissolution, 2) induction of diuresis, which impairs the antimicrobial effects of urine, 3) induction of diuresis, which reduces the concentration of antimicrobial agent in urine and/or 4) reduced clearance of urea, which may impair the antimicrobial effects of urine. However, despite persistence of bacteriuria during therapy, uroliths composed of struvite will dissolve and the associated inflammatory response will subside. Antimicrobial therapy should be continued until the uroliths completely dissolve.

Varying degrees of elevated serum alkaline phosphatase activity frequently occur in dogs fed very low-protein foods such as the veterinary therapeutic food fed to this patient. Studies in dogs indicate that the alkaline phosphatase is of hepatic origin. The greatest increases in serum alkaline phosphatase activity occur in dogs that do not consume an adequate amount of the veterinary therapeutic food. Contrary to the situation in this case, the litholytic food should not be fed with a goal of weight reduction because this practice may contribute to negative nitrogen balance. Weight reduction should be achieved with an appropriate food after resolution of the urocystolith problem.

Endnote

a. Prescription Diet s/d Canine. Hill's Pet Nutrition, Inc., Topeka, KS, USA.

Bibliography

Osborne CA, Lulich JP, Bartges JW, et al. Canine and feline urolithiasis: Relationship of etiopathogenesis to treatment and prevention. In: Osborne CA, Finco DR, eds. Canine and Feline Nephrology and Urology. Baltimore, MD: Williams & Wilkins, 1995; 798-888.

CASE 43-2

Dysuria in a Puppy

Jody P. Lulich, DVM, PhD, Dipl. ACVIM (Internal Medicine)

Carl A. Osborne, DVM, PhD, Dipl. ACVIM (Internal Medicine)
College of Veterinary Medicine
University of Minnesota
St. Paul, Minnesota, USA

Patient Assessment

A nine-week-old, male, mixed-breed puppy was examined for dysuria, anorexia, vomiting and depression of one day's duration. The history was incomplete because the owners had acquired the puppy only five days earlier. Physical examination was unremarkable except for an overdistended, painful urinary bladder. Palpation of the urinary bladder induced a micturition reflex, but the puppy was unable to void. The puppy's body weight (5 kg) and condition (body condition score 3/5) were normal.

Survey abdominal radiographs revealed multiple, radiodense uroliths in the penile urethra. Following decompression of the urinary bladder by abdominal cystocentesis, the urethroliths were returned to the urinary bladder lumen by urohydropropulsion (**Figure 1**). Analysis of an aliquot of urine collected by cystocentesis revealed an inflammatory response associated with bacteriuria (**Table 1**). Quantitative aerobic and anaerobic culture of urine revealed >10^5 colony-forming units/ml of urease-positive *Staphylococcus intermedius*. The bacteria were susceptible to most commonly used antimicrobial agents. Results of a complete blood count were normal except for a stress-induced mature neutrophilic leukocytosis. Results of a serum biochemistry profile were unremarkable (**Table 2**).

A small urolith was spontaneously voided and submitted for quantitative mineral analysis one day later.

Assess the Food and Feeding Method

The dog was fed a commercial dry specialty brand growth food (Science Diet Canine Growth[a]) twice daily.

Questions

1. What is the most likely urolith type in this patient?
2. What additional diagnostic tests might be important?
3. Outline an appropriate treatment and feeding plan for this puppy.

Answers and Discussion

1. The most likely urolith type in this patient is magnesium ammonium phosphate (struvite). This "guesstimate" is based on finding a urinary tract infection with a urease-producing staphylococcal bacteria and radiodense uroliths. Infection-induced struvite uroliths can form within days and may occur in dogs at any age including very young dogs.
2. Anatomic defects of the urinary tract can predispose animals to bacterial infection. Ultrasound and/or contrast radiography should be considered to evaluate the lower urinary tract for such defects.
3. Dietary and medical or surgical protocols can be used to treat this puppy. Dietary and medical therapy designed to induce struvite urolith dissolution includes an appropriate orally administered antimicrobial agent and a food with restricted levels of protein, magnesium and phosphorus that is metabolized to produce an acidic urinary pH. Because foods formulated to aid in dissolution of struvite uroliths contain reduced quantities of protein, calcium, magnesium and phosphorus and thus are not designed to meet the long-term nutritional requirements of immature dogs, the feeding plan should be monitored closely. Monitoring serum biochemistry parameters (albumin, phosphorus, calcium, etc.) is an acceptable means of determining nutritional status in young dogs. An alternate treatment method includes a cystotomy to remove the uroliths; however, anesthesia and surgery in an immature dog are also associated with some degree of risk.

Progress Notes

Quantitative analysis of the voided urolith revealed that it was composed of 95% magnesium ammonium phosphate hexahydrate and 5% carbonate apatite. Retrograde positive-contrast urethrocystography and double-contrast cystography revealed a diverticulum located at the bladder vertex (**Figures 2** and **3**). The urethral lumen was also narrowed just distal to the site normally occupied

Table 1. Urinalyses of an immature male, mixed-breed dog with dysuria.*

Factors	Day 1**	Day 10	Day 25	Day 39	Day 73	Day 226
Specific gravity	1.021	1.005	1.042	1.050	1.030	1.052
pH	6.5	5.5	6.0	6.0	7.0	6.5
Protein***	3+	Trace	1+	1+	Neg	1+
RBC†	TNTC	20-30	20-30	TNTC	0	0
WBC†	TNTC	0	2-3	20-25	0	0
Bacteria†	Many cocci	0	0	0	0	0
Crystals††	0	0	0	0	0	0
Culture	*S. intermedius*	Neg	Neg	Neg	Neg	Neg

Key: Neg = negative, RBC = red blood cells, TNTC = too numerous to count, WBC = white blood cells.
*Samples collected by cystocentesis.
**Dietary and medical therapy for urinary tract infection and urolith dissolution was initiated on Day 2 and discontinued on Day 10. Antibiotic therapy for urinary tract infection was initiated on Day 2 and discontinued on Day 39.
***Values represent semiquantitative evaluations based on a scale of 0 to 4; urine volume was not considered.
†Number per high power field (x450).
††Number per low power field (x100).

Table 2. Serum biochemistry values of an immature male, mixed-breed dog with dysuria.

Factors	Reference values	Day 1*	Day 10	Day 25	Day 39	Day 73	Day 226
SUN (mg/dl)	7-28	28	2	8	20	12	12
Creatinine (mg/dl)	0.5-1.5	1.0	0.7	0.5	0.7	0.9	1.2
Calcium (mg/dl)	9.3-11.4	9.5	11.3	11.3	11.1	11.3	11.0
Phosphorus (mg/dl)	1.9-7.0	8.9	6.7	9.3	9.5	7.6	5.1
Sodium (mEq/l)	143-150	139	148	147	151	147	148
Chloride (mEq/l)	108-125	104	114	110	113	109	111
Potassium (mEq/l)	3.2-5.6	3.9	6.8	5.2	4.8	4.6	4.4
Albumin (g/dl)	2.4-3.8	3.2	2.7	3.1	3.3	3.7	4.1
ALT activity (U/l)	5-62	32	27	58	61	55	68
Alk phos activity (U/l)	10-149	180	349	207	186	113	62
Total bilirubin (mg/dl)	0.1-0.6	0.2	0.6	0.2	0.3	0.2	0.2
Total CO_2 (mEq/l)	17-26	20.5	21.1	20.8	23.4	21.6	20.1

Key: SUN = serum urea nitrogen, ALT = alanine aminotransferase, Alk phos = alkaline phosphatase.
*Dietary and medical therapy for urinary tract infection and urolith dissolution was initiated on Day 2 and discontinued on Day 10. Antibiotic therapy for urinary tract infection was initiated on Day 2 and discontinued on Day 39.

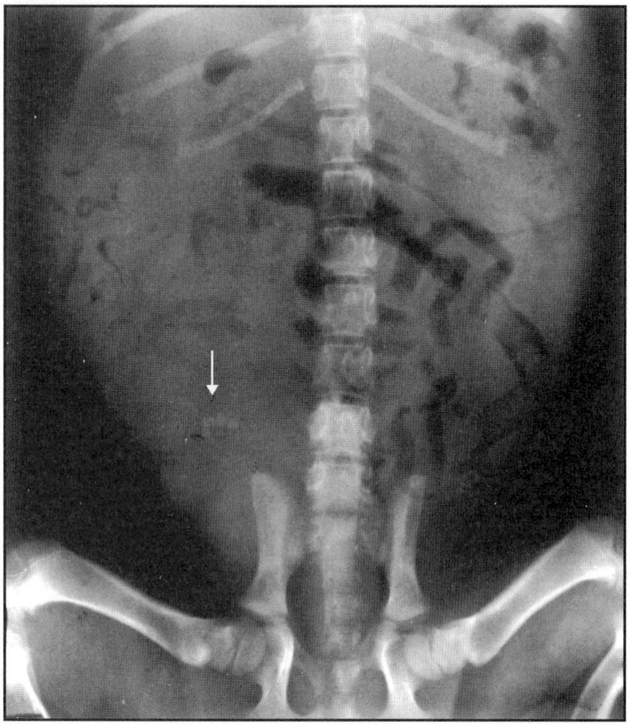

Figure 1. Ventrodorsal survey abdominal radiograph of a nine-week-old male dog with multiple radiodense urocystoliths (arrow).

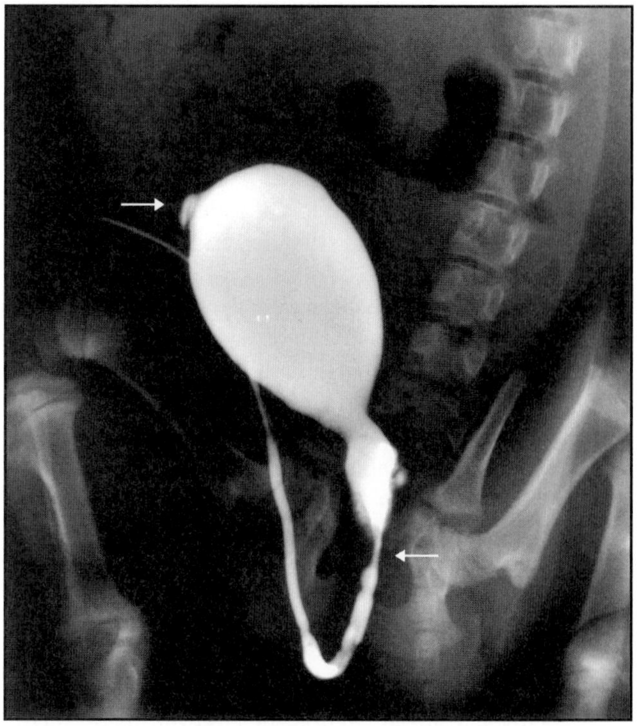

Figure 2. Positive-contrast retrograde urethrocystogram of the same dog described in Figure 1. Note the vesicourachal diverticulum (top arrow) and narrowing of the proximal portion of the urethra (bottom arrow).

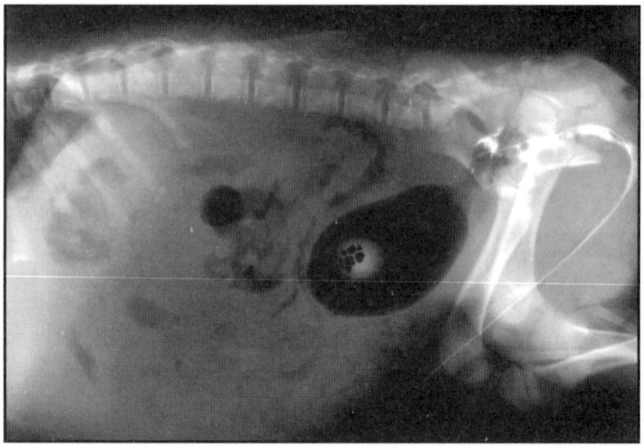

Figure 3. Double-contrast cystogram with at least eight uroliths in the bladder lumen. Radiopaque contrast medium has refluxed into the periurethral tissue in the area of the prostate gland. The urethral lumen contains air bubbles surrounded by contrast medium.

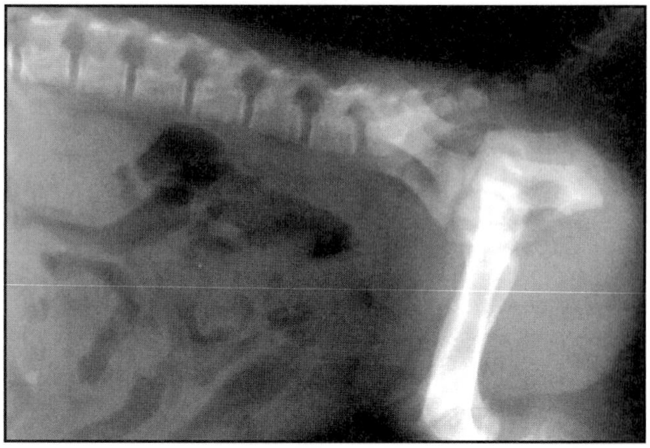

Figure 4. Survey abdominal radiograph obtained 10 days following initiation of therapy with an antibiotic and a food designed to dissolve struvite uroliths. Radiodense uroliths cannot be detected within the urinary tract.

by the prostate gland.

Dietary and medical therapy included a combination of amoxicillin and clavulanic acid (Clavamox[b]) given orally and feeding a food designed to aid in dissolution of struvite uroliths (Prescription Diet s/d Canine[a]). Compared with typical dog foods, Prescription Diet s/d Canine is greatly reduced in protein (7.9% dry matter [DM]), reduced in phosphorus (0.10% DM), calcium (0.31% DM) and magnesium (0.02% DM) and produces a more acidic urine (target urinary pH = 5.9 to 6.1). The puppy was fed one-half can three times daily (700 kcal [2.93 MJ]).

Gross hematuria and dysuria progressively declined. A urine sample collected by cystocentesis 10 days later revealed acidification of the urine and marked reduction in the inflammatory response (**Table 1**). Formation of less concentrated urine (reduction in renal medullary urea concentration) and marked reduction in serum urea nitrogen concentration (**Table 2**) was attributed to the low-protein food. Aerobic culture of urine resulted in no growth. Survey abdominal radiography, positive-contrast urethrocystography and

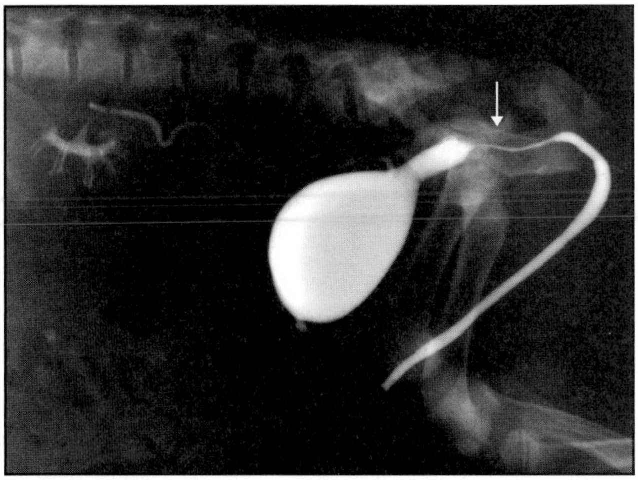

Figure 5. Positive-contrast retrograde urethrocystogram obtained 39 days following diagnosis of uroliths and a vesicourachal diverticulum. There is no evidence of a vesicourachal diverticulum, but narrowing of the lumen of the proximal urethra is still present (arrow).

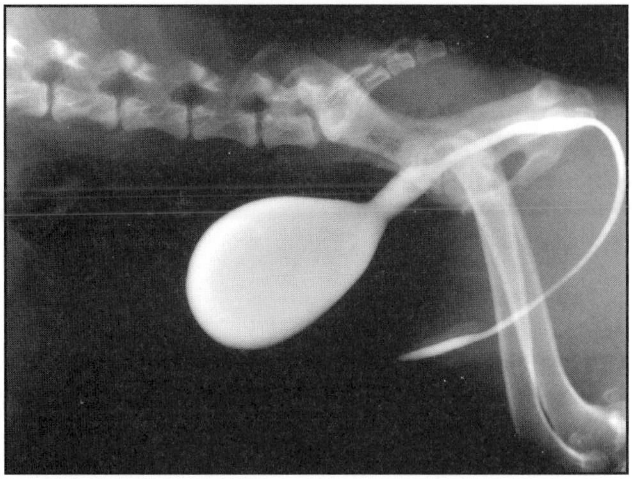

Figure 6. Positive-contrast retrograde urethrocystogram obtained 226 days following initial assessment. The lower urinary tract appears normal.

double-contrast cystography revealed no evidence of uroliths in the lower urinary tract. The vesicourachal diverticulum was still present but reduced in size (**Figure 4**). Serum albumin (2.7 g/dl), phosphorus (6.7 mg/dl) and urea nitrogen (2 mg/dl) concentrations had decreased from initial values (**Table 2**).

Because urolith dissolution was complete and because of diet-related alterations in serum phosphorus and albumin concentrations, the food was changed to a moist product designed for growing dogs (Science Diet Canine Growth), fed twice daily. The oral antimicrobial agent was continued for an additional two weeks.

Reevaluation of the dog 25 days after the initial diagnosis revealed further reduction in the size of the vesicourachal diverticulum. The dog was forming concentrated urine, but still had microscopic hematuria (**Table 1**). Serum albumin and phosphorus concentrations were normal (**Table 2**). Antimicrobial therapy was continued.

Fourteen days later (39 days after the initial diagnosis), survey and contrast radiographs revealed no evidence of the vesicourachal diverticulum or uroliths (**Figure 5**). However, the urethral lumen adjacent to the prostate gland was still reduced. Nevertheless, the dog had no clinical signs of lower urinary tract disease. Although bacteria could not be cultured by aerobic techniques, urinalysis revealed an inflammatory response (**Table 1**).

No clinical or laboratory evidence of disease was present 73 days after the initial diagnosis (**Tables 1** and **2**). Antimicrobial therapy was discontinued. Evaluation at 10 months of age revealed a normal dog with no detectable radiographic abnormalities of the lower urinary tract (**Figure 6**).

Endnotes

a. Hill's Pet Nutrition, Inc., Topeka, KS, USA.
b. Pfizer Animal Health, Exton, PA, USA.

Bibliography

Osborne CA, Lulich JP, Bartges JW, et al. Canine and feline urolithiasis: Relationship of etiopathogenesis to treatment and prevention. In: Osborne CA, Finco DR, eds. Canine and Feline Nephrology and Urology. Baltimore, MD: Williams & Wilkins, 1995; 798-888.

CASE 43-3

Recurrent Urinary Tract Infection in a Rottweiler

Carl A. Osborne, DVM, PhD, Dipl. ACVIM (Internal Medicine)
College of Veterinary Medicine
University of Minnesota
St. Paul, Minnesota, USA

Patient Assessment

A five-year-old, 41-kg, neutered male rottweiler was examined for recurrent dysuria and pollakiuria of six months' duration, presumed to be caused by bacterial urinary tract infection. These clinical signs had been treated intermittently with a variety of orally administered antibiotics given for intervals ranging from 10 to 21 days. Treatment was associated with remission of dysuria and pollakiuria, but these signs recurred a short time following cessation of therapy.

The results of physical examination, including rectal palpation and body condition assessment (body condition score 3/5), were normal. Micturition was normal. Analysis of a urine sample collected by cystocentesis revealed that the urine was slightly concentrated (specific gravity 1.015), had a neutral pH and contained evidence of inflammation, most likely due to an infectious process (**Table 1**). Crystals were not observed. Aerobic culture of an aliquot of urine revealed significant numbers (>10^5 colony-forming units/ml) of urease-producing *Staphylococcus intermedius*, which was susceptible to many antimicrobial agents. Results of a complete blood count and serum biochemistry profile were normal (**Table 1**).

Problems identified on the basis of the animal assessment included bacterial urinary tract infection with staphylococci characterized by dysuria and pollakiuria, possible impaired urine concentrating capacity, and hematuria, pyuria, proteinuria and bacteriuria.

Assess the Food and Feeding Method

The dog was fed a commercial dry adult maintenance food free choice and offered commercial treats/snacks several times each day.

Questions

1. What is the anatomic site or sites of the bacterial urinary tract infection?
2. Are further diagnostic tests justified for this patient?

Answers and Discussion

1. Dysuria and pollakiuria suggest involvement of the lower urinary tract but formation of urine with a specific gravity of 1.015 in absence of azotemia suggests that ascending infection may have involved the medullary portions of the kidney.
2. Additional diagnostic tests should be considered because: 1) the bacterial urinary tract infection appears to be recurrent, 2) the sites of infection and inflammation have not been confirmed and 3) the predisposing causes of infection are unknown. There is no evidence of diabetes mellitus or hyperadrenocorticism, both of which are frequently associated with recurrent bacterial urinary tract infection. Another urinalysis is indicated to assess the concentrating capacity of the kidneys. Survey and contrast abdominal radiography and/or ultrasonography will help evaluate the patient for uroliths, neoplasia and anatomic abnormalities. These imaging procedures will also assist in evaluation of the prostate gland.

Further Assessment

Results of a second urinalysis included a urine specific gravity of 1.021. Hematuria, pyuria, proteinuria and bacteriuria were still present. Survey radiography and ultrasonography of the abdomen revealed a large urolith in the pelvis of the right kidney (**Figures 1** and **2**). Retrograde positive-contrast urethrocystography revealed normal size, shape and position of the lower urinary tract and prostate gland. Double-contrast cystography revealed a few uroliths approximately 1 mm in diameter in the bladder. An intravenous urogram revealed no evidence of outflow obstruction in the ureters (**Figure 2**).

Further Questions

1. On the basis of the available data, what is the most likely mineral composition of this patient's uroliths?
2. Why were crystals not identified in the urine sediment even though the patient had multiple uroliths?
3. Outline a treatment and feeding plan for this dog.

Answers and Discussion

1. The mineral composition of the nephrolith and urocystoliths most likely is infection-induced struvite because: 1) staphylococci may cause formation of struvite uroliths, 2) very large radiodense nephroliths are usually composed of infection-induced struvite, 3) the urinary pH was not acidic and 4) crystals associated with other types of uroliths were not detected.
2. The combination of risk factors necessary for struvite crystals to form was not present at the time urine samples were collected

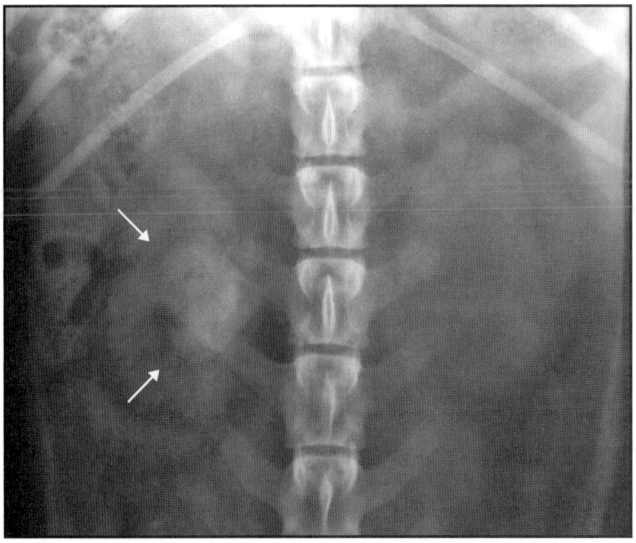

Figure 1. Survey ventrodorsal abdominal radiograph illustrating a large radiodense nephrolith (arrows) in the renal pelvis of the right kidney of a five-year-old neutered male rottweiler.

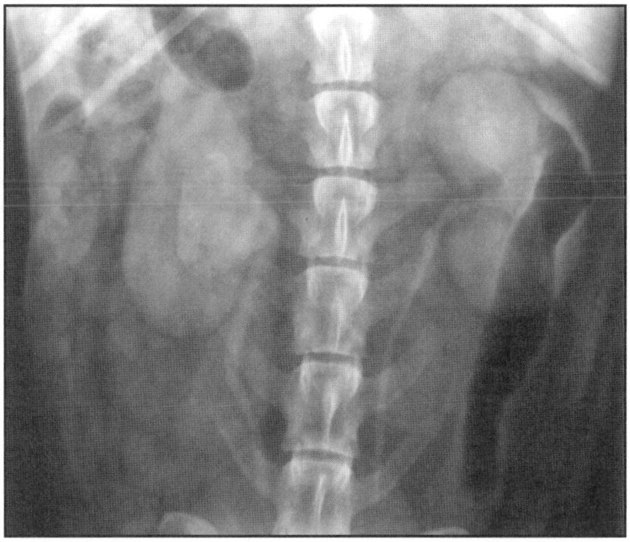

Figure 2. Intravenous urogram of the same dog described in Figure 1 showing both ureters filled with contrast material and no evidence of outflow obstruction.

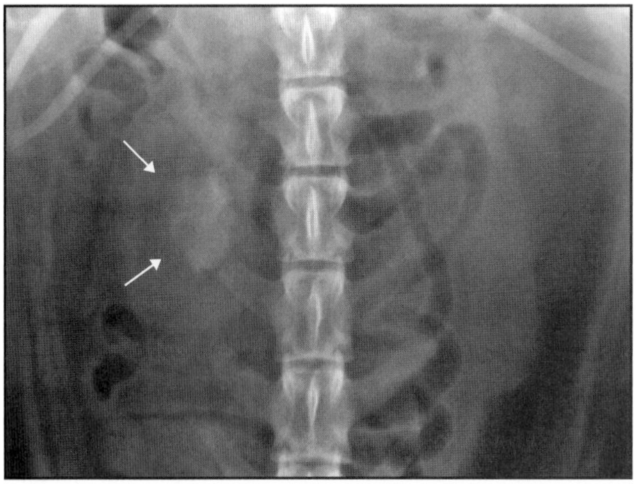

Figure 3. Survey ventrodorsal radiograph obtained five weeks after initiation of therapy with a litholytic food and antibiotics. The nephrolith (arrows) is about 75% of its original size.

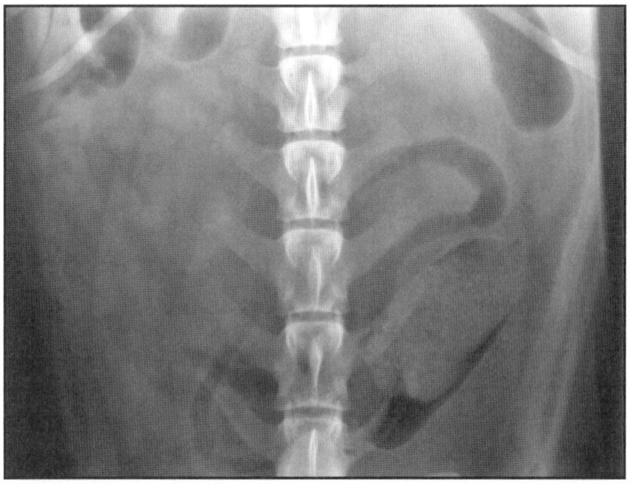

Figure 4. Survey ventrodorsal abdominal radiograph obtained 18 weeks after initiation of therapy. There is no evidence of the nephrolith in the right kidney.

for analysis. Consumption of food that usually results in acidic urine, administration of an antibiotic and formation of poorly concentrated urine may have reduced the likelihood of struvite crystalluria.

3. Dissolution of nephroliths presumed to be composed of infection-induced struvite can be accomplished using a combination of a commercial veterinary therapeutic struvite litholytic food[a] and antimicrobial therapy. In studies conducted at the University of Minnesota, the mean time required for dissolution of infection-induced nephroliths was 26 weeks (range nine to 42 weeks). Nephroliths and/or ureteroliths causing complete outflow obstruction and marked impairment of function in the associated kidney should be managed by surgical intervention. Surgical removal of uroliths has the obvious advantage of rapid correction of the mechanical components of the disease process; however, surgery cannot be relied upon to remove very small uroliths or to prevent their recurrence. Likewise, nephrectomy is always associated with destruction of nephrons, the magnitude of which is influenced by the number of renal end arteries that are transected.

Progress Notes

The owners requested dietary and medical treatment. A combination of a struvite litholytic food and a bactericidal antimicrobial agent (amoxicillin and clavulanic acid[b]), chosen on the basis of antimicrobial susceptibility results, was used. The daily energy requirement was estimated to be approximately 1,800 kcal (7.5 MJ) (1.4 x resting energy requirement) or 1.5 cans of Prescription

Table 1. Results of selected urinalysis and serum biochemistry parameters of a five-year-old neutered male rottweiler with recurrent urinary tract infection.*

Factors	Reference values	Week 0	Week 5	Week 9	Week 13	Week 18	Week 25	Week 29	Week 34
Urine specific gravity	-	1.015	1.007	1.007	1.007	1.015	1.008	1.022	1.015
Urinary pH	-	7	6	6	8	7	7	7.5	6
Hematuria	-	+	+	+	0	0	0	0	0
Pyuria	-	+	0	0	0	0	0	0	0
Bacteriuria	-	+	0	0	0	0	0	0	0
SUN (mg/dl)	7-28	26	5	9	5	6	6	13	11
Creatinine (mg/dl)	0.5-1.5	1.6	1.4	1.4	1.4	1.1	1.1	1.5	1.1
Magnesium (mg/dl)	1.5-2.7	2.3	1.9	1.8	2.0	1.8	1.6	1.8	2.0
Albumin (g/dl)	2.4-3.8	3.5	3.1	3.3	3.3	3.4	2.9	3.5	3.4
Alkaline phosphatase (U/l)	10-149	28	56	67	65	123	164	43	29

Key: + = present, 0 = absent, SUN = serum urea nitrogen.
*Therapy with a litholytic food and antibiotics was initiated during Week 1 and discontinued on Week 25.

Diet s/d Canine[a] twice daily. In order to facilitate dietary compliance, the owners were asked to restrict treats to baked slices of the moist therapeutic food. Therapeutic efficacy was monitored by physical examination and serial evaluation of survey radiographs (a ventrodorsal view is usually best for nephroliths, and a lateral view is usually best for urocystoliths), urinalyses, urine cultures, serum biochemistry profiles and complete blood counts (**Table 1**). Reduction in the serum urea nitrogen concentration and formation of less concentrated urine indicates compliance with the feeding plan.

Survey abdominal radiographs obtained at four- to five-week intervals revealed progressive reduction in the size of the nephrolith (**Figure 3**). Radiodense uroliths could not be detected on Week 18 (**Figure 4**). After initiation of antimicrobial therapy, bacteria could not be cultured from urine samples collected by cystocentesis. Urinalysis revealed progressive reduction in hematuria and pyuria (**Table 1**).

Consumption of the litholytic food was associated with polyuria, formation of less concentrated urine, reduction in the serum concentration of urea nitrogen and magnesium and an increase in serum alkaline phosphatase activity. Clinically significant changes were not observed in serial hemograms. Dietary and antimicrobial therapy was discontinued on Week 25. Most diagnostic parameters returned to baseline values by Weeks 29 and 34 (**Table 1**).

The owners indicated that the dog readily consumed the food and gained 3.5 kg during the treatment period. Decreasing the amount of food offered and consumed during the treatment period may have prevented significant weight gain.

Endnotes

a. Prescription Diet s/d Canine. Hill's Pet Nutrition, Inc., Topeka, KS, USA.
b. Pfizer Animal Health, Exton, PA, USA.

Bibliography

Osborne CA, Lulich JP, Bartges JW, et al. Canine and feline urolithiasis: Relationship of etiopathogenesis to treatment and prevention. In: Osborne CA, Finco DR, eds. Canine and Feline Nephrology and Urology. Baltimore, MD: Williams & Wilkins, 1995, 798-888.

Chapter 44

Canine Silica Urolithiasis: Causes, Detection, Treatment and Prevention

Carl A. Osborne
Jody P. Lulich
Lisa K. Ulrich

"There is a difference between unanswered questions and unquestioned answers."
Carl A. Osborne

TERMINOLOGY

The name silicon (Si) is derived from the Latin word "silicis" meaning flint. Silicon is a naturally occurring nonmetallic element. When combined with oxygen, Si forms SiO_2 and is called silica or silicon dioxide. The term silicate is a noun used to designate a salt derived from silicic acid (as in aluminum silicate and magnesium trisilicate). The term silicon should not be confused with silicone. Silicone refers to any of a group of synthetic resins, oils, greases, plastics, etc. in which the carbon element has been replaced with silicon.

Inorganic Silica

Inorganic silica, whose basic formula is SiO_2, occurs naturally in crystalline, microcrystalline, cryptocrystalline or amorphous forms. The designation SiO_2 as crystalline refers to the orientation of silicon molecules in a fixed, orderly and repetitive pattern resulting in a characteristic shape. Crystals reflect internal order. The term microcrystalline refers to the fact that the crystals are so small that they can only be seen through a microscope. The term cryptocrystalline refers to the fact that the crystals are too small to be seen by light microscopy. The designation as amorphous (without shape) refers to the orientation of SiO_2 molecules in a random or non-periodic pattern. Amorphous minerals are also called mineraloids. Most silica-containing uroliths removed from dogs are composed of amorphous silica.

Inorganic crystalline silica is the basic component of sand, quartz and granite. Microcrystalline silica is found in quartz, chalcedony (agate, onyx, etc.) and chert (flint, jasper, etc.). Amorphous silica is found in glass, opal and diatomaceous earth.

Organic Silica

Although silicate and silica minerals constitute more than 90% of the earth's crust, they occur in very low concentrations in most animals. The low quantities of silica in most animals may be attributable to the low solubility of silica in all but a very few naturally occurring waters. In contrast, plants often contain higher quantities of silica. For example, grasses contain between 1 and 4% silica by dry weight. Plants notable for their high silica content include rice and scouring rushes (genus *Equisetum*), which contain up to 16% silica (Salisbury and Ross, 1985).

EPIDEMIOLOGY AND MINERAL COMPOSITION

Prevalence

Silica accounted for 0.4% of all canine uroliths submitted to the Minnesota Urolith Center from 1981 to 2007, (1,414 of 350,803 [Table 38-8]) and 0.33% of (134 of 40,612) uroliths submitted in 2007. Silica accounted for 0.34% of all upper tract uroliths analyzed at the Minnesota Urolith Center from 1981 to 2007 (19 of 5,591). Silica uroliths were more commonly removed from the lower urinary tract (99%) than the upper urinary tract (1%) (Table 38-9).

Age and Gender

In approximately 310,000 cases of urolithiasis evaluated at our center, only one case of silica urolithiasis was documented in dogs less than 12 months of age. The mean age of dogs at the time of urolith retrieval was 7.7 years (range eight months to 19 years). Males were affected (95%) more commonly than females (5%). However, female dogs may void small silica uroliths before they induce clinical signs, reducing the detection rate.

Breeds

From 2000 to 2006, 82 different breeds were affected including mixed breeds (19%), German shepherd dogs (13%), golden retrievers (6%), Shih Tzus (6%), black Labrador retrievers (6%), rottweilers (2%), miniature schnauzers (2%) and cocker spaniels (1%). A high prevalence of silica uroliths in German shepherd dogs, Yorkshire terriers, Shih Tzus, Lhasa apsos, golden retrievers, miniature schnauzers and old English sheepdogs has been recognized (Aldrich et al, 1997, Ling, 1995). Several of these breeds also appear to be at risk for calcium oxalate uroliths. This association, and the observation that silica uroliths often contain calcium oxalate, prompt questions about the possibility of epitaxy associated with silica and calcium oxalate urolithiasis.

MINERAL COMPOSITION AND ARCHITECTURE

Of 1,414 canine silica uroliths, 982 were composed entirely (100%) of amorphous silica, and 432 were composed of at least 70% of this mineral. Silica uroliths may contain varying quantities of other minerals, especially calcium oxalate. Ammonium urate and calcium phosphate are encountered less frequently in association with silica.

Most canine silica uroliths have a jackstone configuration (Osborne et al, 1981). The name jackstone was selected because their shape is similar to the small, six-pronged metal pieces used in the children's games of "jacks." Protrusions from different uroliths vary in number (usually from 15 to 30), length (from a few mm to more than one cm) and diameter. Some protrusions are long and slender, whereas others are blunt, imparting a mammillary appearance to the urolith. Protrusions from individual uroliths are usually but not invariably similar in length and diameter. These features of silica uroliths often impart a distinctive appearance, which can often be identified by radiography. Cross sections of canine silica jackstones reveal that they are distinctly laminated; however, these laminations cannot be detected by radiography. In most dogs, silica jackstones occurred in multiples with some patients having more than 30. However, a few dogs had solitary uroliths. Silica uroliths ranged in diameter from less than 1 mm to more than 3 cm. Not all uroliths composed primarily of silica had a jackstone configuration. However, all silica uroliths formed by dogs had some form of surface protrusions at more or less regular intervals, imparting a regularly uneven surface contour to the uroliths. Some silica jackstones were coated with layers of struvite, which altered their characteristic shape. In some instances, struvite completely surrounded silica jackstones.

Calcium oxalate monohydrate, calcium oxalate dihydrate and ammonium urate uroliths may also have a jackstone-like appearance as detected by survey and contrast radiography. However, the macroscopic appearance of non-silica jackstones is typically different than that of silica jackstones.

ETIOPATHOGENESIS AND RISK FACTORS

Overview

Naturally occurring silica jackstones were first reported in dogs living in the United States in the mid-1970s (Osborne et al, 1986). An extensive review of the literature revealed a conspicuous absence of this type of canine urolith before that time. In the mid-1970s, silica uroliths were reported to occur only in dogs from the United States and Canada. However, in 1985, canine silica jackstones were recognized in Japan and shortly thereafter in Europe. Calcium magnesium aluminum silicate uroliths without a jackstone configuration were identified in dogs native to Kenya in 1977 (Brodey et al, 1977).

Relationship of Silica Uroliths to Food

Hypothesis

Several observations prompt the hypothesis that development of canine silica uroliths may be related to hyperexcretion of silica in urine following consumption of an absorbable form of silica in various foods. It is noteworthy that silicic acid is readily absorbed across the intestinal wall (Ammerman et al, 1980; Sutor et al, 1970; White and Porter, 1969). The fact that ingested silica is rapidly cleared by the kidneys from plasma of dogs and other animals following absorption into the body also supports the "dietary risk factor" hypothesis (Benke and Osborn, 1979; King et al, 1933).

Possible Dietary Sources of Silica or Silicate

Silicate minerals occur in very low concentrations in most animals. Therefore, ingredients in pet foods derived from animal sources are an unlikely source of this mineral. In contrast, plants contain larger quantities of silica. As mentioned above, grasses contain between 1 and 4% silica by dry weight and rice and scouring rushes (horsetails, genus *Equisetum*) contain up to 16% silica (Salisbury and Ross, 1985).

One plausible explanation as to why canine silica uroliths began to be recognized in the mid-1970s is that at that approximate time, the pet food industry initiated use of an increased quantity of plant-derived ingredients in moist and especially dry dog foods. Silicon is taken up by the roots of plants and deposited in their cell walls as silica, soluble silicates and organic combinations. Although unlikely, another factor could have been the addition of fillers, which contain relatively large quantities of silica (e.g., rice or soybean hulls), to some pet foods designed for reduction in obesity (Underwood, 1977).

Corn gluten feed, a by-product of the wet milling and distilling process designed to separate shelled corn into various components, was another suspected source of silica in some pet foods. Corn gluten feed remains after extraction of starch, gluten and germ from shelled corn. The term gluten, meaning "glue" in Latin refers to the sticky characteristic of substances derived from corn, wheat and other grains. Corn gluten feed contains about 40% protein and is contained in some low quality pet foods. We emphasize that corn gluten feed is not the same as corn gluten meal. Corn gluten meal is contained in many higher quality manufactured foods designed for dogs because it is readily digestible and a relatively inexpensive form of protein (approximately 60%), vitamins, minerals and energy. Corn gluten meal is an unlikely source of the silica in uroliths.

Contamination of various types of plants with soil during harvesting is also conceivable. Another possibility that may apply to some dogs is consumption of soil secondary to diet-associated pica.

Caution: studies performed in rats indicate that the type of silica compound ingested influences its absorption from the gastrointestinal tract (Yoko and Saboro, 1979). In addition, other factors (e.g., pH) may be involved (Pyrah, 1979; Yoko and Saboro, 1979). Therefore, detection of a relatively large quantity of silica in food is not itself synonymous with intestinal absorption and urinary excretion of silica.

Dogs and People

Silica uroliths developed in male dogs fed experimental foods containing a high concentration of silicic acid and talc [$Mg_3SiO_{10}(OH)_2$] for several months (Ehrhart and McCullagh, 1973; McCullagh and Ehrhart, 1974). Replacement of dietary silicic acid with purified cellulose prevented further urolith development. In a pilot study, we detected multiple tiny silica uroliths in the urinary bladder of an adult male beagle dog after it was given magnesium trisilicate orally for approximately four months.

Silica uroliths have been reported in several people who consumed large quantities of antacids containing magnesium trisilicate to alleviate signs of peptic ulcers (Farrer and Rajfer, 1984; Forman et al, 1959; Herman and Goldberg, 1960; Levison et al 1982; Pyrah,1979).

The high prevalence of silica urolithiasis in native Kenyan dogs has been hypothesized to be related to consumption of unprocessed Kenyan corn, a common ingredient in their diet garnered primarily by scavenging (Brodey et al, 1977). It is also conceivable that Kenyan dogs could have consumed silica contained in the soil as they scavenged for food.

Another potential source is micro-fine silica, which is used in small quantities as an anti-caking agent in the manufacture of many pet foods. Although a cause and effect relationship between micro-fine silica and silica urolithiasis is unlikely, until additional information becomes available, it seems logical to avoid giving foods containing this ingredient to dogs with recurrent silica urolithiasis.

Ruminants

The association of food and silica urolith formation in ruminants is relevant to consideration of diet-related risk factors in dogs. Silica uroliths are common in range cattle and sheep that consume forage grasses with a high concentration of silica (Bailey, 1970; Emerick and Embry, 1960; Emerick et al, 1959; Pyrah, 1979; White and Porter, 1969). In Canada, prairie grass (*Festuca scabrella*) has been found to contain 4 to 8% silica (Bailey, 1966). It is noteworthy, however, that attempts to induce silica uroliths in sheep with inorganic forms of silica (sodium silicate) have been unsuccessful (Beeson et al, 1943; Emerick et al, 1959).

Dietary risk factors for induced silica urolithiasis in sheep include low phosphorus concentrations, a high calcium-phosphorus ratio and factors contributing to alkalinization (Emerick et al, 1959).

Rats and Guinea Pigs

Silica uroliths have been experimentally induced in rats fed diets containing 2% tetraethylorthosilicate (Emerick, 1984; Emerick et al, 1963; Stewart et al, 1993). Siliceous deposits were detected in the renal tubules of guinea pigs given large oral doses of soluble silica (Coe et al, 1991).

Applications of Observations to Diet Hypothesis

Affected dogs that formed silica uroliths submitted to the Minnesota Urolith Center were consuming a large variety of commercially manufactured moist and dry foods in addition to homemade foods. A widespread change in the formulation of commercially manufactured dog food in the U.S. was probably associated with the onset of silica urolithiasis in the mid-1970s and early 1980s, but this assumption has not yet been confirmed.

We consider foods containing large quantities of plant-derived ingredients as risk factors for silica urolithiasis in susceptible dogs. Corn gluten feed, rice hulls and soybean hulls have also been incriminated as dietary risk factors (Osborne et al, 1986).

Concentrations of lithogenic substances in urine are dependent on urine volume. Because dry foods (~10 to 20% water) are often associated with production of more concentrated urine compared with canned formulated diets (~75 to 80% water),

Table 44-1. Key nutritional factors for foods for canine silica urolithiasis prevention.

Factors	Dietary recommendations
Water	Water intake should be encouraged to achieve a urine specific gravity <1.020 Moist food will increase water consumption and formation of less concentrated urine
Protein	Restrict high quality dietary protein to 10 to 18% dry matter
Silica	Avoid foods with corn gluten feed, rice hulls and soybean hulls listed on the ingredient panel of the product label
Urinary pH	Feed a food that maintains an alkaline urine (urinary pH = 7.1 to 7.7)

consumption of dry diets may also be considered as a risk factor for silica urolith formation.

BIOLOGIC BEHAVIOR

The time required for naturally occurring silica uroliths to develop in susceptible dogs is unknown. Silica uroliths were induced in dogs four months after consuming foods containing large quantities of silicic acid (McCullagh and Ehrhart, 1974). Silica uroliths have been produced in rats within eight weeks after consumption of tetraethylorthosilicate (Forman et al, 1959; Emerick, 1984; Emerick et al, 1963). Silicious uroliths have also been observed in calves by the time they were approximately four months old (Forman et al, 1959). Evaluation of case reports of people who developed silica uroliths while consuming silicate-containing antacids suggests that the uroliths developed over a period of years (Farrer and Rajfer, 1984; Levinson et al, 1982).

We have observed recurrence of silica uroliths in five dogs following surgical removal of silica uroliths from the lower urinary tract. Struvite urocystoliths developed in at least two dogs as a consequence of infection with urease-producing staphylococci following surgical removal of silica urocystoliths. Formation of struvite uroliths in this situation is not surprising because urease-producing staphylococci are lithogenic in dogs.

KEY NUTRITIONAL FACTORS

Because initiating and perpetuating causes of silica urolithiasis are unknown, only supportive and symptomatic measures designed to reduce the degree of supersaturation of urine with lithogenic substances can be recommended for prevention. These key nutritional factors are discussed below and summarized in **Table 44-1**.

Water

Concentrations of lithogenic substances in urine depend on urine volume. For dogs with recurrent silica urolithiasis, increasing the volume of urine produced by increasing water consumption will increase the volume of urine in which lithogenic substances are dissolved or suspended. Moist foods rather than dry foods should be considered. Oral administration of sodium chloride has been a favored empirical method to induce diuresis in dogs with uroliths. However, the use of sodium chloride to promote diuresis in dogs that form silica uroliths cannot be routinely recommended without evidence of safety and efficacy because of the unpredictable but marked occurrence of calcium oxalate in silica uroliths and because orally administered sodium chloride is associated with hypercalciuria. Strive to promote formation of urine with a specific gravity value less than 1.020.

Protein

Moderate restriction of dietary protein (10 to 18% dry matter) has the advantage of contributing to obligatory polyuria by decreasing renal medullary urea concentration and is therefore, recommended.

Besides the amount of protein, the predominant protein source can be important. Some protein supplying ingredients for pet foods are higher in silica than others. Animal-derived protein ingredients are an unlikely source of silica. In contrast, some plant-derived protein sources contain larger quantities of silica. As mentioned above, corn gluten feed is an example. On the other hand, many higher quality commercial pet foods contain corn gluten meal because it is readily digestible and is a relatively inexpensive source of protein. Corn gluten meal is an unlikely source of the silica in uroliths. Check the ingredient label. Foods listing "corn gluten feed" as one of the first four non-water ingredients should be avoided.

Silica

Foods with large quantities of plant-derived ingredients are suspected to be risk factors for silica uroliths in susceptible dogs. Consumption of dry foods may also be considered a risk factor for silica urolith formation. Corn gluten feed, rice hulls and soybean hulls have been incriminated (Osborne et al, 1986). Although an unlikely source, ingestion of micro-fine silica used as a de-caking agent in the manufacture of some foods is a possibility. Avoid foods whose product label ingredient panel lists corn gluten feed, rice hulls or soybean hulls.

Urinary pH

Silica is less soluble in acidic than alkaline water, and currently available information suggests that silica is less soluble in acidic than alkaline biologic environments. It is noteworthy that the urinary pH of eight non-infected dogs with silica uroliths was acidic to neutral at the time of diagnosis (mean = 6.0; range = 5.0 to 7.0). Whether or not alkalinization of urine is beneficial in increasing the solubility of silica or silicates in urine is unknown. However, until more research evidence is available, we recommend that the urinary pH produced by a food or a food and urine alkalinizing agents be in the range of 7.1 to 7.7.

FEEDING PLAN

Effective dietary and medical protocols to induce dissolution of canine silica jackstones have not yet been developed. At this time, surgery is the only practical option to remove large silica uroliths. Voiding urohydropropulsion may be used to remove small urocystoliths (Figure 38-5 and Table 38-7) (Lulich et al, 1993). Lithotripsy may be considered to remove urethroliths. Litholytic foods that do not contain large quantities of plant ingredients and that induce diuresis may prevent further growth of silica uroliths.

At this time, our recommendations include change of diet, augmentation of urine volume and consideration of altering urinary pH (**Table 44-1**) (Osborne et al, 1986; Osborne et al, 1999).

Assess and Select the Food

Although the role of food in the genesis of canine silica uroliths is still somewhat speculative, it seems reasonable to recommend that food(s) of affected patients be changed, especially if the problem is recurrent. Although empirical, this maneuver is unlikely to be harmful and may be helpful. Based on the assumption that the primary source of excessive silica in foods is vegetable in origin, selection of a food with reduced quantities of specific vegetable protein and other plant-based ingredients is recommended. Our empirical experience with this method of prevention has been favorable. **Table 44-2** lists selected veterinary therapeutic foods that can be considered for prevention of silica urolithiasis and compares their key nutritional factor content to the recommended levels. Select the food that is most similar to the key nutritional factor profile. Because these foods are intended for long-term feeding, they should also be approved by the Association of American Feed Control Officials (AAFCO), or some other credible regulatory agency. Dogs consuming dry foods may be at greater risk for urolithiasis than dogs consuming moist foods. Dry foods are often associated with higher urine concentrations of urolith constituents (in the case of silica urolithiasis, more plant origin ingredients) and more concentrated urine. Therefore, when possible, moist foods should be selected.

Assess and Determine the Feeding Method

A few dogs with silica uroliths have a history of pica and coprophagia associated with consumption of dirt and/or compost in one form or another. The relationship of the onset of pica with the diet history should be investigated with the goal of correcting this problem.

Transitioning a patient from the current food to a new food selected for the prevention of silica urolithiasis should be done gradually over a period of a few days. Begin the transition by feeding 75% of the current food and 25% of the new food on Day 1. On Day 2, feed half of each food. On Day 3, feed 75% new food and 25% old food. By Day 4 or 5, feed only the new food.

Because moist foods tend to increase water intake and produce a less concentrated urine, recommend the client feed specific amounts (meal fed) two to three times per day rather than free-choice feeding. Moist foods can spoil if left at room temperature for several hours (Chapter 11). Opened containers of moist foods should be refrigerated and the feeding bowl should be kept clean.

Table 44-2. Levels of key nutritional factors in selected commercial foods used to minimize recurrence of silica uroliths in dogs compared to recommended levels.*

Dry food	Protein (%)	Urinary pH**
Recommended levels	**10-18**	**7.1-7.7**
Hill's Prescription Diet u/d Canine	11.2	7.70
Moist food		
Hill's Prescription Diet u/d Canine	13.3	7.40

*Manufacturer's published values; protein expressed as % dry matter; when possible recommend moist foods; where possible, check the ingredient panel of the product label and avoid foods that list corn gluten feed, rice hulls or soybean hulls.
**Protocols for measuring urinary pH may vary.

Besides offering moist foods, there are several additional ways to facilitate increased water intake. These include: 1) Ensuring multiple water bowls are available in prominent locations in the dog's environment; this may mean providing several bowls outside in a large enclosure or a bowl on each level of the house. 2) Bowls should be clean and, if possible, kept full of fresh water. 3) Small amounts of flavoring substances (e.g., salt-free bouillon) can be added to water sources to increase consumption. 4) Ice cubes can be offered as treats or snacks. 5) If a dry food is selected, advise the client to add liberal quantities of water; however, as with moist foods left at room temperature for too long, be aware that there are also potential food safety issues that might arise from leaving moistened dry foods out for prolonged intervals (Chapter 11).

If the patient has a normal body condition score (BCS 2.5/5 to 3.5/5), the amount of the previous food being fed was probably appropriate. On an energy basis, a similar amount of the new food would be a good starting point.

Oral administration of sodium chloride has been a favored empirical method to induce diuresis in dogs with uroliths. However, the use of sodium chloride to promote diuresis in dogs that form silica uroliths cannot be routinely recommended without evidence of safety and efficacy because of the unpredictable but marked occurrence of calcium oxalate in silica uroliths and because orally administered sodium chloride is associated with hypercalciuria.

ADJUNCTIVE MEDICAL MANAGEMENT

Urine Alkalinizing Agents

Silica is apparently less soluble in acidic than alkaline water, and currently available information suggests that silica is less soluble in acidic than alkaline biologic environments. It is noteworthy that the urinary pH of eight non-infected dogs with silica uroliths was acidic to neutral at the time of diagnosis (mean = 6.0; range = 5.0 to 7.0). Whether or not alkalinization of urine is beneficial in increasing the solubility of silica or silicates in urine is unknown. Likewise, the effects of orally administered alkalinizing agents (e.g., sodium bicarbonate) on the absorbability of silica from the gastrointestinal tract have not been evaluated. Nonetheless, it seems prudent to recommend that efforts

Table 44-3. Summary of recommendations for prevention of canine silica uroliths.

1. Perform appropriate diagnostic studies including complete urinalysis, quantitative urine culture and diagnostic radiography. Determine precise location, size and number of uroliths.
2. If uroliths are available, determine their mineral composition. If unavailable, determine their composition by evaluation of appropriate clinical data.
3. Small urocystoliths may be removed by voiding urohydropropulsion (Figure 38-5 and Table 38-7). Consider surgical removal of larger uroliths causing clinical disease.
4. To prevent further growth of existing silica uroliths or to prevent recurrence of silica uroliths after surgical removal:
   a. Avoid use of foods containing large quantities of plant proteins, and especially avoid those containing rice hulls, soybean hulls or corn gluten feed.
   b. Enhance diuresis by adding moisture to the food.
   c. Avoid efforts to deliberately acidify urine.
5. If necessary, eradicate or control urinary tract infections with appropriate antimicrobial agents.

to deliberately acidify the urine of dogs with recurrent silica uroliths be avoided. The observation that silica may occur in uroliths in association with calcium oxalate is additional support for the recommendation to avoid acidification of urine. Mild alkalinization (pH range 7.1 to 7.7) of the urine (but not of the digestive system) might be considered for dogs affected by silica uroliths that recur frequently. Prevention of systemic acidosis is recommended to minimize calcium oxalate urolith formation.

REASSESSMENT

Therapy should be initiated in a stepwise fashion (**Table 44-3**). The goal of therapy is to prevent silica urolith recurrence. Dietary management should minimize exposure to minerals predisposing to silica uroliths and result in formation of less concentrated urine; strive to promote formation of urine with a specific gravity less than 1.020. A urinalysis and lateral abdominal radiograph should be evaluated periodically. Initially, every three to four months seems reasonable. Depending on results, the interval may be increased or decreased. The goal is to detect recurrent urocystoliths when they are small enough to be removed by voiding urohydropropulsion (Lulich et al, 1993) or lithotripsy.

REFERENCES

The references for **Chapter 44** can be found at www.markmorris.org.

Chapter

45

Canine Compound Urolithiasis: Prevalence, Significance and Management

Carl A. Osborne

Jody P. Lulich

Lisa K. Ulrich

"The best veterinary teaching hospitals in the world not only use contemporary data, they create it."
Carl A. Osborne

Compound uroliths (nucleus composed of one mineral type and shells of a different mineral type) occurred in approximately 7% of the canine uroliths analyzed at the University of Minnesota (Table 38-8). Examples include: 1) a nucleus of 100% calcium oxalate monohydrate surrounded by a shell of 80% magnesium ammonium phosphate and 20% calcium phosphate, 2) a nucleus composed of 95% magnesium ammonium phosphate and 5% calcium phosphate surrounded by a shell of 95% ammonium acid urate and 5% magnesium ammonium phosphate and 3) a nucleus composed of 95% silica and 5% calcium oxalate monohydrate surrounded by a shell of 100% calcium oxalate monohydrate.

Voiding urohydropropulsion may be used to remove small compound urocystoliths (Figure 38-5 and Table 38-7) (Lulich et al, 1993). Lithotripsy may be considered to remove uroliths lodged in the urethra. For most practitioners, surgery remains the most reliable method to remove large compound urocystoliths.

Because risk factors that predispose patients to precipitation (nucleation) of different minerals vary, the occurrence of compound uroliths poses a unique challenge in terms of preventing recurrence. In the absence of clinical evidence to the contrary, it seems logical to recommend management protocols designed primarily to minimize recurrence of minerals composing the nucleus (rather than those in shells) of compound uroliths (Lulich and Osborne, 2000; Osborne, 2003). (See specific chapters for recommendations [Chapters 39 through 44]). Followup studies designed to evaluate efficacy of preventive protocols should include complete urinalyses, radiography or ultrasonography and if available, evaluation of the urine concentration of lithogenic metabolites.

REFERENCES

The references for **Chapter 45** can be found at www.markmorris.org.

CASE 45-1

Inappropriate Urination in a Yorkshire Terrier Cross

Jody P. Lulich, DVM, PhD, Dipl. ACVIM (Internal Medicine)

Carl A. Osborne, DVM, PhD, Dipl. ACVIM (Internal Medicine)
College of Veterinary Medicine
University of Minnesota
St. Paul, Minnesota, USA

Patient Assessment

An 11-year-old, neutered female Yorkshire terrier cross weighing 5 kg was examined for inappropriate urination. The dog had been urinating in the house during the day while the owners were at work. Sometimes the urine appeared red. Physical examination was normal except for dental calculus and gingivitis. Body condition was normal (body condition score 3/5).

Urinalysis of a voided sample revealed alkaline urine with hematuria, proteinuria, pyuria, bacteriuria and a few struvite crystals (**Table 1**). A presumptive diagnosis of bacterial urinary tract infection was made. Urine collected by cystocentesis was submitted for aerobic bacterial culture. Pending culture results, the dog was given a combination of amoxicillin and clavulanic acid (14 mg/kg body weight, per os, q12h). Urine culture results identified *Staphylococcus intermedius*, which was susceptible to the prescribed antimicrobial.

One week later the dog was examined for continued hematuria and dysuria. Bacterial culture of urine was negative indicating that antimicrobial therapy was successful. Survey abdominal radiographs (**Figure 1**) revealed a large solitary radiodense urocystolith with a distinct central core (outside diameter = 2.9 cm, core diameter = 1.3 cm). The urolith core was denser than the outer layer. A urinalysis was not performed.

Assess the Food and Feeding Method

The dog ate a commercial moist grocery brand food supplemented with milk, turkey and chicken meat.

Questions

1. What is the probable mineral composition of this dog's urolith?
2. What are the advantages and disadvantages of surgical vs. dietary and medical management of this urolith?

Answers and Discussion

1. Based on the clinical findings, the outer portion of the urolith was probably composed of magnesium ammonium phosphate (struvite) (**Table 2**). Because of the difference in radiodensity, the nidus may be composed of a different mineral salt, likely calcium oxalate.
2. Although struvite urocystoliths are amenable to dietary and medical dissolution, surgical removal is probably the best treatment option in cases of suspected compound uroliths.

Progress Notes

Results of a serum biochemistry profile were normal. The urolith was removed surgically

Table 1. Urinalyses of an 11-year-old female Yorkshire terrier crossbred dog with inappropriate urination.*

Factors**	Day 1	Day 14***	Day 28	Day 60
Specific gravity	1.028	1.035	1.005	1.007
pH	8.0	6.0	7.0	7.5
Protein†	2+	Trace	Trace	Trace
RBC††	3-6	0	0	0
WBC††	30-40	0	0	0
Epithelial cells††	Occ	Occ	None	Few
Bacteria††	Moderate	None	None	None
Crystals†††	Struvite	None	None	Few
Aerobic bacterial culture	*S. intermedius*	Neg	Neg	Neg

Key: RBC = red blood cells, WBC = white blood cells, Occ = occasional, Neg = negative.
*Samples collected by cystocentesis on Days 14, 28 and 60.
**Glucose, bilirubin and acetone were not detected in any specimen.
***Dietary therapy was initiated on Day 14.
†Values represent semiquantitative evaluations based on a scale of 0 to 4; urine volume was not considered.
††Per high power field (x450).
†††Per low power field (x100).

Table 2. The advantages and disadvantages of dietary and medical urolith dissolution and surgical urolith removal can be accurately assessed after the mineral composition of the urolith is known or predicted. This table lists factors used to predict mineral composition of radiodense uroliths when no uroliths are available for quantitative analysis vs. clinical findings in the patient described in this case.*

Factors	MAP	CaOx	CaP	Silica	Cystine
Typical urinary pH	Yes	No	Possible	No	No
Typical crystalluria	Yes	No	No	No	No
Typical urine culture	Yes	No	No	No	No
Typical radiographic density	Yes	Yes	Yes	Yes	No
Typical radiographic contour	Yes	Possible	Possible	No	No
Typical breed	No	Yes	Yes	No	No
Typical gender	Yes	No	No	No	No
Typical age	No	Yes	Yes	No	No

Key: MAP = magnesium ammonium phosphate, CaOx = calcium oxalate, CaP = calcium phosphate.
*Characteristics of urate uroliths were not considered because they are typically radiolucent.

and antimicrobial therapy was continued for an additional two weeks. Quantitative mineral analysis of the urolith by polarizing light microscopy and infrared spectroscopy revealed that the nidus was composed of 100% calcium oxalate monohydrate and the outer layer was composed of 95% magnesium ammonium phosphate and 5% calcium phosphate carbonate.

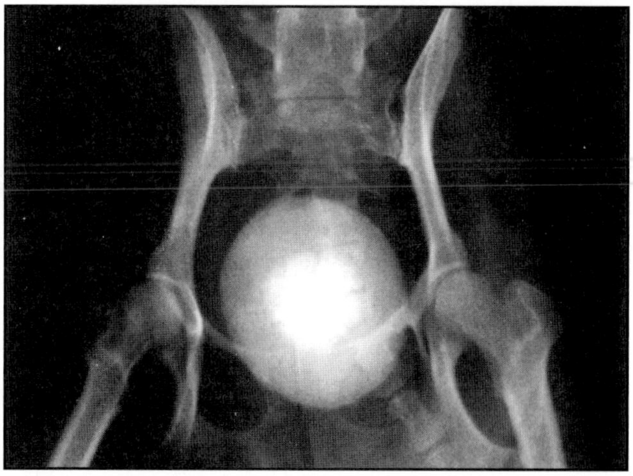

Figure 1. Survey abdominal radiograph (ventrodorsal view) showing a solitary urocystolith. Note that the urolith nidus is radiographically denser than the outer layer.

Further Questions

1. How does a compound urolith develop?
2. How can recurrence of urolithiasis be minimized in this patient?

Answers and Discussion

1. Although the exact mechanisms responsible for calcium oxalate urolith formation are unknown, supersaturation of urine with calcium and oxalic acid is a prerequisite. The calcium oxalate nidus probably disrupted local defense mechanisms predisposing this patient to a staphylococcal bacterial infection of the urinary bladder. These bacteria produce the enzyme urease, leading to urine alkalinity and oversaturation with struvite. The calcium oxalate nidus served as template for struvite crystal deposition (heterogeneous nucleation).
2. Some strategies designed to prevent calcium oxalate urolith formation increase the risk for struvite urolith formation. The reverse is also true. When managing patients with compound uroliths containing both mineral salts, minimizing calcium oxalate urolith recurrence is given priority over minimizing struvite urolith formation because struvite uroliths can be nutritionally and medically dissolved. At present, there is no strategy to dissolve calcium oxalate uroliths.

   Dietary recommendations to minimize recurrence of calcium oxalate uroliths include reducing calcium, oxalate, protein and sodium, providing additional water and citrate and maintaining adequate phosphorus and magnesium. One therapeutic goal to prevent calcium oxalate recurrence is alkalinization of urine, which minimizes calcium excretion and augments citrate excretion. Although urine alkalinization increases saturation for struvite, other factors appear to have a greater impact on struvite urolith formation in dogs. In this patient, struvite formed as a result of a urinary tract infection with bacteria that produce urease. Therefore, it is unlikely that struvite will reform without recurrence of a urease-positive urinary tract infection. Urine cultures should be evaluated periodically to detect and eradicate urinary tract infections early so that struvite uroliths do not form.

Progress Notes

A commercial veterinary therapeutic food (Prescription Diet u/d Canine[a]) was recommended (one-half can per day, 375 kcal [1.57 MJ]) and the owners were instructed to avoid feeding human foods, commercial dog treats and vitamin-mineral supplements (especially those containing vitamins C and D and calcium). Urinalysis, urine culture and survey abdominal radiographs were recommended at regular intervals (i.e., every six months).

Endnote

a. Hill's Pet Nutrition Inc., Topeka, KS, USA.

Bibliography

Osborne CA, Lulich JP, Bartges JW, et al. Canine and feline urolithiasis: Relationship of etiopathogenesis to treatment and prevention. In: Osborne CA, Finco DR, eds. Canine and Feline Nephrology and Urology. Baltimore, MD: Williams & Wilkins, 1995; 798-888.

Section 16

Feline Lower Urinary Tract Diseases

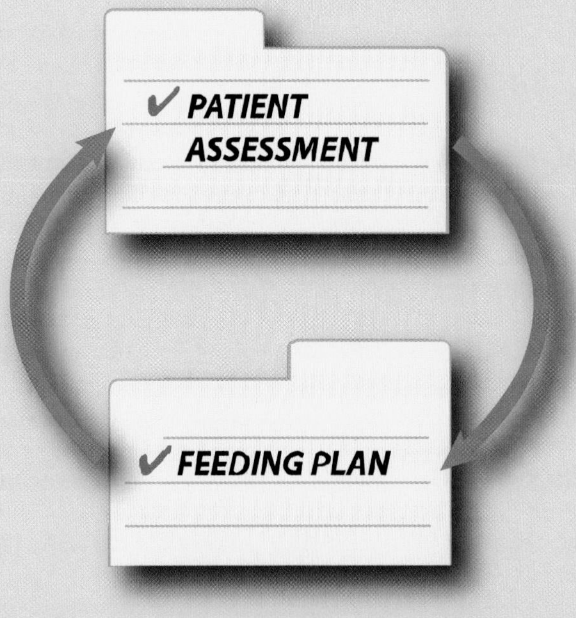

Chapter 46

Feline Lower Urinary Tract Diseases

S. Dru Forrester
John M. Kruger
Timothy A. Allen

"There is a great difference between knowing and understanding: you can know a lot about something and not really understand it."
Charles F. Kettering

CLINICAL IMPORTANCE

Diseases of the feline lower urinary tract involve the urinary bladder or urethra and may be associated with varying combinations of signs including dysuria, hematuria, pollakiuria, stranguria and periuria (i.e., urinating in inappropriate locations). Feline lower urinary tract diseases (FLUTD) encompass many diverse causes; however, this chapter will focus primarily on the three most common: 1) idiopathic lower urinary tract disease, often called feline idiopathic cystitis (FIC), 2) urolithiasis and 3) urethral plugs. Nutritional management is an important component in the treatment of cats with these lower urinary tract disorders. Nutritional management is recommended for cats with FIC together with environmental enrichment and behavioral management. Nutritional management also is indicated for dissolving struvite uroliths and decreasing risk for recurrence of struvite uroliths and urethral plugs and calcium oxalate uroliths.

The true incidence of the various forms of FLUTD is unknown; however, previous estimates in the United States and the United Kingdom have been approximately 0.85 and 1.5% per year, respectively (Lawler et al, 1985; Willeberg, 1984). These estimates were based on presence of clinical signs and did not consider subsets of cats with specific diagnoses, such as struvite urolithiasis or FIC. In a 1995 survey of primary care veterinary hospitals in the U.S., prevalence of lower urinary tract disorders among 15,226 cats was 3% (Lund et al, 1999). The proportional morbidity ratio (i.e., frequency with which cases are seen at a veterinary hospital) of cats with lower urinary tract diseases has been reported to be 4.6% of those evaluated in primary care hospitals and 7 to 8% of those at North American veterinary teaching hospitals (Bartges, 1997; Kirk et al, 2001; Lekcharoensuk et al, 2001). Proportional morbidity ratios, however, are not reliable estimates of disease incidence because they are affected by other parameters including type of veterinary hospital, interest and expertise of veterinarians at the hospital and economic status of clients served by the hospital.

Another measure of the importance of a clinical problem is the degree of owner concern and recognition. In an animal health survey prepared for the Morris Animal Foundation, 1,211 owners indicated that their top feline health concerns were urinary diseases (n = 576; 48%), dental problems (29%), cancer (27%) and feline leukemia virus infection (27%) (MAF, 1998). In a survey of current and previous donors, kidney and urinary disease (43%) were the most common feline health concerns identified by respondents (MAF, 2005). According to

Table 46-1. Prevalence of feline lower urinary tract diseases in four clinical studies.

Diagnosis*	Occurrence among cats with lower urinary tract signs (%)			
Idiopathic (FIC)	63	55	64	57
Urethral obstruction	19	21**	na	58***
Urethral plugs	nr	21	na	10
Uroliths	19	23	15	22
Behavioral disorder	nr	nr	9	0
Incontinence	4	0	0	0
Bacterial UTI	3†	3	1	8
Anatomic anomaly	0.3	nr	11	0
Neoplasia	0.3	0	2	0
Unknown	0	0	0	3
Study characteristics				
Study type	Retrospective††	Prospective†††	Prospective‡	Prospective‡‡
Population	All clinical presentations	All clinical presentations	Non-obstructed clinical presentations	All clinical presentations
Collection period	1980-1997	1982-1985	1993-1995	2000-2002
Cases (n)	22,908	141	109	77

Key: FIC = feline idiopathic cystitis, na = not applicable, nr = not reported, UTI = urinary tract infection.
*Some cats had multiple disorders.
**All cats had urethral obstruction associated with urethral plugs.
***Included 24 cats with FIC, 13 cats with uroliths and eight cats with urethral plugs.
†Another 9% were reported to have undefined infection
††Adapted from Lekcharoensuk C, Osborne CA, Lulich JP. Epidemiologic study of risk factors for lower urinary tract diseases in cats. Journal of the American Veterinary Medical Association 2001; 218: 1429-1435.
†††Adapted from Kruger JM, Osborne CA, Goyal SM, et al. Clinical evaluation of cats with lower urinary tract disease. Journal of the American Veterinary Medical Association 1991; 199: 211-216.
‡Adapted from Buffington CAT, Chew DJ, Kendall MS, et al. Clinical evaluation of cats with non-obstructive lower urinary tract disease: 109 cases (1993-1995). Journal of the American Veterinary Medical Association 1997; 210: 45-50.
‡‡Adapted from Gerber B, Boretti FS, Kley S, et al. Evaluation of clinical signs and causes of lower urinary tract disease in European cats. Journal of Small Animal Practice 2005; 46: 571-577.

Table 46-2. Prevalence of lower urinary tract diseases in 81 cats over 10 years of age evaluated at the University of Georgia Veterinary Teaching Hospital between 1980 and 1995.*

Disorders	Cats (%)
UTI	46
UTI and uroliths	17
Uroliths	10
Urethral plugs	7
Trauma	7
FIC	5
Incontinence	5
Neoplasia	3

Key: UTI = urinary tract infection, FIC = feline idiopathic cystitis.
*Adapted from Bartges JW. Lower urinary tract disease in geriatric cats. In: Proceedings. 15th Annual Veterinary Medical Forum, American College of Veterinary Internal Medicine, Lake Buena Vista, FL, 1997: 322-324.

data from VPI Pet Insurance, lower urinary tract disease was the most common reason pet owners filed a claim for reimbursement of veterinary expenses for their cats in 2006; gastric upsets and kidney disease were the second and third most common reasons (2007). Finally, inappropriate elimination often accompanies FLUTD and is the most common behavioral problem for which pet owners seek professional counsel. It also is the primary behavioral reason why pet owners relinquish their cats to shelters (Beaver, 1989; Neilson, 2003; Salman et al, 2000). Therefore, correct diagnosis and management of underlying causes of periuria are important for maintaining the pet-family bond.

CAUSES OF FLUTD

Many different lower urinary tract diseases occur in cats; however, only a few are common and these may differ depending on the cat's age, presence of concomitant diseases and geographic location. If clinical signs are present and a specific cause is not identified after appropriate evaluation, FIC is the most likely diagnosis. Based on findings from four clinical studies, the three most common lower urinary tract diseases in cats are FIC, urolithiasis and urethral plugs (Lekcharoensuk et al, 2001; Kruger et al, 1991; Buffington et al, 1997; Gerber et al, 2005) (**Table 46-1**). In cats older than 10 years, urinary tract infection (UTI) and uroliths were the most common causes of lower urinary tract signs (**Table 46-2**) (Bartges, 1997). In a study from Norway, 33% of 134 cats with stranguria, dysuria, hematuria and pollakiuria were diagnosed with UTI based on culture of urine obtained by cystocentesis, catheterization or voiding (Eggertsdóttir et al, 2007). No significant difference existed in occurrence of UTI based on methods of sampling in this study. In contrast to previous studies, in which most cats were evaluated at teaching hospitals, 97% of cats in the Norwegian study were first-opinion cases and only 3% were referred. Before the approach to management of cats with signs of FLUTD is modified, further evaluation is needed to determine if UTI is a common occurrence in first-opinion cases, and whether there are geographic differences.

Uroliths and urethral plugs are named based on their mineral composition, which is determined by quantitative analysis.

Usually one mineral type predominates; however, the composition may be mixed in some uroliths and plugs. Different mineral types may be dispersed throughout the urolith (i.e., mixed urolith) or organized into separate, discrete bands or layers (i.e., compound urolith). The most common mineral types identified in feline uroliths are struvite (magnesium ammonium phosphate) (**Figures 46-1** and **46-2**) and calcium oxalate (**Figure 46-3**) (Houston et al, 2003; Cannon et al, 2007).[a] Rarely, uroliths are composed of non-mineral substances (e.g., dried solidified blood) (Westropp et al, 2006). Although there have been changes in trends over the past 25 years, struvite and calcium oxalate have remained the most common uroliths in cats (**Table 46-3**). The most recently collected data reveal that struvite is the most common feline urolith followed by calcium oxalate and purine (e.g., urate) (**Table 46-4**). Since 1981, struvite has consistently been the most common mineral type identified in urethral plugs, representing 81 to 87% of plugs analyzed in the U.S. and Canada (**Table 46-5**) (Houston et al, 2003).[a]

Over the past 25 years, several changing trends have been noted in occurrence of feline uroliths (Cannon et al, 2007; Picavet et al, 2007).[a] In 1981, 78% of feline uroliths evaluated at the Minnesota Urolith Center (University of Minnesota) were struvite and only 2% were calcium oxalate.[a] From 1994 to 2001, however, occurrence of calcium oxalate uroliths increased to 55% and struvite decreased to 33%. In 1994, 77% of uroliths from cats in Benelux (Belgium, The Netherlands and Luxemburg) were struvite and 12% were calcium oxalate; however, by 2003, struvite uroliths had decreased to 32% and calcium oxalate had increased to 61% (Picavet et al, 2007). At the Canadian Urolith Centre (University of Guelph, Ontario), approximately 50% of feline urinary bladder uroliths analyzed from 1998 to 2003 were calcium oxalate and 44% were struvite (Houston et al, 2003). Since 2001, the number of struvite uroliths analyzed at the Minnesota Urolith Center has consistently increased whereas the number of calcium oxalate uroliths has decreased (**Figure 46-4**). At the Gerald V. Ling Urinary Stone Analysis Laboratory (University of California, Davis), struvite-containing uroliths were the predominant mineral type analyzed from 1985 to 1993. Thereafter, calcium oxalate became more common (Cannon et al, 2007). From 2002 to 2004; however, 44% of feline uroliths submitted were struvite and 40% were calcium oxalate. The cause(s) for these changing trends is unknown and needs further study.

Urethral obstruction is a complication of both uroliths and urethral plugs, particularly in male cats (Bovee et al, 1979; Kruger et al, 1991; Gerber et al, 2007). During the past 20 years, the number of perineal urethrostomies performed at veterinary teaching hospitals in the U.S. and Canada has declined, which has paralleled a similar decline in the frequency of urethral obstructions, urethral plugs or urethroliths (**Figure 46-5**) (Lekcharoensuk et al, 2002). These trends coincide with widespread use of specially formulated foods to minimize struvite crystalluria in cats. This is important considering that struvite has consistently been the predominant mineral type in feline urethral plugs during the same time period.

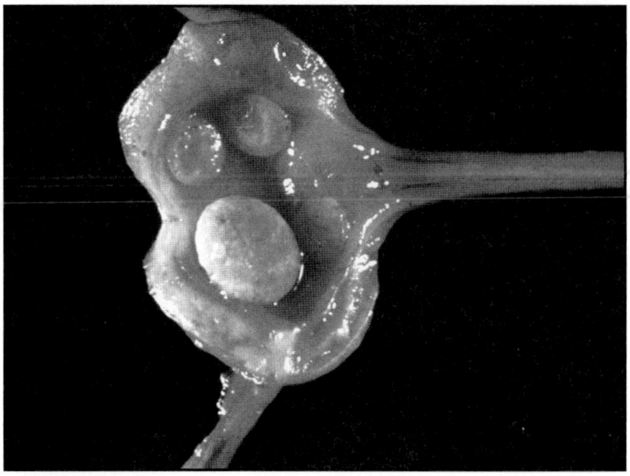

Figure 46-1. Urinary bladder from a cat with struvite urolithiasis. Note the thickened urinary bladder wall and several struvite uroliths within the urinary bladder lumen.

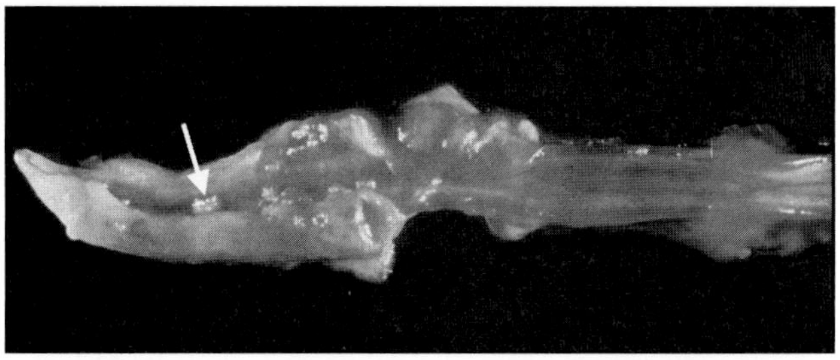

Figure 46-2. Penis and urethra from a cat with urethral obstruction. Note the small struvite urolith (white arrow) in the penile urethra. Uroliths consist of small amounts of matrix and macroscopic crystalline mineral concretions. They are less common causes of urethral obstruction in male cats than urethral plugs (**Figure 46-12**).

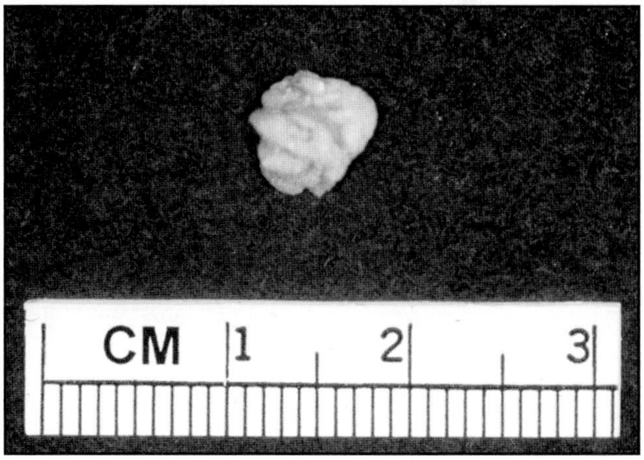

Figure 46-3. Calcium oxalate dihydrate urolith removed from the urinary bladder of a cat with hematuria and dysuria.

Although data from urolith centers are helpful, this information cannot be used to determine incidence (i.e., rate of occurrence of new cases in the population) or prevalence (i.e., total number of urolith cases during a given time) of urolith types. Not all cats with uroliths are diagnosed or treated (e.g., they may not receive veterinary care). In addition, not all uroliths are submitted for quantitative analysis and not all laboratories routine-

Table 46-3. Mineral composition of feline uroliths submitted for quantitative analysis to three centers.

Predominant mineral type	Uroliths submitted during collection period (%)		
Struvite	43.5	43	44
Calcium oxalate	45.4	53	50
Purine	5.0*	10**	3
Compound	3.4	–	–
Mixed	1.0	13***	–
Matrix	0.9	–	–
Calcium phosphate, apatite and brushite	0.3	6	0.1
Cystine	0.1	0.1	–
Silica	0.04	0.4	–
Dry solidified blood	Included with matrix	1	–
Summary information for data sources			
Urolith center	Minnesota Urolith Center†	Gerald V. Ling Urinary Stone Laboratory††	Canadian Urolith Centre†††
Collection period	1981-2008	1985-2004	1998-2003
Uroliths (n)	102,191	5,230	4,866

*Includes uroliths that contained 70 to 100% urate, uric acid or xanthine.
**Includes uroliths that contained any amount of urate.
***Includes mixed and compound uroliths.
†Adapted from Osborne CA, Lulich JP. Unpublished data. Minnesota Urolith Center. University of Minnesota, St Paul, 2009.
††Adapted from Cannon AB, Westropp JL, Ruby AL, et al. Evaluation of trends in urolith composition in cats: 5,230 cases (1985-2004). Journal of the American Veterinary Medical Association 2007; 237: 570-576.
†††Adapted from Houston DM, Moore AE, Favrin MG, et al. Feline urethral plugs and bladder uroliths: A review of 5,484 submissions 1998-2003. Canadian Veterinary Journal 2003; 44(12): 974-977.

Table 46-4. Mineral composition of 11,416 feline uroliths analyzed quantitatively at the Minnesota Urolith Center in 2008.*

Mineral type	Percent
Struvite	49
Calcium oxalate	39
Urate/uric acid	4.9
Compound/matrix/mixed	4.29/0.7/1.0
Calcium phosphate	0.2
Cystine	0.04
Xanthine	<0.01

*Adapted from Osborne CA, Lulich JP. Unpublished data. Minnesota Urolith Center. University of Minnesota, St Paul, 2009.

ly report urolith data annually. In addition, some urolith types are more likely to be submitted for evaluation than others. For example, struvite uroliths can be dissolved with nutritional management; however, calcium oxalate uroliths are more likely to be removed and submitted for quantitative analysis. This could result in an underestimation of the occurrence of struvite uroliths and overestimation for calcium oxalate uroliths.

Regarding trends in occurrence of feline uroliths, several relevant questions remain unanswered: 1) What is the incidence (i.e., rate of occurrence among all cats, not only those presented for veterinary evaluation) of uroliths and has it changed over the past decades? 2) How has the apparent aging feline population affected the relative frequency of different urolith types (e.g., has this contributed to increased diagnosis of calcium oxalate uroliths)? 3) Does the occurrence of calcium oxalate uroliths appear greater because fewer struvite uroliths are submitted for analysis due to the availability of struvite dissolution protocols? 4) What role has nutritional management played in managing or causing uroliths? 5) Are there common factors that explain increased occurrence of calcium oxalate uroliths in cats, dogs and people? 6) During the time that calcium oxalate uroliths were more common in cats from North America, why were struvite uroliths more common elsewhere (e.g., Australia, Japan)? and 7) Why have most urethral plugs been composed of struvite for more than 25 years whereas other mineral types of uroliths have changed?

Table 46-5. Mineral composition of feline urethral plugs submitted for quantitative analysis to two centers.

Predominant mineral type	Urethral plugs submitted during collection period (%)	
Struvite	83.8	81
Calcium oxalate	0.94	6.6
Calcium phosphate	0.55	2.4
Urate	0.13*	1.1
Cystine	0	0.16
Silica	0	0.5
Mixed	2.46	3.6
Matrix (no crystals)	11.11	4.5
Summary information for data sources		
Center location	Minnesota Urolith Center**	Canadian Urolith Centre***
Plugs (n)	6,704	618
Collection period	1981-2008	1998-2003

*Includes eight ammonium acid urate plugs and one xanthine plug.
**Adapted from Osborne CA, Lulich JP. Unpublished data. Minnesota Urolith Center. University of Minnesota, St Paul, 2009.
***Adapted from Houston DM, Moore AE, Favrin MG, et al. Feline urethral plugs and bladder uroliths: A review of 5,484 submissions 1998-2003. Canadian Veterinary Journal 2003; 44(12): 974-977.

PATIENT ASSESSMENT

Each cat presenting with lower urinary tract signs should be thoroughly evaluated to identify the underlying cause(s). To guide initial assessment and need for emergency treatment (e.g., urethral obstruction), it is helpful to categorize patients into one of four clinical presentations, realizing that some cats may have features of several presentations (**Table 46-6**) (Lulich, 2007). A thorough history, physical examination and diagnostic evaluation including urinalysis and some form of diagnostic imaging (i.e., abdominal radiography and/or ultrasound) are indicated for every patient. Individualized treatment recommendations can be made based on these findings.

History

The nutritional history should include information about specific brand(s) of food fed, form (dry, moist, semi-moist or a combination), method of feeding (meal fed, free choice) and whether table food, supplements or treats are offered. Access to other food should also be determined (e.g., other pets in the household that eat different foods, access to food at other households or in the outdoor environment). Trends in water consumption (i.e., increased, decreased, unchanged) should also be noted.

Pet owners should be questioned carefully about: 1) duration and progression of clinical signs (same, better, worse), 2) whether the episode was the patient's first or a recurrence, 3) interval between episodes, 4) previous treatments (medical, surgical, nutritional) and response to therapy, 5) presence of other illnesses, injuries or trauma (current or previous) and 6) presence of systemic signs (e.g., inappetence, vomiting, diarrhea, weight loss). Questions should be asked to determine presence or absence of dysuria, pollakiuria, urinary incontinence, periuria, discolored urine and uroliths or urethral plugs voided during urination. Approximate urine volume and any changes in volume should be determined to distinguish between pollakiuria and polyuria. Owners should be asked about pharmaceutical agents that may be risk factors for urolithiasis (e.g., allopurinol may predispose to xanthine uroliths, excessive use of urinary acidifiers may predispose cats to calcium-containing uroliths).

Physical Examination

The urinary bladder should be palpated carefully to evaluate its size, shape, surface contours and thickness of the bladder wall. The presence of pain or masses within the urinary bladder lumen should also be assessed. Most feline urocystoliths cannot be detected by abdominal palpation; however, hearing a "grating" sound during palpation of the urinary bladder strongly suggests their presence. In male cats, the penis and prepuce should be examined for urethral abnormalities. The kidneys should be evaluated for size, shape, surface contour and symmetry. If possible, the patient should be observed during urination to evaluate the size of its urine stream and detect abnormalities such as discolored urine, pollakiuria, dysuria and stranguria.

Diagnostic Evaluation

Initial diagnostic evaluation of all cats with lower urinary tract signs should include urinalysis and some form of diagnostic imaging (i.e., plain abdominal radiographs, abdominal ultrasound). Additional tests may be indicated in some patients. Because urine sediment examination is an unreliable means of detecting UTI, quantitative urine culture should be performed in all cats with lower urinary tract signs. (See Urine Culture below.) Contrast urethrocystography should be performed to exclude small or radiolucent uroliths, urethral plugs and anatomic defects. If available, cystoscopy can also be used to detect and evaluate disorders of the lower urinary tract (e.g., uroliths, neoplasia). In cats with systemic signs of illness (e.g., inappetence, vomiting, weight loss), a complete blood count and serum biochemistry analysis are indicated; however, these tests are unlikely to be helpful in cats with signs limited to the lower urinary tract.

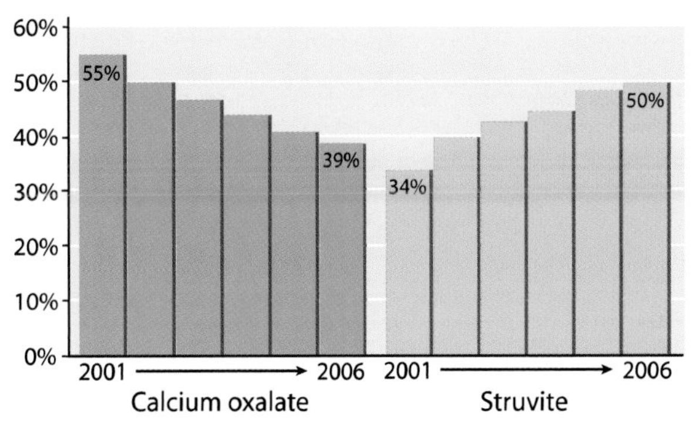

Figure 46-4. Occurrence of calcium oxalate and struvite uroliths analyzed at the Minnesota Urolith Center from 2001-2006. During this six-year period, the number of calcium oxalate uroliths gradually declined with a concomitant increase in struvite uroliths. (Adapted from Osborne CA, Lulich JP. Unpublished data. Minnesota Urolith Center, University of Minnesota, St Paul, 2007.)

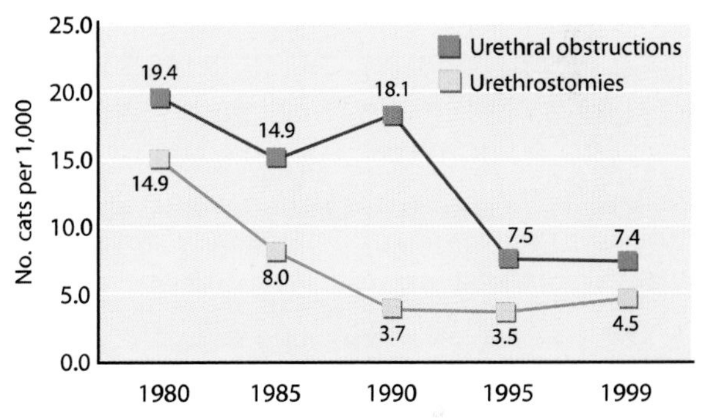

Figure 46-5. The frequency of feline perineal urethrostomies performed at veterinary teaching hospitals in Canada and the United States declined during a 20-year period and paralleled a similar decline in frequency of urethral obstructions and urethral plugs or urethroliths. (Adapted from Lekcharoensuk C, Osborne CA, Lulich JP. Evaluation of trends in frequency of urethrostomy for treatment of urethral obstruction in cats. Journal of the American Veterinary Medical Association 2002; 221: 502-505.)

Urinalysis

Complete urinalysis including determination of specific gravity, dipstick analysis and sediment examination is indicated in all cats with lower urinary tract signs. Because many cats with lower urinary tract diseases have pollakiuria, obtaining an adequate sample for urinalysis may be challenging. Whenever possible, urine should be collected before treatment and evaluated as soon as possible. This is especially important for patients with crystalluria because crystals may begin to form immediately in urine as its temperature decreases. Microscopic examination of urine sediment is essential to confirm the presence of hematuria, pyuria and crystalluria. Examination of unstained urine sediment, however, is an unreliable method of detecting bacteriuria. When compared

Table 46-6. Clinical presentations of cats with various lower urinary tract diseases.*

Presentation	Nonobstructive periuria	Obstructive dysuria	Behavioral periuria**	Urinary incontinence
Probable diagnoses	FIC Uroliths Infection Neoplasia	Urethral plugs Urethroliths Urethral strictures Functional obstruction Blood clots Foreign material	Toileting preferences/ aversions and/or marking with or without medical causes of lower urinary tract disease (e.g., FIC, uroliths, UTI, others)	Neurologic incontinence Anatomic abnormalities Partial obstruction
Initial tests	Urinalysis Diagnostic imaging	Abdominal radiographs Urinalysis	Urinalysis Diagnostic imaging	Neurologic examination Urinalysis Diagnostic imaging
Ancillary tests	Urine culture Abdominal ultrasound Contrast urethrocystography	Serum biochemistry profile Urine culture Contrast urethrocystography Complete blood count	Urine culture Abdominal ultrasound Contrast urethrocystography Coagulation profile Complete blood count	Urine culture Abdominal ultrasound Contrast urethrocystography Intravenous urography Cystoscopy

Key: FIC = feline idiopathic cystitis, UTI = urinary tract infection.
*Adapted from Lulich JP. FLUTD: Are you missing the correct diagnosis? In: Proceedings. Hill's Symposium on Feline Lower Urinary Tract Disease, 2007: 12-19 (www.hillsvet.com/conferenceproceedings).
**May occur with or without hematuria and signs of urinary tract inflammation.

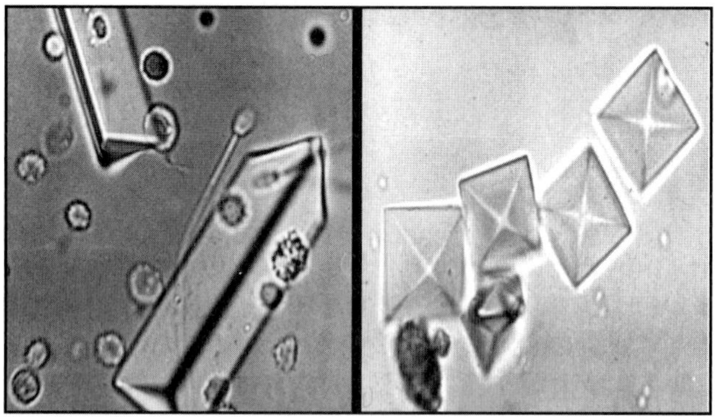

Figure 46-6. Magnesium ammonium phosphate (struvite) crystals (left) typically are colorless, orthorhombic, coffin-like prisms. Struvite crystals may have square or rectangular dimensions, vary in size, may have three to six sides and often have oblique ends. Calcium oxalate dihydrate crystals (right) typically are colorless and have a characteristic octahedral or envelope shape; they resemble small squares with corners connected by intersecting diagonal lines.

with quantitative urine culture, microscopic examination of unstained urine sediment was associated with only an 11% positive predictive value (i.e., the proportion of cats with a positive test that were correctly diagnosed) (Swenson et al, 2004). Bacteria may also be difficult to visualize by routine microscopic examination of urine sediment. Approximately 10,000 rod-shaped bacteria per ml of urine are required for visualization by light microscopy in unstained preparations of urine sediment. Cocci may not be consistently detected if fewer than 100,000 per ml are present. Inability to detect bacteria in urine sediment, therefore, does not exclude their presence. Staining of urine sediment with Wright's, Gram's or new methylene blue stain may significantly improve detection of bacteriuria (Swenson et al, 2004a).

Results of urinalysis are used to: 1) help determine underlying cause(s) of lower urinary tract signs, 2) detect conditions that may predispose to formation of uroliths or urethral plugs, 3) infer mineral composition of uroliths or urethral plugs (**Figure 46-6**) and 4) evaluate response to treatment or preventive measures. Hematuria is a common finding in cats with most lower urinary tract disorders; however, it is uncommon in cats with behavioral periuria (unless it results from a previous medical disorder). Pyuria is uncommon in cats with nonobstructive FIC and behavioral periuria and more often occurs with urolithiasis, urethral obstruction and UTI (Kruger et al, 1991; Osborne et al, 1990).

Several factors influence the number of crystals present in the urine sediment. Because storage at room temperature or refrigeration of urine samples may cause in vitro crystal formation, fresh urine samples should be evaluated ideally within 30 minutes of collection (Sturgess et al, 2001; Albasan et al, 2003). Other factors that affect the presence of crystalluria include volume of urine centrifuged, centrifugation speed and volume of sediment re-suspended and transferred to the microscope slide for evaluation. Consequently, it is difficult to attach clinical significance to the number of crystals observed. In addition to evaluating crystal type, sediment should be evaluated for tendencies of crystals to aggregate. Detection of large aggregates of struvite or calcium oxalate crystals is an important finding when monitoring effectiveness of preventive measures. Crystals only form when urine is supersaturated with crystallogenic materials. Therefore, crystalluria is a risk factor for formation of uroliths and urethral plugs. However, crystalluria alone is not diagnostic for uroliths or urethral plugs (**Box 46-1**). Conversely, urolithiasis is possible without associated crystalluria (Kruger et al, 1991). Crystalluria should be interpreted in the context of the patient's medical history, laboratory methods used and complete diagnostic findings.

Box 46-1. Managing Cats with Crystalluria.

Detection of crystalluria on microscopic examination of urine sediment does not mean a cat subsequently will develop urolithiasis; however, it does indicate increased risk for urolith development. Crystalluria in cats with normal anatomy and physiology of the urinary tract is usually of no clinical significance; these crystals are voided before they grow to sufficient size to interfere with urinary tract function and health.

Crystals that form in vitro after a urine specimen is collected are often of no clinical importance. Temperature, evaporation and pH are in vitro variables that may cause a urine specimen to become oversaturated, leading to crystal formation. Importantly, in vitro conditions may cause crystals to dissolve or grow. It is possible that urine kept at room temperature after collection may lose carbon dioxide into the atmosphere, which could affect pH, and subsequently, presence of crystalluria. However, a recent study found that urinary pH was not affected by storage time or temperature. Analysis of stored urine from cats consuming a mixture of moist and dry food was associated with significant increases in struvite crystalluria compared with evaluation of a fresh urine sample. In another study that included 31 dogs and eight cats, calcium oxalate and struvite crystals formed in vitro in urine that was stored at either room or refrigeration temperature. However, this phenomenon occurred more commonly at refrigeration temperature. In addition, length of crystals that formed in vitro was significantly increased in urine stored at refrigeration temperature compared with samples stored at room temperature.

Bacterial contamination of urine specimens also may affect crystalluria. Urease-producing bacteria (e.g., *Staphylococcus* spp., *Proteus* spp.) alkalinize urine, possibly altering crystal composition and disrupting cellular components in urine (e.g., red and white blood cells). Other bacteria produce acid metabolites with similar consequences. To prevent bacterial overgrowth, urine samples should be refrigerated if they cannot be evaluated promptly. However, this is not ideal for evaluation of crystalluria.

The nutritional history, including water intake, must be considered when evaluating significance of crystalluria. Cats consuming moist food are less likely to have crystalluria than those eating dry food exclusively. In addition, results of urine sediment examination may not accurately reflect what occurs in the home environment if cats are fed different foods in the hospital before urine collection.

Crystalluria should not be used as the sole criterion to predict mineral type of confirmed uroliths; only quantitative analysis of a retrieved urolith can provide that information. However, crystalluria can be used along with other factors (e.g., history, age, breed, urinary pH, radiographic appearance, other urinalysis findings and biochemistry profile results) to predict mineral type. Uroliths may be present in cats without crystalluria. In this case, factors that influenced formation and growth of crystals may be absent transiently. Factors typically responsible for this phenomenon include food changes, anorexia, increased water intake, different urinary pH values and in vitro changes in urine specimens that are not fresh. The crystal type may be different from the urolith type in some cases. This dichotomy exists when cats are assumed to have one urolith type, which is not confirmed by quantitative analysis (e.g., assumed to have struvite uroliths and fed according to struvite dissolution or preventive protocols, when in reality the cat has calcium oxalate uroliths and calcium oxalate crystalluria). Finally, cats may have more than one crystal type concurrently (e.g., struvite and calcium oxalate crystals may be identified in the same urine sample).

Struvite crystals may occur in: 1) normal cats, 2) cats with infection-induced struvite uroliths, 3) cats with sterile struvite uroliths, 4) cats with non-struvite uroliths, 5) cats with uroliths of mixed mineral type and 6) cats with urinary tract disease other than uroliths (e.g., feline idiopathic cystitis). Calcium oxalate dihydrate crystals occur uncommonly in normal cats. Large quantities of these crystals alone or in combination with calcium oxalate monohydrate crystals in fresh urine specimens probably indicate a hypercalciuric or hyperoxaluric disorder (e.g., ethylene glycol toxicity, calcium oxalate urolithiasis).

Should all cats with crystalluria be treated? In the absence of urolithiasis or a history of urolithiasis, cats with struvite or calcium oxalate crystalluria should be monitored serially. Cystine, ammonium urate or xanthine crystalluria should be investigated and the cause treated. Frequent detection of large crystals and aggregates of crystals in a fresh urine sample may be clinically important, especially if the cat has a history of urolith formation. In this case, preventive nutritional management should be implemented, and the cat should be encouraged to increase water intake. Finally, urine sediment examination should be performed periodically to monitor effectiveness of preventive therapy in patients with a history of uroliths.

The Bibliography for **Box 46-1** can be found at www.markmorris.org.

Urinary pH

Urinary pH influences formation of several crystal types. Although exceptions occur, crystal types tend to form and persist at certain urinary pH ranges (**Table 46-7**) (Osborne et al, 1995). In general, struvite uroliths are associated with more alkaline urinary pH values (>6.4) and calcium oxalate uroliths are associated with lower urinary pH values. Overlapping values can be detected; however, in cats with either urolith type. The method of measuring urinary pH should be considered because the urine dipstick method is not as accurate as a pH meter. In addition, urinary pH varies throughout the day due to the influence of food, time of eating, method of feeding and amount of food consumed. Consequently, it is difficult to interpret a single urinary pH value, especially if the type of food and time of eating are unknown. Furthermore, it has been reported that simply putting a cat in a carrier and traveling to a veterinary hospital can increase urinary pH (Buffington and Chew, 1996).

In laboratories, pH meters with glass and reference electrodes are used to make pH measurements. The electrode must be calibrated periodically against buffers of known pH. For clinical purposes, urinary pH can be measured with pH meters or indicator paper. Most multi-test reagent strips and test tapes use indicator paper impregnated with two indicator dyes: methyl red and bromthymol blue. The typical pH range is

Table 46-7. Clinical and diagnostic findings associated with the most common feline uroliths.*

Parameters	Struvite	Calcium oxalate	Purine (urate)
Breed predisposition	Chartreux Domestic longhair Domestic shorthair Foreign shorthair Himalayan Manx Oriental shorthair Ragdoll Siamese	Burmese British shorthair Exotic shorthair Foreign shorthair Havana brown Himalayan Persian Ragdoll Scottish fold Domestic shorthair	Siamese
Gender predisposition	Female >male Neutered >intact	Male >female	Neutered >intact
Common age (years)	Younger (<7 years)	Middle-aged to older (>7 years)	Young (if associated with portosystemic shunt)
Serum biochemistries	Normal	Hypercalcemia Acidemia (decreased TCO_2)	Normal (idiopathic) Evidence of hepatic disease (low urea nitrogen, increased ammonia)
Urinary pH**	Slightly acidic (>6.5) or alkaline	Acidic to neutral	Acidic to neutral
Bacteria	Usually sterile Occasionally associated with urease-producing bacteria	Usually sterile May be present in cats with infection secondary to uroliths	Usually sterile May be present in cats with infection secondary to uroliths
Typical crystals	Colorless, coffin-lid prisms, sometimes shaped like squares	Monohydrate–oval, dumbbell shaped Dihydrate-squares with diagonal lines	Spherical, tan in color May be green/brown Thorn apple appearance
Radiopacity	1+ to 4+	3+ to 4+	0 to 2+
Radiographic appearance	Rough or smooth, round or faceted, sometimes disk-shaped	Rough or smooth, usually small, occasionally jackstone shaped	Smooth, occasionally irregular

*Adapted from Osborne CA, Kruger JM, Lulich JP, et al. Disorders of the feline lower urinary tract. In: Osborne CA, Finco DR, eds. Canine and Feline Nephrology and Urology. Baltimore, MD: Williams & Wilkins 1995; 651.
**Concomitant infection with urease-producing bacteria may cause alkaline urine in cats with uroliths.

Table 46-8. Possible risk factors for urinary tract infection in cats.

Age (≥10 years)
Female gender
Urinary tract procedures
Urethral catheterization
Perineal urethrostomy
Urolithiasis
Systemic diseases
Chronic kidney disease
Hyperthyroidism
Diabetes mellitus

roughly from 5.0 (orange) to 9.0 (blue). According to most manufacturers, pH values measured with indicator paper are only accurate to within 0.5 pH units. For best results, indicator squares on reagent strips should be compared with the manufacturer's color standards in well-illuminated areas, as directed by product instructions. Urine reagent strips may be used to estimate pH for routine urinalysis; however, they should not be relied on when accurate pH measurements are needed for diagnosis, prevention and management of disease (Johnson et al, 2007).

Relatively inexpensive microprocessor-based, pocket-sized pH meters[b] have become available and are more accurate for measuring urinary pH than reagent strips (Heuter et al, 1998; Raskin et al, 2002; Johnson et al, 2007). These instruments can be used in veterinary hospitals or by pet owners at home. A study in cats revealed that portable pH meters were more accurate than pH paper or reagent test strips for measuring urinary pH in healthy cats (Raskin et al, 2002). Another study of hospitalized dogs compared hand-held pH meters, pH paper and reagent strips with a bench top pH meter, considered the gold standard for measuring pH. Results revealed that pH paper and reagent strips had poor to moderate agreement with the reference method, whereas, hand-held pH meters had nearly perfect agreement (Johnson et al, 2007). Based on these studies, a portable or bench top pH meter should be used when accurate urinary pH measurements are crucial for diagnosis or treatment.

Urine Culture

Urine culture should be done in all cats with lower urinary tract signs or in asymptomatic cats when there is increased risk of UTI (**Table 46-8**). Quantitative bacterial culture of urine collected by cystocentesis is the gold standard for diagnosis of UTI. For most accurate results, urine should be cultured within 30 minutes of collection or refrigerated because multiplication or destruction of bacteria may occur within one hour. If urine samples cannot be processed immediately, other alternatives such as inoculating culture plates in the hospital or using special storage media should be considered (Bartges, 2004). Growth of any bacteria from a sample of urine collected by cystocentesis is abnormal; contamination during collection should be suspected if multiple organisms are cultured. If a UTI is diagnosed, antimicrobial susceptibility testing is indicated to select appropriate treatment, especially in cats with pyelonephritis, recurrent infections or those that have been receiving antimicrobials.

Radiography

Radiography of the urinary tract (including the entire urethra in male cats) is a valuable diagnostic procedure that allows for detection of most feline uroliths and crystalline-matrix urethral plugs (Johnston et al, 1996). Radiography can determine the size, shape, location and number of uroliths. Relative radiodensity of uroliths can be used to make a rough guess of mineral composition (**Table 46-7**). Struvite and calcium oxalate uroliths are usually radiodense, whereas urate uroliths often are radiolucent. Radiographic shape, contour and size can be used as an inexact predictor of mineral composition. Struvite uroliths can be smooth or rough, round or faceted. Calcium oxalate dihydrate uroliths are usually small, rough and round to oval. Calcium oxalate monohydrate uroliths are usually small, smooth and round. Occasionally, calcium oxalate monohydrate uroliths have a "jackstone" appearance. The size and number of urocystoliths does not predict whether medical dissolution (if applicable) will be successful. Survey radiography or ultrasonography may fail to detect small uroliths (i.e., less than three mm in diameter); however, uroliths greater than one mm in diameter usually can be detected with double-contrast cystography if excessive contrast medium is not infused (Osborne et al, 1996).

Radiographic abnormalities also may be detected in the kidneys and ureters, especially in feline patients with calcium oxalate urolithiasis. The overwhelming majority of feline nephroliths are composed of calcium salts; only a small percentage of nephroliths are struvite (Kyles et al, 2005; Cannon et al, 2007).[a] Nephroliths must be differentiated from dystrophic or metastatic calcification of renal parenchyma, calcified mesenteric lymph nodes and ingesta or medications in the intestinal tract.

Contrast radiography is indicated in cats with recurrent or persistent clinical signs that do not respond to appropriate treatment. Contrast studies can be used to identify radiolucent uroliths, small uroliths or space-occupying lesions of the urinary tract such as neoplasia. Double-contrast radiography is helpful in evaluating urinary bladder wall thickness. Retrograde urethrography may be necessary in cases of urethral disease or obstruction. Patients with FIC may have normal findings or abnormalities including focal or diffuse thickening of the urinary bladder wall, irregularities of the urinary bladder mucosa or filling defects (Scrivani et al, 1998).

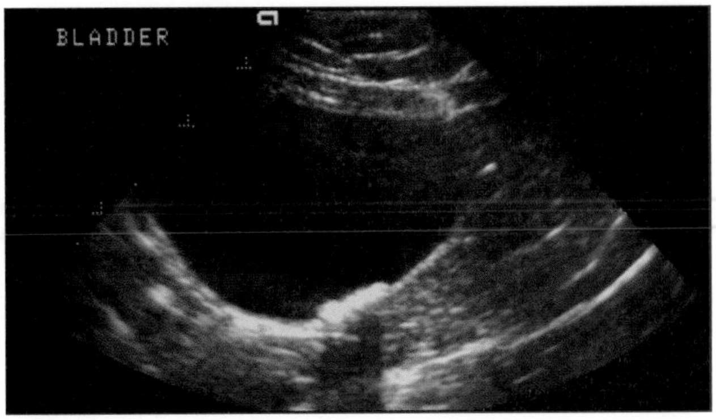

Figure 46-7. Sagittal plane urinary bladder sonogram of a cat with a history of lower urinary tract signs and several previous episodes of urethral obstruction. Note the presence of several hyperechoic densities in the urinary bladder, with acoustic shadowing below. These findings are typical of urinary bladder uroliths. After surgical removal, the uroliths were confirmed to be composed of calcium oxalate.

Ultrasonography

Ultrasonography is a rapid, safe, noninvasive imaging technique for evaluating the urinary bladder. Results often are unique, or at least complementary, compared with other diagnostic procedures; however, ultrasonography should not be viewed as a replacement for other tests including survey radiography (Widmer et al, 2004; Lulich, 2007). Factors affecting accuracy of ultrasonographic evaluation of the lower urinary tract include size and superficial location of the urinary bladder, inaccessible location of much of the urethra within the bony pelvis, degree of urinary bladder distention and presence of urinary bladder disease. Caudal abdominal structures are most readily visualized when the urinary bladder is full. In addition, when there is minimal distention, the urinary bladder mucosa develops folds that misrepresent wall thickness and mucosal contour (Widmer et al, 2004). Minimal transducer pressure should be used when scanning the urinary bladder to avoid displacement away from the transducer; this is especially important in cats with minimal urinary bladder distention.

Urinary bladder ultrasonography may be used to identify uroliths, masses or signs of chronic inflammation. Radiopaque and radiolucent uroliths in the urinary bladder have high echogenicity with characteristic acoustic shadowing (**Figure 46-7**). They tend to gravitate to the most dependent part of the urinary bladder with movement of the patient. Small uroliths may be difficult to distinguish from mineralization of the urinary bladder wall and should be displaced by shaking the urinary bladder during ultrasonography (Widmer et al, 2004). Blood clots also shift location with patient movement; however, they do not cause acoustic shadowing. Diffuse thickening of the urinary bladder mucosa is typical of chronic inflammation from any cause; however, it also may occur with neoplasia, especially lymphoma in cats. Thickening of the mucosa must be interpreted carefully in patients that have a partially filled urinary bladder because mucosal folds may appear in this situation in the absence of disease. Discrete

Table 46-9. Contact information for urolith analysis laboratories.

Antech Diagnostics - East
111 Marcus Ave.
Lake Success, NY 11042
800.872.1001

Antech Diagnostics - West
17672 Cowan Ave.
Irvine, CA 92614
800.745.4725

Canadian Veterinary Urolith Centre
Laboratory Services Division
University of Guelph
95 Stone Road West
P.O. Box 3650
Guelph, ON N1H8J7

Gerald V. Ling Urinary Stone Analysis Laboratory
Department of Medicine
Room 3106 MSI-A
School of Veterinary Medicine
Davis, CA 95616
Phone: 530.752.3228
Fax: 530.752.0414
www.vetmed.ucdavis.edu/vme/labs.htm

Laboratory for Stone Research
81 Wyman Street
P.O. Box 129
Newton, MA 02168

Louis C. Herring and Company
1111 South Orange Ave.
Orlando, FL 32806-1236
P.O. Box 2191
Orlando, FL 32802
Phone: 407.841.770
Fax: 407.422.8896
www.herringlab.com

Minnesota Urolith Center
University of Minnesota
1352 Boyd Ave.
St. Paul, MN 55108
Phone: 612.625.4221
Fax: 612.624.0751
www.cvm.umn.edu/depts/minnesotaurolithcenter

Urolithiasis Laboratory
P.O. Box 25375
Houston, TX 77265-5375
800.235.4846
www.urolithiasis-lab.com

masses, often located in the apex of the body of the urinary bladder, suggest urinary bladder neoplasia, which is rare in cats (Forrester, 2006; Wilson et al, 2007).

Urethrocystoscopy
Transurethral cystoscopy (or urethrocystoscopy) is becoming an increasingly important diagnostic method for evaluating the urethra and urinary bladder of cats. However, its availability may be limited to certain specialty hospitals. Patients with recurrent or persistent lower urinary tract signs despite normal findings on routinely available diagnostic tests (i.e., urinalysis, urine culture and diagnostic imaging) are candidates. The lower urinary tract of nearly all female cats weighing more that 3.0 kg can be evaluated with one of several small rigid cystoscopes. Urethrocystoscopy may be the method of choice for evaluating female cats with signs of periuria, pollakiuria, dysuria or stranguria. Observation of submucosal petechial hemorrhages (glomerulations), in the absence of other lesions, supports a diagnosis of FIC.

Serum Biochemistry Profiles
Serum biochemistry profiles are not generally helpful in most cats with FLUTD unless there are systemic signs of illness, urolithiasis or frequent recurrences of FLUTD with no obvious cause (**Table 46-7**). Hypercalcemia has been reported to occur in 14 to 35% of cats with calcium oxalate uroliths (Osborne et al, 1996a; Kyles et al, 2005). These patients should be evaluated for underlying causes of hypercalcemia (e.g., hyperparathyroidism, neoplasia and hypervitaminosis D); in most cases, however, a cause is not evident and idiopathic hypercalcemia is diagnosed (McClain et al, 1999; Midkiff et al, 2000; Savary et al, 2000). Presumably, persistent hypercalcemia increases the risk of forming calcium-containing uroliths by increasing excretion of calcium in urine. However, it is possible that processes involved with formation of calcium-containing uroliths and hypercalcemia are unrelated. Acidemia and serum total CO_2 less than 18 mEq/l, were reported in 64% of non-azotemic cats with calcium oxalate uroliths and 92% of cats with concurrent azotemia and uroliths (Osborne et al, 1996a). Metabolic acidosis may contribute to calcium-containing urolith formation because it promotes mobilization of calcium from bone and inhibits renal tubular reabsorption of calcium. Most urate uroliths in cats do not have an identifiable cause; however, serum biochemistry abnormalities (e.g., low urea nitrogen, increased ammonia) may occur in those with concurrent hepatic disease or portosystemic shunts.

Urolith Analysis
Recommendations for urolith dissolution and prevention are based on mineral composition of uroliths; therefore, it is important to analyze uroliths whenever possible. In addition to surgical removal, several less invasive techniques for obtaining uroliths should be considered. These methods include retrieval with a urinary catheter, voiding urohydropropulsion and voiding into an empty or plastic bead-filled litter box (Lulich et al, 1993). Ideally, all uroliths retrieved from a cat should be analyzed by a urolith diagnostic laboratory to determine specific mineral type(s) (**Table 46-9**).

Uroliths can be analyzed qualitatively or quantitatively. Qualitative analysis uses spot tests to identify radicals and ions; however, these tests do not reveal the proportion of mineral types and do not detect certain mineral crystals (e.g., silica) and drug crystals (e.g., sulfadiazine). Qualitative tests lack sensitivity and specificity for analyzing feline and canine uroliths (Osborne et al, 1996; Bovee and McGuire, 1984; Ruby and Ling, 1986). Investigators at the Minnesota Urolith Center examined 223 uroliths by qualitative and quantitative methods

Table 46-10. Reported risk factors for selected feline lower urinary tract diseases.*

Parameters	Feline idiopathic cystitis	Struvite uroliths	Calcium oxalate uroliths
Patient characteristics	Four to 10 years old Breeds (purebred, longhaired, Persian) Neutered Overweight Lazy/little exercise	Younger cats (<7 years) Breeds (**Table 46-7**) Female Neutered Urinary tract infection (urease positive)	Older cats (>7 years) Breeds (**Table 46-7**) Male Neutered
Environmental conditions	Multi-cat household Less freedom to leave house Provided with litter box Living in conflict with another cat Moving within last three months High number of rainfall days in month before signs		Indoor environment
Nutritional factors	Fed dry cat food Decreased water intake	Alkalinizing foods (urinary pH >6.5) Magnesium content 0.14 to 0.56% (0.36 to 1.4 mg/kcal) Phosphorus content 1.27 to 1.88% (3.17 to 4.70 mg/kcal) Sodium content 0.57 to 1.48% (1.43 to 3.7 mg of Na/kcal) Fiber content ≥2.7 (≥0.71 g/100 kcal)	Dry foods 7 to 7.9% moisture Excessively acidifying foods (urinary pH = 5.8 to 6.29) Feeding single brand Sodium content 0.2 to 0.3% (0.48 to 0.77 mg/kcal) Potassium content 0.04 to 0.06% (0.95 to 1.6 mg/kcal) Protein content 21 to 32% (5.15 to 7.98 g/100 kcal) Magnesium content 0.04 to 0.07% (0.09 to 0.18 mg/kcal) or 0.14 to 0.56% (0.36 to 1.4 mg/kcal) Phosphorus content 0.34 to 0.70% (0.85 to 1.76 mg/kcal) or 1.27 to 1.88% (3.17 to 4.70 mg/kcal) Calcium content 0.39 to 0.82% (0.97 to 2.05 mg/kcal) or 1.5 to 2.0% (3.76 to 5.06 mg/kcal)

*Nutrient values expressed on a percent dry matter basis and assume a food energy density of 4 kcal metabolizable energy/g (17.6 kJ/g); however, dry matter nutrient content of foods with energy densities substatially higher or lower than 4 kcal/g will be under- or overreresented, respectively. Thus, the energy basis nutrient values in this table (parenthetical values) are more accurate.

and found that qualitative methods yielded false-negative results in 38.1% of the uroliths and false-positive results in 6.7% (Ulrich et al, 1996). These two methods agreed in only 43.1% of the analyses. Uroliths, therefore, should be analyzed quantitatively to obtain the most accurate information about mineral content.

Quantitative analytical methods include optical crystallography, x-ray diffraction, infrared spectroscopy and electron scanning microscopy (Ulrich et al, 1996). In optical crystallography, crystalline material is removed from representative areas of the urolith using a dissecting microscope. The optical characteristics (e.g., refractive index and birefringence) of the crystalline material then are determined by polarizing microscopy and compared with known standards to determine mineral composition. Methods such as infrared spectroscopy are used if results of optical crystallography are inconclusive.

Different minerals may be deposited in layers (i.e., compound) or mixed throughout the urolith. Although one mineral type predominates, the composition of uroliths frequently is mixed. Thus, sampling and reporting results from different parts of the urolith become important when considering urolith dissolution and prevention. The following terms are sometimes used: the "nidus" is where growth of the urolith apparently started; it is not necessarily the geometric center. "Shells" are one or more complete outer layers of the urolith. "Surface crystals" refer to an incomplete outermost layer. Grossly visible layers do not always mean different mineral composition. The layers represent different phases of deposition and may be composed of the same or different minerals.

Risk Factors

Many studies have evaluated risk factors for FLUTD including patient characteristics, environmental conditions and various nutritional factors (**Table 46-10**) (Buffington et al, 1997, 2006; Houston et al, 2003; Kirk et al, 1995; Cameron et al, 2004; Lekcharoensuk et al, 2000, 2001, 2001a; Walker et al, 1977; Jones et al, 1997; Thumchai et al, 1996). For some risk factors, findings are consistent between studies, whereas others are different (e.g., living in a multi-cat household has been associated with increased risk of FIC in some studies but not in others). It is important to keep in mind that risk factors identified in epidemiologic studies show associations between certain factors and the disease of interest; additional study is necessary to show a cause-and-effect relationship. For exam-

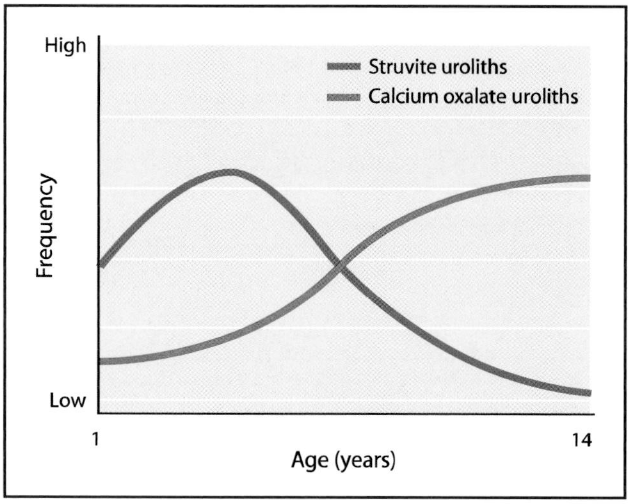

Figure 46-8. Relationship between urolith mineral type and age in cats. Note that struvite urolithiasis occurs more frequently in younger cats, whereas calcium oxalate urolithiasis occurs more frequently in older cats.

ple, it is likely that feeding a therapeutic renal food is associated with (i.e., is a risk factor for) chronic kidney disease; however, this does not mean it causes kidney disease. Finally, individual cats in a population are rarely exposed to a single risk factor; it is likely that FIC is a multifactorial disease and effects of interaction between multiple risk factors are challenging to evaluate (Willeburg, 1984).

Patient Characteristics

Patient factors that may affect risk for various types of FLUTD include age, breed, gender, neuter status, body condition and miscellaneous factors.

AGE

Review of data from the Veterinary Medical Database (1980-1990) revealed that lower urinary tract disease is most prevalent in cats between one and 10 years of age (Bartges, 1997). Another study using information from the same database (1980-1997) revealed that cats between four and seven years of age had the highest risk of lower urinary disease in general (Lekcharoensuk et al, 2001). Cats between four and 10 years of age had increased risk for urocystolithiasis, urethral obstructions and FIC, whereas, cats older than 10 years were at increased risk for UTI and neoplasia (Lekcharoensuk et al, 2001). Compared with younger to middle-aged cats, UTI is more commonly diagnosed in older cats (Lees, 1984; Bartges, 1997; Lekcharoensuk et al, 2001). In one study of cats with lower urinary tract disease that were 10 years of age and older, 63% had UTI (46% had UTI only and 17% had UTI combined with uroliths) (Bartges, 1997).

In general, cats with struvite uroliths tend to be younger and those with calcium oxalate uroliths older (**Figure 46-8**) (Thumchai et al, 1996; Cannon et al, 2007). In one study, cats with struvite uroliths (5.75 ± 3.12 years [mean age ± standard deviation]) were significantly younger than cats with calcium oxalate uroliths (7.5 ± 3.42 years) (Lekcharoensuk et al, 2000). Cats four years of age and older but younger than seven years had the highest risk of developing struvite uroliths. Cats older than seven years, but younger than 10 years, had the highest risk of developing calcium oxalate uroliths.

BREED

Several breeds of cats have increased risk for lower urinary tract disorders; however, there is so much overlap that it is difficult to draw meaningful conclusions (**Tables 46-7** and **46-10**) (Thumchai et al, 1996; Lekcharoensuk et al, 2000; Cannon et al, 2007). In one study, Persian, Himalayan and manx cats had increased risk for lower urinary tract diseases in general, whereas Siamese cats had decreased risk (Lekcharoensuk et al, 2001). Breeds with increased risk of developing urocystoliths were Persian, Himalayan and Russian blue (Lekcharoensuk et al, 2001). No breed predilection was observed for urethral obstruction (Lekcharoensuk et al, 2001). Breeds reported to have decreased risk for struvite uroliths include Burmese, Persian, Himalayan, Rex, Abyssinian, Russian blue, Birman, Siamese and mixed-breed cats (Thumchai et al, 1996; Lekcharoensuk et al, 2000). However, Siamese cats were reported to have significantly more struvite uroliths than other breeds in another study (Cannon et al, 2007). Birman, Abyssinian, Siamese and mixed-breed cats had significantly lower risk of developing calcium oxalate uroliths in one study (Lekcharoensuk et al, 2000). Persian cats had significantly fewer urate uroliths than other breeds in another study (Cannon et al, 2007).

GENDER

Neutered males and females had increased risk of lower urinary tract diseases overall and intact females had decreased risk in one epidemiologic study (Lekcharoensuk et al, 2001). Male cats are at increased risk for calcium oxalate uroliths, whereas females are at greater risk for struvite uroliths (Thumchai et al, 1996; Lekcharoensuk et al, 2000; Houston et al, 2003; Cannon et al, 2007). In one study, however, there was no gender predilection for cats with calcium oxalate uroliths (Kirk et al, 1995). Neutered cats are reported to have increased risk for both struvite and calcium oxalate uroliths compared with sexually intact cats (Lekcharoensuk et al, 2000). Neutered males are at increased risk for urethral obstruction (Lekcharoensuk et al, 2001). UTI is more common in female than male cats (Bailiff et al, 2006; Lekcharoensuk et al, 2001).

BODY CONDITION

Being overweight or obese has been a risk factor for lower urinary tract diseases in older and more recent studies (Walker et al, 1977; Cameron et al, 2004; Willeburg, 1984). Overweight cats (defined as ≥6.8 kg) had increased risk for lower urinary tract diseases when compared with cats weighing less than 6.8 kg (Lekcharoensuk et al, 2001). In a study of more than 8,000 cats in the U.S., nearly 29% were overweight, which was associated with urinary tract disease (Lund et al, 2005).

MISCELLANEOUS FACTORS

Cats described as lazy, or that exercise little, appear at increased risk for lower urinary tract disorders (Walker et al, 1977; Jones et al, 1997). It may be that these cats are overweight, which also is a risk factor for lower urinary tract diseases. In a study of indoor-housed cats, significantly more owners of those with lower urinary tract signs observed gastrointestinal signs, scratching and fearful, nervous or aggressive behaviors than owners of healthy cats (Buffington et al, 2006).

Environment

Living in a multi-cat household has been identified as a risk factor for lower urinary tract disorders in some studies (Walker et al, 1977; Jones et al, 1997). Cats that live indoors (or have restricted access to the outdoors) and/or are provided a litter box are also at increased risk for lower urinary tract diseases (Walker et al, 1977; Jones et al, 1997; Kirk et al, 1995). Conditions that may cause increased stress (e.g., living in conflict with another cat or moving to another home) have been associated with FIC (Jones et al, 1997; Cameron et al, 2004).

Nutritional Factors

Decreased moisture content of foods (feeding dry food) and/or decreased water intake have been associated with increased risk of FIC and calcium oxalate uroliths but not struvite uroliths (Walker et al, 1977; Kirk et al, 1995; Lekcharoensuk et al, 2001a). In one study, cats fed foods with a high moisture content (74.4 to 81.2%) were about a third as likely to develop calcium oxalate uroliths as were cats fed foods low in moisture (7 to 7.9%) (Lekcharoensuk et al, 2001a). In another study, cats with FIC were significantly more likely to eat dry pet food exclusively (59%) compared with cats in the general population (19%); however, this study did not include a control group (Buffington et al, 1997). Instead, results of a survey conducted by another organization regarding feeding practices of pet owners were used. These survey results differ from other studies, which show 95 to 99% of cat owners feed either dry food exclusively or a mixture of dry and moist (Habits and Practices, 2002; Gunn-Moore and Shenoy, 2004). Eating dry cat food has been associated with increased occurrence of FIC, whereas eating food with higher moisture content (e.g., canned food) has been associated with decreased occurrence (Walker et al, 1977; Jones et al, 1997; Willeberg, 1984). In addition, feeding moist food to cats with FIC has been associated with reduced recurrence of clinical signs compared with feeding dry food (Markwell et al, 1999). Additional study, however, is needed to determine if dry food causes FIC. As noted previously, more than 95% of owners feed their cats dry food exclusively or a combination of dry and moist food, yet the reported incidence of lower urinary tract diseases overall is less than 2% (Habits and Practices, 2002; Gunn-Moore and Shenoy, 2004; Lawler et al, 1985; Willeberg, 1984).

The source of water (e.g., tap vs. well) is not believed to be a contributing factor in cats with lower urinary tract disorders; however, it has not been carefully evaluated. In an epidemiologic study, water sources for cats with calcium oxalate uroliths (i.e., municipal, well or bottled) were similar to those for hospital control cats; more than 80% of cats in both groups received water from municipal supplies (Kirk et al, 1995). Mineral content of water is expressed as parts per million whereas mineral content of food is expressed as parts per hundred. Therefore, even water with high mineral content (i.e., "hard water") would contribute little to the total daily mineral intake compared with the amount supplied in food (Kirk et al, 1995).

A case-control study was performed to identify nutritional factors associated with struvite and calcium oxalate uroliths in cats (Lekcharoensuk et al, 2001a). Data were collected from cats whose uroliths were submitted to the Minnesota Urolith Center between 1990 and 1992. A content-validated questionnaire was mailed to owners to obtain information about their cat's food (e.g., types and quantities fed), feeding methods, mineral and vitamin supplements and source of drinking water. Nutrient information and expected urinary pH ranges for each food were obtained from pet food manufacturers. Data from 290 cats with magnesium ammonium phosphate uroliths and 216 cats with calcium oxalate uroliths were compared with data from 827 control cats without urinary tract disease. Distributions for breed, age, gender, body condition and living environment were significantly different between case and control cats; therefore, multivariate analyses were performed to adjust for potential confounding variables. The authors identified several associations between food components and occurrence of uroliths. Cats fed foods with high amounts of magnesium, phosphorus, fiber, calcium, sodium, chloride or potassium, or moderate protein content had increased risk of struvite uroliths (Lekcharoensuk et al, 2001a). In addition, cats fed foods formulated to produce urinary pH values between 6.5 and 6.9 were two times as likely to develop struvite uroliths as cats fed foods formulated to produce a urinary pH between 5.99 and 6.15. Cats fed foods with low amounts of sodium, potassium or protein, low or high amounts of magnesium, phosphorus or calcium, or those formulated to produce an overly acidified urinary pH had increased risk for calcium oxalate uroliths (Lekcharoensuk et al, 2001a) (**Table 46-10**). Increased dietary magnesium was previously associated with struvite urolith formation; however, presence of a concomitant alkaline urinary pH was likely a more important factor (Taton et al, 1984; Buffington et al, 1985, 1990).

To date, the strongest association with occurrence of calcium oxalate urolithiasis has been use of acidifying foods (Kirk et al, 1995; Lekcharoensuk et al, 2001a). It has been hypothesized that uniform use of these foods for managing struvite disease may be the cause for increased occurrence of calcium oxalate uroliths in cats (Buffington et al, 1994; Kirk et al, 1995; Thumchai et al, 1996; Lekcharoensuk et al, 2001a). In one epidemiologic study, cats with calcium oxalate urolithiasis were more than three times as likely as hospital control cats to have been fed foods that typically promote urinary pH equal to or lower than 6.29 (Kirk et al, 1995). In another study, cats fed foods formulated to produce urinary pH values between 5.99 and 6.15 were three times as likely to develop calcium oxalate uroliths as cats fed foods formulated to produce urinary pH values ranging from 6.5 to 6.9 (Lekcharoensuk et al, 2001a). Although two studies have identified that feeding acidifying foods is associated with calcium oxalate uroliths in cats, additional evaluation is necessary to show a cause-and-effect relationship and to determine what specific nutritional factors (e.g., magnesium content, degree of acidifying potential) are involved. It is of interest to note that normal urinary pH values in feral cats are reported to be 5.97 ± 0.10 (range, 5.54 to 6.57) in females and 6.37 ± 0.07 (range, 5.73 to 7.39) in males (Cottam et al, 2002). Both studies described above evaluated data collected from 1990 to 1992, when occurrence of calcium oxalate uroliths was increasing. Since 2001, occurrence of struvite uroliths has been increasing and calcium oxalate has been decreasing. Therefore, additional study is needed to identify more current risk factors and causes for recent trends of feline urolithiasis. It seems likely that multiple factors (e.g., nutritional, presence and function of urolith inhibitors, genetic predisposition) play a role in formation of calcium oxalate uroliths in susceptible cats.

Pathogenesis

Feline Idiopathic Cystitis

The clinical course of FIC is characterized by episodes of lower urinary tract signs that usually resolve spontaneously within three to five days, with or without treatment (Barsanti et al, 1982; Gunn-Moore and Shenoy, 2004). Although not evaluated in a large number of cases, it appears that 39 to 65% of cats with FIC will have recurrence of signs within a six- to 12-month period (Barsanti et al, 1982; Markwell et al, 1999; Kruger et al, 2003; Gunn-Moore and Shenoy, 2004). Many cats have multiple recurrences within a year. In a study involving 70 cats with FIC, 63 (90%) had multiple episodes of lower urinary tract signs; 30 (43%) cats had at least three episodes in the year before diagnosis (Buffington et al, 1997). In a study of 15 untreated cats with acute FIC, eight (53%) had one or more episodes of recurrent signs of lower urinary tract disease with 22 events reported over a period of 7,942 days at risk (Kruger et al, 2003). The overall incidence rate was 2.6 events per 1,000 days at risk. Survival analysis revealed that increasing number of prior episodes of lower urinary tract signs was associated with a significantly higher risk, whereas increasing age was associated with a significantly lower risk of recurrence of clinical signs. In another study, cats with FIC experienced a mean of five recurrences in six months (Gunn-Moore and Shenoy, 2004).

FIC shares many features in common with human interstitial cystitis and has been called feline interstitial cystitis when cystoscopic examination reveals characteristic findings (Buffington et al, 1997, 1996a, 1996b). Comparisons are based on clinical signs and diagnostic features. All of the National Institutes of Health (NIH) criteria (i.e., history, laboratory evaluation, cystoscopy and cystometrics) for interstitial cystitis in human patients have been applied to cats (Gao et al, 1994). Affected people and cats present as adults with symptoms/signs of variable severity that are influenced by stress. Spontaneous remissions occur in people and cats. According to NIH criteria, the diagnosis in people also requires cystoscopic lesions, either glomerulations or Hunner's ulcer. Glomerulations are submucosal petechial hemorrhages, whereas Hunner's ulcer is a small area of brownish-red mucosa, surrounded by a network of radiating vessels. Veterinary investigators report that lesions indistinguishable from glomerulations are observed commonly during cystoscopic examination of cats with FIC (Osborn et al, 1994; Buffington et al, 1997). A single case report describes a cat with FIC and findings of Hunner's ulcer (Clasper, 1990).

The pathogenesis of FIC appears to involve a variety of abnormalities affecting the urinary bladder, nervous system and hypothalamic-pituitary-adrenal axis (Westropp et al, 2004, 2005). One study of patients with FIC revealed abnormally low amounts of urinary glycosaminoglycans (GAG) compared with normal controls (Buffington et al, 1996b). In contrast, studies of urinary GAG in human patients with interstitial cystitis have yielded variable results (Akcay et al, 1999; Erickson et al, 1997; Hurst et al, 1993). The surface layer covering the urinary bladder mucosa includes GAG. A defective GAG layer or damaged urothelium may allow irritating substances in the urine to contact sensory nerve endings, which transmit action potentials through the spinal cord to the brain, resulting in perception of pain. In addition, there may be local release of neurotransmitters (e.g., substance P) and other inflammatory mediators (e.g., histamine) within the urinary bladder mucosa, which interact with receptors on vessel walls causing vascular permeability and leakage (i.e., neurogenic inflammation) (Westropp et al, 2005). Studies have shown that patients with FIC have increased urinary bladder permeability and leakage of ions across the urothelium compared with normal cats (Lavalle et al, 2000; Gao et al, 1994; Westropp et al, 2006a). Histologic changes associated with FIC generally are nonspecific and may include an intact or damaged urothelium with submucosal edema, dilatation of submucosal blood vessels, submucosal hemorrhage and sometimes increased mast cell density (Westropp et al, 2005). There is no correlation between histologic lesions, cystoscopic findings and clinical signs in patients with FIC. Cats may have remission of clinical signs but persistently abnormal cystoscopic findings (Westropp et al, 2005).

Several neurohormonal abnormalities have been described in patients with FIC and may play a role in its pathogenesis. A significant increase in tyrosine hydroxylase immunoreactivity was identified in the locus coeruleus (a nucleus in the brainstem) of patients with FIC compared with findings in healthy control cats (Reche Júnior and Buffington, 1998; Welk et al, 2003). Urinary bladder distention stimulates neuronal activity in the locus coeruleus, the origin of the descending excitatory pathway to the urinary bladder. Tyrosine hydroxylase is the rate-limiting enzyme involved in synthesis of catecholamines (e.g., norepinephrine). Chronic stress can increase tyrosine hydroxylase activity in the locus coeruleus with subsequent increases in autonomic outflow. It is possible this may play a role in the waxing and waning of clinical signs observed in patients with FIC, particularly in response to environmental stressors (Westropp et al, 2005). Patients with FIC also have increased plasma norepinephrine concentrations (Buffington and Pecak, 2001; Westropp et al, 2006a). In a study evaluating effects of stress, patients with FIC had significantly increased plasma concentrations of catecholamines, including norepinephrine, compared with healthy cats (Westropp et al, 2006a).

Abnormalities also have been identified in the hypothalamic-pituitary-adrenal axis of cats with FIC. Those with FIC had significantly decreased cortisol response to administration of synthetic adrenocorticotropic hormone compared with that of healthy cats (Westropp et al, 2003). In the same study, adrenal gland volume was significantly lower in cats with FIC compared with healthy cats; however, there were no correlations between adrenal size and cortisol production (Westropp et al, 2003, 2005). In another study of the effects of stress, there was no significant difference in urinary cortisol:creatinine ratios between patients with FIC and healthy cats (Westropp et al, 2006a). Based on studies conducted to date, it appears there is dissociation between the response of the sympathetic nervous system and the hypothalamic-pituitary-adrenal axis to stress in patients with FIC.

Although many risk factors have been identified in patients with FIC, additional evaluation is likely needed to identify its definitive cause(s). Based on current understanding of pathogenesis, it appears that abnormalities are not limited to the urinary bladder and interactions between other systems (e.g., nervous and endocrine) are likely involved. This possibility must be considered when formulating a treatment plan, which should include a multimodal approach (i.e., decreasing environmental stress, nutritional management, behavioral modification, pain management) for all patients with FIC.

Urolithiasis

Uroliths, or urinary calculi, are composed primarily of crystalline mineral concretions with a small amount of organic matrix. Urolithiasis is a multifaceted process that begins with microcrystals in urine and ends with mature uroliths somewhere in the urinary tract (Osborne and Kruger, 1984). Urolith formation occurs in two separate phases-initiation of the crystal nidus and continued growth to form a urolith. In general, there are four factors involved in formation of uroliths: 1) oversaturation of urine with calculogenic crystalloids, which may result from increased urinary excretion of these substances or increased urine concentration (e.g., due to decreased water intake), 2) decreased solubility of crystalloids in urine (e.g., struvite is less soluble in alkaline urine), 3) presence or absence of crystallization inhibiters or promoters in urine and 4) retention of crystals/uroliths within the urinary tract.

In its simplest form, initiation and growth of uroliths involves chemical precipitation of dissolved ions or molecules from a solution that has become oversaturated with respect to those components (**Figure 46-9**). From a physiochemical perspective, the degree of saturation or undersaturation of urine influences the probability that precipitates will form, or if already present, will dissolve. Relatively simple diagrams depict states of saturation of any solution (**Figures 46-10** and **46-11**). These diagrams provide the framework for understanding the concept of how nutritional management influences probability of urolith formation or dissolution. Units and numerical values

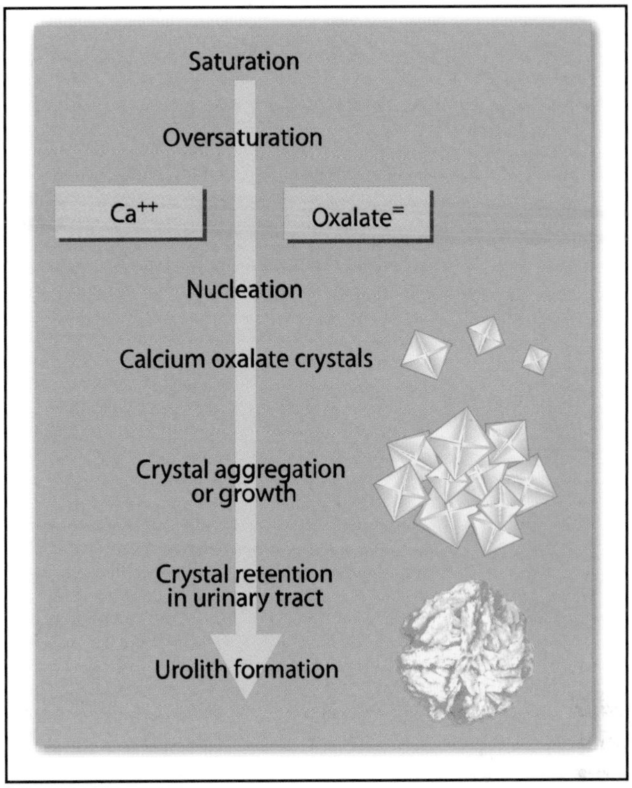

Figure 46-9. Increasing saturation of urine with urolith-forming constituents (e.g., calcium, oxalate) results in crystal growth, aggregation and ultimately urolith formation, if the components are retained in the urinary tract. (Adapted from Bartges JW, Osborne CA, Lulich JP, et al. Methods for evaluating treatment of uroliths. Veterinary Clinics of North America: Small Animal Practice 1999; 29: 46.)

are not included in these diagrams because they differ for each of the urolith components and measurement technique; however, the general features apply to all crystalline materials. At concentrations below the solubility product (i.e., in the undersaturation zone), it is impossible for crystals to form and crystals added to such a solution would dissolve. However, crystals may grow if added to a solution with a concentration greater than the solubility product. The formation product is the concentration at which crystals will begin to spontaneously precipitate in the absence of preformed crystalline material. Although the solubility product is constant for a pure crystalline material, the formation product is much more difficult to demonstrate; therefore, this area is illustrated by a shaded band rather than a line (**Figure 46-11**). Strictly speaking, the ionic activities (not concentrations) of the species govern the described solubility principles. Ionic activities are influenced by the presence of other ions in solution (i.e., ionic strength) and by the presence of other species that form complex ions, thereby reducing their "free" concentrations in solution.

The metastable zone is of most interest clinically; in this concentration range crystal growth and aggregation may occur or other factors (e.g., crystallization inhibitors) may impede or prevent crystallization (**Figure 46-11**). Risk factor reduction

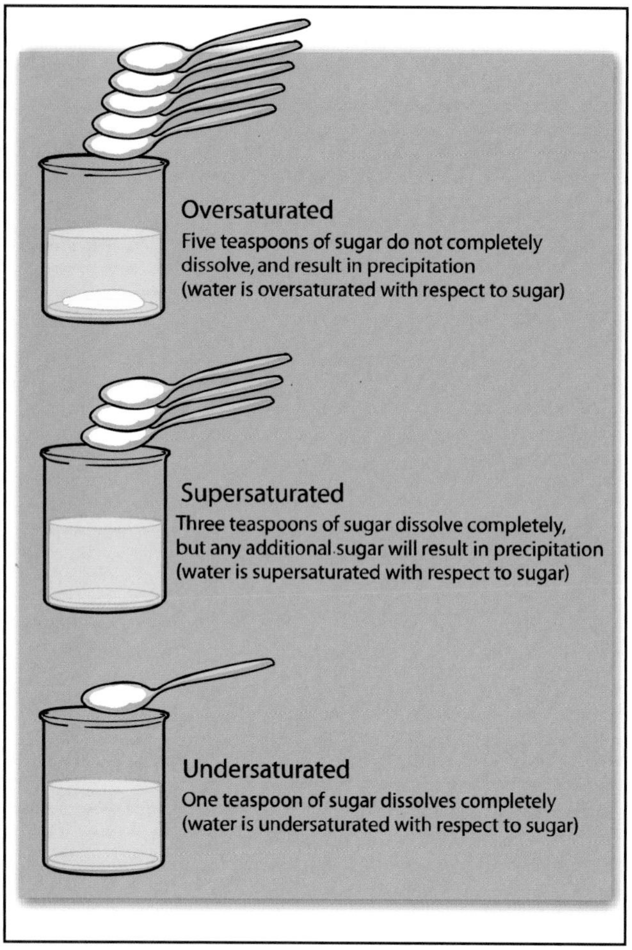

Figure 46-10. This diagram depicts a simplified explanation of effects of different levels of urine saturation (oversaturation, supersaturation [metastable] or undersaturation) on formation of uroliths. In this example, the liquid is tea and the mineral or crystalloid is sugar. As the amount of added sugar increases, the solution (tea) goes from being undersaturated (all the sugar completely dissolves) to being oversaturated (some of the sugar precipitates). Similar phenomena occur with mineral salts in urine. However, just as there are different outcomes when dissolving sugar in iced vs. hot tea, other factors (e.g., temperature, pH, crystalloid inhibitors) also affect saturation of urine with crystalloids. (Adapted and modified from Bartges JW, Osborne CA, Lulich JP, et al. Methods for evaluating treatment of uroliths. Veterinary Clinics of North America: Small Animal Practice 1999; 29: 47.)

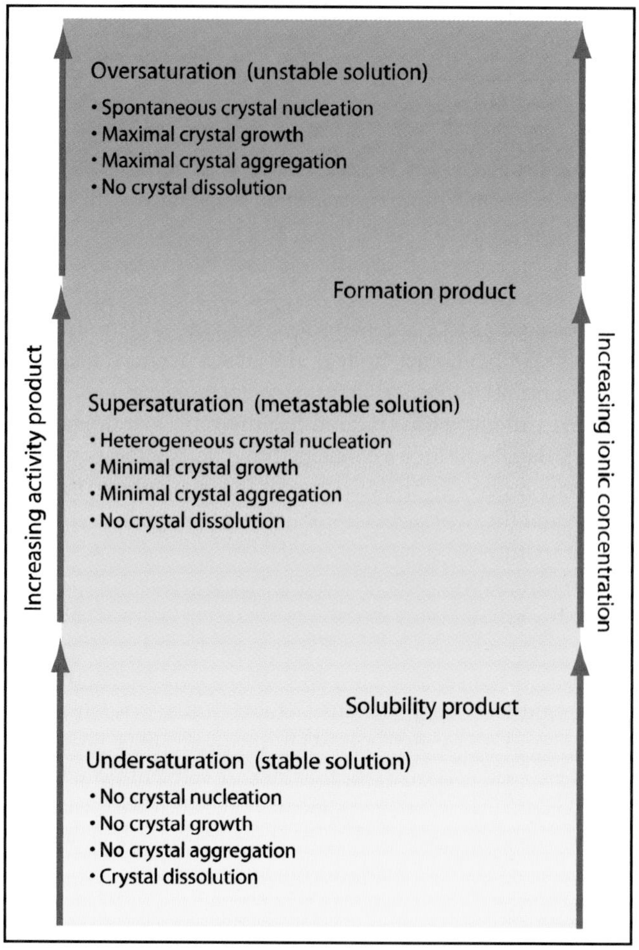

Figure 46-11. This diagram illustrates effects of differing degrees of urine saturation on risk of urolith formation. Increasing concentrations of urolith-forming substances result in metastable (supersaturated) and eventually, oversaturated urine. Crystal growth and aggregation may occur in the metastable zone. Presence of a nidus promotes nucleation (i.e., heterogeneous nucleation) and subsequent crystal formation. Inhibitors in urine may impede or prevent crystallization in the metastable zone. Spontaneous or homogenous nucleation occurs, however, when concentrations of urolith-forming substances increase to the point of oversaturation. After oversaturation occurs, inhibitors of crystal formation generally are ineffective. (Adapted from Bartges JW, Osborne CA, Lulich JP, et al. Methods for evaluating treatment of uroliths. Veterinary Clinics of North America: Small Animal Practice 1999; 29: 48.)

and nutritional intervention may be most beneficial with urine in this region. A precarious balance exists between crystal formation and inhibition in the metastable zone. Anatomic defects within the urinary tract that allow for stasis of metastable urine will lead to formation and growth of crystals. Urine containing microscopic impurities will facilitate crystal formation and growth. This process is called "heterogeneous nucleation." Crystal formation is much less likely in urine without impurities (i.e., homogeneous solution) (Bartges et al, 1999). **Box 46-2** discusses laboratory techniques used to measure these changes in urine. A more detailed description of this entire process is found in Chapter 38.

STRUVITE UROLITHS

Struvite uroliths form as a result of oversaturation of urine with magnesium ammonium phosphate. This oversaturation can occur in the presence of infection with a urease-producing organism. However, in contrast to the situation in dogs, most struvite uroliths in cats form in sterile urine (Osborne et al, 1996a). Urinary magnesium levels are related to dietary intake; as the amount of dietary magnesium increases, urinary magnesium excretion increases linearly (Sauer et al, 1985; Pastoor, 1993). **Box 46-3** provides more information about the effects of urinary pH on struvite urolith formation.

Box 46-2. Determining Risk for Urolith Formation or Recurrence.

Analytical data indicate that urine often is supersaturated with respect to most common urolith components. Thus, the question is not why a specific patient formed a urolith, but rather why doesn't every patient form uroliths? Inhibitors in urine probably explain the less than predicted prevalence of urolith formation. The current therapeutic strategy is to reduce risk factors by decreasing the degree of supersaturation because we know less about changing urinary inhibitors. One way to express urinary saturation is to determine the relative supersaturation (RSS) of a calculogenic substance (e.g., struvite or calcium oxalate). RSS is determined by measuring the concentration of a number of urinary analytes, including sodium, calcium, oxalate, magnesium and potassium. The concentrations of these analytes are entered into a computer program that calculates the saturation of the urolith elements compared with a standard human urine sample. RSS has limitations because it is highly dependent on urine volume and involves comparison with standard values for human urine.

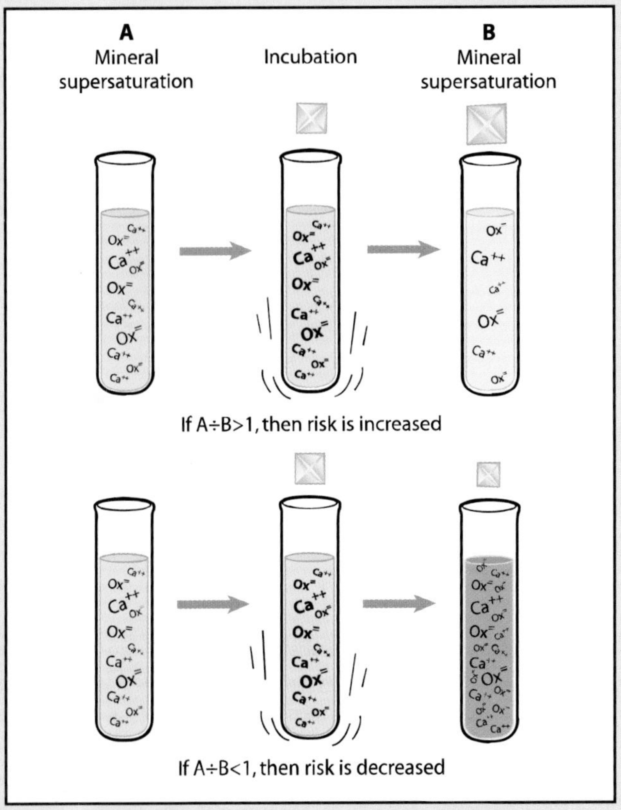

Figure 1. Schematic depicting how APRs are calculated. Urine from a cat is analyzed for pertinent minerals (Tube A) and then is incubated with a seed crystal. After incubation, the urine is analyzed for the same mineral constituents (Tube B). Dividing the pre-incubation activity product by the post-incubation activity product yields the APR. The risk of urolith formation increases with an APR greater than 1. This means the seed crystal has grown and the urine is supersaturated and/or contains inadequate concentrations of crystal inhibitors. The risk of urolith formation decreases with an APR less than 1. This means the seed crystal became smaller during the incubation process and the urine is undersaturated or contains adequate concentrations of crystal inhibitors.

Another technique for predicting likelihood of crystal formation is the activity product ratio (APR) (**Figure 1**). The APR for calcium oxalate is the mathematical product of the activity of calcium and the activity of oxalate. Activity is different than simple concentration of the substance of interest in an aqueous solution. Activity refers to the ionic activity, which is influenced by the concentration of the substance of interest, other substances in urine and factors such as pH and temperature. Like RSS, APR involves measurement of a number of analytes (e.g., sodium, potassium, calcium, oxalate, magnesium) in urine that are entered into a computer program. Unlike RSS, however, the APR technique requires incubation of seed crystals (e.g., calcium oxalate) in an aliquot of urine. After incubation, urinary analytes are measured again and the post-incubation activity product is determined. Dividing the pre-incubation activity product by the post-incubation activity product yields the APR. An APR less than one indicates that crystals dissolved during incubation. The APR provides a better indication of risk of crystal formation than RSS because APR considers the influence of unmeasured inhibitors and promoters and is not unduly influenced by urine volume. APRs can be used to evaluate quantitatively the influence of nutrients, complete foods and drugs on the risk of crystal formation.

Several studies have reported effects of various foods on urinary saturation values for calcium oxalate and struvite (APR and/or RSS) in healthy cats; however, only one has reported these values in cats with a history of forming uroliths. Although decreasing values for urine saturation indicate decreased risk for urolith formation, these values serve as surrogate markers. There are no reported studies correlating urine saturation values (APR or RSS) in urolith-forming cats with rate of urolith recurrence.

The Bibliography for **Box 46-2** can be found at www.markmorris.org.

CALCIUM OXALATE UROLITHS

Based on a small study of cats with calcium oxalate uroliths and information extrapolated from canine and human patients, it seems reasonable that factors promoting hypercalciuria and/or hyperoxaluria are involved in the pathogenesis of calcium oxalate urolithiasis in cats (Lulich et al, 1991, 2004; Stevenson et al, 2004; Seiner et al, 2003, 2005). Hypercalciuria was identified in 10 cats with calcium oxalate uroliths; feeding a therapeutic food[C] formulated to prevent urolith recurrence was associated with a significant decrease in urine calcium excretion and urine calcium oxalate saturation compared with feeding their regular food. Hypercalcemia promotes urinary excretion of calcium and therefore may increase the risk of calcium oxalate urolithiasis. Mild hypercalcemia (11.1 to 13.5 mg/dl) has been identified in approximately 35% of cats with calcium oxalate uroliths (Osborne et al, 1996a). Radiopaque uroliths were diagnosed in seven of 20 cats (35%) with idiopathic hypercalcemia in one study; uroliths were removed from two

Box 46-3. Urinary pH, Ammonium and Anionic Phosphate.

Normal urinary concentration of total phosphate ions is high and not subject to great variation by dietary manipulation. Although complexes are formed between phosphate ions and calcium and magnesium ions, these complexes do not markedly decrease free phosphate ion concentration. The urinary variable that has the greatest impact on trivalent phosphate ion concentration is urinary pH. Urinary pH influences formation of struvite precipitates because it influences the amount of total urinary phosphorus present as the free trivalent phosphate ion. Concentration of the free trivalent ion depends on the position of the acid-base equilibria of the two principal phosphate species that exist in the normal urinary pH range: HPO_4^{2-} and $H_2PO_4^-$. As urinary pH increases, concentration of free trivalent ions increases, as monobasic and dibasic phosphates are deprotonated.

$$H_2PO_4^- = HPO_4^{2-} + H^+$$

$$HPO_4^{2-} = PO_4^{3-} + H^+$$

According to the above equations, an increase in hydrogen ion concentration will shift both equilibria to the left, resulting in lower concentrations of free trivalent phosphate (PO_4^{3-}). Decreasing urinary pH from 8.5 to 5.5, the approximate physiologic range for cats, results in a 14,000-fold decrease in free trivalent ion concentration, with no change in total urinary phosphate.

Urinary pH also influences concentration of ammonium ions. Ammonia generated by urease enzymes provides necessary ions that react with available hydrogen ions to increase urinary pH:

$$NH_3 + H^+ = NH_4^+$$

Reduction in urinary pH from the upper to the lower end of the physiologic range changes the ratio of NH_4^+ to NH_3 from 3.4:1 to 3,400:1. Thus, foods that produce moderately acidic urine increase urinary ammonium concentration. However, because the effect on free trivalent phosphate ion concentration is greater, the net effect of moderate urinary acidification is a reduced likelihood of struvite precipitation.

The Bibliography for **Box 46-3** can be found at www.markmorris.org.

cats and were confirmed to be calcium oxalate (Midkiff et al, 2000). In another study of 71 cats with hypercalcemia, eight of 11 had calcium oxalate uroliths; nine of the 11 cats with uroliths also had chronic kidney disease (Savary et al, 2000). The role of hypercalcemia in the pathogenesis of calcium oxalate uroliths requires further study; it is appropriate to screen patients for hypercalcemia and, when possible, manage the underlying cause.

Hyperoxaluria may result from increased dietary intake or endogenous production of oxalate from metabolism of ascorbic acid (vitamin C), glycine, glyoxylate or other substances. A study in healthy cats fed differing amounts of vitamin C ranging from 40 to 193 mg vitamin C/kg of food for approximately one month found no significant change in urinary oxalate excretion (Yu and Gross, 2005). However, the effects of vitamin C supplementation have not been studied in cats at risk for calcium oxalate urolithiasis. A large part of the metabolic pool of glyoxylate is transaminated to glycine by the enzyme alanine glyoxylate aminotransferase, which requires pyridoxine (vitamin B_6) as a cofactor (Menon and Koul, 1992). Pyridoxine deficiency has been associated with increased oxalate production and urinary excretion in cats but has not been associated with calcium oxalate uroliths in cats (Bai et al, 1989, 1991). Primary hyperoxaluria, due to reduced activity of hepatic D-glycerate dehydrogenase, has been recognized in a family of cats; however, the role of primary hyperoxaluria in cats with calcium oxalate uroliths is unknown (McKerrell et al, 1989).

Urinary oxalate is an important determinant of urinary calcium oxalate saturation because small increases in oxalate excretion profoundly influence the activity product ratio. Oxalate forms a number of complexes and salts in solution; the calcium salt is relatively insoluble and pH does not influence its solubility over the physiologic range. The calcium salt of oxalate is just as insoluble in the luminal content of the intestinal tract as in other complex solutions. Consequently, dietary calcium is an important determinant of oxalate availability and intestinal absorption. Sufficiently available dietary calcium in the intestinal lumen combines with oxalate to form insoluble complexes of calcium oxalate. This phenomenon reduces intestinal absorption and subsequently less renal excretion of calcium oxalate. In contrast, if dietary calcium is reduced without a concomitant reduction in dietary oxalate, intestinal absorption and urinary excretion of oxalate may increase.

Urine normally contains substances that modify and inhibit nucleation, growth and aggregation of crystals. This likely explains, in part, why urine of most human beings is continuously saturated with calcium oxalate, yet only a small percentage of the human population will form calcium oxalate uroliths during their lifetime. Inhibitors such as citrate, magnesium and pyrophosphate can form soluble complexes with calcium or oxalic acid, making them unavailable to form insoluble salts such as calcium oxalate (Khan et al, 1993). Low concentrations of urinary citrate are common in human patients with calcium oxalate uroliths and some recurrent urolith formers may have defective inhibitory substances (Hess et al, 1991; Parks and Coe, 1986). Magnesium is a potent inhibitor of calcium oxalate crystallization in vitro. Low excretion of magnesium in urine has been suggested as a possible risk factor for development of calcium-containing uroliths. In an experimental study in rats, administration of magnesium oxide prevented renal deposition of calcium oxalate crystals in hyperoxaluric rats (Khan et al, 1993). Magnesium presumably increased urinary pH and excretion of citrate and decreased urinary oxalate excretion. This effect of magnesium depends on which specific salt is used (e.g., magnesium oxide has an alkalinizing effect, whereas magnesium sulfate has an acidifying effect). Other substances such as mucoproteins (e.g., Tamm-Horsfall mucoprotein), nephrocalcin and osteopontin (uropontin) also may inhibit crystal nucleation, growth and/or aggregation; however, their role in preventing calcium oxalate uroliths in cats has not been evalu-

Table 46-11. Potential factors associated with formation of uncommon feline uroliths.

Factors	Causes	Pathogenesis
Urate		
Hyperuricosuria	Portosystemic shunt or severe hepatic disease	Decreased hepatic conversion of uric acid to allantoin, which is more soluble in urine
	Excessive purine intake	Promotes hyperuricemia with subsequent hyperuricosuria
Hyperammonuria	Excessive protein intake	Additional urea and glutamine available for conversion to ammonium (NH_4)
	Metabolic acidosis	Promotes metabolism of glutamine to NH_4
	Acidic urine	Ammonia (NH_3) is converted to NH_4, which is excreted in urine
	Hypokalemia	Results in intracellular acidosis (potassium exchanged for hydrogen) and subsequent excretion of NH_4
	Urinary tract infection with urease-producing organism	Converts urea in urine to NH_3 and NH_4
Aciduria	Acidic urine	Decreased solubility of uric acid in urine
Decreased urine volume	Decreased water intake	Increased urine concentration and saturation with uric acid Decreased urination causes retention of crystals and uroliths
Calcium phosphate		
Hypercalciuria	Hypercalcemia	Increased urinary calcium excretion
	Excessive vitamin D	Increased intestinal calcium absorption and suppressed parathyroid hormone secretion, which promotes calcium excretion
	Hypophosphatemia	Stimulates vitamin D production, which augments intestinal absorption of calcium
	Acidosis	Promotes skeletal release of calcium and inhibits renal tubular reabsorption of calcium
	Excessive calcium intake	Increases urinary calcium excretion
	Excessive sodium intake	Increases urinary calcium excretion
Hyperphosphaturia	Excessive phosphorus intake	Increased urinary phosphorus excretion
	Alkaline urine	Increases urine concentration and saturation of phosphate
Alkaline urine	Alkaline urine	Reduces solubility of calcium phosphates, especially brushite
Decreased urine volume	Decreased water intake	Increased urine concentration and saturation with calcium phosphate Decreased urination causes retention of crystals and uroliths

ated (Nakagawa et al, 1987; Hess, 1991; Asplin et al, 1991).

Although a cause-and-effect relationship remains to be established, feeding foods formulated to maintain an acidic urinary pH (≤6.29 in one study and between 5.99 and 6.15 in another study) has been associated with calcium oxalate uroliths in two epidemiologic studies of cats (Kirk et al, 1995; Lekcharoensuk et al, 2001a). Acidosis may cause mobilization of calcium from bone (along with buffers), resulting in increased urinary calcium excretion. In addition, metabolic acidosis is associated with decreased urinary citrate excretion and increased citrate metabolism by renal tubular cells.

OTHER UROLITHS

Pathogenesis of less commonly diagnosed urolith types is not well understood, although several factors may be involved in formation of uroliths composed of purine (e.g., ammonium acid urate, uric acid) or calcium phosphate (**Table 46-11**). An underlying metabolic disorder is likely in these patients; however, often one is not identified. Detection of certain crystals (i.e., ammonium urate, cystine and xanthine), even in patients without clinical signs, suggests an important underlying metabolic defect, but not all cats with these crystals will develop uroliths. UTI may be associated with uncommon urolith types, but there is little evidence to support that UTI is the cause of these uroliths. Xanthine uroliths have been reported to occur in seven cats that had not received allopurinol; an underlying cause was not obvious (Osborne et al, 1996a). Cystinuria, presumably due to a defect in renal tubular transport of certain amino acids including cystine, has been identified in a small number of cats with cystine uroliths (DiBartola et al, 1991; Osborne et al, 1996a).

Urethral Plugs

It is likely that urethral plugs result from different pathogenic mechanisms than uroliths. In contrast to uroliths, urethral plugs typically contain large amounts of matrix and tend to be soft, compressible and friable (**Figure 46-12**). Although most plugs contain crystalline minerals, some do not. On occasion, plugs can be composed almost completely of matrix, blood cells, inflammatory cells and sloughed tissue (**Table 46-5**). Matrix is the nondialysable portion of urethral plugs that remains after mild solvents have dissolved crystalline components. Matrix may provide the "glue" for urolith and plug formation (Osborne et al, 1996b). The exact composition of feline urethral plug matrix is unknown. It is possible that a major component of matrix is Tamm-Horsfall mucoprotein based on the observation that the urinary concentration of Tamm-Horsfall mucoprotein is increased in cats with a history of forming uroliths (Rhodes et al, 1992). Tamm-Horsfall mucoprotein may be a local host defense against bacterial and viral UTIs. Excess mucus may be secreted by cells within the urinary bladder and urethra in response to an irritant or inflammatory stimulus.

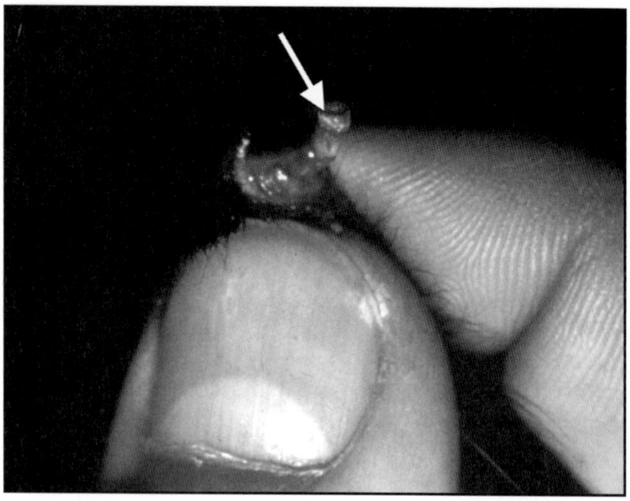

Figure 46-12. Note urethral plug (white arrow) extruding from the tip of the penis in a cat with urethral obstruction. Most urethral plugs are soft, compressible, friable and composed of large amounts of matrix mixed with smaller amounts of crystalline minerals. Although urethral plugs are diagnosed more often in male cats, due to occurrence of urethral obstruction, they also may occur in female cats.

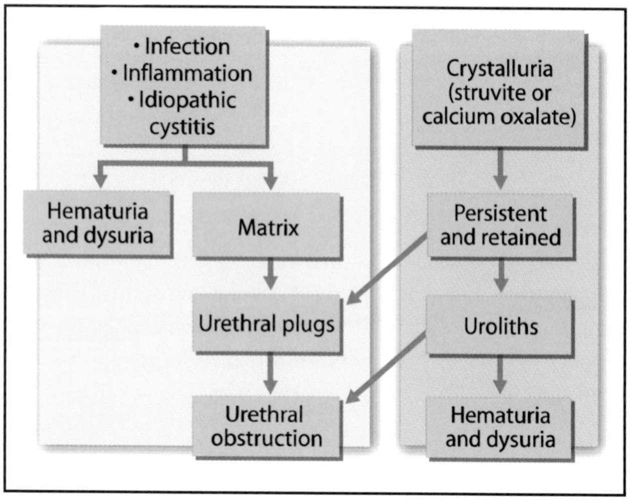

Figure 46-13. Unifying concept for pathogenesis of feline lower urinary tract disease. Infection or inflammation (e.g., idiopathic cystitis) results in clinical signs of lower urinary tract disease and production of excess matrix. Persistent crystalluria can combine with matrix to form urethral plugs or contribute to urolith formation and typical clinical signs. (Adapted from Osborne CA, Kruger JM, Lulich JP. Feline lower urinary tract disorders: Definition of terms and concepts. Veterinary Clinics of North America: Small Animal Practice 1996; 76: 169-179.)

Formation of matrix-crystalline urethral plugs hypothetically requires two simultaneous but unrelated events (**Figure 46-13**) (Osborne et al, 1992, 1996b, 1996c). One event is the formation of matrix that may result from some inflammatory process (e.g., idiopathic, bacterial or viral UTI). The other event is the formation of crystalline precipitates, most often struvite. If matrix forms without concomitant crystals, the noncrystalline gel is voided; however, nonobstructive dysuria and hematuria result. A more rigid plug forms in the presence of crystals that may cause urethral obstruction. The mineral composition of crystals can serve as the basis for preventive efforts. This process of plug formation has been compared with the formation of casts in renal tubular lumina. Urinary mucoprotein provides a gel that traps intact cells (producing cellular casts) or disintegrating cellular elements (producing granular casts). A more trivial analogy is the creation of fruit gelatin (**Figure 46-14**). The "gelatin" (i.e., matrix) traps pieces of "fruit" (i.e., crystals) as it forms.

Urinary Tract Infection

BACTERIAL INFECTION

Infection with urease-producing bacteria (e.g., *Staphylococcus* spp. and *Proteus* spp.) causes persistently alkaline urine, which may be associated with formation of struvite uroliths. It appears that most cats with struvite uroliths do not have UTI; however, urolith-induced changes in host-defense mechanisms may lead to bacterial colonization of the urinary tract (Osborne et al, 1996a). Thirty percent of feline patients with urocystoliths in one study had positive urine cultures (Osborne et al, 1990). In a study of uroliths from 150 cats, investigators cultured bacteria from a urolith or urine in 30 (41%) of 74 cats. Coagulase-positive staphylococci were cultured from uroliths or urine in 17 cats, representing 45% of bacteria isolated (Ling et al, 1990). In some cases, culture of urine may be negative or yield the same or different organisms than cultures from uroliths.

Although a cause-and-effect relationship has not been established, there is an increased occurrence of UTI in cats with systemic diseases. Of cats with chronic kidney disease, 10 to 50% are reported to have UTI; it isn't known if kidney disease causes UTI or if other factors (e.g., older age) are responsible (Lulich et al, 1992; McMahon et al, 2006; Mayer-Roenne et al, 2007). UTI also has been reported to occur in 12 to 13% of cats with diabetes mellitus and 12% of cats with hyperthyroidism (Bailiff et al, 2006; Mayer-Roenne et al, 2007).

Perineal urethrostomies are associated with significant postoperative sequelae, including urethral strictures, bacterial UTI and struvite urolithiasis (Osborne et al, 1991; Griffin et al, 1992; Bass et al, 2005). These postoperative sequelae can produce lower urinary tract signs. In a prospective clinical study of 30 male cats with intraluminal urethral obstruction and negative urine cultures, investigators randomly assigned cats to receive one of three treatments following relief of the obstruction: 1) nutritional management with a struvite dissolution food, 2) perineal urethrostomy or 3) nutritional management and perineal urethrostomy. During the one-year followup period, none of the cats receiving nutritional management alone had episodes of UTI, whereas episodes of bacterial UTI were documented in 50% of the group managed by surgery alone, and 40% of the group receiving nutritional management and surgery. Three of the infected cats from the urethrostomy-only group subsequently developed urocystoliths (Osborne et al, 1991). In a more recent study, one-year followup of 39 cats that had perineal urethrostomy revealed that 51.3% had complications (UTI in nine, stricture in two) or recurrent signs due to urolithiasis (five cats) or FIC (four cats) (Bass et al, 2005).

Several factors associated with perineal urethrostomies have been incriminated as risk factors for bacterial UTI. These include decreased length of the urethra after surgery, loss of normal penile urethral mucosal defense mechanisms, transurethral catheterization, wider external urethral orifices, impaired function of the striated urethralis muscle and decreased intraluminal pressure. Some cats have decreased postprostatic urethral pressure and decreased activity of the striated muscle sphincter after perineal urethrostomy, as determined by urethral pressure profiles and electromyographic changes (Gregory and Vasseur, 1983). These changes were linked to extensive tissue dissection and damage to the pudendal nerve during surgery.

A modified surgical procedure, designed to preserve function of the striated urethral sphincter, was evaluated in a group of healthy neutered male cats and a group of cats with persistent or recurrent urethral obstruction. All cats had normal urethral pressure profiles and electromyographic results postoperatively. Twenty-two percent of the cats with persistent or recurrent urethral obstruction had bacterial UTIs vs. none of the normal cats. These findings suggest that decreased urethral pressure does not predispose cats to ascending UTI (Griffin et al, 1989).

Vesicourachal diverticula were reported to occur in one of every four cats with dysuria, hematuria and/or urethral obstruction (Osborne et al, 1987). Vesicourachal diverticula can be congenital or acquired. Diverticula alter the normal flow of urine; thus in theory, they may predispose patients to UTI, infection-related urolithiasis and formation of urinary precipitates. It has been suggested that acquired diverticula occur as a result of increased intraluminal pressure due to urethral obstruction or hyperactivity of the detrusor muscle associated with inflammation. Spontaneous resolution of diverticula has been observed in cats (Osborne et al, 1987, 1989).

VIRAL INFECTION

Although not a consistent finding in cats with lower urinary tract signs, viral infections have been implicated as causative agents based on isolation of feline cell-associated herpesvirus, feline calicivirus (FCV) and syncytia-forming virus from cats with hematuria and dysuria alone or in combination with urethral obstruction (Kruger and Osborne, 1990). Calicivirus-like viral particles have been identified in crystalline/matrix urethral plugs from cats with obstructive lower urinary tract disease. Although standard cell culture inoculation methods with urine were negative for virus, investigators were able to induce bovine herpesvirus type 4 (BHV-4) infections experimentally in feline urinary bladders using tissue explantation techniques. However, the pathogenic role of BHV-4 in FLUTD remains unclear because the prevalence of BHV-4 antibodies in affected cats was not significantly different from that of clinically normal control cats (Kruger et al, 1991). In a study of 40 cats, researchers identified FCV in one female cat with FIC and one male cat with obstructive FIC; the FCV (FCV-U1 and FCV-U2) were genetically different from known field and vaccine strains (Rice et al, 2002). In a more recent epidemiologic study

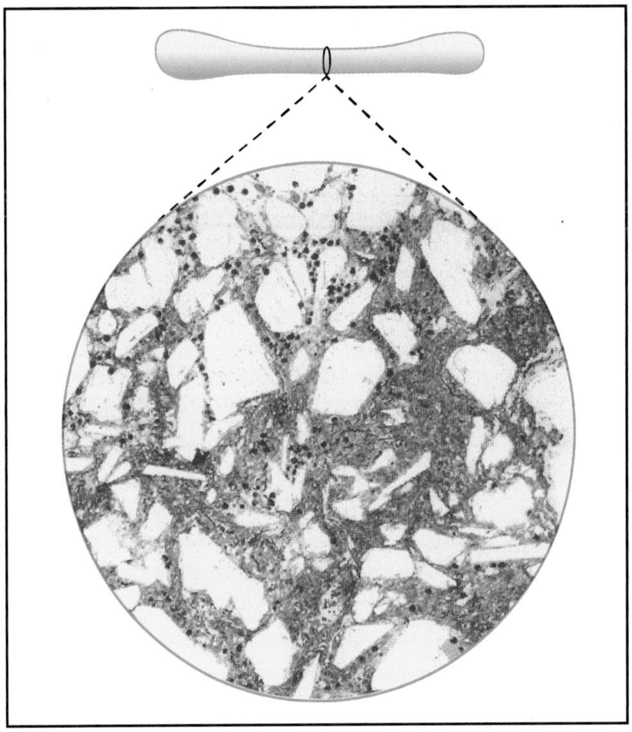

Figure 46-14. Diagram showing a cross-section of a matrix-crystalline urethral plug. Note the spaces previously occupied by struvite crystals are surrounded by matrix containing amorphous material, cellular debris and a small number of inflammatory cells. This phenomenon is analogous to a gelatin salad that contains various fruits or vegetables (depicting crystals, cells, cellular material) embedded in a gelatin matrix.

of 47 cats with nonobstructive FIC, 22 cats with obstructive FIC, 56 cats with signs of upper respiratory tract disease and 46 asymptomatic cats, FCV was detected by reverse transcription-polymerase chain reaction (RT-PCR) in urine from approximately 6% of cats with FIC or upper respiratory tract disease. FCV was not detected in urine from any asymptomatic cat. Mean FCV virus neutralizing antibody titers for cats with nonobstructive FIC, obstructive FIC and upper respiratory tract disease were significantly higher than the mean titers of asymptomatic control cats (Larson et al, 2007). Despite increasing evidence that FCV invades the urinary system and that cats with FIC have increased exposure to FCV, establishing a cause-and-effect relationship between FCV and FIC requires further investigation.

FUNGAL INFECTION

Fungal UTI is rarely diagnosed in cats; *Candida* spp. are the organisms most often isolated (Pressler et al, 2003; Jin and Lin, 2005). *Candida* spp. are considered a normal part of the genital mucosal flora and most patients with fungal UTI have underlying disorders that alter host defenses against opportunistic infection. Some treatments and concomitant disorders diagnosed in cats with fungal UTI have included administration of antimicrobials or corticosteroids, diabetes mellitus, kidney disease, indwelling urinary catheters, perineal urethrostomy and

Table 46-12. Key nutritional factors and recommended levels for managing cats with common lower urinary tract diseases.*

Factors	Dietary recommendations				
	FIC	Struvite dissolution	Struvite prevention	Calcium oxalate uroliths	Combined FIC, struvite and calcium oxalate prevention
Water	Moist foods are best	Moist foods are best	Moist foods are best	Moist foods are best	Moist foods are best
Magnesium (%)	–	0.04 to 0.09	0.04 to 0.14	0.07 to 0.14	0.07 to 0.14
Phosphorus (%)	–	0.45 to 1.1	0.5 to 0.9	0.5 to 1.0	0.5 to 0.9
Calcium (%)	–	–	–	0.6 to 1.0	0.6 to 1.0
Protein (%)	–	30 to 45	30 to 45	≥32	32 to 45
Sodium (%)	–	0.3 to 0.6	0.3 to 0.6	0.3 to 0.6	0.3 to 0.6
Urinary pH	–	5.8 to 6.2	6.0 to 6.4	≥6.2	6.2 to 6.4
Total omega 3 (%)	0.35 to 1.0	–	–	–	0.35 to 1.0

Key: FIC = feline idiopathic cystitis, Total omega 3 = total omega-3 fatty acids.
*Nutrients expressed on a dry matter basis unless otherwise stated.

Table 46-13. Key nutritional factors for preventing uncommon feline uroliths.

Factors	Dietary recommendations
Purine uroliths (urate, uric acid)	
Water	Promote water intake by using a moist food or other measures
Protein	Avoid excess dietary protein Recommend foods with 28 to 30% DM protein Recommend foods with low purine content Avoid proteins with high purine content such as liver, sardines and anchovies
Urinary pH	Use foods that maintain less acidic urine (6.6 to 6.8)
Calcium phosphate uroliths	
Water	Promote water intake by using a moist food or other measures
Calcium	Avoid excess dietary calcium Recommend foods with 0.6 to 0.8% DM calcium
Phosphorus	Avoid excess dietary phosphorus Recommend foods with <0.8% DM phosphorus
Sodium	Avoid excess dietary sodium Recommend foods with <0.30% DM sodium
Vitamin D	Avoid excess dietary vitamin D Recommend foods with <2,000 IU of vitamin D/kg DM

Key: DM = dry matter.

Table 46-14. Water intake and urine volume in cats fed dry or moist food.*

Volume (ml/day)	Moist food	Dry food
Water (in food)	246	6
Water (in addition to food)	32	221
Total water intake	278	227
Fecal water	27	44
Urine	166	79

*Adapted from Burger IH, Smith PM. Effects of diet on the urine characteristics of the cat. In: Proceedings. International Symposium on Nutrition, Malnutrition and Dietetics in the Dog and Cat, 1987: 71-73.

other lower urinary tract disorders (e.g., uroliths).

Key Nutritional Factors

Nutritional management plays a key role in successful treatment and/or prevention of the most common FLUTDs. Nutrition may be helpful for decreasing urine concentration of crystallogenic minerals and inflammatory mediators, increasing solubility of crystalloids in urine, promoting increased concentrations of crystallization inhibiters in urine and decreasing retention of crystals and/or uroliths within the urinary tract. When designing a therapeutic regimen for patients with FIC, struvite uroliths or urethral plugs, or calcium oxalate uroliths, consider the key nutritional factors discussed below. **Table 46-12** summarizes these key nutritional factors and recommended nutrient ranges for managing patients with common lower urinary tract disorders. **Table 46-13** summarizes key nutritional factors for cats with less common urolith types. Recommended ranges of nutrient levels of the key nutritional factors were determined by: 1) considering nutrient levels in foods evaluated in cats with various lower urinary tract diseases, 2) using information about risk factors from epidemiologic studies of cats with lower urinary tract signs and 3) extrapolation from studies in other species. Available evidence supporting effectiveness of different foods should be considered when planning treatment as well as each patient's response to treatment.

Water

The volume of water cats consume daily depends on the composition and quantity of food ingested and possibly feeding frequency. Although somewhat variable, most dry cat foods contain less than 10% water and moist foods (most often packaged in cans or pouches) contain more than 72% water. Healthy cats drink more water when eating dry food compared with moist food. The total volume of water ingested (i.e., drinking water plus water in food); however, is significantly greater and more water is excreted in urine than in feces when cats are fed moist food (**Table 46-14**) (Gaskell, 1989; Burger and Smith, 1987). The solute load of food also influences water consumption; urea is a major contributor to the renal solute load. Increasing the protein content of food increases the solute load (e.g., urea). Therefore, foods with higher protein content are associated with higher water intake. Metabolism of energy substrates yields endogenous water but the daily volume of endogenously produced water is small (approximately 10 to 15%) compared with the total daily water intake. Metabolism of fats provides the most water per gram whereas carbohydrate metabolism results in the most water per calorie. The amount of water generated differs slightly depending on the source of fat, chain length and degree of saturation. Feeding frequency also appears to affect water intake in cats. In a study of healthy adult cats, water intake (in addition to that consumed in the food) increased significantly when cats were fed two or three meals compared with a single meal each day. However, the study did not note whether the food was dry or moist (Kirschvink et al, 2005).

Of all treatments evaluated in controlled studies, the only one that has been associated with a statistically significant difference in recurrence of clinical signs in cats with FIC is feeding moist food (Barsanti et al, 1982; Gunn-Moore and Shenoy, 2004; Gunn-Moore and Cameron, 2004; Kruger et al, 2003; Kraijer et al, 2003; Osborne et al, 1996d; Markwell et al, 1999). During a one-year nonrandomized clinical study of cats with FIC, clinical signs recurred less often in cats fed moist food compared with cats fed the dry formulation of the same food[c] (**Figure 46-15**) (Markwell et al, 1999). In a six-month FIC study evaluating glucosamine hydrochloride[d] vs. placebo, cats receiving either treatment improved significantly compared with evaluations at the beginning of the study (**Figure 46-16**) (Gunn-Moore and Shenoy, 2004). Before the study, 95% of cats were fed either dry food exclusively or at least half of their daily intake was dry food. After starting the study, however, 36 (90%) owners increased the amount of moist food given to their cats, so that at least 50% of their daily intake was moist food. Owners began feeding moist food exclusively to 33 (82.5%) cats. In both studies described above, it is likely that increased consumption of moist food caused urine dilution, which was associated with clinical improvement in cats with FIC. However, other beneficial effects of feeding moist food (e.g., increased owner/cat interactions associated with delivery of canned meals) cannot be excluded.

Moist foods also are recommended in the management of urolithiasis and urethral plugs because they lead to production of less concentrated urine that is less saturated with crystalloids. Increased water consumption has been used as an effective strategy for controlling calcium oxalate uroliths in people, dogs and cattle. A case-controlled study of nutritional factors associated with urolithiasis in cats unexpectedly found no association between high-moisture foods and decreased risk for struvite uroliths (Lekcharoensuk et al, 2001a). However, cats fed high-moisture (74.4 to 81.2%) foods were about a third as likely to develop calcium oxalate uroliths as were cats fed low-moisture (7.0 to 7.9%) foods. The authors concluded that it is possible that increases in urine volume produced by moisture content of food may have less influence on struvite urolith formation than on calcium oxalate urolith formation.

Based on available information, patients with FIC and calcium oxalate uroliths should be fed foods that contain more than 74% moisture, as fed (e.g., foods in cans or pouches). Current evidence is less clear regarding beneficial effects of moist food for cats with struvite disease. However, it seems reasonable to also recommend moist foods for these cats as well, especially if

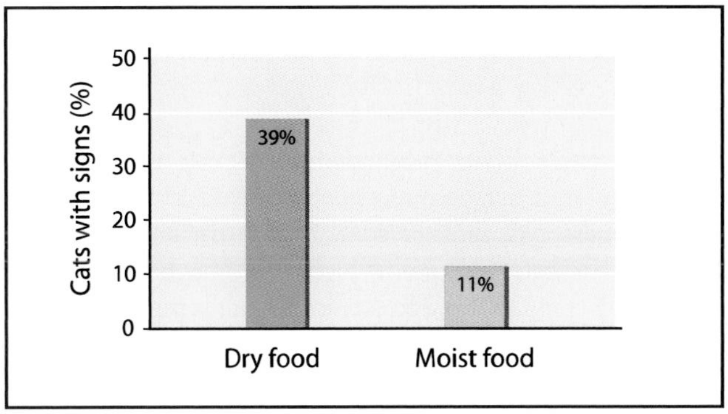

Figure 46-15. Results of a one-year study of 46 cats with feline idiopathic cystitis showed that recurrence of clinical signs was significantly greater in cats fed a dry food[c] (n = 28) compared with cats fed the moist version of the food (n = 18) (p = 0.04). After feeding the dry food, mean urine specific gravity values (measured at 2 weeks, 16 weeks, 6 months and 12 months) ranged from 1.050 to 1.051 whereas mean urine specific gravity values in cats eating moist food ranged from 1.032 to 1.041. (Adapted from Markwell PJ, Buffington CA, Chew DJ, et al. Clinical evaluation of commercially available urinary acidification diets in the management of idiopathic cystitis in cats. Journal of the American Veterinary Medical Association 1999; 214: 361-365.)

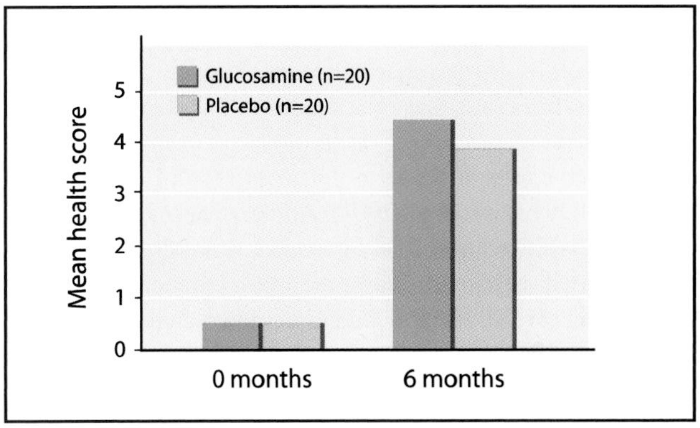

Figure 46-16. Mean health scores (0 = very severe cystitis, 5 = normal) from owner ratings at the beginning (0 months) and end (6 months) of a clinical study evaluating effects of glucosamine[d] compared with placebo in cats (n = 40) with feline idiopathic cystitis (FIC). There was no significant difference between groups (glucosamine or placebo) at baseline or after six months of treatment; however, mean health scores were significantly higher in both groups of cats at six months compared with baseline (p <0.001). Mean urine specific gravity at the beginning of the study was 1.050 and it was significantly lower (1.036) when reassessed one month later. Most owners switched from feeding dry food to moist food after receiving educational material at the beginning of the study that included benefits of feeding moist food to cats with FIC. (Adapted from Gunn-Moore DA, Shenoy CM. Oral glucosamine and the management of feline idiopathic cystitis. Journal of Feline Medicine and Surgery 2004; 6: 219-225.)

there is recurrent disease in the face of feeding a dry struvite preventive food.

Magnesium

Avoiding excess dietary magnesium intake can reduce urinary concentration of magnesium, which decreases risk for struvite disease. In an epidemiologic study, risk of struvite uroliths was increased in cats fed foods higher in magnesium (Lekcharoensuk et al, 2001a). Excess magnesium is present in some commercial cat foods because they contain ingredients high in magnesium (e.g., high-ash meat and bone, fish and poultry meals). The recommended range of dietary magnesium for dissolving struvite uroliths in cats is 0.04 to 0.09% (dry matter [DM]). For preventing recurrence of struvite uroliths or urethral plugs, the recommended range of magnesium is 0.04 to 0.14% DM (**Table 46-12**).

Magnesium is considered to be an inhibitor of calcium oxalate crystal formation. Potential mechanisms for this inhibitory effect include increased urinary pH, increased urinary excretion of citrate and formation of magnesium oxalate complexes in urine, which are more soluble than calcium oxalate. Formation of magnesium oxalate, in theory, reduces the concentration of oxalate available for precipitation as calcium oxalate. Low urinary magnesium concentration has been suggested as a potential risk factor for formation of calcium-containing uroliths in cats (Lekcharoensuk et al, 2000, 2001). Clinical studies evaluating effectiveness of magnesium supplementation on recurrence of calcium oxalate uroliths in people have yielded conflicting results (Johansson et al, 1980; Ettinger et al, 1988; Schwartz et al, 2001). Addition of magnesium was associated with reduced calcium oxalate saturation in urine as demonstrated with in vitro studies using synthetic human urine (Kohri et al, 1988). In vitro studies demonstrated that physiologic concentrations of magnesium decreased rate of nucleation and growth of calcium oxalate crystals (Kohri et al, 1988; Li et al, 1985). However, excessive dietary magnesium may result in hypercalciuria, a risk factor for calcium oxalate urolithiasis (Fetner et al, 1978).

An epidemiologic study of nutritional factors associated with urolithiasis in cats demonstrated that foods with the lowest magnesium content (0.04 to 0.07% DM; 0.09 to 0.18 mg/kcal) were associated with increased risk of forming calcium oxalate uroliths when compared with foods that had moderate magnesium content (0.08 to 0.14% DM; 0.19 to 0.35 mg/kcal) (Lekcharoensuk et al, 2001a). Foods with the highest magnesium content (0.14 to 0.56% DM; 0.36 to 1.40 mg/kcal) also were associated with increased risk of developing calcium oxalate uroliths when compared with foods containing moderate amounts of magnesium. In another study of cats with calcium oxalate uroliths, the mean magnesium content (0.19 mg/kcal) of the food being fed at the time of urolith diagnosis was similar to that of the magnesium content of a urolith-prevention food[e] (0.2 mg/kcal), which significantly decreased urine calcium oxalate saturation compared with the regular food (Lulich et al, 2004). To minimize risk of calcium oxalate uroliths, foods should contain a moderate amount of magnesium (0.07 to 0.14% DM). Individual foods intended to reduce the recurrence of both struvite and calcium oxalate urolithiasis should also be within this range.

Phosphorus

Varying dietary phosphorus levels can alter urinary phosphate concentrations in cats, thereby influencing likelihood of urinary struvite precipitates. High-phosphorus foods have been associated with increased risk of struvite uroliths in cats (Lekcharoensuk et al, 2001a). The recommended range of dietary phosphorus for dissolving struvite uroliths is 0.45 to 1.1% DM phosphorus; for struvite prevention the recommended range is 0.5 to 0.9% DM (**Table 46-12**).

Urinary phosphate can exist in several states; anionic phosphate (PO_4^{-3}) is the important form in precipitation and dissolution of struvite. Urinary concentration of anionic phosphate is reversibly influenced by pH. (See Urinary pH below and **Box 46-3.**) Thus, as urine becomes more acidic, anionic phosphate is converted to monobasic and dibasic phosphate, thereby reducing the concentration of anionic phosphate available for forming struvite precipitates. As urine becomes more alkaline, the reaction proceeds in the opposite direction and concentration of anionic phosphate increases.

Compared with foods containing moderate amounts of phosphorus, both low- and high-phosphorus foods are associated with increased risk of calcium oxalate uroliths in cats. Reduction in dietary phosphorus may cause activation of vitamin D, which promotes intestinal absorption of calcium and subsequent urinary calcium excretion. Rats fed a very low-phosphorus food (0.07% DM) had marked hypercalciuria (Werness et al, 1981). Feeding this level of phosphorus for one week resulted in urine that was oversaturated with calcium oxalate and contained large amounts of calcium oxalate crystals. A possible explanation for increased risk of calcium oxalate uroliths associated with increased phosphorus intake is that excessive dietary phosphorus could form insoluble salts with dietary calcium, which in turn could increase availability of noncomplexed oxalic acid for intestinal absorption and renal excretion (Lekcharoensuk et al, 2001a).

The recommended range of dietary phosphorus for decreasing risk of calcium oxalate urolithiasis is 0.50 to 1.0% DM phosphorus (**Table 46-12**). The recommended range for the phosphorus content of foods intended for prevention of both struvite and calcium oxalate should be between 0.5 and 0.9% DM.

Calcium

Calcium availability from the gastrointestinal tract may be influenced by non-dietary and dietary factors. Intestinal absorption of calcium occurs primarily in the duodenum; transport of calcium across the gut is a saturable process that is vitamin D-dependent. In general, calcium absorption from the intestinal tract is inversely proportional to dietary intake. In other words, absorption is high from low-calcium foods and low from high-calcium foods. Other dietary factors (e.g., vitamin D, sucrose, fructose, glucose, xylose, dietary fiber, oxalic acid, phytic acid, protein and phosphorus) reportedly affect calcium availability.

Excessive dietary calcium should be avoided to prevent recurrence of calcium oxalate uroliths. The most important sources of excess calcium are commercial foods and mineral supplements containing high calcium levels. High intake of dietary calcium may lead to hypercalciuria and urolith formation in patients with intestinal hyperabsorption of calcium. Calcium-rich human foods (**Table 46-15**) should be avoided in patients at risk for calcium oxalate uroliths. In addition to foods naturally high in calcium, a number of different human foods (e.g., breads and breakfast cereals) and beverages are fortified with calcium. The amount of calcium added to these foods can be found on the product label.

Another potential unrecognized source of excess dietary calcium is vitamin-mineral supplements, especially calcium supplements. A wide variety of calcium supplements are available over the counter. These supplements differ in the amount of elemental calcium provided. Calcium carbonate, for example, contains 40% calcium (by weight), whereas calcium lactate and calcium gluconate contain 13 and 9% calcium, respectively. Little is known about the relative availability of calcium from different supplements. Calcium supplements differ not only in their calcium content, but also in their solubility. Increasing dietary calcium intake prevents dietary hyperoxaluria in human patients eating oxalate-rich foods (Pak, 1990). This finding presumably is due to decreased intestinal absorption of oxalate. However, women taking calcium supplements had a 79% increased risk of calcium oxalate uroliths (Curhan et al, 1995). The increased risk associated with calcium supplements may be due to timing of ingestion. If not taken with meals, calcium supplements may lead to increased urinary calcium excretion, without decreasing oxalate absorption in the gastrointestinal tract.

Excessive restriction of calcium should also be avoided; it may cause negative calcium balance and contribute to hyperoxaluria, which increases risk for calcium oxalate uroliths. Cats fed foods containing moderate amounts of calcium had decreased risk of developing calcium oxalate uroliths compared with cats fed either low or high amounts of calcium (Lekcharoensuk et al, 2001a). The recommended range of dietary calcium for decreasing risk of calcium oxalate uroliths is 0.6 to 1.0% DM. This is also the recommended range for the calcium content of foods intended for prevention of both struvite and calcium oxalate urolithiasis.

Table 46-15. Calcium-rich foods that should be avoided in cats at risk for calcium oxalate urolithiasis.*

Food item	Serving size	Calcium (mg)
Yogurt	1 cup (8 oz.)	415
Whole milk	1 cup (8 oz.)	291
Cheese	1 oz.	200-270
Ice cream or ice milk	1 cup (8 oz.)	176
Cottage cheese, creamed	1 cup (8 oz.)	136
Broccoli, cooked	1 large stalk	88

*Mineral supplements and some commercial cat foods contain much more calcium than these foods; therefore, a thorough and complete nutritional history is important for managing these patients.

Protein

Excessive dietary protein intake should be avoided in patients at risk for struvite uroliths. Protein provides additional urea and glutamine, which are metabolized to ammonia and ammonium, respectively. Urinary excretion of ammonia and ammonium increases their availability to combine with magnesium and phosphate to form struvite crystals and uroliths. In addition, foods that have increased amounts of protein also tend to have increased phosphorus, which is a component of struvite uroliths. The recommended amount of dietary protein for struvite dissolution and prevention ranges from 30 to 45% DM protein.

The risk of calcium oxalate urolithiasis in people and dogs generally is considered to increase with ingestion of foods that are high in protein. During the last century, the predominant urolith type in people in the U.S. has shifted from struvite to calcium oxalate (Goldfarb, 1994). Cross-cultural studies have shown a shift from struvite to calcium oxalate uroliths with increasing industrialization (Samuel and Kasidas, 1995). The reason for the increased incidence of calcium oxalate in these human populations is unknown. However, dietary habits are thought to play a major role. Nutritional epidemiologic studies have emphasized the role of increased dietary intake of animal protein. This link seems plausible because the amount of animal protein in the diet correlates with industrialization. Dietary protein increases calcium, uric acid and possibly oxalate excretion and decreases urinary pH. Animal proteins are rich in sulfur-containing amino acids, which are metabolized to sulfate and thus may reduce urinary pH and increase urinary calcium and uric acid concentrations. High dietary protein intake reportedly increases urinary calcium excretion in dogs. The 24-hour urinary calcium excretion almost doubled when dogs were fed a food containing 31% DM protein compared with calcium excretion for dogs fed a food containing 10% DM protein (Bartges et al, 1995). The type of protein, duration of protein intake and phosphorus intake influence the effect of protein on calcium.

At present, available evidence does not support that excessive dietary protein is associated with calcium oxalate uroliths in cats. Healthy cats eating a high-protein food (13.7 g/100 kcal; 55% DM protein for a food with 4 kcal metabolizable energy [ME]/g DM) had increased water intake, urine volume and urinary pH; however, they did not have increased urinary calcium excretion (Funaba et al, 1996). In a case-controlled study of nutritional factors associated with urolithiasis, cats fed foods containing more than 7.98 g of protein/100 kcal (32% DM protein for a food with 4 kcal ME/g DM) were less likely to form calcium oxalate uroliths than cats fed low-protein foods (5.15 to 7.98 g/100 kcal; 21 to 32% DM protein for a food with 4 kcal ME/g DM) (Lekcharoensuk et al, 2001a). It is possible that increased urine volume associated with increased protein intake plays a role in decreasing risk of urolith formation. On the basis of current information, cats at risk for calcium oxalate uroliths should be fed foods with at least 32% DM protein. The protein content of foods intended for prevention of both struvite and calcium oxalate should be between 32 and 45% DM.

Sodium

Increasing the salt (i.e., sodium chloride) content of food is an effective method for increasing water intake and causing subsequent urine dilution in healthy cats (Hawthorne and Markwell, 2004; Luckshander et al, 2004). However, most factors that promote natriuresis tend to increase urinary calcium excretion, which could increase risk for calcium oxalate uroliths. Calcium and sodium are reabsorbed at common sites in the renal tubules. Hypercalciuric people who form calcium-containing uroliths appear to have a proportionally greater increase in urinary calcium excretion than non-urolith formers. Increasing dietary sodium intake from 140 to 310 mmol/day increased urinary calcium excretion by 34% and decreased urinary citrate by 10% (Kok et al, 1990). However, urinary calcium and sodium excretion was not correlated in healthy people with low dietary calcium intake (Dawson-Hughes et al, 1996).

Effects of increased sodium intake on urinary excretion of calcium or urinary calcium oxalate saturation in cats with calcium oxalate uroliths have not been reported. Increased urinary excretion of calcium was identified in cats with mild, naturally occurring chronic kidney disease consuming a food with 1.2% DM sodium compared with consumption of a food containing 0.4% DM sodium (Kirk et al, 2006). Additional study of effects of increased sodium intake on urinary calcium excretion in cats with kidney disease is indicated because nephroliths and ureteroliths, which are most often calcium oxalate, are being diagnosed more often in cats with chronic kidney disease (Ross et al, 2005, 2007).

In healthy cats fed a high-salt food, urine calcium concentration and calcium oxalate saturation were not increased, although there was a significant increase in 24-hour urine calcium excretion (Biourge et al, 2001). This was likely due to dilution of calcium and other substances in urine associated with increased urine volume. In another study of healthy cats, increased dietary sodium was associated with increased water intake and urine volume and significantly decreased values for calcium oxalate urine saturation (Hawthorne and Markwell, 2004).

In an epidemiologic study, feeding foods containing less sodium (0.48 to 0.77 mg sodium/kcal; 0.19 to 0.31% DM, for a food with 4 kcal ME/g DM) was associated with calcium oxalate uroliths in cats (Lekcharoensuk et al, 2001a). Despite this finding, feeding a veterinary therapeutic food containing 0.67 mg sodium/kcal (0.27% DM for a food with 4 kcal ME/g DM) to calcium oxalate urolith-forming cats was associated with a significant decrease in urine calcium excretion and calcium oxalate saturation compared with eating their regular food (Lulich et al, 2004). The recommended range for dietary sodium intake in cats at risk for calcium oxalate uroliths is 0.3 to 0.6% DM sodium.

Varying levels of sodium have been used in foods[f,g] that have been shown to be effective for struvite dissolution in feline patients (Osborne et al, 1990; Houston et al, 2004). In lieu of other data, based on the sodium levels in these foods, a recommended range for sodium content for foods for struvite dissolution could be developed by simply bracketing the levels in these foods (e.g., 0.37 to 1.27% DM sodium). However, research indicates that urinary calcium excretion increases when healthy cats are fed a high-salt food (Biourge et al, 2001). Also, as mentioned above, cats prone to the development of calcium oxalate urolithiasis benefit from avoiding increased sodium intake (Lulich et al, 2004). Thus, to avoid excess calcium excretion and the possibility of formation of calcium oxalate crystals while feeding these types of foods, a sodium range of 0.3 to 0.6% DM is recommended in foods intended for struvite dissolution.

Cats fed foods containing 1.43 to 3.7 mg of sodium/kcal (0.57 to 1.48% DM, for a food with 4 kcal ME/g DM) were 4.1 times as likely to develop struvite uroliths as cats consuming foods with less sodium (0.48 to 0.77 mg/kcal; 0.19 to 0.31% DM, for a food with 4 kcal ME/g DM) (Lekcharoensuk et al, 2001a). In this epidemiologic study there was a significant correlation between high sodium and high phosphorus content in foods. It is possible that increased risk for struvite uroliths in cats eating high-sodium foods is related to the type of sodium salt (e.g., monosodium phosphate, sodium tripolyphosphate) used in foods. However, additional study is needed to confirm this. There are no reported studies evaluating effects of increased sodium intake in cats with naturally occurring struvite uroliths. The recommended range of dietary sodium intake for prevention of struvite disease in cats is 0.3 to 0.6% DM.

In order to cause production of dilute urine, food must contain more than 1% DM sodium. Many foods formulated for cats with lower urinary tract diseases contain between 0.3 and 0.6% DM sodium, whereas, some contain 1 to 1.4% DM sodium. The minimum recommended allowance of sodium for adult cats is 0.068% DM (NRC, 2006). According to the most recent information published by the National Research Council (NRC), it is difficult to suggest a safe upper limit of sodium for healthy adult cats (NRC, 2006). The NRC has concluded that as long as unlimited amounts of water are available, cats probably can tolerate reasonably high concentrations of dietary sodium; the safe upper limit for adult cats has been defined as greater than 1.5% DM. However, the safe upper limit of sodium for cats with chronic kidney disease, lower urinary tract disorders and other conditions (e.g., hypertension) is unknown. One study revealed that six cats with early kidney disease had significant increases of serum creatinine, urea nitrogen and phosphorus when consuming a food with 1.2% DM sodium for three months vs. when fed a food with 0.4% DM sodium (Kirk et al, 2006). Additional evaluation of effects of increased sodium intake is needed because most studies have either been of short duration (<6 months) or were performed in healthy cats. Pending availability of additional data (e.g., effects of high sodium intake in cats with calcium oxalate uroliths), orally administered sodium chloride should be used cautiously and with careful monitoring because of the potential for increased risk of calcium oxalate urolith formation in some patients (Bartges and Kirk, 2006).

Urinary pH

The kidneys eliminate acid that is produced as a result of normal metabolism, including digestion of food. Therefore, to

Box 46-4. Determining the Effect of Food on Urinary pH.

Several important effects of food on acid-base balance can be described by the anion-cation balance (ACB). Calculation of a food's ACB has been evaluated as a practical method for predicting the effect of a food on urinary pH. In this method, the ACB is calculated from the concentrations of alkaline and acid compounds in the food, expressed as mmol/kg dry matter, using the formula:
ACB = 49.9 (Calcium) + 82.3 (Magnesium) + 43.5 (Sodium) + 25.6 (Potassium) – 64.6 (Phosphorus) – 13.4 (Methionine) – 16.6 (Cysteine) – 28.2 (Chloride). Factors take into account atomic/molecular weight and valence (2 for phosphorus).

This method was evaluated in a study involving 10 commercial foods (moist and dry) and several additives. Feeding trials involved four to six cats per trial. Cats were fed the foods for two days and urine was collected for at least five days. During the eight hours after feeding, urinary pH was measured immediately after urination and urine excreted during the remainder of the day was tested the following morning. A highly significant correlation was seen between ACB of the food and the mean urinary pH. In the amounts used in this study, the addition of calcium carbonate and calcium lactate significantly increased urinary pH; dibasic calcium phosphate and ascorbic acid had no effect; and calcium chloride, ammonium chloride and phosphoric acid decreased urinary pH.

Another study was conducted recently to determine if urinary pH could be predicted using the nutrient components of feline foods. One-hundred-fifty foods (90 dry, 60 wet) were fed to groups of 10 adult cats to determine urinary pH of cats fed each food. Each food was fed for seven days and pH was determined on freshly voided urine on Days 5 to 7 of the study. Using stepwise regression, it was determined which cations, anions and sulfur-containing amino acids were of importance for predicting urinary pH. Separate formulas had to be used for dry and wet foods to maintain accuracy.

Although calculation of ACB may roughly estimate urinary pH and formulas can be used to predict urinary pH based on nutrient content of food, the most accepted method of comparing foods is to feed the food to a group of cats and compare urinary pH values. However, although most reputable cat food manufacturers provide urinary pH data for their products, no standard urinary pH testing protocol has been developed. Consequently, it is important to know the protocol used to measure urinary pH before comparing results from different companies or laboratories.

The Bibliography for **Box 46-4** can be found at www.markmorris.org.

define "normal" urinary pH, it is necessary to consider the "normal" or habitual diet. On a volume basis, the gastric content of feral cats is approximately 90% small mammals (e.g., mice, rats) (Coman and Brunner, 1972). In one study, the average urinary pH was approximately 6.3 when cats were fed a diet of rat carcasses (Vondruska, 1987). In another study, mean urinary pH was reported to be 5.97 for feral female cats and 6.37 for feral male cats eating a natural diet (Cottam et al, 2002).

The kidneys provide long-term defense against acid and alkali deviations; this process occurs continuously as endogenous acids are generated. The kidneys must conserve bicarbonate in the glomerular filtrate and regenerate bicarbonate degraded by the reaction with metabolic acids to maintain normal plasma bicarbonate levels. The kidneys can increase the amount of net acid excretion in urine and generate bicarbonate in response to exogenous acid loads. Normally, the kidneys synthesize urinary ammonia (NH_3) and thus ammonium (NH_4^+) almost exclusively. With chronic metabolic acidosis, more NH_3 is produced and urinary NH_4^+ ion concentration is increased. The kidneys excrete hydrogen ions (H^+) in the form of titratable acid (e.g., phosphoric acid) and NH_4^+ ions. Reduction of urinary pH greatly increases the ratio of NH_4^+ to NH_3. Acidifying foods, therefore, increase urinary concentration of NH_4^+ ions, one component of struvite. Although decreasing urinary pH theoretically increases urinary NH_4^+ concentration, the same change in urinary pH decreases anionic phosphate levels in urine. Thus, as urine becomes more acidic, precipitation of struvite becomes less likely.

The effect of a food on urinary pH is the net effect of its constituent nutrients (**Box 46-4**). Dietary acid is derived from several nutrients (**Table 46-16**) (Halperin and Jungas, 1983).

Table 46-16. Urine acidifying and alkalinizing pet food ingredients.

Protein sources that are acidifying ingredients
Poultry meal
Corn gluten meal
Other acidifying ingredients
Ammonium chloride*
Calcium chloride
Calcium sulfate
dl-methionine
Phosphoric acid
Alkalinizing ingredients
Calcium carbonate
Potassium citrate
Magnesium oxide

*Not approved in the United States as a food additive.

Sulfuric acid is formed when sulfur-containing amino acid (e.g., methionine and cysteine) residues of proteins are oxidized to sulfate. In general, animal-source protein ingredients contain more sulfur-containing amino acid residues than do plant-source proteins. Phosphorus has strong effects on acid-base balance, depending on its chemical form. Inorganic phosphorus can be ingested as phosphoric acid, monobasic and dibasic or anionic phosphate. Phosphoric acid is used in cat foods to enhance palatability, either separately or as a component of topically applied animal digests. Phosphoric acid has a strong acidifying effect. Monobasic phosphate also is acidifying, whereas dibasic phosphate has little effect on urinary pH (Kienzle et al, 1991). Anionic phosphate is alkalizing.

Mineral salts vary in their effect on urinary pH and thus are potential acid or base sources. Oxides and carbonates are alka-

Table 46-17. Effect of urinary pH on urine saturation values in healthy cats (n = 6).*

Food	Urinary pH	CaOx RSS	Struvite RSS
$NaHCO_3$	6.81 ± 0.33[b]	0.78 ± 0.53[a]	7.98 ± 4.62[b]
Control	6.18 ± 0.26[a]	0.71 ± 0.28[a]	1.61 ± 1.11[a]
NH_4Cl	5.81 ± 0.14[a]	1.66 ± 0.58[b]	1.16 ± 0.25[a]

Key: $NaHCO_3$ = sodium bicarbonate, NH_4Cl = ammonium chloride, CaOx = calcium oxalate, RSS = relative supersaturation.
*Significant differences within columns indicated by different superscripts. Adapted from Stevenson AE, Wrigglesworth DJ, Markwell PJ. Urine pH and urinary relative supersaturation in healthy adult cats In: Rodgers AL, Hibbert BE, Hess B, et al, eds. IXth International Symposium on Urolithiasis. Cape Town, South Africa, 2000: 818-820.

Table 46-18. Oxalate content of selected human foods.*

Product categories	Moderate to high oxalate	Low oxalate
Milk and dairy products	–	Milk** Cheese**
Meats	Liver Sardines	Beef Bacon Ham Lamb Shellfish Poultry
Fruits	Apples (green) Apricots Bananas Cherries Berries (most) Oranges/tangerines Pears Peel (lemon/lime/orange) Pineapple	Apples (red) Coconut (fresh) Cranberries Melons Peaches
Vegetables	Beans Carrots Celery Green beans Green peppers Greens (collards, mustard, turnips) Peas Soybean products Spinach Sweet potatoes Tofu Tomatoes	Asparagus Avocado Broccoli** Cabbage Corn (sweet) Cucumber
Breads/ grains/nuts	Bagels Bread (whole wheat) Cornbread Fig newtons Fruitcake Grits Oatmeal Most nuts Rice (brown)	Bread (white) Tortilla (corn) Pasta (boiled) Popped popcorn Rice (white)

*For information about oxalate content of additional foods see www.ohf.org
**High in calcium, therefore, may not be ideal for cats with calcium oxalate uroliths.

lizing. Differences in absorption of the cation and anion portion of a salt are important. Intestinal absorption of calcium and magnesium is relatively low. However, absorption of accompanying anions can be high and influences urinary pH. Nonmetabolizable anions (e.g., chloride, phosphate and sulfate) absorbed in excess of their accompanying cations are acidifying. For example, ammonium chloride, calcium chloride and calcium sulfate decrease urinary pH, and magnesium oxide and calcium carbonate increase urinary pH.

Urinary pH plays a critical role in managing cats with struvite disease but appears less important in cats with calcium oxalate uroliths. Struvite is highly soluble and is, therefore, less likely to precipitate in acidic urine (pH <6.5). Alterations in urinary pH have a proportionally greater effect on changing struvite activity product than changes in crystalloid (e.g., magnesium) concentrations. Decreasing urinary pH, therefore, is the most reliable means of producing urine undersaturated for struvite. Although acidifying foods have been associated with occurrence of calcium oxalate uroliths in cats, changes in urinary pH values over the physiologic range appear to have little effect on solubility of calcium oxalate (**Figure 46-17**) (Verplaetse et al, 1985; Yu and Gross, 2007; Stevenson et al, 2000). One study showed that pH changes between 4 and 11 had minimal effect on calcium oxalate solubility (Verplaetse et al, 1985). In a study of healthy cats fed three foods to produce different urinary pH values, reducing urinary pH from 6.81 to 6.18 had no significant effect on urine saturation for calcium oxalate (0.78 vs. 0.71) but significantly decreased struvite saturation (**Table 46-17**) (Stevenson et al, 2000).

The recommended urinary pH range for dissolving struvite uroliths is 5.8 to 6.2. To decrease risk for recurrence of struvite uroliths or urethral plugs, urinary pH should be 6.0 to 6.4; however, to decrease risk for recurrence of calcium oxalate uroliths, urinary pH should be at least 6.2. Thus, foods for prevention of both struvite and calcium oxalate urolithiasis should produce a urinary pH between 6.2 to 6.4.

Fatty Acids

Urinary bladder inflammation is characteristic of most lower urinary tract disorders including FIC and urolithiasis. Long-chain omega-3 (n-3) fatty acids such as eicosapentaenoic acid (EPA) and docosahexaenoic acid (DHA) have potent antiinflammatory properties. These dietary fatty acids are absorbed and incorporated into cell membranes, including those of the urinary bladder, where they may alter production of inflammatory mediators. Antiinflammatory effects of omega-3 fatty acids such as EPA have been demonstrated in dogs with osteoarthritis and patients with dermatitis. Effects of omega-3 fatty acids have not been evaluated in cats with various lower urinary tract disorders; however, they appear to have beneficial urinary effects in studies of other species. Administration of EPA to rats prevented experimentally induced nephrocalcinosis and significantly decreased urinary calcium excretion compared with a placebo (Buck et al, 1991). In a second part of the study, 12 human patients with recurrent calcium oxalate uroliths and hypercalciuria had significantly decreased urinary calcium and oxalate excretion when treated with EPA for eight weeks. In another study, administration of EPA for three months to 88 people with recurrent urinary stones, primarily calcium oxalate, was associated with significantly decreased urinary calcium in those with hypercalciuria (Yasui et al, 2001).

The recommended range of dietary total omega-3 fatty acids (i.e., DHA and/or EPA) for managing inflammation associated with lower urinary tract diseases is 0.35 to 1.0% DM. This range was extrapolated from levels associated with antiinflammatory effects in other species. Additional study is needed to better define the therapeutic range of omega-3 fatty acids for managing patients with FIC and calcium oxalate uroliths.

Other Nutritional Factors

Antioxidants

Vitamin E has antioxidant properties that have been shown to decrease oxidative stress and damage caused by free radicals. Because oxidative stress is often associated with inflammation, antioxidants may help create an unfavorable environment for the development of uroliths. However, this has not been evaluated in cats with naturally occurring urolithiasis.

Vitamin C is also an antioxidant. However, a portion of urinary oxalate is derived from endogenous metabolism of vitamin C. In a controlled study of healthy cats fed differing amounts of vitamin C ranging from 40 to 193 mg vitamin C/kg of food for four weeks, there was no significant change in urinary oxalate excretion (Yu and Gross, 2005). Effects of vitamin C supplementation have not been studied in cats with calcium oxalate uroliths. Because cats do not have a dietary requirement for vitamin C, supplementation should be avoided in cats at risk for calcium oxalate uroliths (Bartges and Kirk, 2006). One source of vitamin C that should be avoided is cranberry concentrate tablets.

Oxalate

Excessive intake of oxalate is unlikely in dogs and cats eating most commercial foods but it could occur in pets receiving excessive amounts of certain human foods as treats. Foods that contain relatively high amounts of oxalate (e.g., spinach, carrots, liver, sardines) should be avoided in patients with a history of calcium oxalate uroliths. **Table 46-18** provides more information about the oxalate content in selected human foods.

Potassium

Transient negative potassium balance has been reported to occur in adult cats receiving long-term dietary acidification (i.e., for struvite urolith prevention) with phosphoric acid and NH_4Cl; potassium balance returned to normal by the end of both studies (Fettman et al, 1992; Ching et al, 1990). In an epidemiologic study, cats fed foods with higher amounts of potassium (2.17 to 3.20 mg/kcal; 0.87 to 1.28% DM for a food with 4 kcal ME/g DM) had decreased risk of calcium oxalate uroliths compared with cats that were eating foods with less potassium (0.95 to 1.60 mg/kcal; 0.35 to 0.64% DM for a food with 4 kcal ME/g DM) (Lekcharoensuk et al, 2001a). Additional study is needed to determine if potassium supplementation benefits cats with calcium oxalate uroliths. Based on current information, dietary potassium intake should exceed 0.65% DM in cats at risk for struvite disease and calcium oxalate uroliths. Most commercial foods are replete with potassium.

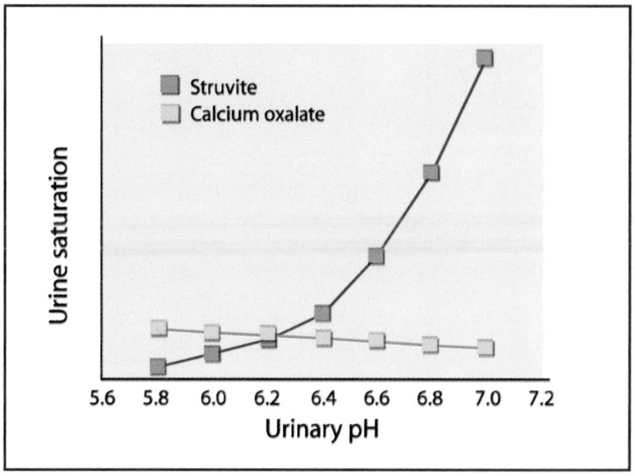

Figure 46-17. This graph demonstrates the relationship between urinary pH and urine saturation values for struvite and calcium oxalate. Data were collected from 21 adult cats (10 healthy and 11 urolith-forming cats) during consumption of a food (Hill's Prescription Diet c/d Multicare Feline) formulated to manage both struvite and calcium oxalate uroliths. Mineral type was not available for uroliths in most cats; however, calcium oxalate was presumed most likely due to location (eight cats had nephroliths), radiographic appearance and results of quantitative analysis for uroliths that were removed. Urine constituents (e.g., calcium oxalate, magnesium, phosphate) and pH were measured for each cat and used to calculate values for relative supersaturation (RSS). This was followed by a computer-modeling procedure to predict effect that changing only urinary pH would have on RSS values. Results were similar for both healthy and urolith-forming cats; therefore, all data are shown in one graph. Note that as urinary pH increases, urine saturation for struvite increases; however, as urinary pH decreases over the physiologic range, there is only a slight change in calcium oxalate saturation. In this model, reducing urinary pH from 7.4 to 6.4 decreased struvite saturation by 122 units but only increased calcium oxalate saturation by 0.9 units. (Adapted from Yu S, Gross KL. Dietary management of the three most common lower urinary tract diseases in cats. In: Proceedings. Hill's Symposium on Lower Urinary Tract Disease. Educational Concepts, 2007: 53-57.)

Vitamin B_6 (Pyridoxine)

Increases in urinary oxalic acid excretion have been observed in kittens fed pyridoxine-deficient foods. However, no studies have evaluated effects of vitamin B_6 in cats with calcium oxalate uroliths (Bai et al, 1989, 1991). No evidence suggests that supplementing vitamin B_6 beyond nutritional requirements benefits cats with calcium oxalate urolithiasis. Because most commercially available pet foods are well supplemented with vitamin B_6, it seems unlikely that additional supplementation would be helpful unless the primary food is homemade.

Vitamin D

Increased vitamin D intake should be avoided because it can lead to increased intestinal absorption of calcium with subse-

Table 46-19. Comparison of key nutritional factors in selected commercial veterinary therapeutic foods for reducing the recurrence of feline idiopathic cystitis, struvite disease (uroliths or urethral plugs) and/or calcium oxalate uroliths in cats.*

Moist foods**	**Mg (%)**	**P (%)**	**Ca (%)**	**Protein (%)**	**Na (%)**	**Urinary pH**	**Total omega 3 (%)**
Recommended levels	**0.07-0.14**	**0.5-0.9**	**0.6-1.0**	**32-45**	**0.3-0.6**	**6.2-6.4**	**0.35-1.0**
Hill's Prescription Diet c/d Multicare with Chicken Feline	0.052	0.68	0.72	43.8	0.32	6.35	0.96
Hill's Prescription Diet c/d Multicare with Seafood Feline	0.054	0.71	0.62	44.8	0.33	6.4	0.62
Medi-Cal Urinary SO	na	1.20	1.20	43.5	1.1	6.4	na
Purina Veterinary Diets UR Urinary St/Ox Feline Formula	0.07	0.97	0.96	50.6	0.62	6.0-6.4	na
Royal Canin Veterinary Diet Urinary SO in gel	0.10	1.36	1.02	41.3	1.02	6.0-6.3	na
Dry foods	**Mg (%)**	**P (%)**	**Ca (%)**	**Protein (%)**	**Na (%)**	**Urinary pH**	**Total omega 3 (%)**
Recommended levels	**0.07-0.14**	**0.5-0.9**	**0.6-1.0**	**32-45**	**0.3-0.6**	**6.2-6.4**	**0.35-1.0**
Hill's Prescription Diet c/d Multicare Feline	0.06	0.65	0.74	36.1	0.35	6.3	0.65
Hill's Prescription Diet c/d Multicare with Chicken Feline	0.06	0.65	0.76	34.6	0.33	6.3	0.64
Purina Veterinary Diets UR Urinary St/Ox Feline Formula	0.07	1.08	1.1	44.9	1.17	6.0-6.4	na

Key: Mg = magnesium, P = phosphorus, Ca = calcium, Na = sodium, total omega 3 = total omega-3 fatty acids, na = not available from manufacturer.
*Nutrients expressed on a dry matter basis unless otherwise stated.
**In general, it is recommended that moist foods be fed to cats with lower urinary tract disorders, especially those with feline idiopathic cystitis or calcium oxalate uroliths.

Table 46-20. Descriptions of grades used to classify evidence supporting treatments for cats with lower urinary tract diseases.*

Grade	**Description of evidence**
I	At least one properly designed, randomized, controlled clinical study performed in patients of the target species
II	Evidence from properly designed, randomized, controlled studies in animals of the target species with spontaneous disease in a laboratory or research animal colony setting
III	Appropriately controlled studies without randomization Appropriately designed case-control epidemiologic studies Studies using models of disease or simulations in the target species Dramatic results from uncontrolled studies Case series
IV	Studies conducted in other species Reports of expert committees Descriptive studies Case reports Pathophysiologic justification/rationale Opinions of respected experts

*Adapted from Roudebush P, Allen TA, Dodd CE, et al. Application of evidence-based medicine to veterinary clinical nutrition. Journal of the American Veterinary Medical Association 2004; 224: 1765-1771.

quent hypercalciuria and increased risk for oxalate uroliths. The minimum recommended allowance for vitamin D for adult cats is 280 IU/kg food (DM; for a food with 4 kcal ME/g DM) (NRC, 2006). However, cats at risk for calcium oxalate urolithiasis and those with hypercalcemia associated with calcium oxalate urolithiasis should be fed foods that do not exceed 2,000 IU/kg of food. Dietary supplements containing vitamin D should not be fed to at-risk cats.

Fiber

The role of dietary fiber has not been carefully evaluated in cats with lower urinary tract disorders. In an epidemiologic study of cats with uroliths, those fed high-fiber foods (0.71 to 11.57 g/100 kcal) were 2.12 times more likely to develop struvite uroliths than cats fed low-fiber foods (0.06 to 0.30 g/100 kcal) (Lekcharoensuk et al, 2001a). In the same study there was no association between dietary fiber and development of calcium oxalate uroliths. Dietary fiber may bind calcium in the small intestine, preventing its absorption. There are anecdotal reports that feeding foods with increased fiber helps control hypercalcemia in cats with concomitant calcium oxalate uroliths (McClain et al, 1999).

FEEDING PLANS

Successful management of cats with various lower urinary tract diseases requires a multifaceted approach and effective communication between health care team members and owners. Nutritional management plays a key role in the treatment of patients with FIC, struvite disease (uroliths and urethral plugs) and calcium oxalate uroliths. Environmental enrichment (e.g., stress reduction, litter box management) also should be implemented in patients with FIC and may be helpful for cats with other lower urinary tract disorders. For cats with persistent clinical signs, especially periuria, behavioral modification may also be needed to correcting the underlying medical disorder. Finally, other treatments such as pain management may be needed for some cats, especially during acute episodes.

Feeding plans for cats with various lower urinary tract diseases continue the iterative process and include the following steps: 1) assess and select the food, 2) assess and determine the feeding method and 3) reassess and modify the feeding plan, as

Table 46-21. Summary of evidence for treatments used to manage cats with idiopathic cystitis, struvite uroliths or urethral plugs and calcium oxalate uroliths.*

Feline idiopathic cystitis
Grade III
- Environmental enrichment/stress reduction
- Feeding moist food
- Long-term treatment with amitriptyline (6 to 9 months) for severe cases

Grade IV
- Increased salt intake to stimulate urine dilution
- Additional methods to stimulate water intake
- Analgesics and nonsteroidal antiinflammatory drugs during acute episodes
- Feline facial pheromone
- Glycosaminoglycans (pentosan polysulfate, glucosamine/chondroitin sulfate)
- Propantheline during acute episodes

Dissolution of struvite uroliths
Grade III
- Hill's Prescription Diet s/d Feline
- Medi-Cal Dissolution Formula

Grade IV
- Other therapeutic foods formulated to dissolve uroliths

Prevention of struvite urolith or urethral plug recurrence
Grade III
- Hill's Prescription Diet s/d (for urethral plug prevention)

Grade IV
- Other therapeutic foods formulated to prevent struvite disease

Decreasing risk of calcium oxalate recurrence**
Grade III
- Feeding moist food
- Hill's Prescription Diet x/d Feline (currently available as c/d Multicare Feline)

Grade IV
Other therapeutic foods formulated to prevent calcium oxalate
- Potassium citrate
- Thiazide diuretics
- Vitamin B_6
- Using other methods (in addition to moist food) to increase water intake

*Adapted from Forrester SD, Roudebush P. Evidence-based management of feline lower urinary tract disease. Veterinary Clinics of North America: Small Animal Practice 2007; 37: 533-558.
**Based on decreased urine calcium oxalate saturation or decreased risk in epidemiologic studies.

necessary. Four feeding plans are reviewed below, including treatment and prevention of FIC, dissolution of struvite uroliths, prevention of struvite urolithiasis and urethral plugs and managing cats with calcium oxalate urolithiasis.

Regarding the food assessment/selection step: more recently, several foods have been developed that are intended to simultaneously manage the combination of risk factors associated with FIC-, struvite- and calcium oxalate-based FLUTD. These foods are listed in **Table 46-19** and are compared to the composite key nutritional factors for these three forms of lower urinary tract disease. The use of this type of food is intended to simplify and improve the effectiveness of FLUTD prevention strategies. The following sections provide guidelines for successful implementation of feeding plan recommendations and

Table 46-22. Comparison of key nutritional factors in selected commercial veterinary therapeutic foods for reducing the recurrence of feline idiopathic cystitis.*

Moist foods**	**Omega 3 (%)**
Recommended levels	**0.35-1.00**
Hill's Prescription Diet c/d Multicare with Chicken Feline	0.96
Hill's Prescription Diet c/d Multicare with Seafood Feline	0.62
Iams Veterinary Formula Urinary S Low pH/S Feline	na
Medi-Cal Veterinary Diet Urinary SO	na
Purina Veterinary Diets UR Urinary St/Ox Feline Formula	na
Royal Canin Veterinary Diet Feline Urinary SO in Gel	na
Dry foods	**Omega 3 (%)**
Recommended levels	**0.35-1.00**
Hill's Prescription Diet c/d Multicare Feline	0.65
Hill's Prescription Diet c/d Multicare with Chicken Feline	0.64
Medi-Cal Veterinary Diet Urinary SO	na
Purina Veterinary Diets UR Urinary St/Ox Feline Formula	na

Key: Omega 3 = total omega-3 fatty acids, na = not available from manufacturer.
*Nutrients expressed on a dry matter basis.
**Moist foods are best because increased water intake is considered important in the management of feline idiopathic cystitis.

other treatments that may improve outcome and enhance quality of life for cats and their owners. In addition to considering key nutritional factors, the quality of evidence supporting different treatments and foods should be evaluated (Roudebush et al, 2004; Forrester and Roudebush, 2007). **Tables 46-20** and **46-21** provide more information about evidence for treatments of cats with FLUTD.

Feline Idiopathic Cystitis

FIC is characterized by recurrent episodes of lower urinary tract signs that usually resolve within three to five days. Because of the nature of this disorder, complete elimination of episodes is unlikely. Therefore, goals of treatment are to improve quality of life by decreasing frequency of episodes and their severity. Environmental enrichment (e.g., stress reduction, litter box management) should also be implemented in patients with FIC. In cats with persistent clinical signs, especially periuria, behavioral modification may be needed in addition to correcting the underlying medical disorder. Other treatments such as pain management may be needed for some cats, especially during acute episodes. **Boxes 46-5**, **46-6**, and **46-7** include information about environmental enrichment, behavioral modification and pain management.

Assess and Select the Food

Moist foods are recommended for patients with FIC. Feeding moist food has been associated with increased daily water intake and urine volume in cats compared with feeding dry food (**Table 46-14**) (Burger and Smith, 1987; Gaskell, 1989). Beneficial effects have been observed in patients with FIC when urine specific gravity decreased from values around 1.050

Box 46-5. Ancillary Management for Patients with Feline Idiopathic Cystitis: Environmental Enrichment.

In addition to nutritional management, currently recommended treatment for patients with feline idiopathic cystitis (FIC) includes environmental enrichment, stress reduction and appropriate litter box maintenance. Recently, a prospective, uncontrolled study evaluated the effects of multimodal environmental modification in 46 client-owned cats with FIC. Significant reductions in lower urinary tract signs, fearfulness and nervousness were seen after treatment for 10 months, compared with the signs noted before using environmental enrichment.

Environmental enrichment includes providing opportunities for play/resting (e.g., horizontal and vertical surfaces for scratching, hiding places and climbing platforms). Food and water bowls should be clean and kept in safe places (e.g., not next to noisy appliances). Litter boxes should be clean and kept in locations that do not increase stress. An adequate number of litter boxes (generally defined as one more than the number of cats in the home) should be available. Most cats prefer clumping, unscented litter but individual preferences may differ for some cats and different strategies can be used to determine a cat's particular preference. More detailed and helpful information about environmental enrichment and litter box management is available elsewhere.

BEHAVIORAL MANAGEMENT

Even after successful implementation of strategies described above, some patients with FIC (or other lower urinary tract disorders) may continue to urinate in inappropriate locations. This undesirable behavioral pattern may be maintained for several reasons. Classic conditioning may play a role in persistent periuria. The litter box is associated with pain and discomfort that occurred when the cat urinated in the box previously; therefore, the cat might associate this experience with the litter box and avoid using it in the future. In this situation, it may help to change the location or physical characteristics of the litter box. It also is possible for cats to develop a litter box aversion secondary to lack of cleanliness, because the litter box may be used more frequently during episodes of FIC. If this happens, it may help to provide additional litter boxes and/or increase frequency of cleaning the litter box or changing litter. If a cat develops a litter box aversion secondary to FIC or experiences an urgency that causes elimination elsewhere, the possibility exists for development of a secondary location or substrate preference. In this situation, the litter box is not necessarily the problem; however, the cat may discover a better toileting option (e.g., a substrate that is softer, more absorbent, more accessible or cleaned more readily). To resolve this problem, the preferred inappropriate site should be made less attractive or unavailable while the litter box is improved to meet the preferences of the cat. Finally, the pain associated with an episode of FIC may result in increased irritability and subsequent social strife between previously friendly cats in the household. When signs of FIC resolve, cats may not return to their previously friendly relationship. In serious cases, full segregation and gradual reintroduction using desensitization and counter-conditioning may be necessary. Cats with persistent periuria can be very frustrating to manage and may be relinquished to a shelter if not handled appropriately. Therefore, consulting with a veterinary behaviorist (sooner rather than later) should be considered to increase chances of improving quality of life for the cat and the owner. **Boxes 46-6** and **46-7** provide more information about behavioral management of cats with inappropriate urination.

PAIN MANAGEMENT

Analgesics are indicated to manage patient discomfort during acute episodes of FIC. Drugs that have been used include buprenorphine[a] (0.03 mg/kg body weight administered topically via buccal mucosa every six to eight hours), butorphanol[b] (0.5 to 1 mg/kg body weight orally every six to eight hours) and meloxicam[c] (0.1 mg/kg body weight orally once daily for three to four days). Although other analgesics and nonsteroidal antiinflammatory agents may be appropriate, selection is often based on clinician preference or experience and whether the patient has concomitant conditions (e.g., kidney disease) that might preclude their use. No clinical studies have evaluated opioid analgesics (e.g., butorphanol, buprenorphine) or nonsteroidal antiinflammatory agents in patients with FIC.

FELINE FACIAL PHEROMONE

Synthetic feline facial pheromone therapy has been recommended to decrease signs of stress in patients with FIC. In a double-blind, placebo-controlled clinical study of 20 hospitalized cats (13 with lower urinary tract disease and seven apparently healthy), exposure to feline facial pheromone[d] was associated with significant increases in grooming, interest in food and food intake; these results suggested an anxiolytic effect in some cats. Another study evaluated effects of feline facial pheromone in 12 patients with FIC. Although no significant difference was seen between treatment of the environment with placebo and feline facial pheromone for two months, a trend was identified for cats exposed to facial pheromone. Exposed cats had fewer days with clinical signs of cystitis, a reduced number of episodes and reduced negative behavioral traits (e.g., less aggression and fear). Further study is needed; however, it seems reasonable to consider treatment with facial pheromones in cats with signs of stress or when clinical signs persist after implementing environmental enrichment and methods to increase water intake.

GLYCOSAMINOGLYCANS

Glycosaminoglycan (GAG) replacers such as pentosan polysulfate have been used in people with interstitial cystitis and have been recommended for patients with FIC. Anecdotally, these agents have

to values ranging from 1.032 to 1.041 (Markwell et al, 1999; Gunn-Moore and Shenoy, 2004). It is not known if FIC predisposes to urolith formation, but the presence of inflammatory cells and other products of inflammation could conceivably pose such a risk. Foods that are most similar to the key nutritional factor target ranges and/or have the best evidence for managing these uroliths should be considered for cats with FIC. **Tables 46-19** and **46-22** provide key nutritional factor information about selected veterinary therapeutic foods for managing patients with FIC compared with recommended levels of key nutritional factors. When possible, moist foods should be selected over dry foods.

been mentioned as useful. However, only one GAG has been critically evaluated. In a randomized, double-blinded, controlled clinical study, administration of glucosamine hydrochloride[e] (125 mg orally once daily) was not associated with any difference in clinical signs compared with cats that received placebo. If signs of FIC persist despite other treatments, GAGs (such as pentosan polysulfate[f] [8 mg/kg body weight orally q12h] or a combination of glucosamine and chondroitin sulfate[g] [250 mg/200 mg orally q24h]) may be attempted.

AMITRIPTYLINE

Amitriptyline[h] is a tricyclic antidepressant with anticholinergic, antihistaminic, sympatholytic, analgesic and antiinflammatory properties that has been used in treating people with interstitial cystitis and cats with FIC. In an uncontrolled study of cats with severe, recurrent FIC that failed to respond to other treatments, administration of amitriptyline for 12 months was associated with decreased clinical signs in nine (60%) of 15 cats during the last six months of treatment. A randomized, controlled clinical trial of amitriptyline treatment for seven days revealed no significant difference in rate of recovery from pollakiuria or hematuria; overall, clinical signs recurred significantly faster and more frequently in cats that had been treated with amitriptyline compared with control cats. In a similar study, amitriptyline combined with amoxicillin was no more effective than placebo and amoxicillin when given to cats with FIC for seven days. Based on current information, amitriptyline does not appear to be beneficial for short-term management of cats with FIC. It is possible that longer use (i.e., several months) may be helpful; however, this has not yet been demonstrated in a controlled, long-term clinical study.

ENDNOTES

a. Buprenex. Reckitt Benckiser Pharmaceuticals, Inc., Richmond, VA, USA.
b. Torbutrol and Torbugesic. Fort Dodge Animal Health, Fort Dodge, IA, USA.
c. Metacam. Boehringer Ingelheim Vetmedica, Inc., Saint Joseph, MO, USA.
d. Feliway. Veterinary Product Laboratories, Phoenix, AZ, USA.
e. Cystease. Ceva Animal Health, Chesam, United Kingdom.
f. Elmiron. Ortho McNeil Pharmaceutical, Inc., Raritan, NJ, USA.
g. Cosequin for Cats. Nutramax Laboratories, Inc., Edgewood, MO, USA.
h. Elavil. Astra-Zenaca, Wilmington, DE, USA.

The Bibliography for **Box 46-5** can be found at www.markmorris.org.

Assess and Determine the Feeding Method

Gradual transition to moist food and recommending other strategies to increase water intake should be part of initial management of patients with FIC. Cat owners may be hesitant to switch from dry to moist food and some believe their cat will not eat moist food. However, switching to moist food is possible in most situations if the change is made gradually; for some cats this many require a period of several weeks. Failure to make a gradual transition may result in refusal to eat the moist food or increased stress, which may cause recurrence of clinical signs. Therefore, moist food should be offered initially as a food option in a second dish next to the usual food (two-pan approach) (Westropp and Buffington, 2004; Buffington, 2007). If the cat consumes the moist food, the amount of moist food can be increased gradually while decreasing the amount of dry food correspondingly. **Table 46-23** lists tips for increasing water consumption.

Increasing frequency of feeding (i.e., dividing the daily amount of food into several meals) may increase daily water intake in cats. In a study of healthy cats with free access to water, feeding two or three meals per day was associated with a significant increase in total water intake compared with feeding a single meal (Kirschvink et al, 2005).

Reassessment

Clinicians should use their best judgment regarding the most appropriate times for reevaluating patients with FIC. Because of stress associated with hospital visits, it may be preferable to conduct evaluations by talking with owners more often than examining the patient. This allows for discussing effectiveness of current treatments and recommendations for changes if needed. If there are changes in the cat's clinical findings (e.g., increased severity or frequency of episodes) despite appropriate treatment, additional patient evaluation including urinalysis, urine culture and diagnostic imaging is indicated to detect other disorders (e.g., uroliths, UTI).

Feeding Plan for Struvite Urolith Dissolution

Treatment options for cats with struvite uroliths include dissolution by nutritional management and physical removal of uroliths (e.g., cystotomy, voiding urohydropropulsion, catheter retrieval, laser lithotripsy). Treatment selection depends on clinician experience, expertise and preference, availability of necessary equipment, patient factors and client preferences. Considering all factors, it is generally preferred to select the least invasive treatment that has the most evidence for effectiveness.

Two studies reported effects of feeding a dissolution food to cats with struvite uroliths (Osborne et al, 1990; Houston et al, 2004). In one study, 25 cats (13 males, 12 females) with 28 occurrences of struvite uroliths were fed a struvite dissolution food[f] (Osborne et al, 1990). Among cats in the study, there were 20 occurrences of sterile uroliths and eight with UTI (five urease-positive infections, three urease-negative infections). Mean time for sterile struvite urolith dissolution was 36 days (range, 14 to 141 days), while the average time for dissolution of uroliths associated with UTI was 44 days (range, 14 to 92 days). Clinical signs (gross hematuria and dysuria/pollakiuria) were present in 90% or more of urolith occurrences before nutritional management and were absent by the time of first reevaluation in two weeks. None of the cats developed urethral obstruction but perineal urethrostomy had been performed

Box 46-6. Behavioral Screen for Cats with Inappropriate Urination.*

All cats that urinate outside the litter box or in inappropriate places should receive a medical evaluation to identify and address underlying medical disease(s). In some cases, a primary medical reason for inappropriate urination will be identified, treatment implemented and the problem resolved. However, in other cases there will be no primary medical problem identified or even after resolution/control of an identified medical issue, inappropriate urination continues. In the latter case, the medical problem may have been the initiating cause but behavioral issues maintain inappropriate urination, despite successful control/resolution of primary medical problems. For cats with continued inappropriate urination despite diagnosis and management of all primary medical issues, the following questions should be considered:

Question**	Answer
1. Does your cat urinate on vertical surfaces outside the litter box?	☐YES ☐NO
2. Does your cat urinate on horizontal surfaces outside the litter box?	☐YES ☐NO
3. Does your cat seek out certain targets for urination?	☐YES ☐NO
4. Do these targets have a common quality (e.g. all soft, absorbent materials, certain room, always slick surfaces)?	☐YES ☐NO
5. Is the quantity of urine deposited very small?	☐YES ☐NO
6. Does your cat defecate outside the litter box?	☐YES ☐NO
7. Does your cat ever use the litter box?	☐YES ☐NO
8. Does your cat dig in its litter when it uses the litter box?	☐YES ☐NO
9. Is there more than one cat in the household?	☐YES ☐NO
10. Does your cat ever fight or appear frightened of other pets or people in the household?	☐YES ☐NO
11. Are the litter boxes all in the same site/room/area/floor of the home?	☐YES ☐NO
Total number of litter boxes in the house	______

Indicate number of boxes with each characteristic:

Box style:
- Covered . . . . ____
- Uncovered . . . . ____
- Large . . . . ____
- Medium . . . . ____
- Small . . . . ____
- With plastic liner . . . . ____

Litter type:
- Unscented . . . . ____
- Scented . . . . ____
- Clumping (sand-like) . . . . ____
- Recycled paper (pellets) . . . . ____
- Crystal (silica) . . . . ____
- Non-clumping clay . . . . ____
- Wheat clumping . . . . ____
- Corn clumping . . . . ____
- Pine . . . . ____
- Other . . . . ____

Cleaning schedule for litter boxes	**Check rate**
Scooping:	
Multiple times per day	☐
Once per day	☐
Once every other day	☐
Twice a week	☐
Once a week or less often	☐
Complete box change (wash, new litter):	
Daily	☐
Weekly	☐
Every two weeks	☐
Monthly	☐
Every 2-3 months	☐
Every 3-6 months	☐
Every year or more	☐
Never	☐

*Adapted from Neilson JC. FLUTD: When should you call the behaviorist? In: Proceedings. Hill's Symposium on Feline Lower Urinary Tract Disease, 2007: 20-28 (www.hillsvet.com/conferenceproceedings).
**"YES" answers for Questions 1 and 5 may indicate urine marking.

previously in 10 of the male cats. In another study, 32 cats (10 males, 22 females) with struvite uroliths were fed either a dry or moist version of a dissolution food[g] (Houston et al, 2004). Mean time for dissolution in cats eating moist food (3.73 weeks) was not significantly different from those eating dry food (4.82 weeks) ($p = 0.066$). Clinical signs resolved in an average of 19 days after beginning nutritional management. No occurrences of urethral obstruction were reported. Approximately 30% of cats had radiographic evidence of urolith disappearance after two weeks of feeding the dissolution food. Time to resolution of clinical signs or urolith dissolution did not differ significantly with the number of uroliths.

Box 46-7. Behavioral Management for Cats with Inappropriate Urination.*

Cats that urinate and/or defecate outside the litter box can do so for a variety of reasons including disease, communication (e.g., marking) and toileting preferences/aversions. Sometimes the medical problem can be an initiating factor for toileting problems. For example, medically triggered urgency to urinate causes the cat to select a convenient location like the bed; but even with resolution of the medical problem, the new behavior persists. These cats develop a new preference for toileting. (e.g., the bed is convenient, nicely absorbent and is cleaned readily) or have such negative associations with the litter box (e.g., painful urination when they were ill) that they persist in using a new, alternative, inappropriate site. Issues that should be addressed in cases of inappropriate elimination are listed below.

Resources	Recommendations	Explanations/consequences
Number of litter boxes	Number of litter boxes = number of cats +1	Too few litter boxes may result in problems that cause a cat to seek alternative toileting sites. These problems may include: volume of excrement in the litter box; box occupied by another cat; box being guarded by another cat.
Location of litter boxes	Should be spread throughout environment in easily accessible locations	Clustering litter boxes in one location may create access problems. These problems may include: guarding by another cat and physical challenges (e.g., stairs/distance) with getting to the litter box location.
Litter box style	Large	Boxes that are too small may be uncomfortable for cats to use, causing them to seek out other sites.
	Uncovered	Boxes that are covered may trap odors, creating an unpleasant environment and causing the cat to seek other toileting sites.
Litter	Clumping (sand-like) Unscented	Although individual preferences exist, the majority of cats prefer unscented clumping (finely particulate matter–similar to sand) litter.
Litter box hygiene	Daily litter box scooping Complete litter box cleaning/ change every 1 to 4 weeks	Cats tend to be fastidious and prefer clean toileting locations. Frequency of full box cleaning (wash/new litter) will depend on litter type; clumping type litters that allow owners to remove urine may require less frequent changes.
Scratching posts/pads	Multiple, sturdy, tall, prominently located	Scratching is a form of marking behavior. Encouraging scratch marking on appropriate targets may reduce the likelihood of other forms of marking and prevent destruction of household items.
Resting perches	Multiple, single cat sized, elevated, upholstered surfaces	Creative use of vertical space in the home can reduce inter-cat tension/aggression. Cats tend to prefer upholstered surfaces over slick surfaces but individual preferences may exist.
Feeding/water stations	Number of stations = number of cats	Providing adequate resources spread throughout the environment allows cats to self-segregate; this may help to reduce social tension in multi-cat households.
Play/social interaction	At least 2 to 3 daily short sessions (5 to 10 minutes)	Cat age and personality may affect type and duration of interaction but it is important to recognize that domesticated cats are social and will often benefit from play/interaction. Indoor-only cats can especially benefit from owner-initiated activity such as play with toys for overall stress reduction and exercise. Play activity also enhances the family-pet bond and is useful for overweight cats.

*Adapted from Neilson JC. FLUTD: When should you call the behaviorist? In: Proceedings. Hill's Symposium on Feline Lower Urinary Tract Disease, 2007: 20-28 (www.hillsvet.com/conferenceproceedings).

Despite evidence for effectiveness of nutritional management for dissolving struvite uroliths, many veterinarians still prefer to surgically remove uroliths because of perceptions that surgical management is more effective, is less expensive overall when considering monitoring and aftercare, controls clinical signs quicker and will not be associated with urethral obstruction as uroliths decrease in size, especially in male cats. Although surgical removal of uroliths has not been critically evaluated in cats, a retrospective study of 37 dogs and 29 cats with urinary bladder uroliths revealed that four cats (14%) and eight dogs (22%) had incomplete removal of uroliths by cystotomy in a veterinary teaching hospital (Lulich et al, 1993a; Lulich and Osborne, 2007).

Assess and Select the Food

Table 46-24 provides nutrient information about foods compared with recommended levels of key nutritional factors for dissolution of struvite uroliths. Generally the food that most closely matches the recommendations should be selected; however, only two foods[f,g] have published clinical evidence of effectiveness. Treatment with a struvite dissolution food is contraindicated in growing kittens, reproducing queens and

Table 46-23. Tips for increasing water consumption in cats.

Food
Feed moist food
Add small amount of water to moist food
Add warm water to dry food
Divide daily food amount into several smaller meals
Add flavor enhancers to food
Low-sodium chicken or beef broth
Clam juice
Tuna juice (low sodium)
Water
Use fresh, clean water at all times (change at least once daily)
Try water from different sources
Tap water
Filtered water
Bottled water
Distilled water
Place ice cubes in water or provide cold water
Offer frozen cubes of water mixed with low-sodium tuna juice, etc.
Containers
Use non-reflective bowls for food and water
Use wide bowl so whiskers do not touch sides
Ensure ideal location of water and food bowls
Quiet, draft-free environment (avoid noisy appliances, near vents)
In areas where cats can escape if needed
Not in same area as litter boxes
On different levels of multi-floor house
Provide access to other sources of water
Water fountains with circulating water
Dripping faucet

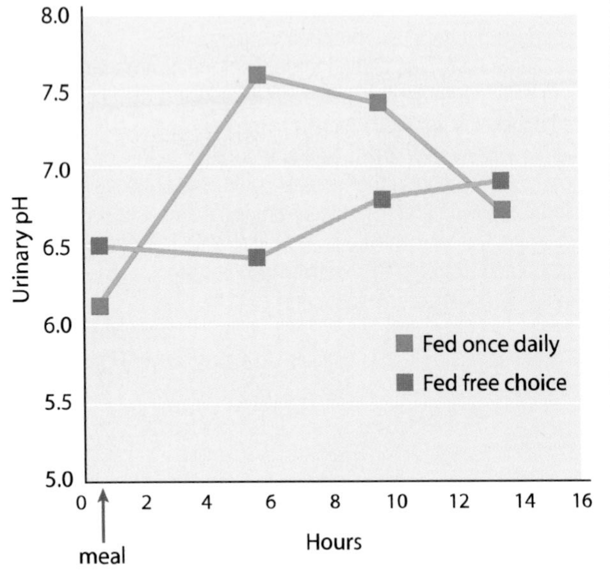

Figure 46-18. Mean urinary pH of cats fed a commercial food either free choice (i.e., ad libitum) or once daily. Note how once daily feeding results in a significant increase in urinary pH (i.e., postprandial alkaline tide). (Adapted from Taton DF, Hamar D, Lewis LD. Evaluation of ammonium chloride as a urinary acidifier in the cat. Journal of the American Veterinary Medical Association 1984; 184: 433-436.)

patients with metabolic acidosis or hypokalemia. In addition, struvite dissolution foods with increased amounts of sodium may not be ideal for patients with concomitant conditions including chronic kidney disease, hypertension or congestive heart failure.

Assess and Determine the Feeding Method

Cats with suspected struvite uroliths (usually <7 years of age, often with alkaline urinary pH, struvite crystalluria and/or radiopaque uroliths) can usually be transitioned to a dissolution food over a seven-day period. The method of feeding influences urinary pH values throughout the day and therefore may affect the success of the struvite dissolution protocol. When fed free choice, most cats will eat small amounts every few hours, resulting in a smaller but more prolonged alkaline tide than with meal feeding (**Figure 46-18**) (Taton et al, 1984). The smaller alkaline urinary pH excursions observed with free-choice feeding may improve dissolution of struvite uroliths and thus may be the preferred method of feeding. However, this has not been confirmed. Also, dry foods are most likely to be fed free-choice; nevertheless, feeding moist food is preferred for dissolution of struvite uroliths and managing most other types of uroliths and FIC.

If a UTI has been diagnosed, an appropriate antimicrobial drug should be administered for two to four weeks beyond removal or radiographic disappearance of uroliths. Although most cats do not have UTI, infection with urease-producing organisms may cause struvite uroliths in some cases and other bacteria may cause UTI secondary to uroliths in others.

Reassessment

During the time a dissolution food is being fed, cats should be reevaluated every two to four weeks. A thorough nutritional history should be collected, including amounts of all foods and supplements given; this is especially helpful when uroliths do not decrease in size as expected. Urinalysis is indicated to evaluate urinary pH and examine urine sediment for presence of abnormalities (e.g., crystalluria, pyuria). When interpreting pH of a spot or random urine sample, consider when the sample was collected relative to the time of eating. Samples obtained early in the morning, before food is offered, tend to be more acidic, whereas samples obtained within several hours of eating tend to be more alkaline (because of the postprandial alkaline tide). When evaluating effects of a food change on urinary pH, standardize the time of collection relative to the time of eating. For most accurate results, urinary pH should be measured using a pH meter. Urine culture should be done in cats with UTI to confirm the absence of infection during treatment with antimicrobial drugs and one week after completion of treatment to confirm eradication of UTI. Abdominal radiographs should be taken to evaluate number and size of uroliths compared with previous results. Nutritional management should be continued for one month beyond radiographic evidence of urolith(s) dissolution. If uroliths do not dissolve completely or decrease in size after two months of feeding a dissolution food exclusively, a different treatment (urolith removal) should be considered.

Figure 46-19 is an algorithm to assist in managing patients with struvite urolithiasis (Lulich, 2007a).

The rate of urolith recurrence has not been critically evaluated in cats. However, a recently published abstract described the rate of urolith recurrence in cats that had uroliths submitted for quantitative analysis at the Minnesota Urolith Center in 1998 (Albasan et al, 2006). Recurrence (defined as subsequent urolith submission) was detected in 2.7% of 1,821 cats with struvite uroliths; 0.2% of cats had a second recurrence. Mean time to initial recurrence was 27 months. Urolith recurrence was 1.6 times higher in females than males. Because some uroliths associated with recurrent episodes were likely not submitted for analysis, the actual recurrence rate for struvite uroliths was likely higher.

Table 46-24. Comparison of key nutritional factors in selected commercial veterinary therapeutic foods for dissolution of struvite uroliths in cats.*

Moist foods	**Mg (%)**	**P (%)**	**Protein (%)**	**Na (%)**	**Urinary pH**
Recommended levels	**0.04-0.09**	**0.45-1.1**	**30-45**	**0.3-0.6**	**5.8-6.2**
Hill's Prescription Diet s/d Feline	0.056	0.56	39.9	0.37	6.08
Medi-Cal Veterinary Diets Dissolution Formula	na	1.1	46.5	1.1	6.2
Purina Veterinary Diets UR Urinary St/Ox Feline Formula	0.07	0.97	50.6	0.62	6.0-6.4
Royal Canin Veterinary Diet Dissolution Formula	0.052	1.0	49.9	1.21	5.9
Royal Canin Veterinary Diet Urinary SO in Gel	0.097	1.36	41.3	1.02	6.0-6.3
Dry foods	**Mg (%)**	**P (%)**	**Protein (%)**	**Na (%)**	**Urinary pH**
Recommended levels	**0.04-0.09**	**0.45-1.1**	**30-45**	**0.3-0.6**	**5.8-6.2**
Hill's Prescription Diet s/d Feline	0.059	0.77	34.4	0.4	5.9
Medi-Cal Veterinary Diets Feline Dissolution Formula	na	1.0	35.7	0.4	5.8
Purina Veterinary Diets UR Urinary St/Ox Feline Formula	0.07	1.08	44.9	1.17	6.0-6.4
Royal Canin Veterinary Diet Urinary SO 33	0.065	0.88	37.1	1.45	6.0-6.3

Key: Mg = magnesium, P = phosphorus, Na = sodium, na = not available from manufacturer.
*Nutrients expressed on a dry matter basis unless otherwise stated.
**In general, moist foods should be fed to cats with FLUTD.

Table 46-25. Comparison of key nutritional factors in selected commercial veterinary therapeutic foods for decreasing risk of recurrence of struvite disease (uroliths or urethral plugs) in cats.*

Moist foods**	**Mg (%)**	**P (%)**	**Protein (%)**	**Na (%)**	**Urinary pH**
Recommended levels	**0.04-0.14**	**0.5-0.9**	**30-45**	**0.3-0.6**	**6.0-6.4**
Hill's Prescription Diet c/d Multicare with Chicken Feline	0.052	0.68	43.8	0.32	6.35
Hill's Prescription Diet c/d Multicare with Seafood Feline	0.054	0.71	44.8	0.33	6.4
Hill's Prescription Diet r/d with Liver & Chicken Feline	0.075	0.62	37.5	0.29	6.25
Hill's Prescription Diet w/d with Chicken Feline	0.064	0.68	39.6	0.38	6.26
Iams Veterinary Formula Urinary S Low pH/S/Feline	0.088	0.75	41.8	0.26	na
Medi-Cal Veterinary Diets Feline Dissolution Formula	na	1.1	46.5	1.1	6.2
Medi-Cal Veterinary Diets Feline Preventive Formula	na	0.9	47.1	0.4	6.3
Medi-Cal Veterinary Diets Feline Reducing Formula	na	1.6	54.3	1.0	6.5
Medi-Cal Veterinary Diets Feline Urinary SO in Gel	na	1.2	43.5	1.1	6.4
Medi-Cal Veterinary Diets Feline Weight Control	na	1.1	40.0	0.5	6.6
Purina Veterinary Diets UR Urinary St/Ox Feline Formula	0.07	0.97	50.6	0.62	6.0-6.4
Royal Canin Veterinary Diet Feline Control Formula	0.082	1.03	43.0	0.45	6.0-6.3
Royal Canin Veterinary Diet Feline Urinary SO in Gel	0.097	1.36	41.3	1.02	6.0-6.3
Dry foods	**Mg (%)**	**P (%)**	**Protein (%)**	**Na (%)**	**Urinary pH**
Recommended levels	**0.04-0.14**	**0.5-0.9**	**30-45**	**0.3-0.6**	**6.0-6.4**
Hill's Prescription Diet c/d Multicare Feline	0.06	0.65	36.1	0.35	6.30
Hill's Prescription Diet c/d Multicare with Chicken Feline	0.061	0.65	34.6	0.33	6.35
Hill's Prescription Diet r/d Feline	0.073	0.81	36.9	0.35	6.38
Hill's Prescription Diet r/d with Chicken Feline	0.067	0.84	37.7	0.35	6.33
Hill's Prescription Diet w/d Feline	0.059	0.77	39.0	0.3	6.27
Hill's Prescription Diet w/d with Chicken Feline	0.068	0.86	39.9	0.35	6.22
Iams Veterinary Formula Urinary S Low pH/S/Feline	0.096	0.93	36.5	0.45	na
Medi-Cal Veterinary Diets Feline Dissolution Formula	na	1.0	35.7	0.4	5.8
Medi-Cal Veterinary Diets Feline Preventive Formula	na	0.9	33.4	0.4	6.1
Medi-Cal Veterinary Diets Feline Reducing Formula	na	1.2	41.8	0.3	6.1
Medi-Cal Veterinary Diets Feline Urinary SO 30	na	0.9	34.6	1.4	6.2
Medi-Cal Veterinary Diets Feline Weight Control	na	1.0	34.4	0.3	6.0
Purina Veterinary Diets UR Urinary St/Ox Feline Formula	0.07	1.08	44.9	1.17	6.0-6.4
Royal Canin Veterinary Diet Feline Control Formula	0.065	0.65	33.7	0.71	6.0-6.3
Royal Canin Veterinary Diet Feline Urinary SO 33	0.065	0.88	37.1	1.45	6.0-6.3

Key: Mg = magnesium, P = phosphorus, Na = sodium, na = not available from manufacturer.
*Nutrients expressed on a dry matter basis unless otherwise stated.
**In general, moist foods should be fed to cats with FLUTD.

Box 46-8. Regulatory Claims Related to Feline Urinary Foods in the United States, Canada and the European Union.

The United States Food and Drug Administration, Center for Veterinary Medicine (FDA-CVM) has issued guidelines for pet-food companies to establish the following claims: "reduces urinary pH," "low magnesium" and "improves urinary tract health." The FDA-CVM suggests that submissions requesting permission to make "reduces urinary pH" or "improves urinary tract health" claims include supportive utility data demonstrating efficacy (i.e., the ability of the food to produce appropriately acidic urine compared with a non-acidifying control food) and safety data.

Foods with label claims such as "helps maintain urinary tract health" are low in magnesium and produce appropriately acidic urine. The FDA-CVM has promulgated guidelines for protocols to support urinary tract health claims. The guidelines focus on prevention of struvite urinary precipitates, but do not address the question of calcium oxalate precipitate formation.

Guidelines suggest safety studies for a minimum of six months. These studies should include physical examinations and the following observations: food consumption, body weight measurements, urinalyses (including sediment examinations), serum biochemistry and blood gas analyses and mineral (calcium, phosphorus, magnesium and potassium) balance studies. Foods claiming to promote urinary tract health and reduce urinary pH must be nutritionally complete and balanced, as demonstrated by the Association of American Feed Control Officials (AAFCO) feeding protocols. It is noteworthy that the "improves urinary tract health" claim focuses on documentation of safety, urine acidification and restricted dietary intake of magnesium and does not in any way address the issue of calcium oxalate urolith formation.

The guideline for a low-magnesium claim is a magnesium level guaranteed less than 0.12% dry matter, using the maximum magnesium and maximum water guarantee. The magnesium must also be less than 25 mg/100 kcal, with energy content based on the AAFCO-approved calculation method or an actual digestibility study. Analysis of multiple batches is required. The FDA-CVM does not allow the claim of "low ash" on cat food labels. Current scientific information does not demonstrate that ash per se is related to the incidence of lower urinary tract disease. Ash content can only be included in the guaranteed analysis of the food.

The Canadian Veterinary Medical Association (CVMA) Pet Food Certification Program has established guidelines for nutrient standards for magnesium-restricted/pH-controlling cat foods. These foods must meet the following requirements:

Magnesium levels must be no more than 0.1% and no less than 0.05%, dry matter basis.

Magnesium levels per 100 kilocalories (kcal) of metabolizable energy (ME) shall be no more than 20 milligrams.

The average resting urinary pH shall be 6.5 or less, and the average postprandial peak pH shall not exceed 7.0.

In July 1995, labeling of veterinary therapeutic foods in Europe (termed "dietetic pet foods") became strictly regulated (Chapter 9). European regulations require only certain indications for therapeutic foods, termed "Particular Nutritional Purposes." Indications permitted for feline lower urinary tract disease include: 1) dissolution of struvite uroliths, 2) reduction of struvite urolith recurrence, 3) reduction of oxalate urolith formation, 4) reduction of urate urolith formation and 5) reduction of cystine urolith formation. Essential nutritional characteristics of the corresponding foods and specific label declarations must be met.

The Bibliography for **Box 46-8** can be found at www.markmorris.org.

After dissolution or removal of struvite uroliths, further nutritional management is indicated to prevent recurrence. (See Feeding Plan for Prevention of Struvite Urolithiasis and Urethral Plugs.) If UTI with urease-producing bacteria was the cause of uroliths, controlling infections may prevent urolith recurrence; however, most uroliths in cats are either sterile or cause secondary infections. It is unknown how long struvite preventive foods should be fed. Struvite disease is more common in young- to middle-aged cats; however, as cats age, the risk of calcium oxalate urolithiasis increases. Cats eating struvite preventive foods should be monitored periodically for crystalluria and urinary pH values. If no episodes of struvite uroliths occur for several years, consider recommending a high-quality wellness food that avoids excessive magnesium and phosphorus, as cats get older. Cats should still be monitored periodically for occurrence of alkaline urinary pH, struvite crystalluria and urolith recurrence.

Struvite uroliths may recur months to years after removal or dissolution, particularly if preventive measures are not implemented (Osborne et al, 1990). Interpretation of recurrence of uroliths (of any mineral type) and interval until recurrence should be based on answering a number of questions (Lulich et al, 1993). 1) *Were all uroliths removed from the urinary tract at the time of surgery or other procedure?* Recurrence of uroliths following surgery is commonly attributed to failure of medical therapy to prevent urolith formation. However, this hypothesis is based on the premise that all stones were completely removed from the urinary tract before beginning preventive measures. Incomplete surgical removal of uroliths probably occurs more frequently than recognized, even when performed by experienced surgeons (Lulich et al, 1993a; Lulich and Osborne, 2007). 2) *Did nonabsorbable suture materials left exposed in the lumen of the urinary bladder during surgery provide a nidus for precipitation of crystalline material?* In 2005, the Minnesota Urolith Center analyzed uroliths from more than 32,000 dogs; non-mineral, foreign material was identified in uroliths from 96 dogs and 86 of these submissions contained a nidus of suture material (Lulich and Osborne, 2007). Uroliths from an additional 235 dogs contained a hollow cylindrical track consistent with formation around suture material. On the basis of these findings, approximately 1% of canine uroliths would be best prevented by more appropriate selection and placement of sutures. Similar data for cats have not been reported; however, it seems reasonable that inappropriate surgical techniques also could predispose to development of feline uroliths. 3) *What diagnostic methods were used to detect recurrence?* 4) *How often was the patient evaluated for recurrence?* 5) *Were recommendations to decrease likelihood of recurrence given and was the owner able to follow them?* 6) *Has infection with a urease-producing microorganism persisted or recurred?* Most uroliths in cats are not associated

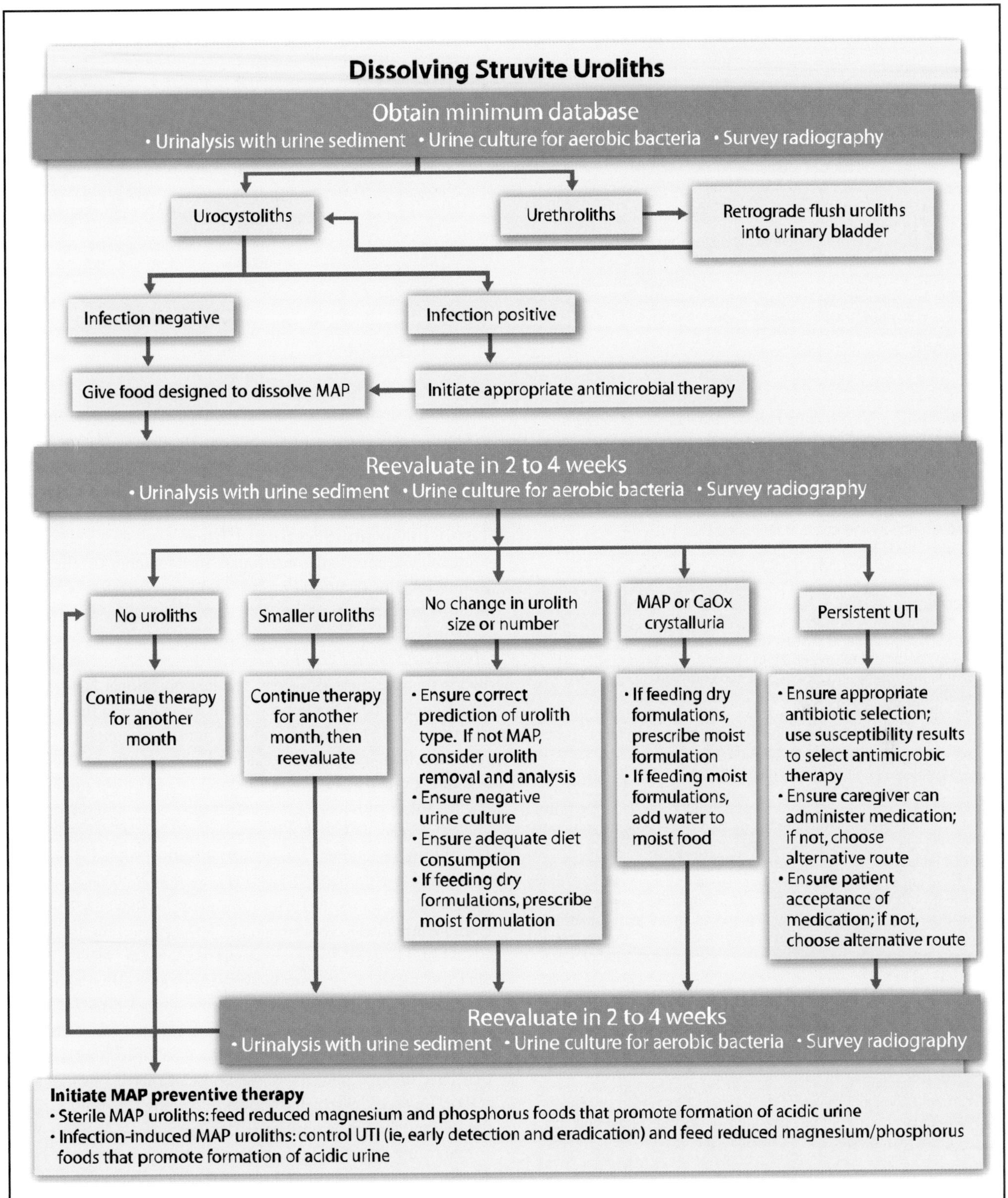

Figure 46-19. Algorithm for management and reassessment of cats with struvite urolithiasis. Key: MAP = magnesium ammonium phosphate (struvite), CaOx = calcium oxalate, UTI = urinary tract infection. (Adapted from Lulich JP. FLUTD: Are you choosing the right therapy? Part 1. Urolithiasis. In: Proceedings. Hill's Symposium on Feline Lower Urinary Tract Disease, 2007a: 29-36).

Table 46-26. Comparison of key nutritional factors in selected commercial veterinary therapeutic foods for decreasing risk of recurrence of calcium oxalate uroliths in cats.*

Moist foods**	Mg (%)	P (%)	Ca (%)	Protein (%)	Na (%)	Urinary pH
Recommended levels	**0.07-0.14**	**0.5-1.0**	**0.6-1.0**	**≥32**	**0.3-0.6**	**≥6.2**
Hill's Prescription Diet c/d Multicare with Chicken Feline	0.052	0.68	0.72	43.8	0.32	6.35
Hill's Prescription Diet c/d Multicare with Seafood Feline	0.054	0.71	0.62	44.8	0.33	6.4
Iams Veterinary Formula Urinary O - Moderate pH/O	0.085	0.77	1.11	43.4	0.34	na
Medi-Cal Urinary SO in Gel	na	1.2	1.2	43.5	1.1	6.4
Purina Veterinary Diets UR Urinary St/Ox Feline Formula	0.07	0.97	0.96	50.6	0.62	6.0-6.4
Royal Canin Veterinary Diet Urinary SO in Gel	0.097	1.36	1.02	41.3	1.02	6.0-6.3
Dry foods	**Mg (%)**	**P (%)**	**Ca (%)**	**Protein (%)**	**Na (%)**	**Urinary pH**
Recommended levels	**0.07-0.14**	**0.5-1.0**	**0.6-1.0**	**≥32**	**0.3-0.6**	**≥6.2**
Hill's Prescription Diet c/d Multicare Feline	0.06	0.65	0.74	36.1	0.35	6.3
Hill's Prescription Diet c/d Multicare with Chicken Feline	0.061	0.65	0.76	34.6	0.33	6.3
Iams Veterinary Formula Urinary O - Moderate pH/O	0.098	0.91	1.24	36.5	0.46	na
Medi-Cal Urinary SO	na	0.9	1.1	34.6	1.4	6.2
Purina Veterinary Diets UR Urinary St/Ox Feline Formula	0.07	1.08	1.1	44.9	1.17	6.0-6.4
Royal Canin Veterinary Diet Urinary SO 33	0.065	0.88	0.96	37.1	1.45	6.0-6.3

Key: Mg = magnesium, P = phosphorus, Ca = calcium, Na = sodium, na = not available from manufacturer.
*Nutrients expressed on a dry matter basis unless otherwise stated.
**In general, moist foods should be fed to cats with FLUTD.

Table 46-27. Stepwise approach for management of calcium oxalate urolithiasis in cats.*

1. Obtain baseline data (post-removal radiographs, complete urinalysis, serum concentrations of calcium, urea nitrogen and creatinine) to evaluate effectiveness of removal procedure, renal function and calcium homeostasis.
2. If the patient is hypercalcemic, correct underlying cause. If no cause is identified (i.e., idiopathic hypercalcemia exists) consider high-fiber foods and potassium citrate to decrease urine acidity.
3. If the patient is normocalcemic, consider foods with reduced oxalate, sodium and protein that do not promote formation of overly acidic urine (pH <6.2). Ideally foods should contain additional water and citrate and have adequate phosphorus and magnesium. Avoid excess vitamins C and D.
4. Reevaluate patient in two to four weeks to verify compliance with nutritional recommendations (urine specific gravity and pH) and amelioration of crystalluria (urine sediment examination). For most accurate results, urinary pH should be measured using a pH meter.
5. If calcium oxalate crystals or concentrated urine (specific gravity >1.030) persist, consider moist foods or additional water added to current food. If calcium oxalate crystals or aciduria persist (urinary pH <6.2), consider additional potassium citrate.
6. Reevaluate patient in two to four weeks to verify compliance with nutritional recommendation (urine specific gravity and pH) and amelioration of crystalluria (urine sediment examination). If calcium oxalate crystalluria persists, and patient is consuming a homemade food, consider vitamin B_6 supplementation (2 to 4 mg/kg every 24 hours).
7. After three to six months, reevaluate patient to verify compliance with nutritional recommendations, amelioration of crystalluria and lack of urolith recurrence (abdominal radiography). If no uroliths are present, continue present therapy and reevaluate in three to six months. If uroliths have recurred, consider nonsurgical urolith removal. Consider using voiding urohydropropulsion in females or male cats with a previously performed perineal urethrostomy. If unsuccessful, surgery can be considered if clinical signs referable to urocystolithiasis persist. If clinical signs are not present, continue therapy to minimize urolith growth.

*Adapted from Lulich JP. FLUTD: Are you choosing the right therapy? Part 1. Urolithiasis. In: Proceedings. Hill's Symposium on Feline Lower Urinary Tract Disease, 2007: 29-36.

with UTI; however, some cats will develop struvite uroliths associated with urease-producing organisms. 7) *Has an underlying anatomic defect gone uncorrected?*

Feeding Plan for Prevention of Struvite Urolithiasis and Urethral Plugs

Generally, appropriate nutritional management is the most important consideration for prevention of recurrence of struvite uroliths and urethral plugs.

Assess and Select the Food

Foods that are most similar to the key nutritional factor target ranges and/or have the best evidence for managing the patient's disorder should be selected. Information about content of many nutrients (e.g., magnesium, calcium, phosphorus and sodium) and target urinary pH ranges are not required on pet food labels. **Tables 46-19** and **46-25** provide lists of selected veterinary therapeutic foods marketed for prevention of struvite urolithiasis (and urethral plugs) and compare their key nutritional factor content to the recommended levels of key nutritional factors. The foods listed in **Table 46-19**, in addition to struvite-associated disease, are intended to co-manage FIC- and calcium oxalate-based FLUTD. These foods are compared to composite key nutritional factors for the aforementioned types of lower urinary tract disease. For foods under consideration that are not listed in **Tables 46-19** and **46-25**, contact the manufacturer or review published information to determine key nutritional factor content. For cats that have urethral plugs composed only of matrix or other substances (e.g., epithelial cells or mucus), feeding the moist form of the selected food is recommended.

Regarding urethral plugs, a struvite dissolution food (**Table 46-24**) may be appropriate for initial management (i.e., one to three months) after relieving obstruction. (See Feeding Plan for Struvite Urolith Dissolution, above.) However, such a food should not be fed long term because of risks associated with prolonged, excessive urinary acidification (urinary pH <6.0).

Several commercially available foods have claims for struvite prevention; however, only one has been evaluated in cats with urethral plugs. In a randomized, prospective study of cats with urethral plugs, effectiveness of feeding this food was compared with perineal urethrostomy alone and perineal urethrostomy plus the calculolytic food[f] (Osborne et al, 1991). During the one-year study, urethral obstruction was not observed in any group. This study did not include an untreated control group; however, recurrence rates for urethral obstruction in two other studies were 35 and 36% (Bovee et al, 1979; Gerber et al, 2007). Bacterial UTI occurred in 40 to 50% of cats that had perineal urethrostomies, but was not observed in cats managed by the calculolytic food alone. Several foods formulated for struvite prevention have been evaluated by measuring values for struvite saturation in healthy cats (Bartges et al, 1998; Abood et al, 2000; Devois et al, 2000; Xu et al, 2006).

Urinary tract health claims on pet food labels may be of some help in evaluating foods (**Box 46-8**). In the U.S., a food with a "low magnesium" claim contains a maximum of 0.12% DM magnesium or 25 mg magnesium/100 kcal ME.

Depending on the amount fed, treats and other supplements can significantly alter the key nutritional factor profile of the desired dietary regimen and may decrease the effectiveness of appropriately formulated therapeutic foods. Some commercial cat treats or foods, and processed human foods may have very high levels of magnesium or phosphorus and their effect on urinary pH is hard to predict. Most pet owners give their pets treats or supplement their pets' primary food with other foods, either another cat food or human food. Therefore, it is important for veterinary health care team members to educate owners about the importance of compliance to the successful outcome. This is especially true for cats that are at risk for urethral obstruction. Owners aware of the risks may be more willing to avoid feeding other foods or products and encourage their cats only to eat the recommended therapeutic food.

Assess and Determine the Feeding Method

Cats should be transitioned gradually to a food formulated to decrease occurrence of struvite crystalluria. The method of feeding influences urinary pH values throughout the day and therefore may affect success of the dietary management protocol. Ingestion of food stimulates secretion of acid by gastric parietal cells with subsequent secretion of bicarbonate into the blood in exchange for chloride ions. This alkali load transiently increases urinary bicarbonate and pH (i.e., postprandial alkaline tide) unless offset by absorption of acidifying ingredients. When offered food free choice, most cats will eat small amounts every few hours, resulting in a smaller but more prolonged alkaline tide than with meal feeding (**Figure 46-18**) (Taton et al, 1984). The smaller alkaline urinary pH excursions observed with free-choice feeding may reduce the likelihood of struvite precipitate formation, and thus may be the preferred method of feeding to prevent struvite associated disease; however, this has not be confirmed in clinical studies. Free-choice feeding may be associated with obesity; however, which in turn is a risk factor for lower urinary tract diseases in general. In addition, free-choice feeding is most likely to be done using dry food, and moist food is preferred for managing urolithiasis and FIC.

Based on information currently available, meal-feeding moist food would seem to be best for most cats with struvite disease because of increased water intake and reduced concentration of crystal-forming elements. However, less evidence supports this benefit compared with cats that have calcium oxalate uroliths. If meal feeding is associated with increased urinary pH throughout the day and significant struvite crystalluria or recurrent uroliths or urethral plugs, another feeding method should be considered (e.g., feeding dry food or feeding multiple small meals of moist food).

Reassessment

Cats eating struvite preventive foods should be monitored periodically for evidence of crystalluria and urinary pH values. If no episodes of struvite uroliths occur for several years, it would be appropriate to consider switching to a high-quality wellness food that maintains an appropriate urinary pH and avoids excessive magnesium and phosphorus.

Feeding Plan for Calcium Oxalate Urolithiasis

Calcium oxalate uroliths are not amenable to medical dissolution and must be removed by surgery, voiding urohydropropulsion, lithotripsy or other techniques. An alternative to cystotomy is voiding urohydropropulsion if urocystoliths are small enough to pass through the urethra (Lulich et al, 1993). Voiding urohydropropulsion is generally more successful in queens than in tomcats because the urethra is larger in females than in males. Voiding urohydropropulsion is usually ineffective in cats with uroliths lodged in the urethra. After urolith removal, medical protocols to minimize recurrence should be implemented. Goals of nutritional management include decreasing urine calcium and oxalate concentrations, promoting high concentrations of urolith inhibitors, decreasing urine acidity and decreasing urine specific gravity (i.e., urine dilution).

Assess and Select the Food

Several commercially available therapeutic foods are marketed for prevention of calcium oxalate uroliths in cats. No foods have been studied to determine if they prevent urolith recurrence and only one food[e] has been evaluated in cats with naturally occurring calcium oxalate uroliths (Lulich et al, 2004). In a study of 10 cats with confirmed calcium oxalate uroliths, urinary calcium oxalate saturation was measured before beginning the study and after feeding the therapeutic food. Using a cross-over design, half of the cats were randomly assigned to continue their regular food and the other half were assigned to eat the therapeutic food. After eight weeks, the foods were switched and fed for another eight weeks. Urinary calcium oxalate saturation values (i.e., activity product ratios and relative supersaturation values) were determined and compared between groups (regular vs. therapeutic food). Results revealed that hypercalciuria was a consistent abnormality in urolith-forming cats and urinary calcium oxalate saturation was significantly lower in cats fed the therapeutic food compared with regular food. This study concluded that feeding the therapeutic food decreased the risk of urolith recurrence.

Tables 46-19 and **46-26** list selected veterinary therapeutic foods marketed for prevention of calcium oxalate urolithiasis and compare their key nutritional factor content to the recommended levels. The foods listed in **Table 46-19** are also intended to co-manage FIC- and struvite-based FLUTD. These foods are compared to composite key nutritional factors for all three of these types of lower urinary tract disease. For foods under consideration that are not listed, contact the manufacturer or review published information to determine levels of key nutritional factors. Foods that are most similar to the key nutritional factor target ranges and/or have published evidence of efficacy for managing calcium oxalate urolithiasis should be selected. Owners of cats that form calcium oxalate crystals and uroliths should be cautioned about grocery brand foods with urinary tract health claims because these foods are formulated for healthy cats to avoid struvite crystals and uroliths. Feeding such foods may actually increase the risk of developing calcium oxalate uroliths. The standard of care for decreasing risk of calcium oxalate urolith recurrence is to feed moist food and encourage water intake (**Table 46-23**). In addition, owners should be advised to avoid giving treats with increased amounts of calcium or oxalate (**Tables 46-15** and **46-18**). These foods/products may increase urinary excretion of calcium and oxalate, which increases the risk for development of uroliths.

Therefore, veterinary health care team members need to educate owners about the importance of nutritional management in the treatment of cats with calcium oxalate disease, especially cats at risk of urethral obstruction. Increasing owners' awareness may lead to better compliance.

Assess and Determine the Feeding Method

Based on information currently available, meal feeding moist food is appropriate to manage cats with calcium oxalate uroliths. Moist foods increase water intake and reduce concentrations of crystal-forming elements. The method of feeding influences urinary pH throughout the day and therefore may affect success of managing cats with calcium oxalate urolithiasis. Although calcium oxalate crystalluria is not as pH dependent as is struvite crystalluria formation, management of urinary pH is still important. As discussed above, ingestion of food stimulates a postprandial alkaline tide, unless offset by acidifying ingredients in the food. When offered food free choice, most cats will eat small amounts every few hours, resulting in a smaller but more prolonged alkaline tide than with meal feeding (**Figure 46-18**) (Taton et al, 1984). Thus, it has been suggested meal feeding, rather than feeding multiple small meals per day (as in free-choice feeding), might lower the risk of calcium oxalate urolith formation because of the production of a more alkaline urinary pH (Bartges and Kirk, 2006).

Reassessment

Of cats with calcium oxalate uroliths submitted to the Minnesota Urolith Center in 1998 (n = 2,393), 169 (7.1%) had a recurrence (i.e., subsequent urolith submission), 15 (0.6%) had a second recurrence and two (0.1%) had a third recurrence (Albasan et al, 2006). Mean recurrence times were 23, 38 and 48 months, respectively. Urolith recurrence rate was not different between males and females. It is likely that uroliths from some cats with recurrences were not submitted for subsequent evaluation; therefore, the actual recurrence rate was probably higher. Further study is needed to better define recurrence rates for calcium oxalate uroliths in cats.

All cats should be monitored for recurrence, including urinalysis every three months to detect calcium oxalate crystalluria and diagnostic imaging every six months to detect uroliths. Serum calcium concentration should be monitored in cats with hypercalcemia. If uroliths recur, less-invasive procedures (e.g., voiding urohydropropulsion) are more likely to be effective when uroliths are smaller. **Table 46-27** summarizes the steps for managing cats with calcium oxalate urolithiasis. **Box 46-9** reviews other treatments for calcium oxalate urolithiasis

CONCLUSION

The most common forms of FLUTD include FIC, struvite disease (uroliths and urethral plugs) and calcium oxalate uroliths. Trends in occurrence of urolith types have changed in the past 25 years. Many risk factors have been identified for FLUTD, in general; however, additional study is needed to determine pathogenesis and show a cause-and-effect relationship. Although many treatments have been recommended for FIC, only a few have been evaluated by controlled, randomized clinical trials in cats with naturally occurring disease. When evaluating treatment, consider those options that have the highest level of evidence for effectiveness (**Tables 46-20** and **46-21**) (Roudebush et al, 2004; Forrester and Roudebush, 2007). Feeding moist food and recommending other methods to increase water intake are appropriate for the most common forms of FLUTD including FIC, urolithiasis and urethral plugs. In addition, implementing environmental enrichment and stress reduction is indicated for patients with FIC. Feeding a therapeutic food for one to two months is a very effective method for dissolving struvite uroliths in cats. Foods formulated to prevent recurrence of struvite uroliths or urethral plugs are indicated after urolith dissolution or removal of urethral plugs. Treatment for calcium oxalate uroliths involves urolith removal, followed by feeding moist food formulated to decrease risk of urolith recurrence. Cats with lower urinary tract disorders should be monitored periodically by performing urinalyses and diagnostic imaging to detect recurrence of their original disease, development of a different lower urinary tract disorder or occurrence of adverse events associated with therapeutic interventions. The therapeutic regimen can then be modified as needed.

ENDNOTES

a. Osborne CA, Lulich JP. Minnesota Urolith Center, University of Minnesota, St Paul, USA. Unpublished data. 2007.

b. Oakton pHTestr 1, Model 35624-00. Oakton Instruments, Vernon Hills, IL, USA.

Box 46-9. Additional Treatments for Calcium Oxalate Urolithiasis.

VITAMIN B_6

Deficiency of vitamin B_6 has been associated with increased urinary oxalate excretion; however, it has not been shown to cause calcium oxalate uroliths. Additional vitamin B_6 is unlikely to benefit cats eating most commercial foods; however, if a cat with calcium oxalate uroliths is being fed a homemade food, it would be appropriate to supplement with vitamin B_6 (2 to 4 mg/kg body weight orally once daily).

THIAZIDE DIURETICS

Thiazide diuretics are known to cause renal tubular reabsorption of calcium, resulting in decreased urine calcium excretion, which may decrease likelihood of calcium oxalate urolith recurrence. Thiazide diuretics have been used for treatment of calcium oxalate urolithiasis in people but no studies have been reported in cats with calcium oxalate uroliths. In a blinded, placebo-controlled crossover study performed with healthy cats, administration of hydrochlorothiazide suspension (1 mg/kg orally q12h) was associated with significantly decreased urinary saturation of calcium oxalate compared with placebo. For cats with recurrent calcium oxalate uroliths despite feeding a therapeutic food and increasing water intake, thiazide diuretics may be considered. Thiazide diuretics should not be used in cats with hypercalcemia.

POTASSIUM CITRATE

Increased urinary citrate may form soluble complexes with calcium, making it unavailable to form calcium oxalate uroliths. Citrate inhibits calcium oxalate crystal formation by promoting formation of alkaline urine and by forming complexes with calcium (**Figure 1**). When citrate complexes with calcium, ionic calcium concentration and urine saturation with calcium oxalate are reduced.

Hypocitraturia is reported to occur in 19 to 63% of human patients with calcium oxalate urolithiasis; however, frequency of hypocitraturia in cats with calcium oxalate urolithiasis is unknown. Changes in acid-base status influence renal handling of citrate. Metabolic acidosis virtually eliminates urinary citrate excretion by promoting citrate oxidation. Acidosis favors influx of citrate into renal mitochondria and inhibits efflux of citrate from mitochondria. Tubular and peritubular citrate uptake increases when cytosolic citrate concentration decreases. Increased reabsorption of citrate reduces urinary citrate excretion. The citrate in urine is the small quantity that escapes reabsorption. In metabolic alkalosis, urinary citrate increases because mitochondrial uptake and thus oxidation of citrate is reduced, cytosolic citrate concentration increases, reabsorption decreases and urinary excretion of citrate increases.

Thus, depending in part on the acid-base status of the patient, dietary citrate may have little effect on urinary citrate. Feeding up to 100 mg of citric acid/kg body weight to cats has been shown to have little effect on urine citrate concentrations. Effects of potassium citrate alone on urinary calcium oxalate saturation or urolith recurrence have not been evaluated in healthy cats or cats with calcium oxalate uroliths. One therapeutic food[a] containing potassium citrate was associated with decreased urinary calcium oxalate saturation in cats with calcium oxalate uroliths. Potassium citrate (50 to 75 mg/kg body weight orally q12h with food) should be considered in cats that have recurrent calcium oxalate uroliths despite using other measures (e.g., feeding moist food or therapeutic food, increased water intake).

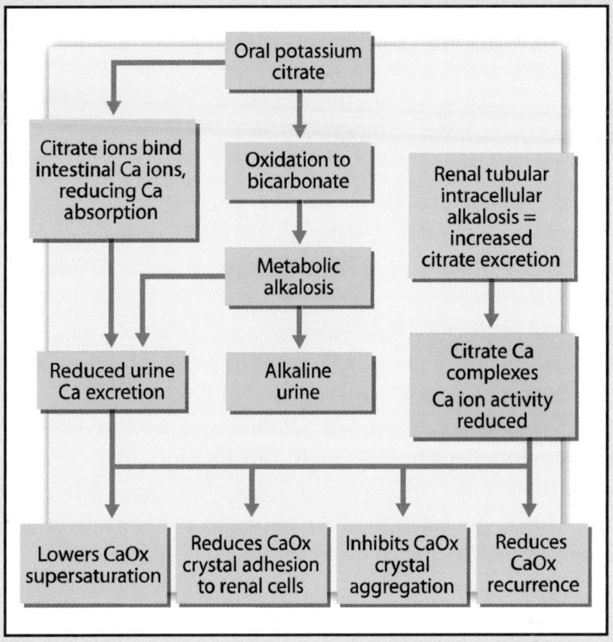

Figure 1. Schematic depicting the role of citrate in binding intestinal calcium (Ca) ions and reducing calcium absorption, promoting formation of alkaline urine and preventing calcium oxalate (CaOx) urolith formation.

ENDNOTE

a. Hill's Prescription Diet x/d Feline. Hill's Pet Nutrition Inc., Topeka, KS, USA.

The Bibliography for **Box 46-9** can be found at www.markmorris.org.

c. Feline Control pHormula Waltham Veterinary Diet. Waltham, Vernon, CA, USA.
d. Cystease. Ceva Animal Health, Chesam, United Kingdom.
e. Hill's Prescription Diet x/d Feline. Hill's Pet Nutrition Inc., Topeka, KS, USA.
f. Hill's Prescription Diet s/d Feline. Hill's Pet Nutrition Inc., Topeka, KS, USA.
g. Medi-Cal Dissolution Formula. Veterinary Medical Diets, Guelph, Ontario, Canada.

REFERENCES

The references for **Chapter 46** can be found at www.markmorris.org.

CASE 46-1

Obstructive Uropathy in a Cat

John M. Kruger, DVM, PhD, Dipl. ACVIM (Small Animal Internal Medicine)
College of Veterinary Medicine
Michigan State University
East Lansing, Michigan, USA

Patient Assessment

A four-year-old, castrated male, mixed-breed cat was examined for acute dysuria, pollakiuria and stranguria. The cat had one previous episode of obstructive uropathy approximately 18 months earlier. No other historical problems were identified.

Physical examination revealed that the cat was depressed, lethargic and approximately 5% dehydrated. Temperature was normal. Heart and respiratory rates were increased. The cat weighed 6.4 kg and was considered overweight (body condition score 4/5). Abdominal palpation revealed a firm, painful and overly distended urinary bladder. A small plug of tan, gritty material was identified at the level of the external urethral orifice.

Analysis of a urine specimen collected by cystocentesis revealed moderately concentrated urine with a neutral pH, struvite crystalluria and findings typical of inflammation (i.e., hematuria, pyuria and proteinuria). Aerobic bacteria were not detected by quantitative urine culture. Results of a hemogram were within normal limits. A serum biochemistry profile revealed mild azotemia. Venous blood gas measurement identified a mild metabolic acidosis. Survey abdominal radiographs revealed increased amounts of intraabdominal fat and an overly distended urinary bladder.

Assess the Food and Feeding Method

The cat had been fed a dry commercial maintenance food free choice, which was supplemented with a small amount of moist commercial maintenance food (one tablespoon, once daily). The cat had unlimited access to fresh water.

Questions

1. What are potential causes of urethral obstruction in male cats?
2. What differences exist between uroliths and urethral plugs?
3. What are risk factors for formation of struvite crystals?
4. Can nutritional management dissolve urethral plugs?
5. What is the effectiveness of perineal urethrostomy vs. medical therapy for preventing recurrent urethral obstruction due to struvite-containing urethral plugs?

Answers and Discussion

1. Urethral obstruction may be caused by one or more intramural, mural or extramural abnormalities located at one or more sites. In a prospective study of urethral obstruction in 51 male cats, investigators identified crystalline-matrix urethral plugs in 59% of cats; urethroliths were identified in 12% of cats and a specific cause could not be identified in 29% of affected cats. In a prospective study of European cats, 45 of 67 male cats with signs of lower urinary tract disease had urethral obstruction; most common causes included feline idiopathic cystitis (FIC) (24 cats), uroliths (13 cats) and urethral plugs (eight cats). Other possible causes of urethral obstruction include sloughed tissue fragments originating from the bladder or urethra, acquired urethral strictures, prostatic lesions, urethral neoplasms, periurethral neoplasms, congenital urethral anomalies and functional urethral obstruction (e.g., reflex dyssynergia).
2. There are distinct physical and probable etiopathogenic differences between feline uroliths and urethral plugs; therefore, these terms should not be used synonymously. Uroliths are highly organized polycrystalline concretions composed primarily of minerals (organic and inorganic crystalloids) and smaller quantities of nonmineral matrix. In contrast, most feline urethral plugs are composed of relatively large quantities of matrix mixed with mineral crystals. However, some urethral plugs are composed primarily of matrix, some consist of sloughed tissue, blood and/or inflammatory reactants and a few are composed primarily of aggregates of crystalline minerals. In general, feline crystalline-matrix urethral plugs appear as cylindrical concretions that conform to the diameter of the urethra and vary from a few mm to several cm. They usually are soft, friable, easily compressed and have no visible organized external structure. Urethral plugs contain varying quantities of minerals in proportion to large quantities of matrix. Struvite is the most common mineral type identified in feline urethral plugs. However, a variety of different mineral types (e.g., calcium oxalate, ammonium urate, calcium phosphate) have been identified in urethral plugs of cats, suggesting that multiple risk factors are involved in their formation.

   The matrix component of feline urethral plugs is less well defined. Studies in cats and other species suggest that matrix is heterogeneous and may be composed of mucoproteins, albumin, globulins, cells (e.g., erythrocytes, leukocytes, epithelial cells and spermatozoa) and microorganisms (e.g., bacteria and viruses).

One hypothesis suggests that formation of matrix by infectious or inflammatory agents in cats with concomitant crystalluria of any type may lead to formation of matrix-crystal urethral plugs. Crystalluria per se is unlikely to cause production of large quantities of matrix because classic uroliths, which are composed of at least 90% crystalline material, contain relatively little matrix.

3. Risk factors associated with formation of struvite crystals found in urethral plugs are probably similar to those associated with formation of struvite uroliths. Factors of major therapeutic importance include nutritional factors affecting urine magnesium concentration and urinary pH and anything that predisposes to urinary tract infection with urease-producing microorganisms.
4. In general, the immediate need to remove urethral plugs within hours precludes attempts to induce their dissolution over a period of days or weeks. However, it is often possible to repulse urethral plugs into the urinary bladder lumen. Although urethral plugs contain markedly greater quantities of matrix than do uroliths, medical protocols that dissolve sterile struvite uroliths would probably also be effective for dissolving the struvite crystalline component of urethral plugs located in the urinary bladder lumen. However, such therapy may not result in dissolution of plug matrix. In addition, it must be emphasized that calcium oxalate, calcium phosphate and ammonium urate crystals are occasionally identified in some naturally occurring feline urethral plugs.

   Attempts to dissolve struvite crystals by promoting formation of acidic urine should not be initiated in cats with postrenal azotemia. The metabolic sequela of urethral obstruction, particularly severe metabolic acidosis, should be corrected before pharmacologic agents or foods designed to acidify urine are used.
5. Perineal urethrostomies can minimize recurrent obstruction of the penile urethra of patients unresponsive to nonsurgical therapeutic and prophylactic management. In a prospective study of 30 cats with struvite crystalline-matrix urethral plugs, perineal urethrostomy and nutritional management were equally effective in their ability to prevent recurrent urethral obstruction. However, 16 episodes of bacterial urinary tract infection developed in nine cats with perineal urethrostomies; bacterial urinary tract infections were not observed in cats treated only with nutritional management. Furthermore, staphylococcal-induced struvite urocystoliths developed in two cats with perineal urethrostomies. In another study of cats that had perineal urethrostomy, over half developed complications (urinary tract infection, stricture) or had recurrent clinical signs due to urolithiasis or FIC. These observations emphasize that perineal urethrostomies may be associated with significant short-term and long-term complications. Localization of the site(s) and cause(s) of urethral obstruction is especially important if urethrostomy is considered.

Progress Notes

To further characterize the composition of the urethral plug and identify potential etiopathologic factors, a portion of the urethral plug was obtained and submitted for light and electron microscopic examination and quantitative mineral analysis. Light microscopic evaluation of the urethral plug revealed that it was composed of numerous unorganized crystals, occasional white blood cells and large quantities of amorphous matrix (**Figure 1**). Electron microscopy did not reveal any specific etiologic agents. Subsequent quantitative mineral analysis revealed that the crystalline component of the plug was composed of 100% struvite.

Urethral patency was reestablished with a combination of procedures that included: 1) gentle massage of the distal urethra followed by gentle compression of the urinary bladder, 2) partial decompression of the bladder by cystocentesis and 3) flushing of the urethral lumen with sterile 0.9% saline solution. After urine flow was restored, particulate material in the urinary bladder was removed by lavage of the bladder lumen with sterile saline solution. Because the large quantity of urine precipitates in the bladder lumen represented a potential risk factor for reobstruction, a sterile indwelling red-rubber urinary catheter was placed and connected to a closed sterilized drainage system. Systemic fluid and acid-base imbalances associated with obstructive uropathy were corrected over a 24-hour period by intravenous administration of lactated Ringer's solution.

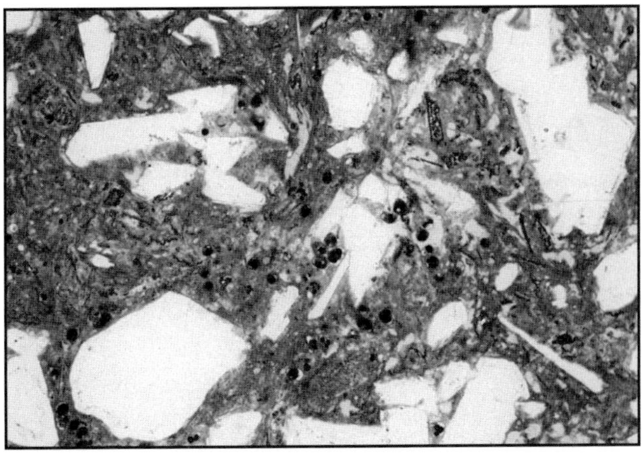

Figure 1. Photomicrograph of a urethral plug removed from a four-year-old, castrated male, mixed-breed cat with obstructive uropathy. Note spaces previously occupied by struvite crystals surrounded by large quantities of amorphous matrix containing white blood cells (toluidine blue stain; 100X original magnification).

Gross hematuria gradually subsided over 48 hours. The indwelling urinary catheter was removed and the cat was observed for signs of reobstruction. Aerobic bacteria were not detected on followup quantitative culture of urine collected via the indwelling catheter before its removal.

The cat was fed a commercial veterinary therapeutic food designed to promote dissolution of the struvite crystal component of the urethral plug (Prescription Diet s/d Feline[a]). When the cat was discharged from the hospital, its owner was instructed to feed the food in sufficient quantity to maintain stable body weight (approximately 320 kcal [1,339 kJ]; 2/3 cup). Analysis of a urine sample collected 20 days after initiation of nutritional therapy revealed a pH of 6.0 and no crystalluria. After approximately three weeks of calculolytic therapy, the food was changed to a commercial veterinary therapeutic food that has lower energy density, decreased fat, increased fiber, reduced magnesium concentration and that produces a normal acidic urine (Prescription Diet w/d Feline[a]). Therapeutic goals were to: 1) promote formation of acidic urine (pH 6.2 to 6.4) at approximately four to eight hours after feeding, 2) reduce or eliminate struvite crystalluria and 3) promote gradual weight reduction. Therapeutic efficacy was monitored by serial urinalyses and physical examinations. Over the next several months the cat lost approximately 1.2 kg and remained free of signs of lower urinary tract disease. The quantity of food was adjusted to maintain a stable body weight of 5 kg.

Endnote
a. Hill's Pet Nutrition, Inc., Topeka, KS, USA.

Bibliography
Bass M, Howard J, Gerber B, et al. Retrospective study of indications for and outcome of perineal urethrostomy in cats. Journal of Small Animal Practice 2005; 46: 227-231.
Corgozinho KB, de Souza HJ, Pereira AN, et al. Catheter-induced urethral trauma in cats with urethral obstruction. Journal of Feline Medicine and Surgery 2007; 9: 481-486.
Gerber B, Boretti FS, Kley S, et al. Evaluation of clinical signs and causes of lower urinary tract disease in European cats. Journal of Small Animal Practice 2005; 46: 571-577.
Kruger JM, Osborne CA, Goyal SM, et al. Clinical evaluation of cats with lower urinary tract disease. Journal of the American Veterinary Medical Association 1991; 199: 211-216.
Osborne CA, Caywood DD, Johnston GR, et al. Perineal urethrostomy versus dietary management in prevention of lower urinary tract disease. Journal of Small Animal Practice 1991; 32: 296-305.
Osborne CA, Kruger JM, Lulich JP. Feline matrix-crystalline urethral plugs: A unifying hypothesis of causes. Journal of Small Animal Practice 1992; 33: 172-177.

CASE 46-2

Recurrent Urolithiasis in a Himalayan Cat
S. Dru Forrester, DVM, MS, Dipl. ACVIM (Small Animal Internal Medicine)
Scientific Affairs
Hill's Pet Nutrition, Inc.
Topeka, Kansas, USA

Timothy A. Allen, DVM, Dipl. ACVIM (Small Animal Internal Medicine)
Lawrence, Kansas, USA

Carl A. Osborne, DVM, PhD, Dipl. ACVIM (Small Animal Internal Medicine)
College of Veterinary Medicine
University of Minnesota
St. Paul, Minnesota, USA

Patient Assessment
A five-year-old, neutered male Himalayan cat was examined for a six-week history of pollakiuria, stranguria, gross hematuria and licking the perineal area. Multiple urocystoliths (bladder uroliths) had been removed one year earlier. The uroliths had been given to the owner at that time and were not submitted for analysis. The current clinical signs had not improved after treatment with an oral antimicrobial agent (sulfadiazine/trimethoprim).

Physical examination revealed a thin 3-kg cat (body condition score [BCS] 2/5) with a small and painful urinary bladder and erythematous penile mucosa. Evaluation of these problems included a complete blood count (normal), serum biochemistry profile (normal), urinalysis (red color, proteinuria, hematuria, pH = 6.5, no crystals visualized), aerobic urine culture (negative) and abdominal radiographs. Multiple radiodense uroliths (3 mm diameter) with rough edges were found in the urinary bladder. The owner had uroliths that had been previously removed, which were submitted for quantitative analysis. Results revealed the uroliths were composed of 100% calcium oxalate (monohydrate and dihydrate).

Assess the Food and Feeding Method

The cat was given a variety of commercial dry and moist cat foods before the urocystoliths were removed one year ago. After surgery, the food was changed to a commercial dry veterinary therapeutic food[a] formulated to avoid excessive magnesium and phosphorus and to allow production of normal acidic urine. These nutritional attributes are important for prevention of struvite crystalluria. This food was offered free choice.

Questions

1. Why were no crystals identified in urine from this patient?
2. What is the probable composition of the recurrent uroliths in this cat?
3. How should this cat be treated and how can urolith recurrence be minimized?

Answers and Discussion

1. Crystals were not seen in the urine sample because the urine was not supersaturated with crystal-forming substances at the time the sample was collected and examined. This finding suggests an absence of the typical combination of factors that lead to the initiation, nucleation, growth and aggregation of crystals. Some factors that influence the variable presence of crystals include time since the last meal, how concentrated or dilute the urine is, how the urine sample is handled after collection, fluctuations in urinary pH and differences between the food consumed at home vs. that in the hospital.
2. The urocystoliths are probably composed of calcium oxalate, based on the signalment (calcium oxalate occurs more commonly in neutered male, middle-aged cats with a higher prevalence in Burmese, Himalayan and Persian breeds) and clinical findings (i.e., aciduria, radiodense uroliths and analysis of the previous uroliths).
3. Medical protocols to promote dissolution of calcium oxalate uroliths in cats are currently unavailable. Urocystoliths small enough to pass through the urethra may be removed by voiding urohydropropulsion. Very small urocystoliths may be retrieved with the aid of a urinary catheter. At present, cystotomy is the only practical alternative for removing larger calcium oxalate uroliths. Following urolith removal, medical protocols should be considered to minimize urolith recurrence. In general, medical therapy should be formulated in a stepwise fashion, with the initial goal of reducing urine concentration of lithogenic substances.

   A food that provides adequate protein (>32% dry matter), avoids excessive calcium and sodium chloride and does not promote formation of overly acidic urine (urinary pH <6.2) should be considered to help minimize recurrence of calcium oxalate uroliths in this cat. Potassium citrate helps promote increased urinary pH and may inhibit formation of calcium oxalate crystalluria; it is present in some therapeutic urinary foods.[b,c] The food should not contain restricted or increased levels of phosphorus or magnesium. Excessive intake of vitamin D (which promotes intestinal absorption of calcium) and ascorbic acid (a precursor of oxalate) should be avoided by not offering vitamin supplements. The food should be adequately fortified with vitamin B_6 (pyridoxine) because pyridoxine deficiency may promote endogenous production and subsequent urinary excretion of oxalic acid. Most commercial foods contain more than adequate levels of pyridoxine; however, homemade foods might be deficient if they are not supplemented.

   Other preventive measures include increasing urine volume and maintaining less concentrated urine by feeding moist (canned) rather than dry food. Drugs (e.g., furosemide, glucocorticoids) that may increase hypercalciuria should be avoided. Hydrochlorothiazide diuretics may decrease urinary calcium oxalate saturation in healthy cats; however, there currently are no data to indicate their effectiveness in cats with calcium oxalate uroliths. Serial monitoring (e.g., radiographs, urinalyses, serum biochemistry profiles) should be performed every six months to detect underlying metabolic problems, and to aid detection of recurrent uroliths when they are small enough to be removed by nonsurgical techniques.

Progress Notes

Abdominal radiographs were reviewed to ensure that radiodense nephroliths were not overlooked. The urocystoliths were removed via cystotomy. Because the number of uroliths could not be determined from the pre-surgery radiographs, postsurgical radiographs were taken to confirm that all of the uroliths had been removed. Evaluating postsurgical radiographs is important because failure to remove all urocystoliths during surgery is possible and may result in the appearance of recurrence of clinical signs and uroliths despite preventive measures. A moist veterinary therapeutic food[b] that provided the appropriate nutritional benefits discussed above was prescribed; the nutritional benefits of this food currently are available in different food.[d] Because the cat was thin (BCS 2/5), the daily energy requirement (DER) was estimated to be 1.4 x the resting energy requirement at the ideal weight of 4 kg (DER = 265 kcal [1,109 kJ]). The owners were instructed to divide the amount of food supplying the DER into two daily feedings and monitor the food intake closely until optimal weight was achieved.

Serial monitoring consisted of periodic urinalyses (with emphasis on urine specific gravity, urinary pH, crystalluria and evidence of urinary tract infection), survey radiographs and serum biochemistry profiles (serum calcium and electrolytes). Initially, routine urinalyses were performed every two to four weeks and the owners were carefully interviewed to assess compliance with feeding recommendations.

Endnotes

a. Prescription Diet c/d Feline, Hill's Pet Nutrition, Inc., Topeka, KS, USA.
b. Prescription Diet x/d Feline, Hill's Pet Nutrition, Inc., Topeka, KS, USA.
c. Iams Veterinary Formula Urinary O Moderate pH/O/Feline, P&G Pet Care, Dayton, OH, USA.
d. Prescription Diet c/d Multicare Feline, Hill's Pet Nutrition, Inc., Topeka, KS, USA.

Bibliography

Bartges JW, Kirk CA. Nutrition and lower urinary tract disease in cats. Veterinary Clinics of North America: Small Animal Practice 2006; 36: 1361-1376.

Forrester SD, Roudebush P. Evidence-based management of feline lower urinary tract disease. Veterinary Clinics of North America: Small Animal Practice 2007; 37: 533-558.

CASE 46-3

Struvite Urolithiasis in a Cat

S. Dru Forrester, DVM, MS, Dipl. ACVIM (Small Animal Internal Medicine)
Scientific Affairs
Hill's Pet Nutrition, Inc.
Topeka, Kansas, USA

Jody P. Lulich, DVM, PhD, Dipl. ACVIM (Small Animal Internal Medicine)
College of Veterinary Medicine
University of Minnesota
St. Paul, Minnesota, USA

Patient Assessment

An eight-year-old, spayed female domestic shorthair cat was evaluated for pollakiuria of three days' duration. Although the cat was using the litter box, its caregivers suspected that it also was urinating in other locations in the house. Physical examination was unremarkable (body condition score 3/5) and the urinary bladder was small. The cat remained in the hospital until there was sufficient urine to collect for analysis.

Urine subsequently obtained by cystocentesis had a specific gravity of 1.043, pH of 6.5, hematuria (>200 RBCs/hpf) and struvite crystalluria. Survey abdominal radiographs revealed two radiopaque uroliths in the urinary bladder (**Figure 1**). Subsequent aerobic bacterial culture of the urine sample revealed no growth. With a tentative diagnosis of struvite urolithiasis, the attending veterinarian discussed treatment options with the owners including medical dissolution and surgical removal.

Assess the Food and Feeding Method

Before urolith diagnosis, the cat was fed a commercial moist food twice daily and a dry commercial maintenance food was available at all times. Water was available free choice.

Questions

1. What urolith types are most likely in cats and how does one determine their mineral composition?
2. What treatment should be recommended for cats with struvite uroliths?
3. What recommendations should be made to prevent struvite urolith recurrence?

Answers and Discussion

1. Approximately 90% of uroliths in cats are composed of either magnesium ammonium phosphate (struvite) or calcium oxalate. Using information from the history, signalment, urinalysis and diagnostic imaging, it is possible to estimate the mineral type. The textbook case of struvite uroliths involves a younger (<7 years), spayed female cat with slightly acidic to alkaline urine (pH >6.5), struvite crystalluria and round or disk-shaped radiopaque uroliths. Cats with calcium oxalate uroliths usually are older (>7 years), male, have acidic to neutral urinary pH, calcium oxalate crystalluria and radiopaque uroliths that may be small and/or have pointed edges. Some cats with uroliths may not have all findings (e.g., there may be no urine crystals) or there may be findings consis-

tent with both urolith types. Findings consistent with struvite uroliths in this cat include female gender, presence of struvite crystalluria and round, radiopaque uroliths whereas the age and urinary pH could occur with calcium oxalate uroliths. A definitive diagnosis requires quantitative urolith analysis, which is particularly helpful when there are mixed or compound uroliths. For this cat, one option would be to attempt nutritional dissolution therapy for four weeks; if the uroliths decrease in size or disappear, struvite urolithiasis is likely and treatment should be continued. If the uroliths do not decrease in size or they become larger, other treatment (e.g., physical removal of uroliths) is indicated because the uroliths are likely composed of another mineral type.

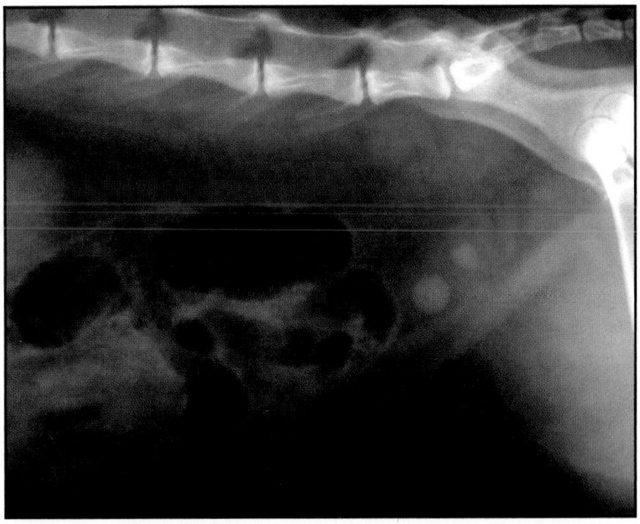

Figure 1. Lateral abdominal radiograph reveals two radiopaque uroliths in the urinary bladder.

2. At this time, the most common treatments for managing cats with struvite uroliths are surgical removal via cystotomy and medical dissolution with nutritional management. The choice between these options may depend on the clinician's preference and expertise as well as the pet owner's preferences. Many veterinarians prefer to surgically remove uroliths because they believe that surgical management is more effective, controls clinical signs quicker and will not be associated with urethral obstruction as uroliths decrease in size, especially in male cats. However, effectiveness of surgical removal of uroliths has not been critically evaluated in cats. A retrospective study including 20 cats with urinary bladder uroliths revealed that five cats (20%) had incomplete removal of uroliths by cystotomy in a veterinary teaching hospital. In the absence of appropriate studies, it should not be assumed that surgical management of uroliths is 100% effective. In addition, there have been no reported studies documenting the time required for resolution of clinical signs after surgical removal of uroliths or that urethral obstruction does or does not occur postoperatively.

   Medical management using dissolution foods[a,b] has been evaluated in two studies of cats with struvite uroliths. The mean time required for urolith dissolution was around four weeks; however, some cats had radiographic resolution of uroliths two weeks after beginning nutritional management. Urethral obstruction has not been reported to occur in male cats with struvite uroliths that were dissolved with nutritional management. In most cats, clinical signs are no longer evident within two weeks of beginning dissolution foods.

   In summary, when selecting treatment for cats with struvite uroliths it may help to ask and answer the following questions: 1) Which treatment is the least invasive?, 2) Which treatment would I prefer if I had uroliths? and 3) Which treatment is the most effective based on currently published evidence?

3. After dissolution or removal of struvite uroliths, nutritional management is indicated to decrease risk of urolith recurrence. Based on current evidence, foods used for prevention of struvite disease should avoid excessive protein, magnesium, phosphorus and sodium and should maintain a mildly acidic urinary pH. Cats eating struvite preventive foods should be monitored periodically for urinary pH values and evidence of crystalluria. The goal of treatment is to prevent occurrence of struvite crystalluria and maintain urinary pH ≤ 6.4.

Progress Notes

After considering treatment options and the owner's preferences, the veterinarian recommended a struvite dissolution fooda for this patient. The daily caloric requirement was calculated and divided into two meals. It was recommended that the patient return in two weeks for reevaluation to include physical examination, urinalysis and abdominal radiographs. During the first followup examination two weeks later, the patient was eating the prescribed food exclusively. Analysis of urine collected by cystocentesis revealed specific gravity = 1.034, pH = 6.0 and mild hematuria (7 RBCs/hpf); there was no pyuria, crystalluria or bacteriuria. Survey abdominal radiographs confirmed that uroliths were smaller (**Figure 2**); therefore, nutritional management was continued. Radiographic evaluation performed four weeks after initiation of the dissolution food revealed no visible uroliths (**Figure 3**). The dissolution food was prescribed for an additional month after which it was recommended that the patient be transitioned to a maintenance food with reduced magnesium and phosphorus to prevent struvite urolith recurrence.

Endnotes

a. Prescription Diet s/d Feline, Hill's Pet Nutrition, Inc., Topeka, KS, USA.
b. Dissolution Formula, Medi-Cal Royal Canin, Guelph, ON, Canada.

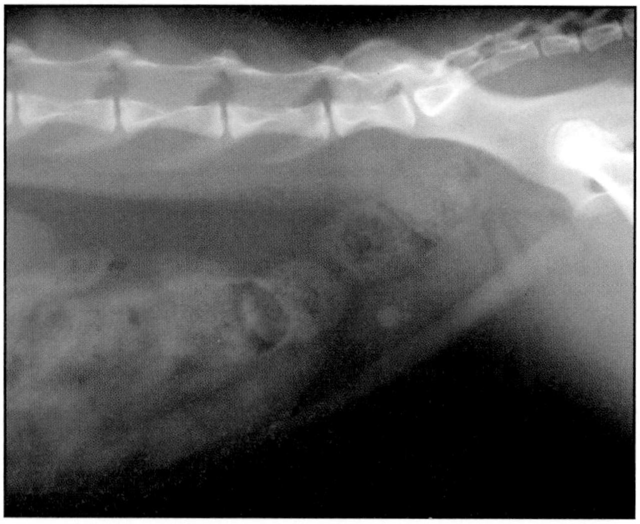

Figure 2. Radiographic image obtained two weeks after beginning nutritional management for struvite urolithiasis. Radiopaque uroliths have decreased in size.

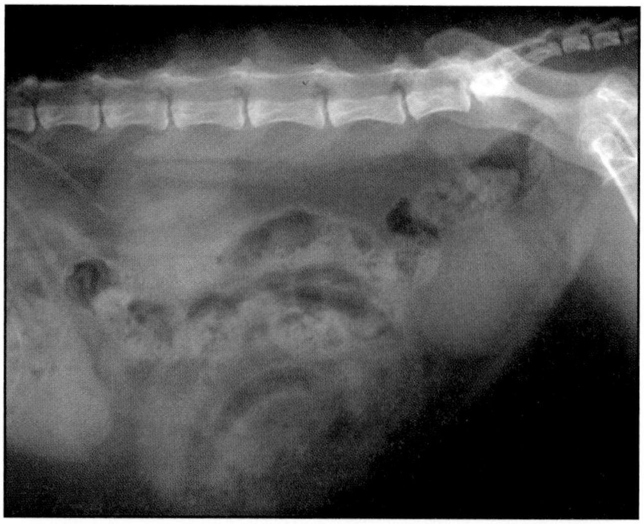

Figure 3. Radiographic image obtained four weeks after initiation of dissolution therapy reveals no evidence of uroliths. The struvite dissolution food should be continued for an additional four weeks to ensure that small uroliths (below the level of radiographic detection) are dissolved.

Bibliography

Houston DM, Rinkardt NE, Hilton J. Evaluation of the efficacy of a commercial diet in the dissolution of feline struvite bladder uroliths. Veterinary Therapeutics 2004; 5: 187-201.

Lulich JP, Osborne CA, Polzin DJ, et al. Incomplete removal of canine and feline urocystoliths by cystotomy (abstract). Journal of Veterinary Internal Medicine 1993; 7: 124.

Osborne CA, Lulich JP, Kruger JM, et al. Medical dissolution of feline struvite urocystoliths. Journal of the American Veterinary Medical Association 1990; 196: 1053-1063.

CASE 46-4

Inappropriate Urination in a Cat

S. Dru Forrester, DVM, MS, Dipl. ACVIM (Small Animal Internal Medicine)
Scientific Affairs
Hill's Pet Nutrition, Inc.
Topeka, Kansas, USA

Patient Assessment

A four-year-old, spayed female domestic shorthair cat was presented for evaluation of inappropriate urination that occurred intermittently over the past four to six months. The owner reported that the cat urinates in the litter box but also in various locations throughout the home (e.g., bathtub, laundry basket). For the past three days the owner also noted increased frequency of urination and the urine appeared pink. The cat lives indoors with two other cats that are healthy. Physical examination revealed a body weight of 5.5 kg and body condition score of 4/5.

Initial evaluation included a urinalysis and diagnostic imaging. Analysis of urine collected by cystocentesis revealed a red/hazy appearance with a specific gravity of 1.052. Dipstick analysis revealed a urinary pH of 6.0, 2+ protein and 3+ occult blood. There were numerous red cells and three to five white cells/hpf noted during urine sediment examination. Aerobic urine culture was negative for bacterial growth. Results of abdominal ultrasound and radiographs were normal. Based on all findings, feline idiopathic cystitis (FIC) was considered most likely.

Assess the Food and Feeding Method

Before the diagnostic evaluation the cat was fed primarily dry commercial food that was available at all times with occasional canned food as a treat. Water was available free choice.

Questions

1. What disorders are associated with inappropriate urination and why is it important to identify the underlying cause?
2. How is FIC diagnosed?
3. What is the most effective approach for controlling clinical signs in patients with FIC?

Answers and Discussion

1. Inappropriate urination (i.e., periuria) may occur as a result of behavioral and/or medical disorders. Any medical condition that causes inflammation of the lower urinary tract (e.g., FIC, urolithiasis, urinary tract infection) may cause urination outside the litter box. Behavioral periuria typically results from toileting problems or urine marking (spraying). Cats with toileting problems have elected to use an alternate location other than the litter box because they have an aversion to or preference for a particular substrate (e.g., litter) or litter box characteristics such as location, style and cleanliness. Cats with lower urinary tract diseases may develop secondary toileting problems that may persist after correction of the underlying medical disorder and this must be distinguished from primary behavioral periuria. Urine marking is a means of communication and often is characterized by expelling urine on vertical surfaces although cats may mark by depositing urine on horizontal surfaces from a squatting position. Finally, aging cats with osteoarthritis may urinate inappropriately in the absence of primary behavioral disorders or urinary tract diseases due to difficulty accessing the litter box (e.g., the sides are too high or the cat must travel up or down stairs to reach the litter box).

   Inappropriate elimination is the most common behavioral problem for which pet owners seek professional counsel. It also is a common reason why owners relinquish their cats to shelters. To prevent the negative impact of inappropriate urination on the pet-family bond, it is important to educate pet owners about potential causes of inappropriate urination so they seek help before relinquishing their cat. When medical causes are excluded, a veterinary behaviorist should be consulted so that appropriate evaluation and treatment can be recommended. This should be done sooner rather than later in the course of the disease, when the chances are greater for having a successful outcome with behavioral modification.
2. The presence of pollakiuria and hematuria indicates that inappropriate urination in this patient is probably due to a medical disorder of the lower urinary tract. In a young to middle-aged female cat, the most likely causes for these signs are FIC and struvite urolithiasis; less likely causes include uroliths of other mineral type (e.g., calcium oxalate, urate), urinary tract infection, anatomic anomalies and neoplasia. At a minimum, all cats with signs of lower urinary tract disease should have a urinalysis and diagnostic imaging performed. Selection of the initial diagnostic imaging procedure (i.e., plain abdominal radiographs or abdominal ultrasonography) may depend on equipment availability; however, using both modalities can be helpful. For radiographs, it is critical to include the entire urinary tract; otherwise, abnormalities such as urethral uroliths may be overlooked. On the basis of initial findings, additional tests such as urine culture and contrast urethrocystography may be indicated for some patients. FIC is diagnosed by excluding all other causes of lower urinary tract disease; therefore, thorough diagnostic evaluation is necessary.
3. A multimodal approach including nutritional management, environmental enrichment, pain management and in some cases, behavioral modification, is recommended to control clinical signs in patients with FIC. Many treatments have been suggested for managing affected cats; however, only a few have been evaluated in clinical studies. To date, the treatments that have been associated with improvement in patients with FIC are feeding moist food and implementing environmental enrichment. Gradual transition to moist food should be part of initial management. It is believed that increased urine volume associated with increased water intake results in dilution of inflammatory mediators in the urinary bladder of patients with FIC; however, other effects of feeding moist food (e.g., increased interaction with owners) cannot be excluded.

   Although being overweight or physically inactive has not been shown to cause urinary tract disease, both are risk factors for FIC. Recent research findings have confirmed that obesity is characterized by a state of systemic inflammation and other negative consequences such as insulin resistance. Therefore, to improve this cat's overall health, a weight-reduction program should be recommended with a goal of reaching ideal body weight and condition. This should include nutritional management and environmental enrichment (e.g., increased exercise and interaction with the owner).

Progress Notes

The owner was given additional information about environmental enrichment to help manage clinical signs of FIC and assist with achieving ideal body condition. A moist veterinary therapeutic food[a] was initially recommended until the cat achieved ideal body weight (4.5 kg). The resting energy requirement (RER) for ideal body weight was calculated as follows: RER = $70(4.5)^{0.75}$ = 218 kcal. In order to lose weight, it was initially recommended to feed approximately 175 kcal per day. The owners were instructed to transition the food change over seven days by feeding 0.75 can of the therapeutic food (87 kcal) twice daily and monitoring food intake closely until optimal weight was achieved. Body weight was measured every two weeks and recorded on a progress chart; the cat achieved ideal body weight five months later and was transitioned to another moist therapeutic food[b] formulated for management of cats with FIC. In order to maintain body condition, the owners were instructed to initially feed 0.75 can of the therapeutic food twice daily (147 kcal per can), which provided slightly less than the daily energy requirement (1.4 x RER) for the cat's ideal body weight. The owner was counseled that this amount of food was a starting point and that adjustments should be made as needed to maintain body weight.

Endnotes

a. Prescription Diet r/d Feline, Hill's Pet Nutrition, Inc., Topeka, KS, USA.
b. Prescription Diet c/d Multicare Feline, Hill's Pet Nutrition, Inc., Topeka, KS, USA.

Bibliography

Buffington CAT. The indoor cat initiative. www.vet.ohio-state.edu/indoorcat (accessed September 2008).

Neilson JC. Feline housesoiling: Elimination and marking behaviors. Veterinary Clinics of North America: Small Animal Practice 2003; 33: 287-301.

Westropp JL, Buffington CAT. Feline idiopathic cystitis: Current understanding of pathophysiology and management. Veterinary Clinics of North America: Small Animal Practice 2004; 34: 1043-1055.

Section 17

Periodontal Disease

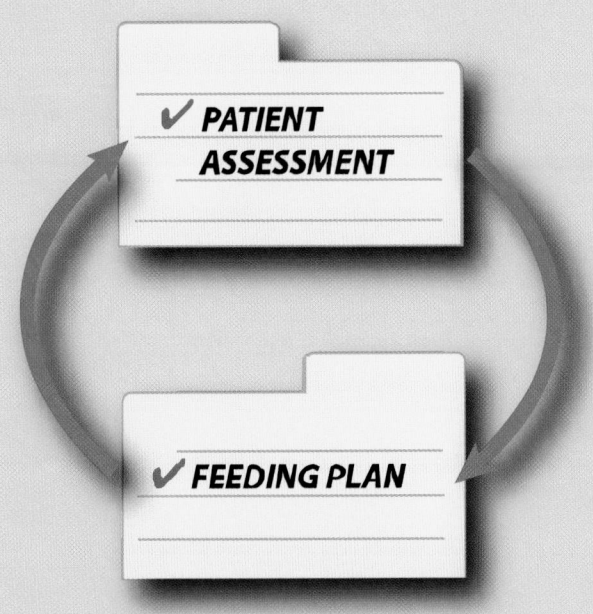

Chapter 47

Periodontal Disease

Ellen I. Logan
Robert B. Wiggs
Dale Scherl
Paul Cleland

"Because periodontal disease is the most common problem affecting dogs and cats of all age groups, programs to prevent periodontal disease should be considered among the most important prophylactic services we can offer."
Gregg A. Dupont

INTRODUCTION

Primary oral diseases can be subdivided into conditions affecting the tooth, the periodontium or other oral tissues (**Table 47-1**). Diseases that affect tooth structure (**Figure 47-1**) may result in lesions of the periodontal apparatus, oral mucosa or both. Diseases affecting the periodontium may result in exfoliation of teeth. Additionally, primary diseases of other organs may cause oral lesions and are important considerations in formulating differential diagnoses. Furthermore, oral disease can contribute to diseases of other organs and body systems.

Periodontal disease is the principal cause of tooth loss in dogs and cats. Food can influence periodontal disease through control of plaque and thus is the primary focus of this chapter. Oral health is achieved through professional care and effective homecare; however, compliance is a significant issue in veterinary dentistry (**Box 47-1**). Traditional methods of plaque control such as toothbrushing may be difficult for clients to accomplish. Therefore use of an effective dental food can be an appropriate and effective means of daily plaque control and oral health maintenance for dogs and cats.

The steps in promoting oral health in dogs and cats include: 1) controlling plaque, the cause of periodontal disease, 2) assessing the level of plaque control necessary to prevent gingivitis in each patient, 3) determining each pet owner's ability to control substrate accumulation and selecting methods most likely to ensure compliance, 4) feeding a food with an appropriate texture and nutritional profile and 5) recognizing that oral health may affect systemic health; therefore, a healthy oral cavity may affect longevity and quality of life.

CLINICAL IMPORTANCE

Prevalence of Periodontal Disease

Periodontal disease is the most common disease of adult dogs and cats. As early as 1899, Eugene Talbot described "interstitial gingivitis or so-called pyorrhoea alveolaris" found in dogs at necropsy (1899). In 1939, Wright noted that "the incidence of

Table 47-1. Conditions affecting the oral cavity.

Conditions primarily affecting teeth	Conditions primarily affecting the periodontium/oral mucosa
Abrasion	Chemical or thermal burns
Attrition	Gingival hyperplasia
Erosion	Gingivitis
Fracture	Gingivostomatitis
Intrinsic staining	Neoplasia
Odontoclastic resorption	Periapical abscess
Pulpitis	Periodontitis
	Ulcers

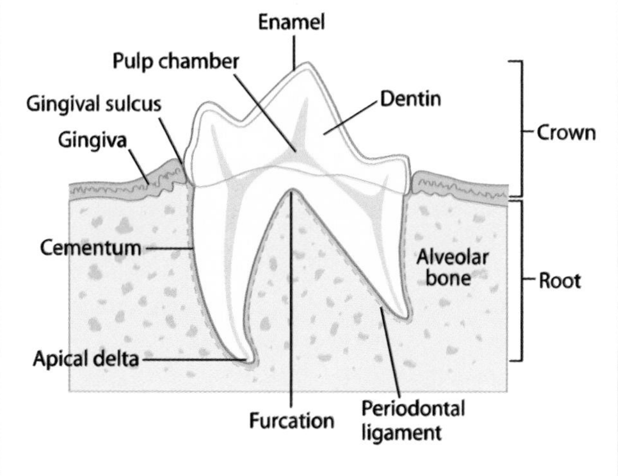

Figure 47-1. Normal tooth and periodontal anatomy.

disease of the teeth in the dog is so high that dental surgery occupies a prominent place in the work of the veterinarian engaged in small-animal practice. The most common affection necessitating surgical interference is paradontal disease" (1939).

Periodontal disease has been observed in dogs and cats of varying breed, gender and age. Surveys from several countries report prevalence rates of periodontal disease that range from 60 to more than 80% of dogs and cats examined (Gray, 1923; Bell, 1965; Rosenberg et al, 1966; Saxe et al, 1967; Gad, 1968; Hamp et al, 1975; Hamp and Lindberg, 1971; Sorensen et al, 1980; Page and Schroeder, 1979; Golden et al, 1982; Reichart et al, 1984; Isogai et al, 1989; Harvey, 1992; Hoffman and Gaengler, 1996).

Data from the National Companion Animal Study representing 54 veterinary practices across the United States confirmed that oral disease was the most frequent diagnosis in all age categories of 39,556 dogs and 13,924 cats (Lund et al, 1999).

PATIENT ASSESSMENT

History

A complete history is important to diagnosis and treatment planning and is an integral tool for developing a complete health maintenance program for pets. An adequate health history must include: 1) information about previous medical and surgical procedures, 2) current preventive measures such as vaccination status and heartworm medication administration, 3) the pet's general environment, including confinement, 4) information about other household pets and 5) who in the household is responsible for primary care.

Inquiries specific to nutrition and oral care should include past and present information about: 1) oral hygiene and level of compliance, 2) presence of any signs that may be related to oral dysfunction, 3) chewing behavior, 4) access to rocks and other materials that may cause occlusal trauma, 5) access to dental treats and toys, 6) eating behavior and 7) foods eaten, with special attention given to texture and other factors.

Box 47-1. Compliance and Dental Homecare.

Oral health is achieved through an effective periodontal management program that includes professional care and client-provided homecare. Appropriate homecare recommendations consider the client and patient preferences and specifically address the degree of oral pathologic change present and client and patient compliance.

Compliance is critical to effective homecare. Clients must be willing and able to perform the recommended hygiene and the patient must accept oral hygiene procedures. Noncompliance may result from lack of an effective recommendation by the veterinary health care team. A comprehensive study of compliance demonstrated that appropriate periodontal therapy was not provided for approximately 15.5 million dogs and cats with recorded periodontal disease scores of 2, 3 or 4. No recommendation for periodontal management was given in 66% of cases with a recorded periodontal disease score of 1. In the same study, 19% of patients lacked any notation of periodontal examination or score in health records.

Even with client education and good pet compliance, some owners are unable to provide routine and effective plaque control. Compliance failure may be due to: 1) lack of skill, 2) lack of perceived benefit, 3) unpleasantness of procedure, 4) lack of noticeable impact and 5) lifestyle constraints. Emphasizing the benefits, including improved oral and systemic health, less breath odor, cost effectiveness and strengthening of the owner-pet bond, may increase compliance.

The most important part of periodontal therapy is how well a patient maintains oral health. Long-term success depends on the degree of plaque control the client is capable of providing between professional visits.

Physical Examination

Initial Oral Examination

Examination of the skull and oral cavity should be a regular part of every physical examination. An extraoral examination should be done before opening the mouth to inspect the skull and facial areas for any abnormalities, such as muscle atrophy, swelling, draining tracts and ocular or nasal discharge. Extraoral examination should also include inspection for facial symmetry, palpation of the temporomandibular joints, regional lymph nodes and salivary glands and thorough inspection of the skin and lips. Extraoral abnormalities related to oral dysfunction may include mucopurulent discharge from the eyes or nostrils, soft or hard swellings, crepitus, salivation and an inability to open or close the mouth (Marretta, 1987, 1992; Kapatkin et al, 1991; Ramsey et al, 1996).

After the extraoral examination, the lips should be gently parted or retracted to allow inspection of the oral mucosa. Patients experiencing severe oral pain may not tolerate even a cursory oral examination without sedation. The facial surfaces of the teeth and gingivae (**Figure 47-2**) should be examined for substrate accumulation (i.e., plaque, calculus and stain [See Etiopathogenesis.]), inflammation, trauma and capillary refill time. Tooth position and occlusion should be evaluated. The lingual surfaces of the teeth and gingivae should be inspected, as well as the palates, tongue (ventral and dorsal), frenulum, oropharyngeal area and tonsils.

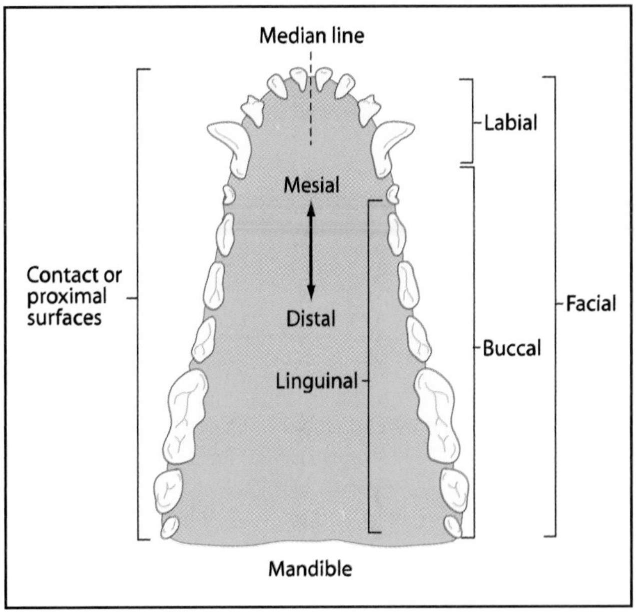

Figure 47-2. Directional nomenclature used to describe anatomic position of tooth surfaces. (Adapted from Wiggs RB. Canine oral anatomy and physiology. Compendium on Continuing Education for the Practicing Veterinarian 1989; 11: 1476.)

Comprehensive Oral Examination

A definitive oral examination must be done with the patient heavily sedated or anesthetized, and is often done immediately before periodontal therapy. The general examination should be used as a starting point in client communication with the understanding that the definitive oral examination may uncover other lesions that require treatment.

The examination should begin with a thorough inspection of all oral tissues. An overall assessment of oral health should consider the amount and location of substrate accumulation. Substrate location and accumulation provide valuable information about the frequency and effectiveness of oral hygiene (Woodall, 1990). Common substrate and periodontal indices used to measure oral health have been described (Logan et al, 1992; Logan and Boyce, 1994) and were adopted by participants of the 1994 International Symposium on Veterinary Oral Care (Logan and Boyce, 1994; SVOC, 1994). Modifications and refinements to substrate indices have been published (Hennet, 1999; Harvey, 2002; Hennet et al, 2006). Furthermore, a recognized system (Veterinary Oral Health Council [VOHC]) exists for validating product claims.

The remainder of the periodontal indices (e.g., probe depth, attachment loss, furcation exposure and tooth mobility) are usually charted after prophylaxis or periodontal therapy to ensure accurate assessment after removal of subgingival debris that may impede measurement. Each tooth and its associated periodontium should be evaluated using a dental explorer-probe to examine the tooth for defects, lesions or both. The same instrument should be used to evaluate periodontal health by measuring the extent of gingival inflammation, attachment loss and alveolar bone loss. Any abnormalities in tooth or periodontal structures should be noted on the dental chart. Detailed dental charting allows for disease assessment and provides a record for future reference. The results should become part of the patient's permanent medical record.

Radiographic Examination

Oral radiography may be indicated to identify lesions that cannot be detected visually or manually, and to determine the extent of pathology. Root fractures, periapical abscesses, alveolar bone loss, acute resorption lesions and anatomic anomalies are difficult to assess without radiography. Additionally, oral radiographs are useful in selecting a definitive treatment plan and assessing the outcome of a dental procedure. Oral radiographic techniques have been well described elsewhere (Wiggs and Lobprise, 1997; Niemiec, 2005; Niemiec and Furman, 2004, 2004a; Niemiec et al, 2004, 2004a). In addition, digital radiography is becoming more common (DuPont and DeBowes, 2002).

Laboratory Studies

A complete blood count, serum biochemistry profile, bacterial culture, virus isolation, cytologic examination and biopsy may add useful information. Other diagnostic tests such as urinalyses and cardiac examinations may complement a standard panel as part of a preanesthetic profile. Patients with suspected renal or cardiac disease may be compromised by bacteremia associated with dental manipulations.

Risk Factors

All mammals are susceptible to periodontal disease. The primary etiologic agents associated with periodontal disease are bacterial plaque and bacterial by-products (Löe et al, 1965; Theilade et al, 1966; Socransky, 1979; Lindhe et al, 1973; Lindhe and Rylander, 1975). Bacterial plaque is also directly involved in the pathogenesis of enamel caries and may be a contributing factor in the development and progression of

Box 47-2. Digestible Carbohydrates and Their Role in Oral Health of Dogs and Cats.

The role of digestible (soluble) carbohydrates (sugars) in the development of dental caries has been well documented in people and rodents. Dental caries, however, occurs infrequently in dogs and cats. One study demonstrated that dogs do not develop carious lesions even after long periods of consuming carbohydrate-rich foods. Carlsson and Egelberg reported that the addition of sucrose to a soft food resulted in no difference in plaque accumulation and gingival inflammation in a group of 12 mongrel dogs. Human studies have demonstrated that larger amounts of plaque were formed when sucrose was the primary sugar consumed. Commercial and homemade pet foods typically contain large quantities of digestible carbohydrates, usually in the form of starch.

The Bibliography for **Box 47-2** can be found at www.markmorris.org.

tooth resorption and other oral inflammatory lesions. Any factor that enhances bacterial accumulation or affects the resistance of the periodontium may influence the disease process. Specific risk factors that contribute to the severity and progression of periodontal diseases include: 1) breed, 2) age, 3) immunocompetence, 4) nutrition and food characteristics, 5) chewing behavior and 6) systemic health (Wiggs, 1995).

Breed

Breed plays a major role in the development of dental disease. Small, toy and brachycephalic breeds are prone to malocclusive disorders including overcrowding and rotation of teeth, retained deciduous teeth and supernumerary teeth. Occlusal abnormalities provide plaque retentive areas and increase the difficulty of oral hygiene procedures. Brachycephalic breeds are also predisposed to mouth breathing, which tends to dry and irritate oral tissues (West-Hyde and Floyd, 1995). Periodontal disease, tooth resorption and gingivostomatitis have been reported to occur with relatively greater frequency in purebred cats, particularly Asian breeds such as Siamese and Abyssinians (Van Wessum et al, 1992). Ulcerative stomatitis has been documented to occur in family clusters of Maltese dogs (Harvey and Emily, 1993).

Age

Several surveys have reported that older pets have a greater frequency and an increased severity of dental disease. One report of a survey of owners of 1,350 dogs noted that calculus deposition, gingival inflammation, tooth mobility, furcation exposure, attachment loss and missing teeth all increased significantly with increasing age (Harvey et al, 1994). In an evaluation of 4,776 cats aged seven to 25 years and 8,692 dogs aged 10 to 25 years, oral disease was the most frequent diagnosis reported (Lund et al, 1999).

It has long been reported that periodontal disease in people increases in severity with increasing age. Recent data suggest that the severity may represent a lifetime disease accumulation and not necessarily be an age-specific condition (Page, 1984; Van der Velden, 1984; Johnson et al, 1989). There may be some age-related changes that could negatively affect oral health, such as decreased salivary flow and antioxidant capacity (Dodds et al, 2005; Aejmelaeus et al, 1997; Navazesh, 2002). It is not surprising that geriatric pets with little history of oral hygiene or veterinary oral care demonstrate an increased prevalence and severity of periodontal disease.

Immunocompetence

The host immune response protects against systemic infection from periodontal pathogens. An over exaggerated immune response can cause severe local periodontal destruction. An inadequate immune response may predispose pets to opportunistic or overwhelming systemic infection (Genco, 1992).

Nutrition and Food Characteristics

The dramatic difference in food form represented by commercial dog and cat foods as compared with the natural prey of wild canids and felids is often implicated as a significant cause of the degree of periodontal disease diagnosed in domestic dogs and cats (Gray, 1923; Colyer, 1990; Watson, 1994). Colyer examined 1,157 wild canid skulls and reported that periodontal disease as suggested by alveolar bone destruction was present in only 2% of specimens (1990). The subject of how well specific commercial food types promote oral health is discussed below.

Box 47-2 reviews a common concern of pet owners regarding food sugar content and dental caries and **Box 47-3** discusses the role of topical coatings of dry cat foods in feline tooth resorption. Although not associated with periodontal disease, these text boxes are included because the topics relate to food and dental diseases.

Etiopathogenesis

Tooth-Accumulated Materials

Several materials accumulate on tooth surfaces and participate in the pathophysiology of dental and periodontal disease. These substances are commonly referred to as tooth-accumulated materials or dental substrates and are categorized as: 1) acquired enamel pellicle, 2) microbial plaque, 3) materia alba/debris, 4) calculus and 5) stain. These substrates accumulate in a dynamic continuum, initiated by the adsorption of salivary constituents onto tooth surfaces (Fedi, 1985; Schwartz et al, 1971).

Saliva is a critical oral fluid primarily recognized for its digestive functions. However, saliva also bathes the oral cavity with a fluid rich in proteins (e.g., enzymes), glycoproteins, electrolytes, lipids, antioxidants, antimicrobial peptides (defensins), immunoglobulins, bicarbonate ions and mucins that provide an initial protective barrier to pathogenic invasion, lubricate and clean the oral cavity and aid in the transportation of solids (Lingström and Moynihan, 2003; Mizukawa et al, 1999). In people, diminished salivary function (xerostomia) is associated with increased prevalence of caries and periodontal disease, mucosal irritation, difficulties in chewing and swallowing and impaired taste. Saliva initiates film formation on all oral surfaces (Scannapieco and Levine, 1990; Navazesh, 2002).

ENAMEL PELLICLE

Enamel pellicle is a thin film or cuticle. Early enamel pellicle is composed of proteins and glycoproteins deposited from saliva and gingival crevicular fluid. Early enamel pellicle protects and lubricates. However, as pellicle ages, existing constituents are modified and additional salivary, crevicular and bacterial components are incorporated. Enamel pellicle and its components provide a framework for initial bacterial colonization and also function in the maturation of dental plaque (Scannapieco and Levine, 1990; Rolla, 1983).

DENTAL PLAQUE

Pellicle deposition and subsequent bacterial colonization occur almost immediately after a dental prophylaxis. Studies have demonstrated that within minutes after polishing, approximately one million organisms are deposited per mm^2 of enamel surface (Lindhe, 1989). Aggregates of bacteria combine with salivary glycoproteins, extracellular polysaccharides and occasionally epithelial and inflammatory cells to form a soft adherent plaque that covers tooth surfaces. Dental plaque is not easily removed by normal tongue actions, water drinking or forced water spray, but can be affected by mechanical and chemical means.

Dental plaque has a specific composition and structure that changes with time (DuPont, 1997). Supragingival dental plaque forms above and along the free gingival margin; subgingival dental plaque is formed entirely within the gingival sulcus. Growth and maturation of supragingival plaque are necessary for subsequent colonization of subgingival surfaces by dental plaque (Kornman, 1986). Supragingival and subgingival plaque are distinct compositional masses that influence the inflammatory reaction of gingival tissues. Studies in people have demonstrated an organized progression of microbial colonization and growth that leads to the development of mature pathogenic dental plaque (Lindhe, 1989).

Canine and feline studies characterizing the microbial composition of supragingival and subgingival plaque have been reported. Supragingival plaque in dogs with clinically healthy gingivae is primarily composed of gram-positive aerobic organisms. As plaque matures, the bacterial composition shifts to a predominately gram-negative anaerobic flora (Courant et al, 1968; Soames and Davis, 1974; Wunder et al, 1976; Syed et al, 1980, 1981; Svanberg et al, 1982; Isogai et al, 1988; Mallonee et al, 1988; Hennet and Harvey, 1991, 1991a, 1991b; Boyce et al, 1995; Harvey et al, 1995). Several sources have detailed lists of specific bacteria associated with periodontal diseases of dogs (Hardham et al, 2005; Syed et al, 1980; Wunder et al, 1976; Hennet and Harvey, 1991, 1991a, 1991b; Allaker et al, 1997; Isogai et al, 1989; Svanbert et al, 1982) and cats (Mallonee et al, 1988). The inflammation and destruction that accompanies periodontal disease results from the direct action of bacteria and their by-products on periodontal tissues and the indirect activation of the host immune response (Genco, 1990). Thus, bacterial plaque is the most important substrate in the development of periodontal disease.

Box 47-3. Do Commercial Cat Foods Cause Tooth Resorption?

Although the etiology of tooth resorption in cats is unknown, examination of skulls that pre-date the 1960s revealed a lower prevalence of tooth resorption than current estimates, which suggests a relatively recent increase. Commercial foods have been implicated as a causative factor in the increased detection of tooth resorption in cats based on several physical and chemical properties of these foods.

Questions have been raised that relate to the common practice of applying an acidic coating to dry cat foods (i.e., feline digest) to enhance palatability. Human studies have demonstrated that consumption of a food or beverage with an acidic pH contributes to erosive lesions. Additionally, chronic vomiting/regurgitation have been associated with these lesions because vomitus is acidic. To address this issue, Zetner and Steurer investigated the tooth surface pH of cats with 1) tooth resorption, 2) chronic oral inflammatory disease and 3) cats with no oral lesions. These researchers also measured tooth surface pH after cats consumed either a commercial moist food or a commercial acid-coated dry food. Results from this study demonstrated that cats with tooth resorption had lower tooth-surface pH values than healthy cats, but that consumption of the dry food was not associated with the pathogenesis of odontoclastic resorptive lesions.

It has also been suggested that hard dry cat foods cause microfractures that predispose teeth to infection and initiate the inflammatory cascade leading to odontoclastic activation. However, it must also be noted that teeth that are not normally associated with mechanical forces related to consuming dry foods are also susceptible to tooth resorption.

Finally, recent work has implicated dietary vitamin D in the etiology of tooth resorption. Evidence in support of this theory includes the correlation between cats with tooth resorption and increased blood levels of 25-hydroxyvitamin D, and histologic comparisons of the effects of excessive intake of vitamin D to the effects of tooth resorption. Because cats cannot synthesize vitamin D, they must rely on their diet to supply the nutritional requirement.

Definitive studies that document a cause-and-effect relationship implicating a single etiologic factor have not yet been done, and care must be taken to maintain distinctions between casual and causal relationships when evaluating current information. In addition, it is possible that tooth resorption has a multifactorial etiology, highlighting the complexity of the problem and emphasizing the need for additional research.

The Bibliography for **Box 47-3** can be found at www.markmorris.org.

MATERIA ALBA AND OTHER ORAL DEBRIS

Materia alba is a soft mixture of salivary proteins, bacteria, desquamated epithelial cells and leukocyte fragments. Materia alba and dental plaque are two distinct materials. Materia alba does not have the organized bacterial structure or the adherence properties of dental plaque (Schwartz et al, 1971); it can generally be washed off with a forced water spray. The role of materia alba in the etiopathogenesis of plaque accumulation and periodontal disease remains unclear.

Other debris commonly observed in the oral cavity of dogs and to some extent in cats includes food, impacted hair and miscellaneous foreign materials acquired through chewing behaviors. Food debris retained in the mouth after eating can usually be removed by the action of the tongue and saliva.

Dogs and cats fed soft, sticky foods, particularly those breeds compromised by occlusal abnormalities, may retain more food debris. No reports directly correlate retention of food debris with increased plaque accumulation and periodontal disease in dogs and cats. Egelberg reported that neither the frequency of feeding nor bypassing the oral cavity by tube feeding affected the accumulation of plaque and the development of gingivitis in a group of six mixed-breed dogs with medium to large body size (1965). The effect of food retention in small and brachycephalic breeds is unknown. Retained or impacted debris may act as a nidus for plaque accumulation and exacerbate gingival inflammation. The role of food type and texture in oral health and disease is discussed below.

DENTAL CALCULUS

Dental calculus is mineralized plaque. Calculus is a hard substrate formed by the interactions of salivary and crevicular calcium and phosphate salts with existing plaque. Dental calculus is observed frequently in dogs and cats (Harvey, 1992; Harvey et al, 1994; Richardson, 1965; Coignoul and Cheville, 1984) but differs in its composition. Feline calculus is comprised mostly of carbonate-containing hydroxyapatite, whereas canine calculus is comprised mostly of calcium carbonate (calcite) (Clarke, 1999; Legeros and Shannon, 1979). Calculus accumulates supragingivally and subgingivally; calculus deposits thicken with time. Undisturbed calculus is always covered by vital dental plaque. Aged calculus may chip or break off with mastication; however, a film of plaque remains that is rapidly mineralized. Calculus provides a roughened surface to enhance plaque attachment and accumulation and chronically irritates gingival tissues (Lindhe, 1989a; Mandel, 1990; Schroeder, 1969). A study in dogs demonstrated that calculus control in the absence of plaque control is cosmetic only; thus, preventive or therapeutic protocols to control periodontal disease should always include anti-plaque measures (Warrick et al, 2003).

DENTAL STAIN

Acquired dental stain (extrinsic stain) is initially stained pellicle that becomes part of the mineralized, layered laminate of pellicle, plaque and calculus. Dental stain occurs frequently in dogs (Schemehorn et al, 1982). Various nutritional, chemical and bacterial factors affect the presence and intensity of stain. Although nonpathogenic, dental stain is of aesthetic concern to pet owners and may signal teeth abnormalities.

Enamel staining (intrinsic stain) occurs due to trauma or antibiotic administration during development or before tooth eruption. Erupted teeth may also be injured with resulting discoloration due to hemorrhage into the dentinal tubules.

Enamel staining varies in intensity and distribution of discoloration and is distinguished from acquired stain by its irreversible nature (Robinson et al, 1983).

Pathophysiologic Basis of Clinical Signs

PERIODONTAL DISEASE

In susceptible patients, plaque accumulation along the gingival margin induces inflammation in adjacent gingival tissues. Without plaque removal or control, gingivitis progresses in severity to include local changes that allow subsequent bacterial colonization of subgingival sites. Inflammatory mediators damage the integrity of the gingival margin and sulcular epithelium, allowing further infiltration of bacteria. The immune response of the host attempts to localize the invasion of periodontal tissues; the result may be further destruction of local tissues due to cytokines released from inflammatory cells (Grove, 1982; Genco, 1984, 1990; DeBowes, 2000; Harvey, 2005).

Periodontal disease is episodic with periods of active tissue destruction followed by periods of inactivity and healing (**Figure 47-3**). Additionally, not all teeth are affected at the same rate or to the same degree. Periodontal disease begins with gingivitis and progresses through increased destruction of the periodontal apparatus, resulting in tooth mobility and eventual tooth loss. Generally, a stage classification system is used, beginning with a healthy periodontium and ending with tooth exfoliation (**Table 47-2** and **Figure 47-4**) (Wiggs and Lobprise, 1997a).

Periodontal disease is often a silent process that progresses without detection. Even in severe cases, dogs and cats may not demonstrate obvious discomfort. One signal often noticed by pet owners is oral malodor (Hennet et al, 1995), but even then, pet owners may not link bad breath to periodontal disease. Oral disease is a primary cause of offensive breath odor, but other metabolic processes may be involved (Tonzetich, 1977, 1978; Preti et al, 1992; Chen et al, 1970). A positive correlation between periodontal disease and malodor has been found in beagles (Simone et al, 1997).

Other signs of periodontal disease include: 1) accumulation of dental substrates on tooth surfaces, 2) gingival redness, 3) swelling and bleeding of the gingival margin, 4) gingival recession, 5) periodontal pocket formation, 6) accumulation of purulent material in the gingival sulcus or periodontal pocket and 7) tissue destruction with loss of attachment, furcation exposure and tooth mobility (**Table 47-3**).

Systemic Complications of Periodontal Disease

Periodontal disease may predispose affected pets to systemic complications. In people, periodontal disease has been linked to arthritis, low birth weight and pre-term birth, cardiovascular disease, stress and anxiety, diabetes, obesity and stroke (Hamilton, 2005; Mandel, 2004; Newman, 1996; O'Reilly and Claffey, 2000; Rutkauskas, 2000; Gaffar and Volpe, 2004; Klages et al, 2005; Roman, 2003; Dorfer et al, 2004).

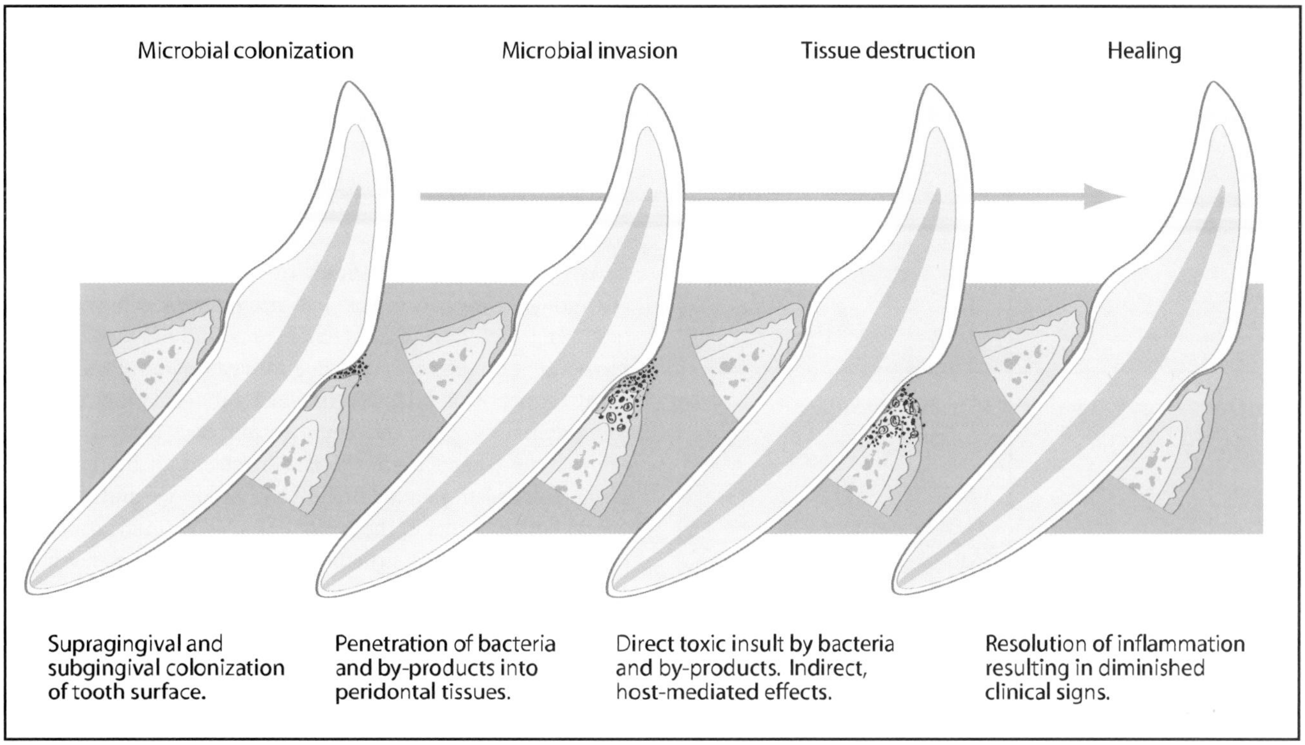
Microbial colonization
Microbial invasion
Tissue destruction
Healing
Supragingival and subgingival colonization of tooth surface.
Penetration of bacteria and by-products into peridontal tissues.
Direct toxic insult by bacteria and by-products. Indirect, host-mediated effects.
Resolution of inflammation resulting in diminished clinical signs.

Figure 47-3. Host-bacterial interactions in the pathogenesis of periodontal disease. Periodontal disease is cyclic with bursts of tissue destruction followed by periods of healing and relative quiescence. Four stages in the pathogenesis of periodontal disease have been proposed: 1) Microbial colonization. Salivary pellicle is deposited on the enamel surface and is soon colonized by oral bacteria that multiply forming plaque. 2) Microbial invasion. Plaque bacteria and their by-products invade the gingival tissues and initiate a host inflammatory response. 3) Tissue destruction. Direct toxic effects of bacteria and their by-products and indirect host-mediated toxic responses lead to destruction of periodontal tissue. 4) Healing. Periods of disease remission are characterized by a reduction in the inflammatory response and gingival healing. (Adapted from Genco RJ, Goldman HM, Cohen WD, eds. Contemporary Periodontics. St Louis, MO: CV Mosby Co, 1990; 189.)

Although much of the evidence is based on documentation of correlations between oral and systemic health, and the effect of systemic diseases on the health of the oral cavity (particularly in the case of diabetes) (Mealey, 1998; Levin et al, 1996), data are emerging that suggest a more causal and two-way relationship that makes a case for periodontal therapy as an adjunctive treatment to classic disease therapies (D'Aiuto et al, 2004; Montebugnoli et al, 2005; Montebugnoli, 2004; Farooqi et al, 2004; Kiran et al, 2005; Mealey, 2000; Miller et al, 1992; Pucher and Stewart, 2004; Taylor et al, 2004; Rahman et al, 2005; Mercanoglu et al, 2004).

In dogs, numerous reports speculate on the association between chronic periodontal disease and conditions affecting the heart valves and pulmonary airways (Hamlin, 1990; Prueter and Sherding, 1985; Calvert and Dow, 1990; Bonagura, 1981). Furthermore, a positive correlation has been found between the severity of periodontal disease and histopathologic changes in the kidneys, myocardium and liver (DeBowes et al, 1996). Periodontal infections allow bacterial migration into lymphatic and blood vessels, resulting in bacteremia and are associated with increased levels of many of the systemic markers associated with the diseases described above, including C-reactive protein, proinflammatory cytokines, serum cholesterol, plasma fibrinogen, white blood cells and blood glucose (Harari et al, 1993, 1991; Slade et al, 2000; Ide et al, 2004; D'Aiuto et al, 2004, 2005; Joshipura et al, 2004; Lowe, 2004; Holzhausen et al, 2004). The host defenses of normal healthy pets can effectively clear transient bacteremia; however, blood-borne bacteria may colonize distant sites in patients impairing immune function and/or compromising organ function, including development of atherosclerotic lesions (Calvert and Green, 1986; Glurich et al, 2002).

Table 47-2. Stages of periodontal disease.*

Stage 0	**Clinically normal** No gingival inflammation or periodontitis clinically evident.
Stage 1	**Gingivitis only** No attachment loss. Height and architecture of the alveolar margin are normal.
Stage 2	**Early periodontitis** Less than 25% attachment loss or Stage 1 furcation involvement in multirooted teeth.
Stage 3	**Moderate periodontitis** 25 to 50% attachment loss or Stage 2 furcation involvement in multirooted teeth.
Stage 4	**Advanced periodontitis** Greater than 50% attachment loss or Stage 3 furcation involvement in multirooted teeth.

*Adapted from AVDC.org. Wolf HF, Rateitschak EM, Rateitschak KH, et al. Color atlas of dental medicine: Periodontology, 3rd ed. Stuttgart, Germany: Georg Thieme Verlag, 2005.

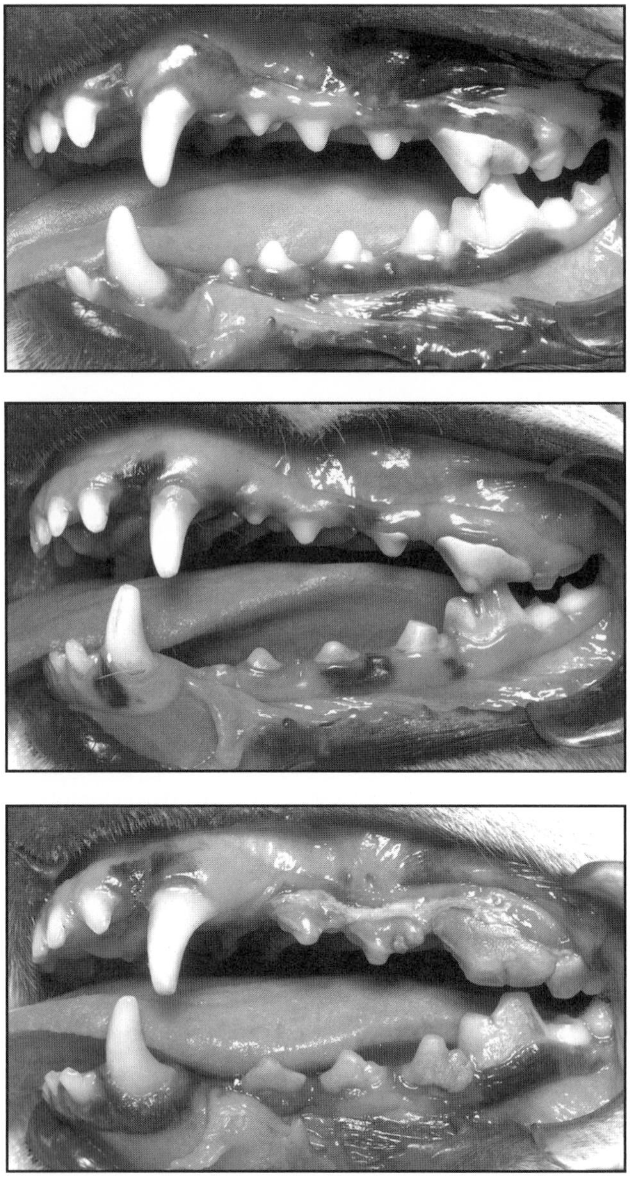

Figure 47-4. Photographic representations of mild, moderate and severe periodontal disease in dogs. (Top) Mild periodontal disease. Some accumulation of plaque and calculus is evident on tooth crowns. There is slight gingival recession around the maxillary canine tooth and the gingival margins are slightly rounded, particularly around the caudal premolar teeth. (Middle) Heavy plaque and calculus accumulation is evident on most teeth. Accumulations are abundant on the maxillary fourth premolar and first molar. A distinct margin of gingival inflammation is present around the maxillary fourth premolar. Inflammatory changes including swelling, reddening and recession are evident around most teeth. (Bottom) Gross plaque and calculus accumulation is present on premolar and molar teeth. Distinct marginal gingivitis with severe gingival recession and periodontal tissue loss is present. Impaction of hair and foreign material occurs commonly at sites of severe tissue destruction.

Key Nutritional Factors

The key nutritional factors for oral health should provide a sufficient level of plaque control to prevent periodontal disease and gingivitis. Proper food texture and composition can directly affect the oral environment through: 1) maintenance of tissue integrity, 2) alteration of bacterial plaque metabolism, 3) stimulation of salivary flow, 4) cleansing of tooth and oral surfaces by appropriate physical contact and/or 5) chelation of calculogenic constituents (**Box 47-4**). However, control of calculus is a secondary consideration because calculus control by itself has not been shown to decrease gingivitis and periodontal disease. Calculus along with stain and malodor are more of a cosmetic concern.

Assessing the relative efficacy of an oral health related key nutritional factor is complex. It is more practical to determine the overall benefit of these constituents in a finished product. However, it can be very confusing for veterinarians, and particularly for pet owners, to discern which products provide significant dental benefits and thus warrant use as oral hygiene agents. The Center for Veterinary Medicine of the Food and Drug Administration (CVM-FDA) monitors and regulates dental health claims in the United States. Cosmetic claims are not objectionable and structure-function claims are not stringently regulated; thus, the wide availability of products that make some type of plaque or calculus claim with little or no research to document their effectiveness. Phrases such as "cleans teeth, freshens breath" are commonplace on commercial food and treats packages. Because "crunchy" texture provides little dental benefit, the purported ability of these types of products to provide any significant level of oral hygiene is a misrepresentation to pet owners.

However, standardized scientific methods by which plaque (and calculus) accumulation are measured in dogs and cats for evaluating product efficacy have been established by the international veterinary dental community (Boyce, 1992; Logan and Boyce, 1994; SVOC, 1994; Harvey, 1995; Logan et al, 1995; Logan, 1996, 1996a; Hennet, 1999; Harvey, 2002; Hennet et al, 2006). **Box 47-5** discusses these methods and the VOHC Seal of Acceptance. The presence of a VOHC Seal of Acceptance for plaque or plaque and calculus and/or published evidence-based studies helps determine which products are effective.

Because foods that provide dental health benefits replace regular maintenance foods, several key nutritional factors are included because of their relationship to general health rather than specific benefits for periodontal disease. The key nutritional factors for dental foods for dogs and cats are summarized in **Table 47-4** and discussed in more detail below.

Food Texture

The physical consistency, or texture, of foods and treats has long been thought to affect the oral health of dogs and cats. Many of the recommendations made about the effect of food texture on oral health are unsubstantiated and several have turned out to be untrue when exposed to rigorous study, including "natural foods" (**Box 47-6**). However, food texture can be a very effective means of controlling dental plaque and ultimately periodontal disease.

Numerous studies have reported that dogs and cats fed soft foods have increased accumulation of plaque and calculus and a higher prevalence or severity of periodontal disease when com-

Table 47-3. Clinical signs associated with periodontal disease.

Anorexia	Red, swollen or bleeding gingivae
Behavioral changes	Substrate accumulation (plaque, calculus, stain)
Difficulty eating	Tooth mobility
Halitosis	Ulcerations on gingivae or oral mucosa
Head shaking	
Ptyalism	

Box 47-4. Hexametaphosphate and Tartar Control.

Calcium chelators such as hexametaphosphate (HMP) are sequestrants that bind salivary calcium, making it unavailable for incorporation into the plaque biofilm to form calculus. HMP is delivered as a coating on various treats, dental chews and foods. The purported benefits of these compounds are that they are released during chewing and remain for prolonged periods of time in the oral cavity. It has been demonstrated that the addition of HMP to the surface of baked biscuit treats, rawhide chews and dry foods results in reduced calculus accumulation. However, there is also evidence that shows no significant differences in plaque or calculus accumulation in dogs fed dry foods plus HMP-coated biscuits. Polyphosphates like HMP have no known direct effect on oral microflora populations or plaque accumulation. An effective plaque control regimen should always be the primary recommendation for prevention or post-therapeutic care of periodontal disease.

The Bibliography for **Box 47-4** can be found at www.markmorris.org.

pared with the same parameters in pets fed hard foods. These studies are difficult to compare because different methods were used to assess substrate accumulation and gingival health, and different populations of patients were studied.

Feeding recommendations for oral health commonly include feeding a dry pet food. Hard food purportedly increases mastication, which aids oral health by exercising the gums, increasing keratinization of the gingivae and reducing accumulation of plaque and calculus (O'Rourke, 1947). But many of the studies traditionally cited to substantiate claims that dry foods reduce accumulation of plaque and calculus are old reports that used small numbers of subjects, had varying evaluation methods and did not report data analysis (Burwasser and Hill, 1939; Egelberg, 1965a; Krasse and Brill, 1960; Studer and Stapley, 1973).

Consumption of soft foods may promote plaque accumulation. However, the general belief that dry foods provide significant oral cleansing should be regarded with skepticism. A moist food may perform similarly to a typical dry food in affecting plaque, stain and calculus accumulation (**Figure 47-5**) (Boyce and Logan, 1994). In a large epidemiologic survey, dogs consuming dry food alone did not consistently demonstrate improved periodontal health when compared with dogs eating moist foods (Harvey et al, 1996). Also, periodontal disease is the most common disease in dogs and cats (Lund et al, 1999); however, most dogs and cats eat dry foods.

Thus, typical commercial dry dog and cat foods contribute

Table 47-4. Key nutritional factors for foods for dogs and cats for prevention of periodontal disease and maintenance of overall health.*

Factors	Dogs	Cats
Food texture	VOHC Seal for plaque control	VOHC Seal for plaque control
Antioxidants		
Vitamin E (IU/kg)	≥400	≥500
Vitamin C (mg/kg)	≥100	100-200
Selenium (mg/kg)	0.5-1.3	0.5-1.3
Phosphorus (%)	0.4-0.8	0.5-0.8
Sodium (%)	0.2-0.4	0.2-0.5
Magnesium (%)	-	0.04-0.1
Average urinary pH	-	6.2-6.4

Key: VOHC = Veterinary Oral Health Council Seal of Acceptance for plaque control.
*All values are amounts in food on a dry matter basis unless otherwise stated.

Box 47-5. Veterinary Oral Health Council: A System for Recognizing Effective Veterinary Dental Products.

The Veterinary Oral Health Council (VOHC) was established in 1997 after 10 years of open meetings, which included representatives from the American Veterinary Dental College, Academy of Veterinary Dentistry, American Veterinary Dental Society, American Veterinary Medical Association, American Animal Hospital Association, United States Food and Drug Administration, private practice and industry. The purpose of the VOHC is to provide an independent, objective and credible means of recognizing veterinary dental products that effectively control accumulation of plaque and/or calculus (tartar). The VOHC system is similar to the American Dental Association (ADA) Seal of Acceptance system and is recognized worldwide.

The VOHC does not conduct efficacy testing; the council reviews results of tests performed in accordance with approved protocols set by the VOHC. The VOHC awards the Seal in two claim categories: 1) Helps control plaque and 2) Helps control tartar. It is important to recognize the difference between the two claims; plaque is the primary cause of periodontal disease and tartar control in the absence of plaque control is primarily cosmetic. If a product with the "helps control tartar" claim is recommended it is critical to recommend a proven plaque control method. In addition to noting the type of Seal awarded, it is important to be aware of the study design and application (feeding) recommendations associated with meeting the claim requirements. A product that is awarded the Seal based on a specific application (daily) may not perform similarly when applied less frequently.

The first canine and feline dental products to receive the VOHC Seal of Acceptance were Hill's Prescription Diet t/d Canine and t/d Feline, respectively. A complete list of products that have been awarded the VOHC Seal of Acceptance is available at vohc.org.

Box 47-6. Natural Food Sources and Periodontal Disease.

Early literature reported that the typical foods of wild canids and felids had a plaque-retardant effect and that wild canids and felids were not afflicted with the generalized form of periodontal disease seen in domesticated pets. Pet food commercialization is often implicated as a contributing factor to the increased prevalence and severity of periodontal disease in domestic dogs and cats (**Box 47-3**). The constituents of natural foods for wild canids and felids probably depend on geographic location, environmental season and individual hunting capabilities. However, historically a natural food refers to small rodents/mammals that would typically fall prey to wolves, coyotes, etc. Colyer specifically refers to "flesh that the animals must rend with their teeth." Wild canids in particular probably eat fruits and vegetables and an array of tissues including blood, intestines plus contents, muscle, cartilage, bone marrow and bones.

Despite these assertions, there are no published data that compare controlled populations of domestic dogs or cats consuming natural food sources with those consuming a commercial food. In addition, even if it were possible to make such comparisons, confounding variables might include dramatic changes in food form (moist, semi-moist, dry and evolving pet owner preferences) through development of commercial pet foods, specific nutrient variation and selective breeding, which has resulted in dramatic differences in body size and head types of dogs and cats.

Reports exist about the oral condition of small populations of dogs and cats consuming natural foods. One study involved 67 English foxhounds, one to nine years of age that were routinely fed raw carcasses consisting of the bony skeleton, muscle and associated tissues. Oral examinations revealed that all dogs had varying signs of periodontal disease as well as a high prevalence of tooth fractures. Another study examined 45 small feral cats from an Australian national park and reported conditions including calculus deposits, periodontal disease, fractured teeth, attrition and tooth resorption. Examination of gastrointestinal contents of these cats revealed the presence of natural food sources including small mammals, birds, lizards and insects. These findings cast skepticism on the long-held view that a natural food source prevents development of oral disease, particularly periodontal disease, in dogs and cats. **Box 47-8** describes the role of chew toys in periodontal health.

The Bibliography for **Box 47-6** can be found at www.markmorris.org.

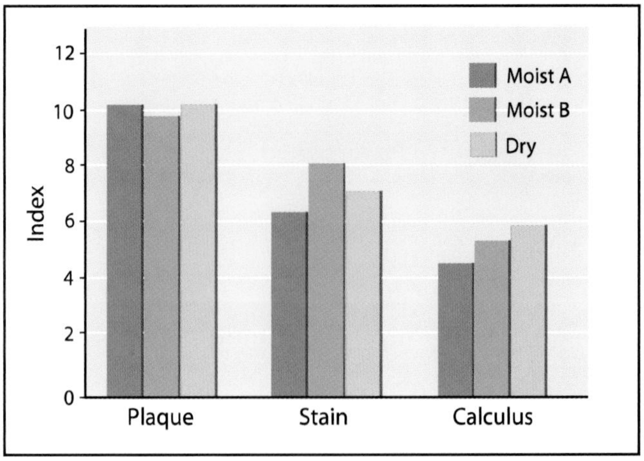

Figure 47-5. Comparison of plaque, stain and calculus accumulation in dogs fed a specialty brand moist food (Moist A), a grocery brand moist food (Moist B) and a grocery brand dry food. There is no significant difference in substrate accumulation among dogs fed the three foods. Moist foods do not always promote increased plaque and calculus formation in comparison to dry foods.

little dental cleansing. As a tooth penetrates a kibble or treat the initial contact causes the food to shatter and crumble with contact only at the coronal tip of the tooth surface (**Figure 47-6**). To provide effective mechanical cleansing, a food should promote chewing and maximize contact with the tooth surface (**Figure 47-6**).

Foods with enhanced textural characteristics promote oral health. Several maintenance pet foods are available that provide clinically significant oral cleansing compared with regular commercial dry or moist foods and/or snacks. Numerous studies have demonstrated that foods possessing an appropriate combination of shape, size and mechanical structure provide significant plaque, calculus and stain control in dogs and cats (Logan, 1996, 1996a; Boyce, 1992; Jensen et al, 1995; Logan et al, 1995; Finney, 1996). A six-month study investigating the effects of food on plaque accumulation and gingival inflammation in 40 adult mongrel dogs reported that dogs fed the test food had 39% less plaque accumulation and 36% less gingival inflammation than dogs fed the control food (**Figure 47-7**). These studies used a clean-tooth model in which plaque, calculus and stain were evaluated at a specified time following a dental prophylaxis.

One study reported that feeding a food with appropriate physical characteristics to beagles with existing plaque, calculus and gingivitis resulted in a significant decrease in mean plaque and calculus indices after two weeks and in the gingival index after six weeks (**Figure 47-8**). Beagles eating the control food had a significant increase in plaque and calculus accumulation and no change in gingival inflammation over the 16-week test period (Finney et al, 1996).

Fiber-containing foods have long been viewed as "nature's toothbrush." Investigators have theorized that fibrous foods: 1) exercise the gums, 2) promote gingival keratinization and 3) clean the teeth. Fiber in foods, especially as it relates to texture, has been shown to affect plaque and calculus accumulation and gingival health in dogs and cats (Watson, 1994; Boyce and Logan, 1994; Logan, 1996). Certain types of fiber combined with specific manufacturing processes can affect a food's texture. Fiber characteristics that maximize tooth contact time (e.g., orientation within the kibble matrix), combined with a size and shape that promote chewing, are critical to obtaining a dental benefit. A typical dry food does not possess the mechanical characteristics for adequate dental cleansing. Simply enlarging the kibble or varying the shape of the product is likewise inadequate. In the absence of effective plaque control

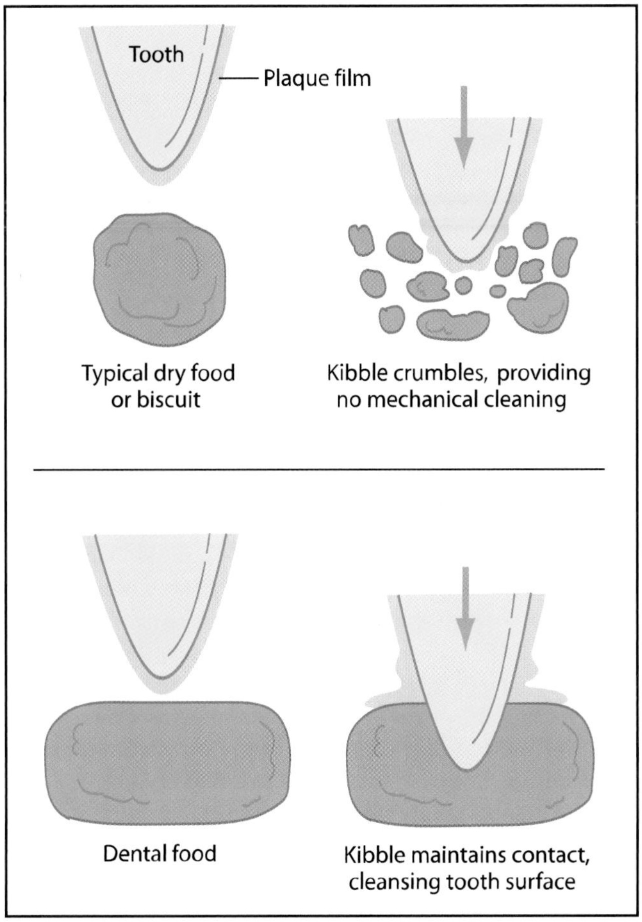

Figure 47-6. This illustration depicts the mechanical cleansing properties of commercial dog and cat foods. The top illustration demonstrates what occurs when a dog or cat chews a typical dry food. The kibble crumbles providing little to no mechanical cleansing. The bottom illustration demonstrates what happens when a dog or cat chews a dental food. The kibble stays together, maintaining contact with the tooth surface and providing mechanical cleansing.

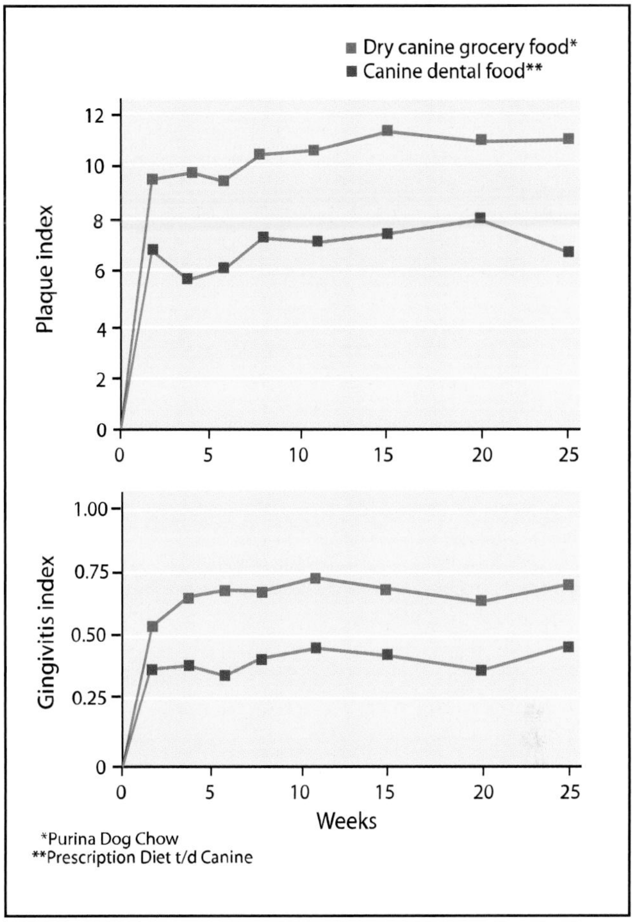

Figure 47-7. The effects of commercial dog foods on plaque accumulation and gingival health in dogs. These graphs compare plaque accumulation and gingival inflammation in dogs fed two different foods for six months. Each group of dogs began the study with a plaque index of zero and clinically healthy gingivae. At all time points, the dogs consuming the test food (Prescription Diet t/d Canine) had significantly lower scores for plaque accumulation and gingival inflammation than the dogs consuming the control food (Purina Dog Chow).

through other measures, or in cases demanding adjunctive plaque control, mechanical attenuation of plaque and calculus accumulation daily with a maintenance dental food is a reasonable alternative. Given the prevalence of periodontal disease in dogs and cats, effective homecare products that improve owner compliance can be a valuable addition to an oral health maintenance regimen.

One way to assess whether the texture of a specific dog or cat food is effective in preventing accumulation of dental plaque (or calculus) is whether or not the product's label carries the VOHC Seal of Acceptance, specifically stating that the product is effective in controlling plaque. Published Grade 1 or 2 evidence-based studies are also reliable indicators of product efficacy.

Antioxidants

Oxidative stress may be important in the etiology of periodontal disease. In one study, dogs with severe periodontitis had gingival crevicular fluid and serum with lower total antioxidant capacity than dogs with gingivitis or mild periodontitis (Pavlica et al, 2004). The body synthesizes many antioxidants but relies on food for others. Vitamins E and C and selenium are proposed as antioxidant key nutritional factors for foods for periodontal disease because: 1) they are biologically important, 2) they act synergistically (e.g., vitamin C and selenium-containing glutathione peroxidase regenerate vitamin E after it has reacted with a free radical) and 3) much is known about their safety.

VITAMIN E

Vitamin E (α-tocopherol) is the main lipid-soluble antioxidant in plasma, erythrocytes and tissues (NRC, 2006). It is one of the most effective antioxidants for protecting cell membrane constituent polyunsaturated fatty acids from oxidation. Vitamin E inhibits lipid oxidation by scavenging lipid peroxyl radicals faster than these radicals can react with adjacent fatty acids or membrane proteins (Gutteridge and Halliwell, 1994).

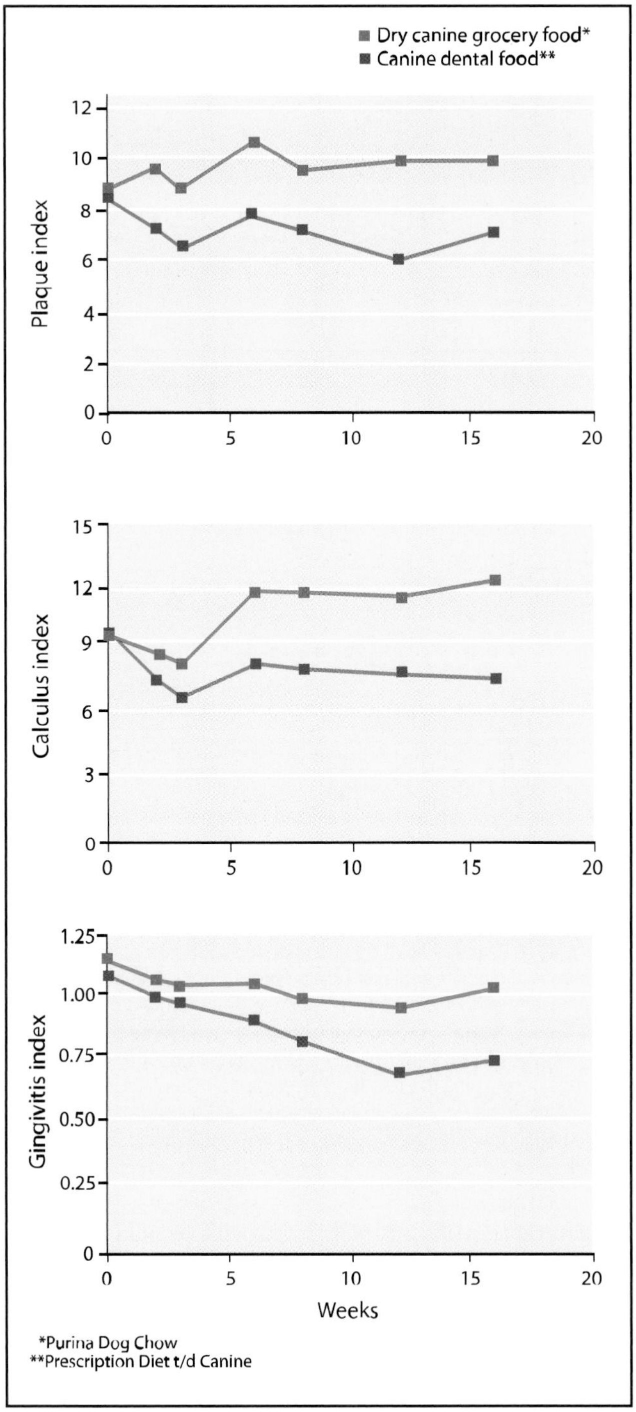

Figure 47-8. The effects of commercial dog foods on existing plaque, calculus and gingivitis in dogs. Each group of dogs entered the study with similar amounts of plaque, calculus and gingivitis. Dogs were fed either a control food (Purina Dog Chow) or a test food (Prescription Diet t/d Canine). Plaque, calculus and gingivitis were evaluated over a four-month period. Dogs eating the test food demonstrated a highly significant reduction in plaque, calculus and gingival inflammation whereas dogs eating the control food had a significant increase in plaque, a highly significant increase in calculus and no significant change in gingivitis.

Research indicates that a level of vitamin E higher than the requirement confers specific biologic benefits (Hayes et al, 1969; Hall et al, 2003; Meydani et al, 1998; Jewell et al, 2002). Based on antioxidant biomarker studies in dogs and cats, for improved antioxidant performance, foods for oral health should contain at least 400 IU/kg dry matter (DM) (dog foods) and at least 500 IU/kg DM (cat foods) (Jewell et al, 2000).

VITAMIN C

Vitamin C (ascorbic acid), is the most powerful reducing agent available to cells. Ascorbic acid: 1) regenerates oxidized vitamin E, glutathione and flavonoids, 2) quenches free radicals intra- and extracellularly, 3) protects against free radical-mediated protein inactivation associated with oxidative bursts of neutrophils, 4) keeps transition metals in reduced form and 5) may quench free radical intermediates of carcinogen metabolism.

Although dogs and cats can synthesize enough vitamin C to fulfill minimum requirements (Naismith, 1958), in vitro studies indicated that dogs and cats have from one-quarter to one-tenth the ability to synthesize vitamin C as other mammals (Chatterjee et al, 1975). Whether or not this translates to a reduced ability in vivo is unknown. For improved antioxidant performance, and in conjunction with recommended levels of vitamin E, foods for adult dogs and cats should contain at least 100 and 100 to 200 mg vitamin C/kg DM, respectively.

SELENIUM

Glutathione-peroxidase is a selenium-containing antioxidant enzyme that defends tissues against oxidative stress by catalyzing the reduction of H_2O_2 and organic hydroperoxides and by regenerating vitamin E. The minimum requirement for selenium in foods for dogs and cats is 0.13 mg/kg DM (Wedekind et al, 2003, 2003a). Animal studies and clinical intervention trials in people have shown selenium to be anticarcinogenic at levels much higher (five to 10 times) than the recommended allowances for people or the minimal requirements for dogs and cats (Combs, 2001; Neve, 2002). Therefore, for increased antioxidant benefits, the recommended range of selenium for dog and cat foods is 0.5 to 1.3 mg/kg DM.

Phosphorus, Sodium, Magnesium and Urinary pH

Phosphorus and sodium are considered key nutritional factors for apparently healthy adult dogs and cats for purposes of ameliorating or slowing the progression of subclinical kidney disease and/or hypertension. The recommended allowances for phosphorus and sodium in foods for adult dogs are 0.4 to 0.8% and 0.2 to 0.4% DM, respectively. For foods for adult cats, the recommended allowances for phosphorus and sodium are 0.5 to 0.8% and 0.2 to 0.5% DM, respectively. In addition, for adult cats, magnesium and urinary pH are also key nutritional factors, based on their role in feline lower urinary tract disease. The recommended allowance for magnesium in foods for adult cats is 0.04 to 0.1% DM. Foods for adult cats should produce a urinary pH in the range of 6.2 to 6.4. For more information see Chapters 13 and 20.

Other Nutritional Factors

Calcium

Foods deficient in calcium and excessive in phosphorus may lead to secondary nutritional hyperparathyroidism and significant loss of alveolar bone (Bawden et al, 1995; Becks and Weber, 1931). Experiments in dogs have demonstrated resorption of alveolar bone following consumption of a food with a low ratio of calcium to phosphorus (Henrikson, 1968). Krook and colleagues proposed that periodontal disease results from a nutritional deficiency of calcium, an excess of phosphorus or both (1972, 1972a). Svanberg and colleagues reported that nutritional secondary hyperparathyroidism occurred in a group of beagles fed a food deficient in calcium. The food did not have any effect on the initiation or rate of progression of periodontal disease when compared with findings in a control group fed a nutritionally adequate food (1973). It is unlikely that dietary deficiencies in calcium and phosphorus are primary causes of periodontal disease; however, they may contribute to the progression of the disease process and exacerbate bone loss. Calcium deficiency occurs rarely in dogs and cats that consume commercial pet foods that contain calcium levels that meet Association of American Feed Control Officials' (AAFCO) allowances (2007). Improperly formulated homemade foods are more likely to be deficient in calcium.

Vitamin Deficiencies

Adequate vitamin content can be a problem in improperly formulated homemade foods. Vitamins that have been studied in relation to periodontal disease include A, B, C, D and E. Vitamin A deficiencies have been reported to cause marginal gingivitis, gingival hypoplasia and resorption of alveolar bone (King, 1940; Reifen, 2002). Deficiencies of B-complex vitamins (including folic acid, niacin, pantothenic acid and riboflavin) have been associated with gingival inflammation, epithelial necrosis and resorption of alveolar bone (Becks et al, 1943). Vitamin C, besides functioning as an antioxidant (discussed above), also plays a key role in collagen synthesis. Ascorbic acid deficiencies reportedly affect periodontal tissues adversely in people, including gingival inflammation (Ismail, 1983; Leggott et al, 1986). Vitamin D helps regulate serum calcium concentrations. Vitamin D deficiencies affect calcium homeostasis and reportedly affect the gingivae, periodontal ligament and alveolar bone (Becks and Weber, 1931). Deficiencies of these vitamins are highly unlikely to occur in dogs and cats fed commercial foods that contain levels that meet AAFCO allowances.

Vitamin E is an antioxidant and in one study, dogs with more severe periodontitis also had lower total antioxidant capacity of their gingival crevicular fluid and serum than dogs with gingivitis or mild periodontitis (Pavlica et al, 2004).

FEEDING PLAN

How to Feed Dogs and Cats for Optimal Oral Health

If properly fed as puppies and kittens (**Box 47-7**), most dogs and cats enter adulthood with healthy mouths. In most cases, periodontal disease can be prevented with appropriate plaque control. The level of plaque control necessary to maintain oral health must be assessed for each individual patient. Frequent plaque removal (daily, if possible) is widely recommended. Brushing, when done correctly and conscientiously, is a very effective method for achieving the level of plaque control necessary to control gingivitis.

After oral disease is present, it should be treated with appropriate professional therapy. However, aftercare, or continued dental hygiene provided by the pet owner, will determine the overall success of professional therapy. A regimen of soft food may be recommended after invasive or advanced procedures during the initial healing phase. Chemical plaque control should be provided in these instances until mechanical plaque control can be resumed. However, many pets can resume their normal food regimen immediately after receiving professional care, provided the client has been instructed in appropriate plaque control procedures (**Box 47-1**).

If the pet owner is able to provide effective plaque control through toothbrushing, then an oral benefit from foods and/or treats may be of less concern (Lindhe and Rylander, 1975; Tromp et al, 1986, 1986a). Realistically, however, compliance with toothbrushing is a problem for many pet owners. In addition, certain patients may require aggressive plaque control combined with frequent professional care to maintain optimal oral health. Thus, in many cases, a food/treat approach to plaque control is necessary. The feeding plan includes assessing and selecting the best food and feeding methods for the individual patient.

Assess and Select the Food

After the oral and general health status of the patient has been assessed and the key nutritional factors and their target levels have been determined, the adequacy of the food can be assessed. The steps to assessing foods include: 1) assuring the nutritional adequacy of the food by a credible regulatory agency such as AAFCO and 2) comparing the food's key nutritional factors with the recommended levels. Because dental foods are used in place of regular maintenance foods, the key nutritional

Box 47-7. Feeding Puppies and Kittens for Optimal Dentition.

Puppies and kittens are born edentulous. However, the nutrition they receive from the bitch or queen can affect oral development. The bitch or queen should receive an appropriate growth/lactation food during lactation to ensure adequate milk production and to meet ongoing needs. Deciduous teeth begin to erupt at about three weeks of age. Most puppies and kittens can be given access to soft food at this age. Full deciduous dentition should be present in puppies by 12 weeks of age and in kittens by six weeks of age. The permanent tooth bud will already be formed, so it is essential to dental health that puppies and kittens receive appropriate nutrition during the early weeks of development. This is also the ideal time to train a pet to accept oral hygiene.

Table 47-5. Key nutritional factor content of selected dry commercial dog foods marketed for dental health compared to recommended levels.*

Factors	VOHC Seal for plaque control (Yes/No)	Vitamin E (IU/kg)	Vitamin C (mg/kg)	Selenium (mg/kg)	Phosphorus (%)	Sodium (%)
Recommended levels	**Yes**	**≥400**	**≥100**	**0.5-1.3**	**0.4-0.8**	**0.2-0.4**
Hill's Prescription Diet t/d Canine	Yes	652	79	0.50	0.40	0.22
Hill's Prescription Diet t/d Small Bites Canine	Yes	652	79	0.50	0.40	0.22
Hill's Science Diet Adult Oral Care	Yes	564	175	0.62	0.65	0.24
Medi-Cal Dental Formula	No	na	na	na	0.90	0.40
Purina Veterinary Diet DH Dental Health	No	1,171	na	na	1.25	0.57
Purina Veterinary Diet DH Dental Health Small Bites	No	1,169	na	na	1.24	0.61
Royal Canin Veterinary Diet Dental DD 20	No	604	na	0.44	0.66	0.38
Royal Canin Veterinary Diet Dental DS 23 Small Breed	No	725	na	0.44	0.66	0.77

Key: VOHC = Veterinary Oral Health Council Seal of Acceptance for plaque control, na = information not available from manufacturer.
*All values are amounts in food on a dry matter basis unless otherwise stated.

Table 47-6. Key nutritional factor content of selected dry commercial cat foods marketed for dental health compared to recommended levels.*

Factors	VOHC Seal for plaque control (Yes/No)	Vitamin E (IU/kg)	Vitamin C (mg/kg)	Selenium (mg/kg)	Phosphorus (%)	Sodium (%)	Magnesium (%)	Urinary pH
Recommended levels	**Yes**	**≥500**	**100-200**	**0.5-1.3**	**0.5-0.8**	**0.2-0.5**	**0.04-0.1**	**6.2-6.4**
Hill's Prescription Diet t/d Feline	Yes	811	83	0.59	0.80	0.33	0.065	6.34
Hill's Science Diet Adult Oral Care	Yes	670	171	0.55	0.75	0.37	0.058	6.30
Medi-Cal Dental Formula	No	na	na	na	0.70	0.60	na	na
Purina Veterinary Diets DH Dental Health	Yes	722	na	na	1.50	0.63	0.10	na
Royal Canin Veterinary Diet Dental DD 27	No	710	na	0.34	0.81	0.65	0.097	na

Key: VOHC = Veterinary Oral Health Council Seal of Acceptance for plaque control, na = information not available from manufacturer.
*All values are amounts in food on a dry matter basis unless otherwise stated.

factors include those for promoting long-term general health by managing certain other important disease risk factors.

Besides providing the recommended levels of key nutritional factors, **Tables 47-5** and **47-6** provide key nutritional factor profiles for selected commercial foods marketed to provide a dental benefit for dogs and cats, respectively. Special emphasis should be given to the presence of the VOHC Seal of Acceptance for plaque control. If the food in question cannot be found in this table, contact the manufacturer. Manufacturers' addresses, websites and toll-free customer service numbers are listed on pet food labels. If the manufacturer cannot provide the necessary information, consider switching to a food for which this information is available. Optimal nutrient balance is critical to overall health and should not be overlooked when assessing whether a food or treat is appropriate for periodontal health. Thus, it is important that a dental food or treat provide optimal nutritional balance for dogs and cats for their lifestage. Comparing a food's key nutritional factor content with the recommended levels is fundamental to food selection.

Another criterion for selecting a food that may become increasingly important in the future is evidence-based clinical nutrition. Practitioners should know how to determine risks and benefits of nutritional regimens and counsel pet owners accordingly. Currently, veterinary medical education and continuing education are not always based on rigorous assessment of evidence for or against particular management options. Still, studies have been published to establish the nutritional benefits of certain pet foods. Chapter 2 describes evidence-based clinical nutrition in detail and applies its concepts to various veterinary therapeutic foods. Evidence Grade 1 (the highest level) and Grade 2 exist for foods that confer dental benefits for cats and dogs, respectively.[a,b]

Treats are often considered for their purported dental benefits, as well as a reward. From a strictly nutritional standpoint, small amounts of treats (less than 10% of the total food intake) will not importantly affect a pet's overall daily nutrient intake. Excessive feeding of treats, however, can markedly affect a food's cumulative nutritional profile. Therefore, it is important to assess the impact of treats with respect to the dietary needs of individual dogs or cats.

The impact of treats on daily nutrient intake depends on three factors: 1) the nutrient profile of the treat, 2) the number

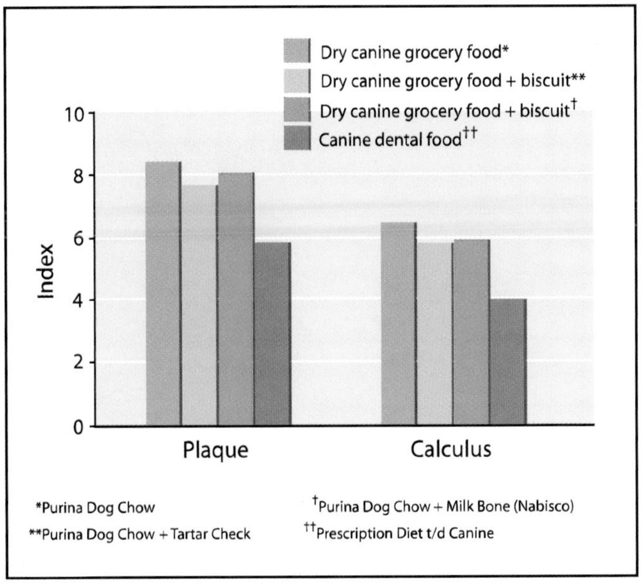

Figure 47-9. The effects of four different food regimens on plaque and calculus accumulation in dogs. Forty mongrel dogs were fed one of four food regimens: 1) Control (Purina Dog Chow), 2) Control plus two hexametaphosphate-coated biscuits/day (Tartar Check), 3) Control plus seven medium or four large (based on manufacturer's feeding directions) plain biscuits/day (Milk Bone) or 4) Prescription Diet t/d Canine. There was no significant difference in plaque or calculus accumulation in dogs fed Purina Dog Chow or Purina Dog Chow plus Milk Bone or Tartar Check biscuits. Dogs fed Prescription Diet t/d Canine had significantly less accumulation of plaque and calculus than dogs fed Purina Dog Chow or Purina Dog Chow plus Milk Bone or Tartar Check biscuits.

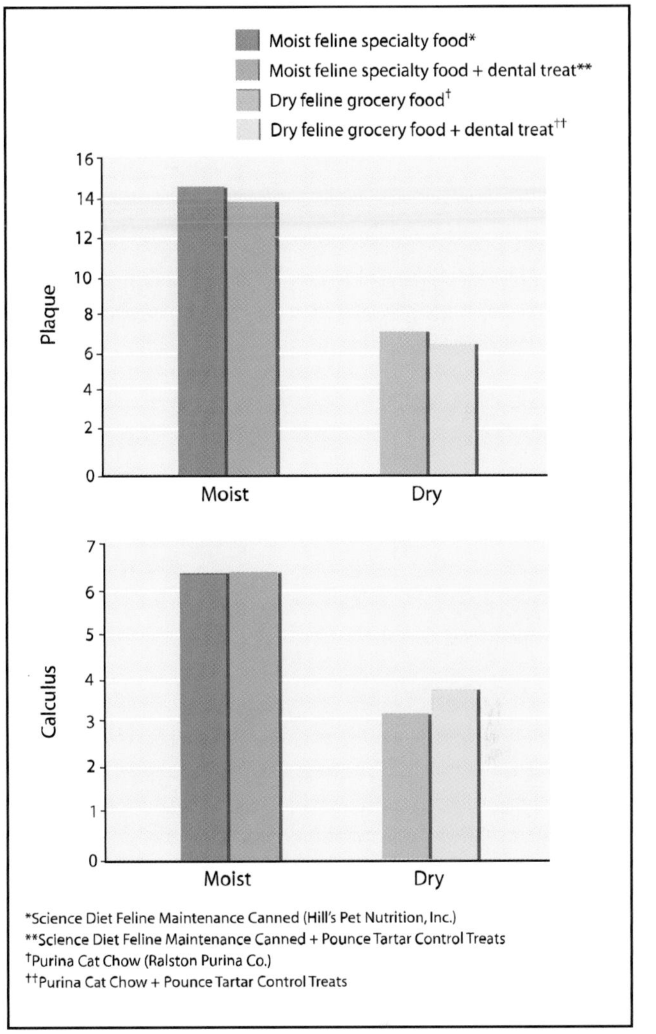

Figure 47-10. The effects of "dental" treats in cats fed commercial dry or moist foods. The top graph illustrates plaque accumulation in cats fed a moist or dry cat food or the same food plus dental treats. The bottom graph illustrates calculus accumulation in cats fed moist cat food or the same food plus dental treats. There was no significant difference in plaque or calculus accumulation with the addition of dental treats to either a dry or a moist cat food.

of treats provided daily and 3) the nutrient composition of the patient's regular food. Because meeting nutrient requirements is not the primary reason pet owners provide treats, commercial treats often are not complete and balanced. (See package labels.) If treats are fed, recommend that they be commercial treats that match the key nutritional factor profile recommended for the patient's lifestage. Generally, feeding excessive amounts (>10% of the total food intake on a volume or calorie basis) of any treat is not recommended. Ideally, the nutritional composition of treats and food should be combined and assessed as the entire dietary regimen. From a dental benefit standpoint, the efficacy of treats and non-food items such as rawhide chews should be evaluated just like dental foods. The safety of such products should also be considered.

Plain baked biscuits, although long thought of as "dental" treats, provide little additional plaque and calculus reduction when compared with feeding dry dog food alone (**Figure 47-9**). Additionally, manufacturers of some feline treats make a calculus control claim;[c,d] however, two studies have failed to demonstrate an effect on plaque and calculus accumulation compared with feeding dry or moist foods alone (Logan, 1996a; Logan et al, 1997). **Figure 47-10** describes the effect of dental treats on plaque and calculus accumulation in cats fed dry and moist foods with and without supplemental treats.

The addition of hexametaphosphate (HMP) (**Box 47-4**) to the surface of baked biscuits[e] significantly reduced calculus accumulation in beagles over a four-week period compared with a regimen of plain baked biscuits and dry food alone (Stookey et al, 1995, 1996). One three-week study, however, demonstrated no significant differences in plaque and calculus accumulation in dogs fed dry food, dry food plus baked biscuits or dry food plus HMP-coated biscuits.[f] A treat made of rice and whey and formed into a bone shape[g] to promote chewing activity has been reported to reduce plaque and calculus accumulation in small dogs over a four-week period (Gorrel and Rawlings, 1996). The disadvantages of these products may include pet acceptance, potential for gastrointestinal side effects, cost of the recommended feeding dosage and nutritional influences such as caloric excess and nutrient imbalances (Crane, 1990).

Box 47-8. Chew Toys and Periodontal Disease in Dogs and Cats.

Chew toys are a category of products that claim an oral benefit for dogs (**Figure 1**). Many varieties are available with claims ranging from "flosses teeth" to "reduces harmful plaque;" however, few data in the literature substantiate these claims. One report claimed less calculus accumulation in 14 of 20 client-owned dogs when dogs were allowed access to a urethane chewing device[a] for one month. Anecdotal reports of oral trauma (e.g., gingival lacerations and tooth fractures) resulting from aggressive chewing of some dental toys can also be found in the veterinary dental literature.

ENDNOTE

a. Nylabone. Nylabone Products, Neptune, NJ, USA.

The Bibliography for **Box 47-8** can be found at www.markmorris.org.

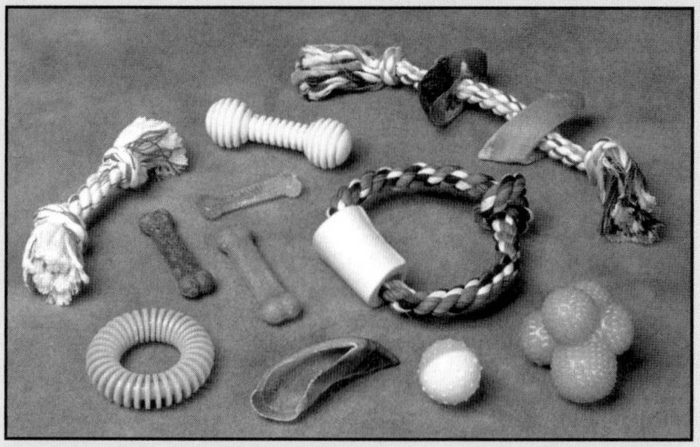

Figure 1. Manufacturers of many toys and devices make dental claims. Some of these claims include, "removes/reduces tartar, massages gums and flosses teeth." In most cases, no scientific studies substantiate these claims and pet owners can easily be misled. There is clinical evidence, however, that suggests gum lacerations and fractured teeth may result from inappropriate use of toys and devices, including failure to match toy size to pet size, use of hard toys, particularly with puppies and toy use with pets that chew aggressively.

Besides commercial treats, rawhide strips have been reported to control calculus accumulation, provided the dog actively chews the strips daily (Lage et al, 1990). Two rawhide chews each day are typically recommended.[h] Compacted rawhide treats in the shape of balls and bones can cause tooth fractures if chewed aggressively or if used as "catch" toys. Flat rawhide chews coated with an enzymatic system[i] are also available commercially; however, there are no published data demonstrating that these products are any more effective than plain rawhide strips. Although not foods, chew toys are a category of chewable products that claim an oral benefit for dogs. Box 47-8 provides a brief discussion of the potential benefits vs. risks of these products.

Assess and Select the Feeding Method

The method of feeding is often not altered in the nutritional management of periodontal disease. If a new food is fed, the amount to feed can be determined from the amount of the previous food being fed (calorie basis), particularly if the patient is in optimal body condition (body condition score of 2.5/5 to 3.5/5). The food dosage may need to be changed if the caloric density of the new food differs from that of the previous food. Otherwise product labels or other supporting materials can be used as starting points. The food dosage and feeding method should be altered if the patient's body weight and condition are suboptimal. Initially, the patient should be weighed every two weeks or so to ensure the food dosage is correct. Although most healthy dogs and cats do not experience digestive upsets with typical food changes, a gradual transition to a new food may benefit some patients. Progressively exchanging the new food for the usual food over four to seven days will minimize untoward effects and food refusal. Chapter 1 contains more in depth information about feeding methods and food transitions.

Good compliance is necessary for effective clinical nutrition. Enabling compliance includes limiting access to other foods and knowing who feeds the pet. Communicating the need for and the methods of effective plaque control may improve oral hygiene compliance.

REASSESSMENT

Monitoring depends on the: 1) degree of oral pathology, 2) level of periodontal therapy and 3) ability of the owner to provide routine oral hygiene. An annual oral examination and professional prophylaxis should be adequate for adult dogs and cats with good oral health and normal occlusion. As the severity of oral disease increases, the degree of periodontal therapy required to treat the condition will increase as well. An increased level of oral hygiene will be necessary to prevent disease progression toward advanced stages of periodontal disease (e.g., periodontitis, etc.).

Initially, patients should be rechecked weekly to monitor healing and oral hygiene. If both are satisfactory, the time between recalls can increase to three-month intervals. If the patient has severe pathology affecting plaque retention or if the owner is unable to provide effective plaque control, the time between periodontal therapies will need to be adjusted to maintain oral health. These recommendations are initial guidelines. Veterinarians must decide appropriate recall for each case, depending on the degree of oral pathology, periodontal therapy and owner compliance.

ACKNOWLEDGMENTS

The authors and editors acknowledge the contributions of Drs. Karl Zetner and John J. Hefferren in the previous edition of Small Animal Clinical Nutrition.

ENDNOTES

a. Prescription Diet t/d Feline. Hill's Pet Nutrition, Inc., Topeka, KS, USA.
b. Prescription Diet t/d Canine. Hill's Pet Nutrition, Inc., Topeka, KS, USA.
c. Pounce Tartar and Plaque Control. Del Monte Pet Products, Pittsburgh, PA, USA.
d. Whisker Lickin's Tartar Control Treats. Nestle Purina Pet Care Products, St. Louis, MO, USA.
e. Tartar Check. Del Monte Pet Products, Pittsburgh, PA, USA.
f. Logan EI. Unpublished data. December 1996.
g. Pedigree Dentabone. Kal Kan Foods, Vernon, CA, USA.
h. Purina Chew-eez. Nestle Purina Pet Care Products, St. Louis, MO, USA.
i. C.E.T. Chews. Virbac Animal Health, Ft. Worth, TX, USA.

REFERENCES

The references for **Chapter 47** can be found at www.markmorris.org.

CASE 47-1

Oral Foreign Body in a Doberman Pinscher

Robert B. Wiggs, DVM, Dipl. AVDC
Coit Road Animal Hospital
Dallas, Texas, USA

Patient Assessment

A five-year-old, 30-kg, male Doberman pinscher was presented for removal of a large beef knucklebone that was lodged in its mouth. The dog was excited, salivating profusely and difficult to handle. The bone was lodged caudal to the canine teeth between the dental arcades and was holding the dog's mouth open to the point of causing strain upon the jaws. Attempts to remove the bone while the patient was awake were unsuccessful. The dog's excited condition and the obstructing bone made a complete physical and oral examination impossible before sedation. After the dog was sedated, it was possible to gradually extricate the bone without further damaging the teeth or oral tissues (**Figures 1A** and **1B**). The dog was intubated and anesthetized to allow a comprehensive oral examination.

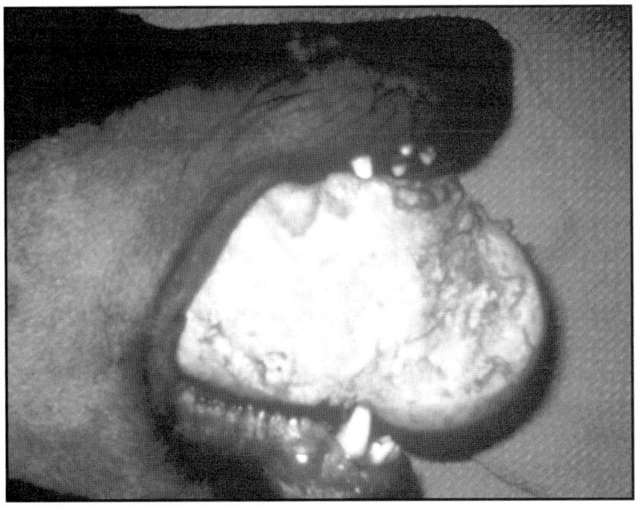

Figure 1A. A large bone lodged in the oral cavity of a Doberman pinscher.

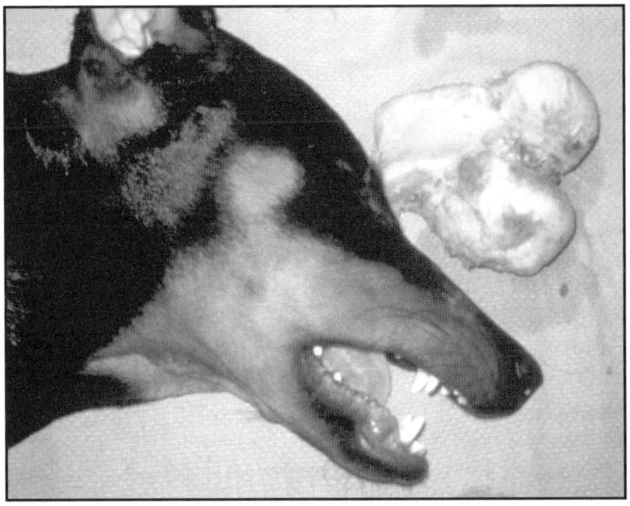

Figure 1B. The same patient after the bone was removed. Note the size of the bone in relation to the patient's head and mouth.

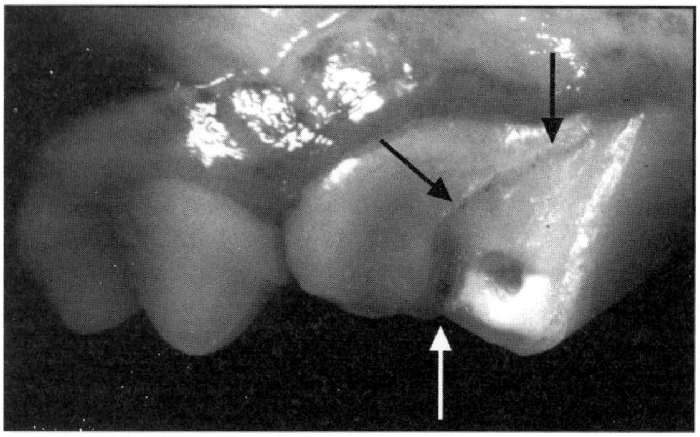

Figure 2. Slab fracture (dark arrows) of the maxillary fourth premolar with an exposed pulp chamber (white arrow).

The jaw had a full range of movement and no crepitation was detected over the temporomandibular joints. A laceration about 7 mm long and of moderate depth was found ventrally on the right side of the tongue in the proximity of the distal premolars. This laceration probably occurred as a result of the tongue pressing against the lower premolars.

The right carnassial teeth (maxillary fourth premolar and mandibular first molar) had Class VI/VI, cusp-type slab fractures. A slab of tooth was lost from the buccal side of the maxillary fourth premolar (**Figure 2**) and from the lingual side of the mandibular first molar. This type of injury commonly affects these tooth surfaces. Both fractures involved the pulp chamber; the exposed sites were dark and open. The pulp of these teeth was nonvital. Calculus accumulation and gingivitis were present on both arcades.

Assess the Food and Feeding Method

The owner had been feeding the dog various dry commercial dog foods sometimes mixed with water or moist foods. When the dog was examined and vaccinated by the referring veterinarian approximately seven months earlier, the owner had been informed that the teeth were in generally good shape but there was slight calculus accumulation. The veterinarian had recommended a dental prophylaxis, which the owner declined. Shortly thereafter, the owner had begun feeding bones to the dog at the suggestion of a friend who said that bones could clean the dog's teeth. All bones had been cooked before they were given to the dog. This was the first time the dog had received a large knucklebone.

Questions

1. What are the treatment options for the two fractured teeth?
2. What safety concerns are associated with feeding bones to dogs?
3. What recommendations should be made concerning the dog's food?
4. When should a dog's teeth be cleaned?

Answers and Discussion

1. There are typically six options for treating fractured teeth: 1) leave them as they are, 2) smooth the fractured edges and seal the dentinal tubules, 3) place a restoration, 4) perform a pulp capping, 5) perform a root canal or 6) extraction. Small enamel chips of vital teeth may be left as is; however, the jagged edges of these teeth should be smoothed. In this case, the pulp was exposed; therefore, leaving the teeth untreated could lead to abscessation or more likely to a chronic active granuloma at the root apex or tip. Chronic shedding of bacteria into the bloodstream may gradually damage organs such as the heart, kidneys and liver. It would be medically unsound to leave these teeth untreated. The most common repair technique for fractures of vital teeth that extend into the dentin is to smooth the fracture edges and seal the dentinal tubules with a dentinal bonding agent and possibly apply a restorative agent. This technique is also used in association with a pulp capping or root canal procedure. For this patient, this treatment would be appropriate only if done in conjunction with an endodontic procedure. Restoratives, such as a metal, composite, glass, porcelain or porcelain fused to a metal crown or inlay, are also used to repair fractures of vital teeth that extend into the dentin. These are also used in association with a pulp capping or endodontic procedure. Treatment with a restorative would be appropriate for this dog only in conjunction with an endodontic procedure. Pulp capping procedures are used for repair of fractured teeth with pulp exposure in which the pulp is still vital or alive. Successful pulp capping procedures inconsistently maintain the vitality of the tooth. At least 20% of the procedures fail even when performed under optimal circumstances. The severity of the trauma, amount of contamination, elapsed exposure time and degree of pulp exposure all play a crucial role in the success of pulp capping procedures. In this case, the teeth have Class VI/VI fractures and the pulp is nonvital, so a pulp capping procedure would be inappropriate.

   Root canal or complete endodontic procedures are used when fractured teeth have pulp cavity exposure and the pulp is either in a state of irreversible pulpitis or already nonvital. A root canal procedure is an option for this patient. The determining factors for selecting this treatment include the extent of damage to the tooth crown, the state of the external root structure, the condition of the pulp cavity, the status of the periodontal tissues and the ability of the owner to eliminate or nullify causative agents. If these conditions are all favorable, this procedure plus some form of restoration would be the treatment of choice to maintain the function of the carnassial teeth.

   The above procedures require advanced training and dental equipment. Extraction (exodontia) is a treatment option for damaged teeth, teeth affected by severe periodontal disease, highly mobile teeth that cannot be stabilized and teeth with root fractures. The tooth type and location, number of roots, status of surrounding periodontal tissues and supporting bone and indications of root abnormalities (i.e., dilacerated, ankylosed, etc.) determine the type of extraction process. Extraction is a reasonable alternative for veterinarians who lack the training or equipment to perform the treatments discussed above.

2. Some pet owners believe that feeding cooked bones to domesticated pets helps control calculus accumulation. However, there are no reliable, published studies showing dental benefits derived from bone chewing. This practice has gradually fallen into disfavor among many veterinarians because bone consumption often results in health problems such as fractured teeth, bone lodgments, constipation, intestinal or rectal blockages and esophageal, gastric and intestinal perforations.

   Recently, some veterinarians have again begun recommending the feeding of bones. However, the recommendation is to feed raw bones with meat attached, sometimes designated "raw and meaty bones." Current theory proposes that uncooked bones are not as hard as cooked bones and do not fracture teeth or cause other problems associated with cooked bones. However, anecdotal reports suggest the health concerns presented with cooked bones also occur commonly with raw, meaty bones. Feeding raw, whole chicken or chicken parts has been suggested as providing dental benefits without the risk of dental fractures because chicken bones are smaller. However, feeding raw meats, particularly chicken, raises food safety concerns (Chapter 11). The safety and efficacy of feeding bones, regardless of type, remain undetermined. Veterinarians should be cautious about recommending bones for dental benefits.

3. There is little reliable scientific information about the dental benefits of most commercial dog and cat foods or about the dental benefits of one food compared with those of another. In general, dry foods have been accepted as causing less calculus and plaque accumulation than moist foods, even though controversies and inconsistencies exist in the literature. A commercial canine veterinary therapeutic food, Prescription Diet t/d Canine[a] has valid data documenting effective dietary cleansing. Research has demonstrated this food influences the control or reduction of plaque, calculus, stain and gingivitis. Prescription Diet t/d Canine would be an appropriate food for this dog.

4. Teeth cleaning and professional dental prophylaxis are not always synonymous. The term prophylaxis means to prevent disease, whereas teeth cleaning means to prevent or treat disease. Teeth should be cleaned when calculus accumulations occur, or when stomatitis and periodontal disease develop. The professional dental prophylaxis, if taken literally, must be performed at intervals needed to prevent stomatitis or periodontal disease from developing. There are no definitive time intervals for the veterinary professional dental prophylaxis. The veterinarian must combine information about the pet's health status, oral and tooth pathology, degree of successful homecare, foods offered to the pet and the pet's chewing behavior to customize a professional dental prophylaxis program. A reasonable starting point is every six to 12 months for large-breed dogs.

Progress Notes

The tongue laceration was sutured and a comprehensive oral examination was completed at the initial visit. The clinical findings and treatment options were discussed with the owner. Three days after the original incident, a root canal procedure was performed on the dog's two fractured carnassial teeth and the tooth crowns were prepared for restoration. A dental prophylaxis was also performed at that time. About two weeks later the crowns were cemented, seated and adjusted. Initial owner instructions included restricting the dog's access to all bones and excessively hard chew toys. After endodontic treatment and crown preparation, the dog was fed a soft food to avoid injury to the prepared teeth. Following crown placement the dog was fed Prescription Diet t/d Canine.

The tongue had healed well when examined at the time of crown placement. When the dog was reexamined six months after the incident, no calculus accumulation was present and the gingivitis had resolved. The dog's general condition was very good. Its current weight was 31 kg with a body condition score of 3/5.

Endnote

a. Hill's Pet Nutrition, Inc., Topeka, KS, USA.

Bibliography

Emily P, Penman S. Endodontics. In: Handbook of Small Animal Dentistry. New York, NY: Pergamon Press, 1990: 65-80.

Emily P. Problems associated with diagnosis and treatment of endodontic disease. Problems in Veterinary Medicine: Dentistry 1990; 2: 152-182.

Gorrell C, Robinson J. Endodontics in small carnivores. In: Crossley DA, Penman S, eds. Manual of Small Animal Dentistry, 2nd ed. London, UK: British Small Animal Veterinary Association, 1995; 168-192.

Holmstrom SE, Frost P, Gammon RL. Veterinary Dentistry Techniques for the Small Animal Practitioner. Philadelphia, PA: WB Saunders Co, 1992; 207-266.

Shipp AD, Farhenkrug P. Practitioners' Guide to Veterinary Dentistry. Beverly Hill's, CA: Dr. Shipp's Lab, 1992; 77-94.

Wiggs RB, Lobprise HB, eds. Basic endodontic therapy. In: Veterinary Dentistry: Principles and Practice. Philadelphia, PA: Lippincott-Raven, 1997; 280-324.

CASE 47-2

Inappetence in a Cat

Robert B. Wiggs, DVM, Dipl. AVDC
Coit Road Animal Hospital
Dallas, Texas, USA

Patient Assessment

A three-year-old, 3.4-kg, neutered female domestic shorthair cat (body condition score 3/5) was referred for inappetence, salivation, periodic gagging and resistance to oral examination. The condition began suddenly two days earlier. The cat's abdomen was painful when palpated. Cervical lymph nodes and the thyroid glands were normal, although the patient resented palpation of the lower neck region. Eyes and ears were normal.

The cat's resistance to the oral examination limited the initial assessment. Moderate calculus accumulation and gingivitis were noted, however. A raised, non-inflamed mass of gingival tissue was present where the crown of the lower left third premolar should have been located. Due to the cat's agitation, the teeth and their associated sulci could not be examined with a dental explorer/probe. The lips, alveolar mucosa, dorsal surface of the tongue and hard and soft palate appeared normal. Examination of the ventral tongue base revealed a string foreign body.

Following sedation, the string was found to extend across the base and caudally around the lateral sides of the tongue into the pharyngeal region. The two leaders of the string extended into the esophagus. The tongue was lifted and the string grasped with Brown-Adson thumb forceps and gently pulled rostrally out of the mouth with no resistance. The string appeared to be a cotton-like material, 32 cm long. Endoscopic and radiographic examination of the esophagus and stomach were recommended.

The cat was intubated and anesthetized with isoflurane. Radiography showed the left mandibular gingival mass covered the roots of the lower third molar and that the majority of the crown was absent. The mass appeared to be a Stage V feline tooth resorption (**Table 1**). Other findings included moderate calculus accumulation and mild gingivitis.

A dental prophylaxis was performed and the cat was given antibiotics for 10 days.

Assess the Food and Feeding Method

The cat was fed a variety of moist foods purchased from grocery outlets.

Questions

1. What are the safety concerns of string-type chew toys?
2. What should be done concerning the gingival mass?
3. What recommendations should be made concerning the cat's food?

Answers and Discussion

1. The foreign body was similar to material from one of the cat's toys. When purchased, the toy was a ball made from loops of a cotton-like string, which purportedly would help clean and floss the teeth when the cat chewed on the toy. The toy came with a package of coarsely ground dried catnip with instructions to sprinkle the catnip on the toy to entice the cat to play with and chew on it. The owners said that it was one of the cat's favorite toys, especially when the catnip was applied. String, thread and pieces of fabric commonly cause problems when ingested by cats. Apparently, the type, diameter and length of fiber and the proportional length of fiber to cat size all play an important role in whether these fibers cause problems or pass through the gastrointestinal tract. No studies concerning these factors have been published. Short lengths of a multi-stranded, absorbable material would seem more appropriate, but more research is needed to determine safety requirements. Some string and rope chew toys are promoted for their "flossing effect." However, no research documents these claims. Additionally, some packages instruct the owner to use the toys in a tug-of-war with the pet to attain the flossing action. Strings tangled around teeth can avulse or fracture teeth. Therefore, these types of chew toys for dogs and cats should be recommended with extreme care, particularly for patients with moderate to advanced periodontal disease and mobile teeth. Clients who use string and rope-type chew toys should be encouraged to supervise their use and dispose of them at the first sign of unraveling or fraying.
2. The gingival mass was a Stage V feline tooth resorption (**Table 1**). There are three options for treating these lesions: 1) restoration of the tooth, 2) extraction of the tooth and 3) no treatment (leave the lesion as it is). Restorations, usually with glass ionomers, are generally used in repair of Stage I and, to a limited degree, Stage II lesions. Success of restoration for Stage II lesions is generally poor, but is an option the client should be given. Stage II to IV lesions can be extremely painful and should be treated. Careful extraction of tooth roots should be considered in Stage V lesions if inflammation is present in the gingival area overlying the retained roots. If inflammation is not present and the lesion is not painful or sensitive to the patient, the roots may be left in place. Often the roots will completely resorb with no further problems. In this case, there was no inflammation associated with

the mass and no treatment was performed.

3. Commercial cat foods are available that provide effective dietary cleansing through mechanical reduction of plaque and calculus accumulation (Prescription Diet t/d Feline[a], Friskies Dental Diet[b] and Purina Veterinary Diets DH Dental Health Brand Feline Formula.[c]

Table 1. Staging feline dental resorptive lesions.

Stage I	Lesion extends into cementum or enamel only
Stage II	Lesion extends into the dentin
Stage III	Lesion extends into the pulp cavity
Stage IV	Extensive structural damage to tooth, root or both
Stage V	Root retention with complete loss of crown

Progress Notes

Fiberoptic and radiographic examination of the esophagus and stomach revealed no abnormalities. The cat's food was changed to Prescription Diet t/d Feline. The cat was reexamined three weeks after the initial presentation. The gingival mass appeared unchanged to slightly smaller with no inflammation. The cat was eating well and no calculus accumulation was present.

Endnotes

a. Hill's Pet Nutrition, Inc., Topeka, KS, USA.
b. Friskies Pet Care Co., Glendale, CA, USA.
c. Nestlé Purina PetCare Co., St Louis, MO, USA.

Bibliography

Harvey CE, Emily PP. Atlas of oral pathology of the dog and cat. In: Small Animal Dentistry. St. Louis, MO: Mosby-Year Book, Inc, 1993; 48-56.

Wiggs RB, Lobprise HB, eds. Domestic feline oral and dental disease. In: Veterinary Dentistry: Principles and Practice. Philadelphia, PA: Lippincott-Raven, 1997; 482-517.

Wiggs RB, Lobprise HB. Dental disease. In: Norsworthy GD, ed. Feline Practice. Philadelphia, PA: JB Lippincott Co, 1993; 290-304.

CASE 47-3

Periodontal Disease in a Geriatric Miniature Schnauzer

Robert B. Wiggs, DVM, Dipl. AVDC
Coit Road Animal Hospital
Dallas, Texas, USA

Patient Assessment

A 12-year-old, 10-kg male miniature schnauzer was examined for severe halitosis and reluctance to eat dry food. Physical examination revealed a grade 1/6 heart murmur and a body condition score of 3/5. Abnormal oral findings included moderate accumulations of plaque and calculus on both dental arcades, gingivitis, furcation exposure and attachment loss, most prominent around the mandibular caudal premolar and molar teeth.

After the initial oral examination, the dog was given enrofloxacin (Baytril[a]) to control infection while further evaluations were performed. Results of a complete blood count were normal. Results of a serum biochemistry profile were normal except for mild azotemia (BUN = 42 mg/dl, normal = 10 to 25). A cardiac evaluation indicated mild valvular endocardiosis.

Assess the Food and Feeding Method

The owner had been feeding various commercial dry and moist grocery brand dog foods. Approximately six months earlier the dog became reluctant to eat dry foods and was currently eating only moist foods.

Questions

1. At what age should periodontal therapy be discontinued due to anesthetic risks?
2. When are antibiotics appropriate in periodontal therapy?
3. What medications may have adverse oral effects, particularly in geriatric dogs?
4. Is maintenance of alveolar bone under the tooth (alveolar ridge) a concern when extracting permanent teeth?
5. Outline an appropriate feeding plan for this geriatric patient.

Answers and Discussion

1. Many owners and veterinarians are reluctant to anesthetize geriatric patients for periodontal procedures. There is no specific age, however, when a patient cannot be anesthetized. An appropriate preanesthetic assessment should be made in all cases to identify potential risks and define an appropriate anesthetic regimen. Placing an intravenous catheter and administering fluids during periodontal procedures reduces the risk of anesthetic complications. Periodontal disease is associated with bacterial infection. The potential for systemic disease due to chronic showering of the bloodstream with oral bacteria may pose a greater risk to the patient than the anesthesia required for appropriate periodontal therapy.
2. Antibiotics may be used before, during or after dental procedures. Each period has specific justification. Antibiotics used before dental procedures help control the existing periodontal infection, thereby decreasing inflammation, which allows for more accurate clinical assessment and helps when making therapeutic choices. Antibiotics used during dental procedures are generally administered to protect the body from infection resulting from bacteremia. Healthy immunocompetent patients clear this bacteremia within 20 minutes. However, patients with organ pathology or a compromised immune system may be predisposed to sequential infection. Antibiotics given after dental procedures are generally prescribed to prevent oral reinfection during the healing stages.
3. Many medications can affect oral physiology, particularly salivary flow. Saliva is rich in proteins, glycoproteins, electrolytes and lipids and provides a protective barrier to oral tissues. Reduced salivary flow is associated with an increased prevalence of caries, periodontal disease and oral irritation in people. Patients receiving medications that alter the oral environment may need additional professional or homecare to maintain oral health. Examples of such drugs include narcotic analgesics, anticonvulsants, antihistamines, antiarrhythmics, antineoplastics, antiemetics, diuretics and tranquilizers.
4. Alveolar ridge maintenance is a concern, particularly if the mandibular incisor, canine or carnassial teeth are extracted. Atrophy of the alveolar ridge and mandibular weakening are common following extraction of these teeth, and may result in future pathologic or iatrogenic fractures. Packing extraction sites with osseopromotive material may reduce and in some cases prevent alveolar ridge atrophy.
5. Because aging affects all body systems, there is a high likelihood of multiple problems in older pets. A thorough systems review, which should include a complete history, physical examination and extended laboratory database, is important in older pets. This review enables the veterinarian to define problems accurately, prioritize the problems and establish appropriate diagnostic, therapeutic and feeding plans. Chronic valvular heart disease (endocardiosis) and renal failure are common causes of morbidity and mortality in older dogs. Because these conditions are so common, geriatric dogs may benefit from a food that avoids excess levels of phosphorus, protein, sodium and chloride (Chapters 36 and 37). Other nutrient levels and the feeding method may need to be adjusted based on body condition of the patient and results of the comprehensive systems review.

   This dog has clinical and laboratory evidence of dental disease, chronic valvular heart disease and renal disease. Accordingly, it may benefit from a food that avoids excess levels of phosphorus, protein, sodium and chloride. In addition, oral care at home should be initiated to prevent accumulation of dental substrates and further periodontal disease. A food or dental treat that enhances mechanical cleansing or teeth would be appropriate.

   Prescription Diet t/d Canine[b] is a dry veterinary therapeutic food formulated to reduce accumulation of plaque and calculus and reduce gingivitis. This food is most effective when fed as the sole maintenance food for adult dogs. However, some pets with dental disease should receive food(s) with different nutrient profiles because of concurrent disease.

Progress Notes

The dog was given a vasodilator (isosorbide dinitrate) and a moist veterinary therapeutic food that avoids excess phosphorus, protein, sodium and chloride (Prescription Diet k/d Canine[b]).

Therapeutic options for the oral problems were discussed with the owner and the decision was made to proceed with periodontal therapy. The dog was anesthetized with isoflurane (administered via mask and intubation), and supragingival scaling followed by root planing and subgingival curettage was performed. Severe periodontal disease was present around the left mandibular fourth premolar and first molar teeth. Advanced bone loss was noted around the distal roots (**Figure 1**); a mobility index of 3/3 (severe mobility) was present. Both teeth were extracted by crown sectioning and elevation. The alveolar sockets were curetted and bony spicules were smoothed. An osseopromotive bioactive material (Bioglass[c]) was placed into the sockets to aid in alveolar ridge maintenance. The extraction sites were closed with sutures and the remaining teeth were polished. Oral clindamycin (Antirobe[d]), an oral ascorbic acid/zinc gluconate rinse (Maxiguard[e]) and the moist veterinary therapeutic food (Prescription Diet k/d Canine) were prescribed for two weeks. After two weeks, the dog was reexamined. The extraction sites were healing well and the owner commented that the dog was more active than it had been for many months. The dog was fed the dry form of the same renal food (Prescription Diet k/d Canine) and the owner was instructed to provide daily oral care through toothbrushing and feeding four kibbles of Prescription Diet t/d Canine/day. The combined foods were calculated to deliver approximately 500 kcal/day (2.1 MJ/day).

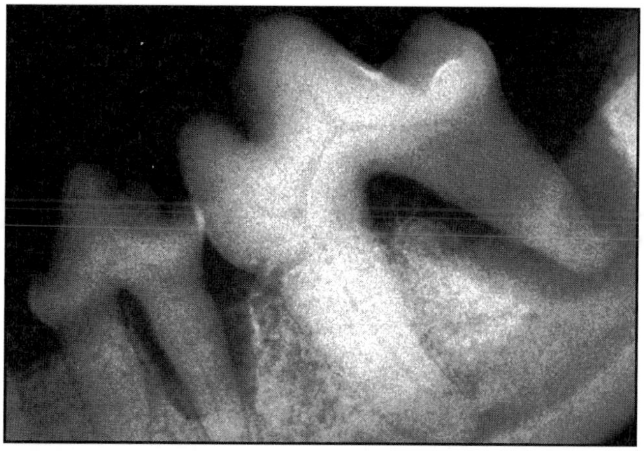

Figure 1. Radiographic evaluation indicating severe alveolar bone loss around the distal roots of the mandibular fourth premolar and first molar.

Endnotes

a. Bayer Animal Health, Shawnee, KS, USA.
b. Hill's Pet Nutrition, Inc., Topeka, KS, USA.
c. Nutramax Laboratories, Inc., Baltimore, MD, USA.
d. Upjohn Veterinary Products, Kalamazoo, MI, USA.
e. Addison Laboratories, Fayette, MO, USA.

Bibliography

Edgar WM, O'Mullane DM, eds. Factors influencing salivary flow rate and composition. In: Saliva and Dental Health. British Dental Association, 1990.

Maretta SM. Oropharynx. In: Birchard SJ, Sherding RG, eds. Manual of Small Animal Practice. Philadelphia, PA: WB Saunders Co, 1994; 607-629.

Wiggs RB, Lobprise HB, eds. Periodontology. In: Veterinary Dentistry: Principles and Practice. Philadelphia, PA: Lippincott-Raven, 1997; 186-231.

Section 18

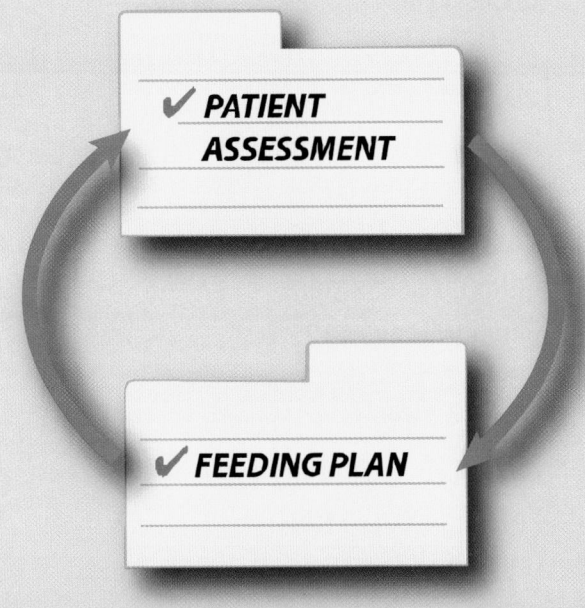

Gastrointestinal Disorders

Gastrointestinal Disorders

Chapter 48

Introduction to Gastrointestinal and Exocrine Pancreatic Diseases

Deborah J. Davenport
Rebecca L. Remillard

". . . food should be . . . frequently administered, for food soothes the soul."
Aretaeus, the Cappadocian

CLINICAL IMPORTANCE

"What should I feed?" is one of the most common questions addressed by veterinarians managing gastrointestinal (GI) and exocrine pancreatic disorders in dogs and cats. Owners of affected pets often intuitively understand that the feeding plan plays an important role in the treatment of their animals and expect guidance regarding specific foods and nutrients to avoid or change in their pet's diet.

Many GI and exocrine pancreatic diseases are amenable to dietary management (**Table 48-1**). Altering food ingredients, nutrient profiles, food form and feeding method can be powerful tools in managing GI and exocrine pancreatic diseases. Drug therapy instituted without concomitant dietary therapy often yields less than desirable results. Occasionally, foods or ingredients may function as diagnostic tools in evaluating patients with GI and pancreatic disorders. Herbs (**Box 48-1**), oligosaccharides and medium-chain triglycerides have also been used to treat certain of these diseases.

A multitude of factors, including trophic hormones, adequate blood flow, neurologic input and nutrient composition of digesta, are involved in maintaining intestinal integrity (mass and function). The presence or absence of certain nutrients and ingredients can positively or negatively affect the bowel (**Table 48-2**). For example, effects of starvation include decreased pancreatic enzyme production and secretion, intestinal mucosal atrophy and reduced gastric emptying rates. The resultant diarrhea and malassimilation further exacerbate the malnutritive state (Guilford, 1996). In addition, starvation can markedly affect bowel immune response and mucosal integrity.

Discussion of the dietary management of patients with GI and exocrine pancreatic disease can be organized in many ways. This chapter and the ones that follow assume the reader has already identified the major clinical problems of the patient as dysphagia (i.e., oropharyngeal disease), regurgitation (i.e., esophageal disease), vomiting (i.e., many causes including primary gastric, intestinal and exocrine pancreatic diseases), small bowel diarrhea, large bowel diarrhea, constipation or flatulence. Thus, rather than being organized around clinical problems, the following GI and exocrine pancreatic chapters focus on specific diseases allowing formulation of better feeding plans for individual patients.

The individual chapters for GI and exocrine pancreatic diseases include:

- Oral Diseases (Chapter 49)
- Pharyngeal and Esophageal Disorders (Chapter 50)
- Introduction to Gastric Diseases (Chapter 51)
- Gastritis and Gastroduodenal Ulceration (Chapter 52)
- Gastric Dilatation and Gastric Dilatation-Volvulus in Dogs (Chapter 53)
- Gastric Motility and Emptying Disorders (Chapter 54)

Table 48-1. Gastrointestinal and exocrine pancreatic diseases amenable to dietary management.

Oral
Inflammatory disorders (stomatitis, radiation-induced mucositis)
Physical abnormalities (trauma, neoplasia, congenital malformations)
Pharynx and esophagus
Inflammatory disorders (esophagitis)
Motility disorders (cricopharyngeal achalasia, megaesophagus)
Obstructive disorders (vascular ring anomalies, strictures, neoplasia)
Stomach
Gastric dilatation/gastric dilatation-volvulus
Gastric motility/emptying disorders
Gastritis
Gastroduodenal ulceration
Hairballs
Small intestine
Acute enteritis
Inflammatory bowel disease
Intestinal neoplasia
Lymphangiectasia
Protein-losing enteropathy
Short bowel syndrome
Small intestinal bacterial overgrowth
Wheat-sensitive enteropathy
Large intestine
Colitis
Constipation
Flatulence
Irritable bowel syndrome
Pancreas
Exocrine pancreatic insufficiency
Pancreatitis

- Introduction to Small Intestinal Diseases (Chapter 55)
- Acute Gastroenteritis and Enteritis (Chapter 56)
- Inflammatory Bowel Disease (Chapter 57)
- Protein-Losing Enteropathies (Chapter 58)
- Short Bowel Syndrome (Chapter 59)
- Small Intestinal Bacterial Overgrowth (Chapter 60)
- Introduction to Large Intestinal Diseases (Chapter 61)
- Large Bowel Diarrhea: Colitis (Chapter 62)
- Large Bowel Diarrhea: Idiopathic Bowel Syndrome in Dogs (Chapter 63)
- Constipation/Obstipation/Megacolon (Chapter 64)
- Flatulence (Chapter 65)
- Exocrine Pancreatic Insufficiency (Chapter 66)
- Acute and Chronic Pancreatitis (Chapter 67)

Vomiting and diarrhea have a myriad of causes and feeding plans vary according to the underlying condition. The feeding plans for acute gastroenteritis are most appropriate when a specific cause of acute vomiting or diarrhea is unknown. When a specific cause of chronic small bowel diarrhea is not identified, then feeding plans as outlined for exocrine pancreatic insufficiency are most appropriate. Finally, when a specific cause of chronic large bowel diarrhea is not identified, then feeding plans for colitis are most appropriate.

Each patient should be seen as an individual variant of the norm; therefore, multiple dietary manipulations should be considered, as needed, for each patient (**Box 48-2**). Because of the

Box 48-1. Herbal Remedies for Gastrointestinal Disorders.

Herbal remedies have become a major factor in human health care. Various botanicals have become household words, and sales of herbal remedies are increasing dramatically. As herbs move out of health food stores and into mainstream supermarkets, drug stores and even pet stores, use of these products in pets will also increase.

A wide variety of herbal or botanical products are advocated for patients with gastrointestinal (GI) disorders, including individuals with diarrhea, vomiting, constipation, stomatitis, colitis and flatus. There are also long lists of herbs and botanicals that are described as "gastrointestinal agents." Although today's herbal remedies exhibit varying degrees of therapeutic value, most have not been investigated thoroughly for safety and efficacy. It is beyond the scope of this textbook to list all the herbal and botanical remedies that may have use in pets. Interested readers are referred to books listed in the Bibliography for further information about human herbal remedies that might be used in pets with GI disorders.

The Bibliography for **Box 48-1** can be found at www.markmorris.org.

Box 48-2. Performing Dietary Trials in Patients with Gastrointestinal Disease.

Nutritional therapies are extremely useful for treating gastrointestinal (GI) disease in dogs and cats. Several commercial and homemade foods are available to practitioners and pet owners for this purpose. Unfortunately, there is no historical or clinical finding that will predict the success of a specific food type. Therefore, selection of the most appropriate food for an individual patient is often based on results of a dietary trial.

Dietary trials are easily performed in most clinical and home settings. Oral food consumption is preferred for managing GI diseases, except in those rare situations in which the patient is intolerant of enteral feeding.

After the veterinarian identifies those foods to be included in the trial, selection of the initial test food is often based on clinical experience and the patient's nutritional history. In general, foods that have been used unsuccessfully in the past to manage the patient should be avoided. Typically, highly digestible GI or elimination foods are good first choices for patients with gastric or small intestinal disorders. Fiber-enhanced foods are often the initial selection when large bowel signs predominate.

No other foods, supplements, table foods or treats should be offered during the dietary trial. Dietary trials are most useful if continued for at least seven to 10 days. In certain settings (e.g., adverse reactions to food), trials lasting two to four weeks (12 weeks in cases with dermatologic signs) may be necessary to determine efficacy (Chapter 31). Successful dietary trials are marked by partial or complete resolution of clinical signs.

The Bibliography for **Box 48-2** can be found at www.markmorris.org.

Box 48-3. Food Types Useful in the Management of Gastrointestinal and Exocrine Pancreatic Diseases.

GASTROINTESTINAL FOODS

Several commercial veterinary therapeutic foods have been specially formulated for managing gastrointestinal (GI) disease in dogs and cats. Typically, these products are highly digestible and have consistent ingredient and nutrient profiles.

The term highly digestible is not defined in a regulatory sense. However, highly digestible has generally been reserved for products with protein digestibility ≥87% and fat and carbohydrate digestibilities ≥90%. The average digestibility coefficients for popular commercial foods are 78 to 81%, 77 to 85% and 69 to 79% for crude protein, crude fat and carbohydrate, respectively. Commercial veterinary therapeutic foods formulated for GI disease usually contain highly refined meat and carbohydrate sources to increase digestibility.

Carbohydrates make up the largest nonwater fraction of foods formulated for managing GI diseases. Carbohydrate digestibility of pet foods is influenced by source and processing. Dogs digest most properly cooked starches very well, including starch components in corn, rice, barley and wheat. Other starches, including potato and tapioca, are less digestible, particularly when inadequately cooked. Although cats also efficiently digest carbohydrates, some clinicians feel that cats with small bowel disorders are less tolerant of dietary carbohydrate than dogs with similar causes of malassimilation.

There is a link between particle size and carbohydrate digestibility of moist foods. As a result, carbohydrate ingredients (e.g., rice, corn, etc.) should be chopped or ground before they are incorporated into moist foods. This relationship apparently is not an issue for extruded dry products. There is almost complete ileal carbohydrate digestibility in dogs consuming extruded grains (dry products).

The requirements for many macro- and microminerals in the face of GI disease are not well understood. However, sodium, potassium and B-vitamin losses are expected with vomiting and diarrhea. Therefore, foods formulated for managing GI diseases should contain sodium, potassium and B vitamins in excess of maintenance allowances. Patients with fat malabsorption are at risk for developing fat-soluble vitamin deficiencies. Highly digestible foods formulated for feeding steatorrheic patients should, therefore, be fortified with fat-soluble vitamins.

It is unusual for GI foods to contain crude fiber levels greater than 5% dry matter (DM) because fiber reduces dry matter digestibility and decreases pancreatic enzymatic activity in vitro. More recently, manufacturers of some highly digestible commercial veterinary therapeutic foods have added small amounts (<5% DM) of soluble or mixed fibers because short-chain fatty acids produced by intestinal microbial fermentation of fiber may positively affect the large intestinal mucosa.

Veterinarians recommend GI foods most often for managing acute gastroenteritis or malassimilation associated with small bowel disease or exocrine pancreatic insufficiency. The utility of highly digestible foods has been demonstrated through anecdotal reports and by the use of such foods in clinical trials involving animals with spontaneous and experimental exocrine pancreatic insufficiency. Some gastroenterologists also recommend these foods for patients with certain colonic disorders to reduce exposure of the colonic mucosa to ingesta. This therapeutic strategy has been suggested for management of inflammatory colitides and constipation.

FIBER-ENHANCED FOODS

Commercial veterinary therapeutic foods contain varying levels and sources of fiber. Based on the combined knowledge obtained from research in people, ongoing research in dogs and cats and clinical experience, fiber is beneficial in managing many large and some small bowel diseases.

Soluble fibers (e.g., pectins and gums) increase the viscosity of intestinal contents, which delay gastric emptying and slow small bowel transit time. Viscosity markedly affects the extent of intraluminal mixing of digesta and digestive enzymes, which can shift sites of absorption and subsequently the rate of nutrients entering the bloodstream. Bacteria in the colon ferment soluble fiber to short-chain fatty acids, including acetic, propionic and butyric acids. Colonocytes apparently use butyrate, whereas propionic and acetic acids are absorbed. Short-chain fatty acids are nutritive to the colonic mucosa and foster normal colonic flora while discouraging pathogenic flora. These properties result in an acidic colonic pH and increased colonic bacterial numbers, colonic mucosal mass and fecal dry matter and water content. Soluble fiber may bind and decrease macronutrient absorption and decrease protein digestibility. Certain fiber types, especially gels and gums, may be of benefit in GI disease because they bind toxins and irritating bile acids. This binding effect prevents these substances from further damaging the intestinal mucosal surface.

Insoluble fiber is primarily composed of cellulose and structural polysaccharides that are relatively resistant to digestion and that ferment slowly, increase intestinal residue and normalize intestinal transit time. These fibers have little or no effect on gastric emptying, mineral absorption or colonic microflora unless fed in high concentrations (>20% DM). One of the most profound effects of fiber on the GI tract is the normalization of gut motility, particularly in the stomach, proximal small bowel and colon. This effect appears to be greatest for insoluble fibers such as cellulose. In general, increasing the insoluble fiber content of the food resolves or modulates most cases of colitis. There are several plausible mechanisms by which insoluble fiber controls large bowel diarrhea. Undigested residues absorb water and increase bacterial mass, which increases fecal bulk. Fecal bulk provides physical intraluminal stimulation to reestablish neuromuscular-endocrine coordinations and normalize intestinal transit times. Fecal bulk increases intestinal residue, which absorbs toxins and offending agents. For more basic information about fiber see Chapter 5.

RESTRICTED- AND MODERATE-FAT FOODS

In general, dietary fat is more digestible than digestible carbohydrate and protein and provides 2.25 times more calories by weight. Average fat digestibility in commercial dog food is approximately 90%. Average fat digestibility of commercial cat foods ranges from 74

Box 48-3 continued

to 91%. Patients with GI or pancreatic disease may not tolerate high-fat foods (>25% DM), which may contribute to diarrhea and steatorrhea. Foods containing moderate amounts of fat (12 to 15% DM for dogs and 15 to 22% DM for cats) are generally tolerated and have sufficient caloric density for most patients. Commercial veterinary therapeutic foods containing less than 10% DM fat need to be fed in larger volumes to meet the patient's caloric requirement. Some patients may not tolerate this volume of food.

Restricted-fat foods are often recommended for patients with gastroenteritis in which the complex process of fat digestion and absorption may be disrupted. Unabsorbed fat in the bowel lumen may cause secretory diarrhea. Dietary fat should be reduced when fat maldigestion or malabsorption is present due to exocrine pancreatic insufficiency or reduced bowel surface area. The latter occurs in short bowel syndrome and other conditions in which inflammation, infectious agents, neoplasia or surgery markedly reduces the intestinal villus surface area. For example, intestinal malabsorption of fat is seriously impaired in primary and secondary lymphangiectasia. Fat restriction is also useful in small intestinal bacterial overgrowth in which many of the side effects of the condition can be ameliorated by removing the inciting cause of the secretory diarrhea.

ELIMINATION FOODS

Elimination foods are most often recommended for patients with GI signs due to suspected food intolerance or food hypersensitivity. Protein sources and amounts are of key importance for elimination foods. Chapter 31 discusses adverse food reactions and elimination foods in more detail.

GLUTEN- AND GLIADIN-FREE FOODS

Several potential antigens are found in flour when cereal grains are processed. One polypeptide, gliadin, is found in wheat, barley, rye, buckwheat and oat flours. Gliadin is responsible for gluten-sensitive enteropathies in people and dogs. Homologous gliadin polypeptides are not present in whole grains and flours produced from rice and corn.

In people, gluten-induced enteropathy or celiac disease is an important malabsorptive disorder. An analogous condition, termed wheat-sensitive enteropathy, has been identified in Irish setter dogs and is suspected to affect dogs of other breeds. Affected animals develop small bowel diarrhea due to malabsorption secondary to villous atrophy. Gluten- and gliadin-free foods are most commonly recommended for managing dogs suspected of having wheat-sensitive enteropathy. In most cases, withdrawal of the offending gliadin antigen from the diet results in resolution of the villous atrophy and clinical signs.

MONOMERIC FOODS

Monomeric foods are water-soluble, liquid foods containing nutrients in their simplest absorbable form. Amino acids are most commonly provided by a mixture of di- and tripeptides and/or individual amino acids. Fats are present as triglycerides or as fatty acids. Carbohydrates are generally present as mono- or disaccharides. Minerals and vitamins are present to meet requirements. These foods minimize GI and pancreatic secretions and allow nutrient usage with minimal requirements for digestion. In addition, relative to complete proteins, the small size of amino acids, dipeptides and tripeptides in monomeric products ensures delivery of a truly "hypoallergenic" food. Monomeric foods should be considered for patients with severe malabsorption or short bowel syndrome and in initial refeeding of patients with acute pancreatitis. In addition, these foods may provide "bowel rest" for patients with severe inflammatory bowel disease. Monomeric foods are often unpalatable and are not well accepted by cats. Thus, these foods are usually administered for several days via indwelling feeding tubes. Chapter 25 lists monomeric foods.

The Bibliography for **Box 48-3** can be found at www.markmorris.org.

Table 48-2. Potential dietary influences on the gastrointestinal tract.*

Food may alter:
Absorption
Cellular turnover rate
Luminal ammonia concentration
Luminal volatile fatty acid content
Microflora
Motility
Secretory rate
Villous height
Food may be a source of:
Chemical/bacterial toxins
Dietary antigens
Food may correct:
Nutritional deficiencies

*Modified from Guilford WG. Feline gastrointestinal tract disease. In: Wills JM, Simpson KW, eds. The Waltham Book of Clinical Nutrition of the Dog & Cat. London, UK: Pergamon Press, 1994; 221-238.

diverse nature of GI and exocrine pancreatic disorders, a number of food types may be appropriate (**Box 48-3**). Nutrient profiles should be considered as *starting points* on a continuum of possible nutrient concentrations that can be adjusted for each patient as necessary. All too often, relative terms such as "low" vs. "high" are used without stating the point of reference. The reference point should be the current food that the owner feeds. Changes include increases or decreases, usually in 5 to 10% increments, of nutrient concentrations relative to the previous food.

REFERENCES

The references for **Chapter 48** can be found at www.markmorris.org.

Chapter 49

Oral Diseases

Deborah J. Davenport
Rebecca L. Remillard
Ellen I. Logan

"If you have no Honey in your Pot, have some in your mouth."
Benjamin Franklin, Poor Richard's Almanac

CLINICAL IMPORTANCE

The oral cavity is susceptible to a number of acquired and congenital disorders. In comparison to the high incidence of dental disease, however, these conditions are relatively uncommon. Chapter 47 discusses periodontal disease in detail. Among the more common conditions affecting the oral cavity are inflammatory lesions and physical abnormalities such as neoplasia, trauma and congenital malformations (e.g., cleft palate).

Acquired inflammatory lesions of the oral cavity and tongue are relatively uncommon in dogs and cats but appear to be increasing in frequency (Lyon, 2005). These conditions include eosinophilic granuloma complex, gingivostomatitis, labial granuloma immune-mediated diseases (e.g., pemphigus) and mucositis due to radiation therapy of the head and neck (Ulbricht, 2008; Quimby, 2007). Infectious oral disorders (e.g., candidiasis or fusospirochetal infections) are rare and usually occur in immunocompromised animals. Oral ulcerations may be seen in cats in association with herpesvirus and calicivirus infections. Oral neoplasia is relatively common in dogs and cats (Theilen and Madewell, 1987; Smith, 2005). Malignant melanoma, squamous cell carcinoma and fibrosarcoma are the most commonly reported oral malignancies. Trauma to the oral cavity may arise from fights among animals, falls (high-rise syndrome), motor vehicle accidents, chemical and electrical burns and penetrating foreign bodies. Oral congenital anomalies such as cleft palate are uncommon but may have nutritional causes (e.g., copper deficiency in pregnant queens) or profound consequences due to malnutrition and secondary aspiration pneumonia in growing animals.

PATIENT ASSESSMENT

History and Physical Examination

Dogs and cats with oral disease have variable clinical signs depending on the type and location of the lesions. Patients may exhibit dysphagia or pain associated with eating. Owners may report excessive salivation, oral hemorrhage, halitosis and reluctance to eat resulting in loss of body weight and condition. In some cases, careful questioning of the owner will reveal ingestion of foreign bodies or caustic materials or a history of trauma. Puppies and kittens with congenital anomalies such as cleft palate may be presented to veterinarians for ineffectual suckling, poor weight gain and coughing or gagging following attempts at nursing.

Sedation may be required to facilitate examination of the oropharynx and tongue. Various conditions may present with specific signs. Congenital defects may be noted in the soft or hard palate. Epulides originate from periodontal stroma and are most commonly located in the gingiva near the incisor teeth and appear as pedunculated or smooth, non-ulcerated masses. Odontogenic tumors (e.g., ameloblastoma and odontoma) are

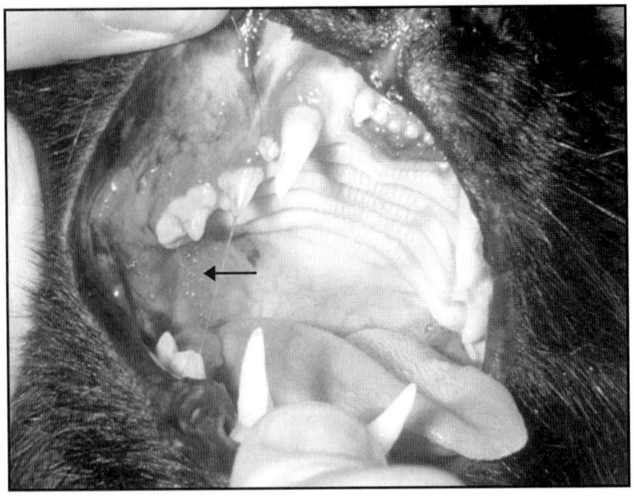

Figure 49-1. Severe lymphoplasmacytic gingivitis and stomatitis in a cat. Note the raised, cobblestone-like lesions (arrow) at the right glossopalatine arch. (Courtesy Dr. Michael Leib, Virginia-Maryland Regional College of Veterinary Medicine, Blacksburg, VA.)

Box 49-1. Feeding Patients Undergoing Radiation Therapy.

Dogs and cats undergoing radiation therapy for oral and nasal tumors often develop mucositis within the third week of a four- to five-week therapeutic protocol. This oral mucosal inflammation is painful; therefore, most animals will stop eating during this time but will drink voluntarily. A change in food form from moist or dry to a liquid is necessary for most animals to continue consuming at least their daily resting energy requirement. Most patients will consume variable quantities of a palatable chilled liquid veterinary therapeutic food during this time even if they won't consume a mixture of their regular food and water. Mixing the liquid with the patient's regular food one week before the expected onset of mucositis allows acclimation to the liquid food. Patients usually voluntarily consume their regular food as the mucositis resolves.

Some patients stop eating and drinking voluntarily when they develop mucositis and may require intravenous administration of fluids and nutrients. Discontinuing radiation therapy for a few days is also beneficial. Nasogastric or orogastric feeding tubes are not appropriate, whereas pharyngeal or esophageal feeding tubes may be useful if placed in advance and if they are not in the field to be irradiated (Chapter 25). Most patients recover quickly from mucositis (i.e., within three to four days) and consume food and water again, eliminating the need for a gastrostomy tube. Radiation treatments can usually then be continued uneventfully.

The Bibliography for **Box 49-1** can be found at www.markmorris.org.

typically expansile, slow-growing odontogenic masses that often form in the incisor region. Malignant tumors (e.g., squamous cell carcinoma, malignant melanoma and fibrosarcoma) grow rapidly and are characterized by early invasion of the gingiva and bone. Pets with suspected oral or tonsillar tumors should be carefully evaluated for peripheral lymphadenopathy.

Gingivostomatitis is characterized by raised, erythremic cobblestone-like lesions at the glossopalatine arches (**Figure 49-1**), whereas feline eosinophilic granuloma complex manifests as ulcers, plaques and granulomas on the maxillary lips, tongue and palate. In dogs, inflammatory lesions are most often present on the tongue or palatine and labial mucosa.

Head trauma in pets often results in mandibular symphyseal fractures, maxillary fractures, displaced teeth and separation of the hard palate. These injuries may result in reluctance or inability to eat.

Chemical, electrical and thermal burns are characterized by ulceration and necrosis of affected tissues. Animals with oral burns may suffer life-threatening consequences such as pulmonary edema or cardiogenic shock.

Laboratory and Other Clinical Information

Laboratory values are often unremarkable in patients with oral disease and generally reflect underlying conditions when present. Leukocytosis and a polyclonal hyperglobulinemia are frequent findings in cats with lymphoplasmacytic stomatitis. Radiography is often of value in cases with suspected trauma to assess the extent of bony injury. Radiography is invaluable for tumor staging in patients with oral neoplasia. Generally, both skull and thoracic films are evaluated. In addition, thoracic films allow assessment of aspiration pneumonia in young animals with cleft palate. Diagnosis of lesions within the oral cavity often requires biopsy and histopathologic examination.

Risk Factors

Age and breed are risk factors for several oral disorders. Young patients are more likely to present with congenital and traumatic lesions, whereas older dogs and cats are more likely to suffer from oral neoplasia and inflammatory disorders. Patients undergoing radiation therapy of the head and neck for cancer are susceptible to radiation-induced mucositis (**Box 49-1**). In addition, certain breeds are predisposed to various oral disorders (**Table 49-1**).

Etiopathogenesis

Pets with oral disease often exhibit dysphagia or reluctance to eat resulting in malnutrition. Often this nutritional state is compounded by inflammatory, traumatic or neoplastic processes. The etiology of oral inflammatory lesions such as gingivostomatitis and faucitis, and eosinophilic granuloma complex is unknown. Gingivostomatitis in cats has been theorized to be an aberrant immunologic response to antigenic stimuli. Various bacterial, viral, periodontal, dietary and immune factors have been implicated (Quimby, 2008). There is a strong association between this disorder and infection with feline immunodeficiency virus (FIV) or calicivirus (DeBowes, 1997). Approximately 50% of cats with FIV infection and 60% of cats with calicivirus infection have chronic oral disease (DeBowes, 1997). These findings do not prove causality, however. The response of some cats with the disorder to radical extraction of teeth and the isolation of antibodies to plaque bacteria (*Actinobacillus* and *Bacteroides* spp.) from affected cats also suggest the potential of "plaque intolerance" (DeBowes, 1997).

Key Nutritional Factors

The key nutritional factors for foods for oral diseases are discussed below and summarized in **Table 49-2.**

Water

Dehydration is a frequent problem in dogs and cats with oral disorders that interfere with consumption of water. Whenever possible, fluid balance should be maintained via oral consumption of fluids. However, parenteral fluid administration is often needed for dehydrated patients and those unable or unwilling to drink adequate amounts of water.

Energy Density

A food with a relatively high energy density concentration is helpful in meeting the patient's caloric requirement in a small volume of food. Foods with energy densities in excess of 4.5 kcal/g (18.8 kJ/g) dry matter (DM) for dogs and 5 kcal/g (20.9 kJ/g) DM for cats are recommended.

Food Form

The veterinarian or owner should experiment with foods of differing consistency. Often liquid foods or slurries made from moist pet food and water are more readily accepted. A dilute consistency is often associated with less discomfort and is less likely to accumulate in oral lesions or adhere to surgical sites within the oral cavity.

Table 49-1. Breed-associated oral disorders.

Disorders	Breeds
Cleft palate	Brachycephalic dogs and cats
Epulides	Boxer
Gingivitis/stomatitis	Maltese dog
	Siberian husky
Lymphoplasmacytic stomatitis	Abyssinian cat
	Burmese cat
	Himalayan cat
	Maltese cat
	Persian cat
	Siamese cat
Neoplasia	Cocker spaniel
	German shepherd dog
	German shorthaired pointer
	Golden retriever
	Weimaraner

Table 49-2. Key nutritional factors for foods for patients with oral diseases.

Factors	Dietary recommendations
Water	Maintain fluid balance with oral, and if necessary, parenteral fluids
Energy	For dogs: >4.5 kcal/g (>18.8 kJ/g) dry matter For cats: >5 kcal/g (>20.9 kJ/g) dry matter
Food form	Liquid foods and slurries made from moist food are often more readily accepted

FEEDING PLAN

The goals of dietary management for patients with oral disease are to provide adequate nutrition while minimizing discomfort to the pet and enhancing resolution of the oral lesions.

Assess and Select the Food

The key nutritional factors recommended for foods for patients with oral diseases should be compared with the levels in the foods under consideration for feeding. Underweight patients may need a nutrient profile similar to that found in a growth or recovery-type formula to regain normal body condition. In addition, the food should be suitable for any other conditions present that are amenable to dietary management.

Patients with extensive oral injuries or inflammation of the oral cavity may benefit from foods designed for assisted feeding or recovery (Chapter 25). Patients with oral neoplasia may benefit from foods specifically formulated for patients with cancer (Chapter 30).

Assess and Determine the Feeding Method

Because the feeding method is often altered in patients with oral disease, a thorough assessment should include verification of the feeding method currently being used. Items to consider include feeding frequency, amount fed, how the food is offered, access to other food sources including table food and who feeds the animal. All of this information should have been gathered when the history of the animal was obtained.

Dogs and cats with oral disease should initially be fed several small meals daily if they are able and willing to consume food voluntarily. After each meal, the oral cavity should be flushed with water to remove particulate matter adhered to the oral mucous membranes. In many cases, tube-feeding methods are preferred until oral discomfort is reduced, oral lesions are healed and voluntary food consumption resumes (Chapter 25).

REASSESSMENT

Body condition scores and hydration status should be evaluated to determine adequacy of food and water consumption. Assisted feeding should be instituted if oral feeding is inadequate to maintain body weight and condition (Chapter 25).

REFERENCES

The references for **Chapter 49** can be found at www.markmorris.org.

Chapter

50

Pharyngeal and Esophageal Disorders

Deborah J. Davenport

Michael S. Leib

Rebecca L. Remillard

"The Chinese do not draw any distinction between food and medicine."
Lin Yutang

CLINICAL IMPORTANCE

Compared with vomiting and diarrhea, swallowing disorders are relatively uncommon in dogs and cats. However, these conditions are often profoundly debilitating due to undernutrition (i.e., lack of adequate food intake) and recurrent pulmonary infections resulting from aspiration. Pharyngeal and esophageal disorders most commonly encountered include: 1) motility disorders (e.g., cricopharyngeal achalasia, megaesophagus), 2) inflammatory disorders (e.g., esophagitis, gastroesophageal reflux) and 3) obstructive lesions (e.g., vascular ring anomalies, strictures and foreign bodies).

PATIENT ASSESSMENT

History and Physical Examination

Congenital pharyngeal and esophageal disorders are typically diagnosed in young animals soon after weaning. In some young dogs, clinical and subclinical esophageal dysmotility may improve with age, whereas the disorder progresses in other patients (Bexfield et al, 2006). Rarely, dogs with congenital malformations of the aortic arches, also known as vascular ring anomalies, may present with late-onset regurgitation as adults (Fingeroth and Fossum, 1987; Muldoon et al, 1997).

Acquired pharyngeal and esophageal disease can affect dogs and cats of any age. Owners of pets presenting for suspected pharyngeal and esophageal disorders should be asked about feeding dental chew treats (Leib and Sartor, 2008), bones or bone and raw food diets, which can result in esophageal foreign bodies. The history of a recent anesthetic procedure may suggest reflux esophagitis (Wilson et al, 2005). Owners of cats presenting with signs of esophageal disease should be asked about recent oral antibiotic administration (Westfall et al, 2001; Beatty et al, 2006; German et al, 2005).

Owners of dogs with dysphagia due to pharyngeal disease typically report coughing or gagging as the dog chews and swallows its food. In dogs and cats, the hallmark of an esophageal disorder is regurgitation (**Box 50-1**). Additional clinical signs include ptyalism, frequent swallowing, gurgling esophageal noises, halitosis and apparent pain on swallowing. Affected cats may vocalize in conjunction with gagging or regurgitation. The frequency of regurgitation is variable. Owners may report immediate postprandial regurgitation of undigested food, water or saliva or describe signs manifested several hours after feeding. Affected dogs and cats often have a voracious appetite despite regurgitation unless they have secondary aspiration pneumonia. Dyspnea, coughing, weakness and fever may be referable to severe respiratory compromise associated with aspiration pneumonia.

Esophageal disorders may be associated with neuromuscular diseases and endocrinopathies. Owners may describe their pets as being weak or uncoordinated. The evidence for association of megaesophagus and hypothyroidism is tenuous and uncommon.

Poor body condition is often evident (body condition score [BCS] 1/5 or 2/5). Body condition should be monitored close-

Box 50-1. Regurgitation vs. Vomiting.

Differentiating regurgitation from vomiting is important in distinguishing esophageal from gastric disease. Characteristics of vomiting include expulsion of digested and bile-stained food and retching with involuntary abdominal contractions. Gastric contents are often highly acidic, which may be reflected in the pH of the vomitus. However, vomiting often involves reflux of bicarbonate-rich fluid into the stomach from the duodenum, which buffers gastric acid. The vomited material may then have a neutral or near-neutral pH.

Regurgitation involves less forceful casting up of tubular, bile-free, undigested food. Mucoid secretions mixed with the undigested food will usually have a pH of 6.5 to 7.0. Copious salivation may also be a confusing sign; it may be a primary sign of esophageal diseases (e.g., foreign body) or it may be part of the nausea that often accompanies vomiting.

The Bibliography for **Box 50-1** can be found at www.markmorris.org.

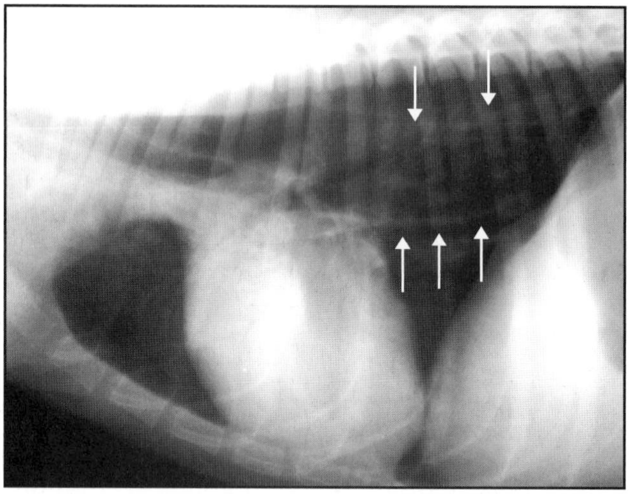

Figure 50-1. Lateral thoracic radiograph demonstrating esophageal dilatation in a dog with acquired megaesophagus. The arrows depict the dorsal and ventral margins of the dilated esophagus. (Courtesy Dr. Joanne Burns, Veterinary Imaging Services, Topeka, KS.)

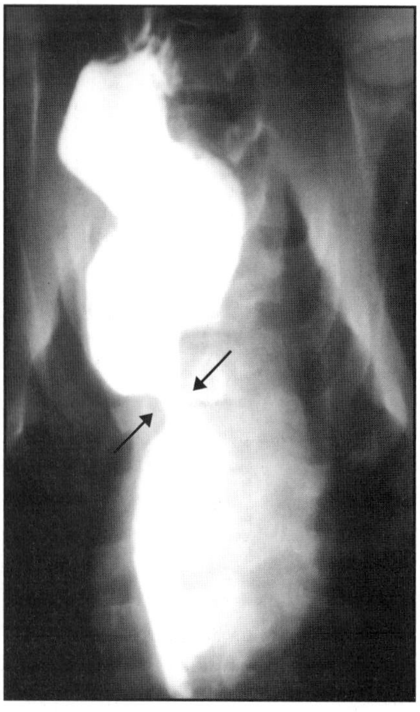

Figure 50-2. Ventrodorsal thoracic radiograph with a positive-contrast esophagram demonstrating an esophageal stricture due to a persistent right aortic arch in a puppy. Note the narrowed esophageal lumen at the base of the heart (arrows) and dilatation of the esophagus on either side of the obstruction.

ly during reassessment and the BCS should be recorded. Young patients with congenital megaesophagus, vascular ring anomalies or cricopharyngeal dysphagia are often stunted compared to littermates.

Auscultatory findings often indicate secondary aspiration pneumonia and may include crackles and prominent bronchovesicular sounds. Dogs with aspiration pneumonia may be febrile and have a mucopurulent nasal discharge.

A complete neurologic examination should be performed on adult dogs with swallowing disorders because acquired megaesophagus is often associated with neuromuscular disorders. Signs of lower motor neuron disease may provide evidence of a generalized polymyopathy, polyneuropathy or neuromuscular junctionopathy (e.g., myasthenia gravis).

Laboratory and Other Clinical Information

A complete blood count may provide evidence of aspiration pneumonia and some sense of the severity of infection. In chronically affected patients, serum protein and albumin concentrations may provide an indication of nutritional status. Additionally, other serum biochemical abnormalities may provide evidence for an underlying disorder (e.g., hypoadrenocorticism, hypothyroidism).

Radiography is a vital diagnostic aid for evaluating dogs and cats with suspected swallowing and esophageal disorders. Survey films may provide definitive information in cases of megaesophagus and esophageal foreign bodies (**Figure 50-1**). Radiographic findings in dogs and cats with megaesophagus include a dilated, air-filled esophagus. In the case of vascular ring anomalies, characteristic esophageal dilatation proximal to the heart base can be identified. Thoracic radiography also allows the clinician to assess the patient for aspiration pneumonia. Additionally, thoracic films may reveal a cranial thoracic mass. Thymoma and thymic lymphosarcoma have been associated with secondary acquired megaesophagus and generalized inflammatory myopathies.

An esophagram offers additional diagnostic information, especially in cases of obstructive lesions, esophagitis and esophageal hypomotility without megaesophagus (**Figure 50-2**). When coupled with video fluoroscopy, an esophagram allows sensitive evaluation of the swallow reflex and esophageal motility (Bexfield et al, 2006) (**Figure 50-3**).

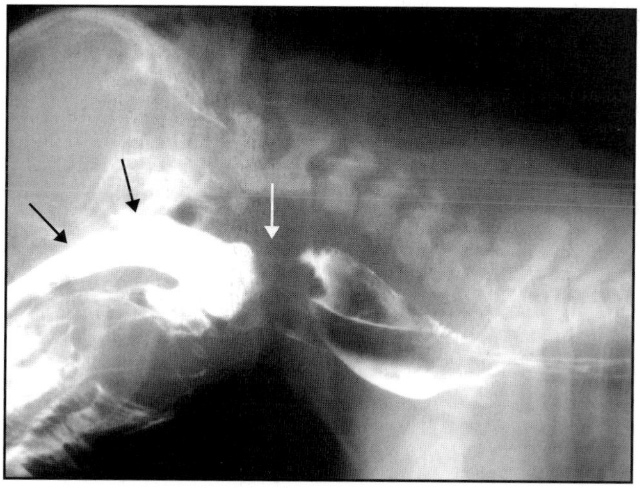

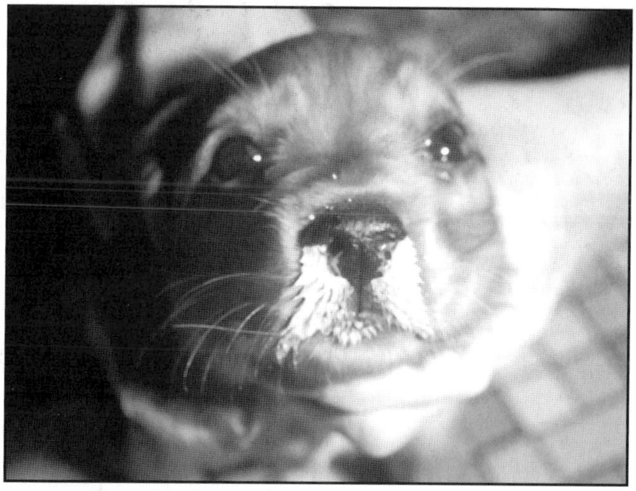

Figure 50-3. Cricopharyngeal achalasia in a cocker spaniel puppy presented for dysphagia. A barium swallow (Left) demonstrated that the cricopharyngeal region (white arrow) did not relax normally during swallowing, which resulted in reflux of barium into the nasopharynx (black arrows). Only a small amount of barium entered the esophagus. The puppy had a difficult time swallowing liquids as shown by regurgitation of milk back through the nose (Right). (Courtesy Dr. Philip Roudebush, Topeka, KS.)

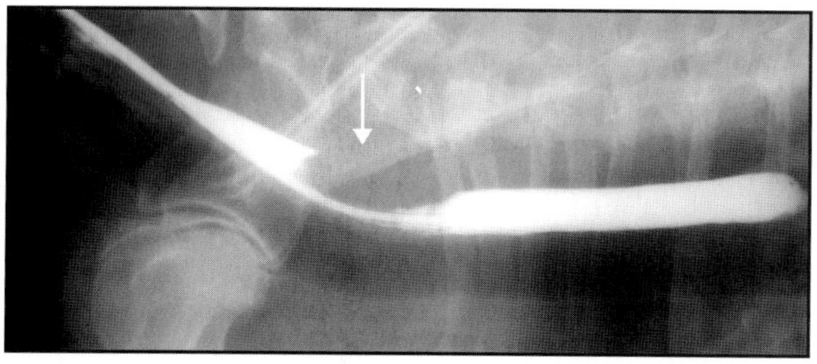

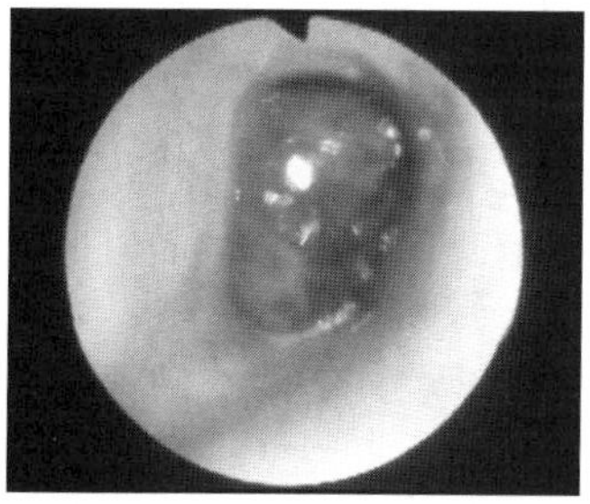

Figure 50-4. Positive-contrast esophagram (Left) from a 12-year-old mixed-breed dog presented for worsening regurgitation. A filling defect is noted in the dorsal wall of the esophagus (arrow). Endoscopy demonstrated a mass lesion (Right) that was confirmed by examination of biopsy specimens as a squamous cell carcinoma. This lesion developed at the site of an acquired esophageal stricture secondary to an episode of postsurgical gastroesophageal reflux. (Courtesy Dr. Michael Leib, Virginia-Maryland Regional College of Veterinary Medicine, Blacksburg, VA.)

Esophagoscopy is a valuable tool for evaluating dogs and cats with suspected obstructive, neoplastic or inflammatory lesions of the esophagus and pharynx (**Figure 50-4**). This tool allows visualization of the entire area and collection of tissue specimens for microbiologic and histopathologic examination, if indicated. Additionally, in cases of esophageal foreign bodies or strictures, the flexible endoscope can provide definitive treatment of the lesion. Foreign bodies can be retrieved or pushed into the stomach using a variety of forceps, whereas esophageal strictures are best managed with endoscopic bougienage, balloon dilatation or both procedures (Weyrauch and Willard, 1998; Leib et al, 2001).

Acquired megaesophagus can occur secondary to several neuromuscular disorders such as myasthenia gravis, dysautonomia, hypothyroidism, hypoadrenocorticism, systemic lupus erythematosus and other causes of generalized myopathy or neuropathy (Dewey et al, 1995; Shelton, 1996, 1996a; Gaynor et al, 1997; Bartges and Nielson, 1992; Harkin et al, 2002).[a] Consult internal medicine and gastroenterology textbooks for a more complete discussion of the diagnosis of these disorders.

Risk Factors

Swallowing disorders have been thought to occur rarely in cats. However, several recent reports have described esophagitis and esophageal strictures in cats after administration of oral antibiotics (tetracycline, doxycycline and clindamycin) (Leib et al, 2001; Beatty et al, 2006; German et al, 2005). Cats may also develop esophageal disease as a result of anesthesia-associated gastroesophageal reflux (Pearson et al, 1978; Leib et al, 2001), gastroesophageal reflux disease (Han et al, 2003) and foreign bodies (Augusto et al, 2005).

In dogs, risk factors for swallowing disorders are primarily breed and age related. Several breeds appear to be predisposed to the development of congenital disorders such as cricopharyngeal dysphagia, congenital megaesophagus and vascular ring anomalies (**Table 50-1**).

No gender predisposition for idiopathic acquired swallowing disorders is apparent. The condition, however, occurs more often in large-breed dogs (Leib and Hall, 1984). One report indicated that Great Dane, golden retriever, German shepherd and Irish setter dogs are at risk for the disease (Gaynor et al,

Table 50-1. Breed-associated disorders of the pharynx and esophagus.

Conditions	Breeds
Cricopharyngeal dysphagia	Cocker spaniel
Congenital esophageal dysmotility and/or megaesophagus	Bouvier des Flandres Chinese Shar-Pei Fox terrier and other terrier breeds German shepherd dog Great Dane Irish setter Labrador retriever Miniature schnauzer Newfoundland Siamese cat
Idiopathic acquired megaesophagus	German shepherd dog Golden retriever Great Dane Irish setter
Vascular ring anomalies	Boston terrier English bulldog German shepherd dog Irish setter Labrador retriever Poodle

Table 50-2. Mechanisms of pharyngeal and esophageal disorders.

Mechanisms	Disorders
Aberrant motility	Congenital megaesophagus Cricopharyngeal dysphagia Dysautonomia Endocrinopathies (hypothyroidism, hypoadrenocorticism) Esophageal dysmotility in young dogs Extraluminal obstruction (mediastinal or hilar lymphadenopathy) Idiopathic megaesophagus Infectious diseases (canine distemper) Myasthenia gravis Paraneoplastic syndromes (lymphosarcoma, thymoma) Polymyopathies Polyneuropathies Secondary megaesophagus Toxin ingestion (lead)
Inflammatory conditions	Foreign body esophagitis Pharyngitis Reflux esophagitis
Obstructive lesions	Foreign bodies Neoplasia *Spirocerca lupi* granulomas Strictures Vascular ring anomalies

1997). Middle-aged to older dogs are more likely to develop myasthenia gravis and other neuromuscular disorders resulting in esophageal disease. Nearly 90% of dogs with focal or generalized myasthenia gravis develop megaesophagus (Shelton et al, 1990). In addition, those breeds predisposed to endocrinopathies (e.g., hypothyroidism and hypoadrenocorticism) are at risk for development of megaesophagus as a rare manifestation of their disease. Dogs with laryngeal paralysis are also at risk for development of megaesophagus (Gaynor et al, 1997). In certain areas (e.g., northeastern United States), exposure to lead has been linked to cases of secondary acquired megaesophagus. In the Midwest, dysautonomia may be associated with acquired megaesophagus (Harkin et al, 2002).

Etiopathogenesis

Pharyngeal and esophageal disorders can generally be attributed to one of three basic pathophysiologic mechanisms: aberrant motility, obstructive lesions or inflammatory degenerative conditions that cause esophagitis/gastroesophageal reflux (**Table 50-2**) (Twedt, 1995).

Aberrant Motility

Cricopharyngeal dysphagia is characterized by asynchrony of the swallowing reflex (Papazoglou et al, 2006). In this condition, the cricopharyngeal muscle fails to relax in coordination with pharyngeal muscle contractions, thus preventing passage of a food bolus from the oropharynx to the esophagus.

Historically, dogs with megaesophagus were presumed to have esophageal achalasia. In this condition, the lower esophageal sphincter fails to relax as esophageal peristaltic activity delivers food to the gastroesophageal junction (GEJ). However, lower esophageal sphincter pressure is normal and activity is synchronous with esophageal motility in dogs with congenital and acquired megaesophagus. The work of several investigators suggests that the efferent pathway in many dogs with megaesophagus is functional, whereas the afferent pathway is dysfunctional (Tan and Diamant, 1987; Holland et al, 1993, 1994). Using intraluminal balloon distention, investigators demonstrated that dogs with idiopathic megaesophagus have a defect in their afferent neural pathway (Washabau, 1992). Other investigators have suggested a defect in esophageal compliance (Holland et al, 1993). These findings have clinical implications because they suggest that foods containing more bulk or prepared in larger boluses may have the capacity to stimulate esophageal motility in mildly affected animals (**Box 50-2**).

Obstructive Lesions

Persistent right aortic arch is the most common vascular ring anomaly recognized in dogs and cats (Muldoon et al, 1997). This anomaly results in constriction of the esophagus at the level of the heart base by the right fourth aortic arch and the ligamentum arteriosum. Esophageal dilatation develops proximal to the vascular ring, leading to regurgitation. Esophageal motility defects may persist if the obstructive lesion is not surgically corrected before irreversible damage to esophageal function occurs.

Esophageal obstruction due to stricture formation may occur as a consequence of recurrent or severe esophageal injury. Strictures occur most commonly due to esophageal foreign bodies or as sequelae to gastroesophageal reflux during general anesthesia. Rarely, infectious (e.g., pythiosis), parasitic (e.g., *Spirocerca lupi*) or neoplastic conditions can result in obstructive esophageal lesions (Mylonakis et al, 2008).

Box 50-2. Swallowing Reflex.

In animals with simple stomachs, deglutition is a sequential, complex, coordinated action that transports food and liquid from the oral cavity to the stomach. It has been divided into three phases: oropharyngeal, esophageal and gastroesophageal.

The oropharyngeal phase begins with the formation of a bolus in the mouth and ends as the bolus passes through the cricopharyngeal area. Pharyngeal contraction is coordinated with relaxation of the upper esophageal sphincter. Following passage of the bolus, the upper esophageal sphincter contracts to close the upper esophagus and to initiate the esophageal phase of swallowing.

The esophageal phase of deglutition begins with the arrival of the bolus in the cranial esophagus. This phase encompasses passage of the bolus from the cranial esophagus to the gastroesophageal junction (GEJ). Four sequences of events that might occur during the esophageal phase have been described.

1. A swallow is followed immediately by an esophageal peristaltic wave, which progresses uninterrupted to the GEJ (primary peristalsis).
2. Liquid and some solid boluses remain in the proximal esophagus until a second or third swallow occurs, then a peristaltic wave carries the combined boluses to the GEJ (primary peristalsis). Other solids immediately move down the esophagus.
3. A bolus temporarily pauses in the proximal esophagus, then a stimulated peristaltic wave carries it to the GEJ (secondary peristalsis).
4. Several boluses accumulate in the proximal esophagus, then a stimulated peristaltic wave carries them to the GEJ (secondary peristalsis).

Direct stimulation of the esophageal wall by a bolus initiates a second peristaltic wave. This is also the pathway for perpetuation of the primary wave; sensory stimulation from the bolus continues as it moves down the esophagus. Progression of primary or secondary peristaltic contractions depends on the presence, size and location of the bolus in the esophagus. In the absence of a bolus, peristalsis in the esophagus does not follow the act of swallowing. In the thoracic esophagus, contractions are facilitated by, but do not depend on a bolus. Thus, two mechanisms are involved in the regulation of esophageal contraction: 1) a central regulatory mechanism (swallowing center) in the brainstem and 2) afferent nerve impulses that originate in the esophagus in the presence of a bolus.

The lower esophageal sphincter (LES) is not a true anatomic sphincter, but rather a physiologic high-pressure zone. This zone is found in the most distal portion of the esophagus and separates the esophagus from the stomach. The LES is the functional term used for this region, but many authors use the anatomic term GEJ. During peristalsis, the LES relaxes and allows the bolus to pass into the stomach (gastroesophageal phase). A prevalent misunderstanding is that LES relaxation and opening are synonymous. Relaxation and opening of the LES are related but distinct events. LES opening is a passive mechanical event affected by the force of an oncoming bolus, whereas LES relaxation occurs as an active reflex process mediated neurologically. The average canine LES begins to relax several seconds before the esophageal pressure wave peaks in the distal esophagus. Even if the LES opens and closes normally, synchronization of LES with the esophageal wave is still required for normal passage of a bolus. It closes after passage of the bolus to prevent gastroesophageal reflux.

The GEJ is the only area of the gastrointestinal tract in which luminal structures having opposite cavitary pressures are in continuity. Mechanical factors and intrinsic LES tone serve as the major control mechanisms to prevent reflux of gastric contents. Whatever external force or positive pressure is applied to the stomach is also exerted on the terminal abdominal esophagus; therefore, no pressure gradient occurs between the stomach and thoracic esophagus. Other mechanical factors that prevent gastroesophageal reflux include: 1) interdigitating gastric rugal folds, 2) focal thickening of the distal esophageal muscle coat (in the dog there is an inner section of smooth muscle), 3) oblique implantation of the distal esophagus into the stomach and 4) the flap-like cardiac incisura, which is pushed against the GEJ by the enlarging gastric fundus. Gastrin and other gastrointestinal hormones at pharmacologic doses appear to increase LES tone. Whether these hormones function to increase LES tone when released physiologically during normal food ingestion is still speculative.

The Bibliography for **Box 50-2** can be found at www.markmorris.org.

Inflammation/Degeneration

Esophagitis arises most often as a consequence of gastroesophageal reflux or foreign body ingestion (Sellon and Willard, 2003). The GEJ serves as a barrier preventing reflux of gastric contents including pepsin and hydrochloric acid into the lumen of the esophagus. Postprandially, GEJ pressure increases in response to neural and hormonal stimuli. Certain gastrointestinal (GI) hormones, including gastrin, pancreatic polypeptide, motilin and substance P increase GEJ pressure, whereas others (i.e., secretin, cholecystokinin) reduce GEJ pressure. Dietary influences on the GEJ pressure are presumably mediated via GI hormone release. High-protein meals increase GEJ pressure through gastrin release, whereas high-fat foods reduce GEJ pressure via cholecystokinin release.

The most common cause of esophagitis in dogs and cats appears to be anesthesia-associated reflux of gastric contents into the esophagus (Sellon and Willard, 2003). Certain sedatives, including acepromazine, xylazine and diazepam reduce GEJ pressure and may predispose an animal to reflux esophagitis following anesthetic episodes (Strombeck and Harrold, 1985; Hall et al, 1987). Recently, anesthetic-associated gastroesophageal reflux has been demonstrated to occur equally in dogs maintained under anesthesia for orthopedic procedures with isoflurane, halothane or sevoflurane (Wilson et al, 2006). Fifty-one of 90 dogs studied developed acid reflux within 30 to 90 minutes following induction and 13 of 90 patients regurgitated.

Foreign body ingestion is most commonly reported in young patients. However, certain feeding practices can result in esophageal foreign bodies in adult patients. Feeding vegetable-based dental chews and treats, bones and rawhide

Table 50-3. Key nutritional factors for foods for patients with swallowing disorders due to obstructive lesions or aberrant motility.*

Factors	Recommended levels
Energy density	≥4.5 kcal/g (≥18.8 kJ/g)
Fat	≥25%
Protein	≥25% for dog foods ≥35% for cat foods

*Nutrients expressed on a dry matter basis; food form is also a key nutritional factor but varies with individual patients (see text).

Table 50-4. Key nutritional factors for foods for dogs and cats with esophagitis/gastroesophageal reflux.*

Factors	Recommended levels
Energy density	≥4 kcal/g (≥16.7 kJ/g)
Fat	≤15% for dog foods ≤20% for cat foods
Protein	≥25% for dog foods ≥35% for cat foods

*Nutrients expressed on a dry matter basis; food form is also a key nutritional factor, but varies with the disease and individual patients (see text).

chews have resulted in esophageal foreign bodies (Rousseau et al, 2007; Leib and Sartor, 2008). In a recent retrospective review, 46 of 60 esophageal foreign bodies removed from dogs were bones (Rousseau et al, 2007). Occasionally, consumption of irritative substances such as strong acids or alkalis may cause serious esophagitis. Drug-induced esophageal disease is common in people (Sellon and Willard, 2003) and has been reported to occur in cats receiving antibiotic tablets or capsules via a "dry swallow." In cats, esophageal transit times are prolonged following the administration of dry capsules as compared to capsules followed by a water bolus (Westfall et al, 2001). Administration of oral antibiotics to cats should be accompanied by wet food and/or a water bolus (Westfall et al, 2001; Beatty et al, 2006).

Iatrogenic esophagitis may occur as a sequela to nasoesophageal intubation when the feeding tube crosses the GEJ, resulting in incompetence of the sphincter (Lantz et al, 1983). Hiatal hernias are rarely reported in dogs and cats, but can interfere with the function of the GEJ.

Key Nutritional Factors

Key nutritional factors for patients with swallowing disorders are summarized in **Tables 50-3** and **50-4** and discussed in detail below. Patients with swallowing disorders are often debilitated and growth of very young patients is often stunted. In addition to the key nutritional factors discussed here, other nutritional factors may be important depending on the lifestage and body condition of the patient.

Energy and Fat

In patients with motility and obstructive disorders, a relatively high energy density is helpful in meeting the patient's caloric requirement in a small volume of food relative to lower fat foods. Foods with at least 25% dry matter (DM) fat and energy densities of at least 4.5 kcal/g (18.8 kJ/g) DM are recommended. However, a lower fat content (≤15% DM for dogs and ≤20% DM for cats) is a better option for cases of esophagitis due to gastric reflux. High dietary fat delays gastric emptying and reduces lower esophageal sphincter pressure, which promotes reflux of food and gastric secretions into the esophagus (Washabau and Hall, 1997). However, these patients also need relatively energy dense foods (at least 4 kcal/g DM [16.7 kJ/g]). An energy dense, moderate fat food is recommended for patients with esophagitis/gastroesophageal reflux. Foods with these characteristics tend to be highly digestible.

Protein

Protein is required in amounts adequate for tissue repair and to support growth in young patients. Additionally, dietary protein may play an important role in reducing episodes of gastroesophageal reflux because protein stimulates an increase in gastroesophageal sphincter pressure. This effect is linked to dietary protein's stimulatory effect on gastrin and gastric acid secretion (Guilford, 1996). By increasing the lower esophageal sphincter pressure, episodes of gastroesophageal reflux are decreased, thus limiting the potential for further esophageal injury or aspiration pneumonia. For these reasons, dietary protein content should be at least 25% DM for foods for adult dogs and at least 35% DM for foods for adult cats.

Food Form

Foods of differing consistency should be used to determine the best texture for individual patients. A liquid or gruel consistency is usually best for patients with cricopharyngeal dysphagia, esophageal obstructive lesions and/or esophagitis and may be effective in patients with megaesophagus. Esophageal performance may improve in patients with megaesophagus when the swallowing reflex is maximally stimulated by the texture of dry foods or when moist foods are formed into large boluses. Dry food or boluses of moist food may act as a stimulus (secondary peristalsis) to any remaining normal esophageal tissue. Gruels or liquids may not stimulate secondary peristalsis, thereby increasing the risk of aspiration pneumonia.

FEEDING PLAN

The goals of dietary management for patients with megaesophagus are to minimize regurgitation, avoid secondary aspiration pneumonia and to provide adequate nutrition to regain or maintain proper body weight and condition.

Assess and Select the Food

The appropriate key nutritional factor profile and the form of the food recommended for use in patients with pharyngeal/esophageal disorders depend on whether the problem is due to obstructive lesions/aberrant motility or underlying inflammatory conditions.

Table 50-5. Key nutritional factor content of selected commercial veterinary therapeutic foods for dogs with esophagitis/gastroesophageal reflux compared to recommended levels.*

Dry foods	Energy density (kcal/cup)**	Energy density (kcal/g)	Fat (%)	Protein (%)
Recommended levels	**-**	**≥4**	**≤15**	**≥25**
Hill's Prescription Diet i/d Canine	379	4.2	14.1	26.2
Iams Veterinary Formula Intestinal Low-Residue	257	3.8	10.7	24.6
Medi-Cal Gastro Formula	330	na	13.9	22.9
Purina Veterinary Diets EN GastroENteric Formula	397	4.2	12.6	27.0
Royal Canin Veterinary Diet Intestinal HE	389	4.5	22.0	33.0
Moist foods	**Energy density (kcal/can)****	**Energy density (kcal/g)**	**Fat (%)**	**Protein (%)**
Recommended levels	**-**	**≥4**	**≤15**	**≥25**
Hill's Prescription Diet i/d Canine	485/13 oz.	4.4	14.9	25.0
Iams Veterinary Formula Intestinal Low-Residue	413/14 oz.	4.6	13.2	35.9
Medi-Cal Gastro Formula	455/396 g	na	11.7	22.1
Purina Veterinary Diets EN GastroENteric Formula	423/354 g	4.0	13.8	30.5
Royal Canin Veterinary Diet Intestinal HE	446/396 g	4.3	11.8	23.1

Key: na = information not available from manufacturer.
*From manufacturers' published information or calculated from manufacturers' published as-fed values; all values are on a dry matter basis unless otherwise stated.
**Energy density values are listed on an as fed basis and are useful for determining the amount to feed; cup = 8-oz. measuring cup. To convert to kJ, multiply kcal by 4.184.

Obstructive Lesions and Aberrant Motility

Feeding a high-calorie, high-fat balanced growth or recuperative food (a working/sporting food for dogs) is appropriate for most patients with megaesophagus, cricopharyngeal achalasia or obstructive lesions. The food consistency that best promotes flow through the esophagus to the stomach is determined in each case by trial and error.

Gruels often work well, which necessitates using foods with high water content (>80%). Moist foods are typically made with ingredients that blenderize easily with water. For example, meat ingredients containing connective tissue and bone do not blenderize as easily as skeletal muscle and organ protein sources. Therefore, using nutrient-dense products made from highly digestible ingredients is more likely to meet the nutrient requirements of the patient in the smallest volume possible. Recommending larger cans of calorically dense cat food can help reduce the volume and cost of feeding a large dog.

However, esophageal performance may improve in megaesophagus patients when the swallowing reflex is maximally stimulated by the texture of dry foods or moist foods formed into large boluses. These food forms may act as a stimulus (secondary peristalsis) to any remaining normal esophageal tissue whereas, gruels or liquids may not stimulate secondary peristalsis, thereby increasing the risk of aspiration pneumonia.

Comparing the key nutritional factor content of a food being considered with the recommendations in **Table 50-3** will facilitate the selection process. Tables 17-4, 18-12, 24-3, 25-8 and 25-9 are also useful.

Inflammatory Conditions

Foods with lower levels of dietary fat are recommended for managing patients with esophagitis and gastroesophageal reflux. Higher dietary fat levels may precipitate gastroesophageal reflux by delaying gastric emptying and reducing lower esophageal sphincter pressure. Increased dietary protein enhances lower esophageal sphincter tone. **Tables 50-5** and **50-6** compare the key nutritional factor content of selected veterinary therapeutic foods to the recommended levels for canine and feline patients, respectively, with esophagitis and gastroesophageal reflux. As mentioned above, moist foods are usually more readily liquefied.

Assess and Determine the Feeding Method

Patients with swallowing disorders often require specialized feeding methods because the current feeding protocol of one to three meals per day fed in a bowl on the floor is rarely appropriate. In addition to a change to the appropriate food (including form), the key tools of nutritional management in these cases are a change in the feeding method.

Small-volume, frequent meals are recommended when feeding patients with swallowing disorders. Gruel-type foods are often necessary because the liquid form is more amenable to gravity fill of the stomach. Feeding a high-calorie food to a patient in an upright position and maintaining this position for 20 to 30 minutes after feeding provides ample time for gravitational flow of the food through the esophagus to the stomach. Upright feeding can be accomplished by several methods. The most common technique is to elevate the food bowl so that the dog or cat has to sit down or stand on its hind legs to eat. Pets can be trained to eat on stairs or from a counter or stool. Alternatively, small dogs and cats can be cradled in an upright position in the owner's arms while eating (**Figure 50-5**). Large dogs can be trained to sit after eating or lie in sternal recumbency on an inclined board for the required period of time. Several companies manufacture devices to facilitate upright feeding (**Figure 50-6**).

In some patients, upright feeding is inadequate to control regurgitation or is impractical because of the pet's temperament or

Table 50-6. Key nutritional factor content of selected commercial veterinary therapeutic foods for cats with esophagitis/gastroesophageal reflux compared to recommended levels.*

Dry foods	Energy density (kcal/cup)**	Energy density (kcal/g)	Fat (%)	Protein (%)
Recommended levels	**-**	**≥4**	**≤20**	**≥35**
Hill's Prescription Diet i/d Feline	483	4.3	20.2	40.3
Iams Veterinary Formula Intestinal Low-Residue	348	3.9	13.7	35.8
Medi-Cal Hypoallergenic/Gastro	350	na	11.5	29.8
Purina Veterinary Diets EN GastroENteric Formula	572	4.4	18.4	56.2
Royal Canin Veterinary Diet Intestinal HE 30	396	4.4	23.7	34.4
Moist foods	**Energy density (kcal/can)****	**Energy density (kcal/g)**	**Fat (%)**	**Protein (%)**
Recommended levels	**-**	**≥4**	**≤20**	**≥35**
Hill's Prescription Diet i/d Feline	161/5.5 oz.	4.2	24.1	37.6
Iams Veterinary Formula Intestinal Low-Residue	169/6 oz.	4.0	11.7	38.4
Medi-Cal Hypoallergenic/Gastro	184/170 g	na	35.9	35.5
Medi-Cal Sensitivity CR	162/165 g	na	35.1	34.5

Key: na = information not available from manufacturer.
*From manufacturers' published information or calculated from manufacturers' published as-fed values; all values are on a dry matter basis unless otherwise stated.
**Energy density values are listed on an as fed basis and are useful for determining the amount to feed; cup = 8-oz. measuring cup. To convert to kJ, multiply kcal by 4.184.

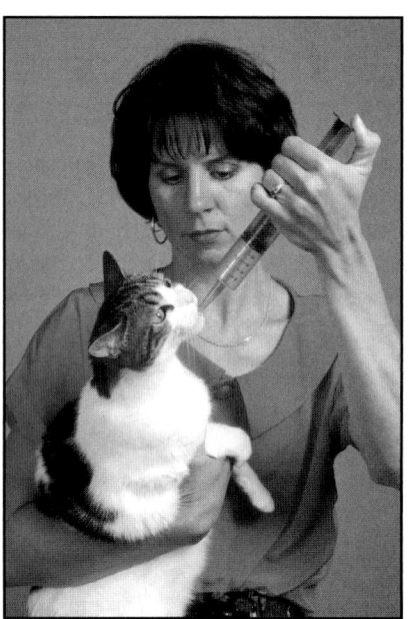

Figure 50-5. Upright feeding position that can be used for cats and small dogs with megaesophagus.

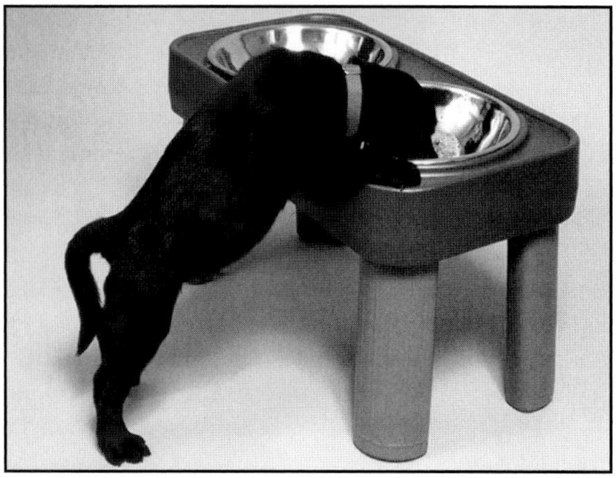

Figure 50-6. Feeding device that can be used to maintain an upright feeding position for patients with megaesophagus.

the owner's schedule. In those cases, placement of a gastrostomy or enterostomy tube is recommended to bypass the esophagus entirely. Nasoesophageal, nasogastric and esophagostomy tubes are not appropriate in this situation because they deliver food into the esophagus where it can be regurgitated. Patients with ongoing signs of malnutrition at presentation should receive a large-bore gastrostomy feeding tube, if possible, and immediate alimentation via the tube until adequate oral intake can be achieved. Gastrostomy tubes have been used successfully for long periods to maintain the nutritional status of dogs with megaesophagus. A permanent button-type gastrostomy tube should be considered in cases in which owners are willing to feed their pet long-term via gastrostomy tube. Even with the use of gastrostomy tubes, regurgitation of saliva and food refluxed from the stomach may still occur, which can result in aspiration pneumonia. Some clinicians prefer feeding via enterostomy tube because of the potential for gastroesophageal reflux and recurrent aspiration. Owners should be made aware that regurgitation might not completely cease even if all food and water is administered through the gastrostomy tube. Many patients will continue to regurgitate fluid, which is most likely salivary secretions. However, the likelihood of aspiration pneumonia is reduced greatly.

Pharyngeal and esophageal tissues heal slowly and are susceptible to secondary bacterial infections. Therefore, surgeons have traditionally recommended withholding oral feedings of regular pet foods for three to four days for patients with inflammation, trauma or surgery to these tissues. Patients with no history or evidence of malnutrition may be safely held off food (but not water) for two to three days if necessary, but should receive nutrition by the fourth day. Percutaneous endoscopic gastrostomy tube placement may be useful in patients after dilatation of esophageal strictures or in pets with severe esophagitis secondary to foreign body removal. The tubes can be placed at the time of an endoscopic esophageal examination. Dietary goals in these patients are to provide adequate nutrition to the patient using foods that minimize irritation and trauma to sensitive pharyngeal and esophageal tissues.

CONCURRENT THERAPY

The feeding plan is often used in conjunction with other therapeutic modalities including surgery (e.g., cricopharyngeal myotomy, esophageal stricture, vascular ring anomaly, esophageal foreign bodies), bougienage (e.g., esophageal stricture), endoscopy (e.g., foreign body removal) and drugs (e.g., antibiotics, prokinetic agents, corticosteroids, antacids, H_2-receptor blockers, mucosal protective agents).

REASSESSMENT

Nutritional reassessment of patients with swallowing disorders includes: 1) monitoring changes in body weight and condition, 2) evaluating owner compliance regarding feeding the proper amount of food to the patient, 3) determining the extent of ongoing dysphagia or regurgitation and 4) monitoring resolution of other concurrent disease processes (e.g., pneumonia, myopathies, endocrinopathies). Daily food dosage should be adjusted as indicated by changes in the patient's body weight and condition.

ENDNOTE

a. Davenport DJ, Ware W. The Ohio State University, Columbus. Unpublished data. 1986.

REFERENCES

The references for **Chapter 50** can be found at www.markmorris.org.

CASE 50-1

Regurgitation in a Collie

Deborah J. Davenport, DVM, MS, Dipl. ACVIM (Internal Medicine)
Hill's Science and Technology Center
Topeka, Kansas, USA

Patient Assessment

A six-year-old, neutered female collie dog was examined for regurgitation and coughing of two weeks' duration. The owners had first noticed what they described as vomiting two weeks earlier. Further questioning confirmed that the problem was probably regurgitation because the process involved casting up undigested food in a tubular form with little or no force, rather than forceful expulsion of digested food with retching and involuntary abdominal contractions. Soft coughing and a mucoid nasal discharge began about a week after the onset of regurgitation. The dog was also somewhat lethargic.

Physical examination revealed a quiet, thin (body condition score [BCS] 2/5), mildly febrile (39.1°C [102.5°F]), 23-kg dog with an increased respiratory rate (45 breaths/min.). Slight mucopurulent discharge was noted in both external nares. Low-pitched, coarse crackles were heard over the entire lung field, but were loudest in the ventral half of the thorax. The coat appeared dry and lusterless. When this finding was mentioned to the owners, they confirmed that a change in coat quality had occurred more than a year ago.

Initial diagnostic evaluation included a complete blood count (neutrophilic leukocytosis), serum biochemistry profile (normal), urinalysis (normal), fecal flotation (whipworm ova) and thoracic radiography (changes consistent with megaesophagus and mild bronchopneumonia).

Further testing was done to rule out secondary or acquired causes of megaesophagus. A thorough neurologic examination failed to reveal neurologic deficits. Tests for myasthenia gravis (i.e., acetylcholine receptor antibody test) and lead toxicosis were negative. A positive-contrast esophagram revealed no evidence of strictures, granulomas, foreign bodies, neoplasia or extraesophageal compression. Results of a thyroid-screening panel included decreased serum concentrations of total thyroxine (T_4) and free T_4, and increased serum concentrations of thyrotropin (TSH).

The tentative diagnoses were hypothyroidism, megaesophagus and aspiration pneumonia.

Assess the Food and Feeding Method

The dog was normally fed a dry specialty brand food twice daily mixed with a small amount of various moist grocery brand foods. A homemade mixture of chicken and rice had also been offered during the past week in an effort to control the regurgitation.

Questions
1. What are the key nutritional factors to consider for this patient?
2. Outline an appropriate feeding plan (foods and feeding method) for this dog.

Answers and Discussion
1. Key nutritional factors for patients with megaesophagus and other motility or obstructive-type swallowing disorders include energy, fat, protein and food form. These patients are often debilitated because of inadequate food intake and secondary aspiration pneumonia. A relatively high-fat (≥25% dry matter [DM] fat) energy-dense (≥4.5 kcal/g [18.8 kJ/g] DM) food helps meet the patient's caloric requirement in small volumes. Protein is required in amounts adequate to support tissue repair and help reduce episodes of gastroesophageal reflux. Dietary protein should generally be at least 25% DM. The food form may influence esophageal motility and subsequent clinical signs. Esophageal performance in patients with congenital or acquired esophageal dilatation may improve when the swallowing reflex is maximally stimulated by the texture of coarse, dry foods. Dry food boluses may stimulate any remaining normal esophageal tissue; therefore, dry foods are the form of choice because gruels may increase the risk of aspiration pneumonia.
2. The goals of dietary management for patients with megaesophagus are to minimize regurgitation, avoid secondary aspiration pneumonia and provide adequate nutrition to regain or maintain proper body weight and condition. In this case, the feeding plan was used in conjunction with thyroid hormone replacement and treatment of the aspiration pneumonia. (See Progress Notes below.) The acquired esophageal motility defect may or may not be reversible. A high-fat, high-calorie recuperative, working/sporting dog or growth-type food is appropriate for this patient. The food should be given in small-volume, frequent meals and offered so the dog eats in an upright position. The food consistency and feeding method that best promote flow through the esophagus to the stomach in individual patients are often determined by trial and error.

Progress Notes
Thyroid hormone replacement therapy was started using 0.6 mg per day of oral synthetic levothyroxine sodium[a] (L-thyroxine). The pneumonia was treated with one injection of enrofloxacin (Baytril[b]) followed by oral enrofloxacin tablets (68 mg, b.i.d.) for three weeks. The whipworm infection was treated with a broad-spectrum anthelmintic (Drontal Plus[b]). The food was changed to a commercial dry veterinary therapeutic food designed for stress and recovery. This food has increased fat levels (25% DM) and energy density (4.8 kcal/g [20.1 kJ] DM) and increased protein levels (38.1% DM) to support recovery and weight gain. Daily energy requirement was estimated to be 1,400 kcal (5.86 MJ) for an ideal body weight of 27 kg. The food was given in small, frequent meals and offered from a bowl placed on the edge of a table.

The coughing and nasal discharge gradually improved so the antibiotic was discontinued. Regurgitation continued but gradually lessened in frequency. Radiographs six weeks later revealed no evidence of aspiration pneumonia, but the megaesophagus was still evident. Body weight (26.5 kg) and body condition (BCS 3/5) had improved. The food was changed to the commercial dry specialty brand food originally fed to the dog but it was offered from an elevated position. This feeding plan successfully reduced the regurgitation to a few episodes per week.

Endnotes
a. Soloxine. Daniels Pharmaceuticals Inc., St Petersburg, FL, USA.
b. Baytril. Bayer Animal Health, Shawnee, KS, USA.

Bibliography
Guilford WG, Strombeck DR. Diseases of swallowing. In: Guilford WG, Center SA, Strombeck DR, et al, eds. Strombeck's Small Animal Gastroenterology, 3rd ed. Philadelphia, PA: WB Saunders Co, 1996; 211-238.

Jaggy A, Oliver JE. Neurologic manifestations of thyroid disease. Veterinary Clinics of North America: Small Animal Practice 1994; 24: 487-494.

Peterson ME, Melian C, Nichols R. Measurement of serum total thyroxine, triiodothyronine, free thyroxine and thyrotropin concentrations for diagnosis of hypothyroidism in dogs. Journal of the American Veterinary Medical Association 1997; 211: 1396-1402.

Chapter 51

Introduction to Gastric Diseases

Deborah J. Davenport
Rebecca L. Remillard

"Content the stomach and the stomach will content you."
Thomas Walker (1784-1836)

CLINICAL IMPORTANCE

Vomiting is the hallmark of gastric disorders in dogs and cats (Box 52-1). Vomiting may be acute or chronic with a long list of possible etiologies (Twedt, 2005; Simpson, 2005). Vomiting requires a forceful coordinated musculoskeletal effort to eject food from the stomach to the mouth.

Table 51-1 lists breed-associated gastric disorders. Certain gastric diseases (gastritis, gastroduodenal diseases and gastric motility/emptying diseases) may also require management with pharmacologic agents (**Table 51-2**).

Dietary goals are to meet the nutritional requirements of the patient with foods that minimize gastric irritation, promote gastric emptying and normalize gastric motility. In most vomiting cases of less than 48 hours' duration, withholding water for 24 hours and food for 24 to 48 hours generally controls the episode. The patient's regular food should then be gradually reintroduced in small frequent meals over two to three days. Episodes of acute vomiting that occur for longer than three days and cases of chronic vomiting (i.e., persisting longer than 21 days) with signs of malnutrition require more intensive nutritional and medical management.

Chapters 52 through 54 include feeding plans for patients with gastric disorders. Tables in those chapters list the key nutritional factors for such patients as well as tables that include the levels of key nutritional factors of commercial veterinary therapeutic foods marketed for patients with gastric disorders. For comparative purposes, these tables also include the recommended levels of key nutritional factors for patients with gastric disorders.

REFERENCES

The references for **Chapter 51** can be found at www.markmorris.org.

Table 51-1. Breed-associated gastric disorders.

Disorders	Breeds
Atrophic gastritis	Lundehund
Chronic hypertrophic gastritis	Basenji Drentse patrijshond
Chronic hypertrophic pyloric gastropathy	Lhaso apso Maltese dog Pekingese Shih Tzu
Gastric dilatation-volvulus	Basset hound Doberman pinscher Gordon setter Great Dane Irish setter Saint Bernard Weimaraner
Gastric neoplasia	Beagle Belgian shepherd Rough collie Staffordshire bull terrier
Hemorrhagic gastroenteritis	Dachshund Miniature schnauzer Toy poodle
Pyloric stenosis	Boston terrier Boxer Siamese cat

Table 51-2. Pharmacologic agents useful in managing gastritis, gastroduodenal ulceration and gastric motility/emptying disorders.

Antacids	
Mylanta (Al + Mg)	1 to 2 tabs or 5 to 10 ml PO every four to six hours
Amphojel (AlOH)	
Tums ($CaCO_3$)	
Antiemetic agents	
Chlorpromazine	0.2 to 0.5 mg/kg body weight, PO, SC, IM every six to eight hours
Prochlorpromazine	0.5 mg/kg body weight, PO, SC, IM every six to eight hours
Odansetron	0.1 to 0.2 mg/kg body weight, SC every eight hours or 0.5 mg/kg body weight, IV (loading dose) followed by 0.5 mg/kg body weight as a constant IV infusion or 0.5 to 1.0 mg/kg body weight, PO every six to eight hours
Metoclopramide	0.2 to 0.4 mg/kg body weight, IM, SC every eight hours or 1.0 mg/kg body weight/day as a constant IV infusion
Butorphanol	0.4 mg/kg body weight, IM or 0.1 mg/kg body weight/hour as a constant IV infusion
Antihistamines	
Diphenhydramine	2 to 4 mg/kg body weight, PO
Dimenhydrinate	25 to 50 mg PO per dog or 12.5 mg PO per cat
Anti-prostaglandin agent	
Misoprostol	1 to 3 µg/kg body weight, PO every eight to 12 hours (dogs)
H_2-receptor blockers	
Cimetidine	5 to 10 mg/kg body weight, PO, SC every six to eight hours
Ranitidine	1 to 4 mg/kg body weight, PO, SC, IV every eight to 12 hours
Famotidine	0.5 to 1.0 mg/kg body weight, PO, IV every 12 to 24 hours
Nizatidine	2.5 to 5.0 mg/kg body weight, PO every 24 hours
Prokinetic agents	
Metoclopramide	0.2 to 0.4 mg/kg body weight, IM, SC every eight hours or 1.0 mg/kg body weight/day as a constant IV infusion
Cisapride	0.25 to 0.5 mg/kg body weight, PO every eight hours*
Erythromycin	0.5 to 1.0 mg/kg body weight, PO every eight hours (dogs)
Proton pump inhibitors	
Omeprazole	0.2 to 0.7 mg/kg body weight, PO every 24 hours (dogs)
Mucosal protectants	
Sucralfate	1 g/25 kg body weight, PO every six to eight hours
Colloidal bismuth	

Key: PO = per os, SC = subcutaneously, IM = intramuscularly, IV = intravenously.
*Available from compounding pharmacies.

Chapter 52

Gastritis and Gastroduodenal Ulceration

Deborah J. Davenport
Rebecca L. Remillard
Christine Jenkins

"If your stomach disputes you, lie down and pacify it with cool thoughts."
Satchel Paige

CLINICAL IMPORTANCE

Gastritis is one of the most common causes of vomiting in dogs and cats (Van der Gaag, 1988). Acute gastroenteritis is covered in Chapter 56. The prevalence of gastritis in the pet population is unknown, but is thought to be high because many different insults can result in gastric mucosal inflammation (**Table 52-1**). In one survey, 9% of research beagles had histologic evidence of gastritis in the absence of clinical signs (Hottendorf and Hirth, 1974). Gastritis has been diagnosed in 35% of dogs presented for chronic vomiting and has been identified in 26 to 48% of asymptomatic dogs. The prevalence in cats is unknown (Simpson, 2006). The National Companion Animal Study was developed in the early 1990s to determine the most common disorders affecting dogs and cats examined at private veterinary practices in the United States. In 1995, 31,484 dogs and 15,226 cats were examined at 52 private veterinary clinics in 31 states. In this study, the prevalence of vomiting was 2.1% for dogs and 2.2% for cats (Lund et al, 1999). Acute gastritis often accompanies acute enteritis and is called acute gastroenteritis.

Previously, the prevalence of gastroduodenal ulcers in dogs and cats was thought to be low compared with the prevalence reported in people. In many cases, the historical infrequent diagnosis of gastroduodenal ulceration was possibly due to the absence of obvious clinical signs. For example, in experimental studies involving dogs, extensive gastroduodenal ulceration was present, whereas only mild clinical signs were evident (Dow et al, 1990). However, gastroduodenal ulceration is now diagnosed more frequently in veterinary patients. While advances in diagnostics (endoscopy) have provided improved capability to identify gastroduodenal ulcers, the apparent increase in prevalence has been associated with the use of nonsteroidal antiinflammatory drugs (NSAIDs) for pain management and treatment of inflammatory conditions. The actual incidence of gastroduodenal ulceration related to NSAID use in dogs is unknown (Hinton et al, 2002; Lascelles et al, 2005; Dowers et al, 2006).

PATIENT ASSESSMENT

History and Physical Examination

Although some patients are asymptomatic, vomiting is the most common presenting complaint for patients with acute or chronic gastritis. Typically, owners report intermittent vomiting of food or bile-stained fluid. Fresh or digested blood appearing as "coffee grounds" may be present in the vomitus. Associated signs may include diarrhea, abdominal pain and melena. Anorexia is the presenting sign in many patients with gastritis. The clinician should obtain details regarding frequency, duration and progression of the vomiting episodes. In addition, the vomitus should be characterized (e.g., color, contents). It is important to differentiate vomiting from regurgitation (Simpson, 2005; Willard, 2005). Some owners may report that their dog

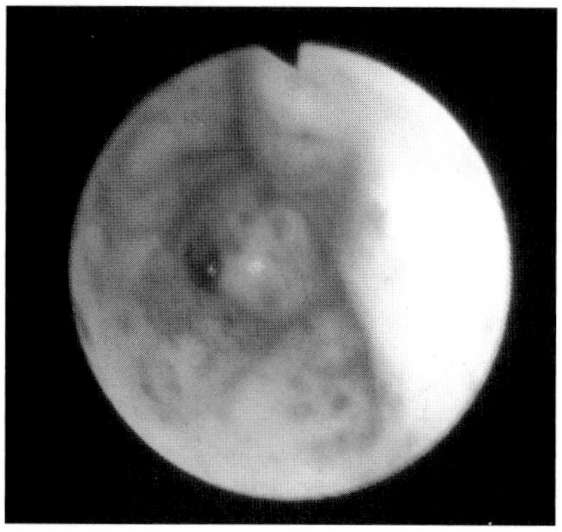

Figure 52-1. Endoscopic appearance of antral gastritis in a dog with chronic vomiting. Note the multiple hemorrhagic erosive lesions of the gastric mucosa. (Courtesy Dr. Michael Leib, Virginia-Maryland Regional College of Veterinary Medicine, Blacksburg, VA.)

assumes a "praying posture," which is considered a manifestation of upper abdominal pain.

Patient history often is adequate to provide a presumptive diagnosis of gastritis. Owners should be questioned closely about potential for toxin exposure (e.g., lead, arsenic) and foreign body ingestion (e.g., bones, coins, garbage) by the patient. A history of NSAID administration provides a presumptive diagnosis of drug-induced gastroduodenal erosions or ulcerations. The veterinarian should question the owner specifically about the use of over-the-counter agents (e.g., aspirin, ibuprofen) in addition to prescription NSAIDs.

Physical examination is often unremarkable in dogs and cats with gastritis or gastroduodenal ulcerations. Reduced skin turgor and tacky mucous membranes indicate dehydration. Abdominal pain may be recognized, particularly in those patients that develop peritonitis as a consequence of a perforated ulcer. In chronic cases, weight loss and poor body condition may be noted. Pallor and weakness may be present in patients with significant gastrointestinal (GI) blood loss. Other findings may reflect the underlying cause of gastritis (e.g., cutaneous masses or hepatosplenomegaly associated with mastocytosis).

Laboratory and Other Clinical Information

Routine hematology, serum biochemistry profiles and urinalyses help rule out metabolic causes of gastritis. These tests readily identify renal disease, hepatopathies and hypoadrenocorticism. The hematocrit and hemogram are useful in assessing severity and chronicity of gastric disease. Inflammatory leukograms may be identified in animals with neoplasia, perforated GI ulcers, inflammatory bowel disease (IBD) and pythiosis. Eosinophilia may indicate parasitism or eosinophilic gastritis. In cats, extreme eosinophilia is suggestive of hypereosinophilic syndrome or systemic mastocytosis. Identification of circulating mast cells is generally diagnostic for mast cell tumors, which are associated with GI ulcer disease due to hyperhistaminemia.

Fecal examinations for parasites and occult blood are important screening tests. Parasites are an unlikely cause of gastritis, but should be considered. Gastric parasites, such *Ollulanus tricuspis* or *Physaloptera* spp., are identified more readily in vomitus or gastric juice or on endoscopic visualization. The accuracy of fecal occult blood testing has been confirmed in dogs consuming dry foods (Dow et al, 1990; Gilson et al, 1990). Moist meat-based foods often yield false-positive results. Both the modified guaiac and orthotoluidine tests are sensitive and specific for detecting occult blood in feces (Gilson et al, 1990).

Imaging modalities (e.g., survey and contrast radiography and ultrasonography) are noninvasive diagnostic techniques for evaluating pets with gastritis or GI ulceration. Abdominal radiographs frequently are normal in patients with gastritis (Simpson, 2005). Survey radiography may be useful in the diagnosis of radiopaque foreign bodies. Abnormalities in renal size or shape may suggest renal insufficiency as the cause of gastritis. Hepatosplenomegaly in cats suggests systemic mastocytosis or alimentary lymphosarcoma. Free air in the abdomen is diagnostic for viscus rupture associated with a perforated GI ulcer and indicates the need for immediate exploratory surgery.

Contrast radiographic examinations may be useful. Iodinated contrast agents[a] should be used if GI perforation is suspected. Otherwise, barium sulfate is the contrast agent of choice for GI studies because of its superior ability to coat the GI mucosa. More complete descriptions of radiographic findings in gastric disease are available (Moon and Myer, 1986).

Endoscopic examination is the most sensitive test for detection of gastritis and gastroduodenal ulcerative disease. Gastric fluid can be collected for parasitic and microbiologic examination. Endoscopic evaluation allows for the identification of mucosal and submucosal hemorrhages, erosions and ulcers, tumors and foreign bodies (**Figure 52-1**). Gastric and duodenal biopsy specimens for histopathologic examination and brush cytology samples can be collected endoscopically (Jergens et al, 2000). *Helicobacter* spp. can be identified in impression smears prepared from such samples (Simpson, 2005). Gastric biopsy specimens can be evaluated for *Helicobacter* spp. using the rapid urease test[b] (Leib and Duncan, 2005).

Risk Factors

Dogs with liver or kidney disease, hypoadrenocorticism, spinal cord disease, shock, stress, neoplasia, mastocytosis and systemic disease are at increased risk for gastroduodenal ulceration (Lascelles et al, 2005; Simpson, 2005; Henderson and Webster, 2006).

Older pets are more likely to be suffering from metabolic or neoplastic causes of gastritis. Dogs of any age receiving NSAIDs, corticosteroids, or both, for management of osteoarthritis are at risk for gastritis and gastroduodenal ulceration.

Younger dogs and cats and unsupervised pets are more likely to suffer from gastritis secondary to foreign bodies or dietary indiscretion. Several breed-associated causes of gastritis have been recognized (Table 51-1). Dachshunds, miniature schnauzers, toy poodles and other small- and toy-breed dogs are most commonly affected with hemorrhagic gastroenteritis (Guilford and Strombeck, 1996). Several breeds are at risk for chronic gastritis including the basenji, Norwegian lundenhund and Drentse patrijshond (Slappendel et al, 1997; Hart, 2004; Simpson, 2005, 2006; Berghoff et al, 2007). Racing sled dogs in competition are at increased risk for gastroduodenal erosions and ulceration although dogs in training are not (Davis et al, 2006). Nearly 50% of dogs completing the Iditarod race were found to have gastric lesions (Davis et al, 2003, 2003a).

Etiopathogenesis

Acute Gastritis and Gastroduodenal Ulceration

Acute gastritis is characterized by sudden-onset vomiting, resulting from gastric mucosal insult or inflammation. Hematemesis usually indicates that gastroduodenal erosions or ulcerations are present (Willard, 2005). Gastroduodenal ulceration occurs following disruption of the gastric mucosal barrier. The gastric mucosal barrier is a group of physical and chemical defense mechanisms designed to protect the gastric mucosa from insults leading to erosions or ulcers. Disruption of the gastric mucosal barrier may involve direct injury, decreased mucosal blood flow, alterations in protective prostaglandins (prostaglandin E_2 [PGE_2]) or hypersecretion of gastric acid (e.g., gastrinoma) (Simpson, 2005; Henderson and Webster, 2006).

Several metabolic disorders are associated with acute gastritis and gastroduodenal ulceration (**Table 52-1**). Uremia may result in diffuse GI tract hemorrhage. GI erosions and ulcers are thought to result from effects of uremic toxins on the gut mucosa. Additionally, increased circulating concentrations of gastrin have been identified in patients with uremia. The kidneys normally excrete up to 40% of circulating gastrin. Clearance of gastrin is decreased with chronic kidney disease. The resulting hypergastrinemia leads to increased acid production. Studies suggest that hypersecretion of gastrin may contribute to gastric ulceration in chronic kidney disease (Thornhill, 1983; Peters et al, 2005; Polzin et al, 2005; Henderson and Webster, 2006).

GI signs and histopathologic changes are seen in dogs with chronic kidney disease. A retrospective study was done to determine the prevalence of gastric histopathology in necropsy samples from 28 dogs with chronic kidney disease and to characterize the histopathologic changes. All dogs presented with GI signs, including anorexia and vomiting. Twenty-two (79%) of the 28 dogs had gastric pathology. The most common pathology included edema, vasculopathy, glandular atrophy and mineralization. No evidence of ulceration was seen histopathologically and only one dog had ulceration noted on gross necropsy. Dogs with higher serum biochemistry scores (i.e., blood urea nitrogen, creatinine and calcium-phosphorus product) were more likely to have gastric pathology. The authors concluded that gastric ulceration may be uncommon in dogs with chronic kidney disease (Peters et al, 2005).

Liver disease is a common cause of GI ulcerations, which may be manifested as hematemesis. Liver disease was one of the two most common risk factors (the other being treatment with NSAIDs) in a retrospective study of 43 dogs with gastroduodenal ulceration (Henderson and Webster, 2006). The pathogenesis of mucosal ulceration associated with hepatopathies is multifactorial and associated coagulopathies may worsen clinical manifestations. Potential mechanisms include altered gastric blood flow due to portal hypertension, delayed epithelial turnover, gastric hyperacidity and hypergastrinemia. Experimental evidence suggests that hypergastrinemia is a less important mechanism than previously suspected (Booth, 1990; Henderson and Webster, 2006).

A variety of adverse drug reactions have been reported following the use of NSAIDs in dogs. These include GI bleeding, ulceration or both and hepatotoxicity and nephrotoxicity (Sennello and Leib, 2006). The adverse GI effects occur because some NSAIDs have a topical irritant effect on the gastric mucosa and can inhibit protective prostaglandins (McCarthy, 1999; Enberg et al, 2006). Experimentally induced and spontaneous gastritis and gastroduodenal ulcerations have been reported to occur in dogs in conjunction with the use of NSAIDs, including aspirin, indomethacin, naproxen, ibuprofen, phenylbutazone, flunixin meglumine, piroxicam, sulindac and meclofenamic acid (Dow et al, 1990; Lipowitz et al, 1986; Wallace et al, 1990; Davenport, 1992). The ulcerogenicity of NSAIDs is attributed to inhibition of the enzyme cyclooxygenase (COX) in the prostaglandin synthesis pathway, resulting in the loss of the gastric protective effects of prostacyclin and prostaglandin E (Davenport, 1992).

Table 52-1. Potential causes of gastritis and/or gastroduodenal ulceration.

Adverse reactions to food
Food allergy (hypersensitivity)
Food intolerance
Dietary indiscretion
Chemicals
Foreign bodies
Garbage toxicosis
Gluttony
Heavy metal toxicosis
Plants
Drug administration
Corticosteroids
Nonsteroidal antiinflammatory agents
Idiopathic gastritis
Infectious agents
Fungi
Parasites
Spiral bacteria
Inflammatory bowel disease
Neoplasia
Gastrinoma
Mastocytosis
Primary gastric neoplasia
Reduced gastric blood flow
Disseminated intravascular coagulopathy
Neurologic disorders
Sepsis
Shock
Reflux gastritis
Systemic disease
Hypoadrenocorticism
Kidney disease
Liver disease
Pancreatitis

Table 52-2. Key nutritional factors for dogs and cats with gastritis and/or gastroduodenal ulceration.*

Factors	Recommended levels
Potassium	0.8 to 1.1%
Chloride	0.5 to 1.3%
Sodium	0.3 to 0.5%
Protein	***Highly digestible food approach:*** ≤30% for dogs and ≤40% for cats ***Elimination food approach:*** Limit dietary protein to one or two sources Use protein sources that the patient has not been exposed to previously or feed a protein hydrolysate (Chapter 31) 16 to 26% for dogs 30 to 40% for cats
Fat	<15% for dogs <25% for cats
Fiber	≤5% crude fiber; avoid foods with gel-forming fiber sources such as pectins and gums (e.g., gum arabic, guar gum, carrageenan, psyllium gum, xanthan gum, carob gum, gum ghatti and gum tragacanth)
Food form and temperature	Moist foods are best; warm foods to between 70 to 100°F (21 to 38°C)

*Nutrients expressed on a dry matter basis.

Isoforms of COX have been identified. COX-1 is a constitutive form that is found in many tissues (e.g., gastric mucosa), where it is involved in the production of protective prostaglandins. COX-2 is primarily an inducible enzyme that is involved in the production of inflammatory mediators, including proinflammatory prostaglandins. Newer NSAIDs have been developed to minimize the effects on COX-1 and thereby, to decrease the adverse effects on gastric mucosa. The newer NSAIDs are selective inhibitors of COX-2 and generally are considered to be "gastric sparing." However, despite the selective inhibition of COX-2, these newer NSAIDs still carry risk of GI ulceration and perforation. Newer veterinary-approved selective COX inhibitors include flunixin meloxicam, carprofen, etodolac, ketoprofen, tepoxalin, previcox and deracoxib (McCarthy, 1999; Enberg et al, 2006; Dowers et al, 2006; Sennello and Leib, 2006). The use of NSAIDs in patients with underlying renal or hepatic insufficiency may increase the risk of GI ulcerative disease. Concurrent NSAID and corticosteroid use should also be avoided due to the risk of gastric injury.

GI ulcers are recognized complications of critical illnesses (e.g., hypotension, coagulopathy, sepsis) in people. They are thought to develop as a response to the stress of the critical illness and are termed "stress ulcers" (Henderson and Webster, 2006). Stress ulcerations are poorly defined entities in veterinary patients. However, gastroduodenal ulcerations have been noted in companion animals in conjunction with severe burns, heat stroke, multiple trauma, head injuries and spinal cord disorders. In addition, hypovolemic shock and sepsis may be complicated by development of GI ulcers. Experimentally, endotoxin in septic dogs decreases gastric blood flow resulting in mucosal ischemia. Histamine release stimulated by catecholamines worsened the mucosal damage (Henderson and Webster, 2006).

Gastrin-producing pancreatic tumors, histamine-producing tumors (e.g., mast cell tumors, basophilic leukemia) and a polypeptide-producing pancreatic tumor have been associated with gastric or duodenal ulceration in dogs and cats. Persistent gastric hyperacidity stimulated by gastrin, histamine or pancreatic polypeptide was thought to induce ulcers in these patients.

Helicobacter pylori has a recognized association with gastritis, gastroduodenal ulcers and gastric neoplasia in people. The role of *Helicobacter* spp. in GI disease in dogs is unclear although the prevalence is high. These spiral bacteria have been found in 67 to 100% of clinically healthy dogs and 74 to 90% of vomiting dogs. Gastric inflammation has been present in some, but not all, infected dogs. No significant relation has been demonstrated between *Helicobacter* spp. infection and clinical signs or GI ulceration in dogs. *Helicobacter* spp. have been identified in 40 to 100% of healthy and sick cats (Simpson, 2005; Henderson and Webster, 2006; Happonen et al, 2001; Rohrer et al, 1999; Simpson et al, 1999; Peters et al, 2005; Lecoindre et al, 2000).

Chronic Gastritis

Chronic gastritis generally is defined as intermittent vomiting that occurs for more than one to two weeks' duration (Hart, 2004) (**Box 52-1**). Vomiting of food or bile is the primary clinical manifestation of chronic gastritis. Other signs include decreased appetite, weight loss, hematemesis or melena (Simpson, 2005, 2006). Chronic gastritis is diagnosed based on histopathologic examination of gastric biopsy specimens. The histopathology (e.g., cellular infiltrate, architectural abnormalities and severity) and etiology, if identified, determine the type of chronic gastritis affecting the patient (Simpson, 2006).

The etiopathogenesis of chronic gastritis in dogs and cats is not fully understood. In some cases, an underlying etiology, such as parasitism or a metabolic disorder (e.g., uremia, liver disease), can be identified. In most cases, however, an immune-mediated response is hypothesized to be responsible for inflammatory infiltrates within the gastric mucosa (Simpson, 2005, 2006). Experimentally, chronic gastritis can be produced in dogs via mucosal irritants, systemic administration of gastric juices or prenatal thymectomy (Smith et al, 1958; Hennes et al, 1962; Krohn and Finlayson, 1973; Fukuma et al, 1988). Each of these treatments disturbs oral tolerance to antigens.

Chronic idiopathic gastritis is probably a subset of the IBD syndrome or may arise as an adverse reaction to food antigens. Chronic idiopathic gastritis may be localized or can occur with more diffuse IBD of the small or large bowel. Chapters 31 and 57 discuss adverse food reactions and IBD, respectively. Once present, inflammation interferes with gastric motility and reservoir function leading to vomiting. Nutrients including proteins are lost through the inflamed mucosal surface.

Key Nutritional Factors

Key nutritional factors for patients with gastritis and gastroduodenal ulceration are listed in **Table 52-2** and discussed in detail below.

Box 52-1. Hairballs.

Hairballs occur commonly in cats because of their normal grooming behavior and sharp barbs on the tongue that enhance hair ingestion. Cats with longer, thicker coats and those with fastidious grooming behavior usually have more problems with hairballs. Swallowed hair initially accumulates as loose aggregates or more compacted, soft aggregates mixed with mucus. Hairballs are regurgitated periodically from the oropharynx or esophagus or vomited from the stomach, or they pass into the intestinal tract, where they are voided in the feces. Owners observe periodic gagging, retching and regurgitation or vomiting of hair and mucus (usually not containing food or bile). Hairballs are often tubular.

Trichobezoars are harder concretions within the stomach or intestines formed of hair, mucus and other material. Trichobezoars probably begin as simple aggregates of hair, but progress to larger and harder concretions. They are less common in cats than typical hairballs, but are more likely to cause severe clinical signs. Trichobezoars are a common cause of anorexia in pet rabbits (Chapter 70). Large trichobezoars may obstruct pyloric outflow or the intestines and must be removed by surgery or endoscopy.

How cats eliminate aggregates of hair is probably similar to how they eliminate the pelts of small mammals that are ingested as part of a natural diet. Cats that hunt frequently may be seen vomiting the pelts of voles, mice, small rabbits and other mammals. This may be a protective mechanism for eliminating less digestible portions of prey.

Although hairballs do not usually cause significant clinical disease, their associated clinical signs are considered to be a nuisance by many cat owners. Hairballs generally can be controlled. Various laxatives, lubricants, treats and foods are available for routine management of these problems. Several commercial foods are available to help reduce the frequency with which cats vomit hairballs. Most of these foods have increased amounts of dietary fiber. Insoluble fiber, specifically cellulose, increases fecal hair content as compared to other fibers when incorporated in complete foods. Kibble size is another important feature of foods designed to reduce vomiting associated with hairballs. Radiographic gastrointestinal transit studies indicate that a larger kibble size is associated with an increased tendency for hairballs to exit the stomach and be eliminated in the feces, thereby reducing the frequency of vomiting. There is little or no evidence to support the use of lubricants (e.g., petroleum jelly) or papain for the treatment of hairballs in cats. If used, laxatives and lubricants should be given intermittently because large daily doses may interfere with normal digestion and nutrient absorption.

Frequent regurgitation or vomiting of hairballs (i.e., every day) with or without diarrhea, weight loss, anorexia or abdominal pain usually indicates an underlying problem (e.g., gastric motility defect or lymphoplasmacytic enteritis). Cats with severe or frequent clinical signs should be evaluated more extensively with diagnostics including hematology, serum biochemistry profiles, radiography and upper gastrointestinal endoscopy.

The Bibliography for **Box 52-1** can be found at www.markmorris.org.

Water

Water is the most important nutrient for patients with acute vomiting because of the potential for life-threatening dehydration due to excessive fluid loss and inability of the patient to replace those losses. Patients with persistent nausea and vomiting should be supported with subcutaneous or intravenous rather than oral fluids. Moderate to severe dehydration should also be corrected with appropriate parenteral fluid therapy.

Electrolytes

Gastric and intestinal secretions differ from extracellular fluids in electrolyte composition, so their loss can result in systemic electrolyte abnormalities. Dogs and cats with vomiting and diarrhea may have low, normal or high serum potassium, chloride and sodium concentrations. The derangement that predominates in a particular animal depends on several factors, such as the severity of the disease, nutritional status of the patient and site of the disease process. Serum electrolyte concentrations are helpful in tailoring appropriate fluid therapy and nutritional management of these patients. Mild hypokalemia, hypochloremia and either hypernatremia or hyponatremia are the electrolyte abnormalities most commonly associated with acute vomiting (and diarrhea).

Total body depletion of potassium is a predictable consequence of severe or chronic GI disease because the potassium concentration of gastric and intestinal secretions is high. Hypokalemia in association with GI disease will be particularly profound if losses are not matched by sufficient intake of potassium.

Electrolyte disorders should be corrected initially with appropriate parenteral fluid and electrolyte therapy. Foods for patients with acute gastroenteritis should contain levels of potassium, chloride and sodium above the minimum allowances for normal dogs and cats. Recommended levels of these nutrients are 0.8 to 1.1% potassium (dry matter [DM]), 0.5 to 1.3% DM chloride and 0.3 to 0.5% DM sodium.

Protein

Foods for patients with acute gastritis and/or gastroduodenal ulcers should probably not provide excess protein (no more than 30% for dogs and 40% for cats). Products of protein digestion (peptides, amino acids and amines) increase gastrin and gastric acid secretion (Feldman and Grossman, 1980; Delvalle and Yamada, 1990).

Some authors recommend "hypoallergenic" or elimination foods for patients with chronic idiopathic gastritis because dietary antigens are suspected to play a role in the etiopathogenesis (Guilford, 1997). In some cases, elimination foods may be used successfully without pharmacologic intervention because mild to moderate chronic gastritis may respond to dietary management alone. Ideal elimination foods should: 1) avoid protein excess (16 to 26% for dogs; 30 to 40% for cats), 2) have

Table 52-3. Key nutritional factors in selected commercial veterinary therapeutic foods compared to recommended levels for dogs with gastritis and/or gastroduodenal ulceration.*

Moist foods**	Potassium (%)	Chloride (%)	Sodium (%)	Protein (%)***	Fat (%)	Crude fiber (%)
Recommended levels	**0.8-1.1**	**0.5-1.3**	**0.3-0.5**	**≤30**	**<15**	**≤5**
Hill's Prescription Diet i/d Canine	0.95	1.22	0.44	25.0	14.9	1.0
Iams Veterinary Formula Intestinal Low-Residue	0.84	0.84	0.53	35.9	13.2	3.9
Medi-Cal Gastro Formula	0.6	na	0.6	22.1	11.7	1.0
Purina Veterinary Diets EN GastroENteric Formula	0.61	0.78	0.37	30.5	13.8	0.9
Royal Canin Veterinary Diet Digestive Low Fat LF	0.74	1.06	0.39	31.9	6.9	3.0
Royal Canin Veterinary Diet Intestinal HE	0.80	0.92	0.57	23.1	11.8	1.4
Dry foods	**Potassium (%)**	**Chloride (%)**	**Sodium (%)**	**Protein (%)*** **	**Fat (%)**	**Crude fiber (%)**
Recommended levels	**0.8-1.1**	**0.5-1.3**	**0.3-0.5**	**≤30**	**<15**	**≤5**
Hill's Prescription Diet i/d Canine	0.92	1.04	0.45	26.2	14.1	2.7
Iams Veterinary Formula Intestinal Low-Residue	0.90	0.66	0.35	24.6	10.7	2.1
Medi-Cal Gastro Formula	0.8	na	0.5	22.9	13.9	1.9
Purina Veterinary Diets EN GastroENteric Formula	0.66	0.85	0.60	27.0	12.6	1.5
Royal Canin Veterinary Diet Digestive Low Fat LF 20	0.88	1.10	0.49	24.2	6.6	2.3
Royal Canin Veterinary Diet Intestinal HE 28	0.88	0.99	0.55	33.0	22.0	1.6

Key: na = information not available from manufacturer.
*From manufacturers' published information or calculated from manufacturers' published as fed values; all values are on a dry matter basis unless otherwise stated.
**Moist foods are best and ideally they should be offered at temperatures between 70 to 100°F (21 to 38°C).
***Dietary protein may need to be limited to one or two sources that the patient has not been exposed to previously. Table 31-5 contains foods with these characteristics.

high protein digestibility (≥87%) and 3) contain a limited number of novel protein sources to which the patient has never been exposed. Alternatively a food containing a protein hydrolysate may be fed (Chapter 31).

Fat

Solids and liquids higher in fat are emptied more slowly from the stomach than similar foods with less fat. Fat in the duodenum stimulates the release of cholecystokinin, which delays gastric emptying. Foods with less than 15% DM fat for dogs and less than 25% DM fat for cats are appropriate for dietary management of gastritis and gastroduodenal ulcers.

Fiber

Many grocery brand moist foods contain gelling agents such as gums or hydrocolloids to enhance the aesthetic characteristics of the food. Foods containing gel-forming soluble fibers should be avoided in patients with gastric emptying and motility disorders because they increase the viscosity of ingesta and slow gastric emptying. Such fibers include pectins and gums (e.g., gum arabic, guar gum, carrageenan, psyllium gum, xanthan gum, carob gum, gum ghatti and gum tragacanth). However, increased levels (>8% DM crude fiber) of insoluble fiber (powdered cellulose) in dry foods fed to cats had no effect on gastric emptying (Armbrust et al, 2003). Other reports show that the ratio of slowly to rapidly fermentable fibers is important. Because of the variability of fiber types on gastric emptying, in general, the crude fiber content of foods for patients with gastritis and gastroduodenal ulcers should probably not exceed more than 5% DM.

Food Form and Temperature

Moist foods are best because they reduce gastric retention time. For the same reason, clients should warm foods to between room and body temperature (70 to 100°F [21 to 38°C]).

Other Nutritional Factors

Vitamins and Trace Minerals

Iron, copper and B vitamins may benefit patients with gastroduodenal ulceration and GI blood loss. Hematinics should be used in patients with nonregenerative, microcytic/hypochromic anemias attributable to iron deficiency. Hematinics probably are unnecessary in most animals that receive blood transfusions.

Acid Load

Alkalemia should be expected if vomiting patients lose hydrogen and chloride ions in excess of sodium and bicarbonate. Hypochloremia perpetuates the alkalosis by increasing renal bicarbonate reabsorption. Mild alkalemia is common, but profound alkalemia is more likely to occur with pyloric or upper duodenal obstruction rather than with acute gastritis.

Acidemia may occur in vomiting patients if the vomited gastric fluid is relatively low in hydrogen and chloride ion content (e.g., during fasting) or if concurrent loss of intestinal sodium and bicarbonate occurs. Severe acid-base disorders are best corrected with parenteral fluid and electrolyte therapy. Foods for

Table 52-4. Key nutritional factors in selected commercial veterinary therapeutic foods compared with recommended levels for cats with gastritis and/or gastroduodenal ulceration.*

Moist foods**	Potassium (%)	Chloride (%)	Sodium (%)	Protein (%)***	Fat (%)	Crude fiber (%)
Recommended levels	**0.8-1.1**	**0.5-1.3**	**0.3-0.5**	**≤40**	**<25**	**≤5**
Hill's Prescription Diet i/d Feline	1.06	1.18	0.33	37.6	24.1	2.4
Iams Veterinary Formula Intestinal Low-Residue	0.93	0.69	0.40	38.4	11.7	3.7
Medi-Cal Hypoallergenic/Gastro	1.1	na	0.7	35.5	35.9	1.2
Medi-Cal Sensitivity CR	1.1	na	1.1	34.5	35.1	2.5
Dry foods	**Potassium (%)**	**Chloride (%)**	**Sodium (%)**	**Protein (%)*****	**Fat (%)**	**Crude fiber (%)**
Recommended levels	**0.8-1.1**	**0.5-1.3**	**0.3-0.5**	**≤40**	**<25**	**≤5**
Hill's Prescription Diet i/d Feline	1.07	1.11	0.37	40.3	20.2	2.8
Iams Veterinary Formula Intestinal Low-Residue	0.66	0.63	0.25	35.8	13.7	1.8
Medi-Cal Hypoallergenic/Gastro	0.8	na	0.4	29.8	11.5	3.1
Purina Veterinary Diets EN GastroENteric	0.99	0.58	0.64	56.2	18.4	1.3
Royal Canin Veterinary Diet Intestinal HE 30	0.97	0.97	0.65	34.4	23.7	5.8

Key: na = information not available from manufacturer.
*From manufacturers' published information or calculated from manufacturers' published as fed values; all values are on a dry matter basis unless otherwise stated.
**Moist foods are best and ideally they should be offered at temperatures between 70 to 100°F (21 to 38°C).
***Dietary protein may need to be limited to one or two sources that the patient has not been exposed to previously. Table 31-6 contains foods with these characteristics.

patients with acute vomiting and diarrhea should avoid excess dietary acid load. Foods that normally produce alkaline urine are less likely to be associated with acidosis.

FEEDING PLAN

The first objective in managing vomiting patients should be to correct dehydration and electrolyte and acid-base imbalances, if present. The dietary goals are to provide a food that meets the patient's nutrient requirements, allows normalization of gastric motility and function and controls vomiting. In most cases of acute vomiting, initial fasting for 24 to 48 hours, with parenteral fluid administration, reduces or resolves vomiting by simply removing the effects of undigested food and the offending agents from the stomach and duodenum. Chronic vomiting cases generally require a more detailed diagnostic and therapeutic (i.e., combined medical and nutritional) approach.

Assess and Select the Food

Bland foods often are recommended for veterinary patients with gastritis. This recommendation probably originated from physicians' orders for people recovering from GI upsets to eat bland foods. The term "bland" is poorly defined, but it is most often applied to easily digested/absorbed and nonirritating, non-spicy foods. Most pet foods fall within this category. The use of topical digests on dry foods may be construed as potentially irritating because many digests contain high concentrations of reactive amines (Guilford et al, 1994). The term "bland" is not a useful recommendation to pet owners; instead specific ingredients or nutrients to avoid should be clearly stated.

Tables 52-3 and 52-4 include the key nutritional factor content of selected commercial veterinary therapeutic foods marketed for GI diseases and compare them to the recommended levels for vomiting patients (dogs and cats, respectively). Food selection should be based on a product closely matching the key nutritional factor target levels.

Liquids are emptied from the stomach more quickly than solids due to lower digesta osmolality. Water is emptied most quickly, whereas liquids containing nutrients are emptied more slowly. High-osmolality fluids are emptied more slowly than dilute fluids. Solids are the slowest to be emptied from the stomach. Dry foods empty more slowly than moist foods in cats (Goggin et al, 1998). Thus, foods for patients with gastritis and gastroduodenal ulcers should have a liquid or semi-liquid consistency. Cold meals slow gastric emptying so food should be between room and body temperature (70 to 100°F [21 to 38°C]). Refrigerated or frozen foods should be warmed before being fed.

Assess and Determine the Feeding Method

Two feeding methods have been described for patients with acute gastric disorders. The more classic feeding method for patients with acute gastritis begins by discontinuing oral intake of food and water (i.e., nothing per os [NPO]) for 24 to 48 hours. After this period, patients should be offered small amounts of water or ice cubes every few hours. If water is well tolerated, small amounts of food can be offered several times (i.e., six to eight times) a day. In cats and probably dogs, larger meals are emptied more slowly than smaller meals (Goggin et al, 1998); thus, smaller meals promote gastric emptying. If the patient eats food without vomiting, the amount fed can be increased gradually over three to four days until the patient is receiving its estimated daily energy requirement in two to three meals per day. Food should be withdrawn and offered again after a few hours if the patient begins to vomit during this period.

In some cases, persistent vomiting may complicate refeeding. If so, metoclopramide or other antiemetic agents are recommended after GI obstruction has been ruled out (Table 51-2). Rarely, some patients may require parenteral feeding (Chapter 26).

The second approach, known as "feeding through vomiting," has been a successful alternative to NPO therapy in some vomiting patients. Pregnant women suffering hyperemesis reported feeling less nausea and preferred the placement of a nasogastric tube with slow frequent self feeding of small liquid meals to eating small regular meals or NPO therapy (MacBurney, 1993). This feeding method has also been used successfully in dogs with parvoviral enteritis (Mohr et al, 2003). A possible explanation for persistent vomiting is that the normal motility pattern throughout the length of the bowel cannot be reestablished without strong intraluminal stimulation. In fact, vomiting and mucosal atrophy probably perpetuate bowel dysfunction. Feeding restarts normal patterns of motility beginning in the esophagus and food may reestablish motility patterns as it passes down the bowel. The physical presence of food and nutrients serves as mechanical and chemical stimuli to normalize bowel motility and function.

Simply refeeding dogs (orally) and cats (via nasoesophageal tube) has stopped protracted vomiting (i.e., lasting more than seven days) successfully without using antiemetic drugs.[c] Feedings are continued although the patient may vomit. Most cases of protracted vomiting cease within 24 hours of administering liquid food. These patients then are offered small frequent meals of a highly digestible, moderate-fat food 24 hours after the last episode of vomiting (**Tables 52-3** and **52-4**).

CONCURRENT MEDICAL THERAPY

Nutritional management often is used in conjunction with other therapeutic modalities including parenteral fluids, antacids, histamine (H_2)-receptor antagonists, cytoprotective drugs, PGE_2 analogs, antibiotics and anthelmintics (Table 51-2).

REASSESSMENT

Nutritional reassessment of patients with gastritis or gastroduodenal ulcers includes monitoring changes in body weight and condition and determining the extent of vomiting. Daily food dosage should be adjusted as indicated by changes in body weight and condition.

If vomiting persists in the face of appropriate medical and nutritional therapy, further diagnostics are warranted. Additionally, different foods should be tried (**Tables 52-3** and **52-4**). If anemia was identified as a problem in pets with GI ulcers, reassessment of the hemogram is recommended to ensure adequate repletion of iron and copper. In addition, frequent monitoring of fecal occult blood loss is recommended.

ENDNOTES

a. Gastrografin. Squibb Diagnostics, New Brunswick, NJ, USA.
b. CLOtest, Ballard Medical Products, Draper, UT, USA.
c. Remillard RL. Personal observation. 1998.

REFERENCES

The references for **Chapter 52** can be found at www.markmorris.org.

Chapter 53

Gastric Dilatation and Gastric Dilatation-Volvulus in Dogs

Deborah J. Davenport
Rebecca L. Remillard
Christine Jenkins

"Size counts. That's all."
Gina Gershon

CLINICAL IMPORTANCE

Gastric dilatation (GD) is distention of the stomach with a mixture of air, food and fluid. GD often occurs intermittently, usually in young dogs, particularly as a result of overeating or some other dietary indiscretion. Gastric dilatation-volvulus (GDV) is characterized by rotation of the stomach on its mesenteric axis, entrapping gastric contents and compromising vascular supply to the stomach, spleen and pancreas. Acute GDV is a medicosurgical emergency with high morbidity and mortality (Monnet, 2003; Buber et al, 2007). Rarely, chronic, intermittent GDV may occur associated with a partial (i.e., <90 degree) rotation of the stomach.

GDV most commonly affects large-breed, deep-chested dogs and has been estimated to affect 40,000 to 60,000 dogs annually (Lantz et al, 1992). Based on necropsy findings, GDV accounted for 3.4% of deaths of military dogs (Jennings, 1992) and has been reported to occur at a monthly rate of 2.5 cases/1,000 military dogs (Herbold et al, 2002). A review of data from the Veterinary Medical Database, Purdue University, West Lafayette, IN, suggests a 1,500% increase in the frequency of GDV from 1964 to 1974 within cases presented to veterinary teaching hospitals (Glickman, 1996).

PATIENT ASSESSMENT

History and Physical Examination

Clinical signs of GD include nausea, belching and vomiting. Conversely, there may be no effort to vomit, but instead lethargy, reluctance to move and grunting sounds with respiratory effort. The onset of GDV is usually acute and often occurs at night or in the early morning. Owners often report some precipitating stressful event. Boarding, hospitalization, travel and participation in shows have been associated with GDV. Affected dogs exhibit restlessness, progressive abdominal distention with tympany, abdominal pain, hypersalivation and repeated, nonproductive attempts to vomit. Occasionally, owners will find affected dogs dead or in shock.

Chronic GDV is a rare manifestation of the syndrome. Dogs present with intermittent, progressive signs including vomiting, borborygmus, inappetence and weight loss. Periods of illness are interspersed with periods of normalcy. If untreated, these dogs often progress to acute GDV.

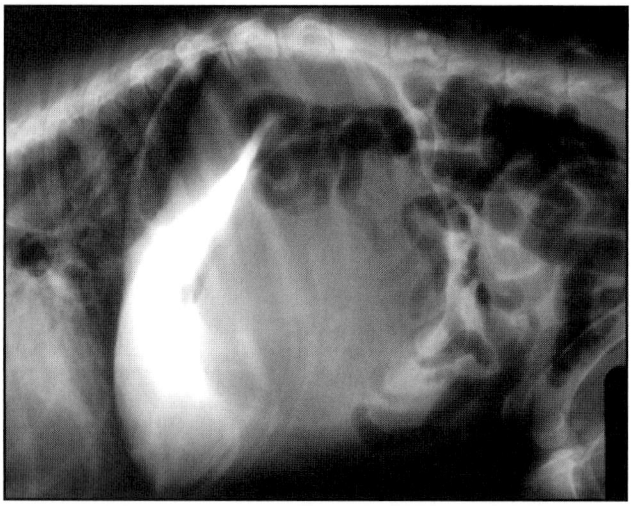

Figure 53-1. Lateral abdominal radiograph from a nine-year-old neutered male Doberman pinscher with a 180-degree gastric dilatation-volvulus. (Courtesy Dr. Joanne Burns, Veterinary Imaging Services, Topeka, KS.)

The most prominent sign of GD and GDV is abdominal distention. In some dogs, concurrent splenomegaly may be identified by abdominal palpation. Clinical manifestations of cardiovascular shock include tachycardia, delayed capillary refill time, pallor and weak pulses.

Laboratory and Other Clinical Information

Laboratory assessment of patients with GD or GDV should include a complete blood count, serum biochemistry profile, urinalysis and blood gas analysis. The complete blood count often reflects stress and can provide early evidence of disseminated intravascular coagulopathy if thrombocytopenia is present. If faced with thrombocytopenia, a complete coagulation panel is recommended before surgery.

Hypokalemia is common in patients with GDV and should be managed with intravenous potassium supplementation because hypokalemia can potentiate cardiac dysrhythmias. Metabolic acidosis, metabolic alkalosis, respiratory acidosis and mixed acid-base disorders have been reported to occur in dogs with GDV (Muir, 1987). Routine use of alkalinizing fluids and sodium bicarbonate, therefore, is not recommended.

Radiography is critical to the diagnosis of GD and GDV. Dorsoventral and right lateral views should be evaluated to distinguish simple GD from GDV (**Figure 53-1**). In most cases, gastric rotation is clockwise (i.e., with the dog in a dorsoventral position, viewed from above) and ranges from 90 to 360 degrees. Other significant findings may include splenomegaly and free abdominal air, which indicates gastric rupture.

Electrocardiographic recordings should be monitored in patients with GDV pre- and postoperatively because cardiac dysrhythmias occur in approximately half of patients (Muir, 1982; Brockman et al, 1995; Buber et al, 2007). The distended, malpositioned stomach compresses the caudal vena cava and portal vein resulting in cardiovascular compromise. Reduction in venous return and cardiac output leads to myocardial ischemia and cardiovascular shock. Cardiac dysrhythmias, gastric necrosis and multiple organ ischemia are potential consequences if gastric decompression is not performed expeditiously. Generally, dysrhythmias are ventricular in origin and can be life-threatening.

Risk Factors

Considerable effort has been expended over the last 30 years in attempts to identify the cause or causes of GD and GDV. Despite these efforts, no definitive cause for the syndrome has been identified. However, a number of predisposing and precipitating risk factors have been demonstrated through epidemiologic studies (**Table 53-1**).

GD and GDV occur most frequently in large-breed, deep-chested dogs, but may occur rarely in smaller dogs and in cats. A number of breeds including Great Danes, Irish setters, Gordon setters, Weimaraners, Saint Bernards, Doberman pinschers and basset hounds appear to be at risk. Other large breeds, notably the retriever breeds, have much smaller odds ratios. Attempts to assess the GDV risk in individual breeds demonstrated a lifetime incidence of 25% in Irish setters and a risk of 10% in Great Danes by the age of 2.6 years (Glickman, 1996). In a prospective cohort study, the likelihood of large- (bloodhounds, Akitas, Weimaraners, Irish setters, standard poodles, collies and rottweilers) or giant-breed dogs (Great Danes, Irish wolfhounds, Saint Bernards and Newfoundland dogs) developing GDV during their lifetime ranged from 21 to 24%, with the highest incidence occurring in Great Danes (Glickman et al, 2000).

Within breeds, certain anatomic and conformational factors increase the risk of GDV (Glickman et al, 1994). Increased adult body size compared with breed standards and specific types of thoracic conformation as determined radiographically appear to be related to the incidence of GDV. A chest depth-width ratio greater than 1.5 is associated with increased risk for developing GDV in certain breeds (Glickman et al, 1996; Schaible et al, 1997; Schellenberg et al, 1998). Dogs with GDV were found to have elongated hepatogastric ligaments as compared with control dogs of similar breeds (Hall et al, 1995). A longer hepatogastric ligament may allow increased gastric mobility or stretch as a consequence of GDV (Monnet, 2003).

GD or GDV appears not to have an age predisposition, but both occur more commonly in middle-aged dogs. The syndrome is also more common in male dogs (Glickman et al, 1997). Having a first-degree relative (sibling, sire, dam, offspring) with GDV also increases the risk by 63% (Glickman et al, 2000). This finding has led to the recommendation for prophylactic incisional, laparoscopic-assisted or endoscopically-assisted gastropexy for such dogs (Watson and Tobias, 2006; Ward et al, 2003; Rawlings et al, 2002; Dujowich and Beimer, 2008). These procedures can be performed in young female dogs (six to eight months) at the time of ovariohysterectomy. Percutaneous endoscopic gastrostomy is not recommended for prophylactic gastropexy because it is does not create consistently strong pexy sites and is associated with higher morbidity than incisional or laparoscopic techniques (Waschak et al, 1997).

Other dog-related risk factors include a nervous or fearful temperament and being underweight. The incidence of GDV in dogs characterized by their owners as fearful was increased 257% compared to those considered non-fearful. Conversely, the owner-perceived personality trait of "happiness" appears to reduce the incidence of GDV by 78% (Glickman et al, 1997, 2000). Physiologic differences between happy and fearful dogs might influence gastrointestinal motility. These findings suggest that behavioral modification should be considered as part of a GDV preventive program in aggressive, nervous dogs.

A retrospective study identified intestinal lesions consistent with inflammatory bowel disease in approximately 25% of dogs with GDV (Braun et al, 1996). Splenectomy for treatment of hemangiosarcoma and splenic torsion has also been recognized as a risk factor for GDV in dogs (Monnet, 2003; Marconato, 2006; Millis et al, 1995; Neath et al, 1997). For that reason, large- and giant-breed dogs undergoing splenectomy should be recommended for a prophylactic gastropexy (Monnet, 2003).

Several dietary risk factors have been identified in one or more epidemiologic studies (Raghavan et al, 2006, 2004; Glickman et al, 2000, 2000a, 1994, 1997; Elwood, 1998; Theyse et al, 1998). Feeding from an elevated bowl, feeding a large volume of food per meal, feeding only one meal a day, feeding only one type of food, rapid eating, episodes of overeating, consumption of large volumes of water, postprandial exercise and a food particle diameter less than 5 mm have been implicated. Factors that appeared to decrease the risk of GDV in one case-control study were the inclusion of moist food or table foods as part of the diet (Glickman et al, 1997). In another study, consuming foods with a particle size greater than 30 mm was protective (Theyse et al, 1998).

In the past, consumption of dry dog food, unmoistened dry food, nutritional supplements and cereal- or soy-based foods were incriminated as dietary risk factors for GDV. More recent epidemiologic studies have not found these factors to increase the risk of GDV (Raghavan et al, 2004, 2006). In a European study of GDV cases, 40% of patients consumed dry food, 26% ate moist food and 25% received fresh meat diets, reflecting no increased risk associated with food form (Nagel and Neumann, 1992).

Attempts to reproduce GDV by dietary manipulation have been unsuccessful. In one study, researchers found no difference in gastric motility or emptying in large-breed dogs fed either a moist, meat-based food free of soybean meal or a dry, extruded, cereal-based food containing soybean meal with and without moistening (Burrows et al, 1985). A similar study evaluating Irish setters fed either a commercial dry food or a meat and bone mixture again showed no difference in gastric emptying or gastric acid secretion between diet types (Van Kruiningen et al, 1987). Investigators concluded that most large dogs are fed dry cereal-based food for reasons of cost and convenience, and that these foods may have been wrongly incriminated as a predisposing factor in GDV (Burrows et al, 1985; Raghavan et al, 2004).

In a nested case-control study of a group of dogs consuming dry foods as more than 95% of their diet, investigators found an association between dietary fat and GDV (Raghavan et al, 2006). If a vegetable oil or animal fat source was included as one of the first four label ingredients, dogs were at 2.4-fold increased risk of GDV. In such foods, the percent of metabolizable energy of the food derived from fat was higher than that in control foods. This unexpected finding contradicts the authors' earlier work in the same population of dogs, which demonstrated that patients with and without GDV consumed similar fat intakes (Raghavan et al, 2004). At this time, it is unclear which set of results from this population are most significant, suggesting the need for further investigation (Kass, 2006).

Table 53-1. Risk factors for canine gastric dilatation-volvulus.*

Consuming a food with vegetable oil or animal fat listed as one of the first four ingredients
Eating a large volume of food per meal
Eating from an elevated food bowl
Eating only one meal per day
Excluding moist food, table food and treats from the diet
Exclusive feeding of one food type
Exercising more than two hours per day
Fearful, nervous or aggressive temperament
Feeding food with a mean particle size <5 mm
Having an affected first-degree relative
Increased adult weight, based on breed standards
Increased chest or abdominal depth:width ratio
Increasing age
Large- or giant-breed status
Great Danes, Weimaraners, Saint Bernards, Gordon setters, Irish setters, standard poodles, basset hounds, Doberman pinschers, Old English sheepdogs, German shorthaired pointers
Lean body condition (body condition score ≤2/5)
Male gender
Purebred status
Rapid eating
Stressful events (boarding in kennel or travel)

*Adapted from Glickman LT, Glickman NW, Schellenberg DB, et al. Multiple risk factors for the gastric dilatation-volvulus syndrome in dogs: A practitioner/owner case-control study. Journal of the American Animal Hospital Association 1997; 33: 197-204. Theyse LFH, Van Den Brom WW, Van Sluijs FJ. Diet and other risk factors for gastric dilatation-volvulus in Great Danes. Journal of Veterinary Surgery 1997; 26: 260. Theyse LFH, Van Den Brom WE, Van Sluijs FJ. Small size food particles and age as risk factors for gastric dilatation-volvulus in Great Danes. Veterinary Record 1998; 143: 48-50. Raghavan M, Glickman NW, Glickman LT. The effects of ingredients in dry dog foods on the risk of gastric dilatation-volvulus in dogs. Journal of the American Animal Hospital Association 2006; 42: 28-36.

Etiopathogenesis

A single cause of GDV will probably not be found. GDV is more likely a condition that arises because of the interaction of two or more risk factors. The gastric distention manifested in GDV is associated with an as yet uncharacterized functional or mechanical gastric outflow obstruction. This obstruction results in loss of the normal means for removing air from the stomach (i.e., eructation, vomiting and gastroduodenal flow). In some dogs, gastric volvulus apparently develops as a consequence of gastric distention, but, in others, gastric volvulus may precede the dilatation. Because gastropexy prevents recurrence of GDV, some authors have postulated that volvulus is the initial event.

Table 53-2. Key nutritional factor for dry foods for dogs for the prevention of gastric dilatation and volvulus.

Factor	Recommendation
Kibble size	Large particle size: >30 mm was protective against GDV in giant-breed dogs (Great Danes). Somewhat smaller kibble dimensions may be effective in medium- and large-breed dogs as long as the size of the kibble is sufficiently large to prevent rapid eating.

Table 53-3. Kibble size comparison of selected large-kibble dry commercial foods to consider for feeding medium-, large- and giant-breed dogs to reduce the risk of gastric dilatation and volvulus.*

Factor	Kibble cross sectional dimension(s)**
Recommendation	**>30 mm for giant-breed dogs** Somewhat smaller kibbles (<30 mm) may be effective in medium- and large-breed dogs as long as the kibble is sufficiently large to prevent rapid eating
Hill's Prescription Diet t/d Canine	28.3 x 26.4 mm
Medi-Cal Dental Formula	23.3 x 20.3 mm
Purina Veterinary Diets DH Dental Health	21.9 x 21.2 mm
Royal Canin Giant Adult 28	29.72 x 28.88 mm

*For additional key nutritional factors of importance for canine maintenance, see appropriate lifestage recommendations (Chapters 13 through 17).
**Kibble size represents the mean of measurements (diameter or width X thickness) made on three randomly selected kibbles from one bag of each product listed.

GD episodes may persist after gastropexy (Monnet, 2003).

Gas in the stomach of dogs with GDV is primarily atmospheric air, which differs greatly in composition from the gas produced by bacterial fermentation (Caywood et al, 1977). For that reason, aerophagia is believed to be the primary source of gastric gas in dogs with GDV. In some cases, carbon dioxide concentrations in the trapped stomach gas approached 10% (Caywood et al, 1977). The most likely source for this gas is the interaction between gastric acid and bicarbonate secretions. Normally, swallowed air is eructated and does not accumulate in excessive quantities. It has been hypothesized that dogs with GDV have defective eructation mechanisms. In one study, esophageal motility abnormalities were observed in 60% of dogs with GDV (Van Sluijs and Wolvekamp, 1993). It is possible that such abnormalities are linked to defective eructation complicated by the anatomic relationship of the stomach and esophagus in deep-chested, large-breed dogs, which also may interfere with effective eructation of air (Guilford, 1996). Aerophagia increases with rapid food consumption, excitement, stress and exercise; thus, controlling these factors is recommended in high-risk dogs.

Hypergastrinemia is present in dogs with acute GDV and persists after treatment and recovery, suggesting that dogs with GDV have a pre-existing hypergastrinemia (Leib et al, 1984). Gastrin increases gastroesophageal junction pressure and some investigators have postulated that hypergastrinemia may be a factor in the pathogenesis of GDV (Leib et al, 1984). However, further investigations revealed no relationship between the degree of gastric distention and the magnitude of plasma gastrin increase (Leib et al, 1985). Others suggest that hypergastrinemia in dogs with GDV is a result of the syndrome rather than a cause (Hall et al, 1989).

Key Nutritional Factor

The only key nutritional factor that may be of concern for dogs with an increased risk for GDV is food particle size. Fat content may play a role as described in the Risk Factor section above and the Other Nutritional Factor section below. The key nutritional factors for postoperative patients are similar to those for patients with acute gastritis (Chapter 52).

Kibble Size

Commercial dry extruded dog food particles having a diameter of less than 5 mm have been implicated as a risk factor for GDV. Also, in a study involving Great Danes, consuming foods with a particle size greater than 30 mm was protective (Theyse et al, 1998). The study included dry foods, moist chunky foods and homemade foods. The working assumption is that larger particles require more extensive and prolonged mastication, and in most dogs, probably prevents rapid eating of food. Somewhat smaller food particles might have a similar beneficial effect in medium- and large-breed dogs at risk for GDV, as long as the food particles are large enough to sufficiently slow eating. Thus, a practical consideration for medium-, large- and giant-breed dogs at risk for GDV would be to offer large kibble foods to slow eating (**Table 53-2**).

Other Nutritional Factor

Fat

Dietary fat can delay gastric emptying. One study found an association between dietary fat and GDV (Raghavan et al, 2006). If a vegetable oil or animal fat source was included as one of the first four label ingredients, dogs were at 2.4-fold increased risk of GDV. Unfortunately, percent dry matter content of fat was not recorded in the report. Ingredient order doesn't always reflect dietary fat content. Splitting ingredients on the first part of the product label can result in high fat ingredients being moved further down the label (Chapter 9). Thus, a food could be relatively high in dietary fat content but have a fat source ingredient at fifth or sixth place on the ingredient label. Until more information regarding dietary fat content and its relationship to GDV is available, this information cannot be reliably used. However, the data do suggest that lower fat is better.

FEEDING PLAN

Without early diagnosis and appropriate treatment, GDV is usually fatal. Initial management includes cardiovascular stabi-

Box 53-1. Recommendations from the 1990 Morris Animal Foundation Panel on Bloat in Dogs.

The following measures may reduce the incidence and recurrence of acute gastric dilatation-volvulus ("bloat"). These measures are especially important when managing purebred dog kennels and individual pet animals of the most susceptible breeds.

1. Large dogs should be fed two or three times daily, rather than once a day, and at times when the owner can observe post-feeding behavior.
2. Owners of susceptible breeds should be aware of prodromal signs (i.e., actions from the dog that signal abdominal discomfort). These signs include evidence of abdominal fullness after meals, whining, pacing, getting up and lying down, stretching, looking at the abdomen, anxiety and unproductive attempts to vomit. A veterinarian should examine animals with these signs as soon as possible.
3. Owners of susceptible breeds should establish a good working relationship with their local veterinarian and should discuss emergency measures in the event of bloat, including administration of antacids (e.g., Mylanta[a] and Di-Gel[b]), passing a stomach tube or piercing the abdomen with a hypodermic needle to relieve bloat.
4. Water should be available to dogs at all times, but should be limited immediately after feeding if overconsumption is a problem.
5. Vigorous exercise, excitement and stress should be avoided one hour before and two hours after meals. Walking, however, is permissible because it may help stimulate normal gastrointestinal function.
6. Food changes should be made gradually over three to five days.
7. Susceptible dogs should be fed individually and, if possible, in a quiet location.
8. Special attention should be paid to the above measures after animals return home from veterinary hospitals and boarding facilities.
9. Dogs that have survived bloat are at increased risk for future episodes; therefore, prophylaxis in the form of preventive surgery or medical management should be discussed with the veterinarian.

ENDNOTES

a. Stuart Pharmaceuticals, Wilmington, DE, USA.
b. Schering-Plough, Corp. Madison, NJ, USA.

lization (i.e., treatment of shock and cardiac dysrhythmias), gastric decompression (i.e., orogastric intubation, gastric trocharization), surgery (i.e., gastric repositioning and permanent gastropexy) and appropriate postsurgical care (Monnet, 2003). If a permanent gastropexy is not performed after gastric repositioning, the recurrence rate of GDV approaches 80% (Wingfield et al, 1975) and median survival times fall from 547 to 188 days (Glickman et al, 1998). The feeding plan is implemented as part of a preventive strategy or after rapid, aggressive emergency management.

Assess and Select the Food

Foods that have relatively large kibble size and that are appropriate for the patient's current lifestage and activity level should be provided. Selected foods that have large kibble size are listed in **Table 53-3** along with their typical kibble dimensions. Other feeding practices can be used to slow eating. (See Assess and Determine a Feeding Method below.) Because foods are fed for adult maintenance, foods should be chosen that are appropriate for the dog's lifestage and activity level (Chapters 13 through 17). In the postoperative period, foods should be used that provide levels of the key nutritional factors outlined for acute gastritis (Chapter 52).

Assess and Determine the Feeding Method

Because feeding methods are often altered in postoperative patients and patients at risk for GD and GDV, a thorough assessment should include verification of the feeding method currently being used. Items to consider include feeding frequency, amount fed, how the food is offered, access to other food (e.g., access to other pets' food, table food, treats, etc.), relationship of feeding to exercise and who feeds the dog. All of this information should have been gathered when the history of the animal was obtained. If the animal has a normal body condition score (2.5/5 to 3.5/5), the amount of food it was fed previously (energy basis) was probably appropriate.

It appears prudent to recommend feeding a dog at risk for GDV two to three times per day in an environment that decreases competitive eating. At risk dogs should not be fed from an elevated platform or feeder. If the dog typically eats too fast, placing large balls or rocks in the food bowl or feeding the dog from a muffin tin may slow consumption of food and decrease aerophagia. A specially made food bowl[a] that has three large vertical cylinders protruding from the bottom to slow food consumption is available for dogs at risk for GDV. Feeding a mixture of moist and dry food appears to reduce the risk of GDV (Glickman et al, 1997). Alternatively, feeding foods with kibble sizes greater than 30 mm is also thought to reduce the risk of GDV (Theyse et al, 1998). To deliver foods with particle sizes this large, a mix of chunked moist food and dry food, a canine dental food,[b] formed complete meals[c] or a food formulated for giant breeds[d] may be used. However, none of these commercial products have been demonstrated to prevent or reduce the risk of GDV. Although no definitive link between exercise and GDV has been found, limiting exercise within three to four hours of eating (i.e., corresponds to normal gastric emptying time) is prudent. The Morris Animal Foundation Canine Bloat Panel recommends avoiding vigorous exercise at least one hour before and two hours after feeding (1990) (**Box 53-1**).

REASSESSMENT

Postoperative patients should be monitored closely for cardiac dysrhythmias, coagulopathies, surgical dehiscence, electrolyte and acid-base abnormalities and infections. Treatment with H_2-receptor blockers and sucralfate is indicated for most dogs with gastric mucosal damage. In most cases, food can be reintroduced within 24 to 36 hours postoperatively. Postoperative patients are best fed small meals frequently. Judicious use of antiemetics and/or metoclopramide in conjunction with continuous feeding may allow adequate caloric intake by patients with persistent vomiting. If tube gastrostomy was chosen as the method of permanent gastropexy, this indwelling catheter should be used for feeding (Chapter 25).

After the patient is discharged, the owner should monitor its appetite, activity level and attitude. Rechecks should include body weight and body condition assessment. Food dosages should be adjusted to maintain the dog at ideal body condition. The ultimate marker of success in GDV patients is the prevention of recurrent disease. Rarely, GD will develop in dogs that have had a gastropexy. Any episode of dilatation and precipitating factors should be reported and evaluated.

Persistent vomiting in a postoperative patient may indicate an outflow obstruction arising from an improperly positioned gastropexy site. If the angle between the pyloric antrum and duodenum is too acute, a functional obstruction may occur (Watson and Tobias, 2006).

ENDNOTES

a Brake-Fast Dog Food Bowl. Brake-Fast LLC., Virginia Beach, VA, USA.
b. Prescription Diet t/d Canine. Science Diet Oral Care Adult Canine. Hill's Pet Nutrition, Inc., Topeka, KS, USA.
c. WholeMeals. Mars Petcare U.S. Inc., Franklin, TN, USA.
d. Royal Canin Giant Adult 28. Royal Canin USA, Inc., St. Charles, MO, USA.

REFERENCES

The references for **Chapter 53** can be found at www.markmorris.org.

CASE 53-1

Acute Vomiting in an Irish Setter

Michael S. Leib, DVM, MS, Dipl. ACVIM (Internal Medicine)
Virginia-Maryland Regional College of Veterinary Medicine
Blacksburg, Virginia, USA

Patient Assessment

A seven-year-old neutered female Irish setter was examined for vomiting and retching of two hours' duration. The dog vomited approximately 20 times during the hour before presentation, producing small amounts of phlegm each time. Earlier in the morning the dog had escaped from the yard and wandered freely. The owner reported no previous gastrointestinal (GI) problems.

Physical examination revealed a 28-kg dog with normal body condition (body condition score [BCS] 3/5) and a firm, distended abdomen. Vital signs (mucous membrane color, pulse rate and strength, capillary refill time, respiratory rate) were normal. Abdominal radiographs revealed a dilated stomach that was full of ingesta but appeared to be in its normal position. The ingesta contained a large amount of calcified material.

A tentative diagnosis of gastric dilatation (GD) was made and emergency treatment instituted. An orogastric tube was easily passed into the stomach but only a small amount of gas, fluid and nonspecific debris was recovered. Total decompression was not achieved even after warm water lavage. Intravenous fluids and a sedative were administered; gastric lavage with suction was continued. Large pieces of a plastic bag were removed and the lavaged gastric contents contained a large amount of shellfish debris. Sufficient decompression was still not obtained; therefore, an exploratory celiotomy was performed.

During surgery, the stomach was found to be in a normal position and a gastrotomy was performed. A large volume of shrimp and crab legs was removed and the stomach was lavaged with saline solution. The stomach was sutured closed and attached to the abdominal wall using a modified gastropexy technique. The abdomen was closed routinely and recovery from anesthesia was uneventful.

Assess the Food and Feeding Method

The dog was normally fed a combination of a commercial dry grocery brand dog food mixed with various commercial moist grocery brand dog foods and table foods. This food combination was offered in the early evening when the owner returned home from work. Water was available free choice.

Questions

1. What are risk factors for GD and gastric dilatation-volvulus (GDV) in dogs?
2. Outline a feeding plan (foods and feeding method) for this patient.

Answers and Discussion

1. Several risk factors for development of GD and GDV have been identified. These risk factors include large breed (i.e., Great Danes, Weimaraners, Saint Bernards, Gordon setters, Irish setters, standard poodles, Newfoundlands, basset hounds, Doberman pinschers), purebred dogs, older age (mean six to seven years old), heavier body weight (greater than 23 kg), rapid eating, feeding less moist dog food, feeding once daily rather than multiple times, feeding less table foods, feeding fewer snacks, gulping water, feeding small kibbles (<5 mm diameter; feeding large kibbles [>30 mm] is protective), excessive belching or flatulence, esophageal motility disorders, previous GI disease (e.g., inflammatory bowel disease) and personality (fearful or aggressive vs. happy and easy going). Other risk factors for GDV identified in Irish setter dogs included feeding a single food form, recent car journey (i.e., within preceding 24 hours), recent time in a boarding kennel (within preceding 24 hours), a history of aerophagia and thin body condition (BCS 1/5 or 2/5).
2. Dietary indiscretion obviously played an important role in development of GD in this dog and should be avoided. However, strategies to avoid other dietary risk factors for GD and GDV should also be considered, including offering a highly digestible food in multiple small meals. Meals should be avoided in association with exercise or traveling in a motor vehicle. Multiple small meals may also help eliminate rapid eating and significant aerophagia. Excessive or recurrent belching, flatus, vomiting, regurgitation and diarrhea may indicate underlying GI disease and warrant further diagnostic evaluation before implementing a feeding plan.

Progress Notes

The dog was offered a small amount of water and a moist highly digestible commercial veterinary therapeutic food (Prescription Diet i/d Canine[a]) the day following surgery. The amounts of water and food were gradually increased over the next couple of days. The dog was released to the owner's care with instructions to continue the therapeutic food in an amount to meet the daily energy requirement at home (1.6 x resting energy requirement = 1,450 kcal [6.07 MJ]). The food was to be offered in three separate meals (one can each meal) during the day (morning, immediately after work, late evening before bed). The owner was warned about the increased risk of GDV in Irish setter dogs, the potential for a fatal outcome, associated clinical signs and the need for emergency treatment if the problem recurred. Restricted exercise and avoiding rides in a motor vehicle in close association with meals were suggested. The owner was advised to make all attempts to avoid dietary indiscretion. Three months following surgery, the owner reported the dog was normal and doing well.

Endnote

a. Hill's Pet Nutrition Inc., Topeka, KS, USA.

Bibliography

Elwood CM. Risk factors for gastric dilatation in Irish setter dogs. Journal of Small Animal Practice 1998; 39: 185-190.

Glickman LT, Glickman NW, Perez CM, et al. Analysis of risk factors for gastric dilatation and dilatation-volvulus in dogs. Journal of the American Veterinary Medical Association 1994; 204: 1465-1471.

Leib MS, Blass CE. Acute gastric dilatation in the dog: Various clinical presentations. Compendium on Continuing Education for the Practicing Veterinarian 1984; 6: 707-712.

Chapter 54

Gastric Motility and Emptying Disorders

Deborah J. Davenport
Rebecca L. Remillard
Christine Jenkins

"Dyspepsia is the remorse of a guilty stomach."
A. Kerr

CLINICAL IMPORTANCE

Normally, the stomach should be emptied following an average meal in six to eight hours for dogs and four to six hours for cats (Twedt, 2005). The rate of gastric emptying is influenced by formulation and nutrient content of the food, size of the meal and body size (Nelson et al, 2001).

Gastric motility disorders arise from conditions that directly or indirectly disrupt three of the basic functions of the stomach: 1) storage of ingesta, 2) mixing and dispersion of food particles and 3) timely expulsion of gastric contents into the duodenum. Various processes can affect gastric emptying; however, some may not lead to clinical signs (Twedt, 2005). Delayed gastric emptying may be involved in the etiopathogenesis of gastric dilatation-volvulus (Wyse et al, 2001, 2003; Twedt, 2005; Burger et al, 2006).

Species differences in gastric emptying have been identified (Wyse et al, 2003). In addition, differences may be seen between breeds of dogs. A recent study of the long-term measurement of gastric motility using passive telemetry found significant differences in the postprandial motility patterns between the Labrador retriever test group and the beagle test group. Further studies in breed-related gastric motility are needed (Burger et al, 2006).

Table 54-1 outlines a number of primary and secondary causes of gastroparesis reported to occur in dogs and cats. The importance of these disorders in the general pet population is unknown, but primary gastric motility disorders are probably rare.

PATIENT ASSESSMENT

History and Physical Examination

Delayed gastric emptying due to any cause results in vomiting. Owners may report vomiting of undigested or partially digested food more than 12 hours after the pet eats. The onset of clinical signs may be gradual in acquired cases of chronic hypertrophic pyloric gastropathy or acute in the case of foreign body ingestion. Clinical signs may have been present since weaning in dogs and cats with congenital pyloric stenosis.

Weight loss and poor body condition are often present in chronic cases. Other manifestations may include intermittent gastric bloating, nausea, partial or complete inappetence and

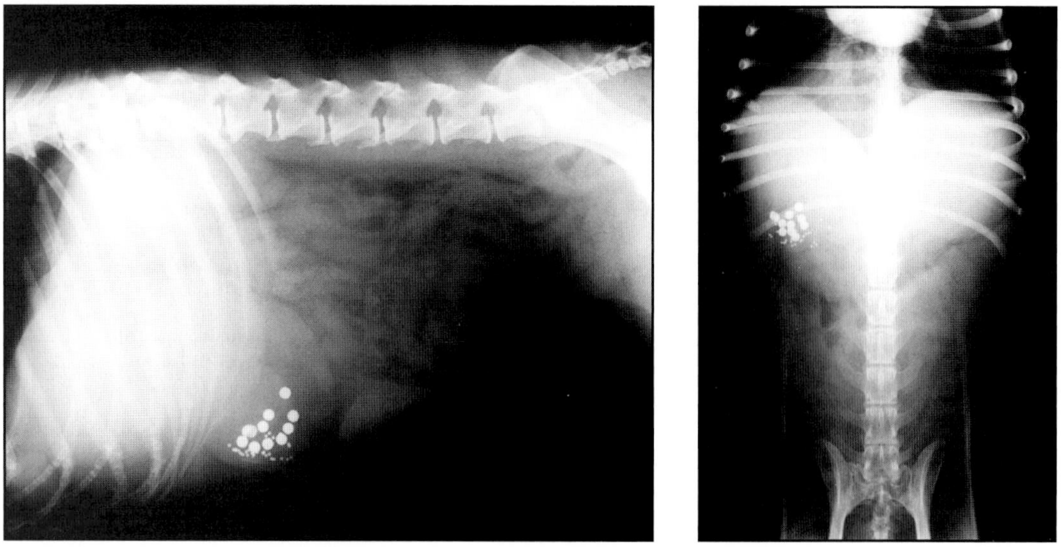

Figure 54-1. Lateral and ventrodorsal abdominal radiographs from an 11-year-old neutered female fox terrier with projectile vomiting demonstrating use of barium-impregnated polyethylene spheres (BIPS). A gastric emptying disorder was confirmed because the spheres were detected in the pyloric antrum 16 hours postadministration. (Courtesy Dr. Grant Guilford, Massey University, New Zealand.)

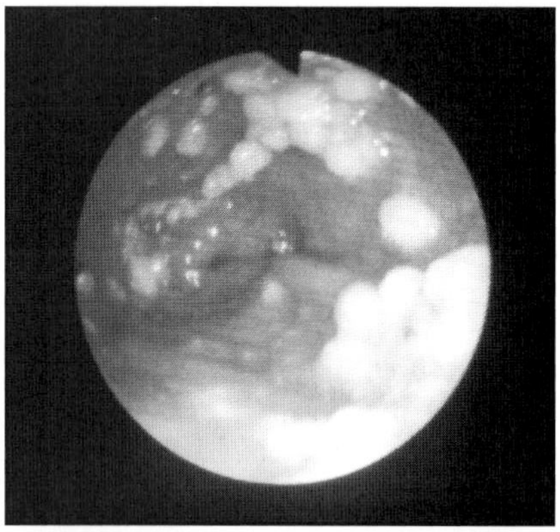

Figure 54-2. Endoscopic view of retained food in the stomach of a 12-year-old neutered female Scottish terrier presented for chronic intermittent vomiting. Food was found in the stomach 20 hours after consumption of a meal, which confirms delayed gastric emptying.

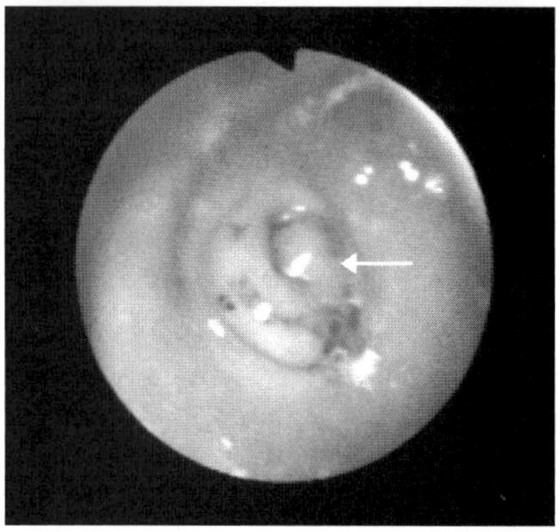

Figure 54-3. Gastroscopic photograph demonstrating hyperplastic mucosal folds (arrow) typical of chronic hypertrophic gastropathy in a 13-year-old neutered male Shih Tzu. (Courtesy Dr. Mike Matz, Southwest Veterinary Specialty Center, Tucson, AZ.)

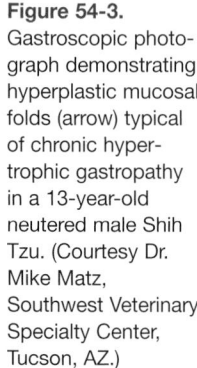

belching. Occasionally, patients will present with unrelenting or projectile vomiting; complete gastric outflow obstruction should be suspected in such cases.

Physical examination findings are often unremarkable beyond evidence of weight loss. Body condition should be assessed and used as a reassessment tool. Gastric distention and tympany may be evident in some cases. Patients with unrelenting vomiting may present with dehydration, depression and malaise. In rare cases, severe electrolyte abnormalities resulting from persistent vomiting may manifest as weakness.

Laboratory and Other Clinical Information

Hematologic and serologic findings in patients with gastroparesis or gastric obstruction are nonspecific and may be more reflective of the underlying disorder. Chronic, persistent vomiting may precipitate dehydration and electrolyte (hypokalemia, hypochloremia) and acid-base abnormalities. Prerenal azotemia is common. Hypochloremic metabolic alkalosis with paradoxical aciduria may be present in dogs and cats with complete pyloric outflow obstruction.

Survey abdominal radiographs are often helpful for evaluating dogs and cats with gastric motility disorders. Typical findings include a stomach distended by fluid, air or food. The presence of food in the stomach 12 to 18 hours after the last meal is evidence of an emptying disorder. Occasionally, gastric wall thickening may be recognized on survey radiographs. Rarely, extraluminal masses causing pyloric obstruction may be identified.

Gastrointestinal (GI) contrast studies confirm delayed gastric emptying. If liquid contrast media (i.e., barium sulfate) remains in the stomach for more than four hours in dogs or 30 minutes in cats, gastroparesis or mechanical obstruction should be suspected (Moon and Myer, 1986). Liquid contrast media, however, is not representative of a typical meal. For that reason, feeding barium mixed with food or administering radiopaque particles (e.g., barium-impregnated polyethylene spheres, BIPS)[a] mixed with food[b] more completely assesses gastric function (**Figure 54-1**). Studies have demonstrated that radiopaque markers exit the stomach at a rate proportional to the disappearance of food (dry matter [DM]) in dogs (Sparkes et al, 1997; Wyse et al, 2001, 2003; Nelson et al, 2001; Twedt, 2005; Simpson, 2005). GI contrast studies also may identify thickened gastric walls, intraluminal foreign bodies and extraluminal masses.

Endoscopy frequently is preferred over radiographic studies in evaluating delayed gastric emptying and gastric outflow obstruction. Barium in the stomach can make endoscopy more difficult; therefore, endoscopy should be performed before administration of barium contrast media (Simpson, 2005).

Gastric emptying disorders may be suspected at the time of upper GI endoscopy. Food in the stomach after a 12- to 18-hour fast is good evidence of the condition (**Figure 54-2**). In some cases, endoscopic findings may be diagnostic. Chronic hypertrophic pyloric gastropathy, for example, has a typical endoscopic appearance, including hyperplastic mucosal folds surrounding the pylorus, protuberance of the pylorus and polyps (**Figure 54-3**) (Leib et al, 1993). In the case of antropyloric or proximal duodenal foreign bodies, endoscopy can be both diagnostic and curative.

Ultrasonography can be used to evaluate delayed gastric emptying. The rate of liquid- and solid-phase gastric emptying measured by ultrasonography is correlated closely with measurements by scintigraphy in people. Gastric contractions can be visualized in dogs using ultrasonography and prolonged retention of fluid in the stomach may indicate delayed gastric emptying. Studies suggest that ultrasonography may be a noninvasive method of evaluating liquid- and solid-phase gastric emptying in dogs (Wyse et al, 2003). Ultrasonography may be useful in the evaluation of pyloric masses and extraluminal sources of pyloric compression (Biller et al, 1994).

Fluoroscopy and nuclear scintigraphy can help assess gastric emptying rate. Radioscintigraphy is considered the gold standard method for evaluating gastric emptying. Correlation with results of radioscintigraphy is necessary to validate other methods of determining gastric motility (Wyse et al, 2003; Nelson et al, 2001). Other means of evaluating gastric motility include a variety of tracer studies and breath tests that have been developed for use in research settings (Wyse et al, 2001, 2003).

Risk Factors

Several breeds are associated with gastric motility disorders (Table 51-1). Congenital pyloric stenosis most often is encountered in brachycephalic dogs and Siamese cats. Chronic hypertrophic pyloric gastropathy usually affects small, purebred, middle-aged dogs, such as the Lhasa apso, Maltese, Shih Tzu and Pekingese (Matthieson and Walter, 1986; Simpson, 2005). Young animals are more at risk for gastric foreign bodies, whereas older pets are more likely to have neoplastic lesions that may obstruct gastric outflow. Young, large-breed dogs living in states bordering the Gulf of Mexico may be infected with *Pythium insidiosum*, resulting in gastric pythiosis and possible gastric outflow obstruction (Simpson, 2005, 2006; Grooters and Taboada, 2004).

Etiopathogenesis

Gastric motility disorders may arise from functional or mechanical obstruction of gastric outflow. Functional disorders of gastric emptying arise from abnormal or asynchronous gastric motility. Myenteric neuronal or gastric smooth muscle function or antropyloroduodenal coordination may be impaired.

A number of benign and malignant anatomic lesions of the stomach and proximal duodenum may result in mechanical gastric outflow obstruction (**Table 54-1**). The most common of these is chronic hypertrophic pyloric gastropathy, which refers to an acquired hypertrophic mucosal or muscular lesion of the pyloric antrum. In addition, congenital pyloric stenosis occurs in young dogs and cats as a consequence of benign muscular hypertrophy of the pylorus. Certain gastric and proximal duodenal neoplasms and granulomatous conditions (e.g., pythiosis, eosinophilic gastritis) can result in pyloric obstruction.

Table 54-1. Potential causes of gastric emptying disorders in dogs and cats.

Functional obstruction (primary motility defects)
Gastric ulcers
Idiopathic asynchronous motility
Idiopathic hypomotility
Infectious gastroenteritis
Postoperative ileus
Functional obstruction (secondary motility defects)
Drug therapy
Anticholinergics
Beta-adrenergic agonists
Narcotic analgesics
Electrolyte disturbances
Hypercalcemia
Hypocalcemia
Hypokalemia
Hypomagnesemia
Inflammation
Acute pancreatitis
Peritonitis
Metabolic disorders
Diabetes mellitus
Hepatic encephalopathy
Hypothyroidism
Mechanical obstruction
Congenital or acquired antral pyloric hypertrophy
Extraluminal compression
Gastric or duodenal foreign bodies
Gastric or duodenal granulomatous lesions
Gastric or duodenal neoplasia or polyps

Key Nutritional Factors

Key nutritional factors for patients with gastric motility and emptying disorders are listed in **Table 54-2** and discussed in detail below.

Water

Dehydration is a common problem in patients with persistent vomiting. Dehydration should be corrected with appropriate parenteral fluid therapy. Thereafter, water should be available free choice. Water should be offered between room and body temperature. Colder water delays gastric emptying.

Energy

Patients with chronic vomiting are often underweight due to longstanding inadequate caloric intake. The energy density of the food should be moderate to increased (4.0 to 4.5 kcal/g [16.7 to 18.8 kJ/g] [DM]) to ensure intake of sufficient energy with small amounts of food. Higher energy densities may help patients maintain or regain body weight and condition, but would require higher dietary fat levels. As discussed below, increased levels of dietary fat adversely affect gastric emptying and should be avoided.

Table 54-2. Key nutritional factors for foods for dogs and cats with gastric motility and emptying disorders.*

Factors	Recommended levels
Energy density	4.0 to 4.5 kcal/g (16.7 to 18.8 kJ/g)
Potassium	0.8 to 1.1%
Chloride	0.5 to 1.3%
Sodium	0.3 to 0.5%
Fat	≤15% for dogs ≤25% for cats
Crude fiber	≤5% crude fiber; avoid foods with gel-forming fiber sources such as pectins and gums (e.g., gum arabic, guar gum, carrageenan, psyllium gum, xanthan gum, carob gum, gum ghatti and gum tragacanth)
Food form consistency	Moist is best; initially liquid or semi-liquid
Food temperature	70 to 100°F (21 to 38°C)

*Nutrients expressed on a dry matter basis.

Electrolytes
Abnormalities in serum electrolyte concentrations, especially potassium, sodium and chloride, are common in patients with chronic vomiting and can adversely affect gastric motility and emptying. Initial abnormalities should be corrected with appropriate parenteral fluid therapy. Foods for patients with gastric motility should contain levels of potassium, chloride and sodium above the minimum allowances for normal dogs and cats. Recommended levels of these nutrients are 0.8 to 1.1% DM potassium, 0.5 to 1.3% DM chloride, and 0.3 to 0.5% DM sodium. Thereafter, the food should contain levels of minerals appropriate for the patient's lifestage.

Fat
Patients with chronic vomiting are often underweight due to longstanding inadequate caloric intake. The energy density of foods is related to dietary fat content and increasing dietary fat typically results in increased caloric intake. However, both solid and liquid foods containing increased fat levels generally are emptied more slowly from the stomach than similar foods with lower fat content. Fat in the duodenum stimulates release of cholecystokinin, which delays gastric emptying. Thus, foods for cats and dogs with gastric emptying or motility disorders should not provide excess fat. Foods with 15% or less (dogs) or 25% or less (cats) DM fat are probably appropriate for patients with gastric emptying or motility disorders.

Fiber
Many grocery brand moist foods contain gelling agents such as gums or hydrocolloids to enhance the aesthetic characteristics of the food. Foods containing gel-forming soluble fibers should be avoided in patients with gastric emptying and motility disorders because they increase the viscosity of ingesta and slow gastric emptying (Russell and Bass, 1985; Prove and Ehrlein, 1982; Sandhu et al, 1987; Burger et al, 2006). Such fibers include pectins and gums (e.g., gum arabic, guar gum, carrageenan, psyllium gum, xanthan gum, carob gum, gum ghatti and gum tragacanth). However, increased levels (>8% DM) of insoluble fiber (powdered cellulose) in dry foods fed to cats had no effect on gastric emptying (Armbrust et al, 2003). Other reports show that the ratio of slowly to rapidly fermentable fibers is important (Kritchevsky, 2001). Therefore, the crude fiber content of foods for patients with gastric motility or emptying disorders should be limited to no more than 5% DM.

Meal Size, Food Form and Food Temperature
In cats and probably dogs, larger meals are emptied more slowly from the stomach than smaller meals (Goggin et al, 1998). Liquids are emptied from the stomach more quickly than solids due to lower digesta osmolality. Water is emptied most quickly, whereas liquids containing nutrients are emptied more slowly. High-osmolality fluids are emptied more slowly than dilute fluids. Solids are the slowest to be emptied from the stomach (Fleming, 1997). A study in cats noted that dry foods emptied more slowly than moist foods (Goggin et al, 1998).

The ideal food form for patients with gastric emptying disorders has a liquid or semi-liquid consistency. Cold meals slow gastric emptying. Therefore, food should be offered between room and body temperature (70 to 100°F [21 to 38°C]).

FEEDING PLAN

Dehydration, electrolyte and acid-base abnormalities and gastric outflow obstruction should be corrected with appropriate fluid therapy and surgical intervention, respectively, before the feeding plan is initiated. For dogs or cats with functional gastric motility disorders, several prokinetic agents are available (Table 51-1) and should be considered if dietary management is insufficient to control clinical signs.

Assess and Select the Food
The form and levels of key nutritional factors should be assessed in the current food and compared with the recommendations outlined in the key nutritional factors section (**Table 54-2**). Most importantly, the food should be complete and balanced for the current lifestage of the patient. The food may not need to be altered for patients with mild disease or few clinical signs.

Tables 54-3 for dogs and **54-4** for cats provide information about key nutritional factor content of selected commercial veterinary therapeutic foods marketed for GI diseases and compares them to the recommended levels. Moist foods are preferred and partially or fully liquefying the food may help promote gastric emptying. These techniques should be used initially in patients with gastric motility or emptying disorders. Add water to a moist veterinary therapeutic food and hand mix or blend to produce a liquid or semi-liquid consistency. Alternatively, liquid enteral products with appropriate key nutritional factor content may be used.

Feed or offer buffering foods rather than foods that contain acidifying salts to most patients with acute or chronic vomiting. Hypochloremic metabolic alkalosis may occur in patients with

Table 54-3. Key nutritional factors in selected moist commercial veterinary therapeutic foods compared to recommended levels for dogs with gastric motility and emptying disorders.*

Factors	Energy density (kcal/g)	Potassium (%)	Chloride (%)	Sodium (%)	Fat (%)	Crude fiber (%)
Recommended levels	**4.0-4.5**	**0.8-1.1**	**0.5-1.3**	**0.3-0.5**	**≤15**	**≤5**
Hill's Prescription Diet i/d Canine	4.4	0.95	1.22	0.44	14.9	1.0
Iams Veterinary Formula Intestinal Low-Residue	4.6	0.84	0.84	0.53	13.2	3.9
Medi-Cal Gastro Formula	na	0.6	na	0.6	11.7	1.0
Purina Veterinary Diets EN GastroENteric	4.0	0.61	0.78	0.37	13.8	0.9
Royal Canin Veterinary Diet Digestive Low Fat LF	4.0	0.74	1.06	0.39	6.9	3.0
Royal Canin Veterinary Diet Intestinal HE	4.3	0.8	0.92	0.57	11.8	1.4

Key: na = information not available from manufacturer.
*From manufacturers' published information or calculated from manufacturers' published as fed values; all values are on a dry matter basis unless otherwise stated. Moist foods, foods with liquid or semi-liquid consistency are preferred. Foods should be offered at temperatures between 70 to 100°F (21 to 38°C).

Table 54-4. Key nutritional factors in selected moist commercial veterinary therapeutic foods compared to recommended levels for cats with gastric motility and emptying disorders.*

Factors	Energy density (kcal/g)	Potassium (%)	Chloride (%)	Sodium (%)	Fat (%)	Crude fiber (%)
Recommended levels	**4.0-4.5**	**0.8-1.1**	**0.5-1.3**	**0.3-0.5**	**≤25**	**≤5**
Hill's Prescription Diet i/d Feline	4.2	1.06	1.18	0.33	24.1	2.4
Iams Veterinary Formula Intestinal Low-Residue	4.0	0.93	0.69	0.40	11.7	3.7
Medi-Cal Hypoallergenic/Gastro	na	1.1	na	0.7	35.9	1.2
Medi-Cal Sensitivity CR	na	1.1	na	1.1	35.1	2.5

Key: na = information not available from manufacturer.
*From manufacturers' published information or calculated from manufacturers' published as fed values; all values are on a dry matter basis unless otherwise stated. Moist foods, foods with liquid or semi-liquid consistency are preferred. Foods should be offered at temperatures between 70 to 100°F (21 to 38°C).

unrelenting vomiting secondary to gastric outflow obstruction. In such patients, oral consumption of food is not possible and intravenous fluid administration with electrolyte therapy should be used to correct this profound acid-base disturbance. A highly digestible food formulated for GI disease should be fed after the gastric outflow obstruction has been resolved by surgical or endoscopic means.

Foods with lower energy density require larger or more frequent meals to meet the patient's daily energy requirement. Larger meals may promote more vomiting and can slow gastric emptying. Optimal energy and fat levels should be determined according to the patient's ability to tolerate meal size and maintain optimal body condition.

Assess and Determine the Feeding Method

Patients with gastric motility disorders often require specialized feeding methods; the current feeding protocol is rarely appropriate. A thorough assessment includes verification of the feeding method currently used. Items to consider include feeding frequency, amount fed, how the food is offered, access to other food, relationship of feeding to exercise and who feeds the pet. All of this information should have been gathered when the history of the patient was obtained. If the patient has a normal body condition score (BCS of 2.5/5 to 3.5/5), the amount of food fed previously was probably appropriate.

Offer foods between room and body temperature (70 to 100°F [21 to 38°C]). Frequent small meals (at least three per day) are preferred. In some cases of complete pyloric outflow obstruction, parenteral nutritional support may be necessary to meet the patient's needs before surgical alleviation of the obstruction. This is indicated when the patient's body condition is poor (BCS of 1/5 or 2/5) and the patient is deemed at increased risk for postsurgical complications.

Late evening feedings are recommended for dogs with the so-called "bilious vomiting" syndrome. Gastroduodenal reflux in these patients probably arises secondarily to a gastric motility disorder. Late evening meals with or without prokinetic therapy may resolve clinical signs in affected dogs (Simpson, 2005).

Most patients can be fed using a feeding method similar to that used for normal pets, if normal gastric function is restored after surgery. The best feeding method will need to be individualized for each patient and determined by trial and error based on remaining gastric function.

REASSESSMENT

Body weight and condition should be assessed every two to four weeks. Document the presence or absence of vomiting. If vomiting continues, alter the food or feeding pattern. Dividing the daily food intake into additional meals also may increase GI tolerance. Use of prokinetic agents (e.g., metoclopramide, cisapride) should be considered if vomiting persists despite implementation of these therapeutic strategies.

Gradual attempts to normalize the feeding regimen can be made if the patient is doing well on the recommended therapy. Feeding more solid foods and larger, less frequent meals are more convenient for pet owners.

The prognosis for dogs and cats with gastric motility disorders varies with the underlying cause. Mechanical obstructions often can be managed effectively through surgical or endoscopic (e.g., foreign body retrieval) means, resulting in an excellent prognosis (Matthieson and Walter, 1986). Occasionally, dogs and cats with longstanding gastric outflow obstruction with gastric distention may have residual gastric motility abnormalities (Leib, 1997). These patients may benefit from the use of prokinetic agents.

ENDNOTES

a. BIPS. Barium impregnated polyethylene spheres. Med-I.D., Medical I.D. Systems, Inc., Grand Rapids, MI, USA.
b. Hill's Prescription Diet i/d, d/d or r/d are the foods recommended to be used with BIPS by the manufacturer.

REFERENCES

The references for **Chapter 54** can be found at www.markmorris.org.

Chapter 55

Introduction to Small Intestinal Diseases

Deborah J. Davenport
Rebecca L. Remillard

"From the gut, comes the strut, and where hunger reigns, strength abstains."
Francois Rabelais

CLINICAL IMPORTANCE

Disorders of the small intestine are encountered frequently in veterinary practice. A number of acute and chronic enteropathies are recognized (**Tables 55-1** and **55-2** and **Boxes 55-1** through **55-3**) and must be distinguished from diseases of other organ systems resulting in gastrointestinal (GI) signs. Typical clinical manifestations of small intestinal disease include diarrhea, weight loss, poor body condition, vomiting, borborygmus and flatulence. **Table 55-3** lists breed-associated small intestinal disorders.

Diarrhea is defined as a change in the frequency, consistency or volume of bowel movements and stools. Diarrhea is the most common manifestation of small intestinal disease. The diarrhea associated with small intestinal conditions differs from that typically associated with large intestinal disorders (**Table 55-4**).

Chapters 56 through 60 include feeding plans for patients with small intestinal disorders. Tables in those chapters list the key nutritional factors for such patients as well as tables that include the levels of key nutritional factors of commercial foods marketed for patients with small intestinal diseases. For comparative purposes, these tables also include the recommended levels of key nutritional factors for patients with small intestinal diseases. Box 60-1 discusses the use of certain oligosaccharides in small intestinal disease.

MECHANISMS OF DIARRHEA

An understanding of normal gut physiology and the common pathophysiologic mechanisms responsible for diarrhea in companion animals allows for a rational approach to evaluation and treatment of patients with small intestinal disorders. There are four major mechanisms for diarrhea: 1) osmotic, 2) altered mucosal permeability, 3) abnormal motility and 4) secretory (Moon, 1978).

Osmotic Diarrhea

Osmotic diarrhea, also referred to as diarrhea of malabsorption, is the most common cause of diarrhea in dogs and cats (Moon,

1978). Osmotic diarrhea may occur in conjunction with other pathophysiologic processes. The presence of unabsorbed nutrients (solutes) in the bowel results in passive diffusion of water into the gut lumen (**Box 55-3**). This process continues until the osmolality of the intestinal chyme is approximately that of plasma. Osmotic diarrhea may occur as a result of maldigestion, malabsorption, administration of osmotic laxatives and overeating. Clinical manifestations of osmotic diarrhea include passage of large volumes of fluid or soft stools. Stools may appear greasy if steatorrhea is present. The diarrhea usually resolves following a 24- to 36-hour fast.

Diarrhea Due to Altered Mucosal Permeability

Altered mucosal permeability (i.e., exudative diarrhea) is another common cause of diarrhea in dogs and cats. The large or small bowel may be affected. The intestinal permeability barrier is composed of epithelial tight junctions, mucosal lymphatics and capillaries and the local immune system. Failure of any one of these components can result in diarrhea. Intestinal diseases that result in erosions, ulcerations and mucosal inflammation or infiltration are potential causes of gut permeability changes and diarrhea. Diarrhea associated with increased gut permeability may present as a protein-losing enteropathy (i.e., hypoproteinemia, hypoalbuminemia, weight loss). Fresh and/or melenic blood may be present in the stool. Fecal examination may reveal inflammatory cells. Often these diarrheas do not completely resolve if food is withheld.

Diarrhea Due to Abnormal GI Motility

Diarrhea may be associated with deranged intestinal motility. It is often difficult to determine whether abnormal GI motility is a primary entity or a consequence of another disorder. In general, deranged intestinal motility is not a common cause of small bowel diarrhea in dogs and cats. The most common motility

Table 55-1. Potential causes of acute small bowel diarrhea in dogs and cats.

Dietary	**Infectious agents**	**Miscellaneous**	**Toxin or drug induced**
Dietary indiscretion	Bacteria	Hemorrhagic gastroenteritis	Chemotherapeutic agents
Foreign bodies	*Bacillus* spp.		Digoxin
Garbage toxicity	*Campylobacter* spp.		Heavy metals
Raw meat consumption	*Clostridium* spp.		Laxatives (magnesium oxide, lactulose)
	Escherichia coli		Nonsteroidal antiinflammatory drugs
	Salmonella spp.		
	Staphylococcus spp.		
	Yersinia spp.		
	Parasites		
	Helminths (roundworms, hookworms, *Strongyloides* spp.)		
	Protozoa (*Giardia* spp., *Isospora* spp., *Cryptosporidium* spp.)		
	Rickettsia		
	Salmon poisoning		
	Viruses		
	Canine distemper		
	Coronavirus		
	Panleukopenia		
	Parvovirus		
	Rotavirus		

Table 55-2. Potential causes of chronic small bowel diarrhea in dogs and cats.

Dietary	**Infectious agents**	**Inflammatory bowel disease**	**Miscellaneous**	**Neoplasia**
Adverse reactions to food	Algae	Eosinophilic gastroenteritis	Juvenile diarrhea of cats	APUD cell tumors
Food allergy (hypersensitivity)	Protothecosis	Lymphocytic enteritis	Lymphangiectasia	Lymphosarcoma
Lactose intolerance	Bacteria	Lymphoplasmacytic enteritis		Mast cell tumor
	Campylobacter spp.	Regional enteritis		
	Mycobacterium spp.	Suppurative gastroenteritis		
	Salmonellosis			
	Small intestinal bacterial overgrowth			
	Fungi			
	Histoplasmosis			
	Pythiosis			
	Zygomycosis			
	Parasites			
	Helminths (roundworms, hookworms)			
	Protozoa (*Isospora* spp., *Giardia lamblia*, *Cyrptosporidium* spp.)			
	Viruses			
	Coronavirus			
	Feline immunodeficiency virus			
	Feline infectious peritonitis			
	Feline leukemia virus			

Key: APUD = amine precursor uptake and decarboxylation.

derangement is rapid intestinal transit associated with a decreased frequency of rhythmic segmental contractions, also termed ileus. The reduction in segmental contractions results in a "pipe" effect with little resistance to ingesta flow. Ileus may occur in conjunction with infiltrative diseases, severe abdominal pain, parvoviral enteritis or may develop postoperatively. In many cases, iatrogenic ileus complicates the management of patients treated inappropriately with anticholinergic agents. Increased frequency of peristaltic contractions is probably not an important cause of diarrhea in dogs and cats. However, it may play a role in the irritable bowel syndrome. A reduction in peristaltic or interdigestive motility may result in small intestinal bacterial overgrowth. Response to dietary manipulation is variable.

Secretory Diarrhea

Secretory diarrhea is relatively uncommon in companion animals vs. people (cholera is the prototypical example) and food animal species. Crypt epithelial cells produce intestinal fluid, whereas enterocytes lining the villous tips are responsible for absorption. Normally, absorption exceeds intestinal secretion. Most secretagogue effects are mediated via a second messenger (e.g., cyclic AMP, cyclic GMP, calmodulin). Secretagogues include GI hormones, bacterial enterotoxins, certain pharmacologic agents, deconjugated bile acids and hydroxy fatty acids. Clinical manifestations of secretory diarrhea are often extreme. Patients have large volumes of fluid diarrhea and often become dehydrated rapidly. Generally, fasting is not successful in alleviating clinical signs.

REFERENCE

The reference for **Chapter 55** can be found at www.markmorris.org.

Table 55-3. Breed-associated small intestinal disorders.

Eosinophilic gastroenteritis	German shepherd dog Irish setter
Hemorrhagic gastroenteritis	Dachshund Miniature poodle Miniature schnauzer
Immunoproliferative small intestinal disease	Basenji Ludenhund
Intestinal adenocarcinoma	Siamese cat
Lymphoplasmacytic enteritis	German shepherd dog Chinese Shar-Pei Soft-coated wheaten terrier Domestic shorthair cat
Parvoviral enteritis	American pit bull terrier Doberman pinscher Rottweiler Labrador retriever (black)
Small intestinal bacterial overgrowth	German shepherd dog Beagle
Lymphangiectasia*	Yorkshire terrier Golden retriever Dachshund Basenji (IPSID) Ludenhund (IPSID)
Wheat-sensitive enteropathy	Irish setter

Key: IPSID = immunoproliferative small intestinal disease.
*Soft-coated wheaten terriers may be affected by a protein-losing enteropathy that may occur in conjunction with a protein-losing nephropathy.

Box 55-1. Small Intestinal Neoplasia.

Lymphosarcoma, adenocarcinoma and mast cell tumors are the most common intestinal tumors recognized in cats, whereas adenocarcinomas and leiomyomas are more common in dogs. Adenocarcinomas occur most commonly in the jejunum and ileum of cats and in the duodenum and colon of dogs. Lymphosarcoma arising from gut-associated lymphoid tissue is the most common extranodal form. A number of other tumor types occur, including plasma cell tumors, leiomyosarcomas, hemangiosarcomas and carcinoid tumors, but are less common.

The diffuse nature of lymphosarcomas and mast cell tumors often results in maldigestion of carbohydrates and some proteins, malabsorption and subsequent malnutrition and provides the greatest opportunity for dietary therapy.

Nutritional support is of critical importance in managing patients with intestinal neoplasia. Providing optimal nutrition helps the clinician return the patient to ideal body condition, provides some protection against the toxic side effects of antineoplastic chemotherapy and improves the patient's quality of life (Chapter 30). As with many small bowel disorders, use of highly digestible foods is recommended with nutrient levels adjusted for each patient as tolerated.

In cases of intestinal neoplasia, assisted-feeding techniques (enteral or parenteral) may be required initially to meet nutritional, fluid and electrolyte needs as the patient recovers from surgery or receives chemotherapy. In particular, early nutritional support (i.e., parenteral or enteral) in debilitated cats is very advantageous in the initial management of gastrointestinal lymphosarcoma. Parenteral administration of nutrients can be added to oral intake to fully meet the patient's requirements. Reestablishing normal intestinal function and stimulating adaptation should begin as soon as the patient tolerates oral food intake.

Multiple (i.e., six to eight) small meals per day are recommended in a form best tolerated by the patient. Occasionally, a liquid form of the food may be necessary for patients undergoing various forms of treatment.

The Bibliography for **Box 55-1** can be found at www.markmorris.org.

Box 55-2. Wheat-Sensitive (Gluten-Sensitive) Enteropathy.

Wheat-sensitive enteropathy is a chronic small bowel disorder recognized primarily in Irish setter dogs. The condition is believed to have an autosomal recessive mode of inheritance. The condition, also termed gluten-sensitive enteropathy, is comparable in some ways to celiac disease of people. The disorder results from a hypersensitivity to gliadin, a glycoprotein found in many grains including wheat, barley, rye, buckwheat and oats. Gliadin is not found in rice, corn or potatoes.

Affected dogs usually develop clinical signs by six months of age, including weight loss, failure to thrive and chronic, intermittent small bowel diarrhea. Some dogs may outgrow the condition and fail to respond to wheat-gluten exposure as adults despite being affected as young dogs. There are no consistent laboratory findings in dogs with wheat-sensitive enteropathy. The results of intestinal function tests such as D-xylose absorption and serum folate/cobalamin concentrations are often normal. Intestinal biopsy can be a useful diagnostic aid. Typical histopathologic findings include partial villous atrophy and intraepithelial lymphocyte infiltration with inflammatory infiltrates within the lamina propria.

Diagnosis of this condition is usually based on signalment, history and response to a therapeutic food trial. Clinical signs usually resolve within two to four weeks after gliadin-containing grains are eliminated from the food. Definitive diagnosis can be made if the clinical signs recrudesce upon re-exposure to gliadin-containing foods or purified gluten.

The pathogenesis of gluten- or wheat-sensitive enteropathy is not completely understood. Hypersensitivity to gliadin has been theorized to develop in dogs due to an age-related delay in expression of a brush border peptidase (i.e., aminopeptidase N) or to increased intestinal permeability. Affected Irish setters have increased serum IgA levels and circulating CD4+ lymphocytes compared to normal dogs. Compared to celiac disease in man, there is no link to major histocompatibility genes (Chapter 31).

The feeding plan includes eliminating all sources of gliadin from the diet including commercial foods, homemade foods, table foods, commercial treats, supplements and chewable medications containing wheat, barley, rye, buckwheat or oats as ingredients. The carbohydrate portion of the food should be composed of potatoes, rice or corn.

Affected dogs should be fed to meet their daily energy requirement. Young growing dogs should be fed foods suitable for growth, whereas young adult and mature adult dogs should receive foods suitable for their lifestage and lifestyle.

The Bibliography for **Box 55-2** can be found at www.markmorris.org.

Box 55-3. Disaccharide Intolerance.

Lactose intolerance is the most common carbohydrate intolerance in people and possibly in dogs and cats. Lactose intolerance results from a relative or absolute deficiency of the enzyme lactase. If brush border lactase fails to hydrolyze lactose into galactose and glucose, the unabsorbed sugar will induce an osmotic diarrhea when it reaches the colon. In addition, colonic bacteria ferment lactose, producing volatile fatty acids, hydrogen and carbon dioxide, resulting in flatulence and pain.

The intestinal brush border mucosa and the disaccharidase enzymes that it contains (i.e., lactase, sucrase, maltase and α-dextrinase) are often lost due to enteritis from any cause. These enzymes are essential for digestion of disaccharides (i.e., lactose, sucrose, maltose and α-dextrins) and subsequent absorption of their constituent monosaccharides. As mentioned above, unabsorbed disaccharides result in a colonic osmotic diarrhea.

Often, one to two weeks are needed to fully restore intestinal lactase and sucrase brush border disaccharidase activity after the cause for their loss is corrected. Diarrhea may, therefore, occur during this period with the ingestion of carbohydrates requiring disaccharidase digestion. For example, jejunal and ileal lactase and sucrase activity were significantly less in piglets fed nothing per os; however, maltase activity in the jejunum and ileum was not different from that of enterally fed piglets after four weeks. Therefore, during and for several days after a diarrheic episode, foods containing maltodextrins should be fed but not those containing lactose and sucrose.

Inadequate intestinal disaccharidase activity is also the mechanism responsible for causing diarrhea after excessive milk consumption. Puppies and kittens normally have small but adequate amounts of intestinal lactase. After weaning age, lactase decreases to about 10% of peak activity in dogs and cats, and continued consumption of milk does not alter the decline in lactase activity. Diarrhea occurs if more lactose is consumed than the animal can digest. Bitch's milk contains only 3.1% lactose and queen's milk 4.2% vs. cow's and goat's milk (4.5 to 5%) as fed. This difference explains why puppies and kittens commonly have diarrhea when given cow's or goat's milk as a milk replacer.

Healthy adult dogs and cats may also develop diarrhea when fed milk. Adult dogs and cats have low levels of brush border lactase activity compared with levels present in pre-weaning animals and levels of other disaccharidases. Most newborn mammals have negligible maltase and sucrase activities, which develop during the first few weeks of life; however, lactase activity is high at birth and decreases with age. In one study, dogs developed diarrhea while consuming more than 1 g of lactose/kg body weight, an amount equivalent to about 20 ml milk/kg body weight or three-fourths cup of milk for a 10-kg dog. Thus, milk-based enteral diets and milk drinks for dogs and cats are commonly treated with enzymes (β-galactosidase) to hydrolyze lactase. However, this increases the osmolality of the product, which may cause diarrhea.

Altered intestinal disaccharidase activity also is hypothesized to be one of the factors responsible for diarrhea subsequent to rapid change in foods and feeding methods. Lactase and sucrase are food-inducible enzymes, whereas, maltase is not. Several days are required for intestinal disaccharidase enzyme activity to respond to a change in dietary carbohydrates.

The Bibliography for **Box 55-3** can be found at www.markmorris.org.

Table 55-4. Characteristics of small and large bowel diarrhea.

Characteristics	**Small bowel**	**Large bowel**
Blood in feces	Melena	Hematochezia
Fecal quality	Loose, watery, “cow-pie”	Loose to semi-formed, “jelly-like”
Fecal volume	Large quantities	Small quantities
Frequency of defecation	Normal to slightly increased	Increased
Malaise	May be present	Rare
Mucus in feces	Usually absent	Usually present
Steatorrhea	May be present	Absent
Tenesmus	Absent	Usually present
Urgency	Absent	Usually present
Vomiting	May be present	Absent
Weight loss	May be present	Rare

Chapter 56

Acute Gastroenteritis and Enteritis

Deborah J. Davenport
Rebecca L. Remillard

"When the Humour falls upon the intestines, it produces a Diarrhea with a sense of heat, and sometimes a Griping...and sometimes with hot stools...so that most of the nutricious juices run off that way, which greatly wastes and sinks the patient."
Williams Hillary 1759, Observations on Changes of the Air

CLINICAL IMPORTANCE

Acute gastroenteritis (enteritis often accompanied by acute gastritis; called gastroenteritis) is one of the most common illnesses of dogs and cats. A number of infectious, toxic and dietary factors can trigger the sudden onset of diarrhea with or without vomiting (Table 55-1). This chapter addresses the diagnosis and management of dogs and cats with an acute onset of diarrhea with or without vomiting.

PATIENT ASSESSMENT

History and Physical Examination

Patients are usually presented for the sudden onset of diarrhea, vomiting or both. In many cases, the owner will report that the pet acts depressed and has a poor appetite. The number and character of the defecations should be assessed. Large fluid stools are typical of small bowel disorders. Melenic or hemorrhagic stools may indicate a potentially life-threatening disorder (**Table 56-1**).

The dietary history is critical. Food-induced diarrhea is relatively common; therefore, a recent change to a moist high-fat or meat-based food may be the source of the patient's diarrhea.[a,b] Often, it is possible to elicit a history of dietary indiscretion, feeding table foods over a holiday or access to garbage, carrion or abrasive materials. Cats that hunt birds may have been exposed to *Salmonella* spp. and dogs eating raw salmon are at risk for salmon poisoning (Scott, 1988; Hibler and Greene, 1986).

Feeding uncooked meat in homemade foods and racing greyhound rations is linked to bacterial enteritis (Chapter 11). Greyhound rations often contain raw ground beef and have been identified as fomites for salmonellosis and colibacillosis (Chengappa et al, 1993; Stone et al, 1993; Morley et al, 2006). Incorporation of raw poultry in foods has been linked to campylobacteriosis and salmonellosis (Davenport, 1989) (Chapter 11).

Other husbandry issues are also important. Records of vacci-

Table 56-1. Clinical signs associated with life-threatening acute gastroenteritis.

Abdominal pain	Fecal leukocytes
Dehydration	Fever
Depression	Melena or hematochezia

nations and anthelmintic treatments should be reviewed. Questions should be asked about the health of other pets and people in the household. A positive answer to these questions raises the likelihood that an infectious organism was involved.

Often, affected dogs and cats are depressed and dehydrated. Typically, the diarrhea is most consistent with small bowel disease (Table 55-4). Occasionally, patients may present with signs reflective of small and large bowel involvement. Abdominal discomfort may be recognized on palpation. Patients should be carefully evaluated for evidence of septic shock. Animals exhibiting systemic signs of illness such as fever and congested mucous membranes in addition to gastrointestinal (GI) signs should be treated more aggressively.

Laboratory and Other Clinical Information

Because there are many potential causes of acute gastroenteritis and enteritis, achieving a definitive diagnosis can be difficult. It is more important to determine whether the patient's condition is self-limiting or if it is potentially life-threatening. This decision, based on historical and physical findings, is critical. **Table 56-1** lists factors that suggest a potentially life-threatening condition. Cases of a serious nature should be pursued aggressively with the use of hematology, serum biochemistry profiles, urinalyses and fecal examinations for parasites and other infectious pathogens. Abdominal films or GI contrast radiographs are recommended to rule out obstruction. Self-limiting cases are usually approached more conservatively. Diagnostics are often limited to assessment of hydration status (i.e., packed cell volume, total protein concentration and body weight) and thorough examination of feces for evidence of parasites, bacterial pathogens (e.g., spores of *Clostridium* spp.), viruses (e.g., fecal ELISA for parvovirus) and enterotoxins (e.g., *C. difficile* fecal ELISA) (Chouicha and Marks, 2006).

Risk Factors

Risk factors for acute gastroenteritis and enteritis include age, breed, immune status and environment. Young animals are more susceptible to a variety of infectious pathogens including parasites, viruses and bacteria (De Santis-Kerr et al, 2006). Hemorrhagic gastroenteritis is reported most commonly in miniature schnauzers, dachshunds, toy poodles and other toy and small dogs (Guilford and Strombeck, 1996). Rottweilers, American pit bull terriers and Doberman pinschers appear to be at increased risk for parvoviral enteritis (Mantione and Otto, 2005; Houston et al, 1996).

Several canine breeds (e.g., Chinese Shar-Pei, German shepherd dog, beagle) may have IgA deficiency; therefore, these dogs may be more susceptible to develop a number of GI conditions, including giardiasis and small intestinal bacterial overgrowth (Table 55-1) (Batt et al, 1991; Whitbread et al, 1984). Likewise, immunocompromised animals are at risk for contracting viral and bacterial enteritides. For example, an outbreak of *C. difficile*-associated enteritis was reported in hospitalized dogs (Weese and Armstrong, 2003). Several conditions including cancer, diabetes mellitus, feline leukemia and feline immunodeficiency virus infections may result in deranged immune function.

Environment also plays an important role in exposure to pathogens. Dogs and cats kept in unsanitary or overcrowded conditions are much more likely to develop infectious enteropathies (De Santis-Kerr, 2006). In addition, animals kept in poorly controlled environments have higher risk for exposure to high-fat table foods, garbage containing spoiled food and toxins. Dogs in particular eat indiscriminately. Consumption of rotten garbage, decomposing carrion or abrasive materials (e.g., hair, bones, rocks, plastic, aluminum foil) can result in severe enteritis. Poor husbandry practices including inadequate parasite control and vaccination programs and overcrowding put pets at risk for acute gastroenteritis and enteritis.

Consumption of raw food diets has been associated with bacterial enteritides (Chengappa et al, 1993; Stone et al, 1993; Morley et al, 2006). Cultures of home-prepared and commercially available raw foods have demonstrated bacterial pathogens including *Salmonella* spp., *Campylobacter* spp., *Escherichia* spp. and *Yersinia* spp. (Weese, 2006; Strohmeyer et al, 2006). Dogs consuming such foods shed bacterial pathogens at a much higher rate than those consuming conventionally cooked commercial foods (Weese and Armstrong, 2006). A thorough dietary history should elicit details of potential exposure to raw meats.

Etiopathogenesis

In acute enteritis, diarrhea may occur as a result of any or all of the four mechanisms of diarrhea described in Chapter 55. Many viral organisms and cancer chemotherapeutic agents destroy intestinal villi. Consequently, diarrhea may occur due to altered gut permeability and/or osmotic mechanisms. Ileus may arise due to abdominal pain in patients with parvoviral enteritis. Finally, bacterial pathogens may elaborate enterotoxins that serve as potent secretogogues.

Small bowel atrophy begins within days in the absence of luminal stimulation. Atrophy, the small intestinal response to disuse, occurs in several species with simple stomachs, including foals (Oikawa et al, 1992), cats (Lippert et al, 1989), dogs (Remillard and Thatcher, 1989) and pigs (Schulman, 1988) and is similar morphologically. The hallmarks of small bowel atrophy are decreased villus height (about 50% in the jejunum and 25% in the ileum) with an overall reduced absorptive surface area and brush border enzyme activity (Remillard et al, 1998, 1998a; Levine et al, 1974).

Food in the lumen of the small bowel stimulates intestinal integrity (mass and function) by several mechanisms. Ingested nutrients mechanically and chemically stimulate the

Table 56-2. Key nutritional factors for dogs and cats with acute gastroenteritis or enteritis.*

Factors	Recommended levels
Sodium	0.3 to 0.5%
Chloride	0.5 to 1.3%
Potassium	0.8 to 1.1%
Fat	12 to 15% for dogs (highly digestible foods) 15 to 25% for cats (highly digestible foods) 8 to 12% for dogs (increased-fiber foods) 9 to 18% for cats (increased-fiber foods)
Energy density	4.0 to 4.5 kcal/g (16.7 to 18.8 kJ/g) (highly digestible foods) ≥3.2 kcal/g (≥13.4 kJ/g) for dogs and ≥3.4 kcal/g (≥14.2 kJ/g) for cats (increased-fiber foods)
Fiber	≤5% in highly digestible foods (mixed fiber sources are best) 7 to 15% in fiber-enhanced foods (insoluble fiber sources are best)
Digestibility	≥87% for protein and ≥90% for fat and carbohydrate (highly digestible foods) ≥80% for protein and fat and ≥90% for carbohydrate (fiber-enhanced foods)

*Nutrient levels are on a dry matter basis.

Table 56-3. Selected commercial oral rehydration solutions available for use in dogs and cats.

	Nutrient content (mEq/l)								
Products (manufacturers)	Na	K	Cl	Mg	Ca	P	Citrate	ME (kcal/l)	Comments
Electramine (Life Science Products)	69.8	15.4	69.7	–	–	–	–	–	Contains glycine
Enfamil Enfalyte (Mead Johnson)	50	25	45	–	–	–	34	126	mOsm/l = 167
Pedialyte Solution unflavored (Abbott Nutrition)	45	20	35	–	–	–	30	100	mOsm/l = 250-270
Rebound OES (Virbac)	52.2-65.2	20.5-25.6	10-20	–	–	–	–	253	–

Key: mEq/l = milliequivalents per liter, Na = sodium, K = potassium, Cl = chloride, Mg = magnesium, Ca = calcium, P = phosphorus, ME = metabolizable energy.

intestine, increasing intestinal secretory and endocrine activity. The type and amount of ingested nutrients mechanically alter the mucosal cell mass by affecting the rate of stem cell division and the rate of mucosal cell renewal. Gastric, duodenal and pancreato-biliary secretions, which normally accompany eating, digestion and absorption, promote mucosal structure and function (Yamada, 1985; Castillo et al, 1990). Refeeding the atrophied small bowel should consider altered function. Limited enteral feeding of milk (i.e., 2 ml/kg body weight, per os, twice daily) to piglets, providing only 10% of the resting energy requirement, resulted in significantly greater jejunal lactase and sucrase activities with taller villi and deeper crypts vs. findings in animals fed nothing per os (Remillard et al, 1998).

Glutamine is the preferred fuel for enterocytes. Glutamine is a conditionally essential amino acid necessary during intestinal recovery to stimulate enterocyte-DNA synthesis and increase enterocyte mucosal mass (Windmueller and Spaeth, 1974). In dogs, there is an increased intestinal requirement for glutamine during the immediate postoperative phase (i.e., less than seven days postsurgery). Glutamine uptake returns to normal later during the recovery phase (i.e., more than 10 days postsurgery) (Souba et al, 1990, 1987).

Key Nutritional Factors

Table 56-2 lists key nutritional factors for patients with acute gastroenteritis or enteritis, which are discussed in detail below.

Water

Water is the most important nutrient for patients with acute diarrhea with or without vomiting because of the potential for life-threatening dehydration due to excessive fluid loss and inability of the patient to replace those losses. Moderate to severe dehydration should be corrected with appropriate parenteral fluid therapy rather than using the oral route. Intraosseous fluid administration may be used in patients with limited venous access, but the subcutaneous route is not recommended in moderate to severely dehydrated patients.

Oral fluid therapy is typically reserved for non-vomiting patients with minor fluid deficits or to supply maintenance fluid requirements. Oral rehydration solutions have been used commonly in people and food production animals with acute diarrhea. Oral rehydration solutions have also been advocated for use in dogs and cats (Zenger and Willard, 1989). Oral rehydration solutions contain glucose, amino acids and electrolytes in addition to water. The physiologic basis for these solutions is the coupled transport of sodium and glucose and other actively transported small organic molecules (Avery and Snyder, 1990). The maximum uptake of water and electrolytes occurs when the ratio of glucose to sodium approaches 1:1 (Avery and Snyder, 1990). An oral rehydration solution containing rice carbohydrate-based glucose polymers developed by the World Health Organization has been licensed for the small animal market (**Table 56-3**). Such solutions are most useful in secretory diarrheas, which are uncommon in small animals. However, oral rehydration solutions can be useful as an alternate fluid source, if readily consumed by the patient.

Electrolytes: Sodium, Chloride and Potassium

The electrolyte composition of intestinal (and gastric) secretions differs from that of extracellular fluids; therefore, loss of intestinal (and gastric) secretions may result in systemic electrolyte abnormalities. Dogs and cats with diarrhea and vomiting may have low, normal or high serum sodium, potassium and chloride concentrations. The derangement that predominates in a particular animal depends on the severity of the disease, nutritional status, site of the disease process, etc. For these reasons, serum electrolyte concentrations are helpful in tailoring the fluid therapy and nutritional management. Mild hypokalemia, hypochloremia and either hypernatremia or hyponatremia are the electrolyte abnormalities most commonly associated with acute diarrhea and vomiting.

Depletion of total body potassium is a predictable consequence of severe or chronic GI disease because the potassium concentration of gastric and intestinal secretions is high. Hypokalemia in association with GI disease will be particularly profound if losses are not matched by sufficient intake of dietary potassium.

Electrolyte disorders should be corrected initially with appropriate parenteral fluid and electrolyte therapy. Foods for patients with acute gastroenteritis should contain levels of sodium, chloride and potassium above the minimum allowances for normal dogs and cats. Recommended levels of these nutrients for dogs and cats are 0.30 to 0.5% dry matter (DM) sodium, 0.5 to 1.3% DM chloride and 0.8 to 1.1% DM potassium.

Fat and Energy Density

In comparison to processes involved with other macronutrients, fat digestion and absorption are relatively complex and may be disrupted in patients with GI disease. Ingestion of a fatty meal decreases gastroesophageal tone, slows gastric emptying and is a potent stimulus for pancreatic secretion.

On the other hand, dietary fat is a concentrated source of calories; higher fat foods allow smaller amounts of food to be ingested to meet the patient's daily energy requirement (DER). This is an important consideration in many patients because limiting the amount of food entering the GI tract helps control clinical signs. Fat also improves the palatability of food, which is important in patients with nausea.

For these reasons, foods for patients with acute gastroenteritis and many other GI diseases should contain moderate amounts of fat. Recommended dietary DM fat levels are 12 to 15% for dogs and 15 to 25% for cats. Dietary fat within these ranges should ensure the energy density of the food falls between 4.0 to 4.5 kcal/g (16.7 to 18.8 kJ/g) DM, thus providing sufficient energy with small amounts of food. Foods with higher energy densities may help restore or maintain body weight and condition in patients but would require higher dietary fat levels. Increased levels of dietary fat delay gastric emptying and therefore should usually be avoided. When feeding foods with increased fiber, the food's DM fat content will typically be lower (eight to 12% for dogs and nine to 18% for cats), as will energy density. Energy densities for these foods should be at least 3.2 kcal/g (13.4 kJ/g) DM for dogs and at least 3.4 kcal/g (14.2 kJ/g) DM for cats.

Fiber

Although dietary fiber predominantly affects the large bowel of dogs and cats, fiber can also affect gastric, small intestinal and pancreatic structure and function. Effects of dietary fiber include: 1) modifying gastric emptying, 2) normalizing intestinal motility and intestinal transport rate, 3) buffering toxins in the GI lumen, 4) binding or holding excess water, 5) supporting growth of normal GI microflora, 6) buffering gastric acid and 7) altering viscosity of GI luminal contents. Dietary fiber also adds indigestible bulk and decreases the DM digestibility of the food.

Various types and levels of dietary fiber have been advocated for patients with acute gastroenteritis. The traditional approach is to recommend low-fiber foods (≤5% DM mixed fiber) that are highly digestible and provide "low residue" in the GI tract. Mixed fibers include beet pulp, brans (rice, wheat or oat), pea, soy fibers, soy hulls and mixtures of soluble and insoluble fibers. Insoluble fibers include purified cellulose and peanut hulls. Soluble fiber sources include fruit pectins, guar gums and psyllium.

Another approach used by one of the authors (RLR) is to use foods containing insoluble fiber sources at levels between 7 to 15% DM. Each of these strategies can be successful in managing selected patients with acute gastroenteritis and enteritis.

Digestibility

The term "highly digestible" is not defined in a regulatory sense. However, the term has generally been reserved for products with protein digestibility ≥87%, and fat and carbohydrate digestibility ≥90%. Fiber-enhanced foods will typically have somewhat lower protein and fat digestibilities but carbohydrate should be about the same. Digestibility targets for fiber-enhanced foods are at least 80% for protein and fat and 90% or above for carbohydrate. The average digestibility coefficients for popular commercial dog and cat foods are 78 to 81%, 77 to 85% and 69 to 79% for crude protein, crude fat and digestible (soluble) carbohydrate, respectively (Kendall et al, 1982; Kendall, 1981). Veterinary therapeutic foods formulated for patients with GI disease usually contain meat and carbohydrate sources that have been highly refined to increase digestibility. Meat ingredients in many therapeutic foods are usually composed of muscle and organ sources rather than meat and bone meals. Typical meat/animal source ingredients in commercial GI foods include egg, cottage cheese, chicken,

Table 56-4. Key nutritional factors in selected highly digestible commercial veterinary therapeutic foods marketed for dogs with acute gastroenteritis or acute enteritis.*

Dry foods	Na (%)	Cl (%)	K (%)	Fat (%)	Energy density (kcal/g)	Fiber (%)**	Protein digestibility (%)	Fat digestibility (%)	Carbohydrate digestibility (%)	Ingredient comments
Recommended levels	**0.3-0.5**	**0.5-1.3**	**0.8-1.1**	**12-15**	**4.0-4.5**	**≤5**	**≥87**	**≥90**	**≥90**	**-**
Hill's Prescription Diet i/d Canine	0.45	1.04	0.92	14.1	4.2	2.7	92	93	94	–
Iams Veterinary Formula Intestinal Low-Residue	0.35	0.66	0.90	10.7	3.8	2.1	na	na	na	FOS, MOS prebiotics
Medi-Cal Gastro Formula	0.5	na	0.8	13.9	na	1.9	na	na	na	OS prebiotic, *Bacillus subtilis* dried fermentation extract
Purina Veterinary Diets EN GastroENteric Formula	0.6	0.85	0.66	12.6	4.2	1.5	84.5	91.4	94.4	MCT
Royal Canin Veterinary Diet Digestive Low Fat LF 20	0.49	1.10	0.88	6.6	3.7	2.3	na	na	na	FOS, MOS prebiotics
Royal Canin Veterinary Diet Intestinal HE 28	0.55	0.99	0.88	22.0	4.5	1.6	na	na	na	FOS, MOS prebiotics
Moist foods	**Na (%)**	**Cl (%)**	**K (%)**	**Fat (%)**	**Energy density (kcal/g)**	**Fiber (%)****	**Protein digestibility (%)**	**Fat digestibility (%)**	**Carbohydrate digestibility (%)**	**Ingredient comments**
Recommended levels	**0.3-0.5**	**0.5-1.3**	**0.8-1.1**	**12-15**	**4.0-4.5**	**≤5**	**≥87**	**≥90**	**≥90**	**-**
Hill's Prescription Diet i/d Canine	0.44	1.22	0.95	14.9	4.4	1.0	88	94	93	–
Iams Veterinary Formula Intestinal Low-Residue	0.53	0.84	0.84	13.2	4.6	3.9	na	na	na	–
Medi-Cal Gastro Formula	0.6	na	0.6	11.7	na	1.0	na	na	na	FOS prebiotic
Purina Veterinary Diets EN GastroENteric Formula	0.37	0.78	0.61	13.8	4.0	0.9	85.1	95.6	92.2	MCT
Royal Canin Veterinary Diet Digestive Low Fat LF	0.39	1.06	0.74	6.9	4.0	3.0	na	na	na	–
Royal Canin Veterinary Diet Intestinal HE	0.57	0.92	0.80	11.8	4.3	1.4	na	na	na	Inulin prebiotic

Key: Na = sodium, Cl = chloride, K = potassium, fiber = crude fiber, na = information not available from manufacturer, FOS = fructooligosaccharide, MOS = mannanoligosaccharide, MCT = medium-chain triglyceride.
*Nutrients expressed on a dry matter basis. To convert kcal to kJ, multiply kcal by 4.184.
**Mixed fiber sources are best in highly digestible foods (see text).

low-ash poultry by-product meal and ground beef.

Carbohydrates make up the largest non-water fraction (i.e., 60 to 80% DM) of commercial and homemade foods formulated for managing patients with GI diseases. In pet foods, carbohydrate digestibility is influenced by source and processing. Dogs digest most properly cooked starches very well including corn, rice, barley and wheat (Walker et al, 1994; Bissett et al, 1998). Other starches (e.g., potato and tapioca) are less digestible, especially when inadequately cooked (Wolter, 1993; Schunemann et al, 1994; Baker and Czarnecki-Maulden, 1991; Kienzle, 1993; Morris et al, 1977). Cats, despite their obligate carnivorous nature, also efficiently digest carbohydrates. However, the opinion of some clinicians is that cats with small bowel disorders are less tolerant of dietary carbohydrate than dogs with similar causes of malassimilation (Buddington et al, 1991; Kienzle, 1993; Sherding, 1989; Washabau et al, 1986). More recently, a feeding trial in cats with diarrhea demonstrated no difference in response to foods containing moderate carbohydrate levels (31.7% DM) or low levels (15% DM) (Laflamme and Long, 2004).

A link has been established between particle size and carbohydrate digestibility in moist foods (Bissett et al, 1997). These findings support chopping or grinding carbohydrate ingredients (e.g., rice, corn, etc.) before they are incorporated into moist foods. These findings are probably not applicable to extruded dry products because the extrusion process allows for a more complete cook than the canning process. Studies have demonstrated almost complete ileal carbohydrate digestibility in normal dogs consuming extruded grains (Harmon et al, 1999).

In general, dietary fat is more digestible than digestible carbohydrates and protein. Depending on the fat source, the ap-

Table 56-5. Key nutritional factors in selected fiber-enhanced commercial veterinary therapeutic foods marketed for dogs with acute gastroenteritis or acute enteritis.*

Dry foods	Na (%)	Cl (%)	K (%)	Fat (%)	Energy density (kcal/g)	Fiber (%)**	Protein digestibility (%)	Fat digestibility (%)	Carbohydrate digestibility (%)	Primary sources of fiber**
Recommended levels	**0.3-0.5**	**0.5-1.3**	**0.8-1.1**	**8-12**	**≥3.2**	**7-15**	**≥80**	**≥80**	**≥90**	**-**
Hill's Prescription Diet w/d Canine	0.22	0.46	0.70	8.8	3.3	16.4	84	92	95	Cellulose, soybean mill run, beet pulp
Medi-Cal Fibre Formula	0.3	na	1.0	10.6	na	14.3	na	na	na	Tomato pomace, rice hulls, oat hulls, flax meal, apple pomace
Purina Veterinary Diets DCO Dual Fiber Control	0.34	0.82	0.70	12.4	3.7	7.6	79.9	80.4	90.6	Beet pulp, pea fiber
Purina Veterinary Diets OM Overweight Management Formula	0.31	0.97	0.83	7.2	2.9	10.3	81.9	78.9	72.3	Soybean hulls, pea fiber, cellulose
Royal Canin Veterinary Diet Calorie Control CC 26 High Fiber	0.33	0.77	0.90	10.4	3.1	17.6	na	na	na	Cellulose, pea fiber, rice hulls, beet pulp, psyllium husk
Royal Canin Veterinary Diet Diabetic HF 18	0.27	0.88	0.88	9.9	3.3	12.1	na	na	na	Cellulose, rice hulls, guar gum

Moist foods	Na (%)	Cl (%)	K (%)	Fat (%)	Energy density (kcal/g)	Fiber (%)**	Protein digestibility (%)	Fat digestibility (%)	Carbohydrate digestibility (%)	Primary sources of fiber**
Recommended levels	**0.3-0.5**	**0.5-1.3**	**0.8-1.1**	**8-12**	**≥3.2**	**7-15**	**≥80**	**≥80**	**≥90**	**-**
Hill's Prescription Diet w/d Canine	0.24	0.76	0.64	12.7	3.6	12.4	88	90	92	Cellulose
Medi-Cal Fibre Formula	0.5	na	0.7	9.1	na	15.0	na	na	na	Tomato pomace, guar gum, flax meal, carrageenan
Purina Veterinary Diets OM Overweight Management Formula	0.28	0.51	1.06	8.4	2.5	19.2	80.9	89.8	62.9	Pea fiber, beet pulp, carrageenan
Royal Canin Veterinary Diet Calorie Control CC 26 High Fiber	0.53	0.70	0.82	12.5	3.6	8.8	na	na	na	Tomato pomace, guar gum, flax meal, carrageenan

Key: Na = sodium, Cl = chloride, K = potassium, fiber = crude fiber, na = information not available from manufacturer.
*Nutrients expressed on a dry matter basis. To convert kcal to kJ, multiply kcal by 4.184.
**Insoluble fiber sources are best in fiber-enhanced foods (see text).

parent digestibility of fat by dogs can vary from approximately 81 to 95%; fats with higher levels of unsaturated fatty acids are more digestible (NRC, 2006). The apparent digestibility of dietary fat by cats is between 85 to 99%. Fat digestibility also depends on saturation of constituent fatty acids and age of cats. Older cats and kittens have lower fat digestibility (NRC, 2006). Digestibility of protein, carbohydrates and fat in foods for patients with acute GI disease should be high because normal digestion and absorption of nutrients are often compromised. Moderate amounts of fiber decrease the DM digestibility of the overall food; however, digestibility of the non-fiber macronutrients is usually unaffected (Harmon et al, 1999).

Other Nutritional Factors

Glutamine

The amino acid, glutamine, is considered a conditionally essential nutrient for pets with severe GI disorders. As the preferred energy substrate for enterocytes, glutamine is necessary for maintaining gut mucosal integrity (Windmueller and Spaeth, 1974, 1978). Commercial and homemade pet foods containing meat ingredients provide glutamine. Unfortunately, an analytical method for determining glutamine levels in foods is not widely available, making selection of foods based on glutamine content impractical (Kuhn et al, 1996). Glutamine intake can be increased by orally administering a 2% solution of glutamine in water; 0.5 g of glutamine per kg body weight should be provided daily. Many pets will readily consume a glutamine solution, or these solutions can be administered by dose syringe or indwelling feeding tubes. Such glutamine dosing regimens have been used for treating canine patients with parvoviral enteritis. Alternatively, commercial liquid or moist homogenized enteral foods (Chapter 25) enhanced with glutamine may be offered.

Table 56-6. Key nutritional factors in selected highly digestible commercial veterinary therapeutic foods marketed for cats with acute gastroenteritis or acute enteritis.*

Dry foods	Na (%)	Cl (%)	K (%)	Fat (%)	Energy density (kcal/g)	Fiber (%)**	Protein digestibility (%)	Fat digestibility (%)	Carbohydrate digestibility (%)	Ingredient comments
Recommended levels	**0.3-0.5**	**0.5-1.3**	**0.8-1.1**	**15-25**	**4.0-4.5**	**≤5**	**≥87**	**≥90**	**≥90**	**-**
Hill's Prescription Diet i/d Feline	0.37	1.11	1.07	20.2	4.3	2.8	88	92	90	–
Iams Veterinary Formula Intestinal Low-Residue	0.25	0.63	0.66	13.7	3.9	1.8	na	na	na	FOS, MOS prebiotics
Medi-Cal HYPOallergenic/ Gastro	0.4	na	0.8	11.5	na	3.1	na	na	na	FOS prebiotic, *Bacillus subtilis* dried fermentation extract
Purina Veterinary Diets EN GastroENteric	0.64	0.58	0.99	18.4	4.4	1.3	94.0	93.1	79.7	–
Royal Canin Veterinary Diet Intestinal HE 30	0.65	0.97	0.97	23.7	4.4	5.8	na	na	na	FOS, MOS prebiotics
Moist foods	**Na (%)**	**Cl (%)**	**K (%)**	**Fat (%)**	**Energy density (kcal/g)**	**Fiber (%)****	**Protein digestibility (%)**	**Fat digestibility (%)**	**Carbohydrate digestibility (%)**	**Ingredient comments**
Recommended levels	**0.3-0.5**	**0.5-1.3**	**0.8-1.1**	**15-25**	**4.0-4.5**	**≤5**	**≥87**	**≥90**	**≥90**	**-**
Hill's Prescription Diet i/d Feline	0.33	1.18	1.06	24.1	4.2	2.4	91	89	91	–
Iams Veterinary Formula Intestinal Low-Residue	0.40	0.69	0.93	11.7	4.0	3.7	na	na	na	FOS prebiotic
Medi-Cal HYPOallergenic/Gastro	0.7	na	1.1	35.9	na	1.2	na	na	na	FOS prebiotic
Medi-Cal Sensitivity CR	1.1	na	1.1	35.1	na	2.5	na	na	na	–

Key: Na = sodium, Cl = chloride, K = potassium, fiber = crude fiber, na = information not available from manufacturer, FOS = fructooligosaccharide, MOS = mannanoligosaccharide.
*Nutrients expressed on a dry matter basis. To convert kcal to kJ, multiply kcal by 4.184.
**Mixed fiber sources are best in highly digestible foods (see text).

Acid Load

Acidemia is common in pets with diarrhea because fluid secreted in the caudal small intestine and large intestine contains bicarbonate concentrations higher than those in plasma and sodium in excess of chloride ions. The acidosis is compounded in some patients by development of hypovolemia (i.e., severe dehydration). Severe acid-base disorders are best corrected with appropriate parenteral fluid therapy. Foods for patients with acute diarrhea accompanied by vomiting should also avoid excess dietary acid load and preferably contain buffering salts (e.g., potassium gluconate and calcium carbonate). Ideally, foods that normally produce a urinary pH greater than 6.8 should be selected.

FEEDING PLAN

The first objective in managing acute gastroenteritis or enteritis should be to correct dehydration and electrolyte, glucose and acid-base imbalances, if present. Colloidal solutions or plasma transfusions may be necessary for those patients with hypoalbuminemia (Buriko and Otto, 2007). The dietary goals are to provide a food that meets the patient's nutrient requirements and allows normalization of intestinal motility and function. Medical therapy may include antibiotics, antidiarrheals, antiemetics, nonsteroidal antiinflammatory agents (e.g., flunixin meglumine), anti-endotoxin sera, analgesics, interferon and anthelmintics.

Assess and Select the Food

Levels of the key nutritional factors should be evaluated in foods currently fed to patients with acute gastroenteritis or enteritis and compared with recommended levels. Information from this aspect of assessment is essential for making any changes to foods currently provided. Changing to a more appropriate food is indicated if key nutritional factors in the current food do not match recommended levels.

There are several plausible dietary strategies for managing small bowel diarrhea after a 24- to 36-hour fast and they may be attempted in any order. The traditional approach is to first feed a highly digestible, low-residue food with moderate levels of fat. Small amounts of soluble or mixed fiber sources may be included in such foods. Including low levels of fiber does not usually impair digestibility or increase fecal volume. This approach can be accomplished by feeding commercial veterinary therapeutic

Table 56-7. Key nutritional factors in selected fiber-enhanced commercial veterinary therapeutic foods marketed for cats with acute gastroenteritis or acute enteritis.*

Dry foods	Na (%)	Cl (%)	K (%)	Fat (%)	Energy density (kcal/g)	Fiber (%)**	Protein digestibility (%)	Fat digestibility (%)	Carbohydrate digestibility (%)	Primary sources of fiber**
Recommended levels	**0.3-0.5**	**0.5-1.3**	**0.8-1.1**	**9-18**	**≥3.4**	**7-15**	**≥80**	**≥80**	**≥90**	**-**
Hill's Prescription Diet w/d Feline	0.30	0.84	0.84	9.8	3.5	7.6	90	87	86	Cellulose
Hill's Prescription Diet w/d with Chicken Feline	0.35	0.82	0.80	9.9	3.5	7.6	91	85	94	Cellulose
Medi-Cal Fibre Formula	0.5	na	0.9	12.2	na	14.9	na	na	na	Pea fiber, beet pulp, flax meal
Purina Veterinary Diets OM Overweight Management	0.57	0.84	0.89	8.5	3.6	5.6	91.1	87.7	66.8	Oat fiber, cellulose
Royal Canin Veterinary Diet Calorie Control CC 29 High Fiber	0.51	0.92	0.88	10.2	3.3	14.0	na	na	na	Cellulose, pea fiber, rice hulls, beet pulp, psyllium

Moist foods	Na (%)	Cl (%)	K (%)	Fat (%)	Energy density (kcal/g)	Fiber (%)**	Protein digestibility (%)	Fat digestibility (%)	Carbohydrate digestibility (%)	Primary sources of fiber**
Recommended levels	**0.3-0.5**	**0.5-1.3**	**0.8-1.1**	**9-18**	**≥3.4**	**7-15**	**≥80**	**≥80**	**≥90**	**-**
Hill's Prescription Diet w/d with Chicken Feline	0.38	0.89	0.89	16.6	3.5	10.6	92	na	na	Cellulose, oat fiber, guar gum, locust bean gum, carrageenan
Medi-Cal Fibre Formula	0.4	na	0.8	17.1	na	16.7	na	na	na	Pea fiber, flax meal, guar gum
Purina Veterinary Diets OM Overweight Management	0.31	0.93	0.91	14.6	3.9	10.2	87.3	88.6	84	Pea fiber, oat fiber, guar gum
Royal Canin Veterinary Diet Calorie Control CC High Fiber	0.38	0.51	0.77	21.3	4.1	7.7	na	na	na	Cellulose, guar gum, flaxseed

Key: Na = sodium, Cl = chloride, K = potassium, fiber = crude fiber, na = information not available from manufacturer.
*Nutrients expressed on a dry matter basis. To convert kcal to kJ, multiply kcal by 4.184.
**Insoluble fiber sources are best in fiber-enhanced foods (see text).

foods formulated for GI disease (**Tables 56-4** and **56-5** for dogs and **56-6** and **56-7** for cats) or properly prepared homemade foods (Chapter 10). Foods for puppies and kittens with GI disease should also meet requirements for growth.

As mentioned above, dietary fiber content may be increased to normalize intestinal motility, water balance and GI microflora. Fiber has several physiologic characteristics that are beneficial in managing small bowel diarrhea. Moderate amounts of fiber (7 to 15% DM) add indigestible bulk, which buffers toxins, holds excess water and, perhaps more important, provides intraluminal stimuli to reestablish the coordinated actions of hormones, neurons, smooth muscles, enzyme delivery, digestion and absorption. Fiber normalizes transit time through the small bowel, which means fiber slows a hypermotile state, but also improves a hypomotile state to reestablish normal peristaltic action. **Tables 56-5** (dogs) and **56-7** (cats) list selected fiber-enhanced commercial veterinary therapeutic foods.

For cases in which protracted small bowel disuse (i.e., three to five days) is expected, a third strategy may be used. This involves providing early enteral nutrition intermittently by the oral route or continuously by a nasoesophageal tube. This strategy of feeding through vomiting and diarrhea rather than providing a period of bowel rest has been studied prospectively in dogs with parvoviral enteritis (Will et al, 2005; Mohr et al, 2003). The combination of an orally administered highly digestible food (previously incubated with pancreatic enzymes) every eight hours plus total parenteral feeding was compared to total parenteral feeding alone (Will et al, 2005). Dogs in the combined therapy group had a lower mortality rate than those receiving total parenteral nutrition alone, but the intermittent oral administration of food was complicated by marked nausea and vomiting in 90% of patients. The effect of early enteral nutrition using a polymeric enteral food administered continuously by a nasoesophageal tube was evaluated in dogs with parvoviral enteritis as compared to dogs held NPO (nothing per os) (Mohr et al, 2003). Early enteral nutrition resulted in a more rapid clinical improvement including increased body weight, resolution of vomiting and diarrhea and a lower mortality rate. The precise mechanisms responsible for these benefits are unknown but may include reduced protein/calorie malnutrition, more rapid intestinal villous recovery, enhanced integrity of epithelial tight junctions, normalization of intestinal microflora and enhanced gut immunity (Mohr et al, 2003; Will et al, 2005).

For dogs held NPO for acute gastroenteritis, reintroduction to oral feeding may be accomplished by offering small amounts of a highly digestible food formulated for GI disease. Alternatively, initially feeding small amounts of a monomeric liquid food containing maltodextrins and glutamine may ease the transition to other foods (Chapter 25). Feeding puppies recovering from parvoviral enteritis a monomeric, iso-osmotic liquid food containing maltodextrins (no lactose) plus glutamine reduces nausea and vomiting, and subsequently eases the transition to feeding other commercial veterinary therapeutic foods.[c]

Assess and Determine the Feeding Method

A thorough assessment should include verification of the feeding method currently used. Items to consider include feeding frequency, amount fed, how the food is offered, access to other food and who feeds the pet. All of this information should have been gathered when the history of the patient was obtained. If the animal has a normal body condition score (2.5/5 to 3.5/5), the amount of food previously fed (energy basis) was probably appropriate.

Withholding oral intake of food and water for 24 to 48 hours is the first step in the feeding method for dogs and cats with acute gastroenteritis or enteritis. After this period, patients should be offered small amounts of water or ice cubes every few hours. If water is well tolerated, small amounts of food can be offered several times (i.e., six to eight times) a day. If the pet can eat food without episodes of diarrhea or vomiting, the amount fed can be increased over three to four days until the patient is receiving its estimated DER in two to three meals per day. During this period, if the patient begins to vomit, food should be withdrawn and offered again after several hours. As discussed above, continuous feeding can be used to deliver early enteral nutrition or monomeric liquid foods can be offered.

Persistent vomiting in some cases of parvoviral enteritis may complicate refeeding; some puppies develop gastroparesis and may require prokinetic drugs to facilitate feeding. In such cases, intravenous infusion of metoclopramide (at a rate of 1.0 mg/kg body weight/day) is recommended. Alternatively, metoclopramide can be administered to well-hydrated patients subcutaneously or intramuscularly at a dose of 0.5 mg/kg body weight q8h. Some patients may require partial parenteral or total parenteral feeding (Chapter 26).

REASSESSMENT

The prognosis for recovery in most cases of acute gastroenteritis and enteritis is good. Body weight should be recorded daily until recovery is complete. Changes in body weight from day to day usually reflect changes in hydration status rather than loss or gain of body tissue. Further diagnostic testing is warranted if severe diarrhea or vomiting persists. Acute worsening of clinical signs especially when accompanied by abdominal pain in a young dog with gastroenteritis may be a result of intestinal intussusception (Patsikas et al, 2003; Rallis et al, 2000). In such cases, abdominal radiography and/or ultrasonography are indicated.

Dogs and cats presenting with multiple or recurrent episodes of small bowel diarrhea require further diagnostic workup and, most probably, a combination of dietary and medical therapies. Parasitic causes, however, should be ruled out or treated empirically before pursuing further diagnostics. The diagnostic approach to patients with chronic small bowel diarrhea is beyond the scope of this book; readers are referred to internal medicine and gastroenterology texts for more information.

ENDNOTES

a. Davenport DJ. Unpublished data. 1996.
b. Remillard RL. Personal observation. 1998.
c. Remillard RL. Personal experience. 1998.

REFERENCES

The references for **Chapter 56** can be found at www.markmorris.org.

CASE 56-1

Acute Diarrhea in a Young Cat

Deborah J. Davenport, DVM, MS, Dipl. ACVIM (Internal Medicine)
Hill's Pet Nutrition Center
Topeka, Kansas, USA

Patient Assessment

A six-month-old intact male domestic shorthair kitten was examined for acute onset of vomiting, watery diarrhea, anorexia and lethargy. The kitten had been found as a stray two months previously and vaccination status was unknown. The kitten lived in a barn and the owners were concerned that it had been poisoned. A dog also lived in the house and there were several horses on the property. None of these animals were ill.

Physical examination revealed depression and dehydration. Excessive amounts of fluid and gas were palpable in the intestinal tract. Abdominal palpation stimulated vomiting; the vomitus was clear fluid with flecks of blood. Body weight was 2.5 kg and the kitten appeared thin (body condition score [BCS] 2/5).

Evaluation included a fecal flotation (negative), complete blood count (leukopenia) and serum biochemistry profile (normal except for changes associated with dehydration). A tentative diagnosis of panleukopenia due to feline parvovirus infection was made.

Treatment included aggressive intravenous fluid therapy to correct dehydration and systemic antibiotics. The kitten improved clinically within a few days and the leukocyte count returned to normal. The kitten began drinking water and eating small amounts of a moist homogenized recovery formula (Prescription Diet a/d Canine/Feline[a]). There was no further vomiting but diarrhea continued. The feces were no longer watery but were semi-formed and voluminous.

Assess the Food and Feeding Method

The kitten was fed a commercial dry grocery brand food formulated for growth (Purina Kitten Chow[b]). The food and water were available free choice in the barn. The kitten had access to other animal feed (commercial dry dog food, grain mixture for the horses) but had never been seen eating these foods.

Questions

1. What is the likely cause for the persistent diarrhea?
2. What are the key nutritional factors for this patient?
3. Outline a feeding plan for this kitten.

Answers and Discussion

1. Feline parvovirus infection destroys intestinal crypt cells in the jejunum and ileum. This results in shortened, blunt intestinal villi and also malabsorption. Villi will normally regrow very quickly after viremia resolves and crypt cells are reestablished. However, some cats have a prolonged recovery period with chronic enteritis and diarrhea. This may occur because villi are slow to recover or because of concurrent parasite, viral or bacterial infection. The recovery food may also contain excessive amounts of fat (29% dry matter [DM] fat) for the recovering gastrointestinal (GI) tract.
2. Key nutritional factors for patients with infectious enteritis include water, electrolytes, fat, energy, fiber and digestibility.

   Water. Water is the most important nutrient for patients with acute vomiting or diarrhea because of the potential for life-threatening dehydration due to excessive fluid loss and inability of the patient to replace losses. Oral fluid therapy is reserved for cats with minor fluid deficits or to supply maintenance fluid requirements.

   Electrolytes. Hypokalemia, hypochloremia and either hypernatremia or hyponatremia are the electrolyte abnormalities most commonly associated with acute vomiting and diarrhea. Electrolyte disorders should be corrected initially with appropriate parenteral fluid therapy. Foods for cats with acute gastroenteritis should contain levels of sodium, chloride and potassium above the minimum allowances for normal kittens and adult cats.

   Fat/energy density. Dietary fat is a concentrated source of calories; higher fat foods allow smaller amounts of food to be ingested to meet the cat's daily energy requirement (DER). This is important for many patients with GI disease because limiting the amount of food entering the GI tract helps control clinical signs. Fat also helps improve the palatability of food, which is important for patients with nausea. For these reasons, foods for cats with acute gastroenteritis should contain moderate amounts of fat (i.e., 15 to 25% DM).

   Fiber. Dietary fiber is beneficial because it: 1) modifies gastric emptying, 2) normalizes intestinal motility, 3) buffers toxins in the GI lumen, 4) binds or holds excess water, 5) supports growth of normal GI microflora, 6) buffers gastric acid and 7) alters viscosity of GI luminal contents. Cats with gastroenteritis may benefit from small amounts (i.e., crude fiber ≤5% DM) of a mixed (i.e., soluble/insoluble) fiber type in conjunction with a highly digestible food.

Digestibility. Digestibility of foods for cats with acute gastroenteritis should be high (fat and digestible carbohydrate ≥90% and protein ≥87%) because normal digestion and absorption of nutrients is often impaired.

3. Small amounts of water and food should be gradually reintroduced to the kitten. The food should reflect the nutrient profile discussed above. Veterinary therapeutic foods designed for patients with GI disease have appropriate nutrient levels and usually have high digestibility. Levels of nutrients in these products are also usually appropriate for growing cats. The DER should reflect the needs of a growing cat (i.e., at least 2.5 x resting energy requirement or 360 kcal [1.51 MJ]).

Progress Notes

Multiple fecal flotations were negative for intestinal parasites. A fecal culture was negative for bacterial pathogens. Tests for feline leukemia and feline immunodeficiency virus infection were negative. A commercial moist veterinary therapeutic food (Prescription Diet i/d Feline[a]) was mixed with the recovery food (approximately 50:50) and gradually introduced to the kitten. This food is highly digestible, contains a mixed fiber source and is formulated to meet the nutritional needs of kittens. The kitten readily ate this mixture for two days in the hospital and was sent home with the dry formula of i/d Feline (three-fourths cup daily to be increased as the cat grew and gained weight). Semi-formed feces persisted for several weeks but then gradually returned to normal. The food was changed to a commercial dry product appropriate for adult cats when the cat was neutered at nine months of age.

Endnotes

a. Hill's Pet Nutrition Inc., Topeka, KS, USA.
b. Ralston Purina Co., St. Louis, MO, USA.

Bibliography

Pollock RVH, Postorino NC. Feline panleukopenia and other enteric viral diseases. In: Sherding RG, ed. The Cat: Diseases and Clinical Management, 2nd ed. New York, NY: Churchill Livingstone, 1994; 479-487.

Chapter 57

Inflammatory Bowel Disease

Deborah J. Davenport
Albert E. Jergens
Rebecca L. Remillard

"With good digestion all can be turned to health."
George Herbert

CLINICAL IMPORTANCE

The term inflammatory bowel disease (IBD) refers to a group of chronic, idiopathic gastrointestinal (GI) disorders characterized by histopathologic lesions of mucosal inflammation. Each IBD variant is named by the predominant cellular infiltrate within the lamina propria. Currently, IBD is considered the most common cause of chronic diarrhea and vomiting in dogs and cats (Guilford, 1996; Jergens, 1999). The generic term, IBD, encompasses lymphoplasmacytic enteritis, lymphocytic gastroenterocolitis, eosinophilic gastroenterocolitis, segmental granulomatous enterocolitis (regional enteritis), suppurative enterocolitis and histiocytic colitis. The lymphoplasmacytic form is probably the most common type of IBD (Leib, 1997; Craven et al, 2004; Hall, 2005, Hall and German, 2005).

The severity of IBD varies from relatively mild clinical signs to life-threatening protein-losing enteropathies. In particular, the Basenji and Ludenhund breeds may present with a very severe variant that has been termed immunoproliferative small intestinal disease (Breitschwerdt, 1992; Flesja and Yri, 1977; Williams, 1997).

Inflammatory infiltrates may involve the stomach, small bowel and colon. In cats, the stomach and small bowel are affected most often. In dogs, IBD is common in both the small and large intestines. In many cases, multiple segments of the bowel are involved and clinical signs may be mixed, reflecting the broad distribution of mucosal lesions.

PATIENT ASSESSMENT

History and Physical Examination

The most common clinical signs in dogs and cats with IBD are chronic vomiting, diarrhea and weight loss. The predominant GI sign varies with the portion or portions of bowel affected. Vomiting tends to be the predominant clinical sign when the stomach and proximal duodenum are affected. Loose, fluid or steatorrheic stools are most common when the small intestine is involved. Diarrhea marked by tenesmus, mucus and small scanty stools is noted with colonic lesions. Clinical signs may be intermittent or persistent. Clinical signs tend to increase in frequency and intensity as IBD progresses temporally. The presence of systemic signs is also variable. Some animals present with a history of depression, malaise and inappetence. Others are alert and active at the time they are examined.

The frequency and character of the vomitus and stools are important features. At times, vomiting will be temporally related to food intake and the vomitus will contain food particles. In other cases, animals may vomit only fluid or froth. Owners should be questioned closely about the appearance of the vomited material. Dark black or coffee grounds material may indicate gastric ulceration or erosions. The diarrhea may be small or large bowel in origin. The color of the stools should be assessed to determine the presence of GI bleeding.

Physical examination findings in dogs and cats with IBD are variable. Many patients have no abnormalities. Others present

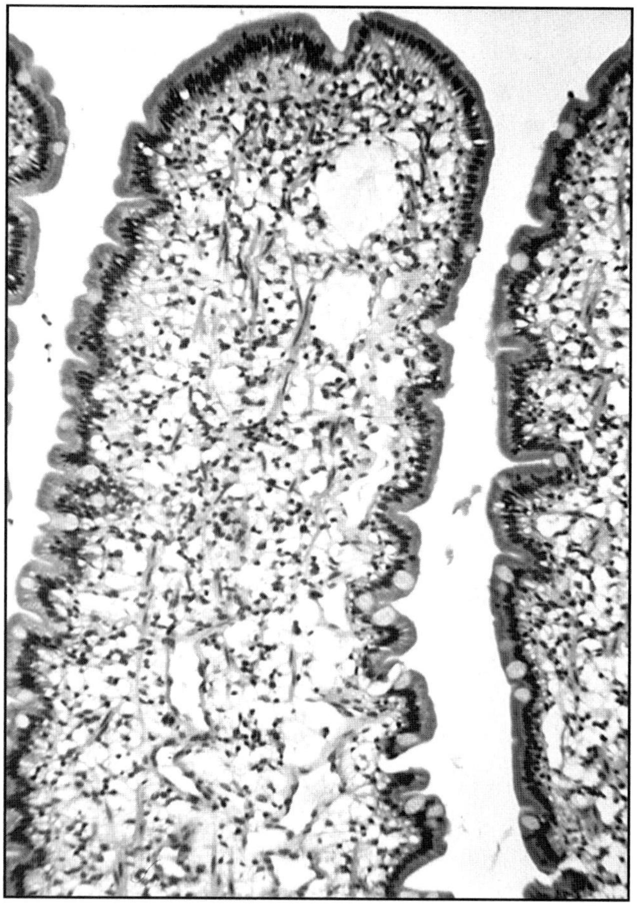

Figure 57-1. Photomicrograph of an intestinal villus showing typical monocellular infiltrates recognized in lymphoplasmacytic enteritis (original magnification 400X).

only with evidence of weight loss and poor body condition. Weight loss may be severe in longstanding cases. Mild peripheral lymphadenopathy may be detected in rare cases of IBD. This finding is most often recognized in cats with eosinophilic gastroenteritis and hypereosinophilic syndrome, which is characterized by multisystemic eosinophilic infiltrates (Moore, 1983).

Occasionally, thickened loops of bowel may be detected by abdominal palpation. This finding is more easily detected in cats. A segmental thickening of bowel may be suggestive of eosinophilic gastroenteritis in cats or granulomatous enteritis in dogs. This finding should also be distinguished from intestinal intussusceptions, foreign bodies, histoplasmosis and neoplastic lesions. Occasionally, pets with IBD present with abdominal pain, which suggests gastroduodenal ulceration (Jergens et al, 1992; Jergens, 1992).

Evidence of hemorrhage or hypoproteinemia may be noted in very severe cases. A vitamin K-dependent coagulopathy has been reported to occur in animals with marked steatorrhea but is rare. At times, IBD may cause protein-losing enteropathy. When severe, hypoalbuminemia and external manifestations of hypoproteinemia (i.e., pitting edema, ascites) may be present. Surprisingly, some animals with protein-losing enteropathy may present with only mild or no diarrhea.

Laboratory and Other Clinical Information

Laboratory findings in patients with IBD are often nonspecific. Hematologic findings are variable and may include blood loss anemia, anemia of chronic disease and/or eosinophilia. In cats with eosinophilic gastroenteritis and hypereosinophilic syndrome, eosinophil counts may exceed 100,000/µl (Moore, 1983). Patients with chronic diarrhea should be assessed with serum biochemistry profiles and urinalyses to determine the systemic effects of the GI disorder and to rule out concurrent disease. Electrolyte abnormalities, including hypokalemia, may be identified. Hypoproteinemia and hypoalbuminemia may be recognized in severe cases with protein-losing enteropathy. Prerenal azotemia may be present in dehydrated patients. In cats, IBD may be associated with pancreatitis and hepatitis, a syndrome that has been termed triaditis (Weiss et al, 1996; Steiner, 2007). In such cases, neutrophilia, increased hepatic enzyme activities, hyperbilirubinemia and increased serum pancreatic lipase immunoreactivity may be noted. IBD is often associated with a protein-losing nephropathy in soft-coated wheaten terriers. Varying degrees of azotemia and proteinuria are also common in these dogs (Vaden et al, 1998; Littman and Giger, 1990).

Fecal examinations are very important in the evaluation of patients with chronic diarrhea. Multiple fecal examinations using concentration techniques are necessary to rule out parasitism. Radiographic findings in IBD are usually nonspecific and nondiagnostic. Occasionally, thickened bowel loops with fluid and/or ingesta are observed on survey abdominal films. In addition, ultrasonographic examination may reveal enlarged mesenteric lymph nodes, focal thickening of the gut and poor definition of the intestinal wall (Baez et al, 1999).

Endoscopic abnormalities in IBD include mucosal granularity, hyperemia, friability and inability to visualize colonic submucosal blood vessels (Jergens et al, 1992). Multiple biopsy specimens should be collected from several bowel segments because histologic changes may be present despite a normal appearance (Jergens et al, 1992; Roth et al, 1990; Marks and LaFlamme, 1998).

The definitive diagnosis of IBD is based on histopathologic examination of biopsy specimens (**Figure 57-1**) collected by endoscopic or surgical techniques (Wilcock, 1992). Expected findings include lymphocytic and plasmacytic infiltrates within the lamina propria as well as architectural abnormalities such as crypt distortion and villous blunting. Histologic grading systems have been proposed to allow objective assessment of intestinal biopsy specimens and to reduce inter-observer variation (Jergens et al, 1992; Roth et al, 1990; Yamasaki et al, 1996; Willard et al, 2002). Despite the use of formal classification schemes, interpretation of histologic changes can be difficult when the lesions are mild or suggest lymphosarcoma (Roth et al, 1990; Wilcock, 1992; Willard et al, 2002; Evans et al, 2006). The latter finding is a serious concern in cases of lymphoplasmacytic enteritis and lymphocytic enteritis.

Quantification of mucosal inflammatory markers found in colonic lavage fluid (e.g., IgG, nitrite) has been suggested for evaluation of dogs with suspected IBD (Gunawardana et al,

1997). The use of a clinical scoring index for disease activity and measurement of C-reactive protein can provide value for assessing disease burden (Jergens et al, 2003; Garcia-Sancho et al, 2007).

Risk Factors

There does not appear to be an age or gender predisposition for IBD. The condition usually arises in adult dogs and cats, but has been diagnosed in puppies and kittens (i.e., less than six months of age). In people, there is a well-recognized familial tendency toward IBD (Fiocchi, 1998). A genetic influence has also been recognized in some dog breeds: 1) the German shepherd dog, Chinese Shar-Pei and soft-coated wheaten terrier for lymphoplasmacytic enteritis, 2) the German shepherd dog and Irish setter for eosinophilic gastroenteritis, 3) the boxer and French bulldog for ulcerative colitis and 4) the Basenji and Ludenhund for immunoproliferative enteropathy (Table 55-3).

The environment may also play an important role in IBD. Animals maintained in overcrowded, contaminated quarters are at risk for development of parasitic infections, viral and bacterial enteritis and small intestinal bacterial overgrowth, all of which are speculated to play a role in the pathogenesis of IBD. The role of parasites in the pathogenesis of IBD is poorly understood; however, occult parasitism has been suggested as a cause for these disorders. For example, in German shepherd dogs, visceral larval migrans has been linked to eosinophilic gastroenteritis (Hayden and van Kruiningen, 1973). In cats, feline infectious peritonitis has been associated with granulomatous and suppurative enterocolitis (Leib et al, 1986; Tebeau, 2007). In addition, small intestinal bacterial overgrowth has been reported in association with lymphoplasmacytic infiltrates and enteritis (Rutgers, 1996). Cats with IBD have been found to have higher fecal concentrations of *Desulfovibrio* spp. and lower numbers of *Bifidobacterium* spp. as compared to healthy cats (Inness et al, 2007).

Etiopathogenesis

Despite intensive study by veterinary and medical researchers, the pathophysiology of inflammatory bowel disorders is not fully understood (Fiocchi, 1998; Hanauer, 1996; German et al, 2003; Hall and German, 2005). The disorder is undoubtedly immune-mediated, yet the pathogenesis of the various forms of IBD is poorly defined. Increased populations of plasma cells producing IgA and IgG as well as T lymphocytes have been recognized in dogs with IBD as compared to normal dogs (Jergens, 1996 et al, 1999 et al; German et al, 2001). In addition, altered cytokine expression has been demonstrated in dogs with small and large intestinal IBD (German et al, 2001). Abnormal cytokine mRNA expression has been identified within intestinal biopsy specimens from cats with IBD (Nguyen Van et al, 2006).

The fundamental pathway for the development of IBD involves hypersensitivity. However, the underlying cause for hypersensitivity reactions is unknown. Two related theories have been proposed. The first speculates that IBD patients develop a defect in the intestinal mucosal barrier. This loss of mucosal integrity results in increased gut permeability and hypersensitivity responses to antigens that are normally tolerated (**Figure 57-2**) (Guilford, 1996). Alternatively, IBD may result from aberrant immunologic responses to luminal antigens. It has been hypothesized that defects in gut-associated lymphatic tissue (GALT) suppressor function may predispose patients to development of hypersensitivity to normally tolerated luminal antigens (**Figures 57-3** and 31-2 through 31-4) (Guilford, 1996). Parasites, pathogenic organisms, normal gut flora and dietary antigens may all serve as the trigger for these immunologic reactions. Both potential pathways culminate in release of inflammatory mediators. These substances may then further damage the intestinal mucosal surface and set up a vicious cycle of inflammation and loss of barrier function.

It is likely that the pathogenetic pathway is influenced by environmental (i.e., exposure to dietary antigens or GI parasites) and genetic factors that modulate disease expression (German et al, 2003). The predisposition for IBD in certain breeds (e.g., Basenjis, soft-coated wheaten terriers) suggests a likely role for genetic influences.

Mucosal inflammatory infiltrates and soluble factors are responsible for the clinical manifestations of IBD. Mucosal

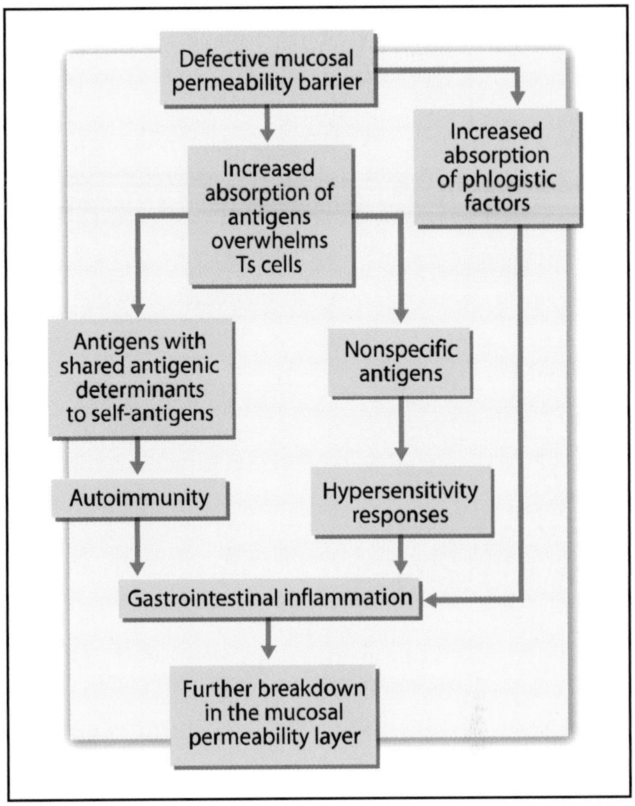

Figure 57-2. A proposed pathway for a defect in the mucosal permeability barrier as a cause of inflammatory bowel disease. (Adapted from Guilford WG. Idiopathic inflammatory bowel diseases. In: Guilford WG, Center SA, Strombeck DR, et al, eds. Strombeck's Small Animal Gastroenterology, 3rd ed. Philadelphia, PA: WB Saunders Co, 1996; 457.)

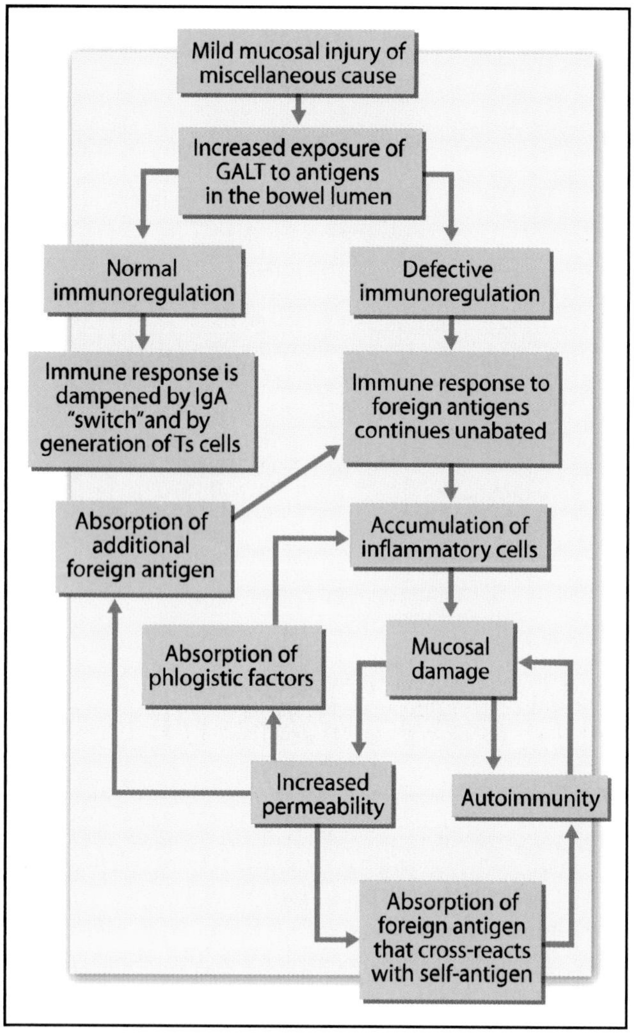

Figure 57-3. A proposed pathway for a defect in the suppressor function of the gut-associated lymphoid tissue (GALT) as a cause of inflammatory bowel disease. (Adapted from Guilford WG. Idiopathic inflammatory bowel diseases. In: Guilford WG, Center SA, Strombeck DR, et al, eds. Strombeck's Small Animal Gastroenterology, 3rd ed. Philadelphia, PA: WB Saunders Co, 1996; 453.)

inflammation disrupts normal absorptive processes resulting in malabsorption and osmotic diarrhea. Altered gut permeability can result in leakage of fluid, protein and blood into the gut lumen. Malabsorbed fats, carbohydrates and bile acids result in secretory diarrhea. Inflammatory mediators may also directly trigger intestinal secretion and mucus production by goblet cells. Mucosal inflammatory infiltrates may alter intestinal and colonic motility patterns, a mechanism attributed to the influence of prostaglandins and leukotrienes on smooth muscle. Inflammation of the proximal bowel (stomach and small bowel) may stimulate visceral afferent receptors that trigger vomiting. Delayed gastric emptying associated with gastroparesis or ileus may exacerbate vomiting.

Key Nutritional Factors

Key nutritional factors for patients with IBD are listed in **Table 57-1** and discussed in more detail below.

Water

Dehydration is a frequent problem in patients with IBD. Reduced water consumption is often aggravated by fluid losses from vomiting and/or diarrhea. Whenever possible, fluid balance should be maintained via oral consumption of fluids. However, dehydrated patients and those with persistent vomiting often need parenteral fluid administration.

Electrolytes

Serum electrolyte concentrations should be assessed regularly to allow early detection of abnormalities as vomiting and diarrhea persist. Hypokalemia is particularly common in patients with IBD. Thus, foods containing 0.8 to 1.1% dry matter (DM) potassium are preferred for dogs and cats with IBD. Initially, potassium levels should be restored with intravenous potassium supplementation. In addition, affected patients often lose large amounts of sodium through fluid feces; however, sodium deficits may be masked by dehydration.

Energy Density and Fat

Energy dense foods are preferred for managing patients with chronic enteropathies. Such foods allow the provision of smaller volumes of food, which minimizes GI distention and secretions. Unfortunately, energy dense foods are also high in fats. High-fat foods may contribute to osmotic diarrhea and GI protein losses, which complicate IBD. Thus, it is often advantageous to initially provide a food with moderate energy density (4.0 to 4.5 kcal/g [16.7 to 18.8 kJ/g] DM) for dogs and cats and fat levels of 12 to 15% for dogs and 15 to 25% for cats DM). Foods with higher fat levels can be offered if the patient tolerates them.

Fiber-enhanced foods typically have lower energy density levels than highly digestible foods because fiber-enhanced foods are usually lower in fat. The DM energy density of fiber-enhanced foods for IBD should be at least 3.2 kcal/g (13.4 kJ/g) for dog foods and at least 3.4 kcal/g (14.2 kJ/g) for cat foods. Fat content for fiber-enhanced foods for dogs and cats with IBD should be 8 to 12% and 9 to 18% DM, respectively.

There appears to be a difference in how dogs and cats are able to tolerate dietary fat in the face of GI disease. Normal cats can tolerate much higher concentrations of dietary fat than dogs (Lewis et al, 1979). Anecdotal information suggests that foods with increased fat content may actually benefit cats with small bowel disease (Guilford, 1996a). Recently, low-fat and high-fat foods were fed to cats with naturally occurring chronic diarrhea in a randomized six-week trial. Fecal scores in more than 65% of cats consuming both high- and low-fat foods improved over the course of the feeding period (Laflamme et al, 2007). The underlying cause of diarrhea in the cats was not investigated. More controlled evaluations are needed to confirm these observations.

Protein

Protein malnutrition may occur in dogs and cats with IBD due to fecal losses. High biologic value, highly digestible (≥87%) protein sources should be used. Protein should be provided at levels sufficient for the appropriate lifestage for patients not experienc-

Table 57-1. Key nutritional factors for dogs and cats with inflammatory bowel disease.*

Factors	Recommended levels
Potassium	0.8 to 1.1%
Energy density	4.0 to 4.5 kcal/g (16.7 to 18.8 kJ/g) for highly digestible foods for dogs and cats ≥3.2 kcal/g (≥13.4 kJ/g) for fiber-enhanced foods for dogs and ≥3.4 kcal/g (≥14.2 kJ/g) for cats
Fat	12 to 15% for dogs and 15 to 25% for cats for highly digestible foods For fiber-enhanced foods: 8 to 12% for dogs 9 to 18% for cats
Protein	≥25% for dogs ≥ 35% for cats If using a limited protein (elimination food) approach, restrict protein to one or two sources and use protein sources to which the patient has not been exposed previously or feed a protein hydrolysate (Chapter 31); also use lower protein levels (16 to 26% for dogs and 30 to 45% for cats)
Crude fiber	≤5% for highly digestible foods (mixed fiber) for dogs and cats 7 to 15% for increased-fiber foods (insoluble fibers are best) for dogs and cats
Digestibility	≥87% for protein and ≥90% for fat and digestible carbohydrate for highly digestible foods ≥80% for protein and fat and ≥90% for carbohydrate for fiber-enhanced foods

*Nutrients expressed on a dry matter basis.

ing excessive GI protein loss (at least 25% for adult dogs and 35% for adult cats [DM]). Suggested protein levels for patients being managed with "hypoallergenic foods" can be lower.

Because dietary antigens are suspected to play a role in the pathogenesis of IBD, "hypoallergenic" novel protein elimination foods or foods containing a protein hydrolysate are often recommended (Nelson et al, 1984; Nelson and Stookey, 1988; Davenport et al, 1987; Guilford, 1996a; Guilford et al, 2001). In some cases, elimination foods may be used successfully without pharmacologic intervention (Hall and German, 2005; Allenspach et al, 2006). Ideal elimination foods should: 1) avoid protein excess (16 to 26% for dogs and 30 to 45% for cats), 2) have high protein digestibility (≥87%) and 3) contain a limited number of novel protein sources to which the patient has never been exposed or contain a protein hydrolysate. Chapter 31 discusses elimination foods in detail. The suspected pathogenesis of IBD involves an increase in gut permeability; therefore, the use of "sacrificial" dietary antigens in the treatment of IBD has been also suggested, but proof of the concept using controlled dietary trials is lacking (Guilford, 1996) (**Box 57-1**).

The evidence regarding the efficacy of elimination foods in people with IBD is conflicting (Husain and Korzenik, 1998). Although specific foods provoking symptoms may be identified in as many as 80% of human patients with Crohn's disease, double-blinded rechallenges suggest that food hypersensitivity may be identified consistently in fewer than 10% (Husain and Korzenik, 1998). Similarly, positive reactions to food antigens applied topically to the gastric mucosa (i.e., gastroscopic food sensitivity test) have been recognized in canine patients with IBD (Vaden, 2000; Vaden et al, 1998a; Guilford et al, 1994; Elwood et al, 1994). Gastroscopic food sensitivity test findings, however, often do not correlate with the results of provocative food challenges or clinical responses (Guilford et al, 1994).[a] A protein hydrolysate-based elimination food has been used successfully in refractory canine IBD cases (Marks and LaFlamme, 1998; Hannah et al, 2000).

Box 57-1. Sacrificial Proteins in Inflammatory Bowel Disease.

Oral tolerance is difficult to maintain in the inflammatory milieu; therefore, animals with inflammatory bowel disease (IBD) are at risk for becoming rapidly sensitive to undigested food proteins entering the lamina propria. This theoretical concern has led to the concept of feeding a "sacrificial protein" source. The first novel protein fed to patients in the early phase of therapy is referred to as a sacrificial protein because it is being offered when the bowel is inflamed and the mucosal barrier porous. The dietary protein source is then changed after the first six weeks of therapy. For animals receiving concurrent prednisone therapy, this diet change is made just before the prednisone dose is decreased from the immunosuppressive to the antiinflammatory range, by which time it is hoped that the mucosal inflammation has been controlled and the mucosal barrier has markedly recovered. As a result, the second dietary protein source is less likely to result in acquired food hypersensitivity and delayed recovery from IBD. The potential benefit of this recommendation is currently under investigation. This type of nutritional management is likely to be of most value in those patients in which IBD has resulted from a transient injury to the gut-associated lymphoid tissue or the mucosal barrier (e.g., from a viral infection) rather than those in which IBD is due to an inherent (i.e., permanent) defect in these structures.

Grant Guilford, BSVSC, PhD, Dipl. ACVIM (Internal Medicine)
Massey University
New Zealand

The Bibliography for **Box 57-1** can be found at www.markmorris.org.

Fiber

It has been recommended that people with IBD eat small quantities of soluble or mixed fiber sources (Fiocchi, 1998). In fact, short-chain fatty acid and butyrate enemas induce clinical improvement in people with ulcerative colitis (Harig et al, 1989; Breuer et al, 1991). A number of substrates including beet pulp, soy fiber, inulin and fructooligosaccharides have been demonstrated by in vitro fermentation to produce volatile fatty acids that may be beneficial in IBD that involves the distal small intestine and colon (Sunvold et al, 1995, 1995a, 1995b; Jamikorn et al, 1999). In addition, these fermentable fibers may serve as prebiotics and foster the growth of beneficial bacterial organisms such as *Bifidobacterium* and *Lactobacillus* at the expense of more pathogenic microbes such as *Desulfovibrio* and *Clostridium* spp. (Chapter 5). These fibers are usually incorporated at rates of 1 to 5% DM in commercial products.

A second approach is to increase dietary fiber content to normalize intestinal motility, water balance and microflora. Fiber has several physiologic characteristics that are beneficial in managing small bowel diarrhea. Moderate levels (7 to 15% DM) of insoluble fiber (e.g., cellulose) add nondigestible bulk, which buffers toxins, holds excess water and, perhaps more important, provides intraluminal stimuli to reestablish the coordinated actions of hormones, neurons, smooth muscle, enzyme delivery, digestion and absorption. Fiber can help normalize transit time through the small bowel, which means slowing a hypermotile state, but also improving a hypomotile state to reestablish normal peristaltic action. However, this level of fiber reduces the energy density and digestibility of a food.

Digestibility

Feeding highly digestible (fat and digestible [soluble] carbohydrate at least 90% and protein at least 87%) foods provides several advantages in the management of dogs and cats with IBD. Nutrients from low-residue foods are more completely absorbed in the proximal gut. Furthermore, these highly digestible foods are associated with: 1) reduced osmotic diarrhea due to fat and carbohydrate malabsorption, 2) reduced production of intestinal gas due to carbohydrate malabsorption and 3) decreased antigen loads because smaller amounts of protein are absorbed intact. Ideal foods for IBD patients are free of lactose to avoid the complication of lactose intolerance. If fiber-enhanced foods are used, the digestibility will be reduced. Digestibility of protein, fat and carbohydrate of fiber-enhanced foods should be at least 80, 80 and 90%, respectively.

The use of monomeric liquid foods and total parenteral nutrition to provide a period of "bowel rest" for people and animals with IBD is controversial (Griffiths et al, 1995; Ling and Griffiths, 2000). Bowel rest has been recommended as a means of reducing or eliminating antigenic stimuli while minimizing GI secretions. The greatest benefit appears to be for human patients with Crohn's disease (Lewis and Fisher, 1994; Jeejeebhoy, 1995). Placebo controlled trials of monomeric foods have not been performed in people but response rates in clinical practice have been convincing (Ling and Griffiths, 2000). Monomeric feedings provide energy and nitrogen in a readily available, nonantigenic form. Monomeric liquid foods are also supplemented with glutamine. In pediatric human patients, a recent meta-analysis demonstrated that enteral nutritional support was as efficacious as corticosteroid therapy in acute Crohn's disease (Henschkel et al, 2000). Parenteral nutrition does not appear to provide any advantage over monomeric foods and is not recommended except in those patients unable to tolerate enteral feeding (Hanauer, 1996). Complete bowel rest may theoretically worsen GI mucosal lesions by depriving mucosal epithelial cells of nutrients such as glutamine and short-chain fatty acids (Husain and Korzenik, 1998). Veterinary experience with parenteral feeding and monomeric and hydrolysate-based foods in the management of IBD is limited (Marks and LaFlamme, 1998; Guilford, 1996a; Hannah et al, 2000). Most often, these therapies have been used in refractory cases in which other therapeutic modalities have failed.

Other Nutritional Factors

Vitamins

Adequate intake of water-soluble and fat-soluble vitamins is critical for patients with IBD. In many cases, the limited stores of water-soluble vitamins have been depleted by diarrheic losses and the large fluid flux through the animal. Thiamin deficiency, in particular, occurs commonly and can profoundly affect appetite. Cobalamin (vitamin B_{12}) deficiency has been recognized in dogs and cats with chronic enteropathies and can result in severe metabolic abnormalities including increased serum methylmalonic acid and disturbances in serum amino acid levels (Ruaux et al, 2001). Dogs and cats appear to more susceptible to cobalamin depletion than people because they have a more rapid cobalamin turnover as a consequence of biliary excretion of cobalamin (Simpson et al, 2001; Simpson, 2003). In addition, dogs and cats lack cobalamin binding protein TC1, which facilitates long-term cobalamin storage in people (Simpson, 2003). Hypocobalaminemia typically occurs when specific cobalamin receptors in the ileum are damaged as a consequence of inflammatory disease (Suchodolski and Steiner, 2003). Deficiency is accelerated by reduced cobalamin consumption and ongoing GI losses. A recent case control study demonstrated that parenteral cobalamin supplementation in cats with undetectable serum cobalamin values (<100 ng/l) normalized serum cobalamin and methylmalonic acid values and improved clinical indices such as body weight, vomiting and diarrhea (Ruaux et al, 2005). For that reason, serum cobalamin should be assessed in patients with chronic small intestinal disease and those with hypocobalaminemia (<300 ng/l) should receive weekly subcutaneous cobalamin therapy (250 µg in cats and 500 µg in dogs) for four to six weeks or until serum levels return to the normal range (Ruaux et al, 2005). Once or twice monthly therapy may be required for longer term maintenance. Disease of the proximal small intestine can inhibit absorption of dietary folate, which is present in foods in the polyglutamate form. Folate absorption requires the jejunal brush border enzyme, folate deconjugase, and specific folate monoglutamate carriers

(Suchodolski and Steiner, 2003). Chronic inflammatory disease of the small bowel can result in low serum folate values due to jejunal mucosal damage, reduced folate absorption and depletion of folate stores.

Loss of fat-soluble vitamins can be significant in patients with steatorrhea (e.g., vitamin K-deficient coagulopathies may occur in patients with IBD). Initially, parenteral administration of fat-soluble vitamins may be necessary. Administering 1 ml of a vitamin A, D and E solution,[b] divided into two intramuscular sites, is simple and cost effective. This should supply fat-soluble vitamins for approximately three months. Vitamin K_1 at a dosage of 0.5 to 1 mg/kg subcutaneously is recommended if a vitamin K-responsive coagulopathy is suspected. Dietary intake of vitamins is often sufficient when the disease responds to treatment and fat absorption is reestablished.

Zinc

Zinc deficiency is well recognized in people as a complication of IBD (Hendricks and Walker, 1988). The small intestine is the primary site of zinc homeostasis and there are several potential mechanisms for zinc deficiency in IBD (**Table 57-2**). In Crohn's disease, oral zinc supplementation improves clinical signs and normalizes intestinal permeability (Sturniolo et al, 2001). Zinc may provide benefits by enhancing brush border enzyme activity, water and electrolyte absorption and regeneration of the gut epithelial surface. Supplemental dietary zinc intake should be considered if dogs and cats with IBD have poor coat quality or dermatitis (Chapters 6 and 32).

Table 57-2. Potential causes of zinc deficiency in patients with inflammatory bowel disease.*

Decreased absorption
Intestinal inflammation
Supplemental iron and/or copper
Surgical resection of distal duodenum
Inadequate dietary intake
Anorexia
High fiber or phytate intake
Parenteral nutrition
Increased losses
Chronic blood loss
Increased metabolism
Increased requirements
Growth
Lactation
Pregnancy
Wound healing

*Adapted from Hendricks KM, Walker A. Zinc deficiency in inflammatory bowel disease. Nutrition Reviews 1988; 46: 401-408.

Magnesium

Hypomagnesemia has been reported to occur in 30% of dogs and cats hospitalized for GI disorders (Martin, 1994; Toll et al, 2002). Anorexia and malabsorption complicated by the use of magnesium-free fluids are likely causes of low serum magnesium. Magnesium repletion can be accomplished via the use of intravenous fluids.

Omega-3 Fatty Acids

Omega-3 (n-3) fatty acids derived from fish oil or other sources have been hypothesized to have a beneficial effect in controlling mucosal inflammation in IBD. The rationale for the use of omega-3 fatty acids in inflammatory GI disorders first arose from the epidemiologic observation that Japanese and Eskimo populations consuming diets rich in fish sources of these fatty acids have a low prevalence of IBD (Ling and Griffiths, 2000). Some clinical evidence suggests that dietary supplementation with these fatty acids can modulate the generation and biologic activity of inflammatory mediators. More recently, it has been suggested that omega-3 fatty acids may act as competitive agonists of bacterial Toll-like receptor 4 (lipopolysaccharide receptor complex). Because aberrant immune responses to enteric flora have been speculated to play a role in the pathogenesis of IBD, this inhibitory effect may provide another rationale for the use of omega-3 fatty acids in IBD (Lee et al, 2003).

Foods supplemented with fish oil have been used in a limited number of human trials with mixed results (Belluzi et al, 1996, 2000; Mate et al, 1991; Lorenz-Meyer et al, 1996; Lorenz et al, 1989; Stenson et al, 1992). To date, there are no published therapeutic trials investigating the efficacy of omega-3 fatty acid supplementation in dogs or cats with IBD. Although use of omega-3 fatty acids warrants further consideration in veterinary gastroenterology, there is no well-established effective dose for dogs and cats. A reasonable starting dose estimated from human and animal trials is approximately 175 mg (range 50 to 300 mg) omega-3 fatty acids/kg body weight/day.

FEEDING PLAN

The justification for nutritional management of IBD is twofold. First, dietary factors may contribute to the initiation or perpetuation of the disease. Second, malnutrition is a common sequela to IBD due to anorexia, malabsorption and increased nutrient losses. Thus, dietary intervention should be aimed at controlling clinical signs while providing adequate nutrients to meet requirements and compensate for ongoing losses through the GI tract. Some dogs and cats with IBD may only require dietary manipulation (Hall and German, 2005; Allenspach et al, 2006). In other cases, dietary therapy is better used in concert with pharmacologic agents. Antibiotics (e.g., tylosin, tetracycline, enrofloxacin, metronidazole), anthelmintics (e.g., fenbendazole) and immunosuppressive agents (e.g., corticosteroids, budesonide, cyclosporine, azathioprine, cyclophosphamide) are often used for managing IBD.

Assess and Select the Food

Selection should focus on foods that reduce intestinal irritation/inflammation and normalize intestinal motility. Three types of foods may be useful in managing diarrhea associated with IBD: 1) highly digestible, low-residue foods formulated

Table 57-3. Key nutritional factors in selected highly digestible veterinary therapeutic foods marketed for dogs with inflammatory bowel disease compared to recommended levels.* (See Table 31-5 if foods with novel protein sources or protein hydrolysates are desired.)

Dry foods	K (%)	Energy density (kcal/g)	Fat (%)	Protein (%)	Fiber (%)	Protein digestibility (%)	Fat digestibility (%)	Carbohydrate digestibility (%)
Recommended levels	**0.8-1.1**	**4.0-4.5**	**12-15**	**≥25**	**≤5**	**≥87**	**≥90**	**≥90**
Hill's Prescription Diet i/d Canine	0.92	4.2	14.1	26.2	2.7	92	93	94
Iams Veterinary Formula Intestinal Low-Residue	0.90	3.8	10.7	24.6	2.1	na	na	na
Medi-Cal Gastro Formula	0.8	na	13.9	22.9	1.9	na	na	na
Medi-Cal Vegetarian Formula	0.8	na	10.5	20.9	3.2	na	na	na
Purina Veterinary Diets EN GastroENteric Formula	0.66	4.2	12.6	27.0	1.5	84.5	91.4	94.4
Royal Canin Veterinary Diet Digestive Low Fat LF 20	0.88	3.7	6.6	24.2	2.3	na	na	na
Royal Canin Veterinary Diets Intestinal HE 28	0.88	4.5	22.0	33.0	1.6	na	na	na

Moist foods	K (%)	Energy density (kcal/g)	Fat (%)	Protein (%)	Fiber (%)	Protein digestibility (%)	Fat digestibility (%)	Carbohydrate digestibility (%)
Recommended levels	**0.8-1.1**	**4.0-4.5**	**12-15**	**≥25**	**≤5**	**≥87**	**≥90**	**≥90**
Hill's Prescription Diet i/d Canine	0.95	4.4	14.9	25.0	1.0	88	94	93
Iams Veterinary Formula Intestinal Low-Residue	0.84	4.6	13.2	35.9	3.9	na	na	na
Medi-Cal Gastro Formula	0.6	na	11.7	22.1	1.0	na	na	na
Medi-Cal Vegetarian Formula	0.7	na	11.5	26.4	1.9	na	na	na
Purina Veterinary Diets EN GastroENteric Formula	0.61	4.0	13.8	30.5	0.9	85.1	95.6	92.2
Royal Canin Veterinary Diet Digestive Low Fat LF	0.74	4.0	6.9	31.9	3.0	na	na	na
Royal Canin Veterinary Diet Intestinal HE	0.80	4.3	11.8	23.1	1.4	na	na	na

Key: K = potassium, Fiber = crude fiber, na = information not available from manufacturer.
*Manufacturers' published values. Nutrients expressed on a dry matter basis. To convert kcal to kJ, multiply kcal by 4.184.

for GI disease, 2) fiber-enhanced foods and 3) elimination foods. Unfortunately, no physical examination finding, laboratory test result or historical fact will dictate which method will be successful in any one patient. Dietary trials are often needed to find which food type works best.

The most commonly used strategy is to feed a highly digestible, low-residue GI food. There are several commercial veterinary therapeutic foods marketed for treatment of GI diseases. **Tables 57-3** and **57-5** list selected highly digestible foods for dogs and cats, respectively, and compare them to the recommended levels of key nutritional factors for IBD. When possible, choose the food that most closely matches the recommendations for key nutritional factors. Recipes for highly digestible homemade foods are also available (Table 10-6). Besides being the most common initial approach for dietary management of IBD, this strategy has also been effective in cats with chronic nonspecific diarrhea (Laflamme and Long, 2004).

A second approach is to increase dietary fiber content to normalize intestinal motility, water balance and microflora. **Tables 57-4** and **57-6** list selected fiber-enhanced commercial veterinary therapeutic foods for dogs and cats with IBD, respectively, and compare them to the recommended key nutritional factors for this approach. These foods typically have a lower energy density and IBD patients may have difficulty maintaining a normal body weight and body condition. Also, foods with 10 to 15% DM fiber usually have lower digestibility. The third dietary option in IBD cases is the use of an elimination food with a limited number of highly digestible, novel protein sources or one containing a protein hydrolysate. Commercial veterinary therapeutic foods (Tables 31-5 and 31-6) or homemade foods that contain novel protein sources often combine lamb, rabbit, venison, duck, fish or game meats with a highly digestible or novel carbohydrate source. All other possible dietary sources of protein and carbohydrate should be eliminated including treats, snacks, table foods, vitamin-mineral supplements and chewable/flavored medications. Clinical signs should abate within the first three weeks of strict dietary management (e.g., feeding only the novel ingredient or protein hydrolysate food). After signs abate, owners may add individual specific ingredients previously fed in an effort to identify the allergen. Clinical GI signs may recur within 12 hours after the offending ingredient is fed. In many cases, owners elect to continue feeding the elimination food if clinical signs abate.

Assess and Determine the Feeding Method

If the patient has a normal body condition score (BCS [2.5/5 to 3.5/5]), the amount of food previously fed (energy basis) was

Table 57-4. Key nutritional factors in selected fiber-enhanced veterinary therapeutic foods marketed for dogs with inflammatory bowel disease compared to recommended levels.* (See Table 31-5 if foods with novel protein sources or protein hydrolysates are desired.)

Dry foods	K (%)	Energy density (kcal/g)	Fat (%)	Protein (%)	Fiber (%)	Protein digestibility (%)	Fat digestibility (%)	Carbohydrate digestibility (%)
Recommended levels	**0.8-1.1**	**≥3.2**	**8-12**	**≥25**	**7-15**	**≥80**	**≥80**	**≥90**
Hill's Prescription Diet w/d Canine	0.70	3.3	8.8	18.9	16.4	84	92	95
Medi-Cal Fibre Formula	1.0	na	10.6	26.2	14.3	na	na	na
Purina Veterinary Diets DCO Dual Fiber Control	0.7	3.7	12.4	25.3	7.6	79.9	80.4	90.6
Purina Veterinary Diets OM Overweight Management	0.83	2.9	7.2	31.1	10.3	81.9	78.9	72.3
Royal Canin Veterinary Diet Calorie Control CC 26 High Fiber	0.9	3.1	10.4	30.9	17.6	na	na	na
Moist foods	**K (%)**	**Energy density (kcal/g)**	**Fat (%)**	**Protein (%)**	**Fiber (%)**	**Protein digestibility (%)**	**Fat digestibility (%)**	**Carbohydrate digestibility (%)**
Recommended levels	**0.8-1.1**	**≥3.2**	**8-12**	**≥25**	**7-15**	**≥80**	**≥80**	**≥90**
Hill's Prescription Diet w/d Canine	0.64	3.5	12.7	17.9	12.4	88	90	92
Medi-Cal Fibre Formula	0.7	na	9.1	24.8	15.0	na	na	na
Purina Veterinary Diets OM Overweight Management	1.06	2.5	8.4	44.1	19.2	80.9	89.8	62.9
Royal Canin Veterinary Diet Calorie Control CC High Fiber	0.82	3.6	12.5	25.9	8.8	na	na	na

Key: K = potassium, Fiber = crude fiber, na = information not available from manufacturer.
*Manufacturers' published values. Nutrients expressed on a dry matter basis. To convert kcal to kJ, multiply kcal by 4.184.

Table 57-5. Key nutritional factors in selected highly digestible veterinary therapeutic foods marketed for cats with inflammatory bowel disease compared to recommended levels.* (See Table 31-6 if foods with novel protein sources or protein hydrolysates are desired.)

Dry foods	K (%)	Energy density (kcal/g)	Fat (%)	Protein (%)	Fiber (%)	Protein digestibility (%)	Fat digestibility (%)	Carbohydrate digestibility (%)
Recommended levels	**0.8-1.1**	**4.0-4.5**	**15-25**	**≥35**	**≤5**	**≥87**	**≥90**	**≥90**
Hill's Prescription Diet i/d Feline	1.07	4.3	20.2	40.3	2.8	88	92	90
Iams Veterinary Formula Intestinal Low-Residue	0.66	3.9	13.7	35.8	1.8	na	na	na
Medi-Cal Hypoallergenic/Gastro	0.8	na	11.5	29.8	3.1	na	na	na
Purina Veterinary Diets EN GastroENteric Formula	0.99	4.4	18.4	56.2	1.3	94.0	93.1	79.7
Royal Canin Veterinary Diet Intestinal HE 30	0.97	4.4	23.7	34.4	5.8	na	na	na
Moist foods	**K (%)**	**Energy density (kcal/g)**	**Fat (%)**	**Protein (%)**	**Fiber (%)**	**Protein digestibility (%)**	**Fat digestibility (%)**	**Carbohydrate digestibility (%)**
Recommended levels	**0.8-1.1**	**4.0-4.5**	**15-25**	**≥35**	**≤5**	**≥87**	**≥90**	**≥90**
Hill's Prescription Diet i/d Feline	1.06	4.2	24.1	37.6	2.4	91	89	91
Iams Veterinary Formula Intestinal Low-Residue	0.93	4.0	11.7	38.4	3.7	na	na	na
Medi-Cal Hypoallergenic/Gastro	1.1	na	35.9	35.5	1.2	na	na	na
Medi-Cal Sensitivity CR	1.1	na	35.1	34.5	2.5	na	na	na

Key: K = potassium, Fiber = crude fiber, na = information not available from manufacturer.
*Manufacturers' published values. Nutrients expressed on a dry matter basis. To convert kcal to kJ, multiply kcal by 4.184.

probably appropriate. If the patient has a low BCS (1/5 or 2/5), the amount of food previously fed may have been inappropriate or significant malassimilation may be occurring due to IBD.

Initially, IBD patients should be fed multiple small meals per day as indicated by their acceptance and tolerance for the food. Meal size can be increased and meal frequency can be reduced as tolerated by the patient after the clinical signs have been successfully managed for several weeks.

REASSESSMENT

Regaining or maintaining optimal body weight and condition, normal levels of activity and alertness and absence of clinical signs are measures of successful dietary and medical management. Serial measurement of the clinical IBD activity index (CIBDAI) offers a more rigorous method of assessing response

Table 57-6. Key nutritional factors in selected fiber-enhanced veterinary therapeutic foods marketed for cats with inflammatory bowel disease compared to recommended levels.* (See Table 31-6 if foods with novel protein sources or protein hydrolysates are desired.)

Dry foods	K (%)	Energy density (kcal/g)	Fat (%)	Protein (%)	Fiber (%)	Protein digestibility (%)	Fat digestibility (%)	Carbohydrate digestibility (%)
Recommended levels	**0.8-1.1**	**≥3.4**	**9-18**	**≥35**	**7-15**	**≥80**	**≥80**	**≥90**
Hill's Prescription Diet w/d Feline	0.84	3.5	9.8	39.0	7.6	90	87	86
Hill's Prescription Diet w/d with Chicken Feline	0.80	3.5	9.9	39.9	7.6	91	85	94
Medi-Cal Fibre Formula	0.9	na	12.2	34.2	14.9	na	na	na
Purina Veterinary Diets OM Overweight Management	0.89	3.6	8.5	56.2	5.6	91.1	87.7	66.8
Royal Canin Veterinary Diet Calorie Control CC 29 High Fiber	0.88	3.3	10.2	33.5	14.0	na	na	na
Moist foods	**K (%)**	**Energy density (kcal/g)**	**Fat (%)**	**Protein (%)**	**Fiber (%)**	**Protein digestibility (%)**	**Fat digestibility (%)**	**Carbohydrate digestibility (%)**
Recommended levels	**0.8-1.1**	**≥3.4**	**9-18**	**≥35**	**7-15**	**≥80**	**≥80**	**≥90**
Hill's Prescription Diet w/d with Chicken Feline	0.89	3.5	16.6	39.6	10.6	92	na	na
Medi-Cal Fibre Formula	0.8	na	17.1	40.0	16.7	na	na	na
Purina Veterinary Diets OM Overweight Management	0.91	3.9	14.6	44.6	10.2	87.3	88.6	84.0
Royal Canin Veterinary Diet Calorie Control CC High Fiber	0.77	4.1	21.3	33.5	7.7	na	na	na

Key: K = potassium, Fiber = crude fiber, na = information not available from manufacturer.
*Manufacturers' published values. Nutrients expressed on a dry matter basis. To convert kcal to kJ, multiply kcal by 4.184.

to treatment (Jergens et al, 2003; Garcia-Sancho et al, 2007). Endoscopically obvious gastric and intestinal lesions often respond to therapy (Garcia-Sancho et al, 2007), but underlying histopathologic changes typically remain unchanged (Schreiner et al, 2005; Allenspach et al, 2006; Garcia-Sancho et al, 2007). Laboratory tests to assess serum cobalamin and folate levels are recommended for patients receiving parenteral cobalamin injections for hypocobalaminemia and/or have a history of low serum folate levels to assess the adequacy of and necessity for continued supplementation. The feeding method and amount fed can be adjusted as needed to maintain body weight and condition.

The prognosis for IBD varies with the specific entity present, severity of the condition at the time of presentation and owner compliance. The hypereosinophilic form of eosinophilic gastroenteritis in cats and segmental granulomatous enterocolitis (regional enteritis), immunoproliferative enteropathy and histiocytic colitis in dogs may be refractory to treatment (Breitschwerdt, 1992; Moore, 1983; van Kruiningen, 1967). Likewise, response to therapy may be poor when animals present late in the course of disease and with evidence of protein-losing enteropathy.

In most cases, judicious use of dietary and medical regimens controls the disease. Often, medical measures can be withdrawn after three to six months; thereafter, animals maintain remission with appropriate foods. In some cases, however, pharmacologic treatment may be required for the life of the patient.

The most common causes for failure to respond include noncompliance on the part of the owner and failure of the clinician to tailor a program incorporating dietary and pharmacologic measures for each patient (Guilford, 1996). Intercurrent illnesses such as triaditis in cats, small intestinal bacterial overgrowth or exocrine pancreatic insufficiency may also result in a poor response to treatment. Occasionally, treatment failures occur because of misdiagnosis of alimentary lymphosarcoma or progression of IBD to lymphosarcoma. This progression has been previously reported to occur in dogs (Breitschwerdt, 1982) and cats (Davenport, 1987, 1991).

ENDNOTES

a. Davenport DJ. Unpublished data. 1991.
b. Vital E-A+D containing 100 IU of D and 300 IU of alpha-tocopherol per ml. Schering-Plough Animal Health Corp., Kenilworth, NJ, USA.

REFERENCES

The references for **Chapter 57** can be found at www.markmorris.org

CASE 57-1

Chronic Diarrhea in a Cat

Deborah J. Davenport, DVM, MS, Dipl. ACVIM (Internal Medicine)
Hill's Pet Nutrition Center
Topeka, Kansas, USA

Patient Assessment

A 10-year-old castrated male domestic shorthair cat was examined for a three-month history of intermittent diarrhea. The owner described the feces as being abnormal, three to five times per week; feces were usually fluid to semi-formed and occasionally black. No tenesmus or blood or mucus in the feces had been noted. The cat had not vomited although the owner felt that its appetite had decreased in the last few days. The cat lived in an apartment and no other pets were in the household.

Physical examination was normal except for mild accumulation of dental calculus and a somewhat "doughy" abdomen. Body weight was 4.4 kg with normal body condition (body condition score [BCS] 3/5). The medical record indicated that a body weight of 4.6 kg was recorded six months previously.

Diagnostic evaluation included a complete blood count (mild eosinophilia, 1,170/µl), serum biochemistry profile (normal), urinalysis (normal), serum T_4 concentration (normal), zinc sulfate fecal flotation (negative for *Giardia* cysts but positive for coccidia ova) and a Sudan black stain for fecal fat (positive). Two weeks of treatment with sulfadimethoxine for coccidiosis improved the diarrhea.

The owner returned with the cat six weeks after completion of sulfadimethoxine treatment because the diarrhea had worsened. The cat was thinner (BCS 2/5) and weighed 3.8 kg. Feces were soft and still positive for fat; however, fecal flotation was negative for coccidia and other parasites. A complete blood count revealed more severe eosinophilia (3,500/µl).

Endoscopic examination of the upper gastrointestinal (GI) tract revealed a normal esophagus and stomach but a coarse, granular, friable mucosa in the duodenum. Histopathologic examination of biopsy specimens collected during endoscopy revealed a normal esophagus, mild lymphoplasmacytic infiltration of the stomach and severe lymphoplasmacytic infiltration in the duodenum. Diagnosis was inflammatory bowel disease (IBD) (lymphoplasmacytic gastroenteritis).

Assess the Food and Feeding Method

The cat was fed a commercial dry grocery brand cat food. The food and water were offered free choice.

Questions

1. Outline a feeding plan for this cat.
2. What other medical therapy can be used in this patient?

Answers and Discussion

1. Several different types of foods may benefit patients with IBD. One strategy involves using a highly digestible, low residue food in conjunction with medical management to control inflammation. (See Answer 2.) Another strategy uses foods with mild to moderate levels of fiber to alter intestinal motility in conjunction with medical management. A third strategy uses an elimination ("hypoallergenic" or one containing a protein hydrolysate) food to decrease mucosal exposure to potential antigens. Although the etiopathogenesis of IBD is unknown, limiting exposure of the GI mucosa to potential antigens is considered an important part of the feeding plan. Use of an elimination food is often the first choice in these cases although a combination of various dietary strategies can also be tried. Access to table food and snacks should be avoided. Therapeutic trials with several different food types and careful monitoring are necessary for optimal case management. The food should be fed in an appropriate amount for the patient's body condition and activity level. For this cat, the daily energy requirement (DER) was estimated to be 1.4 x resting energy requirement for an ideal body weight of 4.5 kg (DER = 290 kcal [1.21 MJ]).
2. Medical therapy is indicated along with dietary management in most moderate to severe cases of IBD. Mild to moderate cases may respond to dietary management alone. Although clinical remission can be obtained in some cases without medical therapy, many gastroenterologists believe that remission will be more rapid, complete and prolonged if the patient is given a short course of antiinflammatory drugs. The rationale for this recommendation is that the more rapidly intestinal inflammation can be controlled, the more rapidly the intestinal permeability barrier will be restored and the less exposure the animal will have to intestinal luminal antigens, including the antigens in the new food. A large variety of medications have been used in cats with this condition including oral corticosteroids, parenteral corticosteroids (i.e., nonresponsive patients with severe disease), azathioprine, cyclophosphamide, metronidazole, tylosin, miscellaneous antibiotics and motility modifiers.

Progress Notes

The owner was offered several therapeutic options but elected to try an elimination food alone. The cat was started on a commercial moist veterinary therapeutic food (Prescription Diet Feline d/d[a]) that contained highly digestible ingredients (lamb and rice) to which the cat had not been exposed previously. The food was offered as two meals per day (one-fourth of a 14.25-oz. can twice daily). Four weeks later, the owner reported that the diarrhea had resolved completely and the cat weighed 4.2 kg. The feeding plan was continued.

The cat did well for more than a year; however, lethargy, vomiting and weight loss were noted 16 months after the initial diagnosis of IBD. Physical examination revealed a thin cat (body weight 3.5 kg, BCS 2/5) with palpably thickened bowel loops. Persistent eosinophilia and elevated liver enzyme activity were present. Evaluation of intestinal biopsy specimens obtained endoscopically revealed GI lymphosarcoma. The cat was euthanized at the owner's request.

Endnote

a. Hill's Pet Nutrition Inc., Topeka, KS, USA. This product is currently available as Prescription Diet d/d Feline.

Bibliography

Dimski DS. Therapy of inflammatory bowel disease. In: Bonagura JD, ed. Current Veterinary Therapy XII. Philadelphia, PA: WB Saunders Co, 1995; 723-728.

Chapter 58

Protein-Losing Enteropathies

Deborah J. Davenport
Albert E. Jergens
Rebecca L. Remillard

"Lymph, v.: to walk with a lisp."
From a Washington Post reader submission word contest

CLINICAL IMPORTANCE

Protein-losing enteropathy (PLE) is a broad term encompassing intestinal disorders characterized by gastrointestinal (GI) protein loss of such magnitude as to result in hypoalbuminemia. Lymphangiectasia is one form of PLE. Lymphangiectasia is characterized by abnormalities of the intestinal lymphatic system, which cause lymphatic hypertension. Lymphangiectasia may occur as a primary lymphatic defect or as a consequence of severe intestinal infiltrative disease (e.g., inflammatory bowel disease, alimentary lymphosarcoma, fungal enteritis). Lymphangiectasia is a common cause of PLE in dogs. PLE in cats is rare. Collectively, PLE is a relatively uncommon manifestation of diarrheic disorders in dogs and cats.

PATIENT ASSESSMENT

History and Physical Examination

Typically, signs of lymphangiectasia are insidious in onset and follow a waxing and waning course over several weeks to months before becoming overt. The clinical manifestations of lymphangiectasia are generally attributable to the loss of lymph constituents (i.e., albumin, lymphocytes, fat) or to the underlying enteric disease. Many patients present with chronic intermittent diarrhea or vomiting; however, not all have GI signs. Progressive weight loss, often in the face of a good appetite, is a consistent finding in longstanding cases. Excessive protein loss from leaky intestinal lymphatics results in hypoalbuminemia and loss of colloidal oncotic pressure. External manifestations of hypoalbuminemia may include pitting edema, ascites and pleural effusion. In some cases, chylous effusions of the abdomen, subcutis or thoracic cavity may occur in conjunction with primary or congenital lymphangiectasia (Fossum et al, 1987, 1990, 1992) Rarely, affected dogs may present with thromboembolic phenomena (e.g., pulmonary thromboembolism) as a consequence of antithrombin III deficiency. Severe hypocalcemia due to malabsorption in affected dogs can cause tetany and rarely seizures.

Physical examination findings may be unremarkable in dogs with PLE. Patients with severe hypoproteinemia may present with dyspnea and abdominal enlargement due to accumulation of fluid in the thoracic or abdominal cavities, respectively. Pitting edema of the limbs may be noted. Body condition

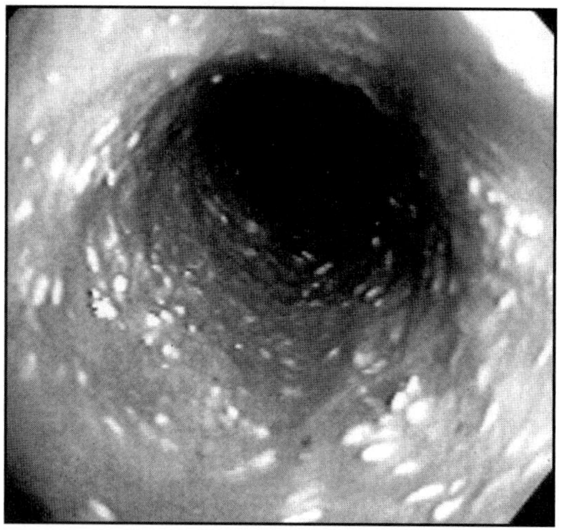

Figure 58-1. Endoscopic view of lymphangiectasia in the duodenum of a three-year-old Yorkshire terrier with diarrhea. Note the raised, white miliary structures along the mucosal surface. These structures are grossly dilated lacteals (intestinal lymphatics) filled with chylomicron-rich fluid. (Courtesy Dr. Chris Ludlow, Veterinary Internal Medicine Specialists of Kansas City, Kansas City, MO.)

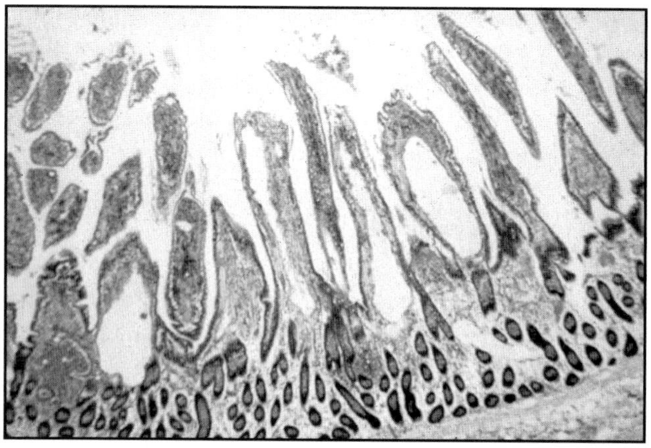

Figure 58-2. Photomicrograph of an intestinal biopsy specimen from a patient with lymphangiectasia. Note the distended intestinal lacteals (original magnification 100X). (Courtesy Dr. Lois Roth, Angell Memorial Animal Hospital, Boston, MA.)

assessment of body fat loss vs. muscle wasting should be performed because many patients are underweight at the time of presentation.

Laboratory and Other Clinical Information

There is a consistent pattern of laboratory results in many dogs with PLE. Panhypoproteinemia (i.e., hypoglobulinemia and hypoalbuminemia) and hypocholesterolemia are classic findings of lymphangiectasia and reflect the loss of lymphatic fluid into the gut lumen. A unique feature of PLE in Basenji dogs is an IgA-associated hyperglobulinemia. In lymphangiectasia, lymphopenia is an important finding that can be used to differentiate this condition from other causes of PLE (Tams and Twedt, 1981). Other laboratory findings may include anemia of chronic disease, a stress leukogram and hypocalcemia. Hypocalcemia is caused by malabsorption of calcium and/or vitamin D. Symptomatic hypocalcemia is rare; therefore, ionized calcium levels should be assessed before initiating intravenous calcium supplementation.

Fecal α-1-protease inhibitor assays have been developed for dogs and cats and offer a sensitive and specific technique for detection of increased intestinal protein loss (Melgarejo et al, 1998; Murphy et al, 2003). Fecal α-1-protease inhibitor is a plasma protein that is lost at the same rate as albumin. As a proteinase inhibitor, this protein is resistant to digestion and reaches the distal colon and rectum intact thus lending itself to a fecal immunoassay. Measuring fecal α-1-protease inhibitor is a particularly useful diagnostic tool for patients with PLE that do not have panhypoproteinemia.

Endoscopic examination in patients with PLE can be helpful to confirm a diagnosis. Mucosal granularity and glistening white patches, which indicate dilated lacteals may be noted (**Figure 58-1**). Feeding small amounts (10 to 20 ml) of corn oil or cream eight to 12 hours before endoscopy can enhance detection of dilated lacteals. Endoscopy also provides a noninvasive route for obtaining intestinal biopsy specimens. A definitive diagnosis of lymphangiectasia and other types of PLE is made through histologic demonstration of characteristic mucosal lesions. In lymphangiectasia, these lesions include dilated, chyle-engorged lacteals and submucosal lymphatics (**Figure 58-2**). Often, mucosal edema is present. In some cases, lipogranulomas may be identified adjacent to intestinal and mesenteric lymphatics. The pathogenesis of these lipogranulomas is unknown, but they are hypothesized to result from extravasation of chyle into perilymphatic tissue. Surgical techniques (e.g., laparoscopy) can be used to collect full-thickness intestinal biopsy specimens. The potential for surgical dehiscence should be considered before biopsy specimens are taken from patients with PLE. Full-thickness biopsy specimens should be obtained if a diagnosis cannot be made based on evaluation of endoscopic biopsy specimens. Care must be taken to use serosal patch grafts and to preserve abdominal fluid accumulation to reduce the potential for dehiscence and further decreases in total body albumin, respectively (Peterson and Willard, 2003).

Risk Factors

Several dog breeds appear to be at risk for development of PLE; Chinese Shar-Peis and rottweilers were identified as at risk at one university teaching hospital (Peterson and Willard, 2003). Primary lymphatic defects appear to be most common in Yorkshire terriers (Kimmel et al, 2000), poodles (Peterson and Willard, 2003), golden retrievers and dachshunds. Lymphangiectasia secondary to severe mucosal inflammatory infiltrates is a common sequela to immunoproliferative enteropathy in Basenjis and Lundenhunds (Breitschwerdt, 1992; Flesja and Yri, 1977; Williams, 1997). In one study, about 50% of the North American Lundenhund population had evidence of PLE (Berghoff et al, 2004). PLE may occur in conjunction with protein-losing nephropathy in soft-coated wheaten terriers; 10 to 15% of the population may be affected (Littman and Giger, 1990; Littman et al, 2000).

Etiopathogenesis

Normally, plasma proteins are lost into the GI lumen daily. This loss is attributed to protein leakage at the time of villous tip extrusion. Typically, these plasma proteins are re-assimilated through digestive and absorptive processes. Certain GI disorders can disturb protein balance. Intestinal protein loss can accelerate when the mucosal barrier is disrupted or disorders interfere with lymphatic drainage. Altered intestinal lymphatic drainage results in reflux of protein-rich lymph into the gut lumen. Excess protein can be lost through exudation or hemorrhage when the intestinal mucosa is damaged. Hypoproteinemia develops in either case after protein losses exceed compensatory synthesis.

Intestinal lymphangiectasia can arise as a primary disorder of the lymphatic system or secondary to chronic inflammatory bowel disease. Severe inflammatory infiltrates and lipogranulomas can obstruct lymphatic drainage. Normally, the intestinal lymphatics transport absorbed fats from enterocytes to the venous circulation via the thoracic duct. Lacteals become distended with chyle if lymphaticovenous flow is impaired. Over-distended lacteals rupture and release intestinal lymph (containing protein, lymphocytes, fat and cholesterol) into the lumen. In some patients with primary lymphangiectasia, the lymphatic defects are not limited to the GI tract. In these animals, abnormal lymph flow may result in chylothorax, chylous abdominal effusions and subcutaneous chyle accumulations (Fossum et al, 1987, 1990, 1992).

Key Nutritional Factors

Key nutritional factors for patients with lymphangiectasia and other types of PLE are listed in **Table 58-1** and discussed in detail below.

Table 58-1. Key nutritional factors for foods for patients with lymphangiectasia/protein-losing enteropathy.*

Factors	Recommended levels
Energy density	>3.5 kcal/g (>14.6 kJ/g)
Fat**	<15% for dogs and cats
Protein	≥25% for dogs ≥35% for cats
Crude fiber	≤5%
Digestibility	≥87% for protein and ≥90% for fat and digestible carbohydrate

*Nutrients expressed on a dry matter basis.
**Inclusion of medium-chain triglycerides is desirable.

Energy Density and Fat

Controlling dietary fat intake is important in PLE patients. For many pet foods, most of the fat content is from long-chain triglycerides. After digestion and lymphatic absorption, reconstituted long-chain triglycerides in the form of chylomicrons provide a major stimulus for intestinal lymph flow (Chapter 5). The chylomicrons are transported from the mucosal epithelium via lacteals to the thoracic duct and into the systemic circulation. Long-chain triglyceride absorption increases lymph protein content and lymph flow two- to threefold for four to six hours postprandially (Simmonds, 1954). The protein content of lymph tends to increase with dietary fat intake (Simmonds, 1954). If lymphatic flow is impaired, lacteals become distended with lymph. These over-distended lacteals can rupture and release lymph into the intestinal lumen. This process can damage the intestinal mucosa and, as a result, even more protein is lost through exudation or hemorrhage into the small intestine. Limiting fat intake (i.e., <15% dry matter (DM) for dogs and cats) minimizes lymph flow, reduces lacteal and lymphatic distention and minimizes protein loss.

PLE patients may be cachectic and including medium-chain triglycerides (MCT) as a source of calories has been recommended (**Box 58-1** and **Table 58-2**). MCT are water-soluble, and readily and rapidly hydrolyzed. They were previously thought not to require micellarization for absorption so that they would be absorbed directly into the portal vasculature and thus would not affect lymph flow as do long-chain triglycerides. However, a study in dogs showed that some MCT absorption does occur via the lymphatics (Jensen et al, 1994). The oil is best used when it is incorporated into foods rather than as a supplement added to foods because MCT supplementation negatively affects palatability. Also, because MCT oils do not contain essential fatty acids, it is important to ensure adequate intake when MCT oils are supplemented for prolonged periods. In addition, supplemental use of MCT oils in cats has been linked to hepatic lipidosis (MacDonald et al, 1984).

From a dietary energy and fat perspective, the best option is to feed a balanced, highly digestible low-fat food (fat <15% DM for dogs and cats) with adequate energy density (>3.5 kcal/g [>14.6 kJ/g DM]). If MCT oils are used, they are best incorporated into the food.

Protein

Foods for patients with PLE should contain enough high biologic value proteins to support hepatic protein synthesis and replace depleted tissue proteins. In general, food protein content should be at least 25% DM for canine patients and at least 35% DM for feline patients. Feeding high-protein or all-meat foods without other appropriate dietary alterations has not been successful (Finco et al, 1973; Matteeuws et al, 1974). If severe inflammatory bowel disease is the underlying cause of PLE, the use of a low-fat, elimination food containing lower levels (16 to 26% DM for dogs and 30 to 45% DM for cats) of highly digestible, novel protein sources or hydrolysate-based foods should be considered.

Fiber

Foods containing increased levels of insoluble fiber (>7%) are not routinely recommended for the dietary management of PLE. Fiber-containing foods do not seem to be directly detrimental for these patients. The assumption that the "rough" texture of fiber might mechanically traumatize the intestinal mucosa is not supported by clinical evidence (Guilford, 1996) and there are cases in the veterinary literature in which a high-fiber (20% DM) food was successfully fed because of the food's particularly low fat content (Tams and Twedt, 1981; Erickson,

Box 58-1. Medium-Chain Triglycerides.

Triacylglycerides (TAG) are the most common form of fat found in foods and stored in body fat depots. TAG are primarily composed of long-chain fatty acids (i.e., 16 to 24 carbons long). Medium-chain triglycerides (MCT) are eight to 10 carbons long and are typically minor constituents of a food. Increased levels of dietary MCT have theoretical advantages over long-chain triglycerides (LCT) for the treatment of some forms of gastrointestinal disease.

The most striking difference between MCT and LCT is the former are more water-soluble than the latter. MCT are normally absorbed by mechanisms independent of those used by LCT. MCT are hydrolyzed more rapidly and can rely on the small amount of intestinal lipase available, rather than on pancreatic lipase. The products of hydrolysis are easily dispersed and absorbed in the absence of bile acids. Like short-chain fatty acids, medium-chain fatty acids are absorbed at a faster rate, are not re-esterified with glycerol in enterocytes and are primarily transported from the gut via the portal vein directly to the liver. However, some MCT also appear to be incorporated in chylomicrons and transported to some degree in the thoracic duct.

MCT may have a place in the nutritional management of patients with defects in intraluminal hydrolysis of fat (e.g., decreased pancreatic lipase, decreased bile salts), fat malabsorption or defective lymphatic transport of fat (lymphangiectasia). MCT are prepared commercially by hydrolysis and fractionation of coconut oil to create an oil (MCT Oil[a]) that contains approximately 67% caprylic acid (C8) and 23% capric acid (C10). The oil provides 8.3 kcal/g (34.7 kJ/g); one tablespoon (15 ml) weighs 14 g and provides 115 kcal (481 kJ). The oil can be included in commercial foods, homemade recipes or used to supplement commercial foods. Empiric recommendations are to provide 25 to 30% of calories as MCT.

MCT are also available as part of a nutritionally complete formula for human infants and children (Portagen[a]). This dry powder is composed of corn syrup solids, MCT oil, casein, sucrose, corn oil, soy lecithin, vitamins and minerals. Caloric distribution is 14% protein, 40% fat and 46% carbohydrate. The fat content is 95% MCT. The powder is mixed with water to produce a solution providing 1 kcal (4.2 kJ) per ml. Alternatively, the powder can be included in a homemade food or mixed with a commercial pet food.

Potential side effects of using supplemental MCT in foods for patients with gastrointestinal disease include reduced palatability, vomiting and osmotic diarrhea. In cats, experimental MCT oil administration has been linked to hepatic lipidosis. MCT products are expensive and their use supplementally is generally reserved for those patients that are refractory to more traditional dietary approaches.

ENDNOTE

a. Mead Johnson Nutritionals, Evansville, IN, USA.

The Bibliography for **Box 58-1** can be found at www.markmorris.org.

1988; Remillard, 1989; Sherding, 1987). Higher levels of dietary fiber bind digestive enzymes and bile acids, decrease pancreatic secretion of lipase and reduce pancreatic enzyme activity. Insoluble fiber, through these mechanisms, decreases intraluminal fat digestion and micelle formation, which selectively inhibits long-chain fatty acid absorption (Remillard, 1989). Therefore, fiber may play a secondary role in reducing long-chain fatty acid absorption and decreasing lymphatic flow and subsequent lymph fluid losses. However, increased levels of fiber (>10% DM) also reduce the caloric density and digestibility of a food; both factors are deemed important to the appropriate management of patients with PLE. Thus, lower fiber levels (≤5% DM), which support higher caloric density and improved digestibility are recommended for foods for these patients.

Digestibility

Feeding highly digestible (fat and digestible [soluble] carbohydrate ≥90% and protein ≥87%) foods provides several advantages for managing lymphangiectasia in dogs and cats. Nutrients (including the energy-supplying nutrients just mentioned) in highly digestible foods are more completely absorbed in the proximal gut. Furthermore, highly digestible foods are associated with: 1) reduced osmotic diarrhea related to fat and carbohydrate malabsorption, 2) reduced production of intestinal gas due to carbohydrate malabsorption and 3) decreased antigen loads because smaller amounts of protein are absorbed intact.

Other Nutritional Factors

Vitamins

Vitamin supplementation is rarely necessary when feeding commercially prepared foods. Dogs and cats usually have body stores of vitamins A, D, E and K to last several months. However, parenteral supplementation with fat-soluble vitamins may be needed if marked steatorrhea persists. Fat-soluble vitamin supplementation is warranted in cases of long-term fat malabsorption. It is simple and cost effective to administer 1 ml of a vitamin A, D and E solution,[a] divided into two intramuscular sites. This should supply fat-soluble vitamins for approximately three months. Patients with vitamin K deficiency should be treated appropriately. Vitamin K_1, at a dosage of 0.5 to 1 mg/kg, subcutaneously, is recommended if a vitamin K-responsive coagulopathy is suspected.

Minerals

Patients with fat malabsorption fed foods containing higher levels of fat may have increased divalent cation losses (i.e., calcium, magnesium, zinc and copper) because of intraluminal saponification. Calcium supplementation is generally not needed because serum calcium levels usually increase in conjunction with serum albumin concentrations. However, intravenous calcium supplementation should be instituted if hypocalcemic tetany develops. Hypomagnesemia has been reported to occur in Yorkshire terriers with lymphangiectasia (Kimmel et al,

Table 58-2. Summary of digestion and absorption of long- and medium-chain triglycerides.

Characteristics	Long-chain triglycerides	Medium-chain triglycerides
Digestion		
Hydrolysis by gastric lipase	Slow	Fast
Hydrolysis by pancreatic lipase	Fast	Very fast
Luminal transport		
Paracellular absorption	None	Some
Re-esterification and chylomicron formation	Yes	No
Requires bile acid micellarization	Yes	No
Transport route from gut	Lymphatics	Portal blood; some via lymphatics
Water solubility of essential fatty acids	Low	High

2000). Anorexia and malabsorption complicated by the use of magnesium-free fluids are likely causes of low serum magnesium levels in these dogs. If necessary, magnesium repletion can be accomplished by the use of appropriate intravenous fluids. Supplementation with other minerals should also be based on evidence of deficiency rather than given pro forma.

FEEDING PLAN

The goal of therapy for patients with lymphangiectasia or PLE is to decrease the enteric loss of plasma protein. In some cases, dietary manipulation alone is adequate. In others, concurrent medical management is necessary.

Assess and Select the Food

Levels of key nutritional factors in foods currently fed to patients with lymphangiectasia or PLE should be evaluated and compared with recommended levels (**Table 58-1**). Information from this aspect of assessment is essential for making any changes to foods currently fed. Changing to a more appropriate food is indicated if the key nutritional factors in the current food do not match recommended levels. However, it is unlikely that a suitable food is being fed if clinical signs are present. **Tables 58-3** and **58-4** list selected veterinary therapeutic foods marketed for lymphangiectasia or PLE for dogs and cats, respectively, and compare them to recommended levels. It is usually best to choose the food that most closely matches the key nutritional factor recommendations. Home-prepared foods (Chapter 10) can also be considered (Peterson and Willard, 2003).

If a patient cannot maintain normal body weight and condition when fed an appropriate food, supplemental MCT oil may be added to the food. This supplement, however, should be used with caution, introduced gradually and should not exceed 25% of the caloric requirement (<1 ml/lb [<0.5 ml/kg] body weight). **Box 58-1** provides more information about MCT, including potential problems with the use and misuse of supplemental MCT.

Some patients with PLE may require additional protein. Dogs may be fed a low-fat (<10% fat DM) cat food that has a higher protein (>35% DM) content (**Table 58-4**) than a comparable dog food. Protein may also be added in the form of cooked egg whites. Egg whites contain 90% of a very high biologic value protein, which can be a useful supplement for some patients with PLE to increase serum albumin levels. Provide a minimum of one to two cooked large egg whites per 10 kg body weight as needed to maintain serum albumin levels above 2 g/dl.

If severe inflammatory bowel disease is the underlying cause of PLE, a highly digestible, low-fat elimination food containing lower levels (16 to 26% DM for dogs and 30 to 45% DM for cats) of novel protein sources or hydrolysate-based foods should also be considered. Chapters 31 and 57 provide information about these foods.

Assess and Determine the Feeding Method

Initially, patients with lymphangiectasia or PLE should be fed multiple small meals per day as indicated by acceptance and tolerance of the food. Meal size can be increased as tolerated by the patient after the clinical signs have been successfully managed for several weeks. Anorectic patients can be fed by nasoesophageal or esophagostomy tube using liquid monomeric or polymeric foods. Longstanding hospitalized patients in poor body condition should be given a parenteral solution containing calories, protein and essential micronutrients (Chapter 26). Calories can also be easily administered peripherally to dogs and cats using an isomolar 20% lipid solution piggybacked with standard fluid therapy at volumes sufficient to meet the patient's resting energy requirement.[b]

CONCURRENT THERAPY

Immunosuppressive therapy as described for inflammatory bowel disease is indicated when lymphangiectasia or PLE occurs as a consequence of mucosal inflammatory infiltrates. Drugs with reported efficacy include glucocorticoids and cyclosporine. In addition to treating the underlying enteric lesions, corticosteroid therapy has the added advantage of controlling the inflammatory lesions of lymphangiectasia, lymphangitis and lipogranulomas.

When hypoalbuminemia is severe, plasma, concentrated human albumin, dextran or hetastarch infusions may be necessary to restore colloidal oncotic pressure. In general, aggressive nutritional support will be more successful than plasma transfusions for restoring normoalbuminemia. Plasma transfusions may, however, benefit those patients with hypercoagulability resulting from panhypoproteinemia; plasma serves as a rich source of coagulation factors and antithrombin III.

Table 58-3. Key nutritional factors in selected veterinary therapeutic foods for dogs with lymphangiectasia/protein-losing enteropathy compared to recommended levels.* (See Table 31-5 if foods with novel protein sources or protein hydrolysates are desired.)

Dry foods	**Energy density (kcal/g)**	**Fat (%)**	**Protein (%)**	**Fiber (%)**	**Protein digestibility (%)**	**Fat digestibility (%)**	**Carbohydrate digestibility (%)**
Recommended levels	**>3.5**	**<15**	**≥25**	**≤5**	**≥87**	**≥90**	**≥90**
Hill's Prescription Diet i/d Canine	4.2	14.1	26.2	2.7	92	93	94
Iams Veterinary Formula Intestinal Low-Residue	3.8	10.7	24.6	2.1	na	na	na
Medi-Cal Low Fat LF 20	na	6.6	24.2	5.2	na	na	na
Purina Veterinary Diets EN GastroENteric Formula**	4.2	12.6	27.0	1.5	84.5	91.4	94.4
Royal Canin Veterinary Diet Digestive Low Fat LF 20	3.7	6.6	24.2	2.3	na	na	na
Moist foods	**Energy density (kcal/g)**	**Fat (%)**	**Protein (%)**	**Fiber (%)**	**Protein digestibility (%)**	**Fat digestibility (%)**	**Carbohydrate digestibility (%)**
Recommended levels	**>3.5**	**<15**	**≥25**	**≤5**	**≥87**	**≥90**	**≥90**
Hill's Prescription Diet i/d Canine	4.4	14.9	25.0	1.0	88	94	93
Iams Veterinary Formula Intestinal Low-Residue	4.6	13.2	35.9	3.9	na	na	na
Medi-Cal Low Fat LF	na	9.0	32.8	3.1	na	na	na
Purina Veterinary Diets EN GastroENteric Formula**	4.0	13.8	30.5	0.9	85.1	95.6	92.2
Royal Canin Veterinary Diet Digestive Low Fat LF	4.0	6.9	31.9	3.0	na	na	na

Key: Fiber = crude fiber, na = information not available from manufacturer.
*Manufacturers' published values. Nutrients expressed as % dry matter.
**Food contains medium-chain triglycerides.

Table 58-4. Key nutritional factors in selected veterinary therapeutic foods for cats with lymphangiectasia/protein-losing enteropathy compared to recommended levels.* (See Table 31-6 if foods with novel protein sources or protein hydrolysates are desired.)

Dry foods	**Energy density (kcal/g)**	**Fat (%)**	**Protein (%)**	**Fiber (%)**	**Protein digestibility (%)**	**Fat digestibility (%)**	**Carbohydrate digestibility (%)**
Recommended levels	**>3.5**	**<15**	**≥35**	**≤5**	**≥87**	**≥90**	**≥90**
Hill's Prescription Diet i/d Feline	4.3	20.2	40.3	2.8	88	92	90
Iams Veterinary Formula Intestinal Low-Residue	3.9	13.7	35.8	1.8	na	na	na
Medi-Cal Hypoallergenic/Gastro	na	11.5	29.8	3.1	na	na	na
Purina Veterinary Diets EN GastroENteric Formula	4.4	18.4	56.2	1.3	94.0	93.1	79.7
Royal Canin Veterinary Diet Intestinal HE	4.4	23.7	34.4	5.8	na	na	na
Moist foods	**Energy density (kcal/g)**	**Fat (%)**	**Protein (%)**	**Fiber (%)**	**Protein digestibility (%)**	**Fat digestibility (%)**	**Carbohydrate digestibility (%)**
Recommended levels	**>3.5**	**<15**	**≥35**	**≤5**	**≥87**	**≥90**	**≥90**
Hill's Prescription Diet i/d Feline	4.2	24.1	37.6	2.4	91	89	91
Iams Veterinary Formula Intestinal Low-Residue	4.0	11.7	38.4	3.7	na	na	na
Medi-Cal Hypoallergenic/Gastro	na	35.9	35.5	1.2	na	na	na
Medi-Cal Sensitivity CR	na	35.1	34.5	2.5	na	na	na

Key: Fiber = crude fiber, na = information not available from manufacturer.
*Manufacturers' published values. Nutrients expressed as % dry matter.

REASSESSMENT

Initially, patients with PLE should be reassessed weekly following discharge from the hospital. Each reexamination should include assessment of body weight and condition. Assessment of serum albumin and calcium concentrations and lymphocyte counts every two weeks is useful. In addition, serial radiography can be used to assess the resolution of abdominal or thoracic effusion.

If the patient's condition improves, dietary therapy should continue until the underlying enteropathy is resolved. Failing that, dietary management should continue for the lifetime of the pet. Over time, it may be possible to increase dietary fat intake; however, this should be done cautiously and only for patients having difficulty maintaining ideal body weight or those manifesting evidence of essential fatty acid deficiency (e.g., poor skin or coat quality).

ENDNOTES

a. Vital E-A+D containing 100 IU of D and 300 IU of alpha-tocopherol per ml. Schering-Plough Animal Health Corp., Kenilworth, NJ, USA.
b. Remillard RL. Unpublished data. 1998.

REFERENCES

The references for **Chapter 58** can be found at www.markmorris.org.

Chapter 59

Short Bowel Syndrome

Deborah J. Davenport
Chris L. Ludlow
Rebecca L. Remillard

"Who needs such a long intestine, anyway?"
Moshe Dayan

CLINICAL IMPORTANCE

Short bowel syndrome is a malabsorptive state that may develop after massive resection of the small intestine (Vanderhoof and Langnas, 1997). Short bowel syndrome is an important clinical entity in people but is uncommon in dogs and cats. This difference probably reflects the relative frequency with which predisposing conditions occur. In people, the most common reasons for extensive bowel resection are inflammatory and neoplastic conditions in which the residual bowel is often compromised. In dogs and cats, a number of intestinal conditions may warrant the removal of large segments of the bowel, including linear foreign bodies, intussusception, volvulus, infarction, neoplasia, entrapment, gastrointestinal (GI) surgical site dehiscence and fungal infections. In many of these conditions, the remaining intestine is healthy. The syndrome is characterized by malabsorption due to lack of gut surface area resulting in diarrhea, malnutrition and weight loss. Short bowel syndrome may occur whenever large segments of the small intestine (≥50%) are excised surgically (Gorman et al, 2006; Yanoff and Willard, 1989; Yanoff et al, 1992; Pawlusiow and McCarthy, 1994; Williams and Burrows, 1981; Joy and Patterson, 1978; Feldman et al, 1976; Uchiyama et al, 1996). However, one retrospective study was unable to correlate the percentage of resected bowel with the development of short bowel syndrome (Gorman et al, 2006).

PATIENT ASSESSMENT

History and Physical Examination

Dogs with short bowel syndrome typically develop diarrhea one or more days after a large portion of the small bowel is resected (Gorman et al, 2006; Yanoff et al, 1992). The diarrhea may be intermittent or persistent. Stools range from soft, cowpie consistency to explosive, watery diarrhea. In longstanding cases, the patient may have weight loss, polyphagia and evidence of malnutrition.

Occasionally, patients present weeks to months after surgery with small bowel diarrhea, flatulence and borborygmus. A delayed onset of clinical signs is associated with small intestinal bacterial overgrowth, which can develop as a sequela to resection of the ileocolic valve. Physical examination findings are usually unremarkable. Body condition assessment may demonstrate poor condition (body condition score 1/5 or 2/5). Most patients are bright, alert and active with an increased appetite.

Laboratory and Other Clinical Information

Hematologic and biochemical findings are variable, often reflecting the underlying condition that led to the bowel resection. Hypoproteinemia and hypoalbuminemia may be present in long-term cases. Mild, normocytic, normochromic nonregenerative anemia may be recognized as a consequence of chronic disease. Patients in which the ileum has been resected

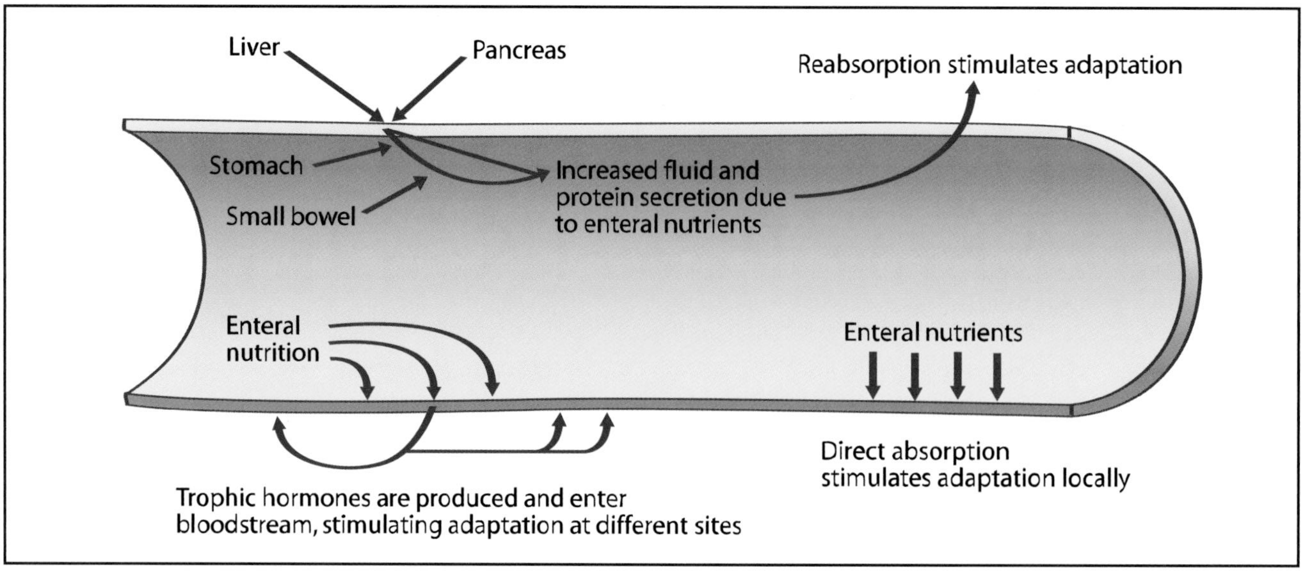

Figure 59-1. Schematic representation of the pathways by which enteral nutrients stimulate intestinal adaptation. (Adapted from Vanderhoff JA, Langnas AN. Short-bowel syndrome in children and adults. Gastroenterology 1997; 113: 1767-1778.)

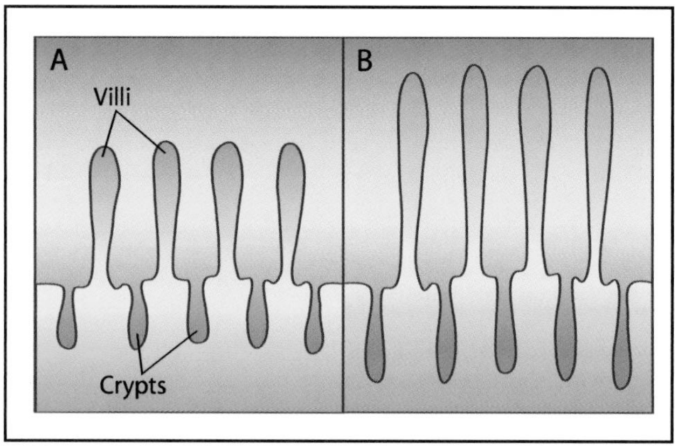

Figure 59-2. Diagrammatic comparison of normal (A) and adapted (B) gastrointestinal epithelium in patients with short bowel syndrome. Note the increased villous length and crypt depth. Increased muscle mass may also be observed. (Adapted from Vanderhoff JA, Langnas AN. Short-bowel syndrome in children and adults. Gastroenterology 1997; 113: 1767-1778.)

may have microcytic anemia consistent with that caused by cobalamin deficiency.

Radiographic findings are usually not helpful. Contrast films may demonstrate rapid transit of ingesta from the stomach to the colon. Contrast radiography can also be used to estimate the length of bowel remaining. In normal dogs, the small intestinal length is approximately four times the distance from the crown of the head to the rump. The percentage of small intestine remaining can be calculated by comparing the length of bowel remaining to this standard (Yanoff et al, 1992).

Risk Factors

Puppies and young adult dogs are most likely to suffer from GI conditions that may require extensive small bowel resection. Young cats, in particular, are at risk for linear foreign bodies (Gorman et al, 2006). GI conditions that may require resection include intestinal intussusception, volvulus, fungal infections (e.g., histoplasmosis), neoplasia and foreign bodies. Larger breeds, especially German shepherd dogs, are more likely to suffer from intussusception and mesenteric volvulus.

Etiopathogenesis

A surgeon may be faced with the need to resect a large portion of the small intestine in the management of a number of obstructive small intestinal diseases. Generally, as mentioned above, the potential for the syndrome exists any time 50% or more of the small bowel is resected. Remarkably, dogs with as little as 30 to 40 cm and cats with 18 to 20 cm of residual small intestine may achieve nutritional autonomy (Yanoff and Willard, 1989; Yanoff et al, 1992). Short bowel syndrome arises due to a lack of sufficient mucosal absorptive surface area. The reduced gut surface results in incomplete digestion and absorption of nutrients. Unabsorbed nutrients in the gut lumen lead to osmotic diarrhea. In addition, unabsorbed bile acids and fatty acids may result in secretory diarrhea in the large bowel.

Massive intestinal resection causes morphologic and functional adaptation in the remaining small bowel. Adaptation is stimulated by: 1) exposure to luminal nutrients, 2) endogenous GI secretions, 3) trophic effects of gut hormones, especially epidermal growth factor, enteroglucagon and gastrin, 4) intraluminal polyamines, 5) neural factors and 6) changes in blood flow to the remaining bowel (**Figure 59-1**) (Kouti et al, 2006; Chan and Klein, 1997). During adaptation, the intestine dilates and hyperplasia occurs in villi and crypts; however, the absorptive capacity of individual enterocytes does not change (Kouti et al, 2006; Williamson and Chir, 1978; Dowling, 1988). Therefore, the net increase in absorptive function in the remaining small bowel occurs because of increased total surface area.

In general, jejunal resections are tolerated better than removal of the ileum or the ileocolic valve. An intact ileum markedly enhances fluid, bile acid, cobalamin and electrolyte resorption. Loss of the ileocolic valve removes the physical barrier that separates the profuse bacterial flora of the colon from the relatively sparse population of the small bowel. Loss of the valve predisposes patients to development of small intestinal bacterial overgrowth or colonization of the remaining small bowel with bacterial pathogens.

Over time, the colon may begin to play an important role in maintaining nutritional homeostasis in patients with short bowel syndrome (Aghdassi et al, 1994; Nightingale et al, 1992). Following massive small bowel resection, colonic fermentation of malabsorbed carbohydrate may provide significant calories in the form of short-chain fatty acids. Short-chain fatty acids also promote mucosal hyperplasia. The mechanisms that lead to intestinal adaptation are not completely understood. However, a number of GI hormones including enteroglucagon, gastrin, cholecystokinin and secretin are involved, as are other pancreatobiliary secretions. Intraluminal foodstuffs including protein, protein hydrolysates, fats and glutamine stimulate release of these substances. Thus, intestinal adaptation appears to rely on exposure of the remnant bowel to intraluminal nutrients.

Intestinal adaptation is marked by enterocyte hyperplasia and increases in bowel diameter, villous height, crypt depth and number of enterocytes per length of the villous/crypt unit (**Figure 59-2**). Ideally, these physical changes will increase the bowel's absorptive capacity. Mucosal changes begin to occur within one to two days and can result in a fourfold increase in mucosal surface area within 14 days, if intraluminal nutrients are provided (Vanderhoof et al, 1992).

Table 59-1. Key nutritional factors for foods for dogs and cats with short bowel syndrome.*

Factors	Recommended levels
Digestibility	≥87% for protein and ≥90% for fat and digestible carbohydrate
Fat	12 to 15% for dogs 15 to 25% for cats
Fiber	≤5% (soluble or mixed fiber)
Carbohydrate	Lactose free
Food form	Dry foods are preferred due to slower gastric emptying vs. moist foods

*Nutrients expressed on a dry matter basis.

Key Nutritional Factors

Key nutritional factors for patients with short bowel syndrome are listed in **Table 59-1** and discussed in more detail below.

Digestibility

Because this is a malassimilative condition, highly digestible foods (fat and digestible [soluble] carbohydrate ≥90% and protein ≥87%) are recommended. The use of monomeric foods has been investigated in people with the syndrome; however, clinical evidence suggests that these foods are no more effective than polymeric foods (McIntyre et al, 1986). In addition, use of monomeric foods has been associated with villous atrophy (McIntyre et al, 1986; Levy et al, 1998). Polymeric foods are preferred because of their cost, palatability and trophic effects on the gut.

Fat

There are sound reasons for including fat in foods for dogs and cats with short bowel syndrome. Many patients with long-standing short bowel syndrome are underweight at the time of evaluation (Yanoff and Willard, 1989; Yanoff et al, 1992). Therefore, high-fat, energy-dense foods are recommended. Dogs and cats readily use most fats and oils of either animal or plant origin; therefore, fat should be included in the food for animals with short bowel syndrome up to the point of causing steatorrhea. Dietary fat levels of 12 to 15% dry matter (DM) in dogs and 15 to 25% DM in cats are often well tolerated. Intraluminal fat is probably the most influential nutrient in stimulating small bowel adaptation. Fat exerts profound effects on enterocyte growth, villous morphology, mucosal enzyme activity and segmental absorptive functions (Lentze, 1989). Fat also slows gastric emptying of digesta, which may better match the nutrient load to the compromised digestive capabilities of the shortened small bowel.

Replacing 50 to 75% of dietary fat with medium-chain triglycerides (MCT) has been reported to improve nutritional status in human patients with short bowel syndrome (Bochenek et al, 1970). Unfortunately, use of MCT in veterinary patients is limited due to cost, reduced palatability and poor GI tolerance. For these reasons, it is uncommon for MCT to be incorporated in excess of 30% of calories in homemade foods and 10% of calories in commercial foods. Whether MCT in foods are beneficial at these levels in veterinary patients is unknown.

Fiber

Although highly digestible foods are generally recommended for patients with short bowel syndrome, foods with moderate levels (10 to 15% DM) of insoluble fiber (e.g., cellulose) have been successfully used in refeeding patients with short bowel syndrome. Insoluble fiber included in foods at these levels is thought to help modulate intestinal motility and better control fecal water. Maintaining intraluminal bulk may stimulate the adaptive process through the release of GI trophic factors, including enteroglucagon, gastrin, cholecystokinin, secretin and other pancreatobiliary secretions.

Soluble fiber in foods may also benefit patients with short bowel syndrome by modulation of intestinal transit rate, absorption of intestinal water and production of short-chain fatty acids, which stimulate mucosal hyperplasia. Gel-forming fibers (e.g., pectins, gums) may slow gastric emptying rates (Russell and Bass, 1985; Prove and Ehrlein, 1982; Sandhu et al, 1987). Fermentable fiber supplementation (e.g., pectins, green banana) increases gut mass and colonic villous length, resulting in increased capacity for water reabsorption (Rabbini et al, 2001; Sales et al, 1998; Koruda et al, 1986). The most desirable approach is highly digestible, low-fiber foods with no more than 5% of a mixed fiber source DM. Mixed fiber sources include combinations of soluble (citrus and apple pectins and most gums) and insoluble (cellulose and peanut hulls) fiber

Table 59-2. Key nutritional factors in selected commercial veterinary therapeutic foods for dogs with short bowel syndrome compared to recommended levels.*

Dry foods	Protein digestibility (%)	Fat digestibility (%)	Carbohydrate digestibility (%)	Fat (%)	Fiber (%)**	Primary sources of fiber**	Lactose free (Yes/No)
Recommended levels	**≥87**	**≥90**	**≥90**	**12-15**	**≤5**	**–**	**Yes**
Hill's Prescription Diet i/d Canine	92	93	94	14.1	2.7	Cellulose, beet pulp	Yes
Iams Veterinary Formula Intestinal Low-Residue	na	na	na	10.7	2.1	Beet pulp	Yes
Medi-Cal Gastro Formula	na	na	na	13.9	1.9	Flax meal, pea fiber	Yes
Medi-Cal Low Fat Formula	na	na	na	6.6	5.2	Beet pulp, cellulose	Yes
Purina Veterinary Diets EN GastroENteric Formula	84.5	91.4	94.4	12.6	1.5	–	Yes
Royal Canin Veterinary Diet Digestive Low Fat LF 20	na	na	na	6.6	2.3	Beet pulp, cellulose	Yes
Royal Canin Veterinary Diet Intestinal HE 28	na	na	na	22.0	1.6	Beet pulp, psyllium husks	Yes

Moist foods	Protein digestibility (%)	Fat digestibility (%)	Carbohydrate digestibility (%)	Fat (%)	Fiber (%)**	Primary sources of fiber**	Lactose free (Yes/No)
Recommended levels	**≥87**	**≥90**	**≥90**	**12-15**	**≤5**	**–**	**Yes**
Hill's Prescription Diet i/d Canine	88	94	93	14.9	1.0	Soy fiber	Yes
Iams Veterinary Formula Intestinal Low-Residue	na	na	na	13.2	3.9	Beet pulp	Yes
Medi-Cal Gastro Formula	na	na	na	11.7	1.0	Oat bran, guar gum, flax meal	No
Medi-Cal Low Fat Formula	na	na	na	9.0	3.1	Cellulose, beet pulp, guar gum, carrageenan	Yes
Purina Veterinary Diets EN GastroENteric Formula	85.1	95.6	92.2	13.8	0.9	Gum arabic	Yes
Royal Canin Veterinary Diet Digestive Low Fat LF	na	na	na	6.9	3.0	Cellulose, guar gum	Yes
Royal Canin Veterinary Diet Intestinal HE	na	na	na	11.8	1.4	Oat bran, guar gum, carrageenan, flaxseed	No

Key: Fiber = crude fiber, na = information not available from manufacturer.
*Manufacturers' published values; nutrients expressed as % dry matter; dry foods are preferred because they have slower gastric emptying compared to moist foods.
**Foods with soluble or mixed fiber sources are best (see text).

sources or mixed fiber sources (rice, oat and wheat brans; soy fibers; soy hulls and beet pulp). Patients that have undergone ileal resection do not absorb bile acids well, which may cause secretory diarrhea. In such cases, dietary intake of mixed fibers may bind bile salts. Several manufacturers include small amounts of a mixed fiber source in their highly digestible foods intended for GI diseases. This is the most desirable option if it can be done without negatively affecting digestibility. Lower levels of fiber (≤5% [DM]) are generally recommended and facilitate high digestibility and higher energy density while providing the benefits described above.

Digestible Carbohydrate

The digestible carbohydrate fraction of the selected food should be highly digestible (≥90%). Lactose-containing ingredients should be avoided because extensive small bowel resection results in loss of lactase and other brush border disaccharidases.

Food Form

Dry foods may be preferred because they may increase gastric retention time; it takes longer to lower the digesta osmolality of dry foods compared to moist foods.

Other Nutritional Factors

Prebiotic Fibers

Fructooligosaccharides and other prebiotic fibers have been proposed for use in the management of dogs with small intestinal bacterial overgrowth and, therefore, may be useful in cases of short bowel syndrome in which the ileocolic valve has been resected. However, clinical evidence to support use of these ingredients remains sparse in dogs and cats.

Vitamins

Fat-soluble vitamins are malabsorbed in many canine and feline patients with steatorrhea. Although commercial foods are supplemented with fat-soluble vitamins, fat-soluble vitamins may need to be administered by intramuscular or subcutaneous routes until intestinal adaptation occurs and diarrhea resolves. It is simple and cost effective to administer 1 ml of a vitamin A, D and E solution,[a] divided into two intramuscular sites. This should supply fat-soluble vitamins for approximately three months. Vitamin K_1 at a dosage of 0.5 to 1 mg/kg subcutaneously is recommended if a vitamin K-responsive coagulopathy is suspected.

If the distal ileum has been surgically removed, cobalamin

Table 59-3. Key nutritional factors in selected commercial veterinary therapeutic foods for cats with short bowel syndrome compared to recommended levels.*

Dry foods	Protein digestibility (%)	Fat digestibility (%)	Carbohydrate digestibility (%)	Fat (%)	Fiber (%)**	Primary sources of fiber**	Lactose free (Yes/No)
Recommended levels	**≥87**	**≥90**	**≥90**	**15-25**	**≤5**	**-**	**Yes**
Hill's Prescription Diet i/d Feline	88	92	90	20.2	2.8	Cellulose, beet pulp	Yes
Iams Veterinary Formula Intestinal Low-Residue	na	na	na	13.7	1.8	Beet pulp	Yes
Medi-Cal Hypoallergenic/Gastro	na	na	na	11.5	3.1	Beet pulp, rice bran	Yes
Purina Veterinary Diets EN GastroENteric Formula	94.0	93.1	79.7	18.4	1.3	Cellulose	Yes
Royal Canin Veterinary Diet Intestinal HE 30	na	na	na	23.7	5.8	Cellulose, beet pulp	Yes

Moist foods	Protein digestibility (%)	Fat digestibility (%)	Carbohydrate digestibility (%)	Fat (%)	Fiber (%)**	Primary sources of fiber**	Lactose free (Yes/No)
Recommended levels	**≥87**	**≥90**	**≥90**	**15-25**	**≤5**	**-**	**Yes**
Hill's Prescription Diet i/d Feline	91	89	91	24.1	2.4	Beet pulp, cellulose, guar gum	Yes
Iams Veterinary Formula Intestinal Low-Residue	na	na	na	11.7	3.7	Beet pulp	Yes
Medi-Cal Hypoallergenic/Gastro	na	na	na	35.9	1.2	Cellulose, carrageenan, guar gum, flax meal	Yes
Medi-Cal Sensitivity CR	na	na	na	35.1	2.5	Cellulose, guar gum, carrageenan, carob gum	Yes

Key: Fiber = crude fiber, na = information not available from manufacturer.
*Manufacturers' published values; nutrients expressed as % dry matter; dry foods are preferred because they have slower gastric emptying compared to moist foods.
**Foods with soluble or mixed fiber sources are best (see text).

deficiency will develop because this portion of the bowel is solely responsible for B_{12} absorption. In such cases, parenteral supplementation of B_{12} is necessary. In dogs, cobalamin should be administered at 600 µg to 1 mg weekly for six weeks followed by injections every other week for six weeks then monthly doses until serum B_{12} levels normalize.[b] In cats, a dose of 250 µg weekly for four to six weeks is recommended. When short bowel syndrome is complicated by small intestinal bacterial overgrowth, bacterial uptake of vitamin B_{12} may exacerbate cobalamin deficiency.

Glutamine

Glutamine is the preferred fuel for enterocytes (Chan, 2006; Windmueller and Spaeth, 1974, 1978). Enteral administration of 2% glutamine solutions may benefit patients with short bowel syndrome (Frankel et al, 1993). Research in short-term (one-week) rat models has shown that adding glutamine to intravenous nutritional solutions reduces some aspects of disuse intestinal atrophy and enhances intestinal immune function (Burke et al, 1989; Alverdy et al, 1992; Jacobs et al, 1989). Glutamine administered intravenously for six to seven days prevents decreased intestinal weight, DNA content, villous height (O'Dwyer et al, 1989) and prevents decreased sucrase and lactase activities (Grant and Snyder, 1988) in adult rats fed parenterally. However, administering glutamine via foods (Vanderhoof et al, 1992a) and intravenous solutions (Remillard et al, 1998; Scott and Moellman, 1992) to research animals for more than one week was not shown to improve intestinal morphology. Glutamine may be a conditionally essential amino acid only during early periods of physiologic stress to stimulate DNA synthesis and increase mucosal mass early in recovery (Lacey and Wilmore, 1990). For example, rats undergoing abdominal radiation and fed glutamine orally the subsequent eight days had significant increases in jejunal villous numbers and height and an increase in the number of mitoses per crypt. Non-irradiated control rats fed the same glutamine-enriched food had no significant increase in mucosal cell activity (Klimberg et al, 1990). In one study performed in cats with methotrexate-induced intestinal injury, glutamine supplementation of a purified food failed to provide a benefit (Marks et al, 1996). Additional studies are needed to assess the benefits of glutamine supplementation in dogs and cats with GI disease including short bowel syndrome.

FEEDING PLAN

The goals of dietary and medical therapy for patients with short bowel syndrome are to provide adequate nutritional support during the period of intestinal adaptation and to stimulate adaptive changes that increase function in the remaining bowel segments. Diarrhea should be controlled as soon as possible because most pet owners will not tolerate persistent diarrhea. Changes required in the feeding management of short bowel syndrome are primarily determined by the function of the remaining small intestine. The feeding plan is often used in conjunction with medical therapy. (See below.)

Assess and Select the Food

Parenteral nutritional support is often required initially to meet nutritional, fluid and electrolyte needs as patients with short bowel syndrome recover from surgery. This is of particular benefit in situations in which the remaining intestine does not have normal function (e.g., infiltrative disease), in patients that have a low body condition score (1/5 to 2/5) at the time of surgery and in patients with complete or partial anorexia postoperatively. Reestablishing normal intestinal function and stimulating adaptation should begin as soon as the patient tolerates food enterally. Experimentally, intestinal adaptation did not occur in dogs with short bowel syndrome fed only parenterally (Feldman et al, 1976). Intestinal adaptation depends on using the remnant bowel, and not "bowel rest."

Parenteral administration of nutrients can be used in conjunction with enteral refeeding to meet the patient's requirements. The combination of continuous enteral nutrition through a feeding tube (nasoesophageal, esophageal, gastrostomy or enterostomy) and partial parenteral nutrition can be used in anorectic patients. A reduced fraction of the nutrient requirements (typically up to 30%) are given enterally, which provides nutrients and trophic factors for the adapting intestine. The remaining nutrient requirements are provided parenterally. This combination of feeding methods can be used in referral and primary care hospitals.

Continuous enteral nutrition consists of providing the calculated food volume at a constant rate over a prolonged period of time (12 to 24 hours). Studies in normal dogs and cats show that continuous enteral nutrition is well tolerated (Abood and Buffington, 1992; Chandler et al, 1996). Gravity drip, an intravenous infusion pump or an enteral feeding pump can be used to administer the food. The remaining nutrients are provided parenterally. Because only part of the patient's protein and caloric needs are being met parenterally, partial parenteral nutrition solutions are less hypertonic and may be administered through a peripheral vein (cephalic or saphenous) if less than 550 mOsm/l. This technique is less cumbersome and expensive than parenteral nutrition, which provides full caloric and protein needs, but requires central venous access. Partial parenteral nutrition may provide 30 to 70% of the patient's protein and caloric requirements assuming the remaining requirements are met through enteral nutrition. The solutions used in partial parenteral nutrition are similar to those used for parenteral nutrition, but more dilute glucose solutions are required. Providing 20% calories as glucose and 80% as lipid reduces the osmolality of the final solution and thus reduces endothelial irritation. Studies evaluating the use of partial parenteral nutrition demonstrate that complications are infrequent (Chan et al, 2002).

Refeeding should begin with a food that has the appropriate levels of key nutritional factors for patients with short bowel syndrome. **Tables 59-2** and **59-3**, provide the key nutritional factor content of selected veterinary therapeutic foods marketed for malabsorptive-type GI diseases in dogs and cats, respectively. These tables also include recommended levels of key nutritional factors for comparison. Appropriate formulations will be energy dense enough to meet the daily energy requirement of the patient in a reasonable volume of food and stimulate adaptation of remaining small bowel segments. Dry foods may be preferred because they may increase gastric retention time; it takes longer to lower the digesta osmolality of dry foods compared to moist foods (Chapter 54).

A liquid monomeric food containing glutamine and soluble fiber can be mixed with dry food during the first few days of recovery (Chapter 25). Such foods contain nutrients in readily absorbable forms and glutamine to fuel enterocyte hyperplasia.

Assess and Determine the Feeding Method

In contrast to feeding frequency commonly recommended for healthy animals (i.e., once or twice daily), patients with short bowel syndrome usually require multiple smaller meals per day to improve digestibility and prevent intestinal overload. Multiple (i.e., six to eight) small meals per day are recommended during the period of intestinal adaptation.

The amount of food may need to be increased to help animals regain or maintain ideal body condition. Aggressive nutritional support is recommended for patients with body condition scores less than 3/5. Additionally, supplemental parenteral feeding should be considered if the patient continues to lose weight despite consumption of what would normally be adequate calories. If parenteral support is used, infusion rates should be calculated to meet the patient's total caloric needs (Chapter 26). In some cases, total or partial parenteral nutritional support should be considered as an interim feeding method until the patient can meet its needs orally. Parenteral nutrition can be withdrawn gradually as intestinal function recovers and enteral feeding provides at least 70% of the patient's caloric needs. As mentioned above, intestinal adaptation did not occur in experimental dogs with short bowel syndrome when they were fed only parenterally (Feldman et al, 1976). Oral feedings or enteral infusions of glutamine-containing foods should continue throughout the parenteral feeding period to facilitate intestinal adaptation.

CONCURRENT MEDICAL THERAPY

Drugs commonly used in patients with short bowel syndrome include opiate antidiarrheal agents (e.g., loperamide, diphenoxylate), antibiotics (e.g., tetracycline, tylosin) and bile salt binding agents (e.g., cholestyramine, ursodeoxycholic acid). In addition, octreotide, a long-acting analogue of somatostatin (Nehra et al, 2001) has been recommended for use by some physicians in short bowel syndrome. This agent inhibits GI secretions and prolongs intestinal transit thus reducing diarrhea and fecal fluid loss. Glucagon-like peptide 2 has also been recommended due to its trophic effect on the GI mucosa (Jeppesen et al, 2001). The use of these compounds has not been investigated in veterinary patients with short bowel syndrome.

REASSESSMENT

Weekly determinations of body weight and condition and stool evaluations are useful for assessing dogs with short bowel syndrome. Medical therapies mentioned above should be considered if dietary therapy alone does not sufficiently improve stool quality and maintain body weight. Well-compensated patients should be evaluated immediately if a decline in body condition is noted. This presentation suggests concurrent GI disease or the onset of small intestinal bacterial overgrowth in dogs without an ileocolic valve.

The prognosis for recovery from short bowel syndrome is variable and cannot be based solely on the extent of resection (Gorman et al, 2006; Yanoff et al, 1992). The patient's preoperative condition, the functional integrity of the remnant bowel, degree of intestinal adaptation and the site of the resection are also important (Yanoff et al, 1992). For example, secondary complications (i.e., small intestinal bacterial overgrowth and large bowel diarrhea due to bile acid overload) may be avoided if the ileocolic valve can be preserved. In cases of surgical excision of intestinal neoplasia, adjuvant cytotoxic chemotherapy may be detrimental to remaining mucosa. In general, intestinal adaptation occurs in most dogs within one to two months and diarrhea may resolve in that time (Guilford and Strombeck, 1996). However, adaptation may continue for years; thus, stool quality may improve with time. In the meantime, the veterinarian and owner must work closely together to ensure optimal postoperative care.

ENDNOTES

a Vital E-A+D containing 100 IU of D and 300 IU of alpha-tocopherol per ml. Schering-Plough Animal Health Corp., Kenilworth, NJ, USA.

b. Steiner J. College of Veterinary Medicine, Texas A&M University, College Station, TX, USA. Personal communication. 2006.

REFERENCES

The references for **Chapter 59** can be found at www.markmorris.org.

CASE 59-1

Vomiting in a Labrador Retriever Crossbred Dog

Douglas Brum, DVM
Angell Memorial Animal Hospital
Boston, Massachusetts, USA

Patient Assessment

An 18-month-old neutered male Labrador retriever crossbred dog was examined for a 12-hour period of vomiting. The dog had no previous medical problems. The night before presentation, the dog ate a rawhide chew and began to vomit several hours later. The vomitus initially contained undigested food but then rapidly changed to a more liquid consistency. The dog weighed 22.3 kg (body condition score [BCS] 3/5) and was extremely depressed and weak. Rectal body temperature was 37.2°C (99°F). Mucous membranes were pale gray and the capillary refill time was three seconds. The heart rate was 180 beats/min. and femoral pulses were fair to poor. The dog's abdomen was tense and extremely painful. Significant clinical pathologic abnormalities included hyperglycemia (glucose 217 mg/dl, normal 65 to 110), thrombocytopenia ($19.0 \times 10^3/\mu l$, normal 122 to 475) with clotting dysfunction (i.e., prolonged prothrombin time [8.7 sec., normal 4.5 to 7.6] and activated partial thromboplastin times [19.8 sec., normal 10.3 to 17.0]). Changes consistent with a small intestinal obstruction were apparent radiographically.

Exploratory celiotomy performed within two hours of presentation revealed a mesenteric volvulus involving the jejunum. Most of the jejunum was purple to black due to occlusion of mesenteric vessels. Resection of all questionable bowel was performed resulting in a final anastomosis of the remaining 10 cm of proximal jejunum to the ileum. The duodenum, pancreatic/bile duct, ileum and ileocecal junction were preserved.

Assess the Food and Feeding Method

The dog was normally fed a commercial dry grocery brand food (Purina Dog Chow[a]) once daily. Water was available free choice. Treats, snacks and table foods were given to the dog occasionally.

Questions

1. What preoperative, intraoperative and postoperative care is important for this dog?
2. What complications might occur subsequent to intestinal resection in this patient?
3. What are the key nutritional factors and feeding plan for this dog?

Answers and Discussion

1. Most dogs with mesenteric volvulus present in hypovolemic or endotoxic shock and therefore require immediate aggressive fluid therapy and broad-spectrum antibiotics preoperatively. Rapid surgical intervention is required in cases of small bowel obstruction. Intraoperative blood loss and hemorrhage due to coagulopathies may complicate recovery. Postoperative concerns include fluid losses, electrolyte imbalances, infection control and caloric intake. These problems can be addressed through aggressive fluid therapy, electrolyte replacement, continued broad-spectrum antibiotics and assisted feeding.
2. Short bowel syndrome often occurs when a large portion of the small intestine is removed, resulting in maldigestion and malabsorption causing diarrhea, steatorrhea, malnutrition and weight loss. The remaining length of small intestine will hypertrophy and absorptive capability will significantly increase; however, the functional capacity of the remaining intestine is difficult to predict and varies from case to case. Generally, complete adaptation takes months.
3. The key nutritional factors for this dog in the immediate postoperative days are water, electrolytes, energy (fat) and protein. Longer-term management of dogs with short bowel syndrome includes providing nutritional support to the patient until the intestine adapts, the diarrhea is controlled and weight can be maintained. A highly digestible food fed in small frequent feedings (i.e., six to eight meals/day) is recommended. Food characteristics should be individually modified to meet each patient's specific needs. Eventually, the patient may be fed its normal or similar food.

Progress Notes

The packed cell volume decreased to 19% during surgery; therefore, the dog was given one unit (500 ml) of packed red cells and one unit (50 ml) of fresh frozen plasma during surgery. Postoperatively, the dog had large amounts of bloody diarrhea, became hypoproteinemic and continued to have significant fluid losses through vomiting and diarrhea.

Crystalloid solutions supplemented with potassium were administered in quantities sufficient to meet fluid requirements and replace ongoing losses. The dog was given a parenteral mixture designed to meet daily fluid, electrolyte, resting energy and protein requirements. This mixture was administered via a peripheral catheter for the first five days after surgery (Chapter 26). After four days, the vomiting had resolved and a nasoesophageal tube (8 Fr.) was placed for a continuous infusion of a commercial liquid monomeric food (Peptamen[b]). This homogenized food contains protein, carbohydrates and fat in small, readily absorbable forms, has a caloric density of 1 kcal (4.2 kJ)/ml and contains glutamine. To meet the daily energy requirement of this dog, 720 ml of the monomeric food were infused via nasoesophageal tube continuously over 24 hours. This liquid food accounted for approximately 720 ml of the patient's daily water requirement, thus infusion of the intravenous crystalloid fluid was appropriately reduced.

After seven days in the hospital, the patient was discharged with instructions for the owner to feed a mixture of a commercial moist growth food (Science Diet Canine Growth[c]), the monomeric liquid food and small amounts of a moist high-fiber veterinary therapeutic food (Prescription Diet Feline r/d[c]). The moist growth food (521 kcal/can [2.18 MJ/can]) provided a nutrient-dense, highly digestible food to promote nutrient absorption and weight gain or maintenance. The monomeric food provided nutrients that were immediately absorbable with little or no digestion, and was to be used in decreasing amounts as the remaining small bowel adapted. Feline r/d (30% dry matter fiber) was used in small amounts to help control the diarrhea. Initially, the dog went home with instructions for the owner to feed 250 kcal (1.05 MJ) of the monomeric liquid food with each half can (260 kcal [1.09 MJ]) of the growth formula and to add 2 tbs of the high-fiber veterinary therapeutic food as needed to manage diarrhea. This mixture was offered every two to three hours for the first week and then less frequently as the dog tolerated larger meals. The proportions of these foods were varied over the next several weeks, depending on the dog's appetite, body weight and condition and stool quality.

The dog's body weight and condition declined initially; however, as stool quality gradually improved, the body weight and condition improved so that the dog was essentially normal eight weeks after surgery. The dog was fed the moist growth food only until its weight stabilized. After six months, the dog was fed a commercial dry maintenance-type food (Science Diet Canine Maintenance[c]) free choice. Four years postoperatively, the dog continued to do well, was maintaining a normal weight of 22.7 kg and body condition score (BCS 3/5) and had reasonably normal stools. The dog was fed two meals daily.

Endnotes

a. Ralston Purina Co., St Louis, MO, USA.
b. ClinTec, Chicago, IL, USA.
c. Hill's Pet Nutrition Inc., Topeka, KS, USA. These products are available under different names.

Bibliography

Shealy PM, Henderson RA. Canine intestinal volvulus. A report of nine new cases. Veterinary Surgery 1992; 21: 15-19.
Yanoff SR, Willard MD, Boothe HW, et al. Short-bowel syndrome in four dogs. Veterinary Surgery 1992; 21: 217-222.

Chapter 60

Small Intestinal Bacterial Overgrowth

Deborah J. Davenport
Chris L. Ludlow
Karen L. Johnston
Rebecca L. Remillard

*"The microbe is so very small you cannot make him out at all.
But many sanguine people hope to see him through a microscope."
Hilaire Belloc, More Beasts for Worse Children (1897)*

CLINICAL IMPORTANCE

Small intestinal bacterial overgrowth (SIBO), a diarrheic disorder characterized by excessive numbers of small intestinal bacteria, has received much attention (Willard et al, 1994; Simpson, 1994; Johnston, 1999, 1999a; Davenport et al, 1994). Although the incidence of SIBO is unknown, some authors have suggested that it is present in up to 50% of dogs with chronic small bowel diarrhea (Rutgers et al, 1995), whereas others suggest that it occurs rarely in clinical practice (Johnston, 1999a; German et al, 2003). Controversy exists as to whether SIBO is a synonym for or a subset of a group of chronic enteropathies termed antibiotic- or tylosin-responsive diarrhea (Westermarck et al, 2005; Hall and Simpson, 2000).

PATIENT ASSESSMENT

History and Physical Examination

Affected dogs usually present with a history of weight loss and intermittent small bowel diarrhea. Borborygmus and flatulence are also common complaints. Physical examination findings are often unremarkable. Poor body condition (body condition score [1/5 or 2/5]) and unthriftiness may be present if the condition is longstanding.

Laboratory and Other Clinical Information

The gold standard for diagnosing SIBO is quantitative aerobic and anaerobic culture of undiluted duodenal juice. Samples can be collected via endoscopy or direct needle aspiration at surgery (Davenport, 1996; Papasouliotis et al, 1998; Johnston, 1999b). In dogs and cats, the small intestine normally contains a relatively sparse bacterial flora compared with the densely populated oral cavity and large bowel. Historically, the accepted upper limit for small intestinal bacterial flora has been 10^5 colony-forming units (CFU)/ml based on work done before 1984 (Batt and Needham, 1983). Subsequent studies have demonstrated that the small bowel of healthy dogs may contain bacteria in excess of 10^5 CFU/ml (Davenport et al, 1994, 1994a; Ludlow and

Box 60-1. Oligosaccharides.

Oligosaccharides are naturally-occurring carbohydrates found in some fruits, vegetables and grains. Structurally, oligosaccharides are sugar polymers that contain up to six sugars. Oligosaccharides containing fructose are termed fructooligosaccharides (FOS). Those that contain mannose are termed mannanoligosaccharides or MOS and so on. Typically found in low concentrations in foods, these complex carbohydrates can also be manufactured for commercial purposes using microbial or plant-derived enzymatic digestion of sugars.

Oligosaccharides resist digestion by mammalian digestive enzymes. Thus, they are classified as fibers or resistant starches. Because they resist digestion, oligosaccharides enter the large bowel in an intact form where they are readily fermented by certain colonic bacteria such as *Bifidobacterium* and *Bacteroides* spp. Based on in vitro studies, the fermentability of oligosaccharides is intermediate between that of cellulose and lactulose. Other organisms such as lactobacilli, eubacteria and clostridia do not readily use oligosaccharides. This preferential fermentation pattern suggests dietary supplementation with oligosaccharides may help foster beneficial gut bacteria.

The addition of oligosaccharides to pet foods has been studied with variable results. The inclusion of FOS at 0.75% (dry matter) did not influence the duodenal flora of healthy cats quantitatively or qualitatively. However, the fecal flora of cats was affected, resulting in increased numbers of lactobacilli and reduced numbers of *Escherichia coli.* Similar findings have been reported to occur in healthy cats consuming another oligosaccharide (i.e., lactosucrose). The clinical significance of these findings is unknown.

Investigators studied FOS supplementation in a group of healthy German shepherd dogs thought to have small intestinal bacterial overgrowth based on bacterial counts of specimens obtained by needle aspiration of the proximal small bowel at the time of surgery. In these dogs, the inclusion of FOS at 1.0% (as fed) was associated with changes in duodenal bacterial flora. However these changes were of less magnitude than normal dog variability for these parameters. Again, the clinical significance of these findings is unknown.

In some species, MOS derived from yeast cell walls binds to intestinal pathogens such as *Salmonella* spp. MOS inhibits attachment of salmonella to the intestinal mucosa by preferentially binding lectins. This effect has not been demonstrated to occur in companion animals to date.

The Bibliography for **Box 60-1** can be found at www.markmorris.org.

Davenport, 2000; Johnston, 1999a). Normal cats also have small intestinal bacterial counts in excess of 10^5 CFU/ml (Papasouliotis et al, 1998; Johnston et al, 1993). These findings suggest that laboratories should establish their own control or reference ranges for duodenal juice using their own sampling and microbiologic techniques. Furthermore, quantitative microbiology is cumbersome, invasive and not readily available to practitioners. Therefore, a number of other diagnostic modalities have been explored.

Other tests useful in diagnosing SIBO include serum folate and cobalamin concentrations, breath hydrogen measurements (with or without lactulose administration), serum total unconjugated bile acids and intestinal permeability tests. Determination of fasting serum folate and cobalamin concentrations is a rapid, noninvasive and simple method for evaluating dogs with suspected SIBO. Folate and cobalamin analyses have been useful in an experimental model of SIBO (Davenport, 1986) and in naturally occurring cases (Simpson, 1994; Batt and Morgan, 1982; Williams, 1991). However, these assays have low sensitivity and specificity (Rutgers, 1996; Simpson, 1994; German et al, 2003). Diet can influence serum folate and cobalamin concentrations. An analytical survey of commercial foods performed in 1994 revealed a wide range of dietary folate levels (Davenport et al, 1994a). Serum folate and cobalamin concentrations obtained from healthy dogs consuming foods containing high folate and cobalamin levels often exceed the upper limits of the reference ranges established for these vitamins (Davenport et al, 1994a; Williams, 1991). The influence of food on folate and cobalamin concentrations is responsible in part for the poor sensitivity of these assays for the diagnosis of SIBO.

Breath hydrogen testing has been used in human and veterinary medicine to diagnose SIBO. This technique is based on the fact that hydrogen is produced as a by-product of bacterial rather than mammalian metabolism. When given a carbohydrate substrate such as a sugar solution or ^{14}C-d-xylose, bacteria produce hydrogen, which can be measured in expired breath. Intestinal transit time can influence this technique; therefore, it is best considered a tool for assessment of carbohydrate assimilation (Johnston, 1999a). Recently, a ^{13}C-glycocholic acid blood test was validated for use in dogs. This test, which is based on the bacterial deconjugation of glycocholic acid, has the potential to recognize increased numbers of small intestinal bacteria through the early detection of ^{13}C-glycocholic acid (Suchodolski et al, 2005). Clinical data in affected animals, however, are lacking.

Intestinal permeability tests are nonspecific tools useful for evaluating animal patients with suspected small intestinal disease. These tests are most commonly available at referral centers and veterinary teaching hospitals.

Response to therapy with antibiotics should not be overlooked as an effective diagnostic tool. A therapeutic trial may be particularly useful in situations when quantitative cultures are not possible (Westermarck et al, 2005).

Risk Factors

A number of risk factors have been identified for SIBO. German shepherd dogs appear to be predisposed to this enteropathy (Willard et al, 1994; Batt and Needham, 1983) possibly because of IgA deficiency (Batt et al, 1991; Whitbread et al, 1984; Willard et al, 1994). The recent development of fecal IgA assays has made detection of IgA deficiency more convenient as compared to measurement of IgA levels in intestinal biopsy samples (Tress et al, 2006; Littler et al, 2006).

Exocrine pancreatic insufficiency is also a predisposing factor for SIBO, and this condition can complicate management of exocrine pancreatic insufficiency (Williams et al, 1987).

Investigators have hypothesized that kenneled dogs (especially beagles) may be more likely to have duodenal fluid bacterial counts in excess of 10^5 CFU/ml (Batt et al, 1992).[a] Kennel-housed beagles, German shepherd dogs, Yorkshire terriers and poodles have subsequently been found to have increased counts (Willard et al, 1994; Davenport et al, 1994, 1994a). Quantitative counts in these apparently healthy dogs have ranged up to 10^8 CFU/ml. Potential causes for abnormal bacterial counts in kennel-housed dogs include environment (i.e., cleanliness), coprophagia and breed-specific characteristics (e.g., IgA deficiency). The bacterial flora of healthy colony cats, healthy pet cats and cats with gastrointestinal (GI) disease has been investigated (Johnston, 1996b). Both healthy colony and pet cats had small intestinal bacterial counts exceeding 10^5 CFU/ml duodenal fluid. Clinically abnormal cats had similar bacterial counts but had lower levels of anaerobic and microaerophilic bacteria.

Etiopathogenesis

SIBO can develop any time normal host defenses are impaired. Loss of gastric acid secretion, normal intestinal peristalsis, interdigestive ("housekeeper") motility, ileocolic valve function or local IgA production can result in SIBO. In people, intestinal stasis is the most common cause of SIBO; however, this particular underlying cause is far less common in dogs.

Key Nutritional Factors

Key nutritional factors for patients with SIBO are listed in **Table 60-1** and discussed in more detail below.

Digestibility

Feeding highly digestible (fat and digestible [soluble] carbohydrate ≥90% and protein ≥87%) foods provides several advantages for managing dogs with SIBO. Nutrients from these low-residue foods are more completely absorbed in the proximal gut. Highly digestible foods are also associated with reduced osmotic diarrhea due to fat and carbohydrate malabsorption and reduced production of intestinal gas due to carbohydrate malabsorption. The ideal food for SIBO patients is lactose free to avoid the complication of lactose intolerance due to loss of brush border disaccharidases.

Fat

Energy-dense foods are preferred for managing patients with chronic enteropathies. Calorie-dense products allow the clinician to provide smaller volumes of food at each meal, which minimizes GI stretch and secretions. Unfortunately, energy-dense foods tend to be high in fat. High-fat foods may contribute to osmotic diarrhea and GI protein losses, which complicate SIBO. Therefore, it is often advantageous to initially provide a food with moderate energy density (3.5 to 4 kcal/g [14.6 to 16.7 kJ/g] dry matter [DM]) that contains moderate levels of fat (12 to 15% DM for dogs and 15 to 25% DM for cats). Higher fat and more energy-dense foods can be offered if the patient tolerates these fat levels.

Table 60-1. Key nutritional factors for foods for dogs and cats with small intestinal bacterial overgrowth.*

Factors	Recommended levels
Digestibility	≥87% for protein and ≥90% for fat and digestible carbohydrate
Fat	12 to 15% for dogs 15 to 25% for cats

*Nutrients expressed on a dry matter basis.

Other Nutritional Factor

Prebiotic Fibers

Fructooligosaccharides (FOS) and other prebiotic resistant starches have been proposed for use in managing patients with SIBO. These indigestible sugars are thought to promote beneficial bacteria at the expense of bacterial pathogens (Fishbein et al, 1988; Hidaka et al, 1990; Hussein et al, 2005) (**Box 60-1**). When FOS was fed (1.0% as fed) to a group of German shepherd dogs with asymptomatic SIBO, total bacterial counts were reduced within the duodenum (Willard et al, 1994a). However, this reduction was smaller than the change in bacterial numbers demonstrated within the same dogs at different sampling intervals. Therefore, the clinical utility of FOS and other oligosaccharides in the treatment of SIBO remains unproven in dogs. In cats, feeding the non-digestible trisaccharide lactosucrose increased fecal counts of the favorable bacteria lactobacilli and bifidobacteria and decreased numbers of potential pathogens such as clostridia and Enterobacteriaceae (Terada et al, 1993).

FEEDING PLAN

The feeding plan is often used in conjunction with other medical therapy. Underlying causes of SIBO (e.g., partial intestinal obstruction) should be identified and treated before specific medical and dietary therapy is instituted. Antibiotic therapy is usually required for effective management of SIBO. Antibiotic selection should be based on culture and antimicrobial sensitivity testing of specific pathogens identified in duodenal aspirates. Tetracycline or tylosin should be used if no pathogen is isolated (Westermarck et al, 2005).

Assess and Select the Food

Levels of key nutritional factors should be evaluated in foods currently fed to patients with SIBO and compared with recommended levels (**Table 60-1**). Key nutritional factors include food digestibility and fat content. Information from this aspect

Table 60-2. Key nutritional factors in selected highly digestible commercial veterinary therapeutic foods marketed for dogs with small intestinal bacterial overgrowth compared to recommended levels.*

Dry foods	Fat (%)	Protein digestibility (%)	Fat digestibility (%)	Carbohydrate digestibility (%)	Ingredient comments
Recommended levels	**12-15**	**≥87**	**≥90**	**≥90**	**–**
Hill's Prescription Diet i/d Canine	14.1	92	93	94	–
Iams Veterinary Formula Intestinal Low-Residue	10.7	na	na	na	FOS, MOS prebiotics
Medi-Cal Gastro Formula	13.9	na	na	na	FOS prebiotic, *Bacillus subtilis* dried fermentation extract
Medi-Cal Low Fat LF 20	6.6	na	na	na	MCT
Purina Veterinary Diets EN GastroENteric Formula	12.6	84.5	91.4	94.4	Sodium silico aluminate, FOS, MOS prebiotics
Royal Canin Veterinary Diet Digestive Low Fat LF 20	6.6	na	na	na	FOS, MOS prebiotics
Moist foods	**Fat (%)**	**Protein digestibility (%)**	**Fat digestibility (%)**	**Carbohydrate digestibility (%)**	**Ingredient comments**
Recommended levels	**12-15**	**≥87**	**≥90**	**≥90**	**–**
Hill's Prescription Diet i/d Canine	14.9	88	94	93	–
Iams Veterinary Formula Intestinal Low-Residue	13.2	na	na	na	–
Medi-Cal Gastro Formula	11.7	na	na	na	FOS prebiotic
Medi-Cal Low Fat LF	9.0	na	na	na	–
Purina Veterinary Diets EN GastroENteric Formula	13.8	85.1	95.6	92.2	MCT
Royal Canin Veterinary Diet Digestive Low Fat	6.9	na	na	na	Inulin prebiotic

Key: na = information not available from manufacturer, FOS = fructooligosaccharide, MOS = mannanoligosaccharide, MCT = medium-chain triglyceride.
*Manufacturers' published values. Nutrients expressed as % dry matter.

Table 60-3. Key nutritional factors in selected highly digestible commercial veterinary therapeutic foods marketed for cats with small intestinal bacterial overgrowth compared to recommended levels.*

Dry foods	Fat (%)	Protein digestibility (%)	Fat digestibility (%)	Carbohydrate digestibility (%)	Ingredient comments
Recommended levels	**15-25**	**≥87**	**≥90**	**≥90**	**–**
Hill's Prescription Diet i/d Feline	20.2	88	92	90	–
Iams Veterinary Formula Intestinal Low-Residue	13.7	na	na	na	FOS, MOS prebiotics
Medi-Cal Hypoallergenic/Gastro	11.5	na	na	na	FOS prebiotic, *Bacillus subtilis* dried fermentation extract
Purina Veterinary Diets EN GastroENteric Formula	18.4	94.0	93.1	79.7	–
Royal Canin Veterinary Diet Intestinal HE	23.7	na	na	na	FOS, MOS prebioti sodium silico aluminate
Moist foods	**Fat (%)**	**Protein digestibility (%)**	**Fat digestibility (%)**	**Carbohydrate digestibility (%)**	**Ingredient comments**
Recommended levels	**15-25**	**≥87**	**≥90**	**≥90**	**–**
Hill's Prescription Diet i/d Feline	24.1	91	89	91	–
Iams Veterinary Formula Intestinal Low-Residue	11.7	na	na	na	FOS prebiotic
Medi-Cal Hypoallergenic/Gastro	35.9	na	na	na	FOS prebiotic
Medi-Cal Sensitivity CR	35.1	na	na	na	–

Key: na = information not available from manufacturer, FOS = fructooligosaccharide, MOS = mannanoligosaccharide.
*Manufacturers' published values. Nutrients expressed as % dry matter.

of assessment is essential for making any changes to foods currently provided. Changing to a more appropriate food is indicated if key nutritional factors in the current food do not match recommended levels.

Commercial veterinary therapeutic foods that are highly digestible and designed for patients with GI disease are recommended for patients with SIBO (**Tables 60-2** and **60-3** for dogs and cats, respectively). Many of these foods contain moderate levels of dietary fat. Young growing dogs and cats with SIBO should receive a food that meets the optimal levels of key nutritional factors for growth.

Assess and Determine the Feeding Method

Because the feeding method is often altered in patients with SIBO, a thorough assessment should include verification of the feeding method currently being used. Items to consider include feeding frequency, amount fed, how the food is offered, access to other food and who feeds the animal. All of this information should have been gathered when the history of the animal was obtained. If the animal has a normal body condition score (2.5/5 to 3.5/5), the amount of food previously fed was probably appropriate.

Ideally, patients with SIBO should be fed multiple small meals per day as indicated by animal acceptance and tolerance for the food. Meal size can be increased as tolerated by the patient after clinical signs have been successfully managed for several weeks.

REASSESSMENT

Owners of affected animals should be asked about frequency of diarrhea, borborygmi and flatus. Body weight and condition should be evaluated frequently to assess resolution of malabsorption. In general, SIBO can be managed effectively with a combination of medical (e.g., antibiotic) and nutritional therapies.

ENDNOTE

a. Williams DA, School of Veterinary Medicine, Purdue University, West Lafayette, IN. Personal communication. 1993.

REFERENCES

The references for **Chapter 60** can be found at www.markmorris.org.

Chapter 61

Introduction to Large Intestinal Diseases

Deborah J. Davenport
Rebecca L. Remillard

"Never ignore a gut feeling, but never believe that it's enough."
Robert Heller

CLINICAL IMPORTANCE

Disorders of the large intestine are frequently encountered in veterinary practice. A number of potential causes of acute and chronic large bowel diarrhea (**Tables 61-1** and **61-2**) must be distinguished from diseases of other organ systems resulting in gastrointestinal signs. Diarrhea associated with large intestinal conditions differs from that associated with small intestinal disorders (Table 55-4). Typical clinical manifestations of large bowel disease include frequent small scanty stools, tenesmus, dyschezia, urgency and passage of mucus and blood. **Table 61-3** lists breed-associated large intestinal disorders.

Chapters 62 through 65 include feeding plans for patients with large intestinal disorders including colitis, idiopathic (irritable) bowel syndrome, constipation/obstipation/megacolon and flatulence. Tables in those chapters list the key nutritional factors for such patients as well as tables that compare the levels of key nutritional factors of commercial foods marketed for patients with large intestinal diseases.

Table 61-1. Potential causes of acute large bowel diarrhea in dogs and cats.

Dietary
Dietary indiscretion
Foreign bodies
Garbage toxicity
Drugs
Cyclophosphamide
Doxorubicin
Infectious agents
Bacteria
- *Campylobacter* spp.
- *Clostridium* spp.
- *Salmonella* spp.

Parasites
- *Giardia lamblia*
- *Trichuris vulpis*
- *Tritrichomonas foetus*

Viruses
- Panleukopenia
- Parvovirus

Miscellaneous
Hemorrhagic gastroenteritis
Colon volvulus

Table 61-2. Potential causes of chronic large bowel diarrhea in dogs and cats.

Infectious causes
- Parasitic
  - *Giardia lamblia*
  - *Trichuris vulpis*
- Bacteria
  - *Campylobacter* spp.
  - *Salmonella* spp.
- Viral
  - Feline immunodeficiency virus
  - Feline leukemia virus
- Fungal
  - Histoplasmosis
  - Pythiosis

Inflammatory bowel disease
- Eosinophilic colitis
- Lymphocytic colitis
- Lymphoplasmacytic colitis
- Regional enterocolitis
- Suppurative colitis

Dietary (adverse reactions to food)
- Food allergy (hypersensitivity)
- Food intolerance

Neoplasia
- Adenocarcinoma
- Adenoma/polyps
- Lymphosarcoma
- Mast cell tumor

Table 61-3. Breed-associated colonic disorders.

Disorders	Breeds
Flatulence	Brachycephalic dogs and cats
Hemorrhagic gastroenteritis	Dachshund, miniature schnauzer, toy poodle
Irritable bowel syndrome	Working breeds, toy breeds
Ulcerative colitis	Boxer, French bulldog

Chapter 62

Large Bowel Diarrhea: Colitis

Deborah J. Davenport
Rebecca L. Remillard
Maureen Carroll

"The physician strengthens nature, and employs food and medicine, for which nature makes use for the intended end."
Thomas Aquinas, Summa Theologica, 1270

CLINICAL IMPORTANCE

Colitis is a common disorder of dogs and cats. A number of infectious, toxic, inflammatory and dietary factors can trigger an episode of large bowel diarrhea (Tables 61-1 and 61-2). This chapter addresses the diagnosis and management of dogs and cats with acute and chronic colitis.

Currently, inflammatory bowel disease (IBD) is thought to be the most common cause of chronic large bowel diarrhea in dogs and cats (Guilford, 1996), although large bowel IBD appears to be more prevalent in dogs (Washabau, 2004). The generic term, IBD, encompasses lymphoplasmacytic enterocolitis, lymphocytic enterocolitis, eosinophilic enterocolitis, segmental granulomatous enterocolitis, suppurative enterocolitis and histiocytic colitis. Specific types are categorized based on the type of inflammatory cells found in the lamina propria. Lymphoplasmacytic colitis is thought to be the most common form of colitis (Leib, 1997, 2005). The severity of the condition varies from relatively mild clinical signs to life-threatening protein-losing enteropathy (PLE), although PLE is seen more commonly with severe small bowel disease. The boxer breed may present with an especially severe variant termed histiocytic or ulcerative colitis (Leib and Matz, 1995).

PATIENT ASSESSMENT

History and Physical Examination

The most common clinical sign in dogs and cats with acute or chronic colitis is large bowel diarrhea characterized by tenesmus, dyschezia, urgency and passage of mucus and blood (Table 55-4). Clinical signs may be intermittent or persistent. The clinical signs tend to increase in frequency and intensity as colitis progresses. The presence of systemic signs is also variable. Some patients present with a history of depression, malaise and inappetence; however, most are alert and active when examined. Hemorrhagic stools indicate a potentially life-threatening disorder (Table 56-1).

When evaluating colitis cases, careful attention should be paid to the dietary history. Food-induced diarrhea is common; a recent change to a moist high-fat or meat-based food may be the source of the patient's diarrhea.[a,b] Often, it is possible to elicit a history of food change, indiscretion, feeding table foods over a holiday or access to garbage, carrion or abrasive materials, such as bones.

Other husbandry issues are also important; for example, records of anthelmintic treatments should be scrutinized. The likelihood that an infectious organism is involved is increased if other animals or people in the household are similarly affected.

Dogs and cats with acute colitis may act depressed and be dehydrated and may exhibit pain on abdominal palpation. Patients should be carefully evaluated for evidence of septic shock. Those patients with systemic signs of illness (i.e., fever and congested mucous membranes) in addition to gastrointestinal (GI) signs should be treated more aggressively.

Physical examination findings vary in dogs and cats with chronic colitis. Many patients have no abnormalities. Rarely, dogs and cats with colitis present with weight loss and poor body condition. In such cases, serious infiltrative colonic disorders (e.g., histoplasmosis, neoplasia, histiocytic colitis or large intestinal disease complicated by small intestinal disease) should be suspected.

Occasionally, thickened loops of bowel may be palpated, especially in cats. Segmental thickening of bowel is consistent with eosinophilic gastroenterocolitis in cats and granulomatous enteritis in dogs (Moore, 1983; Lecoindre et al, 2007). This finding should also be distinguished from intussusceptions, foreign bodies, histoplasmosis and neoplastic lesions.

Laboratory and Other Clinical Information

Because there are many potential causes of acute colitis, achieving a definitive diagnosis can be difficult. In acute cases, it is most important to determine whether the patient's condition is self-limiting or potentially life-threatening. This determination, based on historical and physical findings is critical. Some factors suggest a potentially life-threatening condition (Table 56-1). Cases of a serious nature should be pursued aggressively with diagnostics (i.e., hematology, serum biochemistry profiles, urinalyses and fecal examinations for parasites and other infectious pathogens such as *Giardia* and *Tritrichomonas foetus*) (Leib, 2002; Washabau, 2004a). An abundance of inflammatory cells in a fecal smear is an important finding and justifies a fecal culture. Self-limiting cases are usually approached more conservatively. Diagnostics are often limited to assessing hydration status (i.e., packed cell volume, total protein concentration and body weight) and a thorough examination of feces for parasites and bacterial pathogens (e.g., spores of *Clostridium* spp. or clostridial enterotoxins).

Laboratory findings in patients with chronic colitis are often nonspecific. Hematologic findings are variable and may include blood loss anemia, anemia of chronic disease, eosinophilia and lymphopenia. Serum biochemistry profiles and urinalyses should be performed on samples from patients with chronic diarrhea to assess the systemic affect of the GI disorder and to rule out concurrent disease. Decreased cholesterol values may be seen in patients with colitis. Electrolyte abnormalities, including hypokalemia and hypochloremia, may be identified. Acid-base derangements may occur with diarrhea, but are more common with small bowel disease. Hypoproteinemia and hypoalbuminemia may be recognized in severe cases of PLE. Dehydrated patients may have prerenal azotemia.

Fecal examinations are very important in the evaluation of patients with chronic large bowel diarrhea. Multiple fecal parasite examinations using concentration techniques are necessary to rule out parasitism and infection with organisms such as *Giardia* and *T. foetus*.

Endoscopic abnormalities in chronic colitis may include mucosal granularity, hyperemia, increased friability and inability to visualize colonic submucosal blood vessels (Jergens et al, 1992). Multiple biopsy specimens should be collected from multiple bowel segments. Even if these areas appear normal endoscopically, histologic changes may still be present (Jergens et al, 1992; Roth et al, 1990; Marks and LaFlamme, 1998). The definitive diagnosis of IBD is based on histopathologic examination of endoscopic or surgical biopsy specimens (Wilcock, 1992).

Risk Factors

The risk factors for acute colitis include age, breed, immune status and environment. Puppies and kittens are more susceptible to a variety of infectious pathogens including parasites (Gookin et al, 2004), viruses and bacteria. Likewise, immunocompromised dogs and cats are at risk for contracting viral and bacterial enteritides. Hospitalization and administration of cancer chemotherapeutic drugs are associated with nosocomial infection with *Clostridium* (Twedt, 1992) and *Campylobacter* (Davenport, 1989) spp.

Environment also plays an important role in exposure to pathogens. Dogs and cats kept in unsanitary or overcrowded conditions are much more likely to develop infectious enteropathies. In addition, pets kept in poorly controlled environments have a higher risk for exposure to high-fat table foods, garbage and toxins. Dogs in particular eat indiscriminately. Consumption of rotten garbage, decomposing carrion and abrasive materials (e.g., hair, bones, rocks, plastic, aluminum foil, etc.) can result in severe colitis. Poor husbandry practices including inadequate parasite control and overcrowding also put pets at risk for acute colitis. Feeding raw foods may predispose dogs and cats to infectious enteropathies (Chapter 11).

There does not appear to be an age or gender predisposition for any of the forms of IBD. Certain breeds appear to be at risk for specific colonic disorders (Table 61-3). For example, the boxer breed is linked to histiocytic colitis (van Kruiningen, 1967). Other breeds at risk for chronic inflammatory colonopathies include German shepherd dogs and French bulldogs (Guilford, 1996).

Etiopathogenesis

Chapter 55 describes four mechanisms of diarrhea. In acute colitis, diarrhea may occur as a result of altered gut permeability or osmotic mechanisms. Many of the bacterial pathogens elaborate enterotoxins that serve as potent secretogogues.

Despite intensive study by veterinary and medical researchers, the pathophysiology of IBD is not completely understood (Fiocchi, 1998; Hanauer, 1996). IBD may have a genetic origin in several animal species. Crohn's disease and ulcerative colitis are more common in certain human genotypes; a mutation leads to the development of colitis in mice (Watanabe et al, 2006). Genetic influences have not yet been identified in canine or feline IBD, but certain breeds (e.g., German shepherd dogs, boxers) appear to be at increased risk for the disease (Washabau, 2004) (Chapter 57).

Histiocytic colitis, also termed ulcerative or boxer colitis, is characterized by infiltration of the lamina propria with PAS-positive histiocytes. Some authors have suggested that the presence of these macrophages indicates an infectious etiology, especially in light of the occasional recognition of intralesional pathogens and the marked improvement many of these cases experience with fluoroquinolone therapy. However, to date no organisms have been consistently identified in tissues from affected canine and feline patients and immunohistochemical examination of samples from affected dogs suggests an immunologically-mediated pathogenesis for the disorder (Leib and Matz, 1995; German et al, 2000; Stokes et al, 2001).

Key Nutritional Factors

Key nutritional factors for acute and chronic colitis are listed in **Table 62-1** and discussed in more detail below.

Water

Water is the most important nutrient in patients with acute large bowel diarrhea because of the potential for life-threatening dehydration due to excessive fluid losses and inability of the patient to replace those losses. Moderate to severe dehydration should be corrected with appropriate parenteral fluid therapy rather than using the oral route.

Protein

Protein should be provided at levels sufficient for the appropriate lifestage of colitis patients unless PLE is present. Thus, dry matter (DM) protein levels in foods for adult dogs and cats should be between 15 to 30% and 30 to 45%, respectively (Chapters 13 and 20). Protein levels for growing puppies and kittens should be in the ranges of 22 to 32% and 35 to 50% DM, respectively (Chapters 17 and 24). High biologic value, highly digestible (≥87%) protein sources are preferred.

Some authors recommend the use of elimination foods because of the suspected role of dietary antigens in the pathogenesis of chronic colitis (Nelson et al, 1984; Nelson and Stookey, 1988; Guilford, 1997; German, 2006). In some cases, elimination foods may be used successfully without pharmacologic intervention. Mild to moderate lymphoplasmacytic and eosinophilic colitis are the forms most likely to respond to dietary management (Nelson and Stookey, 1988; Davenport et al, 1987). Chapter 31 discusses elimination foods and protein hydrolysates in more detail. The suspected pathogenesis of IBD involves an increase in gut permeability; therefore, the use of "sacrificial" dietary antigens has been suggested in the treatment of IBD (Box 57-1) (Guilford, 1996).

Table 62-1. Key nutritional factors for dogs and cats with colitis.*

Factors	Recommended levels
Protein	Adult dogs: 15 to 30% Growing puppies: 22 to 32% Adult cats: 30 to 45% Growing kittens: 35 to 50% Option: consider elimination foods or protein hydrolysates (Table 31-5 for dogs and Table 31-6 for cats)
Fat	Dogs: 8 to 15% Cats: 9 to 25%
Digestibility	Highly digestible foods: ≥87% for protein and ≥90% for fat and digestible carbohydrate Fiber-enhanced foods: ≥80% for protein and fat and ≥90% for digestible carbohydrate
Fiber	Highly digestible foods: ≤5% Fiber-enhanced foods: ≥7%
Electrolytes	Sodium: 0.3 to 0.5% Chloride: 0.5 to 1.3% Potassium: 0.8 to 1.1%

*All values expressed on a dry matter basis.

Fat

Compared with the processes involved with other macronutrients, fat digestion and absorption are relatively complex and may be disrupted in patients with GI disease. The action of bacterial flora on unabsorbed fats in the colon resulting in hydroxy fatty acid production is an important cause of large bowel diarrhea. Thus, foods indicated for patients with colitis and many other GI diseases often contain low to moderate amounts of fat (i.e., 8 to 15% DM for dogs and 9 to 25% DM for cats). However, dogs and cats digest fat very efficiently and the process is rarely disrupted except in malassimilative disorders. Therefore, colitis patients can be fed foods containing higher concentrations of fat when greater caloric density is required.

Digestibility

Feeding highly digestible (fat and digestible [soluble] carbohydrate ≥90% and protein ≥87%) foods provides several advantages for managing dogs and cats with longstanding inflammatory colitis. Nutrients from highly digestible, low-residue foods are more completely absorbed from the proximal gut. Low-residue foods are associated with: 1) reduced osmotic diarrhea due to fat and carbohydrate malabsorption, 2) reduced production of intestinal gas due to carbohydrate malabsorption and 3) decreased antigen loads because smaller amounts of protein are absorbed intact. Fiber-enhanced foods inherently have somewhat lower digestibility values. These foods should have protein and fat digestibilities of at least 80% and carbohydrate digestibility of at least 90%.

Fiber

Dietary fiber predominantly affects the large bowel of dogs and cats. Beneficial effects of dietary fiber include: 1) normalizing colonic motility and transit time, 2) buffering toxins (e.g., bile acids and bacterial enterotoxins) in the GI lumen, 3) binding or holding excess water, 4) supporting growth of normal GI microflora, 5) providing fuel for colonocytes and 6) altering viscosity of GI luminal contents.

Fibers are often categorized as soluble, insoluble or mixed. Mixed fibers include beet pulp, brans (rice, wheat or oat), pea and soy fibers, soy hulls and mixtures of soluble and insoluble fibers. Insoluble fibers include purified cellulose and peanut hulls. Soluble fiber sources include fruit pectins, guar gums and psyllium.

Various types and levels of dietary fiber have been advocated for use in patients with colitis. Some veterinarians recommend low-fiber foods (≤5% DM crude fiber) to enhance DM digestibility and reduce quantities of ingesta presented to the colon. Other authors have had success using moderate levels (10 to 15% DM crude fiber) to high levels (>15% DM crude fiber) of insoluble fiber (Dennis et al, 1993). If a food with an increased fiber level is being considered, a crude fiber content of at least 7% DM is advisable. All three strategies have been used successfully in managing patients with colitis and each strategy is patient dependent.

Small amounts (1 to 5% DM fiber) of a mixed- (i.e., soluble/insoluble) fiber type can also be added to a highly digestible food. Some authors have suggested that feeding insoluble or slowly fermentable fibers is detrimental to the management of colonopathies; these suggestions are based on the results of a small, uncontrolled feeding trial comparing cellulose-containing foods with foods containing beet pulp (Reinhart et al, 1994). However, larger, controlled trials incorporating pre- and poststudy histopathology and electron microscopic examination of tissues have not identified any negative effects of slowly fermentable fiber on the colon (Campbell, 1993; Leib, 1992).[c] In fact, many clinicians select foods enhanced with insoluble fiber as their first food option in the management of acute and chronic colitis (Leib, 1989, 2000; Leib and Matz, 1995).[d]

Feeding soluble- or mixed-fiber sources in small quantities to human patients with chronic inflammatory colitis has been advocated (Fiocchi, 1998). Short-chain fatty acid and butyrate enemas induce clinical improvement in patients with ulcerative colitis (Harig et al, 1989; Breuer et al, 1991). Several substrates including beet pulp, soy fiber, inulin and fructooligosaccharides have been demonstrated by in vitro fermentation to produce volatile fatty acids that may be beneficial in inflammatory colonopathies (Sundvold et al, 1995, 1995a, 1995b; Jamikorn et al, 1999). Manufacturers of commercial products usually incorporate these fibers at 1 to 5% DM.

Electrolytes

Potassium depletion is a predictable consequence of severe and chronic enteric diseases because the potassium concentration of intestinal secretions is high. Hypokalemia in association with colitis will be particularly profound if losses are not matched by sufficient dietary intake of potassium.

Electrolyte disorders should be corrected initially with appropriate parenteral fluid and electrolyte therapy. Foods for patients with colitis should contain levels of sodium, chloride and potassium above the minimum allowances for normal dogs and cats. Recommended levels of these nutrients are 0.3 to 0.5% DM sodium, 0.5 to 1.3% DM chloride and 0.8 to 1.1% DM potassium.

Other Nutritional Factors

Acid Load

Acidemia (i.e., normal anion gap hyperchloremic acidosis) is common in patients with acute large bowel diarrhea because fluid secreted in the caudal small intestine and large intestine contains bicarbonate concentrations higher than those in plasma and sodium in excess of chloride ions. Hypovolemia (i.e., severe dehydration) compounds the acidosis in some patients. Severe acid-base disorders are best corrected with appropriate parenteral fluid therapy. Foods for patients with acute colitis should normally produce an alkaline urinary pH. These foods preferably contain buffering salts such as potassium gluconate and calcium carbonate.

Omega-3 Fatty Acids

Omega-3 (n-3) fatty acids derived from fish oil or other sources may have a beneficial effect in controlling mucosal inflammation in patients with chronic inflammatory colitis (Simopoulos, 2002; Barbosa et al, 2003). There is some clinical evidence that dietary omega-3 fatty acid supplementation may modulate the generation and biologic activity of inflammatory mediators. Chapter 57 provides more information.

Vitamins

Folic acid supplementation is recommended for patients receiving long-term sulfasalazine therapy (Linn and Peppercorn, 1992).

FEEDING PLAN

Initially, the objectives for managing acute colitis should be to correct dehydration and electrolyte, glucose and acid-base imbalances, if present. Medical therapy may include antibiotics, anthelmintics, motility modifying agents (e.g., loperamide) and immunosuppressant agents (e.g., corticosteroids and azathioprine). Local-acting antiinflammatory drugs such as sulfasalazine and olsalazine/mesalamine may also be used.

The feeding plan goal is to provide a food that meets the patient's nutrient requirements and allows normalization of colonic motility and function, and fecal water balance. In most cases of acute large bowel diarrhea, initial fasting for 24 to 48 hours, with access to water, either reduces or resolves the diarrhea by simply removing the effects of unabsorbed food and offending agents from the colon. Often, the patient's previous food can be gradually reintroduced over several days.

In chronic colitis, dietary intervention should be aimed at controlling clinical signs while providing adequate nutrients to meet requirements and compensate for ongoing losses through the GI tract. Optimal management of some dogs and cats with chronic colitis may require only dietary manipulation. In other cases, dietary therapy is better used in concert with appropriate

Table 62-2. Key nutritional factors in selected fiber-enhanced veterinary therapeutic foods marketed for dogs with acute or chronic colitis compared to recommended levels.* (See Table 31-5 if foods with novel protein sources or protein hydrolysates are desired.)

Dry foods	Protein (%)	Fat (%)	Protein digestibility (%)	Fat digestibility (%)	Carbohydrate digestibility (%)	Fiber (%)	Na (%)	Cl (%)	K (%)
Recommended levels	**15-30**	**8-15**	**≥80**	**≥80**	**≥90**	**≥7**	**0.3-0.5**	**0.5-1.3**	**0.8-1.1**
Hill's Prescription Diet w/d Canine	18.9	8.8	84	92	95	16.4	0.22	0.46	0.70
Medi-Cal Fibre Formula	26.2	10.6	na	na	na	14.3	0.3	na	1.0
Purina Veterinary Diets DCO Dual Fiber Control	25.3	12.4	79.9	80.4	90.6	7.6	0.34	0.82	0.70
Purina Veterinary Diets OM Overweight Management Formula	31.1	7.2	81.9	78.9	72.3	10.3	0.31	0.97	0.83
Royal Canin Veterinary Diet Calorie Control CC 26 High Fiber	30.9	10.4	na	na	na	17.6	0.33	0.77	0.90
Royal Canin Veterinary Diet Diabetic HF 18	22	9.9	na	na	na	12.1	0.27	0.88	0.88
Moist foods	**Protein (%)**	**Fat (%)**	**Protein digestibility (%)**	**Fat digestibility (%)**	**Carbohydrate digestibility (%)**	**Fiber (%)**	**Na (%)**	**Cl (%)**	**K (%)**
Recommended levels	**15-30**	**8-15**	**≥80**	**≥80**	**≥90**	**≥7**	**0.3-0.5**	**0.5-1.3**	**0.8-1.1**
Hill's Prescription Diet w/d Canine	17.9	12.7	88	90	92	12.4	0.24	0.76	0.64
Medi-Cal Fibre Formula	24.8	9.1	na	na	na	15.0	0.5	na	0.7
Purina Veterinary Diets OM Overweight Management Formula	44.1	8.4	80.9	89.8	62.9	19.2	0.28	0.51	1.06

Key: Fiber = crude fiber, Na = sodium, Cl = chloride, K = potassium, na = information not available from manufacturer.
*Nutrients expressed on a dry matter basis.

pharmacologic agents. Antibiotics (e.g., metronidazole, tylosin, fluoroquinolones [for histiocytic colitis]), anthelmintics, antiinflammatory agents (e.g., sulfasalazine) and immunosuppressive agents (e.g., prednisone, budesonide, azathioprine, cyclosporine) have all been used. Lifelong dietary therapy is often required to control clinical signs in longstanding colitis cases.

Assess and Select the Food

Levels of key nutritional factors in foods currently fed to patients with colitis should be evaluated and compared with recommended levels. Information from this aspect of assessment is essential for making any changes to foods currently provided. Changing to a more appropriate food is indicated if the current food does not match recommended levels.

Withholding food for one to two days and then reintroducing either a highly digestible or fiber-enhanced food is often palliative in managing acute colitis. After feeding the highly digestible or fiber-enhanced food for another three to four days, the pet's regular food may be reintroduced over another three-day period. Further workup is recommended if colitis recurs when the regular food is reintroduced.

Three types of food can be used to manage chronic colitis and they may be attempted in any order: 1) fiber-enhanced foods 2) highly digestible, low-residue foods formulated for GI disease and 3) elimination foods. Alternatively, fiber supplementation can be used in conjunction with the patient's original food. The optimal fiber level is determined by trial and error. There is no physical examination finding, laboratory test or historical fact to predict which method will be successful in any one patient. Dietary trials are often needed to determine which food type works best for individual patients. **Tables 62-2** through **62-5** list selected veterinary therapeutic foods for colitis management for dogs and cats, respectively. These tables compare the key nutritional content of selected veterinary therapeutic foods to the key nutritional factor target levels. Alternatively, homemade foods can be prepared. Foods for extended feeding of puppies and kittens with colitis should also meet the nutritional requirements for growth.

Another option in chronic colitis is to use an elimination food with a limited number of highly digestible, novel protein sources or a protein hydrolysate (Tables 31-5 and 31-6 for dogs and cats, respectively). Commercial veterinary therapeutic foods and homemade foods that contain novel protein sources are often formulated from lamb, rabbit, venison, duck or fish and a highly digestible or unusual carbohydrate source or protein hydrolysates. All other possible dietary sources of protein and carbohydrate should be eliminated including treats, snacks, table foods, vitamin-mineral supplements and chewable/flavored medications (Chapter 31).

Assess and Determine the Feeding Method

A thorough assessment should include verification of the feeding method currently being used. Considerations include feeding frequency, amount fed, how the food is offered, access to other

Table 62-3. Key nutritional factors in selected highly digestible veterinary therapeutic foods marketed for dogs with acute or chronic colitis compared to recommended levels.* (See Table 31-5 if foods with novel protein sources or protein hydrolysates are desired.)

Dry foods	Protein (%)	Fat (%)	Protein digestibility (%)	Fat digestibility (%)	Carbohydrate digestibility (%)	Fiber (%)	Na (%)	Cl (%)	K (%)
Recommended levels	**15-30****	**8-15**	**≥87**	**≥90**	**≥90**	**≤5**	**0.3-0.5**	**0.5-1.3**	**0.8-1.1**
Hill's Prescription Diet i/d Canine	26.2	14.1	92	93	94	2.7	0.45	1.04	0.92
Iams Veterinary Formula Intestinal Low-Residue	24.6	10.7	na	na	na	2.1	0.35	0.66	0.90
Medi-Cal Gastro Formula	22.9	13.9	na	na	na	1.9	0.5	na	0.8
Purina Veterinary Diets EN GastroENteric Formula	27.0	12.6	84.5	91.4	94.4	1.5	0.60	0.85	0.66
Royal Canin Veterinary Diet Intestinal HE 28	33.0	22.0	na	na	na	1.6	0.55	0.99	0.88
Moist foods	**Protein (%)**	**Fat (%)**	**Protein digestibility (%)**	**Fat digestibility (%)**	**Carbohydrate digestibility (%)**	**Fiber (%)**	**Na (%)**	**Cl (%)**	**K (%)**
Recommended levels	**15-30****	**8-15**	**≥87**	**≥90**	**≥90**	**≤5**	**0.3-0.5**	**0.5-1.3**	**0.8-1.1**
Hill's Prescription Diet i/d Canine	25.0	14.9	88	94	93	1.0	0.44	1.22	0.95
Iams Veterinary Formula Intestinal Low-Residue	35.9	13.2	na	na	na	3.9	0.53	0.84	0.84
Medi-Cal Gastro Formula	22.1	11.7	na	na	na	1.0	0.6	na	0.6
Purina Veterinary Diets EN GastroENteric Formula	30.5	13.8	85.1	95.6	92.2	0.9	0.37	0.78	0.61
Royal Canin Veterinary Diet Intestinal HE	23.1	11.8	na	na	na	1.4	0.57	0.92	0.80

Key: Fiber = crude fiber, Na = sodium, Cl = chloride, K = potassium, na = information not available from manufacturer.
*Nutrients expressed on a dry matter basis.
**22 to 32% are recommended levels for growing puppies.

Table 62-4. Key nutritional factors in selected fiber-enhanced veterinary therapeutic foods marketed for cats with acute or chronic colitis compared to recommended levels.* (See Table 31-6 if foods with novel protein sources or protein hydrolysates are desired.)

Dry foods	Protein (%)	Fat (%)	Protein digestibility (%)	Fat digestibility (%)	Carbohydrate digestibility (%)	Fiber (%)	Na (%)	Cl (%)	K (%)
Recommended levels	**30-45**	**9-25**	**≥80**	**≥80**	**≥90**	**≥7**	**0.3-0.5**	**0.5-1.3**	**0.8-1.1**
Hill's Prescription Diet w/d Feline	39.0	9.8	90	87	86	7.6	0.30	0.84	0.84
Hill's Prescription Diet w/d Feline with Chicken	39.9	9.9	91	85	94	7.6	0.35	0.82	0.80
Medi-Cal Fibre Formula	34.2	12.2	na	na	na	14.9	0.5	na	0.9
Purina Veterinary Diets OM Overweight Management Formula	56.2	8.5	91.1	87.7	66.8	5.6	0.57	0.84	0.89
Royal Canin Veterinary Diets Calorie Control CC 29 High Fiber	33.5	10.2	na	na	na	14.0	0.51	0.92	0.88
Moist foods	**Protein (%)**	**Fat (%)**	**Protein digestibility (%)**	**Fat digestibility (%)**	**Carbohydrate digestibility (%)**	**Fiber (%)**	**Na (%)**	**Cl (%)**	**K (%)**
Recommended levels	**30-45**	**9-25**	**≥80**	**≥80**	**≥90**	**≥7**	**0.3-0.5**	**0.5-1.3**	**0.8-1.1**
Hill's Prescription Diet w/d Feline with Chicken	39.6	16.6	92	na	na	10.6	0.38	0.89	0.89
Medi-Cal Fibre Formula	40.0	17.1	na	na	na	16.7	0.4	na	0.8
Purina Veterinary Diets OM Overweight Management Formula	44.6	14.6	87.3	88.6	84.0	10.2	0.31	0.93	0.91
Royal Canin Veterinary Diets Calorie Control CC High Fiber	33.5	21.3	na	na	na	7.7	0.38	0.51	0.77

Key: Fiber = crude fiber, Na = sodium, Cl = chloride, K = potassium, na = information not available from manufacturer.
*Nutrients expressed on a dry matter basis.

Table 62-5. Key nutritional factors in selected highly digestible veterinary therapeutic foods marketed for cats with acute or chronic colitis compared to recommended levels.* (See Table 31-6 if foods with novel protein sources or protein hydrolysates are desired.)

Dry foods	Protein (%)	Fat (%)	Protein digestibility (%)	Fat digestibility (%)	Carbohydrate digestibility (%)	Fiber (%)	Na (%)	Cl (%)	K (%)
Recommended levels	**30-45****	**9-25**	**≥87**	**≥90**	**≥90**	**≤5**	**0.3-0.5**	**0.5-1.3**	**0.8-1.1**
Hill's Prescription Diet i/d Feline	40.3	20.2	88	92	90	2.8	0.37	1.11	1.07
Iams Veterinary Formula Intestinal Low-Residue	35.8	13.7	na	na	na	1.8	0.25	0.63	0.66
Medi-Cal Hypoallergenic/Gastro	29.8	11.5	na	na	na	3.1	0.4	na	0.8
Purina Veterinary Diets EN GastroENteric Formula	56.2	18.4	94.0	93.1	79.7	1.3	0.64	0.58	0.99
Royal Canin Veterinary Diets Intestinal HE 30	34.4	23.7	na	na	na	5.8	0.65	0.97	0.97
Moist foods	**Protein (%)**	**Fat (%)**	**Protein digestibility (%)**	**Fat digestibility (%)**	**Carbohydrate digestibility (%)**	**Fiber (%)**	**Na (%)**	**Cl (%)**	**K (%)**
Recommended levels	**30-45****	**9-25**	**≥87**	**≥90**	**≥90**	**≤5**	**0.3-0.5**	**0.5-1.3**	**0.8-1.1**
Hill's Prescription Diet i/d Feline	37.6	24.1	91	89	91	2.4	0.33	1.18	1.06
Iams Veterinary Formula Intestinal Low-Residue	38.4	11.7	na	na	na	3.7	0.40	0.69	0.93
Medi-Cal Hypoallergenic/Gastro	35.5	35.9	na	na	na	1.2	0.7	na	1.1
Medi-Cal Sensitivity CR	34.5	35.1	na	na	na	2.5	1.1	na	1.1

Key: Fiber = crude fiber, Na = sodium, Cl = chloride, K = potassium, na = information not available from manufacturer.
*Nutrients expressed on a dry matter basis.
**35 to 50% are recommended levels for growing kittens.

food and who feeds the pet. In cases in which colitis is caused by exposure to garbage or inappropriate amounts or types of foods, avoiding foods other than the pet's regular food is recommended and will often prevent further occurrences. If the animal has a normal body condition score (2.5/5 to 3.5/5), the amount of food previously fed (energy basis) was probably appropriate.

Initially, patients with acute colitis should have all food withheld for 24 to 48 hours. After this period, patients should be offered small amounts of food several times (i.e., six to eight times) a day. If the pet tolerates food without a recurrence of diarrhea, the amount fed can be increased over three to four days until the animal is receiving its estimated daily energy requirement in two to three meals per day.

Initially, chronic colitis patients should be fed multiple small meals per day as indicated by acceptance and tolerance of the food. Meal size can be increased and meal frequency can be decreased as tolerated by the patient after clinical signs have been successfully managed for several weeks.

REASSESSMENT

The prognosis for recovery in most cases of acute colitis is good. Bouts of acute colitis often resolve within two to four days with conservative medical and nutritional management. Body weight should be recorded daily until recovery is complete. Changes in body weight from day to day usually reflect changes in hydration status rather than loss or gain of lean or adipose tissue. Further diagnostic testing is warranted if severe large bowel diarrhea persists, or if clinical signs indicative of concurrent small bowel disease become apparent, such as vomiting, hypoalbuminemia and melena.

Weekly recordings of body weight and condition and stool evaluations are useful for assessing patients with chronic colitis. Regaining or maintaining optimal body weight and condition, normal level of activity and alertness and absence of clinical signs are measures of successful dietary and medical management. The feeding method and amount fed can be adjusted as needed to maintain body weight and condition. Additional medical therapies should be considered if dietary therapy alone fails to improve stool quality and maintain body weight.

Dogs and cats presenting with multiple or recurrent episodes of large bowel diarrhea require further diagnostic workup and, most probably, a combination of dietary and medical therapies; however, parasitic causes should be ruled out or treated empirically before pursuing further diagnostics.

ENDNOTES

a. Davenport DJ. Unpublished data. 1996.
b. Remillard RL. Unpublished data. Personal observation. 1996.
c. Kappel L. Louisiana State University, Baton Rouge. Personal communication. 1998.
d. Remillard RL. Unpublished data. 1999.

REFERENCES

The references for **Chapter 62** can be found at www.markmorris.org.

CASE 62-1

Chronic Diarrhea in an Irish Setter

Michael S. Leib, DVM, MS, Dipl. ACVIM (Internal Medicine)
Virginia-Maryland Regional College of Veterinary Medicine
Blacksburg, Virginia, USA

Patient Assessment

A two-and-one-half-year-old neutered female Irish setter was examined for a five-month history of worsening diarrhea. Initially, the dog produced one abnormal stool every four or five days but now had two abnormal stools daily. Diarrhea was accompanied by tenesmus, hematochezia and excess fecal mucus. Hookworm ova were found in a fecal flotation; however, therapy with an appropriate anthelmintic did not improve the clinical signs. No other parasites or ova were identified in three additional fecal flotations. The owner reported no obvious weight loss.

The dog was obtained as a stray after being hit by a car more than a year ago. It sustained an acetabular fracture that was managed conservatively. Three other dogs and four cats housed with this dog were clinically normal. The dog lived inside and was well supervised in a fenced yard.

Physical examination was normal except for the healed pelvic fracture noted on rectal palpation. Rectal mucosa felt normal and there was no evidence of sublumbar lymphadomegaly or intraluminal masses. Body weight was 30 kg with normal body condition (body condition score [BCS] 3/5).

Assess the Food and Feeding Method

A commercial dry grocery brand food (Ken-L-Ration Biskit[a]) and a commercial dry veterinary therapeutic food (Prescription Diet Canine i/d[b]) had been fed during the previous five months. No difference in the diarrhea was noted when the dog ate either food. Table food and other snacks were not offered. Water was available free choice.

Questions

1. Prepare a list of differential diagnoses for this patient.
2. Outline a diagnostic plan for this dog.

Answers and Discussion

1. The following conditions should be strongly considered: lymphoplasmacytic colitis (inflammatory large bowel disease), irritable bowel syndrome, histiocytic ulcerative colitis, neoplasia and whipworm infection. Idiopathic colitis or inflammatory bowel disease involving the colon is a common diagnosis made after biopsy specimens are obtained from dogs with chronic large bowel diarrhea and examined microscopically. The cause is unknown. The causes of irritable bowel syndrome are poorly understood but the disorder may result from psychological influences on the colon resulting in abnormal motility and signs of large bowel diarrhea. This dog was introduced into the household as a stray. Although the dog seemed to interact well with the seven other household pets, group-related social factors may have caused stress that contributed to the diarrhea. Histiocytic ulcerative colitis has been seen most commonly in boxers but can occur in other breeds. It is much less common than lymphoplasmacytic colitis. Neoplasia would be uncommon in a dog of this age although colonic lymphosarcoma may occur in young dogs. Whipworm infection is still possible despite the negative fecal evaluations for parasites. Other causes of chronic large bowel diarrhea include *Giardia* infection, eosinophilic colitis, cecal inversion, bacterial infection (*Yersinia* spp., *Salmonella* spp., others), histoplasmosis, pythiosis and protothecosis. These disorders should only be considered after exclusion of the more likely diagnoses listed above.
2. The diagnostic plan for this dog should include the following: fecal flotation with zinc sulfate, complete blood count, serum biochemistry profile, urinalysis and colonoscopy with collection of multiple mucosal biopsy specimens. The laboratory database will evaluate the dog's anesthetic risk and identify systemic diseases that may produce chronic diarrhea. However, the history and physical examination make systemic disease unlikely. Flexible colonoscopy allows visualization and biopsy of the entire colonic mucosa. Although four routine fecal flotations only identified hookworm ova on one occasion, this procedure is not sensitive for identification of *Giardia* cysts. *Giardia* infection commonly produces small bowel diarrhea but can occasionally cause large bowel signs. Zinc sulfate flotation or formol-ether sedimentation is necessary to identify *Giardia* cysts in feces. Whipworms shed ova intermittently; therefore, infection may be present despite multiple negative fecal examinations.

Progress Notes

Two fecal flotations using zinc sulfate failed to identify *Giardia* cysts or other parasite ova. Results of the complete blood count, serum biochemistry profile and urinalysis were normal except for mild eosinophilia (2,200/µl). The cecum, ascending, transverse and majority of the descending colon were normal during endoscopic examination. A small 0.5-cm bleeding erosion was noted 15 cm from the anus. Biopsy specimens were obtained from the ascending and transverse colon, from three normal appearing areas in the descending colon and from the eroded area 15 cm from the anus. Microscopically, the eroded region had mucosal ulceration and moderate mucosal infiltration with plasma cells and lymphocytes. All other biopsy specimens had moderate lymphoplasmacytic infiltration into the mucosa. Final diagnosis was lymphoplasmacytic colitis.

Further Questions

1. Outline a feeding plan for this dog.
2. What other therapy should be considered for this patient?

Answers and Discussion

1. Several different types of foods can be used in patients with large bowel disease. One strategy involves using a highly digestible, low-residue food to minimize the amount of ingesta entering the colon. Another strategy uses foods with moderate levels of fiber to alter colonic motility, increase production of volatile fatty acids and control pathogen growth by helping maintain normal colonic pH. A third strategy uses an elimination ("hypoallergenic") food (or one containing a protein hydrolysate) to decrease the amount of potential antigens absorbed by the colon. Ideal elimination foods have moderate levels of protein (i.e., avoid protein excess); have reduced numbers of novel, highly digestible protein sources; and avoid excess food additives and biogenic amines. A combination of these dietary strategies can also be tried. Although the etiopathogenesis of lymphoplasmacytic colitis is unknown, limiting exposure of the colonic mucosa to potential antigens is considered an important part of the feeding plan. Use of an elimination food (or one containing a protein hydrolysate) is often the first choice in these cases. Access to table food, snacks and food for other household pets should be avoided. Therapeutic trials with several different food types and careful monitoring are necessary for optimal case management. The food should be fed in an appropriate amount for the animal's body condition and activity level. For this dog, the daily energy requirement was estimated to be 1.6 x resting energy requirement (1,550 kcal [6.49 MJ]).
2. Medical management of chronic colitis also includes antiinflammatory and immunosuppressive drugs (mesalamine, sulfasalazine [sulfapyridine and mesalamine], olsalazine, prednisone, azathioprine) and antimicrobial agents (metronidazole, sulfasalazine, tylosin, other antibiotics). Changing the environment to alleviate stressful situations may also benefit some patients in which irritable bowel syndrome is a complicating factor.

Progress Notes

The dog was fed a commercial dry veterinary therapeutic food, i.e., a novel protein food (Prescription Diet Canine d/d Rice and Duck[b]) for six weeks. The dog was fed two cups twice daily. The owner reported only two bouts of diarrhea during this period. The dog was eating the food readily and maintaining normal body weight and condition.

Flexible colonoscopy was again performed. Friable, granular mucosa was observed around the ileocolic junction and in the descending colon. Erosions were not seen. Histopathologic evaluation of biopsy specimens revealed moderate lymphoplasmacytic colitis with an increased eosinophilic component compared with specimens from previous biopsy sites. The feeding plan was not changed but therapy with sulfasalazine[c] (1 g, t.i.d.) was instituted. Although clinical signs were eliminated, tear production gradually decreased over the next six months. Keratoconjunctivitis sicca is a common side effect of prolonged therapy with sulfa drugs. The dose of sulfasalazine was tapered and increased tear production occurred but intermittent diarrhea also returned. Therapy with oral prednisone was initiated (40 mg every 24 hours) and the dose slowly tapered. Oral administration of 10 mg prednisone every 48 hours in conjunction with the feeding plan controlled most of the clinical signs. Stressful circumstances still caused intermittent diarrhea.

Endnotes

a. Quaker Oats, Chicago, IL, USA.
b. Hill's Pet Nutrition Inc., Topeka, KS, USA. These products are available under different names.
c. Azulfidine. Pharmacia, Dublin, OH, USA.

Bibliography

Leib MS. Chronic diarrhea in a dog. Veterinary Medicine Report 1989; 1: 346-350.

Leib MS, Matz ME. Diseases of the intestines. In: Leib MS, Monroe WE, eds. Practical Small Animal Internal Medicine. Philadelphia, PA: WB Saunders Co, 1997; 685-760.

Nelson RW, Stookey LJ, Kazaxcos E. Nutritional management of idiopathic chronic colitis in the dog. Journal of Veterinary Internal Medicine 1988; 2: 133-137.

Chapter 63

Large Bowel Diarrhea: Idiopathic Bowel Syndrome in Dogs

Deborah J. Davenport
Maureen Carroll
Rebecca L. Remillard

"The colon is an organ of expression."
Dr. Bernhard Berliner (1938)

CLINICAL IMPORTANCE

Idiopathic (irritable) bowel syndrome (IBS) is a poorly defined functional bowel disorder of people and animals believed to be caused by gastrointestinal (GI) dysmotility. IBS is also called spastic colon, nervous colon, spastic colitis and mucous colitis. In people, IBS is a disease entity characterized by recurrent abdominal pain or discomfort associated with altered bowel movements (constipation and diarrhea), in which no obvious histopathologic lesion is identifiable (Halvorson et al, 2006). The postulated pathogenesis for IBS includes abnormalities of GI motility, visceral sensations, the brain and gut complex, personality and postepisodic infections in the colonic mucosa (Hongo and Sato, 2006). It is one of the most common GI complaints in human medicine with random population surveys indicating 12 to 15% of adults are affected (Jones and Lydeard, 1992; Talley et al, 1992; Camilleri and Choi, 1997). In veterinary medicine, IBS is a catchall term for a chronic large bowel disorder of presumed functional origin (Willard, 2003). This disorder is thought to occur far less commonly in pets than in people; however, it has been reported to account for 5 to 17% of large bowel disorders in dogs (Guilford, 1996; Henroteaux, 1990). IBS has not been recognized in cats.

PATIENT ASSESSMENT

History and Physical Examination

Dogs with IBS have chronic, intermittent bouts of diarrhea that are predominantly large bowel in character. Frequent, small-volume, fluid stools containing mucus are reported. Occasionally, explosive bouts of diarrhea and flatus may occur, often in association with abdominal pain. The intermittent diarrhea is often accompanied with varying signs of bloating, nausea, vomiting, dyschezia and tenesmus. Rarely, hematochezia may be seen. Some dogs have abdominal pain that is relieved by eating, eructation or defecation. Borborygmus, belching and flatus are frequent complaints in IBS. Typically, signs are variable and may change from bout to bout.

In some cases, GI signs can be linked to identifiable stressors. A thorough history may elicit such stress-causing variables as showing, work, boarding or changes in the home environment (e.g., owner anxiety, new spouse, child, pet, house or apartment).

Table 63-1. Diagnostic criteria for the irritable bowel syndrome in people.*

Abdominal pain or discomfort, relieved by defecation and/or associated with a change in stool frequency and/or consistency
Altered stool form
Altered stool frequency
Altered stool passage
An irregular pattern of defecation at least 25% of the time
Bloating or feeling of abdominal distention
Passage of mucus
Continuous or recurrent symptoms for at least three months

*Adapted from Thompson WG, Longstreth GF, Drossman DA. Functional bowel disorders and functional abdominal pain. In: Drossman DA, Corrazziara E., Talley NJ, et al, eds. The Functional Gastrointestinal Disorders: Diagnosis, Pathophysiology, and Treatment, 2nd ed. McLean, VA: Degnon, 2000; 351-375.

Table 63-2. Myoelectric and motility abnormalities prominent in people with irritable bowel syndrome.*

Clustered contractions in the small bowel
Delayed but prolonged colonic hypermotility in response to ingestion of food, particularly fats
Increased colonic motility and abdominal pain in response to cholecystokinin
Increased colonic motor activity in response to low concentrations of bile acids
Increased frequency of basal electrical rhythm
Lowered gastroesophageal sphincter pressure
Pronounced colonic hypermotility in response to cholinergic agents
Small bowel transit rate is faster when diarrhea is predominant
Small bowel transit rate is slower when constipation is predominant
Spastic response to rectal distention

*Adapted from Guilford WG. Motility disorders of the bowel. In: Guilford WG, Center SA, Strombeck DR, et al, eds. Strombeck's Small Animal Gastroenterology, 3rd ed. Philadelphia, PA: WB Saunders Co, 1996; 533.

Table 63-3. Key nutritional factors for foods for dogs with idiopathic bowel syndrome.*

Factors	Recommended levels
Soluble fiber**	1 to 5%
Mixed fiber**	5 to 10%
Insoluble fiber**	10 to 15%
Crude fiber***	≥8%

*All values are on a dry matter basis.
**Any one of the three types of fiber listed at the recommended levels can be effective, depending on patient response. See Chapter 5 and Figures 5-12 and 5-13 for more information about dietary fiber types and associated ingredient sources.
***Crude fiber is the only fiber value readily available for pet foods.

Generally, dogs with IBS are in good physical condition and do not exhibit weight loss or poor body condition as is often associated with organic GI disorders (e.g., inflammatory or infectious causes). Affected dogs may exhibit discomfort during abdominal palpation if examined during an acute episode of GI distress. Rectal examination may reveal mucoid feces.

Laboratory and Other Clinical Information

In IBS, colonic dysfunction exists in the absence of structural, biochemical or microbiologic lesions and therefore is a diagnosis of exclusion following an appropriate diagnostic workup (Leib, 2004). Results of routine laboratory tests are usually normal in dogs with IBS. Radiography and colonoscopy are rarely useful in the diagnosis of IBS other than as a tool to rule out organic disorders, because the findings are usually within normal limits. A consistent set of diagnostic criteria has been established for people based on numerous epidemiologic and pathophysiologic investigations (**Table 63-1**) (Zighelboim and Talley, 1993; Horwitz and Fisher, 2001). Clinical criteria have not been standardized in dogs. The diagnosis of IBS is applied to those dogs with the clinical signs and history in which other, more common organic causes have been ruled out.

Risk Factors

In people, IBS occurs three times as commonly in women than men and is often associated with diagnoses of other conditions such as fibromyalgia, interstitial cystitis and psychiatric disorders (Horwitz and Fisher, 2001). In veterinary patients, there is no known gender predilection for IBS. The condition is recognized most commonly in large working breeds (police and military dogs, drug- and bomb-sniffing dogs, search and rescue dogs and handicap assistance dogs) and small, nervous toy breeds. Any dog with a nervous, excitable temperament and/or a behavioral disorder such as separation anxiety seems predisposed to IBS. Abnormal personality traits, nervousness or stressors have been identified as preceding bouts of chronic idiopathic large bowel diarrhea in approximately 40% of IBS cases (Leib, 2000). The diagnosis of IBS should be strictly reserved for those cases in which no abnormalities have been found histologically. Intestinal biopsy specimens are normal in IBS patients (Tams, 2001).

Etiopathogenesis

The etiology of IBS is not defined; however, balloon distention, manometric and motility studies in people suggest disordered GI motility and visceral hyperresponsiveness to stimuli. Recent studies have suggested that neurotransmitter imbalances may be involved in IBS pathogenesis (Horwitz and Fisher, 2001). Additionally, IBS has been reported to occur as a sequelae to infectious enteritis (i.e., salmonellosis, dysentery) (Horwitz and Fisher, 2001). Comparable research has not been performed in dogs. The relationship of stress to the myoelectric and motility abnormalities present in IBS is not completely understood (**Table 63-2**). However, psychological stress can trigger hypermotility. In addition, the effect of central nervous system neuropeptides (e.g., cholecystokinin, serotonin, acetylcholine, vasoactive intestinal peptide and substance P) on GI motility and visceral sensitivity has been recognized (Tache et al, 1990). For example, cholecystokinin infusions promote colonic hypermotility and abdominal pain in patients with IBS.

Key Nutritional Factor: Fiber

Reports suggest that many canine and feline patients with IBS improved clinically when dietary fiber intake was increased

Box 63-1. Medical Therapy to be Considered for Concurrent Use with Appropriate Dietary Management for Dogs with Idiopathic Bowel Syndrome.

Most patients diagnosed with idiopathic bowel syndrome (IBS) respond favorably to increased intake of dietary fiber and can be managed successfully long term with appropriate food and intermittent pharmacotherapy. Medical treatment generally includes, either individually or in combination, antidiarrheal drugs, anticholinergics and tranquilizers.

Pharmacotherapy for diarrhea-predominant IBS includes use of motility-modifying drugs such as loperamide at 0.2 to 0.5 mg/lb, per os, or diphenoxylate at 0.1 to 0.22 mg/lb, per os, b.i.d. Loperamide is a potent antidiarrheal drug that decreases intestinal secretions, enhances absorption, stimulates rhythmic segmental contractions and increases anal sphincter tone. Stool consistency often improves significantly and pain and urgency abate after loperamide therapy. Although loperamide can be used safely on a long-term basis, several days to one to two weeks of therapy is often sufficient to normalize stools. After the first several days of therapy, it may be possible to decrease administration to once or twice daily.

Patients with signs of abdominal pain (e.g., cramping, bloating, assuming an arched-back stance, reluctance to move, loud abdominal gurgling sounds) or those with signs of general distress (e.g., pacing) can be treated with antispasmodics or combination antispasmodic-tranquilizer preparations. Antispasmodics reduce smooth muscle contractility. Abdominal pain can often be relieved by antispasmodic agents and the effects of stressors can be reduced by sedatives. Librax[a] contains the sedative chlordiazepoxide (5 mg) and an anticholinergic agent clidinium bromide (2.5 mg). The dose of Librax is 0.2 to 0.5 mg/lb of clidinium, per os, b.i.d. or t.i.d. Chlordiazepoxide is a benzodiazepine with peripheral smooth-muscle relaxant properties and central nervous system effects. This combination seems to be especially effective in relieving the discomfort that may be associated with increased colonic motor function. The drug can be given when the owner first notices that the patient has signs of abdominal pain or diarrhea or when stressful conditions are encountered and can usually be discontinued after a few days. Long-term use may be necessary (one to two doses daily) in patients affected by unpredictable flare-ups of abdominal distress.

Other anticholinergics such as propantheline (0.25 mg/kg, per os, b.i.d. or t.i.d.), hyoscyamine (0.003 to 0.006 mg/kg, per os, b.i.d. or t.i.d.) or dicyclomine (0.15 mg/kg, per os, b.i.d. or t.i.d.) have been suggested. Anticholinergics can decrease or inhibit gastrointestinal motility, which may worsen diarrhea. In people, side effects include xerostomia, urinary retention, blurred vision, headache, psychosis, nervousness and drowsiness.

Combination therapy (e.g., loperamide plus clidinium/chlordiazepoxide) may be necessary in some patients with diarrhea and abdominal pain. Sulfasalazine, especially when used in combination with loperamide or clidinium, sometimes provides symptomatic relief in patients with significant dyschezia and increased evacuation of small volumes of loose, mucoid stool. This response has been observed in patients in which multiple colon biopsy specimens and careful evaluation for pathogenic intestinal organisms have proved negative. Likewise, H_2-receptor blockers such as famotidine at dosages of 0.25 to 0.5 mg/lb, per os, every 24 hours, used in combination with clidinium or isopropamide, may provide better control of IBS-related nausea or vomiting than either drug alone.

The novel use of peppermint oil for the relief of pain in pediatric human patients with IBS has been reported. In randomized, placebo-controlled trials, enteric-coated peppermint oil capsules were found to relieve pain in 75% of affected patients. This treatment has not been evaluated in veterinary medicine.

ENDNOTE

a. Roche Laboratories, Inc., Nutley, NJ, USA.

The Bibliography for **Box 63-1** can be found at www.markmorris.org.

(Leib, 1997, 2004; Guilford, 1996; Leib et al, 1997; Tams, 1992, 2001; Willard, 2003). Increasing dietary fiber alters fecal water content, colonic motility, intestinal transit time and gut microbial populations, all of which may benefit patients with IBS. Patients have been reported to respond to foods containing small amounts of soluble fiber (1 to 5% dry matter [DM]) or moderate amounts of insoluble fiber (10 to 15% DM) (Leib, 1997; Leib and Matz, 1995; Guilford, 1996; Leib et al, 1997; Tams, 2001; Willard, 2003). Foods with 5 to 10% DM mixed (insoluble and soluble) fiber sources are also recommended. However, from a practical matter, obtaining food content of the various fiber types is difficult. Typically, crude fiber values and ingredient lists are all that are available. Thus, it is recommended that foods for patients with IBS contain moderate amounts (≥8% DM) of crude fiber. Ingredient lists may provide information about the predominate type of fiber. Insoluble fiber sources include cellulose and peanut hulls. Soluble fiber sources include citrus and apple pectins, psyllium and gums. Rice bran, oat bran, wheat bran, soy fibers, soy hulls, pea fiber and beet pulp are sources of mixed fibers. Combinations of insoluble and soluble fiber sources would also be considered as mixed fibers. For a more detailed discussion of fiber types, see Chapter 5 and Figures 5-12 and 5-13. **Table 63-3** summarizes the recommended fiber types and levels for dogs with IBS.

FEEDING PLAN

Dietary management may not completely control IBS but is integral to comprehensive management of the condition. Appropriate dietary management can reduce the frequency and severity of clinical signs, either alone or in combination with medical treatment (psychotropic and GI antispasmodic drugs may be beneficial [**Box 63-1**]. Along with dietary and medical management, stressful events that trigger diarrheic episodes should be eliminated or reduced.

Table 63-4. Key nutritional factors in selected veterinary therapeutic foods for dogs with idiopathic bowel syndrome.*

Dry foods	Crude fiber (%)	Primary sources of fiber
Recommended levels	**≥8**	**-**
Hill's Prescription Diet w/d Canine	16.4	Cellulose, soybean mill run, beet pulp
Hill's Prescription Diet w/d with Chicken Canine	17.1	Cellulose, soybean mill run, beet pulp
Medi-Cal Fibre	14.3	Tomato pomace, rice hulls, oat hulls, flax meal, apple pomace
Purina Veterinary Diets DCO Dual Fiber Control	7.6	Soybean hulls, pea fiber, cellulose
Purina Veterinary Diets OM Overweight Management	10.3	Soybean hulls, pea fiber, cellulose
Royal Canin Veterinary Diet Calorie Control CC 26 High Fiber	17.6	Cellulose, pea fiber, rice hulls, beet pulp, psyllium husk
Royal Canin Veterinary Diet Diabetic HF 18	12.1	Cellulose, rice hulls, guar gum
Moist foods	**Crude fiber (%)**	**Primary sources of fiber**
Recommended levels	**≥8**	**-**
Hill's Prescription Diet w/d Canine	12.4	Cellulose
Iams Veterinary Formula Intestinal Low-Residue	3.9	Beet pulp
Medi-Cal Fibre Formula	15.0	Tomato pomace, guar gum, flax meal, carrageenan
Purina Veterinary Diets OM Overweight Management Formula	19.2	Pea fiber, beet pulp, carrageenan
Royal Canin Veterinary Diet Calorie Control CC High Fiber	8.8	Tomato pomace, guar gum, flax meal, carrageenan

*All values expressed on a dry matter basis.

Assess and Select the Food

The principle key nutritional factor for dogs with IBS is dietary fiber. **Table 63-4** lists selected veterinary therapeutic foods with increased levels of fiber that should be considered for dogs with IBS. Changing to a more appropriate food is indicated if the current food's level of fiber is low and/or the type of fiber it contains (i.e., soluble, insoluble or mixed) is unknown. In the event that the fiber content of the food currently being fed is within the recommended ranges, changing to a different food should still be considered. However, the most effective combination of fiber type and level cannot be predicted. These factors are determined by trial and error, on a patient-by-patient basis.

The veterinary therapeutic foods listed in **Table 63-4** include a variety of fiber types and concentrations. Clinicians should become familiar with several of these foods and work closely with the owner to determine the food composition that works best for each individual patient. One approach is to begin with a product containing mixed-fiber types (combination of insoluble and soluble fibers, e.g., brans, soy fibers, pea fiber, beet pulp). If the patient is unresponsive, other food choices should be considered with either soluble or insoluble types of fiber. Figures 5-12 and 5-13 provide information about the solubility of various fiber ingredients. Foods other than those determined to control the clinical signs should be strictly avoided for dogs in which recurring bouts are initiated by food changes, access to garbage or feeding table foods, treats or snacks.

If it is impractical to change the patient's food (e.g., pet owner bias) or if the food currently being fed is necessary for the management of concurrent medical conditions, fiber can be added to the current food. Moist foods are more suitable for fiber supplementation. Separation of fiber sources from kibbles of dry foods can be problematic. Moistening a fiber supplement before adding it to dry food or wetting a dry food before adding the fiber supplement may help. Excessively high levels of fiber added to a food may make the food unpalatable and/or unbalanced. Do not exceed recommended supplemental levels.

Soluble fiber supplementation can be achieved by adding psyllium-husk powder (e.g., Metamucil[a]) to the patient's regular food. The recommended daily starting dose is 1.3 g psyllium powder/kg body weight. This is equivalent to approximately 6 tsp of psyllium powder per 30 lb (13.9 kg) body weight/day (Leib, 2000, 2004). Soluble fiber improves stool quality and supports butyrate production for colonocyte health. However, soluble fiber may not sufficiently alter the underlying motility abnormalities thought to be involved in IBS. Exceeding more than 20%, or one part fiber supplement to five parts food, is not advisable.

High-fiber human breakfast cereals (e.g., Fiber One Bran Cereal[b]) can be used to increase the patient's insoluble fiber intake (Chapter 5, Case 5-1). The recommended starting dose of this fiber source is 0.5 g/kg body weight/day or 1 level tsp/30 lb (13.6 kg) body weight/day. Exceeding more than 5 tsp/30 lb body weight/day is not advisable. Insoluble fiber binds water, increases the bulk of the stool and improves intestinal motility.

Regardless of the supplemental fiber source, adding fiber should be done systematically based on a recommended fiber dose and the patient's response. The supplemental fiber source should be added in small amounts and increased by increments of 25% of the starting dose, every two weeks, until clinical signs improve or resolve. In some cases, the initial addition of a fiber supplement may increase the severity of clinical signs. If this happens, the fiber supplement should be discontinued immediately because clinical signs are unlikely to improve with time.

Assess and Determine the Feeding Method

When switching to a new food, do so gradually over a period of several days. When meal feeding, offering the food once or twice daily is usually sufficient; however, three to four meals per day may be necessary in some cases to minimize the amount of digesta passing into the large bowel at one time. If the patient has a normal body condition score (2.5/5 to 3.5/5), the amount of food previously fed (energy basis) was appropriate. Thus, the same amount of calories of the new food would be a good starting place for the amount to feed.

REASSESSMENT

Regular body weight and condition assessment and stool evaluations are useful for monitoring patients with IBS. Well-compensated patients should be evaluated immediately if a change or decline in condition is noted. Maintaining optimal body weight and condition, normal activity level and behavior and absence of clinical signs are measures of successful dietary and medical management. The feeding method and amount fed can be adjusted as needed to maintain body weight and condition. Additional medical therapy (**Box 63-1**) should be considered if dietary therapy alone is insufficient to improve stool quality and maintain body weight and condition. Finally, the patient's home life should be evaluated in an effort to identify the stressors, if any exist, and then these should be alleviated whenever possible. Clinicians are reminded that being available for communication and providing guidance to clients whose pets are afflicted by the unpredictable clinical signs of IBS are essential to successful management (Tams, 2001).

ENDNOTES

a. Proctor & Gamble, Cincinnati, OH, USA.
b. General Mills Cereals, LLC, Minneapolis, MN, USA.

REFERENCES

The references for **Chapter 63** can be found at www.markmorris.org.

Chapter 64

Constipation/ Obstipation/Megacolon

Deborah J. Davenport
Rebecca L. Remillard
Maureen Carroll

"Austerity causes constipation; excess, diarrhea."
Mason Cooley, City Aphorisms, Twelfth Selection, New York, 1993

CLINICAL IMPORTANCE

The term constipation is applied to those patients that pass stools infrequently or exhibit tenesmus in association with defecation. Constipation is a clinical sign, not a disease, and may result from several disorders, separately or in combination. Constipation is not easily assessed in dogs and cats because it is often difficult to obtain accurate information about their defecation habits. However, constipation appears to be far less common in veterinary medicine than in human medicine. In people, it is the number one gastrointestinal (GI) complaint, accounting for more than 2 million physician visits each year in the United States (Sweeney, 1997; Lembo and Camilleri, 2003).

Obstipation is severe constipation that requires medical therapy in addition to dietary management for relief. The term megacolon refers to anatomic dilatation of the colon. Feline idiopathic megacolon is a frustrating, chronic, recurring problem that often results in euthanasia of affected patients. A similar condition occurs in dogs although it is relatively rare. Megacolon in dogs is usually seen as a consequence of severe chronic constipation resulting from obstruction (e.g., perineal hernias, stenosis of the pelvic canal or pelvic fracture malunion) and/or an underlying innervation defect. In cats, the pathogenesis of idiopathic megacolon remains unclear but appears to result from a generalized abnormality of colonic smooth muscle function (Washabau and Sammarco, 1996; Washabau et al, 2002; Byers et al, 2006).

PATIENT ASSESSMENT

History and Physical Examination

Dogs and cats with constipation typically exhibit tenesmus, dyschezia and abdominal pain. Chronically affected animals may present with systemic signs of illness including weight loss, inappetence, vomiting and depression.

Constipated cats are usually presented for reduced, absent or painful defecation for a period ranging from days to weeks or months. Some cats are observed making multiple, unproductive attempts to defecate in the litter box, whereas other cats may sit in the litter box for prolonged periods without assuming a defecation posture. Dry, hardened feces are seen inside and outside of the litter box. Occasionally, chronically constipated cats have

Table 64-1. Drugs associated with constipation.*

Antacids	Bismuth subsalicylate
Anticholinergics	Diuretics
Anticonvulsants (phenytoin)	Hematinics
Antidepressants	Opiates
Barium sulfate	Sucralfate

*Dimski DS. Constipation: Pathophysiology, diagnostic approach and treatment. Seminars in Veterinary Medicine and Surgery: Small Animal 1989; 4: 247-254.

intermittent episodes of hematochezia or diarrhea due to colonic mucosal irritation, which may give the owner the erroneous impression that diarrhea is the primary problem.

Cats with megacolon are usually presented for repeated episodes of constipation or obstipation. Although it is common for obese cats to present for constipation, chronically obstipated animals often exhibit weight loss and poor body condition. Prolonged inability to defecate may result in other systemic signs, including anorexia, lethargy, vomiting and poor coat quality (Washabau, 2001, 2005; Washabau and Holt, 1999; Bertoy, 2002). Owners of constipated pets should be questioned about medications their pet is receiving because a number of commonly used drugs are associated with constipation (**Table 64-1**). In addition, consumption of bones and raw foods has been associated with constipation and obstipation in dogs. Lastly, owners should be questioned regarding potential exposure to lead because lead poisoning can result in constipation. Consumption of lead-based paint chips and glazed ceramic food bowls are potential sources.

Depression and dehydration may be noted at physical examination of constipated animals. Abdominal palpation often reveals colonic distention and the presence of dry hard feces. Digital rectal examination may also confirm dry hard feces. Rectal examination may also reveal foreign bodies, rectal neoplasia or a reduction in the pelvic inlet due to a previous pelvic fracture. Anal sac disease, perianal fistulas and perineal hernias may be visualized upon examination of the perineum. In dysautonomia, constipation will be accompanied by other autonomic signs including mydriasis, distended urinary bladder, dysphagia, prolapsed nictitans and dry mucous membranes (Lyons, 1998).

Laboratory and Other Clinical Findings

Most constipated pets do not require diagnostic evaluation beyond a careful history and physical examination and the appropriate exclusion of systemic and GI causes. However, all obstipated and chronically constipated pets should have a workup that includes a complete blood count, biochemistry profile, urinalysis, thyroxine analysis and abdominal radiography. Further diagnostic evaluation may require abdominal ultrasound, GI contrast studies and/or colonoscopy.

Risk Factors

In cats, constipation occurs most commonly in middle-aged (mean = 5.8 years), male cats (70%) of domestic shorthair (46%), domestic longhair (15%) or Siamese (12%) breeding. A review of obstipation in cats (Washabau, 2001) revealed 62% of cases were due to idiopathic megacolon, 23% to pelvic canal stenosis and 6% to nerve injury with most related to Manx sacral spinal cord deformity. The remaining cases (4%) were due to complications of colopexy (1%), colonic neoplasia (1%) and suspected colonic hypo- or aganglionosis (2%). Inflammatory, pharmacologic and environmental/behavioral causes were not cited as predisposing factors in any of the original case reports in this review (Washabau, 2001). Endocrine factors including obesity were noted in several cases, but were not acknowledged as the etiology of megacolon. Although it is important to consider an extensive list of differential diagnoses in individual cats, it should be kept in mind that most cases are idiopathic, orthopedic or neurologic in origin.

The use of opioid narcotics for pain or control of GI transit time has long been recognized to cause constipation. The constipating effect of narcotic analgesics is well known but its mechanisms are poorly understood. Postulated mechanisms include decreased intestinal water, increased rhythmic segmentation and delayed colonic transit. Several other commonly used medications, including barium sulfate, bismuth subsalicylate and anticonvulsants, also have constipating effects.

Dietary indiscretion is frequently associated with constipation in dogs. Consumption of bones, rocks and clay may trigger an episode. Constipation and obstipation have been reported to occur in dogs consuming bones and raw food diets due to the large contribution bones make to such foods. Although not generally prone to dietary indiscretion, cats may develop constipation as a consequence of trichobezoar formation.

Perineal and perianal disorders (e.g., perineal hernias, perianal fistulas and anal sacculitis) often predispose pets to constipation because of the pain associated with defecation (**Box 64-1**). Suppression of defecation results in increased fecal retention time, increased water absorption and inspissated feces. Orthopedic disorders may have a similar effect if the animal experiences pain when it assumes the defecation stance. Improperly healed pelvic fractures may reduce the size of the pelvic inlet and impinge on the rectal lumen.

Lastly, lead exposure may lead to constipation in affected animals presumably due to autonomic nervous system damage.

Etiopathogenesis

It is important to consider an extensive list of differential diagnoses (e.g., neuromuscular, mechanical, inflammatory, metabolic/endocrine, pharmacologic, environmental and behavioral causes) for the obstipated patient (Byers et al, 2006; Bertoy, 2002; Washabu and Holt, 1999). The parasympathetic nervous system and intrinsic myenteric and submucosal plexuses innervate the colon. Destruction or damage to either pathway results in reduced colonic motility and potentiates constipation. Normal colonic motility involves both propulsive and non-propulsive patterns. Ingesta, digesta and associated somatic activity stimulate propulsive contractions, which serve to move colonic contents distally. Non-propulsive motility, also termed rhythmic segmentation, mixes colonic contents and promotes absorption of water and electrolytes.

Box 64-1. Dietary Management of Perianal Fistulas in Dogs.

The perianal fistula syndrome (anal furunculosis) is a frustrating problem for pet owners and veterinarians. Although uncommon in the general canine population, it is commonly seen in the German shepherd dog. This condition is often recurrent or refractory to treatment and may lead to elective euthanasia. The etiology of perianal fistulas is unknown, although it is suspected to be immune-mediated. Immunohistochemical studies of tissues from affected dogs support this concept. These tissues had T-helper cell cytokine mRNA profiles and increased expression of matrix metalloproteinases 9 and 13, which are primarily produced in macrophages. Reports of the successful use of immunosuppressive drugs, including prednisone and cyclosporine, and elimination foods in affected dogs lend credence to the idea that the condition is immune mediated. Concurrent lymphoplasmacytic colitis is found in the majority of dogs with perianal fistulas, although it is unknown if these conditions are causally linked.

Dietary treatments for perianal fistula patients are highly case specific and dependent on the degree of diarrhea, constipation, tenesmus and rectal stricture that may be present. Success with dietary therapy can be unpredictable, and it is often trial and error to discover which dietary maneuver will succeed in a particular patient. The feeding plan is used in conjunction with immunosuppressive agents and stool softeners, depending on the degree of rectal stricture. The preferred therapy for perianal fistula is immunosuppressive therapy, with the greatest success occurring with cyclosporine therapy. This is the preferred therapy in severe disease and when rectal stricture is present. Other options include systemic prednisone and azathioprine or topical tacrolimus administration. The reader is referred to medical texts for more information. When medical management is not successful or there are residual fistulas, surgical resection of necrotic, inflamed tracts is necessary. The most successful surgical procedures involve cryotherapy or the use of the Nd:YAG laser; other surgical techniques have high complication and recurrence rates. Interested readers are referred to surgical texts for more information.

The signs of large bowel diarrhea associated with perianal fistula are sometimes managed successfully by increasing the insoluble fiber content of the food. If the current food contains less than 5% dry matter (DM) crude fiber, insoluble fiber is the first treatment of choice because it increases fecal bulk and improves transit time. However, it is prudent to increase the DM fiber concentration in increments of 5% per week until clinical signs resolve; increasing fiber intake too rapidly may result in pain and obstipation. This can be done by mixing the patient's current food with a high-fiber food, in a manner recommended for a gradual transition from one food to another. Another successful approach, especially when rectal stricture is present, is to use a lower residue food containing a mixed-fiber source. Low-residue foods may contain either little or no (<2% DM) crude fiber or use predominately soluble or fermentable fiber (<5% DM total dietary fiber).

Novel antigen diets have been suggested for managing dogs with perianal fistulas. This approach was used successfully in 18 of 27 (67%) dogs also receiving immunosuppressive doses of corticosteroids. Chapter 31 discusses elimination foods.

Some investigators have speculated that omega-3 (n-3) fatty acids derived from fish oil or other sources may have a beneficial effect in controlling inflammation associated with perianal fistulas. Chapter 57 provides more information about omega-3 fatty acids.

Some dogs with perianal fistulas may benefit from small, frequent meals in conjunction with exercise to encourage more frequent defecation.

Body weight and condition determinations and stool evaluations are useful for assessing patients with perianal fistulas. Patients should be evaluated immediately if a change or decline in body weight or condition is noted. Regaining or maintaining optimal body weight and condition, normal activity level, normal behavior and absence of clinical signs are measures of successful management. Feeding method and amount fed, as tolerated by the patient, can be adjusted as needed to maintain body weight and condition. If dietary therapy alone is insufficient to improve stool quality and maintain body weight, additional medical or surgical therapy should be considered. Unfortunately, recurrence is common and prolonged medical therapy and multiple surgeries may be necessary. Many affected dogs are eventually euthanized because of client frustration with repeated bouts of the disease or the cost of continuous medical therapy.

The Bibliography for **Box 64-1** can be found at www.markmorris.org.

The pathogenesis of feline idiopathic megacolon has been variably attributed to primary neurogenic or degenerative neuromuscular disorders. Although a small number of cases (11%) result from neurologic disease, the vast majority (>60%) of cases have no evidence of neurologic disease (Washabau, 2001; Washabau and Holt, 1999). These cases may involve disturbances of colonic smooth muscle; in vitro studies suggest that colonic smooth muscle function is impaired in cats affected with idiopathic megacolon (Washabau and Sammarco, 1996; Washabau et al, 2002).

Isometric stress measurements (in vitro) were performed on colonic smooth muscle segments obtained from cats suffering from idiopathic dilated megacolon. Megacolonic smooth muscle developed less isometric stress in response to neurotransmitters (acetylcholine, substance P, cholecystokinin), membrane depolarization (potassium chloride) and electrical field stimulation, when compared to muscle from healthy controls. These differences were observed in longitudinal and circular smooth muscle from both the ascending and descending colon. No significant abnormalities of smooth muscle cells or of myenteric neurons were observed histologically. These studies suggested that feline idiopathic megacolon is a generalized dysfunction of colonic smooth muscle, and that treatments aimed at stimulating colonic smooth muscle contraction might improve colonic motility (Washabau and Sammarco, 1996).

Dehydration and electrolyte imbalances may induce constipation. Dehydration enhances colonic water absorption and leaves a dry, hard fecal mass. For example, cats with chronic

Table 64-2. Key nutritional factors and their recommended levels for foods for patients with chronic constipation or obstipation.*

Factors	Recommended levels
Water	>75% for cats and dogs with constipation or obstipation (moist foods)
Fiber	≥7% crude fiber (insoluble or mixed is best) for cats and dogs with chronic constipation and intermittent obstipation ≤5% for cats with chronic obstipation (megacolon)
Digestibility	Highly digestibility for cats with chronic obstipation (megacolon) (fat and digestible carbohydrate ≥90% and protein ≥87%)
Energy density	≥4 kcal/g for cats with chronic obstipation (megacolon)

*All values are on a dry matter basis except water; to convert kcal to kJ, multiply kcal by 4.184.

kidney disease may have intermittent constipation associated with dehydration. Electrolyte disturbances (e.g., hyponatremia, hypokalemia, hypocalcemia and hypercalcemia) may alter colonic muscular activity resulting in constipation.

Mechanical obstruction may result in constipation due to intraluminal or extraluminal masses, rectal strictures and narrow pelvic outlets (e.g., improperly healed pelvic fractures). Additionally, a number of neurologic disorders may result in reduced colonic motility. These include cauda equina syndrome, dysautonomia (Key-Gaskell syndrome) and diabetic or hypothyroid polyneuropathy.

Key Nutritional Factors

Key nutritional factors for chronic constipation differ from key nutritional factors for obstipation. **Table 64-2** summarizes key nutritional factors for constipation and obstipation.

Water

Maintaining normal hydration status is important for managing patients with chronic constipation or obstipation. Water is a key nutrient and its intake is often overlooked. A variety of methods should be used to encourage water intake. These include providing multiple bowls of potable water in prominent locations in the pet's environment, feeding moist (>75% water) rather than dry forms of foods, adding small amounts of flavoring substances such as bouillon or broth to water sources and offering ice cubes as treats or snacks. Addition of canned pumpkin and/or sweet potato to the current food has been successfully used in some cases of constipation.[a] These canned vegetables consist primarily of water (90%), which adds a significant quantity of water to the digesta. Beneficial effects resulting from canned pumpkin or sweet potato are likely the result of an increase in total daily water consumption, although fiber intake is also increased.

Fiber

Many patients with constipation improve clinically when the fiber content of their food is increased. Dietary fibers are poorly digestible polysaccharides, derived from a variety of sources. Fiber sources typically used in commercial pet foods include sugar beet pulp, cereal grains, cellulose, soy hulls, peanut hulls and pea fiber. Increasing fiber intake usually increases fecal water content, colonic motility and intestinal transit rate, all of which may benefit patients with constipation. Both fermentable and non-fermentable fiber sources have been advocated for the management of constipation (Dimski, 1989; Zoran, 1999). Fiber acts as a bulk-forming laxative. Insoluble (poorly fermentable) fibers (e.g., purified cellulose, peanut hulls) normalize colonic motility by distending the colonic lumen, increasing colonic water content, diluting luminal toxins (e.g., bile acids, ammonia and ingested toxins) and increasing the rate of passage of digesta. This change in colonic transit time reduces colonocyte exposure to toxins while softening the stool and increasing the frequency of defecation. Several gel-forming fibers have been recommended as an aid in managing constipation in people (Wald, 1998) and animals (Dimski, 1989). Soluble (fermentable) fibers (fruit pectins, guar gum, psyllium) are readily fermented by bacteria, producing short-chain fatty acids, which benefit colonic health. These fibers, whether added to or incorporated into food, are reported to swell to form emollient gels and facilitate passage of fecal matter (Dimkski, 1989; Lembo and Camilleri, 2003). However, fermentable fibers may not be as laxative as insoluble or mixed fibers because they have little ability to increase fecal bulk or dilute luminal toxins (Washabau, 2005a). Flatulence, diarrhea and abdominal cramping are potential side effects to fermentable, gel-forming fibers. These side effects can be reduced by a gradual transition to fiber supplementation, slowly increasing the level of added fermentable fiber until efficacy is achieved with minimal side effects. Such fibers should be added at no more than 5% of the total food because soluble fibers can significantly reduce the availability of minerals, including zinc, calcium, iron and phosphorus (Wedekind et al, 1995, 1996, 1996a) (Chapter 5).

Ingredients such as beet pulp, brans (rice, wheat or oat), pea fiber, soy fibers, soy hulls or mixtures of soluble and insoluble fiber sources are intermediate in their fermentability and have moderate attributes of both fermentable and poorly fermentable fibers (Figure 5-13). They are referred to as mixed fibers.

For patients with chronic constipation that still have some level of colonic motility, the crude fiber content of a food should be at least 7% dry matter (DM) initially and the fiber source should be insoluble or mixed.

Fiber sources can be added to a patient's current food (**Box 64-2**), but it is generally better to switch to a fiber-enhanced food. Feeding additional dietary fiber is preferable to the use of laxative medications alone. Dietary fiber is more physiologic, better tolerated and often more effective than non-fiber laxatives.

The motility patterns of patients with obstipation are completely abolished (e.g., severe endstage megacolon in cats). In these patients, fiber-enhanced foods and fiber supplements are no longer effective stimulants of colonic motility and, worse, can contribute to obstipation. Foods for patients with megacolon should have no more than 5% DM crude fiber.

Box 64-2. A Safe and Practical Method for Providing Supplemental Fiber to a Patient's Current Food and Limitations of Using Canned Pumpkin as a Supplemental Fiber Source.

Adding fiber supplements is the least desirable approach for increasing fiber intake in patients with chronic constipation. In most constipation cases, dietary fiber intake can be increased by switching to a balanced food with the desired fiber content (**Tables 64-3** and **64-4**) or a mixture of two balanced foods can be fed using the Pearson square method to determine the amounts of constituent foods in the mixture (Chapter 1). If fiber supplements are used, they should be added to moist foods to ensure the fiber is mixed with the food and doesn't settle out in the bowl.

For this method, a practical source of fiber is Fiber One Bran Cereal[a] breakfast cereal. Although it is a human breakfast cereal and is not nutritionally balanced for dogs and cats, it does contain carbohydrate, protein, minerals and vitamins. Thus, relative to other readily available fiber supplements such as psyllium, wheat bran or canned pumpkin, Fiber One breakfast cereal is a more balanced source of fiber. It is somewhat palatable (depending on the individual patient's preferences and amount used) and contains a good amount of insoluble fiber (almost 50% dry matter [DM] crude fiber). **Table 1** provides a dose schedule for moist food.

Use the Pearson square method for determining how much Fiber One to add to a dry pet food to achieve a specific crude fiber level. Variability in the weight density per 8-oz. measuring cup makes it difficult to create a similar reliable table for dry pet foods.

Besides not being a balanced food, canned pumpkin as a fiber source has an important volume limitation. Canned pumpkin contains 90% water and on an as fed basis has only a fraction of the crude fiber of Fiber One cereal. As noted below, to obtain a fiber level of 10 to 11%, 2 tsp of Fiber One breakfast cereal are added to an 8-oz. cup of moist food. To achieve the same amount of fiber, more than 8 oz. of canned pumpkin would have to be added to the 8 oz. of moist food, more than doubling the amount of food the patient would have to eat to ingest the same amount of crude fiber.

ENDNOTE

a. Fiber One Bran Cereal. General Mills Cereals, LLC, Minneapolis, MN, USA.

Table 1. Dose schedule for Fiber One Bran Cereal to add to a typical moist food* and resultant crude fiber level.

Added Fiber One	Total crude fiber in mixture (DM)
1 tsp	7 to 8%
2 tsp	10 to 11%
3 tsp	13 to 14%
4 tsp	16 to 17%
5 tsp	18 to 19%

Key: tsp = rounded teaspoon (~5 g).
*8 volume oz. measuring cup of a typical moist food; assumed crude fiber content of approximately 3% DM, before Fiber One cereal is added. To improve acceptance by the patient and allow the colon and colonic microflora to adapt to the increase in fiber intake, gradually increase the amount of fiber added.

Digestibility and Caloric Density

For patients suffering from obstipation (including feline megacolon), in which colonic motility patterns are completely abolished, feeding a highly digestible food (fat and digestible [soluble] carbohydrate ≥90% and protein ≥87%) with an increased energy density (≥4.0 kcal/g [≥16.7 kJ/g] DM) will provide adequate nutrition and markedly reduce the fecal mass. A food's energy density and digestibility are inversely related to its fiber content. Reducing fiber results in increased caloric density, which helps meet the patient's requirements in a small volume of food. Calorically dense foods can markedly reduce the burden of home management (i.e., administering stool softeners and enemas) for pet owners. In such cases, fecal production is reduced to such an extent that owners can generally remove feces by cleansing enemas once or twice weekly. In many cases, this food transition is made as the owner considers the surgical option of subtotal colectomy.

The energy density and digestibility of a food are less important in constipated patients.

FEEDING PLAN

Initial management of chronic constipation includes owner education, encouraging increased water intake, appropriate dietary changes and judicious use of laxatives and enemas. If the affected animal is overweight, a weight-reduction program should be considered. Obstipation often requires multiple cleansing enemas with or without mechanical removal of impacted feces before dietary changes are instituted.

Assess and Select the Food

The key nutritional factor content of the food currently being fed should be evaluated in patients with constipation. Information from this aspect of assessment is essential for making any changes to foods currently provided. Changing to a more appropriate food is indicated if levels of key nutritional factors of the current food do not closely match recommended levels. **Tables 64-3** and **64-4** list selected commercial veterinary therapeutic foods for dogs and cats, respectively, affected with chronic constipation and compare the key nutritional content of these foods to recommended levels.

Many constipated cats respond favorably when fed a fiber-enhanced food, particularly if it is a moist food. Cats should be well hydrated before increasing fiber intake to maximize the therapeutic effect of fiber and to minimize the potential for fiber impaction in the constipated colon (Scherk, 2003; Washabau and Sammarco, 1996). Also, it is prudent to increase the fiber concentration gradually (e.g., 5%, 10%, 15%, 20%) over several weeks until clinical signs improve or resolve.

While less convenient, the fiber intake can also be increased by adding a higher fiber food to the current food. Most commercial grocery and specialty brand pet foods contain less than 5% DM crude fiber. Fiber-enhanced foods contain between 8

Table 64-3. Key nutritional factors in selected veterinary therapeutic foods for dogs with constipation and intermittent obstipation compared to recommended levels.*

Moist foods	Crude fiber (%)	Primary sources of fiber**
Recommended levels	**≥7**	**-**
Hill's Prescription Diet w/d Canine	12.4	Cellulose
Iams Veterinary Formula Intestinal Low-Residue	3.9	Beet pulp
Medi-Cal Fibre Formula	15.0	Tomato pomace, guar gum, flax meal, carrageenan
Purina Veterinary Diets OM Overweight Management Formula	19.2	Pea fiber, beet pulp, carrageenan
Royal Canin Veterinary Diet Calorie Control CC High Fiber	8.8	Tomato pomace, guar gum, flax meal, carrageenan
Dry foods	**Crude fiber (%)**	**Primary sources of fiber****
Recommended levels	**≥7**	**-**
Hill's Prescription Diet w/d Canine	16.4	Cellulose, soybean mill run, beet pulp
Iams Veterinary Formula Intestinal Low-Residue	2.1	Beet pulp
Medi-Cal Fibre Formula	14.3	Tomato pomace, rice hulls, oat hulls, flax meal, apple pomace
Purina Veterinary Diets DCO Dual Fiber Control	7.6	Beet pulp, pea fiber
Purina Veterinary Diets OM Overweight Management	10.3	Soybean hulls, pea fiber, cellulose
Royal Canin Veterinary Diet Calorie Control CC 26 High Fiber	17.6	Cellulose, pea fiber, rice hulls, beet pulp, psyllium husk
Royal Canin Veterinary Diet Diabetic HF 18	12.1	Cellulose, rice hulls, guar gum

*Moist foods are best. Manufacturers' published values. Values expressed on a dry matter basis.
**Fiber sources should be insoluble or mixed. Increased levels of soluble fiber are not recommended (see text).

Table 64-4. Key nutritional factors in selected veterinary therapeutic foods for cats with constipation and intermittent obstipation compared to recommended levels.*

Moist foods	Crude fiber (%)	Primary sources of fiber**
Recommended levels	**≥7**	**-**
Hill's Prescription Diet w/d with Chicken Feline	10.6	Cellulose, oat fiber, guar gum, locust bean gum, carrageenan
Iams Veterinary Formula Intestinal Low-Residue	3.7	Beet pulp
Medi-Cal Fibre Formula	16.7	Pea fiber, flax meal, guar gum
Purina Veterinary Diets OM Overweight Management	10.2	Pea fiber, oat fiber, guar gum
Royal Canin Veterinary Diet Calorie Control CC High Fiber	7.7	Cellulose, guar gum, flaxseed
Dry foods	**Crude fiber (%)**	**Primary sources of fiber****
Recommended levels	**≥7**	**-**
Hill's Prescription Diet w/d Feline	7.6	Cellulose
Hill's Prescription Diet w/d Feline with Chicken	7.6	Cellulose
Iams Veterinary Formula Intestinal Low-Residue	1.8	Beet pulp
Medi-Cal Fibre Formula	14.9	Pea fiber, beet pulp, flax meal
Purina Veterinary Diets OM Overweight Management	5.6	Oat fiber, cellulose
Royal Canin Veterinary Diet Calorie Control CC High Fiber	14.0	Cellulose, pea fiber, rice hulls, beet pulp, psyllium

*Moist foods are best. Manufacturers' published values. Values expressed on a dry matter basis.
**Fiber sources should be insoluble or mixed. Increased levels of soluble fiber are not recommended (see text).

Table 64-5. Key nutritional factors in selected veterinary therapeutic foods for cats with chronic obstipation (megacolon) compared to recommended levels.*

Moist foods	Crude fiber (%)	Protein digestibility (%)	Fat digestibility (%)	Carbohydrate digestibility (%)	Energy density (kcal/g)**
Recommended levels	**≤5**	**≥87**	**≥90**	**≥90**	**≥4**
Hill's Prescription Diet a/d Canine/Feline	1.3	90	89	96	4.8
Hill's Prescription Diet i/d Feline	2.4	91	89	91	4.2
Iams Veterinary Formula Intestinal Low-Residue	3.7	na	na	na	4
Iams Veterinary Formula Stress/Weight Gain Formula Maximum-Calorie	2.7	na	na	na	5.8
Medi-Cal Hypoallergenic/Gastro	1.2	na	na	na	na
Medi-Cal Recovery Formula	3.4	na	na	na	na
Medi-Cal Sensitivity CR	2.5	na	na	na	na
Royal Canin Veterinary Diet Recovery RS	3.4	na	na	na	4.4
Dry foods	**Crude fiber (%)**	**Protein digestibility (%)**	**Fat digestibility (%)**	**Carbohydrate digestibility (%)**	**Energy density (kcal/g)****
Recommended levels	**≤5**	**≥87**	**≥90**	**≥90**	**≥4**
Hill's Prescription Diet i/d Feline	2.8	88	92	90	4.3
Iams Veterinary Formula Intestinal Low-Residue	1.8	na	na	na	3.9
Medi-Cal Hypoallergenic/Gastro	3.1	na	na	na	na
Purina Veterinary Diets EN GastroENteric Formula	1.3	94.0	93.1	79.7	4.4
Royal Canin Veterinary Diet Intestinal HE 30	5.8	na	na	na	4.4

Key: na = information not available from manufacturer.
*Moist foods are best. Manufacturers' published values. All values expressed on a dry matter basis.
**To convert to kJ, multiply kcal by 4.184.

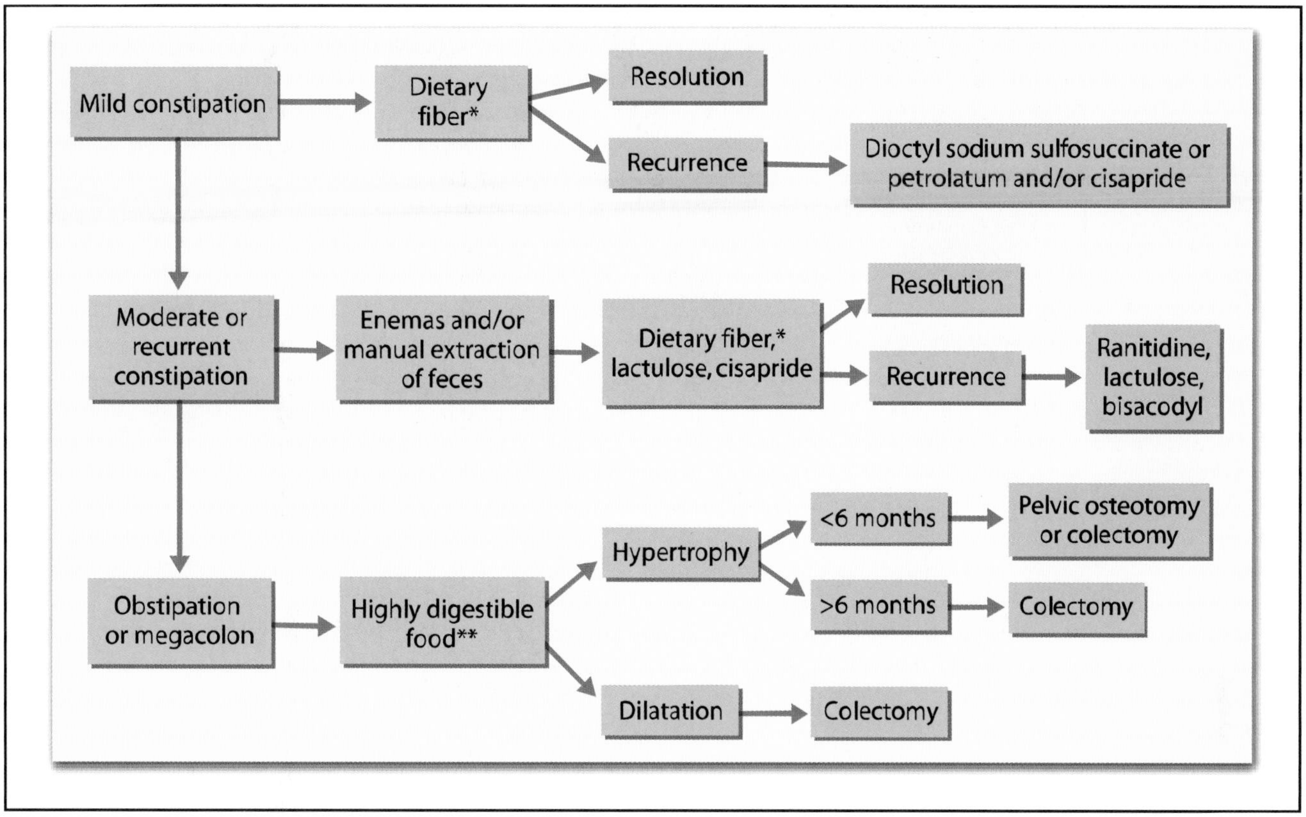

Figure 64-1. An algorithm for combined dietary and medical management for constipation and obstipation.
*__Tables 64-3__ and **64-4**.
**__Table 64-5__.
(Adapted from Washabau RJ, Sammarco J. Alterations in colonic smooth muscle function in cats with idiopathic megacolon. American Journal of Veterinary Research 1996; 57: 580-587. Scherk MA. Feline megacolon. In: Proceedings. 21st Annual American College of Veterinary Internal Medicine Forum 2003, Charlotte, NC: 911-913.)

and 25% DM crude fiber. The source of fiber may be determined by reviewing the ingredient list (Chapter 9). Almost any intermediate fiber concentration can be achieved by combining foods (dry or moist) that have different levels of fiber. The amounts of the constituent foods for the mixture can be determined using the Pearson square (Chapter 1). When making this calculation, be sure to use the same method of expressing the foods' fiber content (i.e., as fed or DM basis).

Adding fiber supplements such as psyllium, coarse wheat bran, bran cereals and canned pumpkin to the pet's regular food is another method of increasing the fiber intake of constipated patients. However, this is a less desirable approach. Fiber supplements can be awkward to use, may make the food unpalatable and in some instances can significantly reduce mineral bioavailability and create an unbalanced food. Fiber supplements work best when added to moist foods. **Box 64-2** provides a safe method for increasing the fiber content of a moist pet food by using a high-fiber human breakfast cereal as the fiber source.

Obstipated patients that have lost colonic motility should be fed foods that are highly digestible and have increased energy density. **Table 64-5** lists the key nutritional factor contents for foods for feline patients with chronic obstipation (megacolon) and compares them to recommended levels. Patients with severe megacolon may need veterinary therapeutic foods for stress/recovery (Tables 25-8 and 25-9) or homemade foods.

Assess and Determine the Feeding Method

Because the feeding method may be altered in patients with constipation, a thorough assessment should include verification of the feeding method currently being used, including feeding frequency, amount fed and access to other food.

In some cases, smaller more frequent meals may aid colonic motility patterns. Dogs should be walked immediately after feeding; both mild exercise and the gastrocolic reflex will often result in defecation during the immediate postprandial period. Feeding three to four meals per day also minimizes the amount of ingesta entering the large bowel at one time. As discussed above, water intake should be encouraged and drinking water should be readily available (i.e., multiple locations in the pet's environment) at all times.

ADJUNCTIVE MEDICAL THERAPY

The specific therapeutic plan will depend upon the severity of constipation and the underlying cause (**Figure 64-1**). First epi-

Table 64-6. Non-dietary medical therapies.

Emollient/lubricant laxatives/stool softeners
Dioctyl sodium succinate (Colace, Regulax SS, Surfak)
Dioctyl calcium sulfosuccinate (Sufax)
Mineral oil (Fleet mineral oil)
Hyperosmolar laxatives
Glycerin
Lactulose (Cephulac, Chronulac, Duphalac)
Polyethylene glycol (Miralax) (toxic to cats)
Polyethylene glycol with electrolytes (Colyte, GoLYTELY, NuLYTELY)
Sugar alcohols
Sorbitol (potentially toxic to small dogs and cats)
Mannitol
Saline laxatives
Magnesium citrate (Evac-Q-Mag)
Magnesium hydroxide (Phillip's Milk of Magnesia)
Magnesium sulfate
Sodium phosphate (Fleet enema, Fleet Phospho-Soda, Visicol)
Stimulant laxatives
Aloe
Anthraquinones
Cascara sagrada (Colamin, Sagrada-lax)
Senna (Senokot, Ex-Lax)
Castor oil (Purge, Neoloid, Emulsoil)
Diphenylmethanes
Phenolphthalein
Bisacodyl (Dulcolax, Correctol)
Sodium picosulfate (Lubrilax, Sur-Lax)
GI prokinetic therapy
Cisapride
Prucalopride (Resolor) (not approved in the U.S.)
New applications of existing drug classifications
Acetylcholinesterase inhibitors (ranitidine, nizatidine, neostigmine)
Erythromycin
Metoclopramide
Prostaglandin E_1 analogues (misoprostol)

sodes are often transient and resolve without medical therapy. Mild to moderate or recurrent episodes of constipation usually require medical intervention. In addition to dietary management, these cases may be managed, often on an outpatient basis, with water enemas, oral or suppository laxatives, and/or colonic prokinetic agents. Obstipation usually requires hospital admittance to correct metabolic abnormalities and to evacuate impacted feces using water enemas, manual extraction of retained feces, or both. Followup therapy in such cases is directed at correcting predisposing factors and preventing recurrence (Washabau and Sammarco, 1996). Medical therapies for mild to moderate constipation include enemas, stool softeners, laxatives (**Table 64-6**) and colonic motility modifiers (e.g., cisapride[b], 0.25 mg/kg body weight, t.i.d. to q.i.d.). A number of poorly absorbed carbohydrates may prove useful as laxatives. These sugars, including polyethylene glycol, sorbitol, lactulose and lactitol are hydrolyzed to fatty acids by the colonic microflora. The metabolites of these sugars exert osmotic pressure and draw fluid into the colon lumen. Additionally, laxative therapy may occasionally be needed to promote fecal hydration and lubrication.

Cats suffering from bouts of obstipation or idiopathic dilated megacolon are, by definition, unresponsive to medical therapy. Surgery (subtotal colectomy) may become necessary to remove the affected portion of the bowel in cases of idiopathic megacolon. In most cases, subtotal colectomy with ileorectal or cecocolic-rectal anastomosis is the treatment of choice.

REASSESSMENT

Body weight and condition assessments and stool evaluations are useful for monitoring patients with constipation. Well-compensated patients should be evaluated immediately if a change or decline in condition is noted. Regaining or maintaining optimal body weight and condition, normal activity level, normal behavior and absence of clinical signs are measures of successful dietary management. The feeding method and amount fed can be adjusted as needed to maintain body weight and condition. Additional medical therapies should be considered if dietary management alone is insufficient to improve stool quality and maintain body weight. Although treatment is highly case specific, many cases can eventually be managed with diet alone after initial medical therapies are gradually discontinued.

Occasionally, a patient may develop constipation, obstipation or flatulence while being fed moderate- (8 to 15% DM fiber) or high-fiber (>15% DM fiber) foods. The prudent recommendation in such cases is to decrease the fiber content by one-half, reevaluate the patient in one week and decrease the fiber content again if necessary. This situation occurs more commonly in older overweight and obese cats consuming dry, high-fiber, low-calorie foods for weight control than in cats being treated for constipation with fiber.

ENDNOTES

a. Maureen Carroll, Angell Animal Medical Center, Boston, MA. Personal observation.

b. Available from compounding pharmacies.

REFERENCES

The references for **Chapter 64** can be found at www.markmorris.org.

CASE 64-1

Constipation in a Domestic Shorthair Cat

Deborah J. Davenport, DVM, MS, Dipl. ACVIM (Internal Medicine)
Hill's Science and Technology Center
Topeka, Kansas, USA

Patient Assessment

A six-year-old, neutered male exclusively indoor domestic shorthair cat was examined for tenesmus and apparent constipation. The owners had noticed the cat making multiple unproductive attempts to defecate in the litter box. The cat was also seen sitting in the litter box for prolonged periods without making attempts to urinate or defecate. Two other cats in the household were normal. The owners cleaned the litter box daily and noticed both normal and dry, hardened feces. Because the cat had been constipated in the past, the owners were giving a flavored petrolatum product (Laxatone[a]) each day by mouth.

Physical examination revealed a normal-appearing, overweight, 5.5-kg cat. The cat's body condition score (BCS) was 4/5. Abdominal palpation elicited a painful response and the entire colon was distended with firm feces.

Warm tap water and mineral oil enemas were given to the cat; some of the fecal material was subsequently passed. The cat was anesthetized and warm tap water was infused into the colon while the remaining fecal material was manually expressed by abdominal palpation. The cat was discharged the same day with instructions for the owners to increase the amount of flavored petrolatum given each day.

Ten days later, the cat was reexamined for similar problems. Abdominal radiographs revealed a markedly distended colon impacted with feces. No foreign material, mass lesions, healed pelvic fractures or spinal abnormalities were noted radiographically. The fecal material was removed by enemas and manual extraction. A tentative diagnosis of chronic constipation and possible megacolon was made.

Assess the Food and Feeding Method

All of the cats in the house were fed a commercial dry specialty brand adult cat food free choice. Canned tuna or a variety of commercial moist grocery brand foods were offered once or twice weekly as a treat. Water was available free choice although all three cats liked to drink from faucets and toilet bowls.

Questions

1. What are the key nutritional factors to consider for this patient?
2. Outline an appropriate feeding plan (foods and feeding method) for this cat.
3. What other therapy can be used in conjunction with the feeding plan?

Answers and Discussion

1. The key nutritional factors for this patient are water and fiber intake. Fiber is classified as a bulk-forming laxative although it has many other properties. Fiber's beneficial effects in treating animals with constipation include increasing fecal water content, increasing intestinal motility, altering intestinal transit rate and increasing frequency of defecation. Feeding more moist food and less dry food would also increase water intake.
2. Fiber supplements such as psyllium husk fiber, wheat bran or pumpkin can be added to the moist foods. Alternatively, commercial, fiber-enhanced moist foods can make up part or all of a patient's diet. This cat will need to be fed separately from other cats in the household. Several smaller meals during the day rather than one large meal may be beneficial and will be similar to the free-choice feeding method used previously.
3. Therapy for chronic constipation includes: 1) removing impacted feces, 2) administering laxatives, 3) assessing the diet and 4) administering prokinetic agents. Laxatives are classified as emollient (dioctyl sodium sulfosuccinate), lubricant (mineral oil, petrolatum), hyperosmotic (lactulose, magnesium salts, polyethylene glycols) and stimulant (bisacodyl). All these may be used in cats with mild to moderate constipation, but they should be avoided in cases with functional or mechanical bowel obstruction (obstipation). Studies suggest that stimulating colonic smooth muscle contraction may improve colonic motility in cats with idiopathic dilated megacolon. In vitro studies have shown that cisapride[b] stimulates propulsive motility in the colon, and anecdotal experience suggests that cisapride also effectively stimulates colonic propulsive motility in cats with mild to moderate idiopathic constipation. Cats with longstanding obstipation and megacolon are not likely to improve with dietary, laxative and prokinetic therapy alone. Subtotal colectomy should be considered in these cases.

Progress Notes

Metamucil[c] (0.5 tsp) was added to the moist food (1-1/4 5.5-oz. cans) and offered to the cat daily in addition to the regular commercial dry food fed free choice. The moist food plus fiber supplement made up approximately half of the daily food intake. Little improvement was noted after one month. The cat was then exclusively fed a commercial moist veterinary therapeutic food (Prescription Diet w/d Feline[d]) with moderate fiber levels (9.3% dry matter crude fiber). One 5.5-oz. can was divided into three meals per day for slow weight loss. There was some improvement after one month (i.e., increased frequency of defecation and moister feces). However, constipation remained an intermittent problem. Cisapride, 2.5 mg, two to three times daily per os, was added to the therapeutic protocol and, subsequently, the cat had only occasional problems with constipation.

Endnotes

a. EVSCO Pharmaceuticals, Buena, NJ, USA.
b. Available from compounding pharmacies.
c. Procter & Gamble, Cincinnati, OH, USA.
d. Hill's Pet Nutrition, Inc., Topeka, KS, USA.

Bibliography

DeNovo RC, Bright RM. Chronic feline constipation/obstipation. In: Kirk RW, Bonagura JD, eds. Current Veterinary Therapy XI. Philadelphia, PA: WB Saunders Co, 1992; 619-626.

Washabu RJ, Hasler AH. Constipation, obstipation and megacolon. In: August JR, ed. Consultations in Feline Internal Medicine 3. Philadelphia, PA: WB Saunders Co, 1997; 104-112.

Chapter 65

Flatulence

Philip Roudebush
Deborah J. Davenport
Rebecca L. Remillard

"He couldn't ad-lib a fart after a baked-bean dinner."
Johnny Carson

CLINICAL IMPORTANCE

Flatulence is excessive formation of gases in the stomach or intestine, but the term is often used incorrectly. Excessive flatulence is usually associated with noticeable flatus, belching, borborygmus or a combination of these signs. Flatus, rather than flatulence, is gas expelled through the anus. Belching is the noisy voiding of gas from the stomach through the mouth. Borborygmus is a rumbling noise caused by the propulsion of gas through the intestines.

Excessive flatus is a chronic objectionable problem that occurs often in dogs and less commonly in cats. Although belching and borborygmus are rarely chief complaints of pet owners, routine questioning may elicit their presence. Flatus, belching and borborygmus occur in normal pets but often develop as a consequence of small intestinal or colonic disorders. At times, flatus is the primary reason pet owners seek veterinary advice.

PATIENT ASSESSMENT

History and Physical Examination

Pet owners often describe an increase in frequency of belching, audible flatus or an objectionable odor associated with flatus (Jones et al, 1998). At times, it may be possible to elicit a history of dietary change or dietary indiscretion in association with flatus. Occasionally, belching and flatus develop in conjunction with other gastrointestinal (GI) signs including weight loss, diarrhea and steatorrhea. This type of history is very suggestive of an underlying small intestinal disorder.

In most cases, physical examination findings are unremarkable in dogs and cats with flatulence, although abdominal distention is sometimes noted in cats. Intestinal gas can often be detected during abdominal palpation; however, it is difficult to assess the quantity of gas by palpation alone. Animals having poor body condition and objectionable flatus may have an underlying GI condition.

Laboratory testing is usually not indicated. However, further evaluation is in order if concomitant GI signs are present. Readers are referred to earlier chapters involving small and large bowel disorders for further information.

Risk Factors

Excessive aerophagia is a risk factor for flatulence and is seen with brachycephalic, working and sporting canine breeds and pets with aggressive and competitive eating behaviors. Dietary indiscretion and ingestion of certain pet food ingredients may be risk factors for certain individuals.

Etiopathogenesis

Gas in the GI tract is normal and may be derived from three sources: air swallowing, intraluminal gas production and diffusion of gas from the blood to the GI tract.

Regarding flatus, the rate of excretion of gas per rectum varies greatly in people and animals. Excretion rates in people range from 400 to 1,500 ml/day (mean 705 ml/day). People, eating their usual foods, passed gas per rectum an average of eight to 10 times per day with an upper normal limit of 20 times per day (Strocchi and Levitt, 1997). Swallowed air is thought to contribute the most to gas in the digestive tract. This may be the cause of flatus commonly seen in many brachycephalic breeds. Vigorous exercise and rapid and competitive eating situations may exacerbate aerophagia. Studies using ultrafast computed tomography in people show that a mean of 17 ml of air accompanies the swallowing of 10 ml of water. In people, air introduced into the stomach can result in flatus within 15 to 35 minutes and it has been estimated that gases can move 10 cm/second through the GI tract (Levitt, 1980). In a study using an in vivo methodology of flatulence assessment in dogs, flatus developed as soon as two hours post-feeding (Yamka et al, 2006).

A large amount of gas is formed from colonic bacterial fermentation of poorly digestible carbohydrates and certain fibers. Fiber-containing foods contribute to flatus indirectly through reduced dry matter (DM) digestibility. Certain fibers (soluble or fermentable) used in pet foods are fermented by colonic microflora and may contribute to flatus directly. Foods that contain large amounts of nonabsorbable oligosaccharides (e.g., raffinose, stachyose and verbascose) are likely to produce large amounts of intestinal gas (Levitt, 1980). Dogs and cats lack the digestive enzymes needed to split these sugars into absorbable monosaccharides. Therefore, bacteria in the colon ferment these sugars producing hydrogen and carbon dioxide. Soybeans, beans and peas contain large quantities of nonabsorbable oligosaccharides (Yamka et al, 2003, 2006). Soybean meal is commonly used in pet foods as a protein source. The stachyose and raffinose content of soybean meal is variable ranging from 32 to 112 g/kg and 6 to 14 g/kg DM, respectively, which could contribute to flatulence if they compose more than 22 g/kg of food DM (Yamka et al, 2006).

Diseases that cause maldigestion or malabsorption are often associated with excessive flatus because excessive amounts of malassimilated substrates are delivered to the colon where bacterial fermentation occurs. Flatus may be present in animals with lactose intolerance.

The interaction between hydrochloric acid and alkaline food and saliva produces carbon dioxide in the stomach. The reaction between gastric acid and pancreatic bicarbonate in the duodenum also generates carbon dioxide. In addition, carbon dioxide enters the GI tract via diffusion from the blood. Belched gas is largely swallowed air (nitrogen and oxygen) plus variable quantities of carbon dioxide.

Odorless gases (i.e., nitrogen, oxygen, carbon dioxide, hydrogen and methane) compose as much as 99% of flatus (Strocchi and Levitt, 1997). The residual 1% is composed of odoriferous gases that contain sulfur, such as hydrogen sulfide, methanethiol and dimethylsulfide (Roudebush, 2001; Collins et al, 2001). These gases contribute the objectionable odors associated with flatus. Excessive quantities of odorless gases provide a vehicle for the odoriferous gases and volatiles and probably worsen objectionable flatus. Onions, nuts, spices, cruciferous vegetables (e.g., broccoli, cabbage, cauliflower, Brussels sprouts) and high protein ingredients often increase production of odiferous gases.

Key Nutritional Factors

Table 65-1 summarizes the key nutritional factors, discussed below, for foods for dogs and cats with objectionable excessive flatulence.

Digestibility

Digestibility, especially of the carbohydrate fraction of food, is an important nutritional factor in patients with excessive flatulence. Feeding a highly digestible food reduces the residues available for bacterial fermentation in the large intestine. Thus, foods with high digestibility (fat and digestible [soluble] carbohydrate ≥90% and protein ≥87%) are recommended for patients with objectionable flatus).

Carbohydrate

Certain carbohydrate sources may affect flatus production in individual patients. Changing the source of carbohydrate in the food may benefit some animals (Suarez et al, 1999). Anecdotal reports in people suggest that a food in which all carbohydrate is supplied by white rice reduces flatus output. Studies in dogs have also shown that foods containing rice as a carbohydrate source result in less intestinal gas formation than foods containing wheat or corn (Washabau et al, 1986). This suggests that animals with flatus may benefit from foods with rice as the sole or predominant carbohydrate source.

Protein

Dietary protein sources and amount may affect flatus odor. Changing the sources of protein in the food may benefit some patients (Suarez et al, 1999). Ammonia and volatile amines are odorous and could result from microbial fermentation of food protein residues reaching the large intestine. Therefore, protein digestibility (discussed above) and amount should be considered if flatus is a problem. Dietary protein should probably not exceed 30% for dogs and 40% for cats DM. Leguminous protein sources such as soybean meal should be avoided in pets with excessive flatulence.

Fiber

Soluble or fermentable fiber-enhanced foods may contribute to excessive flatus in some patients. Soluble fibers including fruit pectins and gums (e.g., guar gum, carrageenan) are readily fermentable by gut microbes resulting in gas production (Chapter 5). Even some mixed fibers in adequate amounts (brans, soy fiber, soy hulls, pea fiber and beet pulp) can be a source of flatulence. Some of these sources of fiber also contain non-fiber ingredients that can contribute to objectionable flatus (e.g., soy hulls and pea fiber). For patients with excessive flatus, the amount of fiber should probably be limited to no more than 5% DM.

Table 65-1. Key nutritional factors for foods, treats and snacks for dogs and cats with excessive flatulence.*

Factors	Recommendations
Digestibility	Increased digestibility Fat and carbohydrate digestibility ≥90% Protein digestibility ≥87%
Carbohydrate	Change source: rice is preferred
Protein	Avoid high-protein foods Adult dogs: limit to ≤30% Adult cats: limit to ≤40% Avoid legumes (see below)
Fiber	Dogs and cats: limit to ≤5% fiber (most important aspect regarding fiber) Avoid high-fiber foods, especially soluble/fermentable and mixed fibers (soy fiber, soybean hulls, pea fiber, psyllium, pectin, carrageenan, guar gum, bran and beet pulp)
Legumes	Avoid all beans (including soybeans), peas, lentils, peanuts
Lactose sources	Avoid milk, ice cream, cheese, yogurt
Sulfur-containing vegetables	Avoid broccoli, cauliflower, Brussels sprouts, cabbage
Onions	Avoid
Nuts	Avoid
Spices	Avoid
Fructose	Avoid fruits and high-fructose corn syrup
Vitamin-mineral supplements	Avoid; unnecessary with most commercial foods

*Nutrient values are on a dry matter basis.

Food Ingredients

As discussed above, certain protein, carbohydrate and fiber ingredients or levels may affect flatus production in individual animals. Of the numerous foods alleged to enhance flatus in people, baked beans is the only natural food that has been carefully studied. A diet regimen deriving half of its calories from pork and beans increased flatus elimination in people from a basal level of 15 to 176 ml/hour (Steggarda, 1968).

Changing the sources of protein or carbohydrate in the food may benefit some animals (Suarez et al, 1999). For example, changing from a commercial dry food that contains corn, chicken meal and soybean meal to a dry food that contains lamb meal, rice and barley may be helpful. Vegetarian-based foods can be problematic because they often include potentially odiferous sulfur-containing vegetables and legumes. The lactose content of foods and treats (e.g., cheese, ice cream, milk) may be a factor in adult dogs and cats, especially those with lactase deficiency or in animals with underlying GI disease. A series of dietary trials is often successful in finding a food that lessens flatulence in individual pets. **Table 65-1** lists several categories of human foods and food ingredients to avoid or limit.

FEEDING PLAN

Dietary management of flatulence is primarily concerned with decreasing intestinal gas production by bacterial fermentation of undigested food. Changes in the feeding plan can be used in conjunction with other therapy. Recently, commercial products have been introduced that claim to reduce flatulence (**Box 65-1**).

Assess and Select the Food

Obtaining a thorough dietary history is of paramount importance in evaluating patients with excessive flatulence. Specific foods, major food ingredients, treats, supplements and opportunities for dietary indiscretion should be evaluated.

In general, pets with excessive flatulence will benefit from highly digestible foods. Consumption of such foods may reduce the amount of residue reaching the large intestine, thereby decreasing substrate availability for bacterial fermentation and subsequent gas production. Commercial foods and treats fed to pets that have excessive flatulence should also be evaluated for specific ingredients that might be further contributing to the problem. To accomplish this, compare the food's ingredient list on the package or label (Chapter 9) to the ingredients recommended to avoid or limit as listed in **Table 65-1**. If a food's major ingredients are potentially offensive, change to a food that has a nutrient profile and ingredient list that more closely compares to the recommendations in **Table 65-1**. Several veterinary therapeutic foods marketed for GI diseases or adverse food reactions are often suitable for feeding to patients with excessive flatulence (**Tables 65-2** and **65-3**, for dogs and cats, respectively). Most of these foods are complete and balanced for long-term feeding. Dietary trials may be necessary to select a food that reduces flatus. **Table 65-1** also lists human foods to avoid as treats or snacks or as ingredients for homemade foods for patients that have a history of excessive flatulence.

Assess and Determine the Feeding Method

A thorough assessment should include verification of the feeding method currently being used. Considerations include feeding frequency, amount fed, how the food is offered, access to other food, relationship of feeding to exercise and who feeds the animal. All of this information should have been gathered when the history of the animal was obtained. If the animal has a normal body condition score (2.5/5 to 3.5/5), the amount of food previously fed (energy basis) was probably appropriate.

Reducing aerophagia is important in the control of flatulence in dogs, especially in brachycephalic breeds. Feed several small

Box 65-1. Carminatives.

INTRODUCTION
Carminatives are medicines or preparations that relieve flatulence. Various herbal and botanical preparations have been used for thousands of years as carminatives. More recently, commercial products have been introduced that claim to reduce or control flatulence. These products can be used in conjunction with changes in the feeding plan and usually contain activated charcoal, bismuth subsalicylate (BSS), zinc acetate, simethicone, *Yucca schidigera* preparations, α-galactosidase, pancreatic enzyme supplements and various herbal preparations. Nonabsorbable antibiotics such as neomycin reduce flatulence and the number of flatus episodes in healthy people and dogs. However, routine use of nonabsorbable antibiotics in otherwise healthy pet animals with flatulence is not indicated.

ACTIVATED CHARCOAL
Dry activated charcoal adsorbs virtually all odoriferous gases when mixed directly with human feces and flatus gas. However, ingestion of activated charcoal by human subjects has been ineffective in reducing the number of flatus events, volume of intestinal gas released, odor of feces or breath hydrogen excretion after bean ingestion. In vitro studies suggest that the failure of ingested charcoal to reduce liberation of volatile sulfur compounds is due to the saturation of charcoal binding sites during passage through the gut. Wetting activated charcoal slows uptake of sulfur-containing gases considerably. Activated charcoal is found in a number of commercial canine treats purported to control flatulence.

BISMUTH SUBSALICYLATE
BSS reduces fecal and flatus odor in people when given frequently (four times daily). Bismuth is the active ingredient and avidly adsorbs hydrogen sulfide, forming insoluble bismuth sulfide. Bismuth sulfide imparts a characteristic black color to feces. Bismuth also has antibacterial activity, which may account for some of its effects. BSS contains 50% bismuth by weight and is found in various commercial veterinary antidiarrheal-adsorbent products and in over-the-counter antidiarrheal products for human use (e.g., Pepto-Bismol). There appears to be a striking dose-dependent response with BSS in that a dose of 400 mg of BSS/100 g of dry food completely suppresses cecal hydrogen sulfide release in rats, whereas one-fifth this concentration has no demonstrable effect. BSS may be effective in controlling objectionable flatus in pet animals but probably needs to be given multiple times per day, which precludes its practical, long-term use. BSS should be used with caution in cats because of concerns with salicylate toxicosis.

ZINC ACETATE
Similar to bismuth, zinc acetate binds sulfhydryl compounds and reduces volatile sulfur compounds when exposed directly to gas from human flatus. Addition of zinc acetate to food (1%) decreased fecal hydrogen sulfide concentrations and improved flatus odor in rats. One report showed that an oral treat containing zinc acetate, activated charcoal and *Yucca schidigera* extract reduced highly odoriferous episodes of flatus in dogs.

SIMETHICONE
Simethicone (dimethylpolysiloxane) is an antifoaming agent that reduces surface tension of gas bubbles and is found in commercial veterinary products and over-the-counter products for human use. Why simethicone would be beneficial in patients with flatulence is not obvious; however, one could speculate that altered gas bubbles might be more effectively eliminated. A few controlled trials of treatment with simethicone have been conducted in people. In general, simethicone had no effect on total daily flatus volume, number of

Table 65-2. Key nutritional factors in selected commercial veterinary therapeutic foods for dogs with excessive flatulence compared to recommended levels.*

Dry foods	Protein digestibility (%)	Fat digestibility (%)	Carbohydrate digestibility (%)	Protein (%)	Crude fiber (%)
Recommended levels	**≥87**	**≥90**	**≥90**	**≤30**	**≤5**
Hill's Prescription Diet i/d Canine	92	93	94	26.2	2.7
Iams Veterinary Formula Intestinal Low-Residue	na	na	na	24.6	2.1
Medi-Cal Gastro Formula	na	na	na	22.9	1.9
Purina Veterinary Diets EN GastroENteric Formula	84.5	91.4	94.4	27.0	1.5
Royal Canin Veterinary Diet Digestive Low Fat LF 20	na	na	na	24.2	2.3
Royal Canin Veterinary Diet Intestinal HE 28	na	na	na	33.0	1.6

Moist foods	Protein digestibility (%)	Fat digestibility (%)	Carbohydrate digestibility (%)	Protein (%)	Crude fiber (%)
Recommended levels	**≥87**	**≥90**	**≥90**	**≤30**	**≤5**
Hill's Prescription Diet i/d Canine	88	94	93	25.0	1.0
Iams Veterinary Formula Intestinal Low-Residue	na	na	na	35.9	3.9
Medi-Cal Gastro Formula	na	na	na	22.1	1.0
Purina Veterinary Diets EN GastroENteric Formula	85.1	95.6	92.2	30.5	0.9
Royal Canin Veterinary Diet Digestive Low Fat LF	na	na	na	31.9	3.0
Royal Canin Veterinary Diet Intestinal HE	na	na	na	23.1	1.4

Key: na = information not available from manufacturer; see **Table 65-1** for specific ingredients to avoid.
*Protein and crude fiber levels are on a dry matter basis.

flatus episodes or average volume per flatus event in people. Simethicone may help reduce gastric accumulation of gas and alleviate upper gastrointestinal (GI) signs. The effectiveness of simethicone in controlling flatulence in pet animals is unknown. It would not be expected to control objectionable flatus odors.

Yucca schidigera

Extracts of the *Yucca schidigera* plant have been used to control fecal malodor in animal waste lagoon systems and may help decrease fecal aroma. The mechanisms of action are poorly understood and may include "binding" ammonia or altering microbial activity. In the United States, *Yucca* preparations are only approved as flavoring agents in pet foods and it is unknown whether they effectively control flatulence or objectionable flatus odors when ingested by pet animals. An oral treat containing *Yucca schidigera* extract, activated charcoal and zinc acetate reduced highly odoriferous episodes of flatus in dogs.

α-GALACTOSIDASE and β-MANNANASE

Products containing α-galactosidase are available as human (Beano) and veterinary (CurTail) products. They reduce flatus volume by improving digestion of nonabsorbable oligosaccharides found in soybeans, beans, peas and other legumes. These products would not be expected to improve excessive flatus due to other causes (e.g., aerophagia) or improve the odor of flatus. Anecdotal reports suggest that these products may be beneficial in some animals. β-mannanase is another enzyme that may improve digestion of nonabsorbable oligosaccharides in legumes. β-mannanase has been used to increase feed conversion and dry matter digestibility of soy-based diets in poultry and swine. In dogs, however, supplemental β-mannanase was not shown to increase digestibility of food or reduce flatulence.

PANCREATIC ENZYMES

Pancreatic enzyme supplementation decreases abnormal intestinal gas production in dogs with exocrine pancreatic insufficiency. Pancreatic enzyme preparations have also been widely used for bloating and abdominal distention in people. Because ingestion of these preparations should add little to the enzyme output of the pancreas in otherwise normal individuals, no solid rationale exists for their use in flatulent patients without pancreatic disease. Nevertheless, a recent study in people showed that a microencapsulated pancreatic enzyme preparation significantly reduced postprandial symptoms of bloating and abdominal distention experienced by healthy people ingesting a high-calorie, high-fat meal. This finding suggests that pancreatic enzyme supplements might benefit some patients with flatulence.

HERBS AND BOTANICALS

More than 30 herbal and botanical preparations have been listed as carminatives. Grape seed extract containing proanthocyanidins is one botanical preparation that alters GI microflora and decreases fecal release of volatile sulfur compounds in human patients. The dosage, safety and efficacy of grape seed extract and other botanical preparations in pets with flatulence have not been established.

SUMMARY

To date, the best evidence exists for short-term use of bismuth subsalicylate, zinc acetate and nonabsorbable antibiotics as carminatives. Less evidence exists for use of activated charcoal, simethicone, digestive enzyme preparations, *Yucca* extract and grape seed extract. Changing the feeding plan (food and feeding method), rather than using carminatives, offers the best opportunity for successful long-term management of flatulence in pet animals.

Table 65-3. Key nutritional factors in selected veterinary therapeutic foods for cats with excessive flatulence compared to recommended levels*

Dry foods	Protein digestibility (%)	Fat digestibility (%)	Carbohydrate digestibility (%)	Protein (%)	Crude fiber (%)
Recommended levels	**≥87**	**≥90**	**≥90**	**≤40**	**≤5**
Hill's Prescription Diet i/d Feline	88	92	90	40.3	2.8
Iams Veterinary Formula Intestinal Low-Residue	na	na	na	35.8	1.8
Medi-Cal Hypoallergenic/Gastro	na	na	na	29.8	3.1
Purina Veterinary Diets EN GastroENteric Formula	94.0	93.1	79.7	56.2	1.3
Royal Canin Veterinary Diet Intestinal HE 30	na	na	na	34.4	5.8
Moist foods	**Protein digestibility (%)**	**Fat digestibility (%)**	**Carbohydrate digestibility (%)**	**Protein (%)**	**Crude fiber (%)**
Recommended levels	**≥87**	**≥90**	**≥90**	**≤40**	**≤5**
Hill's Prescription Diet i/d Feline	91	89	91	37.6	2.4
Iams Veterinary Formula Intestinal Low-Residue	na	na	na	38.4	3.7
Medi-Cal Hypoallergenic/Gastro	na	na	na	35.5	1.2
Medi-Cal Sensitivity CR	na	na	na	34.5	2.5

Key: na = information not available from manufacturer; see **Table 65-1** for specific ingredients to avoid.
*Protein and crude fiber levels are on a dry matter basis.

Table 65-4. Feeding plan summary for patients with excessive flatulence.

Control aerophagia Discourage rapid or competitive eating Feed a mixture of moist and dry foods Feed several small meals daily Surgically correct stenotic nares and elongated soft palate in brachycephalic dogs
Decrease production of obnoxious intestinal gas Select a food with the appropriate key nutritional factors (**Table 65-1**) Walk the dog outdoors within 30 minutes of meals to encourage defecation and the elimination of intestinal gas. In general, more activity and exercise result in fewer problems with flatus.
Carminatives If changes in the feeding plan do not result in significant improvement, consider the use of carminatives. To date, the best evidence exists for short-term use of bismuth subsalicylate, zinc acetate and nonabsorbable antibiotics. Less evidence exists for use of activated charcoal, simethicone, digestive enzyme preparations, *Yucca* extract and grape seed extract (**Box 65-1**).

meals daily in an effort to discourage rapid eating and gulping of air. Feeding small frequent meals also improves digestibility and reduces food residues available for bacterial fermentation in the large intestine. A recent study in dogs demonstrated that feeding twice daily resulted in fewer episodes of flatus (9.9/day) than feeding once daily (13.5/day) (Yamka et al, 2006). Feeding in a quiet, isolated location will eliminate competitive eating and reduce aerophagia. Walking dogs outdoors within 30 minutes of eating encourages defecation and elimination of intestinal gas (**Table 65-4**).

REASSESSMENT

Patients should be evaluated for evidence of malassimilation if the methods outlined above are not successful in reducing or controlling flatulence, including objectionable flatus. Relapses in animals that have been controlled often indicate dietary indiscretion. The prognosis for control of flatulence is good in most cases. However, owners should be educated about normal intestinal gas production and should not expect complete cessation of flatulence (Cho, 1994).

If changes in the feeding plan do not result in significant improvement, consider use of carminatives (**Box 65-1**).

REFERENCES

The references for **Chapter 65** can be found at www.markmorris.org.

CASE 65-1

Flatulence in a Young Puppy

Philip Roudebush, DVM, Dipl. ACVIM (Small Animal Internal Medicine)
Hill's Scientific Affairs
Topeka, Kansas, USA

Patient Assessment

A 16-week-old intact male beagle puppy was examined for routine health maintenance procedures. The owners obtained the puppy from a local animal shelter six weeks ago. The puppy had been active and healthy with no apparent problems. However, the owners complain the puppy passes excessive amounts of intestinal gas with an offensive odor, especially after meals. There has been no evidence of vomiting, diarrhea or other gastrointestinal (GI) problems. Physical examination revealed an active puppy with no abnormalities. A fecal sample was negative for intestinal parasites.

Assess the Food and Feeding Method

The patient was fed a commercial dry puppy food containing the following ingredients: corn, chicken meal, soybean meal, animal fat, beet pulp, rice, fish oil, flaxseed, vitamins and minerals. The daily feeding amount was divided into two equal meals, offered in the morning and evening. The puppy's appetite was very good and the food was usually consumed at each meal within a few minutes. The puppy also enjoyed small amounts of fresh fruit and vegetables as snacks.

Questions

1. What are the common clinical manifestations of flatulence?
2. What are the most common causes of excessive intestinal gas formation?
3. Are there ingredients in the current diet that could be contributing to excessive intestinal gas formation?
4. Outline a feeding plan for this puppy that will help control the problem with flatulence.

Answers and Discussion

1. Flatulence is excessive formation of gases in the stomach or intestine. Excessive flatulence is usually associated with noticeable flatus, belching, borborygmus, abdominal distention or a combination of these signs. Flatus, rather than flatulence, is the term that should be used for gas expelled through the anus. Dog owners often complain of excessive amounts of flatus, with or without an objectionable odor.
2. The quantitatively important gases in the intestinal tract are nitrogen, oxygen, hydrogen, carbon dioxide and methane. These gases comprise more than 99% of the intestinal gas volume and are odorless. The characteristic unpleasant odor of intestinal gas appears to result primarily from the presence of trace gases that contain sulfur. Gas in the GI tract is derived from four sources: 1) air swallowing (oxygen and nitrogen), 2) interaction of bicarbonate and acid (carbon dioxide), 3) diffusion from the blood (carbon dioxide, nitrogen and oxygen) and 4) bacterial metabolism (carbon dioxide, hydrogen, methane and a variety of trace gases). Swallowed air and bacterial fermentation in the colon contribute most of the intestinal gas volume.
3. Foods that contain ingredients with nonabsorbable oligosaccharides (e.g., raffinose, stachyose, verbacose) are likely to produce large amounts of intestinal gas. Dogs and cats lack the digestive enzymes needed to split these sugars into absorbable monosaccharides. Therefore, bacteria in the colon ferment these sugars producing hydrogen and carbon dioxide. Soybeans, beans, peas and other legumes contain large quantities of nonabsorbable oligosaccharides. Fiber-containing foods may contribute to flatus indirectly through reduced dry matter digestibility. Many fibers used in pet foods are fermented by the colonic microflora and may contribute to flatus directly. Rapidly fermentable fibers in pet foods include pectins and most gums. Intestinal gas production is also increased by fresh or dried foods containing fructose and fermentable fiber (e.g., apples, prunes, bananas). The food fed to this puppy contains soybean meal, a source of nonabsorbable oligosaccharides, which is likely contributing to excessive gas formation. The fresh fruits and vegetables used as snacks may also be contributing to the problem. Rice is the most highly digestible carbohydrate source used routinely in pet foods. Pets with flatulence will often improve when fed foods with rice as the sole or predominant carbohydrate source.
4. Feeding plans for animals with flatulence should focus on the food, feeding method, efforts to control aerophagia and management after meals. For this puppy, another commercial dry food that is complete and balanced for growth should be found that does not contain legumes (especially soybean meal), vegetables or fruits. A snack or treat should also be recommended that is not a vegetable or fruit. Aerophagia is most likely associated with rapid eating. Food can be offered more frequently to decrease the amount of air ingested at each meal or other methods can be tried to slow food ingestion and prevent gulping. Finally, the puppy should be walked or allowed to exercise within 30 minutes of each meal to encourage defecation or passage of intestinal gas outdoors.

Progress Notes

A different commercial dry puppy food was recommended (Science Diet Puppy Lamb Meal & Rice Formula[a]). This food contains the following major ingredients: lamb meal, rice, corn gluten meal, wheat, animal fat, egg, beet pulp, fish oil, vitamins and minerals. It does not contain soybean meal and uses rice as the major carbohydrate source; this change in ingredients should help minimize intestinal gas formation from bacterial fermentation. The food was still offered twice daily, but large rubber balls were put in the food bowl in an attempt to slow the rate of food ingestion. Fruits and vegetables were replaced as snacks with an appropriate commercial puppy treat (Science Diet Puppy Treats with Real Chicken[a]). The puppy was allowed to exercise in the fenced yard for 30 to 60 minutes after each meal. During the next health maintenance examination four weeks later, the owners reported a noticeable reduction in objectionable flatus.

Endnote

a. Hill's Pet Nutrition, Inc., Topeka, KS, USA.

Section 19

Pancreatic Disorders

,

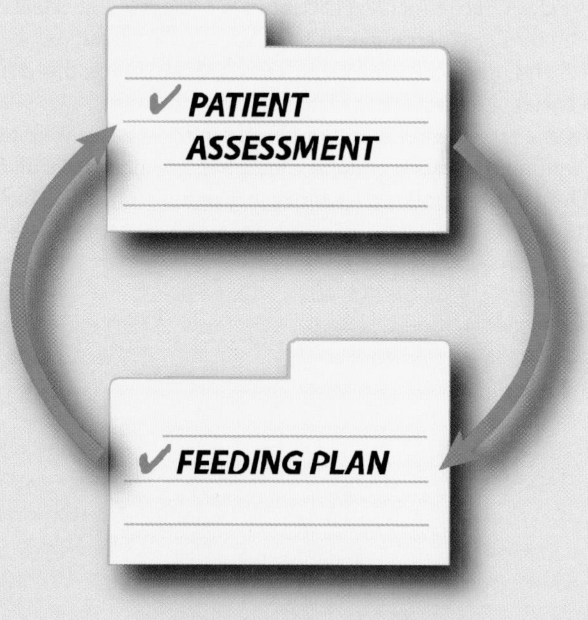

Chapter 66

Exocrine Pancreatic Insufficiency

Deborah J. Davenport
Rebecca L. Remillard
Kenny W. Simpson

"To eat is human, to digest divine."
Charles Copeland

CLINICAL IMPORTANCE

Malassimilation is failure of nutrients to pass across the intestinal wall in quantities sufficient to maintain body weight and condition (Jacobs et al, 1989). Malassimilation can be caused by either maldigestive or malabsorptive diseases. Malabsorption occurs with diseases that alter the structure and function of the small intestinal mucosa including the lymphatics. Maldigestion occurs with defects in intraluminal digestion and may result from gastric, pancreatic or biliary dysfunction. Exocrine pancreatic insufficiency (EPI) refers to a partial or complete deficiency of pancreatic enzymes and is the most common cause of maldigestion in dogs (Williams, 1994). Occurring most commonly in young dogs as a congenital disorder, pancreatic acinar atrophy, EPI may also develop as a sequela to acute and chronic pancreatitis (Williams, 1994) or pancreatic neoplasia (Westermarck and Wiberg, 2003). EPI is rare in cats but has been reported to occur in juvenile and acquired forms (Williams, 1994a; Steiner and Williams, 2000).

PATIENT ASSESSMENT

History and Physical Examination

Dogs and cats with EPI have a history of chronic small bowel diarrhea, weight loss and failure to thrive (Raiha and Westermarck, 1989). Pets with EPI defecate frequently (six to 10 bowel movements per day) and stools are typically voluminous, greasy, foul smelling and pale in color. When stained with Sudan III and examined microscopically, fat droplets are readily identified in such feces (**Figure 66-1**). Polyphagia, borborygmus, flatulence, pica and coprophagia are often reported. Vomiting and polydipsia occur less commonly (Raiha and Westermarck, 1989; Westermarck and Wiberg, 2003).

Affected dogs and cats generally have a normal appearance except for poor body condition (body condition score [BCS] 1/5 to 2/5) and poor coat quality. Cats with EPI may soil the coat in the perineal region (Steiner and Williams, 2000). Animals with pancreatic atrophy will be stunted in comparison to unaffected littermates or breed standards. Severely affected

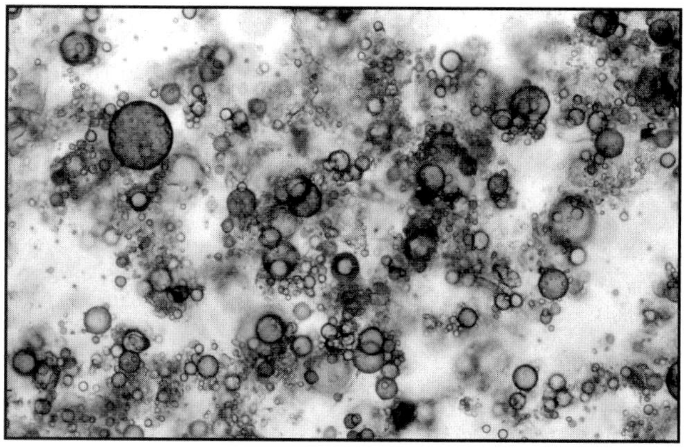

Figure 66-1. Feces stained with Sudan stain demonstrating increased amounts of fat (note globules) typical of exocrine pancreatic insufficiency. (Courtesy Dr. Robert Sherding, College of Veterinary Medicine, The Ohio State University, Columbus.)

patients may have hemorrhages due to a vitamin K-deficient coagulopathy (Perry et al, 1991).

Laboratory and Other Clinical Information

A presumptive diagnosis of EPI is often based on the signalment and patient history. Definitive diagnosis is achieved by radioimmunoassay of serum trypsin-like immunoreactivity (TLI). Low fasting TLI values (<2.5 µg/l) indicate EPI in dogs and cats (Williams and Batt, 1983, 1988; Steiner and Williams, 1996, 2000; Williams, 2006). This sensitive, specific, easy to perform serologic assay has replaced older tests including the bentiromide-PABA challenge, assay of fecal proteolytic activity, x-ray film digestion test and oral fat challenges. TLI measures serum levels of pancreatic trypsin and trypsinogen. Trypsinogen leaks out of pancreatic acini in trace amounts in healthy animals (normal canine serum TLI values = 5.0 to 35.0 µg/l, normal feline serum TLI values = 17.0 to 50.0 µg/l). In EPI, pancreatic acinar atrophy and fibrosis result in reduced serum TLI values. Serum amylase, isoamylase and lipase concentrations are of little value in diagnosing EPI due to pancreatic atrophy (Steiner et al, 2006). These tests may be of benefit when EPI occurs in conjunction with pancreatitis (Meyer and Williams, 1992).

Risk Factors

EPI due to pancreatic acinar atrophy is most common in young, large-breed dogs. German shepherd dogs, Eurasians and rough-coated collies appear to have a genetic predisposition to pancreatic acinar atrophy; however, any breed can be affected (Williams, 1994; Westermarck and Wiberg, 2003; Proschowsky and Fredholm, 2007). In the German shepherd dog and rough-coated collie, the pancreatic acinar atrophy appears to be an autosomal recessive disorder (Moeller et al, 2002) with an estimated disease prevalence of 1% (Westermarck and Wiberg, 2003). In the Eurasian dog breed, the inheritance pattern also appears to be autosomal recessive, but no candidate genes could be identified (Proschowsky and Fredholm, 2007). It is likely that the condition is multifactorial.

Acquired EPI may occur as a consequence of severe or recurrent pancreatic inflammation and resultant fibrosis. Thus, risk factors for acquired EPI are the same as for pancreatitis (Chapter 67).

Etiopathogenesis

Juvenile EPI results from atrophy of pancreatic acinar tissue rather than from congenital hypoplasia (Westermarck and Wiberg, 2003; Steiner, 2008). The disease has been subdivided into subclinical and clinical phases (Wiberg et al, 1999). Reports suggest that histopathologic evidence of atrophy is present before the onset of clinical signs (Westermarck et al, 1993; Wiberg et al, 1999). In the subclinical phase, atrophied and normal acinar cells are present in the pancreatic parenchyma along with a lymphocytic inflammatory infiltrate. The lymphocytic infiltrate suggests an autoimmune reaction. A prospective, placebo-controlled trial of an immunosuppressive drug (azathioprine) in dogs with subclinical EPI demonstrated the natural course of the pancreatic acinar atrophy to be extremely variable with some dogs remaining in the subclinical phase for many years without immunosuppressive therapy (Wiberg and Westermarck, 2002). Unfortunately, the authors were unable to identify markers predictive of disease progression.

Clinical signs do not develop until 85 to 90% of functional exocrine tissue is lost (Jacobs et al, 1989), usually when patients are six to 18 months old (Westermarck et al, 1993). Subnormal serum TLI levels may be present in the subclinical phase even when clinical signs are not present (Wiberg et al, 1999a).

In the juvenile form of EPI, endocrine function is usually normal and diabetes mellitus does not develop. In rare cases, EPI and diabetes mellitus may occur concurrently in young dogs and cats (Sherding, 1979; Boari et al, 1994).

The acquired form of EPI arises as a consequence of the inflammation and fibrosis of endstage chronic pancreatitis (Watson, 1995). Diabetes mellitus may develop concurrently because pancreatic islet cells are similarly affected. EPI may occur as a consequence of pancreatic adenocarcinoma or cholecystoduodenostomy (Williams, 1994).

Several mechanisms are responsible for the severe nutrient malassimilation that occurs in EPI. Most important, the deficiency of pancreatic enzymes results in a failure of intraluminal digestion and inability of the patient to effectively use nutrients. In addition, the lack of other pancreatic secretory products, including bicarbonate, gastrointestinal (GI) trophic factors, antimicrobial factors and intrinsic factor contribute to impaired GI function and nutrient malassimilation. Intestinal mucosal enzyme activity is impaired in experimental and naturally occurring EPI (Williams, 1996). Impaired mucosal enzyme function results in abnormal sugar, amino acid and fatty acid transport. The cause for the intestinal mucosal abnormality is unknown but is suspected to result from the absence of trophic pancreatic secretions and concurrent small intestinal bacterial overgrowth (SIBO).

Dogs with EPI commonly have SIBO because they lack the antibacterial factors present in pancreatic secretions and have changes in immunity secondary to malnutrition (Williams et al, 1987; Westermarck et al, 1993a; Simpson et al, 1990). In addition, many German shepherd dogs with EPI also have IgA deficiency (Batt et al, 1991; Whitbread et al, 1984). Bacterial overgrowth contributes to malnutrition in EPI by destroying exposed brush border enzymes and consuming unabsorbed intraluminal nutrients. In addition, bacterial hydroxylation of fatty acids may exacerbate fat malabsorption and contribute to osmotic and secretory diarrhea.

Diarrhea in EPI is usually characterized as osmotic. Distal ileal and colonic microflora ferment undigested sugars and fats, releasing osmotically active particles. These particles drive fluid into the gut lumen, which overwhelms the colonic capacity for water reabsorption. Additionally, hydroxy fatty acids formed from bacterial metabolism of undigested fats can trigger secretory diarrhea.

Key Nutritional Factors

Key nutritional factors for patients with EPI are listed in **Table 66-1** and are discussed in more detail below.

Table 66-1. Key nutritional factors for foods for patients with exocrine pancreatic insufficiency.*

Factors	Recommended levels
Digestibility	≥87% for protein and ≥90% for fat and digestible carbohydrate
Fat	10 to 15% for dogs 15 to 25% for cats
Fiber	≤5%**

*Nutrients expressed on a dry matter basis.
**Lower is better.

Digestibility

The primary nutritional factor in the management of EPI is food digestibility. The use of highly digestible foods (fat and digestible [soluble] carbohydrate ≥90% and protein ≥87%) should be coupled with the addition of pancreatic enzyme preparations to the food. In one study, the combination of a highly digestible commercial veterinary therapeutic food plus pancreatic enzymes provided more metabolizable energy to dogs with EPI than a grocery brand food with pancreatic enzyme supplementation (Pidgeon, 1982). Further studies using naturally occurring EPI cases also demonstrated the benefits of feeding highly digestible foods (Westermarck et al, 1990, 1995).

Highly digestible veterinary therapeutic foods contain meat and carbohydrate sources that have been highly refined to increase digestibility. Typical ingredients in such commercial foods include egg, cottage cheese and muscle and organ meats. Carbohydrates in highly digestible foods are primarily starches of corn, rice, barley and wheat, which are readily digested if properly cooked.

Fat

Steatorrhea is the most prominent clinical sign in patients with EPI. As discussed above, feeding a highly digestible food in conjunction with pancreatic enzyme supplementation is more effective than simply decreasing the fat content of the current food (Pidgeon, 1982; Westermarck et al, 1995). Dry matter (DM) dietary fat levels for patients with EPI should be in the range of 10 to 15% for dogs and 15 to 25% for cats. Overall fat digestion of a highly digestible food with added pancreatic enzymes can exceed 70% in dogs with EPI (Pidgeon, 1982). The addition of medium-chain triglycerides (MCT) to the food can result in increased total fat assimilation because they are more water soluble and are digested and absorbed by mechanisms independent of those used for long-chain triglycerides. However, supplementation of foods with MCT generally decreases the food's palatability, which may decrease total food intake and thus be counterproductive. This is not necessarily true for commercial foods that contain MCT. Addition of MCT is unnecessary in most cases (Rutz et al, 2004) (Box 58-1).

Feeding high-fat growth-type foods (>27% DM fat) in conjunction with pancreatic enzymes has been associated with increased frequency of defecation, poor fecal consistency and higher fecal fat content in canine EPI as compared to results obtained from feeding lower fat diets (Westermarck et al, 2006).

Fiber

Foods for patients with EPI should contain very little fiber (≤5% DM, lower is better) to maximize food digestibility. Dietary fiber impairs pancreatic enzyme activity in vitro. Decreasing the fiber content from 4% to less than 1% in a study of people with EPI decreased fecal weight and fat excretion by one-third and reduced bloating and flatus (Dutta and Hlasko, 1985). In a three-week dietary trial in dogs with EPI, feeding a low-fat (7% DM), high-fiber (25% DM) food in conjunction with pancreatic enzymes resulted in mild weight loss, increased consumption of food and increased fecal mass and defecation frequency (Westermarck and Wiberg, 2006). These findings are likely attributable to the low fat and caloric content of the food and the effect of high fiber levels on food digestibility. Interestingly, stool quality in these patients was considered good (firmer) as compared to feces produced when the dogs were fed higher fat foods.

Other Nutritional Factors

Vitamins

Micronutrients should be considered in the dietary management of patients with malassimilation. In EPI, the lack of pancreatic lipase results in failed solubilization and absorption of the fat-soluble vitamins A, D, E and K. Vitamins A and D may be initially administered intramuscularly (0.5 to 1 ml divided into two intramuscular sites every three months), if fat absorption remains impaired. Supplementation of vitamins A and D should be reserved for patients with demonstrably low levels of these vitamins or ongoing fat malabsorption because oversupplementation may be harmful.

Vitamin E supplementation (400 to 500 IU, per os, q24h) may be beneficial when serum concentrations are very low. Clinically, vitamin K deficiency has been described (Perry et al,

Table 66-2. Key nutritional factors in selected commercial veterinary therapeutic foods for dogs with exocrine pancreatic insufficiency compared to recommended levels.*

Dry foods	Protein digestibility (%)	Fat digestibility (%)	Carbohydrate digestibility (%)	Fat (%)	Crude fiber (%)
Recommended levels	**≥87**	**≥90**	**≥90**	**10-15**	**≤5****
Hill's Prescription Diet i/d Canine	92	93	94	14.1	2.7
Iams Veterinary Formula Intestinal Low-Residue	na	na	na	10.7	2.1
Medi-Cal Gastro Formula	na	na	na	13.9	1.9
Purina Veterinary Diets EN GastroENteric Formula***	84.5	91.4	94.4	12.6	1.5
Purina Veterinary Diets HA Hypoallergenic Formula***	90.7	93.1	95.7	10.54	1.58
Royal Canin Veterinary Diet Low Fat LF 20	na	na	na	6.6	2.3
Royal Canin Veterinary Diet Hypoallergenic HP 19	na	na	na	20.9	2.3

Moist foods	Protein digestibility (%)	Fat digestibility (%)	Carbohydrate digestibility (%)	Fat (%)	Crude fiber (%)
Recommended levels	**≥87**	**≥90**	**≥90**	**10-15**	**≤5****
Hill's Prescription Diet i/d Canine	88	94	93	14.9	1.0
Iams Veterinary Formula Intestinal Low-Residue	na	na	na	13.2	3.9
Medi-Cal Gastro Formula	na	na	na	11.7	1.0
Purina Veterinary Diets EN GastroENteric Formula***	85.1	95.6	92.2	13.8	0.9
Royal Canin Veterinary Diet Low Fat LF	na	na	na	6.9	3.0

Key: na = information not available from manufacturer.
*All values are on a dry matter basis; values obtained from manufacturer.
**Lower is better.
***Contains medium-chain triglycerides; see text.

1991). Severe hemorrhage may occur when vitamin K stores are depleted because of the vitamin's pivotal role in the post-translational carboxylation of coagulation factors. Parenteral supplementation of vitamin K_1 is recommended (5 to 20 mg, q12h) if coagulopathies are detected in dogs and cats with EPI.

Folate and cobalamin are also of concern. Dogs and cats with EPI often have low serum cobalamin concentrations (Williams, 1996). Reports have identified cobalamin deficiency in 82% of dogs (Batchelor et al, 2007) and 60% of cats (Steiner and Williams, 2000) with EPI. Cobalamin deficiency has been associated with poor outcomes in canine EPI (Batchelor et al, 2007). Several mechanisms may play a role in the development of cobalamin deficiency in EPI. The absence of pancreatic bicarbonate secretion may reduce the intestinal luminal pH and the affinity of cobalamin for intrinsic factor (Simpson et al, 1989). Additionally, the pancreas appears to be the primary source of intrinsic factor in dogs and cats rather than the gastric mucosa (Simpson et al, 1989; Fyfe, 1993). Finally, when SIBO is present, the proximal gut microflora may consume dietary cobalamin before it can be absorbed (Batt and Morgan, 1982; Williams, 1991). If serum levels of cobalamin are low, weekly supplementation by subcutaneous or intramuscular routes is recommended (100 to 250 µg for cats; 250 to 1,200 µg for dogs) for six weeks or until serum cobalamin concentration normalizes (Williams, 1996; Steiner, 2008). Long-term monitoring of serum cobalamin levels is recommended in dogs and cats with EPI to avoid a recurrence (Williams, 2006).

Serum folate levels are elevated in most dogs with EPI probably due to SIBO and bacterial elaboration of folate (Williams, 1996). Serum folate concentration may be decreased, however, in dogs with EPI and concurrent enteropathies involving the ileum (Williams, 1996). In such cases, parenteral supplementation of folate (0.5 to 1 mg, per os q24h) is recommended until the ileal pathology is resolved. Folate deficiency inhibits pancreatic exocrine function in rats (Balaghi and Wagner, 1995).

Minerals

Dogs with experimentally induced EPI had reduced serum and tissue levels of zinc and copper (Adamama-Moraitour et al, 2001). Similar findings have been recognized in some human patients with EPI (Watson et al, 1988) and are speculated to be due to a deficiency in a pancreatic zinc-binding factor, which facilitates zinc transport and absorption within the intestinal epithelium. However, zinc and copper levels have been investigated in spontaneous cases of EPI and were not found to be low (Williams, 1992). Thus, routine supplementation of these minerals does not seem to be warranted in EPI.

FEEDING PLAN

Dietary management is an essential component in the medical management of patients with maldigestive diseases. Dietary intake should meet the patient's nutrient needs in a form that promotes nutrient absorption. The organs of the GI tract have very large reserve capacities and the small intestine has a very large and efficient absorptive area. About 90% of the pancreas must be dysfunctional before clinical signs of maldigestion are seen (Jacobs et al, 1989). Consequently, patients with clinical signs of maldigestion have very little digestive capacity remaining.

Assess and Select the Food

Levels of key nutritional factors should be evaluated in foods currently fed to patients with EPI and compared with recom-

Table 66-3. Key nutritional factors in selected commercial veterinary therapeutic foods for cats with exocrine pancreatic insufficiency compared to recommended levels.*

Dry foods	Protein digestibility (%)	Fat digestibility (%)	Carbohydrate digestibility (%)	Fat (%)	Crude fiber (%)
Recommended levels	**≥87**	**≥90**	**≥90**	**15-25**	**≤5****
Hill's Prescription Diet i/d Feline	88	92	90	20.2	2.8
Iams Veterinary Formula Intestinal Low-Residue	na	na	na	13.7	1.8
Medi-Cal Hypoallergenic/Gastro	na	na	na	11.5	3.1
Purina Veterinary Diets EN GastroENteric Formula	94.0	93.1	79.7	18.4	1.3
Royal Canin Veterinary Diets Hypoallergenic HP 23	na	na	na	21.5	4.8

Moist foods	Protein digestibility (%)	Fat digestibility (%)	Carbohydrate digestibility (%)	Fat (%)	Crude fiber (%)
Recommended levels	**≥87**	**≥90**	**≥90**	**15-25**	**≤5****
Hill's Prescription Diet i/d Feline	91	89	91	24.1	2.4
Iams Veterinary Formula Intestinal Low-Residue	na	na	na	11.7	3.7
Medi-Cal Hypoallergenic/Gastro	na	na	na	35.9	1.2

Key: na = information not available from manufacturer.
*All values are on a dry matter basis; values obtained from manufacturer.
**Lower is better.

mended levels. Information from this aspect of assessment is essential for making any changes to foods currently provided. Changing to a more appropriate food is indicated if key nutritional factors in the food currently provided do not match recommended levels.

Selected commercial veterinary therapeutic foods that are highly digestible and designed for canine and feline patients with GI disease are listed in **Tables 66-2** and **66-3**, respectively. These foods are marketed for patients with EPI. For comparative purposes, these tables include recommended levels of key nutritional factors. Feeding these foods to patients with EPI often allows smaller amounts of pancreatic enzyme preparations to be used, which results in significant cost savings for pet owners, especially those with large-breed dogs. Foods for young, growing dogs and cats with EPI should also meet the optimal levels of key nutritional factors for growth (Chapters 17 [puppies] and 24 [kittens]).

Assess and Determine the Feeding Method

Because the feeding method is often altered in patients with EPI, a thorough assessment should include verification of the feeding method currently being used. Items to consider include feeding frequency, amount fed, how the food is offered, access to other food and who feeds the pet. All of this information should have been gathered when the dietary history was obtained.

Patients presenting with signs of malnutrition due to chronic maldigestion should be given parenteral nutritional support during the diagnostic workup. Parenteral nutrition in the management of these patients is primarily supportive, may be essential in the initial stages of case management and improves the patient's disposition. Parenteral nutrition also improves caloric, protein and micronutrient balances in veterinary patients, thereby decreasing risks associated with diagnostic procedures including exploratory surgery. Continued administration of parenteral nutrition (more than three days) is necessary in debilitated patients as a supportive procedure until nutrients can be adequately absorbed. Parenteral nutrition can be performed at most practices in a manner similar to other fluid therapies (Chapter 26).

Patients with EPI usually should be fed multiple small meals per day with pancreatic enzyme supplementation to improve digestibility. At home, feeding at least two to three times daily helps prevent dietary overload and osmotic diarrhea. The daily energy requirement of underweight patients should be increased above that for healthy patients (2 x resting energy requirement for their estimated ideal weight) until ideal body weight and condition (BCS 2.5/5 to 3.5/5) are reached. Even after patients reach ideal body weight, it may be necessary to offer an above average amount of food to offset the persistent degree of malabsorption. Pancreatic enzymes should be added immediately before feeding. (See below.)

ADJUNCTIVE MEDICAL MANAGEMENT

Supplemental Pancreatic Enzymes

In addition to dietary management, effective treatment of EPI requires oral administration of pancreatic enzymes. Most often, pancreatic enzymes are supplied as dried, powdered extracts of bovine or porcine pancreas (**Table 66-4**). Such powder extracts are typically more effective than tablets or capsules (Westermarck, 1987; Steiner, 2008). Tablets, capsules and enteric-coated preparations are not recommended. Lipase activity of pancreatic enzyme preparations varies markedly. Generally, the more expensive preparations have better lipase activity.

If available, raw bovine, porcine or ovine pancreas can be effective (Westermarck et al, 1990). Raw pancreas can be frozen in individual doses for several months without losing enzyme activity. Dogs should receive 30 to 90 g (1 to 3 oz.) of freshly thawed, chopped pancreas, whereas cats should

Table 66-4. Enzyme preparations used in patients with exocrine pancreatic insufficiency.*

Products (manufacturers)	Lipase	Protease	Amylase	Formulation
Viokase-V Powder (Fort Dodge)	71,400	388,000	460,000	Powder
Viokase-V Tablets (Fort Dodge)	9,000	57,000	64,000	Tablets
Viokase Powder (Axcan Scandipharm)	16,800	70,000	70,000	Powder
Pancrezyme Powder (Daniels Pharmaceuticals)	71,400	388,000	460,000	Powder
Pancrezyme Tablets (Daniels Pharmaceuticals)	9,000	57,000	64,000	Tablets
Pancrease MT16 Capsules (McNeil)	18,000	18,000	48,000	Enteric-coated microtablets
Pancrease MT20 Capsules (McNeil)	20,000	44,000	56,000	Enteric-coated microtablets
Pancreatic Plus Powder (Butler)	71,400	388,000	460,000	Powder
Pancreatic Plus Tablets (Butler)	9,000	57,000	64,000	Tablets
Pancrelipase Capsules (Mutual)	18,000	18,000	48,000	Enteric-coated pellets
Lypex Pancreatic Enzyme Capsules (Vio-Vet)	30,000	18,750	1,200	Capsules

*Enzymatic contents (IU) per capsule, tablet or tsp of powder (2.8 g).

receive 30 g (1 oz.) of chopped pancreas per meal (Steiner, 2008).

Pancreatic enzyme supplementation for dogs should be initiated at a dose of 1 tsp of powdered pancreatic extract per 10 kg body weight at each meal. For cats, a starting dose of 1 tsp should be administered with each meal (Suzuki et al, 1997). Enzymes should be mixed with food immediately before the meal is fed. Owners may be able to decrease the dose of pancreatic enzymes based on their pet's response. Most dogs require at least 1 tsp of enzymes per meal (Williams, 1996).

Despite the administration of pancreatic enzyme preparations, fat digestion does not return to normal in dogs with EPI. Inactivation of pancreatic lipase by the acidic pH of the stomach is likely responsible for failure to normalize fat digestion (Williams, 1994).

Antacids and H_2-Receptor Blockers

Antacids and H_2-receptor blockers have been recommended in the therapeutic regimen to reduce gastric acid-induced destruction of orally administered enzymes. This practice, however, is costly and does not increase efficacy of pancreatic enzyme supplementation (Williams, 1994). Concurrent oral administration of sodium bicarbonate or bile salts and pre-incubation of the meal with pancreatic enzymes are also unnecessary (Williams, 1994, 1996). In one study, adding digestive enzymes to food 20 to 30 minutes before feeding did not improve the response to dietary management (Pidgeon, 1980).

Antibiotics

Oral antibiotics may be necessary to resolve clinical signs in dogs and cats with concurrent SIBO. Tetracycline (20 mg/kg body weight, per os, t.i.d. for 21 days) or tylosin (25 mg/kg body weight, per os, b.i.d. for six weeks) is most often recommended for this purpose; however, metronidazole (10 to 20 mg/kg body weight, per os, every 24 hours for seven to 14 days) may be more effective if SIBO with anaerobic organisms is suspected.

Insulin

Concurrent diabetes mellitus in EPI cases must be managed with insulin. Unfortunately, the fiber-enhanced foods often recommended for diabetic pets are contraindicated for those with EPI (Remillard and Thatcher, 1989). Dietary management of patients with concurrent diabetes mellitus and EPI often requires a modified profile of key nutritional factors. In many cases, foods containing 10 to 15% DM fat, 50 to 55% DM complex, digestible (soluble) carbohydrate and 5 to 10% total dietary fiber can be used.

REASSESSMENT

The prognosis for long-term response to treatment is good in dogs with EPI. In one study, 19% of affected dogs were euthanized within one year of diagnosis due to cost of treatment and/or persistence of clinical signs; however, the median survival time was more than 60 months (Batchelor et al, 2007).

Clinical signs usually resolve within three to five days with proper dietary and enzyme therapy, and weight gain is evident by five to 10 days. Successfully managed canine cases of EPI are recognized by weight gain (0.5 to 1 kg per week) and improved body condition and stool consistency. The food and enzyme dose should be reevaluated if less satisfactory results are obtained. In a retrospective study of dogs with EPI, approximately 10% of patients still had soft to diarrheic stools and 20% were considered underweight (owners' assessment) after 12 months of treatment (Batchelor et al, 2007). Often, the initial dose of pancreatic enzymes is inadequate and must be increased. Every effort should be made to rule out concurrent small bowel disease (e.g., eosinophilic gastroenteritis, lymphoplasmacytic enteritis, SIBO) or diabetes mellitus when clinical response is unsatisfactory. In addition, serum cobalamin levels should be assessed to ensure that cobalamin nutriture is adequate. If not, parenteral cobalamin supplementation should be initiated as described above.

Pancreatic enzyme extract may cause oral mucosal irritation resulting in hemorrhage and reluctance to eat (Rutz et al, 2002; Snead, 2006). If this occurs, decreasing the dose and mixing the pancreatic enzyme powder well in the food may resolve the issue. If not, feeding raw pancreas should be considered.

Well-compensated patients should be evaluated immediately if a change or decline in condition is noted. Feeding more food than expected may be necessary to compensate for decreased digestibility and to maintain optimal body weight and condition. Regaining or maintaining optimal body weight and condition, normal activity level, improved disposition and absence of clinical signs are measures of successful dietary management.

REFERENCES

The references for **Chapter 66** can be found at www.markmorris.org.

CASE 66-1

Chronic Diarrhea in a German Shepherd Crossbred Dog

Jörg M. Steiner, med vet, Dr med vet, Dipl. ACVIM (Internal Medicine) and ECVIM (Companion Animal)
College of Veterinary Medicine
Texas A&M University
College Station, Texas, USA

Patient Assessment

A two-and-one-half-year-old neutered male German shepherd crossbred dog was examined for chronic diarrhea, polyphagia and weight loss of six months' duration. The feces were characteristic of small bowel disorders: watery to semi-formed consistency, clay-colored, large volumes passed two to three times per day, no melena or hematochezia and only small amounts of mucus. Body weight had decreased over the past six months from 34 kg to 22 kg and body condition was now poor (body condition score [BCS] 1/5). The dog's coat was dull and brittle.

Diagnostic evaluation included a complete blood count (normal), serum biochemistry profile (normal except for mild elevations in liver enzyme activity), urinalysis (normal), direct fecal smear and fecal flotation for parasites (negative), fecal stain for fat (positive) and testing for serum concentrations of canine trypsin-like immunoreactivity (TLI), cobalamin and folate. Serum canine TLI concentration was decreased (0.6 mg/l, normal 5 to 35), serum cobalamin concentration was decreased (150 ng/l, normal 225 to 1,680) and serum folate concentration was increased (23.4 mg/l, normal 6.7 to 17.4).

Assess and the Food and Feeding Method

The dog had been fed several commercial dry foods free choice during the past six months. A veterinary therapeutic food (Limited Ingredient Diet: Canine Whitefish and Potato[a]) had been fed for the last two months as an elimination trial for suspected food allergy. The dog was fed five cups per day (1,645 kcal [6.88 MJ]).

Questions

1. What is the tentative diagnosis?
2. What are the key nutritional factors for this dog?
3. Outline a feeding plan (foods and feeding method) for this patient.
4. What ancillary therapy is indicated to complement the feeding plan?

Answers and Discussion

1. A history of chronic diarrhea, steatorrhea and weight loss in a young German shepherd dog suggests exocrine pancreatic insufficiency (EPI) or some other cause of malassimilation (i.e., maldigestion or malabsorption). The decreased serum TLI concentration confirms that EPI is present. Mild increases in hepatic enzyme activity are often seen in patients with EPI. Liver disease does not need to be evaluated further unless hepatic enzyme activity continues to increase or if response to therapy is suboptimal. The decreased serum cobalamin concentration and increased serum folate concentration are consistent with small intestinal bacterial overgrowth (SIBO). Increased numbers of many species of bacteria generate large quantities of folate, which is available for absorption via specific carriers in the proximal small intestine. In contrast, most bacteria compete for available intraluminal cobalamin and thereby reduce its uptake in the distal small intestine. SIBO commonly occurs as a secondary problem associated with EPI. The poor coat probably reflects protein-calorie malnutrition and essential fatty acid deficiency.
2. Key nutritional factors to consider in patients with EPI include food digestibility and fat and fiber content. Selected vitamins are sometimes important. The use of highly digestible foods (fat and digestible carbohydrate ≥90% and protein ≥87%) in conjunction with pancreatic enzyme supplements provides more metabolizable nutrients to dogs with EPI than use of foods with average digestibility and comparable supplementation. Although steatorrhea due to fat malassimilation is a prominent sign in patients with EPI, fat restriction is unnecessary. Moderate dietary fat levels in conjunction with pancreatic enzyme supplementation are more effective than simply decreasing the fat content of the food. Some forms of dietary fiber impair pancreatic enzyme activi-

ty in vitro and may have similar effects in animals. Therefore, excess dietary fiber should be avoided (≤5% fiber, dry matter basis) in these patients. Fat-soluble vitamins, cobalamin and folate are sometimes nutrients of concern in patients with EPI complicated by SIBO. Such patients may develop deficiencies in one or more fat-soluble vitamins. Clinical signs of vitamin K deficiency (vitamin K-responsive coagulopathy) have been described in patients with EPI. Several mechanisms may play a role in cobalamin deficiency including alterations in intestinal luminal pH, decreased levels of intrinsic factor and SIBO. Serum folate concentrations are often elevated in EPI patients with SIBO but may be decreased in patients with concurrent enteropathies.

3. Dogs with EPI should be fed commercial or homemade foods that are highly digestible, moderate in fat and low in fiber (**Table 66-2**). The initial daily energy requirement (DER) should be estimated as 2 x resting energy requirement using an ideal body weight of 34 kg (DER = 2,180 kcal [9.12 MJ]). The DER should be adjusted based on weekly assessments of fecal quantity/quality and body weight and condition. Parenteral administration of fat-soluble and B-complex vitamins is also appropriate.
4. Pancreatic enzyme supplementation is necessary using either dried pancreatic extracts (1 tsp/10 kg body weight with meal) or raw bovine, porcine or ovine pancreas (30 g/10 kg body weight with meal). Powdered extracts are usually preferred to tablets and capsules. The amount can be gradually decreased to find the minimum effective dose after clinical improvement occurs. Broad-spectrum antimicrobial therapy is appropriate for most cases of SIBO; oral oxytetracycline or tylosin is often recommended. However, SIBO is often self-limiting in patients with EPI if dietary alterations and pancreatic enzyme supplementation are successful in controlling clinical signs. SIBO is clinically significant in some patients with EPI, so recovery will not be complete unless antimicrobial therapy is given.

Progress Notes

The food was changed to a commercial dry veterinary therapeutic food that was highly digestible, moderate in fat and low in fiber (Prescription Diet i/d Canine[b]). Two tsp of dried pancreatic extract (Pancrezyme[c]) were mixed thoroughly with two cups of slightly moistened food just before feeding. This mixture was fed three times daily.

The dog ate this mixture well and the diarrhea gradually decreased over the next six to eight weeks. As the dog's stool improved, body weight increased, body condition improved and the dog's coat became shinier and less brittle. A body weight of 31 kg and BCS of 3/5 were reached approximately 12 weeks after initiating therapy. At that time the dosage of dried pancreatic extract was reduced to 1.5 tsp with each meal and plans were made to further reduce the dosage if clinical signs did not return.

Endnotes

a. Innovative Veterinary Diets, Newport, KY, USA.
b. Hill's Pet Nutrition, Inc., Topeka, KS, USA.
c. Daniels Pharmaceuticals Inc., St Petersburg, FL, USA.

Bibliography

Pidgeon G. Effect of diet on exocrine pancreatic insufficiency in dogs. Journal of the American Veterinary Medical Association 1982; 281: 232-235.

Williams DA. Exocrine pancreatic disease. In: Ettinger SJ, Feldman EC, eds. Textbook of Veterinary Internal Medicine, 4th ed. Philadelphia, PA: WB Saunders Co, 1995; 1372-1392.

Williams DA. Small intestinal bacterial overgrowth. In: Guilford WG, Center SA, Strombeck DR, et al, eds. Strombeck's Small Animal Gastroenterology, 3rd ed. Philadelphia, PA: WB Saunders Co, 1996; 370-373.

Chapter 67

Acute and Chronic Pancreatitis

Deborah J. Davenport
Rebecca L. Remillard
Kenny W. Simpson

"What do you want–an adorable pancreas?"
Jean Kerr, The Snake Has All the Lines

CLINICAL IMPORTANCE

Pancreatitis has been recognized as a clinical entity in dogs for more than a century (Simpson, 1993). In dogs, acute pancreatitis is an important differential diagnosis for vomiting and abdominal pain. Because of difficulties in diagnosis, pancreatitis is a less common diagnosis in cats. Based on clinical and pathologic reports, diagnosis of feline pancreatitis is apparently increasing (Akol et al, 1993; Hill and Van Winkle, 1993; Steiner and Williams, 1997; Hines et al, 1996; De Cock et al, 2007; Maddison, 2008). One study reported an incidence of 0.57 to 3.5% in cats (Mansfield and Jones, 2001). Another pathology study reported that exocrine pancreatic lesions are present in approximately 1.5% of patients presented for necropsy and that 59% of dogs and 46% of cats with exocrine pancreatic lesions had evidence of pancreatitis (Hanichen and Minkus, 1990).

PATIENT ASSESSMENT

History and Physical Examination

As many as 90% of dogs with pancreatitis present with acute vomiting (Hess et al, 1998). Vomiting may be sporadic and mild or very severe. Other clinical signs include abdominal pain, depression, anorexia, fever and diarrhea. Icterus and pale-colored stools may be reported if pancreatic inflammation and edema are severe enough to result in common bile duct obstruction. If present, diarrhea is usually of large bowel origin because the transverse colon passes dorsal to the pancreas and is susceptible to local inflammation at that site.

An episode of dietary indiscretion often occurs during the 24 hours before the onset of vomiting. The owner commonly relates consumption of high-fat human food. Occasionally, the onset of clinical signs is preceded by administration of drugs associated with pancreatitis. Corticosteroids, in particular, have been linked to pancreatitis in dogs (Simpson, 1993).

Cats with pancreatitis have highly variable clinical signs. In some cats, the disease may mimic the typical canine presentation (i.e., acute vomiting, lethargy, anorexia, diarrhea and abdominal pain). In others, a more indolent, smoldering course occurs, resulting in a mild chronic illness (Steiner and Williams, 1997). The most common clinical signs in cats are anorexia, lethargy, dehydration and weight loss. Abdominal pain may be difficult to recognize and vomiting occurs in fewer than 50% of cases (Washabau, 2001). Other cats may present with a palpable abdominal mass. In some cats, pancreatitis may be linked to diabetes mellitus and clinical signs may include polydipsia/polyuria and weight loss (Steiner and Williams, 1997). In others, hepatic lipidosis or cholangiohepatitis may occur concurrently resulting in icterus (Akol et al, 1993; Weiss et al, 1996). In some cats, pancreatitis, cholangiohepatitis and inflammatory bowel disease (IBD) may be present simultaneously (triaditis).

Depression, fever and dehydration may be the most prominent physical examination findings. Abdominal palpation may elicit splinting and discomfort that can be localized to the right cranial quadrant. Icterus, shock and coagulopathies may be detected in severe cases.

Clinical manifestations are variable in chronic pancreatitis. Weight loss and poor body condition may be the only signs noted in cats. An abnormal thickening or hardness of the falciform fat pad may be palpated in some cats, suggesting saponification and fat necrosis.

Laboratory and Other Clinical Information

The laboratory diagnosis of acute and chronic pancreatitis can be very frustrating. Diagnosis is hampered by the poor specificity of available laboratory tests and the inaccessibility of tissue for cytologic or histopathologic examination. Serum amylase and lipase activities are the most commonly used laboratory tests for the diagnosis of pancreatitis in dogs and cats. Unfortunately, these tests are not very specific because they are influenced by a number of other disease conditions (e.g., renal failure, dehydration, hyperlipidemia). In addition, the short half-life of amylase and lipase often precludes their use as diagnostic aids unless the patient is presented promptly after the onset of clinical signs. If present, hyperamylasemia and hyperlipasemia support a diagnosis of pancreatitis if azotemia and hyperlipidemia are not present. In cats, pancreatic amylase secretion is only 10% of that in dogs and serum amylase is usually low in cats with pancreatitis (Zoran, 2007).

Serum trypsin-like immunoreactivity (TLI) concentration has been suggested as a diagnostic aid for evaluating dogs and cats with suspected pancreatitis. Because TLI is specifically pancreatic in origin, high serum TLI concentrations were hoped to be a more reliable indicator of clinical pancreatitis than high amylase or lipase activities (Simpson et al, 1989). However, the sensitivity of TLI assays in dogs and cats with acute pancreatitis appears to be very low (30 to 60%) (Williams, 2006).

More recently, assays for canine and feline specific pancreatic lipase have come into clinical use. In healthy dogs and cats, very little pancreatic lipase is present in blood. In pancreatitis, the inflamed organ leaks larger amounts of lipase into the blood, which is measurable by immunoassay. These species-specific assays appear to be more sensitive (>80%) than TLI concentrations for the diagnosis of pancreatitis in dogs and cats (Steiner, 2006; Forman et al, 2002). Additionally, these assays are not falsely elevated in renal disease (Steiner et al, 2001) or by corticosteroid administration (Steiner et al, 2003).

A complete blood cell count, serum biochemistry profile and urinalysis should be done for any dog or cat suspected to have pancreatitis to rule out other potential causes for the clinical signs. Additionally, these tests may aid in the diagnosis of concurrent medical conditions such as diabetes mellitus, hepatic lipidosis, interstitial nephritis and cholangiohepatitis.

Anorectic or vomiting canine and feline patients with pancreatitis may become hypokalemic. In one retrospective study, hypocalcemia was recognized in 40% of cats with acute pancreatitis and was considered indicative of a poor prognosis (Kimmel et al, 2001). Hypocalcemia may be attributable to conditions such as hypoalbuminemia, parathormone resistance or to the saponification of calcium by fatty acids (Kimmel et al, 2001; Washabau, 2001).

An inflammatory leukogram is typically identified in patients with pancreatitis. A degenerative left shift may indicate severe necrotic pancreatitis. In cats, leukopenia appears to occur more commonly than in dogs and is associated with a poor prognosis (Washabau, 2001). If thrombocytopenia is noted on the hemogram, a complete coagulation screen should be performed to rule out disseminated intravascular coagulation.

Imaging can be useful for diagnosing pancreatitis in dogs and cats. Findings consistent with pancreatic inflammation on survey abdominal radiographs may include haziness and widening of the gastroduodenal angle in the right cranial quadrant. Often, segmental gas distention of the proximal duodenum is noted. In the hands of an experienced operator, abdominal ultrasonography appears to be a sensitive test for the diagnosis of acute pancreatitis in dogs (Mansfield et al, 2008). Typical findings include enlargement of the pancreas, hypoechogenicity, dilatation of the pancreatic duct and hyperechogenicity of the mesentery. Peripancreatic fluid accumulation is a common finding in dogs and cats (Williams, 2006). Ultrasonography may reveal fluid-filled cysts, pseudocysts or abscesses within the pancreatic parenchyma and can be used to guide needle aspiration of pancreatic masses (Salisbury et al, 1988; VanEnkevort et al, 1999). In cats, the reported sensitivity of abdominal ultrasonography ranges from 20 to 67% (Rademacher et al, 2008). Typical ultrasonographic findings in cats are similar to those described in dogs. More sophisticated contrast-enhanced power and color Doppler ultrasonographic procedures also distinguish between normal cats and cats with pancreatitis (Rademacher et al, 2008). When coupled with measurement of serum pancreatic lipase immunoreactivity, abdominal ultrasonography was more sensitive than computed tomography in the diagnosis of acute pancreatitis in cats (Forman et al, 2004).

The gold standard for diagnosing acute and chronic pancreatitis is histopathology. Unfortunately, pancreatic biopsies are rarely performed because of the invasive nature of the procedure and because many patients with pancreatitis are poor anesthetic risks. However, laparoscopic techniques for the diagnosis of pancreatic disease in dogs and cats have been described; these provide a minimally invasive method for collection of pancreatic biopsy specimens (Marmoinen et al, 2002; Webb and Trott, 2008). Unfortunately, laparoscopy does not provide good visualization of the entire pancreas, which can result in failure to biopsy affected areas of the organ (Steiner, 2008).

Risk Factors

Several risk factors have been associated with pancreatitis in dogs and cats (**Table 67-1**). Most patients with these risk factors, however, do not develop pancreatitis.

A number of endocrinopathies such as diabetes mellitus, hypothyroidism and hyperadrenocorticism have been linked to pancreatitis in dogs (Hess et al, 1999). These endocrine conditions are often associated with hyperlipidemia and obesity, two other risk factors for acute pancreatitis.

An association has been made between hyperlipidemia and acute pancreatitis in dogs and people that has led to speculation that disturbances in lipid metabolism may be involved (Simpson, 1993). The exact relationship is unknown in dogs and cats and information is often extracted from human cases. Hyperlipidemia is thought to precede and cause the development of pancreatitis; however, it can also be evident during and after such episodes (Simpson, 1993). The rate of hyperlipidemia in people with pancreatitis has been estimated between 3 and 12% when alcoholics are not included in the case study. The incidence of hyperlipidemia in dogs or cats with pancreatitis is generally thought to be high. In a retrospective study of fatal acute pancreatitis in dogs, 26% of patients were hyperlipidemic (Hess et al, 1998). However, experimentally induced pancreatitis in dogs has not resulted in lipemia or hypertriglyceridemia (Bass et al, 1976; Whitney et al, 1987). Hypertriglyceridemia is present in some but not all naturally occurring cases of canine pancreatitis as determined by serum lipid and electrophoretic patterns (Whitney et al, 1987; Rogers et al, 1975). Most people with pancreatitis do not have hyperlipidemia; however, those that do and who are not alcoholics more often have preexisting hyperlipoproteinemia types I and V; more specifically hypertriglyceridemia. Serum triglyceride levels (>900 mg/dl) increase the risk of pancreatitis in dogs (Xenoulis et al, 2006).

Several pet breeds are predisposed to pancreatitis (e.g., miniature schnauzers, briards, Shetland sheepdogs, Siamese cats). This predisposition may be attributed to the fact that these breeds are also frequently hypertriglyceridemic. Recently, mutations in the pancreatic secretory trypsin-inhibitor gene (SPINK gene) have been described in miniature schnauzers, which may explain this breed's increased risk for pancreatitis (Bishop et al, 2007; Steiner, 2008). A number of other breeds also appear to be at risk for pancreatitis including boxers, cavalier King Charles spaniels, cocker spaniels, collies and Yorkshire terriers (Watson et al, 2007; Hess et al, 1999; Lem et al, 2008). Feeding a high-fat (>20% dry matter [DM]) food, treat or human food has often been associated with the onset of acute pancreatitis and a history of dietary indiscretion of high-fat human foods increases the risk of acute pancreatitis (Steiner, 2008). Ingestion of table scraps, garbage and new/unusual foods has been linked to pancreatitis in a case control study (Lem et al, 2008). Experimentally, feeding high-fat, low-protein foods was associated with the development of pancreatitis and hepatic lipidic changes in dogs (Lindsay et al, 1948; Goodhead, 1971). The most widely repeated explanation for the association between hypertriglyceridemia and acute pancreatitis is that hydrolysis of serum triglycerides by lipase within the pancreatic microvasculature releases free fatty acids locally. Free fatty acids cause microthrombi and/or bind with calcium to cause further capillary damage, which, in turn, releases more pancreatic lipase (Havel, 1969). Consumption of calorically dense, high-fat foods also contributes to obesity in pets, which is also considered a risk factor for pancreatitis (Lem et al, 2008). In one report, 43% of dogs with acute pancreatitis were considered overweight or obese (Hess et al, 1998). Obese patients develop more severe experimental pancreatitis than dogs with lower body condition scores (Relford et al, 2006).

Table 67-1. Risk factors for pancreatitis in dogs and cats.

Breed
Boxer
Briard
Cavalier King Charles spaniel
Cocker spaniel
Collie
Miniature schnauzer
Sheltie
Yorkshire terrier
Himalayan cat
Dietary factors
High-fat, low-protein foods
Ingestion of garbage or table scraps
Drug administration
Azathioprine
Corticosteroids
L-asparaginase
Organophosphate insecticides (cats)
Fasting hyperlipidemia
Gender
Castrated males
Spayed females
Hepatobiliary disease
Feline suppurative cholangiohepatitis
Triaditis (IBD, cholangiohepatitis, pancreatitis)
Hypercalcemia
Hyperparathyroidism
Intravenous calcium infusion
Increasing age
Intervertebral disk disease
Ischemia or reperfusion
Postgastric dilatation-volvulus
Obesity

Pancreatitis has been associated with hypercalcemia in several dogs with hyperparathyroidism or cancer and in a dog receiving a calcium infusion (Simpson, 1993; Relford et al, 2006). Experimentally, elevated ionized calcium concentrations can induce pancreatitis in cats (Frick et al, 1990). The pathophysiologic mechanism for pancreatitis in association with hypercalcemia has not been determined.

Drug-induced pancreatitis in people is very common; alcohol consumption is recognized as the most common cause of the disease. Reports of drug-induced pancreatitis in companion animals are uncommon but the following compounds have been implicated: calcium, azathioprine, vinca alkaloids, l-asparaginase, phenobarbital and potassium bromide in dogs and tetracyclines, sulfonamides and organophosphates in cats.

Anecdotal reports suggest that corticosteroids are the most common drug associated with pancreatitis in dogs. Pancreatitis

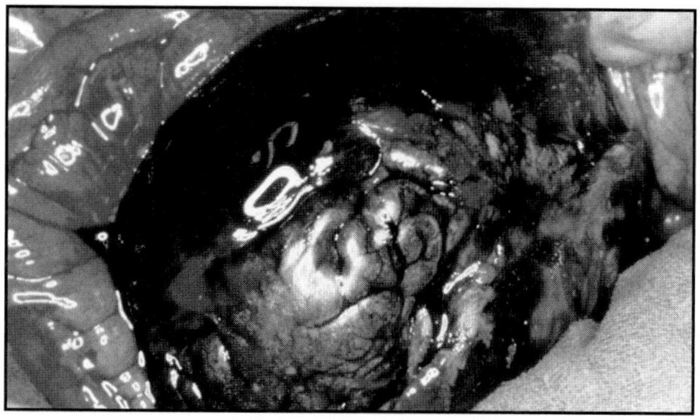

Figure 67-1. Intraoperative photograph of a dog with acute necrotizing pancreatitis. (Courtesy Dr. Dan Smeak, College of Veterinary Medicine, The Ohio State University, Columbus.)

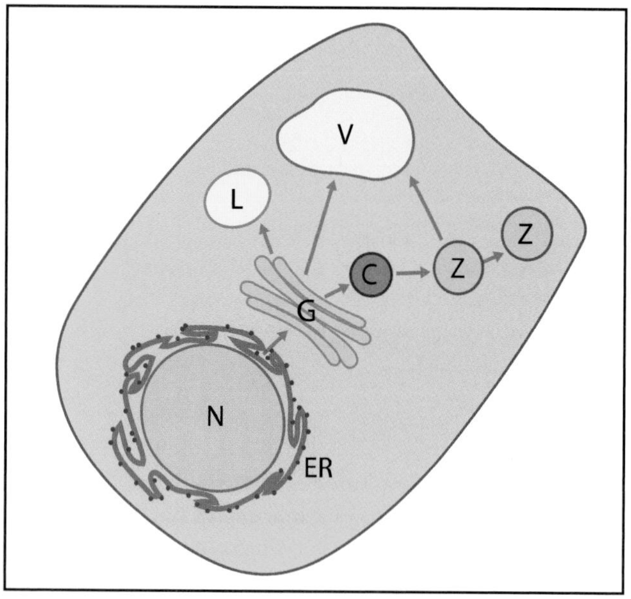

Figure 67-2. Schematic representation of zymogen and lysosomal fusion in acute pancreatitis. Digestive and lysosomal enzymes are synthesized in the rough endoplasmic reticulum (ER) and transferred to the Golgi apparatus (G) next to the nucleus (N). Normally, digestive and lysosomal enzymes are separated. Digestive enzymes are concentrated in zymogen granules within acinar cells and lysosomal enzymes are stored separately in lysosomes (L). Digestive enzymes are concentrated in condensing vacuoles (C) and in zymogen granules (Z) that fuse with luminal-plasma membranes. Hyperstimulation of the pancreas results in mixing of lysosomal and digestive enzymes in large vacuoles (V). (Adapted from Simpson KW. Current concepts of the pathogenesis and pathophysiology of acute pancreatitis in the dog and cat. Compendium on Continuing Education for the Practicing Veterinarian 1993; 15: 247-254.)

is common in dogs with hyperadrenocorticism and in dogs receiving corticosteroids for management of intervertebral disk disease (Moore and Withrow, 1982). Experimentally, corticosteroids increase the sensitivity of dispersed acinar cells to cholecystokinin and stimulate proliferation of the pancreatic ductular epithelium (Simpson, 1993). However direct evidence is lacking for a role of corticosteroids in the development of pancreatitis in dogs and cats (Steiner, 2008).

In dogs, potassium bromide and phenobarbital administration has been associated with elevations in serum pancreatic lipase immunoreactivity and acute pancreatitis (Podell and Fenner, 1993; Gaskill and Cribb, 2000; Steiner et al, 2008). Pancreatitis occurs in as many as 6 to 7% of dogs treated for seizures with potassium bromide.

Ischemia and reperfusion injury have been linked to acute pancreatitis (Williams, 1996; Simpson, 1993). Hypovolemic shock, gastric dilatation-volvulus and abdominal trauma have been reported to precede acute pancreatitis (Williams, 1996; Simpson, 1993). In addition, abdominal surgery marked by inept manipulation of the pancreas can result in pancreatitis (Williams, 1996; Simpson, 1993).

In cats, pancreatitis does not seem linked to obesity, hyperlipidemia, hypertriglyceridemia or to dietary triggers (Mansfield and Jones, 2001; Zoran, 2007). Instead, a number of infectious diseases have been implicated including calicivirus, toxoplasmosis, feline infectious peritonitis, feline immunodeficiency virus, panleukopenia, the fluke, *Amphimerus pseudofelieus*, (Relford et al, 2006) and enterococci (Lapointe et al, 2000).

Etiopathogenesis

Acute pancreatitis is the sudden onset of inflammation of the pancreatic acinar tissue. Typically, the primary histopathologic lesion is edema. After resolution, there is usually no residual pancreatic lesion. However, in more severe cases, the pancreatic lesion may become hemorrhagic or may progress to necrosis (**Figure 67-1**). Mortality is high in acute necrotizing pancreatitis. Acute edematous or hemorrhagic pancreatitis may occur as a singular or recurrent event in dogs and cats.

Pancreatitis occurs as a consequence of intracellular pancreatic acinar enzymatic activation and resultant autodigestion of the pancreas. In the normal pancreas, safeguards ensure that harmful pancreatic enzymes are not activated until they reach the intestinal lumen (**Table 67-2**) (Stewart, 1994). Pancreatic enzymes are synthesized in endoplasmic reticuli, modified in Golgi apparatuses and stored in zymogen granules within acinar cells. Evidence suggests that intracellular pancreatic enzyme activation occurs as a result of abnormal zymogen activation. Normally, zymogens and lysosomes are segregated intracellularly. In pancreatitis, lysosomes containing proteases fuse with zymogen granules (**Figure 67-2**) (Simpson, 1993). The lysosomal contents (e.g., proteases such as cathepsin B) activate trypsinogen. In addition, the acidic environment of lysosomes interferes with self-regulating trypsin inhibitors stored with pancreatic enzymes in zymogen granules.

Cholecystokinin and acetylcholine are widely recognized as the principal physiologic mediators of pancreatic enzyme secretion (Simpson, 1993). Normally, these substances initiate fusion of zymogen granules with the acinar cell membrane. Hyperstimulation of the pancreas with supraphysiologic doses of cholecystokinin appears to cause pancreatitis in experimental animals by interfering with the intracellular movement of zymogens resulting in fusion of zymogens and lysosomes (Simpson, 1993). The lysosomal enzyme cathepsin B is then thought to activate trypsinogen and precipitate pancreatitis

(Simpson, 1993). Pancreatic duct obstruction also appears to facilitate fusion of zymogens and lysosomal enzymes. Foods high in fat and protein (particularly the amino acid arginine) stimulate production and release of cholecystokinin, gastrin and secretin (Simpson, 1993). Organophosphate insecticides and intravenous calcium infusions are hypothesized to cause hyperstimulation via cholecystokinin (Simpson, 1993).

Bile acid and enteric reflux into the pancreatic duct can also activate pancreatic enzymes interstitially (i.e., within the pancreatic duct system and interstitium) (Simpson, 1993). This mechanism is thought to be involved in the development of pancreatitis in cats in conjunction with suppurative cholangiohepatitis and enteritis (Simpson, 1993). The anatomic configuration of the common bile duct and pancreatic duct in cats facilitates this mechanism. Experimentally, free fatty acids generated by the action of lipase on triglycerides damage acinar cell membranes, releasing lecithin, which causes marked necrosis of acinar cells when converted to lysolecithin by phospholipase A_2 (Simpson, 1993).

Regardless of the initiating cause, active pancreatic enzymes (trypsin, phospholipase, collagenase and elastase) and inflammatory mediators are released into the pancreatic tissues and blood vessels. These factors apparently activate coagulation, fibrinolytic, kinin and complement cascades (Simpson, 1993). Circulating defense mechanisms include α_1-antitrypsin and α_2-macroglobulin, which bind to active enzymes to contain local damage and prevent systemic damage (Simpson, 1993). After these defenses are overwhelmed, increased pancreatic permeability leads to fluid loss into the pancreas and the abdomen, a decline in pancreatic blood flow and an increase in the local concentrations of pancreatic enzymes and inflammatory mediators (Simpson, 1993). Large numbers of leukocytes migrate to the inflamed pancreas and serve as a source of free radicals, inflammatory mediators and enzymes (Simpson, 1993). This vicious, self-perpetuating cycle may ultimately lead to thrombosis of pancreatic blood vessels and pancreatic necrosis. Systemic complications may develop, including hypovolemic shock and disseminated intravascular coagulation.

Chronic pancreatitis is less commonly recognized in companion animals vs. people in whom alcohol can serve as a constant stimulus for smoldering acinar inflammation. Some authors suggest that chronic mild interstitial pancreatitis is the most common form of pancreatitis recognized in cats (Williams, 1996; Maddison, 2008). Histopathologic examination of tissues from dogs and cats with chronic pancreatitis reveals irreversible fibrotic changes resulting from the persistent inflammatory condition. Chronic and recurrent pancreatitis may result in acquired exocrine pancreatic insufficiency.

Key Nutritional Factors

Key nutritional factors for patients with pancreatitis are listed in **Table 67-3** and discussed in more detail below.

Water

Water is the most important nutrient in patients with acute vomiting because of the potential for life-threatening dehydration due to excessive fluid loss and inability of patients to replace those losses. Moderate to severe dehydration should be corrected with appropriate parenteral fluid therapy rather than using the oral route. Further nutritional support should be postponed until electrolyte, fluid and acid-base abnormalities have been corrected.

Table 67-2. Protection against pancreatic autodigestion.

Enterokinase, produced by the duodenal brush border, is required for activation of proenzymes
Pancreatic enzymes are synthesized as proenzymes (zymogens)
Serum protease inhibitors bind free trypsin
The pancreas secretes a trypsin inhibitor in pancreatic juice that binds free trypsin
Zymogens and lysosomal enzymes are stored in different intracytoplasmic membranes

Table 67-3. Key nutritional factors for foods for canine and feline patients with pancreatitis.*

Factors	Recommended levels
Fat	≤15% for non-obese and non-hypertriglyceridemic dogs
	≤ 25% for non-obese and non-hypertriglyceridemic cats
	≤10% for obese and/or hypertriglyceridemic dogs
	≤15% for obese and/or hypertriglyceridemic cats
Protein	15 to 30% for dogs
	30 to 40% for cats

*Nutrients expressed on a dry matter basis.

Protein

Free amino acids (i.e., phenylalanine, tryptophan and valine) in the duodenum are a strong stimulus for pancreatic secretion, in fact, more so than fat (Go et al, 1970). Therefore, excess dietary protein should be avoided, while providing adequate protein for recovery and tissue repair. DM protein levels of 15 to 30% for dogs and 30 to 40% for cats are appropriate.

Fat

Obese and hypertriglyceridemic patients recovering from pancreatitis should receive low-fat foods (≤10 and ≤15% DM for dog and cat foods, respectively). Other patients can be fed moderate-fat foods (≤15 and ≤25% DM for dog and cat foods, respectively). The most clinically relevant form of hypertriglyceridemia in veterinary patients is hyperchylomicronemia because triglycerides make up 84 to 89% of the lipids in chylomicrons (Chapter 28). Plasma chylomicrons are derived from two sources. Large (12-carbon) triglycerides are present for a few hours after ingestion of dietary fat, whereas smaller triglycerides, secreted from the liver, are always present and independent of dietary fat intake.

Other Nutritional Factors

Antioxidants

Recently, results of a randomized controlled clinical trial in people with chronic pancreatitis demonstrated a 50% reduction in painful days per month with oral antioxidant administration as compared to placebo (Bhardwaj et al, 2009). One third of patients receiving an antioxidant preparation containing selenium, vitamin C, vitamin E, β-carotene and methionine became pain free as compared to 12% of those receiving placebo. Markers of oxidative stress including lipid peroxidation products were higher in chronic pancreatitis than in healthy patients and improved after antioxidant administration. Similar trials have not been performed in chronic or acute pancreatitis in veterinary patients.

Cobalamin

Assessment of serum cobalamin is recommended in cats with pancreatitis complicated by IBD or triaditis. If levels are depleted, parenteral supplementation is recommended. Cats should receive weekly subcutaneous parenteral cobalamin therapy (250 µg/cat) for four to six weeks or until serum levels return to the normal range (Ruaux et al, 2005). Once or twice monthly therapy may be required for longer-term maintenance.

FEEDING PLAN

Dietary management goals for patients with pancreatitis are to decrease stimuli to pancreatic secretion (thus preventing pancreatic autodigestion) and still provide adequate nutrient levels to support tissue repair and recovery. Acute hemorrhagic or necrotizing pancreatitis should be considered a medical emergency. Initially, appropriate parenteral fluid therapy should be provided to correct dehydration and electrolyte and acid-base disturbances.

Oral food intake stimulates pancreatic secretions by several mechanisms. Likewise, the physical presence of food in the stomach stimulates gastrin, which in turn stimulates pancreatic secretion. In addition, many patients with pancreatitis will exhibit abdominal pain and/or vomit when fed, which increases the risk of aspiration. Therefore, nothing per os (NPO) therapy is the initial treatment of choice for a limited time period (≤ three days including days of anorexia pre-presentation). The advent of potent antiemetics (e.g., dolansetron, ondansetron) has led some clinicians to initiate immediate enteral nutritional support (Relford et al, 2006).

Therapy used in conjunction with the feeding plan includes intravenous fluids, antiemetics, plasma transfusions, nasogastric suctioning of gastric secretions and air, control of gastric acidity with H_2-receptor blockers or proton pump inhibitors, anticholinergic agents, somatostatin analogues (octreotide), antibiotics and surgical exploration of the abdomen for extirpation or drainage of pancreatic abscesses or pseudocysts (Johnson and Mann, 2006). Aggressive pain control with single agents or combination therapy with opioids, lidocaine, ketamine or epidurals is also recommended for canine and feline patients with pancreatitis (Whittemore and Campbell, 2005).

Assess and Select the Food

Levels of protein and fat should be evaluated in foods currently fed to patients with pancreatitis and compared with recommended levels. Information from this aspect of assessment is essential for making any changes to foods currently provided. Changing to a more appropriate food is indicated if protein and fat levels in the food currently fed do not match recommended levels. Owners of dogs at risk for acute pancreatitis fed struvite litholytic foods should be counseled about potential adverse events that require medical attention (Chapter 43).

Small amounts of water, ice cubes, oral rehydration solutions or monomeric foods can be offered after vomiting and abdominal discomfort subside. Monomeric foods are liquid foods containing nutrients in their simplest absorbable form. Thus, nutrients in these foods minimally stimulate pancreatic secretion (Green and Guan, 1993). Some monomeric products also contain glutamine to stimulate enterocyte hyperplasia after several days of NPO therapy, which may have induced intestinal mucosal atrophy. In general, 1 to 2 ml/kg body weight q.i.d. are well tolerated and rarely induce vomiting.

If liquids are well tolerated for one to two days, solid food may be slowly reintroduced. Highly digestible, commercial veterinary therapeutic foods designed for patients with gastrointestinal (GI) disease are often used initially (**Tables 67-4** and **67-5**, for dogs and cats, respectively). These foods also contain moderate levels of protein and fat. If vomiting recurs, NPO therapy should be reinstituted and feeding attempted again after 12 to 24 hours. A veterinary therapeutic food formulated for patients with GI diseases should be fed for another seven to 10 days before reintroducing the patient's regular food, if it is to be used at all.

Low-fat (<10% DM fat) foods are often used if obesity or hyperlipidemia was a contributing factor (**Tables 67-6** and **67-7**, for dogs and cats, respectively). High-fat commercial foods (>20% DM fat), table foods and snacks should be avoided. It may be necessary to remind clients of this around the holiday season, when many owners succumb to the desire to share family meals with pets.

Assess and Determine the Feeding Method

Because the feeding method is often altered in patients with pancreatitis, a thorough assessment should include verification of the feeding method currently being used. Items to consider include feeding frequency, amount fed, how the food is offered, access to other food sources including human food and garbage and who feeds the pet. All of this information should have been gathered when the dietary history was obtained. In cases in which acute pancreatitis is associated with eating garbage or other inappropriate foods (most often during a holiday), strict avoidance of foods other than the pet's regular food is recommended.

Discontinuing oral intake of food and water (NPO) has been the cornerstone of initial therapy for acute pancreatitis. Factors (GI distention and hormone release [gastrin, secretin, cholecystokinin]) that would normally stimulate pancreatic secretions, nausea, vomiting and abdominal discomfort are reduced when food and water are withheld. Most patients respond within two to three days. After vomiting and abdominal discomfort resolve or lessen in severity, liquids and food can be reintroduced grad-

Table 67-4. Key nutritional factors in selected commercial veterinary therapeutic foods for dogs with pancreatitis compared to recommended levels.* (See **Table 67-6** if patient is obese or hypertriglyceridemic.)

Moist foods	**Fat (%)**	**Protein (%)**
Recommended levels	**≤15**	**15-30**
Hill's Prescription Diet i/d Canine	14.9	25.0
Iams Veterinary Formula Intestinal Low-Residue	13.2	35.9
Medi-Cal Gastro Formula	11.7	22.1
Purina Veterinary Diets EN GastroENteric Formula	13.8	30.5
Royal Canin Veterinary Diet Digestive Low Fat LF	6.9	31.9
Royal Canin Veterinary Diet Intestinal HE	11.8	23.1
Dry foods	**Fat (%)**	**Protein (%)**
Recommended levels	**≤15**	**15-30**
Hill's Prescription Diet i/d Canine	14.1	26.2
Iams Veterinary Formula Intestinal Low-Residue	10.7	24.6
Medi-Cal Gastro Formula	13.9	22.9
Purina Veterinary Diets EN GastroENteric Formula	12.6	27.0
Royal Canin Veterinary Diet Digestive Low Fat LF 20	6.6	24.2
Royal Canin Veterinary Diet Intestinal HE 28	22.0	33.0

*Manufacturers' published values. Nutrients expressed as % dry matter.

Table 67-5. Key nutritional factors in selected commercial veterinary therapeutic foods for cats with pancreatitis compared to recommended levels.* (See **Table 67-7** if patient is obese or hypertriglyceridemic.)

Moist foods	**Fat (%)**	**Protein (%)**
Recommended levels	**≤25**	**30-40**
Hill's Prescription Diet i/d Feline	24.1	37.6
Iams Veterinary Formula Intestinal Low-Residue	11.7	38.4
Medi-Cal HYPOallergenic/Gastro	35.9	35.5
Medi-Cal Sensitivity CR	35.1	34.5
Dry foods	**Fat (%)**	**Protein (%)**
Recommended levels	**≤25**	**30-40**
Hill's Prescription Diet i/d Feline	20.2	40.3
Iams Veterinary Formula Intestinal Low-Residue	13.7	35.8
Medi-Cal HYPOallergenic/Gastro	11.5	29.8
Purina Veterinary Diets EN GastroENteric	18.4	56.2
Royal Canin Veterinary Diet Intestinal HE 30	23.7	34.4

*Manufacturers' published values. Nutrients expressed as % dry matter.

ually over several days. Normal feeding methods can be reintroduced after several days without clinical signs, unless dietary indiscretion or inappropriate foods or feeding methods initially contributed to the problem.

After three days (including periods of inappetence before admission) of the NPO protocol, patients with severe pancreatitis should receive enteral or parenteral nutritional support. The method deemed most desirable is the least invasive, supports the patient nutritionally and minimally stimulates pancreatic secretions. Some clinicians suggest feeding anorectic cats even earlier because of the risk of hepatic lipidosis (Zoran, 2007).

Protracted cases of pancreatitis with intractable vomiting often require parenteral nutrition to meet the patient's energy, protein, electrolyte and B-vitamin requirements while minimizing pancreatic secretions (Chapter 26). This is particularly true for patients for which the general anesthesia required for tube placement is considered too risky. Parenteral administration of nutritional solutions (including lipid solutions) has been associated with pancreatic atrophy; thus, pancreatic stimulation is minimal or nonexistent (Relly and Nahrwold, 1976; Betzhold and Howard, 1986). Both total parenteral and partial parenteral nutritional feeding have been used in patients with pancreatitis (Zsombor-Murray and Freeman, 1999; Zoran, 2007). In one review, pancreatitis was the most common diagnosis in hospitalized patients receiving partial parenteral nutrition (Chan et al, 2002). Intravenous administration of nutrients to support patients with pancreatitis through a five- to 14-day course of vomiting is possible, safe and economical in most practices (Chapter 26). Parenteral solutions are of particular benefit for managing pancreatitis in cats, especially when complicated by hepatic disorders, IBD or interstitial nephritis (Akol et al, 1993; Weiss et al, 1996).

Selection of parenteral solutions for feeding patients with pancreatitis is controversial because of the association between hyperlipidemia and pancreatitis. Some authors suggest that selection of parenteral solutions be based on amino acid and dextrose content only, whereas others advocate the use of lipid solutions in the admixture if the patient is not hyperlipidemic.

Table 67-6. Key nutritional factors in selected commercial veterinary therapeutic foods for obese or hypertriglyceridemic dogs with pancreatitis compared to recommended levels.*

Moist foods	Fat (%)	Protein (%)
Recommended levels	**≤10**	**15-30**
Hill's Prescription Diet w/d Canine	12.7	17.9
Medi-Cal Fibre Formula	9.1	24.8
Purina Veterinary Diets OM Overweight Management Formula	8.4	44.1
Dry foods	**Fat (%)**	**Protein (%)**
Recommended levels	**≤10**	**15-30**
Hill's Prescription Diet w/d Canine	9.0	18.9
Medi-Cal Fibre Formula	10.6	26.2
Purina Veterinary Diets DCO Dual Fiber Control	12.4	25.3
Purina Veterinary Diets OM Overweight Management Formula	7.2	31.1
Royal Canin Veterinary Diet Calorie Control CC 26 High Fiber	10.4	30.9
Royal Canin Veterinary Diet Diabetic HF 18	9.9	22

*Manufacturers' published values. Nutrients expressed as % dry matter.

People with pancreatitis have a decreased capacity to oxidize glucose, peripheral resistance to insulin and hyperglycemia. Administering glucose as the sole nonprotein energy source perpetuates hyperglycemia and increases the risk of hepatic steatosis (Helton, 1993). Lipids in total nutrient admixtures (Chapter 26) have been used successfully in dogs and cats with pancreatitis.[a] Lipid emulsions administered intravenously are synthetic 0.5-µm chylomicrons that appear to be well used by rats, people and dogs with pancreatitis (Raasch et al, 1983; Silberman et al, 1982; Kawaura et al, 1976; Zieve, 1968). People with pancreatitis and concurrent hypertriglyceridemia or hyperlipoproteinemia types I and V are not given lipids intravenously until levels of these parameters have decreased (Helton, 1993). Plasma lipid data from dogs with naturally occurring pancreatitis are sparse; however, not all canine patients with pancreatitis are hypertriglyceridemic (Whitney et al, 1987; Rogers et al, 1975). Therefore, serum triglyceride levels should be assessed before lipids are administered intravenously. Although isolated cases of pancreatitis in people have been linked to lipid infusion, these cases are considered rare and were complicated by concurrent diseases such as alcoholism and IBD (Wolfe and Ney, 1986). Second, respiratory quotients in people with pancreatitis are between 0.76 and 0.91, indicating mixed fuel (glucose and lipid) use. Finally, adding fat to dextrose infusions improves nitrogen balance (Sitzmann et al, 1989). Although respiratory quotients have not been measured in dogs and cats with pancreatitis, lipid administration is well tolerated, most likely because the liver would be using endogenous fat stores if lipid were not supplied exogenously as in people.

Enteral nutritional support by nasoesophageal, esophagostomy, gastrostomy or jejunostomy tubes should also be considered in prolonged cases of pancreatitis. Human reports suggest that enteral feeding after a short period of NPO (two days) may be superior to parenteral feeding in acute pancreatitis. Intra-jejunal feeding reduced complications and shortened hospital stays as compared to total parenteral nutrition (Windsor et al, 1998; Meier and Beglinger, 2006). Similar findings have been reported in experimental canine pancreatitis; enteral feeding was found to improve gut barrier function without increasing enteric hormone release (Qin et al, 2002, 2007). Studies have not been performed in spontaneous pancreatitis in dogs or when enteral routes proximal to the jejunum were used (Watson, 2007; Mansfield, 2007).

Jejunostomy tubes bypass the stomach and duodenum but are best placed when patients must undergo general anesthesia and abdominal surgery for other reasons (Swann et al, 1997). Studies have demonstrated the efficacy of nasojejunal feeding in people with mild and complicated acute pancreatitis (McClave et al, 1997; Kudsk et al, 1990). Jejunal feedings in people and dogs stimulate pancreatic secretion no more than parenteral feedings (Ragins et al, 1973; Cassim and Allardyce, 1974). In veterinary patients, however, a practical technique for nasojejunal feeding has not been developed; thus, jejunal feeding requires abdominal surgery. For that reason, some clinicians prefer parenteral feeding or the use of minimally invasive techniques such as nasoesophageal or percutaneous gastrostomy tube placement in patients with prolonged, refractory pancreatitis (Zoran, 2007).

Monomeric liquid foods infused directly into the duodenum of dogs stimulate some pancreatic output, whereas oral administration of the same monomeric foods stimulated a greater volume of pancreatic secretion (Relly and Nahrwold, 1976). If jejunal tube feeding is selected, a liquid food supplemented with glutamine to maintain intestinal integrity that minimally stimulates the pancreas and meets the patient's resting energy requirement (RER) is most suitable. Directly infusing a readily absorbable monomeric liquid food (vs. a polymeric product) into the jejunum should also reduce pancreatic secretions because whole nutrients elicit a greater response from the pancreas than monomeric nutrient forms. Monomeric liquid foods may be infused into the jejunum by slow continuous gravity drip (1 to 2 ml/kg body weight/hour) or, preferably, by an enteral pump. This rate of enteral feeding meets the RER of most patients and precludes other forms of nutritional support until oral intake is possible. If patients tolerate this rate of administration, solid food in small frequent meals may be given

Table 67-7. Key nutritional factors in selected commercial veterinary therapeutic foods for obese or hypertriglyceridemic cats with pancreatitis compared to recommended levels.*

Moist foods	Fat (%)	Protein (%)
Recommended levels	**≤15**	**30-40**
Hill's Prescription Diet w/d Feline with Chicken	16.6	39.6
Medi-Cal Fibre Formula	17.1	40.0
Purina Veterinary Diets OM Overweight Management Formula	14.6	44.6
Royal Canin Veterinary Diets Calorie Control CC High Fiber	21.3	33.5
Dry foods	**Fat (%)**	**Protein (%)**
Recommended levels	**≤15**	**30-40**
Hill's Prescription Diet w/d Feline	9.8	39.0
Hill's Prescription Diet w/d Feline with Chicken	9.9	39.9
Medi-Cal Fibre Formula	12.2	34.2
Purina Veterinary Diets OM Overweight Management Formula	8.5	56.2
Royal Canin Veterinary Diets Calorie Control CC 29 High Fiber	10.2	33.5

*Manufacturers' published values. Nutrients expressed as % dry matter.

for several days in addition to the liquid feedings. Liquid feedings may cease and the number of oral meals per day increased when solid food is well tolerated. Hydrolyzed or novel protein foods may be of value in cats with concurrent pancreatitis and inflammatory bowel disease (Zoran, 2009). These foods are typically highly digestible and may be beneficial for managing intestinal and pancreatic disorders (Chapter 31).

REASSESSMENT

Hospitalized patients with pancreatitis should be assessed frequently. Assessment of body weight and condition are recommended to ensure adequate hydration and caloric intake, if feeding is instituted. Electrolyte and acid-base status should be monitored to assess adequacy of therapy. If parenteral nutrition is used, daily monitoring of electrolytes, glucose and triglycerides is necessary to allow adjustment of parenteral solution composition (Whittemore and Campbell, 2005). Certain laboratory parameters (leukogram and serum concentrations of amylase, lipase, pancreatic lipase immunoreactivity and bilirubin) are helpful markers of progress. However, the patient's attitude, appetite and presence or absence of vomiting and abdominal pain are often the most important predictors of progress. In addition, it is imperative that sera be evaluated for triglyceride concentration initially and then monitored daily for lipemia. It is important to distinguish between lipemia from endogenous sources vs. exogenous fat emulsions when parenteral nutrition is administered.

Discharged patients should be reevaluated in a number of weeks. If a low-fat, high-fiber food was recommended to control obesity or hyperlipidemia, body weights should be recorded and serum triglyceride concentrations determined (or the sample should be inspected visually for lipemia) to assess compliance with the dietary management program. Regaining or maintaining optimal body weight and condition, normal activity level and absence of clinical signs are measures of successful dietary management.

Patients that relapse should be reevaluated and assessed for evidence of pancreatic pseudocysts, pancreatic necrosis or abscesses because these are potential sequelae to acute pancreatitis (Coleman and Robson, 2005).

ENDNOTE

a. Remillard RL. Personal experience. 1999.

REFERENCES

The references for **Chapter 67** can be found at www.markmorris.org.

CASE 67-1

Anorexia in a German Shepherd Crossbred Dog

Philip Roudebush, DVM, Dipl. ACVIM (Small Animal Internal Medicine)
Hill's Scientific Affairs
Topeka, Kansas, USA

Patient Assessment

A five-year-old neutered male German shepherd crossbred dog was examined on an emergency basis for acute onset of anorexia and depression. The owners found the dog outside hiding under a large shrub. The dog seemed lethargic and refused food and water. Past clinical problems included multiple seizures, hyperlipidemia and recurrent superficial staphylococcal pyoderma. The dog was receiving phenobarbital for seizures and had just completed six weeks of therapy with cephalexin for superficial pyoderma.

Physical examination revealed a very depressed, febrile (rectal temperature 40.0°C [104.0°F]) dog. Pain was elicited when the cranial abdomen was palpated and the dog vomited a small amount of clear liquid. Oral mucous membranes were brick red. The dog was overweight (body condition score [BCS] 4/5, body weight 45 kg).

Blood was drawn for a complete blood count and serum biochemistry profile. Therapy for shock was initiated with intravenous fluids, antibiotics and corticosteroids. Results of diagnostic studies included leukocytosis with a marked left shift (**Table 1**, Day 1) and very lipemic serum. Fluid therapy and antibiotics were continued through the night.

Intermittent vomiting continued. The next morning, abdominal radiographs were taken. Loss of serosal detail in the cranial abdomen consistent with focal fluid accumulation or peritonitis was noted. Results of a complete blood count were still consistent with severe inflammation (**Table 1**, Day 2) and the serum was still lipemic. Results of a serum biochemistry profile included increased serum amylase and lipase activities and increased liver enzyme activity (**Table 1**, Day 2). Fluid recovered by abdominal lavage was evaluated cytologically. The abdominal lavage fluid contained many nondegenerative neutrophils with no evidence of bacteria. Pancreatitis with non-septic peritonitis was diagnosed.

Assess the Food and Feeding Method

The dog was fed a commercial dry premium brand dog food free choice plus a variety of leftover foods from the owner's meals.

Questions

1. What are potential complications of pancreatitis?
2. What are the key nutritional factors for this patient?
3. Outline a short-term (i.e., next few days) and long-term (i.e., next several months) treatment and feeding plan for this dog.

Answers and Discussion

1. Life-threatening complications of pancreatitis include shock, pulmonary edema, cardiac dysrhythmias, peritonitis, sepsis, disseminated intravascular coagulopathy, hepatic lipidosis (cats) and extrahepatic bile duct obstruction. Other complications include diabetes mellitus and exocrine pancreatic insufficiency.
2. Key nutritional factors for patients with pancreatitis include water, protein and fat. Aggressive intravenous fluid therapy to correct water, electrolyte and acid-base deficits is a cornerstone of successful treatment for acute pancreatitis. Potassium supplementation in fluids is often indicated because of potassium losses in vomitus. Dietary protein and fat are the major stimuli for pancreatic secretions; therefore, excessive levels should be avoided. Excess dietary fat should also be avoided in patients with hyperlipidemia.
3. Initially, oral food and water are withheld for three to five days to minimize pancreatic secretions and help control vomiting. Parenteral fluid therapy is used to correct fluid deficits and electrolyte and acid-base disturbances and to meet maintenance water requirements. Colloids (e.g., dextrans, hetastarch) may be needed initially to maintain blood volume and pancreatic microcirculation. After replacement of deficits, additional fluids are given to match the patient's maintenance requirements and ongoing losses. Drug therapy usually includes corticosteroids (only in shock), antiemetics, antibiotics and analgesics. Food and water are gradually introduced in multiple small feedings while clinical signs, especially vomiting, are monitored. Foods for patients with pancreatitis should avoid excessive levels of protein and fat, and contain balanced levels of other nutrients. Some clinicians suggest using a "bland," low-protein, low-fat, high-carbohydrate food such as cooked rice for the initial few days of feeding. Parenteral nutritional support should be considered if clinical signs persist beyond five days (Chapter 26). Long-term use of foods that avoid excess dietary fat (i.e., <10% dry matter fat) may be especially important in this overweight dog with a history of hyperlipidemia (Chapter 28).

Table 1. Selected laboratory parameters from a dog with pancreatitis.

Parameters	Day 1	Day 2	Day 6	Day 107	Day 121	Day 154	Reference values
Packed cell volume (%)	68	57	53	45	45	56	37-55
Total white blood cells (/µl)	20,900	22,500	12,900	12,500	10,800	26,200	8,000-17,000
Total segmented neutrophils (/µl)	9,614	9,450	11,868	8,750	7,236	19,388	3,600-13,100
Total band neutrophils (/µl)	5,852	8,775	258	0	1,944	1,834	0-400
Total juvenile neutrophils (/µl)	1,254	112	0	0	0	0	0
Amylase (IU/l)	ND	1,608	563	897	2,340	2,640	350-1,200
Lipase (U/l)	ND	107	133	64	ND	260	0-100
ALT (IU/l)	ND	99	77	42	ND	120	0-75
Alkaline phosphatase (IU/l)	ND	333	309	30	ND	757	0-80

Key: ND = not done, ALT = alanine aminotransferase.

Progress Notes

Intravenous fluids, antibiotics and phenobarbital were continued for several days. The dog apparently felt much better by the sixth day of hospitalization and the hemogram indicated that the peripheral inflammatory response had improved (**Table 1**, Day 6). No vomiting had occurred for 24 hours and the dog readily ate cooked rice. The dog continued to improve and was released to the owner's care four days later.

A commercial low-fat, moderate-fiber veterinary therapeutic food (Prescription Diet w/d Canine[a]) was dispensed for use at home. The dog began eating this food during its last two days in the hospital. The daily energy requirement (DER) was calculated to achieve mild weight loss (1.2 x resting energy requirement [RER] [RER = $30Wt_{kg}+70$] for an ideal body weight of 39 kg) while supporting recovery from pancreatitis and peritonitis. DER equals approximately 1,500 kcal (6.28 MJ), which was met by feeding three and one-half cups of food twice daily. The owners were asked to eliminate table food and other snacks from the diet.

Three months later, the dog was examined for recurrent pyoderma. Blood parameters were normal and the serum was not lipemic (**Table 1**, Day 107). The dog's weight remained stable. Antibiotics were dispensed, oral phenobarbital was continued and the amount of food offered was reduced to two and two-thirds cups of food twice daily. Two weeks later, the dog developed anorexia, vomiting and mild abdominal pain after eating fried chicken. Serum was lipemic and blood parameters were consistent with recurrent pancreatitis (**Table 1**, Day 121). Five days of therapy with intravenous fluids, antibiotics and nothing per os resulted in clinical improvement. The dog was released to the owner's care with instructions to strictly follow the previously developed feeding plan.

A month later, the dog was again examined for anorexia, vomiting, icterus and severe cranial abdominal pain. Laboratory parameters were consistent with pancreatitis and bile duct obstruction (**Table 1**, Day 154). Exploratory celiotomy revealed severe, chronic, fibrosing pancreatitis with entrapment and compression of the extrahepatic bile duct. The fibrotic portion of the pancreas was excised and the gallbladder was attached to the duodenum (cholecystoduodenostomy). The dog recovered uneventfully from anesthesia and surgery and was released from the hospital seven days later. The low-fat, moderate-fiber food was fed for the next three years until the dog died from other causes. Significant weight loss did not occur but body weight was stabilized at 43 kg and there was no evidence of hyperlipidemia or further pancreatitis.

Endnote

a. Hill's Pet Nutrition Inc., Topeka, KS, USA.

Bibliography

Williams DA. Acute pancreatitis. In: Kirk RW, Bonagura JD, eds. Current Veterinary Therapy XI. Philadelphia, PA: WB Saunders Co, 1992; 631-639.

Section 20

Hepatobiliary Disorders

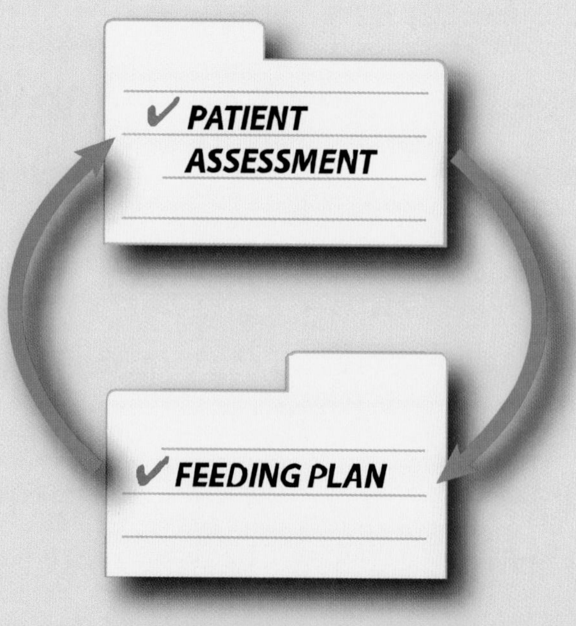

Chapter 68

Hepatobiliary Disease

Hein P. Meyer
David C. Twedt
Philip Roudebush
Elizabeth Dill-Macky

"Life loves the liver of it."
Maya Angelou

CLINICAL IMPORTANCE

Among the most challenging problems in medicine are those that involve failure of a metabolically active organ such as the liver. The liver is the second largest organ of the body and performs an estimated 1,500 essential biochemical functions (Zakim, 1985). In addition to its role in drug metabolism, the removal of environmental and endogenous noxious substances and synthesis of important substances (e.g., albumin and blood clotting factors), the liver plays a key role in food digestion and nutrient metabolism. The liver influences nutritional status through its elaboration of bile salts and central role in intermediary metabolism of protein (amino acids), carbohydrate, fat and vitamins. **Table 68-1** lists the most important hepatic functions.

Patients with hepatobiliary disease are often seen in companion animal practice. An estimated 2 to 3% of all animals presented at a veterinary teaching hospital have some form of hepatobiliary disease (Meyer, 2000). Hereditary portosystemic shunts (PSS), tumors (metastasis, malignant lymphoma and primary liver tumors) and chronic hepatitis account for more than 60% of these patients (Rothuizen and Meyer, 2000). Hereditary PSS occur in 2 to 5% of investigated breeds (Meyer et al, 1995). The liver may also be damaged secondarily by other disease processes. Resultant changes are often classified as a reactive hepatopathy. Because the liver plays an essential role in the metabolism of protein, carbohydrate and fat, nutritional support plays an essential role for many patients with hepatobiliary disease.

The liver has tremendous storage capacity, functional reserve and regenerative capabilities. All of these functions protect the body from profound metabolic alterations. However, these same characteristics complicate the clinical recognition of serious liver disease. Consequently, hepatobiliary disease must be severe before clinical signs occur. As a result, the patient may be suffering longstanding and profound metabolic alterations by the time a diagnosis is made and an appropriate management plan is implemented.

The liver is also unique in that it derives its nutrient blood supply from venous and arterial sources (Anderson and

Table 68-1. Major hepatobiliary functions related to nutrient digestion and metabolism.

Metabolic functions
Converts glucose to glycogen and triglycerides during absorptive state
Converts glycogen to glucose in postabsorptive period
Synthesizes glucose from glucogenic precursors such as glycerol and amino acids in postabsorptive period (gluconeogenesis)
Transforms amino acids (transamination and deamination), synthesizes nonessential amino acids as needed for metabolism
Synthesizes triacylglycerols and secretes them as lipoproteins
Synthesizes and releases cholesterol into blood
Forms ketones from degraded fatty acids during fasting
Synthesizes urea from ammonia (sole site in body)
Synthesizes plasma albumin, fibrinogen and various other coagulation factors
Biliary functions
Synthesizes bile salts from cholesterol, which are secreted into bile for lipid emulsification and absorption in the small intestine
Secretes a bicarbonate-rich solution to help neutralize acid in the duodenum
Secretes plasma cholesterol into bile
Conjugates and excretes bilirubin in bile
Detoxifies substances by biotransformation before biliary excretion
Excretes endogenous and foreign organic molecules in bile
Storage functions
Stores glucose as glycogen and triglycerides
Stores vitamins, particularly A but also D, E, K, B_{12} and to a lesser extent other B vitamins
Stores minerals such as iron, copper, manganese and zinc
Stores blood, especially with pressure increases in the hepatic vein or posterior vena cava
Endocrine functions
Activates (partial) vitamin D by dehydroxylation
Converts thyroxine to triiodothyronine
Secretes IGF-1 in response to growth hormone
Metabolizes (deactivates) and excretes hormones
Miscellaneous functions
Removes bacteria and food antigens that regularly cross the intestinal epithelial barrier (Kupffer cells of mononuclear-macrophage system in the sinusoids)

Anderson, 1994). The portal vein provides 70 to 75% of total hepatic blood flow (Center and Strombeck, 1996). Portal venous blood is nutrient rich in the absorptive state but oxygen poor. The hepatic artery provides about 25 to 30% of blood flow with oxygen-rich blood (Center and Strombeck, 1996). Hepatotropic factors especially from portal venous blood modulate the functional and structural integrity of the liver (Diehl, 1991). Concentrations of several hormones, including hepatocyte growth factor, insulin, glucagon, glucocorticoids, thyroid hormones, parathyroid hormone, calcitonin, α- and, β-adrenergic agents and insulin-like growth factors I and II, increase after hepatic injury or resection and affect the ensuing hepatic regenerative growth (Bucher and Malt, 1971; Stolz et al, 1999; Nishino et al, 2008).

Unlike most terminally differentiated cells, hepatocytes in adult liver retain the capacity to proliferate. After partial (70%) hepatectomy, compensatory hyperplasia begins within minutes of resection and is typically completed within two weeks in rats and in less than one month in people (Higgins and Anderson, 1931; Francavilla et al, 1990). The unique regenerative ability of the liver should be a consideration in the management of many hepatic diseases (Bauer and Schenck, 1989).

Hepatobiliary diseases can be categorized depending on their cause (**Table 68-2**). (See Common Hepatobiliary Diseases below.) Irrespective of the primary liver disease, the hepatic reaction pattern is similar; thus, most of these disorders, if severe and/or longstanding, often lead to a few syndromes with potentially serious metabolic consequences (e.g., cholestasis, icterus, portal hypertension, ascites and hepatic encephalopathy [HE]). **Table 68-3** lists the frequency distribution of liver diseases in dogs and cats.

Cholestasis is decreased bile flow and can happen at any level of the complex interplay of bile formation, excretion, hepatic re-uptake or intracellular transport. Cholestasis is present to some degree in most patients with hepatobiliary disease. Severe cholestasis becomes apparent as icterus. Moreover, deposition of increased amounts of extracellular collagen and reorganization of the hepatic architecture (i.e., cirrhosis) may lead to an increase in hepatic vascular resistance, which results in portal hypertension. Portal hypertension in turn may lead to formation of multiple portosystemic collaterals and ascites. Portosystemic shunting in combination with a decrease in functional liver mass may lead to the development of HE, the complex of neurologic and behavioral signs due to gastrointestinal (GI) toxins bypassing the liver.

Malnutrition is a common finding in patients with advanced hepatic disease and is an independent risk factor for predicting clinical outcome in human patients with chronic hepatic disease (Qiao et al, 1988). In human patients with nonalcoholic cirrhosis, 14% had significant weight loss (O'Keefe et al, 1980), 50% had mild to moderate steatorrhea and 40% had deficiencies of fat-soluble vitamins (Morgan et al, 1976). Food intake was normal and was unrelated to the degree of malnutrition, suggesting that factors other than decreased food intake are involved in the malnutrition of human patients with hepatic disease. Potential causes of malnutrition in animals with hepat-

Table 68-2. Diseases of the liver and biliary tract commonly seen in dogs and cats.*

Disease categories	Etiology
Liver	
Hepatitis**	Immune mediated
	Viral
	Bacterial
	Drug induced
	Reactive
	Toxins
	Lobular dissecting
Storage disorders**	Copper toxicosis
	Lipidosis
	Amyloidosis
	Steroid-induced hepatopathy
Circulatory disorders**	Hereditary portosystemic shunt
	Portal vein hypoplasia
	Portal vein thrombosis
	Arteriovenous fístula
Neoplasia	Metastases
	Malignant lymphoma
	Hemangiosarcoma
	Hepatocellular carcinoma
Biliary tract	
Cholangitis**	Bacterial/immune mediated
(Neutrophilic/lymphocytic)	Drug induced
Cholecystitis	Bacterial
Choleliths	Bilirubin
	Cholesterol
Neoplasia	Cholangiocarcinoma
Extrahepatic cholestasis	Pancreatitis
(Not covered by above)	Pancreatic/intestinal tumor

*Adapted from Meyer HP. Hepatic encephalopathy: An overview. In: Proceedings of the Hill's European Symposium on Canine and Feline Liver Disease, Amsterdam, 2000, ISBN 0-9540567-0-1, pp 24-28.
**Hepatic encephalopathy may be present.

ic disease include: 1) anorexia, nausea and vomiting, 2) impaired nutrient digestion, absorption and metabolism, 3) increased energy requirements and 4) accelerated protein catabolism with impaired protein synthesis (Marks et al, 1994).

Nutritional management of hepatobiliary disease is usually directed at clinical manifestations of the disease rather than the specific cause. The goals of nutritional management for hepatobiliary disease include: 1) maintaining normal metabolic processes and homeostasis, 2) avoiding and managing HE, 3) providing substrates to support hepatocellular repair and regeneration, 4) decreasing further oxidative damage to damaged liver tissue and 5) correcting electrolyte disturbances (Center, 1998; Blackburn and O'Keefe, 1989).

PATIENT ASSESSMENT

History and Physical Examination

Recognition of liver disease based on history and clinical signs is usually difficult. Signs are often nonspecific and few indications of liver disease are found on physical examination. Consequently without appropriate laboratory evaluation, liver disorders are often overlooked and either the patient recovers without treatment or becomes worse despite symptomatic treatment. This section considers the expected clinical signs of liver disease and the difficulties in interpreting them.

Table 68-3. Frequency distribution of liver diseases in dogs and cats.

Dogs*	**Frequency (%)**
Reactive hepatitis	25
Chronic hepatitis/cirrhosis	17
Portosystemic shunts	16
Liver tumors (primary, metastases)	14
Malignant lymphoma	14
Other conditions	12
Extrahepatic cholestasis	2
Cats**	
Lipidosis (idiopathic and secondary)	26
Cholangitis	25
Neoplasia (malignant and benign)	20
Reactive hepatopathies	16
Other conditions	8
Vascular anomalies	5

*Adapted from Rothuizen J, Meyer HP. History, physical examination, and signs of liver disease. In: Ettinger SJ, Feldman EC, eds. Textbook of Veterinary Internal Medicine: Diseases of the Dog and Cat, 5th ed. Philadelphia, PA: WB Saunders Co, 2000; 1272-1277.
**Twedt DC. 175 consecutive liver biopsies in cats: Unpublished data. College of Veterinary Medicine and Biomedical Sciences, Colorado State University, Fort Collins, Colorado.

Table 68-4. Clinical signs that most often accompany primary liver disease in dogs.*

Signs	Frequency of occurrence (%)
Apathy and listlessness	60
Reduced appetite	59
Vomiting	58
Weight loss	50
Polydipsia/polyuria	45
Diarrhea	27
Reduced endurance	27
Ascites	25
Neurologic signs	12
Icterus	12
Acholic feces	7

*Adapted from Rothuizen J, Meyer HP. History, physical examination, and signs of liver disease. In: Ettinger SJ, Feldman EC, eds. Textbook of Veterinary Internal Medicine: Diseases of the Dog and Cat, 5th ed. Philadelphia, PA: WB Saunders Co, 2000; 1272-1277.

Table 68-4 lists the most important clinical signs and the frequencies with which they occur in primary liver diseases. These signs occur in a variety of combinations in many liver diseases. Physical findings are often similar and include lethargy, neurologic signs, low body condition score (BCS), icterus and ascites.

GI abnormalities include anorexia, vomiting and diarrhea (Center, 1995). Ptyalism (hypersalivation) is especially common in cats (**Figure 68-1**) with HE. Hematemesis suggests GI ulceration, which can also be a complication of hepatobiliary disease. The anorexia, GI disturbances and metabolic alterations associated with liver disease often contribute to chronic

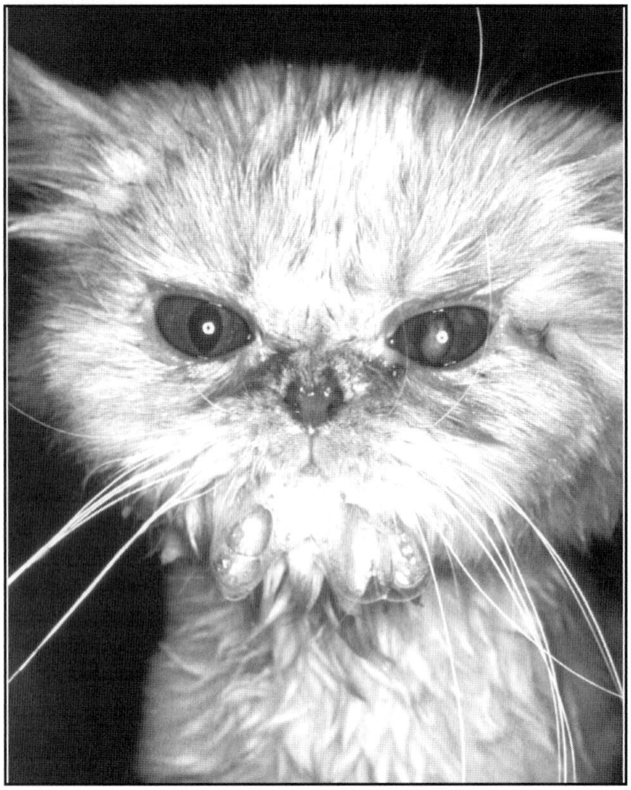

Figure 68-1. A 14-year-old Persian cat with ptyalism due to liver disease.

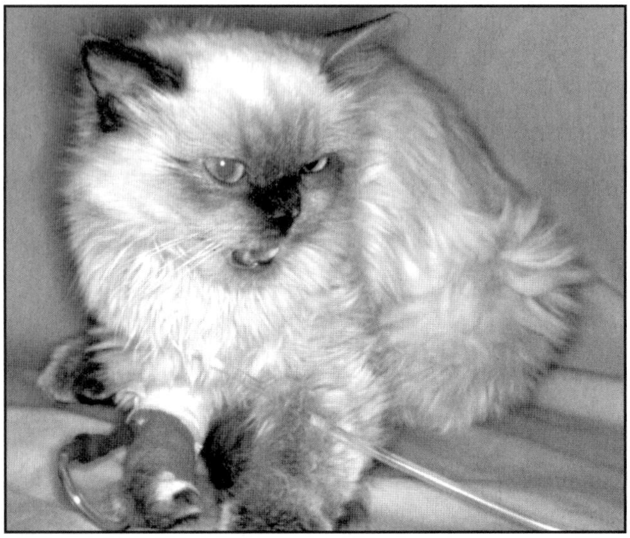

Figure 68-2. An eight-month-old Himalayan cat with clinical signs of aggression associated with hepatic encephalopathy due to a congenital portosystemic shunt.

weight loss. Bleeding tendencies (which are rarely noted clinically) may develop due to a decrease in hepatic production of clotting factors, to consumption coagulopathy (disseminated intravascular coagulation) (Rothuizen and Meyer, 2000) or malabsorption of vitamin K, which is essential for production of vitamin K-dependent factors in patients with prolonged extrahepatic bile duct obstruction (Center, 1995). Subclinical blood clotting abnormalities may become clinically evident during liver biopsy procedures or surgery. Icterus may be observed with severe cholestasis. Acholic feces due to total bile duct obstruction occur rarely in dogs and cats. Consequently, serious disturbances in fat digestion and absorption, which rely on functional biliary excretion, are rare in hepatobiliary disease (Rothuizen and Meyer, 2000).

Neurobehavioral signs of HE develop in animals with portosystemic vascular anomalies and a decreased functional liver mass. Typical signs include aggression (cats) (**Figure 68-2**), aimless wandering, manic barking (dogs), ataxia, lethargy, episodic weakness, ptyalism (cats especially), altered consciousness (disorientation, stupor or rarely coma), head pressing (**Figure 68-3**), sudden blindness, circling, pacing and seizures (Center, 1995). These signs may be episodic and may be linked to meals, dietary changes, GI hemorrhage or some other event.

A normal liver can be difficult to palpate in dogs and cats; the edges are normally sharp and the liver resides cranial to the ribcage. Hepatomegaly, however, is readily palpated in most cases. Hepatomegaly may be caused by passive venous congestion, inflammation, neoplasia, nodular hyperplasia and infiltration by fat, amyloid or glycogen. On the other hand, reduced liver size is difficult to palpate in dogs and cats. Abdominal enlargement associated with ascites usually develops slowly and insidiously. Small amounts of effusion may go undetected, whereas moderate to severe abdominal effusion becomes obvious. Hyperadrenocorticism may also cause distention from abdominal wall muscle weakness and hepatomegaly from steroid hepatopathy.

When liver disease is included in the differential diagnosis based on one or more of the historical or physical findings, additional diagnostics are required. **Figure 68-4** presents a diagnostic algorithm for liver diseases.

Laboratory Evaluation

It is beyond the scope of a nutrition textbook to discuss in detail, specific laboratory tests and imaging techniques (i.e., ultrasound, nuclear imaging techniques, laparoscopy) used to detect and confirm hepatobiliary disease. Readers are referred to small animal internal medicine, GI and surgical texts for these details. However, routine tests that help establish parameters for developing feeding and reassessment plans are summarized below.

Liver disease is most often discovered during hematologic, serum biochemistry and urine tests performed either as part of a routine wellness screen or diagnostic evaluation of sick dogs and cats. Hematologic changes may include anemia, abnormal erythrocyte morphology, reduced platelet numbers or function and detection of icteric or lipemic plasma (Center, 1995, 1996e; Dial, 1995). A regenerative anemia caused by blood loss due to GI hemorrhage and/or a bleeding diathesis may by present. More commonly, a nonregenerative anemia is found and is associated with chronic disease, chronic blood loss, malnutrition and reduced erythrocyte survival (Center, 1995, 1996e). Target cells, poikilocytes and spur cells, Heinz bodies (cats) and microcytosis are erythrocytic abnormalities seen in animals with liver disease (Center, 1995, 1996e; Dial, 1995). Erythrocyte microcytosis is associated with acquired and congenital portosystemic vascular shunts in dogs.

Measurement of plasma enzyme activities (usually but not entirely correctly called "liver enzymes") is based on the concept that certain enzymes are released and enter the bloodstream when changes occur in the liver or bile ducts. The most important enzymes for dogs and cats are discussed below.

Alkaline Phosphatase

Alkaline phosphatase (AP) is found in almost all organs but primarily in bone, liver, kidney, small bowel mucosa, placenta and bile duct epithelium. The plasma half-life of intestinal, renal and placental AP is only a few minutes; their contribution to total serum AP is negligible. In dogs, measurable serum AP arises from bone, liver or corticosteroid induction.

The half-life of AP from liver and bone in dogs is about 70 hours. Bone AP increases from osteoblastic activity in young growing dogs or occasionally from osteoblastic bone tumors. AP increases from cholestatic disorders resulting in induction of a liver AP and subsequent enzyme solublization and elution from damaged membranes into the blood (Gary and Twedt, 2009). Abnormal bile acid concentrations may play a role in AP production and release. Thus, significant extrahepatic cholestasis usually causes very high plasma AP activity. Finally, in dogs but not cats, corticosteroids, either endogenous or exogenous, can induce specific corticosteroid AP isoenzyme produced in the liver, leading to higher AP activity. The corticosteroid fraction of AP can be determined by heating plasma to 65°C (149°F) for two minutes, which inactivates AP of liver and bone origin, but not that induced by corticosteroids. Clinically determining the percent fraction arising from corticosteroids is generally not helpful in determining hyperadrenocorticism from other diseases.

In cats, AP is of less diagnostic importance because the half-life is very short (i.e., 5.8 hours); thus, it is only elevated in severe hepatobiliary diseases. In addition, feline hepatic AP concentrations are low; therefore, the sensitivity of AP in detecting feline liver disease is low. The highest concentrations of plasma AP in cats often occurs with hepatic lipidosis.

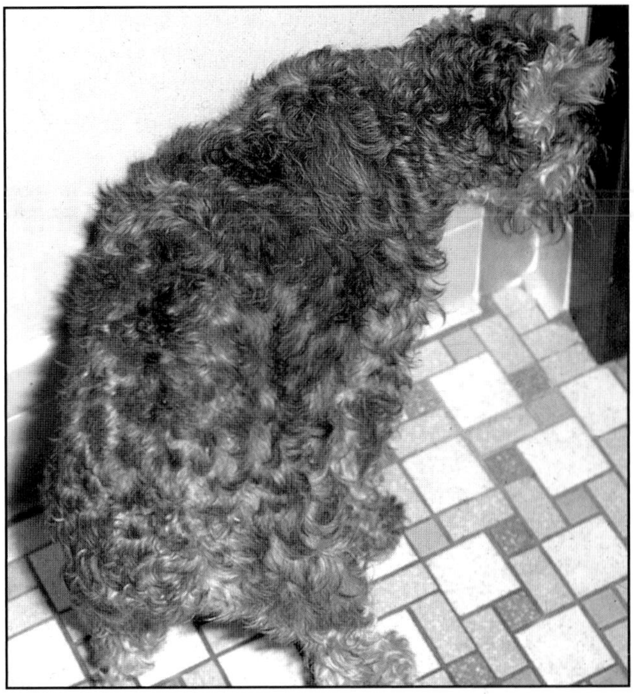

Figure 68-3. A miniature schnauzer with head pressing due to hepatic encephalopathy as a result of chronic hepatitis and cirrhosis.

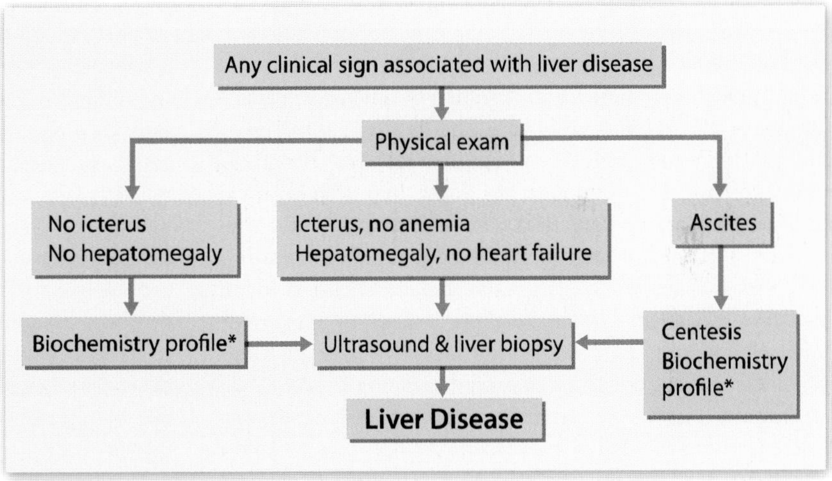

Figure 68-4. Algorithm for the diagnosis of hepatobiliary disease. (Adapted from Rothuizen J, Meyer HP. History, physical examination, and signs of liver disease. In: Ettinger SJ, Feldman EC, eds. Textbook of Veterinary Internal Medicine: Diseases of the Dog and Cat, 5th ed. Philadelphia, PA: WB Saunders Co, 2000; 1272-1277.)
*Alkaline phosphatase, alanine aminotransferase, bile acids, ammonia.

Gamma Glutamyl Transferase

Hepatic γ-glutamyl transferase (GGT) is associated with hepatocyte canalicular membranes and bile ducts. Highest concentrations generally are associated with disease of biliary epithelium such as bile duct obstructions or cholangitis. Cats with cholangitis, biliary tract disease or hepatobiliary disease generally have higher GGT concentrations than AP. GGT concentrations are usually only mildly elevated in feline idiopathic hepatic lipidosis (Center et al, 1986).

Alanine Aminotransferase and Aspartate Aminotransferase

Alanine aminotransferase (ALT) and aspartate aminotransferase (AST) were known in the older nomenclature as GPT and GOT, respectively. They are often collectively referred to as "hepatic leakage" enzymes. ALT is very liver-specific in dogs and cats. It is localized in the cytoplasm of hepatocytes and released with even mild damage to cell membranes. Hepatocytes, however, do not need to be irreversibly damaged and a number of metabolic or systemic conditions can alter membrane function without being a primary liver disorder. The biologic half-life of ALT is about two and one-half days in dogs and approximately six hours in cats (Webster and Cooper, 2009). ALT is fairly sensitive and specific in dogs and cats and thus a good parameter for use in screening for liver disease.

AST is not liver specific. In dogs, it is mainly present in cardiac and skeletal muscle and other tissues and to a lesser degree in the liver. In cats, AST is more limited to the liver. Although not liver specific, AST is useful because it is chiefly located in the mitochondria and thus only released by cell death. The half-life of serum AST in dogs is five to 12 hours and 77 minutes in cats (Webster, 2005). Increased activities of AST and ALT generally indicate more severe hepatocellular damage than does an increase in ALT alone. However, this reasoning has proved to have no real diagnostic meaning, hence AST is not used.

Other Blood Examinations

Laboratory tests found in most biochemistry profiles that can reflect, in part, hepatic function include bilirubin, albumin, cholesterol, glucose and urea nitrogen. Other specialized tests of hepatic function include serum bile acid concentrations. Because the liver is involved in a multitude of functions, no single test can reflect its functional state and interpretation of function must be made in light of the clinical and laboratory testing results. Chronic hepatic dysfunction can cause hypoalbuminemia and clotting disorders. The liver exclusively produces albumin and coagulation factors except factor VIII. A number of non-hepatic conditions cause hypoalbuminemia; however, albumin synthesis declines with the loss of approximately 70% of hepatic function. Serum albumin concentrations may fall even lower with concurrent ascites and third-spacing in the ascitic fluid. The biologic half-life of albumin is approximately two weeks. Glucose and clotting factor concentrations decline when more than 75% of hepatic function is lost.

Abnormal blood coagulation generally reflects significant hepatic dysfunction due to reduced protein synthesis. Rarely, chronic bile duct obstruction can deplete intestinal bile acid concentrations required for adequate vitamin K absorption and can result in depletion of hepatic production of vitamin K-dependent clotting factors (factors II, VII, IX and X). When this situation occurs, clotting times are quickly corrected following parenteral vitamin K administration.

Ammonia is an important parameter to consider when HE is suspected. Elevated ammonia concentrations generally reflect the presence of portosystemic circulation abnormalities (e.g., congenital PSS or acquired shunts from portal hypertension). Plasma ammonia concentration is less sensitive and specific in reflecting hepatocellular function but is the method of choice when HE is suspected. Most in-house dry chemical methods provide reliable results (Sterczer et al, 1999). Care should be taken when handling samples because a number of factors may interfere with accurate results. When results are equivocal, an ammonia tolerance test can be performed. Bile salts (primarily taurocholate in dogs and cats), also erroneously called bile acids, are produced by the liver and excreted in the bile. After uptake in the portal blood, the liver re-extracts bile salts (i.e., enterohepatic circulation). Concentration of bile salts increases in the systemic circulation in cholestasis (either intrahepatic or extrahepatic), hepatocyte dysfunction (failure to extract bile acids from the sinusoidal circulation) and when vascular portosystemic shunting is present. Thus, determination of the venous concentration of total bile salts is a specific and an early, sensitive indicator of liver function. Bile salts are stable and easy to measure (Webster and Cooper, 2009). An eight-hour fasted sample should be obtained followed by a postprandial sample two hours later in dogs and cats. After hemolysis has been ruled out, bilirubin elevations reflect hepatic or extrahepatic cholestasis. The ratio between conjugated and unconjugated bilirubin fractions is not useful for differentiating among various hepatic disorders; other diagnostic testing is required. Also, urinary urobilinogen concentrations have a very low diagnostic accuracy for supporting a diagnosis of extrahepatic cholestasis.

Imaging the Liver

Radiographs are useful to determine the size and shape of the liver and to identify other concurrent abdominal disorders. Advanced studies of the hepatobiliary system include ultrasonographic imaging (Szatmari and Rothuizen, 2006). Hepatic ultrasonography is useful for initially identifying disease and monitoring its progression (Partington and Biller, 1995, 1996; Barr, 1990; Nyland et al, 1995; Lamb, 1998). Ultrasonography can detect and differentiate focal and diffuse hepatic parenchymal disorders and changes in the hepatobiliary (gallbladder and bile ducts) system. The evaluation should also include the hepatic vascular system because portosystemic anomalies are extremely common. Ultrasonography is highly operator dependent and imaging expertise takes time to develop. Readers are referred to diagnostic imaging textbooks and manuals for detailed descriptions and classifications of hepatic lesions identified by ultrasonography (Barr, 1990; Nyland et al, 1995; Partington and Biller, 1996; Lamb, 1998).

Nuclear imaging procedures (e.g., hepatic scintigraphy) and magnetic resonance imaging are used to further assess hepatic structure and vasculature or measure the degree of portosystemic vascular shunting. These techniques are usually only available at specialty referral centers.

Liver Biopsy

Histopathologic tissue examination is essential for definitive diagnosis of hepatobiliary disease (Center, 1995; Meyer, 1996; Kerwin, 1995). Liver biopsy is an invasive procedure that must be carefully considered before implementation. Common options for securing liver tissue include ultrasonographic-guided needle biopsy, "blind" biopsy techniques, laparoscopic needle or pinch biopsy and celiotomy for wedge biopsy (Center, 1995). A minimum of three full 16-gauge needle samples should be collected if a needle procedure is used. Small sample size decreases the diagnostic accuracy of the histologic diagnosis (Rothuizen et al, 2006). One study showed a poor histologic correlation when only two 18-gauge needle biopsy specimens were compared to a wedge biopsy (Cole et al, 2002).

The advantage of fine-needle aspiration cytology (**Figure 68-5**) is decreased risk of complications or bleeding. However, a representative sample might not be obtained with this technique because of the very small amount of tissue that is obtained and the fact that liver architecture is not left intact during fine-needle aspiration procedures. Interpretation of hepatic cytology should be used in light of all clinical findings because hepatic cytology does not always correlate with histopathology. Ideally, liver tissue should be submitted for histopathologic and cytologic evaluation, aerobic and anaerobic bacterial cultures and copper quantification when copper toxicosis or chronic hepatitis is suspected. Specific stains for collagen, lipid, copper, iron and infectious agents may be required in some cases (**Figure 68-6**).

Abnormal concentrations of copper can occur from either a primary metabolic defect in copper metabolism reported to occur in certain dog breeds or secondarily as a result of chronic cholestatic liver disease. Abnormal copper levels damage hepatocytes. Hepatic copper content can be determined using either fresh or formalin-fixed liver tissue (Meyer, 1996; Thornburg et al, 1985). Most laboratories require one gram or less of tissue for analysis (Center, 1996a; Thornburg et al, 1990, 1996, 1985a). Normal canine hepatic copper concentrations should be 400 µg/g dry weight (DW) or less. Concentrations ranging from 750 to 2,000 µg/g DW may result from primary or secondary causes. The disease most likely results from a breed-associated copper accumulation disorder when hepatic copper concentrations exceed 2,000 µg/g DW. Hepatic copper concentrations can also be subjectively estimated using a histochemical copper stain grading system. Copper grading ranges tends to correlate with quantitative copper analysis (Teske et al, 1992).

Fine-needle aspiration of the liver using special copper staining correlates with histochemical grading but the extent of liver pathology cannot be adequately determined (Stockhaus et al, 2004). Genetic markers have been made available for testing Bedlington terriers (Yuzbasiyan-Gurkan et al, 1997).

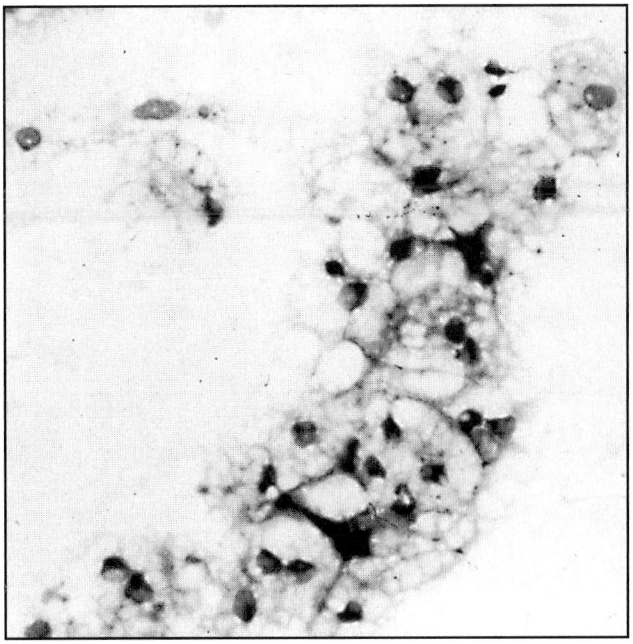

Figure 68-5. A cytologic specimen obtained by fine-needle aspiration of the liver from a cat with hepatic lipidosis. Note the lipid-laden hepatocytes. (Photograph courtesy Dr. Joseph Taboada, Louisiana State University, Baton Rouge.)

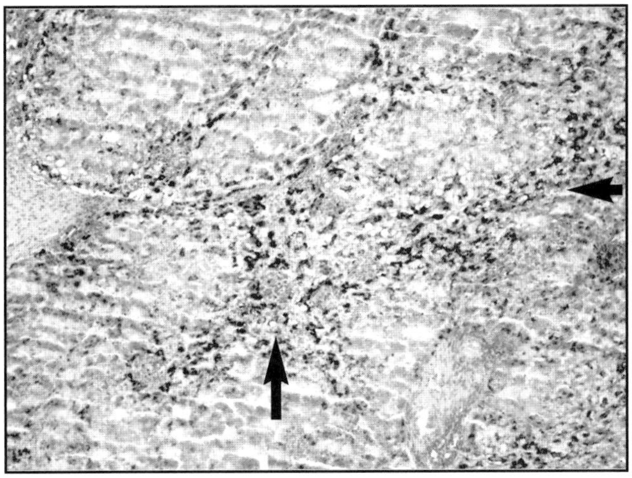

Figure 68-6. Photomicrograph of a liver biopsy specimen from a Doberman pinscher with chronic hepatitis. Note the accumulation of copper (arrows) as detected with rubeanic acid stain. In such cases, the hepatic copper content should be determined by quantitative methods.

Common Hepatobiliary Diseases

Feline Hepatic Lipidosis

Hepatic lipidosis in cats is a well-recognized syndrome characterized by accumulation of excess triglycerides in hepatocytes with resulting cholestasis and hepatic dysfunction (**Figures 68-7 and 68-8**) (Biourge et al, 1990, 1993; Center et al, 1993; Cornelius and Jacobs, 1989; Dimski and Taboada, 1995). Lipidosis can occur secondary to diabetes mellitus, diseases resulting in anorexia and weight loss (such as pancreatitis or inflammatory bowel disease) or as an idiopathic disorder of unknown etiology. Cats with idiopathic hepatic lipidosis often present with a history of prolonged anorexia after a stressful event. The biochemical mechanisms responsible for inducing hepatic lipidosis during fasting are not completely understood (Biourge et al, 1990, 1994; Center, 1996c). Potential causes include protein deficiency, excessive peripheral lipolysis, excessive lipogenesis, inhibition of lipid oxidation and inhibition of the synthesis and secretion of very low-density lipoproteins. The prognosis for this life-threatening disorder has improved dramatically during the past several years as a result of long-term enteral feeding (i.e., three to eight weeks or longer) (Biourge et al, 1990, 1994a; Dimski and Taboada, 1995). Hepatic lipidosis is a reversible process but resolution of hepatic lipidosis secondary to pancreatitis, infection or other causes depends on the success of treating the underlying disorder (Cornelius and Jacobs, 1989) and providing appropriate nutritional support.

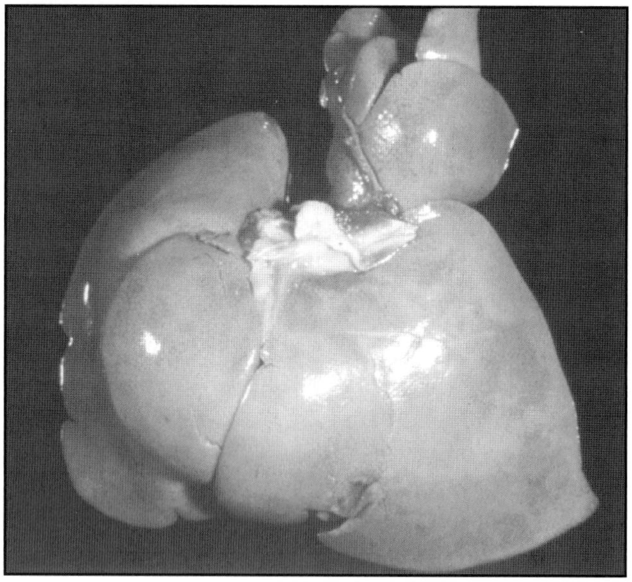

Figure 68-7. An enlarged, pale yellow liver from a cat with hepatic lipidosis.

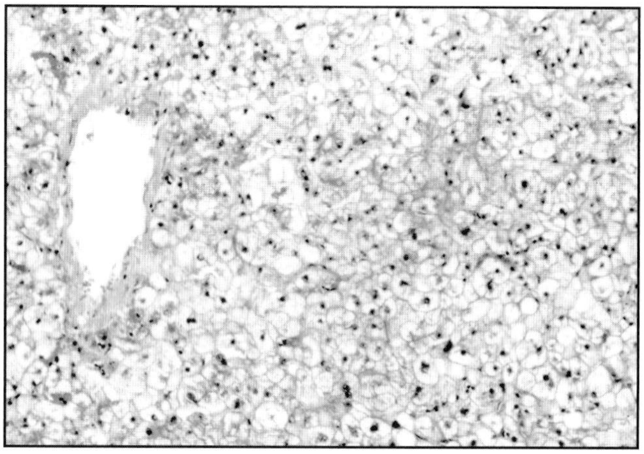

Figure 68-8. Photomicrograph of a liver specimen from a cat with hepatic lipidosis. Hepatocytes containing lipid appear empty with an inconspicuous nucleus when processed routinely with formalin fixation and hematoxylin and eosin stain.

Canine Chronic Hepatitis and Cirrhosis

Chronic hepatitis in dogs is a poorly defined group of clinicopathologic entities characterized by parenchymal necrosis, particularly piecemeal and/or bridging necrosis, with associated lymphoplasmacytic inflammation (Meyer, 1996; Thornburg, 1998; Speeti et al, 1998). Chronic hepatitis can result from many different causes including copper accumulation (See below.), infectious diseases, drugs, breed-associated hepatitis and possibly autoimmune disease. An etiology is never determined in most cases (Watson, 2004).

Lymphoplasmacytic inflammation suggests an immune-mediated mechanism. Autoantibodies have been recognized in dogs with chronic hepatitis but it is unknown if such an immune reaction is the cause or result of the disease (Weiss et al, 1995; Andersson and Sevelius, 1992; Thornburg, 1998). The insidious onset contributes to the poor understanding of the pathogenesis because most patients have an advanced stage of the disease when it is recognized.

Hepatic fibrosis is an accumulation of extracellular collagen and connective tissue within the liver (Center, 1996c) and is a sequela to hepatic inflammation. Fibrosis not only results in distortion of normal hepatic architecture, but also becomes a barrier to movement of substances back and forth between blood and hepatocytes. Cirrhosis is defined as fibrosis with loss of normal acinar liver architecture and with regenerative nodules (**Figure 68-9**) (Meyer, 1996). The architectural changes in cirrhosis impair blood and bile flow and nutrient exchange, thus perpetuating hepatocellular injury.

Canine Copper-Associated Hepatotoxicosis

Hepatic copper storage disease was first described in the Bedlington terrier breed. The disease has some similarities to Wilson's disease in people (Hultgren et al, 1986). It is an inherited autosomal recessive trait that impairs biliary excretion of copper (Su et al, 1982, 1982a). Affected dogs progressively accumulate copper. Evidence of hepatic necrosis is observed when copper concentrations exceed approximately 2,000 ppm (µg/g) DW liver (normal copper concentrations are <400 µg/g DW (Twedt et al, 1979; Twedt, 1990). As copper concentrations increase, damage progresses to chronic hepatitis and ultimately cirrhosis (Hultgren et al, 1986; Twedt et al, 1979; Twedt, 1990). Rarely, massive widespread hepatic necrosis can result in some dogs presenting with acute liver failure. Without appropriate treatment with dietary management and copper chelation, affected dogs usually succumb to their liver disease by approximately seven to 10 years of age (Hultgren et al, 1986; Twedt et al, 1979; Twedt, 1990). The gene responsible for this defect has been identified (Van De Sluis et al, 2002) and it has become possible to distinguish affected, homozygous normal and carrier Bedlington terrier dogs using DNA markers (Yuzbasiyian-Gurkan et al, 1997). It was once estimated that about 25% of Bedlington terriers were affected with copper toxicosis and another 50% were carriers. Now, through genetic testing and responsible breeding programs, the incidence of this disease is significantly lower.

Hepatic mitochondria are important intracellular targets of copper toxicosis. Functional abnormalities of mitochondria associated with oxidative injury (i.e., lipid peroxidation) have been documented to occur in people, rats and Bedlington terriers with copper-induced hepatic injury (Sokol et al, 1993, 1994). Oxidative injury and abnormal hepatic mitochondrial respiration may be involved in the pathogenesis of copper toxicosis. This theory forms the basis for using vitamin E and other antioxidants as potential therapeutic agents in addition to chelation therapy.

The role of copper in hepatic diseases observed in other dog breeds is less clear. Abnormal concentrations of copper in the liver can result secondary to cholestatic liver disease (Center, 1996c; Haywood et al, 1988; Johnson et al, 1982) or as a primary defect in hepatic copper excretion resulting in hepatic injury (Thornburg et al, 1984, 1985, 1986, 1996). Breeds that are currently thought to have primary copper-associated hepatopathies include Skye terriers (Haywood et al, 1988; McGrotty et al, 2003), West Highland white terriers (Thornburg et al, 1996), Doberman pinschers (Specti et al, 1998), Dalmatian dogs (Webb et al, 2002) and Labrador retrievers (Hoffman et al, 2006).

The liver diseases in these dogs are distinct from copper toxicosis in Bedlington terriers in that hepatic copper concentrations are generally lower and do not always increase with age. Other factors may be responsible for hepatic damage in some breeds. The exceptions might be Doberman pinschers and Dalmatian dogs because they tend to accumulate hepatic copper in concentrations similar to Bedlington terriers, suggesting defects in hepatic copper excretion (Mandigers, 2005).

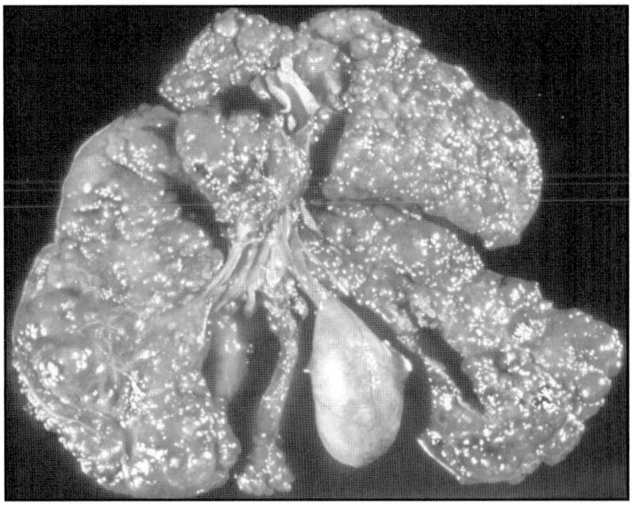

Figure 68-9. Cirrhotic liver from an eight-year-old female Doberman pinscher with chronic hepatitis. (Photograph courtesy Dr. Susan Johnson, The Ohio State University, Columbus.)

Cholangitis in Cats

Cholangitis (i.e., inflammation of the biliary ducts, especially the intrahepatic ducts and the surrounding liver tissue) is the most common feline inflammatory liver disease (Gagne et al, 1999; Armstrong et al, 1997; Day, 1995). The World Small Animal Veterinary Association Liver Pathology Standardization Working Group categorized the two most common forms of cholangitis into neutrophilic and lymphocytic forms (2006). Bacterial infection from enteric bacteria (especially *Escherichia coli*) ascending through the bile ducts is thought to be the cause of most neutrophilic forms, whereas immunologic mechanisms may be involved in the lymphocytic type. Chronic cholangitis may progress to biliary cirrhosis.

Many cats with cholangitis develop significant cholestasis and may have sludged or inspissated bile, causing partial or complete biliary obstruction (Armstrong et al, 1997; Day, 1995). Concurrent cholecystitis, pancreatitis and inflammatory bowel disease are common in feline cholangitis patients (Armstrong et al, 1997; Day, 1995).

Portosystemic Shunts in Dogs and Cats

PSS are vascular communications between the portal and systemic venous circulation. PSS can be either congenital or acquired. Congenital shunts can be further subdivided into intrahepatic shunts, occurring mostly in large-breed dogs or extrahepatic shunts, occurring mostly in smaller dog breeds and cats. Intrahepatic shunts are the remnant of a ductus venosus that did not completely close after birth. Extrahepatic shunts are seen as anomalous embryonic vessels between the portal vein and the systemic circulation (mostly to caudal vena cava or azygos vein) (Moon, 1990; Lamb, 1998; Center, 1996b). A hereditary basis for congenital shunts has been established in Irish wolfhounds (Meyer et al, 1995) and a number of other breeds have a significant risk for development of congenital shunts, supporting a hereditary etiology. Acquired PSS may develop as multiple shunts in response to portal hypertension caused by cirrhosis or other causes (e.g., tumors or portal vein thrombosis). Both congenital and acquired PSS are more common in dogs than in cats.

Primary portal vein hypoplasia (also referred to as microvascular dysplasia) is a second congenital vascular anomaly occurring in dogs, but rarely in cats. This anomaly is a consequence of portal vein hypoperfusion that results in hepatic arterialization in the portal triad and the development of microscopic intrahepatic shunts. Commonly affected breeds include cairn terriers, Yorkshire terriers and Maltese (Schermerhorn et al, 1996). Affected dogs have abnormal bile acid concentrations and variable liver enzymes but rarely have clinical signs. A less common variant of portal vein hypoplasia associated with fibrosis in the portal triads results in portal hypertension, ascites and PSS (Christiansen et al, 2000; Bunch et al, 2001).

Clinical signs of HE usually predominate in patients with PSS (**Box 68-1**). Polydipsia and polyuria are also commonly seen. Ammonium urate and other purine uroliths occur in some animals because of high urinary excretion of ammonia and uric acid (Chapter 39). Stunted growth or failure to gain weight may occur in young animals with congenital shunts. Surgical closure is the treatment of choice for congenital PSS but not for acquired PSS. Dietary management is the cornerstone of successful case management and prevention of HE in the pre- and immediate postoperative phase and in partially closed shunts (Meyer and Rothuizen, 1996).

Neoplasia

The most commonly encountered hepatic malignancies in dogs and cats are metastases, lymphoma, hemangiosarcoma, hepatocellular carcinoma and cholangiocarcinoma (Cullen and Popp, 2002). The appearance may be localized or diffuse. Because the liver has such a tremendous reserve capacity, tumors, especially localized malignancies may be undetected for long periods. In advanced stages, tumors may be visible or palpable during physical examination. Severe liver dysfunction with icterus, coagulopathies and portal hypertension may occur especially in diffusely distributed malignancies (e.g., malignant lymphoma and hemangiosarcoma).

Box 68-1. Hepatic Encephalopathy.

Hepatic encephalopathy (HE) is a neurologic syndrome that may arise due to liver dysfunction and portosystemic shunting (**Figure 1**). HE is categorized as acute or chronic, based on duration of signs and relative importance of the two main etiologic factors. Striking differences exist in the pathogenesis of acute and chronic HE. Because acute HE occurs rarely in dogs and cats, this summary will focus on chronic HE. Chronic HE results from disturbances in various neurotransmitter systems caused by a variety of gut-derived toxins and compounds. These toxins and compounds reach the systemic circulation when liver function is compromised and collateral circulation develops (**Figure 2**).

The pathogenesis of HE remains partly unknown due to the complex interplay between various pathogenetic factors and neurotransmitter systems. However, there seems to be consensus that the main neurotransmitter systems involved in HE are the GABA-ergic (the most abundant inhibitory neurotransmitter system in the brain) and the glutamatergic (the most important excitatory neurotransmitter system in the brain). Other neurotransmitters that may play a role include catecholamines, serotonin and opioids. Without doubt, ammonia is the main causative agent behind neurologic changes. Other contributing factors may include accumulation of manganese (Mn), increased concentrations of neurosteroids and peripheral benzodiazepine receptor ligands and changes in the molar ratio between branched-chain amino acids (BCAA) and aromatic amino acids (AAA) in plasma and cerebrospinal (CSF) fluid.

An abundance of evidence suggests that GABA-ergic tone is increased in HE. Although the nature of this increase is partly unknown, ammonia plays a key role. The role of increased concentrations of endogenous benzodiazepine receptor ligands in HE, an attractive hypothesis postulated in the late 1990s, has been abandoned. However, neurosteroids, which increase in people with HE, may have a direct influence on the GABA-ergic tone.

Although total brain glutamate is decreased in HE, intrasynaptic glutamate is increased, leading to down regulation of various postsynaptic glutamatergic receptor types.

Methionine, degraded by gut bacteria to the mercaptans methanethiol and dimethyldisulfide, has been implicated in the pathogenesis of HE, alone or synergistically with ammonia and free fatty acids. However, previous diagnostic methods overestimated the importance of these compounds; in rats and dogs, there was no correlation between the severity of HE and the concentrations of methanethiol and dimethyldisulfide. Thus these compounds do not play an important role in the pathogenesis of HE. On the other hand, S-adenosylmethionine (SAMe), an important precursor of liver glutathione, may play a role in the treatment of chronic liver disease because liver glutathione, an important antioxidant compound, is depleted in liver disease.

In human HE patients, a relation was found between high Mn concentrations in blood and/or the globus pallidus and hyperintensity of the magnetic resonance imaging signal in the globus pallidus. High Mn concentrations in the globus pallidus were accompanied by a loss of dopamine binding sites. Binding of Mn to dopamine receptors may have resulted in auto-oxidation of dopamine and formation of free radicals that caused tissue damage. No studies have been done to confirm increased Mn concentrations in the brains of dogs and cats with HE.

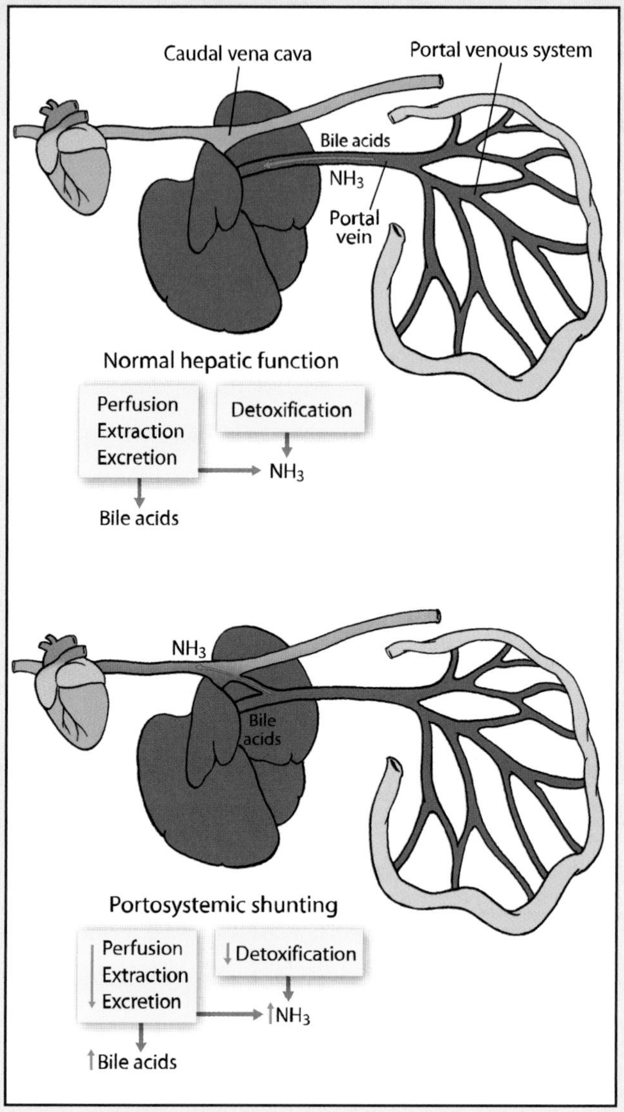

Figure 1. The effect of portosystemic shunting on hepatic extraction of bile acids and ammonia. (Adapted from Center SA. Hepatic vascular diseases. In: Guilford WG, Center SA, Strombeck DR, et al, eds. Strombeck's Small Animal Gastroenterology, 3rd ed. Philadelphia, PA: WB Saunders Co, 1996; 805, 813.)

Although a consistent decrease in the molar ratio between BCAA and AAA in plasma and in CSF has been reported in longstanding HE in many species, the importance of this molar ratio change in the pathogenesis of HE remains unclear. It may play a role in the reported dopaminergic dysfunction in HE, but others have not confirmed this hypothesis. The main beneficial effect of correction of the BCAA:AAA ratio by infusions or diet is reversal of the catabolic state in patients with HE.

Cats develop HE if fed foods deficient in arginine. Cats affected with hepatic lipidosis have low serum arginine concentrations. Because animal-origin protein is generally rich in arginine, most commercial cat foods and foods for stress and recovery are well

Box 68-1 continued

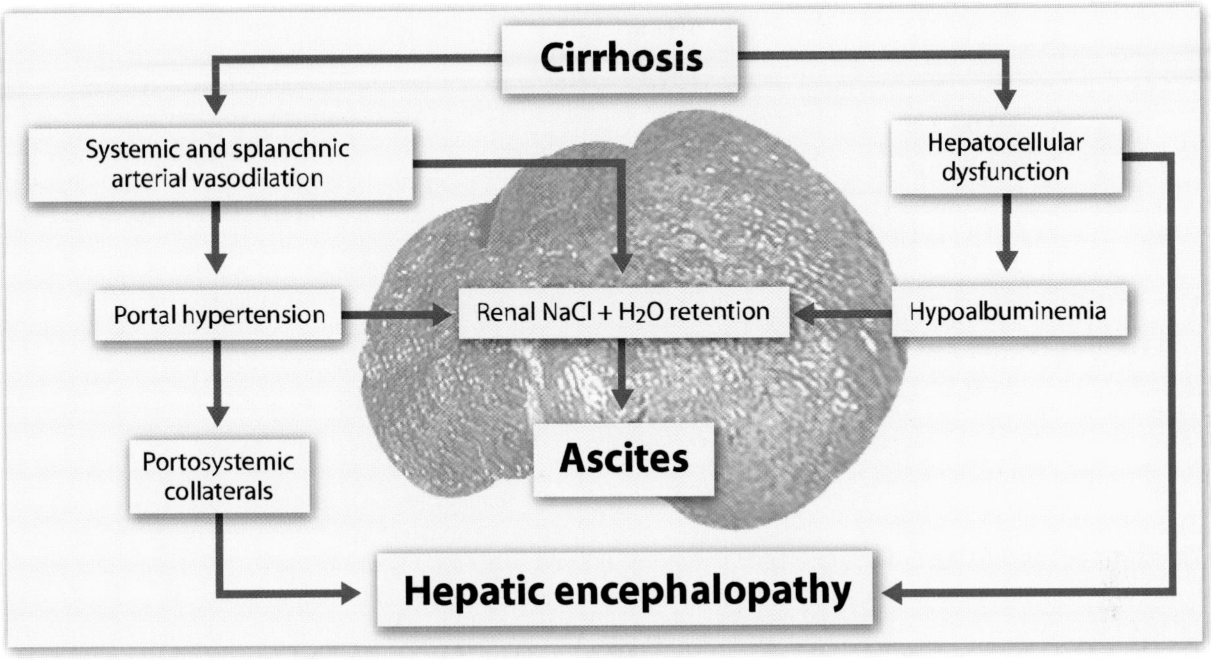

Figure 2. Interrelationships between the complications of cirrhosis. (Adapted from Abrams GA, Fallon MB. Cirrhosis of the liver and its complications. In: Andreoli TTE, Bennett JC, Carpenter CCJ, et al, eds. Cecil Essentials of Medicine, 4th ed. Philadelphia, PA: WB Saunders Co, 1997; 341.)

fortified with this amino acid. Homemade vegetable-based foods and human enteral foods fed to cats with encephalopathic clinical signs should be supplemented with arginine. Arginine levels in food should always be above the minimum dietary allowance for adult maintenance (>0.5% dry matter [DM] in dogs, >1.0% DM in cats). A dietary arginine level of 1.2 to 2.0% DM in dogs and 1.5 to 2.0% DM in cats seems appropriate for most patients with liver disease.

The Bibliography for **Box 68-1** can be found at www.markmorris.org.

Bile Duct Obstruction in Dogs and Cats

Extrahepatic bile duct obstruction, which is rarely seen in companion animals, can be caused by a number of conditions and pancreatitis is thought to be the most common cause in dogs (**Table 68-5**) (Neer, 1992). Cholestasis associated with occlusion of the major bile ducts leads to serious hepatobiliary injury within a few weeks (Center, 1996d). Obstructed bile flow and the resulting stagnation of bile acids and other compounds injure cell membranes and organelles. Bacterial cholecystitis may develop due to biliary reflux of intestinal bacteria or lymphohematogenous dissemination. Biliary injury is associated with cytokine-mediated inflammation and free radical injury. Long-term changes include biliary epithelial hyperplasia, cholangitis, multifocal parenchymal necrosis, fibrosis and cirrhosis (Center, 1996d). Coagulopathies associated with vitamin K deficiency may develop within three weeks.

Most patients with bile duct obstruction are candidates for exploratory celiotomy and corrective surgery. Enteral- or parenteral-assisted feeding is often used before and after surgery while the patient recovers (Chapters 25 and 26). Appropriate adult maintenance-type foods are generally indicated after recovery. Patients with inflammatory bowel disease, exocrine pancreatic insufficiency or concurrent pancreatitis may require a food with an altered nutrient profile (Chapters 57, 66 and 67, respectively).

Metabolic Alterations in Hepatocellular Dysfunction

Hepatocellular dysfunction is responsible for a number of metabolic disturbances that alter usage of various nutrients (**Table 68-6**). Changes in protein, carbohydrate and fat metabolism are particularly prominent in the fasting state (Marks et al, 1994; McCullough and Tavill, 1991; Latfi et al, 1991; Bauer, 1986, 1996; Chang et al, 1996). Attempts to correct these alterations by manipulating nutrient supply represent an important strategy in the management of patients with significant hepatic disease.

Impaired hepatic metabolism and storage may result in vitamin and mineral deficiencies. A combination of these metabolic and storage problems usually exists in patients with hepatic

Table 68-5. Causes of extrahepatic bile duct obstruction.*

Cholelithiasis
Cholecystitis (choledochitis)
Neoplasia
Bile duct adenocarcinoma
Pancreatic adenocarcinoma
Malignant lymphoma
Local tumor invasion
Malformation (polycystic liver disease)
Parasitic (trematode infection)
Extrinsic compression
Lymph nodes
Pancreatic mass
Entrapment in diaphragmatic hernia
Fibrosis or stricture
Blunt trauma
Peritonitis
Pancreatitis
Iatrogenic (postsurgical)

*Adapted from Center SA. Diseases of the gallbladder and biliary tree. In: Guilford WG, Center SA, Strombeck DR, et al, eds. Strombeck's Small Animal Gastroenterology, 3rd ed. Philadelphia, PA: WB Saunders Co, 1996; 870.

disease; each problem should be considered before appropriate dietary therapy is begun.

Carbohydrate Alterations

The liver plays a key role in the metabolism of the major monosaccharides glucose, fructose and galactose (Owen et al, 1981). Glucose can be used for energy production or to synthesize other substrates (e.g., amino acids, fatty acids), or it can be stored as glycogen. Liver glycogen can be readily mobilized when glucose is in demand. Hepatic glycogen can normally meet glucose needs (primarily for the brain) for 24 to 36 hours (Center, 1996). In human patients with hepatic cirrhosis, glycogen stores are more rapidly depleted (in 10 to 12 hours), which results in premature protein catabolism to supply amino acids for gluconeogenesis (Zakim, 1982). Gluconeogenesis, the production of glucose from amino acids, glycerol or lactate, is carried out only in the liver and the renal cortex. Glycolysis is the pathway by which glucose can be metabolized anaerobically with production of ATP. Regulation of glycolysis in the liver is highly integrated with that of gluconeogenesis, lipogenesis, glycogen synthesis and glycogenolysis.

Fasting hypoglycemia is uncommon in patients with liver disease because euglycemia can be maintained with as little as one-fourth to one-third of normal liver parenchymal mass (Zakim, 1982). However, hepatogenic hypoglycemia can occur in dogs with cirrhosis, congenital portosystemic vascular anomalies, fulminant hepatic failure, septicemia and extensive hepatic neoplasia (Center, 1996).

Glucose intolerance is more common than hypoglycemia in people with severe hepatic dysfunction; as many as 80% of cirrhotic patients have this abnormality (Zakim, 1982). The importance and causes of glucose intolerance in dogs and cats with liver disease are poorly documented. Hyperglycemia has been observed in some dogs with cirrhosis and portosystemic vascular shunts and in some cats with hepatic lipidosis and cholangitis (Center, 1996).

Protein and Amino Acid Alterations

The liver synthesizes the majority of circulating plasma proteins. The most abundant is albumin, which represents 55 to 60% of the total plasma protein pool (Center, 1996). Albumin serves as a binding and carrier protein for hormones, amino acids, steroids, vitamins, calcium and fatty acids, as well as exogenous compounds, drugs, toxins, etc. Albumin also helps maintain normal plasma oncotic pressure. The other proteins synthesized and secreted by the liver are usually glycosylated proteins (i.e., glycoproteins) that function in hemostasis, protease inhibition, transport and ligand binding. Hypoalbuminemia and increased bruising/bleeding tendencies result from decreased plasma protein production due to liver disease and/or increased usage (consumption coagulopathy) (Center, 1996). Ascites results from a combination of hypoalbuminemia and portal hypertension.

Protein regulatory events in the liver include amino acid storage and deamination of amino acids for intermediary metabolism. Generally, the liver degrades essential amino acids (including the aromatic amino acids [AAA], but not the branched-chain amino acids [BCAA]) and some of the nonessential amino acids (Center, 1996; Skeie et al, 1990). When dogs and other omnivores consume a minimal amount of dietary protein, the activities of key degradative enzymes are typically down regulated to ensure amino acid availability for protein synthesis. Alternatively, when omnivores ingest excess dietary protein, the activities of these key metabolic enzymes rapidly increase. This down regulation does not occur in carnivores such as cats (Chapter 19). Amino acids not required for protein synthesis are deaminated and oxidized or will be converted to carbohydrate and lipid. In this way, the liver plays an important role in energy balance and regulation of plasma concentrations of important amino acids (Chapter 5).

The deamination of amino acids is linked to carbohydrate and lipid metabolism by a number of common intermediates. These intermediates (e.g., pyruvate, fumarate, succinyl-CoA, oxaloacetate and acetyl-CoA) are entry points for amino acid carbon skeletons into the tricarboxylic acid (TCA or Krebs) cycle after deamination (Chapter 5). Intermediates are used primarily for energy production, gluconeogenesis and storage of excess dietary energy as triglycerides.

Alterations in nitrogen metabolism are one of the most prominent biochemical changes in chronic liver failure. Hyperammonemia is a common finding and results from a combination of factors including: 1) impaired ureagenesis due to decreased functional mass, 2) inadequate delivery of ammonia to the liver because of portosystemic vascular shunting and 3) increased ammoniagenesis due to amino acid deamination and gluconeogenesis (Meyer, 1998) (**Box 68-2**).

Plasma amino acid concentrations may be altered in patients with liver disease (Center, 1996; Strombeck and Rogers, 1978; Strombeck et al, 1983, 1984; Rutgers et al, 1987; Aguirre et al, 1974). Plasma amino acid concentrations differ depending on

Table 68-6. Metabolic alterations in hepatic failure.*

Alterations	Mechanisms
Hyperglucagonemia	Portosystemic shunting Impaired hepatic degradation Increased plasma aromatic amino acid levels Hyperammonemia
Hyperinsulinemia	Increased peripheral insulin resistance Decreased insulin to glucagon ratio Impaired hepatic degradation
Increased plasma cortisol levels	Deranged feedback mechanism
Decreased liver and muscle carbohydrate stores	Accelerated glycogenolysis Impaired glycogenesis
Increased gluconeogenesis	Hyperglucagonemia
Hyperglycemia (fasting and postprandial)	Portosystemic shunting Increased gluconeogenesis Decreased insulin-dependent glucose uptake Decreased insulin-hepatic glycolysis
Increased plasma aromatic amino acid levels	Decreased hepatic clearance and incorporation into proteins Increased release into the circulation
Decreased plasma branched-chain amino acid levels	Hyperinsulinemia and excessive uptake Increased usage as an energy source
Increased plasma methionine, glutamine, asparagine and histidine levels	Decreased hepatic clearance

*Adapted from Marks SL, Rogers QR, Strombeck DR. Nutritional support in hepatic disease. Part I. Metabolic alterations and nutritional considerations in dogs and cats. Compendium on Continuing Education for the Practicing Veterinarian 1994; 16: 972.

the type of hepatic failure present. In health, the AAA (i.e., tyrosine, phenylalanine and tryptophan) are efficiently extracted from the portal circulation and metabolized by the liver. Reduced liver function is associated with an increase in circulating levels of AAA because of continued mobilization of amino acids for gluconeogenesis and impaired hepatic AAA metabolism (Center, 1996; Strombeck and Rogers, 1978). Plasma concentrations of BCAA (i.e., leucine, isoleucine and valine), and most other amino acids metabolized in peripheral tissues are reduced because of an increased rate of usage by muscle and adipose tissue (Center, 1996; Strombeck and Rogers, 1978). The molar ratio between BCAA and the AAA (BCAA:AAA ratio) in healthy dogs usually ranges between 3.0 to 4.0. This ratio is often reduced to 1.0 or less in dogs with portosystemic vascular anomalies and chronic hepatitis (Meyer, 1998; Center, 1996e; Strombeck et al, 1983, 1984; Rutgers et al, 1987). Conversely, massive, acute hepatic necrosis in dogs (which is a rare disorder in dogs and cats) increases the plasma concentrations of all amino acids except arginine (Strombeck and Rogers, 1978). Increased circulating catecholamines, insulin and glucagon concentrations are thought to contribute to the altered amino acid metabolism seen in patients with liver disease (Center, 1996; Strombeck et al, 1983). Because all neutral amino acids (which includes BCAA, AAA and glutamine) use the same carrier to cross the blood-brain barrier, the decreased BCAA:AAA ratio is even more pronounced in cerebrospinal fluid than in plasma. Alterations in plasma amino acid profiles may also play a role in the pathogenesis of HE (Fischer et al, 1975; Maddison, 1992; Meyer, 1998a). Increased cerebral AAA levels have been hypothesized to form "false neurotransmitters," leading to decreased dopaminergic tone. Dopaminergic disinhibition at the pituitary level has been documented to occur in dogs with PSS (Rothuizen and Mol, 1987). Attempts to show that normalization of the BCAA:AAA ratio in cerebrospinal fluid would restore dopaminergic inhibition at the pituitary level have failed in dogs with induced HE (Meyer, 1998a).

Lipid Alterations

Lipid metabolic processes in the liver include: 1) fatty acid and triglyceride synthesis, 2) phospholipid and cholesterol synthesis, 3) lipoprotein metabolism and 4) bile salt synthesis. The liver synthesizes fatty acids from carbohydrate precursors by converting these precursors to acetyl-CoA. Fatty acids are generally stored in the liver as triglycerides. After hepatic glycogen stores are depleted, fatty acids are mobilized from adipose tissue and their rate of hepatic oxidation increases. The ketone bodies produced are an important energy source for peripheral tissues (i.e., brain, skeletal muscle) and decrease the rate of glucose usage.

The liver is a site for β-oxidation of fatty acids, producing energy from fatty acid substrates (Chapter 5 and 6). L-carnitine functions to transport long-chain fatty acids across the inner mitochondrial membrane to the mitochondrial matrix for β-oxidation. The liver is also a major site of cholesterol synthesis from acetyl-CoA. Cholesterol is found throughout the body as a structural component of cell membranes, a substrate for synthesis of steroid hormones and is important in the liver as the precursor for bile acid synthesis. The liver secretes lipoprotein particles and is an essential organ for their uptake and metabolism.

The composition of plasma lipids and lipoproteins is altered in patients with liver disease. These abnormalities are associated with changes in lipoprotein and cholesterol synthesis, lec-

Box 68-2. Ammonia Metabolism and the Urea Cycle.

Ammonia is highly toxic and lethal. Therefore, excretion of excess ammonia is necessary for life. Animals have developed different approaches to this problem. Mammals use the urea cycle and glutamine synthesis as ammonia disposal mechanisms.

UREA SYNTHESIS

Urea is synthesized in the liver via the urea cycle (**Figure 1**). The initial step in urea production is synthesis of carbamoyl phosphate from bicarbonate and ammonia. Carbamoyl phosphate synthetase I catalyzes carbamoyl phosphate formation in mitochondria. This reaction requires free Mg^{++} and magnesium adenine triphosphate, the rate-limiting step of the urea cycle.

Next, citrulline is formed from carbamoyl phosphate and ornithine. Ornithine transcarbamoylase, another mitochondrial enzyme, catalyzes this reaction. This step is followed by the cytosolic portion of the urea cycle, beginning with a reaction catalyzed by argininosuccinate synthetase that combines citrulline with aspartate, a second nitrogen donor, to form argininosuccinate. Argininosuccinate is cleaved to arginine and fumarate via the action of argininosuccinate lyase. Finally arginine is cleaved by arginase to form urea and ornithine. Urea is released into the circulation and ornithine reenters the urea cycle.

THE UREA CYCLE IN NONCARNIVOROUS ANIMALS

In noncarnivorous mammals (i.e., herbivores and omnivores), the urea cycle is controlled by the activities of constituent enzymes, which in turn are controlled by the substrates they act upon. Additionally, during periods of normal protein intake, most enzymes involved in urea synthesis in noncarnivorous animals operate only at 20 to 50% capacity, allowing for adaptation to high or low protein foods. These mechanisms conserve nitrogen during periods of food deprivation, but slow the response time for ammonia detoxification after ingestion of a high protein meal.

The amino acid intermediates used in the urea cycle (i.e., ornithine, citrulline and arginine) are formed within the cycle itself and are provided by dietary sources of amino acids. In noncarnivorous mammals, amino acids for the urea cycle can be synthesized via alternative pathways; for example, rats can synthesize ornithine via proline or glutamate, a process that doesn't occur in obligate carnivores. Therefore, noncarnivorous animals can better adapt to foods containing protein of lower quality that may not contain all of the amino acids required for urea cycle function or foods that vary in protein content over time.

THE UREA CYCLE IN CARNIVOROUS ANIMALS

In contrast to noncarnivorous animals, carnivores (e.g., cats and ferrets) have not developed adaptive mechanisms to conserve nitrogen during periods of low protein intake. Only minimal changes in enzymatic activity are seen in cats fed either high or low protein foods. Thus, urea cycle enzymes act continuously, independent of dietary protein intake. Because enzymatic activity is constant, carnivores control the urea cycle via concentrations of urea cycle intermediates, which allows for rapid detoxification of ammonia.

Carnivores are also unable to synthesize ornithine from proline and glutamate. Therefore, ornithine for the urea cycle must be synthesized exclusively from arginine. Although the kidneys synthesize a small amount of arginine from citrulline, the high activity of

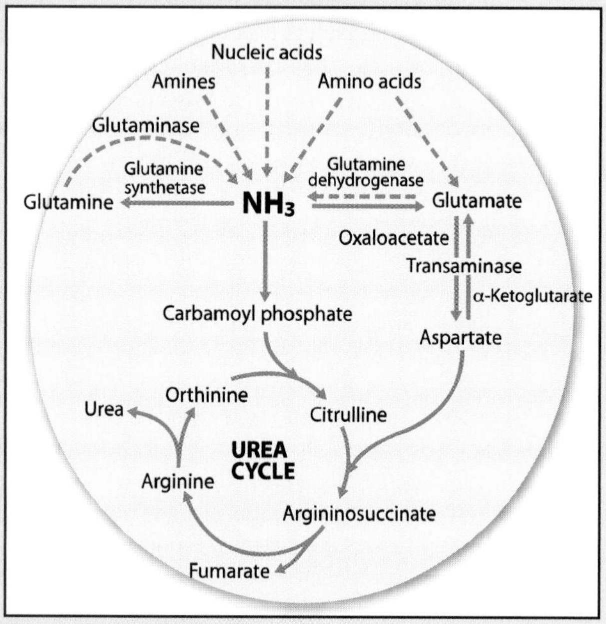

Figure 1. General scheme of hepatic ammonia metabolism, illustrating the pathways of ammonia usage (solid arrows) and ammonia formation (broken arrows). (Adapted from Ampola MG. The urea cycle: Enzymes and defects. In: Arias IM, Boyer JL, Fausto N, et al, eds. The Liver: Biology and Pathobiology, 3rd ed. New York, NY: Raven Press, 1994; 366.)

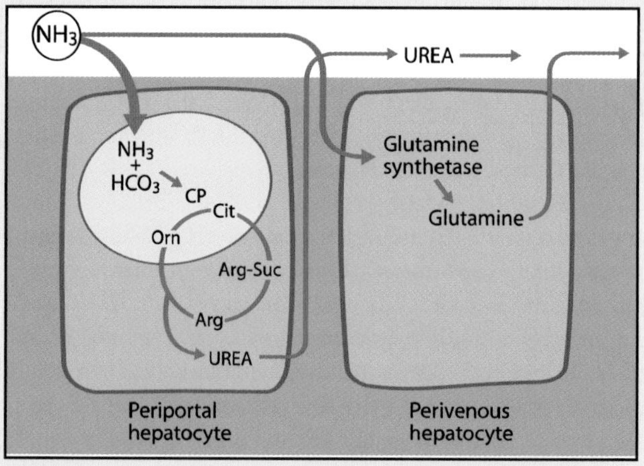

Figure 2. The scavenger role of perivenous hepatocytes. Most ammonia is metabolized to urea in the periportal hepatocytes. Ammonia not metabolized to urea is metabolized to glutamine by the perivenous hepatocytes (catalyzed by glutamine synthetase). This prevents ammonia from entering the systemic circulation and allows for uncoupling of urea production, which may be useful in acid-base regulation. Key: CP = carbamoyl phosphate, Cit = citrulline, Arg-Suc = argininosuccinate, Arg = arginine, Orn = ornithine. (Adapted from Dimski DS. Ammonia metabolism and the urea cycle: Function and clinical implications. Journal of Veterinary Internal Medicine 1994; 8: 75.)

Box 68-2 continued

hepatic arginase dictates that food primarily supply arginine for the urea cycle. To illustrate this point, adult cats and ferrets develop hyperammonemia and hepatic encephalopathy when fed foods devoid of arginine.

GLUTAMINE SYNTHESIS

Glutamine synthesis is the second primary mechanism by which mammals can metabolize excess ammonia. Hepatic glutamine synthetase is compartmentalized in a small area surrounding the centrilobular vein; thus, perivenous cells serve as "scavengers" for any ammonia that has not been converted to urea by periportal hepatocytes (**Figure 2**). Approximately one-third of the total ammonia from portal blood is detoxified by glutamine synthesis, although this percentage varies depending on acid-base status.

The glutamine synthetase pathway is a high affinity system, ensuring that ammonia does not reach the systemic circulation in toxic concentrations. In contrast, urea production is a low affinity, high capacity system for detoxifying ammonia. Thus, glutamine synthesis acts as a backup system for ammonia detoxification, allowing urea production to be decreased as required for acid-base regulation, while preventing hyperammonemia.

Glutamine synthetase activity is also high in brain astrocytes, which detoxify ammonia that may reach the brain. However, this system has limited capacity. Thus, increases in brain ammonia cannot be prevented in cases of severe hyperammonemia.

The Bibliography for **Box 68-2** can be found at www.markmorris.org.

ithin-cholesterol acyltransferase deficiency, defective lipolysis, abnormal recognition and uptake of lipoproteins by the liver and regurgitation of biliary lipids into plasma (Center, 1996). Obstructive icterus may lead to hypercholesterolemia and hypertriglyceridemia (Center, 1996). Hypocholesterolemia has been recognized in animals with portosystemic vascular anomalies and acquired hepatic insufficiency (Center, 1996). Hypotriglyceridemia has been recognized in dogs with PSS and hepatic necrosis (Center, 1996). Little is known about changes in lipoprotein fractions in dogs and cats with liver disease. Because the well-known relationship between plasma lipid and lipoprotein disturbances and cardiovascular disease in people is lacking in dogs and cats, the clinical relevance of the aforementioned disturbances in liver disease in these species may be limited.

Vitamin and Mineral Alterations

The liver serves as a storage reservoir for certain vitamins and minerals. Vitamin A can be stored in quantities sufficient for several months. The other fat-soluble vitamins (D, E and K) and vitamin B_{12} are also stored in the liver. The rest of the B vitamins are found in high concentrations in hepatic tissue, but the liver is not generally considered as their storage reservoir. Iron from dietary sources and from erythrocyte degradation is sequestered in hepatic tissue. Copper, manganese, selenium and zinc are trace elements normally present in high concentrations in the liver (Chapter 6).

Changes may occur in the patterns of storage and availability of all of these micronutrients in patients with significant liver disease. Malabsorption and alterations in hepatic blood flow may decrease availability and liver concentrations of certain vitamins and minerals. Vitamin B_{12} appears to be important in cats and subnormal concentrations of vitamin B_{12} have been reported in cats having liver disease. An adequate supply of B-complex vitamins is essential for the liver to perform a myriad of metabolic activities.

Copper is an essential trace metal required for diverse and numerous metabolic functions. The liver is essential for regulating copper concentrations and excreting excess copper via bile. Hepatic copper concentrations increase as a result of a primary metabolic defect in hepatic copper metabolism noted in some breeds of dogs. In dogs, the concentration of accumulated copper caused by cholestatic disease is less than the concentrations occurring from breed-associated copper hepatotoxicity (Spee et al, 2006). Subcellular damage to hepatocytes can result from significant copper accumulation. Copper is referred to as a transitional metal and is a catalyst (through the Fenton reaction). Free copper can directly damage hepatocyte mitochondria resulting in electron leak with free radical formation leading to lipid membrane peroxidation (Sokol et al, 1989).

Iron accumulates in the liver of canine patients with chronic hepatitis/cirrhosis, congenital portosystemic shunting and possibly other types of liver disease (Schultheiss et al, 2002; Simpson et al, 1997). Iron accumulation is thought to result from three mechanisms: 1) dietary iron uptake from the intestine, which is then deposited in the liver, 2) hepatic sequestration of iron released during hepatic inflammation and 3) abnormal hepatic retention secondary to cholestasis. Most hepatic iron is sequestered as hemosiderin and found in Kupffer cells or as lipogranulomas. Iron in hepatocytes occurs as ferritin or hemosiderin. Kupffer cell damage from iron results in cytokine release with subsequent inflammation and fibrosis. Because iron is a transition metal much like copper, abnormal levels of iron can catalyze the generation of free radicals and initiate lipid peroxidation of hepatocyte membranes and damage cellular proteins (Britton, 1996; Sokol and Hoffenberg, 1996).

Key Nutritional Factors

The specific nutrient requirements of patients with various naturally occurring hepatobiliary diseases are not well understood or documented. Most key nutritional factor recommendations for these patients are based on understanding normal hepatic function, studies in animals with experimentally induced disease, results in human patients with comparable diseases and

Table 68-7. Key nutritional factors for cats with hepatic lipidosis or cholangitis.*

Factors	Recommended levels
Energy density (kcal/g)	≥4.4
Energy density (kJ/g)	≥18.4
Protein (%)	30 to 45
Arginine (%)	1.5 to 2.0
Taurine (%)	≥0.3
Potassium (%)	0.8 to 1.0
L-carnitine (%)	≥0.02

*Nutrients expressed on a dry matter basis.

Table 68-8. Key nutritional factors for dogs and cats with hepatobiliary disease.*

Factors	Dogs	Cats
Energy density (kcal/g)	≥4.0	≥4.2
Energy density (kJ/g)	≥16.7	≥17.6
Protein (%)	15-20**	30-35**
Arginine (%)	–	1.5 to 2.0
Taurine (%)	≥0.1	≥0.3
Sodium (%)	0.08 to 0.25	0.07 to 0.3
Copper (mg/kg)	≤5	–
Zinc (mg/kg)	>200	>200
Iron (mg/kg)	80 to 140	80 to 140
Vitamin E (IU/kg)	≥400	≥500
Vitamin C (mg/kg)	≥100	100 to 200

*Nutrients expressed on a dry matter basis.
**For liver disease patients with signs of hepatic encephalopathy, dry matter dietary protein levels should be limited to 10 to 15% for dogs and 25 to 30% for cats until signs resolve.

clinical experience. The key nutritional factors discussed below support a common nutrient profile that will benefit most liver disease patients. However, it should be noted that due to the wide range of hepatobiliary diseases and their differing severity, one nutrient profile might not always be ideal for all patients. The following section will discuss these key nutritional factors in more detail and outline specific recommendations for the most common hepatobiliary disorders. **Tables 68-7** (feline hepatic lipidosis and cholangitis) and **68-8** (canine and feline hepatobiliary diseases) summarize these key nutritional factors.

Energy

Provision of adequate daily energy intake is the cornerstone of successful medical management of cats with hepatic lipidosis (Biourge et al, 1990, 1994a; Center, 1996c; Biourge, 1997; Marks et al, 1994a). An adequate supply of energy is needed to: 1) prevent catabolism of amino acids for energy, 2) inhibit peripheral lipolysis and 3) avoid excess energy consumption, which will promote hepatic triglyceride accumulation. Cats with hepatic lipidosis are often fed commercial veterinary therapeutic products via assisted-feeding techniques (Chapter 25). Foods with energy densities of at least 4.4 kcal metabolizable energy (ME/g) (18.4 kJ ME/g) (dry matter [DM]) are well tolerated by most cats and result in clinical improvement when fed in appropriate amounts. Energy density recommendations for cats with cholangitis are similar to those outlined for cats with hepatic lipidosis. Achieving this level of energy density typically requires at least 25% DM dietary fat.

Providing adequate daily energy intake is also important in managing dogs and cats with chronic hepatitis, portal hypertension and PSS and dogs with copper-associated hepatotoxicosis. An adequate supply of energy is needed to allow protein synthesis and prevent tissue catabolism that generates ammonia. Foods for patients with these diseases should provide at least 4.0 and 4.2 kcal ME/g DM (16.7 and 17.6 kJ ME/g), for dogs and cats, respectively.

The role of dietary fat in patients with hepatic disease has not been specifically determined. Dietary lipids are beneficial because they have a protein-sparing effect, reduce carbohydrate intolerance, augment fat-soluble vitamin absorption, enhance palatability and are an important source of energy and essential fatty acids.

A minor decrease in fat digestibility (i.e., from 92 to 85%) was found in dogs with experimentally created PSS (Laflamme et al, 1993). Other studies showed that dogs with experimental shunts tolerate foods containing 20 to 25% DM fat (Center, 1996b). Clinically significant impaired fat digestion may occur in animals with severe biliary disease with subtotal or total biliary obstruction.

There appears to be no reason for routinely restricting dietary fat in dogs and cats with liver disease. One of two different situations may be occurring if steatorrhea is a problem in patients with hepatobiliary disease. First, the patient may have concurrent disease that is contributing to fat malassimilation, such as exocrine pancreatic insufficiency. Second, the patient may have subtotal or total biliary duct obstruction.

Medium-chain triglycerides (MCT; i.e., carbon chain lengths <12) have theoretical advantages over long-chain triglycerides (LCT) for the treatment of GI and some forms of hepatobiliary disease (Guilford, 1996). MCT may be more easily hydrolyzed and absorbed than LCT; however, these advantages have yet to be proved. Caloric supplementation with MCT is useful for malnourished human cirrhotic patients with steatorrhea and those with advanced cholestatic hepatic disease (Munoz, 1991). Controlled clinical trials using MCT in animals with cirrhotic or cholestatic liver disease have not been reported.

The inflammatory component of hepatic disease may be attenuated by omega-3 (n-3) fatty acid supplementation. However, the specific amounts to include in foods and the optimal ratio of omega-6 (n-6) to omega-3 fatty acids have not been determined. Some veterinary therapeutic foods for liver disease are enhanced with omega-3 fatty acids (Remillard and Saker, 2005).

Protein and Amino Acids

Dietary protein and the amino acids arginine and taurine are important in cats with hepatic lipidosis. Cats are less efficient in sparing protein during fasting than other animals. As such, protein deficiency may play a major role in the development of feline idiopathic hepatic lipidosis. Cats with hepatic lipidosis have signs of protein malnutrition include hypoalbuminemia, anemia, muscle wasting and negative nitrogen balance (Biourge et al, 1994; Barsanti et al, 1977). Specific amino acids (e.g., methionine and arginine) become limiting during fasting in obese cats (Biourge et al, 1994). Protein or amino acid deficiency may induce lipid accumulation in the liver by limiting lipoprotein synthesis needed for normal lipid metabolism and transport (Biourge et al, 1994). Protein supplementation at only one-fourth of the daily requirement (22 g protein/day) significantly reduced lipid accumulation in the liver and promoted positive nitrogen balance during long-term fasting in obese cats (Biourge et al, 1994a).

Cats with hepatic lipidosis will usually tolerate moderate amounts of dietary protein unless they are suffering from concurrent HE, which is uncommon. Commercial veterinary therapeutic foods containing 30 to 45% DM protein are well tolerated by cats with hepatic lipidosis and have been used successfully in many cases. Protein needs for cats with cholangitis are similar to those for cats with hepatic lipidosis.

Adult cats and ferrets developed hyperammonemia and HE when fed foods devoid of arginine (**Boxes 68-1** and **68-2**). Foods for cats with hepatic lipidosis should provide adequate arginine. Arginine levels in food should always be above the minimum dietary allowance for adult maintenance (≥0.77% DM [NRC, 2006]). More arginine is required in cat foods that contain more than 20% DM protein (NRC, 2006). Arginine levels in foods for cats with liver disease should be between 1.5 to 2.0% DM. Good quality commercial foods are typically adequate in arginine. Homemade vegetable-based foods and human enteral foods fed to cats with encephalopathic clinical signs should be supplemented with arginine.

Ensuring adequate taurine intake is important for anoretic cats with hepatic lipidosis. Cats and dogs primarily synthesize taurine in the liver and bile salts are mainly conjugated with taurine. Compared to cats, dogs have a high capacity to synthesize taurine; therefore, dietary taurine is usually not essential. Food-induced bile salt excretion into the gut can result in significant loss of taurine, particularly when normal enterohepatic recycling is interrupted. Taurine synthesis is limited in cats; therefore, dietary taurine is essential. Adequate taurine nutriture is important in patients with enterohepatic circulation abnormalities and possibly in liver disease. In certain species, taurine also stimulates synthesis and turnover of bile independent of its role as a bile acid conjugate. Taurine appears to aid choleresis in dogs and possibly cats. This role may explain the observation that taurine prevents cholestasis in certain models of liver disease. Most commercial cat foods and foods for stress and recovery for dogs and cats are fortified with taurine. However, homemade and human enteral foods fed to cats should be supplemented with taurine (250 to 500 mg/day) (Chapter 10). The minimum recommended allowance for dry expanded and moist foods for adult cats is 0.10 and 0.17% DM, respectively (NRC, 2006). Foods for cats with hepatic lipidosis and other liver diseases should probably contain at least 0.3% DM taurine. Although no minimum recommended allowances for taurine for healthy dogs have been defined, foods for dogs with liver disease should contain at least 0.1% DM taurine.

Appropriate amounts of high quality dietary protein are also important in patients with chronic hepatitis and/or cirrhosis, portal hypertension and dogs with copper-associated hepatotoxicosis. Hypoalbuminemia, which reflects depleted body stores and reduced protein synthesis, is a frequent and serious problem in patients with chronic liver disease. Protein plays a leading role in hepatic regeneration; therefore, patients with liver disease require adequate protein intake to remain anabolic and support regeneration of hepatocytes. On the other hand, dietary protein restriction may be important in patients with endstage cirrhosis, hyperammonemia and HE. Protein, or more accurately, nitrogen excess, is a major contributor to neurotoxic precursors formed when amino acids are metabolized to ammonia. For patients with liver disease, the goal is to provide adequate dietary protein to support hepatic regeneration while avoiding excess dietary protein that might contribute to HE.

The protein requirements for patients with PSS have been roughly estimated from a nutritional study in adult dogs with surgically created shunts (Laflamme et al, 1993). This study showed that ingestion of 2.11 g crude protein/kg body weight/day with an 80% or greater availability was adequate to maintain body protein reserves without producing HE. In the absence of other data, this recommendation for dietary protein intake seems appropriate. This equates to approximately 14 to 16% protein calories (15 to 20% DM protein) for dogs and 25 to 30% protein calories (30 to 35% DM protein) for cats. These protein levels are also appropriate for dogs and cats with most other forms of liver disease, except hepatic lipidosis (described above) and HE. Patients with evidence of HE will often need restricted dietary protein levels for the short term (10 to 15% DM for dogs and 25 to 30% DM for cats). For a point of reference, the minimum recommended protein allowances for foods for normal adult dogs and cats are 10 and 20% DM, respectively (NRC, 2006).

In addition to the absolute amount of protein fed, the amino acid profile and digestibility are important for optimal protein usage. Amino acids from poor-quality protein sources are deaminated and metabolized to a greater extent than amino acids from higher quality protein sources and exacerbate hyperammonemia. Intestinal bacteria may degrade poorly digested proteins and add to the body's ammonia burden.

The importance of the dietary protein source has been studied in human patients with HE and in several experimental studies in dogs with PSS (Center, 1996b). Vegetable and dairy protein sources have produced the best results in maintaining positive nitrogen balance with minimal encephalopathic signs in human patients with liver disease (Uribe, 1990; Bianchi et al, 1993; Weber et al, 1985). Foods containing soybean meal averted encephalopathic signs in dogs with experimentally created shunts (Center et al, 1997; Thompson et al, 1986; Schaeffer et al, 1986). In addition, dairy products (especially cottage cheese) have been recommended for use in homemade foods for dogs and cats with PSS and chronic hepatic insufficiency (Center,

Box 68-3. Adjunctive Use of Copper Chelating Agents for Patients with Hepatic Copper Toxicosis.

For Bedlington terriers with subclinical or clinical liver disease, in addition to selection of a low-copper (<5 mg/kg, [dry matter]) veterinary therapeutic food (**Table 68-11**), adjunctive treatment with copper chelating agents is clearly indicated. Chelator treatment is used for breeds of dogs with copper-associated chronic hepatitis and cirrhosis and other breeds in which copper accumulation is documented by liver histopathology and/or elevated hepatic copper concentrations (generally >1,000 to 2,000 ppm dry weight).

Adjunctive treatment of hepatic copper toxicosis involves use of zinc or copper chelating agents such as D-penicillamine or trientine (**Figure 1**). Zinc blocks copper absorption. Chelating agents bind to copper and increase its excretion in urine. D-penicillamine, the copper chelating agent most frequently recommended for use in dogs, should be given at a dosage of 10 to 15 mg/kg body weight twice daily, on an empty stomach. Vomiting is the most common side effect in dogs, but can be alleviated by giving the agent more frequently in reduced doses. D-penicillamine therapy also has been associated with pyridoxine deficiency in people. However, this problem has not been recognized in dogs.

Trientine[a] (2,2,2-tetramine) is another chelating agent. In a clinical trial, chelation results with trientine (10 to 15 mg/kg body weight, per os, twice daily) were comparable to those of D-penicillamine and fewer side effects were noted. Modification of 2,2,2-tetramine to 2,3,2-tetramine increases the potency as a copper chelating agent. Use of 2,3,2-tetramine in affected Bedlington terrier dogs significantly reduced liver copper concentrations after 200 days of treatment at a dose of 15 mg/kg body weight. This drug is not commercially available but can be obtained from chemical supply companies in the form of N,N'-bis(2-aminoethyl)-1,3-propanediamine and prepared as a salt for oral administration.

Oral zinc therapy blocks copper absorption from the intestine. In early human studies, therapy with combined zinc and copper chelators found no benefit over single chelator therapy suggesting the chelator most likely binds zinc in the intestinal tract. However, more recently, human patients having Wilson's disease who are intolerant to penicillamine are sometimes treated with a combination trientine and zinc regimen with apparently good results. Affected dogs should be fed copper-restricted foods and be given the faster acting copper chelator. When hepatic copper concentrations approach normal levels, switching to zinc therapy alone may prevent further copper accumulation.

The initial report in dogs used 100 mg of elemental zinc acetate b.i.d. for one to two months during an induction phase followed by a maintenance dose of 50 mg of elemental zinc b.i.d., thereafter. Serum zinc concentrations should be monitored with a goal of approximately a twofold increase in serum concentrations (<200 µg/ml). Hemolysis can occur if serum zinc concentrations increase significantly (>750 µg/ml). Zinc can be given as an acetate, sulfate, gluconate or methionine salt but should be administered on an empty stomach to ensure adequate absorption. Common problems encountered with zinc therapy include anorexia, nausea and vomiting shortly following administration. If concurrent chelator therapy is used, dosing should be staggered to ensure adequate absorption of the chelator.

ENDNOTE

a. Syprine. Merck & Company, Inc., Rahway, NJ, USA.

The Bibliography for **Box 68-3** can be found at www.markmorris.org.

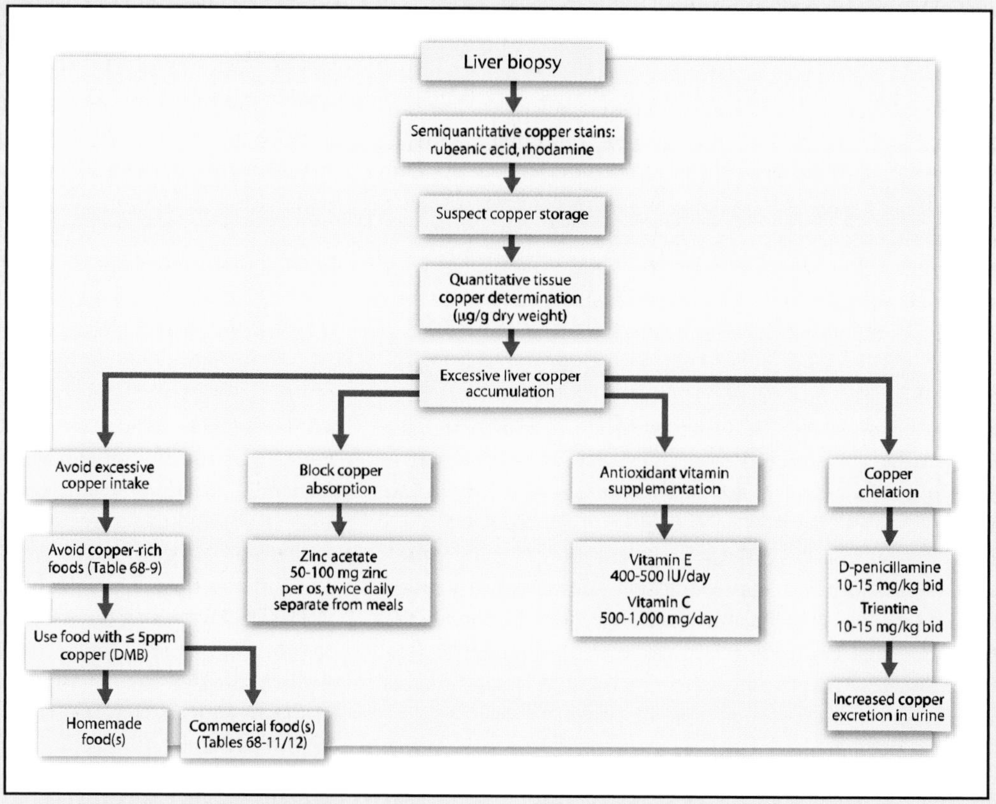

Figure 1. Algorithm for treating copper hepatotoxicosis in dogs. (Adapted from Center SA. Chronic liver diseases. In: Guilford WG, Center SA, Strombeck DR, et al, eds. Strombeck's Small Animal Gastroenterology, 3rd ed. Philadelphia, PA: WB Saunders Co, 1996; 749.)

1996b; Marks et al, 1994a). The amino acid composition of these protein sources is not significantly different from that of meat sources, suggesting that other food factors such as digestibility and levels of digestible (soluble) carbohydrate and fermentable fiber are important. Fermentable carbohydrates increase microbial nitrogen fixation, reduce intraluminal ammonia production in the gut and promote colonic evacuation (Center, 1996b). (See Fiber below.)

Superficial necrolytic dermatitis (hepatocutaneous syndrome) is an uncommon skin disease associated with systemic metabolic disease. Afflicted dogs commonly have concurrent skin erosions and ulcerations with alopecia, exudation and thick adherent crusts on the footpads and around mucocutaneous junctions. The hepatopathy grossly has the appearance of macronodular cirrhosis but is characterized by regenerative hyperplastic nodules separated by fibrous septa containing ductular structures and is void of inflammation. Some authors believe this condition results from exaggerated amino acid catabolism and the resultant hypoaminoacidemia is responsible for the skin and liver lesions (Gross et al, 1990, 1993). Most affected dogs also have low plasma amino acid concentrations and parenteral amino acid replacement with nutritional protein supplementation may resolve the skin lesions (Gross et al, 1993). In these cases, high protein foods, various protein supplements and intravenous amino acid solution administration is recommended. Note that rapid amino acid infusion can result in HE. Repeated amino acid infusions are given weekly as needed if a clinical response is observed using this protocol.

Potassium

Cats with hepatic lipidosis may develop hypokalemia due to inadequate potassium intake, vomiting, polydipsia and polyuria, magnesium depletion and concurrent chronic renal failure. In one study, hypokalemia was present in 19 of 66 cats (29%) with severe hepatic lipidosis (Center et al, 1993). Hypokalemia was significantly related to nonsurvival in this group of cats. Dogs with chronic liver disease and HE also frequently develop hypokalemia due to vomiting and alkalosis (Meyer, 1998). Hypokalemia is exacerbated by ascites due to activation of the renin-angiotensin-aldosterone axis. Hypokalemia, especially in combination with alkalosis (which is also a common feature in the same patients due to decreased use of bicarbonate in the urea cycle and vomiting), is dangerous because it may prolong anorexia and exacerbate expression of HE. This is due to intracellular trapping of ammonia in hypokalemic alkalosis. Foods for cats with hepatic lipidosis should be potassium replete (0.8 to 1.0% DM potassium), or potassium supplementation (2 to 6 mEq potassium gluconate per day) should be considered.

Sodium and Chloride

Excessive dietary sodium chloride should be avoided in liver disease patients with ascites, portal hypertension and/or significant hypoalbuminemia. Dietary sodium chloride restriction to levels recommended for patients with renal and cardiac failure is appropriate. Thus, sodium levels should be restricted to 0.08 to 0.25% DM for dogs and 0.07 to 0.3% DM for cats. Recommended DM chloride levels are typically 1.5 times sodium levels (NRC, 2006).

Table 68-9. Relative copper content of selected human foods.

Foods with very high copper content
Liver
Shellfish
Foods with high copper content
Cocoa
Heart
Kidney
Legumes
Mushrooms
Nuts
Skeletal muscle (meat)
Foods with low copper content
Cheese
Cottage cheese
Rice
Tofu

Copper

Avoiding excessive copper intake is important for dogs with copper-associated hepatotoxicosis, especially when serious hepatic injury has not yet occurred. The minimum recommended allowance for dietary copper in foods for healthy adult dogs is 6 mg/kg DM (NRC, 2006). However, studies have shown that Bedlington terriers achieve copper balance when consuming approximately 0.4 mg copper/day (Brewer et al, 1989). This equates to approximately 2.6 mg/kg of food. Foods for dogs with suspected or confirmed copper-associated hepatotoxicosis should not provide more than 5.0 mg/kg DM copper from an available copper source. Hepatic copper content is also increased (although not to the levels found in patients with inherited copper-related hepatotoxicosis) in patients with cholestasis. Therefore, moderate copper restriction is recommended for most patients with cholestatic liver disease. The role of copper in cats with liver disease has not been adequately investigated but it is generally considered that copper plays a minimal part, if any, in feline liver diseases.

Feeding selected commercial veterinary therapeutic (i.e., those formulated for patients with liver disease) or homemade foods to patients with liver disease can control copper intake, especially those with cholestasis. For patients with copper-associated hepatotoxicosis, copper restriction should be more aggressive and copper chelating agents (**Box 68-3**) or dietary zinc supplementation (See below.) should be used. Dogs should not be fed supplements containing copper or table foods that have a high copper content (**Table 68-9**). Certain fiber sources and minerals in food inhibit copper absorption (Chapters 5 and 6). The appropriate levels of these nutrients in foods for patients with copper toxicosis have not been determined. Zinc supplementation is important for blocking copper absorption and is discussed below.

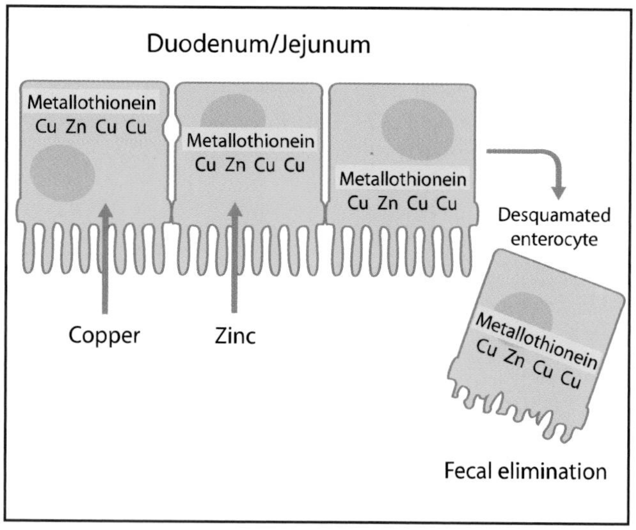

Figure 68-10. Diagrammatic representation of zinc and copper interaction in the intestine. Copper hepatotoxicosis is often treated with zinc supplementation. Zinc appears to induce synthesis of intestinal metallothionein, which has greater affinity for copper than for zinc. Metallothionein binds zinc and copper making them unavailable for systemic absorption. The metals are excreted in the feces with desquamated enterocytes. (Adapted from Center SA. Pathophysiology of liver disease: Normal and abnormal function. In: Guilford WG, Center SA, Strombeck DR, et al, eds. Strombeck's Small Animal Gastroenterology, 3rd ed. Philadelphia, PA: WB Saunders Co, 1996; 596, 599.)

Zinc

Zinc is an important metal involved in intermediary metabolism, enhanced ureagenesis, glutathione concentrations and immune function. The direct hepatoprotective effects of zinc include inhibition of lipid peroxidation and destabilization of lysosomal membranes. Zinc reportedly has antifibrotic activities (Brewer et al, 1992).

Zinc deficiency probably occurs in people with chronic hepatic disease (Riggio et al, 1991). Some dogs with chronic hepatitis or cirrhosis also have subnormal hepatic zinc concentrations (Schultheiss et al, 2002). Urea synthetic capacity may be reduced in zinc-deficient patients because of decreased hepatic ornithine transcarbamoylase activity and increased muscle glutamine synthetase activity (Marks et al, 1994). Zinc deficiency could adversely affect multiple aspects of ammonia metabolism (Mullen and Weber, 1991). Foods for patients with liver disease should contain more than 200 mg/kg DM zinc (Marks et al, 1994). This inclusion level is approximately three times the minimum recommended allowance for foods for healthy dogs and cats (60 and 74 mg/kg DM, respectively) (NRC, 2006), but is probably safe. A study in dogs and cats fed 80 and 200 mg zinc/kg body weight/day, respectively, for several months found no ill effects (Drinker et al, 1927; NRC, 2006). The levels of zinc intake in this study would be at least 60 times higher than would occur with the recommended amount for foods for dogs with liver disease. Similarly, the level is more than 100 times higher than would occur with the recommended amount for foods for feline patients with liver disease.

Dietary zinc blocks intestinal absorption of copper in dogs with copper-associated hepatotoxicosis. Animal and human studies have shown that zinc induces synthesis of intestinal metallothionein, which has greater affinity for copper than for zinc (Brewer, 1993; Friedman, 1993; Yuzbasiyian-Gurkan et al, 1992). In enterocytes, metallothionein acts as an intracellular ligand binding zinc, copper, mercury and cadmium to form mercaptides, thereby rendering them unavailable for systemic absorption. Thus, these metals are excreted in the feces with desquamated epithelial cells (**Figure 68-10**). In people with Wilson's disease, intestinal metallothionein concentrations were significantly elevated during zinc therapy when compared with the concentrations in patients not receiving zinc therapy (Friedman, 1993; Yuzbasiyian-Gurkan et al, 1992). A marked increase in intestinal metallothionein levels was observed in two human patients within a few days after zinc treatment was initiated. This finding was accompanied by suppression of copper uptake (Friedman, 1993; Yuzbasiyian-Gurkan et al, 1992). Discontinuation of zinc therapy was associated with progressive decreases in intestinal metallothionein concentrations and increased copper uptake. Thus, foods for canine patients with copper-associated hepatotoxicosis should also contain more than 200 mg/kg DM zinc, or the food should be supplemented with zinc gluconate (3 mg/kg body weight/day) or zinc sulfate (2 mg/kg body weight/day) divided into three doses (Marks et al, 1994).

Iron

Iron loading by hepatocytes and Kupffer cells has been recognized in some patients with inflammatory liver diseases and hepatic iron content is increased in dogs with cholestasis. Iron is a potent catalyst of oxidative processes (Fenton reaction) and iron-associated hepatic injury may involve lipid peroxidation of membranes and damage to organelles (Center, 1996c). Foods for dogs with chronic hepatitis and those with secondary hemosiderosis documented by evaluation of liver biopsy specimens should avoid excessive iron levels. The minimum recommended iron allowances for foods for normal adult dogs and cats are 30 and 80 mg/kg DM, respectively (NRC, 2006). Iron levels of 80 to 140 mg/kg DM meet the dietary allowance without providing excessive intake. This range is recommended for patients with liver disease. Injectable or oral supplements containing iron should be avoided in these patients.

On the other hand, iron deficiency may also occur in some liver patients with GI ulceration and hemorrhage associated with chronic hepatitis, portal hypertension or bile duct obstruction. Microcytosis, an erythrocyte abnormality associated with iron deficiency, also develops in dogs with portosystemic vascular shunts despite increased hepatic iron stores (Center, 1995, 1996b; Laflamme et al, 1994).

Iron supplementation is only indicated when serum iron concentrations are low, hypochromia is recognized and chronic gastroenteric bleeding or another source of chronic blood loss is recognized (Center, 1996a). Homemade foods, depending on the recipe, may require iron supplementation.

Antioxidant Vitamins E and C

Lipid peroxidation may be involved in the pathogenesis of some forms of acute liver injury and chronic hepatitis (Scalfani et al, 1986). Free radicals are an important component of most forms of liver damage. Abnormal concentrations of bile acids and the accumulation of heavy metals, such as copper and iron, cause free radical generation in the liver (Sokol and Hoffenberg, 1996; Sokol et al, 1994; Twedt et al, 1998). Activated inflammatory cells, damaged hepatocyte mitochondria and release of cytochrome P450 enzymes contribute to the production of reactive oxygen species. As the cascade proceeds, further hepatocyte damage occurs due to subsequent oxidation of cellular lipids, proteins and DNA. Oxidative stress may also activate pro-apoptotic protein kinases, proinflammatory transcription factors and modulators of apoptosis (Medina and Moreno-Otero, 2005).

Vitamin E functions as a cellular membrane-bound antioxidant that protects membrane phospholipids from oxidative damage. Results of vitamin E supplementation studies in human liver disease patients have been inconsistent. Vitamins E and C improved fibrosis scores in patients with nonalcoholic steatohepatitis (Harrison et al, 2003). Results of animal studies have also been mixed, perhaps due study design issues. However, in a study using a rat model of steatocholestasis, subcutaneous vitamin E provided significant protection against bile acid-induced hepatic injury, including a reduction in the release of apoptosis-inducing factor. Bile acid-induced necrotic hepatocyte injury was responsive to vitamin E therapy (Soden et al, 2007). Bedlington terriers with copper-associated hepatopathy have oxidative damage in their mitochondria and reduced mitochondrial vitamin E concentrations (Sokol et al, 1994). Vitamin E has a protective effect in the liver from copper-related oxidant damage and bile acids (Gaetke and Chow, 2003; Sokol et al, 1998). In a study using 20 dogs with naturally occurring chronic hepatitis fed a vitamin E-supplemented food for three months, increases in serum and hepatic vitamin E concentrations were accompanied by an increased hepatic reduced glutathione to oxidized glutathione (GSH: GSSG) ratio, suggesting an improved hepatic redox status. However, no changes in clinical or histologic scores were noted (Twedt et al, 2003).

Vitamin C is an important soluble intracellular antioxidant that helps convert oxidized vitamin E back to its reduced, active form. Vitamin C is also necessary for the synthesis of L-carnitine, which is important for transport of long-chain fatty acids across the mitochondrial membrane. People with liver disease often have low hepatic vitamin C concentrations, in part because human beings are unable to synthesize vitamin C, unlike dogs and cats. Although vitamin C supplementation may be beneficial in treating liver disease, supplementation with excessive amounts of vitamin C may be deleterious in patients with increased hepatic copper or iron concentrations.

No specific dosages of vitamins E and C have been documented to be safe and effective for dogs with liver disease. However, 50 to 400 IU vitamin E/day and 500 to 1,000 mg vitamin C given per os daily have been recommended as supplements for dogs with inflammatory liver disease (Rolfe and Twedt, 1995).

Alkenals (malondialdehyde and 4-hydroxyalkenals) in blood or tissues indicate lipid peroxidation, which may be a result of in vivo oxidative reactions. Alkenals are sometimes measured to determine the effectiveness of antioxidant interventions. Although dietary levels of antioxidant vitamins needed to reduce serum alkenal levels in dogs and cats with liver disease have not been established, a study found that food levels of 445 and 540 IU of vitamin E/kg (as fed basis) were necessary to reduce serum alkenal concentrations in apparently healthy dogs and cats, respectively (Jewell et al, 2000). Until more specific data are available, foods for canine and feline liver patients should provide at least 400 and 500 IU/kg DM, respectively.

Vitamin C is important for regenerating oxidized vitamin E. Foods for canine liver disease patients should contain at least 100 mg vitamin C/kg DM; foods for feline liver disease patients should contain 100 to 200 mg vitamin C/kg DM. This recommendation is based on the vitamin E levels in foods for dogs and cats with liver disease and data that show vitamin C regenerates vitamin E at about a 1:1 molar ratio (Barclay et al, 1985). Also, this range is not a risk for urinary oxalate production (Yu and Gross, 2005).

The earlier antioxidants are used to manage the oxidative damage that accompanies acute and chronic hepatobiliary disease, the more likely they are to be effective.

L-Carnitine

Food and hepatic biosynthesis are the primary sources of L-carnitine for animals. L-carnitine transports long-chain fatty acids across the inner mitochondrial membrane into the mitochondrial matrix for β-oxidation. L-carnitine also removes potentially toxic acyl groups from cells and equilibrates ratios of free CoA/acetyl-CoA between the mitochondria and cytoplasm.

Obesity is a risk factor for feline hepatic lipidosis; several studies have investigated the relationship between L-carnitine, weight loss in obese cats and feline hepatic lipidosis. Mean concentrations of L-carnitine in plasma, liver and skeletal muscle were significantly greater in cats with idiopathic hepatic lipidosis than in control cats (Jacobs et al, 1990). These findings suggest that systemic L-carnitine deficiency does not appear to contribute to the pathogenesis of feline idiopathic hepatic lipidosis. However, other studies have shown that feline foods supplemented with L-carnitine benefit obese cats undergoing rapid weight loss. Dietary L-carnitine supplementation protected obese cats from hepatic lipid accumulation during caloric restriction and rapid weight loss (Armstrong et al, 1992). Foods supplemented with L-carnitine can safely facilitate rapid weight loss in obese cats (Center et al, 1997). Based on these studies, the use of L-carnitine supplements or L-carnitine supplemented foods seems appropriate for obese cats undergoing weight reduction.

Besides being of value in preventing hepatic lipidosis, L-carnitine supplementation may also benefit cats with hepatic lipidosis (Center, 1996c). One author has recommended a dose of 250 to 500 mg L-carnitine/day for cats with hepatic lipidosis (Center, 1996c). Others have found that lower doses

(7 to 14 mg/kg body weight) also benefit weight loss, obesity prevention and hepatic lipidosis (Blanchard, 1998). Foods for cats with hepatic lipidosis should provide at least 0.02% DM L-carnitine.

Other Nutritional Factors

Depending on the type of hepatobiliary disease, some of the following nutritional factors may also be important.

Carbohydrate

Patients with clinical evidence of HE should receive adequate carbohydrate intake. Studies suggest that feeding foods with a high carbohydrate component is advantageous (Zieve and Zieve, 1987). Providing at least 30 to 50% of dietary calories in the form of easily digested, complex digestible carbohydrate (e.g., corn, rice, wheat, barley) may help avert encephalopathic clinical signs (Center, 1996b). Thus, the recommendations for DM digestible carbohydrates in foods for dogs and cats with liver disease are 45 to 55% and 30 to 40%, respectively.

Fiber

Foods with increased dietary fiber levels may benefit patients with hepatobiliary disease. Dietary fiber reduces the availability and production of nitrogenous wastes in the GI tract. Although highly digestible foods were previously advocated to maximize digestion and absorption and reduce colonic residues, considered a major source of encephalopathic toxins, this practice is currently not recommended. Increased amounts of fermentable fiber encourage nitrogen fixation by enteric bacteria, resulting in reduced quantities of nitrogenous substances available for absorption. Increased dietary fiber may bind noxious bile acids, endotoxins and other bacterial products. Dietary fiber is also useful in maintaining euglycemia (Chapter 29) and altering the pH of colonic contents. Total dietary fiber levels should be between 3 and 8% and be primarily soluble fiber. However, pet food labels and available product information list fiber content as crude fiber rather than total dietary fiber. Crude fiber analyses do not represent the soluble or fermentable fiber content of foods. Thus, for all practical purposes, this recommendation cannot be readily evaluated. Crude fiber levels in combination with knowledge of the soluble content of the fiber sources obtained from the foods' ingredient lists could provide imprecise guidelines. Commercial and homemade foods can be supplemented with psyllium husk fiber (1 tsp/5 to 10 kg body weight, added to each meal). If loose stools occur, reduce the supplemental fiber by half.

Branched-Chain Amino Acids

The abnormal plasma amino acid profile in patients with hepatic disease can be improved by feeding a protein with an amino acid composition high in BCAA and low in AAA, or by an intravenous amino acid infusion with a similar profile. However, a causal relationship between a deranged BCAA:AAA ratio in plasma and cerebrospinal fluid and HE has yet to be elucidated. Plasma ammonia levels decrease in dogs with HE after administration of BCAA-enriched intravenous infusions (Meyer, 1998a). The same effect could not be reproduced by feeding a BCAA-enriched food vs. an isonitrogenous control food in dogs with HE. This finding may have been due to reduced consumption of the test diet, leading to a severe catabolic state and increased endogenous ammonia production (Meyer, 1998a). The primary positive effect of dietary and intravenous BCAA enrichment may be the normalization of nitrogen balance, rather than a direct effect on neurotransmitter imbalances per se (Meyer, 1998a).

Vitamins

Vitamin deficiencies are common in patients with chronic hepatic disease. Deficient dietary intake and malabsorption are the principal causes of vitamin deficiency, although decreased storage, metabolic defects and increased requirements also may be involved (Marks et al, 1994).

Deficiency of water-soluble vitamins may occur due to inadequate intake, vomiting and urinary losses. Hepatic concentrations of folate, riboflavin, nicotinamide, pantothenic acid, pyridoxine and vitamin B_{12} are decreased in people with cirrhosis (Leevy et al, 1982). Commercial pet foods usually contain sufficient quantities of water-soluble vitamins to meet the needs of most patients with liver disease. Supplementation with water-soluble vitamins is indicated in patients: 1) receiving aggressive diuretic therapy for ascites, 2) with profound polydipsia and polyuria, 3) with prolonged anorexia and 4) eating homemade foods.

Abnormal blood coagulation tests and excessive bleeding reflect impaired hepatic synthesis, activation of clotting factors and/or a consumptive coagulopathy. Vitamin K stores in the liver are limited and can be rapidly depleted when dietary sources are inadequate or lipid (and therefore fat-soluble vitamin) malabsorption is severe. Among other functions, vitamin K catalyzes the activity of several clotting factors and normally is recycled in the healthy liver back to its active form (this step of vitamin K metabolism is sensitive to inhibition by dicumarol).

Vitamin K deficiency may develop in patients with hepatobiliary disease for several reasons. Oral antibiotic therapy may destroy the intestinal microflora that normally synthesize vitamin K. Chronic bile duct obstruction can interfere with enterohepatic circulation of bile acids causing intestinal bile acid deficiency and fat-soluble vitamin (including vitamin K) malabsorption. Inadequate intake of vitamin K may be a component of overall vitamin K deficiency, particularly if the patient has experienced prolonged anorexia (cats with hepatic lipidosis).

Coagulation abnormalities are common in dogs and cats with hepatobiliary disease. In dogs with naturally occurring liver disease, 50 and 75% had an abnormal prothrombin time (PT) and activated partial thromboplastin time (APTT), respectively. More than 90% of dogs had at least one abnormality (Center, 1996; Webster, 2005). At least one coagulation abnormality was present in 82% of cats with liver disease. Prolonged PT was noted in 73% of cats and factor VII activity was below reference range (<60%) in 68% of cats. When classified according to underlying pathogenesis, vitamin K deficiency was the most common abnormality found (11/22). Other abnormalities were less common and included hepatic

Table 68-10. General therapy for patients with hepatobiliary disease.*

Fluid therapy	
Maintain hydration	Give appropriate parenteral fluid therapy
Prevent hypokalemia	Add KCl to maintenance fluids Use potassium-replete food or potassium supplement
Maintain acid-base balance	Avoid alkalosis in patients with hepatic encephalopathy
Prevent or control hypoglycemia	Add dextrose to parenteral fluids as needed
Nutritional support	
Maintain caloric intake	Ensure that daily energy requirement is being met; if not, begin assisted feeding
Provide adequate vitamins and minerals	Add B vitamins to fluids or give as injection Use complete and balanced food
Modify feeding plan to control complications	See specific complications below
Control hepatic encephalopathy	
Modify food and prevent formation and absorption of enteric toxins	Avoid excess dietary protein Use retention enemas q6h containing lactulose or povidone iodine solution Give lactulose orally
Control GI hemorrhage	Treat GI parasites, treat gastric ulcers, avoid drugs that exacerbate GI hemorrhage (e.g., aspirin, glucocorticoids)
Correct metabolic imbalances	See fluid therapy above
Avoid drugs or therapies that exacerbate hepatic encephalopathy	Do not administer sedatives, analgesics, anesthetics, diuretics, stored blood or methionine-containing products
Control seizures	Use appropriate anticonvulsant drugs (e.g., potassium bromide)
Control infection	Give systemic antimicrobials (see below)
Control ascites and edema	Avoid excess dietary sodium chloride Administer diuretics (e.g., furosemide, spironolactone)
Control coagulation defects and anemia	Give vitamin K_1 parenterally Give fresh plasma or blood transfusion as needed
Control GI ulceration	Give H_2 blockers (e.g., ranitidine) or cytoprotective agents (e.g., sucralfate)
Control infection and endotoxemia	Give systemic antibiotics (e.g., penicillin, ampicillin, cephalosporins, aminoglycosides, metronidazole) Give intestinal antibiotics (e.g., neomycin)
Manage cholestasis	Give bile "altering" or choleretic drugs (e.g., ursodiol) Correct extrahepatic bile duct obstruction

*Adapted from Johnson SE, Sherding RG. Diseases of the liver and biliary tract. In: Birchard SJ, Sherding RG, eds. Manual of Small Animal Practice. Philadelphia, PA: WB Saunders Co, 1994; 730.

synthetic failure (3/22), indeterminate (3/22) and disseminated intravascular coagulation (1/22). Increased AP activity was the only biochemical abnormality statistically correlated with coagulation abnormalities (p = 0.23). Cats with marked increases in AP activity were more likely to have coagulation abnormalities than those with only mild increases in AP activity (Lisciandro et al, 1998). Despite the common presence of coagulation test abnormalities, spontaneous hemorrhage in liver disease patients is rare. However, it should be assumed that liver disease patients have a higher than normal risk of bleeding.

At the very least, foods for patients with liver disease should contain the minimum recommended allowance of vitamin K (menadione) for foods for normal adult dogs and cats: 1.63 and 1.0 mg/kg DM, respectively (NRC, 2006). Supplementing foods with active vitamin K (vitamin K_1) is expensive and the vitamin would likely not survive the heat of processing. The water-soluble form of menadione, menadione sodium bisulfite, is much less expensive, is heat stable and is passively absorbed from the small intestine and colon. However, menadione is biologically inactive, as is vitamin K_1, and requires alkylation by gut microorganisms or animal tissues to biologically active menaquinone-4 (NRC, 2006).

FEEDING PLAN

The universal goals for dietary management of hepatobiliary disease are directed at clinical manifestations of the disease rather than the specific cause itself. The goals of nutritional management for hepatobiliary disease include: 1) maintaining normal metabolic processes and homeostasis, 2) avoiding and managing HE, 3) providing substrates to support hepatocellular repair and regeneration, 4) decreasing further oxidative damage to liver tissue and 5) correcting electrolyte disturbances (Blackburn and O'Keefe, 1989; Center, 1998).

The therapeutic goals for patients with HE also include: 1) recognizing and correcting precipitating causes of encephalopathy (e.g., hypokalemic alkalosis), 2) reducing intestinal production and absorption of neurotoxins, with special emphasis on ammonia and 3) finding the balance between providing too much and too little protein, both of which increase ammonia generation.

Dietary therapy is only beneficial when performed in conjunction with proper medical and surgical management of the specific hepatobiliary disease involved. Medical management often includes use of antiinflammatory agents, immunomodu-

Table 68-11. Levels of key nutritional factors in selected commercial veterinary therapeutic foods marketed for canine patients with hepatobiliary disease compared to recommended levels.*

Dry foods	Energy density (kcal/cup)**	Energy density (kcal ME/g)	Protein (%)***	Taurine (%)	Sodium (%)	Copper (mg/kg)	Zinc (mg/kg)	Iron (mg/kg)	Vit. E (IU/kg)	Vit. C (mg/kg)
Recommended levels	**-**	**≥4.0**	**15-20**	**≥0.1**	**0.08-0.25**	**≤5**	**>200**	**80-140**	**≥400**	**≥100**
Hill's Prescription Diet l/d Canine	399	4.4	18.1	0.08	0.22	4.9	301	170	385	116
Medi-Cal Hepatic LS 14	342	na	17.6	na	0.2	na	300	na	na	na
Medi-Cal Vegetarian Formula	317	na	20.9	na	0.4	na	na	na	na	na
Purina Veterinary Diets EN GastroENteric	397	4.2	27.0	na	0.60	na	na	na	577	na
Royal Canin Veterinary Diet Hepatic LS 14	333	4.4	17.6	0.22	0.21	4.4	253	187	725	na

Moist foods	Energy density (kcal/can)**	Energy density (kcal ME/g)	Protein (%)***	Taurine (%)	Sodium (%)	Copper (mg/kg)	Zinc (mg/kg)	Iron (mg/kg)	Vit. E (IU/kg)	Vit. C (mg/kg)
Recommended levels	**-**	**≥4.0**	**15-20**	**≥0.1**	**0.08-0.25**	**≤5**	**>200**	**80-140**	**≥400**	**≥100**
Hill's Prescription Diet l/d Canine	472/13 oz.	4.5	17.6	0.10	0.20	4.2	258	118	693	190
Iams Veterinary Formula Stress/Weight Gain Formula Maximum-Calorie	333/6 oz.	5.8	41.8	0.33	0.24	na	na	na	na	na
Medi-Cal Vegetarian Formula	319/396 g	na	26.4	na	0.5	na	na	na	na	na
Purina Veterinary Diets EN GastroENteric	423/12.5 oz.	4.0	30.5	na	0.37	na	260	na	505	139

Key: ME = metabolizable energy, Vit. E = vitamin E, Vit. C = vitamin C, na = information not available from manufacturer.
*From manufacturers' published information or calculated from manufacturers' published as fed values; all values are on a dry matter basis unless otherwise stated.
**Energy density values are listed on an as fed basis and are useful for determining the amount to feed; cup = 8-oz. measuring cup. To convert to kJ, multiply kcal by 4.184.
***For liver disease patients with signs of hepatic encephalopathy (HE), dietary protein levels should be limited to 10 to 15% dry matter until signs resolve. In these cases, several commercial veterinary therapeutic foods designed for patients with kidney disease that provide less protein than the foods intended for liver disease may be appropriate (Chapter 37). If these foods are used, the patient should be transitioned to the selected food specifically formulated for liver disease after signs of HE have subsided.

lators, nonabsorbable disaccharides and bile "altering" agents (**Table 68-10**). In acute hepatic failure, correction of fluid and electrolyte imbalances and treatment of other complications such as metabolic acidosis, excessive bleeding, hypotension, hypoglycemia, cardiac dysfunction, renal failure, cerebral edema and infections take precedence over nutritional support. Surgical management can include partial or total ligation of congenital PSS, correction of bile duct obstruction or removal of focal liver masses.

Assess and Select the Food

A wide variety of foods are typically used or recommended for patients with hepatic disease (Marks et al, 1994a; Michel, 1995). **Tables 68-11** and **68-12** list the recommended levels of key nutritional factors for canine and feline hepatobiliary disease patients, respectively, and compare them to the key nutritional factor content of selected veterinary therapeutic foods. This information will help the veterinary health care team select the best food for patients with liver disease. Special consideration should be given to young patients with congenital PSS.

Although the total protein content of some veterinary therapeutic foods formulated for patients with liver disease is lower than that of regular commercial pet foods, protein quality and digestibility are usually high. Also, as discussed above, these foods still exceed minimum requirements. Thus, these foods provide adequate protein to support hepatic function and hepatocyte repair and regeneration while avoiding higher protein levels that exacerbate hyperammonemia. However, further short-term protein reduction may be necessary in patients with HE. In these cases, some commercial veterinary therapeutic foods designed for patients with renal disease that provide less protein than the foods intended for liver disease may be appropriate (Chapter 37). If these foods are used, the patient should be transitioned to the selected food specifically formulated for liver disease after signs of HE have subsided (**Tables 68-11** and **68-12**). Lactulose may be considered for patients with HE. **Box 68-4** provides information about lactulose products, their use and their mode of action.

Supplemental treatment should also be considered for dogs with hepatic copper toxicosis. Copper is considered a key nutritional factor for liver disease in dogs and the recommended DM level in foods is less than 5 mg/kg. This level may still provide too much copper for some patients with hepatic copper toxicosis. In these instances, adjunctive use of copper chelating agents should be considered. Copper chelating agents are discussed in **Box 68-3**. **Box 68-5** reviews other cytoprotective

Table 68-12. Levels of key nutritional factors in selected commercial veterinary therapeutic foods marketed for feline patients with hepatobiliary disease, compared to recommended levels.*

Dry foods	Energy density (kcal/cup)**	Energy density (kcal ME/g)	Protein (%)***	Arginine (%)	Taurine (%)	Sodium (%)	Zinc (mg/kg)	Iron (mg/kg)	Vit. E (IU/kg)	Vit. C (mg/kg)
Recommended levels	**–**	**≥4.2**	**30-35**	**1.5-2.0**	**≥0.3**	**0.07-0.30**	**>200**	**80-140**	**≥500**	**100-200**
Hill's Prescription Diet l/d Feline	505	4.5	31.8	1.98	0.53	0.27	305	173	267	109
Medi-Cal Mature Formula	355	na	29.2	na	0.4	0.4	na	na	na	na
Medi-Cal Reduced Protein	440	na	28.1	na	0.4	0.3	na	na	na	na
Medi-Cal Renal LP 21	409	na	24.7	na	0.2	0.2	na	na	na	na
Purina Veterinary Diets EN GastroENteric	572	4.4	56.2	na	0.32	0.64	na	na	232	na
Royal Canin Veterinary Diet Modified Formula	432	4.7	27.1	1.51	0.23	0.23	320	241	380	na

Moist foods	Energy density (kcal/can)**	Energy density (kcal ME/g)	Protein (%)***	Arginine (%)	Taurine (%)	Sodium (%)	Zinc (mg/kg)	Iron (mg/kg)	Vit. E (IU/kg)	Vit. C (mg/kg)
Recommended levels	**–**	**≥4.2**	**30-35**	**1.5-2.0**	**≥0.3**	**0.07-0.30**	**>200**	**80-140**	**≥500**	**100-200**
Hill's Prescription Diet l/d Feline	183/5.5 oz.	4.7	31.6	2.00	0.52	0.20	336	212	836	124
Medi-Cal Mature Formula	205/170 g	na	41.5	na	0.3	0.3	na	na	na	na
Medi-Cal Reduced Protein	265/170 g	na	33.9	na	0.3	0.2	na	na	na	na
Medi-Cal Renal LP	125/85 g pouch	na	29.3	na	0.8	0.6	na	na	na	na
Royal Canin Veterinary Diet Modified Formula	256/170 g 596/396 g	6.1	34.7	2.07	0.28	0.28	208	545	178	na

Key: ME = metabolizable energy, Vit. E = vitamin E, Vit. C = vitamin C, na = information not available from manufacturer.
*From manufacturers' published information or calculated from manufacturers' published as fed values; all values are on a dry matter basis unless otherwise stated.
**Energy density values are listed on an as fed basis and are useful for determining the amount to feed; cup = 8-oz. measuring cup. To convert to kJ, multiply kcal by 4.184.
***For liver disease patients with signs of hepatic encephalopathy (HE), dietary protein levels should be limited to 25 to 30% dry matter until signs resolve. In these cases, several commercial veterinary therapeutic foods designed for patients with kidney disease that provide less protein than the foods intended for liver disease may be appropriate (Chapter 37). If these foods are used, the patient should be transitioned to the selected food specifically formulated for liver disease after signs of HE have subsided.

agents that are sometimes considered for liver disease patients.

Anorectic cats with cholangitis or hepatic lipidosis will need to be fed via assisted-feeding techniques until they resume eating on their own. This dictates the use of nutrient-dense foods with textures intended for assisted feeding (Chapter 25). These patients should be fed a food intended for dietary management of other hepatic diseases after they start eating (**Table 68-12**).

Another criterion for selecting a food that may become increasingly important in the future is evidence-based clinical nutrition. Practitioners should know how to determine risks and benefits of nutritional regimens and counsel pet owners accordingly. Currently, veterinary medical education and continuing education are not always based on rigorous assessment of evidence for or against particular management options. Still, studies have been published to establish the nutritional benefits of certain pet foods. Chapter 2 describes evidence-based clinical nutrition in detail and applies its concepts to various veterinary therapeutic foods.

Assess and Determine the Feeding Method

Sick, anorectic and severely malnourished patients with hepatobiliary disease should be hospitalized to initiate supportive care and assisted-feeding techniques. Early tube feeding via nasogastric or gastrostomy tube remains the cornerstone of therapy for feline patients with hepatic lipidosis and all other anorectic patients with liver disease. Chapter 25 details foods and enteral feeding techniques commonly used in dogs and cats. Patients that are eating enough food to meet their daily energy requirement (DER) can usually be managed at home.

The DER for cats with hepatic lipidosis should be at least the resting energy requirement (RER) for ideal body weight when cats are managed in the hospital and 1.1 to 1.2 x RER when managed at home. The DER of canine liver disease patients managed at home should be approximately 1.2 to 1.4 x RER. Young patients with congenital shunts may be stunted or underweight. DER calculations for these patients should be based on ideal rather than current body weight. These calorie values can be converted to an amount of food to eat by dividing the energy density of the food (as fed basis) by the DER. The as fed energy density (in cups or cans) of foods for liver disease can be found in **Tables 68-11** and **68-12**.

Multiple daily feedings rather than one or two large meals may benefit patients with hepatobiliary disease. Multiple daily meals minimize the release of free fatty acids from adipose tissue, improve digestibility and reduce the quantity of ingesta at any one time that enters the colon where bacterial fermentation

Box 68-4. Adjunctive Lactulose for Patients with Hepatic Encephalopathy.

Administration of lactulose is considered one of the treatments of choice for hepatic encephalopathy (HE). Lactulose is a synthetic disaccharide that is hydrolyzed by colonic bacteria principally to lactic and acetic acids. Lactulose probably exerts its beneficial effects by: 1) increasing intraluminal nitrogen retention by increasing the colonic flora, 2) increasing intestinal transit rate due to its cathartic properties and 3) decreasing ammonia generation from glutamine in the intestinal wall by providing acetic acid as an alternative energy source. The dosage required to achieve these goals varies greatly, with a range of 2.5 to 25 ml, three times daily for dogs and 1.0 to 3.0 ml, three times daily for cats. The dosage should be titrated to produce a "porridge-like" stool and should be reduced if watery diarrhea develops.

Lactulose also is highly effective when added to water (30% lactulose and 70% water) and given as a retention enema. Approximately 20 to 30 ml/kg body weight are infused and retained in the colon for 20 to 30 minutes before evacuation. Lactulose requires intestinal bacteria for activation. Although neomycin and other nonabsorbable antibiotics are used in the treatment of HE in people, their use is limited to cases that do not respond to lactulose alone. Furthermore, patients should be monitored carefully. Moreover, evidence of their effectiveness in the treatment of dogs and cats with HE is lacking.

The Bibliography for **Box 68-4** can be found at www.markmorris.org.

occurs. Studies involving people with hepatic failure have shown that nitrogen balance can be improved if the food is divided into small, frequent meals, including a snack at bedtime (Swart et al, 1989). Nauseated patients may also better tolerate multiple small meals.

Appetite stimulants and force feeding moist food can be used to encourage caloric intake, but these strategies often fail to ensure enough food is consumed to meet the patient's nutrient requirements and typically frustrate the owner. Appetite stimulants such as anabolic steroids and benzodiazepine derivatives are not recommended and should be used cautiously in patients with hepatic disease, because of the potential for hepatotoxicity and, benzodiazepines may possibly be involved in the pathogenesis of HE (Wilson, 1990; Meyer, 1998).

Many patients may develop learned aversion to the foods they are offered if GI disturbances accompany liver disease. This is the classic scenario in cats with hepatic lipidosis. Cats that refuse to eat a food they associate with nausea may continue to avoid that food even after a complete recovery. Therefore, tube feeding should be started in cats immediately after a diagnosis of hepatic lipidosis is made. Such an approach is preferred to offering several commercial foods and possibly having the cat develop an aversion to them. The prognosis for hepatic lipidosis is influenced largely by the ability of the veterinarian and owner to aggressively meet the nutrient requirements of the cat via enteral feeding.

Managing cats with hepatic lipidosis that are starved or severely malnourished can be complicated by a refeeding syndrome, a condition that results in metabolic electrolyte disturbances that can lead to neurologic, pulmonary, cardiac, neuromuscular and hematologic complications. Cats with hepatic lipidosis often have hypophosphatemia and hypokalemia from low food intake, decreased intestinal absorption or increased renal loss. With the introduction of food and a sudden shift to carbohydrate metabolism, stimulation of insulin secretion promotes intracellular uptake of phosphorus, potassium, magnesium, water and glucose and further lowers serum electrolyte levels within 12 to 72 hours after feeding. Hypophosphatemia can result in muscle weakness, hemolytic anemia, leukocyte dysfunction, platelet dysfunction and decreased tissue oxygenation as a result of decreased levels of 2,3,-diphosphoglycerate. Electrolyte abnormalities should be corrected before feeding hepatic lipidosis patients. Approximately one-fourth of the patient's caloric needs should be provided by tube feeding on Day 1, then the amount should be gradually increased to provide the caloric need within the first week of feeding (Justin and Hohenhaus, 1995; Center et al, 1993).

REASSESSMENT

The owner and veterinarian should monitor the appetite, body weight and condition of the patient, while observing the frequency and severity of GI disturbances (i.e., vomiting, diarrhea), icterus and neurobehavioral signs. One of the most important clinical findings is improvement in the patient's attitude and activity level. This finding is highly correlated with nutritional success. Serial laboratory evaluations (every few days to weeks) of serum liver enzyme activity, bile acids and potassium and blood ammonia concentrations are useful. Serial hepatic biopsy specimens (i.e., every four to six months) can be evaluated for hepatic copper concentrations and assessed for inflammatory hepatopathies. Body weight, abdominal configuration and ultrasonography can be used to monitor patients with ascites.

Assisted-feeding tubes for cats with hepatic lipidosis and/or cholangitis can often be removed after several weeks to months. Enteral tubes are usually removed after the cat has shown clinical improvement and has begun eating two-thirds to three-fourths of its normal DER on its own. Many of these patients can be fed typical adult maintenance-type foods after hepatobiliary disease is resolved. These include patients that have recovered from an acute hepatic insult or hepatic lipidosis and patients that have undergone successful (partial or total) closure of PSS.

Box 68-5. Hepatocytoprotective Agents Considered for Use in Dogs and Cats with Hepatobiliary Disease.

In liver disease, numerous drugs and vitamins could be considered cytoprotective including copper chelators and vitamins E and C. Other cytoprotective agents, such as s-adenosylmethionine (SAMe) and silymarin, are being evaluated for use in dogs and cats with liver disease. Both are reviewed below. Hopefully, in the future, well-designed clinical trials using these and other cytoprotective agents in canine and feline liver disease patients will provide even more evidence regarding their efficacy.

S-ADENOSYLMETHIONINE

The naturally occurring molecule SAMe is synthesized in all living cells, is essential in intermediary metabolism and has hepatoprotective and antioxidant properties. SAMe is produced from the amino acid methionine and subsequently initiates one of three metabolic pathways: 1) The transmethylation pathway is essential in phospholipid synthesis, which is important in membrane structure, fluidity and function. Most (85%) of the SAMe generated, is used in this pathway. 2) The trans-sulfuration pathway generates sulfur-containing compounds, such as glutathione, which participates in many metabolic processes and plays a critical role in cellular detoxification mechanisms. Depletion of glutathione can indirectly cause toxic effects in hepatocytes by increasing oxidative stress. 3) The aminopropylation pathway yields products that have antiinflammatory effects and polyamines important in DNA and protein synthesis.

The liver normally produces abundant SAMe, but evidence also suggests conversion from methionine to SAMe is hindered in liver disease and results in the depletion of glutathione concentration. Orally administered SAMe (but not oral glutathione) increases intracellular glutathione levels in hepatocytes and prevents glutathione depletion when the liver is exposed to toxic substances. Thus, SAMe, in part, acts as an antioxidant by replenishing glutathione stores. Preliminary studies suggest that SAMe supplementation increases hepatic glutathione concentrations in normal cats and prevents glutathione depletion in dogs with steroid-induced hepatopathy. SAMe treatment following acetaminophen administration prevented hepatic glutathione depletion.

SILYMARIN

Silymarin, a flavonolignan from "milk thistle" (*Silybum marianum*), has been used for centuries in human patients with liver disease. Silymarin represents a group of several closely related flavonoids and thus has antioxidant properties. They include silybin, isosilybin, silydianin and silychristin. Among them, silybin is the most active and most commonly used. Silymarin also has antiinflammatory and antifibrotic qualities. In addition, it can increase hepatocyte protein synthesis and accelerate hepatocellular regeneration via increased gene transcription and translation and enhanced DNA synthesis. Silymarin can modulate hepatocyte transport, which is important in its ability to promote choleresis.

Studies in human patients with a wide variety of liver diseases have resulted in conflicting results, probably because of the broad issue of study design problems. As work continues to determine the value of silymarin in the management of human liver disease, better studies will likely bring more cohesive results. However, silymarin has been used successfully in the management of intoxications with acetaminophen and the mushroom toxin phalloidin, both of which exert toxic effects by oxidation. Silymarin appears to be protective against these toxins, which leaves little doubt about its potential therapeutic benefit.

The hepatocytoprotective effects of silymarin (and silybin, an isomer of silymarin) have been shown in a number of in vitro studies as well as studies in animals, including dogs, with induced liver damage. The results have been promising. Studies in dogs with carbon tetrachloride toxicity and dogs with phalloidin toxicity showed that silymarin was protective.

Silymarin, thus far, has been shown to be safe. No serious side effects have been noted in human or animal studies. However, because in vitro studies have shown silymarin to inhibit cytochrome P450 enzyme activities, in the event of concurrent drug therapy, potential adverse interactions should be considered. Unfortunately, the purity of the various commercial products and the ideal therapeutic dose are unknown. Suggested doses for dogs and cats are extrapolated from research in other species.

The Bibliography for **Box 68-5** can be found at www.markmorris.org.

Vomiting is often a problem in patients with hepatobiliary disease, especially cats with hepatic lipidosis or HE. Small frequent meals, continuous tube feeding and antiemetics may be helpful. More aggressive medical treatment of HE may also be needed, such as the use of lactulose.

ACKNOWLEDGMENTS

The authors and editors acknowledge the contributions of Drs. Deborah J. Davenport and Donna S. Dimski in the previous edition of Small Animal Clinical Nutrition.

REFERENCES

The references for **Chapter 68** can be found at www.markmorris.org.

CASE 68-1

Intermittent Vomiting in a Miniature Schnauzer

Deborah J. Davenport, DVM, MS, Dipl. ACVIM (Internal Medicine)
Hill's Science and Technology Center
Topeka, Kansas, USA

Patient Assessment

A three-and-one-half-year-old, neutered female miniature schnauzer was examined for a two-year course of intermittent vomiting. The vomitus rarely contained food and was usually described as a yellow or clear fluid. No diarrhea had been noted. The owners reported that the dog became depressed and lethargic during these vomiting episodes. Antiemetic treatment by another veterinarian had partially controlled the vomiting. Laboratory evaluation, abdominal radiographs and gastrointestinal (GI) contrast radiography four and six months before admission revealed no abnormalities.

Physical examination revealed a thin, nervous dog (body condition score [BCS] 1/5; body weight 7.1 kg). No other abnormalities were noted (**Figure 1**).

A complete blood count revealed erythrocyte microcytosis (i.e., decreased mean corpuscular volume) without hypochromia or anemia. Abnormal results of a serum biochemistry profile included a low serum urea nitrogen level (7 mg/dl, normal 10 to 25 mg/dl), hypoproteinemia (total protein 5.9 g/dl, normal 6.0 to 7.2 g/dl), hypoalbuminemia (2.4 g/dl, normal 3.0 to 4.5 g/dl) and mildly increased alkaline phosphatase activity (125 IU/l, normal 10 to 75 IU/l). Bilirubinuria and many ammonium biurate crystals were found on urinalysis. The stomach appeared cranially displaced radiographically, which suggested a small liver.

The clinical, laboratory and radiographic changes suggested the presence of a portosystemic shunt. Bile acids were elevated (18.6 µmol/l [fasting], 246.1 µmol/l [two hours postprandial]) and an ammonia tolerance test demonstrated elevated baseline and challenge blood ammonia levels.

Abdominal ultrasound demonstrated a small liver and a single large shunt between the portal system and the caudal vena cava external to the liver (**Figure 2**). The final diagnosis was a portocaval shunt with intermittent episodes of hepatic encephalopathy.

Surgical attenuation of the shunt was recommended based on detectable hepatic portal blood flow and the extrahepatic location of the portocaval anastomosis. At the owners' request, the procedure was scheduled for three weeks later.

Assess the Food and Feeding Method

Several dietary changes had been made over the past two years in an effort to control the intermittent vomiting. The most recent food was a commercial dry veterinary therapeutic food for GI problems (Prescription Diet i/d Canine[a]). This food was offered in multiple small meals throughout the day.

Questions

1. What are the key nutritional factors to consider for this dog during the next three weeks?
2. Outline a treatment and feeding plan for this patient before surgery.

Answers and Discussion

1. Numerous key nutritional factors should be considered for patients with portosystemic shunts (**Table 68-8**). Providing adequate daily energy intake is the cornerstone of successful medical management of dogs with hepatobiliary disease, especially underweight animals such as this patient. With respect to protein, the goal is to provide adequate dietary protein to support hepatic regeneration while avoiding excess that might contribute to hepatic encephalopathy. The amount of protein needed by patients with portosystemic vascular shunts has been roughly estimated from a study in dogs with surgically created shunts. This study showed that ingestion of 2.11 g crude protein/kg body weight/day with an 80% or greater availability is adequate to maintain body protein reserves without producing hepatic encephalopathy. The protein should be high quality (i.e., high biologic value) and easily assimilated. Feeding a food with a high carbohydrate to protein component was shown to be advantageous to dogs with experimentally created shunts.
2. A commercial or homemade food that avoids excess dietary protein while providing adequate non-protein calories from fat and carbohydrate is recommended. Foods formulated for renal failure and liver patients generally meet these criteria. The daily energy requirement (DER) should be initially calculated at 1.2 to 1.4 x resting energy requirement (RER) for the estimated ideal body weight (10 kg). Administration of nonabsorbable disaccharides (e.g., lactulose) is also recommended in patients with hepatic encephalopathy. Colonic bacteria hydrolyze lactulose to lactic and acetic acids. Lactulose seems beneficial for several reasons. It: 1) lowers colonic pH with subsequent trapping of ammonium ions, 2) inhibits ammonia generation by colonic bacteria and 3) increases intestinal transit rate via cathartic properties. Neomycin and metronidazole can also be used to decrease ammonia production by inhibiting intestinal bacteria.

Progress Notes

The food was changed to a commercial dry veterinary therapeutic product (Prescription Diet k/d Canine[a]) that contained reduced levels of high quality and easily digested protein while providing a good source of non-protein calories (14.5% dry matter [DM] protein, 19.0% DM fat, 61.1% DM digestible carbohydrate). DER was calculated to be 1.2 x RER for an estimated optimal body weight of 10 kg (DER = 440 kcal [1.84 MJ]). The food was to be offered in at least three separate meals throughout the day. Additional therapy consisted of oral lactulose syrup[b] (10 ml, three times daily).

Three weeks later, the dog had gained 1.2 kg body weight. The owners reported a marked decrease in the number of vomiting episodes and periods of lethargy and depression. No new physical findings were noted. The hypoproteinemia, hypoalbuminemia and ammonium biurate crystalluria persisted. Results of clotting studies done before surgery were normal. During surgery, an anastomotic vessel was easily visualized at the level of the right kidney. This vessel was partially ligated. The dog was released from the hospital five days later with instructions for the owners to continue feeding the veterinary therapeutic food and administering lactulose, as described before surgery.

The dog was reassessed one month later. Body weight had increased to 8.6 kg, the BCS was 2/5 and the owners reported no episodes of malaise or vomiting. The serum urea nitrogen, total protein and albumin concentrations were normal, and ammonium biurate crystals were absent from the urine. The liver size was increased radiographically. Because of the apparent return of normal hepatic function and size, the owners were instructed to change the food to a regular adult maintenance product (25% DM protein, 15.4% DM fat, 53.3% DM digestible carbohydrate) and discontinue the lactulose. The food dosage was continued at 1.2 x RER (440 kcal [1.84 MJ]).

Five months later the dog was examined again. Body weight was 10 kg with a BCS of 3/5. The owners reported that the higher protein food had not precipitated any clinical signs. No changes in foods or feeding methods were recommended.

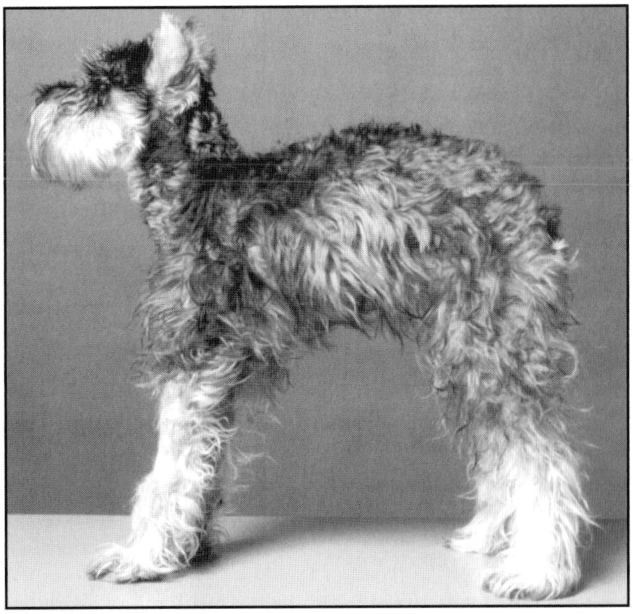

Figure 1. A three-and-one-half-year-old, neutered female miniature schnauzer with chief complaints of intermittent vomiting, depression and lethargy with weight loss and poor body condition.

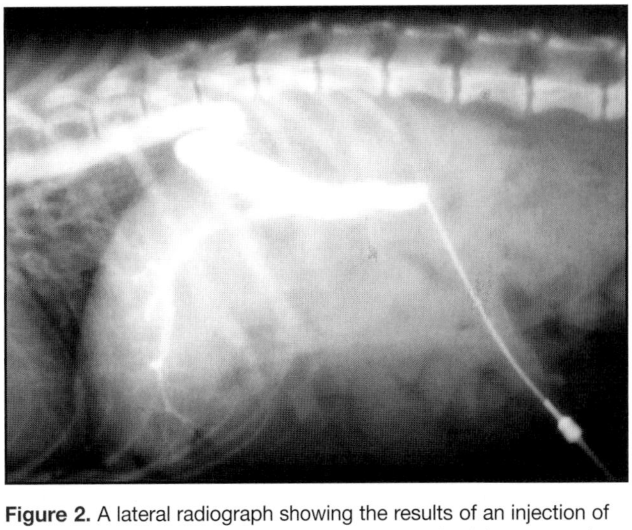

Figure 2. A lateral radiograph showing the results of an injection of positive-contrast medium into the mesenteric vein. A large vascular shunt is communicating from the portal vasculature to the caudal vena cava.

Endnotes

a. Hill's Pet Nutrition, Inc., Topeka, KS, USA.

b. Cholac. Alra Laboratories, Gurnee, IL, USA.

Bibliography

Center SA. Hepatic vascular diseases. In: Guilford WG, Center SA, Strombeck DR, et al, eds. Strombeck's Small Animal Gastroenterology, 3rd ed. Philadelphia, PA: WB Saunders Co, 1996; 802-846.

Laflamme DP, Allen SW, Huber TL. Apparent dietary protein requirement of dogs with portosystemic shunt. American Journal of Veterinary Research 1993; 554: 719-723.

CASE 68-2

Vomiting in a Miniature Poodle

Philip Roudebush, DVM, Dipl. ACVIM (Small Animal Internal Medicine)
Hill's Scientific Affairs
Topeka, Kansas, USA

Patient Assessment

A seven-year-old male miniature poodle was examined for lethargy, excessive panting, elevated liver enzyme activity and intermittent vomiting of six weeks' duration. The vomitus was usually yellow foam or partially digested food. Elevated liver enzyme activity was noted on laboratory work obtained by the referring veterinarian (**Table 1**, Days 0 and 12). A two-week course of oral amoxicillin failed to improve the patient's problems. The dog received a single 2-mg intramuscular injection of triamcinolone[a] for generalized pruritus. The lethargy, panting and vomiting were first noted shortly thereafter.

Physical examination revealed a bright, alert dog that weighed 5 kg, appeared slightly overweight (body condition score [BCS] 4/5) and panted continuously. Other findings included a few subcutaneous lipomas, mild periodontal disease, hepatomegaly, bilateral lenticular sclerosis, right patellar luxation and no evidence of testicles in the scrotum. The owners were given the dog as a young puppy and denied that it had been castrated.

Evaluation of these problems included a complete blood count (mild leukocytosis), heartworm check (negative), serum biochemistry profile (normal except for elevated liver enzyme activity [**Table 1**, Day 19]), urinalysis (normal), fecal flotation (hookworms) and abdominal radiographs. Survey abdominal radiographs revealed an extremely enlarged liver that displaced the axis of the stomach dorsocaudally and displaced the small bowel caudally. Ultrasound demonstrated a segment of terminal jejunum or ileum with a thickened bowel wall. Retained testicles were also identified. Prothrombin and activated partial thromboplastin times were normal. Examination of an ultrasound-guided fine-needle aspirate of the liver revealed vacuolar changes in hepatocytes consistent with steroid hepatopathy. An anthelmintic was administered for the hookworm infection.

The dog was reexamined one week later for an ACTH response test with determination of resting and post-ACTH plasma cortisol concentrations. An exploratory celiotomy was also planned to obtain liver and intestinal biopsy specimens and remove the retained testicles.

The resting cortisol concentration was subnormal and failed to increase after intramuscular administration of ACTH gel (**Table 1**, Day 19). During surgery, a diffusely enlarged, pale liver with rounded margins was noted; biopsy specimens were obtained from the liver, distal small intestine and colon; the retained testicles were identified and removed. Histopathologic examination of these specimens revealed diffuse testicular atrophy, normal intestinal structure except for mild dilatation of lacteals and multifocal hepatic vacuolar change consistent with steroid hepatopathy.

The tentative diagnosis was secondary hypoadrenocorticism and hepatopathy associated with parenteral administration of corticosteroids.

Assess the Food and Feeding Method

The dog was normally fed a combination of commercial grocery brand moist food mixed with broiled chicken and cottage cheese. The commercial food and table food were mixed in approximately a 50:50 ratio. An unspecified amount of this mixture was offered twice daily. The dog preferred to drink either ice water or iced tea.

Questions

1. What are the key nutritional factors to consider for this patient?
2. Outline a feeding plan for this dog including food and feeding method.
3. What other therapy should be considered?
4. How should this dog be monitored for response to therapy?

Answers and Discussion

1. The key nutritional factors for patients with mild to moderate hepatic disease that is expected to be self-limiting are listed in **Table 68-8**. The food should contain appropriate amounts of these key nutrients and other essential nutrients based on the patient's current lifestage. Dramatic changes are not necessary in the nutrient levels of food for patients with mild to moderate hepatic disease and no evidence of hepatic failure, portosystemic vascular shunts, ascites or hepatic encephalopathy.
2. A commercial dog food formulated for older dogs (i.e., senior or geriatric food) would be appropriate for this patient. Such a food would be more balanced and avoid the probable excess protein and fat provided by the current diet of 50% moist commercial grocery brand food and 50% chicken and cottage cheese. The daily energy requirement (DER) should be calculated to maintain current body weight until the liver disease has resolved. The food and water should be offered in multiple small meals throughout

Table 1. Laboratory data from a miniature poodle with steroid hepatopathy.

Parameters	Day 0	Day 12	Day 19	Day 56	Day 110	Day 142	Day 214	Reference values
Alkaline phosphatase (IU/l)	4,990	4,960	3,080	>400	313	106	26	10-80
Alanine aminotransferase (IU/l)	1,380	1,600	1,450	>500	184	236	45	10-70
Cortisol, resting (µg/dl)	na	na	0.3	<1.0	1.8	1.4	12.3	0.5-4.0
Cortisol, post-ACTH (µg/dl)	na	na	0.5	<1.0	1.9	1.7	17.5	8.0-20.0

Key: na = information not available.

the day to help control nausea and vomiting.

3. Physiologic doses of oral hydrocortisone may be given to alleviate glucocorticoid deficiency (and control clinical signs such as lethargy and vomiting) while not exacerbating the liver disease. The patient should also avoid stressful environmental situations because it cannot respond normally to these events.
4. Serum liver enzyme activity and plasma cortisol concentrations (resting and post-ACTH) should be monitored every two months until they return to normal. The clinical signs of lethargy, vomiting and hepatomegaly should resolve as biochemical parameters improve.

Progress Notes

The dog made an uneventful recovery from surgery and was discharged to the owners' care three days later. Other than the single triamcinolone injection, no other sources of exogenous corticosteroids were identified.

In the hospital, the dog began eating a moist specialty brand dog food formulated for senior dogs (Science Diet Canine Senior[b]). This food was nutritionally balanced compared with the combination of commercial dog food, chicken and cottage cheese offered at home. The DER was estimated to be 1.2 to 1.4 x resting energy requirement (RER) for an ideal weight of 4.5 kg (250 to 290 kcal [1.0 to 1.2 MJ]; two-thirds to three-fourths can daily). The food was offered in small frequent meals throughout the day. The owners were also instructed to add water to the food or warm the food in a microwave oven if it was necessary to encourage acceptance.

No other treatment was given because the secondary hypoadrenocorticism and steroid hepatopathy were expected to resolve as the effects of the injectable triamcinolone decreased over the next several months. Recheck examinations over the next six months documented clinical improvement and gradual reduction in liver enzyme activity (**Table 1**, Days 56 to 214). Plasma cortisol concentrations returned to near normal by Day 214. The dog remained normal for the next three years before it died from complications of immune-mediated thrombocytopenia.

Endnotes

a. Vetalog Parenteral. Solvay Animal Health, Mendota Heights, MN, USA.
b. Hill's Pet Nutrition, Inc., Topeka, KS, USA. This food is currently available as Science Diet Mature Adult 7+ Canine.

Bibliography

Center SA. Vacuolar hepatopathy/glucocorticoid hepatopathy. In: Guilford WG, Center SA, Strombeck DR, et al, eds. Strombeck's Small Animal Gastroenterology, 3rd ed. Philadelphia, PA: WB Saunders Co, 1996; 782-788.

CASE 68-3

Anorexia and Icterus in a Domestic Shorthair Cat

Rebecca L. Remillard, PhD, DVM, Dipl. ACVN
MSPCA Angell Animal Medical Center
Boston, Massachusetts, USA

Patient Assessment

A six-year-old neutered female domestic shorthair cat was referred for a one-month history of weight loss and a week-long history of vomiting, icterus and anorexia. The cat was kept exclusively indoors. The family had relocated to the state two months before the cat was presented to the referring veterinarian. The referring veterinarian treated the cat with intravenous fluids.

Physical examination revealed a depressed, cachectic cat (body weight 3.1 kg, body condition score [BCS] 1/5). The cat's mucous membranes, sclera, inner pinnae, lips and nose were icteric. Mild hepatomegaly was detected by abdominal palpation. Dehydration (approximately 5%) was evident based on abnormal skin turgor and tacky mucous membranes.

Results of a complete blood count were consistent with a stress leukogram and mild microcytic normochromic anemia. Results of a serum biochemistry profile included hyperbilirubinemia, elevated liver enzyme activities, mild hyperglycemia, hypoproteinemia, hypoalbuminemia and mild hypokalemia (**Table 1**). Urinalysis results were normal except for marked bilirubinuria. A blood coagulation profile revealed slightly prolonged prothrombin time (13.4 seconds, normal 8.5 to 10.5 seconds). Vitamin K_1 therapy was started (phytonadione, 5 mg/kg body weight, subcutaneously, q12h).

Ultrasonographic evaluation of the liver revealed hepatomegaly with a diffuse increase in echogenicity and no evidence of intrahepatic masses. Hepatic tissue was obtained by ultrasonographic-guided needle biopsy. The hepatic tissue was brown, soft and floated in 10% formalin. Cytologic evaluation revealed an increased number of bile casts, increased amount of bilirubin within hepatocytes and all hepatocytes contained vacuoles filled with lipid. These findings were interpreted as hepatocyte lipid accumulation and cholestasis. Bacterial culture of a portion of the liver biopsy specimen was negative. A diagnosis of feline hepatic lipidosis was made.

Assess the Food and Feeding Method

Historically, since the cat was neutered at nine months of age, it had been slightly overweight (BCS 4/5). Therefore, for several years the cat had been fed a dry commercial specialty brand food with a reduced caloric density (Science Diet Feline Maintenance Light[a]). The food was offered free choice. The exact amount of food consumed by the cat over the last month was unknown but markedly less than normal. A 4-lb bag of food usually lasted a month, but the owners had not purchased a new bag within the last two months. During the past week, the referring veterinarian had been giving vitamin-B supplements and force-feeding an unknown amount of a commercial recovery food (Prescription Diet a/d Canine/Feline[a]) per os. The cat was still vomiting three to four times per day.

Questions

1. Outline an appropriate fluid and feeding plan (food, amount and method of administration) for this cat.
2. What other medical therapy may be appropriate for cats with idiopathic hepatic lipidosis?
3. How should the patient's response to therapy be monitored?

Answers and Discussion

1. Severe dehydration and electrolyte and acid-base disturbances should be corrected with appropriate parenteral fluid therapy before initiating the feeding plan. The single most effective means of treating feline patients with hepatic lipidosis is providing fluid and nutritional support with assisted feeding. This is most easily accomplished using liquid foods administered through a nasoesophageal tube or homogenized/blended foods administered by esophagostomy or gastrostomy tube (Chapter 25). These tubes are well tolerated by cats and help ensure adequate caloric intake and, if necessary, owners can continue feeding the cat at home. A variety of commercial liquid and blended enteral products have been used successfully in patients with hepatic lipidosis.

   Energy requirements, and therefore the daily amount of food, should be calculated to meet the resting energy requirement (RER) for the cat's current body weight. The amount of food should be divided into multiple small feedings (four to six meals daily). Most cats can initially tolerate at least 30-ml bolus feedings and can be given 50- to 80-ml meals after a few days of refeeding. However, vomiting cats, especially those that have not eaten for weeks, may not tolerate bolus feedings initially, but will tolerate continuous rate infusion of a liquid food.

   Vitamin K_1 therapy should be used in cats with abnormal coagulation tests. Some clinical investigators have advocated L-carnitine supplementation for improving recovery based on results in experimental models of feline hepatic lipidosis. At the present time there are no clinical studies demonstrating the effectiveness of L-carnitine supplementation in cats with naturally occurring disease.
2. Vomiting is a common complication of enteral feeding in cats and can be managed with antiemetic drugs given 15 to 30 minutes before each feeding. Cats with hepatic lipidosis rarely develop hepatic encephalopathy. If they do, lactulose, enemas and oral antibiotics may also be needed. Cats that do not eat voluntarily may be given appetite stimulants.
3. The amount of food given each day should be carefully recorded to ensure that an appropriate caloric intake is being achieved. Complications of tube feeding should be monitored. These include epiphora (nasoesophageal tubes), displacement of the tube, vomiting, diarrhea and infection at the site of tube placement. Decreasing icterus, serum bilirubin concentrations, liver enzyme activities and improved activity and mental attitude mark clinical improvement in the hospital. Long-term weight gain, improved body condition and a return of normal appetite indicate improvement. In general, one to three weeks of assisted feeding are necessary, but some patients may require three to seven months of tube feeding. Many patients can be managed at home until normal appetite returns. At home, food and water should be readily available and offered before each tube feeding. Decreasing the amount fed or discontinuing the number of daily tube feedings is recommended when the cat begins to show interest in food again. The feeding tube may be removed when the cat voluntarily consumes an amount equal to its RER for two to three consecutive days.

Progress Notes

An intravenous catheter and nasoesophageal tube were placed the day of hospital admission. The cat was given fluid and nutritional therapy concurrently with vitamin K_1 therapy as diagnostic procedures were performed. Because the cat was still vomiting three to four times per day, a liquid food (CliniCare Feline[b] containing 1 kcal [4.2 kJ]/ml) was given by continuous rate infusion. The cat's RER was 163 kcal (682 kJ)/day [$70(3.1)^{0.75}$]. Fluid requirements were 200 ml/day (3.1 x 60 ml/kg body weight + 5% + ongoing losses). Therefore, the cat initially received 163 ml of liquid food via nasoesophageal tube and 37 ml of Plasmalyte A (with 30 mEq KCl/l), intravenously per day. Dehydration and hypokalemia were corrected, and vomiting ceased by Day 2 of hospitalization. The cat tolerated the continuous rate infusion given by nasoesophageal tube, and its prothrombin time returned to within normal limits after four treatments with vitamin K_1.

A gastrostomy tube (G-tube) was placed on Day 3 of hospitalization. Twelve hours after the tube was placed, the cat began receiving 30-ml bolus feedings of a blended commercial veterinary recovery food (Prescription Diet a/d Canine/Feline) (2 cans plus 50 ml water = 1 kcal/ml). The cat had no problems with the G-tube or the blended food and was discharged to the owners' care on Day 4 with instructions to offer the cat food (Science Diet Feline Maintenance[a]) first and, if the cat did not voluntarily eat, to then feed 55 ml of the blended recovery food followed by a 12-ml water flush, three times daily. This feeding regimen provided the cat with 165 kcal (690 kJ) and 200 ml of water daily.

The owners returned with the cat 11 days later. The G-tube was in place, body weight was 3.3 kg and the cat was more alert with less intense icterus. A complete blood count showed no evidence of anemia. The serum biochemistry profile revealed normoglycemia, increased serum total protein and albumin concentrations and decreased serum total bilirubin concentration. The liver enzyme activities had almost returned to normal (**Table 1**). The cat was still not eating spontaneously; therefore, an appetite stimulant (cyproheptadine[c]) was prescribed (2 mg per os, twice daily). The cat continued to receive 80 ml of the blended food twice daily via the G-tube. The cat began eating the adult maintenance-type food spontaneously after four days of receiving the appetite stimulant. The G-tube was removed three days after the cat began eating voluntarily and the recommendation was made to continue feeding the maintenance-type food free choice until the cat achieved an ideal BCS (3/5) and body weight (approximately 5.0 kg). The owners were instructed to monitor the cat's appetite, body weight and body condition closely and, after the cat had achieved an optimal BCS, to change the feeding method from free choice to meal feeding a specific quantity of food (approximately one-fourth cup, twice daily) to maintain optimal body weight and condition.

Table 1. Laboratory data from a domestic shorthair cat with icterus.

Parameters	Day 1	Day 15	Reference values
Packed cell volume (%)	27.5	31.7	30-45
Hemoglobin (g/dl)	9.2	10	10-15
Glucose (mg/dl)	150	89	70-110
Total protein (g/dl)	5.9	7.2	6.5-7.7
Albumin (g/dl)	2.2	2.4	2.5-4.0
Alanine aminotransferase (IU/l)	264	80	10-33
Alkaline phosphatase (IU/l)	110	45	14-43

Endnotes

a. Hill's Pet Nutrition Inc., Topeka, KS, USA. These foods are available as Science Diet Light Adult Feline and Science Diet Adult Feline.

b. Abbott Laboratories, North Chicago, IL, USA.

c. Periactin. Merck & Company, Inc., Rahway, NJ, USA.

Bibliography

Center SA, Crawford MA, Guida L, et al. A retrospective study of 77 cats with severe hepatic lipidosis: 1975-1990. Journal of Veterinary Internal Medicine 1993; 7: 349-359.

Center SA. Hepatic lipidosis. In: Guilford WG, Center SA, Strombeck DR, et al, eds. Strombeck's Small Animal Gastroenterology, 3rd ed. Philadelphia, PA: WB Saunders Co, 1996; 766-782.

CASE 68-4

Polydipsia/Polyuria in a Doberman Pinscher[a]

Philip Roudebush, DVM, Dipl. ACVIM (Small Animal Internal Medicine)
Hill's Scientific Affairs
Topeka, Kansas, USA

Patient Assessment

A five-year-old neutered female Doberman pinscher was examined for polydipsia and polyuria. The dog's history was uneventful except for treatment of a recurrent interdigital cyst. Physical examination was normal. Body weight was 28.6 kg with a body condition score (BCS) of 3/5. The dog had weighed 32 kg during an examination five months earlier. Blood was obtained for a complete blood count and serum biochemistry profile. Urine was obtained for a urinalysis.

Results of the complete blood count were normal. Serum biochemistry profile abnormalities included elevated liver enzyme activity (**Table 1**, Day 1). Results of the urinalysis were normal except for dilute urine (specific gravity = 1.005). Radiographs of the abdomen were normal except for a small liver silhouette.

Liver specimens were obtained using an ultrasound-guided biopsy needle. Histopathologic changes were consistent with moderate, diffuse, subacute hepatitis. Most of the inflammatory cells were neutrophils and macrophages. Macrophages and some hepatocytes contained focal accumulation of granular pigment. Special stains were positive for accumulating copper, but the quantity of copper was not determined. Bacterial culture of one of the biopsy specimens recovered a coagulase-negative *Staphylococcus* spp. This organism was considered normal flora or an opportunistic pathogen; it was sensitive to most commonly available antibiotics except ampicillin.

Assess the Food and Feeding Method

The dog was normally fed four cups of a dry specialty brand dog food (Iams Minichunks[b]) once daily in the evening.

Questions

1. What is the most likely diagnosis for this patient?
2. Outline an appropriate feeding plan for this dog.
3. In addition to the feeding plan, what other medical therapy is appropriate for this patient?
4. How should the response to therapy be monitored?

Answers and Discussion

1. Middle-aged female Doberman pinscher dogs may develop an aggressive form of chronic hepatitis. Affected dogs may present in fulminant hepatic failure, or the disorder may be detected early based on elevated serum enzyme activity found on routine screening biochemistry profiles. Dogs with advanced liver disease present with weight loss, anorexia, polydipsia/polyuria, icterus, ascites, bleeding tendencies, severe depression and/or signs of hepatic encephalopathy. Dogs presenting in reasonable condition when first examined survive longer. These dogs are typically bright and responsive, have minimal weight loss and do not have ascites or hepatic encephalopathy. Typical laboratory findings include hypoalbuminemia, elevated liver enzyme activity, hyperbilirubinemia, elevated fasting bile acid concentrations and prolonged coagulation studies.

   Histopathologic features of chronic hepatitis in Doberman pinschers include variable degrees of degeneration and necrosis of periportal hepatocytes and mixed inflammatory cell infiltrates. Portal fibrosis may be mild to severe; hepatic cirrhosis occurs in severely affected dogs. The livers of affected dogs have moderately increased copper and increased iron concentrations. The role of copper is not understood but may be associated with cholestasis. Iron accumulation may be associated with hepatic necrosis, hemorrhage and inflammation. Excessive copper and iron accumulation may aggravate ongoing hepatic inflammation.
2. General recommendations for the nutritional management of patients with chronic hepatitis include feeding foods that are energy dense, contain adequate levels of potassium, avoid excess levels of protein, copper, iron, sodium and chloride and contain some fermentable fiber. These goals can be met with either commercial veterinary therapeutic or homemade foods. Highly palatable, energy-dense foods offered in multiple small meals throughout the day may help overcome the nausea and gastrointestinal (GI) complications often associated with liver disease.
3. Definitive medical management of dogs affected with chronic hepatitis is not well established. Medical therapy often includes antibiotics, antiinflammatory and immunosuppressive drugs (e.g., prednisone, azathioprine), choleretic or bile "altering" agents (e.g., ursodeoxycholic acid), vitamin E and other antioxidants, zinc supplementation and copper chelating agents (i.e., D-penicillamine, tetramine). Diuretics may be needed for patients with severe ascites. Hepatic encephalopathy should be treated with reduced protein intake, oral antibiotics, lactulose and retention enemas (**Table 68-10**).

Table 1. Body weight and selected laboratory values from a Doberman pinscher with hepatitis.

Parameters	Day 1	Day 49	Day 73	Day 108	Day 164	Day 288	Day 314	Day 350	Reference values
Body weight (kg)	28.6	28.4	27.3	30.5	30.5	30	29.5	na	na
Glucose (mg/dl)	101	120	95	109	85	132	114	155	60-115
Urea nitrogen (mg/dl)	6	2.5	5	10	5	4.1	3.3	11.6	10-25
Creatinine (mg/dl)	1.2	1.3	2.1	0.5	1.4	1.0	1.0	1.0	0.5-1.2
Total protein (g/dl)	6.4	6.9	6.6	6.6	7.4	6.8	6.7	na	5.5-7.2
Albumin (g/dl)	2.2	3.1	2.8	2.8	3.0	2.7	2.7	2.7	3.0-4.5
Total bilirubin (mg/dl)	0	1.2	2.3	0.4	0.4	0.4	0.2	0.4	0.0-0.6
Alkaline phosphatase (IU/l)	2,655	2,579	1,447	500	215	494	425	541	8.0-75
Alanine aminotransferase (IU/l)	1,080	707	747	417	158	115	136	155	6.0-70

Key: na = information not available.

4. Patients with chronic hepatitis should be monitored frequently (i.e., every few months) with serial physical examinations, body weight and body condition determinations and serum biochemistry profiles that include measurement of albumin concentration and liver enzyme activity. The owner should also be encouraged to document the amount of food eaten daily. If treatment is successful, the dog will maintain body weight, body condition and serum albumin concentrations, have gradually reduced liver enzyme activity and remain alert and active. Serial liver biopsy specimens (i.e., every six to nine months) can also be used to monitor pathologic changes and quantify hepatic copper concentrations.

Progress Notes

The dog was given 500 mg cephalexin, per os, twice daily for the possible secondary bacterial hepatitis. The food was changed to a veterinary therapeutic food that avoids excess levels of protein, sodium, chloride, copper and iron (Prescription Diet u/d Canine[c]). The daily energy requirement (DER) was estimated to be 1.4 to 1.6 x resting energy requirement (RER) for an ideal body weight of 32 kg (DER = 1,440 to 1,650 kcal [6.02 to 6.90 MJ]). The DER was met by feeding 4 to 5 cups of dry u/d Canine daily.

Evaluations six and 10 weeks later revealed slightly reduced liver enzyme activity, continued weight loss and mild hyperbilirubinemia (**Table 1**, Days 49 and 73). The dog was alert and active but not eating well according to the owner. The dietary management was not changed, but more aggressive therapy for liver inflammation and copper accumulation was initiated. This therapy consisted of a bile altering agent (ursodeoxycholic acid [ursodiol[d]] 300 mg per os, daily with food), prednisone (30 mg per os, once daily for two weeks and then 30 mg every other day), vitamin E (400 IU per os, daily) and zinc gluconate (100 mg elemental zinc per os, twice daily).

Further evaluations one month and three months later (**Table 1**, Days 108 and 164) revealed an alert, active dog that had gained weight. The owner reported that the dog seemed to be doing well. Dietary management and medical therapy were continued.

Eighteen weeks later (Day 288) the dog was examined for vomiting, diarrhea and fever. Two other dogs at home were also affected with the same clinical signs. Nonspecific gastroenteritis was suspected. Liver enzyme activity remained increased but lower than the original values (**Table 1**, Day 288). A liver biopsy was recommended to assess the extent of hepatitis, fibrosis and copper accumulation but was declined by the owner. Therapy was not changed.

One month later, the dog was examined because the owner was concerned about weight loss. Mild weight loss was documented, but the dog's serum biochemistry parameters remained stable (**Table 1**, Day 314). Therapy was not changed. Five weeks later the dog was presented in a comatose state. Serum biochemistry parameters were not significantly changed from previous values (**Table 1**, Day 350); however, a resting blood ammonia concentration was elevated (367 µg/dl, normal 0 to 98 µg/dl). Hepatic encephalopathy was diagnosed. The dog was euthanatized at the owner's request.

Endnotes

a. Thanks to Dr. Roy L. Davis, Red Bridge Animal Clinic, Kansas City, MO, USA, for providing the information about this patient.
b. The Iams Co., Dayton, OH, USA.
c. Hill's Pet Nutrition Inc., Topeka, KS, USA.
d. Actigall. CibaGeneva Pharmaceuticals, Summit, NJ, USA.

Bibliography

Center SA. Chronic hepatitis in the Doberman pinscher. In: Guilford WG, Center SA, Strombeck DR, et al, eds. Strombeck's Small Animal Gastroenterology, 3rd ed. Philadelphia, PA: WB Saunders Co, 1996; 742-743.

Speeti M, Eriksson J, Saari S, et al. Lesions of subclinical Doberman hepatitis. Veterinary Pathology 1998; 35: 361-369.

Strombeck DR, Miller LM, Harrold D. Effects of corticosteroid treatment on survival time in dogs with chronic hepatitis: 151 cases (1977-1985). Journal of the American Veterinary Medical Association 1988; 193: 1109-1113.

Thornburg LP. Histomorphological and immunohistochemical studies of chronic active hepatitis in Doberman pinschers. Veterinary Pathology 1998; 35: 380-385.

CASE 68-5

Increased Hepatic Enzyme Activities in a Bedlington Terrier

David C. Twedt, DVM, Dipl. ACVIM (Internal Medicine)
College of Veterinary Medicine and Biomedical Sciences
Colorado State University
Fort Collins, Colorado, USA

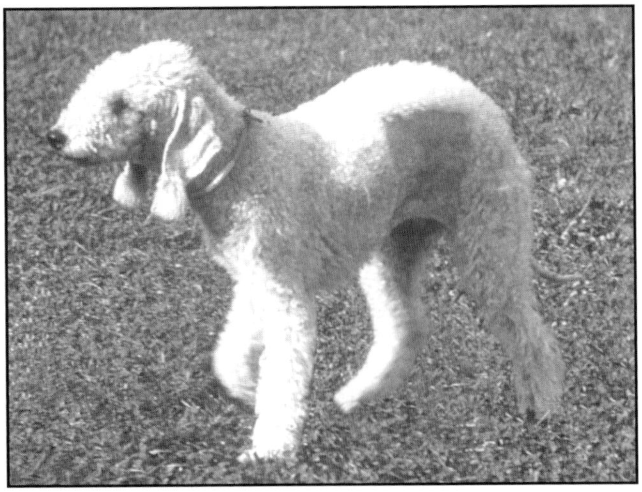

Figure 1. A one-and-one-half-year-old female Bedlington terrier affected with inherited copper hepatotoxicity.

Patient Assessment

A one-and-one-half-year-old female Bedlington terrier (**Figure 1**) was evaluated because a littermate had recently been diagnosed with copper-associated hepatotoxicity. A serum biochemistry profile obtained by the referring veterinarian identified an abnormal alanine aminotransferase (ALT) activity of 161 IU/l (reference range 10 to 120 IU/l). The dog was considered to be normal by the owner and a physical examination was unremarkable. The dog weighed 6.6 kg and had normal body condition (body condition score [BCS] 3/5).

Another serum biochemistry profile confirmed an elevated ALT of 189 IU/l. Serum protein and bile acid concentrations, and clotting times were normal suggesting adequate hepatic function. The liver was grossly normal when biopsy specimens were collected at laparoscopy. Evaluation of the biopsy specimens revealed mild focal necrosis with many hepatocytes containing golden brown granules. These granules stained positive for copper using rhodamine copper stain (**Figure 2**). Hepatic copper quantitation was 4,901 µg/g dry weight liver (normal reference 120 to 400 µg/g dry weight liver). A diagnosis of inherited copper hepatotoxicity was made.

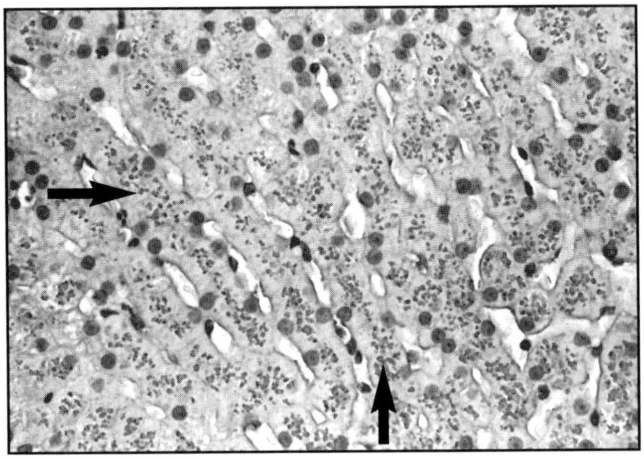

Figure 2. A photomicrograph of a liver specimen from a Bedlington terrier. Granules located in hepatocytes (arrows) stained positive for copper (rhodamine copper stain).

Assess the Food and Feeding Method

The diet was currently a mixture of a commercial dry grocery brand dog food (Purina Dog Chow[a]) and various commercial moist grocery brand foods with occasional table foods. The foods were mixed together at each meal so that approximately two-thirds of the volume came from dry food and one-third from moist food. The exact daily caloric intake was unknown. The patient was eating approximately the same amount of food and there had been no change in body weight during the last year.

Questions

1. What are the key nutritional factors to consider for this patient?
2. What nutritional supplements might benefit patients with copper hepatotoxicity?

Answers and Discussion

1. Key nutritional factors to consider in patients with copper-associated hepatoxicosis include energy, protein, copper, zinc and antioxidant vitamins. Providing adequate daily energy intake is important to allow protein synthesis and prevent tissue catabolism that generates ammonia. The exact caloric needs of these patients have not been determined but would be expected to be similar to those of other dogs of similar age and body condition.

   Most dogs with copper toxicosis develop clinical problems or liver disease is detected during adulthood (i.e., two to six years of age). Protein requirements have not been established for these dogs, but they would be expected to be similar to those of other adult dogs (15 to 30% dry matter [DM]). Patients with evidence of hepatic encephalopathy will often need more restricted dietary protein levels.

   Foods low in copper are recommended for affected dogs that accumulate hepatic copper. Restriction of dietary copper as the primary therapy probably does little to lower abnormal hepatic copper concentrations in diseased dogs. Copper-restricted foods have a minimal depleting effect for hepatic copper.

Commercial dog foods contain supplemental copper to meet or exceed dietary allowances established by the Association of American Feed Control Officials (AAFCO) or similar regulatory agencies. The AAFCO minimum allowance is 7.3 ppm copper (DM) or 2.1 mg copper/1,000 kcal (4.18 MJ) metabolizable energy. Most commercial dog foods exceed these levels of copper. These levels are appropriate for normal dogs but are excessive for dogs with copper-associated liver disease. For affected Bedlington terriers, foods with less than 5 ppm DM copper from available sources are appropriate. A few commercial veterinary therapeutic foods have low copper levels (**Table 68-11**).

Homemade foods can be prepared that do not contain excess copper (Chapter 10). These foods should exclude liver, shellfish, organ meats and cereals because of their high copper content. Vitamin-mineral supplements that do not contain a copper source are recommended. Treats and table food containing copper should also be avoided.

Decreasing the copper content of the food decreases the amount of copper that is absorbed through the intestine and enters the liver. Foods with low copper levels appear to be most useful for managing young dogs diagnosed with an inherited hepatic copper accumulation defect.

2. Oral zinc supplementation decreases intestinal absorption of copper. Zinc induces the increased synthesis of an intestinal mucosal metal-binding protein metallothionein. Copper that enters the intestine binds tenaciously to metallothionein, blocking the transfer of copper to the animal. The copper-metallothionein complex is lost in the feces during normal intestinal epithelial cell turnover.

   Studies suggest that zinc supplementation will prevent copper accumulation and may actually decrease hepatic copper stores in affected patients. This "decoppering" method, however, is a slow process. Therefore, patients with high concentrations of hepatic copper should first receive copper chelating agents to reduce copper levels. Zinc supplementation alone may not be adequate for maintaining affected Bedlington terriers.

   Zinc supplementation (i.e., as acetate, sulfate, gluconate or methionine) given at a dose of 5 to 10 mg/kg body weight every 12 hours has been recommended. Alternatively, 200 mg of elemental zinc given orally for several months for induction, then lowered to a maintenance dose of 100 mg daily, may be used. Serum zinc concentrations should be monitored with the goal of approximately doubling the serum zinc concentrations. Zinc should not be given with meals.

   Experimental studies show that increased concentrations of hepatic copper catalyze hepatocellular oxidative damage and that therapeutic levels of antioxidants have protective properties. Vitamin E (d-α-tocopherol 200 to 400 IU/day) may be used as adjunct therapy. Vitamin C (ascorbic acid) has been suggested to decrease hepatic copper concentrations. However, this practice is not recommended because vitamin C promotes increased oxidative damage in the presence of high copper concentrations.

Table 1. Homemade food for a Bedlington terrier with copper hepatotoxicosis.

Ingredients*	Amounts (g)
Long grain brown rice, cooked	192
Cottage cheese, 4% fat	71
Margarine	8
Calcium carbonate	1
Iodized "lite" salt (KCl/NaCl)	1.7 (1/2 tsp)
Brewer's yeast	1
Other supplements	**

*Provides 350 kcal (1.46 MJ).
**Each day: 175 IU vitamin D, 28 mg iron, 8 µg vitamin B_{12}.

Progress Notes

A low-copper homemade food was recommended, but the owner wanted to continue feeding the dog commercial foods. No major changes to the current feeding plan were made other than eliminating table foods. The estimated daily energy requirement (DER) was 1.6 x resting energy requirement (RER) = 430 kcal (1.8 MJ). The foods were divided into equal portions and fed twice daily. A copper chelating agent, penicillamine[b] (125 mg, twice daily), was also given before meals.

Evaluation at six months found that the liver enzyme activities had returned to the normal reference range. A second liver biopsy was performed 12 months after therapy was instituted. The hepatic copper concentration had declined to 3,900 µg/g dry weight liver, and mild fibrosis, vacuolar degeneration and hepatic copper in centrilobular hepatocytes were evident histologically. Penicillamine therapy was continued.

An elective ovariohysterectomy was performed four years after the onset of penicillamine therapy and a liver biopsy specimen was obtained at that time. Both hepatic histology and hepatic copper concentration (125 µg/g liver) were normal. The penicillamine was discontinued and therapy with zinc gluconate (100 mg, twice daily, for a two-month induction period, followed by 50 mg, twice daily) and vitamin E (200 IU, twice daily) was instituted. Serum zinc concentrations were maintained between 200 and 300 g/ml, which were considered in the therapeutic range. Liver enzyme activities were evaluated at six-month intervals and were normal for three years. At that point, serum ALT concentrations began to increase and remained consistently abnormal when evaluated at six-month intervals for 18 months (i.e., ALT concentrations were 196, 275 and 278 IU/l, respectively). Zinc supplementation was thought not to be maintaining the patient. Therefore, a liver biopsy was suggested to obtain a specimen for evaluation of hepatic copper concentration. The owner declined the biopsy. Zinc therapy was discontinued and penicillamine therapy was reinstituted. The dog was also fed a homemade food, which probably had a lower copper content than the commercial foods that were being fed (**Table 1**). Vitamin-mineral supplements without copper were prescribed and the owner added small quantities of cooked ground beef, chicken or eggs to the basic homemade food recipe. One year following the change to the homemade food and reintroduction of penicillamine therapy, the ALT concentrations returned to the normal reference range.

Further Discussion

This case demonstrates that inherited copper hepatotoxicity can be managed and progression can be stopped by reducing hepatic copper concentrations, if the disease is detected early. The apparent failure of zinc therapy in this case suggests that therapy with copper chelating agents should be instituted in Bedlington terriers with this disease. Penicillamine and trientine[c] are both effective copper chelating agents. It remains unknown whether a low-copper food in conjunction with zinc therapy would have been beneficial in this case. Combination chelating agent and zinc therapy, essentially attacking the problem by two different mechanisms is intriguing, but there are no objective studies evaluating this form of therapy. It is possible that penicillamine may chelate zinc in the gastrointestinal tract making both drugs less effective.

Endnotes

a. Ralston Purina Co., St Louis, MO, USA.
b. Cuprimine. Merck & Company, Inc., Rahway, NJ, USA.
c. Syprine. Merck & Company, Inc., Rahway, NJ, USA.

Bibliography

Brewer GJ, Dick RD, Schall W. Use of zinc acetate to treat copper toxicosis in dogs. Journal of the American Veterinary Medical Association 1992; 201: 564-568.

Guilford WG. Nutritional management of gastrointestinal tract diseases. In Proceedings. Tenth Annual Veterinary Medical Forum, American College of Veterinary Internal Medicine, San Diego, CA, 1992: 66-69.

Rolfe DS, Twedt DC. Copper-associated hepatopathies in dogs. Veterinary Clinics of North America: Small Animal Practice 1995; 25: 399-416.

Section 21

Food-Drug Interactions

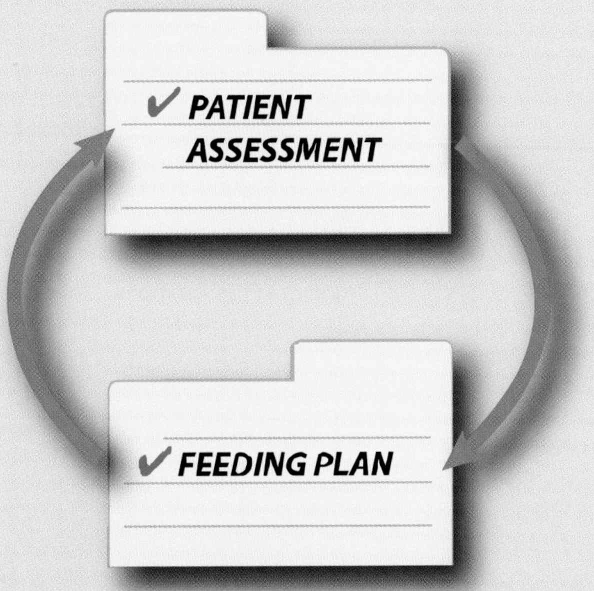

Chapter 69

Effects of Food on Pharmacokinetics

Martin J. Fettman
Butch KuKanich
Robert W. Phillips

"Give me a lever long enough and a fulcrum on which to place it, and I shall move the world."
Archimedes

INTRODUCTION

When the effects of veterinary pharmaceuticals are evaluated and standardized doses are determined, researchers typically use relatively healthy, fasted animals that have been maintained on foods with acceptable nutrient balance. However, in clinical settings, animals receiving a drug often have variable food intake or specific nutrient imbalances, or they must be given a drug in conjunction with a meal, or some combination of these factors may occur. The patient's health status and the nutrient ingredient profile of the diet being consumed may greatly affect drug absorption, distribution, metabolism, elimination, efficacy and toxicity (**Table 69-1**). Concurrent food intake also may markedly affect drug availability and pharmacokinetics (**Tables 69-2** and **69-3**).

Veterinarians should be acquainted with the effects diet can have on drug disposition to anticipate adjustments in the food or drug dose, properly time administration of drugs and allow for changes in the margin for error between efficacy and toxicity of pharmaceutical agents.

GENERAL TYPES OF FOOD AND DRUG INTERACTIONS

Food-drug interactions that occur as a result of the physical form or chemical properties of food may lead to drug binding, precipitation, inactivation or ionization, which alter gastrointestinal (GI) absorption. These interactions may occur in vitro after mixing the drug with food to make administration more convenient, to enhance palatability or to reduce GI irritation. Another concern is adsorption of drugs to synthetic surfaces of the equipment used for nutrient and drug administration (e.g., food containers, feeding syringes and tubing for assisted feeding). Physiochemical interactions may occur in vivo, whereby drug absorption from the GI tract is decreased because of chelation by dietary fiber or minerals, or increased because of favorable changes in ionization or solvent partitioning.

Metabolic Interactions

Both nutrient and non-nutrient substances in foods can alter the metabolism of absorbed drugs. Nutrients are nourishing ingredients of food. Non-nutrient substances are chemicals without metabolic value, including naturally occurring phytochemicals and synthetic chemicals added inadvertently or purposely to food. Protein and energy malnutrition can alter the synthesis of plasma proteins, affecting drug distribution and pharmacokinetics. Individual dietary lipid, carbohydrate, protein, vitamin and mineral levels can effect changes in xenobiotic-metabolizing enzymes, resulting in altered clearance, circulating concentrations and resultant therapeutic efficacy and toxicity. Naturally occurring non-nutrient food ingredients and added synthetic preservatives may similarly

Table 69-1. Factors affecting the disposition of drugs that can be influenced by foods.

Absorption
GI transit time
GI luminal environment
Enterocyte function
Electrochemical gradient across the GI mucosa
pH gradient across the GI mucosa
Distribution
Drug-binding proteins
Blood cells that bind or metabolize drugs
Metabolism
Site of metabolism
  Organ
  Tissue
  Cell type
  Cell organelle
Biotransformation pathways
  Phase I oxidative vs. phase II conjugative pathways
Cofactors required for metabolism
  Vitamins
  Minerals
  Reducing agents
Non-nutrient enzyme inducers
  Phytochemicals
  Synthetic contaminants
  Preservatives
Excretion
Route of excretion
  Biliary
  Fecal
  Mammary
  Pulmonary
  Renal
  Salivary
  Sweat
Electrochemical gradient across mucosa of excretory organs
Rate of excretion

Table 69-2. Selected factors that can determine the effects of nutrients on drug absorption.

Factors	Examples
Physiochemical properties of drugs	Lipophilic or hydrophilic
Drug formulation	Tablet, capsule or liquid
Meal type	Volume, temperature, moisture
Drug dose	Amount and concentration
Route of administration	By mouth, gastric tube, etc.
Order of administration	Pre- vs. postprandial
Time interval between food and drug administration	Phase of digestion
Owner/patient compliance	Mixing drugs and food for ease of administration

alter pharmacokinetics and apparent drug effectiveness.

Indirect Physiologic Effects
The rate of drug elimination is also affected by changes in blood flow and drug delivery to the principal organs of metabolism for that particular agent. Thus, postprandial alterations in blood flow to the liver may affect drug clearance from the portal and systemic circulation, and altered blood flow to the kidneys may change the rate of urinary elimination. Likewise, changes in functional morphology or pathology due to specific nutrient deficiencies or excesses can affect drug clearance.

GENERAL EFFECTS OF FOOD AND DRUG INTERACTIONS

Ameliorating Potential Adverse Effects
The composition and volume of food consumed can modify the degree of GI irritation caused by concurrently administered oral drugs. Enteral and parenteral fluid intake can augment drug absorption and distribution and protect against renal damage induced by nephrotoxic agents. Supplementation with specific nutrients may prevent deficiencies secondary to adverse drug effects on nutrient absorption and metabolism.

Potentiating Drug Action
Specific nutrients can increase drug effects by facilitating GI absorption, improving drug distribution or decreasing drug metabolism and excretion. Furthermore, some nutrients may be necessary for optimal drug effects (e.g., arginine for nitric oxide production, cysteine for nitroglycerin action and carnitine for optimal activity of cardiac glycosides).

Impaired Drug Action
Impaired drug action is the adverse effect most often considered when evaluating nutrient-drug interactions that impair therapeutic efficacy. These adverse effects may result from decreased drug absorption, inadequate amounts of the drug reaching the site of action, or nutrient interference with the drug's action. Drug action may be impaired for variable periods of time after food composition and feeding behavior are altered, if target cell receptor numbers or affinity are suppressed or long-lived biotransforming enzyme systems have been induced.

Adverse Side Effects
Pathologic reactions to nutrient-induced changes in drug distribution and metabolism can be of greater immediate consequence than loss of disease control following impaired drug action. Drug metabolism and excretion routes may be altered, resulting in accumulation of toxic quantities of the agent itself or the products of its biotransformation. This phenomenon is similar in principle to adverse interactions between concurrently administered drugs, but may be more difficult to identify because mental recollection and written records of nutrient intake are not usually as complete as for administration of pharmaceutical agents.

EFFECTS OF NUTRIENTS ON DRUG ABSORPTION

General Observations
The absorption of orally administered drugs may be: 1) decreased, 2) delayed, 3) unaffected or 4) enhanced by the con-

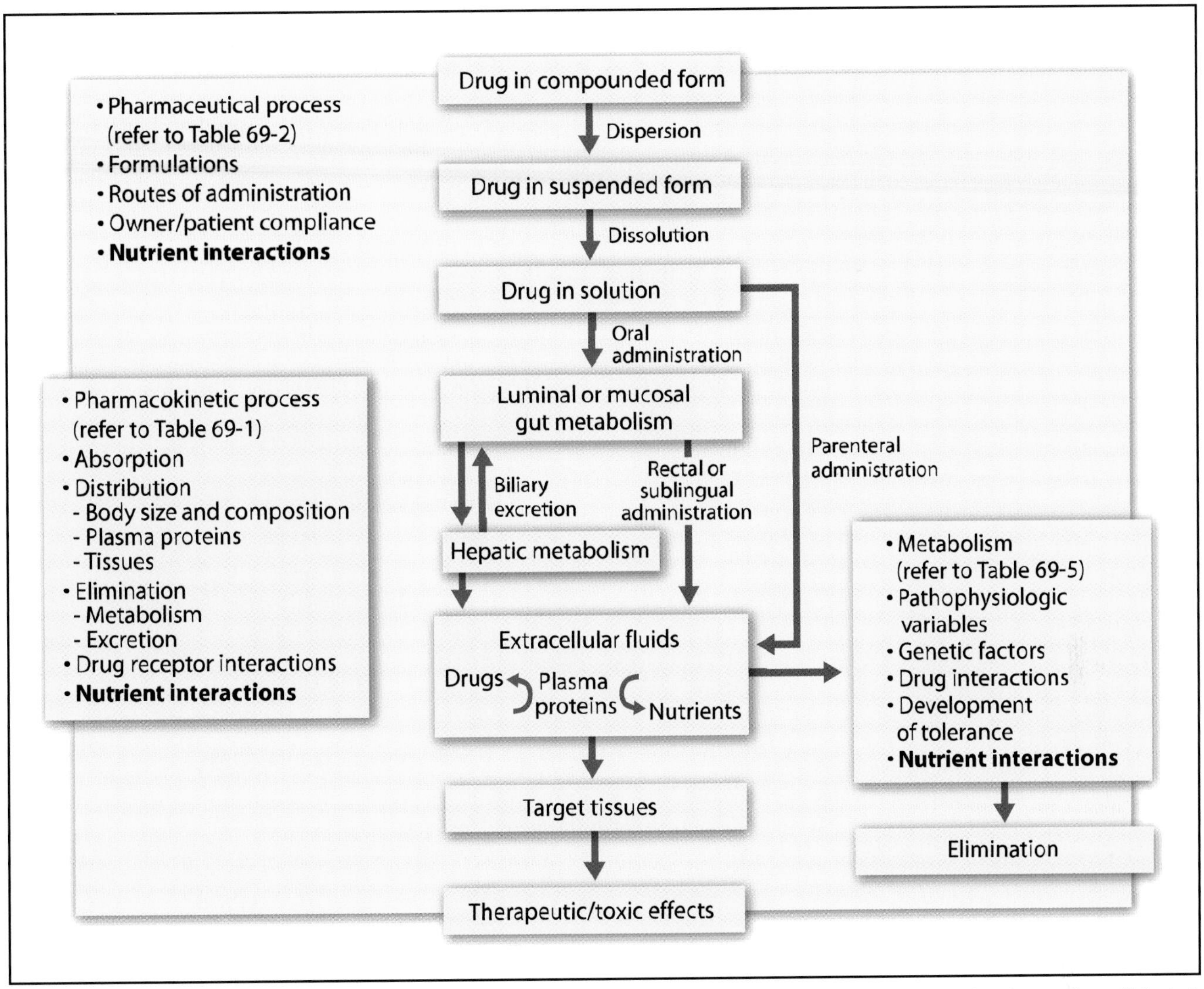

Figure 69-1. Determinants of drug absorption, distribution, metabolism and excretion that may be modified by nutrient interactions. (Adapted from Grahame-Smith DG, Aronson JK. In: The Oxford Textbook of Clinical Pharmacology and Drug Therapy. Oxford, UK: Oxford University Press, 1985.) Rectal absorption in dogs and cats is subject to first-pass hepatic metabolism due to the small relative size of the rectum and the lack of a hemorrhoidal plexus in these species. Transdermal could be substituted for rectal delivery (e.g., fentanyl patches in dogs and cats). A good example of a drug absorbed across oral mucous membranes is buprenorphine in cats.

comitant consumption of food (**Figure 69-1** and **Tables 69-2** and **69-3**). This interaction depends on the physical and chemical nature of the food and the drug, including such things as meal size and type, the formulation in which the drug is administered, the order in which the food and drug are ingested and the interval between their consumption (Roe, 1989).

Any food can reduce drug absorption by creating a barrier that prevents dispersion of the drug and dissolution of the active agent in GI luminal contents. Drugs are better absorbed in dilute vs. concentrated solution because of greater dissolution and more rapid gastric emptying. In people, absorption of erythromycin stearate is reduced by approximately one-half when taken with food or a small fluid volume, as compared with a large fluid volume (Toothaker and Welling, 1980). Absorption of acetylsalicylic acid (aspirin), cephalexin, metronidazole, digoxin, hydralazine and cimetidine are similarly affected (Toothaker and Welling, 1980).

Alternatively, food does not affect absorption of other drugs in people, including erythromycin estolate, oxazepam, propylthiouracil and enteric-coated aspirin granules in caplet form (Toothaker and Welling, 1980). In fact, food enhances the absorption of certain drugs (e.g., erythromycin ethylsuccinate, nitrofurantoin, hydrochlorothiazide and diazepam) (Toothaker and Welling, 1980). The rate and quantity of drug and nutrient delivery are important, as evidenced by studies of hydralazine absorption. A bolus of nutrients impairs hydralazine uptake whereas a constant infusion over several hours does not (Semple et al, 1991). Total hydralazine absorption, however, is similar in both cases, although absorption is delayed by a bolus meal.

Gastric emptying of drugs is delayed when they are administered with a meal. Gastric emptying of drugs is about 15 minutes for fasted dogs, but may take up to three hours if given to dogs fed a full meal. Because the majority of drug absorption occurs in the small intestine, drug administration with food typically results in delayed drug absorption and may or may not affect the extent of absorption. Feeding also stimulates acid secretion in dogs, which markedly increases the absorption of drugs with low pKa (e.g., weak acids, ketoconazole). The rate and extent of absorption of cephalexin are decreased in dogs when this antibiotic is administered with food, but this decrease is clinically irrelevant (a similar example is amoxicillin). In contrast, the extent of absorption of cefadroxil is increased in fed dogs, but its rate of absorption is decreased. Because cefadroxil is a time-dependent antimicrobial, its efficacy is expected to increase when it is administered with food, but this increase may or may not be clinically relevant (Campbell and Rosin, 1998). Feeding also tends to increase GI tract blood flow, increasing both food and drug absorption.

Studies of penicillin absorption in dogs after oral administration have yielded conflicting results. In a study of greyhounds receiving 20 mg/kg body weight ampicillin or amoxicillin per os with no food, moist food or dry food, ampicillin absorption was impeded 60 to 80% by feeding, whereas amoxicillin absorption was unaffected (Watson and Egerton, 1977). In a more recent study involving a variety of breeds, absorption was impaired about 30% when ampicillin (20 mg/kg body weight) was administered immediately or two hours after feeding a dry food as compared with ampicillin administered to fasting dogs or one hour before feeding (Kung et al, 1995). Absorption of ampicillin (20 mg/kg body weight) administered immediately after feeding a moist food was similarly impaired, whereas administration two hours after feeding a moist food had a lesser effect on absorption.

In a comparative study of different penicillin preparations given to dogs, peak plasma concentrations of ampicillin, amoxicillin, penicillin V, phenethicillin and cloxacillin were decreased 40 to 50% by feeding immediately before drug administration; however, time to maximal concentrations was increased 0.5 to 1.5 hours only for ampicillin and amoxicillin (Watson et al, 1986). From these studies, it is recommended that ampicillin be given to fasted dogs and at least one hour before feeding to ensure adequate drug absorption.

Table 69-3. Recommendations for administering medications with or without food.*

Drugs that can be administered with food		
Allopurinol	Hydrocortisone	Mitotane
Amantadine	Isotretinoin	Nitrofurantoin
Aspirin	Itraconazole (capsules)	Olsalazine
Azathioprine	Ketoconazole	Pancrelipase
Betamethasone	Ketoprofen	Paromomycin
Carprofen	Ketorolac	Pentoxifylline
Cefadroxil	Lithium	Phenylbutazone
Cimetidine	Lufenuron	Piroxicam
Clofazimine	Meclofenamate	Praziquantel
Clomipramine	Meloxicam	Prednisolone
Deracoxib	Metformin	Prednisone
Dexamethasone	Methocarbamol (not high fat)	Quinacrine
Diethylcarbamazine	Methylprednisolone	Sulfasalazine
Etodolac	Metoprolol	Tepoxalin
Flunixin	Mexiletine	Triamcinolone
Glyburide	Misoprostol	Ursodiol
Griseofulvin		
Drugs that should not be administered with food (one hour before or three hours after)		
Acetaminophen	Digitoxin	Omeprazole
Ampicillin	Digoxin	Oxacillin
Bethanechol	Dipyridamole	Oxytetracycline
Captopril	Etidronate	Penicillamine
Carbenicillin	Itraconazole (suspension)	Penicillin V
Chlortetracycline	Levodopa	Procainamide
Cloxacillin	Levothyroxine	Quinidine
Codeine	Lincomycin	Rifampin
Cyclophosphamide	Minocycline	Tetracycline
Difloxacin		
No effect = no *clinical* effect, can give to either fed or fasted animals (some of these drugs may have increased absorption in the fasted state but the clinical outcome is unaffected)		
Acepromazine	Diphenoxylate	Methotrexate
Aminophylline	Disopyramide	Metronidazole
Amitriptyline	Dolasetron	Mibolerone
Amlodipine	Doxepin	Milbemycin
Amoxicillin	Doxycycline	Moxidectin
Amoxicillin/clavulanate	Enalapril	Naltrexone
Amprolium	Enrofloxacin	Nandrolone
Atenolol	Ephedrine	Neomycin
Azithromycin	Epsiprantel	Nifedipine
Benazepril	Ergocalciferol	Ondansetron
Bismuth subsalicylate	Erythromycin	Orbifloxacin
Bromide	Famotidine	Ormetoprim/ sulfadimethoxine
Bunamidine	Felbamate	Pamidronate
Buspirone	Fenbendazole	Paroxetine
Busulfan	Finasteride	

Physical Incompatibilities

Specific nutrients (e.g., dietary fiber) can impede drug absorption across the GI mucosa by adsorbing the agent or increasing the unstirred water layer on the mucosal surface (Reppas et al, 1991). Some of these interactions are predictable, based on the behavior of fiber in binding substances such as bile acids or decreasing the absorptive rate of solutes such as monosaccharides. Psyllium mucilloid decreases the absorption of riboflavin, β-carotene, iron, zinc and other trace elements (Roe, 1989).

Both nutritive and non-nutritive cytoprotective agents adsorb drugs and inhibit their absorption. For example, sucralfate binds tetracycline, phenytoin, cimetidine, digoxin and levothyroxine (Havrankova and Lahaie, 1992; McCarthy, 1991). Antacids (e.g., aluminum hydroxide) can precipitate tetracyclines, iron salts, warfarin, digoxin, quinidine, phenothiazines, indomethacin, isoniazid, sulfadiazine, prednisone and levothyroxine (Roe, 1989; Liel et al, 1994). Mineral sup-

Butorphanol	Firocoxib	Phenobarbital
Calcitriol	Florfenicol	Phenoxybenzamine
Carbimazole	Flucytosine	Phenylpropanolamine
Cefaclor	Fludrocortisone	Phytonadione (vitamin K)
Cefdinir	Fluoxetine	Piperazine
Cefixime	Fluconazole	Ponazuril
Cefpodoxime	Furosemide	Potassium
Cephalexin	Gabapentin	Prazosin
Chlorambucil	Granisetron	Primidone
Chloramphenicol	Hydralazine	Promethazine
Chlorothiazide	Hydrochlorothiazide	Propranolol
Chlorpheniramine	Hydrocodone	Pyrantel
Chlorpromazine	Hydroxyurea	Pyridostigmine
Ciprofloxacin	Hydroxyzine	Pyrimethamine
Clenbuterol	Imipramine	Selegiline
Clindamycin	Ipodate	Sotalol
Clonazepam	Isosorbide	Spironolactone
Clorazepate	Ivermectin	Stanozolol
Colchicine	Levamisole	Sulfadiazine
Cyproheptadine	Linezolid	Sulfadimethoxine
Danazol	Lisinopril	Sulfamethazine
Dantrolene	Loperamide	Sulfamethoxazole
Dapsone	Marbofloxacin	Taurine
Dextromethorphan	Mebendazole	Terbutaline
Diazepam	Meclizine	Theophylline
Dichlorvos	Megestrol	Tocainide
Dichlorphenamide	Melphalan	Toltrazuril
Diclazuril	Mercaptopurine	Trimeprazine
Diethylstilbestrol	Mesalamine	Trimethoprim
Dihydrotachysterol	Metaproterenol	Tripelennamine
Diltiazem	Methazolamide	Tylosin
Dimenhydrinate	Methenamine	Valproic acid
Diphenhydramine	Methimazole	Vancomycin
		Warfarin

Prior to = administer 30 to 60 minutes before feeding

Cisapride	Liothyronine	Ranitidine
Domperidone	Metoclopramide	Sucralfate
Gemfibrozil	Propantheline	Trimethobenzamide
Glipizide		

Consistent = can be given to fed or fasted animals, but give in a consistent manner
Cyclosporine

Unknown = data were not available for recommendation
Acetylcysteine
*For no effects, although some of these drugs may have increased absorption in the fasted state, the clinical outcome may be unaffected.

plements, including iron salts such as ferrous sulfate, can decrease the absorption of methyldopa, penicillamine, tetracycline, levothyroxine and quinolone antibiotics (Roe, 1989; Campbell et al, 1992). When orbifloxacin was mixed with a vitamin-mineral supplement in vitro, within four days orbifloxacin concentration was decreased by about 50% of what was expected (KuKanich and Papich, 2003). Calcium salts and calcium-containing foods (e.g., milk, 1 to 2 mg calcium/ml) can precipitate insoluble tetracycline chelates (Williams et al, 1993). Foods of plant origin may contain phytic acid, which inhibits zinc and calcium absorption, and tannins, which inhibit iron uptake. Gelatinization of liquid drug formulations following mixing with enteral formulas has been observed for certain expectorants, elixirs, syrups, concentrates and suspensions.

The potential binding of pharmaceutical agents to equipment used for administration should also be considered. Adsorption of vitamin A and drugs such as phenytoin and insulin to plastic polymers used in nasogastric, gastrostomy and enterostomy tubing has been reported (Fleisher et al, 1990; Spence and Camishion, 1995). Furthermore, precipitation or gelatinization of drugs by nutrients can block feeding tubes. Diazepam binding to intravenous fluid lines is a good example of drugs binding to equipment (Parker and MacCara, 1980). Approximately 45% of diazepam will adsorb to fluid bags within two hours and about 48% of diazepam will bind to intravenous fluid lines during a constant rate infusion.

Physical Factors Affecting GI Absorption of Drugs

The cephalic phase of digestion is normally initiated by the perception, visualization, smell and taste of food. This phenomenon contributes to normal GI motility, secretion, digestion and absorption of food and pharmaceutical agents. For example, when acetaminophen is administered by nasogastric tube postoperatively, its absorption is significantly reduced compared with its absorption following oral administration (Elfant et al, 1992). Decreased GI motility due to stress, pain, luminal obstruction and postsurgical ileus may also contribute to reduced absorption.

Commercial moist and dry foods similarly affect gastric emptying; however, solid food may decrease the emptying of liquids and liquids may decrease the rate and pattern of solid emptying (Burrows et al, 1985; Horowitz et al, 1989). Specific dietary components that affect the rate of GI transit can also alter oral drug assimilation. In dogs, meals containing cellulose or wheat bran increase the frequency of postprandial contractions; yet, only cellulose decreases duodenojejunal flow and prolongs transit time (Bueno et al, 1981). However, bran increases mixing and onward propulsion of ingesta. Addition of guar gum induces continuous low-amplitude contractions in dogs and increases jejunal flow, but still increases transit time because of water adsorption and luminal distention. Soluble fibers (e.g., methylcellulose) increase luminal viscosity, resulting in delayed gastric emptying and increased thickness of the unstirred water layer (Reppas et al, 1991). Thus, both delivery of drug to the intestine and contact with the mucosal surface are impeded.

Addition of fat to a meal changes intragastric distribution of solid material, induces segmental changes in antral and pyloric

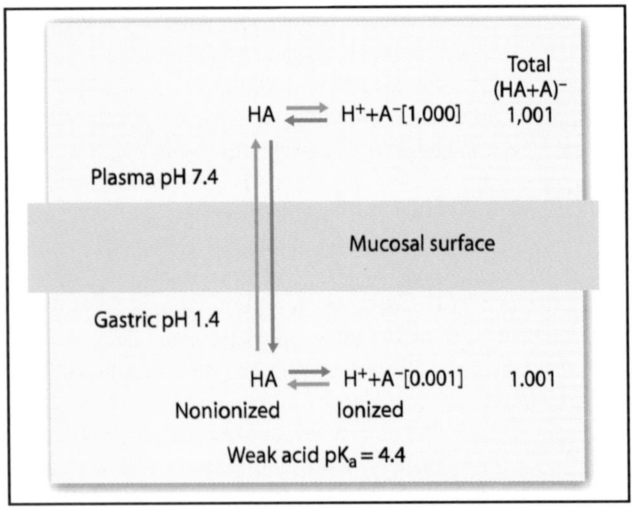

Figure 69-2. Influence of pH on the distribution of a weak acid between gastric contents and blood plasma across the gastric mucosa. The nonionized form of the drug predominates at low pH following gastric acid release. Only the nonionized form has sufficient lipid solubility to diffuse across the gastric mucosa. The ratio of ionized to nonionized drug may be calculated from the Henderson-Hasselbalch equation, and is determined by the pH on either side of the mucosa relative to the pKa of the drug. Dietary factors that increase or decrease gastric acid secretion will promote or inhibit acidic drug absorption. (Adapted from Benet LZ, Kroetz DL, Sheiner LB. The dynamics of drug absorption, distribution, and elimination. In: Hardman JA, Limbird LE, eds. Goodman and Gilman's The Pharmacological Basis of Therapeutics, 9th ed. New York, NY: McGraw-Hill, 1996.)

Table 69-4. Dietary factors that may affect drug metabolism and excretion, principally through induction of phase I biotransformation.

Macronutrients	**Micronutrients**	**Non-nutrients**
Protein	Vitamins	Antioxidants (BHA, BHT)
Carbohydrate	Minerals	Coumarins
Fat	Essential fatty acids	Flavonoids
Fiber		Indoles
		Methylxanthines
		Organonitriles
		Phenols
		Pyrolysis by-products
		Terpenoids

Examples of drugs whose metabolism and excretion is altered by these dietary factors

Acetaminophen	Morphine
Allopurinol	Oxazepam
Aminophylline	Penicillin
Cefoxitin	Pentobarbital
Chloramphenicol	Phenobarbital
Chloroquine	Phenytoin
Diazepam	Prednisolone
Estradiol	Propranolol
Hexobarbital	Theophylline
Isoniazid	Zoxazolamine
Meperidine	

motility and retards gastric emptying (Heddle et al, 1989). Intraduodenal instillation of dilute glucose solutions at a rate in excess of approximately 2 kcal (8.4 kJ)/min., regardless of tonicity, stimulates both phasic and tonic pyloric contractions, thereby inhibiting gastric emptying and delaying oral drug absorption. Propranolol and metoprolol are affected in this manner (Chow and Lalka, 1993; Heddle et al, 1988). Enterohepatic cycling of drugs (e.g., doxycycline) may be affected by rate of passage and by portal blood flow and hepatic metabolism.

Chemical Factors Affecting GI Absorption of Drugs

Beyond the effects of drug binding or precipitation, specific nutrients may compete for absorption by the intestinal mucosa. For instance, phenytoin absorption is impaired by concurrent administration of the B vitamins folic acid and pyridoxine (Roe, 1989). Concurrent food intake and particular food ingredients can alter gastric or intestinal pH, thereby altering drug dissolution, ionization and absorption. In addition to the effect of milk calcium content on tetracycline absorption, milk can increase gastric pH, inducing premature dissolution of enteric-coated tablets, resulting in gastric irritation, altered absorption or both.

Gastric acid secretion associated with food ingestion can assist in the dissolution and ionization of alkaline drugs. Gastric acid secretion, however, limits the rate of absorption of alkaline drugs, while promoting the absorption of dissolved, unionized acidic drugs (**Figure 69-2**). The subsequent release of bicarbonate-rich pancreatic secretions promotes ionization of acidic drugs, but facilitates absorption of dissolved, unionized alkaline drugs. Release of hydrochloric acid in the stomach typically leads to alkalinization of the blood and the postprandial "alkaline tide," establishing an ionization gradient that can affect diffusion of ionizable compounds across the GI mucosa.

By affecting the food's acidification potential, dietary cation-anion balance can alter mineral absorption and drug availability through changes in ionization. Concurrent consumption of fats can affect drug absorption, depending on the polarity and lipid solubility of the individual agent. For example, it has been well documented that lipid-soluble vitamins and the antifungal agent griseofulvin are better absorbed when taken with whole milk or a meal with fat. High-fat foods may promote the absorption of nitrofurantoin, chlorothiazide and riboflavin by delaying gastric emptying, which facilitates dissolution in the stomach before passage into the small intestine for uptake (Roe, 1989).

TRANSPORT FROM THE GI TRACT TO THE SITE OF ACTION OR METABOLISM

Dietary factors that affect blood flow will alter the rate of delivery of absorbed drugs to their site of action or metabolism. Dehydration not only may reduce GI blood flow and absorption, but may also reduce the absorbed drug's subsequent delivery to or removal from particular tissues. Hypovolemia and reduced tissue perfusion may result in target tissue concentrations below the effective concentration. Decreased blood flow may reduce hepatic extraction for metabolism and excretion. Decreased urine formation may increase drug accumulation and toxicity in various organs; aminoglycoside accumulation in the renal proximal tubules is an example. Other dietary ingredients may affect cardiac output (methylxanthines), renal blood flow (protein) or intestinal reperfusion following ischemia (antioxidants), thereby altering drug distribution.

Like many metabolites and hormones, drugs may be transported in the blood in free form or bound to plasma proteins. Thus, changes in nutritional status that affect plasma protein synthesis will likely affect drug binding and distribution. For example, hypoalbuminemia due to low dietary protein quantity or quality can affect the distribution of antibiotics, barbiturates, cardiac glycosides and analgesics. Drugs and nutrients may influence one another's disposition because binding to plasma proteins is competitive. Recent protein-binding interaction studies indicate that drug-drug competition for protein binding sites occurs rarely; the only drug expected to result in an adverse effect is lidocaine administered as an IV infusion (Benet and Hoener, 2002). However, hypoproteinemia may have marked effects that can result in toxicity due to increased free drug (e.g., lidocaine) or decreased efficacy (e.g., cefpodoxime) due to increased elimination by glomerular filtration (i.e., protein-bound drugs are excluded from glomerular filtration). High postprandial free fatty acid levels can displace anionic compounds from cationic binding sites on plasma proteins. Drugs and nutrients that are competitively transported into erythrocytes may be similarly affected. This effect has been documented for the interaction between folic acid and the loop diuretics furosemide and ethacrynic acid (Roe, 1989). Dietary factors that influence acid-base metabolism can alter blood pH and intraerythrocytic pH, thereby affecting drug ionization, protein binding and cell uptake.

DIETARY EFFECTS ON DRUG METABOLISM

The clearance of many drugs from the circulation depends on their biotransformation in the liver, kidneys and other organs with xenobiotic-metabolizing enzymes (**Table 69-4**) (Williams et al, 1993; Anderson and Kappas, 1991). For drugs that are metabolized rapidly, extraction is determined principally by organ blood flow. For example, the rate-limiting step for clearance of indocyanine green and sulfobromophthalein sodium is hepatic blood flow. Lidocaine and fentanyl are examples of currently used drugs, whereas sulfobromophthalein and indocyanine green are typically used for physiologic measurements. For drugs that are metabolized relatively slowly, clearance from the circulation is determined primarily by the quantity and affinity of enzymes responsible for their metabolism.

Hepatic drug metabolism occurs through two predominant biotransformation pathways: 1) phase I (oxidation, reduction and hydrolysis) and 2) phase II (glutathione or glucuronide conjugation, acetylation and sulfation). Phase I reactions are catalyzed principally by a family of cytochrome P-450 enzymes in the microsomal mixed-function oxidase system. Phase I reactions alter the functional groups of a compound (**Figure 69-3**). Phase I reactions increase water solubility. However, phase I reactions do not always alter functional groups (e.g., diazepam→nordiazepam, oxazepam). Furthermore, metabolism increases the conversion of prodrugs to active drugs (e.g., cyclophosphamide→4-hydroxyphosphamide→acrolein, phosphoramide mustard).

Phase II reactions are catalyzed by families of glutathione-S-transferase, glucuronyl transferase and N-acetyltransferase isoenzymes. Phase II reactions result in conjugation and altered water solubility (**Figure 69-4**). The outcome of phase I and II reactions is reduced activity and enhanced drug excretion. Phase I reactions may increase the activity or toxicity of drugs; phase II reactions may alter tissue distribution and subsequent target organs for toxicity or mutagenicity of the drug's metabolites (Guengerich, 1984; Parke and Ioannides, 1981).

Macronutrient Effects on Drug Metabolism

Inappetence due to disease is a common cause of decreased macronutrient intake that can affect drug action. Furthermore,

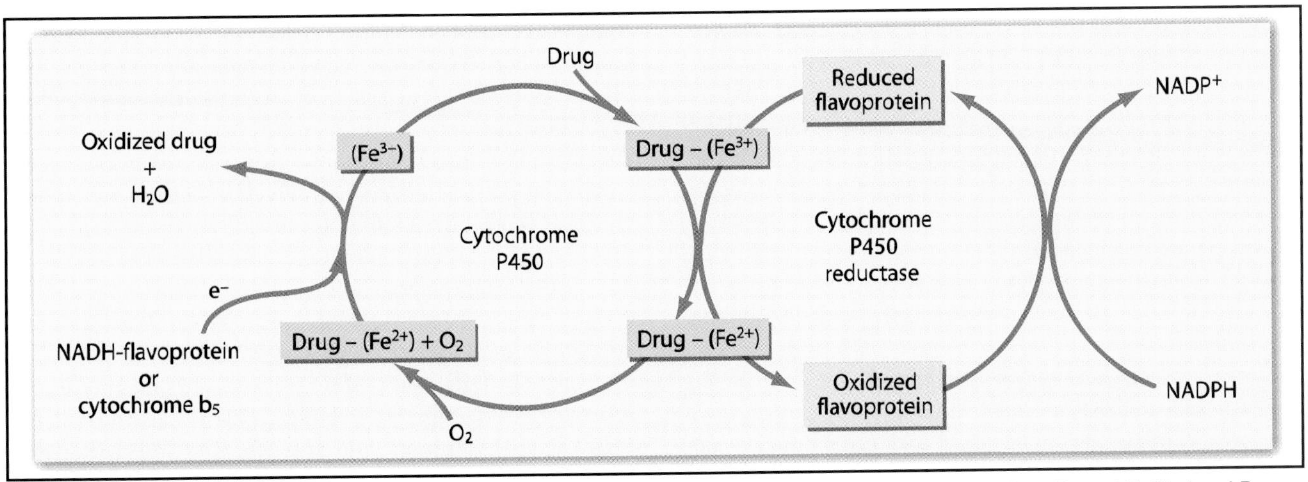

Figure 69-3. The hepatic phase I microsomal mixed-function oxidase system for drug metabolism. (Adapted from Benet LZ, Sheiner LB. Pharmacokinetics: The dynamics of drug absorption, distribution, and elimination. In: The Pharmacological Basis of Therapeutics, 7th ed. New York, NY: McGraw-Hill, 1985.) Key: Fe = iron, $NADP^+$ = the oxidized form of nicotinamide-adenine dinucleotide phosphate, NADPH = the reduced form of NADP.

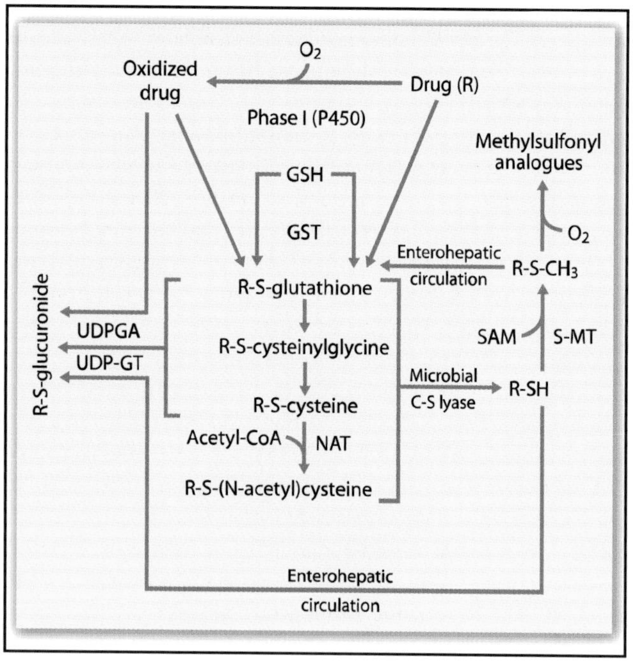

Figure 69-4. The hepatic phase II biotransformation system for drug metabolism. (Adapted from Fettman MJ, Butler RN, McMichael AJ, et al. Metabolic phenotypes and colorectal neoplasia. Journal of Gastroenterology and Hepatology 1991; 6: 81-90.) Key: P-450 = cytochrome P-450, GSH = reduced glutathione, GST = glutathione-S-transferase, acetyl-CoA = acetyl-coenzyme A, NAT = N-acetyltransferase, UDPGA = uridine diphosphoglucuronic acid, UDP-GT = UDP-glucuronyl transferase, SAM = adenosylmethionine, S-MT = S-methyltransferase.

changes in the macronutrient composition of the diet can significantly alter hepatic drug metabolism.

Dietary Protein Intake

In experimental studies in rats, low dietary protein intake reduced the metabolism and increased the toxicity of pentobarbital, strychnine and zoxazolamine (Guengerich, 1984). The activities of the mixed-function oxidase enzymes flavoprotein reductase and cytochrome b5 are decreased by dietary protein restriction. Inducibility of cytochrome P-450 by phenobarbital in rats is also decreased by feeding less dietary protein (Guengerich, 1995).

High-protein (e.g., 44 vs. 10% of kcal, as fed), low-carbohydrate foods (e.g., 35 vs. 70% of kcal, as fed) enhance the hepatic metabolism and excretion of many different drugs in people, including acetaminophen, oxazepam, theophylline, propranolol and estradiol (Guengerich, 1995; Fagan et al, 1987; Pantuck et al, 1991). Conversely, consumption of protein-restricted foods for as few as 10 days significantly decreases elimination of these drugs.

Certain essential amino acids may stimulate hepatic protein synthesis and thereby induce the hepatic mixed-function oxidase system. Sulfur-containing amino acids can promote hepatic drug metabolism by increasing glutathione synthesis and subsequent conjugation reactions (Fettman, 1991). Starvation can reduce the activity of glutathione-S-transferase and the synthesis of glutathione for conjugation; events that also participate in the development of fasting hyperbilirubinemia.

Dietary protein-related changes in renal blood flow and renal tubular transport can simultaneously affect the clearance of drugs eliminated in urine (Park et al, 1989). Increased dietary protein intake in dogs (from 9.4 to 27.3% on a dry matter basis) increases the elimination of gentamicin and reduces the potential for nephrotoxicity, presumably by stimulating renal blood flow (Behrend et al, 1994; Grauer et al, 1994). In people, low-protein diets (19 vs. 268 g/day) decrease the hepatic metabolism of allopurinol to oxypurinol, and decrease renal excretion of oxypurinol (Berlinger et al, 1985). The pharmacokinetics of allopurinol and oxypurinol in dogs do not appear to be affected by dietary protein (Bartges et al, 1997).

One canine study determined the effects of various foods on the pharmacokinetics of phenobarbital and the interactive effects of changes in body composition and metabolic rate (Maguire et al, 2000). Phenobarbital pharmacokinetic studies were performed in 27 healthy, adult, sexually intact female beagles before and two months after they were fed one of three commercially available foods: 1) a maintenance food, 2) a low-protein veterinary therapeutic food for renal failure patients or 3) a low-fat veterinary therapeutic food for weight loss. Phenobarbital, 3 mg/kg body weight orally, twice daily was administered to all three groups. Volume of distribution, mean residence time and half-life ($t_{1/2}$) decreased significantly, whereas clearance rate and elimination rate increased significantly with time in all groups. Dietary protein or fat restriction induced significantly greater changes: $t_{1/2}$ (hours) was lower in dogs fed the renal food (25.9 ± 6.1) and the weight-loss food (24.0 ± 4.7) compared to results from dogs fed the maintenance food (32.9 ± 5.2). Phenobarbital clearance rate (ml/kg/min.) was significantly higher in dogs fed the weight-loss food (0.22 ± 0.05) compared to clearance rates in dogs fed the maintenance food (0.17 ± 0.03) or the renal food (0.18 ± 0.03). Induction of serum alkaline phosphatase activity (IU/l) was greater in dogs fed the renal food (192.4 ± 47.5) and the weight-loss food (202.0 ± 98.2) than in dogs fed the maintenance food (125.0 ± 47.5). The authors concluded that phenobarbital dosage should be reevaluated if a dog's diet, body weight or body composition changes during treatment. Veterinarians in clinical practice, researchers evaluating drug pharmacokinetics (phenobarbital and other drugs) and pet food companies that market veterinary therapeutic foods with nutrient profiles that differ from typical commercial maintenance foods should be aware that a dietary change may markedly affect the pharmacokinetics of concurrent drug therapy.

Dietary Carbohydrate Intake

High carbohydrate intake (70 vs. 35% on a dry matter basis) in people depresses oxidative drug metabolism (Fagan et al, 1987). High dietary fructose, glucose and sucrose levels increase barbiturate sleeping time and decrease in vitro metabolism of barbiturates in mice (Guengerich, 1995). Parenteral glucose has the same effect in dogs and cats; thus, high dietary intake of these carbohydrates may likely modify barbiturate responses in these species as well. Supplemental carbohydrate administration in rats increases liver weight, hepatic fat and glycogen deposition, but decreases hepatic mixed-function oxidase activities. Carbohydrate feeding in rats can similarly decrease the microsomal activation of carcinogens such as benzo(a)pyrene and aflatoxin B_1.

In people, long-term consumption of 70 vs. 35% carbohydrate diets depresses antipyrine and theophylline clearance (Pantuck et al, 1991). The proposed mechanism involves inhibition of the synthesis of d-aminolevulinic acid synthetase, a key enzyme in the synthesis of heme for cytochrome P-450 (Pantuck et al, 1991). However, carbohydrate is also required for UDP-glucuronyl transferase activity for glucuronidation of oxidized drug metabolites; short-term deprivation of carbohydrates can decrease rates of conjugation. This, too, contributes to the hyperbilirubinemia of fasting.

Dietary Fat Intake

In addition to the effects of dietary fat intake on drug absorption and plasma protein binding, lipid intake can affect hepatic xenobiotic-metabolizing enzyme activities (Guengerich, 1995). Foods deficient in essential fatty acids result in decreased rates of drug metabolism. Dietary lipids have been reported to be essential for optimal induction of P-450 enzymes by phenobarbital. Rats fed a 20% corn-oil diet for four days had twofold increases in the activities of several hepatic P-450 isoenzymes (P-450 2, 2A1, 2B1, 2C11, 2E1 and 3A) as compared with enzyme activities in rats fed a fat-free diet (Yoo et al, 1992). However, there is an inverse relationship between lung P-450 2B1 activity and dietary fat intake. In one study in which rats were fed 6% dietary lipid for 40 days as coconut, peanut, corn or fish oil, cytochrome P-450 and epoxide hydrolase activities were highest in the fish-oil group (Mounie et al, 1986). In this same study, UDP-glucuronyl transferase type I activity was increased by fish-oil or corn-oil supplementation, but reduced by coconut oil.

In another study, rats fed 10% dietary lipid for two weeks as soybean oil, lard or fish oil were exposed to pentachlorobenzene (PECB). Blood concentrations of the metabolite pentachlorophenol were highest and tissue concentrations of PECB were lowest after feeding fish oil (Umegaki et al, 1995).

Fish oils are relatively high in polyunsaturated fatty acids, particularly of the omega-3 (n-3) family (eicosapentaenoic and docosahexaenoic acids), but contain relatively less omega-6 (n-6) fatty acids than other sources. Effects of fish-oil supplementation may be due to: 1) altered cell and organelle membrane fluidity, 2) increased propensity towards oxidative damage and/or 3) specific induction of enzyme synthesis. In people, the degree of dietary fatty acid saturation has had little effect on oxidation of antipyrine or theophylline; however, the principal cytochrome P-450 isoenzyme, 3A4, is sensitive to microsomal membrane characteristics (Guengerich, 1995). A dietary deficiency of labile methyl donors (e.g., choline or methionine) increases spontaneous and chemically induced hepatocarcinogenesis in rats because of decreased microsomal enzyme activity (Rogers, 1995). Lipotrope deficiency also impairs methylation of DNA and RNA; however, a considerable portion of microsomal lipid can be removed in vitro without adversely affecting P-450 activity.

Dietary fat restriction alters phenobarbital pharmacokinetics in dogs, as discussed in more detail in the Dietary Protein Intake section (above). Restriction of dietary fat resulted in a significantly shorter phenobarbital half-life, a significantly higher phenobarbital clearance rate and an increased induction of alkaline phosphatase activity vs. the fat levels in the control, maintenance type food (Maguire et al, 2000).

Effects of Feeding Route

The route of nutrient administration may also affect hepatic drug metabolism. Decreased hepatic clearance of indocyanine green in pigs fasted for 12 days returns to normal after enteral feeding for 12 days (Waters et al, 1994). However, intravenous feeding with an identical formula did not improve hepatic clearance despite similar weight gains. Hepatic hydroxylation of pentobarbital and demethylation of meperidine by rats are significantly impaired following seven days of parenteral feeding with a formula that otherwise maintains hepatic drug clearance when administered enterally (Knodell et al, 1984). Lipid-free total parenteral nutrition depresses hepatic phase I and II drug metabolism. Parenteral lipid-free nutrition for 10 days in rats decreased the hepatic activities of cytochrome P-450 oxidase, p-nitroanisole demethylase and p-nitrophenol glutathione-S-transferase by one-half (Raftogianis et al, 1995). Thus, the intake of macronutrients, composition of the food and route of nutritional support interact to modify drug metabolism.

Micronutrient Effects on Drug Metabolism

Dietary Vitamin Intake

The hepatic mixed-function oxidase system requires several vitamins (Anderson and Kappas, 1991; Yang et al, 1992). Niacin and riboflavin participate directly as the principal components of the electron carriers $NADP^+$, NAD^+, FAD and FMN, which are coenzymes for cytochrome P-450 reductase, DT-diaphorase and NADH-cytochrome b_5 reductase (Anderson and Kappas, 1991). Dietary deficiency can lead to a generalized decrease in total P-450 and associated monooxygenase activities (Guengerich, 1984; Catz et al, 1970).

Folate deficiency blocks the induction of cytochrome P-450 by phenobarbital, and pyridoxine (vitamin B_6) deficiency may alter cysteine conjugate β-lyase activity (Guengerich, 1984). Excessive dietary folate can antagonize methotrexate activity, whereas increased pyridoxine intake can increase the metabolism of levodopa, thereby reducing its effectiveness. Thiamin deficiency increases the levels of cytochrome P-450 2E1, NADH-P-450 reductase and cytochrome b5, but decreases the oxidation of N-nitrosodimethylamine, acetaminophen, aminopyrine, ethylmorphine, zoxazolamine and benzo(a)pyrene (Anderson and Kappas, 1991).

The antioxidant vitamins (A, C and E) are required for normal membrane synthesis and stability. Vitamin A deficiency decreases hepatic mixed-function oxidase system activity and depresses oxidation of aminopyrine, ethylmorphine, aniline, benzo(a)pyrene and 7-ethoxycoumarin (Anderson and Kappas, 1991). Vitamin C deficiency decreases NADPH-P-450 reductase activity and prolongs the half-life of antipyrine, acetaminophen and salicylamide. Vitamin E deficiency decreases microsomal metabolism of ethylmorphine, codeine and benzo(a)pyrene (Anderson and Kappas, 1991). Effects of vitamin E deficiency occur without decreases in cytochrome P-450 activity, and probably relate to the antioxidant properties of tocopherol, which may prevent oxidative damage to membrane lipids. Vitamins A and D are substrates for cytochrome P-450 and can competitively block the metabolism of other P-450 substrates.

Dietary Mineral Intake

Many minerals modulate hepatic drug metabolism. Iron is required for heme synthesis in cytochromes and for metal ion-catalyzed oxidative reactions (Parke and Ioannides, 1981). Iron deficiency results in decreased metabolism of hexobarbital and aminopyrine (Anderson and Kappas, 1991). Selenium is a cofactor for glutathione peroxidase; selenium deficiency may promote oxidative damage to the microsomal system. Hypothyroidism resulting from iodide deficiency increases flavoprotein synthesis and cytochrome P-450 oxidative activity (Danforth and Burger, 1989). Deficiencies of zinc, magnesium and potassium decrease drug metabolism, whereas high concentrations of metals (e.g., cobalt and cadmium) may block heme synthesis and thereby lower cytochrome P-450 levels (Anderson and Kappas, 1991).

Non-Nutrient Effects on Drug Metabolism

Non-nutrient dietary factors can profoundly influence drug metabolism by inducing the activity of many hepatic biotransformation enzymes (Guengerich, 1995). Phenols (e.g., hydroxycinnamic, dihydroxycinnamic and ferulic acids) are antioxidants that block chemical carcinogenesis. Methylxanthines, including caffeine, theobromine and theophylline, competitively bind to cytochrome P-450 to block oxidation of other compounds. Coumarin derivatives in vegetables and fruits induce glutathione-S-transferase activity. Organonitriles (1-cyano-2-hydroxy-3-butene, 1-cyano-3,4-epithiobutane) and indole derivatives (indole-3-carbinol, 3,3'-diindolmethane, indole-3-acetonitrile) in cruciferous plants (e.g., broccoli, cauliflower and cabbage) increase hepatic and renal glutathione concentrations and induce hepatic and renal glutathione-S-transferase activities (Fettman, 1991).

Excessive organonitrile exposure induces hepatic and renal toxicity, which may impair drug metabolism, whereas small amounts may have anti-carcinogenic properties (Guengerich, 1995; Fettman, 1991). Flavonoids and terpenoids from citrus fruits can either induce or block cytochrome P-450-related oxidative reactions, and can exert mutagenic or anti-tumorigenic effects, depending on the dose administered (Guengerich, 1995). Flavonoids in grapefruit juice can significantly prolong the half-life of dihydropyridine calcium channel blockers (e.g., nifedipine, felodipine and nisoldipine) and inhibit the metabolism of cyclosporin. St. John's wort is a potent inhibitor of cytochrome P-450 3 families (CYP3A); therefore, it can inhibit metabolism, cause toxicity or lead to decreased efficacy.

Butylated hydroxytoluene (BHT) and butylated hydroxyanisole (BHA) are added to certain processed food products to inhibit lipid oxidation (Guengerich, 1995). These food additives competitively inhibit cytochrome P-450-related oxidases, but induce other enzymes, including glutathione-S-transferase, glucuronyl transferase, DT-diaphorase and quinone reductase. In some experimental systems, they have demonstrated anticarcinogenic properties, presumably by blocking activation of chemical carcinogens (DeLong et al, 1985). In other systems, a hydroperoxide derivative has been shown to have a tumor-promoting effect (Guyton et al, 1991). Polycyclic hydrocarbons and related pyrolysis products of charbroiling are reported to increase cytochrome P-450 oxidase activities and to increase the clearance of such drugs as theophylline, bufuralol, acetaminophen, tacrine and warfarin (Guengerich, 1995). Induction of cytochrome P-450 hydroxylase can lead to activation of arylamine and heterocyclic amines, which are also consumed with food, and have been linked to stimulation of carcinogenesis.

DIETARY EFFECTS ON DRUG EXCRETION

Following P-450 hydroxylation, heterocyclic amines may subsequently undergo N-acetylation, the metabolic phenotype and activity of which affects the organ and route of excretion of the metabolite (Fettman et al, 1991). If there is "slow" N-acetyltransferase activity, most of the hydroxylated amine undergoes hepatic glucuronidation and is returned to the blood for excretion in the urine. In people, so called "slow acetylators" are predisposed to urinary bladder cancer. Those individuals with "fast" N-acetyltransferase activity appear to be predisposed to colorectal cancer, presumably through preferential colonocytic metabolism to mutagenic arylamides and acetoxyarylamines. Thus, metabolic phenotype as determined by genetics, or from enzyme induction due to dietary effects, can influence the site, route and rate of drug excretion. In veterinary patients, dogs are poor acetylators whereas cats are good acetylators.

Because many of the drugs excreted by the kidneys undergo active transport by anion- or cation-specific mechanisms in the renal tubular epithelium, their elimination can be altered through competitive inhibition by other charged solutes. Pharmacologically, this effect has been purposely employed by the co-administration of probenecid with penicillins to block elimination by the anion-specific renal tubular transport mechanism. Nutritionally, this effect may result from consumption of divalent cations (e.g., calcium and magnesium), which decreases renal tubular transport and accumulation of aminoglycosides such as gentamicin (Brinker et al, 1981; Quarum et al, 1984; Schumacher et al, 1991; Wong et al, 1989). As a result, urinary elimination of the antibiotic is increased and nephrotoxicity thereby reduced.

Furthermore, dietary alterations in urinary pH can affect the ionization and trapping of drugs secreted into the tubular lumina. The relatively common practice of formulating commercial feline foods to promote urinary acidification in the prevention and treatment of lower urinary tract diseases (e.g., struvite crystalluria and urolithiasis) may also affect the elimination of pharmaceutical agents excreted in the urine (Fettman et al, 1992). Examples include ion trapping in urine as a treatment for aspirin (salicylate) and amphetamine toxicities. Urine alkalinization increases the elimination of aspirin and urine acidification increases the elimination of amphetamine. However, acid/alkaline changes for these treatments typically occur through fluid and fluid supplementation.

Food ingredients that stimulate bile, fecal or urine flow may affect the excretion of drugs by these routes. For example, dietary fats with choleretic properties will enhance the excretion of drug metabolites in the bile and the return of enterohepatically recycled drugs such as doxycycline. Salts of divalent cations (e.g., magnesium oxide and magnesium hydroxide) can exert a laxative effect that may increase fecal elimination of poorly absorbed oral drugs and enterohepatically recycled drugs. High dietary salt content and other naturally occurring diuretics, including active loop diuretics, can enhance the excretion of drugs and their metabolites in urine.

Table 69-5. Examples of the effects of nutrients on drug action.

Beneficial effects	**Examples**
Enhanced GI drug absorption	Fatty foods enhance absorption of griseofulvin
Prevention of undesirable drug effects	Foods minimize nausea induced by metronidazole
Enhancement of desirable drug effects	Water enhances laxative effects of psyllium
Improved drug metabolism	Enteral feeding supports metabolism of cefoxitin
Altered drug excretion	Protein promotes renal excretion of gentamicin
Detrimental effects	**Examples**
Impaired GI drug absorption	Food interferes with absorption of ampicillin
Antagonism of desirable drug effects	Folate opposes chemotherapeutic effects of methotrexate
	Increased plasma potassium decreases digoxin activity
Potentiation of undesirable drug effects	Potassium increases potential toxicity of captopril
	Decreased plasma potassium increases digoxin activity
Impaired drug metabolism	Fish oil enhances hepatic oxidation of phenobarbital
Altered drug excretion	Calcium increases urinary excretion of gentamicin
	High-chloride diets increase bromide clearance and decrease its half-life

BENEFICIAL EFFECTS OF NUTRIENTS ON DRUG ACTION

The presence of food need not impair drug absorption, and within limits may be indicated to facilitate safe GI uptake of drugs (**Table 69-3**). Food may prevent GI irritation, modify drug-induced nausea or delay drug uptake, increasing the ultimate amount of drug absorbed (**Table 69-5**). For example, food can promote gastric acid secretion to enhance the uptake of an acidic drug such as aspirin while simultaneously protecting the mucosa from irritation by the drug.

Consumption of food can minimize nausea induced by the concurrent administration of hypertonic salt and carbohydrate solutions. In people, micronized preparations of phenytoin are actually better absorbed in the fed rather than the fasted state (Fleisher et al, 1990). In other cases, dietary supplementation with a specific nutrient may be indicated to counteract adverse drug side effects, to prevent drug-induced nutrient imbalances or to potentiate therapeutic effects.

Provision of Nutrients to Prevent Drug-Induced Imbalances

Additional energy and protein may be indicated to combat alterations in drug metabolism associated with prolonged decreases in food intake. A critical example would be the provision of nutrients during enteral- or parenteral-assisted feeding of patients incapable of voluntary food consumption. Effects of individual nutrient deficiencies have already been described. In addition, studies of prolonged starvation and of kwashiorkor in people have demonstrated significant reductions in the metabolism of numerous drugs by phase I and phase II hepatic biotransformation systems (Guengerich, 1995). These drugs include chloroquine, isoniazid, penicillin, chloramphenicol, tobramycin and cefoxitin. In addition, hypoalbuminemia-related decreases in drug binding alter the clearance of cloxacillin, streptomycin, sulfamethoxazole, sulfadiazine, digoxin, thiopental and phenylbutazone (Roe, 1989). Malnutrition-related decreases in renal blood flow and glomerular filtration rate have caused gentamicin toxicity.

Most commercial pet foods are adequately fortified with micronutrients; therefore, supplementation is not necessary unless a homemade food is fed, nutrient intake is decreased or a specific medical indication for prescription of a nutrient as a "neutraceutical" exists. Vitamin supplementation may be indicated to counteract the effects of drugs that specifically antagonize vitamin absorption or function. These include: 1) the use of folacin to manage deficiency induced by folic acid antagonists such as methotrexate, 2) vitamin K vs. antagonists in the coumarin family, 3) tocopherol, retinol and/or ascorbic acid to counter losses due to oxidative drug damage, 4) cholecalciferol for deficiency induced by anticonvulsants such as phenytoin, 5) thiamin to replace that lost to thiaminase activity in raw fish and 6) B vitamins to replace those lost following antibiotic-induced alterations in the GI microflora.

Specific minerals may also become deficient because of binding or precipitation in the GI tract, or following enhanced fecal losses due to laxatives or urinary loss due to diuretics. Urinary electrolyte losses due to loop diuretics can lead to significant physiologic abnormalities. Trace elements such as zinc may bind to fiber or be precipitated by phytates. Oral calcium supplements may block iron absorption. Excessive use of antacids, laxatives and binding resins can result in macroelement deficiencies.

Glutathione precursors (e.g., cysteine or N-acetylcysteine) may be indicated to counter the oxidative damage induced by pharmaceutical agents such as the: 1) analgesic acetaminophen (e.g., S-adenosyl-L-methionine [SAMe] is recommended for oxidative damage in cats caused by acetaminophen as well as hepatotoxicity due to other origins, although definitive efficacy is lacking), 2) urinary antiseptic methylene blue, 3) injectable anesthetic propofol and 4) antitumor agent doxorubicin (Fettman, 1991; Webb et al, 2003). Oxidative damage resulting from administration of oxidized lipid supplements or excessive use of omega-3 fatty acid sources may also necessitate treatment with glutathione precursors or antioxidant vitamins.

Provision of additional water may be indicated for the prevention or treatment of renal damage resulting from nephrotoxic drug administration. Examples of drugs whose administration should routinely be coupled to increased water intake include cisplatin, aminoglycosides, nonsteroidal antiinflammatory drugs, analgesics and diuretics.

Provision of Nutrients to Enhance Drug Effects

Certain nutrients may be prescribed to facilitate a drug's intended effect or to synergistically promote the target physiologic functions. Additional energy or protein can generally facilitate therapeutic drug effects by promoting optimal distribution and hepatic biotransformation activities. These additions will tend to normalize pharmacokinetics to ensure the individual patient's dose response may more closely approximate the anticipated response.

Providing adequate energy and protein to patients receiving exogenous thyroid hormones plays an integral role in the physiologic response to that supplementation (Danforth and Burger, 1989). Undernutrition may result in reduced synthesis of thyroid-binding plasma proteins and subsequent changes in thyroid pharmacokinetics. Reductions in energy or protein intake suppress target tissue monodeiodination of thyroxine to the physiologically active triiodothyronine. Triiodothyronine levels decrease within 24 hours of fasting or caloric restriction, and may decline by 40 to 50% within three days. Should fasting induce increased adrenal glucocorticoid secretion, depressed target tissue triiodothyronine receptor levels may also be observed. Although these reductions in target-cell responsiveness to thyroid hormones represent an appropriate adaptation to conserve energy during starvation, the effect on exogenous thyroid hormone pharmacotherapy may be undesirable.

It is important to maintain a regular feeding schedule and consistent food for animals with diabetes mellitus to stabilize intermediary metabolism. The administration of exogenous insulin to insulin-dependent diabetics and the administration of oral hypoglycemic agents to non-insulin-dependent diabetics should be timed relative to feeding. For both forms of diabetes mellitus, specific dietary formulations are indicated to: 1) modulate GI carbohydrate uptake, 2) meet protein requirements without adversely affecting renal function and 3) moderate overall lipid metabolism to prevent ketoacidosis (Chapter 29).

Dietary intake of specific minerals that modulate hormonal axes should be considered, including calcium and phosphorus intake when cholecalciferol is administered for chronic renal failure, and sodium and potassium when mineralocorticoids are replaced in hypoadrenocorticism. The trace minerals chromium and vanadium may improve glucose tolerance and facilitate management of diabetics with insulin or oral hypoglycemic agents (Anderson et al, 1991; Boden et al, 1996). Specific omega-3 fatty acid therapy may be used to potentiate the effects of antiinflammatory drugs, anticoagulants and antineoplastic agents (Meydani, 1996). Arginine may be provided to improve nitric oxide production and to enhance immune function (Kirk and Barbul, 1990), glutamine to promote enterocyte metabolism (Hall et al, 1996), cysteine to enhance glutathione synthesis (Sellke et al, 1991), carnitine to improve digoxin responsiveness in congestive heart failure (Pepine, 1991) and antioxidant vitamins to protect against oxidative damage.

Dietary fiber may be indicated along with drug therapy for a number of diseases. Increased dietary fiber intake has proved beneficial in the treatment of insulin-dependent and non-insulin-dependent diabetes mellitus by moderating glucose absorption from the GI tract. Fermentable dietary fiber increases colonic short-chain fatty acid concentrations and decreases luminal pH. As a result, these fibers may be used as the primary treatment for canine and feline colitis or as an ancillary therapy to sulfasalazine or metronidazole treatment. Soluble fibers (e.g., psyllium mucilloid) may act in this way in conjunction with other antidiarrheal treatments, or as stool softeners for use with laxatives to treat constipation (Fettman, 1992). Hepatic cytochrome P-450 concentrations and UDP-glucuronyl transferase activities appear to be altered by the type and quantity of fiber in the food (Nugon-Boudon et al, 1996).

Dietary buffers may be indicated in conjunction with other therapies for chronic renal failure to correct metabolic acidosis or to facilitate activity of replacement pancreatic enzymes in exocrine pancreatic disease. They may be used to enhance alkaline drug absorption from the GI tract and to promote acidic drug excretion in the urine. Alkalinization of the urine has been used clinically to reduce the ionization, renal accumulation and toxicity of aminoglycosides (Brown and Riviere, 1991). Finally, buffers (e.g., sodium bicarbonate, aluminum hydroxide) can be used with H_2-receptor antagonists (e.g., cimetidine, ranitidine) or as laxatives (e.g., magnesium oxide, magnesium hydroxide).

ADVERSE EFFECTS OF NUTRIENTS ON DRUG ACTION

In addition to ameliorating undesirable effects on drug absorption or metabolism, specific nutrients may antagonize desired drug effects (**Table 69-5**). Excess caloric intake will complicate weight management in obese patients. Excess protein intake can adversely affect renal handling of drugs by increasing renal blood flow and drug excretion, or by promoting intraglomerular hypertension and reducing glomerular filtration in chronic renal failure. High protein intake can increase the hepatic metabolism of drugs such as the methylxanthines, resulting in reduced therapeutic efficacy.

High mineral intake can complicate drug therapy of specific disorders: 1) sodium and hypertension, 2) potassium and hypoadrenocorticism, 3) magnesium and feline lower urinary tract disease and 4) phosphorus and chronic renal failure.

Excessive dietary intake of iodine can lead to a paradoxical "iodine toxicosis goiter" through what is referred to as the "Wolff-Chaikoff effect." As iodide accumulation by the thyroid gland increases, so does iodination of tyrosyl residues of thyroglobulin. However, very high iodine levels appear to cause auto-inhibition of iodide organification and thyroglobulin proteolysis, leading to thyroid hormone deficiency. This phenomenon has been observed in foals born to mares that received excessive iodine supplementation during gestation, as well as in other species (Drew et al, 1975; Driscoll et al, 1978).

Naturally occurring non-nutritive dietary factors that may influence drug responses include methylxanthines, which may complicate aminophylline therapy, histamine in certain types of fish, which may interfere with antihistamine treatment and tyramine in chicken livers and aged cheeses, which confound the action of monoamine oxidase inhibitors. Alcohols and antioxidants added to certain nutrient sources as preservatives and humectants may have adverse effects as well. Benzoic acid and benzoyl alcohol in commercial fluid and drug preparations, propylene glycol in semi-moist commercial cat food and onion powder in commercial human baby foods may induce oxidative erythrocyte damage and Heinz body anemia in cats (Bedford and Clarke, 1971; Wilkie and Kirby, 1988; Christopher et al, 1989; Kaplan, 1995). These substances are no longer commonly used in commercial product manufacturing.

EFFECTS OF OBESITY ON DRUG DISPOSITION

Although complicated by the metabolic effects of overnutrition during weight gain or restricted food intake during weight loss, numerous studies have documented a significant effect of obesity on drug metabolism in people and other animals (Reidenberg, 1977). Changes in the apparent volume of distribution have been observed because of alterations in the quantity of body fat. Obesity increases the volume distribution of lipophilic drugs such as alprazolam, carbamazepine, diazepam, methotrexate, oxazepam, sufentanil and vancomycin. Increased volume distribution for lipophilic drugs (e.g., thiobarbiturates) necessitates administration of a higher dose to achieve the desired clinical response. Sequestration in body fat may prolong the drug's action. Obesity decreases the volume distribution of polar compounds including acetaminophen, ciprofloxacin, furosemide, gentamicin, isoniazid, sulfisoxazole and tolbutamide (Ducharme et al, 1994; Dunn et al, 1991; Caraco et al, 1992; Abernethy et al, 1984; Shum and Jusko, 1984; Yuk et al, 1988; Fleming et al, 1991; Schwartz et al, 1991; Allard et al, 1993).

Drug clearance may be affected following changes in hepatic microsomal enzyme induction, as well as alterations in the predominant pathways used for phase II conjugation reactions. Several investigations have demonstrated enhanced biotransformation of volatile anesthetics in obese patients, resulting in increased production of the reactive intermediates typically responsible for organ toxicity (Bentley et al, 1982). Enhanced hepatic oxidative metabolism of halothane in obese people has resulted in increased serum levels of fluoride and bromide ions; the former is associated with increased hepatotoxicity. Half-life elimination of triazolam is prolonged in obese subjects, and clearance following oral administration is reduced, presumably because of decreases in hepatic extraction.

Drug toxicity may be enhanced when the dose administered is based on total body mass, but distribution is restricted to lean body mass, resulting in higher plasma drug concentrations and greater exposure to susceptible organs (Corcoran et al, 1989; Corcoran and Salazar, 1989). Obese rats appear to be at increased risk for gentamicin and furosemide nephrotoxicity by this mechanism (Corcoran et al, 1989; Corcoran and Salazar, 1989). Susceptibility to the toxic affects of these drugs remains even when the dose is decreased to reflect lean body mass and to equalize drug exposure. Studies of acetaminophen toxicity in rats have shown that when obese animals are dosed according to fat-free mass, toxicity is increased because of a metabolic shift toward less sulfation and more glucuronidation (Corcoran and Wong, 1987). Obesity likewise appears to increase drug glucuronidation in people. Furthermore, target organs may be predisposed to drug toxicity by pre-existing obesity-related lesions such as hepatic lipidosis.

Obesity increases steroid hormone clearance in people because of enhanced aromatization and interconversion of androgens to estrogens by adipose tissue (Dunn et al, 1991). Prednisolone and methylprednisolone succinate clearance in obese people is also increased, although potential contributions by increased cardiac output, hepatic blood flow, liver size and hydrolysis by extrahepatic carboxyesterases have not been resolved. On the other hand, methylprednisolone clearance appears to be decreased, suggesting that obesity may affect specific oxidative pathways very differently (Dunn et al, 1991).

Although similar studies have not been conducted in companion animals, certain generalizations can be made. Obesity will result in changes in the effective dose administered for drugs given according to total body weight, whether it is increased because of poor lipid solubility or decreased because of lipophilicity. Drug dose or dosing interval may need to be adjusted to maintain therapeutic effect and protect against toxicity. Alterations in body composition concurrent with drug administration may have significant effects on clinical efficacy and margin of safety, and must be considered whenever a patient's body weight changes markedly (Caraco et al, 1992).

SUMMARY

Quantitatively and qualitatively, ingested nutrients have major effects on the biologic activity of pharmacologic agents. This is true not just for orally administered drugs in the GI tract, but also for drugs administered parenterally. Ingested nutrients may modify hepatic and renal metabolic processes, thus altering the action of parenterally administered drugs. Inappetence associated with many chronic diseases may significantly modify drug absorption, metabolism and action.

Specific macronutrients and micronutrients not only support normal physiologic processes necessary for drug delivery and action, but may also modify specific metabolic processes integral to drug activity. For instance, dietary protein must be sufficient to ensure adequate plasma protein synthesis and maintenance of plasma volume for the delivery and action of most systemically administered drugs. Dietary protein may also specifically affect the hepatic metabolism of some drugs, the renal elimination of others and the modification by target tissues of yet others. Specific amino acids can play a role in drug metabolism and action as well. Food is a major modulator of drug activity and food-drug interrelationships must be considered when designing treatment regimens.

Because few studies to determine the effects of food on drug metabolism have been conducted in dogs and cats, it is difficult to delineate specific feeding recommendations for drugs commonly used in veterinary practice. However, it is important to consider potential nutrient-drug interactions whenever the expected action of a prescribed drug is not seen in an individual patient. One may alter the dosing schedule relative to meals or adjust the dietary composition or dose to correct overt nutrient imbalances. Alternatively, one may determine circulating drug concentrations to detect changes in pharmacokinetics and to establish the need for a change in drug type or dose. It is clear that a standardized food, consistent feeding schedule and balanced nutrient intake are prerequisites to successful pharmacologic management of disease.

FOR MORE INFORMATION

See Chapters 25 and 26 for lists of drugs that may affect taste and smell perception, stimulate appetite, are incompatible with B-complex vitamins and are compatible with total nutrient admixtures.

REFERENCES

The references for **Chapter 69** can be found at www.markmorris.org.

CASE 69-1

Epilepsy in a Dachshund

Lauren Trepanier, DVM, Dipl. ACVIM (Internal Medicine)
School of Veterinary Medicine
University of Wisconsin-Madison
Madison, Wisconsin, USA

Patient Assessment

An 11-year-old, neutered female dachshund weighing 10 kg was presented for evaluation of poorly controlled seizures. Idiopathic epilepsy had been diagnosed when the dog was six months old. The dog had received phenobarbital, phenytoin or a combination of both drugs for the past nine years. During the past few months, the dog had been having clusters of seizures each month, despite treatment with phenobarbital. Trough serum phenobarbital concentrations (20.4 µg/ml) were within the therapeutic range (15 to 45 µg/ml).

The results of physical and neurologic examinations were normal. The dog's body condition was 3/5. Serum biochemistry analysis revealed increases in liver enzyme activity (alkaline phosphatase, gamma-glutamyl transferase) and abnormal pre- and postprandial bile acid concentrations. Abdominal ultrasonography revealed mild hepatomegaly with normal hepatic echogenicity. Two small cystic calculi were evident in the urinary bladder.

The presumptive diagnosis was subclinical anticonvulsant-associated hepatopathy. Treatment was initiated with another anticonvulsant, potassium bromide (20 mg/kg body weight, per os, q24h), to control the seizures and allow the dose of phenobarbital to be reduced. The dog had no seizures during the two months after initiation of potassium bromide treatment. Serum bromide concentration had reached 1,100 mg/l (therapeutic range 1,000 to 2,000 mg/l). Alkaline phosphatase and gamma-glutamyl transferase activities had decreased markedly.

On re-examination one month later, the dog was still free from seizures, but had persistent cystic calculi. In the past, the dog had been treated for recurrent struvite crystalluria and cystic calculi with antibiotics and a veterinary therapeutic food. A struvite calculolytic food (Prescription Diet s/d Canine[a]) and antibiotic (Clavamox[b]) were prescribed. Two weeks later, the dog had a cluster of five seizures over a 36-hour period.

Assess the Food and Feeding Method

For the past three years, the dog had been fed a moist veterinary therapeutic food (Prescription Diet c/d Canine[a]) that contains reduced levels of struvite precursor substances and produces an acidic urinary pH. These nutritional characteristics help keep struvite crystalluria and urolithiasis from recurring. Because of the recurrent cystic calculi, the food was changed two weeks ago to a moist veterinary therapeutic food (Prescription Diet s/d Canine[a]) shown to help dissolve struvite uroliths. Nutrient profiles of the two foods are summarized in **Table 1**.

Questions

1. What potential food-drug interactions could be causing the recent increased seizure activity in this dog?
2. What other diagnostic tests should be performed in this patient?
3. How should the treatment and feeding plan be modified?

Answers and Discussion

1. The most likely food-drug interaction in this dog is between the potassium bromide anticonvulsant and the dietary chloride load. Bromide is excreted slowly, but almost exclusively by the kidneys. The amount of bromide excreted depends on the total body halide (i.e., fluorine, chlorine, bromine, iodine) concentration. Bromide and chloride compete for renal tubular reabsorption. An increase in chloride load, in the form of dietary sodium chloride or ammonium chloride, will markedly increase urinary excretion of bromide in several species, including dogs. In addition, high-chloride foods fed experimentally to dogs will significantly shorten the elimination half-life of bromide and lead to decreases in serum bromide concentrations. The veterinary therapeutic food being fed to the dog to help dissolve the cystic uroliths contains increased levels of sodium chloride to increase urine volume thereby decreasing the concentration of struvite-forming constituents in the urine.
2. Serum bromide concentrations can be measured to determine whether therapeutic levels are being maintained. In this patient, the serum bromide concentration the day after the seizures was 410 mg/l, which was much lower than the concentration measured one month earlier (1,100 mg/l) and below the normal therapeutic range (1,000 to 2,000 mg/l). The anticonvulsant dosage or formulation had not been changed, and the owner was adamant that doses of potassium bromide had not been missed.
3. Because high chloride intake enhances bromide elimination and may have reduced the serum bromide concentration, the owner was instructed to discontinue feeding the moist calculolytic food and to resume feeding the moist struvite-preventive food, with the lower chloride content. The dog was fed to maintain a weight of 10 kg (520 kcal [2.18 MJ]; 1.1 cans/day).

   Seven weeks after being fed the lower chloride food again and with daily potassium bromide treatment (20 mg/kg body weight), the dog's serum bromide concentration was 990 mg/l. If a change to a higher chloride food or a food of unknown chloride content is necessary, serum bromide concentrations should be monitored frequently during the weeks to months after the dietary change, and the dosage of potassium bromide should be adjusted as needed to maintain therapeutic bromide concentrations. Eradication of urinary tract infection and monitoring urinary pH to ensure that the urine is continuously acidic are required for successful treatment and prevention of struvite urolithiasis. Serial radiographs and urinalyses should be performed to monitor the cystic uroliths. Surgical removal of uroliths may be indicated if they persist, increase in size or cause clinical problems.

Table 1. Nutrient profiles of veterinary therapeutic foods fed to the patient.

Nutrient (% DM)	c/d Canine, canned[a]	s/d Canine, canned[a]
Protein	23.6	7.9
Fat	24.0	26.0
Carbohydrate (NFE)	46.6	58.9
Crude fiber	1.4	2.1
Calcium	0.68	0.31
Phosphorus	0.51	0.10
Potassium	0.62	0.45
Magnesium	0.08	0.02
Sodium	0.27	1.30
Chloride	0.65	2.41

Key: DM = dry matter, NFE = nitrogen-free extract.

Progress Notes

Serum bromide concentrations remained stable between 1,200 and 1,250 mg/l over the next 21 months. Seizures were not observed since the cluster of seizures that occurred after the change to the high-chloride food.

Endnotes

a. Hill's Pet Nutrition, Inc., Topeka, KS, USA.
b. Pfizer Animal Health, West Chester, PA, USA.

Bibliography

Shaw N, Trepanier LA, Center SA, et al. High dietary chloride content associated with loss of therapeutic serum bromide concentrations in an epileptic dog. Journal of the American Veterinary Medical Association 1996; 208: 234-236.

Trepanier LA, Babish JG. Effect of dietary chloride content on the elimination of bromide by dogs. Research in Veterinary Science 1995; 58: 252-255.

CASE 69-2

Hyperadrenocorticism in a Dachshund

Philip Roudebush, DVM, Dipl. ACVIM (Small Animal Internal Medicine)
Hill's Scientific Affairs
Topeka, Kansas, USA

Patient Assessment

An eight-year-old neutered female dachshund was examined for chronic dermatitis. The owners reported a slowly progressive, non-pruritic dermatopathy and polydipsia and polyuria of three to four months' duration. The dermatitis had been treated with antibiotics and griseofulvin with no response. To the owners' knowledge, the dog had received no corticosteroids.

Physical examination revealed an alert, active 10-kg dog with normal body condition (3/5), a dry coat and a "pot-bellied" appearance. The abdomen was distended and totally devoid of hair. The skin on the abdomen was markedly thinned. Bilateral alopecia and hyperpigmentation were evident on the dorsum, extending from the shoulders to the flank. Focal, circumscribed plaques with peripheral erythema were present in the inguinal and axillary regions. The remainder of the physical examination was normal.

Diagnostic evaluation included a complete blood count (lymphopenia, eosinopenia), serum biochemistry profile (hypercholesterolemia [1,414 mg/dl, normal = 125 to 250 mg/dl] and increased alkaline phosphatase activity [491 IU/l, normal <50 IU/l]), urinalysis (dilute urine with hematuria and bacteriuria) and thoracic and abdominal radiographs (calcification of subcutaneous tissues along the back). Subsequent urine culture yielded large numbers of *Escherichia coli*. Histologic evaluation of skin biopsy specimens confirmed calcinosis cutis. Water consumption in the hospital exceeded 120 ml/kg body weight/24 hours (normal = 40 to 60 ml/kg body weight).

The tentative diagnosis was pituitary-dependent hyperadrenocorticism with secondary calcinosis cutis and bacterial urinary tract infection. Hyperadrenocorticism was confirmed by excessive plasma cortisol response to intramuscular injection of ACTH gel (cortisol, pre 27 mg/dl and cortisol, two hours post-ACTH 60.0 mg/dl; normal pre-cortisol 0.5 to 4.0 mg/dl and post-ACTH 8.0 to 20.0 mg/dl).

Assess the Food and Feeding Method

The dog was fed a combination of a commercial grocery store brand dry food and a grocery store brand moist food. The dry food was available free choice and the moist food was fed once daily in the morning.

Question

Mitotane[a] (o,p'-DDD) was used to treat this patient's hyperadrenocorticism. What food-drug interactions are important to consider in the treatment and feeding plans?

Answer and Discussion

Mitotane is a commonly used drug for treatment of canine hyperadrenocorticism. Mitotane exerts a direct cytotoxic effect on the adrenal cortex, resulting in selective, progressive necrosis and atrophy of the zonae fasciculata and reticularis.

The efficacy of mitotane therapy in patients with hyperadrenocorticism can be improved markedly by dosing with food. Studies have shown that the systemic availability of mitotane is very poor when intact tablets are administered to fasting dogs, whereas availability is much better from intact or powdered tablets given with food (**Table 1**). Mitotane is soluble in fat but poorly soluble in water. The presence of dietary fat during drug administration could assist in dissolution and absorption of lipophilic drugs such as mitotane. Based on these studies, mitotane should always be administered with meals.

The interaction between food and drug probably explains some of the variation in response of pituitary-dependent hyperadrenocorticism patients to mitotane, in relation to the time required to gain initial control with daily administration and the efficacy of weekly maintenance doses. Failure to administer the drug with food may contribute to the apparent "resistance" to the effects of the drug seen in some dogs with hyperadrenocorticism.

Interactions between drugs and ingested food are common. The most common outcome is reduced or delayed absorption of the drug, although absorption is sometimes increased or unaffected by food. In many instances the changes in drug availability are modest and their clinical significance is not great. However, the substantial effect of food on mitotane availability is almost certainly clinically important and should be considered when prescribing adrenolytic therapy with this drug.

Clinical signs that owners should monitor include the dog's attitude, appetite and water intake. A common, early adverse sign of mitotane toxicity is diminished appetite, which usually occurs before other adverse clinical signs develop such as vomiting, weakness and complete anorexia. Therefore, the owners should observe the dog's appetite closely before administering the daily mitotane dose. If the food is consumed rapidly, the owner should administer the mitotane immediately after the dog finishes the meal. If the food is consumed slowly or not at all, the owners should contact the veterinarian before administering the drug.

Progress Notes

Therapy was initiated at home with an induction or loading dose of mitotane (42 mg/kg body weight/day for seven to 10 days). One 500-mg tablet was given each day following the morning meal of moist food. The dog ate the morning meal rapidly over the next 10 days; mitotane was administered each day. By Day 10 of treatment, daily water consumption had decreased from more than 120 ml/kg body weight/day to 31 ml/kg body weight/day. Daily mitotane administration was stopped and weekly therapy initiated. The dog was also treated with sulfisoxazole for the concurrent cystitis.

Endnote

a. Lysodren. Bristol-Myers Oncology Division, Evansville, IN, USA.

Bibliography

Peterson ME, Kintzer PP. Medical treatment of pituitary-dependent hyperadrenocorticism: Mitotane. Veterinary Clinics of North America: Small Animal Practice 1997; 27: 255-272.

Kintzer PP, Peterson ME. Mitotane (o,p'-DDD) treatment of 200 dogs with pituitary-dependent hyperadrenocorticism. Journal of Veterinary Internal Medicine 1991; 5: 182-190.

Watson ADJ, Rijnberk A, Moolenaar J. Systemic availability of o,p'-DDD in normal dogs, fasted and fed, and in dogs with hyperadrenocorticism. Research in Veterinary Science 1987; 43: 160-165.

Table 1. Availability of mitotane in dogs when given in various vehicles.*

Dogs	Dosage method	Maximum plasma drug concentration (mg/l)
Normal	Tablets, fasting	0.4
	Pure drug in emulsion	11.0
	Ground tablets in oil with food	15.4
	Tablets in food	13.0
Hyperadrenocorticism	Tablets in food	24.5

*Adapted from Watson ADJ, Rijnberk A, Moolenaar AJ. Systemic availability of o,p'-DDD in normal dogs, fasted and fed, and in dogs with hyperadrenocorticism. Research in Veterinary Science 1987; 43: 160-165.

CASE 69-3

Traumatic Injury in a Mixed-Breed Dog

Craig D. Thatcher, DVM, MS, PhD, Dipl. ACVN (Veterinary Nutrition)
College of Veterinary Medicine
Virginia-Maryland Regional College of Veterinary Medicine
Blacksburg, Virginia, USA

Patient Assessment

A 10-year-old, female mixed-breed dog weighing 22.2 kg was presented after being attacked by two dogs. Physical examination revealed a temperature of 37.4°C (99.3°F), pulse of 120 beats/min. and a thready, respiratory rate of 140 breaths/min. (panting) and multiple bite wounds associated with severe tearing of the subcutaneous tissues and crushing injuries to the deep musculature of the flank, lumbar and cervical regions. The dog had a flail chest, rib fractures and subcutaneous emphysema over the flank, chest, neck and head. The abdomen was painful on palpation and bruising was noticeable throughout the wound regions. The dog's body condition score was normal (3/5).

Results of a complete blood count and biochemistry profile included marked leukopenia and neutropenia with a degenerative left shift. The dog had panhypoproteinemia and moderate thrombocytopenia, which were consistent with severe sepsis and a poor prognosis. A coagulation panel demonstrated increased activated partial thromboplastin and prothrombin times with a significant decrease in platelet numbers, suggesting disseminated intravascular coagulation. Thoracic radiographs revealed a pneumomediastinum, mild pneumothorax, contusion of the left cranial lung lobe, disseminated emphysema and fractures of the right 11th and 12th ribs. Abdominal radiographs were within normal limits. No fluid was aspirated during abdominocentesis.

Initial treatment consisted of 400 ml of hetastarch (50 ml/hr) followed by lactated Ringer's solution + 20 mEq KCl/l (IV, 80 ml/hr), euroﬂoxacin (IV, 5 mg/kg b.i.d.), ampicillin (IV, 22 mg/kg t.i.d.), metronidazole (IV, 10 mg/kg t.i.d.), plasma (IV, 36 ml/hr administered by pump), sodium heparin (SQ, 1,500 IU t.i.d.), diazepam (IV, 2.1 mg) and 250 ml morphine (3.0 ml/45.6 mg)/lidocaine (27.4 ml/547.2 mg) in 0.9% NaCl at a constant infusion rate (IV, 10 ml/hr). Additionally, one dose of oxymorphone (IV, 1-mg vial) was administered; morphine (IV, 0.2 mg/kg) was provided as needed to control pain.

While the dog was anesthetized, its wounds were surgically débrided, explored and covered. Devitalized tissue and skin were removed, wounds were irrigated, suction tubing was placed in linear incisions over each wound and continuous suction applied. A 20-Fr., 16-in. Argyle thoracostomy tube was placed in the 11th intercostal space because one wound communicated with the thoracic cavity. During surgery, a percutaneous gastrostomy (PEG) tube was placed for nutritional support. The dog was placed in an oxygen cage in the intensive care unit.

Assess the Food and Feeding Method

The dog had been NPO for three days before presenting to the hospital. The dietary goals were to feed a highly digestible, calorically dense diet, with high quality and quantity of protein and high fat content to support wound healing and immune cell function and decrease body catabolism. Because the patient had not eaten for the previous three days, enteral nutritional support was initiated at 75% of the dog's calculated resting energy requirement (510 kcal/day). One 6-oz. can of Maximum-Calorie[a] diet was blended with 60 ml of warm water, which provided 1.4 kcal/ml. The feeding schedule was initiated on Day 1; the dog was fed 63 ml of the blended diet q4h through the PEG tube. Four hours after the first feeding, but before the next scheduled feeding, more than 40 ml of a dark brown granular material was aspirated from the feeding tube. Enteral feeding was discontinued.

Questions

1. What food-drug interaction in this patient resulted in discontinuation of enteral feeding?
2. What alternative feeding route could be used to feed this dog?

Answers and Discussion

1. Morphine is a plant-derived alkaloid of opium and is the most widely used opioid throughout the world. Oxymorphone is produced by modifying the morphine molecule. Both of these opioids produce multiple, major effects on the central nervous, respiratory, cardiovascular and gastrointestinal (GI) systems. Opioids are excellent analgesics but poor to moderately effective sedatives and muscle relaxants. Central nervous system depression occurs in dogs after systemic administration of morphine.

   The dog's first response to morphine is to empty the GI tract. Opioid receptors are found in the myenteric plexus of the GI tract and when stimulated result in constipation. Opioids induce GI stasis, which is associated with increased tone of smooth muscle throughout the GI tract. Morphine decreases biliary and pancreatic secretions, resulting in delayed digestion in the small intestine. Propulsive contractions are markedly decreased throughout the intestinal tract.

   The opioids used to control severe pain in this patient were responsible for GI tract stasis. The enteral feeding route was unsuitable for this patient because food was retained within the stomach and digestion was delayed. The dog may have had GI bleeding as evidenced by the dark brown color of the aspirated material from the PEG tube.
2. Parenteral feeding was selected for this patient.

Progress Notes

Three days after presentation, the dog underwent cardiac arrest and died. Necropsy findings revealed massive trauma, congestion of the heart and lungs and myocardial necrosis. The bite wounds caused severe sepsis that likely led to the death of this patient.

Endnote

a. The Iams Company, Dayton, OH, USA.

Bibliography

Branson KR, Gross ME. Opioid agonists and antagonists In: Adams HR, ed. Veterinary Pharmacology and Therapeutics, 8th ed. Ames, IA: Iowa State University Press, 2001; 272-281.

Hall LW, Clarke KW, Trim CM. Sedation, analgesia and premedication. In: Russell D, Bureau S, eds. Veterinary Anesthesia, 10th ed. New York, NY: WB Saunders Inc, 2001; 93-96.

Section 22

Feeding Small Mammals, Reptiles and Birds

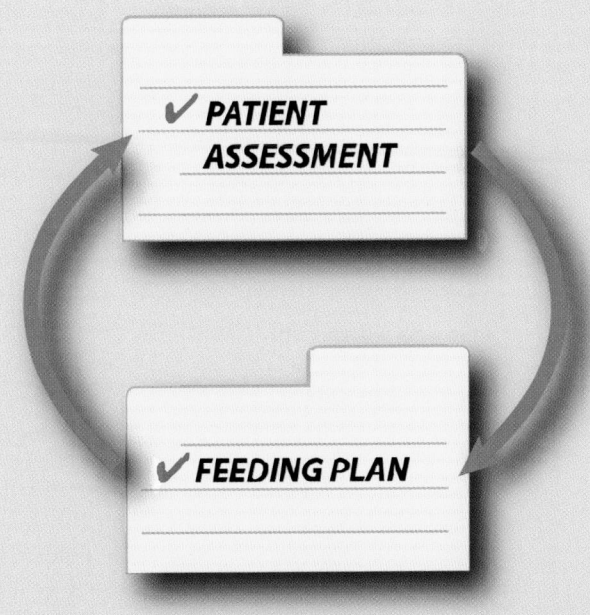

Chapter 70

Feeding Small Pet Mammals

James W. Carpenter
Karen N. Wolf
Christine Kolmstetter

"All the thoughts of a turtle are turtles, and of a rabbit, rabbits."
The Natural History of Intellect, 1893

CLINICAL IMPORTANCE

Ferrets, rabbits and rodents are popular pets that are often presented to veterinarians for advice about their care, including diet and feeding management and treatment of medical disorders. Each species presents nutritional challenges. Dietary management of ferrets, rabbits and rodents may be modified by lifestage, level of physical activity and state of health. Owners may need advice about feeding healthy pets to meet needs for maintenance, growth, reproduction or stress. Patients may present with disorders caused by an imbalanced diet or improper feeding practices. In addition, nutritional support is used for rehabilitation of debilitated animals. This chapter covers the nutritional needs of healthy pet ferrets, rabbits and rodents and those with common disease processes.

Dietary management begins with assessment of the animal, food and feeding method. A feeding plan is formulated based on the results of this assessment (Chapter 1). Although data are lacking for specific exotic species, assessment is similar to that for other mammals. It begins with a thorough history of the animal, including diet, husbandry and environment. Physical examination includes recording body weight and assessing body condition, using body condition scores. Details about body condition scoring systems are unavailable for most small mammals; however, a five-point system (where 1 = cachectic, 3 = optimal, and 5 = obese) can be applied to all species. Body condition scores qualitatively assess amounts of body fat and muscle. Excessive loss of body fat suggests starvation (due to husbandry, diet, or disease), whereas excessive loss of muscling suggests advanced starvation, forced inactivity or altered metabolic states (often due to disease).

Other factors may become part of overall nutritional assessment. Small mammals, for example, can also be evaluated for the condition of their skin and fur and their behavior and attitude. As for other species, serum biochemistry profiles are of limited use in nutritional assessment.

DOMESTIC FERRETS

Husbandry

The domestic or European ferret (*Mustela putorius furo*) is a member of the family Mustelidae, order Carnivora. Other mustelids include the mink (*Mustela vison*) and weasel (*Mustela* spp.). Pet ferrets were domesticated from the wild European polecat and were probably brought to North America by English settlers 300 years ago (Fox, 1988). Two variations are recognized, based on coloration: 1) the fitch ferret is pale yellow buff with black mask, legs and tail, and 2) the albino ferret is white with pink eyes.

Ferrets have become increasingly popular as companion animals due to their small size, ease of care and maintenance and inquisitive personality (Carpenter et al, 1994; Brown, 1993, 2004; Fox, 1988; Bernard et al, 1984; Ryland and Bernard, 1983; McLain et al, 1988).

Key Nutritional Factors

Ferrets are strict carnivores that eat whole, small prey items in the wild. They have a very short, simple gastrointestinal (GI) tract lacking a cecum and ileocolic valve. Ingesta have a rapid intestinal transit time of approximately three to six hours (Bell, 1999; Brown, 2004). Because of the relatively inefficient GI tract, ferrets thrive on highly digestible foods containing large amounts of protein and fat, with minimal digestible (soluble) carbohydrate and fiber (Bell, 1999; Brown, 2004). In nature, the only significant sources of carbohydrates are those obtained from ingesting the gut contents of prey items (Bell, 1999). Although the most appropriate diet for a ferret is whole prey or a balanced fresh or freeze-dried carnivorous diet, this is impractical. Ferrets raised on ranches are often fed pelleted mink diets, which consist of 30 to 35% meat-based protein and 20% animal fat. However, diets for mink depend heavily on fish; mink diets are less palatable to ferrets because mink are naturally fond of fish whereas ferrets are not (Bell, 1999). Because the exact nutritional requirements of pet ferrets are unknown, recommendations for the best food for this species cannot be adequately determined. When evaluating a diet, review the list of ingredients on the package: the crude protein of a maintenance diet should be 30 to 35% and based on high quality meat, not grains; the fat content should be 15 to 20% (Bell, 1999; Brown, 2004). A comparison of constituent nutritional values of some North American commercial foods used for ferrets has been previously published (Bell, 1999; Lewington, 2000).

Commercial foods marketed specifically for ferrets mirror the formulations known to be successful in mink and cats (NRC, 2006, 1982; AAFCO, 2007). Guidelines for cat foods may be used when assessing the completeness and balance of foods intended for ferrets (AAFCO, 2007). Grocery store cat foods are very palatable because of their coating with animal fat and digest, but they are nutritionally inadequate for any stage of ferret's life. Minimally stressed ferrets may live on these foods for years, but nutritional deficiencies may occur especially in breeding animals (Bell, 1999). Pelleted ferret food is the preferred diet, although premium dry kitten food is generally acceptable for meeting the ferret's nutritional requirements for growth and reproduction (Kupersmith, 1998). Canned food should be avoided as the main diet because ferrets may be unable to consume enough protein and fat on a dry matter (DM) basis. Furthermore, periodontal disease may occur earlier if ferrets are fed a moist diet because of the lack of friction to help prevent plaque buildup on the teeth (Bell, 1999; Crossley and Aiken, 2004).

Protein and Amino Acids

Ferrets require foods containing 30 to 35% protein on a DM and metabolizable energy (ME) basis. These levels correspond to label guaranteed analyses of about 27 to 32% for dry food and 6.5 to 8.0% for moist cat food (Bell, 1999; Brown, 2004). Protein quality is as important as quantity. Digestibility must be considered when determining the amount of protein. Poorly digestible protein will not satisfy the animal's nutrient requirements. Premium brands tend to have more digestible protein from meat sources rather than from cereal-based sources. Ferrets fed low-quality cat or dog food have a much higher incidence of struvite urolithiasis and may be susceptible to other complications such as GI diseases, respiratory infections, reproductive failure and poor growth (Bell, 1999; Orcutt, 2003).

Specific amino acid requirements are unknown for ferrets, but are assumed to be similar to requirements for cats. For example, young ferrets fed a single meal of an arginine-free food developed hyperammonemia, as do young cats (Deshmukh and Rusk, 1989). Likewise, cats and other strict carnivores need the high biologic value of proteins found in meat. To ensure high biologic value and maintain high food digestibility, dietary protein for ferrets should originate primarily from animal-based ingredients (poultry meal, meat by-products, eggs).

Fat and Fatty Acids

Ferrets thrive when fed commercial foods containing 15 to 20% DM fat (Bell, 1999; Brown, 2004). These levels correspond to label guaranteed analyses of about 14 to 18% for dry and 3 to 5% for moist cat food.

Specific fatty acid requirements are unknown, but it is assumed that ferrets require linoleic and arachidonic acids. The former is abundant in vegetable oils, whereas the latter is abundant in animal-based ingredients (especially nerve tissue). Fatty acid requirements should be met by providing meat-based commercial cat or mink foods.

Digestible Carbohydrates and Fiber

Other strictly carnivorous species, such as cats and mink, have no dietary requirement for carbohydrates, including fiber. Glucose is provided by hepatic gluconeogenesis, using amino acids. Dietary fiber may play a role in weight control and reduction, and in certain specific GI disorders.

The simple, short digestive tract of strict carnivores dictates hydrolysis of most dietary fuels, with little or no hindgut fermentation of fiber. The ferret intestinal tract is comparatively deficient in brush-border enzymes, thus ferrets are less able to absorb calories from carbohydrates (Bell, 1999). Generally, foods with added fiber should not be fed to healthy ferrets and those in above-maintenance physiologic states, such as growth and lactation, but may be considered for patients with fiber-responsive disorders.

Energy

Metabolic rates for mustelids vary, but generally those with a long thin body shape, short fur, strict carnivorous behavior and high activity (e.g., ferrets and mink) have high metabolic rates, hence high caloric needs, relative to cats and other mustelids with different body shapes and activity levels (Knudsen and Kilgore, 1990). Seasonal metabolic cycles complicate predictions of energy needs. Generally, autumn (shortening daylight) signals fat deposition and weight gain, whereas spring (lengthening daylight) signals fat mobilization and weight loss (Robbins, 1993). Pet ferrets that aren't exposed to variations in photoperiod may not undergo physiologic fluctuations in weight (Bell, 1999).

Ferrets reportedly consume 200 to 300 kcal (837 to 1,255 kJ) ME/kg body weight daily for adult maintenance (**Table 70-1**) (McLain et al, 1988). This amount equals about one-half to three-quarters cup of dry cat food containing about 400 kcal (1,674 kJ) ME per cup (standard eight-oz. measuring cup). This is about three times greater than the food intake of an average cat.

Energy needs increase for growth and reproduction (**Table 70-1**). Caloric requirements may be met by increased intake of an adult maintenance food or by consumption of a diet with increased caloric density. Increasing food intake works to a point, but foods with higher caloric density should be offered in demanding situations. Thus, growing and lactating ferrets should be fed cat foods formulated for growth and reproduction.

A ration with a caloric density of about 5.0 kcal/g (20.9 kJ/g) DM has been recommended for ferrets (McLain et al, 1988). Generally, dry cat foods contain 4.0 to 5.0 kcal ME/g (16.7 to 20.9 kJ ME/g) DM, or about 360 to 450 kcal ME/100 g (1,506 to 1,883 kJ ME/100 g) (about 1 cup). Moist cat foods usually contain 4.0 to 5.0 kcal ME/g (16.7 to 20.9 kJ ME/g) DM, or about 360 to 450 kcal ME/400 g (1,506 to 1,883 kJ ME/400 g) (about one 13-oz. can). Dry foods are generally preferred for ferrets because their texture may help prevent periodontal disease. Furthermore, although moist food may contain more DM protein and fat, ferrets may be unable to consume enough of this formulation to meet their requirements, because the bulk of the high moisture content in the food limits consumption (Bell, 1999).

Obesity is uncommon in ferrets, but may occur in later years as activity decreases. Most ferrets, therefore, are fed successfully by free-choice access to a high quality commercial ferret (or kitten) food. Although ferrets do not need treats, an occasional, judicious addition of natural treats (selected fruits and even vegetables) may be used. Food intake should be regulated for overweight ferrets.

Table 70-1. Average daily metabolizable energy (ME) intakes for ferrets at maintenance (M) and above-maintenance states, based on the recommendation of 200 to 300 kcal ME/kg body weight. For this table, 250 kcal/kg was used. Much variation between individuals should be expected.*

Body weight (g)	Daily energy intake (kcal ME) M	1.5M	2M	2.5M	3M
200	50	75	100	125	150
300	75	112	150	188	225
400	100	150	200	250	300
500	125	188	250	312	375
600	150	225	300	375	450
700	175	262	350	438	525
800	200	300	400	500	600
900	225	338	450	562	675
1,000	250	375	500	625	750
1,200	300	450	600	750	900
1,400	350	525	700	875	1,050
1,600	400	600	800	1,000	1,200
1,800	450	675	900	1,125	1,350
2,000	500	750	1,000	1,250	1,500
2,200	550	825	1,100	1,375	1,650

*To convert to kJ, multiply kcal by 4.184.

Vitamins and Minerals

Dietary guidelines for cats and mink have been established by controlled comparative trials and thus are followed for pet ferrets because of limited research data in this species. Most published reports suggest that ferrets require vitamins and minerals in amounts similar to other carnivores. For example, research suggests that ferrets grow well when fed calcium (0.6 to 0.8% DM) and phosphorus (0.4 to 1.0% DM) in ranges fed to other mammalian carnivores (Edfors et al, 1990). Unlike cats, however, ferrets absorb β-carotene (the plant-based precursor of vitamin A) (Ribaya-Mercado et al, 1989). Despite this interesting finding, the conversion process is inefficient in ferrets: therefore, foods for pet ferrets should contain preformed vitamin A (e.g., retinyl palmitate) and not rely on carotenoids (Lederman et al, 1998).

Generally, deficiencies of specific vitamins and minerals are unlikely to occur in ferrets fed commercial foods formulated for cats, ferrets or mink. Deficiencies are more likely to occur in ferrets fed poorly formulated homemade foods. Imbalanced homemade foods for carnivores are most likely to be deficient in calcium and iodine. Both nutrients are deficient in common ingredients such as meats, most dairy products, rice and vegetables. Homemade foods should contain sources of calcium (bone meal, calcium carbonate) and iodine (iodized salt, kelp). Chapter 10 contains recipes for balanced homemade foods for cats that may be given to owners who insist on cooking for their ferrets (Donoghue and Kronfeld, 1994).

Deficiencies may also occur when excessive amounts of table foods or supplements are added to commercial ferret, cat or mink foods. Supplementation with table foods or single ingredients above about 10% of DM may imbalance previously balanced foods. For example, adding large amounts of corn oil reduces protein and other essential nutrients to deficient levels (on an energy basis). Deficiencies may also arise when large amounts of calcium are added to balanced foods because excess calcium interferes with absorption of trace minerals such as zinc and copper.

Vitamin and mineral toxicities may occur in ferrets overdosed with commercial supplements (e.g., chewable vitamin-mineral preparations given as treats) or with specific ingredients (e.g., vitamin A intoxication from an all-liver diet).

Special Nutritional Needs

Kits from six weeks (weaning) to about 14 weeks of age require a soft, moist food. Growing kits require 35% protein and 20%

fat (Bell, 1999; Brown, 2004). Although a ferret kibble may be most appropriate, a premium quality cat food (formulated for all lifestages or for growth and reproduction) soaked with water may also be adequate for growth. Goat's milk added to softened cat food has been recommended for slow-growing kits (Morton and Morton, 1985). Ferrets achieve 90% of their adult size by 14 weeks of age, thus food consumption is very high.

Providing protein at levels greater than 35% improves the conception rate in jills (Bell, 1999). Pregnant and lactating ferrets also require above-maintenance levels of food. Generally, pregnant animals need about twice the maintenance level, whereas animals at peak lactation need three to four times maintenance amounts. Unrestricted access to premium quality food and a constant supply of water are required during these periods of high metabolic demand.

Food intake varies seasonally. Under natural lighting conditions, ferrets eat more and gain weight in the fall in preparation for the cold winter months (Morton and Morton, 1985). As the photoperiod increases in the spring, ferrets tend to lose most of their body fat, thereby preparing them for summer heat. Weight cycling may occur at other times as a result of unnatural photoperiods (Morton and Morton, 1985). Pet ferrets may not experience these fluctuations if they are not exposed to natural photoperiods.

Selected Nutritional Diseases

Although the prevalence of nutrient deficiencies and toxicities in ferrets is largely unknown, specific diet-related problems are rarely seen in practice. Like dogs and cats, some ferrets with dermatologic problems respond to dietary supplementation with fatty acids (Chapter 32), but direct causal links between diet and disease remain to be established.

Anecdotal reports suggest that some, but not all, ferrets with dermatologic problems may respond to adding meat or liver to their usual diet of commercial cat food. This finding suggests that ferrets may be responding to arachidonic acid in meat or perhaps additional protein. When feeding liver, care must be taken to avoid inducing vitamin A intoxication. Generally, no more than 30 g of liver should be added per 800 kcal (3,347 kJ).

Ferrets fed excessive dietary fat risk protein deficiency. Protein deficiency manifests as slow growth in the young, low conception rates and failed lactation in breeding females and impaired immunity and generalized unthriftiness in ferrets of all ages. The problem may be corrected by feeding a commercial ferret chow or premium kitten chow.

Quality commercial ferret, kitten or cat foods appear to provide adequate levels of vitamins and minerals for ferrets. Most published reports of clinical problems have occurred in large breeding operations or under laboratory conditions.

Vitamin E deficiency results in yellow discoloration of body fat, hemolytic anemia, anorexia and a progressively impaired gait leading to paralysis (McLain et al, 1988). Affected young growing kits are found dead or depressed, cry when handled and are reluctant to move. Diffuse firm swellings under the skin and prominent subcutaneous lumps in the inguinal areas are clinical manifestations of the deficiency (McLain et al, 1988). This disease has been termed yellow fat disease, fatty degeneration of the liver and steatitis. It results from feeding foods containing high levels of polyunsaturated fatty acids with inadequate dietary vitamin E (McLain et al, 1988). Diagnosis is based on clinical signs and a history of feeding a food containing high levels of polyunsaturated fatty acids, deficient levels of vitamin E or both.

Thiamin deficiency resulting from feeding fish containing thiaminase has been reported to occur on ferret farms in New Zealand (McLain et al, 1988). The disease was seen in weanling animals and adults. Clinical signs included anorexia and lethargy followed by dyspnea, prostration and convulsions.

Zinc toxicity has also been reported to occur in ferrets on farms in New Zealand (McLain et al, 1988). The toxicosis resulted from excessive intake of dietary zinc that had leached from galvanized feeding pans and water dishes. Presumptive zinc toxicity was based on clinical signs (anemia, posterior weakness and lethargy), gross pathology and histologic examination of kidney and liver specimens and demonstration of elevated levels of zinc in these tissues.

Copper toxicosis has been reported to occur in sibling pet ferrets (Fox et al, 1994). Signs referred to liver disease; tissue copper concentrations confirmed the diagnosis. A genetic predisposition to copper intoxication was proposed.

Ferrets also can develop lower urinary tract disease similar to that seen in domestic cats. Diet is thought to play an important role. Ferrets fed a diet containing poor quality protein have a higher incidence of struvite urolithiasis (Orcutt, 2003). Metabolism of plant protein creates more alkaline urine, which enhances formation of struvite crystals. Suggestions for prevention mirror recommendations for feline lower urinary tract disease (Chapter 46); however, the disease in ferrets is not well documented.

Feeding Plan

Ferrets require a high-protein, high-fat, low-carbohydrate diet. Foods for ferrets should be a premium quality kibble or chow and should be formulated for strict carnivores–ferrets or kittens (and possibly even adult cats). The diet must contain a high quality animal-source, not plant-source protein, to ensure high digestibility, palatability and protein quality. Protein and fat levels should preferably be 30 to 35% and 20% DM, respectively (Bell, 1999).

Foods may be fed free choice unless the ferret is overweight. Because of their high metabolic rate, ferrets consume more calories, hence more food, than cats.

Healthy ferrets should not be fed high-fiber foods. Dietary fiber, though, may play a role in weight control and in fiber-responsive disorders.

Other dietary recommendations for ferrets include:

- Vitamin-mineral supplements are generally unnecessary for healthy ferrets fed well-formulated commercial ferret or kitten/cat foods. Supplementing foods that are already balanced increases the risk of creating an imbalance and subsequent deficiencies or intoxications.
- Although it was a common practice to supplement a ferret's

diet with table foods such as cooked meat, fish, poultry, and eggs or fresh liver (Bernard et al, 1984; Ryland and Bernard, 1983), this practice is seldom indicated. Foods containing lactose or simple sugars should be avoided to prevent digestive upsets. Fruits and vegetables have also been offered in limited quantities; however, ferrets do not digest the fiber in these foods; therefore, they are generally not required. If a client insists on supplementing a ferret's diet, selected supplements should be used judiciously. Supplements should be limited to no more than 10% of the daily caloric intake. One ml of Linotone[a] or Ferretone[a] is acceptable, and soft-moist meat or liver snacks manufactured for ferrets or cats make good treats (Bell, 1999). Other acceptable snacks include baby food meats that contain no carbohydrates, egg yolk or whole cooked egg or small amounts of raw meat or liver. Pureed raw liver or hamburger mixed with egg yolk is especially appealing to kits and contains amino and fatty acids that may correct deficiencies associated with inadequate diets (Bell, 1999). Ferrets should not be offered carrots or nuts (may rarely cause intestinal obstruction), raisins (high sugar content) and bananas in amounts larger than 1 tsp (Purcell and Brown, 1999).

- Dry foods are generally recommended for ferrets because they may help keep the animal's teeth and gums in good condition, are more energy efficient, cost less and are easier to store and feed than moist foods.
- Ferrets do not need to eat mice or other rodents.
- Because hairballs occasionally occur in ferrets, feline hairball laxatives may be given every other day, following label dosage recommendations for cats (Brown, 1993).
- Bones should be avoided to prevent obstructions in the oral cavity and GI tract.
- Fresh water, in either a heavy crock-type bowl or drinking bottle, should be available free choice.
- Because ferrets are finicky, any food changes should be made gradually.
- Ferrets with insulinomas need constant access to a high-quality protein-based food. If a sugar-based syrup is used for emergency treatment of a hypoglycemic episode, it should be followed by a meat-based supplement after the patient is able to swallow to prevent dramatic fluctuations in glucose concentrations.
- Sick ferrets may be reluctant to eat and often require frequent hand feedings of warmed, moist, highly palatable foods. Examples include meat baby foods or a mixture of meat baby food, premium-quality moist cat food and a high-calorie supplement (e.g., Ensure Plus[b]) blended with the preferred dry diet (ground into a powder) and made into a warm gruel (Bell, 1999).

RABBITS

Husbandry

The domestic rabbit (*Oryctolagus cuniculus*) (Order Lagomorpha) is a descendent of the old world rabbit of western Europe and northwestern Africa (Fox, 1994; Donnelly, 2004a). It has become a popular pet, resulting in an increased demand for veterinary care for this species. Although domestic rabbits are used for commercial meat and fur production, teaching and biomedical research, exhibition by rabbit fanciers and as outdoor pets, most now are probably household pets. As pets, rabbits are small, relatively easy to care for, fastidious, quiet mannered and can be litter-box trained.

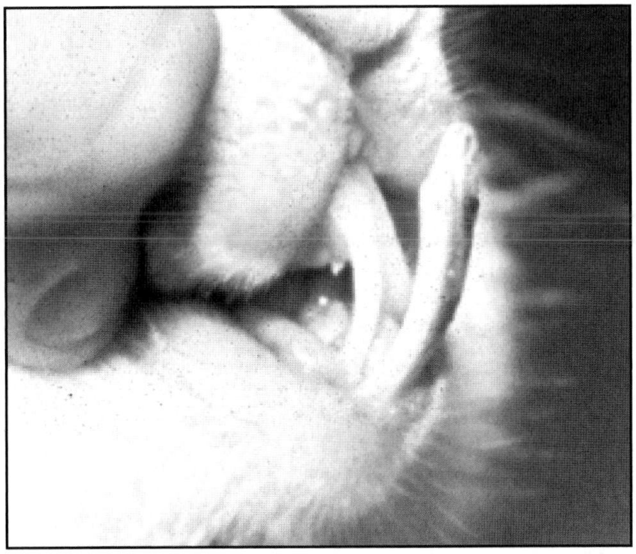

Figure 70-1. Overgrown, maloccluded incisor teeth frequently result in malnutrition or anorexia in rabbits.

As noted by their dental formula (I2/1, C0/0, P3/2, M3/3), lagomorphs can be distinguished from rodents by the presence of two pairs of upper incisor teeth. The smaller, second upper incisors, known as peg teeth, are located directly behind the first and lack a cutting edge. Rabbit teeth are hypsodont or open-rooted (continuously growing). Malocclusion and overgrowth are most likely to occur with the incisor teeth (**Figure 70-1**), which grow 10 to 12 cm a year throughout life, although malocclusion and overgrowth of the molar teeth may also occur (Harkness and Wagner, 1989). Rabbit teeth are developed for a high-fiber, herbivorous diet (Davies and Davies, 2003; Brooks, 2004). Chewing is characterized by up to 120 jaw movements per minute, with a lateral motion, which helps wear the teeth down to the proper occlusal surfaces.

As herbivorous hindgut fermenters, rabbits have a GI system resembling that of horses (Cheeke, 1994). Both species possess a non-compartmentalized stomach and a large cecum. The simple stomach has thin walls and indistinctly separated glandular and nonglandular areas. Rabbits are unable to vomit because of a well-developed cardiac sphincter (Davies and Davies, 2003; Brooks, 2004). The stomach is normally never fully devoid of food and fecal pellets. The terminal ileum expands and forms a thin-walled structure unique to lagomorphs known as the sacculus rotundus. Large amounts of lymphatic tissue are located in the wall of the sacculus, giving it a "honeycomb" external appearance. The thin-walled cecum is

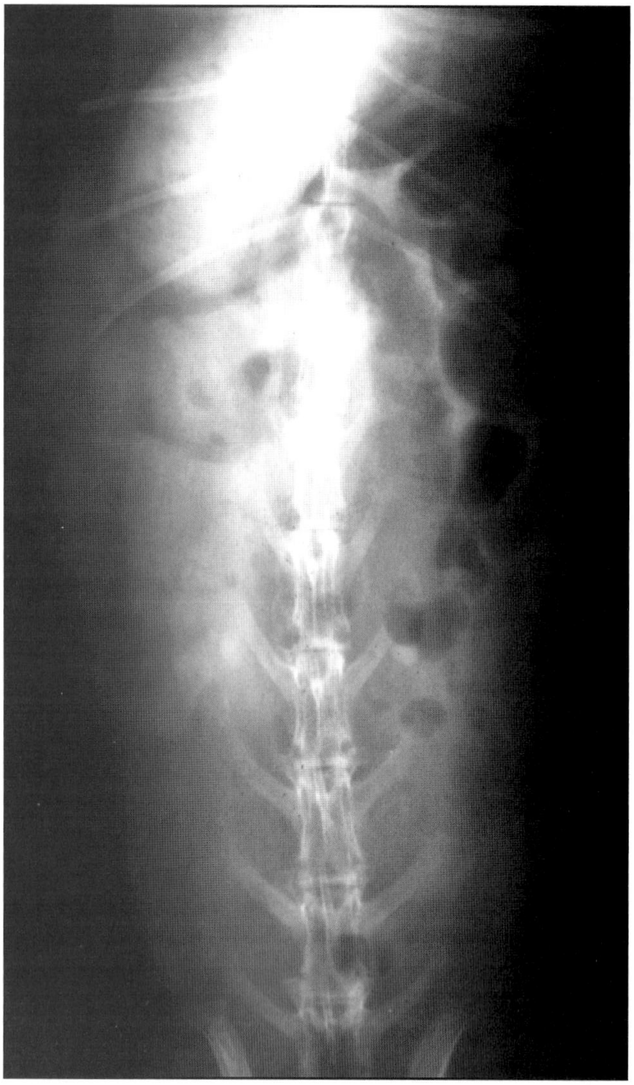

Figure 70-2. A ventrodorsal radiograph of the abdomen of a rabbit with a gastric trichobezoar. Note the tubular distention of the stomach. (Reprinted with permission from Veterinary Medicine 1995; 90: 365-372.)

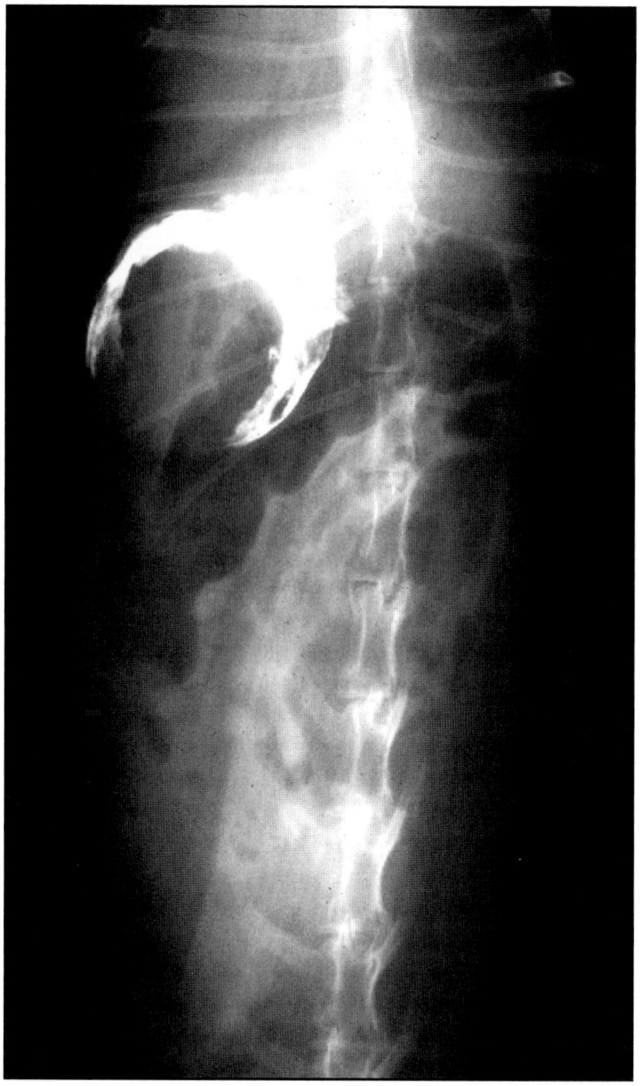

Figure 70-3. A ventrodorsal radiograph of the abdomen of the rabbit in **Figure 70-2** following a barium swallow. Note the contrast medium outlining the mass filling the gastric lumen. (Reprinted with permission from Veterinary Medicine 1995; 90: 365-372.)

a spiral structure and the largest and most prominent organ in the abdominal cavity of rabbits. The cecum has approximately 10-fold the stomach capacity and makes up 40 to 60% of the total volume of the GI tract (Jenkins, 1999). Antiperistaltic action moves small particles and solubles into the cecum, where cellulose is digested and fermented. The GI transit time for fiber is approximately four to five hours.

Instead of chewing cud for improved digestion, as would ruminants, rabbits use cecotrophy or pseudorumination (Brooks, 2004). Muscular contractions in the colon cause indigestible fiber particles to separate from nonfiber components of the gut contents. The fusus coli, another structure unique to lagomorphs, separates the proximal from the distal colon. The fusus coli functions as a pacemaker to control colonic contractions. Peristaltic contractions move fiber through the colon for excretion in hard feces. Antiperistaltic contractions move fluids and particles retrograde through the colon into the cecum for fermentation. After fermentation, the cecal contents are expelled through the colon (Brooks, 2004; Cheeke, 1994; Jenkins, 1999; Irelbeck, 2001). The fermented pellets produced in the cecum are called cecotrophs. Cecotrophs are excreted during the night and early morning, approximately eight hours after consumption of the original food item, as clusters of grapelike material and are consumed (cecotrophy) directly from the anus. Cecotrophs contain twice the protein (25 to 30% DM) of usual fecal pellets, more B vitamins and much less fiber (Tobin, 1996; Lowe, 1998; Brooks, 2004; Davies and Davies, 2003). Cecotrophy is particularly important for efficient digestion of forage proteins. The process also provides the rabbit with microbially synthesized B-complex vitamins, microbial protein and small quantities of volatile fatty acids. The pH of the rabbit's stomach is extremely acidic (<2.0), which may neutralize large numbers of bacteria ingested with cecotrophs.

The most clinically relevant feature, however, of the rabbit's GI system may be that the myoelectrical initiation of peristalsis occurs distal to the stomach. This feature allows hair to accumulate in the stomach and may account for the common occurrence of gastric trichobezoars in rabbits (**Figures 70-2** through **70-4**) (Gentz et al, 1995).

Key Nutritional Factors

Energy

Daily caloric needs for maintenance of healthy adult rabbits are estimated to be $100(BW_{kg})^{0.75}$ (**Table 70-2**) (Tobin, 1996). Thus, a healthy adult rabbit weighing 4 kg consumes almost 300 kcal/day (1,255 kJ). Because energy needs relate to metabolic body size, smaller breeds require a higher caloric intake per unit of body weight.

Daily energy needs increase for growth (190 to $210[BW_{kg}]^{0.75}$), early gestation ($135[BW_{kg}]^{0.75}$), late gestation ($200[BW_{kg}]^{0.75}$) and lactation ($300[BW_{kg}]^{0.75}$) (**Table 70-2**) (Tobin, 1996). Thus, there are two- to threefold increases in energy needs; therefore, food consumption correspondingly increases during growth and lactation (Harkness, 1987; Collins, 1988). Energy needs also increase in cold environmental temperatures.

Production rabbits often adjust feed intake to meet energy needs, when appropriate feed is available. Pet rabbits, however, occasionally overeat and risk obesity.

Protein and Fat

Rabbits require 13 to 18% DM dietary crude protein (**Table 70-3**). Research suggests that 13% is adequate for maintenance, 15 to 16% for maximum growth and 18% for gestating or lactating does. These levels are allowable minimums determined for laboratory and production rabbits. Protein levels of 12 to 16% should be adequate for healthy household rabbits. Protein provided at levels used for production may be excessive for pet rabbits and may lead to reduced appetite for cecotrophs (Harcourt-Brown, 2002).

Rabbits require adequate amounts of relatively high-protein, high-quality foods, which is achieved by efficient use of plant proteins, such as those found in alfalfa and clover (**Table 70-4**). Low-protein foods and nonprotein nitrogen are used poorly. Bacterial protein from the lower bowel contributes little to the amino acid needs of growing rabbits, but may benefit adults fed poor-quality protein at maintenance. Excess dietary protein may allow the proliferation of *Clostridium* spp., which could lead to enteritis (Lebas et al, 1998).

Rabbits require no added dietary fat. Most foods contain 2 to 5% fat, which is sufficient (**Table 70-3**). Excess dietary fat may increase the incidence of arteriosclerosis, although some strains of rabbits may develop arteriosclerotic plaques even on a fat-free diet (Brooks, 2004).

Fiber

Dietary fiber can be divided into indigestible fiber (passes through the digestive tract without entering the cecum) and fermentable fiber (enters the cecum for fermentation). Both indigestible and fermentable fiber are critical to optimal rabbit nutrition. The indigestible fiber stimulates gut motility, provides optimal dental wear and stimulates ingestion of cecotrophs. Fermentable fiber provides a substrate for cecal microflora, allows for volatile fatty acid production and prevents proliferation of pathogenic bacteria in the cecum (Harcourt-Brown, 2002; Brooks, 2004). Rabbits need a minimum of about 12 to 16% dietary crude fiber. The low end of the range, 12%,

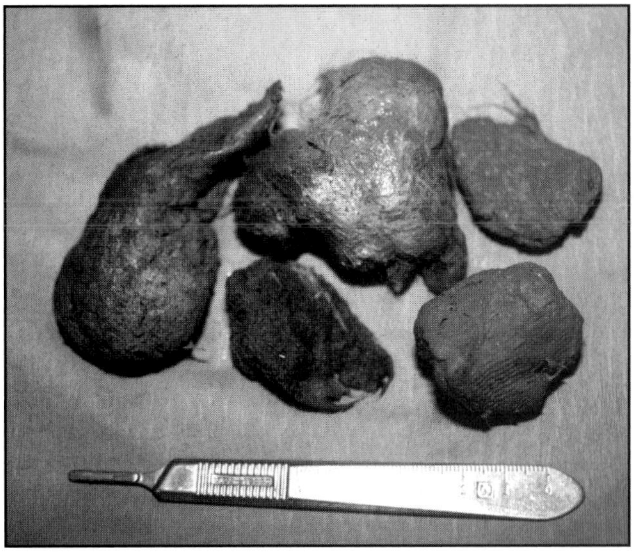

Figure 70-4. The gastric trichobezoar removed in pieces from the rabbit in **Figures 70-2** and **70-3** weighed 102 g. Trichobezoars are frequently associated with a low-fiber diet. (Reprinted with permission from Veterinary Medicine 1995; 90: 365-372.)

Table 70-2. Average daily metabolizable energy (ME) intakes for rabbits at maintenance (M) and above-maintenance states.* Much variation between individuals should be expected.

Body weight (kg)	M	Daily energy intake (kcal ME)** Growth	Early gestation	Late gestation	Lactation
1.4	129	258	174	258	387
1.6	142	284	192	284	426
1.8	156	312	211	312	468
2.0	168	336	227	336	504
2.3	187	374	252	374	561
2.5	199	398	269	398	597
2.7	211	422	285	422	633
3.0	228	456	308	456	684
3.2	239	478	323	478	717
3.4	250	500	338	500	750
3.6	261	522	352	522	783
4.1	288	576	389	576	864
4.5	309	618	417	618	927
5.4	354	708	478	708	1,062
6.4	402	804	543	804	1,206
7.3	444	888	599	888	1,332

*Adapted from Tobin G. Small pets–food types, nutrient requirements and nutritional disorders. Manual of Companion Animal Nutrition & Feeding. London, UK: British Small Animal Veterinary Association, 1996: 208-225.
**To convert to kJ, multiply kcal by 4.184.

Table 70-3. Requirements of selected nutrients for rabbits.*

Nutrients (DM)	Growth (4-12 wks)	Lactation	Gestation	Maintenance	Does and litters fed one food
Crude protein (%)	**15**	**18**	**18**	**13**	**17**
Amino acids					
Methionine + cystine	0.5	0.6	-	-	0.55
Lysine	0.6	0.75	-	-	0.7
Crude fiber (%)	14	12	14	15-16	14
Digestible energy (kcal/kg)**	2,500	2,700	2,500	2,200	2,500
Fat (%)	3	5	3	3	3
Minerals					
Calcium (%)	0.5	1.1	0.8	0.6	1.1
Phosphorus (%)	0.3	0.8	0.5	0.4	0.8
Vitamins					
A (IU/kg)	6,000	12,000	12,000	-	10,000
D (IU/kg)	900	900	900	-	900
E (ppm)	50	50	50	50	50

Key: DM = dry matter.
*Adapted from Cheeke PR. Rabbits. In: Pond WG, Church DC, Pond KR, eds. Basic Animal Nutrition and Feeding. New York, NY: John Wiley & Sons, 1995; 451-459.
**To convert to kJ, multiply kcal by 4.184.

has been recommended for lactating does, 14% for growth and gestation and 15 to 16% for maintenance (**Table 70-3**) (Cheeke, 1995). These levels are minimums established for production rabbits; higher fiber levels may benefit pets. Dietary fiber levels of 18 to 25% have been recommended to maintain optimal GI health and help prevent obesity in pet rabbits (Lowe, 1998; Irlbeck, 2001; Brooks, 2004).

Adequate insoluble dietary fiber is important for rabbit health. In studies, growth rates were reduced in young rabbits fed low-fiber foods. Growth rates of production rabbits are optimal when foods containing 10 to 15% DM crude fiber are fed. Enteritis is more common in rabbits fed less than 10% crude fiber (Cheeke, 1994). Dietary fiber primarily stimulates gut motility rather than serves as a source of nutrition. Fiber promotes intestinal motility, provides nutrition for intestinal microorganisms and minimizes susceptibility to enteritis. Cecal fermentation of fiber produces volatile fatty acids (acetate, butyrate, and propionate), which are absorbed and used for energy. Volatile fatty acids aid in the control of pathogenic organisms by helping to maintain a low cecal pH. Foods with adequate fiber help to prevent obesity and hair chewing (**Table 70-4**) (Harkness, 1987). Diets low in indigestible fiber can lead to decreased GI motility and retention of food and hair in the stomach. Slowed gut motility and increased retention time of food can lead to alterations in the gut flora and development of enterotoxemia (Harcourt-Brown, 2002; Brooks, 2004).

Vitamins

A dietary supply of vitamins A, D and E is an integral part of rabbit nutrition. Bacteria in the gut synthesize B vitamins in adequate quantities. Thus, addition of B vitamins to commercial foods may be unnecessary, although it often occurs. The adequacy of vitamin K synthesis in the gut is questionable; therefore, manufacturers often add this fat-soluble vitamin to commercial foods.

Because vitamins A and E are readily destroyed by oxidation, food preparation and storage methods should prevent losses from excess light or heat. Optimally, feed should be stored at 15°C (60°F) in a vermin proof area and fed within 90 days of milling (Brooks, 2004). Foods containing more than 30% alfalfa meal may provide sufficient vitamin A in the form of the precursor β-carotene (Fraser, 1991). Deficiency may occur, however, if old (more than one year postharvest) alfalfa is fed.

Table 70-3 lists recommended levels of dietary vitamin A for production rabbits. Recommendations for pet rabbits include 7,000 to 18,000 IU vitamin A/kg food, 40 to 70 mg vitamin E/kg food and 2 mg vitamin K/kg food (Tobin, 1996; Lowe, 1998; Harcourt-Brown, 2002). The role of vitamin D in calcium regulation in rabbits differs from that in other species. Intestinal absorption of calcium does not require the presence of vitamin D. In rabbits, vitamin D is important for phosphorus metabolism and deficiencies can lead to hypophosphatemia and osteomalacia (Harcourt-Brown, 2002). Sunlight is necessary for endogenous synthesis of vitamin D in rabbits. Commercial rabbit pellets are also supplemented with vitamin D. A level of 800 to 1,200 IU/kg is recommended for pet rabbits (Lowe, 1998; Harcourt-Brown, 2002).

Minerals

Calcium requirements for rabbits appear to be similar to those for other species (i.e., 0.5 to 1.0 % DM [**Table 70-3**]). Rabbits absorb calcium very efficiently and the excess is excreted in urine, rather than in bile as typically occurs in other species (Cheeke, 1994; Norris, 2001). Normal rabbit urine may have a thick milky appearance due to the excretion of calcium carbonate. Interestingly, rabbits have a higher than normal serum calcium level (12 to 13 mg/dl) compared to that of other mammals. Excess calcium supplementation with certain types of greens or vitamin-mineral mixes may cause urolithiasis or excessive calciuria in some pet rabbits (Irlbeck, 2001; Harcourt-Brown, 2002; Brooks, 2004). Urinary calculi can form in the kidneys, ureters and urinary bladder. **Table 70-5** lists calcium

Table 70-4. Protein and fiber contents (dry matter basis) of forages commonly fed to rabbits.*

Forages	Crude protein (%)	Cellulose (%)	Hemicellulose (%)	Lignin (%)	ADF (%)	Crude fiber (%)
Alfalfa hay	14	26	12	12	39	32
Alfalfa meal	18	24	-	11	35	26
Clover hay	16	26	9	10	-	29
Orchard grass hay	8	39	27	9	45	37
Timothy hay	9	33	31	5	36	31

Key: ADF = acid detergent fiber.
*Adapted from United States–Canadian Tables of Feed Composition, 3rd revision. Washington, DC: National Academy Press, 1982.

and phosphorus contents of commonly fed forages.

Most rabbit foods contain adequate calcium because the formulations include alfalfa meal, which averages about 1.4% calcium, 0.2% phosphorus and at least 300 IU vitamin D_2 (ergocalciferol) per g (DM) (United States-Canadian Tables of Feed Composition, 1982). Prolonged intake of high-calcium foods (4% DM) may cause calcification of soft tissues such as the aorta and kidneys; hypervitaminosis D most likely exacerbates the effect because it aids calcium absorption (Cheeke, 1994). Feeding a food (e.g., possibly a diet lower in alfalfa or alfalfa meal) containing 0.5% calcium prevents soft-tissue calcification.

Table 70-5. Calcium, phosphorus and vitamin D_2 contents (dry matter basis) of forages commonly fed to rabbits.*

Forages	Calcium (%)	Phosphorus (%)	Vitamin D_2 (IU/g)
Alfalfa hay	1.3	0.2	1,411
Alfalfa meal	1.4	0.2	-
Clover hay	1.5	0.3	1,914
Orchard grass hay	0.4	0.4	-
Timothy hay	0.5	0.2	1,930

*Adapted from United States–Canadian Tables of Feed Composition, 3rd revision. Washington, DC: National Academy Press, 1982.

Special Nutritional Needs

The energy requirements of production rabbits fed free choice have been met by feeding dry foods containing 2.2 kcal/g (9.2 kJ/g) of food during maintenance, 2.5 kcal/g (10.5 kJ/g) of food during growth and gestation and 2.7 kcal/g (11.3 kJ/g) during lactation (Cheeke, 1995). Alternatively, feeding a single pelleted commercial rabbit food (hence a single energy density, often about 2.5 kcal/g [10.5 kJ/g] DM) and varying food intake, instead of the food itself, can be used to meet energy goals above maintenance needs.

Ideally, specific foods could be used for different functions: creep, starter, grower, finisher, lactation and maintenance (Cheeke, 1994). In most instances, however, commercial rabbit producers find it impractical to use more than one food. Thus, a single commercial pellet is typically fed to the entire rabbit colony. Adjustments for increased consumption of food above normal must be made for pregnant and lactating animals. Similar techniques may be used for pet rabbits.

Compared with many other mammals, rabbits have a high water intake. Rabbits drink about 120 ml/kg body weight daily (Cheeke, 1994), and even more during lactation and hot weather.

Selected Nutritional Diseases

Although nutrient requirements of rabbits have been summarized in numerous studies (Cheeke, 1987, 1994, 1995; Cheeke et al, 1987; Lebas, 1987; Fraser, 1991), data about specific requirements are limited. However, the major nutritional problems of rabbits are not specific nutrient deficiencies or imbalances, but rather disturbances in digestive tract function (enteric disease) associated with dietary factors (Cheeke, 1994; Harcourt-Brown, 2002; Brooks, 2004) or with malocclusion of teeth.

Malocclusion

Anorexia is a common clinical presentation of pet rabbits. Malocclusion of the teeth is a likely cause. Because rabbit incisor teeth are open-rooted, a developmental defect in the normal appositional anatomy precludes normal wear; thus, overgrowth of the teeth occurs (**Figure 70-1**). Overgrown incisor teeth may limit or prevent prehension of food and can traumatize the oral mucosa. A complete physical examination of rabbits should always include an evaluation of the oral cavity, including the molar teeth. Maloccluded incisor teeth need to be trimmed using either a high- or low-speed dental handpiece every four to six weeks or may need to be extracted (Crossley and Aiken, 2004). Specialized dental equipment, including speculums, mouth gags and long-shank dental burrs are available for use in rabbits. Endoscopic equipment can also be used to examine the oral cavity and teeth (Crossley and Aiken, 2004).

Rabbit molar and premolar teeth may also be maloccluded. Although maloccluded molar teeth are often floated with a fine file or their sharp points clipped off with a rongeur, ideally dental drills (low speed) should be used to remove the points (Crossley, 2003).

Trichobezoars

Gastric obstruction by a trichobezoar is another common cause of anorexia in rabbits (**Figures 70-2 through 70-4**). Hairballs are common incidental findings in rabbit necropsies, even among shorthaired breeds. The rabbit's inability to vomit and the small pyloric lumen predispose to hair accumulation in the stomach. The primary inciting factor for development of trichobezoars is intestinal hypomotility. Diets low in indigestible fiber and high in carbohydrates predispose to GI hypomotility and retention of hair and food in the stomach (Harcourt-Brown, 2002; Jenkins, 2004). A definitive diagnosis can be difficult. Occasionally, the stomach can be palpated in the cranial abdomen as a large, doughy mass. Fecal pellet production is frequently reduced or absent, and those that are passed are smaller than normal. Survey radiography may reveal an enlarged stomach with displaced intestines. Contrast radiography may aid the diagnosis. A large, ingesta-filled stomach in a rabbit that has been anorectic for four to seven days suggests gastric stasis. A definitive diagnosis requires exploratory laparotomy; however, given the risk of surgery in these compromised patients, a presumptive diagnosis is often made based on response to treatment (Jenkins, 2004).

Medical treatment strategies emphasizing rehydration of the patient and stimulation of gastric motility have been developed with very good results (Hernandez-Divers, 2005). Force-feeding fluids, vegetable purees or commercial products (Critical Care for Herbivores[c]) is often indicated, as is administration of subcutaneous fluids, or if the patient is hospitalized, intravenous fluids (Jenkins, 2004). Additional treatments may include administration of an appropriate systemic antibiotic, gastric motility stimulants and surgery if the rabbit fails to respond to medical management. Although feeding fresh pineapple juice (10 ml/day) (which contains the enzyme bromelain), papaya tablets (which contain papain) or proteolytic enzymes have been reported to aid breakdown and passage of trichobezoars, the response to such treatments is equivocal (Jenkins, 2004) and no longer recommended as a treatment strategy. Hairballs or gastric stasis in rabbits can generally be prevented by feeding foods with adequate fiber (>14% DM crude fiber), minimizing stress and boredom, frequent grooming and providing adequate exercise (Carpenter et al, 1995).

Mucoid Enteropathy

Pet rabbits are also commonly presented with diarrhea, for which there are several differential diagnoses. Mucoid enteropathy is a GI disorder that is paradoxically characterized by constipation and diarrhea (Gentz et al, 1995; Jenkins, 2004), and by anorexia, lethargy, weight loss, cecal impaction and excessive production of mucus in the digestive tract (Lelkes and Chang, 1987). The cause of mucoid enteropathy is still under investigation, but the disease appears to be caused by changes in cecal pH that result from disruptions in the normal cecal flora (Lelkes and Chang, 1987; Jenkins, 1993). It likely occurs secondary to microbial alterations caused by hyperacidic cecal pH (Lelkes and Chang, 1987). A food containing about 20% crude fiber seems to maintain an optimal cecal pH to prevent changes in the normal microbial flora.

Mucoid enteropathy generally occurs in young rabbits, typically those just beyond weaning age (seven to 14 weeks) (Jenkins, 1993, 2004). It is rarely encountered in rabbitries that feed a high-fiber ration and avoid grains, simple carbohydrates and excesses of proteins or fats. Treatment includes feeding a high-fiber food (alfalfa hay) or syringe feeding a vegetable baby food (Jenkins, 1993) containing no additional sugars. In some cases, metoclopramide stimulates gastric emptying and apparently improves cecal activity. Fluid therapy to correct fluid and electrolyte imbalances is a priority to counteract losses that accompany the diarrhea (Gentz et al, 1995). Other treatment recommendations have been previously reported (Gentz et al, 1995; Jenkins, 2004).

Enterotoxemia

Enterotoxemia is one of the most common diseases of rabbits seen in clinical practice. Enterotoxemia is caused by the toxin produced by *Clostridium spiroforme* (Jenkins, 2004). Rabbits, particularly those recently weaned, are sensitive to foods high in sugars and starches (Gentz et al, 1995). Feeding these foods has been associated with at least some cases of enterotoxemia. Weanlings have an undeveloped population of normal GI flora and a high gastric pH, which allows proliferation of *C. spiroforme*. Nutritional counseling, therefore, is an important part of rabbit medicine, especially because many rabbit owners think lettuce, carrots and sugary treats are an appropriate diet for their animals.

Obesity

Many household rabbits have limited opportunities for exercise with almost unlimited access to palatable foods. Therefore, obesity is common in pet rabbits.

Because rabbits vary widely in body size, optimal body weights are difficult to estimate. Frequent weighing of each rabbit and recording the results in the medical record are important components of a preventive medicine program. Owners can be shown gradual increases in their rabbit's weight from medical records and the need for intervention. Systems for body condition scoring have not been published for rabbits and would be a welcome addition to preventive medicine programs.

Because rabbits use fiber efficiently, obesity may occur even when high-fiber foods are fed. However, weight control may be achieved by limiting the quantity of food offered. The amount of food offered should be reduced gradually, perhaps 10% every two weeks, until the amount fed maintains the desired body weight and condition.

Vitamin Deficiency and Toxicosis

Although cecal microbes synthesize B-complex vitamins and vitamin K and the rabbit obtains them via cecotrophy, manufacturers may add all of the essential vitamins to commercial foods. The requirement for vitamin D may be low because rabbits readily absorb calcium and phosphorus (Cheeke, 1995).

Signs of vitamin D toxicity include progressive emaciation and weakness, loss of appetite, diarrhea and paralysis. Soft tissues (i.e., liver, kidneys, artery walls and muscle) may become extensively calcified (Cheeke, 1995).

Vitamin A deficiency and excess may lead to reproductive disturbances. Low conception rates, fetal resorption, low survival of newborn kits and hydrocephalus in fetuses occur with toxic levels. Toxicosis is generally associated with adding synthetic vitamin A to foods that contain high levels of good-quality alfalfa

Table 70-6. Energy and nutrient contents of foods commonly fed as snacks to rabbits and rodents.*

Food items	Weight (g)	Water (%)	Energy (kcal/g)** (As fed)	(DM)	Protein	Fat	Carbohydrate	Fiber	Ca	P
Lettuce, romaine	100	94	0.18	3.0	36	7	50	11	1.1	0.4
Spinach, raw	100	91	0.26	2.9	36	3	48	7	1.0	0.6
Mung bean sprouts, raw	100	89	0.35	3.2	31	2	54	6	0.1	0.5
Summer squash, 1/2 cup	100	94	0.18	3.0	17	2	65	9	0.4	0.4
Blueberries, 1 cup	145	85	0.51	3.4	4	2	80	12	0.1	0.1
Strawberries, 1 cup	149	92	0.28	3.5	6	4	77	6	0.2	0.2
Apple, no skin, 1 medium	128	84	0.51	3.2	1	2	86	4	tr	tr
Banana, 1 medium	114	74	0.82	3.2	4	2	86	2	tr	tr
Cantaloupe, 1 cup	160	90	0.32	3.2	8	2	79	4	0.1	0.2

Key: Ca = calcium, P = phosphorus, DM = dry matter, tr = trace.
*Nutrients expressed as % dry matter, except water and as fed energy.
**To convert to kJ, multiply kcal by 4.184.

(Cheeke, 1995). Vitamin A-deficient rabbits exhibit poor growth, leg deformities, increased susceptibility to disease (e.g., enteritis) and hydrocephalus (Cheeke, 1995; Brooks, 2004).

Little information is available about the vitamin E requirements of rabbits. Signs of deficiency include muscular dystrophy, with paralysis of the hind legs, reproductive failure and neonatal death (Cheeke, 1995).

Feeding Plan

A diet commonly recommended by veterinarians for pet rabbits is a commercial high-fiber (at least 18 to 22% DM), pelleted food containing 12 to 16% DM crude protein, fed at the rate of one-fourth cup/2.3 kg body weight, divided into two daily meals (Carpenter, 2003; Cheeke, 1995; Jenkins, 1991). Although alfalfa-based pellets may be appropriate for growing rabbits, timothy hay-based pellets are recommended for adult rabbits because they contain less protein and calcium than alfalfa. Although some rabbits may be offered pellets free choice, many adult rabbits fed in this manner may become obese or fail to consume an adequate amount of loose hay.

Loose hay (mixed grass hay, timothy hay or dried grass clippings), should be provided free choice (Jenkins, 1991; Kupersmith, 1998). Alfalfa hay can be offered throughout the growth stages, but then should be discontinued because it contains higher than needed protein and calcium levels.

The diet should be supplemented with judicious amounts of thoroughly washed leafy greens (romaine lettuce, kale, mustard greens, carrot tops, parsley and dandelion greens) and fresh vegetables (carrots, broccoli, green peppers, cauliflower and cabbage). Dark greens with a low oxalate content should be selected (Kupersmith, 1998). In addition, rabbits may be fed a small amount (up to one tablespoon/2.3 kg body weight) of fresh fruit (strawberries, other berries, apples) daily or several times per week. Amounts of these palatable snacks should be limited because all are nutritionally incomplete and may cause a dietary imbalance (**Table 70-6**). Rabbits should not receive sugary treats, crackers, bread, rolled oats or breakfast cereals, which can cause abnormal fermentation in the gut and an overgrowth of certain bacteria resulting in serious, often fatal diarrhea.

Because rabbits are perhaps the most efficient converters of poorly digestible materials to animal flesh, their nutritional requirements can be met with any good quality hay supplemented with fresh greens (Jenkins, 1999). Therefore, some veterinarians are proposing that a diet of hay and fresh greens may satisfy the nutritional needs of house rabbits and minimizes the chance of diet-induced disease (Jenkins, 1999).

Practitioners often receive telephone calls regarding the feeding of wild orphaned bunnies. Ideally, if the orphaned bunny is deemed healthy, it should be returned to its environment if at all possible. Exceptions to this include if the bunny is smaller than the size of a tennis ball and its mother is known to be dead, or if the patient is not in good health. If hand-rearing is required, the patient should be thoroughly examined and medical problems such as hypothermia and dehydration should be rectified before feeding (Taylor, 2002). Hand-raising of wild bunnies should be done by licensed, trained rehabilitators. Feeding guidelines for orphaned bunnies are available (Sleeman, 2005; Taylor, 2002).

Other dietary recommendations for rabbits include:

- Because of the rabbit's intestinal microflora, food changes should be introduced gradually (over four to five days). For some rabbits with sensitive GI tracts, food changes may need to be made over a 10-day period (Harkness and Wagner, 1989). This is especially true for four- to 12-week-old rabbits. Current and new foods should be mixed 75:25 to begin the conversion. Quantities of the new food can then be increased gradually every few days.
- High-energy foods may increase susceptibility to mucoid enterotoxemia.
- Purchase small quantities of pellets at a time to prevent nutrient losses. Use pellets within 90 days of milling. Pellets can be stored in the freezer to reduce nutrient loss and spoilage.
- Clean, fresh water should be available at all times.

RODENTS

Introduction

The approximately 1,700 species of rodents in existence today represent over one-half of the total species of living mammals. The order Rodentia is divided into three suborders (sciuromorph, myomorph and hystricomorph) based primarily on variations in the origin of the masseter muscle. The word rodent originates from the Latin verb "rodere," to gnaw. Rodents are identified by their four prominent continuously erupting (hypsodontic) incisor teeth, which are frequently orange or yellow. Canine teeth are absent, and a gap, or diastema, exists between the incisor and cheek teeth. All rodents have six upper and six lower molar teeth, which may be either open- or closed-rooted, depending on the species. The presence or absence of premolar teeth is also species dependent.

Understanding rodent dentition is important because malocclusion and overgrowth of open-rooted teeth are common clinical problems, with sequelae such as weight loss, malnutrition and oral mucosal ulcerations. Normal gnawing behavior occurs when a rodent holds an object, frequently with the assistance of the forefeet, against the immobile upper incisor teeth and then shears with lateral to medial movements of the lower incisor teeth and jaw. During the gnawing process, the rodent moves the lower jaw forward, allowing apposition of incisor teeth but preventing occlusion and abrasion of cheek teeth. By withdrawing the cheek into the diastema, the rodent can compartmentalize the gnawed material into the cranial portion of the oral cavity, thus allowing for lengthy periods of gnawing without necessarily swallowing the gnawed material. During the chewing process, the lower jaw moves caudally to bring upper and lower cheek teeth into apposition. The complex muscles and anatomic variations in the associated skull bones, which allow for such specialized jaw movements, are a primary means of classifying rodent species (Sainsbury, 2003).

Although veterinarians may be presented with some very unusual pet rodents for examination, diagnosis and treatment of health problems, the most commonly seen pet rodents are guinea pigs (*Cavia porcellus*), chinchillas (*Chinchilla laniger*), hamsters (multiple species), Mongolian gerbils (*Meriones unguiculatus*), rats (*Rattus norvegicus*) and mice (*Mus musculus*). Rodents are intelligent, relatively inexpensive to purchase and maintain and require little space. Unfortunately, however, owners are frequently unaware of specific husbandry requirements until problems resulting from conditions such as improper caging, poor nutrition and water deprivation become evident. A thorough history about husbandry practices can provide invaluable clues to the clinician when trying to address an owner's concerns.

Cage Requirements

Proper caging is a critical aspect of rodent husbandry. This requirement should be considered when assessing suspected nutritional problems. Inadequate housing, poorly positioned food and water dispensers, dirty cages and a stressful environment can contribute to problems such as anorexia and dehydration. A variety of cages are available in pet stores, and one should be selected carefully, keeping in mind the characteristics of the species for which it will be used. In general, cages must be escape-proof and predator-proof, provide adequate ventilation, minimize the possibility of trauma, have mounted sipper bottles and provide adequate floor space.

Cages are typically constructed of metal, glass or plastic. Wood should not be used for caging rodents because it can be gnawed and is difficult to disinfect. Solid flooring is preferred to wire because it minimizes potential limb trauma and pododermatitis; however, it is more difficult to keep clean. Wire flooring can be used successfully if it is of proper mesh size and a portion of the cage contains solid flooring.

Bedding should be nonabrasive, nontoxic, clean, absorbent, inedible, dust-free and capable of being made into nests. Various medical problems have been associated with some frequently used bedding materials. Cedar shavings have been associated with dermatopathies and pulmonary and hepatic changes. Pine may affect hepatic enzyme activity. Hardwood shavings such as aspen and shredded nontoxic paper are the most commonly recommended bedding materials. Gerbils, hamsters and mice apparently prefer larger amounts of bedding than do guinea pigs, chinchillas and rats (Harkness, 1993). Frequency of cage cleaning and replacement of bedding varies with rodent type and cage.

Environmental enrichment in the form of nesting material, cage toys and different food items can be used to enhance the lives of laboratory and pet rodents, again keeping in mind the behavioral characteristics of the particular animal. Providing opportunities to forage allows animals to engage in natural behavior and can prevent boredom and provide exercise (Baumans, 2005).

Common Aspects of Rodent Nutrition

Although little research has concerned pet rodents specifically, the popularity of rodents as laboratory animals has led to extensive nutritional studies. Nutrient requirements for laboratory rodents serve as initial guides to the nutrient requirements of pet rodents (**Table 70-7**) (NRC, 1978).

Coprophagy

Most rodents are coprophagous, and fecal pellets are frequently ingested directly from the anus. Generally lighter, softer feces (cecotrophs) are selectively ingested. These feces are produced in the cecum and contain important B-complex vitamins and protein. Young rodents ingest maternal feces, thereby inoculating their own intestinal tracts with autochthonous flora (Clark, 1984; Manning et al, 1984).

Anorexia, Weight Loss and Dehydration

Clinical problems related to anorexia, weight loss, dehydration or a combination of these factors are frequently observed in pet rodents. Common etiologies include husbandry-related factors such food and/or water deprivation, inability to reach or manipulate food or water utensils, inappropriate diet, sudden dietary changes, poor hygiene, overcrowding, inadequate temperatures and other environmental stressors (Harkness, 1993).

Careful and tactful questioning by the clinician is necessary for the client to realize or admit to the presence and significance of inadequate husbandry practices. If possible, the client should bring the rodent and its entire cage to the veterinary visit for a more thorough assessment of the animal's environment.

Following a complete physical examination, basic diagnostic

Table 70-7. Estimated nutrient requirements of laboratory rodents.* Some of these values were determined by rigorous comparative trials, others by examination of foods known to suffice for specific species. The data presented here are intended to be used only as starting points. The literature cited should be consulted for more information.

Nutrients	Rats M	Rats Above M	Mice Above M	Gerbils Above M	Hamsters -
Protein as casein (%)**	4.2	12	12.5-18	16-25	15.0
Fat (%)	5.0	5	5	5-20	5
Digestible energy (kcal/g)***	3,800	3,800	-	-	4.2
L-amino acids					
Arginine (%)	-	0.6	0.3	-	0.76
Asparagine (%)	-	0.4	-	-	-
Glutamic acid (%)	-	4.0	-	-	-
Histidine (%)	0.08	0.3	0.2	-	0.40
Isoleucine (%)	0.31	0.5	0.4	-	0.89
Leucine (%)	0.18	0.75	0.7	-	1.39
Lysine (%)	0.11	0.70	0.4	-	1.20
Methionine (%)	0.23	0.60	0.5	-	0.32
Phenylalanine-tyrosine (%)	0.18	0.80	0.4	-	0.83
Proline (%)	-	0.40	-	-	-
Threonine (%)	0.18	0.50	0.4	-	0.70
Tryptophan (%)	0.05	0.15	0.1	-	0.34
Valine (%)	0.23	0.60	0.5	-	0.91
Nonessential (%)	0.48	0.50	-	-	-
Minerals					
Calcium (%)	-	0.50	0.4	0.6-0.8	0.59
Chloride (%)	-	0.05	-	0.2-0.8	-
Magnesium (%)	-	0.04	0.05	0.1-0.2	0.06
Phosphorus (%)	-	0.40	0.4	0.3-0.4	0.30
Potassium (%)	-	0.36	0.2	0.7-0.9	0.61
Sodium (%)	-	0.05	-	0.2-0.4	0.15
Sulfur (%)	-	0.03	-	-	-
Chromium (mg/kg)	-	0.30	2.0	-	-
Copper (mg/kg)	-	5.00	4.5	0.4-4.0	1.6
Fluoride (mg/kg)	-	1.00	-	0-11	0.024
Iodine (mg/kg)	-	0.15	0.25	1-37	1.6
Iron (mg/kg)	-	35.00	25.00	130-470	140
Manganese (mg/kg)	-	50.00	45.00	3-45	3.65
Selenium (mg/kg)	-	0.10	-	-	0.1
Zinc (mg/kg)	-	12.00	30.00	0-8	9.2
Vitamins					
A (IU/kg)	-	4,000	500	18,000-32,000	-
D (IU/kg)	-	1,000	150	2,000-3,250	2,484
E (IU/kg)	-	30	20	9-1,200	3
K (mcg/kg)	-	50	3,000	-	4,000
Choline (mg/kg)	-	1,000	600	750-3,000	2,000
Folic acid (mg/kg)	-	1	0.5	100-1,800	2
Niacin (mg/kg)	-	20	10	22-90	90
Pantothenate (mg/kg)	-	8	10	25-60	40
Riboflavin (mg/kg)	-	3	7	4-20	15
Thiamin (mg/kg)	-	4	5	4-22	20
B_6 (mg/kg)	-	6	1	4-22	6
B_{12} (mcg/kg)	-	50	10	0.18	10

Key: M = maintenance; healthy, non-stressed adults in comfortable surroundings. Above M = ill or stressed adults and growing, pregnant or lactating animals.
*Clark JD, Olfert ED. Rodents (Rodentia). In: Fowler ME, ed. Zoo and Wild Animal Medicine. Philadelphia, PA: WB Saunders Co, 1986; 728-733.
**Minimum protein requirements were determined with animals fed purified and semi-purified diets containing casein as a protein source. For animals fed commercial foods comprised of complex ingredients and relatively lower digestibilities, dietary protein should be higher.
***To convert to kJ, multiply kcal by 4.184.

studies such as complete blood counts, biochemistry profiles, radiographs and fecal examinations should be conducted whenever possible to rule out malocclusion, GI disease and other primary disease problems. Fecal culture and abdominal ultrasound are also often useful.

The prognosis for an anorectic, dehydrated rodent with significant weight loss is guarded. Supportive care includes administering oral, subcutaneous, and/or intraperitoneal fluids and offering a variety of sweetened foods or treats to encourage food intake. Many rodents will also tolerate gentle force-feeding. Pelleted rodent feed may be blenderized with water and appropriate supplements such as yogurt, vegetable baby foods or both. Alternatively, liquid enteral products formulated for people or pets may be fed without supplementation.

Feeding is best accomplished by wrapping the animal gently in a towel, placing the feeding syringe into the diastema, expressing small volumes into the oral cavity and allowing the animal to swallow. One-ml syringes can be used to feed mice, and 3- to 10-ml catheter-tipped syringes used to feed larger rodents. Owners can be shown how to feed their pets at home; however, they must be able to recognize when the animal is responsive enough to allow force feeding, to minimize potential problems with aspiration. Small meals should be fed several times throughout the day.

Malocclusion

Malocclusion is another common clinical problem in pet rodents. The incisor teeth are usually involved, although the cheek teeth may also be maloccluded, depending on the species. Etiologies include genetic, dietary, infectious and traumatic factors. Overgrown teeth can result in tongue and oral ulcers, ptyalism, anorexia and weight loss. An oral examination is an important but often difficult component of a rodent physical examination. An otoscope may help visualize cheek teeth, but the patient may require sedation for the procedure. Skull radiographs are also useful for assessing severe malocclusion and tooth root abscesses. Specialized equipment, including specula, mouth gags and long-shank dental burrs, are available for use in rodents.

Inhalant anesthesia, preferably isoflurane administered through a facemask, is adequate for short dental procedures, such as trimming incisor teeth. The animal is masked down and the mask is removed when the animal attains an appropriate level of anesthesia. Its mouth is held open with a specialized speculum or gauze strips around the upper and lower incisors, and the incisor teeth are cut quickly, preferably with a high-speed dental drill. A variable-speed, rotary power tool with a circular cutting blade (Dremel Moto-Tool[d]) can also be used. Care should be used not to injure the tongue and surrounding tissues. Although sharp clippers have been used to trim the teeth of smaller rodents, teeth may split or shatter with this method; therefore, this technique is not recommended. Inhalant anesthesia delivered by facemask may be challenging for lengthier dental procedures on cheek teeth, which may require clipping with bone rongeurs or, preferably, using a guarded flat or taper fissure burr in a straight, low-speed dental handpiece (Quesenberry, 1994; Harkness and Wagner, 1995; Crossley and Aiken, 2004). Injectable anesthesia may be required for these procedures because small rodents are very difficult to intubate.

Rodents with chronic malocclusion problems may need teeth trimming every few months. Owners should monitor animals for anorexia and drooling. Breeding rodents with malocclusion problems should be discouraged.

Guinea Pigs

Husbandry

Domestic guinea pigs belong in the Caviidae family, which consists of short-tailed or tailless rodents that have one pair of mammary glands, four digits on the forefeet and three digits on the hindfeet. The most commonly seen breeds are: 1) the Shorthair or English, which has very uniform short hair, 2) the Abyssinian, which has a coat arranged in whorls or rosettes and 3) the Peruvian, which can have a coat several inches long. Various coat colors and multicolored patterns also exist for each species. Pet guinea pigs live for five to seven years and weigh 450 to 750 g. Gestation averages 68 days, and litter size ranges from two to four young (Clark, 1984; Anderson, 1987; Quesenberry et al, 2004).

Guinea pigs are herbivores with simple stomachs. Their teeth are open-rooted and erupt continuously. The dental formula is I1/1, C0/0, P1/1 and M3/3. The incisors are white unlike that of other rodents, which normally have yellow incisors. Guinea pigs have a long digestive tract with a gastric emptying time of approximately two hours and a total GI transit time from eight to 20 hours. Normal GI flora consists primarily of *Lactobacillus* and occasionally *Streptococcus* spp., yeast and soil bacteria (Manning et al, 1984; Harkness and Wagner, 1995a). Much of the digestive process occurs in the cecum, which is a thin-walled sac divided into numerous lateral pouches by smooth muscle bands (taenia coli). The cecum is normally found on the central and left side of the abdomen and may contain as much as 65% of the GI contents (Richardson, 1992; Quesenberry et al, 2004). Guinea pigs are coprophagous.

Special Nutritional Needs

Guinea pigs, people and other primates are unable to synthesize vitamin C (ascorbic acid) because they lack the enzyme L-gluconolactone oxidase, which is needed to convert glucose to ascorbic acid. Adequate dietary supplementation is, therefore, critical to prevent hypovitaminosis C (scurvy), as detailed below. (See Feeding Plan.)

Guinea pigs display behavioral characteristics that influence their overall nutritional status. For example, they are extremely susceptible to stressful situations such as inadequate housing, moving into a new household or different cage and changing feeding schedules. Stressed guinea pigs may become anorectic and lose weight. Furthermore, guinea pigs do not tolerate dietary or environmental changes well. Guinea pigs develop dietary preferences early in life and do not adapt readily to change. For this reason, young guinea pigs should be exposed to different dietary items to allow them to become accustomed to variety (Quesenbery et al, 2004).

Proper housing accommodations can be provided by an open-topped enclosure at least 10 inches high, with a floor space of at least 101 square inches for an adult animal, and twice this floor space for a breeding sow. Either solid or wire flooring can be provided. Wire flooring allows for feces and urine to drop to the bottom of the cage. However, it may cause foot injuries and subsequent pododermatitis. Wire flooring should consist of a rectangular mesh 38 by 12 mm. At least a portion of the cage should have a solid bottom (Quesenberry, 1994). Solid floors with a substrate of shredded paper or hardwood shavings generally require more frequent cleaning but are preferable for pet guinea pigs.

Because guinea pigs are easily startled, the cage should be placed in a quiet area in the home to minimize exposure to sudden movements and loud noises. Ideally, a relatively constant temperature between 18 to 24°C (65 to 75°F), and humidity between 40 and 70% should be maintained (Harkness and Wagner, 1995a). Elevated temperatures may cause heat stress. A cool, damp environment can predispose guinea pigs to respiratory diseases.

Additional behavioral characteristics of guinea pigs include their tendency to contaminate food and water dishes with excreta. Sipper bottles are preferred to minimize contamination of drinking water. However, guinea pigs can pass ingesta into sipper tubes. Guinea pigs also play with the end of the sipper tube, which may cause leaks, resulting in wet bedding and an empty water bottle. All food and water utensils should be cleaned and soiled bedding removed daily.

Any changes in access to food and water should be made gradually, over five to 10 days. Owners should also be cautioned to monitor for any signs of anorexia or decreased water intake when husbandry changes are recommended (Peters, 1991).

Common Nutritional Disorders

HYPOVITAMINOSIS C

Although quality commercial guinea pig foods are formulated with adequate vitamin C, hypovitaminosis C (scurvy) is still a common clinical problem because of this nutrient's lability during storage. Also, feeding guinea pigs rabbit food without providing additional vitamin C may cause scurvy. Because guinea pigs are incapable of storing vitamin C, scurvy appears within one to two weeks after a vitamin C deficient diet is fed. Death usually occurs within three weeks (Tobin, 1996; O'Rourke, 2004).

Guinea pigs with scurvy present with anorexia, bruxism, weight loss, an unkempt appearance and gingivitis. Affected animals are reluctant to move because of joint and muscle pain. Discomfort is apparent when limbs are palpated. Ascorbic acid is required for normal collagen formation; therefore, deficiencies primarily affect the musculoskeletal system. Sequelae include enlarged costochondral junctions, hemorrhage into muscles and joints and abnormalities in epiphyseal growth centers with subsequent pathologic fractures. Secondary infections, delayed wound healing and diarrhea may also be present. Subclinical vitamin C deficiency should be considered in any guinea pig presented with generalized illness. Young animals and pregnant sows are most severely affected (Harkness and Wagner, 1995; Peters, 1991).

Diagnosis of vitamin C deficiency is based on the history and clinical signs. Radiographs may reveal enlargement of long bone epiphyses and costochondral junctions.

Treatment involves parenteral supplementation with 50 to 100 mg vitamin C/kg body weight until clinical signs resolve (Quesenberry, 1994) one to two weeks after a vitamin C deficient diet is fed. Death usually occurs within three weeks (Tobin, 1996; O'Rourke, 2004). Oral vitamin C can then be initiated at the same dosage. Owners can supplement the diet with liquid pediatric vitamin C products obtained over-the-counter from pharmacies and supermarkets. (Appropriate dietary supplements are discussed in the Feeding Plan section.) Anorectic and dehydrated animals should receive supportive care such as fluids and forced alimentation as discussed in the Introduction to Rodents section. Client education about dietary requirements of guinea pigs plays a critical role in preventing this disease.

PREGNANCY TOXEMIA

Pregnancy toxemia or ketosis occurs primarily in obese, primiparous, anorectic, stressed guinea pig sows. Boars are also susceptible to ketosis, although obviously pregnancy is not a factor. Obesity and anorexia are the most critical inciting factors for the development of ketosis. Genetics may also play a role. The onset of clinical signs is abrupt and occurs within about five days (before and after) of parturition. Clinical signs include lethargy, ruffled coat, anorexia, prostration, muscle spasms and death.

Diagnostic tests may reveal hypoglycemia (perhaps terminal hyperglycemia), hyperlipidemia, ketonemia, hyperkalemia, hyponatremia, hypochloremia, proteinuria and urinary pH less than six.

Supportive care includes administration of fluids, 5% glucose given orally or intravenously, antibiotics and judicious use of corticosteroids if the animal is in shock. Caesarean section may be attempted to save the fetuses. Prognosis, however, is poor and treatment is generally unsuccessful. Preventing obesity in sows (preferably body weight <500 g), providing a good food, minimizing stress and avoiding fasting or undernutrition in late pregnancy will reduce the risk of pregnancy toxemia.

CECAL IMPACTION

Low fiber intakes (perhaps <10% DM crude fiber) predispose guinea pigs to cecal impaction. Prevention is best accomplished by providing adequate long-stem fiber in the form of chopped grass hay. Hay should be offered free choice, even when fiber-containing guinea pig pellets are fed.

SOFT-TISSUE CALCIFICATION

Guinea pigs are reportedly susceptible to a syndrome involving calcification of soft tissues, especially in the forelimbs. The syndrome is thought to be related to dietary levels of calcium, phosphorus, magnesium, potassium and vitamin D (Tobin, 1996). Means of prevention are unknown, but efforts should be made to restrict use of supplements and to maintain DM vitamin D levels below 2,000 IU/kg (Tobin, 1996).

Feeding Plan

FEEDING ADULTS

Guinea pigs are strict herbivores and should be maintained on a feed specifically labeled for the species. Commercial dry rabbit food, although similar in appearance, should not be used because it contains inadequate levels of protein and vitamin C.

Vitamin C

Adequate dietary vitamin C levels are critical for overall good health, and although commercial guinea pig foods are formulated with approximately 800 mg DM vitamin C/kg, low vitamin C intake is still a common problem due to the vitamin's lability. Heat, moisture and contact with metals hasten its deterioration during storage. Ideally, guinea pig pellets should be stored at 22°C (72°F) and used within 90 days of milling (Quesenberry, 1994; Quesenberry et al, 2004). Consumers may have difficulty determining how long the product has been on the shelf at the time of purchase because: 1) the milling date is frequently not stated on the food container and 2) many pet stores buy feed in bulk and then repackage product for resale. Owners should therefore be encouraged to buy food in small quantities from a reputable pet store that has a relatively high turnover of food products and to store the food properly at home.

Guinea pigs require approximately 10 mg vitamin C/kg body weight daily for maintenance and 30 mg/kg body weight daily for gestation. If the freshness of guinea pig pellets is unknown, 200 mg/ml vitamin C can be added to the drinking water. However, the half life of this nutrient in clean, fresh water is only 24 hours, and shorter if organic debris is present or if metal containers are used. Vitamin C can also be given orally on a daily basis using human pediatric vitamin C formulations (Quesenberry, 1994). Daily feeding small amounts of vegetables with a high vitamin C content such as red or green peppers, tomatoes, spinach and asparagus can augment vitamin C intake. Excess ingested vitamin C is excreted rapidly in the urine, with 80% of the ingested amount being eliminated in three days. Fresh vegetables should be thoroughly rinsed to minimize potential pesticide contaminants and bacterial pathogens such as *Salmonella* spp. (Harkness, 1993a).

Protein, Fiber and Water

Commercial guinea pig pellets contain approximately 20% DM crude protein and 9 to 18% DM crude fiber. For an adult guinea pig, average daily food consumption is 6 g/100 g body weight and average daily water consumption is 10 ml/100 g body weight (Harkness, 1993a). Because guinea pigs are such fastidious eaters, owners should be discouraged from frequently changing brands of food to avoid anorexia. High-quality timothy or grass hay should be available at all times (Quesenberry et al, 2004). Oral lesions may occur if the hay is too coarse. Secondary infection of these lesions with beta-hemolytic *Streptococcus* spp. can lead to cervical lymphadenitis and abscess formation. Owners who allow their guinea pigs access to the yard should also be forewarned about possible herbicide/pesticide exposure. Overgrazing on lush lawns or fresh grass clippings can result in diarrhea. The recommended diet for guinea pigs is comprised of guinea pig pellets and high-quality grass hay supplemented with fresh vegetables.

FEEDING NEONATES

Newborn guinea pigs are precocious, with teeth, a full coat and open eyes. Birth weights vary from 60 to 100 g. Neonates weighing less than 50 to 60 g rarely survive. Birth weight is related to genetic characteristics and maternal nutritional status, and is directly proportional to gestation length and inversely proportional to litter size. Neonatal guinea pigs remain close to the sow but generally will not nurse for the first 12 to 24 hours and, therefore, should not be force fed during this time. Neonates usually begin eating solid food at four to five days of age (i.e., guinea pig chow softened with cow's milk or water). If several lactating sows are present, the young may nurse alternately among them. In this case, the smaller piglets must be monitored to ensure that they nurse adequately. Weaning age varies from 14 to 28 days when body weight reaches 150 to 200 g. Average daily weight gain should be 2.5 to 3.5 g daily until 60 days of age (Manning et al, 1984).

Chinchillas

Husbandry

Chinchillas belong in the Chinchillidae family and are closely related to guinea pigs. Chinchillas originate from the rocky slopes of the South American Andes, where they were nearly hunted to extinction in the early part of the 1900s because of their prized pelts. A small group of chinchillas brought to the United States at that time were successfully bred in captivity and are progenitors for the majority of today's pet population.

Chinchilla breeds are characterized by their coat color, which in the wild is a smoky blue-gray. Other color variations represent mutations. The normal coat is thick and soft, an attribute that often masks problems such as weight loss. Adult chinchillas weigh from 400 to 600 g and have an average life span of 10 years, with a maximum up to 20 years. The average gestation period is 111 days, and average litter size is two, with a range of one to six. The dental formula is I1/1, C0/0, P1/1 and M3/3. All teeth are open-rooted. Incisor teeth grow 6.2 to 7.6 cm per year (Hoefer, 1994; Quesenberry et al, 2004).

Chinchillas are hindgut fermenters and have a long alimentary tract, measuring more than 3.5 m in adult animals. The proximal colon is sacculated and communicates with the large thin-coiled cecum. The longer distal colon is smooth (Williams, 1979). Chinchillas are also coprophagic. Chinchillas ingest more than 70% of their total food intake at night (Quesenberry et al, 2004).

Proper housing is a critical factor for a chinchilla's overall well being. The animal's native environment includes a relatively low temperature and humidity and a sloping, hard, rocky habitat that requires that chinchillas jump from one crevice to another. Chinchillas should therefore be housed in a large (minimum of 1,650 cm^2 floor area per animal), multilevel cage to accommodate normal, active behavior. If wire mesh flooring is used, the mesh size should be small enough to prevent leg entrapment. Some areas of solid flooring should be provided to minimize foot lesions. The optimal temperature range is 16 to 21°C (60 to 70°F). Temperatures as low as 0°C (32°F) can be tolerated if the animal has been acclimated. Temperatures greater than 27°C (80°F) can result in heatstroke, particularly in the presence of high humidity (Quesenberry et al, 2004).

Chinchillas are fastidious groomers and should be provided with a dust bath for a short time (30 to 60 minutes) each day. Keeping the dustpan dish in the cage continuously results in fecal contamination of the dish and subsequently of the coat, and can lead to conjunctivitis. Dust can be obtained commercially and consists of a mixture of 9:1 silver sand to Fuller's earth (Jenkins, 1992; Hoefer, 1994).

Because chinchillas are hindgut fermenters, they have complex digestive processes for fermenting dietary fiber. Any disruption of these processes can result in diarrhea, constipation, mucoid enteritis, bloat, intussusception and rectal prolapse. Inappropriate foods and sudden food changes are common causes of these problems. Inappropriate foods include those that contain high levels of simple carbohydrates and protein or not enough fiber. Such foods alter cecal fermentation processes with subsequent changes in pH, motility and flora, resulting in enteritis. Any change in the normally gram-positive GI flora can lead to overgrowth of bacteria such as *Escherichia coli* and *Clostridium, Proteus* and *Pseudomonas* spp. Therefore, antibiotics such as ampicillin, amoxicillin, penicillin, cephalosporins, clindamycin, lincomycin and erythromycin should be avoided (Ness, 2005). Other causes of enteritis include *Salmonella* spp., *Giardia lamblia, Cryptosporidium* spp., coccidia and nematodes (Williams, 1979; Jenkins, 1992; Hoefer, 1994; Donnelly, 2004b). Unfortunately, the exact cause of gastroenteritis frequently remains undetermined, thus subsequent treatment is symptomatic, including administration of fluids, dietary changes (adding fiber) and appropriate antibiotics.

Few integumentary disorders of chinchillas are directly associated with specific nutrients. Fatty acid deficiency leads to a poor coat, skin flaking and possibly cutaneous ulcers. Zinc deficiency can result in alopecia (Scott et al, 1995).

Feeding Plan

FEEDING ADULTS

Specific nutrient requirements for chinchillas have not been well established. With the exception of being placentophagic, chinchillas are considered to be strict herbivores and subsist in the wild on shrubs and grasses. Controversy exists among various authors as to what type of feeding plan is most suitable for captive animals. All recommendations reflect a high overall dietary fiber requirement. Experts generally agree that good nutritional status can be achieved by feeding a combination of pellets and free-choice, good-quality grass or timothy hay. Commercially available chinchilla pellets are preferred to guinea pig and rabbit pellets because of formulation and size differences. Because chinchillas often use their forefeet to hold their food, the shape and size of the pellets affect ease of food handling and amount of wastage. Pellets should consist of 18 to 20% DM crude protein, 15 to 35% DM crude fiber and 4% DM fat.

Adult chinchillas eat an average of 21 g of food per day. Only one to two tbs of pellets should be fed per day, because overfeeding may cause enteritis. High-quality grass hay should be available free choice. Treats such as fresh fruits, vegetables and nuts can be offered occasionally but should be limited to not more than 1 tsp per day (Harkness, 1993b; Hoefer, 1994; Quesenberry et al, 2004). Fresh water in clean sipper bottles should always be available.

FEEDING NEONATES

Newborn chinchillas are precocious and weigh 30 to 50 g. They generally begin eating pelleted food at one week of age, and are completely weaned by six to eight weeks. Orphaned neonates can be hand-reared or fostered onto other chinchillas, and can survive independently after two to three weeks of age. Two reportedly successful hand-feeding formulas vary markedly. One is a mixture of one part unsweetened condensed milk and two parts water. The other is a mixture of one-half water, one-half evaporated milk, with glucose added to achieve a final concentration of 25% (Williams, 1979; Kraft, 1987). Milk replacers, however, may be a better alternative to condensed or evaporated milk.

Hamsters

Husbandry

Hamsters are rodents in the Cricetidae family. There are many species of hamsters. The most commonly seen are the golden or Syrian hamster (*Mesocricetus auratus*), the Chinese hamster (*Cricetulus griseus*) and the dwarf hamster (*Phodopus sungorus*). Hamsters were introduced into the United States in 1938 for research purposes.

Although hamster species vary markedly, male and female adults weigh 85 to 130 g and 95 to 150 g, respectively. Females tend to be larger and more aggressive than males. Life spans are relatively short and average from 18 to 24 months. The gestation period is 15 to 16 days. Litter size ranges from five to nine. Young are born without hair, with eyes and ears closed, but with erupted incisor teeth. The dental formula is I1/1, C0/0, P0/0 and M3/3. Incisor teeth grow throughout life; however, molar teeth are closed-rooted. Hamsters possess large cheek pouches that are used to transport and store food. When alarmed, hamsters will also temporarily store their young in these pouches. The stomach is divided into glandular and nonglandular portions. The nonglandular forestomach is lined with keratinized epithelium and is the site of pregastric fermentation (Van Hoosier and Ladiges, 1984; Battles, 1991). Like rabbits and many rodents, hamsters are coprophagic.

Hamsters are nocturnal animals. Although they are not true hibernators, hamsters enter a period of "pseudohibernation" from which they can be aroused, when exposed to shorter day lengths and temperatures below 4.4°C (40°F). In the wild, hamsters are solitary animals that live in burrows. Hamsters are very active at gnawing and escape by chewing through cages or by pushing open cage lids. Subsequent ingestion of inappropriate household items can lead to serious GI problems. Therefore, proper caging, as with other rodents, is critical to the overall well being of these animals.

Cages for adult hamsters should have a floor space of at least 125 cm^2 and a height of at least 15 cm. The traditional slotted metal food hoppers that are placed on top of the cage and frequently used for rats and mice are generally inappropriate for hamsters. The flat face of these pets makes it difficult for them to retrieve food items. If slotted metal food hoppers are used, the slots should be at least 7/16 in. wide. Clean water in a sipper bottle should always be available and the bottle should be placed low enough for the hamster to reach. The recommended environmental temperatures for hamsters are 18.3 to 21.1°C (65 to 70°F). Relative humidity should be between 30 and 70%

(Wagner and Farrar, 1987; Harkness, 1993c).

Acute enteric diseases are common problems among hamsters, especially weanlings. Underlying causes often remain unknown; however, stress, inadequate diet and improperly positioned feeders are often contributing factors. Processed feed should have a minimum of 8% crude fiber content to prevent diarrhea. An intracellular bacterium, *Lawsonia intracellularis*, is the causative agent of proliferative ileitis diarrhea or "wet tail;" however, *Escherichia coli*, *Clostridium* spp. or *Bacillus* spp. may also be involved. Rapid weight loss, dehydration and staining of the perineal region are present clinically. Other possible sequelae include intestinal blockage, prolapse and intussusception. Administration of inappropriate antibiotics (e.g., penicillin, ampicillin, lincomycin and bacitracin) can result in overgrowth of *Clostridium difficile* and a subsequent fatal enterocolitis (Harkness, 1993c).

The prognosis for hamsters presenting with signs of enteritis is generally guarded. Treatment involves supportive care such as administration of fluids subcutaneously or intraperitoneally, appropriate antibiotics (e.g., trimethoprim-sulfadiazine, chloramphenicol or enrofloxacin) and oral bismuth salicylate. Hamsters with enteritis should be hand-fed and placed in a warm environment.

Few reports document specific nutrient deficiencies in hamsters. Generalized alopecia and skin problems have been associated with low protein (<16%) and with deficiencies in pantothenic acid, riboflavin, pyridoxine, niacin, fatty acids and copper. Vitamin E deficiency can lead to muscular weakness, ocular secretions and death. Hamsters fed foods high in polyunsaturated fat are more susceptible to vitamin E deficiency and subsequent muscular dystrophy (Harkness, 1993c; Scott et al, 1995).

Feeding Plan
Specific nutrient requirements for hamsters have not been well established. In the wild, hamsters are omnivorous, ingesting a variety of plants, seeds, fruits and meats. Pelleted rodent foods that provide 16 to 20% crude protein appear to provide good growth rates, whereas those containing 8 to 12% crude protein appear to be inadequate. Hamsters tend to ingest fruits, nuts, cereals and prepackaged "rodent treats" preferentially to the more nutritionally balanced rodent foods; therefore, these items should be provided in limited quantities. Adult food consumption averages 15 to 20 g/day (Harkness, 1993c).

Pregnant and lactating females have markedly increased food consumption. A one-week supply of food should be placed in the cage at about the Day 13 of gestation to minimize disturbances during parturition. Food should be placed on the cage floor rather than in a hopper to minimize the dam's distraction with food gathering, which may result in neglect of the young. This practice also allows easier access to food for pups as they approach weaning. Pups should also have easy access to the water bottle, and they should be observed closely to ensure that they can pull hard enough on the sipper tube to obtain water. Neonatal hamsters are altricial, and have birth weights from 2 to 3 g. Young begin gnawing on solid food at seven to 10 days of age and are weaned around 21 days. Weaning weights average 35 g. Attempts at hand raising or cross-fostering of orphaned hamster neonates onto other rodent species are generally unsuccessful (Wagner and Farrar, 1987).

Gerbils
Husbandry
Gerbils are rodents in the Cricetidae family. The Mongolian gerbil is the most common pet species. A frequent color pattern is agouti or brown; however, other color variations such as black, white and cinnamon also exist. Gerbils are social, burrowing animals native to the desert regions of central Asia. As pets, they are generally friendly and easily handled. Because of their water conservation mechanisms, they produce only a few drops of urine daily and are, therefore, virtually odor free. Adult gerbils weigh from 55 to 100 g and have a life span of three to four years. Gerbils generally form monogamous pairs, which is unique among rodents. Gestation length is 24 to 26 days, with a litter of size of four to seven. Neonates are altricial. Approximately half of the pet gerbil population exhibits spontaneous, convulsive seizures that are induced by strange environments or excitement. Fatalities are uncommon and anticonvulsant therapy has not been recommended (Harkness, 1993d, Harkness, 1995a; Donnelly, 2004c).

Gerbils can be housed as described for hamsters. They also actively gnaw so cages need to be escape-proof. Adult gerbils should be provided with a minimum floor space of 230 cm^2 with sides at least 15 cm high. Temperatures should be maintained between 18 to 29°C (65 to 85°F) and humidity levels between 30 and 50%. Gerbils do not tolerate high temperatures and their coat appears greasy under conditions of high humidity (Wagner and Farrar, 1987).

Diarrhea can result from food changes, contaminants or deprivation and protozoal or bacterial infections, such as salmonellosis. Treatment is symptomatic as described for hamsters, because the specific etiology frequently remains undetermined.

Specific nutrient deficiencies are uncommon in gerbils fed commercial dry rodent food. Animals maintained on high-fat diets such as excessive amounts of sunflower seeds develop lipemia and hypercholesteremia with excess fat deposits throughout the body. However, atherosclerosis does not appear to occur under these conditions, which has made gerbils important in cardiac disease research. Weanling animals are especially susceptible to malnutrition and dehydration as a result of poor accessibility to food and water (Wagner and Farrar, 1987).

Feeding Plan
In the wild, gerbils feed on plants, seeds and insects. In captivity, they should be fed a commercial dry rodent food that is suitable for gerbils, offered free choice. Gerbils maintained on a standard rat or mouse diet for longer than six months may develop periodontal disease (Donnelly, 2004c). Gerbils will ingest seeds preferentially, which results in a diet high in fat and low in calcium. Gerbils generally eat about eight meals per day, with a total food consumption of 5 to 8 g/100 g of body weight. Because they eat frequent small meals, rapid weight loss occurs

if food quantities are limited. Clean water in easily accessible sipper bottles should always be available. Young gerbils generally begin eating solid food at 14 to 16 days of age and are weaned at 20 to 26 days. Dry rodent food can be softened with water for weanlings (Harkness, 1993d).

Rats

Husbandry

The common pet rat belongs in the Muridae family and originated in central Asia. Adult female and male rats weigh from 250 to 300 g and 450 to 520 g, respectively. The average life span ranges from 2.5 to 3.5 years. The gestation period is 21 to 23 days, and litter size ranges from six to 12. The rat's dental formula is I1/1, C0/0, P0/0 and M3/3. Incisor teeth erupt continuously, but molar teeth are permanently rooted. Rats have a divided stomach, a large cecum, no gallbladder and a GI transit time of 12 to 24 hours.

A variety of cages, usually constructed of plastic or metal, are available in pet stores. General guidelines for optimal caging were discussed previously. (See Rodents, Cage Requirements.) Cages should be made escape-proof because rats are adept at chewing through cages, lifting lids and opening small cage doors. Adult rats should be provided with a minimum of 250 cm^2 of floor space and a cage height of 18 cm. Ambient temperatures should be 18 to 27°C (65 to 80°F) with an optimum temperature of 22°C (72°F). Relative humidity should be maintained at 40 to 70% (Kohn and Barthold, 1984; Harkness, 1993e).

The formulations of complete rodent diets, including those for rats, have been published, and most animal diet manufacturers have access to computer programs for formulating diets (Knapka, 1999). So, although various nutrient deficiencies have been produced in experimental rats and are described in detail in the literature, they are uncommon in pet rats fed commercial dry rodent food. Protein deficiencies are probably most common and can result in anemia, cataracts, poor growth and impaired reproduction.

Feeding Plan

Rats should be fed a commercial dry rodent food, offered free choice. They are primarily nocturnal feeders. Adult rats consume approximately 10 g of food/100 g of body weight. Treats should not exceed 10% of food intake. Dietary fiber content should be at least 5% to minimize problems with diarrhea. On a dry matter basis, crude protein requirements are approximately 10% for maintenance, and 20% for growth and reproduction. Young rats are weaned at 21 days of age at which time body weight ranges from 40 to 50 g (Harkness, 1993e; Harkness and Wagner, 1995a). Fresh water should be available free choice.

Mice

Husbandry

Mice belong in the Muridae family and originated in Asia. Average life span is 1.5 to 3 years and adult weight ranges from 20 to 40 g. Gestation lasts 19 to 21 days, with litter sizes ranging from 10 to 12. The dental formula is I1/1, C0/0, P0/0 and M3/3. Only the incisor teeth are open-rooted. GI transit time is eight to 14 hours (Jacoby and Fox, 1984; Harkness and Wagner, 1995a).

Cage requirements are similar to those described for rats. (See Rodents, Cage Requirements.) Floor space per adult mouse should be at least 97 cm^2, and 390 cm^2 for breeding females. Ambient temperatures should be maintained between 18 to 29°C (65 to 85°F), with an average of 22°C (72°F). Humidity should range from 30 to 70% (Harkness, 1993f).

Feeding Plan

Mice should be fed a clean, fresh, commercial dry rodent food. Optimal nutrient requirements have not been established and probably vary markedly among various strains of mice. The literature suggests that foods containing 17 to 24% protein, 5% or less fat and 2.5% fiber result in adequate performance levels. Mineral requirements are unknown. Adult mice ingest 4 to 5 g of food daily. Young mice generally begin eating dry food at 10 days of age and are weaned at 21 days (Harkness, 1993f; Harkness and Wagner, 1995a). Clean, fresh water in sipper bottles should always be available.

ENDNOTES

a. Lambert Key, Cranbury, NJ, USA.
b. Abbott Laboratories, Columbus, OH, USA.
c. Oxbow Pet Products, Murdock, NE, USA.
d. Dremel, Racine, WI, USA.

REFERENCES

The references for **Chapter 70** can be found at www.markmorris.org.

CASE 70-1

Calciuria in a Rabbit

Karen N. Wolf, MS, DVM
College of Veterinary Medicine
North Carolina State University
Raleigh, North Carolina, USA

Patient Assessment

A six-year-old, neutered male mini-lop rabbit presented for a one-week history of decreased activity, reduced appetite and spending more time in the litter box. The rabbit was kept indoors, housed in a wire hutch with straw substrate and supervised outdoors one to two hours several times weekly.

On physical examination, the rabbit was overweight, resented abdominal palpation and had gritty material on its fur around the prepuce and on the ventral aspect of its tail. All other physical examination parameters were normal.

Assess the Food and Feeding Method

The diet consisted of free-choice hay and rabbit pellets, one-half cup of leafy green vegetables daily and occasional fruit as a treat. Water was available in a sipper bottle at all times.

Questions

1. What additional questions should be asked about the diet?
2. What is this rabbit's most likely clinical problem?
3. What diagnostic tests should be performed?
4. What are some treatment options?

Answers and Discussion

1. The owner should be asked what type of hay and pellets are being offered to the rabbit. Also, it is important to ask how much the rabbit consumes (proportionately) of each food item offered. Additional information should include how often the water is changed. In this case, the owner was feeding alfalfa hay and alfalfa-based pellets. The rabbit seemed to prefer the pellets but also ate the hay. The water was changed two to three times weekly.
2. The most likely clinical problem based on the dietary history and physical examination is urolithiasis/calciuria. This problem in rabbits is linked to a high concentrate diet, obesity and lack of exercise. Rabbits, unlike most mammals, have a fractional urinary excretion of calcium between 45 to 60%. Increased dietary calcium leads to increased excretion of calcium through the urinary tract. Alfalfa is high in calcium and protein, which contributed to hypercalciuria and obesity in this rabbit. Alfalfa hay and pellets are acceptable for young, growing rabbits but are not recommended for most adult pet rabbits. Chronic, low-grade dehydration may also contribute to the problem. Rabbits have a high water intake (120 ml/kg/day) and need fresh clean water available at all times.
3. Radiographs, urinalyses and blood work (i.e., complete blood counts and serum biochemistry profiles) should be performed to confirm the diagnosis and to assess treatment options. If bacteria are identified, a urine sample collected by cystocentesis should be submitted for culture.
4. The type of treatment is based on the severity of the clinical problem. The presence of large cystic or urethral calculi will mandate either a cystotomy or perineal urethrostomy. If there are nonobstructive calculi or large amounts of dense calcium "sand" filling the bladder, urohydropropulsion or simply administering intravenous or subcutaneous fluid will help flush the bladder. Manual expression of the bladder may aid in the passage of the calcium precipitates. Changing the diet will help prevent recurrence. The diet for an adult pet rabbit should be based on grass hay and green vegetables with limited amounts of timothy hay-based pellets. Fresh water should be available free choice. Ample exercise is also important to prevent obesity.

CASE 70-2

Anorexia in a Guinea Pig

Christine M. Kolmstetter, DVM
Las Vegas, Nevada, USA

Patient Assessment

A one-year-old female Peruvian guinea pig was examined for a two-week history of anorexia and decreased activity. The volume and consistency of the feces were normal. The owner had purchased the guinea pig at two months of age; no other pets were in the household. The animal was housed in a 30-gallon aquarium that contained a shredded paper substrate. The aquarium was located in a quiet area in the living room. The animal was handled daily. No recent changes in environment or husbandry had occurred, and there was no history of trauma.

Physical examination revealed a bright, alert, thin guinea pig with a dull coat. The incisor and cheek teeth and oral mucosa appeared normal. The animal was reluctant to move. Although the guinea pig's joints were not palpably swollen, the animal seemed uncomfortable when the elbow and hock joints were gently flexed and extended. Abdominal palpation was normal.

Assess the Food and Feeding Method

Commercial dry guinea pig food and fresh water in a sipper bottle were provided free choice.

Questions

1. What other questions should be included in the dietary history?
2. What is this patient's most likely nutritional problem?
3. What further diagnostic tests should be offered to the client?
4. What treatment should be recommended?

Answers and Discussion

1. The owner should be questioned about the source of the commercial dry guinea pig food, its length and manner of storage in the home and what other food items the guinea pig consumes. This question revealed that, for the sake of convenience, the owner purchased several bags of food at a local discount grocery store. This supply lasted for two to three months.
2. Hypovitaminosis C is the most likely nutritional problem, based on the history and clinical signs.
3. A complete blood count, serum biochemistry profile and whole body radiographs would reveal the extent of the disease and help disclose other underlying problems that might be present.
4. This patient's food should be supplemented with oral or injectable vitamin C. The client should be educated about proper nutrition and other aspects of husbandry at this time.

CASE 70-3

Dysphagia in a Chinchilla

Karen N. Wolf, MS, DVM
College of Veterinary Medicine
North Carolina State University
Raleigh, North Carolina, USA

Patient Assessment

A five-year-old female chinchilla was examined for a three-month history of dysphagia, decreased appetite and an unkempt appearance. The owner adopted the chinchilla three years earlier and reported that the patient never had any medical problems. The chinchilla was housed indoors in a multi-tiered cage with predominantly wire flooring although areas with solid flooring were available. The patient was provided with a dust bath several times weekly. The chinchilla appeared interested in the normal pelleted food but seemed to not eat as vigorously as before. No changes had been made in the diet. The owner reported that fecal output seemed reduced.

On physical examination, the patient was bright and alert. However, its mandibular fur was moist, matted and discolored. Oral inspection revealed overgrown incisor teeth and the patient was palpably thin. No other abnormalities were detected.

Assess the Food and Feeding Method

Commercial chinchilla pellets and fresh water in a sipper bottle were available free choice and approximately 1/2 cup of mixed leafy greens was provided once or twice weekly.

Questions

1. What other questions should be asked about housing and diet?
2. What is the most likely cause of this chinchilla's clinical signs?
3. What nutritional deficit is likely to have caused this patient's clinical problems?
4. What diagnostic tests should be performed?
5. What treatment options should be considered?

Answers and Discussion

1. The owner should be asked if hay and chew toys were provided. The owner revealed that hay was offered when the chinchilla was first adopted but the patient showed more interest in the pelleted food; therefore, hay was no longer provided regularly. No chew toys were available.
2. Dental malocclusion is the most likely problem based on clinical signs, dietary history and physical examination findings.
3. A lack of hay is the primary factor contributing to this patient's malocclusion. Mastication of hay or other chew items continuously wears cheek teeth; thus, without items to chew, growing teeth are not adequately worn and will become maloccluded.
4. Anesthesia should be administered and the patient's oral cavity examined. Although the incisor teeth are readily visualized in chinchillas without anesthesia, the narrow opening to the oral cavity and the caudal location of the premolars and molars (cheek teeth) preclude adequate visualization even with instruments such as an otoscope. The mucosal surfaces and tongue should be evaluated for abrasions. The occlusal surfaces of the teeth should be assessed. Skull radiographs should be obtained to better evaluate the teeth, including the roots, and to determine if there is evidence of osteomyelitis or apical abscesses. A complete blood count and serum biochemistry profile should also be performed as part of the clinical workup.
5. Overgrown incisor teeth can be trimmed using a high-speed dental hand-piece equipped with a cutting burr. Modifying the diet to include hay may be curative in uncomplicated cases. Malocclusions of the cheek teeth require leveling, and again, dietary changes may be curative in cases that are detected early and are the direct sequela of a poor diet. Advanced cases may require extractions and trimming of the remaining teeth at regular intervals.

Chapter 71

Nutrition of Reptiles

Scott Stahl
Susan Donoghue

"In the parched path I have seen the good lizard (one drop of crocodile) meditating."
Frederico Garcia Lorca, 1921

INTRODUCTION

Diversity among the more than 6,500 species of reptiles challenges a veterinarian's ability to know the feeding management, estimate the nutritional requirements and recommend appropriate diets for every species presented in practice. With the exception of field studies on free-living reptiles, nutritional research is limited. Thus, recommendations are based on knowledge of natural diets, feeding histories, clinical experience and principles of comparative nutrition.

Identification of different species becomes easier with experience, but is often complicated because owners may know only a common name for their reptile. Common names can be colloquial, or assigned to more than one species. Therefore, misidentification of a patient may result in serious errors in nutritional recommendations. Reference texts help identify species and provide information about natural history and diet (Obst et al, 1988; Mattison, 1987; Zimmerman, 1986; Rossi, 1992; de Vosjoli, 1994, 1996; Boyer, 1996; Frye, 1991). This information can guide recommendations for habitat, including requirements for temperature, light, humidity, substrate, furnishings and social interaction. Failure to provide a suitable environment can lead to stress, causing negative effects on food intake and metabolic status of the patient.

For purposes of clinical nutrition, reptiles may be grouped into herbivores, omnivores and carnivores according to broad generalizations about their natural diet (**Table 71-1**). These distinctions serve as initial guides for making recommendations about diet and feeding management.

PATIENT ASSESSMENT

Signalment

Examination of the patient begins with the signalment. After the reptile presented has been properly identified by species, its age and gender should be estimated. Consider its stage of growth, reproductive status and degree of health, because these factors affect dietary recommendations. For example, certain species of aquatic turtles (e.g., the common sliders often kept as pets) change from eating a primarily carnivorous diet to eating a more herbivorous diet with maturity. Thus, feeding recommendations may differ for juvenile and adult reptiles.

Nutritional needs for reproductively active reptiles tend to be greater than for nonreproductive reptiles. This is especially true for females that need energy for development of ovarian follicles, oviductal eggs and embryos and require calcium for egg laying (often multiple clutches in a breeding season). However, some reptiles may become anorectic during phases of reproduction. For example, male snakes may refuse food during courtship and copulation or during times that seasonally correlate with these activities (e.g., ball pythons may not eat during the "dry season"). Likewise, females may not accept food while gravid. Therefore, for reproductively active reptiles, consider

Table 71-1. Foods and fuel sources vary in reptiles, depending on the carnivorous, omnivorous or herbivorous nature of the species.*

	Carnivores	Omnivores	Herbivores
Common pets	Snakes Aquatic turtles Most monitors, tegus Most lizards Leopard geckos Chameleons	Box turtles Bearded dragons Day geckos Forest-dwelling tortoises Anoles Blue tongued skinks	Most tortoises *Iguana* spp. *Uromastyx* spp. *Corucia zebrata*
Foods	Mealworms Flies Crickets Mice Fish Rats	Slugs Snails Crickets Fruits Vegetables Greens	Greens Fruits Vegetables Clover Dandelions Grasses
Dietary contents (% kcal metabolizable energy)			
Protein	25-60	15-40	15-35
Fat	30-60	5-40	<10
Carbohydrate	<10	20-75	55-75

*Adapted from Donoghue S, Langenberg J. Nutrition. In: Mader DR, ed. Reptile Medicine and Surgery. Philadelphia, PA: WB Saunders Co, 1996; 148-174.

Table 71-2. Husbandry questions for reptile owners.

Housing
Description of cage substrate and furniture
Frequency of and routine for cleaning
Location (indoors, outdoors)
Presence of cage mates
Type and size of habitat
Temperature
Measured temperature ranges within habitat (should be gradients of temperature)
Positioning of heat in cage
Safety precautions used to prevent thermal injury
Type of heating (radiant, ventral sources)
Light
Is the light filtered by glass or Plexiglas (these filter out ultraviolet light)
Length of light cycle
Positioning of light source
Type of lighting provided (incandescent, fluorescent, natural sunlight)

recommending heavier feeding during nonreproductive periods to compensate for subsequent nutritional demands.

The nutritional requirements for sick reptiles may also differ from those of healthy reptiles. The overall health status of the patient dictates the need for a change from a traditional diet. Typically, the clinician should recommend diets with greater digestibility and availability (Donoghue and Langenberg, 1996).

History

For reptiles, nutritional disorders are often caused by errors in husbandry; thus, history taking should include specific questions about management. First, a general history is obtained (Boyer, 1996; Divers, 1996). Pertinent information includes the patient's origin (e.g., private breeder, importer, pet shop), whether the patient was born in captivity or caught in the wild, length of ownership, whether there are other reptiles in the home and the disease history for the patient and the entire reptile collection. The history should include specific questions about husbandry (**Table 71-2**).

A dietary history allows the veterinarian to assess the animal's intake of energy and nutrients, and may provide information about the animal's clinical condition and behavior. It also may help in the early detection of nutritional problems before they become serious clinical disorders. Dietary histories may be complex for some reptiles (e.g., iguanas and tortoises) that consume a mix of different foods, including salads and supplements.

One goal of a diet history is to obtain information about all available foods offered to the patient. Foods that may be intentionally offered include commercial foods, homemade salads, snacks, treats and supplements. Foods may also be available unintentionally, such as houseplants for iguanas and tortoises that free range in homes.

Attention should be given to the quality and wholesomeness (absence of potential pathogens) of the food, cleanliness of feeding utensils and the skills and reliability of those responsible for feeding. The veterinarian should also determine whether the reptile has appropriate access to water.

It is best to query those directly responsible for feeding the reptile and not to rely on second-hand information. For complicated feeding programs involving a wide variety of foods, it may be best to ask owners to complete seven- to 10-day diaries, listing all foods offered and estimates of amounts consumed. For both written and oral dietary histories, care must be taken to avoid influencing responses by owners.

When obtaining a dietary history, include specifics about: 1) diet-what is fed, how often and how much, how the food is prepared, where the food is placed in the habitat, when the food is removed and which foods the reptile actually consumes, 2) supplementation-are supplements used, what type, how are they offered, how often, does the animal eat the food when the supplement is offered and 3) water-how is water offered, frequency of water changes and has the owner observed the animal drinking.

For carnivorous reptiles, dietary histories should concern type, source and health of the prey offered and the frequency of feeding. Look for problems with over- or underfeeding, offering malnourished prey, feeding only or mostly invertebrate prey, failure to provide additional supplementation, etc.

For herbivorous reptiles, dietary histories should especially concern the sources of protein, calcium and fiber. Another concern is whether commercially prepared foods are being diluted by excessive amounts of fruits or vegetables. For those patients fed mixed salads, look for sources of protein (romaine lettuce, legumes), calcium (calcium carbonate), fiber (crumbled hay cubes or fresh grasses). For commercial foods, check labels for ingredients.

Physical Examination

Initially observe the undisturbed patient from a distance. Posture, respiratory rate and movement, activity level, agility, strength and symmetry should be noted and compared with the results of the hands-on examination.

The reptile may be evaluated physically after it is appropriately restrained. The physical examination should be consistent and follow a similar pattern with each patient. This process reduces the likelihood that something will be overlooked. A typical approach is to start at the head and work caudally.

Many signs of malnutrition may be evident during the examination and should be noted in the patient's record. Examples include corneal and conjunctival abnormalities and respiratory disease, which may indicate hypovitaminosis A. Enophthalmos may suggest dehydration or inanition and cachexia. Abnormal color in the oral cavity may be due to anemia or icterus. (Note: This finding may be misleading in the bearded dragon, *Pogona vitticeps*, for example, which naturally has yellow oral mucous membranes.) Increased amounts of mucus in the mouth may indicate hypovitaminosis A. Dysecdysis (abnormal shedding) may suggest dehydration or hypo- or hypervitaminosis A.

After a thorough physical examination, the reptile should be weighed. Patients may also be scored for body condition (fat:lean ratio, degree of emaciation or fat loss) and muscle wasting (cachexia, sarcopenia, protein depletion) (Chapter 1). Average weights and morphometrics have not been established for reptiles, but in-house ranges can be established at a practice.

A general guide for reptiles (and mammals) is that an acute loss of 10% or chronic loss of 20% of body weight indicates the need for nutritional intervention. Body weight, however, provides limited quantitative data about lean body mass. All weight loss, even in healthy reptiles, is accompanied by loss of lean and adipose tissue. Losses of body fat and tissue protein will be accelerated in ill reptiles and those recovering from surgery. Muscle wasting is typically characterized clinically by loss of muscle mass and body weight. Protein catabolism results in cumulative losses of skeletal muscle mass and eventually loss of function of enzyme systems. Tissue proteins usually continue to be depleted during initial recovery from illness and surgery. Weight gain immediately after illness or surgery typically represents water and fat replacement whereas tissue protein is restored later.

Diagnostic Testing

In addition to a thorough physical examination, diagnostic testing helps assess nutritional and overall health status. This is especially important because reptiles, like birds, attempt to hide their illnesses. Diagnostic tests such as hematology and serum biochemistry analyses may be helpful.

Reptile blood is fragile. It is best preserved with heparin and should be processed immediately (Frye, 1991a; Bolten et al, 1992). Reptiles tend to have lower normal hematocrit values than other companion animals. Blood samples should be processed in-house or sent to a commercial clinical laboratory that specializes in reptile blood analysis. This is important to obtain consistently accurate total white blood cell and differential counts. Experienced laboratory technicians can describe the morphology of the cells (i.e., toxic, degranulating, shrunken), which can be just as valuable as the white blood cell total and differential counts. Serial samples are helpful for assessing progression of disease and health status.

Kidney disease is common in reptiles; however, uric acid levels may be affected by the most recent meal eaten by the reptile and may not be a sensitive indicator of renal function. In many cases, elevated serum phosphorus and subsequent decreased serum calcium values (usually in an inverse ratio of phosphorus to calcium) may indicate renal disease much earlier than elevated uric acid concentrations.

Deficiencies of calcium and vitamin D are common in reptiles. Radiographs can be a valuable tool to evaluate quality and density of bones. Additionally, radiography and ultrasonography are useful in assessing fat reserves and evaluating reproductive status of females.

Key Nutritional Factors

Reptiles differ from mammalian and avian patients in the metabolism of energy and nitrogen. These differences affect water balance, intake of essential nutrients, prevalence of diet-related diseases and causes of mortality. This section discusses the key nutritional factors that affect reptiles as well as common diseases caused by nutrient excesses and deficiencies.

Energy

Reptiles are ectothermic and heterothermic. Their body temperature depends on ambient environmental temperatures, rather than on internal metabolism, and varies with fluctuating temperatures. This effect of ambient temperature on body temperature affects metabolic rate (hence caloric needs), activity (e.g., food procurement) and digestion. In most cases, reptiles maintain an appropriate core body temperature if provided with a sufficient temperature gradient within their habitat. However, temperatures that are too cold will limit food consumption and impair digestion. Temperatures that are too hot will lead to excessive stress, decreased food intake and weight loss.

Table 71-3. Estimates of standard metabolic rate (MR) in kcal/day and fractional increases for feeding and activity for reptiles at 30°C (86°F).*

Body weight (g)	MR	1.1 MR	1.25 MR	1.5 MR	2.0 MR	2.5 MR
5	0.5	0.6	0.7	0.8	1.1	1.4
10	0.9	1.0	1.2	1.4	1.8	2.3
15	1.3	1.4	1.6	1.9	2.6	3.2
20	1.6	1.7	2.0	2.4	3.2	4.0
25	1.9	2.0	2.3	2.8	3.8	4.8
30	2.2	2.4	2.7	3.2	4.4	5.5
40	2.7	3.0	3.4	4.0	5.4	6.8
50	3.2	3.5	4.0	4.8	6.4	8.0
75	4.4	4.8	5.4	6.5	8.8	11
100	5.4	6.0	6.8	8.2	11	14
125	6.4	7.1	8.1	9.7	13	16
150	7.4	8.2	9.3	11	15	18
175	8.4	9.2	10	12	17	21
200	9.3	10	12	14	19	23
250	11	12	14	16	22	28
300	13	14	16	19	26	32
350	14	16	18	21	28	35
400	16	17	20	24	32	40
450	17	19	22	26	34	42
500	19	21	23	28	38	48
600	22	24	27	32	44	55
700	24	27	30	36	48	60
800	27	30	34	40	54	68
900	30	32	37	44	60	75
1,000	32	35	40	48	64	80
1,250	38	42	47	57	76	95
1,500	44	48	55	66	88	110
1,750	49	54	62	74	98	122
2,000	54	60	68	82	108	135
2,500	65	71	81	97	130	162
3,000	74	82	93	112	148	185
3,500	84	92	105	126	168	210
4,000	93	102	116	140	186	232
4,500	102	112	127	153	204	255
5,000	110	122	138	166	220	275
6,000	127	140	159	191	254	318
7,000	143	157	179	215	286	358
8,000	159	174	198	238	318	398
9,000	174	191	217	261	348	435
10,000	188	207	236	283	376	470
15,000	257	283	322	386	514	642
20,000	321	353	402	482	642	802
25,000	382	420	477	572	764	955
30,000	439	483	549	659	878	1,098
40,000	548	603	685	822	1,096	1,370
50,000	651	716	813	976	1,302	1,628

*MR = $32(BW_{kg})^{0.77}$ where MR = standard metabolic rate in kcal/day and BW = body weight in kg. To convert to kJ, multiply kcal by 4.184. Adapted from Donoghue S, Langenberg J. Nutrition. In: Mader DR, ed. Reptile Medicine and Surgery. Philadelphia, PA: WB Saunders Co, 1996; 148-174.

Because energy is not used to maintain body temperature, reptiles require fewer calories than birds and mammals. Metabolic rates in reptiles relate to metabolic body size-the smaller the animal, the greater its metabolic rate per unit body weight. The metabolic rates of reptiles average about one-fourth those of mammals. Energy requirements increase with eating, activity, reproduction, growth, protein synthesis (i.e., wound healing) and certain disorders (**Table 71-3**). Daily energy intakes should be calculated by multiplying the metabolic rate by a factor (i.e., 1.1 to 2.5) that accounts for activity and other conditions that increase metabolic rate. Unlike birds and mammals, energy requirements for reptiles do not increase with cold ambient temperatures. Estimates of daily calorie intakes are generally derived from experimental studies using a limited number of species, field work on species not often seen in practice and on clinical experiences of knowledgeable herpetoculturists (Frye, 1991; Donoghue and Langenberg, 1996).

Fuel use varies with the feeding ecology of the species. Generally, assumptions can be made based on the species' food preferences. For carnivores (e.g., snakes, most monitors and many aquatic turtles), exogenous fuel sources are fat (providing 8.5 to 9 kcal/g [35.6 to 37.7 kJ/g]) and protein (providing 3.7 to 4 kcal/g [15.5 to 16.7 kJ/g]). Intake of carbohydrate, including fiber, is minimal (**Table 71-1**). Rates of gluconeogenesis are likely to stay relatively high in these species.

For herbivores (e.g., tortoises, green iguanas, prehensile tail skinks [*Corucia zebrata*] and spiny tail lizards [*Uromastyx* spp.]), exogenous fuel sources are primarily carbohydrate (about 3.5 kcal/g [14.6 kJ/g]) and protein (about 3.5 kca1/g [14.6 kJ/g]). Dietary fat (providing about 8.5 kcal/g [35.6 kJ/g]) is usually less than 10% of dry matter (DM) (**Table 71-1**). Fermentation of fiber in the lower bowel of herbivores yields short-chain fatty acids that are also used for energy (perhaps providing about 2 kcal/g [8.4 kJ/g] of fiber).

ENERGY DEFICIENCY AND EXCESS

Low calorie intake leads to underweight and cachectic conditions. Ribs and vertebral processes are prominent or palpable in underweight snakes and lizards. Some exhibit longitudinal folds of skin along the lateral body wall. Thin turtles and tortoises lack heft. Poor body condition may be caused by: 1) improper husbandry, 2) stress, 3) improper temperature, 4) inappropriate diets or too little food and 5) underlying diseases that affect appetite and metabolism.

Excessive caloric intake leads to rapid growth in juveniles and overweight and obese conditions in adults. Especially at risk are those species with a sedentary nature, such as large snakes and lizards. Also at risk are reptiles kept in small habitats and fed high-fat diets, such as aquatic turtles maintained in small tanks. Treatment includes decreasing caloric intake and increasing activity. For example, an obese aquatic turtle that is fed commercial pellets daily can, instead, be fed pellets only three times per week and be offered greens on the other days of the week. Tank size should also be increased to encourage activity.

Water

All captive reptiles should have access to fresh water. Proper delivery of water is important. Turtles and snakes generally drink from bowls. Some lizards such as anoles, chameleons and day geckos lap up droplets sprayed or dripped onto foliage. Other lizards, such as iguanas and monitor lizards learn to drink from bowls and smaller reptiles from lids (e.g., plastic caps for pet food cans). Some reptiles may reject water held in plastic containers, presumably because of odor or taste. A switch to glass, ceramic or stainless steel bowls usually corrects the situation. Tortoises and some snakes soak in large, shallow bowls. Soaking enhances water uptake and stimulates excretion.

Desert animals require less water than temperate and tropical species. Some species receive enough water from food to meet requirements. Empirically, daily parenteral doses of water for rehydration are 10 to 25 ml/kg body weight (Frye, 1991a).

WATER-RELATED PROBLEMS

Water is critically important for reptiles and relates to many of the diseases seen in practice, such as gout and dysecdysis. Aquatic species are at less risk for dehydration, but water quality is critical for these animals. Routine water analyses may be important for maintaining health in aquatic reptiles (Donoghue and Langenberg, 1996). Water should be fresh for all species. Bacterial counts and culture can be included in routine water analyses. The method of providing water to reptiles will influence the humidity in the environment.

Clinical impressions suggest that inadequate humidity may contribute to dehydration, stress and dysecdysis. Likewise, excessive humidity may contribute to skin infections and hyperkeratinization.

Table 71-4. Purine content varies in foods. Low-purine and potentially acidic foods should be selected and high-purine and alkaline foods should be avoided for reptiles predisposed to gout.*

High-purine foods	Low-purine foods
Anchovies	Breads
Asparagus	Cereals
Brains	Cheese
Kidneys	Eggs
Liver	Fats
Mince meats	Fruits
Mushrooms	Milk
Sardines	Most vegetables
	Nuts
Potentially acidic foods	**Potentially alkaline foods**
Brazil nuts	Almonds
Breads	Beet greens
Cereals	Beets
Cheese	Chard
Corn	Chestnuts
Cranberries	Coconut
Lentils	Dairy
Meats	Dandelion
Plums	Fruits**
Prunes	Kale
Rice	Molasses
Walnuts	Mustard
	Spinach
	Turnip greens

*Adapted from Donoghue S, Langenberg J. Nutrition. In: Mader DR, ed. Reptile Medicine and Surgery. Philadelphia, PA: WB Saunders Co, 1996; 148-174.
**Except plums, prunes and cranberries.

Nitrogen

Lizards and snakes excrete mostly uric acid. Aquatic turtles tend to excrete more ammonia and urea than uric acid, whereas terrestrial tortoises excrete relatively more uric acid (Schmidt-Nielsen, 1990). Excretory patterns are clinically important because of difficulties in maintaining positive water balance and the prevalence of dehydration seen in reptiles.

Dehydration is common, especially in sick reptiles. It may result from water provided in improper form or anorexia, or may occur secondary to disease. Uricotelic species require large amounts of water to sustain normal excretion. Dehydration in these species may result in urinary stasis, hyperuricemia and gout, a disease characterized by deposition of urate crystals in soft tissues and joints. Prevention is based on maintaining adequate hydration. Reducing protein levels may restrict purines. Restriction of purines is feasible by avoiding high-purine foods such as liver (**Table 71-4**).

Many reptiles appear to have marked protein requirements. Those that are strict carnivores naturally consume diets consisting of 30 to 60% protein (metabolizable energy [ME] basis).

Table 71-5. Caloric and nutrient content of vertebrate prey.

Food items (g)	Water (%)	Energy (kcal/g)* (As fed)	Energy (kcal/g)* (DM)	Protein (% kcal)	Fat (% kcal)	NFE (% kcal)	Calcium (mg/kcal)	Phosphorus (mg/kcal)
Atlantic herring (100)	69	1.8	5.7	39	58	3	na	1.4
Atlantic smelt (100)	77	1.0	4.3	63	31	6	3.2	4.4
Chick, day old (40)	73	1.3	4.8	52	44	4	2.7	2.0
Mouse, adult (27)	65	1.7	4.8	48	47	5	5.0	3.6
Mouse, pup (1.5)	81	0.8	4.2	57	40	3	3.8	3.7
Mouse, pup (4)	71	1.7	5.9	29	69	2	2.4	2.2
Rat, adult (330)	66	1.6	4.7	55	43	2	4.4	3.2

Key: NFE = nitrogen-free extract (digestible carbohydrate), DM = dry matter, na = not available.
*To convert to kJ, multiply kcal by 4.184.

Table 71-6. Representative energy and nutrient content of invertebrate prey.

Food items	Water (%)	Energy (kcal/g)* (As fed)	Energy (kcal/g)* (DM)	Protein (% kcal)	Fat (% kcal)	NFE (% kcal)	Calcium (mg/kcal)	Phosphorus (mg/kcal)
Acheta domestica (commercial cricket)	62	1.9	4.8	50	44	6	0.2	2.6
Galleria mellonella (wax worm larvae)	63	2.1	5.7	27	73	0	0.1	0.9
Gryllus domesticus (house cricket)	68	1.0	3.1	40	54	6	0.3	2.7
Lumbricus terrestris (earthworm)	84	0.5	3.1	73	13	14	Variable	Variable
Musca domestica (fly larvae)	70	1.5	4.9	48	44	8	0.1	na
Tenebrio molitor (mealworm larvae)	58	2.1	5.0	37	60	3	0.1	1.2

Key: NFE = nitrogen-free extract (digestible carbohydrate), DM = dry matter, na = not available.
*To convert to kJ, multiply kcal by 4.184.

Table 71-7. Caloric and nutrient content of produce on a percent dry matter basis.

Food items	Weight (g)	Water (%)	Energy (kcal/g)* (As fed)	Energy (kcal/g)* (DM)	Protein	Fat	NFE	Fiber	Calcium	Phosphorus
Romaine lettuce	100	94	0.18	3.0	36	7	50	11	1.1	0.4
Spinach (raw)	100	91	0.26	2.9	36	3	48	7	1.0	0.6
Dandelion greens (raw)	100	86	0.44	3.1	18	5	61	11	1.2	0.4
Alfalfa sprouts (raw)	100	88	0.39	3.2	37	4	39	12	0.3	0.8
Bamboo shoots (canned, 1 cup)	133	94	0.18	3.0	28	1	51	13	0.2	0.2
Vegetables (mixed, frozen, 2/3 cup)	100	83	0.47	2.8	16	2	68	7	0.1	0.3
Mushrooms (raw, 10 small)	100	90	0.27	2.7	30	6	49	9	0.1	1.3
Sweet potato (1 large)	180	64	0.82	2.8	5	1	84	2	0.1	0.2
Apple (no skin, 1 medium)	128	84	0.51	3.2	1	2	86	4	tr	tr
Banana (1 medium)	114	74	0.82	3.2	4	2	86	2	tr	tr
Cantaloupe (1 cup)	160	90	0.32	3.2	8	2	79	4	0.1	0.2
Strawberries (1 cup)	149	92	0.28	3.5	6	4	77	6	0.2	0.2

Key: NFE = nitrogen-free extract (digestible carbohydrate), DM = dry matter, tr = trace.
*To convert to kJ, multiply kcal by 4.184.

Herbivorous reptiles consume less protein, but optimal ranges remain to be defined. Feeding trials in green iguanas suggested that dietary protein levels of about 28% DM are needed for optimal growth (Donoghue, 1994, 1997).

Other Nutrients

Intake of nutrients varies with feeding habits. For large carnivorous reptiles, vertebrate prey are assumed to be "complete and balanced" packages that contain all of the essential nutrients. However, neonatal prey (e.g., pinkie [newborn] mice) that are fed to smaller carnivores and omnivores, may lack sufficient calcium and fat-soluble vitamins (Douglas et al, 1994). In adult prey, calcium, phosphorus and magnesium are provided by bone, most trace minerals and vitamins by liver and kidneys, iodine by thyroid glands and zinc by the pancreas. The protein quality is high. Calories are provided almost entirely by fat and protein, and carbohydrate sources are limited to the intestinal content of the prey (**Table 71-5**).

Invertebrate prey also contain much fat and protein but lack a calcium-rich skeleton (**Table 71-6**). The chitinous (amino-cellulose) exoskeleton of most invertebrates contains nonprotein nitrogen. The digestibility of this chitin is questionable (Donoghue and Langenberg, 1996).

Invertebrates are routinely "dusted" with powdery vitamin-mineral supplements to supply calcium and other nutrients lacking in the diet. Dusting can be problematic; it may induce nutrient toxicities if excessive and create deficiencies if too little is provided. Additionally, some reptiles will refuse foods that have been dusted because calcium salts and many vitamins are unpalatable.

Domestic fruits and vegetables available from grocery stores are lower in nutritional value (especially protein and fiber) than fruits and plants consumed in the wild. Among domestic produce, higher protein levels are found in greens (e.g., romaine lettuce, collard greens and spinach), alfalfa and mung-bean sprouts, mushrooms and bamboo shoots. Domestic produce rarely provides enough protein, calcium and fiber, or adequate levels of trace minerals and vitamins to support growth and reproduction in reptiles; therefore, produce needs supplementation (**Table 71-7**) (Donoghue and Langenberg, 1996).

Herbivorous reptiles consume fruits readily, probably because of the bright colors, sweet taste and moist texture. However, fruits contain mostly water, fructose and small amounts of fiber. Even small amounts of fruit can markedly dilute the calories, nutrients and fiber provided by greens.

Nutrient Deficiencies and Excesses

With the exception of those species consuming whole prey, many reptiles suffer from deficiencies and excesses of nutrients. Common among many species are deficiencies of calcium and vitamin D_3.

Vitamin D_3 is problematic. Limited research data, anecdotal evidence and clinical impressions suggest that, at least in some species, dermal synthesis of 1,25-dihydroxycholecalciferol may be more efficient than gastrointestinal absorption of dietary vitamin D_3. Thus, exposure to natural sunlight or ultraviolet (full spectrum) lighting may be critical for adequate vitamin D_3 synthesis in some reptile species. Interactions between vitamin D, calcium and phosphorus, and secondary interactions with vitamin A and several trace minerals, complicate nutritional requirements. For now, general recommendations include consistent but not excessive supplementation of diets (except when feeding whole vertebrate prey) with both calcium and vitamin D_3, exposure to full-spectrum lights and, whenever possible, exposure to direct sunlight.

Diet-related nutritional deficiencies in carnivores include calcium deficiency from feeding primarily unsupplemented invertebrates or muscle meat, vitamin A deficiency from feeding primarily iceberg lettuce and muscle meat and thiamin (vitamin B_1) and tocopherol (vitamin E) deficiency from feeding fish containing thiaminases and high levels of polyunsaturated fatty acids.

Common problems in herbivores include multiple deficiencies, especially calcium deficiency, from feeding unsupplemented produce and protein deficiency from feeding diets containing large amounts of fruit.

Over-supplementation may potentially lead to toxic intakes of vitamins A and D, phosphorus, selenium, iodine and other trace minerals. Some nutrient interactions may occur in reptiles. For example, excess dietary calcium may interfere with the absorption of zinc and copper and affect the thyroidal uptake of iodine.

METABOLIC BONE DISEASE

Metabolic bone disease is probably the most common nutritionally related disease seen in lizards, especially green iguanas. This disease is caused by a dietary deficiency of calcium, excess of dietary phosphorus, deficiency of vitamin D_3 or a combination of these factors. Clinical signs include soft mandibular and maxillary bones, deformed or fractured bones, muscle tremors, poor growth, spinal deviations and paralysis (Frye, 1991a). The disease is most commonly seen in young, growing lizards and adults maintained indoors. Metabolic bone disease is also common in chelonians (tortoises and turtles). Clinical signs include a soft carapace and plastron, improper shell growth and fractured limbs (Frye, 1991a). Treatment includes dietary correction and provision of natural sunlight or full-spectrum ultraviolet light. For severe cases, parenteral injections of calcium, vitamin D_3 and calcitonin may be necessary (Boyer, 1996; Donoghue and Langenberg, 1996; Rossi, 1992; Mader, 1993; Barten, 1995).

HYPOVITAMINOSIS A

Deficiency of vitamin A occurs in lizards fed unsupplemented produce and insects. It is characterized by squamous metaplasia, which causes shedding problems, stomatitis, palpebral edema, conjunctivitis and respiratory disease (Frye, 1991a). Secondary bacterial infections are also common. Treatment includes vitamin A supplementation, parenterally and orally, and dietary correction.

Hypovitaminosis A is likely the most common nutritional disease of chelonia. These animals are typically fed unsupplemented iceberg lettuce, hamburger or other foods deficient in vitamin A. Squamous metaplasia results in palpebral edema and respiratory disease. Common clinical findings include conjunctivitis, nasal discharge, wheezing and stridor (Frye, 1991a). Additionally, respiratory disease may cause water turtles to swim in a lopsided fashion due to fluid buildup in one lung. Secondary bacterial infections are common. Poor skin and shell quality may also be noted.

Treatment of hypovitaminosis A includes dietary correction and oral administration of vitamin A (200 to 300 IU/kg body weight). Secondary bacterial infections are treated with an appropriate antibiotic. Dietary vitamin A should be increased (2,000 to 10,000 IU/kg diet DM).

FAT-SOLUBLE VITAMIN TOXICITIES

Over-supplementation with fat-soluble vitamins may result in renal disease, hepatic disease and metastatic calcification.

The exact requirements of vitamins A and D_3 are currently unknown, but excessive amounts may cause problems in lizards. Clinical signs are consistent with multiple organ failure. The most common example is seen in green iguanas maintained on dog and/or cat food. Renal failure and metastatic calcification of major vessels typically occur. Treatment in most cases involves attempts to reverse organ damage through supportive care, especially fluid therapy. Additionally, calcitonin[a] may be used (2 IU/kg body weight, given intramuscularly q24h) to help reverse metastatic calcification (Frye, 1991; Barten, 1995).

Tortoises and box turtles are very sensitive to injections of vitamin A. When given parenterally, these drugs may cause sloughing of the skin, resulting in severe skin ulceration (Frye, 1991, 1991a). These preparations are best given orally. Treatment for vitamin toxicity in most cases is supportive care and removal of the vitamin source.

Although commercially prepared foods may occasionally be involved, the excessive use of vitamin supplements is more commonly the cause of vitamin toxicities.

THIAMIN DEFICIENCY

Thiamin deficiency is seen occasionally in garter snakes and water snakes fed exclusively frozen fish. Thiaminases, found in many species of fish, deplete available thiamin. Thiamin-deficient snakes typically present with neurologic disease characterized by ataxia, seizures, twisting and rolling. Treatment involves changing the diet to include fresh fish, insects and mice scented with fish, and medicating with oral or parenteral thiamin hydrochloride (25 mg/kg body weight, per os or intramuscularly) (Frye, 1991).

FEEDING PLAN

The advantages and disadvantages of feeding reptiles commercially prepared foods and homemade diets were discussed above. If an individual reptile is healthy and exhibits no signs of deficiency disease, the owner probably is feeding the reptile appropriately and there is no need to change the food.

Although some prepared foods have been available for only a limited time, the overall nutritional quality of commercially prepared foods is rapidly improving as manufacturers consider new scientific information when they prepare their formulations. As commercially prepared foods become more widely used, many of the diet-induced diseases currently observed by veterinarians will become of historical interest only, just as they have for other companion pets.

Assess and Select the Food

Foods appropriately balanced with carbohydrates, proteins, fats, vitamins, minerals and water are essential for all reptiles. Care of captive reptiles must address good nutrition at several levels; the daily satisfaction and health of the reptile as well as the long-term contributions to growth, maturation, defense against disease and reproductive health-the hallmark of good nutrition.

Three methods of providing nutrients and achieving these objectives are commonly used: 1) commercially prepared foods, 2) homemade mixed foods or 3) a combination of commercial and homemade foods, with or without supplements.

Commercially Prepared Foods

Reptiles may be fed commercially prepared foods formulated for the species or the most similar domestic animal. There is little scientific literature about the nutrient requirements of reptiles. However, several reports provide some insight into the levels of dietary nutrients required to result in a nutritionally adequate diet (Allen et al, 1989). These reports make it possible to formulate prepared foods with a high probability of nutritional adequacy for some reptilian species.

Testing protocols for nutritional adequacy have not yet been established for reptile foods, as they have been for commercially prepared canine and feline foods. As commercially prepared reptile foods become more widely used, testing protocols for nutritional adequacy will be established and required.

Commercially prepared foods offer many benefits, including nutrient balance and convenience. A moist, extruded or pelleted food will supply all the nutrients in one particle or form. Thus, the probability of producing a nutritional imbalance by feeding a commercially prepared food is much less than when reptiles are fed individual human foods prepared by uninformed owners.

If commercially prepared food is offered, examine the label for nutrient information or guarantees. The primary nutrients of concern depend on whether the reptile is carnivorous, omnivorous or herbivorous. Protein, fat, digestible (soluble) carbohydrate, fiber, vitamin and mineral levels should be appropriate for the individual reptile. Label space does not allow for detailed nutrient information. Therefore, the manufacturer should be contacted for additional nutritional information. When purchasing or recommending commercial herbivore foods, read labels with extreme care. Some may contain low levels of antibiotics and other growth promotants that have unpredictable and potentially deleterious effects on reptiles. Regardless of the type of food fed, a sample can be submitted to a commercial laboratory for analysis. Consult the laboratory in advance to determine the sample size needed, preservation techniques recommended and shipping instructions.

Compare the nutrient levels of the commercial food to those recommended in this chapter to determine if there are any discrepancies in the nutrient profile. If the food doesn't meet recommended nutrient levels, the owner should change or supplement the diet. The food should not be fed if its label contains no nutrient information and the manufacturer does not provide nutrient levels in other promotional literature or is unavailable to answer questions by phone.

Commercial forages for herbivorous reptiles include legumes, primarily alfalfa, which can be pelleted, cubed and chopped. Unfortunately, most tortoises and herbivorous lizards show limited interest in alfalfa-based meals, eating these items only when disguised with fresh produce or when no other foods are available.

Hay can be purchased from feed stores and farms. Chopped

and cubed hay is sold in pet shops and feed stores. Care should be taken to avoid prolonged storage of these products because about half the vitamin A activity from β-carotene is lost from hay within a year of cutting.

Hay-based pellets range from 12 to 28% DM crude protein and 14 to 19% DM crude fiber. Some success has been noted in the use of hay-based pellets as bedding for juvenile herbivorous reptiles. Although these products are safe if wholesome, pellets can mold quickly and the reptile may then be at risk to develop respiratory disease and digestive upset.

Some commercially prepared foods marketed specifically for iguanas are variable in content. Look for products with at least 18% DM crude protein. Pellets may be soaked in water or fruit juice before feeding. Wet pellets may mold, so they should be offered fresh daily.

Some commercially prepared foods marketed specifically for aquatic species are sold as complete diets and are made from fish and crustacean meals, plant-based ingredients and various additives. Some manufacturers fail to add essential vitamins and minerals. Processes used in extrusion and pelleting involve high temperatures that partially destroy labile vitamins. Mineral and vitamin content of fish meals vary with the species, season of harvest and processing. Examine labels and products carefully. Some foods may not be adequate to sustain growth or even maintenance of carnivorous reptiles. However, the alternative homemade diet is often less desirable.

Protein in dog and cat foods ranges from 16 to 40% of ME; many pet foods provide more than 22% of ME from protein and more than 25% of ME from fat. These protein levels are likely to be adequate for carnivorous reptiles.

Herbivores generally suffer digestive upset when dietary fat exceeds about 12%. Herbivorous reptiles are unlikely to thrive on diets containing more than 12% fat, which limits the use of commercial pet foods to the "light" varieties. Light varieties often contain higher levels of fiber, which is favorable for herbivores.

Homemade Diets

A wide variety of homemade diets have been suggested for reptiles. Although homemade diets may provide adequate nourishment, most reptile owners are unwilling to devote the time necessary to properly prepare these diets. Additionally, owners must be willing to regularly observe which food components are being consumed to prevent reptiles from developing or reverting to preferential selection of specific ingredients. Considering these factors, well-formulated commercially prepared foods are a better alternative for most captive reptiles.

Supplements

Supplements are marketed as containing primarily vitamins and minerals in various amounts. Few if any supply all vitamins and minerals known to be essential for domestic species including reptiles. The tendency is to leave out those that are unpalatable or expensive. Until more work is done about reptile nutrition, no one product should be relied upon to supply all essential nutrients to captive reptiles. Better value may be achieved by using a broad-spectrum micronutrient product designed for people or domestic animals. These products may be used for reptiles, but care must be taken to provide vitamin D_3 (not vitamin D_2) and to avoid overdosage (Donoghue and Langenberg, 1996). A general mammalian guideline that may also be useful in assessing reptile supplements is vitamins A:D:E should be present in a ratio approximating 100:10:1. A review of the nutrient content of many of the commonly used supplements for reptiles has been published (Donoghue and Langenberg, 1996). If a commercially prepared food constitutes more than 50% of total dietary intake, supplements are contraindicated.

Although calcium is often included in commercial vitamin-mineral supplements, it is rarely present in quantities sufficient to meet requirements for reptiles fed mixed salads or invertebrates. Additional calcium may be provided as limestone (38% calcium), or as calcium salts-carbonate (40% calcium), lactate (18% calcium) and gluconate (9% calcium). Calcium and phosphorus are supplied in bone meal (24% calcium, 12% phosphorus) and dicalcium phosphate (18 to 24% calcium, 18% phosphorus). Bone meal tablets vary in size. A small (aspirin size) tablet weighs 0.75 g and provides about 180 mg calcium and 90 mg phosphorus. Products vary, so read labels carefully. Powdered calcium supplements can be dusted on salads and tablet forms can be crushed and mixed with food.

Assess and Select the Feeding Method

It may not always be necessary to change the feeding method when managing reptile patients; however, a veterinarian should verify that an appropriate feeding method is being used. Items to consider include feeding route, amount fed, how the food is offered and who feeds the reptile. All of this information should be gathered when the nutritional history is obtained. If the reptile has normal body condition and weight, the amount of food previously fed (on an energy basis) was probably appropriate.

Lizards

Lizard species (*Sauria*) may be herbivorous, omnivorous or carnivorous. Lizards that are carnivorous may consume either invertebrate or vertebrate prey, or both. Gastrointestinal morphology reflects feeding behavior. Thus, herbivorous lizards have hindguts adapted for fermentation of dietary fiber, and carnivorous lizards have relatively short and simple intestinal tracts suited for hydrolysis in the small intestine.

Herbivores

The green iguana (*Iguana iguana*) is the most common herbivorous lizard seen in veterinary practice. These large, arboreal, diurnal lizards originate from Central and South America and require tropical temperatures (approximately 32°C [90°F]) and humidity (approximately 90% relative humidity). With proper care, green iguanas may live 10 to 15 years in captivity. However, mistakes in husbandry and diet often lead to an early demise.

Other herbivorous lizards occasionally seen in practice include prehensile tail skinks (*Corucia* spp.) and chuckwallas (*Sauromalus* spp.). Others, such as spiny tailed lizards (*Uromastyx* spp.) and rock iguanas (*Cyclura* spp.), use hindgut fer-

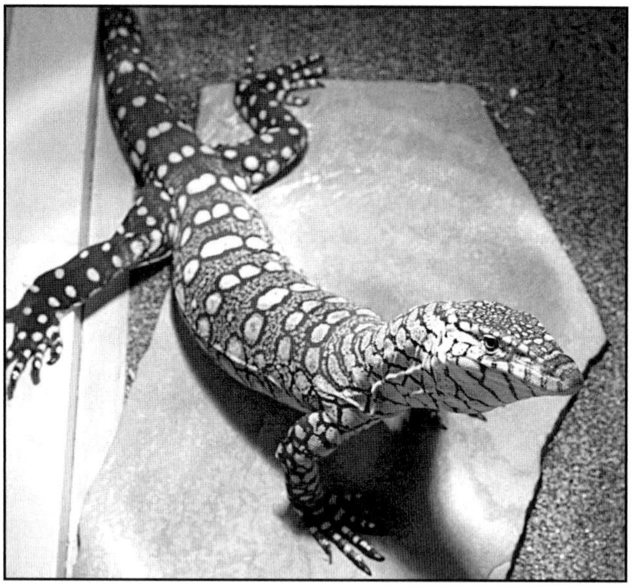

Figure 71-1. Monitor lizards are carnivorous. This large monitor (*Varanus giganteus*) awaits a large pre-killed rat to be dropped into its enclosure.

mentation and are often classified as herbivores, but also are known to consume invertebrate prey.

Diets for herbivorous lizards should include leafy greens such as romaine lettuce and collard greens, mustard greens and endive, dandelion and clover. Vegetables such as green beans, okra, carrots, yellow squash, zucchini and commercial thawed frozen mixed vegetables can make up a small fraction, perhaps 10 to 20%, of the diet.

Spinach, cabbage, peas, potatoes and beet greens contain oxalates that bind calcium and trace minerals, inhibiting their absorption. Trace mineral deficiencies may result if the diet is composed primarily of these foods and mineral intakes are marginal. Goitrogens are found in cabbage, kale, mustard and other cruciferous plants. Large intakes of these foods with marginal iodine intake may lead to hypothyroidism. Small amounts of these oxalate-containing and goitrogenic vegetables may still be fed safely as part of the diet.

Fruits can be used as "treats" or as a very small portion of the diet. Palatable choices include papaya, mango, cantaloupe, grapes and oranges.

Commercially prepared foods may constitute a significant portion of the diet (i.e., up to 50 to 60%). Treats and other nutritionally imbalanced foods should constitute no more than 10% of the diet.

If commercially prepared foods are used for 50% or more of the diet, additional supplementation is usually unnecessary. Homemade diets of vegetables and fruits should be supplemented. Several recipes have been published (Frye, 1991; Donoghue and Langerberg, 1996). Juveniles should be fed bite-sized foods, once or twice daily. Adults should be fed daily or every other day. These diurnal lizards should be offered food at a time that correlates with their need to bask and thermoregulate to allow efficient digestion of food.

Omnivores

Some of the most common omnivorous lizards presented to veterinary practitioners include bearded dragons (*Pogona* spp.), blue-tongued skinks (*Tiliqua* spp.), water dragons (*Physignathus* spp.) and plated lizards (*Gerrhosauras* spp.). In captivity, these omnivores consume prey (often invertebrates) or a meat-based, commercially prepared food mixed with fruits and vegetables.

A commercially prepared food should make up 60 to 75% of the total diet. The remaining portion may include invertebrates such as crickets, mealworms, wax worms, sweepings (insects found by gently sweeping grasses with a net; counsel clients to make sure no pesticides have been used on the grass), earthworms, snails and slugs (especially for skinks). Other prey includes small vertebrates, such as newborn and fuzzy mice, chicks and adult mice and rats. Cooked eggs may also be included as a protein source. Dog food (moist and dry), primate biscuits and trout food can be fed. Cat food is appropriate (up to 50 to 60% of the diet) for blue-tongued and pink-tongued skinks; however, these foods should be fed cautiously to other omnivorous lizards to prevent risks from over-feeding a high-fat diet.

Fresh greens and produce may make up the rest of the diet. Palatable foods include leafy vegetables, squash, carrots, green beans, alfalfa sprouts and thawed frozen mixed vegetables. Fruits should include melon, papaya and oranges.

Nutritionally adequate, commercially prepared foods are available for omnivorous lizards. However, because no long-term feeding trials have been reported, performance of lizards should be monitored to ensure that they are thriving.

In general, the more varied the overall diet, the less supplementation is necessary. If 50% or more of the diet includes dog food, monkey biscuits, cat food or complete omnivore foods, no supplementation is necessary. Otherwise, supplementation of produce and dusting of invertebrates are recommended.

Carnivores

The most common carnivorous lizards kept in captivity are monitors (*Varanus* spp.), tegus (*Tupinambis* spp.) and Gila monsters and beaded lizards (*Heloderma* spp.). These animals eat whole prey items (vertebrate [**Figure 71-1**] and invertebrate), but some also will eat cooked meat and eggs and commercial pet food. Feeding cooked meat and eggs is recommended to avoid exposure to potential pathogenic bacteria such as *Salmonella* spp.

Commercially prepared foods are available for monitors and tegus. As with any dietary regimen, reptiles should be monitored for any dietary-related disease. Supplementation is rarely necessary for adult carnivorous lizards if they are eating whole vertebrate prey items or commercially prepared food or a variety of foods. A calcium and vitamin D_3 supplement can be used twice weekly for juveniles fed a diet of newborn mice and insects.

Insectivorous lizards kept in captivity include species of geckos (*Gekkonidae* and *Eublepharidae*), old-world chameleons (*Chamaeleo* spp.), water dragons (*Physignathus* spp.), anoles

(*Anolis* spp.), small skinks (*Scincidae*), monitors (*Varanus* spp.), girdle-tailed lizards (*Cordylus* and *Pseudocordylus* spp.), lacertas (*Lacertidae*), basilisks (*Basiliscus* spp.), collared lizards (*Crotaphytus* spp.), sailfin dragons (*Hydrosaurus* spp.), ameivas (*Ameiva* spp.) and swifts (*Sceloporus* spp.). These species thrive on a wide variety of well-fed and well-supplemented insects such as crickets, mealworms, wax-moth larvae, king mealworms, cockroaches and fruit flies (for juveniles). Other insects, when available, include butterworms, grasshoppers, earthworms, flies, fly larvae and sweepings.

Insects can be fed a relatively balanced diet to "gut load" them before they are fed to lizards. A variety of whole diets can be used to feed insects including psittacine pellets, tropical fish flakes and commercial invertebrate "gut loading" foods. Also, insects can be fed vegetables that have a high precursor vitamin A content such as collard greens, kale, romaine and red-leaf lettuce, grated carrots and sweet potatoes (Stahl, 1997). Invertebrates should be dusted with a calcium supplement and a multivitamin supplement before they are fed to the reptile. (See Supplements.) Calcium supplement can be used daily for young growing reptiles and three to four times weekly for adults. Multivitamin supplements (which should contain some preformed vitamin A) should be used less frequently (i.e., once or twice weekly) (Stahl, 1997).

Prey should be of the appropriate size for the lizard. A general guide is for prey length to be less than the width of the lizard's head. Insects that are too large may bite the lizard or, if swallowed, cause it to regurgitate. Generally, only enough prey to be consumed at one feeding should be offered. Excess numbers of insects may cause stress or injury to the lizard.

Juveniles should be fed daily. Adults can be fed every second or third day.

Occasionally, larger and adult species of insectivorous lizards can be fed newborn, fuzzy or adult mice. The mice should make up no more than about 25% of the diet.

Several small lizard species, such as anoles and day geckos, readily accept fruit-flavored baby foods and yogurt. Basilisks, sailfin dragons and water dragons may accept a small amount of fruit. These soft foods provide a convenient medium for supplementation of calcium, vitamins and trace minerals.

Fresh water should always be available for lizards. Large soaking bowls should be provided for some species, such as water dragons and water monitors, Nile and Dumeril's monitors, sailfin lizards and basilisks. Misting the environment daily may help increase humidity for tropical species. Chameleons and some smaller species of lizards (e.g., anoles) usually won't drink from standing water. It is usually necessary to visually stimulate these lizards with drip systems, air bubbling systems or by misting the trees and plants in their environment to encourage drinking. These reptiles can also be placed on a clothes-drying rack or large plant, such as a *Ficus* spp., and placed under a spray of water in a shower, in order to simulate a rain shower and encourage drinking.

Some of the desert species (e.g., *Uromastyx* lizards and chuckwallas) need only small water bowls for drinking; however, they may benefit from being soaked in a warm water bath once or twice weekly. Water sources may harbor bacteria so bowls must be kept meticulously clean. Routine disinfection is recommended. Vitamin-mineral supplements should not be added to water sources because they may reduce palatability and result in increased bacterial populations.

Snakes: Serpentes

Snakes that Eat Mammalian and Avian Prey

Most of the snakes seen by private practitioners feed on mammals. Boids (pythons and boas), rat and corn snakes (*Elaphe* spp.) and gopher, bull and pine snakes (*Pituophis* spp.) are some of the more common snakes presented to veterinarians. Their diet consists of rats, mice, gerbils, rabbits and young chicks. These prey items should be fed a high-quality, complete ration to provide adequate nutrition for snakes.

Trauma associated with feeding live prey is common. Therefore, training snakes to eat stunned, dead or frozen-thawed prey is preferred. These reptiles are attracted to prey by the smell, the heat radiating from the prey item and by movement. To help encourage snakes to eat dead food, the prey item should be warm when offered. It can also be wiggled with a long pair of forceps. Eventually, even stubborn snakes become accustomed to eating dead prey.

Frozen rodents should be thawed rapidly in very hot water to minimize bacterial intestinal bloom. Caution should be used when feeding chicks or other birds to snakes because of potential exposure to salmonella. Boiling chicks before feeding may reduce the risk.

Some snakes are finicky feeders. For example, ball pythons prefer gerbils (which are found in their native habitat) or brown or black rodents, rather than white laboratory rodents.

Supplementation is unnecessary when feeding whole vertebrate prey. The only exception is with long-term feeding of newborn mice, which may be deficient in calcium. Allowing newborn mice to obtain milk from the mother for a day or two improves their calcium content. Also, dipping newborn mice in a liquid calcium supplement increases dietary calcium content. Feeding fuzzy mice also improves calcium content. Obese rodents and those that have been frozen for more than six months may have reduced vitamin content.

Snakes that are housed together should be separated for feeding to minimize injuries to each other and to help identify which snake has eaten. If two or more snakes attack the same prey, one snake may inadvertently eat or injure the other.

Feeding frequency varies, depending on the species of snake. Generally, young growing snakes should be fed every five to seven days. Mature, adult snakes may be fed weekly, biweekly or even monthly.

Snakes that Eat Reptiles, Amphibians and Fish

Some snakes feed on ectotherms, including amphibians, fish, crayfish and other reptiles. Snakes that eat these prey items include king snakes (*Lampropeltis* spp.), indigo snakes (*Drymarchon* spp.), water snakes (*Nerodia* spp.), hog-nosed snakes (*Heterodon* spp.), ring-necked snakes (*Diadophis* spp.) and garter snakes (*Thamnophis* spp.). The prey should be frozen for

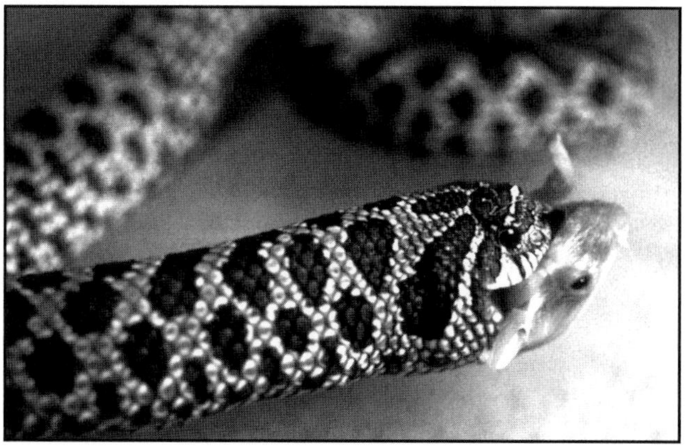

Figure 71-2. Hog-nosed snakes typically feed on amphibians, such as toads, in the wild. In captivity, they can be tricked into eating toad-scented mice. This young Western hog-nosed snake is eating a mouse backwards.

at least three days to minimize exposure to parasites; many of the prey are intermediate hosts to reptile parasites. Freezing may eliminate nematode parasites; however, it will not usually eliminate bacteria and protozoa. Regular fecal examination and deworming may be necessary to control protozoal parasites.

Ectotherm snakes should be trained to eat rodents. Initially, rodents can be scented with a more typical prey item. For example, a hog-nosed snake that typically eats toads and frogs in the wild can be encouraged to eat a rodent whose fur has been rubbed with a toad or frog to impart a familiar scent (**Figure 71-2**). Eventually, most of these snakes will accept rodents as their primary diet. Supplementation is usually unnecessary if a portion of the diet is made up of rodents.

Snakes that eat other snakes in the wild (e.g., king snakes) should be housed alone to prevent cage-mate predation.

Insectivorous Snakes

Insect-eating snakes typically seen by veterinarians include green snakes (*Opheodrys* spp.), worm snakes (*Carphophis* spp.), ring-necked snakes (*Diadophus* spp.), brown snakes (*Storeria* spp.) and other primarily fossorial snakes. Additionally, some ectotherm snakes eat insects, especially as juveniles.

A variety of insects should be offered, including crickets, mealworms, earthworms, nightcrawlers and wax-moth larvae. Insects should be fed a complete diet before they are fed to snakes. Insects should be dusted with a calcium and vitamin supplement weekly. Some of the larger snakes in this group may be weaned onto pinkie mice for added nutrition. Pinkies can be supplemented by dipping them into a liquid calcium supplement.

Many of these snakes also feed on very small amphibians, such as salamanders, tadpoles and frogs. As with feeding ectotherm snakes, cold-blooded prey items should be frozen for at least three days to minimize parasitic infections.

For all snakes, fresh water should be provided at all times. Water bowls should be cleaned and disinfected regularly. A water container that is large enough for soaking should be provided. Vitamin-mineral supplements should not be added to the water. Palatability may be reduced and bacteria in the water may feed on the supplements resulting in a bacterial bloom.

Turtles and Tortoises: Chelonia

Carnivores

The most common carnivorous turtles seen by veterinarians are water turtles, such as snapping turtles (*Chelydra* spp.), mata mata turtles (*Chelys* spp.) and alligator snapping turtles (*Macrochelys* spp.). These turtles usually eat only while in water. They can be fed in their regular aquatic environment or, better yet, in a separate water-filled tank. This practice decreases the amount of fecal material and decaying food in their aquarium, thereby reducing water quality problems.

Most aquatic turtles are fed commercial turtle or fish pellets. Trout food comes in several sized pellets. Large pellets tend to float well and are attractive to large turtles, whereas the smaller pellets tend to sink quickly but are readily accepted by juveniles and small turtles. Trout food may be difficult for reptile owners to find because it is usually only available by special order from feed stores. It is typically sold only in 50-lb bags. Veterinarians who see a large number of reptiles may want to purchase the food, separate it into smaller amounts (store it in a freezer) and make it available to clients who own turtles.

Fish (e.g., goldfish, minnows and guppies) are also fed to aquatic turtles and are available as feeder fish from pet stores. Smelt, mackerel and other oily fish should be fed in limited quantities because their high polyunsaturated fatty acid content may lead to vitamin E deficiency and steatitis. Also, fish may contain thiaminases. Feeding wild-caught fish should also be discouraged because they may be intermediate hosts for reptile parasites. Amphibians (e.g., tadpoles and frogs) can also be fed but they too are safest if captive-born. Crayfish are not recommended because they may harbor the bacterium *Beneckia chitonvora*, which has been implicated in shell diseases of turtles (Boyer and Boyer, 1992).

Other food items include earthworms, snails, slugs, beetles, grasshoppers, moths, crickets, mealworms, giant mealworms, wax worms and other insects. Wild-caught prey should be free of insecticides and pesticides.

Carnivorous turtles may occasionally consume leafy vegetables or fruits, which can be fed as treats. Vitamin-mineral supplementation is not necessary if turtles eat a variety of commercial foods. Cuttlebone may be added as a calcium supplement for juveniles.

Omnivorous Aquatic Turtles

The most common omnivorous water turtles seen by veterinarians are red-eared sliders (*Trachemys* spp.), painted turtles (*Chrysemys* spp.), Reeves turtles (*Chinemys* spp.), diamondback terrapins (*Malaclemys* spp.), map turtles (*Graptemys* spp.) and river cooters (*Pseudemys* spp.). Many omnivorous water turtles are primarily carnivores as juveniles and become more herbivorous as they age. The carnivorous portion of the diet is the same as described for carnivorous water turtles and should make up between 75 and 100% of the diet for juveniles and about 50% of the diet for adults. A wide variety of vegetables should be offered to round out the diet.

Generally, vegetables that float are preferable because turtles can nibble on them throughout the day. Favorites include greens such as romaine lettuce, collard greens, endive, Swiss chard and kale. Fruits tend to disintegrate in water. Supplementation of the diet is usually unnecessary if the diet is varied and includes commercial foods.

Box Turtles

Some of the most popular box turtles include the eastern box turtle (*Terrapene carolina carolina*), the ornate box turtle (*Terrapene ornata ornata*), the three-toed box turtle (*Terrapene carolina triunguis*) and Asian box turtles (*Cuora* spp.).

Box turtles are primarily omnivorous, although some species such as Asiatic box turtles are more carnivorous. Box turtles tend to eat more animal protein as juveniles and become more omnivorous as they mature. The carnivorous portion of the diet is similar to that described for water turtles and should include a wide variety of invertebrates such as earthworms, slugs, mealworms and wax worms.

Commercial box turtle foods, low-fat dog food, trout food, primate biscuits and small amounts of cat food add variety and nutritional balance to the diet. Fruits and vegetables will be more readily accepted as box turtles mature, but should be offered at all ages (**Figure 71-3**). Box turtles seem most interested in eating red, orange and yellow foods. They tend to favor strawberries, tomatoes, raspberries and blueberries. These fruits can be used to entice turtles to eat. Red food dye can be used to convince stubborn animals to try different and more balanced foods.

Water for box turtles should always be available in a shallow, heavy bowl or dish to allow the turtle to enter the water without spilling the contents. Additionally, box turtles should be soaked in a warm water bath once or twice weekly for approximately 30 minutes. Vitamin and mineral supplements should not be placed in water sources because they may reduce palatability and may increase bacterial growth.

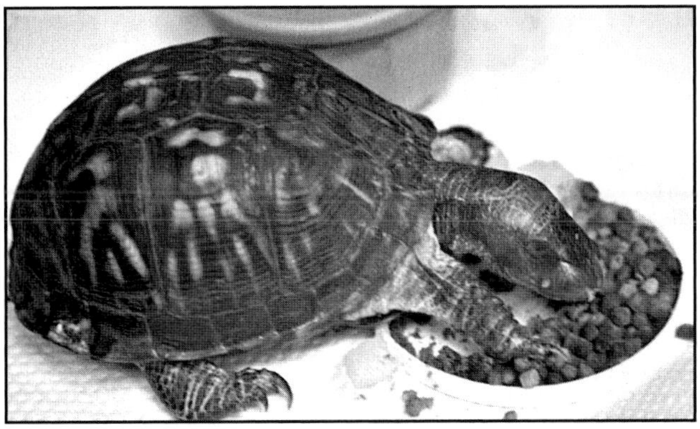

Figure 71-3. Box turtles are omnivorous. This Eastern box turtle is eating a commercial turtle ration with added chopped fruit.

Herbivorous Tortoises

The most common tortoises seen by veterinarians are California desert tortoises (*Gopherus agassizii*), leopard tortoises (*Geochelone pardalis*), South American red-footed tortoises (*Geochelone carbonaria*), yellow-footed tortoises (*Geochelone denticulata*), Greek tortoises (*Testudo graeca*), hingeback tortoises (*Kinexys* spp.) and gopher tortoises (*Gopherus polyphemus*). Most tortoises are strictly herbivorous, although a few accept meat-based foods. All use hindgut fermentation.

The basic diet for most tortoises includes a staple of leafy vegetables, such as collard greens, romaine lettuce, parsley, leaf lettuce, dandelion greens, turnip greens and Swiss chard. Dandelion and clover are excellent forages. These should make up 60 to 70% of the diet. Avoid feeding excessive quantities of produce containing oxalates (e.g., spinach) and goitrogens (e.g., kale). Commercially prepared foods for tortoises and iguanas work well for the other 30 to 40% of the diet because they supply protein, vitamins and minerals not present in vegetables.

Timothy hay, alfalfa hay and pellets and grass clippings may be offered to increase the fiber content of the diet. The remainder of the diet may include small amounts of fruits and vegetables.

For juvenile tortoises, foods should be finely chopped into small, manageable pieces to increase consumption. To minimize ingestion of cage and enclosure substrate, food should be offered on flat trays or plates that juveniles can climb onto. Tortoises are often unable to eat from bowls or raised feeders.

Produce should be supplemented with calcium, vitamins and trace minerals. Usually, diets are supplemented twice weekly for hatchlings and once every seven to 10 days for adults. Supplementation may be unnecessary if 50% or more of the tortoise's diet is comprised of commercial food.

Many tortoises will not drink from water bowls, so all tortoises should be soaked in a tub or large bowl of warm water (up to the plastron) for 15 to 20 minutes to encourage drinking and excretion. Generally, tropical species should be soaked twice weekly, whereas desert species may need to be soaked only once a week. Hatchlings should be soaked daily.

ENDNOTE

a. Calcimar. Rorer Pharmaceutical Corporation, Fort Washington, PA, USA.

REFERENCES

The references for **Chapter 71** can be found at www.markmorris.org.

CASE 71-1

Swollen Eyes and Respiratory Difficulty in a Box Turtle

Scott Stahl, DVM, Dipl. ABVP (Avian)
Stahl Exotic Animal Veterinary Services
Vienna, Virginia, USA

Susan Donoghue, VMD
Nutrition Support Services
Pembroke, Virginia, USA

Patient Assessment

An adult, female Eastern box turtle (*Terrepene carolina carolina*) weighing 357 g was presented for examination. The turtle had a carapace length of 125 mm, and a plastron length of 121 mm. The turtle had been caught and maintained in captivity for one year. It was kept indoors during the winter in a 20-gallon aquarium with one other female Eastern box turtle. In the late spring, it was placed in an outdoor enclosure. The outside environment contained a small wooded area, weeds, grass and leaves. Open areas in the enclosure allowed exposure to sunlight. One male and two other female box turtles also lived in this outdoor enclosure. The turtle was observed laying a clutch of eggs one month earlier.

The owner presented the turtle because its eyes were swollen and sometimes sealed shut. Congestion was noted and mucus bubbled from the turtle's nares. The turtle was anorectic and lethargic.

Physical examination revealed bilaterally swollen eyelids with conjunctivitis and purulent discharge. Visual inspection of the corneas was difficult due to swelling. Mucus was present in both nares, and congestion and mucus were noted in the oral cavity. Increased upper respiratory noises were heard. Skin and shell quality were normal. Body weight was fair.

A culture was taken of the mucus in the nares. A diagnosis of hypovitaminosis A and secondary bacterial conjunctivitis and rhinitis was made based on the historical information and physical examination findings.

Assess the Food and Feeding Method

The turtle's diet for the previous year consisted of a variety of fruits, such as apples, bananas, strawberries, and earthworms and insects found in the outdoor enclosure. The owner had not used any supplements for several months, but previously had used a multivitamin supplement.

Questions

1. What nutrient problems should be suspected based on the dietary history?
2. What should the initial treatment be for this turtle?
3. What long-term changes should be made in the diet?

Answers and Discussion

1. The current diet was probably deficient in vitamin A and other vitamins and minerals, such as calcium. Earthworms are generally a nutritious dietary item, but the fruits offered provided only trace amounts of calcium and inadequate supplementation was provided. Additionally, not feeding a complete food, such as commercial box turtle, trout or dog food as a part of the diet contributed to the problem.
2. The patient was soaked in a warm water bath for 20 minutes then placed in an incubator at 29°C (85°F) and fluid therapy was initiated (20 ml/kg body weight of lactated Ringer's solution given epicoelomically). Vitamin A (200 to 300 IU/kg body weight) was given orally. The turtle was started on enrofloxacin[a] (5 mg/kg body weight, q48h) administered into the musculature of the front legs. One or two gentamicin ophthalmic drops were placed in each eye twice daily.[b]
3. The patient's diet was changed to include foods with higher vitamin A content. A variety of vegetables and fruits, and a commercial box turtle food were provided.

Progress Notes

The following day, the box turtle was soaked in a warm water bath for 15 minutes. Afterward, purulent material was gently removed from the periocular tissues with an eye rinse.[c] Gentamicin ophthalmic drops were placed in both eyes. The patient was then tube fed an enteral diet[d] placed directly into the stomach with a curved metal feeding tube. The following day, the enrofloxacin, gentamicin drops and the warm water bath were repeated.

The turtle was sent home with a two-week course of parenteral enrofloxacin and gentamicin drops. The owner was instructed to apply a vitamin A eye preparation[e] to the eyes daily for 14 days and soak the turtle daily for 15 to 20 minutes. Changes in the diet were recommended and the owner was encouraged to offer food immediately following the soaks.

At a follow-up visit two weeks later, the owner said the turtle had begun to eat well and was much more active. Upon physical examination, the eyes were open and markedly less swollen (**Figure 1**) and no nasal discharge was present. Culture results of the nasal discharge taken earlier revealed *Pseudomonas aeruginosa*. This organism was sensitive to enrofloxacin and gentamicin. The oral dose of vitamin A was repeated, and enrofloxacin, gentamicin and vitamin A drops were continued for another seven days.

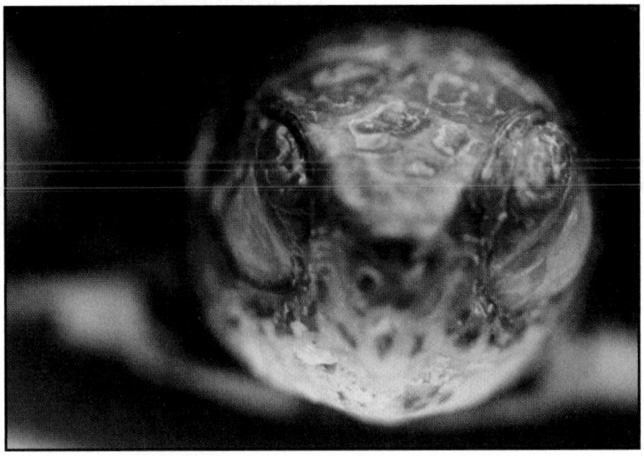

Figure 1. An Eastern box turtle that presented initially for bilaterally swollen eyelids and conjunctivitis with purulent discharge.

Endnotes

a. Baytril. Bayer Corporation, Agricultural Division, Animal Health, Shawnee Mission, KS, USA.
b. Gentocin Durafilm. Schering-Plough Animal Health, Union, NJ, USA.
c. Dacriose Solution. Ciba Vision Ophthalmics, Atlanta, GA, USA.
d. Ensure Liquid Nutrition. Ross Laboratories, Columbus, OH, USA.
e. Turtle Eye Clear. Tetra Terafauna, Morris Plains, NJ, USA.

Bibliography

Boyer TH. Hypovitaminosis A and hypervitaminosis A. In: Mader DR, ed. Reptile Medicine and Surgery. Philadelphia, PA: WB Saunders Co, 1996; 382-385.

Frye FL. Biomedical and Surgical Aspects of Captive Reptile Husbandry. Malabar, FL: Krieger Publishing Co, 1991; 52-53.

CASE 71-2

Lethargy and Bone Swelling in a Green Iguana

Scott Stahl, DVM, Dipl. ABVP (Avian)
Stahl Exotic Animal Veterinary Services
Vienna, Virginia, USA

Susan Donoghue, VMD
Nutrition Support Services
Pembroke, Virginia, USA

Patient Assessment

An 18-month-old green iguana (*Iguana iguana*) was purchased from a local pet store as a farm-raised juvenile and had been in the owner's possession for one year. The iguana was examined for anorexia of 10 days' duration, a swollen mouth and lethargy.

The iguana was housed in a 20-gallon aquarium with indoor/outdoor carpeting, a branch, plastic plant, water bowl and food bowl. A large "hot rock" provided heat. No artificial lighting was provided, but the cage was placed near a window. The iguana was housed alone; the owner had no other reptiles. The iguana had no history of illness and had never been examined by a veterinarian.

The iguana was generally depressed. Its color was a dull yellow-green. At 253 g and 8 inches (snout to vent length) the animal appeared stunted. Under optimal conditions, it should have been three or four times heavier and markedly longer (i.e., 12 to 14 inches). The mandibular bones were severely swollen, the right side significantly more so than the left. Yellow-brown dried material was present along the exposed mandibular mucous membranes. The right forearm, left tibia and right and left femurs were enlarged. The muscle mass over the rear limbs and tailbase was poor. Results of abdominal palpation were normal. The patient exhibited muscle tremors and fasciculations when handled. It was unable to lift its body off the ground to ambulate but would try to slide along the ground.

Radiographs were taken to assess the skeletal system. The right radius and ulna were fractured, but the fractures appeared old (i.e., callous formation). Poor cortical bone density was evident on all long bones and the mandibular and maxillary bones.

A diagnosis of metabolic bone disease was made based on the clinical history, physical examination and radiographic findings.

Assess the Food and Feeding Method

The patient had been raised on a diet of red-tipped and iceberg lettuce, peas, corn, carrots, apples and strawberries. It was fed daily and was offered two or three of these items at a time. The food was always chopped into small pieces and sometimes dusted with a "reptile vitamin." The owner did not know the name of the supplement, only that it came in a yellow container. The supplement hadn't been used for months. Fresh water was always available.

Questions

1. What nutrient problems should be suspected based on the dietary history?
2. What is the initial treatment for metabolic bone disease?
3. What should be the long-term feeding plan?
4. What other husbandry recommendations should be made?

Answers and Discussion

1. The iguana was fed a diet low in calcium and high in phosphorus, with poor and inconsistent calcium and vitamin supplementation. The iguana was not exposed to natural sunlight or ultraviolet light, probably leading to vitamin D_3 deficiency. Sunlight through a glass window does not provide ultraviolet exposure. Other nutrient deficiencies are likely, too.
2. Initially the patient was placed in an incubator at approximately 31°C (88°F). Warm lactated Ringer's solution was given intracoelomically (20 ml/kg body weight). Eight hours later, vitamin D (1,000 IU vitamin D/kg body weight, intramuscularly) and a calcium-containing solution[a] (0.5 ml/kg body weight, subcutaneously) were given. The iguana was kept overnight in the incubator. The following day, fluid therapy was repeated and an enteral nutritional product[b] was administered orally (50% of metabolic requirement, e.g., 5.5 kcal [23 kJ] or 5.5 ml of the liquid enteral product) using a 14-Fr. red rubber urinary catheter. The iguana was started on an oral calcium supplement (1 mg/kg body weight).[c]
3. The iguana's diet was changed to include a wider variety of calcium-rich vegetables. Supplementation included calcium carbonate sprinkled onto the greens, and once weekly sprinkling of a vitamin D_3-containing product onto the greens. Recommendations included placing a full-spectrum fluorescent bulb within 12 to 18 inches of the patient.
4. Iguanas are diurnal basking lizards and must be provided with radiant heat. A temperature gradient should be provided in their environment. The upper end of the temperature range should be 31 to 35°C (88 to 95°F). A "hot rock" does not provide adequate heat for an iguana. A clamp lamp with an incandescent light bulb was placed at one end of the aquarium to keep the hot end of the cage between 31 and 33.5°C (88 and 92°F). In addition, a hide box was provided to help minimize stress and branches were removed to prevent falls until the patient's bones strengthened.

Progress Notes

The iguana's owner was instructed to slowly feed the enteral nutritional product with a syringe (5 to 10 kcal [21 to 42 kJ] daily in small divided doses). The patient was also soaked daily in a warm water bath. The iguana was given the oral calcium supplement (1 ml/kg body weight, b.i.d.) for 30 days.

The iguana returned in one week for a follow-up examination. The owner reported that the iguana was readily accepting the enteral nutritional product and was more alert and active. Upon physical examination, the mandible seemed firmer and the patient was much more responsive. Calcitonin[d] was administered intramuscularly (50 IU/kg body weight). The patient's diet was switched from the enteral product to moistened commercial iguana food. Small meatball-shaped pellets were fed (four to five pieces were fed one or two times daily, depending on the iguana's appetite). Additionally, two tablespoons of chopped dark green leafy vegetables (e.g., collard greens, kale, romaine lettuce) were offered daily. Oral calcium was continued.

The iguana returned weekly for calcitonin injections and a second injection of vitamin D. Three weeks later, a follow-up examination revealed stronger, firmer mandibular and maxillary bones and reduced swelling and increased strength in the long bones. The iguana was able to lift its body off the ground to ambulate. It was eating commercial food vigorously and also eating some of the greens. The owner reported that the iguana was spending time basking and had become more active. The oral calcium supplement was reduced to once daily dosing.

A recheck one month later revealed that the iguana was able to move normally (**Figure 1**). The mandibular and maxillary bones were firm and the patient's appetite was dramatically improved. Rechecks were recommended at three-month intervals over the next year to prevent relapses.

Endnotes

a. Calphosan Solution. Glenwood Inc., Tenafly, NJ, USA.
b. Ensure Liquid Nutrition. Ross Laboratories, Columbus, OH, USA.
c. Neo-Calglucon. Sandoz, East Hanover, NJ, USA.
d. Miacalcin. Schering-Plough, Kenilworth, NJ, USA.

Bibliography

Boyer TH. Metabolic bone disease. In: Mader DR, ed. Reptile Medicine and Surgery. Philadelphia, PA: WB Saunders Co, 1996; 385-392.

Mader DR. Use of calcitonin in green iguanas, *Iguana iguana*, with metabolic bone disease. Bulletin of the Association of Reptilian and Amphibian Veterinarians 1993; 3: 41.

Rossi J. A practical and effective treatment for metabolic bone disease in the green iguana. In: Proceedings. North American Veterinary Conference, Orlando FL, 1992: 707.

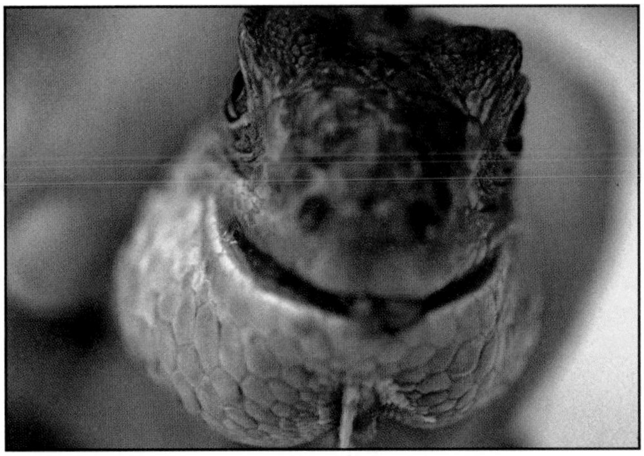

Figure 1. An 18-month-old iguana that presented initially with anorexia, lethargy and a swollen mouth. The iguana's growth had been severely stunted and it had markedly swollen mandibular bones.

CASE 71-3

Anorexia and Lethargy in a Green Iguana

Connie J. Orcutt, DVM, Dipl. ABVP (Avian)
Angell Memorial Animal Hospital
Boston, Massachusetts, USA

Patient Assessment

A two-year-old female green iguana weighing 1.6 kg was presented for anorexia and lethargy of six days' duration. The owner obtained the iguana 18 months ago. The iguana was housed in a 75-gallon aquarium with another iguana. The aquarium was heated with a heating pad under the tank and a 220-watt infrared heat lamp. Ultraviolet-B light was provided by an artificial light source; however, the owner couldn't specify how long the source was provided daily.

When examined, the iguana was lethargic, but moved when stimulated. The overall skin coloration was dark and dull. A firm mass was palpated in the caudodorsal coelomic cavity; deep palpation elicited a response from the patient. The patient's long bones were palpably normal. The mandible was firm and non-compressible.

Abnormal results of a complete blood count and serum biochemistry profile included a heterophilic leukocytosis, hyperproteinemia, marked hyperphosphatemia, hyperuricemia and marked increases in creatine kinase levels and aspartate aminotransferase activity. Radiographs demonstrated bilaterally symmetric soft tissue opacities in the caudodorsal coelomic cavity; these opacities were thought to be the patient's kidneys. A sonogram revealed enlarged hyperechoic kidneys bilaterally.

Assess the Food and Feeding Method

The iguana's diet consisted of a variety of vegetables including greens, broccoli and dandelions as well as an unspecified commercial iguana food, which made up approximately 50% of the total diet. Fruit was given occasionally. The owner had been supplementing the diet with a vitamin-mineral supplement twice daily for several months.

Questions

1. What nutritional problems are suggested by the diet? Could any of these explain the iguana's clinical signs?
2. What is the pathophysiology of the biochemical abnormalities? What is the significance of the abnormalities found by imaging?
3. How can this condition be treated?

Answers and Discussion

1. The owner has been providing large amounts of vitamin D_3 in the form of the vitamin-mineral supplement and the commercially prepared iguana food. Vitamin D_3 is essential for calcium uptake from the intestinal tract; however, it can be toxic when given in large amounts. Either hypervitaminosis D or hypocalcemia could be responsible for the lethargy and anorexia exhibited by the patient.
2. Hyperproteinemia may be due to dehydration. Hyperuricemia and hyperphosphatemia indicate some degree of renal failure. The increase in aspartate aminotransferase activity and elevated creatine kinase value indicate either muscle degeneration and/or hepatic damage. Renomegaly and pain elicited when the kidneys were palpated are signs consistent with nephrosis. The increased opacity in the region of the kidneys seen radiographically and by ultrasound is consistent with mineralization of the renal parenchyma. The combination of these findings is suggestive of renal failure secondary to hypervitaminosis D.

3. Excessive supplementation with vitamin D_3 allows large amounts of calcium to be absorbed from the intestinal tract. The resulting soft tissue mineralization, however, can be widespread and severe. Endstage renal failure is generally unresponsive to treatment; however, diuresis may provide short-term palliative treatment.

Progress Notes

The iguana was diuresed with a mixture of 0.9% saline, 2.5% dextrose and lactated Ringer's solution administered intracoelomically for two days. Unfortunately, the patient died on Day 3. Results of a necropsy examination revealed moderate tubular nephrosis and severe degeneration with mineralization and necrosis of the heart and skeletal muscles. The final diagnosis was vitamin D toxicosis. Vitamin D_3 and calcium metabolism are still not well elucidated in iguanas and vitamin D_3 requirements have not been established. It is unclear how well vitamin D_3 is absorbed in these animals. The risk of over-supplementation can be avoided by providing exposure to adequate amounts of ultraviolet-B light, thus allowing the body to form its own vitamin D_3 instead of giving oral supplementation.

Chapter 72

Feeding Passerine and Psittacine Birds

George V. Kollias
Heidi Wearne Kollias

"Of all forms of life, birds are the most beautiful, most musical, most admired, most watched and most defended. Without them much of our world would seem ominously lifeless and silent."
Roger Tory Peterson

INTRODUCTION

One avian medicine reference states that 75% of the medical problems seen in companion and aviary birds have at least a partial nutritional basis (MacWhirter, 1994). Dietary-induced deficiencies and excesses may lead to immune dysfunction, increased susceptibility to infectious diseases and metabolic and biochemical derangements that manifest clinically as nutritional secondary hyperparathyroidism, thyroid hyperplasia (dysplasia), hemochromatosis and a variety of other problems.

Dietary-induced diseases frequently occur in companion and aviary psittacine and passerine birds for several reasons. First, until recently, specific nutritional requirements for these birds were unknown. Thus, investigators and veterinary practitioners tended to extrapolate the well-known nutrient needs of poultry to other avian species. Although these nutrient needs generally apply, specific nutritional differences of domestic chickens and other avian species have been reported. For example, riboflavin deficiency in broiler chicks manifests itself clinically as "curled-toe paralysis," which is not observed in cockatiel chicks. Cockatiels lack pigmentation (achromatosis) in their primary feathers as a result of riboflavin deficiency (Grau and Roudybush, 1985). Although differences of this type exist experimentally, many prepared foods overcome these differences by supplying levels of nutrients well in excess of the minimum requirement for chickens.

Second, and more important, many people perceive that all-seed diets (particularly diets composed of only one seed type, e.g., millet or sunflower) and diets composed of or are heavily supplemented with, fruits, vegetables and other human foods are complete foods for birds. In reality, most commercially available seeds are deficient in certain limiting nutrients (e.g., specific amino acids, vitamins and trace and macrominerals such as calcium and sodium). Also, seeds are not the primary or natural diet of most species of companion birds. For example, one study revealed that when given the opportunity, the endangered Puerto Rican parrot (*Amazona vittata*) consumed seven species of fruits, seeds and leaves (new foliage), the fruiting structures of 44 species of trees (in addition to bark) and seven species of canopy vines (Synder, 1987). Thus, seeds compose only a small part of their total diet in the wild.

Additionally, evidence suggests that increased protein may be needed during certain points in the reproductive cycle. In the wild, insects supply these increased needs. It is difficult for bird owners to meet these special needs feeding only seed mixtures.

But, perhaps the most common cause of dietary-induced diseases in companion birds is the practice of adding fruits and vegetables sold for human consumption to commercially prepared foods or supplemented seed mixtures. The most readily available fruits and vegetables contain primarily water, carbohydrates and fiber. They are severely deficient in protein, vitamins and minerals (Nutrient Content of Foods, USDA), when compared to the nutrient recommendations for psittacine and passerine birds (Nutrition Expert Panel Report, 1996). Thus, fruits and vegetables primarily dilute key nutrients present in nutritionally balanced commercially prepared foods. Birds often preferentially eat fruits and vegetables due to their high water content instead of dry extruded or pelleted foods and seed mixtures. In fact, birds often select food items based on water content, texture, color or taste, rather than nutrient content (Ullrey et al, 1991), resulting in very imbalanced nutrient intakes.

This common feeding practice leads directly to the third reason captive birds develop nutritional deficiencies, which is the tendency of individual birds to select specific food items from a variety of offerings. Because malnourished birds often tend to overeat the food items presented to them, it is unclear whether this is a cause or an effect of malnutrition. It does lead to the popular misconception that birds are able to preferentially balance their diets. As a result, individual birds may become habituated or fixated on a specific food item (e.g., sunflower, safflower or millet seeds or grapes or oranges). Yet these specific items are usually deficient in several essential nutrients.

This chapter summarizes assessment criteria and feeding plans for healthy birds commonly kept as pets.

PATIENT ASSESSMENT

Signalment

Veterinary practitioners and their health care teams should become familiar with the most common psittacine and passerine species. Psittacine birds are members of the order Psittaciformes, (parrots and parakeets). Passerine birds belong to the order Passeriformes, which includes finches, sparrows, buntings, mynahs, canaries and serins.

Estimation of age and sex is important in nutritional assessment; like dogs and cats, birds have different requirements with varying age and function. Immature psittacine and passerine species characteristically have dull-colored feathers. Beak color varies with age in some species. If adults are dark-billed, immature birds of the same species may have light-colored bills. If adults have pale beaks, those of juveniles are generally dark or have dark markings at the base of the beak. Immature passerine birds are particularly difficult to identify until they go through their first or second molt.

Iris color may help in estimating the age in some species. Young psittacine birds have brown or dark irides. The iris color of macaws fades to gray within one year, appears white from one to three years and then turns yellow in mature birds. The iris color of Amazon parrots may change to red-orange as birds mature. African grey parrots' irides lighten from brown through gray to white. The irides of both genders of immature Moloccan cockatoos (and most all-white cockatoos) are brown; mature males have red irides and mature females have dark brown irides.

History

Because the clinical manifestations of malnutrition in birds are quite variable, the history and physical examination are very important (**Table 72-1**). Before a bird is presented at the veterinary hospital, the client should be instructed to:

1. Bring the bird in its own cage.
2. Not clean the cage.
3. Empty the water dish.
4. Remove all grit (if used) from the cage.
5. Cover the cage and wrap it with a blanket in cold weather.
6. Remove all cage furniture if the bird is weak or injured.
7. Bring any medications and vitamin-mineral supplements the bird has been offered.
8. Bring a sample of the foods offered daily (e.g., seed mixtures, pelleted or extruded food) and a list of fruits, vegetables and other foods regularly fed.

The history should include general questions such as: 1) the origin of the bird, 2) length of ownership, 3) housing arrangements, 4) type of heat and humidity provided, 5) light sources used (e.g., ultraviolet, full spectrum, fluorescent, natural, etc.), 6) exposure to other birds, 7) foods and supplements normally fed, for how long and in what quantities, 8) the owner's assessment of the presenting condition (including changes in food and water consumption, droppings, environment and behavior) and 9) information relative to previous treatment by the owner or another veterinarian.

The history for a newly acquired bird (owned for less than 10 months of age) will often include exposure to infectious diseases (viral, mycoplasmal, bacterial and mycotic) as a result of contact with other birds in a pet shop, aviary or quarantine facility. These problems are among the most difficult to accurately diagnose and treat. Other problems commonly associated with a newly acquired bird include acute malnutrition, trauma, parasitism (hematogenous, gastrointestinal and respiratory), intoxications and secondary immune suppression associated with one or a combination of the above.

Birds owned for more than 10 months can be considered to be from an "uncontaminated" environment unless other birds frequently immigrate and emigrate from the household or collection. Individual birds not exposed to other birds for this period may have chronic malnutrition of dietary origin.

Physical Examination

General Examination

Observation of the patient in its cage or aviary environment is important. The condition of the cage may indicate the type of human-animal bond (e.g., concern, or lack thereof). First

Table 72-1. Clinical manifestations of malnutrition in birds.*

System	Physical or clinical manifestation
Pansystemic or generalized	Behavioral changes
	Epithelial hyperplasia or metaplasia (skin, respiratory, gastrointestinal)
	Gout
	Hypocalcemia
	Immune suppression (lack of infectious disease resistance)
	Low body weight
	Polyphagia/obesity
	Polyuria/polydipsia
	Poor growth
	Subcutaneous edema (vitamin E/selenium deficiency)
Integumentary	
Skin	Dryness
	Exfoliative dermatitis
	Pododermatitis
	Poor wound healing
	Pruritus
	Uropygial gland hypertrophy and duct obstruction
Beak	Excessive or abnormal beak growth, dryness, epithelial exfoliation
Feathers	Abnormal markings in feathers ("stress lines")
	Brittle frayed feathers
	Color or pigment changes (depigmentation, hyperpigmentation, melanosis)
	Curling of feathers
	Feather picking
	Lack of development of contour feathers
	Molting abnormalities
	Retained feather sheaths
Gastrointestinal	Generalized epithelial alterations
Oropharynx	Mucosal ulceration
	Salivary gland abscessation
	White (caseous appearing) plaques involving the oral mucosa
Crop	Lithiasis
	Regurgitation
	Secondary crop stasis or impaction
Esophagus, proventriculus, ventriculus	Altered motility, mucosal erosion, regurgitation
	Koilin abnormalities (erosion, dysgenesis)
Small and large bowel	Diarrhea
	Enteritis (e.g., clostridial infections secondary to high sugar diets)
	Malabsorption
Liver	Hepatopathies (e.g., fatty liver syndrome)
Pancreas	Pancreatic atrophy
Respiratory	Generalized epithelial alterations
	Partial or complete upper or lower airway obstruction causing dyspnea (rhinal cavity, sinuses, syrinx)
Nares	Serous nasal discharge
Eyes	Serous ocular discharge
	Lacrimal duct obstruction (epiphora) secondary to epithelial debris accumulation
	Palpebrae (eyelid) paresis or paralysis
Central and peripheral nervous and neuromuscular	Abnormal gait, "jerky leg movements" (pyridoxine deficiency)
	Behavioral changes (e.g., aggression, cannibalism, self mutilation)
	Cervical paralysis (folic acid deficiency)
	Muscular weakness/paresis (vitamin E deficiency, hyponatremia)
	Seizures (salt toxicity, hypothiaminosis, hypocalcemia, vitamin E deficiency)
	Syncope (hypoglycemia, hypocalcemia)
Musculoskeletal	Hock (tibiotarsal/tarsometatarsal) joint enlargement
	Limb deformities (valgus/varus deformities involving long bones)
	Pathologic fractures (metabolic bone disease)
	Slipped tendon (deficiency of manganese, biotin, pantothenic and/or folic acid in some species)
Urogenital	Egg binding (endocrine or neuromuscular in origin)
	Endocrinopathy affecting fertility/reproductive performance
	Epithelial hyperplasia/metaplasia (renal and/or ureteral obstruction)
	Gout
Cardiovascular	Anemia
	Coagulopathy (vitamin K deficiency, hepatopathy)
	Hemorrhagic diathesis (vitamin E deficiency)
Endocrine	Goiter (thyroid dysplasia), iodine deficiency

*Adapted from MacWhirter P. Malnutrition. In: Ritchie BW, Harrison GJ, Harrison LR, eds. Avian Medicine: Principles and Applications. Lake Worth, FL: Wingers Publishing, 1994; 842-861. Kollias GV. Diets, feeding practices, and nutritional problems in psittacine birds. Veterinary Medicine 1995; 90: 29-39.

observe the bird at a distance (nonthreatening). A healthy bird should appear alert and attentive. Tame birds generally appear relaxed and calm. Some birds vocalize and are very active during examination (macaws, Amazon parrots, African grey parrots and conures). Abnormalities include fluffing of the feathers, head tucking, rhythmic movement of the tail, frequent blinking, lethargy and falling asleep on the examination table.

Trunk and limb asymmetry and skeletal deformities are obvious if the veterinarian is familiar with normal conformation. Drooping wing(s) may indicate paresis or injury. Restlessness, shifting of body weight or favoring one leg may suggest discomfort or dysfunction from pain or injury. Dysequilibrium may be associated with spinal malformation, toxin ingestion, head injury or metabolic derangement affecting the central nervous system that may be associated with malnutrition, especially inadequate intake of calcium or B-complex vitamins. Only minimal restraint should be used during the physical examination.

Oral Examination

The oral cavity should have a neutral odor. Causes of a foul-smelling oral cavity include bacterial pharyngitis, sinusitis or digestive disorders that may be exacerbated by diet or malnutrition. Normal oral epithelium is shiny and has uniform color. Some psittacine and passerine birds (cockatoos, Amazon parrots and macaws) have darkly pigmented oral epithelium, whereas others have a pink oral mucosa.

White caseous lesions on or below the mucosa may suggest inflammatory changes secondary to squamous metaplasia associated with hypovitaminosis A. These types of lesions may also be observed with poxvirus infection, candidiasis, trichomoniasis and coliform abscesses. Sick birds often accumulate mucus in the mouth, under the premaxilla and tongue. Birds that recover from hypovitaminosis A and viral infections may have scar formation around the choanae, or the normal papillae on the choanal boarders may be blunted or absent.

Tongue characteristics vary with the species. Psittacine birds normally have a smooth-surfaced, symmetric, thick and fleshy tongue with a thick layer of epithelium near the tip. The color varies from pink to black depending on the species. Passerine birds have a rigid tongue with a whitish or light gray tip. Unilateral swelling of the tongue may indicate abscess formation.

Beak and Cere Examination

The beak is normally smooth and uniformly colored with a deep sheen. Abnormal, rapid beak growth may be associated with malnutrition, specific viral disease (psittacine beak and feather virus), obesity or hepatopathy. Budgerigars with rapid beak growth often have reddish-black discoloration on the anterior margin of the premaxilla. Twisted beaks (mostly seen in fledglings) are often associated with malnutrition, systemic disease, feeding trauma or genetic-based malformation. Psittacine birds require branches or hardwood to chew on for beak conditioning. Cuttlebones and mineral blocks are inadequate for this purpose. In fact, cuttlebones should *not* be recommended for beak conditioning or as a nutritional supplement. A flaky or rough-looking beak may be associated with malnutrition, lack of proper chewing or systemic disease. The beak should also be examined for fractures, dislocations and erosive lesions that may result from bacterial, fungal and viral infections (e.g., psittacine beak and feather disease).

The cere, a soft cutaneous appendage containing the nares, should normally be firm and smooth, and lack flakes and debris. The nares should be evenly placed in relationship to the cere and be bilaterally symmetric in size and shape. Change in diameter may indicate past or present respiratory infections or neoplasia. Nasal discharge is abnormal and may be indicated by staining of the feathers above the cere.

Eye and Ear Examination

The eyes are best examined with the aid of transillumination externally and from inside the oral cavity. Birds have the ability to voluntarily control pupil size, thus pupillary constriction in response to light is not an accurate indication of vision. A menace response should be present bilaterally.

Symmetry, position and mobility of the globes should be noted. If conjunctivitis is present, culture and sensitivity testing should be done along with a detailed nutritional history. The cornea should be smooth and shiny. Any irregularities should be investigated by staining with fluorescein dye. The anterior chamber of the eye should be examined with indirect or direct ophthalmoscopy. The iris should be flat and thin and have a freely moving pupillary border. Clarity of the lens should be determined when the pupil is dilated.

A normal fundic examination should reveal an evenly reflective, avascular retina. The pecten, a heavily pigmented pleated vascular structure, extends from the optic disk into the vitreous.

The ears normally are free of exudate and debris. Epithelial debris often accumulates in the external auditory meatus of birds as a sign of malnutrition.

Skin and Feather Examination

Injuries and other problems involving the wings are common in birds. Examination should include complete palpation of both wings. Twisted, brittle and deformed wing feathers may be associated with nutritional, genetic, traumatic or a combination of causes. Abnormal feathering is associated with a variety of problems and diseases; malnutrition is the most common cause.

Large areas of feather loss may result from self-mutilation secondary to dermatitis, suggesting possible nutritional and/or systemic disease. The wing web (propatagium) should be evaluated for signs of dermatitis and trauma. The feathers often have to be displaced away from the featherless tracts (apterylae) to examine the skin over the head, dorsum, wings, upper legs and abdomen. Dry exfoliating skin may indicate nutritional problems or a very dry environment.

Primary dermatologic problems in birds are rare; most problems are secondary to trauma or systemic diseases, including malnutrition. Skin overlying cervical and abdominal regions can be assessed for elasticity in an attempt to crudely determine hydration and nutritional status in young birds and to a lesser extent in older birds. The skin of the feet and legs should be shiny and have a uniform scaled pattern. Malnutrition can cause smooth, worn and ulcerated palmar surfaces of the feet. Pododermatitis, with or without ulcer formation, is often associated with improper perches and is exacerbated by malnutrition (e.g., hypovitaminosis A).

Overgrowth of the claws often accompanies beak lesions and is associated with metabolic and nutritional disorders, especially in lories, finches, budgerigars, canaries and Amazon parrots. Some species, such as Frill canaries, normally have long claws.

Contour feathers should adhere tightly together, appear homogeneous and have a bright sheen. The eclectus parrot, however, characteristically has loose, hair-like feathers. The wing and tail feathers should be transilluminated to examine for mites, color abnormalities, structural damage and vane abnormalities (e.g., holes).

Feather lice and mite infestations are common in newly imported birds. Feather picking and mutilation occur commonly in psittacine birds but only occasionally in passerine species. Frequent causes include boredom, stress (change in owner/bird routine), systemic diseases and improper diet.

Feathers of psittacine birds overlying the rump, thigh and crest areas should be examined for signs of viral beak and feather disease. Powder down (a powdery white substance) is present on the feathers of white cockatoo species, African grey parrots and cockatiels. Powder down is a normal finding.

Soiled feathers around the vent may indicate disease of the urogenital or gastrointestinal system. Protrusion of the cloacal mucosa may be associated with mucosal hyperplasia, cloacal papillomas, uterine prolapse (associated with egg binding), irritation due to masturbation, straining due to low intestinal obstruction or inflammation.

Regional Palpation

After examination of the skin and feathers, the intermandibular space should be palpated for swelling (e.g., abscess formation) that may be secondary to hypovitaminosis A in psittacine birds. The crop should normally be partially filled with food. A fluid-filled crop is an abnormal finding, except in recently fed chicks. Normally the ventral borders of the liver are barely evident. Caudally, the ventriculus is palpable between the right and left acetabulum.

The keel or pectoral musculature, a reservoir for large quantities of glycogen, should be palpated as an indicator of overall body condition. No body condition scoring system has been developed for birds. Besides palpation, body weight (mass) is the best criterion.

Cardiopulmonary Examination

Cardiopulmonary examination includes auscultation of the sinuses, trachea and thoracic and abdominal air sacs using a pediatric stethoscope. Normally, only the gentle rush of air should be heard. Audible sounds on inspiration and expiration indicate respiratory disease. Abnormal sounds (e.g., clicking, rattling, wheezing, squeaking and honking) may be associated with hepatopathies, respiratory parasites (air sac mites in passerine birds), malnutrition-induced air sac and tracheal epithelial debris and endocrine disease (e.g., thyroid dysplasia).

Birds normally respire with their mouths closed. Open mouthed breathing may result from: 1) anxiety (stress), 2) hyperthermia, 3) compensation for a plugged nostril, 4) anemia, 5) lung, tracheal and air sac disease, 6) abdominal masses and ascites that compress air sacs and 7) excessive handling and excitement. A bird's respiratory rate should return to normal one to two minutes after handling; if not, cardiopulmonary dysfunction may be present. Auscultation is of value to assess rate and rhythm, but murmurs are rarely heard.

Laboratory and Other Clinical Information

Laboratory data can help in the assessment of avian patients. However, veterinary diagnostic laboratories and practices generally do not offer the expertise necessary to provide reproducible laboratory results unless there is an individual on the staff who has taken a special interest in avian clinical laboratory medicine. A detailed description of avian laboratory evaluations is beyond the scope of this chapter; however, a few clinical biochemistry tests with nutritional implications deserve special comment.

Nitrogen excretion in birds involves the conversion of purines to uric acid via the enzyme xanthine oxidase. Renal tubular water resorption is highly variable in birds (60 to 99%). Avian kidneys are often in a number of primary (e.g., renal gout) and secondary diseases (e.g., bacterial enteritis, acute chlamydiosis) because of their relatively large size (approximately 1% of body weight) and the associated renal portal system. There is no single best test to assess renal function. Single plasma uric acid levels are a relatively insensitive indicator of renal tubular damage. Consequently, plasma creatine values, blood gas analysis, urinalyses in polyuric birds and/or serial plasma uric acid determinations must be used to diagnose and predict the outcome of avian renal disease.

Normal avian serum glucose levels are much higher than those of mammals with equivalent body surface area. Glucose values range from 550 to 600 mg/dl in hummingbirds to 140 to 180 mg/dl in ostriches. Stress associated with handling can rapidly elevate serum glucose levels.

FEEDING PLAN

Assess and Select the Food

The patient history should minimally include a list of foods offered daily. In addition, clients should be encouraged to provide a sample of any commercially prepared foods they feed.

If the food offered is commercially prepared, examine the label for nutrient information or guarantees. The primary nutrients of concern are protein and calcium. Many foods commonly fed to companion birds are composed primarily of carbohydrates and fat. The label of an acceptable commercially prepared food should list a protein guarantee of at least 12%. From the list of ingredients on the label determine if a source of calcium is included in the food. Seeds commonly contain more phosphorus than calcium. Thus, an added calcium source

Table 72-2. Nutrition recommendations for avian foods.*

Nutrient	Psittacine Minimum	Psittacine Maximum	Passerine Minimum	Passerine Maximum
Gross energy (kcal/kg)**	3,200	4,200	3,500	4,500
Total protein (%)	12.0	-	14.0	-
Linoleic acid (%)	1.0	-	1.0	-
Amino acids				
Lysine (%)	0.65	-	0.75	-
Methionine (%)	0.30	-	0.35	-
Methionine + cystine (%)	0.50	-	0.58	-
Arginine (%)	0.65	-	0.75	-
Threonine (%)	0.40	-	0.46	-
Vitamins (fat soluble)				
Vitamin A activity (total) IU/kg	8,000	-	8,000	-
Vitamin D_3 (IU/kg)	500	2,000	1,000	2,500
Vitamin E (ppm)	50	-	50	-
Vitamin K (ppm)	1.0	-	1.0	-
Vitamins (water soluble)				
Thiamin (ppm)	4.0	-	4.0	-
Riboflavin (ppm)	6.0	-	6.0	-
Niacin (ppm)	50.0	-	50.0	-
Pyridoxine (ppm)	6.0	-	6.0	-
Pantothenic acid (ppm)	20.0	-	20.0	-
Biotin (ppm)	0.25	-	0.25	-
Folic acid (ppm)	1.50	-	1.50	-
Vitamin B_{12} (ppm)	0.01	-	0.01	-
Choline (ppm)	1,500	-	1,500	-
Minerals				
Calcium (%)	0.30	1.20	0.50	1.20
Phosphorus (%)	0.30	-	0.50	-
Calcium-phosphorus ratio	1.0-1.0	2.0-1.0	1.0-1.0	2.0-1.0
Potassium (%)	0.40	-	0.40	-
Sodium (%)	0.12	-	0.12	-
Chloride (%)	0.12	-	0.12	-
Magnesium (ppm)	600	-	600	-
Trace minerals				
Manganese (ppm)	65.0	-	65.0	-
Iron (ppm)	80.0	-	80.0	-
Zinc (ppm)	50.0	-	50.0	-
Copper (ppm)	8.0	-	8.0	-
Iodine (ppm)	0.40	-	0.40	-
Selenium (ppm)	0.10	-	0.10	-

*Adapted from the Exotic Bird Nutrition Expert Panel Report, Nutrition and Management Committee of the Association of Avian Veterinarians, 1996.
**To convert to kJ, multiply kcal by 4.184.

such as calcium carbonate, dicalcium phosphate, bone meal, ground limestone or ground oyster shells helps balance the calcium-phosphorus ratio of bird foods. Regardless of the type of food fed, a sample can be submitted to a commercial laboratory for analysis. Consult the laboratory in advance to determine sample size needed, preservation techniques recommended and shipping instructions.

Compare the nutrient levels of the food to those recommended in **Table 72-2** to determine if there are any discrepancies in the nutrient profile. Complete nutrient levels of foods can sometimes be found on the label, in sales materials or from the manufacturer. The food is acceptable if its nutrient levels meet or exceed those levels in **Table 72-2**. If not, recommend that the owner select a food that meets these recommended levels.

The food should not be used for long-term feeding if its label contains no nutrient information or is just a list of ingredients such as seeds or dried fruit. The following discussion describes common strategies used to feed birds. In some instances, it can be very difficult to determine whether an individual bird receives levels of nutrients recommended in **Table 72-2**. (See Food Selection below.)

Foods appropriately balanced with carbohydrates, proteins, fats, vitamins, minerals and water are essential for all birds. Stewardship of confined birds must address good nutrition at several levels: the daily satisfaction and health of the bird as well as the long-term contributions to growth, maturation, defense against disease and reproductive health-the hallmark of good nutrition.

Three methods of providing nutrients and achieving these objectives are commonly used: 1) commercially prepared foods, 2) seeds and seed mixtures and 3) homemade mixed foods.

Table 72-3. Special nutritional needs of emberizids (order Passiformes, family Emberizidae).*

Genus and species	Common name	Special nutritional needs**
Emberzia hortulana	Ortolan bunting	Same as *E. tahapisi*
Emberzia tahapisi	Cinnamon-breasted rock bunting	Canary seed mix, mealworms, ant eggs, weed seeds, milk-soaked bread needed in breeding season
Lophospingus pusillus	Black-crested finch or pygmy cardinal	Live foods (e.g., insects, mealworms) needed during breeding season
Paroaria capitata	Yellow-billed cardinal	Must offer a variety of foods to prevent this species from only eating seeds; diet should consist of live food, fruits (berries, apples, oranges, greens [chickweed]), small mealworms, ant eggs and canary seed mix
Paroaria dominicana	Red-crowned Dominican or Pope cardinal	Live food recommended in addition to canary seed mix as for *S. albigularis*
Passerina lelancheri	Orange-bellied, orange-breasted or rainbow bunting	Canary seed mix, insects, canary color foods or pine and spruce twigs to maintain brilliant coloration
Rhodospingus cruentus	Crimson or rhodospingus finch	Same as *S. albigularis*
Sicalis flaveola	Saffron or Brazilian saffron finch	Need an abundance of insects and some greens in breeding season, in addition to that listed for *E. tahapisi*
Sicalis luteola	Yellow grassquit or little saffron finch	In addition to canary seed mix, insects and greens are required
Sporophila albigularis	White-throated seedeater	Canary seed mix, greens, small mealworms and fruits (apples and bananas are essential)
Sporophilia lineola	Lined seedeater	Same as *L. pusillus*
Tiaris canora	Cuban grassquit or Cuban finch	Same as *S. luteola*
Tiaris olivacea	Yellow-faced grassquit or olive finch	Honeycomb regularly; canary seed mix, ant eggs, hard-boiled egg, insects, mealworms, leaf lice, little spiders, greens (chickweed, etc.), tropical seed varieties
Volatina jacarina	Blue-black grassquit or jacarina finch	Same as *S. albigularis*

*Adapted from Burgmann PM. Feeding Your Pet Bird. New York, NY: Barron's Educational Series, 1993. Lint KC, Lint AM. Feeding Cage Birds-A Manual of Diets for Aviculture. New York, NY: Blanford Press, 1988; 133-175. Vriends MM. Simon and Schuster's Guide to Pet Birds. New York, NY: Simon and Schuster, 1984; 104-118. Woolham F. Diets. In: The Handbook of Aviculture. New York, NY: Blanford Press, 1987; 15-23.
**In addition to commercial foods, these dietary "supplements" or additions are thought to be necessary to stimulate courtship and reproductive behavior or to prevent self-mutilation or feather picking by providing environmental/behavioral enrichment.

Table 72-4. Special nutritional needs of fringillids (order Passeriformes, family Fringillidae).*

Genus and species	Common name	Special nutritional needs**
Carduelis (chloris) chloris	Greenfinch	Canary seed mix, rape seed, small sunflower seed, some hemp, linseed, teasel and greens
Carduelis carduelis	European goldfinch	In addition to the basic finch diet, thistle seeds, other seeds, insects and other invertebrates
Fringilla coelebs	Chaffinch	Need live insects, supplemental commercial softbill diet, sprouted seeds (rape, turnip, radish) and canary seed mixture in breeding season
Serinus alario	Black-headed canary or alario finch	Varied seed mixture needed to induce breeding
Serinus canaria	Wild canary, island canary	Same as *S. mozambicus*
Serinus leucopygia	White-rumped, Layard's seedeater or gray singing finch	Same as *S. mozambicus*
Serinus mozambicus	Yellow-eyed or green singing finch, yellow fronted canary	Canary seed mix, insect diet, greens
Serinus serinus	European serin	Additional small seeds (e.g., lettuce, spray millet, etc.)

*Adapted from Burgmann PM. Feeding Your Pet Bird. New York, NY: Barron's Educational Series, 1993. Lint KC, Lint AM. Feeding Cage Birds-A Manual of Diets for Aviculture. New York, NY: Blanford Press, 1988; 133-175. Vriends MM. Simon and Schuster's Guide to Pet Birds. New York, NY: Simon and Schuster, 1984; 120-130. Woolham F. Diets. In: The Handbook of Aviculture. New York, NY: Blanford Press, 1987; 15-23.
**In addition to commercial foods, these dietary "supplements" or additions are thought to be necessary to stimulate courtship and reproductive behavior or to prevent self-mutilation or feather picking by providing environmental/behavioral enrichment.

Commercially Prepared Foods

The benefits of using commercially prepared, nutritionally complete foods become obvious when the feeding of birds kept as companions is compared to the feeding of other companion animals. Prepared foods supply more than 90% of the nutrients for companion dogs and cats in North America and can contribute markedly to the health of these animals. The gradual transition from diets composed primarily of human food, including table scraps, to commercially prepared complete and balanced foods for dogs and cats has taken approximately 50 years. The same transition will undoubtedly occur for pet birds in a much shorter time as the number and quality of products available increase.

The major benefits of commercially prepared foods are nutrient balance and convenience. Manufacturers commonly formulate commercial foods using sound scientific principles following established nutrient recommendations (**Table 72-2**) (Nutrition Expert Panel Report, 1996). Although adherence to these recommendations and ingredient quality may vary among manufacturers, an extruded or pelleted diet supplies all the nutrients in one particle. Such formulations help prevent alteration of nutrient balance by uninformed owners who feed imbalanced seeds or human foods, or by birds that consume different quantities of imbalanced foods that are fed separately.

A potential disadvantage to feeding commercial foods is that testing protocols for nutritional adequacy have not yet been established for avian foods, as they have been for commercial canine and feline foods. Still, the probability of producing a nutritional imbalance by feeding a commercial avian food is much less than when seeds or human foods prepared by uninformed owners are fed to birds. As the use of commercial avian foods becomes more widespread, such protocols will undoubtedly be established.

Seeds and Seed Mixtures

Seeds are a popular, convenient, inexpensive method of providing nutrients to companion birds. But they are not necessarily the best or even the most natural food for pet birds. A recent renaissance in the pet bird food industry has taken into account the long forgotten holistic views of habitats and natural history of many avian species. Interesting facts have come to light. Food selection in birds is predominantly a learned behavior. Nestling birds accept the appropriate foods brought to them by their parents and once fledged observe where and how to obtain these foods for themselves. In a pet industry where captive breeding and isolation of companion birds are the norm, individual birds have little or no experience with their natural environment or natural food sources and may not have the opportunity to observe feeding behaviors of other birds. Although hundreds of years of domestication in some species have altered feeding behaviors, the associated physiology of nutrient assimilation and use have not changed markedly. The types of seeds present in most commercial mixes are not native to areas where most pet bird species originate. Although seeds may have been used opportunistically in the wild, they would not have been available in large quantities. Considering all these facts, seeds are no more of a "natural" food than any other method of providing nutrients for companion birds.

Other disadvantages of all seed diets are that uninformed owners can alter the diet easily or birds can consume certain seed types, avoiding others, resulting in an imbalanced nutrient intake. With these disadvantages in mind, seeds are much less desirable than commercially prepared foods for feeding birds.

As mentioned, seeds are a common element in many pet bird diets. A well-balanced seed mixture can supply essential nutrients such as fats, carbohydrates and some minerals. However, seeds are rarely, if ever, an appropriate sole nutritional source because they provide inadequate levels of protein, vitamins and minerals. There are numerous commercially available seed mixtures that vary greatly in type and quality. Individual seed types are also sold in most stores, thus formulating seed mixtures is a common practice. The availability of individual seed types promotes nutrient imbalance when uninformed owners create a mixture based primarily on the price and physical appearance of the seeds. Thus, creation or use of homemade seed mixtures should be discouraged.

Commercial mixtures for a particular group of birds may vary greatly in seed types and proportions from one company to another, indicating the lack of scientific sophistication involved in preparing seed mixture diets. Seed mixtures may contain protein and vitamin-mineral supplements in pellet or crumble form. This is the manufacturer's attempt to overcome the nutrient imbalances inherent in a seeds-only diet. The assumption is that birds will consume all of the seeds and supplement pellets, and thus have a nutritionally balanced diet. Unfortunately, this assumption is not always true. If seed mixtures containing supplements are used to feed confined birds, the owner should be advised to leave the food in front of the bird until the entire mixture has been eaten before giving the bird more of the mixture. This practice will ensure that the bird consumes the entire diet, not a nutritionally imbalanced, isolated segment. Because individual birds may not accept some components of a supplemented seed mixture, consuming them irregularly or not at all, an imbalanced nutrient intake is much more likely to occur when a supplemented seed mixture is the sole dietary form fed.

Bird owners feed a variety of live foods as supplements to seeds and seed mixtures. When research showed that even strict seed-eaters opportunistically eat insects as a protein source at certain periods in their reproductive cycle and to improve their condition for migration, insect foods became commercially available. Insect supplements are particularly appropriate for Pekin robins, Indian white eyes, shamas, waxbills and cardinals. Live food must be supplied for other species, most notably chaffinch, avadavats and all Phloceids.

White worms (*Enchytraes* larvae) are available commercially and can be kept for long periods much like earthworms in a cool, damp moss and leaf litter substrate. These worms are especially useful to provide when parent birds are brooding and feeding their young. Ant pupae, which bird fanciers have relied on heavily for their avian diets, are now available commercially in large outlets and by mail order. Water shrimp (*Daphnia* spp.) are relished by some species and greatly enhance red pigments in plumage. Aphids that feed on members of the rose family

Table 72-5. Special nutritional needs of waxbills and allies (order Passeriformes, family Estrildidae).*

Genus and species	Common name	Special nutritional needs**
Amandava amandava	Strawberry finch or red avadavat	Some live food is essential year round
Amandava formosa	Green avadavat	Some live food is essential year round
Amandava subflava	Golden-breasted or zebra waxbill	Some live food is essential year round
Chloebia gouldiae	Gouldian finch	During molting, these birds must be supplied with protein-rich foods, vitamins and minerals, soaked and recently sprouted seeds. Avoid white millet in this species
Estrilda astrild	Common or St. Helene waxbill	Insects and soaked seeds are essential
Estrilda caerulescens	Red-tailed lavender, lavender waxbill	Ant eggs, fine cut mealworms, white worms, greens (lettuce, endive, chicory, chickweed)
Estrilda melpoda	Orange-cheeked waxbill	Require small insects for maintenance and breeding
Estrilda rhodopyga	Crimson or rosy-rumped waxbill	Require insects all year, especially during breeding season
Granatina (U.) granatina	Violet-eared waxbill	In addition to small seeds (grass seeds, spray millet) live food is essential all year for behavioral enrichment
Lagonosticta senegala	Red-bellied firefinch	When chicks are hatched, extra amounts of live food, greens and egg foods are essential for feeding chicks
Longchura caniceps	Gray-headed munia or pearl-headed silverbill	Same as *L. ferruginosa*
Longchura castaneothorax	Chestnut-breasted finch or munia	Same as *L. ferruginosa*
Longchura ferruginosa	Black-headed chestnut or chestnut bellied munia or black-headed nun	Insects, weed seeds, basic passerine seed mix, greens, canary-chick rearing food and bread soaked in milk during breeding season
Longchura malabarica	Indian silverbill or white-throated munia	Same as *L. ferruginosa*
Longchura malacca	Black-headed munia or pearl-headed silverbill	Same as *L. ferruginosa*
Longchura punctulata	Scaly-breasted munia, spice bird or spice finch	Same as *L. ferruginosa*
Longchura striata var. domestica	Bengalese	Same as *L. ferruginosa*
Neochimia modesta	Cherry or plum-headed finch	Ripe and half-ripe seeds, berries, greens, and a variety of live foods are necessary
Neochimia ruficauda	Star finch	During the breeding season, provide a rich variety of insects, seeds, greens and commercial egg and rearing foods
Padda oryzivora	Java sparrow or rice bird	Basic passerine seed mix and greens for breeding
Poephilia acuticauda	Long-tailed finch	Same as *N. modesta*
Poephilia cincta	Black-throated or parson finch	In addition to small ripe and half-ripe seeds, insects, greens, soaked white bread, soaked and germinated seeds and cuttlefish bone are essential
Poephilia personata	Masked finch	Same as *P. cincta*
Pytillia melba	Melba finch or crimson-faced waxbill, green winged pytilia	Need a rich variety of insects and small seeds to prevent hatchling rejection
Taeniopygiaa guttata	Zebra finch	Same as *N. modesta*
Taeniopytia bichenovii	Bicheno's or double-barred finch	Same as *N. modesta*
Uraeginthus angolensis	Blue breasted cordon bleu, Angolan cordon bleu or blue-breasted waxbill	Same as *U. bengalus*
Uraeginthus bengalus	Red-cheeked cordon bleu	Live food important, especially for breeding (aphids, ant eggs, and spiders)

*Adapted from Burgmann PM. Feeding Your Pet Bird. New York, NY: Barron's Educational Series, 1993. Lint KC, Lint AM. Feeding Cage Birds-A Manual of Diets for Aviculture. New York, NY: Blanford Press, 1988; 133-175. Vriends MM. Simon and Schuster's Guide to Pet Birds. New York, NY: Simon and Schuster, 1984; 130-180. Woolham F. Diets. In: The Handbook of Aviculture. New York, NY: Blanford Press, 1987; 15-23.
**In addition to commercial foods, these dietary "supplements" or additions are thought to be necessary to stimulate courtship and reproductive behavior or to prevent self-mutilation or feather picking by providing environmental/behavioral enrichment.

concentrate the same pigments and may be more appropriate for small passerine birds. Moth larvae, commonly known as waxworms, and beetle larvae, called mealworms, supply extra protein and fat, especially at the onset of breeding season. Care should be taken to restrict the intake of these insects or the bird will rapidly gain weight and become obese.

Most true insect-eating birds remove the heads of larvae before the larvae are ingested. Clients should be instructed to remove the head capsules before feeding such larvae, if it is observed that the bird does not perform this function. This practice removes a largely indigestible chitinous mass from the gastrointestinal tract and eliminates the possibility that a live larva could burrow through the crop wall or cause gastrointestinal obstruction.

Homemade Mixed-Food Diets

A wide variety of homemade mixed-food diets have been suggested as alternatives for birds that will not accept commercially prepared foods or seed mixtures even with added fruits and vegetables (Kollias, 1995; Burgmann, 1993; Lint and Lint, 1988; Vriends, 1984; Woolham, 1987). These diets can result in excellent feathering and appropriate body mass for the species, with no discernible signs of nutritional deficiency, if prepared carefully from scientifically developed recipes. These diets often contain varying amounts of ingredients such as seeds, nuts, cooked eggs, low fat yogurt or cheese, vegetables, fruits, grains, bread, pasta, multigrain cereals, legumes, seed mixes, pelleted or extruded psittacine diets, vitamin supplements and calcium supplements. When converting birds to a new homemade diet, have the client offer a mixture containing all the ingredients at one time. This practice usually prevents preferential selection of certain ingredients. Although larger parrots have difficulty eating small seeds such as milo or oat groats, a seed mixture containing 30% hulled safflower, 30% milo, 30% oat groats and 10% peanuts works well for smaller birds.

Although homemade mixed-food diets may provide adequate nourishment, most companion bird owners are unwilling to devote the time necessary to adequately prepare these diets. Additionally, owners must be willing to regularly observe which food components are being consumed to prevent birds from developing or reverting to preferential selection of specific ingredients.

Water

Although feeding a well-balanced food is essential, it is easy to overlook the single most important dietary component: water. As with all animals, water is absolutely essential for birds. Water acts as a food carrier and aids in digestion. Some foods are high in water content whereas others require the addition of free water for efficient digestion and absorption. Some avian species are more physiologically adept at extracting water from their foods. Budgerigars in the wild, for example, are capable of absorbing sufficient water from seeds and green foods to allow them to go without additional sources of water for many days. This observation, however, is not an experiment to be undertaken by pet owners. Birds should never go for more than a few hours without access to fresh clean water. Studies have shown that canaries will die within 48 hours if water is withheld.

Water comprises more than 50% of a bird's body weight (in young birds, the percentage may be even higher). Blood and lymph are largely composed of water. Furthermore, because birds have no sweat glands, water intake plays an important role in thermoregulation. Breeding females may require increased amounts of water for egg production and for heat regulation while incubating eggs.

Water should be provided in containers that are easily accessible but not located in a place that can collect feces, feathers, food particles, etc. For this reason, water bowls should be attached to the wall of enclosures, near or above food bowls. They should not be so large as to invite bathing.

Food Selection

The advantages and disadvantages of feeding birds commercially prepared foods, seeds and seed mixtures and homemade mixed foods are discussed above. If an individual bird is healthy and exhibits no signs of deficiency disease, the owner probably is feeding the bird appropriately and there is no need to change the food. In general, however, fewer deficiency diseases will result from feeding a complete, nutritionally balanced food that meets the nutrient levels listed in **Table 72-2.**

Although some prepared foods have been available for only a limited time, the overall nutritional quality of commercial foods is rapidly improving as manufacturers use new scientific information to create their formulations. As commercially prepared foods become more widely used, many of the diet-induced diseases currently observed by avian veterinarians will become of historical interest only, just as they have for other companion pets.

Owners should be encouraged to experiment with different prepared foods if their bird does not accept a particular product. Often a bird will readily accept an alternative form, shape or formulation of a complete food. When changing the diet of a bird from seeds or fresh human foods to a commercially prepared complete food, the previous foods should be eliminated or substantially restricted to encourage consumption of the complete avian food.

Tables 72-3 through **72-7** list foods that meet the special nutritional or behavioral needs of passerine birds. In addition to commercial foods, these dietary "supplements" or additions are thought to be necessary to stimulate courtship and reproductive behavior or to prevent self-mutilation or feather picking by providing environmental/behavioral enrichment. **Table 72-8** lists homemade mixed-food diets for psittacine birds.

Assess and Determine the Feeding Method

It may not always be necessary to change the feeding method when managing an avian patient, but a thorough assessment includes verification that an appropriate feeding method is being used. Items to consider include feeding route, amount fed, how the food is offered and who feeds the bird. All of this information should have been gathered when the history of the bird was obtained. If the bird has normal body condition, the amount of food it was fed previously (energy basis) was probably appropriate.

Because of the convenience, most owners offer food free choice with additional food added to the bowl as needed. When a seed mixture or homemade diet is offered free choice, it is unknown how much and what components the bird actually consumes. Therefore, the owner may not realize that the bird has not eaten for 24 to 48 hours.

Owners who feed prepackaged seeds, seed mixtures or treats for birds often assume that the product is nutritionally complete and the bird will eat all parts of the product. Both of these

Table 72-6. Special nutritional needs of weavers, wydahs and queleas (order Passiformes, family Ploceidae).*

Genus and species	Common name	Special nutritional needs**
Euplectus afra	Napoleon weaver, yellow-crowned or golden bishop	Live food is essential, as are small seeds, fruits and greens (See *Ploceus* spp.)
Euplectus ardens	Red-collared willow bird or wydah	Same as *P. cucullatus, E. afra*
Euplectus hordeacea	Blackwinged bishop, crimson crowned bishop	Same as *P. cucullatus, E. afra*
Euplectus orix	Grenadier weaver or red bishop	Same as *P. cucullatus, E. afra*
Euplectus progne	Long-tailed willow bird, giant wydah	Same as *P. cucullatus, E. afra*
Ploceus cucullatus	Rufous-necked, black-headed, village weaver or vitelline masked weaver	Live food is essential, in addition to millet, white grass, weed seeds and grains (oats and wheat) for breeding
Ploceus intermedius	Masked weaver	Same as *P. cucullatus*
Ploceus phillippinus	Baya weaver	Same as *P. cucullatus*
Ploceus vitellinus	Half-masked weaver, Zesser-masked weaver	Same as *P. cucullatus*

*Adapted from Burgmann PM. Feeding Your Pet Bird. New York, NY: Barron's Educational Series, 1993. Lint KC, Lint AM. Feeding Cage Birds-A Manual of Diets for Aviculture. New York, NY: Blanford Press, 1988; 133-175. Vriends MM. Simon and Schuster's Guide to Pet Birds. New York, NY: Simon and Schuster, 1984; 182-190. Woolham F. Diets. In: The Handbook of Aviculture. New York, NY: Blanford Press, 1987; 15-23.
**In addition to commercial foods, these dietary "supplements" or additions are thought to be necessary to stimulate courtship and reproductive behavior or to prevent self-mutilation or feather picking by providing environmental/behavioral enrichment.

Table 72-7. Special nutritional needs of babblers and starlings (order Passeriforme, family Timaliidae, family Sturnidae).*

Genus and species	Common name	Special nutritional needs**
Gracula religiosa	Hill mynah	Must be offered a commercial or formulated low-iron food to prevent hemochromatosis; during breeding requires insects and fruit low in or devoid of iron
Leitothrix lutea	Red-billed leiothrix or Pekin robin	Dead, dried or live food are essential for breeding

*Adapted from Kollias GV. Diets, feeding practices, and nutritional problems in psittacine birds. Veterinary Medicine 1995; 90: 29-39. Burgmann PM. Feeding Your Pet Bird. New York, NY: Barron's Educational Series, 1993. Lint KC, Lint AM. Feeding Cage Birds-A Manual of Diets for Aviculture. New York, NY: Blanford Press, 1988; 133-175.
**In addition to commercial foods, these dietary "supplements" or additions are thought to be necessary to stimulate courtship and reproductive behavior or to prevent self-mutilation or feather picking by providing environmental/behavioral enrichment.

assumptions are often incorrect. To correct or avoid these problems, bird owners should offer a nutritionally complete prepared food at regular intervals as a part of the total diet.

Feeding Intervals

An ideal strategy is to ensure that food is offered to companion birds for one to two hours, two or three times daily. The food should be removed during the interim periods, although this is not standard practice for most owners or care providers. Offering food at specific times during the day creates a bond between the owner and bird. This feeding regimen also increases the probability that an owner will examine the contents of the food and water bowls to determine exactly what and how much was consumed and whether the bowls require cleaning.

Changing Foods

Unless commercially prepared nutritionally complete foods are fed, birds fed free choice may develop a habituation to a single type of food (monophagism). This fixation may result in single or multiple nutrient deficiencies. After a deficiency occurs, the owner is faced with changing the food. This can be a formidable challenge depending on the age and species of the bird. Changing foods is generally easier with younger birds and with smaller parrots such as cockatiels and conures. Cockatoos, macaws and African grey parrots are more resistant to change. Most passerine birds switch to new foods easily.

Food changes should not be attempted if the bird is sick or stressed (e.g., recent acquisition, change in environment, exposure to temperature extremes, molting etc.). Conversion to a new balanced food may take weeks to months depending on the degree and length of habituation. Ninety percent of healthy cockatiels can be converted to a new food within seven days.

A variety of strategies can be used to convert birds to a new food. If one of these approaches is unsuccessful, an alternate one should be tried.

1. Gradually add the new food to the current diet, increasing the amount of the new food over days to weeks. Texture and color are important; adding a food that the bird really likes may make the conversion much easier.
2. Unless the new food is extruded or pelleted, warming or cooling it may make a difference in acceptance. The food should be no hotter than 40.6°C (105°F). Alternatively, food can be cooled to refrigerator temperatures (2 to 4°C [35 to 40°F]).
3. Try offering the bird a soft food such as baby cereal, fruits or vegetables, cooked oatmeal or cream of wheat. Birds like the texture of these foods. Then gradually add a prepared diet to these mixtures.
4. If a bird is hand-trained or hand-reared, feeding outside the cage is often helpful. Alternatively, place the new food item

Table 72-8. Homemade mixed-food diets for psittacine birds.*

Diet 1	20-30% seeds and nuts 20-30% dark green, yellow and orange vegetables 10-15% fruit (avoid excess apples and bananas, which have little nutritional value and may contain excessive phosphorus) 20-30% pelleted or extruded psittacine food, which is added to the mixture after thawing and immediately before feeding Much of this diet can be made in advance and frozen in small portions
Diet 2	30% small- or large-parrot seed mix 20% cooked brown rice, dark multigrain bread, pasta and multigrain cereals 15% frozen or fresh vegetables, such as peas, carrots and squash 15% legumes, such as cooked kidney and pinto beans 20% pelleted or extruded psittacine food, which is added to the mixture after thawing and immediately before feeding Much of this diet can be made in advance and frozen in small portions
Diet 3	45% grains, breads and cereal group (whole wheat bread, cooked brown rice, seed mixture) 45% fresh vegetables (broccoli, endive, carrots, pumpkin, winter squash, collard greens, sweet potato) and fruits (limit quantities of papaya, cantaloupe and apricots to 5% of total fruit) 5% from the protein and fat group, including hard-cooked or scrambled eggs and peanuts or other mature legumes (e.g., navy or kidney beans) 5% dairy group (for calcium and protein) Use low-fat non-lactose dairy products, such as low-fat yogurt, cottage cheese and hard cheese; other sources of calcium (although not as good as food sources) may include cuttlebone, oyster shell and mineral blocks; larger psittacine birds may ignore these items or destroy rather than consume them
Diet 4	24% cooked long grain rice 25% cooked kidney beans 24% frozen whole kernel corn 24% pelleted or extruded psittacine diet (total soft diet = 96.63%) Approximately 2% powdered vitamin supplement 1-4% calcium supplement (total supplements = 3.37%) This diet is formulated based on wet weight. Small portions can be frozen (excluding the pelleted or extruded diet) and used as needed. Pay particular attention to food hygiene because these foods decompose fairly rapidly.

*Some species of psittacine birds, such as lorries, have specific dietary requirements for fruit or nectar that differ from that of more common species of New World parrots. When fruit or nectar is used, percentages in the diet should be based on relative proportions by volume, not on a dry or wet weight basis. Avoid including avocado because it is toxic to small psittacine birds. (Adapted from Ullrey DE, Allen MR, Baer DJ. Formulated diets versus seed mixtures for Psittacines. Journal of Nutrition 1991; 121: S193-S205. Kollias GV. Diets, feeding practices, and nutritional problems in psittacine birds. Veterinary Medicine 1995; 90: 29-39.)

in the cage at strategic locations (e.g., by a mirror or favorite toy or attach the food item to the cage bars).

5. Have the owner eat what you want the bird to eat. Some birds mimic their owners by eating foods they see their owners eat.
6. Begin feeding a new food every other day. For larger birds, remove the seeds on that day. If a smaller bird has not eaten the new food by the late afternoon, offer seeds to prevent hypoglycemia overnight. Alternate-day feedings will also prevent excessive weight loss. Increase feedings to four, then five, then seven days a week.
7. Remove all seeds before retiring for the night. In the morning, offer a commercially prepared complete food with new food items instead of the seed. Do not add seed until noon. This strategy presents no danger to the bird because the previous seeds are available later in the day.

The bird's physical condition and body weight should be monitored during the conversion period to prevent starvation. Keep in mind that most birds eating all seeds or "junk food" (e.g., potato chips, peanuts, candy) may be overweight or even obese. If a bird loses excessive body condition during the conversion period, as determined by weighing, it may refuse to eat the previously fed food. Gavage or tube feeding for one to three days will be required to stimulate the bird to eat.

All of these strategies have been successful in enticing companion psittacine birds to eat a more balanced food. Occasionally, however, individual birds cannot be converted. These birds may require specialized water and food supplements to help overcome serious vitamin and mineral deficiencies. In some cases when conversion is unsuccessful, the bird may need to be hospitalized away from the owner. At the hospital, a rigorous dietary protocol can be implemented that may be successful after the behavioral influences of the owner are eliminated.

In multiple-bird households, owners will have an easier time converting birds to a new food if at least one bird has been converted and the other birds can observe it eating the new food. Some companies may provide an "instructor" bird to assist in food conversion if all other methods are unsuccessful.

Client education is crucial to the success of food conversion, especially with companion birds. Owners should be advised to be persistent and patient during this process.

REFERENCES

The references for **Chapter 72** can be found at www.markmorris.org.

CASE 72-1

Feather Loss in a Captive Sulfur Crested Cockatoo

Cheryl L. Dikeman, PhD
Department of Nutrition
Henry Doorly Zoo
Omaha, Nebraska, USA

Patient Assessment

An eight-year-old, male sulfur crested cockatoo was examined for feather loss. The case was brought to the nutrition department after thorough veterinary examination revealed nothing unusual upon fecal testing, radiography and results of biochemistry and hematologic panels. Initial examination by the nutritionist revealed the bird was bright, alert, responsive and vocalizing. The keepers noticed the feather plucking behavior for approximately three weeks. Nothing had changed in the bird's enclosure for the past five weeks. Before that, the bird was moved from a public viewing aviary exhibit to an off exhibit holding area while repairs to the area were being completed. The bird was used in educational programs, and its training and use in educational programs had continued without interruption. Based on the previous examination by the veterinarians and initial screening for the presence of infection and parasites, no additional abnormalities were noted other than the excessive feather picking.

Assess the Food and Feeding Method

The bird's diet consisted of approximately 60% extruded commercial parrot maintenance diet, 20% parrot seed mixture and 20% mixed fruit and (or) vegetables daily (**Table 1**). Water was offered free choice.

Table 1. Guaranteed analysis of the bird's total diet.*

Crude protein (min.)	17.0%
Crude fat (min.)	9.2%
Crude fiber (max.)	10.0%
Zinc	91.0 mg/kg

*(100% dry matter basis)

Questions

1. What nutrients may be problematic and contribute to the etiology of feather plucking?
2. What additional laboratory testing may be beneficial in this case?
3. What additional questions may be useful to ask the keepers about this bird's behavior over the past several weeks?
4. What are the short-term goals to assist in the management of this bird?
5. What are the long-term goals to assist in the management of this bird?

Answers and Discussion

1. Although generalized malnutrition can be a medical cause associated with chronic feather plucking in psittacine birds, malnutrition is rare. Regardless, the diet should be carefully examined and analyzed for key nutrients. One key nutrient for psittacine birds is zinc. Zinc toxicity may be a contributing dietary cause of feather plucking and, therefore, should not be discounted.
2. Although radiographs did not reveal abnormalities or potential ingestion of zinc containing items (pennies, toys, etc.) serum/plasma concentrations of zinc should be determined to rule out potential zinc toxicities. In addition, hormonal abnormalities should be considered.
3. Additional questions should primarily focus on the bird's behavior and environment since its move off exhibit.
   a. What was the social interaction when it was in the aviary; was the bird housed singly or with other birds?
   b. Did it have more human interaction while in the exhibit?
   c. Has the social structure within the area changed (keeper turnover, change in keeper schedules, etc.). Due to the bonding birds have with particular "flock" members, alterations in schedules may disrupt the hierarchy of the "flock" structure and stability.
4. Likely this bird is responding to the environmental changes over the past several weeks. Short-term goals included altering the stimuli in the temporary off exhibit holding area daily. In addition, the seed mixture of the diet was increased to 50%. The complete diet accounted for 30%, and a variety of fruit and vegetables 20% of the diet. The additional seeds were included to supply a source of additional environmental stimuli. The keepers worked to develop a schedule that included only two individuals feeding, and caring for the bird until it was moved back.
5. The long-term goal was to evaluate the bird weekly while off display, then reevaluate it weekly once back on display. The bird's diet would be changed back to the original diet if excessive plucking stopped.

Progress Notes

When the bird was re-checked after one week, it was still plucking; however, the keepers believed the bird's condition had improved. The bird's routine was more consistent. During the following week, the bird was returned to the exhibit aviary that included several other birds and mixed species. By the third week, the keepers did not see any of the excessive plucking behavior observed in the off exhibit area. The bird's diet was changed back to the original formulation.

Bibliography

Chitty J. Feather plucking in psittacine birds 1. Presentation and medical investigation. In Practice 2003; September: 484-493.
Earle RA, Prowse L. Understanding feather plucking in parrots–a behavioral ecological perspective. The Veterinary Times 2000.
Puschner B, St. Leger J, Galey FD. Normal and toxic zinc concentrations in serum/plasma and liver of psittacines with respect to genus differences. Journal of Veterinary Diagnostic Investigation 1999; 11: 522-527.
Romagnano A. Parrot preventative medicine. Proceedings of the International Aviculturists Society 2003.

CASE 72-2

Obesity in Caged Cockatiel

Cheryl L. Dikeman, PhD
Department of Nutrition
Henry Doorly Zoo
Omaha, Nebraska, USA

Patient Assessment

A nine-year-old male cockatiel was examined upon arrival to a foster home from an owner relinquishment. The bird was re-homed after a single home for eight years. The relinquishing owners had reported the cockatiel had been purchased from a local breeder in the area, when the bird was approximately 16 weeks of age. The bird had been housed in the same cage while the owners had the bird. The cage was located in a small bedroom that served as an in-home office that had access to one window for UV light. The owners indicated they interacted with the bird at least once daily. No recent changes had been made to the bird's diet or daily husbandry. Physical examination revealed a healthy and alert bird. Its initial weight was 128 grams. Based on current weight and physical keel palpation, the bird was considered overweight. No additional abnormalities were noted.

Assess the Food and Feeding Method

The owners indicated the bird was fed commercial seed mixtures formulated for cockatiels and purchased from local pet supply stores and (or) grocery stores. The bird reportedly did not readily accept or consume offered fruits, vegetables or complete formulated pelleted diets; therefore, they had not been offered consistently within the previous four years. The most recent fortified commercial seed mixture's ingredient list and guaranteed analysis is included below (**Table 1**). Fresh water and the seed mixtures were changed/offered daily free choice. The bird was not offered additional supplements.

Table 1. Current seed mixture ingredient list.

Canary Grass Seed, White Millet, Striped Sunflower, Safflower, Oat Groats, Red Millet, Wheat, Toasted Corn Flakes, Buckwheat, Corn Gluten Meal, Ground Corn, Ground Wheat, Dehulled Soybean Meal, Flax Seed, Calcium Carbonate, Wheat Middlings, Dicalcium Phosphate, Salt, Soy Oil, Sun-cured Alfalfa Meal, Brewers Dried Yeast, Wheat Germ Meal, Vitamin A Supplement, Choline Chloride, L-Lysine, Ferrous Sulfate, Vitamin B12 Supplement, Manganous Oxide, Vitamin E Supplement, Zinc Oxide, DL-Methionine, Orange Oil, Niacin, Riboflavin Supplement, Menadione Sodium Bisulfite Complex (source of vitamin K activity), Ethoxyquin (a preservative), Cholecalciferol (source of vitamin D3), Copper Sulfate, Calcium Pantothenate, Pyridoxine Hydrochloride, Thiamine Mononitrate, Folic Acid, Calcium Iodate, Biotin, Dried *Bacillus coagulans* Fermentation Product, Dried *Bacillus licheniformis* Fermentation Product, Dried *Bacillus subtilis* Fermentation Product, Cobalt Carbonate, Sodium Selenite, Beta-Carotene, Artificial Color.

Guaranteed analysis (100% dry matter basis)	
Crude protein (min.)	17%
Crude fat (min.)	10.2%
Crude fiber (max.)	15.9%

Questions

1. What would be the benefit to including the ingredient list and guaranteed analysis in the assessment of the commercially formulated seed mixture?
2. What should be considered specifically regarding seed mixes when addressing the guaranteed analysis on the label?
3. What are the short-term goals to assist in the management of this bird?
4. What are the long-term goals to assist in the management of this bird?

Answers and Discussion

1. Commercial seed mixes vary in the quality, quantity and types of ingredients used. In this case, it was valuable to determine the variety of seeds included and which types of seeds the bird was potentially selecting more than others. Typically, granivores, such as cockatiels, select more palatable seeds that typically contain higher concentrations of fat, such as sunflower seeds. Assessing the guaranteed analysis on a dry matter basis, gave the practitioner an idea of overall macronutrient profiles. In this case, the seed mix contained a moderately high fat content of 10.2%, which would be contributing to the bird's weight status.
2. Guaranteed analyses are conducted on the whole diet. In the case of seed mixtures, seeds are analyzed in their entirety. Granivorous birds dehull the seeds before consumption, thereby altering the nutrient profile. In some cases, dehulled seeds may contain twice the analyzed fat content as their hulled counterparts. This should be considered when seed mixes are fed.
3. Short-term goals included not only altering the diet for this bird, but also increasing its level of activity. Birds housed in indoor aviary enclosures, have approximately 15% higher energy requirements, compared with those in indoor cage environments. Therefore, this bird was housed in an indoor aviary that offered three times more room than its original cage. Its food and water dishes were placed on opposite sides of the enclosure to encourage movement. In addition, a lower fat seed mixture was selected along with a commercial extruded diet.
4. The nutritional goal was to transition the bird to an extruded diet. The nutrition plan also included monitoring and recording body weight weekly initially for eight weeks and reassess at that time. The bird's estimated ideal body weight was 110 grams.

Progress Notes

When the bird was weighed seven days later, it had lost 2 grams (1.6% body weight). At this time, it was consuming the new lower fat seed mixture readily. The extruded diet was added at a rate of 10% extruded to 90% seed mixture. At Week 2, the bird weighed 122 grams. The diet was then altered to 20% extruded diet to 80% seed mix. At Week 3, it weighed 121 grams and the diet was changed to 25% extruded to 75% seed mix. By Week 8, the bird weighed 115 grams and was consuming a diet of 50% extruded diet and 50% seed mixture free choice. Due to the 8% body weight loss over eight weeks, this plan was continued and monitored closely. From Week 12 to 16 the bird had maintained an ideal body weight range of 108 to 112 grams. At this time, the bird was consuming a diet of 50% extruded diet and 50% seed mixture. The decision was made to maintain the bird on this diet.

Bibliography

Koutsos EA, Matson KD, Klasing KC. Nutrition of birds in the order psittaciformes: A review. Journal of Avian Medicine and Surgery 2001; 15: 257-275.

Werquin GL, De Cock KS, Ghysels PC. Comparison of the nutrient analysis and caloric density of 30 commercial seed mixtures (in toto and dehulled) with 27 commercial diets for parrots. Journal of Animal Physiology and Animal Nutrition 2005; 89: 215-221.

Section 23

Appendices and Index

Appendices and Index

Appendix 1. Conversions to and from metric measures.

Imperial/U.S. to metric		Metric to imperial/U.S.	
Weights		**Weights**	
1 gr (grain)	64.8 mg	1 g	15.43 gr
1 oz (avoirdupois)	28.4 g	1 g	0.0353 oz
1 lb (avoirdupois)	453.6 g	1 g	0.0022 lb
1 lb	0.454 kg	1 kg	2.2 lb
1 ton (short)	907.2 kg	1 kg	0.0011 (short ton)
1 ton	0.907 ton	1 ton	1.1 ton
Dosages			
1 mg/lb	2.2 mg/kg	1 mg/kg	0.454 mg/lb
1 kcal/lb	2.2 kcal/kg	1 kcal/kg	0.454 kcal/lb
Volumes			
U.S.			
1 fl oz	29.57 ml	1 L	33.82 fl oz
1 cup	0.237 L	1 L	4.221 cup
1 pt	0.473 L	1 L	2.114 pt
1 qt	0.946 L	1 L	1.057 qt
1 gal	3.785 L	1 L	0.264 gal
Imperial			
1 fl oz	28.41 ml	1 L	35.20 fl oz
1 cup	0.284 L	1 L	3.520 cup
1 pt	0.568 L	1 L	1.760 pt
1 qt	1.136 L	1 L	0.88 qt
1 gal	4.546 L	1 L	0.22 gal

Appendix 2. Comparison between U.S. and imperial systems.

Imperial		U.S.	
1 fl oz	28.42 ml	1 fl oz	29.57 ml
1 cup	10 fl oz	1 cup	8 fl oz
1 pt	20 fl oz	1 pt	16 fl oz
1 qt	40 fl oz	1 qt	32 fl oz
1 gal*	160 fl oz	1 gal**	128 fl oz
1 gal*	4 qt	1 gal**	4 qt
1 gal*	4.55 L	1 gal**	3.78 L

*1 gal (imperial) = 4 qt = 8 pt = 160 oz = 4.55 L.
**1 gal (U.S.) = 4 qt = 8 pt = 16 cups = 128 oz = 3.78 L.

Appendix 3. Temperature conversions.*

°C	°F	°C	°F	°C	°F	°C	°F	°C	°F
0	32.0	10	50.0	20	68.0	30	86.0	40	104.0
1	33.8	11	51.8	21	69.8	31	87.8	41	105.8
2	35.6	12	53.6	22	71.6	32	89.6	42	107.6
3	37.4	13	55.4	23	73.4	33	91.4	43	109.4
4	39.2	14	57.2	24	75.2	34	93.2	44	111.2
5	41.0	15	59.0	25	77.0	35	95.0	45	113.0
6	42.8	16	60.8	26	78.8	36	96.8	46	114.8
7	44.6	17	62.6	27	80.6	37	98.6	47	116.6
8	46.4	18	64.4	28	82.4	38	100.4	48	118.4
9	48.2	19	66.2	29	84.2	39	102.2	49	120.2
								50	122.0

*When you know the Fahrenheit temperature, subtract 32 and multiply by 5/9 to obtain °C. When you know the Celsius temperature, multiply by 9/5 then add 32 to obtain °F.

Appendix 4. Equivalent values and conversion factors.

Volumes			
1 gtt*	0.05 ml	1 cup**	16 Tbs
1 tsp	5 ml	1 ml	20 gtt
1 dsp	8 ml	1 cup**	236.6 ml
1 Tbs	15 ml	1 cup***	284.2 ml
Weights			
1 oz	437.5 gr	1 g	1,000 mg
1 lb	16 oz	1 kg	1,000 g
1 ton (short)	2,000 lb	1 ton (metric)	1,000 kg

Key: tsp = teaspoon, dsp = dessertspoon, Tbs = tablespoon, gr = grains.
*Official dropper size for water at 15°C.
**U.S. cup.
***Imperial cup.

Appendix 5. Percent, ppm and ppb.

Percent	ppm	ppb
µg/0.1 mg	1 µg/g	1 ng/g
mg/0.1 g	1 mg/kg	1 µg/kg
g/100 g	0.4545 mg/lb	0.4545 µg/lb
kg/100 kg	1 g/ton (1,000 kg)	1 mg/ton (1,000 kg)
g/0.22 lb	1 kg/1,000 ton	

Appendix 6. Energy conversion units.

Kilocalorie (kcal)	1,000 cal	4.184 kJ
Kilojoule (kJ)	1,000 joule	0.239 kcal
Megajoule (MJ)	1,000 kJ	239.0 kcal

Conversion from:	To:	
mg/MJ	mg/100 kcal	÷ 2.39
mg/100 kcal	mg/MJ	x 2.39
g/MJ	mg/100 kcal	÷ 0.00239
mg/100 kcal	g/MJ	x 0.00239
mg/100 kcal	g/100 kcal	÷ 1,000
g/100 kcal	mg/100 kcal	x 1,000
mg/MJ	g/MJ	÷ 1,000
g/MJ	mg/MJ	x 1,000

Appendix 7. Vitamins A, D and E: Conversions from international units to equivalent activity.*

Vitamins	Units	Substances	
Vitamin A	1 IU	0.300 µg of crystalline retinol (vitamin A alcohol)	0.550 µg of vitamin A palmitate
Vitamin A	1 RE*	1 µg of crystalline retinol	6 µg of β-carotene 12 µg of other provitamin A carotenoids
Provitamin A	1 IU	0.6 µg β-carotene	1.2 µg of other provitamin A carotenoids
Vitamin D	1 IU	0.025 µg of crystalline vitamin D_3	
Vitamin E	1 IU	1 mg of synthetic racemic α-tocopherol acetate	= dl-α-tocopherol acetate = all racemic α-tocopherol acetate

1 mg of synthetic racemic α-tocopherol = 1 mg of synthetic racemic α-tocopherol = 1.1 IU of vitamin E
1 mg of naturally occurring α-tocopherol = d-α-tocopherol = RRR-tocopherol = 1.49 IU of vitamin E
1 mg of naturally occurring α-tocopherol acetate = d-α-tocopherol acetate = 1.36 IU of vitamin E

*On pet food labels and tables with daily nutrient allowances for pets, the vitamins A, D and E are expressed in international units (IU). These units reflect the activity of these vitamins, not their amounts. United States Pharmacopeia Units (USP) are equivalent to IU. In human foods, retinol equivalent (RE) is often used for vitamin A activity.

Appendix 8. Metabolic weight ($BW^{0.75}$) of dogs and cats.*

Body weights kg	lb	Metabolic weights $BW^{0.75}$	Body weights kg	lb	Metabolic weights $BW^{0.75}$
1	2.2	1.000	41	90.2	16.203
2	4.4	1.682	42	92.4	16.498
3	6.6	2.280	43	94.6	16.792
4	8.8	2.828	44	96.8	17.084
5	11.0	3.344	45	99.0	17.374
6	13.2	3.834	46	101.2	17.663
7	15.4	4.304	47	103.4	17.950
8	17.6	4.757	48	105.6	18.236
9	19.8	5.196	49	107.8	18.520
10	22.0	5.623	50	110.0	18.803
11	24.2	6.040	51	112.2	19.084
12	26.4	6.447	52	114.4	19.364
13	28.6	6.846	53	116.6	19.643
14	30.8	7.238	54	118.8	19.920
15	33.0	7.622	55	121.0	20.196
16	35.2	8.000	56	123.2	20.471
17	37.4	8.372	57	125.4	20.745
18	39.6	8.739	58	127.6	21.017
19	41.8	9.100	59	129.8	21.288
20	44.0	9.457	60	132.0	21.558
21	46.2	9.810	61	134.2	21.827
22	48.4	10.158	62	136.4	22.095
23	50.6	10.503	63	138.6	22.362
24	52.8	10.843	64	140.8	22.627
25	55.0	11.180	65	143.0	22.892
26	57.2	11.514	66	145.2	23.156
27	59.4	11.845	67	147.4	23.418
28	61.6	12.172	68	149.6	23.680
29	63.8	12.497	69	151.8	23.941
30	66.0	12.819	70	154.0	24.200
31	68.2	13.138	71	156.2	24.459
32	70.4	13.454	72	158.4	24.717
33	72.6	13.768	73	160.6	24.974
34	74.8	14.080	74	162.8	25.230
35	77.0	14.390	75	165.0	25.486
36	79.2	14.697	76	167.2	25.740
37	81.4	15.002	77	169.4	25.994
38	83.6	15.305	78	171.6	26.246
39	85.8	15.606	79	173.8	26.498
40	88.0	15.905	80	176.0	26.750

*Metabolic weight ($BW^{0.75}$) can be calculated by cubing BW_{kg} and then taking its square root twice.

Appendix 9. Metabolic rate (RER) for animals of different taxonomic groups.

kcal ME/24 hours			(Sub)classes or orders
129	x	$kg^{0.75}$	Passeriformes
78	x	$kg^{0.75}$	Other birds
70	x	$kg^{0.75}$	Placental mammals
48	x	$kg^{0.75}$	Marsupialia
10	x	$kg^{0.75}$	Reptiles at optimal temperature (37°C)

Key: RER = resting energy requirement, ME = metabolizable energy.

Appendix 10. Body surface area (BSA) of cats.

Body weights kg	lb	BSA m^2
1	2.2	0.10
2	4.4	0.17
3	6.6	0.22
4	8.8	0.26
5	11.0	0.30
6	13.2	0.34
7	15.4	0.38

Appendix 11. Body surface area (BSA) of dogs.

Body weights kg	lb	BSA m²	Body weights kg	lb	BSA m²
1	2.2	0.10	36	79.2	1.10
2	4.4	0.16	37	81.4	1.12
3	6.6	0.21	38	83.6	1.14
4	8.8	0.25	39	85.8	1.16
5	11.0	0.30	40	88.0	1.18
6	13.2	0.33	41	90.2	1.20
7	15.4	0.37	42	92.4	1.22
8	17.6	0.40	43	94.6	1.24
9	19.8	0.44	44	96.8	1.26
10	22.0	0.47	45	99.0	1.28
11	24.2	0.50	46	101.2	1.30
12	26.4	0.53	47	103.4	1.32
13	28.6	0.56	48	105.6	1.33
14	30.8	0.59	49	107.8	1.35
15	33.0	0.61	50	110.0	1.37
16	35.2	0.64	51	112.2	1.39
17	37.4	0.67	52	114.4	1.41
18	39.6	0.69	53	116.6	1.43
19	41.8	0.72	54	118.8	1.44
20	44.0	0.74	55	121.0	1.46
21	46.2	0.77	56	123.2	1.48
22	48.4	0.79	57	125.4	1.50
23	50.6	0.82	58	127.6	1.51
24	52.8	0.84	59	129.8	1.53
25	55.0	0.86	60	132.0	1.55
26	57.2	0.89	61	134.2	1.57
27	59.4	0.91	62	136.4	1.58
28	61.6	0.93	63	138.6	1.60
29	63.8	0.95	64	140.8	1.62
30	66.0	0.98	65	143.0	1.63
31	68.2	1.00	66	145.2	1.65
32	70.4	1.02	67	147.4	1.67
33	72.6	1.04	68	149.6	1.68
34	74.8	1.06	69	151.8	1.70
35	77.0	1.08	70	154.0	1.72

Appendix 12. Equations for calculating resting energy requirements of cats and dogs.

BW kg	$70 \times kg^{0.75}$ kcal ME	$0.293 \times kg^{0.75}$ MJ ME	70 + 30 x kg BW kcal ME	0.29 + 0.126 x kg BW MJ ME
5	234	0.98	220	0.92
10	394	1.65	370	1.55
20	662	2.77	670	2.80
30	897	3.75	970	4.06
40	1,113	4.66	1,270	5.31
60	1,509	6.31	1,870	7.82

Key: BW = body weight, ME = metabolizable energy.

Appendix 13. Litter sizes and birth weights of selected canine breeds.*

Breeds**	Average litter sizes	Birth weights (g)
Airedale terrier	9	300
Appenzell mountain dog	10	465
Australian silky terrier	3	-
Bernese mountain dog	5	445
Borzoi	9	450
Boxer	8	440
Cavalier King Charles spaniel	4	230
Chihuahua	2-3	140
Chow chow	6	460
Dachshund	4	215
Dalmatian	5-6	-
Doberman pinscher	7	410
English bulldog	7	295
English cocker spaniel	6	230
English springer spaniel	11	375
Fox terrier	3	260
French bulldog	5	215

Appendix 13 (continued). Litter sizes and birth weights of selected canine breeds.*

Breeds**	Average litter sizes	Birth weights (g)
German shepherd dog	6	445
German shorthaired pointer	7-8	415
Great Pyrenees	≥5	705
Hovawart	11	435
Irish terrier	6	270
Labrador retriever	5	450
Maltese	3	155
Miniature dachshund	3	210
Miniature pinscher	3	-
Miniature poodle	2-3	165
Miniature schnauzer	4	155
Newfoundland	7	595
Norwich terrier	5	225
Papillon	3	120
Pekingese	2-3	-
Pomeranian	2	-
Pug	3	-
Rottweiler	7	-
Saint Bernard	7	640
Scottish terrier	5	240
Shetland sheepdog	4-5	260
Shih Tzu	2-3	-
Sloughi	3	670
Standard schnauzer	6	285
Yorkshire terrier	5	95

*Because of the very large variation in the adult body weight of dogs and number of puppies per litter, there is no direct relationship between birth weight and the body weight of the mother. Puppies from the largest breeds weigh approximately 1% of the bitch's weight, whereas a Chihuahua puppy averages 6.4% of its mother's body weight.
**Breeds listed here are those for which data were available.

Appendix 14. Body weights in kilograms and height at withers in centimeters of selected canine breeds.

Breeds	Body weights (kg)		Height at withers (cm)	
	Females	Males	Females	Males
Affenpinscher	3	4	23	28
Afghan hound	23	27	60-65	65-72.5
Ainu dog	na	na	41-47.5	49-52.5
Airedale terrier	19	25	55-58	58-60
Akita	34	46	60-65	65-70
Alaskan malamute	34	57	57.5-65	62.5-70
American cocker spaniel	11	12.5	34-36	36-39
American Eskimo dog				
Toy	na	na	22.5	30
Miniature	na	na	>30	37.5
Standard	na	na	>37.5	47.5
American water spaniel	11-18	13.5-20.5	37.5-45	37.5-45
Anatolian shepherd dog	41-59	50-64	70-77.5	72.5-80
Anglo-French hound				
Small	22	25	47.5	55
Great	30	32	60	67.5
Appenzell mountain dog	22	25	46-50	55-58
Ariegeois	30	30	52.5-57.5	55-60
Artois hound	18	24	52	59
Australian cattle dog	16	20	42.5-47.5	45-50
Australian kelpie	13.5	13.5	50	50
Australian shepherd	na	na	45-52.5	50-57.5
Australian terrier	6.5	6.5	25	27.5
Basenji	10	11	40	43
Basset hound	18	27	32.5	37.5
Beagle	12	14	32.5	38
Beagle harrier	20	20	42.5	47.5
Bearded collie	18	27	50-52.5	52.5-55
Beauce shepherd (Beauceron)	30	38	60-68	63-70
Bedlington terrier	8	10.5	37.5-41	40-44
Belgian shepherd dog				
Groenendael	28	28	56-60	60-65
Laekenois	28	28	56-60	60-65
Malinois	28	28	56-60	60-65
Tervuren	28	28	56-60	60-65

Appendix 14 (continued). Body weights in kilograms and height at withers in centimeters of selected canine breeds.

Breeds	Body weights (kg)		Height at withers (cm)	
	Females	Males	Females	Males
Bergamasco	26-32	32-38	55	60
Bernese mountain dog (Berner sennenhund)	40-45	50	57.5-65	62.5-70
Bichon frisé	na	na	23	28
Billy	25	30	57.5-62.5	60-65
Bloodhound (St. Hubertus dog)	36-45.5	41-50	57.5-62.5	62.5-67.5
Bolognese	2.5	4	25-27.5	27.5-30
Bordeaux dog (large)	>40	>45	Smaller than male	58-66
Bordeaux dog (medium)	35-40	38-45	na	na
Border collie	13.5	20.5	45-52.5	47.5-55
Border terrier	5-6.4	6-7	25	25
Borzoi	25-41	34-48	≥65	≥70
Boston terrier				
Lightweight class	na	≤6.8	na	na
Middleweight class	na	≤9.0	na	na
Heavyweight class	na	≤11.4	na	na
Bourbonnais setter	18	26	52.5	na
Bouvier des Ardennes	na	na	40-46	42-48
Bouvier des Flandres	27-35	35-40	53-66	61-69
Boxer	24	32	53-59	56-63
Brazilian guard dog	40.5	45	60	74
Briard	34	34	55-64	58-68
Brittany spaniel	13.5	18	44	51
Brussels griffon	2.2	5	17.5	20
Bulldog	18-23	23-25	na	na
Bullmastiff	40-54.5	50-59	60-65	62.5-67.5
Bull terrier	23.5	28	52.5	55
Cairn terrier	6	7.5	24	30
Canaan dog	18	25	49	59
Cao de Castro Laboreiro (Portuguese watchdog)	20-30	30-40	52-57	56-60
Catalonian shepherd	20-30	30-40	43-48	45-50
Cavalier King Charles spaniel	5	8	30	33
Chesapeake Bay retriever	25-32	29.5-36	52.5-60	57.5-65
Chihuahua	≤2.7	≤2.7	16	20
Chinese crested dog	≤5.5	≤5.5	22.5-30	27.5-32.5
Chow chow	20	32	42.5-50	47.5-55
Clumber spaniel	25-32	32-38.5	42.5-47.5	47.5-50
Collie (rough and smooth)	20-30	25-34	55-60	60-65
Coonhound				
Black and tan coonhound	25-34	27-36	57.5-62.5	62.5-67.5
Redbone coonhound	25-34	27-36	57.5-62.5	62.5-67.5
Coton de Tulear	5.5	7	25	30
Curly-coated retriever	32	36	57.5-62.5	62.5-67.5
Czesky terrier	6	9	27.5	35
Dachshund				
Miniature (UK)	4.5	4.5	na	na
Miniature (USA)	≤5	≤5	na	na
Standard (UK)	9.0	12	na	na
Standard (USA)	7.3	14.5	na	na
Dalmatian	22.7	27	47.5	57.5
Dandie Dinmont terrier	8	11	20	27.5
Deerhound (Scottish)	30-43	38.5-50	≥70	75-80
Doberman pinscher	29	40	60-65	65-70
Dogue de Bordeaux	54	65	69	75
Dupuy setter	na	na	64-65	66-67.5
Dutch shepherd	30	30	54-61	57.5-62.5
Elkhound (Norwegian)	20	25	49	51
English cocker spaniel	12-14.5	12.5-15.5	37.5-40	40-42.5
English setter	18	31.5	60	62.5
English springer spaniel	18	22.5	47.5	50
English toy spaniel	3.5	6.5	25	25
Entlebuch mountain dog	25	30	50	50
Eskimo dog	25-41	30-50	50-60	57.5-67.5
Estrela mountain dog	27-41	34-48	50-60	57.5-67.5
Eurasier	18-26	23-32	48-56	52-60
Field spaniel	16	25	42.5	45
Finnish spitz	11.3	16	39-45	44-50
Flat-coated retriever	25-34	25-36	55-59	57.5-61
Foxhound				
American foxhound	na	na	52.5-60	55-62.5
English foxhound	29.5	32	52.5-60	55-62.5

Appendix 14 (continued). Body weights in kilograms and height at withers in centimeters of selected canine breeds.

Breeds	Body weights (kg)		Height at withers (cm)	
	Females	Males	Females	Males
Fox terrier (smooth and wire)	6.8-7.7	7-8.2	≤39	≤39
French bulldog	8	13	30	30
French hound	27	28	61-67.5	61-71
French setter	27	27	60	60
French spaniel	20	25	52.5-57.5	55-60
German hunt terrier	7-8	9-10	40	40
German pointer (Deutscher Vorstehund)				
German shorthaired pointer	20.5-27	25-32	52.5-57.5	57.5-62.5
German wirehaired pointer	20.5-29	25-34	55-60	60-65
German shepherd dog	32	43	55-60	60-65
German spaniel	20	30	39-44	39-49
German spitz				
Small (Kleinspitz)	2.9	3.0	22.5	27.5
Standard (Mittelspitz)	11.3	11.3	29	32.5
Glen of Imaal terrier	16	16	35	35
Golden retriever	25-29.5	29.5-34	54-56	57.5-60
Gordon setter	20.5-32	25-36	57.5-65	60-67.5
Great Dane	55	80	≥72	≥80
Great Gascony blue	32	35	59-64	62.5-70
Greater Swiss mountain dog	na	na	59-67.5	64-71
Greenland dog	≥30	≥30	55	60
Greyhound	27-29.5	29.5-32	67.5-70	70-75
Griffon nivernais	23	25	Smaller than male	52.5-57.5
Griffon Vendéen				
Petit basset	11.5	16	32.5	37.5
Basset	18	20	37.5	42.5
Briquet	16	24	50	55
Grand	30	35	60	65
Hamiltonstövare	23	27	45-56	49-59
Hanover hound	38	45	Smaller than male	50-60
Harlequin pinscher	na	na	30	35
Harrier	22	27	47.5	52.5
Havanese	3	5.5	25	26
Hovawart	25-35	30-40	55-65	60-70
Hungarian coarse-haired vizsla	na	na	52.5-59	56-64
Hungarian greyhound	22.5-27	27-32	na	na
Hungarian Kuvasz	na	≤50	65-69	70-74
Ibizan hound	20.5	23	56-65	59-69
Iceland dog	na	na	38-44	42-48
Irish red and white setter	18	32	59	67.5
Irish setter	27.2	31.7	57.5-62.5	67.5
Irish terrier	11	12	45	45
Irish water spaniel	20.5-26	25-29.5	52.5-57.5	55-60
Irish wolfhound	≥48	≥54	≥75	≥80
Italian greyhound	2.5	4.5	32	38
Italian segugio	18	28	47.5-55	52.5-57.5
Italian setter	25	40	na	na
Italian spinone	28-32	32-37	57.5-64	59-69
Jämthund	na	na	52.5-57.5	57.5-62.5
Japanese chin	1.8	3.2	20	27.5
Japanese fighting dog	45	91	≥59	≥59
Japanese spitz	5.9	5.9	Smaller than male	30-35
Japanese terrier	na	na	30	37.5
Jura hound	na	na	44	55
Keeshond	25	30	42.5	45
Kerry blue terrier	na	15-18	44-47.5	45-49
Komondor	36-50	45-68	≥64	≥69
Kooikerhondje	9	11	37.5	37.5
Kromfohrländer	12	12	37.5	45
Kuvasz (Hungarian shepherd)	32-41	45-52	65-70	70-75
Labrador retriever	25-32	29.5-36	54-59	56-61
Lakeland terrier	7	7.7	34	36
Lancashire heeler	3.5	5.4	25	30
Lapland spitz	20	20	39-44	44-49
Lapponian herder	≤30	≤30	43-48	48-55
Leonberger	36.3	68	65-75	73-80
Lhasa apso	na	na	Smaller than male	25
Löwchen	2	4	20	35
Maltese	1.8	2.7	25	25
Manchester terrier				
Toy (American-bred)	≤3.2	≤3.2	na	na

Appendix 14 (continued). Body weights in kilograms and height at withers in centimeters of selected canine breeds.

Breeds	Body weights (kg)		Height at withers (cm)	
	Females	Males	Females	Males
Toy (English toy terrier)	≤5.4	≤5.4	25	30
Standard (American-bred)	≥5.5	≤7.3	na	na
Standard (open classes)	≥7.3	≤10	37.5	40
Maremma sheepdog	30-40	35-45	60-68	65-73
Mastiff	75	90	≥69	≥75
Mexican hairless dog	na	na	40	50
Miniature bull terrier	4.5	18	25	35
Miniature pinscher	4.5	4.5	25	31
Mudi	8	13	35	47.5
Münsterlander				
Small	15	17	47.5	55
Large	25	25-30	57.5	60
Neapolitan mastiff	50	70	60-68	64-72
Newfoundland	50-55	60-69	65	70
Norfolk terrier	5	5.5	22.5	25
Norwegian buhund	12	18	Smaller than male	42.5-45
Norwich terrier	4.5	5.4	≤25	≤25
Nova Scotia duck tolling retriever	16.5	23	42.5	52.5
Old English sheepdog (bobtail)	25	30	≥52.5	≥55
Otterhound	30-45	34-52	57.5-65	60-67.5
Papillon	1.5	5	20	27.5
Parson Jack Russell terrier	na	na	30-32.5	32.5-35
Pekingese	3-5	3.6-6.5	na	na
Pharaoh hound	na	na	52.5-60	57.5-62.5
Picardy shepherd	23	32	50-60	55-65
Pinscher	na	na	42.5	47.5
Pointer	20.5-29.5	25-34	57.5-65	62.5-70
Poitevin	30	30	62.5	70
Polish lowland sheepdog	na	na	40-46	42.5-50
Pomeranian	1.5	3.2	27.5	27.5
Poodle				
Toy	na	na	≤25	≤25
Miniature	5	5	>25	37.5
Standard	20	32	>37.5	na
Porcelaine	25	28	52.5-55	55-57.5
Portuguese setter	na	na	47.5-55	51-60
Portuguese water dog	16-23	19-27	42.5-52.5	50-57.5
Pudelpointer	25	32	≥60	≥60
Pug	6.5	8	25	30
Puli (Hungarian puli)	10-13	13-15	36-40	40-44
Pumi	8	13	32.5	44
Pyrenean mastiff	55	70	Smaller than male	69-79
Pyrenean mountain dog (Great Pyrenees)	38.5-45	45.5-55	62.5-72.5	67.5-80
Pyrenean shepherd	8	13.5	38-50	39-50
Rafeiro do alentejo	35-45	40-45	64-70	66-74
Rhodesian ridgeback	32	38.5	60-65	62.5-67.5
Romanian shepherd dog	50	50	63.5	65
Rottweiler	40	50	55-62.5	60-67.5
Saint Bernard	50	90.5	≥65	≥70
Saint-Germain setter	18	26	na	na
Saluki	13	30	≥54	58-70
Samoyed	17-25	20-30	47.5-53	53-59
Schapendoes	na	na	40-47	43-50
Schipperke				
Small type	3	5	25-30	27.5-32.5
Large type	5.4	8.2	25-30	27.5-32.5
Schnauzer				
Miniature	5	6.8	30	35
Standard	15	18	45-46	46-50
Giant (Riesenschnauzer)	30	35	60-65	65-70
Scottish terrier	8-9.5	8.5-10	25	na
Sealyham terrier	8-9	10-11	26	≤30
Shar-Pei	18	25	45	50
Shetland sheepdog (sheltie)	na	na	32.5	40
Shiba Inu	9	13.6	34-39	36-41
Shih Tzu	4	8	22.5	26
Siberian husky	16-22.5	20-27	50-55	53-60
Sicilian hound	10-12	12-14	42.5-45	45-50
Silky terrier (Australian)	3.6	4.5	22.5	25
Skye terrier	11.5	11.5	24	25

Appendix 14 (continued). Body weights in kilograms and height at withers in centimeters of selected canine breeds.

Breeds	Body weights (kg)		Height at withers (cm)	
	Females	Males	Females	Males
Sloughi	20	27	58	75
Soft-coated wheaten terrier	13.5-16	16-18	42.5-45	45-47.5
Spanish greyhound	27	30	Smaller than male	64-69
Spanish mastiff	50	60	Smaller than male	65-70
Stabyhoun	15	20	na	≤47.5
Staffordshire bull terrier	11-15	13-17	35	40
Staffordshire terrier (American)	na	na	42.5-45	45-47.5
Sussex spaniel	16	20	32.5	37.5
Swedish vallhund	11.4	16	30-32.5	32.5-34.4
Swiss scent hound (Laufhunde)	na	na	44	55
Tahltan bear dog	6.8	6.8	30	40
Tawny brittany basset	na	na	32.5	42.5
Tibetan mastiff	≥82	≥82	≥60	≥65
Tibetan spaniel	4	6.8	25	25
Tibetan terrier	8	13.6	35	42
Vizsla (Hungarian vizsla)	20	30	52.5-58	56-60
Weimaraner	32	38	57.5-62.5	62.5-67.5
Welsh corgi				
Cardigan	11.4-15.5	13.6-17	26	31
Pembroke	10-12.7	10-13.6	25	30
Welsh springer spaniel	16	20	42.5-45	45-47.5
Welsh terrier	9	9.5	Smaller than male	37.5
West Highland white terrier	7	10	25	27.5
Whippet	13	13	45-52.5	47.5-55
Wirehaired pointing griffon	23	27	50-55	55-60
Yorkshire terrier	≤3.5	≤3.5	22.5	22.5

Key: na = information not available.

Appendix 15. Body weights in pounds and height at withers in inches of selected canine breeds.

Breeds	Body weights (lb)		Height at withers (in.)	
	Females	Males	Females	Males
Affenpinscher	6.5	9	9	11
Afghan hound	50	60	24-26	26-29
Ainu dog	na	na	16.5-19	19.5-21
Airedale terrier	42	55	22-23	23-24
Akita	75	101	24-26	26-28
Alaskan malamute	75	126	23-26	25-28
American cocker spaniel	24	28	13.5-14.5	14.5-15.5
American Eskimo dog				
Toy	na	na	9	12
Miniature	na	na	>12	15
Standard	na	na	>15	19
American water spaniel	25-40	30-45	15-18	15-18
Anatolian shepherd dog	90.5-130	110-141	28-31	29-32
Anglo-French hound				
Small	49	55	19	22
Great	66	71	24	27
Appenzell mountain dog	48.5	55	18.5-20	22-23
Ariegeois	66	66	21-23	22-24
Artois hound	40	53	20.8	23.8
Australian cattle dog	35	45	17-19	18-20
Australian kelpie	30	30	20	20
Australian shepherd	na	na	18-21	20-23
Australian terrier	14	14	10	11
Basenji	22	24	16	17
Basset hound	40	60	13	15
Beagle	26.5	31	13	15
Beagle harrier	44	44	17	19
Bearded collie	40	60	20-21	21-22
Beauce shepherd (Beauceron)	66	85	24-27	25-28
Bedlington terrier	17	23	15-16.5	16-17.5
Belgian shepherd dog				
Groenendael	62	62	22-24	24-26
Laekenois	62	62	22-24	24-26
Malinois	62	62	22-24	24-26
Tervuren	62	62	22-24	24-26

Appendix 15 (continued). Body weights in pounds and height at withers in inches of selected canine breeds.

Breeds	Body weights (lb)		Height at withers (in.)	
	Females	Males	Females	Males
Bergamasco	57-70	70-84	22	24
Bernese mountain dog (Berner sennenhund)	88-100	110	23-26	25-28
Bichon frisé	na	na	9	11
Billy	55	66	23-25	24-26
Bloodhound (St. Hubertus dog)	80-100	90-110	23-25	25-27
Bolognese	5.5	9	10-11	11-12
Bordeaux dog (large)	>88	>99	Smaller than male	23-26.5
Bordeaux dog (medium)	77-88	84-99	na	na
Border collie	30	45	18-21	19-22
Border terrier	11.5-14	13-15.5	10	10
Borzoi	55-90	75-105	≥26	≥28
Boston terrier				
Lightweight class	na	≤15	na	na
Middleweight class	na	≤20	na	na
Heavyweight class	na	≤25	na	na
Bourbonnais setter	40	57	21	21
Bouvier des Ardennes	na	na	16-18.5	17-19
Bouvier des Flandres	60-77	77-88	21-26.5	24.5-27.5
Boxer	53	70	21-23.5	22.5-25
Brazilian guard dog	89	99	24	29.5
Briard	75	75	22-25.5	23-27
Brittany spaniel	30	40	17.5	20.5
Brussels griffon	5	≤12	7	8
Bulldog	40-50	50-55	na	na
Bullmastiff	88-120	110-130	24-26	25-27
Bull terrier	52	62	21	22
Cairn terrier	13	16	9.5	12
Canaan dog	40	55	19.5	23.5
Cao de Castro Laboreiro (Portuguese watchdog)	44-66	66-88	21-23	22-24
Catalonian shepherd	44-66	66-88	17-19	18-20
Cavalier King Charles spaniel	10	18	12	13
Chesapeake Bay retriever	55-70	65-80	21-24	23-26
Chihuahua	≤6	6	6.3	8
Chinese crested dog	≤12	12	9-12	11-13
Chow chow	44.5	70	17-20	19-22
Clumber spaniel	55-70	70-85	17-19	19-20
Collie (rough and smooth)	44-65	55-75	22-24	24-26
Coonhound				
Black and tan coonhound	55-75	60-80	23-25	25-27
Redbone coonhound	55-75	60-80	23-25	25-27
Coton de Tulear	12	15	10	12
Curly-coated retriever	70	80	23-25	25-27
Czesky terrier	13	20	11	14
Dachshund				
Miniature (UK)	10	10	na	na
Miniature (USA)	≤11	11	na	na
Standard (UK)	20	26	na	na
Standard (USA)	16	32	na	na
Dalmatian	50	59.5	19	23
Dandie Dinmont terrier	18	24	8	11
Deerhound (Scottish)	66-95	85-110	≥28	30-32
Doberman pinscher	64	88	24-26	26-28
Dogue de Bordeaux	119	143	27.5	30
Dupuy Setter	na	na	25.5-26	26.5-27
Dutch shepherd	66	>66	21.5-24.5	23-25
Elkhound	44	55	19.5	20.5
English cocker spaniel	26.5-32	27.5-34	15-16	16-17
English setter	40	70	24	25
English springer spaniel	40	50	19	20
English toy spaniel	8	14	10	10
Entlebuch mountain dog	55	66	20	20
Eskimo dog	55-90	66-110	20-24	23-27
Estrela mountain dog	60-90	75-105	20-24	23-27
Eurasier	40-57	51-71	19-22.5	21-24
Field spaniel	35	55	17	18
Finnish spitz	25	35	15.5-18	17.5-20
Flat-coated retriever	55-75	55-80	22-23.5	23-24.5
Foxhound				
American foxhound	na	na	21-24	22-25
English foxhound	65	70	21-24	22-25

Appendix 15 (continued). Body weights in pounds and height at withers in inches of selected canine breeds.

Breeds	Body weights (lb)		Height at withers (in.)	
	Females	Males	Females	Males
Fox terrier (smooth and wire)	15-17	16-18	≤15.5	≤15.5
French bulldog	18	29	12	12
French hound	60	62	24.5-27	24.5-28.5
French setter	60	60	24	24
French spaniel	44	55	21-23	22-24
German hunt terrier	16-18	19.5-22	16	16
German pointer (Deutscher Vorstehund)				
German shorthaired pointer	45-60	55-70	21-23	23-25
German wirehaired pointer	45-64	55-75	22-24	24-26
German shepherd dog	70	95	22-24	24-26
German spaniel	44	66	15.5-17.5	15.5-19.5
German spitz				
Small (Kleinspitz)	6.4	6.6	9	11
Standard (Mittelspitz)	25	25	11.5	13
Glen of Imaal terrier	35	35	14	14
Golden retriever	55-65	65-75	21.5-22.5	23-24
Gordon setter	45-70	55-80	23-26	24-27
Great Dane	121	176	≥29	≥32
Great Gascony blue	71	77	23.5-25.5	25-28
Greater Swiss mountain dog	na	na	23.5-27	25.5-28.5
Greenland dog	≥66	≥66	22	24
Greyhound	60-65	65-70	27-28	28-30
Griffon nivernais	50	55	Smaller than male	21-23
Griffon Vendéen				
Petit basset	25	35	13	15
Basset	40	44	15	17
Briquet	35	53	20	22
Grand	66	77	24	26
Hamiltonstovare	50	60	18-22.5	19.5-23.5
Hanover hound	84	99	Smaller than male	20-24
Harlequin pinscher	na	na	12	14
Harrier	48	60	19	21
Havanese	7	12	10	10.5
Hovawart	55-77	66-88	22-26	24-28
Hungarian coarse haired vizsla	na	na	21-23.5	22.5-25.5
Hungarian greyhound	50-60	60-70	na	na
Hungarian Kuvasz	≤110	≤110	26-27.5	28-29.5
Ibizan hound	45	50	22.5-26	23.5-27.5
Iceland dog	na	na	15-17.5	17-19
Irish red and white setter	40	70	23.5	27
Irish setter	60	70	23-25	27
Irish terrier	25	27	18	18
Irish water spaniel	45-58	55-65	21-23	22-24
Irish wolfhound	≥105	≥120	≥30	≥32
Italian greyhound	5.5	10	13	15
Italian segugio	39	62	19-22	21-23
Italian setter	55	88	na	na
Italian spinone	62-70	71-82	23-25.5	23.5-27.5
Jämthund	na	na	21-23	23-25
Japanese chin	4	7	8	11
Japanese fighting dog	100	200	≥23.5	≥23.5
Japanese spitz	13	13	Smaller than male	12-14
Japanese terrier	na	na	12	15
Jura hound	na	na	17.5	22
Keeshond	55	66	17	18
Kerry blue terrier	na	33-40	17.5-19	18-19.5
Komondor	80	100-150	≥25.5	≥27.5
Kooikerhondje	20	24	15	15
Kromfohrländer	26	26	15	18
Kuvasz (Hungarian shepherd)	70-90	99-110	26-28	28-30
Labrador retriever	55-70	65-80	21.5-23.5	22.5-24.5
Lakeland terrier	15	17	13.5	14.5
Lancashire heeler	8	12	10	12
Lapland spitz	44	44	15.5-17.5	17.5-19.5
Lapponian herder	na	≤66	17-19	19-22
Leonberger	80	150	26-30	29-32
Lhasa apso	na	na	Smaller than male	10
Löwchen	4	9	8	14
Maltese	4	≤6 7	10	10
Manchester terrier				
Toy (American-bred)	na	≤7	na	na
Toy (English toy terrier)	na	≤12	10	12

Appendix 15 (continued). Body weights in pounds and height at withers in inches of selected canine breeds.

Breeds	Body weights (lb)		Height at withers (in.)	
	Females	Males	Females	Males
Standard (American-bred)	≥12	≤16	na	na
Standard (open classes)	≥16	≤22	15	16
Maremma sheepdog	66-88	77-99	24-27	26-29
Mastiff	165	198	≥27.5	≥30
Mexican hairless dog	na	na	16	20
Miniature bull terrier	10	40	10	14
Miniature pinscher	10	10	10	12.5
Mudi	18	29	14	19
Münsterlander				
Small	33	37	19	22
Large	55	55-66	23	24
Neapolitan mastiff	110	154	24-27	25.5-29
Newfoundland	110-120	132-152	26	28
Norfolk terrier	11	12	9	10
Norwegian buhund	26	40	Smaller than male	17-18
Norwich terrier	10	12	na	≤10
Nova Scotia duck tolling retriever	36	51	17	21
Old English sheepdog (bobtail)	55	66	≥21	≥22
Otterhound	65-100	75-115	23-26	24-27
Papillon	3.3	11	8	11
Parson Jack Russell terrier	na	na	12-13	13-14
Pekingese	7-11	8-14.3	na	na
Pharaoh hound	na	na	21-24	23-25
Picardy shepherd	50	70	20-24	22-26
Pinscher	na	na	17	19
Pointer	45-65	55-75	23-26	25-28
Poitevin	66	66	25	28
Polish lowland sheepdog	na	na	16-18.5	17-20
Pomeranian	3	7	11	11
Poodle				
Toy	na	na	≤10	≤10
Miniature	11	11	>10	15
Standard	44.5	70	>15	na
Porcelaine	55	62	21-22	22-23
Portuguese setter	na	na	19-22	20.5-24
Portuguese water dog	35-50	42-60	17-21	20-23
Pudelpointer	55	70	≥24	≥24
Pug	14	18	10	12
Puli (Hungarian puli)	22-28.5	28.5-33	14.5-16	16-17.5
Pumi	17.5	28.5	13	17.5
Pyrenean mastiff	121	154.5	Smaller than male	27.5-31.5
Pyrenean mountain dog (Great Pyrenees)	85-99	100-121	25-29	27-32
Pyrenean shepherd	18	30	15-20	15.5-20
Rafeiro do alentejo	77-99	88-99	25.5-28	26.5-29.5
Rhodesian ridgeback	70	85	24-26	25-27
Romanian shepherd dog	110	110	25	26
Rottweiler	88	110	22-25	24-27
Saint Bernard	110	200	≥26	≥28
Saint-Germain setter	40	57	na	na
Saluki	29	66	≥22	23-28
Samoyed	37-55	44-66	19-21	21-23.5
Schapendoes (Dutch)	na	na	16-19	17-20
Schipperke				
Small type	7	11	10-12	11-13
Large type	11	18	10-12	11-13
Schnauzer				
Miniature	11	15	12	14
Standard	33	40	18-18.5	18.5-20
Giant (Riesenschnauzer)	66	77	24-26	26-28
Scottish terrier	18-21	19-22	10	na
Sealyham terrier	18-20	23-24	10.5	≤12
Shar-Pei	40	55	18	20
Shetland sheepdog (Sheltie)	na	na	13	16
Shiba Inu	20	30	13.5-15.5	14.5-16.5
Shih Tzu	9	18	9	10.5
Siberian husky	35-50	44-60	20-22	21-24
Sicilian hound	22-26	26-30	17-18	18-20
Silky terrier (Australian)	8	10	9	10
Skye terrier	25	na	9.5	10
Sloughi	45	60	23	30
Soft-coated wheaten terrier	30-35	35-40	17-18	18-19

Appendix 15 (continued). Body weights in pounds and height at withers in inches of selected canine breeds.

Breeds	Body weights (lb)		Height at withers (in.)	
	Females	Males	Females	Males
Spanish greyhound	60	66	Smaller than male	25.5-27.5
Spanish mastiff	110	132	Smaller than male	26-28
Stabyhoun	33	44	na	≤19
Staffordshire bull terrier	24-34	28-38	14	16
Staffordshire terrier (American)	na	na	17-18	18-19
Sussex spaniel	35	45	13	15
Swedish vallhund	25	35	12-13	13-14
Swiss scent hound (Laufhunde)	na	na	17.5	22
Tahltan bear dog	15	15	12	16
Tawny brittany basset	na	na	13	17
Tibetan mastiff	≥180	na	≥24	≥26
Tibetan spaniel	9	15	10	10
Tibetan terrier	18	30	14	17
Vizsla (Hungarian vizsla)	44	66	21-23	22.5-24
Weimaraner	70	85	23-25	25-27
Welsh corgi				
Cardigan	25-34	30-38	10.5	12.5
Pembroke	22-28	22-30	10	12
Welsh springer spaniel	35	45	17-18	18-19
Welsh terrier	20	21	Smaller than male	15-15.5
West Highland white terrier	15	22	10	11
Whippet	28	28	18-21	19-22
Wirehaired pointing griffon	50	60	20-22	22-24
Yorkshire terrier	≤8	≤8	9	9

Key: na = information not available.

Appendix 16. Nutrient content of human foods often used as animal treats in North America on a nutrient content/treat basis.

Foods	Weight (g)	Energy (kcal ME)*	DM (g)	Protein (g)	Fat (g)	NFE (g)	Crude fiber (g)	Ca (mg)	P (mg)	K (mg)	Na (mg)	Mg (mg)
Cheese												
American cheese (pasteurized) (1 oz.)	28.4	97.2	17	6.6	8.5	0.5	na	198	219	22.7	322	na
Cheddar cheese (1 oz.)	28.4	105	17.9	7.1	9.1	0.6	na	213	136	23.2	199	12.8
Fruit												
Apples (not pared)	34.5	17.4	5.1	0.1	0.1	4.7	0.2	2.1	3.5	38	0.3	2.8
Apples (pared)	34.5	18.3	5.4	0.1	0.2	4.7	0.3	2.4	3.5	38	0.3	1.7
Ice cream												
Ice cream (10% fat)	66.5	119	24.5	3	7.1	13.8	na	99.1	76.5	120	41.9	9.3
Ice cream (12% fat)	66.5	128	25.2	2.7	8.3	13.7	na	81.8	65.8	74.5	26.6	9.3
Meat												
Bologna	23	64.4	10.1	2.8	6.3	0.3	na	1.6	29.4	52.9	299	na
Frankfurter	66.5	189	29.5	8.3	18.4	1.2	na	4.7	88.4	146	731	na
Others												
Peanut butter	5.3	30.2	5.2	1.5	2.6	0.8	0.1	3.3	21.6	35.5	32.2	na
Popcorn	6	20.9	5.8	0.8	0.3	4.5	0.1	0.7	24.4	na	0.2	na
Popcorn (with fat and salt)	9	37.8	8.7	0.9	2	5.2	0.2	0.7	19.4	na	175	na
Potato chips (1 oz.)	28.4	149	27.8	1.5	11.3	13.7	0.5	11.3	39.4	320	284	na
Pretzels (1 oz.)	28.4	95.6	27.1	2.8	1.3	21.4	0.1	6.2	37.1	36.9	476	na

Key: kcal = kilocalories, ME = metabolizable energy, DM = dry matter, NFE = nitrogen-free extract, Ca = calcium, P = phosphorus, K = potassium, Na = sodium, Mg = magnesium, na = not available.
*Metabolizable energy calculated based on modified Atwater values: protein = 3.5 kcal/g, fat = 8.5 kcal/g, NFE = 3.5 kcal/g dry matter.
To convert to kJ, multiply kcal x 4.184.

Appendix 17. Nutrient content of human foods often used as animal treats in North America on a nutrient level/100 g dry matter basis.*

Foods	Moisture	Energy (kcal ME)**	Protein	Fat	NFE	Crude fiber	Ca	P	K	Na	Mg
Cheese											
American cheese (pasteurized)	40	571	38.7	50	3.2	na	1.2	1.3	0.1	1.9	na
Cheddar cheese	37	585	39.7	51.1	3.3	na	1.2	0.8	0.1	1.1	0.1
Fruit											
Apples (not pared)	85.1	339	1.3	2.0	90.6	4.0	0	0.1	0.7	0	0.06
Apples (pared)	84.4	340	1.3	3.9	86.5	6.4	0.1	0.1	0.7	0	0
Ice cream											
Ice cream (10% fat)	63.2	486	12.2	28.8	56.5	na	0.4	0.3	0.5	0.2	0
Ice cream (12% fat)	62.1	508	10.6	33	54.4	na	0.3	0.3	0.3	0.1	0
Meat											
Bologna	56.2	639	27.6	62.8	2.5	na	0	0.3	0.5	3	na
Frankfurters	55.6	641	28.2	62.2	4.1	na	0	0.3	0.5	2.5	na
Others											
Peanut butter	1.8	581	28.3	50.3	15.6	1.9	0.1	0.4	0.7	0.6	na
Popcorn (plain)	4.0	362	13.2	5.2	77.6	2.3	1.7	0	0.4	na	na
Popcorn (with fat and salt)	3.1	434	10.1	22.5	59.2	1.8	0	0.2	na	2	na
Potato chips***	1.8	536	5.4	40.5	49.3	1.6	0	0.1	1.2	1	na
Pretzels***	4.5	353	10.3	4.7	79.2	0.3	0	0.1	0.1	1.7	na

Key: kcal = kilocalories, ME = metabolizable energy, DM = dry matter, NFE = nitrogen-free extract, Ca = calcium, P = phosphorus, K = potassium, Na = sodium, Mg = magnesium, na = not available.
*Nutrients, except for moisture, are expressed as % dry matter.
**Energy is expressed as kcal metabolizable energy/100 g dry matter. Metabolizable energy calculated based on modified Atwater values: protein = 3.5 kcal/g, fat = 8.5 kcal/g, NFE = 3.5 kcal/g dry matter. To convert to kJ, multiply kcal x 4.184.
***Sodium content varies and may be higher than the levels listed here.

Appendix 18. Nutrient content of human foods often used as animal treats in Europe on a nutrient content/treat basis.

Foods	Weight (g)	Energy (kcal ME)*	DM (g)	Protein (g)	Fat (g)	NFE (g)	Crude fiber (g)	Ca (mg)	P (mg)	K (mg)	Na (mg)	Mg (mg)
Biscuits												
Boudoir (lady finger)	6	20	5.5	0.4	0.2	4.8	0	1.4	5.3	6.3	3.0	0.2
Dry biscuit (average)	5	20	5.0	0.3	0.6	4.0	0	1.6	4.2	8.0	11.6	0.9
Petit beurre	8	30	7.9	0.5	0.8	6.2	0	na	na	na	na	na
Speculoos	8	35	7.9	0.4	1.5	5.8	0	1.3	5.3	6.4	27.0	1.2
Speculoos (all wheat)	8	33	7.9	0.5	1.3	5.5	0.3	2.0	17	18.4	22.4	6.4
Cheese												
Camembert	10	26	4.9	2.5	2.0	0.1	0	60	30	11.0	79	na
Gouda	10	32	5.8	2.5	2.7	0	0	92	52	12.0	60	3.0
Gruyère	10	40.5	6.8	2.9	3.5	0.1	0	90	60	10.0	50	na
Parmesan	10	38	7.4	4.0	2.7	0.2	0	100	90	12.5	100	na
Meat (cold cuts)												
Pâté de foie (liver pâté)	10	33	5.1	1.2	3.3	0.3	0	2.0	15.0	8.0	80	1.0
Salami (one slice)	10	43	6.8	1.9	4.2	0.1	0	2.8	16.7	30.0	152	1.9
Saucisson (average) (one slice)	10	36	5.4	1.4	3.6	0.2	0	2.5	15.4	18.3	102	0.7

Key: kcal = kilocalories, ME = metabolizable energy, DM = dry matter, NFE = nitrogen-free extract, Ca = calcium, P = phosphorus, K = potassium, Na = sodium, Mg = magnesium, na = not available.
*Metabolizable energy calculated based on modified Atwater values: protein = 3.5 kcal/g, fat = 8.5 kcal/g, NFE = 3.5 kcal/g dry matter. To convert to kJ, multiply kcal x 4.184.

Appendix 19. Nutrient content of human foods often used as animal treats in Europe on a nutrient level/100 g dry matter basis.*

Foods	Moisture	Energy (kcal ME)**	Protein	Fat	NFE	Crude fiber	Ca	P	K	Na	Mg
Biscuits											
Boudoir (lady finger)	5.9	369	8.1	4.1	87.1	0	0	0.1	0.1	0.1	0
Dry biscuit (average)	1.0	402	6.7	12.1	80.0	0	0	0.1	0.2	0.2	0
Petit beurre	1.0	378	5.7	10.1	77.8	0	na	na	na	na	na
Speculoos	1.0	437	5.5	19.2	72.8	0	0	0.1	0.1	0.3	0
Speculoos (all wheat)	1.0	411	6.6	17.0	69.7	4	0	0.2	0.2	0.3	0.1
Cheese											
Camembert	51	533	51.0	40.8	2	0	1.2	0.6	0.2	1.6	na
Gouda	42	552	42.9	47.2	0	0	1.6	0.9	0.2	1.0	0.1
Gruyère	32	592	42.7	51.5	1.5	0	1.3	0.9	0.2	0.7	na
Parmesan	26	509	54.1	36.5	2.7	0	1.4	1.2	0.2	1.4	na
Meat (cold cuts)											
Pâté de foie (liver pâté)	49	651	23.7	64.1	6.5	0.4	0	0.3	0.2	1.6	0
Salami (one slice)	32	628	27.4	61.8	1.9	0	0	0.3	0.4	2.2	0
Saucisson (average) (one slice)	46	671	25.9	66.7	3.7	0	0.1	0.3	0.3	1.9	0

Key: kcal = kilocalories, ME = metabolizable energy, DM = dry matter, NFE = nitrogen-free extract, Ca = calcium, P = phosphorus, K = potassium, Na = sodium, Mg = magnesium, na = not available.
*Nutrients, except for moisture, are expressed as % dry matter.
**Energy is expressed as kcal metabolizable energy/100 g dry matter. Metabolizable energy calculated based on modified Atwater values: protein = 3.5 kcal/g, fat = 8.5 kcal/g, NFE = 3.5 kcal/g dry matter. To convert to kJ, multiply kcal x 4.184.

Appendix 20. Nutrient content of common protein sources.*

	Moisture	ME** (kcal)	ME** (kJ)	Protein	Fat	NFE	Fiber	Ca	P	Na	K	Mg	Serving size***
Meats													
Chicken													
Fryers, dark meat, raw, skinless	77.3	112	469	18.1	3.8	0.0	0.0	0.01	0.19	0.07	0.25	na	na
Fryers, fried wings	52.6	268	1,121	29.0	14.8	2.7	0.0	0.01	0.24	na	na	na	na
Fryers, light meat, raw, skinless	77.2	101	423	20.5	1.5	0.0	0.0	0.01	0.22	0.05	0.32	0.02	na
Fryers, raw giblets	78.4	103	431	17.5	3.1	0.1	0.0	0.01	0.22	na	na	na	na
Fryers, raw meat, skinless	77.2	107	448	19.3	2.7	0.0	0.0	0.01	0.20	0.06	0.29	na	na
Fryers, raw wings	73.5	146	611	18.5	7.4	0.0	0.0	0.01	0.20	na	na	na	na
Hens and cocks, dark meat, raw, skinless	71.2	154	644	20.2	7.5	0.0	0.0	0.01	0.19	0.07	0.25	0.02	na
Hens and cocks, light meat, raw, skinless	71.7	133	556	23.4	3.7	0.0	0.0	0.01	0.22	0.05	0.32	0.03	na
Hens and cocks, raw giblets	66.8	191	799	18.6	11.6	1.8	0.0	0.02	0.21	na	na	na	na
Turkey													
Dark meat, raw, skinless	73.6	128	536	20.9	4.3	0.0	0.0	na	na	0.08	0.31	na	na
Light meat, raw, skinless	73.0	116	485	24.6	1.2	0.0	0.0	na	na	0.05	0.32	na	na
Raw, total edible	64.2	218	912	20.1	14.7	0.0	0.0	na	na	na	na	na	na
Duck													
Domesticated, raw meat, skinless	68.8	165	690	21.4	8.2	0.0	0.0	0.01	0.2	0.07	0.29	na	na
Raw, total edible	54.3	326	1,364	16.0	28.6	0.0	0.0	0.01	0.18	na	na	na	na
Beef													
Chuck cuts, raw, lean	70.3	158	661	21.3	7.4	0.0	0.0	0.01	0.21	na	na	0.02	na
Ground beef, raw, lean	68.3	179	749	20.7	10.0	0.0	0.0	0.01	0.19	na	na	0.02	na
Raw, regular	60.2	268	1,121	17.9	21.2	0.0	0.0	0.01	0.16	na	0.24	0.02	na
Raw, total edible	60.8	257	1,075	18.7	19.6	0.0	0.0	0.01	0.19	na	na	0.02	na
Lamb													
Composite of cuts, raw, lean	62.5	247	1,033	16.8	19.4	0.0	0.0	0.01	0.15	na	na	0.02	na
Raw, fat	56.3	310	1,297	15.4	27.1	0.0	0.0	0.01	0.14	na	na	na	na
Raw, regular	61.0	263	1,100	16.5	21.3	0.0	0.0	0.01	0.15	na	na	0.02	na
Pork													
Composite of cuts, lean raw, (avg)	69.0	174	728	19.1	10.2	0.0	0.0	0.01	0.22	na	na	0.02	na
Composite of cuts, total edible raw, fat class (28% fat)	52.6	346	1,448	14.6	31.4	0.0	0.0	0.01	0.16	na	na	na	na
Composite of cuts, total edible raw, medium fat class (23% fat)	56.3	308	1,289	15.7	26.7	0.0	0.0	0.01	0.18	na	na	0.02	na
Composite of cuts, total edible raw, thin class (19% fat)	59.5	276	1,155	16.7	22.7	0.0	0.0	0.01	0.19	na	na	na	na
Horse													
Raw, lean meat	74.0	135	565	19.0	4.5	1.5	0.0	0.01	0.13	0.04	0.29	0.02	na
Rabbit													
Raw, meat	70.0	162	678	21.0	8.0	0.0	0.0	0.02	0.35	0.04	0.39	na	na
Venison													
Raw, lean meat	74.0	126	527	21.0	4.0	0.0	0.0	0.01	0.25	na	na	na	na

Appendix 20 (continued). Nutrient content of common protein sources.*

	Moisture	ME** (kcal)	(kJ)	Protein	Fat	NFE	Fiber	Ca	P	Na	K	Mg	Serving size***
Fish													
Cod, raw	81.2	78	326	17.6	0.3	0.0	0.0	0.01	0.19	0.07†	0.38	0.03	na
Halibut, raw	76.5	100	418	20.9	1.2	0.0	0.0	0.01	0.21	0.05††	0.45	0.03	na
Mackerel, raw (average)	68.5	175	732	20.5	9.8	0.0	0.0	0.01	0.26	na	na	0.03	na
Salmon, raw	63.6	217	908	22.5	13.4	0.0	0.0	0.08	0.19	na	na	na	na
Sardines, in oil (solids and liquid)	50.6	311	1,301	20.6	24.4	0.6	0.0	0.35	0.43	0.51	0.56	na	na
Sardines, raw	70.7	160	669	19.2	8.6	0.0	0.0	0.03	0.22	na	na	na	na
Shrimp, raw	78.2	91	381	18.1	0.8	1.5	0.0	0.06	0.17	0.14	0.22	na	na
Trout, raw	66.3	195	816	21.5	11.4	0.0	0.0	na	na	na	na	na	na
Tuna, canned, in oil	52.6	288	1,205	24.2	20.5	0.0	0.0	0.01	0.29	0.80	0.30	na	na
Tuna, canned, in water	70.0	127	531	28.0	0.8	0.0	0.0	0.02	0.19	0.04‡	0.28	na	na
Tuna, raw	71.0	139	582	25.0	3.6	0.0	0.0	na	na	0.04†††	na	na	na
Other animal products													
Kidneys													
Beef, raw	75.9	130	544	15.4	6.7	0.9	0.0	0.01	0.22	0.18	0.23	na	na
Calf, raw	77.4	113	473	16.6	4.6	0.1	0.0	na	na	na	na	na	na
Lamb, raw	77.7	105	439	16.8	3.3	0.9	0.0	0.01	0.22	0.20	0.23	na	na
Pork, raw	77.8	106	444	16.3	3.6	1.1	0.0	0.01	0.22	0.12	0.18	na	na
Heart													
Beef, raw, lean	77.5	108	452	17.1	3.6	0.7	0.0	0.01	0.20	0.09	0.19	0.02	na
Calf, raw	76.2	124	519	15.0	5.9	1.8	0.0	0.0	0.16	0.09	0.21	na	na
Chicken, raw	74.3	134	561	18.6	6.0	0.1	0.0	0.0	0.16	0.08	0.16	na	na
Lamb, raw	71.6	162	678	16.8	9.6	1.0	0.0	0.0	0.25	na	na	na	na
Pork, raw	77.4	113	473	16.8	4.4	0.4	0.0	0.0	0.13	0.05	0.11	na	na
Turkey, raw	71.3	171	715	16.2	11.2	0.2	0.0	na	na	0.07	0.24	na	na
Liver													
Beef, raw	69.7	140	586	19.9	3.8	5.3	0.0	0.01	0.35	0.14	0.28	0.01	na
Calf, raw	70.7	140	586	19.2	4.7	4.1	0.0	0.01	0.33	0.07	0.28	0.02	na
Chicken, raw	72.2	129	540	19.7	3.7	2.9	0.0	0.01	0.24	0.07	0.17	na	na
Goose, raw	66.9	182	761	16.5	10.0	5.4	0.0	na	na	0.14	0.23	na	na
Lamb, raw	70.8	136	569	21.0	3.9	2.9	0.0	0.01	0.35	0.05	0.20	0.01	na
Pork, raw	71.6	131	548	20.6	3.7	2.6	0.0	0.01	0.36	0.07	0.26	0.02	na
Turkey, raw	70.4	138	577	21.2	4.0	2.9	0.0	na	na	0.06	0.16	na	na
Rumen													
Beef, cleaned	80.0	121	506	12.0	7.0	0.5	0.0	0.02	0.04	0.02	0.04	0.02	na
Beef, uncleaned	72.0	147	615	20.0	5.0	0.6	1.1	0.12	0.13	0.05	0.10	0.04	na
Dairy and egg products													
Milk													
Canned, evaporated, unsweetened	73.8	137	573	7.0	7.9	9.7	0.0	0.25	0.21	0.12	0.30	0.03	249 g/ 8-oz cup
Dried, nonfat	3.0	363	1,519	35.9	0.8	52.3	0.0	1.31	1.02	0.53	1.75	0.14	68 g/ 8-oz cup
Dried, whole	2.0	502	2,100	26.4	27.5	38.2	0.0	0.91	0.71	0.41	1.33	0.10	na
Skim	90.5	36	151	3.6	0.1	5.1	0.0	0.12	0.10	0.05	0.15	0.01	245 g/ 8-oz cup
Whole	87.4	65	272	3.5	3.5	4.9	0.0	0.12	0.09	0.05	0.14	0.01	244 g/8-oz cup
Whey, dried	4.5	349	1,460	12.9	1.1	73.5	0.0	0.65	0.59	na	na	na	na
Buttermilk													
Dried	2.8	387	1,619	34.3	5.3	50.0	0.0	1.25	0.97	0.51	1.61	na	7 g/Tbs
Fluid, cultured (from skim milk)	90.5	36	151	3.6	0.1	5.1	0.0	0.12	0.10	0.13	0.14	0.01	245 g/ 8-oz cup
Yogurt													
From partially skimmed milk	89.0	50	209	3.4	1.7	5.2	0.0	0.12	0.09	0.05	0.14	na	na
From whole milk	88.0	62	259	3.0	3.4	4.9	0.0	0.11	0.09	0.05	0.13	na	227 g/ 8-oz cup
Cottage cheese													
Creamed	78.9	103	431	12.5	4.5	2.7	0.0	0.06	0.13	0.40	0.08	0.01	210 g/ 8-oz cup‡‡
Low fat (1% fat)	82.5	73	305	12.4	1.0	27.4	0.0	0.06	0.13	0.41	0.08	0.01	226 g/ 8-oz cup
Low fat (2% fat)	79.3	90	377	13.8	2.0	3.6	0.0	0.07	0.15	0.41	0.10	0.01	226 g/ 8-oz cup
Cheeses													
Camembert (France)	51.0	284	1,188	25.0	20.0	1.0	0.0	0.60	0.30	0.79	0.11	na	na
Camembert (US)	52.2	299	1,251	17.5	24.7	1.8	0.0	0.11	0.18	na	0.11	na	na
Cheddar (American cheese)	37.0	398	1,665	25.0	32.2	2.1	0.0	0.75	0.48	0.70	0.08	0.05	1 in^3 = 17 g
Gouda	42.0	346	1,448	24.9	27.4	0.0	0.0	0.92	0.52	0.60	0.12	0.03	na
Parmesan	29.5	393	1,644	38.0	26.0	2.3	0.0	1.20	0.90	0.90	0.14	0.05	na

Appendix 20 (continued). Nutrient content of common protein sources.*

	Moisture	ME** (kcal)	(kJ)	Protein	Fat	NFE	Fiber	Ca	P	Na	K	Mg	Serving size***
Eggs													
Dried whole	4.1	592	2,477	47.0	41.2	4.1	0.0	0.19	0.80	0.43	0.46	0.04	5 g/Tbs
White	87.6	51	213	10.9	tr	0.8	0.0	0.01	0.02	0.15	0.14	0.01	33 g/egg
Whole	73.7	163	682	12.9	11.5	0.9	0.0	0.05	0.21	0.12	0.13	0.01	50 g/large egg
Vegetables													
Soy													
Soybean flour, high fat	8.0	380	1,590	41.2	12.1	31.1	2.2	0.24	0.65	tr	1.78	0.27	85 g/8-oz cup
Soybean flour, low fat	8.0	356	1,490	43.4	6.7	34.1	2.5	0.26	0.63	tr	1.86	0.29	88 g/8-oz cup
Soybean milk, liquid	92.4	33	138	3.4	1.5	2.2	0.0	0.02	0.05	0.01	0.14	0.02	240 g/8-oz cup
Soybean milk, powder	4.2	429	1,795	41.8	20.3	27.8	0.2	0.28	na	na	na	na	na
Other													
Baker's yeast	71.0	111	464	16.0	1.2	9.0	0.3	0.03	0.61	0.03	0.65	0.06	na

Key: ME = metabolizable energy, kcal = kilocalories, kJ = kilojoules, NFE = nitrogen-free extract, Ca = calcium, P = phosphorus, Na = sodium, K = potassium, Mg = magnesium, tr = trace, g = grams, Tbs = tablespoons (15 ml), in^3 = cubic inches, na = not available.
*All nutrients are expressed on a percent as fed or as is basis unless otherwise noted.
**Metabolizable energy per 100 g as is.
***g/serving.
†Some fish are treated with brine, in which case the sodium content is markedly increased. Sodium levels of cod treated with brine may approach 0.26%.
††Some fish are treated with brine, in which case the sodium content is markedly increased. Sodium levels of halibut treated with brine may approach 0.36%.
†††Some fish are treated with brine, in which case the sodium content is markedly increased. Sodium levels of tuna treated with brine may approach 0.44%.
‡Some fish are treated with brine, in which case the sodium content is markedly increased. Sodium levels of canned tuna in water treated with brine may approach 0.88%.
‡‡One round tablespoon = 28 g.

Appendix 21. Essential amino acid content of common protein sources.*

	Protein	Arg	Isoleu	Leu	Lys	Met	Cys	Phe	His	Thr	Trp	Val
Meats and fish												
Beef	20	1.34	1.02	1.60	1.82	0.54	0.26	0.90	0.60	0.92	0.26	1.06
Chicken	21	1.30	0.97	1.58	1.89	0.57	0.27	0.95	0.40	0.88	0.23	1.01
Cod, raw	18	1.07	0.82	1.45	1.46	0.53	0.19	0.70	0.52	0.78	0.20	0.92
Halibut, raw	21	1.29	0.96	1.69	1.91	0.62	0.22	0.81	0.61	0.91	0.23	1.07
Lamb	18	1.10	0.83	1.30	1.77	0.47	0.23	0.68	0.40	1.13	0.23	0.86
Pork	15	0.89	0.68	1.05	1.44	0.41	0.20	0.57	0.50	0.65	0.17	0.72
Tuna, raw	25	1.40	1.08	1.90	2.14	0.69	0.25	0.91	0.69	1.02	0.26	1.20
Other animal products												
Beef stomach	15	1.05	0.63	1.01	1.20	0.36	0.20	0.57	0.40	0.65	0.20	0.75
Heart	17	1.09	0.88	1.55	1.46	0.37	0.27	0.78	0.40	0.78	0.22	0.95
Kidney	16	0.90	0.67	1.25	1.31	0.34	0.22	0.80	0.40	0.67	0.21	0.90
Liver	20	1.06	0.86	1.56	1.70	0.48	0.28	1.00	0.50	0.86	0.26	1.16
Dairy and egg products												
Casein	84.4	3.50	5.75	8.84	7.17	2.82	0.31	4.83	2.60	3.93	1.08	6.73
Cottage cheese												
Creamed	12.5	0.57	0.73	1.28	1.0	0.38	0.12	0.67	0.41	0.55	0.14	0.77
Low fat (1% fat)	12.4	0.56	0.73	1.27	1.0	0.37	0.11	0.67	0.41	0.55	0.14	0.77
Low fat (2% fat)	13.8	0.63	0.81	1.41	1.11	0.41	0.13	0.74	0.46	0.61	0.15	0.85
Curd (skim)	36	1.28	2.24	3.43	2.72	0.86	0.31	1.70	0.90	1.61	0.49	2.40
Eggs												
Egg white	11	0.59	0.62	0.90	0.64	0.39	0.20	0.64	0.24	0.53	0.20	0.86
Egg yolk	16	1.15	0.93	1.36	1.15	0.42	0.26	0.64	0.36	0.90	0.29	1.10
Whole egg	13	0.79	0.73	1.08	0.81	0.42	0.23	0.66	0.26	0.66	0.23	0.98
Whole egg, dried	48	3.02	3.06	4.05	2.94	1.44	1.07	2.66	1.10	2.29	0.76	3.42
Milk												
Skim dry milk	36	1.28	2.24	3.43	2.72	0.86	0.31	1.70	0.90	1.61	0.49	2.40
Whole milk	3.5	0.14	0.2	0.36	0.29	0.10	0.04	0.19	0.09	0.18	0.05	0.26
Vegetables												
Soybean meal with hulls	44	3.08	2.34	3.46	2.80	0.61	0.67	2.17	1.13	1.74	0.61	2.16
Soybean meal without hulls	50	3.41	2.43	3.73	3.09	0.69	0.74	2.46	1.22	1.92	0.67	2.50
Soybeans	34	2.58	1.95	3.11	2.08	0.64	0.65	2.15	0.91	1.63	0.49	1.93

Appendix 21 (continued). Essential amino acid content of common protein sources.*

	Protein	Arg	Isoleu	Leu	Lys	Met	Cys	Phe	His	Thr	Trp	Val
Other												
Baker's yeast	16	0.73	0.89	1.30	1.23	0.29	0.14	0.77	0.40	0.82	0.15	1.0

Key: Arg = arginine, Isoleu = isoleucine, Leu = leucine, Lys = lysine, Met = methionine, Cys = cysteine, Phe = phenylalanine, His = histidine, Thr = threonine, Trp = tryptophan, Val = valine.
*Protein and amino acids are expressed in percent as fed or as is. Amino acids are expressed as percent of the food item not in percent of protein.

Appendix 22. Nutrient content of common fat sources.*

	Moisture	ME** kcal	ME** kJ	Protein	Fat	NFE	Fiber	Ca	P	Na	K	Mg	Serving size***
Vegetable sources													
Avocado	74.0	167	699	2.1	16.4	4.7	1.6	0.01	0.04	0.0	0.60	na	173 g/ medium size
Flaxseed	7.2	496	2,075	19.8	38.7	17.2	14.4	0.25	0.55	na	0.70	0.35	na
Margarine	15.5	720	3,012	0.6	81.0	0.4	0.0	0.02	0.02	0.99†	0.02†	na	na
Peanut butter	1.7	589	2,464	25.2	50.6	187.0	1.8	0.06	0.38	0.61	0.63	0.17	16 g/Tbs
Peanuts (roasted)	1.8	582	2,435	26.2	48.7	17.9	2.7	0.07	0.41	0.01	0.70	0.18	na
Pecans	3.4	687	2,874	9.2	71.2	12.3	2.3	0.07	0.19	tr	0.60	0.14	na
Animal sources													
Beef, separable fat	15.2	736	3,079	5.8	78.8	0.0	0.0	0.0	0.05	na	na	na	na
Butter	15.5	716	2,996	0.6	81.0	0.4	0.0	0.02	0.02	0.99††	0.02	0.0	na
Cheddar	37.0	398	1,665	25.0	32.2	2.1	0.0	0.75	0.48	0.70	0.08	0.05	na
Chicken, fryers, fried skin	32.5	419	1,753	28.3	28.9	9.1	0.0	0.01	0.19	na	na	na	na
Chicken, fryers, raw skin	66.3	223	933	16.1	17.1	0.0	0.0	0.01	0.17	na	na	na	na
Cream, heavy whipping	56.6	352	1,473	2.2	37.6	3.1	0.0	0.08	0.06	0.03	0.09	0.01	na
Egg yolk, fresh	51.1	348	1,456	16.0	30.6	0.6	0.0	0.14	0.57	0.05	0.10	1.5	17 g/egg
Pork, separable fat	12.4	770	3,222	3.5	83.7	0.0	0.0	0.0	0.01	0.07	0.28	na	na
Sardines, canned, solids and liquid	50.6	311	1,301	20.6	24.4	0.6	0.0	0.35	0.43	0.51	0.56	na	na
Tuna, canned, solids and liquid	52.6	288	1,205	24.2	20.5	0.0	0.0	0.01	0.29	0.80	0.30	na	na
Whole milk	87.4	65	272	3.5	3.5	4.9	0.0	0.12	0.09	0.05	0.14	0.01	na

Key: ME = metabolizable energy, kcal = kilocalories, kJ = kilojoules, NFE = nitrogen-free extract, Ca = calcium, P = phosphorus, Na = sodium, K = potassium, Mg = magnesium, tr = trace, g = grams, Tbs = tablespoons (15 ml), na = not available.
*All nutrients are expressed on a percent as fed or as is basis unless otherwise noted.
**Metabolizable energy/100 g as is.
***g/serving.
†Values apply to salted margarine. Unsalted margarine contains less than 0.01% of either sodium or potassium.
††Values apply to salted butter. Unsalted butter contains about 0.02% sodium, whereas some salted butter may contain up to 1.5% sodium.

Appendix 23. Fat and fatty acid composition of common fat sources.

	ME* per 100 g (kcal)	ME* per 100 g (kJ)	Total fat** (%)	Linoleic acid*** (%)	Arachidonic acid*** (%)	α-linolenic acid*** (%)	MCT*** (%)	Other***
Fats								na
Beef tallow†	870	3,640	97	2	0.8	0.6	na	na
Beef, separable fat, raw	736	3,079	79	2.2	na	na	na	na
Butter†	716	2,996	81	2.5	0.95	0.7	5.7	na
Chicken fat	900	3,766	100	19	0.75	1.3	1.0	na
Lard†	902	3,774	100	10	1.7	1.0	na	na
Margarine (liquid oil)	720	3,012	81	29	na	na	na	na
Margarine, hydrogenated††	720	3,012	81	14	na	na	1.0	na
Mutton fat	856	3,582	97	4	na	1.3	na	na
Pork, separable fat, raw	770	3,222	84	8	na	na	na	n-6/n-3 ratio: 4 to 1 in muscle fat
Oils†††								
Black currant seed oil	900	3,766	100	48	na	13	na	Total n-6: 77-87%, n-6/n-3 ratio: 5 to 1
Canola oil (rapeseed oil)	900	3,766	100	14-22	na	7-10	na	n-6/n-3 ratio: 2.2 to 1
Coconut oil (coconut milk)	900	3,766	100	2	na	na	55	na
Corn oil	900	3,766	100	55	na	1	na	na
Cottonseed oil	900	3,766	100	53	na	0.5	na	na
Linseed (flax) oil	900	3,766	100	16	na	53	na	na
Menhaden (fish) oil	900	3,766	100	25	na	na	na	n-3: EPA 15%, DHA 9%
Oat oil	900	3,766	100	45	na	0.2	na	na
Olive oil	900	3,766	100	10	na	1	na	na

Appendix 23 (continued). Fat and fatty acid composition of common fat sources.

	ME* per 100 g (kcal)	ME* per 100 g (kJ)	Total fat** (%)	Linoleic acid*** (%)	Arachidonic acid*** (%)	α-linolenic acid*** (%)?	MCT*** (%)	Other***
Palm kernel oil	900	3,766	100	2	na	≥50	na	na
Palm oil	900	3,766	100	10	na	1	na	na
Peanut oil	900	3,766	100	30	2.2	1.5	na	na
Rice bran oil	900	3,766	100	32	na	1.1	na	na
Safflower oil	900	3,766	100	76	na	0.5	na	na
Sesame seed oil	900	3,766	100	42	na	0.2	na	na
Soybean oil	900	3,766	100	54	na	7	na	n-6/n-3 ratio: 7.7 to 1
Soybean oil, hardened	900	3,766	100	26	na	na	na	na
Sunflower seed oil	900	3,766	100	66	na	0.5	na	na
Walnut oil	900	3,766	100	na	0.6	10	na	na
Wheat germ oil	900	3,766	100	na	na	7	na	na
Other fat sources								
Avocados	167	699	16.4	2	na	na	na	na
Cheddar cheese	398	1,665	32.2	1	na	0.4	na	na
Chicken, fryers, fried skin	419	1,753	28.9	5	na	na	na	na
Chicken, fryers, raw skin	223	933	17.1	3	na	na	na	na
Cream, heavy, whipping	352	1,473	37.6	1	na	na	na	na
Egg, whole, hard cooked	na	na	11.5	1	na	na	na	na
Egg, yolk, fresh	348	1,456	30.6	2	0.15	2	na	na
Flaxseed	496	2,075	38.7	5.6	na	19.4	na	Total n-6: 19.8
Peanut butter	589	2,464	50.6	14	na	na	na	na
Peanuts, roasted, shelled	582	2,435	48.7	14	na	na	na	na
Pecans, shelled	687	2,874	71.2	14	na	na	na	na
Sardines, in oil (solids/liquid)	311	1,301	24.4	na	na	na	na	na
Tuna, in oil (solids/liquid)	288	1,205	20.5	8	na	na	na	na
Whole milk‡	65	272	3.5	na	na	0.1	na	na

Key: ME = metabolizable energy, kcal = kilocalories, kJ = kilojoules, MCT = medium-chain triglycerides, na = not available, EPA = eicosapentaenoic acid, DHA = docosahexaenoic acid.
*Metabolizable energy/100 g as is.
**% fat expressed on an as fed or as is basis.
***% of total fatty acids.
†1 tablespoon = about 15 g.
††1 tablespoon = about 11 g.
†††1 tablespoon of most oils = about 14 g, which supplies about 125 kcal ME; 1 teaspoon = about 4.6 g, which supplies about 42 kcal.
‡1 cup = 240 g.

Appendix 24. Nutrient content of common carbohydrate and fiber sources.*

	Moisture	ME** kcal	ME** kJ	Protein	Fat	NFE	Fiber	Ca	P	Na	K	Mg	Serving size***
Vegetables													
Beans, common													
Canned, solids and liquid (red)	76.0	90	377	5.7	0.4	16.4	0.9	0.03	0.11	0.0	0.26	na	na
Raw, white or red (average)	11.1	338	1,414	14.6	1.5	61.0	4.2	0.13	0.41	0.02	1.06	0.16	na
Carrots													
Canned, drained solids	91.2	30	126	0.8	0.3	6.7	0.8	0.03	0.02	0.24	0.12	na	155 g/8-oz cup
Canned, solids and liquid	91.8	28	117	0.6	0.2	6.5	0.6	0.03	0.02	0.24	0.12	na	na
Fresh, raw	88.2	42	176	1.1	0.2	9.7	1.0	0.04	0.04	0.05	0.34	0.02	na
Green beans													
Canned, solids and liquid	92.0	21	88	1.0	0.1	4.2	0.6	0.03	0.02	0.24	na	na	na
Fresh, raw	89.0	39	163	2.4	0.2	7.0	1.4	0.07	0.04	0.0	0.26	0.03	na
Green peas													
Canned, drained solids	77.0	88	368	4.7	0.4	14.5	2.3	0.03	0.08	0.24	0.10	0.02	170 g/8-oz cup
Canned, solids and liquid	82.6	66	276	3.5	0.3	11.0	1.5	0.02	0.07	0.24	0.10	na	na
Raw	78.0	84	351	6.3	0.4	12.4	2.0	0.03	0.12	0.0	0.32	0.04	156 g/8-oz cup
Potatoes													
Boiled, after paring	82.8	65	272	1.9	0.1	14.0	0.5	0.01	0.04	0.0	0.29	na	na
Boiled, in skin	79.8	76	318	2.1	0.1	16.6	0.5	0.01	0.05	0.0	0.41	0.03	na
French fried	44.7	274	1,146	4.3	13.2	35.0	1.0	0.02	0.11	0.01	0.85	na	na
Spinach													
Cooked, boiled, drained	92.0	23	96	3.0	0.3	3.0	0.6	0.09	0.04	0.05	0.32	na	180 g/8-oz cup
Raw	90.7	26	109	3.2	0.3	3.7	0.6	0.09	0.05	0.07	0.47	0.09	56 g/8-oz cup
Cereals and breads													
Bagels	29.1	296	1,238	10.9	2.5	56.2	na	0.04	0.07	0.36	0.07	0.02	55 g/bagel
Barley, pearled	11.1	349	1,460	8.2	1.0	78.3	0.5	0.02	0.19	0.0	0.16	0.04	na
Breads													
White	35.6	270	1,130	8.7	3.2	50.3	0.2	0.08	0.10	0.51	0.11	0.02	25 g/slice
Whole wheat	36.4	243	1,017	10.5	3.0	46.1	1.7	0.10	0.23	0.53	0.27	0.08	28 g/slice

Appendix 24 (continued). Nutrient content of common carbohydrate and fiber sources.*

	Moisture	ME** kcal	ME** kJ	Protein	Fat	NFE	Fiber	Ca	P	Na	K	Mg	Serving size***
Buckwheat													
Flour, light	12.0	347	1,452	6.4	1.2	79.0	0.5	0.01	0.09	na	0.32	0.05	98 g/8-oz cup
Whole grain	11.0	335	1,402	11.7	2.4	63.0	9.9	0.11	0.28	na	0.45	0.23	na
Corn (maize)													
Cornstarch	12.0	362	1,515	0.3	tr	87.5	0.1	0.0	0.0	0.0	0.0	0.0	na
Corn, flour	12.0	368	1,540	7.8	2.6	76.1	0.7	0.01	0.16	tr	na	na	117 g/8-oz cup
Flakes (breakfast cereal)	3.0	393	1,644	7.4	0.5	85.8	2.5	0.01	0.05	0.30†	0.09	0.02	28 g/8-oz cup
Meal (whole ground)	12.0	362	1,515	9.0	3.4	74.5	1.0	0.02	0.22	tr	0.25	0.11	122 g/8-oz cup
Oats													
Oatmeal, cooked	86.5	55	230	2.0	1.0	9.5	0.2	0.01	0.06	0.22	0.06	na	250 g/8-oz cup
Oatmeal, dry	8.3	390	1,632	14.2	7.4	67.0	1.2	0.05	0.40	0.0	0.35	0.11	233 g/8-oz cup
Whole-grain	12.0	332	1,389	11.5	4.7	60.0	10.2	0.06	0.40	0.0	0.44	0.15	na
Pastas													
Macaroni, spaghetti, cooked	63.6	148	619	5.0	0.5	30.0	0.1	0.01	0.07	0.0	0.08	0.02	na
Macaroni, spaghetti, dry	10.4	369	1,544	12.5	1.2	74.9	0.3	0.03	0.16	0.0	0.20	0.05	na
Rice													
Brown, cooked, with salt	70.3	119	498	2.5	0.6	25.2	0.3	0.01	0.07	0.28	0.07	na	na
Brown, raw	12.0	360	1,506	7.5	1.9	67.5	0.9	0.03	0.22	0.01	0.21	0.09	na
Long grain, cooked with salt	73.4	106	444	2.1	0.1	23.2	0.1	0.02	0.06	0.36	0.04	0.01	185 g/8-oz cup
Long grain, parboiled, dry	10.3	369	1,544	7.4	0.3	81.1	0.2	0.06	0.20	0.01	0.15	na	na
White, cooked, with salt	72.6	109	456	2.0	0.1	24.1	0.1	0.04	0.10	0.37	0.03	na	175 g/8-oz cup
White, polished, raw	12.0	363	1,519	6.7	0.4	80.1	0.3	0.02	0.09	0.01	0.09	0.03	112 g/8-oz cup
Rye													
Whole grain	11.0	334	1,397	12.1	1.7	71.4	2.0	0.04	0.38	na	0.47	0.12	na
Flour, light	11.0	357	1,494	9.4	1.0	77.5	0.4	0.02	0.19	na	0.20	0.07	102 g/8-oz cup
Wheat													
Cream of wheat (farina), cooked	89.5	42	176	1.3	0.1	8.7	tr	0.0	0.01	0.14	0.01	0.0	235 g/8-oz cup
Cream of wheat (farina), dry	10.3	371	1,552	11.4	0.9	76.6	0.4	0.02	0.11	0.0	0.08	0.03	11 g/Tbs
Flour (whole)	12.0	333	1,393	13.3	2.0	68.7	2.3	0.04	0.37	0.0	0.37	0.11	125 g/8-oz cup
Wheat bran	11.5	213	891	16.0	4.6	52.8	9.1	0.12	1.28	0.01	1.12	0.49	3.5 g/Tbs
Wheat germ	11.5	363	1,519	26.6	10.9	44.2	2.5	0.07	1.12	0.0	0.83	0.34	na
Whole grain	12.8	331	1,383	11.7	2.1	69.6	2.1	0.04	0.48	0.0	0.39	0.16	na
Fruits													
Apples													
Not pared	84.4	58	243	0.2	0.6	13.5	1.0	0.01	0.01	0.0	0.11	0.01	138 g/apple
Pared	85.1	54	226	0.2	0.3	13.5	0.6	0.01	0.01	0.0	0.11	0.01	128 g/apple
Apricots													
Canned (solids and juice pack)	84.1	54	226	1.0	0.2	13.2	0.4	0.02	0.02	0.0	0.36	0.01	28 g/half
Dried	25	260	1,088	5.0	0.5	63.5	3.0	0.07	0.11	0.03	0.98	0.06	3.5 g/half
Raw	85.3	51	213	1.0	0.2	12.2	0.6	0.02	0.02	0.0	0.28	0.01	35 g/apricot
Cherries													
Sour, raw	83.7	58	243	1.2	0.3	14.1	0.2	0.02	0.02	0.0	0.19	0.01	na
Sweet, raw	80.4	70	293	1.3	0.3	17.0	0.4	0.02	0.02	0.0	0.19	0.01	6.8 g/cherry
Dates, natural, dry	22.5	274	1,146	2.2	0.5	70.6	2.3	0.06	0.06	0.0	0.65	0.06	8.3 g/date
Figs													
Dried	23.0	274	1,146	4.3	1.3	63.5	5.6	0.13	0.08	0.03	0.64	0.07	18.7 g/fig
Raw	77.5	80	335	1.2	0.3	19.1	1.2	0.04	0.02	0.0	0.19	0.02	50 g/fig
Grapes													
American types	81.6	69	289	1.3	1.0	15.1	0.6	0.02	0.01	0.0	0.16	0.01	92 g/8-oz cup
European types	81.4	67	280	0.6	0.3	16.8	0.5	0.01	0.02	0.0	0.17	0.01	160 g/8-oz cup
Nectarines, raw	81.8	64	268	0.6	tr	16.7	0.4	0.0	0.02	0.01	0.29	0.01	136 g/nectarine
Orange, peeled	86.0	49	205	1.0	0.2	11.7	0.5	0.04	0.02	0.0	0.20	0.01	120-140 g/orange
Peaches													
Canned (solids and juice pack)	87.2	45	188	0.6	0.1	11.2	0.4	0.01	0.02	0.0	0.21	0.01	248 g/8-oz cup
Raw	89.1	38	159	0.6	0.1	9.1	0.6	0.01	0.02	0.0	0.20	0.01	87 g/peach
Pears													
Raw, including skin	83.2	61	255	0.7	0.4	13.9	1.4	0.01	0.01	0.0	0.13	0.01	166 g/pear
Canned (solids and juice pack)	87.3	46	192	0.3	0.3	11.0	0.8	0.01	0.01	0.0	0.13	0.01	248 g/8-oz cup
Pineapple													
Canned (solids and juice pack)	84.0	58	243	0.4	0.1	14.8	0.3	0.02	0.01	0.0	0.15	0.01	250 g/8-oz cup
Raw	85.3	52	218	0.4	0.2	13.3	0.4	0.02	0.01	0.0	0.15	0.01	na
Prunes, dried, softened	28.0	255	1,067	2.1	0.6	65.8	1.6	0.05	0.08	0.01	0.69	0.04	8.4 g/prune

Key: ME = metabolizable energy, kcal = kilocalories, kJ = kilojoules, NFE = nitrogen-free extract, Ca = calcium, P = phosphorus, Na = sodium, K = potassium, Mg = magnesium, tr = trace, g = grams, Tbs = tablespoons (15 ml), na = not available.

*All nutrients are expressed on a percent as fed or as is basis unless otherwise designated.

**Metabolizable energy/100 g as is.

***g/serving.

†Low-sodium cereal breakfast is available with about 0.01% sodium.

Appendix 25. Nutrient content of selected mineral sources.*

Mineral sources	Moisture (%)	Ca (%)	P (%)	Na (%)	K (%)	Mg (%)	Cl (%)	Ca/P ratio	Weight (g/tsp)
Bone meal	10	≥28	≥13	0.5	na	0.7	0.0	2.1	4
Calcium carbonate	0	36-39	na	na	na	na	na	na	5
Tums tablets contain 0.50 g calcium carbonate per tablet = 200 mg calcium									
Tums Extra tablets contain 0.75 g calcium carbonate per tablet = 300 mg calcium									
Tums Ultra tablets contain 1.0 g calcium carbonate per tablet = 400 mg calcium									
Dicalcium phosphate, powder	20.9	23	18	na	na	na	na	1.3	4
Salt (NaCl)	0	0	0	39.3	0	0	60.7	0	4
Lite salt (50% NaCl/50% KCl)	0	0	0	17.3	29.4	0	53.3	0	5
Salt substitute (potassium chloride)	0	0	0	0	52.4	0	47.6	0	5

Key: Ca = calcium, P = phosphorus, Na = sodium, K = potassium, Mg = magnesium, Cl = chloride, g = grams, tsp = teaspoons, na = not available.
*All nutrients are expressed on a percent as fed or as is basis.

Appendix 26. Purine content of selected foods.

Foods highest in purines (250-825 mg/100 g as fed)
- Anchovies (363 mg/100 g)
- Kidney (beef: 200 mg/100 g)
- Game meats
- Gravies
- Herring
- Liver (calf/beef: 233 mg/100 g)
- Mackerel
- Meat extracts (160-400 mg/100 g)
- Sardines (295 mg/100 g)
- Scallops
- Sweat breads (825 mg/100 g)

Foods high in purines (50-150 mg/100 g as fed)
- Asparagus
- Whole grain breads and cereals
- Cauliflower
- Eel
- Fish
- Legumes: beans, lentils, peas
- Meat: beef, lamb, pork, veal
- Meat soups and broths
- Mushrooms
- Oatmeal
- Poultry: chicken, duck, turkey
- Shellfish: crab, lobster, oysters
- Spinach
- Wheat germ and bran

Foods low in purines (0-50 mg/100 g as fed)
- Breads and cereals, except whole grain
- Cheese
- Eggs
- Fats
- Fish (roe)
- Fruits
- Milk
- Nuts
- Sugars, syrups, sweets
- Vegetables, except those listed above
- Vegetable and cream soups

Appendix 27. Gluten-containing and gluten-free foods.

Gluten-containing grains
- Barley (hordeins)
- Buckwheat
- Oats (avenins)
- Rye (secalin, prolamins)
- Wheat (gliadin)

Gluten-free grains and products
- Corn, corn flour, cornmeal, cornstarch
- Gluten-free wheat starch
- Beans and bean flour
- Potatoes and potato flour
- Rice and rice flour
- Soybeans and soy flour

Index

Page numbers followed by t indicate tables; f, figures, b, boxes, c, cases, a, appendices.

B

C

E

F

I

J-K

N

O

Q-R

S

T

W-Y

Z

Appendices Directory